OF THE ELEMENTS

PERIODIC TABLE OF THE ELEMENTS

1b	2b	3a	4a	5a	6a	7a	0	Orbit
							2 0 He 4.00260 2	−K
		5 +3 B 10.81 2-3	**6** +2 +4 −4 C 12.011 2-4	**7** +1 +2 +3 +4 +5 −1 −2 −3 N 14.0067 2-5	**8** −2 O 15.9994 2-6	**9** −1 F 18.9984 2-7	**10** 0 Ne 20.17_9 2-8	−K−L
Transition Elements		**13** +3 Al 26.9815 2-8-3	**14** +2 +4 −4 Si 28.086 2-8-4	**15** +3 +5 −3 P 30.9738 2-8-5	**16** +4 +6 −2 S 32.06 2-8-6	**17** +1 +5 +7 −1 Cl 35.453 2-8-7	**18** 0 Ar 39.948 2-8-8	−K−L−M
29 +1 +2 Cu 63.546 −8−18−1	**30** +2 Zn 65.38 −8−18−2	**31** +3 Ga 69.72 −8−18−3	**32** +2 +4 Ge 72.59 −8−18−4	**33** +3 +5 −3 As 74.9216 −8−18−5	**34** +4 +6 −2 Se 78.96 −8−18−6	**35** +1 +5 −1 Br 79.904 −8−18−7	**36** 0 Kr 83.80 −8−18−8	−L−M−N
47 +1 Ag 107.868 −18−18−1	**48** +2 Cd 112.40 −18−18−2	**49** +3 In 114.82 −18−18−3	**50** +2 +4 Sn 118.69 −18−18−4	**51** +3 +5 −3 Sb 121.75 −18−18−5	**52** +4 +6 −2 Te 127.60 −18−18−6	**53** +1 +5 +7 −1 I 126.9045 −18−18−7	**54** 0 Xe 131.30 −18−18−8	−M−N−O
79 +1 +3 Au 196.9665 −32−18−1	**80** +1 +2 Hg 200.59 −32−18−2	**81** +1 +3 Tl 204.37 −32−18−3	**82** +2 +4 Pb 207.2 −32−18−4	**83** +3 +5 Bi 208.9806 −32−18−5	**84** +2 +4 Po (209) −32−18−6	**85** At (210) −32−18−7	**86** 0 Rn (222) −32−18−8	−N−O−P
								−O−P−Q

						Orbit
66 +3 Dy 162.50 −28−8−2	**67** +3 Ho 164.9303 −29−8−2	**68** +3 Er 167.26 −30−8−2	**69** +3 Tm 168.9342 −31−8−2	**70** +2 +3 Yb 173.04 −32−8−2	**71** +3 Lu 174.97 −32−9−2	−N−O−P
98 +3 Cf (251) −28−8−2	**99** Es (254) −29−8−2	**100** Fm (257) −30−8−2	**101** Md (256) −31−8−2	**102** No (254) −32−8−2	**103** Lr −32−9−2	−O−P−Q

TODD-SANFORD

CLINICAL DIAGNOSIS

By Laboratory Methods

15th edition

Edited by

ISRAEL DAVIDSOHN, M.D., F.A.C.P.

Professor of Pathology and Chief, Division of Experimental Pathology,
University of Health Sciences, The Chicago Medical School and
Director, Department of Experimental Pathology,
Mount Sinai Hospital Medical Center, Chicago, Illinois

JOHN BERNARD HENRY, M.D.

Dean, College of Health Related Professions,
Professor of Pathology, College of Medicine, and Director,
Division of Clinical Pathology, University Hospital, State
University of New York, Upstate Medical Center, Syracuse, New York

W. B. SAUNDERS COMPANY • Philadelphia • London • Toronto • 1974

W. B. Saunders Company: West Washington Square
Philadelphia, Pa. 19105

12 Dyott Street
London, WC1A 1DB

833 Oxford Street
Toronto, Ontario M8Z 5T9, Canada

Clinical Diagnosis by Laboratory Methods ISBN 0-7216-2922-9

Print No.: 9 8 7 6 5 4 3 2 1

To our wives,
Clara Davidsohn and Georgette Henry,
who patiently accepted the inconvenience
of our long preoccupation with this work

CONTRIBUTORS

DENNIS L. ALLEN, M.D.
Family Practice Resident, Ball Memorial Hospital, Muncie, Indiana

MYRTON FREEMAN BEELER, M.D.
Professor, Departments of Pathology and Preventive Medicine, Louisiana State University Medical Center, New Orleans; Associate Pathologist, Charity Hospital of Louisiana, Consultant in Clinical Pathology, V.A. Hospital, New Orleans, Louisiana

ELLIS S. BENSON, M.D.
Professor and Head, Department of Laboratory Medicine and Pathology, University of Minnesota Medical School, Minneapolis, Minnesota

G. MARY BRADLEY, M.D.
Associate Professor, Department of Laboratory Medicine and Pathology, University of Minnesota Medical School, Minneapolis, Minnesota

DONALD C. CANNON, M.D., Ph.D.
Director, Bio-Science Laboratories, Van Nuys, California; Visiting Professor of Pathology, The University of New Mexico School of Medicine, Albuquerque, New Mexico

BRADLEY ELLSWORTH COPELAND, M.D.
Chairman, Department of Pathology, New England Deaconess and New England Baptist Hospitals, Boston, Massachusetts

ISRAEL DAVIDSOHN M.D., F.A.C.P.
Professor of Pathology and Chief, Division of Experimental Pathology, University of Health Sciences, The Chicago Medical School, Chicago; Director, Department of Experimental Pathology, Mount Sinai Hospital Medical Center, Chicago, Illinois

ROBERT R. EGGEN, M.D.
Acton, Massachusetts.

RAOUL FRESCO, M.D., Ph.D.
Associate Professor of Pathology, University of Health Sciences, The Chicago Medical School; Head, Division of Electron Microscopy, Mount Sinai Medical Center, Chicago, Illinois

MILTON GOLDIN, Ph.D.
Clinical Associate Professor, University of Health Sciences, The Chicago Medical School, Chicago; Director, Microbiology, Mount Sinai Hospital Medical Center, Chicago, Illinois

JOHN BERNARD HENRY, M.D.
Dean, College of Health Related Professions, Professor of Pathology, College of Medicine, and Director, Division of Clinical Pathology, University Hospital, State University of New York, Upstate Medical Center, Syracuse, New York

YUAN S. KAO, M.D.
Assistant Professor of Pathology, Louisiana State University School of Medicine, New Orleans; Visiting Pathologist, Charity Hospital of Louisiana, New Orleans, Louisiana

ARTHUR F. KRIEG, M.D.
Professor of Pathology, The Pennsylvania State University, Hershey; Director, Division of Clinical Pathology, The Milton S. Hershey Medical Center, Hershey, Pennsylvania

ROBERT G. LANCASTER, M.D.
Assistant Clinical Professor of Pathology, University of Maryland School of Medicine, Baltimore; Director, Department of Pathology and School of Medical Technology, Mercy Hospital, Baltimore, Maryland

ROBERT D. LANGDELL, M.D.
Professor of Pathology, University of North Carolina School of Medicine, Chapel Hill, North Carolina

CHANG LING LEE, M.D.
Professor of Pathology, University of Health Sciences, The Chicago Medical School, Chicago; Director, Charles Hymen Blood Center, Mount Sinai Hospital Medical Center, Chicago, Illinois

JESSE H. MARYMONT, JR., M.D.
Assistant Director of Laboratories, Wesley Medical Center, Wichita, Kansas

RUSSELL M. MCQUAY, Ph.D.
Adjunct Assistant Professor of Microbiology, University of Health Sciences, The Chicago Medical School; Director of Microbiology, Division of Medical Parasitology, Mount Sinai Hospital Medical Center, Chicago, Illinois

DOUGLAS A. NELSON, M.D.
Professor of Pathology, Associate Director of Clinical Pathology, Director Program in Medical Technology, State University of New York, Upstate Medical Center, Syracuse, New York

DANIEL C. NIEJADLIK, M.D.
Assistant Clinical Professor of Pathology, University of Texas Medical School, San Antonio; Assistant Laboratory Director, Wilford Hall Medical Center, U.S.A.F., San Antonio, Texas

ALAN L. ORVIS, Ph.D.
Associate Professor of Biophysics, Mayo Graduate School of Medicine, University of Minnesota, Rochester; Consultant, Department of Therapeutic Radiology, Mayo Clinic and Mayo Foundation, Rochester, Minnesota

ALLEN L. PUSCH, M.D.
Associate Professor, Pathology, State University of New York, Upstate Medical Center, Syracuse; Deputy Director, Clinical Pathology, State University Hospital, Syracuse, New York

JERALD M. ROSENBAUM, M.D.
Pathologist and Director of Clinical Chemistry, Department of Pathology, Springfield Hospital Medical Center, Springfield, Massachusetts

JAMES G. SHAFFER, Sc.D., D.Sc. (Honorary)
Professor of Microbiology and Associate Dean, University of Health Sciences, The Chicago Medical School, Chicago; Consultant in Hospital Epidemiology, Lutheran General Hospital, Park Ridge, and Mount Sinai Hospital Medical Center, Chicago, Illinois

S. THOMAS SHAW, JR., M.D.
Assistant Professor of Obstetrics and Gynecology and of Pathology, Los Angeles County/University of Southern California Medical Center, Los Angeles, California

KURT STERN, M.D.
Professor, Department of Life Sciences, Bar-Ilan University, Ramat-Gan, Israel; Professor Emeritus of Pathology, University of Illinois College of Medicine, Chicago, Illinois

W. NEWLON TAUXE, M.D., M.S. (Pathology)
Associate Professor of Clinical Pathology, Mayo Graduate School of Medicine, University of Minnesota, Rochester; Consultant, Department of Diagnostic Nuclear Medicine, Mayo Clinic and Mayo Foundation, Rochester, Minnesota; Professor of Nuclear Medicine and Clinical Pathology, Division of Nuclear Medicine, University of Alabama, Birmingham, Alabama

HARRY F. WEISBERG, M.D.
Associate Clinical Professor of Pathology and of Medicine, University of Wisconsin Medical School, Madison; Associate Clinical Professor of Health Sciences, University of Wisconsin, Milwaukee; Lecturer in Medical Technology, Carroll College, Waukesha; Associate Director, Department of Pathology, and Director of Division of Biochemistry and of School of Medical Technology, Mount Sinai Medical Center, Milwaukee, Wisconsin

ROBERT E. WENK, M.D.
Acting Pathologist-in-Chief, Sinai Hospital of Baltimore, Inc., Baltimore, Maryland

WEI T. WU, Ph.D.
Clinical Assistant Professor, Louisiana State University School of Medicine, New Orleans; Staff, Charity Hospital of Louisiana, New Orleans, Louisiana

HYMAN J. ZIMMERMAN, M.D.
Professor of Medicine, George Washington University School of Medicine; Clinical Professor, Georgetown University and Howard University Schools of Medicine; Chief, Medical Service, Veterans Administration Hospital, Washington, D.C.

PREFACE

With this 15th edition, Todd and Sanford reaches the mature age of 66 years of service to a third generation of clinical pathologists, medical technologists, medical students, internists and family physicians.

Our objectives or goals in this edition include the following:

1. Identify appropriate measurements and examinations for:
   a. diagnosis.
   b. confirmation of a clinical impression.
   c. screening or detection of disease.
   d. prognosis.
   e. therapeutic or management guideline data.
2. Indicate the order in which such measurements and examinations should be requested.
3. Interpret and translate laboratory findings.
4. Recognize pitfalls, problems and limitations of laboratory data, including discussion of quality control and drug interaction as well as relative merits in terms of methodology, patient preparation and communication.
5. Understand pathophysiology or sequence of disease as reflected by laboratory measurements and examinations.

Since it is virtually impossible to compress all of laboratory medicine into a single volume, we have chosen to emphasize certain topics that have compelling practical application with the patient as the central theme. Thus, the fields of chemical pathology, hematology and medical microbiology have been greatly expanded in the form of a series of chapters.

It is significant that this edition begins with a chapter on statistics and quality control and concludes with a chapter on clinical laboratory computerization: the two subjects identify a basic approach to laboratory science and currently have a pre-eminent role throughout the medical laboratory.

In the appendices, tables of normal values incorporate much data from our own laboratories as well as those of other workers. Body surface area and desirable weights are important in terms of blood volume and measurements of selected organ functions.

Our contributors have been chosen on the basis of great knowledge and current activity in their disciplines. We are grateful to these distinguished scientists who have been faithful to their task and gracious in cooperation.

ISRAEL DAVIDSOHN
JOHN BERNARD HENRY

ACKNOWLEDGMENTS

A work of multiple authorship requires by its very nature the willingness of the contributors to accept the guidance of the editors. We are glad to acknowledge that our collaborators have been most gracious in this respect.

Several individuals have been particularly helpful with suggestions and careful review of selected manuscripts, galley proofs and page proofs: Drs. Frederick Davey, Maurice Furlong, Harold Hawley, Judy Mercer, Daniel Niejadlik, Barry Pearson, Jeffrey Pevnick, Allen Pusch, Charles Rouault, Gloria Sage, Solomon Schreiber, Gerald Simon, Avrum Stein, Howard Weindling, William Welch, Mrs. Shirley Klein, Reginaldo Lauzon, and Miss Bettina Martin, all of Clinical Pathology; Dr. Mary Voorhess, Department of Pediatrics; Drs. Robert Levine and Joan Howanitz, Department of Medicine; Dr. Raja Abdul-Karim, Department of Obstetrics-Gynecology; State University of New York, Upstate Medical Center in Syracuse. Dr. Raymond Troxler at Brooks Air Force Base, Texas, provided invaluable assistance in lipids and Dr. Maurice Furlong provided comparable assistance for proteins in our chemistry chapter, while Dr. F. Donald McGovern assisted in endocrinology. To Dr. George Linke we are particularly grateful for his assistance in the revision of Appendix 2 and his critical analysis of specific portions of the chemistry chapter, particularly on methodology. Dr. Howard Zirkin assisted by critically reviewing several chapters.

For verification of references, we are again indebted to Mr. Clark Rumsey and Mrs. Evelyn Hoey at the Upstate Medical Center Library. Appreciation is also due Mr. Louis Georgianna and Mildred Knowles for photographic assistance and to Mrs. Julia Hammock for contributions in medical illustration.

We should also like to acknowledge the stimulus and efforts of former residents and medical students as well as colleagues who have helped in so many ways to bring this edition to completion.

For sustained devotion and meticulous attention to detail, we are grateful to our secretaries, Miss Carol Mosher, Mrs. Judy Meggesto, Miss Sharon Putney, and Mrs. Marilyn Yarbrough.

To Dr. James N. Patterson, we extend our sincere thanks for bringing us together.

We want to express our appreciation for the cooperation of Mr. Robert B. Rowan, Mr. Herbert Powell, and Mrs. Billie Brick as well as the entire staff of the W. B. Saunders Company.

I.D.

J.B.H.

CONTENTS

Chapter 4

Chapter 1

STATISTICAL TOOLS IN CLINICAL PATHOLOGY

by BRADLEY E. COPELAND, M.D.

Laboratory measurements are used by physicians for two purposes:

(1) to identify the diseased individual, and (2) to follow the progress of the diseased individual under medical therapy. The laboratory itself has two responsibilities to the physician: (1) to provide the physician with an estimate of the variation in the normal human population, and (2) to guarantee the reliability of each individual measurement.

SELECTING THE ABNORMAL INDIVIDUAL

Before the abnormal can be identified, the normal population must be defined. To express the normal values of the human population clearly, one measures a series of individuals who are in normal health. The average value is calculated. The dispersion of values around the average is described by the standard deviation. The complete expression of the normal population will consist of the average, showing the center of the normal distribution, and the standard deviation, which indicates the dispersion of the population about the average.

The standard deviation is a descriptive tool, which condenses the frequency distribution of a population into a single measurement unit. Figure 1–1 shows the normal curve of the frequency distribution of a population. The horizontal axis (x-axis) represents the units of measurement, and the vertical axis (y-axis) represents the frequency or number of times each value occurs. The standard deviation shown in Figure 1–1 describes the distribution of a population as follows:

68 per cent of the population is included within plus or minus (±) one standard deviation from the average.

95 per cent of the population is included

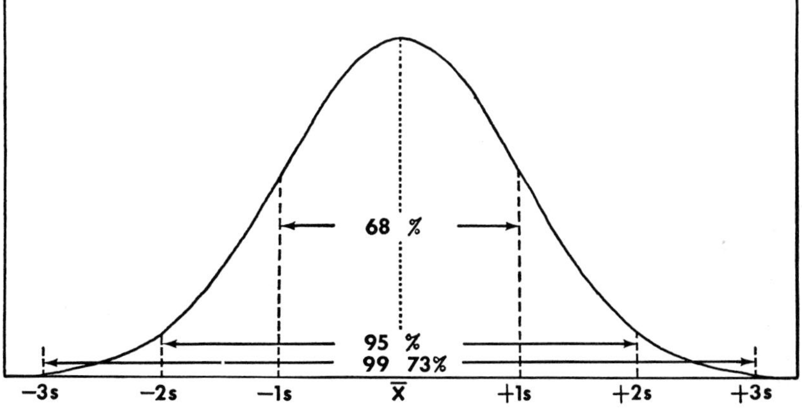

Figure 1–1. Areas under the normal curve between average ($\bar{X}$) and ± 1s = 68%; $\bar{X}$ ± 2s = 95%; and X ± 3s = 99.7% (s means standard deviation; X means average). (Modified from Croxton, F. E.: Elementary Statistics with Applications in Medicine. New York, Prentice-Hall, Inc., 1953.)

within plus or minus (±) two standard deviations from the average.

99.7 per cent of the population is included within plus or minus (±) three standard deviations from the average.

The most frequent measurements cluster around the average, whereas measurements far from the average occur less and less frequently until a point is reached at which, for practical purposes, no normal values occur. This distribution of measurements about an average value has been shown to be true for virtually all types of biologic, chemical, and physical measurements. The measurements may be made upon a population of humans, a population of animals, or a series or population of inanimate objects.

Decision Criterion No. 1. Does the individual differ from the normal population with respect to a particular measurement?

If the value lies outside the ± three standard deviation limits (99.7 per cent), then it is clear that the individual in question does not belong to the normal population. If the value lies outside the two standard deviation limits (95 per cent) and within the three standard deviation limits (99.7 per cent), the individual possibly may not be one of the normal population. The physician would need to give extra thought and attention to this patient.

A typical normal distribution of measured values on a normal human population is shown in Figure 1–2. Hematocrits of 100 normal young women are recorded in the frequency distribution form. The average hematocrit equals 41.0 ml. packed red cells per 100 ml. of whole blood. One standard deviation limit, including 68 per cent of the measurements, is ± 2.4 ml. packed red blood cells per 100 ml. whole blood. The two and three standard deviation limits are 4.8 and 7.2 ml., respectively. Therefore, using the average and the standard deviation value, the complete frequency distribution can be reconstructed as follows: 68 per cent of the young normal women had hematocrit values between 38.6 and 43.4, 95 per cent of the young normal women had hematocrit values between 36.2 and 45.8, and 99.7 per cent of the young normal women had hematocrit values between 33.8 and 48.2.

Normal Values for Each Laboratory. It is necessary for each laboratory to measure its own normal values. Ten to 20 normal samples would give a reasonable approximation of the normal value for the method, the laboratory, and the geographic location. Attention should be given to the age range and to the sex distribution. Two convenient normal population groups are: (1) blood bank donors, and (2) persons who are working and feel healthy. Our true knowledge of normal values is still very limited. It is known that, because of many unknown variables, normal values from the literature cannot be assumed to be valid for any individual laboratory unless checked. When procedures are modified or changed, the normal value should be rechecked. Several texts devoted to normal values are listed at the end of this chapter. These should be used for guidance but the values not actually used until verified for an individual laboratory.

GUARANTEEING RELIABLE MEASUREMENTS

The second laboratory responsibility is to guarantee the reliability of every measurement. Two difficulties should be identified:

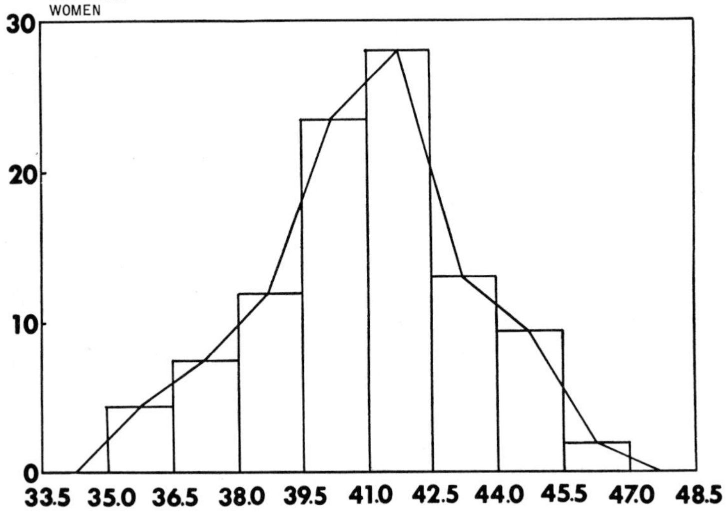

Figure 1–2. Volume of packed red cells per 100 ml. of whole blood for 100 normal young women 18 to 30 years of age. (Data from Osgood, E. E., and Haskins, H. D.: Arch. Intern. Med., *39*:643, 1927. Chart by Croxton, F. E.: Elementary Statistics with Application in Medicine. New York, Prentice-Hall, Inc., 1953.)

First, no method of analysis gives exactly the same result each time it is repeated. There is an *inherent variability* characteristic of each measurement procedure that cannot be avoided. Second, practical considerations limit the amount of sample available for measurement. Each sample is one of a population of possible samples that could have been taken from the subject.

Quality Control System for the Clinical Chemistry Laboratory. Quality control systems have been developed to guarantee reliability of one's procedures and at the same time require only limited blood samples. A large number of identical samples from the same large pool are prepared and are frozen or lyophilized to preserve stability. Every batch of laboratory measurements is accompanied by one of the identical pool samples, the quality control serum. The variability of repeated analyses is measured under regular operating conditions, using the identical samples, and is expressed in standard deviation units. If the quality control sample does not fall within the known limits of inherent variability, the measurements are rejected and the analyses are repeated. In this way each laboratory measurement is accompanied by a known sample, which undergoes exactly the same steps and conditions as the unknown samples.

There are several acceptable methods for setting up quality control. The system described has been found practical, but each laboratory should develop a quality control technique suitable for its own purposes.

Lyophilized Quality Control Serum Pool. REGIONAL QUALITY CONTROL PROGRAMS. In many regions of the United States, regional control programs are in operation. In the regional program a group of 10 to 150 laboratories cooperatively purchase a large volume of lyophilized control serum (enough for a one-year supply). Usually two concentrations are used – normal and abnormal.

Since a large volume is used and since unassayed material is used, the price is lower than could be obtained by individual purchase.

The main advantage of the regional system is the monthly comparison of average values with all other laboratories in the region.

This concept was originated and perfected by Dr. Joseph Preston of Denver. Regional Programs are now available in Massachusetts (including Maine, New Hampshire, Vermont, and Rhode Island), Connecticut, New York State, New York City, New Jersey, Virginia, Oregon-Washington, Louisiana, and Texas.*

*For specific information, contact Dr. Joseph Preston, Colorado Pathologists Reference Laboratory, Denver, Colorado, or Dr. Gerald Rosenbaum, Director of Massachusetts Society of Pathologists Regional Program, Springfield Hospital, Springfield, Massachusetts.

Commercial Lyophilized Serum Pool. It is useful to purchase a supply large enough to last one year. Unassayed material is less expensive and avoids the pitfall of erroneous assay values or assay values which show methodology bias. Repeated observations of the above problems have been made.

In the internal quality control system, one is principally concerned with the within laboratory stability of the methods and instruments in use.

The differences between laboratories due to systematic bias are important but are problems which the individual laboratory should not try to solve at the expense of getting started on an active internal quality control program.

The external quality control material available as part of the Quality Assurance Program of the Standards Committee of the College of American Pathologists* is the most useful program to check the accuracy (closeness to true value) of methodology and also how well one's methodology agrees with that of other laboratories. Four times a year, unknown lyophilized sera are distributed among 5000 U. S. laboratories. Each laboratory receives an individual computer printout with a grading of the accuracy of analyses in comparison with referee laboratories and with other participating laboratories.

Preparation of a Frozen Quality Control Pool. Excess serum is salvaged daily from regular specimens and frozen in a deepfreeze until 2000 to 3000 ml. are collected. Hemolyzed, lipemic, and jaundiced sera are rejected. Fasting human donors may be used if the supply of serum is not available. Beef serum is available commercially and is not expensive. The pool should be thawed, mixed thoroughly, and filtered. Then the pool is divided into samples (aliquots), which are convenient for storage in the deepfreeze. Pyrex screw cap tubes are convenient. Plastic vials capped to prevent evaporation are satisfactory.

It is important to remember that when frozen serum melts, pure water layers out at the top surface. Be sure to mix thoroughly before using each sample. This is the most frequent cause of out-of-control measurements. Changes of 50 to 100 per cent can be caused by incomplete mixing.

A single pool is used for all methods. Special individual pools may be used for PBI (using only analyzed sera), calcium, or enzymes. However, it is useful to have an additional control with values of the constituents in an abnormal range. This is useful for checking the procedure of a range of elevated and depressed values. An abnormal pool with high or ele-

*College of American Pathologists Quality Assurance Program, 230 North Michigan Avenue, Chicago, Illinois.

vated values of constituents may be prepared from known abnormals or additional pool constituent may be added to a normal pool. An abnormal low pool is less common and may be prepared by diluting normal serum with human serum albumin.

Calculation of Average and Standard Deviation Values. The average value and standard deviation for each new pool of quality control serum for each method to be controlled should be established before the pool is put into service. Pool samples are processed with the daily measurements for 15 to 25 days. From the 15 to 25 values an average and a standard deviation are calculated.

EXAMPLE: DAILY POTASSIUM VALUES RUN FOR 15 DAYS PRIOR TO INSTITUTION OF A NEW CONTROL POOL

February 5	5.7
February 6	6.0
February 7	5.9
February 8	5.7
February 9	5.7
February 11	5.9
February 12	5.7
February 13	5.7
February 14	5.8
February 15	5.7
February 16	5.9
February 18	5.7
February 19	6.0
February 20	5.8
February 21	5.6

PROCEDURE FOR CALCULATING AVERAGE AND STANDARD DEVIATION

1. Record analyses in column one.
2. Add column one.
3. Calculate average of column one (step A).
4. Calculate and record in column two the individual differences from the average.
5. Square each individual difference and record in the third column.
6. Add column three (sum of squared differences).
7. Calculate standard deviation (step B). See table in right column.

In the example, the average daily potassium value is 5.8 mEq./liter. The standard deviation is 0.13 mEq./liter.

When beginning quality control, one should set the control limits at ±3 S.D. from the average. The ± three standard deviation limits for the example are ±0.39 mEq./liter or a range of 5.41 to 6.19 mEq./liter. After the control system is well established, the limits may be narrowed to ± two standard deviations, which decreases the overall variability of reported measurements. In the example this would be ±2 S.D. = 5.54 to 6.06.

Figure 1–3 shows a typical month of quality control measurements and the evaluation of these values. Note the out-of-control value on March 12. All measurements were repeated,

DAILY POTASSIUM VALUES

	(mEq/liter)	Difference from Average	Squared Difference from Average
1.	5.7	0.1	0.01
2.	6.0	0.2	0.04
3.	5.9	0.1	0.01
4.	5.7	0.1	0.01
5.	5.7	0.1	0.01
6.	5.9	0.1	0.01
7.	5.7	0.1	0.01
8.	5.7	0.1	0.01
9.	5.8	0.0	0.00
10.	5.7	0.1	0.01
11.	5.9	0.1	0.01
12.	5.7	0.1	0.01
13.	6.0	0.2	0.04
14.	5.8	0.0	0.00
15.	5.6	0.2	0.04
	86.8		0.22

and the second control on March 12 is shown on the following page below.

The reliability of each laboratory measurement is in this way guaranteed to be within the predictable limits of the inherent variability of the method.

What Quality Control Values Should Be Achieved Under Daily Regular Operating Conditions? Because of the importance of the day-to-day quality control values, the following is quoted from Straumfjord and Copeland:

> Laboratories whose day-to-day quality control standard deviation is within the limits of the "most common range" [Table 1–1] are performing work comparable to more than 90 per cent of the reporting university hospital laboratories.
>
> These data are presented to give a preliminary set of reference points for the evaluation of performance in the clinical chemistry laboratory. In the process of evaluation of laboratory performance there are 3 pitfalls. The first is the attempt to be too precise, which often leads to unconscious or conscious bias, as well as unnecessary expense. The second is the acceptance of excessive variability, which may negate the medical usefulness of the measurements. The third difficulty is the definition of the frame of reference, the conditions for the collection of data, and the method of expressing the estimate of precision.
>
> The data presented represent the day-to-day frame of reference which has been adopted extensively in the United States and Canada through the institution of daily quality control programs in hospital laboratories. This frame of reference is: (1) single daily measurements, and (2) measurements made at the same time as regular unknown specimens.
>
> As it is economically wasteful to achieve precision not utilized in the medical decision-making process, the horizon should not be limited to the achievement

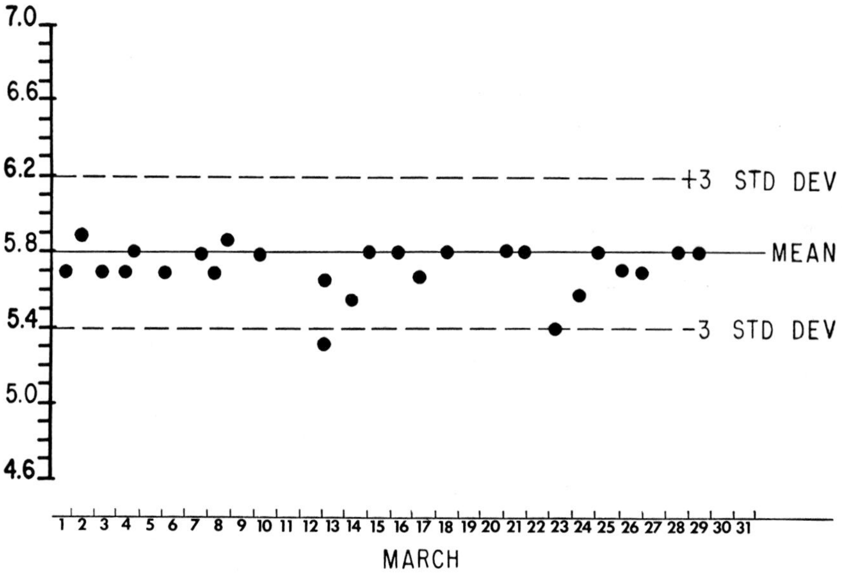

Figure 1–3. Quality control measurements of potassium (mEq./liter) for one month. (From Copeland, B. E., Newell, J., and Dolan, W.: Quality Control Manual. Chicago, American Society of Clinical Pathologists, 1959.)

Calculations

Step A. $\text{Average} = \dfrac{\text{total sum of analyses}}{\text{n}}$

$$\text{n} = \text{number of measurements} = 15$$

$$\text{Average} = \frac{86.8}{15} = 5.78 = 5.8 \text{ mEq./liter}$$

Step B. $\text{Standard deviation} = \sqrt{\dfrac{\text{sum of squared differences from average}^{*}}{\text{n}-1}}$

Sum of squared differences from average = 0.22

n–1 = 15–1 = 14

$$\text{Standard deviation} = \sqrt{\frac{0.22}{14}} = \sqrt{0.0157}^{*}$$

Standard deviation = 0.13 mEq./liter

---

*The square root calculation is easily done by test multiplication or use of a slide rule or calculator. Here $0.13^2 = 0.0169$ is closest to the observed value 0.0157. If further precision is needed, the same process can be used for the next decimal place.

$0.11 \times 0.11 = 0.0122$
$0.12 \times 0.12 = 0.144$
$0.13 \times 0.13 = 0.0169$
$0.14 \times 0.14 = 0.0196$

Table 1–1. DAY-TO-DAY QUALITY CONTROL IN UNIVERSITY HOSPITALS: MEAN AND MOST COMMON RANGE*

ANALYZED COMPONENT	MEAN, 1 STANDARD DEVIATION	MEAN, 1 COEFFICIENT OF VARIATION†	RANGE OF 1 STANDARD DEVIATION‡	SUGGESTED S.D. ACTION LEVEL
Glucose	3.2 mg./100 ml.	3.1	0.5-7.6 (27)	8.0
Urea nitrogen	1.1 mg./100 ml.	5.8	0.15-2.5 (31)	2.0
Carbon dioxide	0.8 mEq./liter	4.3	0.36-2.0 (25)	2.0
Chloride	1.3 mEq./liter	1.0	0.35-2.5 (33)	2.0
Sodium	1.5 mEq./liter	1.1	0.56-3.0 (33)	2.0
Potassium	0.12 mEq./liter	2.5	0.01-0.25 (31)	0.2
Phosphorus	0.19 mg./100 ml.	4.9	0.01-0.40 (32)	0.4
Calcium	0.21 mg./100 ml.	2.3	0.07-0.40 (28)	0.4
Uric acid	0.25 mg./100 ml.	4.8	0.10-0.80 (31)	0.4
Total protein	0.16 gm./100 ml.	2.6	0.03-0.50 (30)	0.25
Creatinine	0.11 mg./100 ml.	7.8	0.03-0.22 (26)	0.25
Cholesterol	8.7 mg./100 ml.	5.1	1.8-23 (30)	1.53
Bilirubin	0.22 mg./100 ml.	7.6	0.03-0.6 (25)	0.3
Amylase	11 units	8.1	1.3-34 (19)	–
Transaminase	4.2 units	11.8	0.7-10 (21)	–
Alkaline phosphatase		10.6		–

*From Straumfjord and Copeland: Am. J. Clin. Path., *44*:252, 1965.

$\dagger CV = \frac{S.D.}{mean} = \frac{S}{X}$

‡Number in parentheses = number of reports included.

of the smallest absolute numerical value. The medical purpose of the measurement should be given primary consideration in order to determine optimal quality control goals. The goals for small hospitals should be the same as those for large hospitals.

Daily, Weekly, and Monthly Review of Quality Control. Quality control data are collected for one purpose. DECISION MAKING–Daily–Weekly–Monthly.

Daily Decisions

1. Is each batch of analyses in control?
2. If out-of-control batches occur, what steps shall be taken to correct the "out-of-control" situation?

Weekly Decisions

1. Are the daily results showing a trend? A useful rule of thumb is that more than five analyses on one side of the mean indicate a trend. Not all trends need action, but often a trend can be used to indicate corrective action before the method goes out of control.

Monthly Decisions. Average values should be observed. Changes may indicate instrument, standard or reagent problems or deterioration or contamination of the pool. The one standard deviation values should be observed for changes from the previous months. A doubling of the value indicates a real change in the standard deviation. Values showing progressive changes or values outside the indicated usual performance (Table 1–1) indicate need for trouble-shooting of instrument, method, reagent, or standards.

Suggested action levels are given for which reparative work is mandatory.

For each method and each level of control concentration, make the following decisions:

1. Has the average changed? compared to previous month? year?
2. Has the standard deviation changed?
3. Are daily values showing a trend?
4. If a regional quality control program serum pool is used, how does the laboratory average compare with that of other laboratories? (Fig. 1–4)
5. How do the laboratory results compare with State or other check samples?

After the initial process of calculation of the average and standard deviation for each value, the values may be inserted in a cumulative record (Table 1–2). Next a photocopy is made which is then ready for evaluation of the comparison of data from the previous month and year (Table 1–2). Note the line showing "Difference from Previous Month" and the next line showing the "Evaluation." Refer to the interpretation of the values in Table 1–2.

The results of the "average and SD evaluation" plus the daily dot chart trend evaluation (Fig. 1–3) and the Regional Quality Control Evaluation (Fig. 1–4) are then recorded in a Quality Control Review report as shown on page 9.

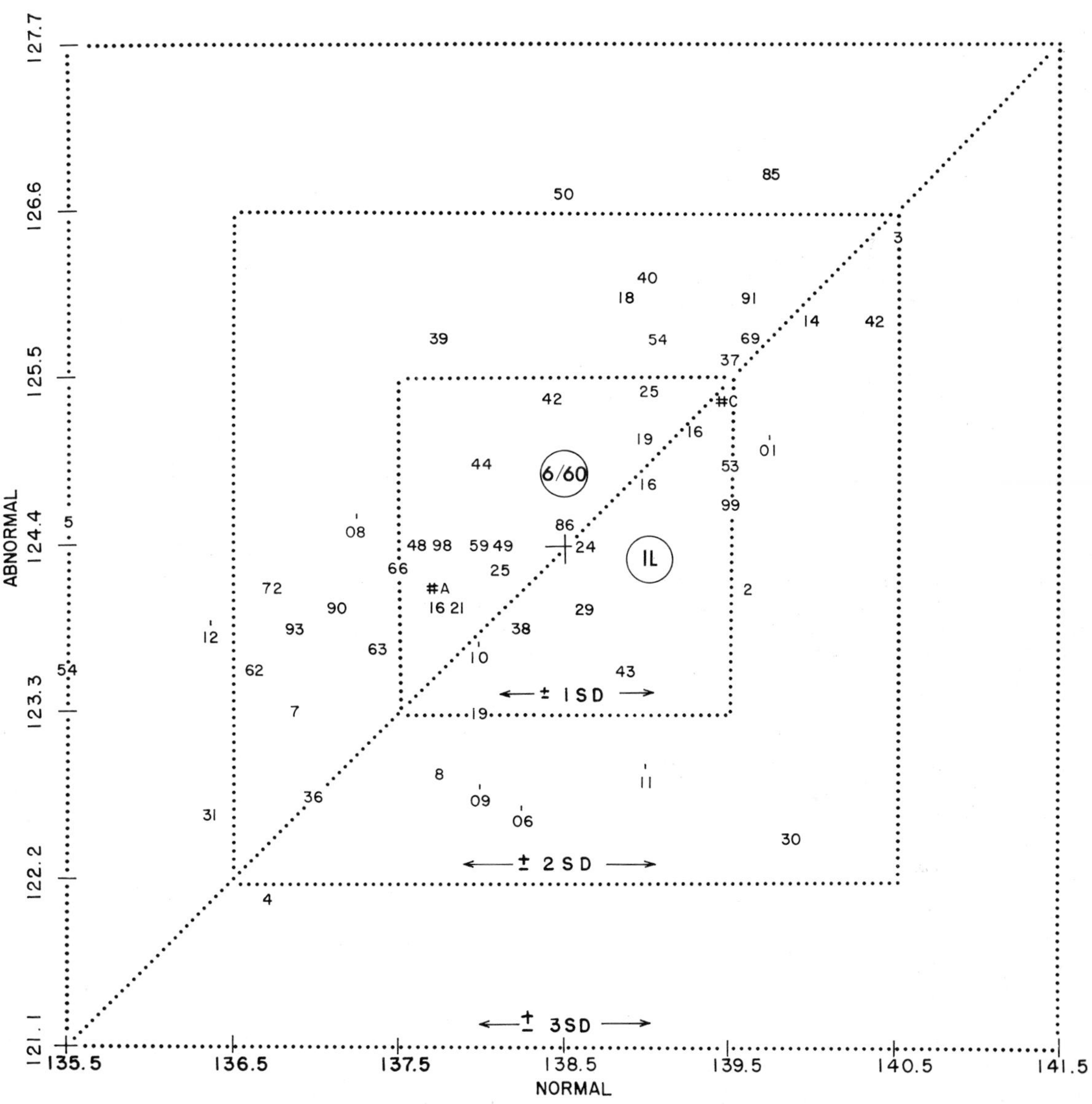

Figure 1-4. Two-way average plot • (Youden) Massachusetts Society of Pathologists Regional Quality Control Report, November, 1971. Each number represents the average value coincidence point of normal and abnormal controls for a single laboratory.

Table 1–2. NEW ENGLAND DEACONESS HOSPITAL PATHOLOGY LABORATORY—CHEMISTRY MASSACHUSETTS SOCIETY OF PATHOLOGISTS' REFERENCE QUALITY CONTROL POOL MONTHLY REVIEW FOR 1971–1972

MONTH	ABNORMAL SGOT Du		ABNORMAL SGOT 12-60		NORMAL SGPT Du		ABNORMAL SGPT Du		NORMAL Sodium IL		NORMAL Sodium 6-60		ABNORMAL Sodium IL		ABNORMAL Sodium 6-60		
	Mean	1 S.D.	Mean	1 S.D.	Mean	1 S.D.	Mean	1 S.D.	Mean	1 S.D.	Mean	1 S.D.	Mean	1 S.D.	Mean	1 S.D.	COMMENTS
PRELIMINARY AVE ± 1 S.D.	87	10.89	101.5	6.26	37.9	6.87	115.1	14.74	139.4	1.99	138.8	1.36	123.1	2.7	125.2	1.46	
JULY	82.1	8.47	96.8	13.84	37.4	10.21	109.4	13.75	139.1	2.26	139.2	1.44	124.7	2.13	125.7	1.20	
AUGUST	78.7	8.5	83.0*	5.1	36.1	5.3	108.1	14.5	138.7	1.7	139.1	0.9	123.6	1.6	125.0	1.2	*Change of reference value
SEPTEMBER	82.8	10.9	80	4.3	34.5	7.19	102.5	16.7	139	1.17	138.6	1.36	124.3	1.51	125.2	1.44	
OCTOBER	79.9	11.7	83.7	3.51	34.6	6.59	106.8	17.4	139.4	1.30	138.4	2.32	124.0	1.68	125.2	1.69	
NOVEMBER	87.0	11.2	82.8	3.85	34.7	7.32	102.0	13.0	138.9	1.30	138.6	1.05	124.1	1.23	124.8	1.41	
DIFFERENCE PREVIOUS MONTH	+7.1	−0.5	−0.9	+0.3	+0.1	+0.7	−4.8	−4.4	−0.5	0.0	+0.2	−1.3	+0.1	−0.4	−0.4	−0.3	
EVALUATION	Note	OK	OK	OK	OK	OK	Note	OK	OK	OK	OK	Improved	OK	OK	OK	OK	BEC, CS, AD
COMMENT	①		②	③	④		⑤			⑥		⑦		⑧			

NOTES OF INTERPRETATION FOR TABLE 1–2

① Note the return to the original average value. Possibly due to change in malic dehydrogenase lot number.

② 12/60 reference material calibrated against kinetic Du method (spectrophotometric). Note first two months were high compared to the reference method. Labeled value on 12/60 reference material was lowered in August. August through November shows good correlation with reference method.

③ Abnormally high 1 S.D. in July corrected in August.

④ Note gradual shift in average to lower values; this needs further observation in future months.

⑤ Note the abnormal range average has decreased significantly since the original month. This may be a reagent or an instrument change. From the pragmatic point of view the average for the dot chart was changed to 105 since the stable average point has been between 102 and 109 for five months.

⑥, ⑦, ⑧. Note 1 S.D. values above the suggested action level (Table 1–1).

Pathology Laboratory
Quality Control Review
Department: Chemistry
Month: November

Reviewed on: December 4, 1972
Reviewed by: C. Shruhan, K. Day, B. E. Copeland

TEST

Test			
SODIUM–IL:	Distribution on dot chart:		
	Normal: Good		
	Abnormal: Good		
	Significant change:	Mean &	1 S.D.
	Normal:	No change	No change
	Abnormal:	No change	Improved
	Position on two-way average plot: Good		
SODIUM–6/60:	Distribution on dot chart:		
	Normal: Good		
	Abnormal: Good		
	Significant change:	Mean &	1 S.D.
	Normal:	No change	Improved
	Abnormal:	No change	Acceptable
	Position on two-way average plot: Good		

Suggested S.D. action levels are given for which reparative work is mandatory. A change in the monthly average greater than 1 S.D. should initiate investigative action.

Decision Criterion No. 2. When is an individual measurement considered reliable? If the quality control sample is in control, the individual sample measurements are reliable because no unusual variables are operating.

EVALUATION OF CHANGE IN A SINGLE PATIENT: THE SIGNIFICANT CHANGE LIMIT

The physician must interpret day-to-day or month-to-month changes in his patient's measurements. He needs tools to distinguish the *inherent variability change* due to methodology from the *real change* in the patient. The information gained from quality control supplies the physician with the tool by which he can follow the progress of the patient under medical therapy from day to day or month to month. **The significant change limit, three times the quality control standard deviation,** is defined as that change which results from a change in the patient and not from the method.

Decision Criterion No. 3. What change in successive measurements indicates a real change in the patient? A change greater than three times the quality control standard deviation is called the significant change limit. The significant change limit enables the physician to follow the course of a disease and its therapy.

Average Versus the Individual: A Note of Caution. In the medical literature, publications frequently indicate a real difference between the average of a normal series of individuals and the average of a series of diseased individuals. Scientifically this is important information. However, this should not lead to the conclusion that such a comparison is useful in identifying the disease in question in a single individual. The diagnosis of disease in an individual depends upon the capacity of a test to show a complete separation of a normal population from a diseased population (Fig. 1–5 A and C). A significant difference between averages can be shown when there is considerable overlap in the two populations

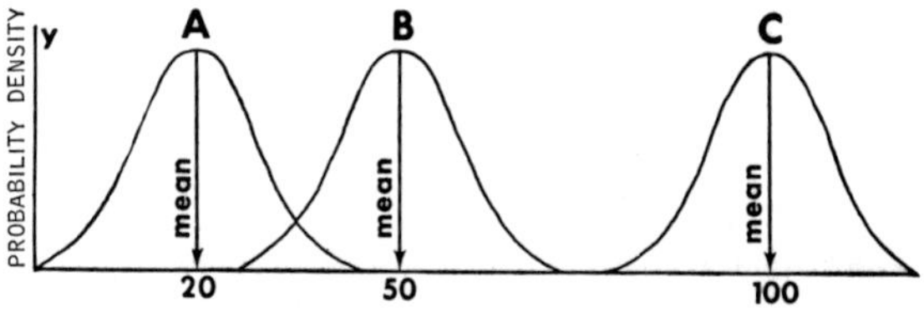

Figure 1–5. Distribution with same standard deviation, or spread, but different mean values. (From Moroney, M. J.: Facts from Figures. London, Penguin Books, 1956.)

(Fig. 1–5 A and B). For example, the difference between the average male height and the average female height is significant. It cannot be inferred that, for the individual, maleness or femaleness can be identified on the basis of height.

Figure 1–5 shows examples of population overlap (A and B) and complete differentiation between populations A and C.

The usefulness of a test to identify a disease state is related to its capacity to help in a problem situation in which the diagnosis is not obvious. Many tests can clearly separate normal populations (Fig. 1–5 A) from the grossly diseased population (Fig. 1–5 C). The crux of the matter is this: How successful is a particular test in indicating disease in the problem case diagnostically, in the presence of other disease states, and in the early stages of the disease when symptoms and physical signs are not present, that is (Fig. 1–5), population A and population B?

A Brief Résumé of Terms Frequently Used To Describe Precision and Accuracy

Precision is the closeness with which measurements agree. Standard deviation is one of the most useful estimates of precision.

Accuracy is the closeness with which results agree with a known true value or a value which is accepted as true.

Standard deviation (Fig. 1–1) describes the distribution of any population of observations.

The standard deviation of individual observations describes the complete distribution (the spread of a distribution) of individuals around the average.

The *relative standard deviation*, also called "coefficient of error" or "coefficient of variation," is the standard deviation related to the concentration level in terms of 100 units of the measured quantity.

$$\frac{\text{Standard deviation}}{\text{Concentration}} \times 100 = \text{relative standard deviation per 100 units}$$

The *standard deviation of the average* is a term which assumes a population of averages when the same experiment is repeated many times. These averages then constitute a population whose distribution has a pattern described by the standard deviation yardstick. By experiment it has been shown that the standard deviation of the average is related to the standard deviation of the individuals in a population. The relationship indicates that as the number of individual observations increases, the validity of the average value increases and its variability decreases.

$$\text{S.D. of av.} = \frac{\text{S. D. of individual}}{\sqrt{\text{no. of individuals}}}$$

The standard deviation of the average is also called the "standard error."

Use of Greek or Latin characters to distinguish known populations from estimates of populations. Statistical jargon differentiates the "estimate of the truth" from the "truth" as follows: the Roman S or S.D. indicates standard deviation (of an estimate), whereas the Greek σ (sigma) indicates true standard deviation (where the complete population has been measured and the actual truth is known). For example, it is possible to know the absolute truth as to the weight of a class of students. It is not possible to know the concentration of glucose in each milliliter of their blood, and therefore we must depend on a sample or estimate of this quantity. For clarification, it can be restated as follows: it is possible to determine the weight distribution of all the children in a school (the population), although we may use a sample of the children to estimate the distribution in the population. In the case of a glucose measurement or a blood sample, one may make several measurements. However, the complete population in this second case consists of an infinity of glucose measurements that could be made on the sample and this clearly is not possible.

Since this fact is usually not clearly indicated in statistics textbooks, the uninitiated frequently make the error of using sigma when an estimate of the standard deviation (S or S.D.) is meant.

Another symbol is the bar over a letter. This means average. $\bar{X}$ (pronounced eks-bar) means the average of all X's measured.

Improvement of Methodology and Instrumentation. It is evident that to reduce the inherent variability of measurements, the major effort should be in the areas of methodology, instrumentation, and primary standards. A method or an instrument that is highly reproducible on a single day may show considerable day-to-day variability over the period of a year. Therefore, it is important to evaluate new methods and new instruments for their inherent variability over a year's time in order to truly evaluate their acceptability in the field. Few methods currently published carry this evaluation nor do any of the new instruments. The tools are readily available for such evaluation and should be utilized. Indeed, workers in the field should demand this information.

The new instruments and new methods constantly being added only create more confusion and increase the variability of this problem, since so few are accompanied by the proper credentials for reproducibility and quality control under regular operating conditions.

TECHNIQUE FOR COMPARING NEW METHODS WITH STANDARD METHODS AND NEW INSTRUMENTS WITH ESTABLISHED INSTRUMENTS.

1. Collect a sample pool large enough to make 20 measurements with each method or instrument.

2. Make the series of 15 to 20 measurements under actual operating conditions, including the effect of different days, technologists, batches of reagents, and so forth.

3. Compute the average and standard deviation for each series of measurements.

Decision Criterion No. 4. Do the methods or instruments under investigation have the same precision, or does one show significantly better precision? If one standard deviation is one-half the other, this method or instrument can be said to be significantly more precise.

Decision Criterion No. 5. Do the methods or instruments give the same average values?

A typical example is given in Table 1–3. Here the Somogyi Nelson reference method is compared with the Beckman Glucose analyzer.

In this case 20 serum samples were analyzed by each method. The instructions for proceeding with the comparison are a simplified form of the average difference relationship (observed versus predicted), also called the "t" test.

Since more than 15 samples are analyzed, evaluation can be made on the basis of the usual two standard deviation limits. Therefore, if the average difference between the two methods is more than two standard deviations of the average from the expected difference of zero, then there is a significant difference between the two methods. When a significant difference is identified, it is important to decide whether it is large enough to be of medical importance. If so, prompt action is indicated, or further evaluation of a new method or instrument should be undertaken.

Criteria for Selection of New Instruments

1. Precision under ideal conditions.

2. Precision under regular working conditions (quality control limits over at least a one-year period).

3. Accuracy (that is, absolute concentration level) and relation to medically accepted values.

4. A complete manual in which all parts are described.

5. Trouble-shooting guide.

6. Approximate cost estimate for yearly maintenance (20 per cent per year has been recommended).

7. Availability of parts and repair service (a four-hour repair time would be ideal).

8. Operating criteria for daily checking.

Criteria for Selection of New Methods

1. Precision under optimal conditions.

2. Precision under regular working conditions.

3. Accuracy (that is, absolute concentration level) and relation to medically accepted values.

4. Quality control limits obtainable over a year's time.

5. Number of analytical runs out of control in a one-year period.

SUMMARY

Laboratory measurements are useful only when interpreted with the knowledge of the normal population variation and an understanding of the inherent variability present in all instruments and methods.

The standard deviation is a descriptive tool, which describes variation in population groups. This property makes it indispensable in quality control systems and in the decision-making process in the laboratory and at the bedside.

CASE HISTORIES

I

A phosphorus procedure had an average pool value of 3.2 mg. per dl. (dl. = deciliter = 100 ml.) and a 1 S.D. of 0.2 mg. per dl. On which of the following days were the quality control samples out of control?

Monday	3.6
Tuesday	2.9
Wednesday	4.1
Thursday	3.3
Friday	3.1

Evaluation: On Wednesday the phosphorus procedure was out of control.

Cause: Review showed that the glassware had been washed with a phosphate cleaner and had not been thoroughly rinsed.

II

A patient was under therapy for kidney damage. The physician observed the BUN daily to detect when kidney function began to improve. The 1 S.D. for day-to-day quality control for the BUN method was 1.5 mg. per dl. The daily BUN values were as follows:

Monday	40.0
Tuesday	41.3
Wednesday	37.6
Thursday	40.3
Friday	35.0
Saturday	31.0

Evaluation: The significant change limit for this BUN method is 4.5 mg. per dl. Therefore, on Friday the change in BUN exceeded the significant change limit. This change represented a real change in the patient's value.

Table 1–3. FORMAT FOR CALCULATION OF AVERAGE DIFFERENCE RELATIONSHIP—OBSERVED AS PREDICTED ("t")

TEST PERIOD

INSTRUMENT A INSTRUMENT B

FRAME OF REFERENCE Time:
Operator:
Sample:

I	II	III	IV	V	VI	VII
Sample n	Instrument A	Instrument B	Diff. A-B Keep Sign*	Observed Ave. Diff. ($\bar{D}$) Insert in each box	Diff. from Ave. Diff. ($D-\bar{D}$)	$(D-\bar{D})^2$
1	95	85	10	-2.5	12.5	156.25
2	102	98	4	-2.5	6.5	42.25
3	101	96	5	-2.5	7.5	56.25
4	104	94	10	-2.5	12.5	156.25
5	79	82	-3	-2.5	-0.5	0.25
6	89	88	1	-2.5	3.5	12.25
7	94	91	3	-2.5	5.5	30.25
8	97	90	7	-2.5	9.5	90.25
9	89	89	0	-2.5	2.5	6.25
10	88	98	-10	-2.5	-7.5	56.25
11	85	95	-10	-2.5	-7.5	56.25
12	85	88	- 3	-2.5	-0.5	0.25
13	103	86	17	-2.5	19.5	380.25
14	96	99	- 3	-2.5	-0.5	0.25
15	90	106	-16	-2.5	-13.5	182.25
16	81	85	- 4	-2.5	-1.5	2.25
17	96	94	2	-2.5	4.5	20.25
18	87	115	-28	-2.5	-25.5	650.25
19	67	100	-33	-2.5	-30.5	930.25
20	96	94	2	-2.5	4.5	20.25
		* Sum + =	61			2849.25
		* Sum − =	110			
		Sum A-B = -49		Sum $(D-\bar{D})^2$ = 2849		

CALCULATION PROCEDURE:
1. Record values in columns 2 and 3
2. Calculate differences A-B. Record in Column 4. (Keep Sign)
3. Calculate average difference from Column 4 - Calculation A (Keep Sign)
4. Record with sign average difference in each box of Column 5.
5. Calculate and record in Column 6 the individual differences from average difference. Observe sign.
6. Square each ($D-\bar{D}$) and record in Column 7.
7. Add Column 7.
8. Calculate standard deviation (SD) of the difference - Line B.
9. Calculate standard deviation of average difference - Line C.

EVALUATION SECTION
10. No difference assumption; if test systems are the same, the average difference will be zero (null).
11. The expected variability around 1 an average difference of zero is plus or minus three times the standard deviation of the average difference (c).
12. Below the diagram insert the calculated value for ± 1,2,3 SD ave diff

CALCULATIONS
A. A-B = each individual difference
n = number of differences
Average difference = $\frac{\text{sum A-B}}{n}$ or $\frac{\Sigma \text{A-B}}{n}$

Observed Ave. Diff. = $\frac{-49}{20}$ = -2.5

B. Standard deviation of the differences A-B = $SD_{A\text{-}B}$ = $\sqrt{\frac{\Sigma(D-\bar{D})^2}{n-1}}$

Standard deviation of the differences A-B = $SD_{A\text{-}B}$ = $\sqrt{\frac{2849}{19}}$ = 149

Standard deviation of the differences A-B = $SD_{A\text{-}B}$ = 12.2

C. Standard deviation of Ave. Difference $\frac{SD_{A\text{-}B}}{\sqrt{n}}$ = $\frac{12.2}{\sqrt{20}}$ = $\frac{12.2}{4.5}$ = 2.7

EVALUATION SECTION
13. Locate observed average difference in the expected distribution around zero.
14. To be no different, obs. ave. diff. should fall within 3 SD of the average difference. If outside 3 SD, there is a statistical difference.

Predicted Distribution

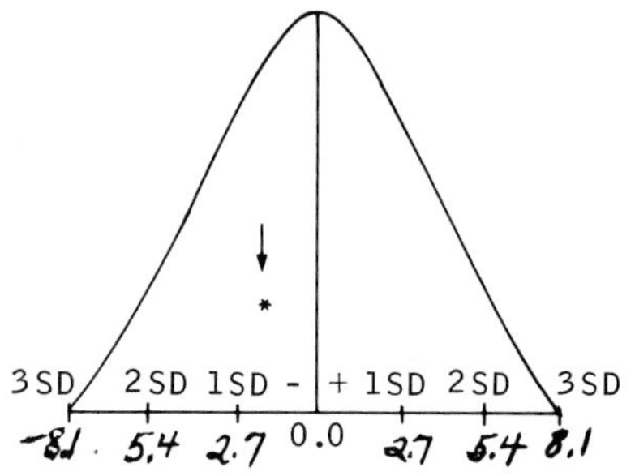

CONCLUSION
15. The difference observed (is, (is not)) statistically significant.
16. The difference observed (is (is not)) medically significant.
17. Evaluated by William Peace 8-1-72
Name Date

This form developed at the New England Deaconess Hospital, Boston
Bradley E. Copeland, M.D.

III

A new model flame photometer is tested and compared with the current model in use. The following results are obtained:

	NEW	CURRENT
Quality control		
Serum pool		
(15 days)		
Average:	135.4	135.9
1 S.D.	1.2	1.5
Normal blood donors		
Twenty subjects		
Average:	140.0	139.0
1 S.D.	2.1	2.4

Questions: (1) Is the new flame photometer as precise as the current model? (2) Is the new flame photometer as accurate as the current model? (3) Will substitution of the new instrument require an announcement to physicians of new normal values?

Evaluation: (1) The day-to-day variability of the two instruments is the same. (2) The current instrument is assumed to be the reference point. With the new instrument, the average values for the pool and normal values are the same as for the current instrument. (3) No notice to the physicians will be required. Normal values for the new and current instrument are the same from two points of view: the average and the standard deviation of the population.

IV

A physician wished to interpret a serum uric acid value of a patient who complained of joint pain in his right hand. The uric acid value was 7.4 mg. per 100 ml. serum. Normal uric acid in an available textbook listed: (1) 4 to 6 mg. per 100 ml. blood, and (2) 5 to 7 mg. per 100 ml. serum as normal. The laboratory reported that on 20 normal male blood donors the average value was 6.4 mg. per 100 ml. serum 1 S.D. = ± 0.6 mg. per 100 ml. serum.

Questions: Which set of normal values should this physician have used? (2) Was the patient normal or abnormal?

Evaluation: (1) The set of normal values determined by the laboratory on serum should have been used. Interlaboratory differences are caused by different methods, different instruments, different reagents. Uric acid methodology is particularly prone to interlaboratory differences. (2) The patient's value fell outside one standard deviation for the normal 7.0 mg. per 100 ml. but within two standard deviations 7.6 mg. per 100 ml. The patient was within the ± 2 S.D. or 95 per cent range of the normal population. A value over 7.6 mg. per 100 ml. would warrant further follow-up in the future. A value over 8.2 mg. per 100 ml. should initiate an immediate search for the cause of hyperuricemia (elevated serum uric acid).

V

The April monthly report of quality control performance is presented for evaluation to the laboratory director and the chief medical technologist.

Questions: (1) Evaluate the stability of each method. (2) Evaluate the precision of each method.

Evaluation: Glucose, Pool is stable. Day-to-day 1 S.D. has increased from 3.0 to 6.1 mg. per dl. since January. *Decision:* Review and renew reagents and check parts of automatic instrument for wear. *BUN,* In this case, pool average has increased. 1 S.D. has increased, which is probably a reflection of the change in the average. *Decision:* Suspect reagent

POOL K		JANUARY	FEBRUARY	MARCH	APRIL
Glucose	Av.	120.0	123.0	119.0	121.0
Automated	1 S.D.	3.0	4.5	4.9	6.1
(ferricyanide)	Number	20	19	21	20
BUN	Av.	18.4	17.8	19.0	21.6
Automated	1 S.D.	1.5	0.9	1.1	2.4
(diacetyl monoxime)	Number	20	21	21	22
CO_2	Av.	24.3	23.1	24.0	23.7
(Van Slyke	1 S.D.	1.2	1.1	0.8	1.3
volumetric)	Number	20	19	21	16
Chloride	Av.	104.0	103.5	104.2	103.8
(electrometric)	1 S.D.	1.2	1.4	1.7	2.2
	Number	19	21	20	21
Transaminase	Av.	150.0	140.0	135.0	128.0
(ultraviolet)	1 S.D.	10.0	12.0	11.0	14.0
	Number	15	17	19	16

or standard deterioration. Prepare new standards and reagents. Check one variable at a time to identify the responsible cause. *Chloride,* Pool stable. 1 S.D. has risen above the usual expected performance (see Table 1–2). *Decision:* Check and clean electrodes. Check instrument for indications of deteriorated components. *CO_2*, Pool stable. 1 S.D. stable. *Transaminase,* Pool deteriorating. *Decision:* Prepare new pool. Maintenance of an elevated transaminase pool is difficult. In the normal range, transaminase pools are quite stable.

Survey Participation as a Quality Control Technique. All laboratories should participate in periodic regional or national surveys. The purpose of the survey is to stimulate interest in precision and accuracy. The survey provides an opportunity for a laboratory to compare itself with referee laboratories of the highest competence and with many hospital laboratories throughout the United States.

Surveys are important in guiding the selection of new instruments and methods. It is the responsibility of all medical laboratories to reduce interlaboratory differences to a minimum. Surveys have played an important role in the past and will be even more important in the future.

Survey samples are available from the Standard Committee of the College of American Pathologists, 230 North Michigan Avenue, Chicago, Illinois 60601, and are also offered by some state public health departments.

REFERENCES

Benenson, A. S., Thompson, H. L., and Klugerman, M. R.: Application of laboratory controls in clinical chemistry. Am. J. Clin. Path. 25:87, 1955.

Bodansky, M., and Bodansky, O.: Biochemistry of Disease. 2nd edition. New York, The Macmillan Company, 1952.

Copeland, B. E.: Quality Control in Clinical Chemistry, Revised edition. Chicago, Commission on Continuing Education. American Society of Clinical Pathologists, 1973.

Freier, E. F., and Rausch, V. L.: Quality control in clinical chemistry. Am. J. Med. Techn. 24:195, 1958.

Spector, W. B. (ed.): Handbook of Biological Data. Philadelphia, W. B. Saunders Company, 1956.

Sunderman, F. W., and Boerner, F.: Normal Values in Clinical Medicine. Philadelphia, W. B. Saunders Company, 1949.

Chapter 2

EXAMINATION OF THE URINE

by G. MARY BRADLEY, M.D.
and ELLIS S. BENSON, M.D.

HISTORY

Inspection of the urine for diagnostic purposes has been practiced for centuries and probably represents the oldest of laboratory procedures used in medicine today.

The ancients paid great attention to the character of the urine in disease (Keele, 1963). The Hippocratic school of medicine (fifth century B.C.) probably relied on earlier teachings. According to the book *Prognostics* (Adams, 1886), a careful examination of all excreta was used as a basis for estimating the course of disease: "If the urine is reddish, the sediment consistent and smooth, the affection will be more protracted but still not fatal. . . . Clouds carried about in the urine are good when white, but bad if black. . . . Fatty substances floating on the surface are to be dreaded, for they are indications of melting."

Hippocrates noted that the volume of urine should be in proportion to the drink that is taken and somewhat thicker than the fluid that is drunk. He differentiated changes in the urine due to local bladder disease from those resulting from generalized disease, an observation later praised by Galen (A.D. 150-190) in his *Commentaries* (Adams, 1886). Unfortunately, however, not all the physicians who followed were so astute, and as a result, for several centuries the systematization of medicine propounded by Galen and the Arabians became grossly overemphasized.

In medieval times a physician or apothecary might examine the urine and not examine the patient. Special vessels with markings representing areas of the body received the urine specimen; these may be seen in medieval paintings and woodcuts depicting uroscopists. Gilles de Corbeil (thirteenth century) used an elaborate system of urinalysis which combines 20 colors, three consistencies, and four zones to predict the course of an illness (Keele, 1963). Johannes Actuarius of Constantinople published his best known work, De Urinis, in the thirteenth century. In it he related urine color to the humors. He was the first to describe paroxysmal hemoglobinuria (Major, 1932). The Italian surgeon William de Saliceto (1210–1280) noted the coincidence of contracted kidney and dropsy, but several hundred years elapsed before his observations were confirmed (Major, 1932).

It was not until the growth of chemistry, physics, and physiology in the seventeenth century began to influence medical thought that urinalysis became more a science and less a mystique. Van Helmont (1572–1644), for example, measured specific gravity and showed that the specific gravity of urine increased during fever and decreased in polyuria (Keele, 1963). The polyuria of diabetes had been noted by ancient physicians, and the sweet taste of diabetic urine was noted by Sasruta, a Hindu physician, in 600 B.C. (Gordon, 1949). However, Thomas Willis was apparently the first to record the sweet taste of diabetic urine in recent times; in 1674 he mentioned that the urine in diabetes had a taste similar to honey (Major, 1932). In 1673 a Dutch physician described a heat and acetic acid urine test which caused a milkiness (or coagulum) in the urine of patients with wasting diseases. The significance of this test was not understood until much later. In 1811 William Wells, and American-born physician working in London, and John Blackall noted the coincidence of proteinuria and dropsy but did not connect the findings with renal disease (Major, 1932). Richard Bright finally elucidated the relationship between edema, proteinuria, and abnormal kidney autopsy findings and published his case reports in 1827. Much of Bright's work on urinalysis was done by a physician-chemist, John Bostock, who reported low specific gravity and large amounts of protein in the urine of patients with renal disease (Osman, 1937).

In the latter part of the nineteenth century, many handbooks on urinalysis were published, the forerunner of these being issued by William Prout, a colleague of Bright's, in 1821 (Foster, 1961). Prout's routine tests included daily urine volume, color, specific gravity, and reaction to litmus paper. Protein was detected by heat and sugar by taste or alternatively by a specific gravity higher than 1.030.

Medicine continued to benefit from the work of chemists: Berzelius analyzed urine for many organic constituents and suggested that the relatively large amounts of urea in the urine compared with blood might indicate that the kidneys remove urea from the blood. Sugar in urine was identified as glucose in 1838, and Fehling's quantitative test for sugars was described in 1848. The biuret test for protein was developed in 1833, and Henry Bence Jones, a physician-chemist, discovered the urinary protein that bears his name in 1848 (Keele, 1963). By this time textbooks of medicine recommended that a routine urinalysis be performed on each patient.

Paralleling the development of chemical tests was the development of medical microscopy. A pioneering course in medical microscopy was taught by Alfred Donné in Paris in 1837 (Foster, 1961). Pus cells were identified in a cloudy urine specimen and distinguished from a variety of crystals and amorphous deposits. Casts—"coagulated albumin sometimes tubular"—were observed in urine in Bright's disease by Golding Bird, a pathologist at Guy's Hospital, London, and others, including Bence Jones.

In the early twentieth century, Thomas Addis developed techniques for the quantitative analysis of urinary sediment (Addis, 1925, 1926). Routine urinalysis changed little in concept, but qualitative tests became easier to perform with the advent of tablets or cellulose strips impregnated with test reagents, and quantitative tests on the urine increased both in number and precision.

Just as Hippocrates in the fifth century B.C. exhorted his followers to examine the urine, the writers of a work on urinalysis in 1863 exhorted the physician to test the urine at the bedside: "Armed with the simplest, newest methods of analysis, the physicians may discover the presence of abnormal constituents" (Neubauer and Vogel, 1863). The same principle applies now.

COMPOSITION OF THE URINE

Nutritional status, the state of metabolic processes, and the ability of the kidney to selectively handle the material presented to it are three principal factors affecting the composition of the urine.

In the normal adult, about 1200 ml. of blood passes through the kidney each minute, exposing the plasma to the semipermeable membrane of each functioning glomerulus. The ultrafiltrate that collects in Bowman's capsule contains all of the substances of the plasma capable of passing through the membrane. The pH of the filtrate (7.4) and its osmolality (about 285 mOsm. per kg. of water) are the same as in plasma. Modification of this filtrate to produce excreted urine occurs in the tubules and collecting duct of the nephron. Glucose, amino acids, and other threshold substances are reabsorbed in the proximal tubules, leaving urea, uric acid, phosphates, and other materials in the filtrate. By the time the fluid reaches Henle's loop in the medulla, the original rate of flow of 130 ml. per minute has been reduced to about 16 ml. per minute because of the absorption of most of the water and electrolytes. In the distal tubule, more water may be absorbed and acidification of urine occurs. Further absorption of water may take place in the collecting duct. The filtrate is now reduced to a flow rate of about 1 ml. per minute, has a pH of about 6, and an osmolality of about 800 to 1200 mOsm. per kg. of water.

A discussion of the volume, appearance and color, hydrogen ion concentration, specific gravity, and osmolality of the urine is presented later in this chapter. A more detailed discussion of the function of the nephron will be found in Chapter 3.

Urine Solute. A large proportion of the urine solute is made up of urea and sodium chloride. On an ordinary diet of about 1 gm. of protein per kg. an average adult excretes in the urine about 10 gm. per day of nitrogen, most of which will be in the form of urea. Other substances, such as uric acid, creatinine, amino acids, ammonia, and traces of proteins, glycoproteins, enzymes, and purines, account for the remaining nitrogen excreted. There is a continuous excretion of uric acid, for example, even when purine intake is absent. Average uric acid excretion in an adult is about 0.5 gm. in 24 hours. Creatinine excretion is higher in children than in adults and higher in males than in females and is not related to dietary protein unless the intake is very high.

Excretions of sodium and chloride are directly related to dietary intake, principally from salt added to food. Since individual intake is quite variable, output may vary from about 5 to about 20 gm. as sodium chloride in a 24-hour period. Potassium is quite ubiquitous in the diet and is found in meats and vegetables. Normally about 70 mEq. of potassium is excreted in a 24-hour period. Sulfate is excreted as inorganic sulfate, organic sulfate, and other sulfur-containing substances, such as sulfides, cysteine, and mercaptan. Urinary inorganic sulfate is derived from the metabolism of cystine and methionine and is thus related to protein intake. Organic sulfates are generally conjugates of steroids and phenols. The proportion of organic sulfate and total sulfate usually remains quite constant; total sulfate excretion in 24-hours is about 0.7 gm. and that of organic sulfate about 0.07 gm. Phosphate excretion is variable and is derived chiefly from nucleic acid in food, casein, and other organic and inorganic phosphates. About 1 gm. of phosphate is excreted as organic phosphate in 24 hours. Phosphate and sulfate are partly responsible for the acidity of urine. For more details on the influence of diet on solute, see Hoffman, 1970. See Appendix 3 for Normal Values.

Other than the nitrogenous material and salts already mentioned, normal urine contains small amounts of sugars, which, for example, like the pentoses, will vary in amount with dietary intake. Intermediary metabolites, such as oxalic acid, citric acid, and pyruvate, are present. Free fatty acids and trace amounts of cholesterol are also found, as are trace amounts of metals.

Hormones such as the ketosteroids, estrogens, aldosterone and pituitary gonadotropins, and the biogenic amines – the catecholamines and serotonin metabolites – are normally found in urine and reflect metabolic and endocrine status. Vitamins such as ascorbic acid are excreted in the urine in amounts that depend on the sufficiency of dietary intake. While hemoglobin and heme pigments are not normally present, trace amounts of porphyrins and related compounds such as delta aminolevulinic acid are found.

In general, the composition of the urine reflects the ability of the normal kidney to retain and reabsorb those substances essential to basic metabolism and homeostasis and to excrete the excess materials from the diet together with the end products of endocrine and metabolic processes.

Normal values for physical properties and cellular constituents of urine are shown in Tables 2–1 and 2–2.

Identification of Urine. Occasionally, following abdominal or pelvic surgery, drainage fluid is submitted to the laboratory for identification as urine. After centrifugation, the supernatant may be tested for urea, creatinine, sodium, and chloride. These levels are usually sufficiently concentrated in urine (even when diluted with wound site effusion) to separate probable urine from plasma or serous exudate.

Table 2–1. PHYSICOCHEMICAL CHARACTERISTICS OF URINE

	NORMAL VALUES	REMARKS	REFERENCE
Dry weight	55.0-70.0 gm./24 hr.		Sunderman, 1949
Freezing-point depression	0.075-2.6° C.		
Osmolality	38-1400 mOsm./kg. water	Average normal urine 500-800 mOsm./kg. water. Ratio of urine to plasma, 3:1.	Maxwell, 1962
pH	4.6-8.0 (mean, 6.1)		Sunderman, 1949
Specific gravity			
Newborn (first few days)	1.012		Rubin, 1964
Infants	1.002-1.006		
Adults	1.001-1.035	Adult normal fluid intake 1.016-1.022.	Sunderman, 1949
Volume			
Newborn (1-2 days old)	30-60 ml./24 hr.		Rubin, 1964
Infants			
3-10 days	100-300 ml./24 hr.		
10-60 days	250-450 ml./24 hr.		
60-365 days	400-500 ml./24 hr.		
Children			
1-3 years	500-600 ml./24 hr.		
3-5 years	600-700 ml./24 hr.		
5-8 years	650-1000 ml./24 hr.		
8-14 years	800-1400 ml./24 hr.		
Adults	600-1600 ml./24 hr.		
Older adults	250-2400 ml./24 hr.		Howell, 1956

Table 2–2. CELLS AND CASTS

	RANGE	MEAN	REFERENCE
Erythrocytes	to 1 million/day 0-473,000/hr., female 0-915,000/hr., male	130,000/day 29,000/hr., female 38,000/hr., male	Addis, 1948 Prescott, 1965
Casts—hyaline and occasional granular	to 5,000/day	2,000/day	Addis, 1948
Leukocytes and nonsquamous epithelial cells	to 2 million/day	650,000/day	
Differential			
Renal tubular cells	5,000-243,000/hr., female 12,000-262,000/hr., male	68,000/hr., female 78,000/hr., male	Prescott, 1965
Leukocytes (PMN)	0-5,042,000/hr., female 0-956,000/hr., male	108,000/hr., female 28,000/hr., male	
Squamous epithelial	variable		

EXAMINATION OF THE URINE: GENERAL COMMENTS

The use of simple tests such as those for proteinuria, sugars, and the examination of the urinary sediment will provide the physician with helpful information concerning the diagnosis and management of renal disease, urinary tract disease, and many systemic diseases. With the introduction of simple techniques in which reagent strips and tablets are used, tests that previously required more complex chemical analysis may now be accomplished with ease. A physician should be able to perform the necessary screening tests himself and know how to interpret them in relation to the health and management of his patient.

Examination of the urine may be considered from two general standpoints—diagnosis and management of renal or urinary tract disease, and the detection of metabolic or systemic diseases not directly related to the kidney.

Among the most important conditions readily detected by chemical means are glycosuria, ketonuria, and the presence of the pigments bilirubin, urobilinogen, hemoglobin, and the porphyrins. The urine may also be screened for metabolites of drugs such as phenothiazines, abnormal amino acid metabolites, calcium, and other substances present in abnormal amounts or not normally present.

Proteinuria is probably the most common indication of renal disease. It is, for example, an early indication of latent glomerulonephritis, toxemia of pregnancy, and diabetic nephropathy. The finding of proteinuria may strongly suggest the presence of renal disease as opposed to lower urinary tract disease when considered with the clinical findings; confirmation of the presence of renal disease can be made by finding casts in the microscopic examination of the urine sediment.

Microscopic examination of the sediment in a properly collected sample of urine may not only provide evidence of renal disease but also indicate the kind of lesion present or the state of activity of a known lesion. It should be included in every complete medical examination because it provides important information concerning the kidneys and urinary tract not readily obtainable in any other way.

For a more detailed discussion of urinary findings in renal disease, the reader is referred to Lippman (1957) and Strauss and Welt (1971).

Procedure for Routine Screening Urinalysis

The Urine Specimen. The volume of urine necessary depends on the number of tests to be performed; as little as 2 ml. will suffice for basic chemical screening, the copper reduction test (5 drops), and specific gravity (1 drop), and a loopful for culture or Gram stain and for sediment examination. However, 15 ml. or more is preferable for routine work.

Specimens must be refrigerated if not examined immediately. All specimens should be free from fecal and vaginal contamination. (See Collection of Urine, p. 79.)

Screening for Bacteriuria. If only one specimen is available for complete urinalysis this should be done first. Alternative procedures include a Gram stain of the uncentrifuged, well-mixed specimen and the quantitative loop culture method or a miniculture method, all of which require a drop or two of urine. The tetrazolium reduction test, a simpler test, is used for mass screening and requires 2 ml. of urine.

Specific Gravity. At this point a drop may be used for refractometer estimation of specific gravity.

Chemical Screening (Basic). Using combination reagent strips, dip and read for all or some of the following:

pH
protein
glucose
ketone
blood } e.g., Labstix*
bilirubin } e.g. Bililabstix*
urobilinogen – e.g., Urobilistix* } Multistix*

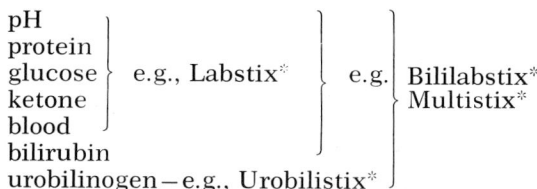

If the multiple reagent strip is not to be used, Ictotest* for bilirubin is as simple, more sensitive, and easier to interpret than Bililabstix reagent strips. The use of reagent strips makes it more certain that tests will be done because of the ease of operation.

Test for Copper-reducing Substances. It is most important that this test be performed on all specimens from infants by either the Benedict or Clinitest* tablet method. The test should be done when the glucose oxidase test is positive to distinguish higher levels of glucose (see Table 2–3).

At this point the specimen should be centrifuged in a disposable centrifuge tube, and the clear supernatant separated from the sediment and refrigerated.

The Sediment. A drop of the concentrated sediment is examined under a coverslip for red blood cells, leukocytes, renal epithelial cells, casts, and excessive numbers of crystals. These are usually graded as to number of cells in an average of 10 high-power fields.

Alternatively, the uncentrifuged, well-mixed specimen may be examined in a counting chamber and reported as cells per cubic millimeter.

The Supernatant. The supernatant is used for the following tests:

1. A confirmatory protein test.
2. Separation of sugars is carried out by thin layer chromatography when Benedict's test is positive and the glucose oxidase test is negative.

The Result. The chemical screening and sediment results should be checked against each other, e.g., for blood and red cells, before reports are issued.

*Ames Co., Inc., Elkhart, Indiana.

Urinary Screening for Inborn Errors of Metabolism

In these diseases an abnormal metabolite or a larger than normal amount of a normal metabolite is excreted in the urine, although the kidney itself is not always involved. Many of these diseases are associated with mental deficiency, degeneration of the nervous system, and "failure to thrive." Early detection is useful in galactosemia and may be helpful in other diseases and for genetic counseling. Mass screening will provide a very low yield; screening of infants at risk and those with slow development will provide higher levels of positive results. However, very careful laboratory and clinical interpretation of the screening tests is required because of the number of false positives, e.g., transient tyrosinuria of the newborn. On the other hand, false negative results will occur if the newborn has not had several days to ingest food or because urine is not the best test material, as in phenylketonuria.

Genetic disease of the kidney is uncommon, and many patients are diagnosed from the history and clinical findings; however, in some instances urinary screening may indicate the presence of a specific disease. Functional genetic abnormalities are usually associated with a transport defect of the proximal renal tubular epithelial cell, and these include renal

Table 2–3. SENSITIVITY OF TESTS FOR GLUCOSE AND REDUCING SUBSTANCES IN URINE

Benedict's Cu reduction	Qual. Interpretation	Neg	Trace	1+	2+		3+	4+
	Approx. mg./100 ml.	0	10–100	250	500–1000		1–2000	>2000
Clinitest* Cu reduction	Qual. Interpretation	—	—	Trace	1+	2+	3+	4+
	Approx. mg./100 ml.	0	—	250	500	750	1000	2000
Glucose oxidase reagent strips								
Clinistix*	Qual. Interpretation		"Light-	Medium-	Dark-		Purple"	
	Approx. mg./100 ml.	0	40–100	250	500+			
Tes-tape†	Qual. Interpretation	0	1+	2+	3+		—	4+
	Approx. mg./100 ml.	0	100	250	500			2000
Diastix*	Qual. Interpretation	0	Trace	1+	2+		3+	4+
	Approx. mg./100 ml.	0	100	250	500		1000	2000

*Ames Co., Elkhart, Indiana.
†Eli Lilly.

glucosuria and cystinuria. Polyuria and low specific gravity are found in vasopressin-resistant diabetes insipidus. Urinary pH measurement is helpful in diagnosis of distal renal tubular acidosis. With structural abnormalities such as polycystic disease and various genetic nephritides, proteinuria, hematuria, increased leukocytes, and renal epithelial cells are found. Frequently there is a urinary tract infection associated with a structural defect in the urinary tract. Urinary findings associated with genetic disease of the kidney may appear on a careful routine examination. For other metabolic diseases additional screening tests are needed. A laboratory offering these screening procedures should have the capability of further investigation or access to a reference laboratory.

SPECIMEN REQUIREMENTS. About 20 ml. of a fresh specimen or refrigerated specimen is required. In older children a concentrated specimen is usually available. The following tests may be used:

1. Benedict's qualitative test – sugars (p. 57).
2. Cyanide-nitroprusside test – for cystine and homocystine (p. 52).
3. Ferric chloride test – for several amino acids (pp. 52, 53).
4. Dinitrophenylhydrazine test – for keto-acids.
5. Nitroso naphthol test – for tyrosine (p. 53).
6. Berry spot test – for mucopolysaccharides.

In these laboratories electrophoretic separation of amino acids is also used as a screening procedure (pp. 50, 71).

Quality Control

This may be difficult to achieve in urinalysis, especially as it relates to the urinary sediment and its interpretation. Whenever possible, positive controls should be run with qualitative tests; this is very important, for example, in the spot test for mucopolysaccharides, to identify a true positive. Standard tubes for the copper reduction test showing trace to 4+ results may be made up in synthetic urine and will store for many months if the tops are corked and sealed. This applies also to standards for the qualitative protein tests. Lyophilized preparations are available for checking reagent strips. These may be diluted and distributed into small vials, stored, and used for each new lot number of test strips. These preparations are also useful for testing the grading of results by new personnel.

To facilitate dissolution, pulverize all dry reagents with a mortar and pestle. Dilute to volume with distilled water. Keep controls in stock bottle at room temperature. Remove 50 to 100 ml aliquots periodically to working control bottle. Solutions are stable 6–9 months at room temperature.

Expected Result

Low Control. Multiple Reagent strip: pH6, protein 2+, glucose med., ketone neg., blood sm. to mod., protein ppt. 2+, Benedict's 1+, Clinitest trace, Diastix 1+, Test-tape 2+, Acetest neg, specific gravity 1.006, osmolality 305 mOsm./kg. water.

High Control. Multiple Reagent Strip: pH 6, protein 4+, glucose dark, ketone small, blood neg., protein ppt. 3–4+, Benedict's 3+, Clinitest 3+, Diastix 3+, Test-tape 3+, Acetest small, specific gravity 1.020, osmolality 660 mOsm./kg. water.

Bilirubin and urobilinogen are negative for each control. Each laboratory will need to establish it's own acceptable range of performance.

NOTE. For teaching purposes, solutions may be made in advance (without chloroform) with varying amounts of reactants, frozen in 10-ml. amounts and stored. Bile may be added. Food coloring to simulate urine may be added. Specimens should be thoroughly thawed before use. Normal hepatitis-free plasma may be substituted for bovine albumin in an appro-

Reagents

QUALITY CONTROL REAGENT

REAGENT	LOW CONTROL		HIGH CONTROL	
	1 liter	concn.	1 liter	concn.
Sodium chloride AR	5.0 g.	500 mg./dl.	10.0 g.	1000 mg./dl.
Urea AR	5.0 gm.	500 mg./dl.	10.0 gm.	1000 mg./dl.
Creatinine AR	0.5 gm.	50 mg./dl.	0.5 gm.	50 mg./dl.
Glucose AR	3.0 gm.	300 mg./dl.	15.0 gm.	1500 mg./dl.
30% Bovine albumin	5.0 ml.	150 mg./dl.	35 ml.	1050 mg./dl.
Whole normal blood (with Hct. 40–45) (Hbg. 13–15 gm.%)	100 μl.	1.3–1.5 mg./dl.	–	–
Acetone AR	–	–	2 ml.	160 mg./dl.
Chloroform AR	5 ml.	0.5 ml./dl.	5 ml.	0.5 mg./dl.
Distilled water qs	to 1 liter		to 1 liter	

priate concentration. It is important to include creatinine to obtain good copper reduction test results.

Precautions in Use of Reagent Strips. Protect reagent strips from moisture and excessive heat to prevent loss of sensitivity. Brownish discoloration may indicate significant loss of reactivity; reagent strips with such discoloration should not be used. Store strips in a cool, dry area but not in a refrigerator. Remove only enough reagent strips for immediate use, and recap bottle immediately.

Avoid contamination of reagent strip. Do not touch test areas with fingers. Do not lay reagent strip on table surface – use clean sheet of paper. Do not use strips in the presence of volatile acid or alkaline fumes.

Properly moisten reagent strip in well-mixed urine when testing specimen. Avoid incomplete dipping; all test areas must be completely moistened. Avoid prolonged dipping; excessive dipping may cause leaching of test reagents.

Exercise care in reading reagent strip. Observe time elements indicated in the directions for their use. Hold reagent strip close to appropriate color chart when reading. Read only under good lighting conditions.

Examination of the Urine Sediment

In order to achieve the best results, a fresh, concentrated, clean-voided urine specimen should be used. The first morning specimen of urine is usually sufficiently concentrated; hypotonic urines may result in lysis of cells and casts. Cleansing and rinsing of the external genital area with soap and water before urination will prevent contamination of the urine with vaginal secretions and cellular debris of the urethral meatus. If examination of the sediment is delayed, the urine sample may be stored in a refrigerator for a short time, but not for more than an hour.

Several techniques have been used to help to delineate the cellular structures and differentiate them from crystals and debris. On careful examination of the unstained sediment, the formed elements of diagnostic significance are usually seen. Subdued light or phase microscopy is needed to delineate translucent elements such as hyaline casts and mucous threads. Other linear structures like bacilli are strikingly apparent with phase. Cellular detail is best seen with stained sediments. A drop of methylene blue solution (Loeffler's) added to the sediment may aid in the recognition of cellular structures and bacteria. A crystal-violet safranine stain is used to help to identify cellular elements; a peroxidase stain will differentiate renal tubular cells that are peroxidase negative and neutrophilic leukocytes that are peroxidase positive.

For most purposes qualitative or semiquantitative examination of the urine sediment is adequate. On qualitative examination of the urine sediment, the relative number and kind of cells and casts present can be assessed. Quantitative enumeration of the formed elements of the urine is time-consuming and unnecessary in most instances. The chief value of quantitative counts, such as the Addis count, lies in following the progress of active renal disease. See p. 39.

Because random urine specimens on the same patient will vary in concentration, only a semiquantitative appraisal of the specimen is possible. With a slide and coverslip, an estimation of the number of cells and casts present may be made by counting them in 10 high-power fields and averaging the results. A semiquantitative result may be obtained by taking a fixed amount of urine (e.g., 10 or 15 ml.), centrifuging for standard time, and reconstituting the sediment to a fixed volume (e.g., 1 ml.). An objection to this method has been that the use of a slide and coverslip allows for considerable variation in the depth of the microscopic field and makes the counts less reliable than is frequently assumed.

A counting chamber may be preferred. Some laboratories prefer to report qualitative results as occasional and 1 to 4+; other laboratories use the terms occasional, moderate, and many.

Microscopic Examination of the Urine Sediment. The method presented uses an unstained and stained sediment (Sternheimer, 1951).

REAGENT

Solution I:	Crystal violet	3.0 gm.
	Ethyl alcohol (95%)	20.0 ml.
	Ammonium oxalate	0.8 gm.
	Distilled water	80.0 ml.
Solution II:	Safranine O	1.0 gm.
	Ethyl alcohol (95%)	40.0 ml.
	Distilled water	400.0 ml.

Three parts of Solution I and 97 parts of Solution II are mixed and filtered. The mixture should be clarified by filtering every two weeks; discard after three months. Separately, Solutions I and II keep indefinitely at room temperature. In highly alkaline urines, the stain will precipitate.

PROCEDURE. The urine specimen must be examined while fresh, since cells and casts will begin to lyse within 1 to 3 hours. Each specimen is concentrated exactly tenfold.

1. Mix the specimen well (casts tend to settle). Pour exactly 10 ml. of urine into a graduated disposable centrifuge tube. Centrifuge at 2000 r.p.m. for 5 minutes. Remove the supernate by decanting into another tube and

resuspend the sediment in exactly 1 ml. of urine. A disposable pipette with rubber bulb is convenient for this.

2. Place a drop of redispersed sediment on one area of a slide and coverslip (avoid bubbles) with a 22-mm. square coverslip. Too much fluid will cause the coverslip to float. (Some workers prefer to examine the sediment in a counting chamber to assure even depth.) To the remaining sediment add 1 drop of crystal-violet safranine stain. Mix with the pipette and place a drop of this suspension on the same slide under a separate coverslip.

3. Examine both fields. Examine with low power (× 100) and subdued light. The fine focus should be varied continuously while scanning. Systematically progress around all four sides of the coverslip. Either the stained or unstained mount may be used, depending on the kind of specimen and the experience of the examiner.

Casts are often found along the edge of the coverslip. Count the number of casts per low-power field in 10 fields. Switch to high power (× 440) and determine the kind of casts present.

Red blood cells, leukocytes and epithelial cells are identified with the high-power objective and counted in 10 fields. Squamous epithelial cells are noted if a large number of them are present. Bacteria and yeasts should be noted.

Crystals are reported if the number is unusually large or they are abnormal; these are counted under low power. The identity of abnormal crystals should be confirmed chemically (see cystine and sulfonamide tests).

REPORT. The following scheme may be used: The counts represent an average of 10 fields. (After viewing 10 representative fields, one may approximate the results to a quantitative count using the table prepared by Kark *et al.*, 1963. See Table 2–4.)

A scale for reporting results of examination of urinary sediment is at the bottom of this page.

Phase Microscopy. Some laboratories prefer the use of phase for unstained material. The same low-power and high-power examination is used as above.

Microscopic Characteristics of Sediment

Table 2–4. A COMPARISON OF ADDIS COUNTS AND ROUTINE EXAMINATION OF THE SEDIMENT*

FORMED ELEMENT	ADDIS COUNT TOTAL EXCRETION PER 12 HRS.	ROUTINE SCREENING EXAMINATION (PER HIGH-POWER FIELD)
Casts	6,700 to 79,000	0 or 1 to 2
	122,000 to 1,000,000	1 to 2
	6,000,000 to 15,000,000	10 to 20
Red cells	220,000 to 2,400,000	0 to 10
	2,500,000 to 8,200,000	1 to 20
	190,000,000 to 570,000,000	5 to 60
Leukocytes and epithelial cells	Less than 1,000,000	0 (occasionally) 3 to 5 (usually)
	1,000,000 to 10,000,000	5 to 10
	10,000,000 to 75,000,000	10 to 20 (clumped)

*From R. M. Kark *et al.*: A Primer of Urinalysis. 2nd edition. New York, Hoeber Medical Division, Harper & Row, Publishers, 1963.

Red Blood Cells. Under high power unstained red blood cells appear as pale discs (see Figs. 2–1 and 2–15). They may vary somewhat in size but are usually about 7 micra in diameter. If the specimen is not fresh when it is examined, the cells will appear as faint, colorless circles or "shadow cells," since the hemoglobin has "dissolved" out. The red blood cells may become crenated and appear as small, rough cells with "crinkly" edges. Smooth, folded, and crenated cells may be seen in the same specimen. Surface crenations may appear as granules. Red blood cells may be con-

SEDIMENT—CONCENTRATION 1:10	NEG.	OCCASIONAL	1+	2+	3+	4+
Erythrocytes (high-power field) × 440	0	less than 4	4–8	8–30	greater than 30, less than packed	packed field
White cells (high-power field) × 440	0	less than 5	5–20	20–50	greater than 50, less than packed	packed field
Casts and abnormal crystals (low-power field) × 100	0	less than 1	1–5	5–10	10–30	greater than 30

fused with oil droplets or yeast cells. Oil droplets, however, exhibit a great variation in size, are highly refractile, and will not "tumble" when the coverglass is touched with a pencil to set the fluid in motion. Yeast cells usually show budding. If there is doubt about identification, two preparations may be made and a few drops of acetic acid added to one. The red cells will be lysed in the acidified preparation.

Red blood cells, stained, may take up no stain or show slight purple staining in acid urine (see Fig. 2–25). Alkaline hematin stains dark purple in alkaline urine.

Neutrophilic Leukocytes. Under high power unstained neutrophilic leukocytes appear as round granular spheres about 12 μ in diameter, larger than red blood cells (see Figs. 2–2 and 2–16). In order to distinguish between a leukocyte and a small renal epithelial cell, the nucleus can be brought more clearly into view by allowing a small drop of glacial acetic acid to run under the coverglass. Epithelial cells have a single, rounded nucleus and leukocytes have a segmented nucleus which may appear as several small rounded nuclei.

When stained, neutrophilic leukocytes have red-purple nuclei and violet granularity of the cytoplasm (see Fig. 2–23). A variety of staining characteristics may appear in the same specimen.

"Glitter" cells stain light blue to almost colorless. These neutrophils are larger than dark-staining cells. Cytoplasmic granules with or without Brownian movement may be noted.

Renal Tubular Epithelial Cells. Unstained renal tubular epithelial cells are about the same size (less than 15 μ) as a leukocyte and contain a large round nucleus (see Fig. 2–3). They are easily confused with degenerating leukocytes. Oval fat bodies are tubular epithelial cells containing fat globules; the nucleus is not visible as a rule.

A renal tubular epithelial cell, when stained, has a dark purple nucleus and a small rim of orange-purple cytoplasm.

Bladder Epithelial Cells. Unstained bladder epithelial cells are larger than renal tubular cells, have a round nucleus (sometimes two nuclei), and vary in size depending on depth of origin in transitional epithelium (see Fig. 2–6). Superficial cells are large and flat with small nucleus. Occasionally clumps or sheets are seen. Some are tailed and are similar to epithelial cells from the renal pelvis (see Fig. 2–4).

When stained, a bladder epithelial cell has a dark blue nucleus with variable amounts of pale blue-staining cytoplasm. Occasional cytoplasmic inclusions are seen.

Squamous Epithelial Cells. Unstained squamous epithelial cells are large, flattened cells with abundant cytoplasm and a small round nucleus (see Fig. 2–5). The cell edge is often folded; occasionally the cell is rolled into a cylinder. These cells originate in the vagina, vulva, or urethra.

When stained, squamous epithelial cells have purple nuclei and abundant pink or violet cytoplasm (see Fig. 2–23).

Casts. Casts are cylindrical and vary in diameter depending on the size of the renal tubule or duct of their origin (see Figs. 2–7 to 2–12). The cylindrical shape can be demonstrated by pressing lightly on the edge of the coverglass and watching the casts roll. The ends are usually rounded but may be flat, irregular, or tapered.

Hyaline casts are colorless, homogeneous, transparent; they stain pink to light purple.

Finely granular casts contain fine granules in all or in part of the cast; the granules stain purple and the matrix pink.

Coarse granular casts contain fat, degenerated cells or protein aggregates, which appear as dark granules. The granules stain deep purple; the matrix is often not visible. If fat is present, it may appear as refractile granules (see Fig. 2–25).

Fatty casts contain highly refractile globules of varying size. The matrix stains pink; the fat is unstained. Fat droplets will stain bright orange with Sudan III (see method, p. 37, and Fig. 2–28).

Red cell casts appear yellow under the low-power objective. If many cells are present in each cast, the matrix will not be visible. On staining, colorless or lavender red blood cells are seen in a pink matrix. *Blood casts* contain hemoglobin from degenerated red blood cells. They have a yellow to orange color which is best seen with the low-power objective. They are best observed in unstained preparations (see Figs. 2–14, 2–19, and 2–20). They may appear dark purple on staining. *Leukocyte casts* contain small granular cells in a clear matrix (Figs. 2–12 and 2–18). The leukocytes may be mixed with red blood cells or epithelial cells. Also granules, free of cells, may be seen in the casts. Small leukocytes stain purple to violet; large leukocytes may be pale blue. The matrix is pink. Clumps of leukocytes may sometimes look like casts. *Tubular epithelial casts* may be difficult to distinguish in unstained sediment from leukocyte casts or mixed cell casts. They often appear as two rows of cells in a narrow cast (Fig. 2–13). On staining, they are shown to contain small cells with purple nuclei in a pink matrix. Mixed cell casts may contain leukocytes and renal epithelial cells or red blood cells. A few cells may be present in a granular cast.

Waxy casts are yellow and homogeneous; they have sharper outlines than hyaline casts. They usually have irregular ends and cracks

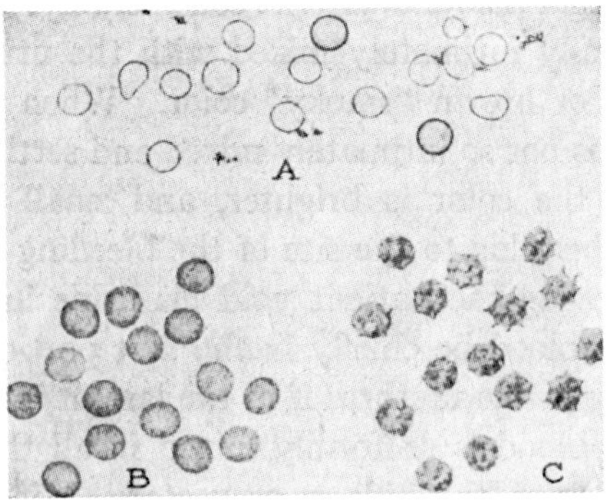

Figure 2–1. Red blood cells. A, Ghost cells. B, Fresh. C, Crenated (×475).

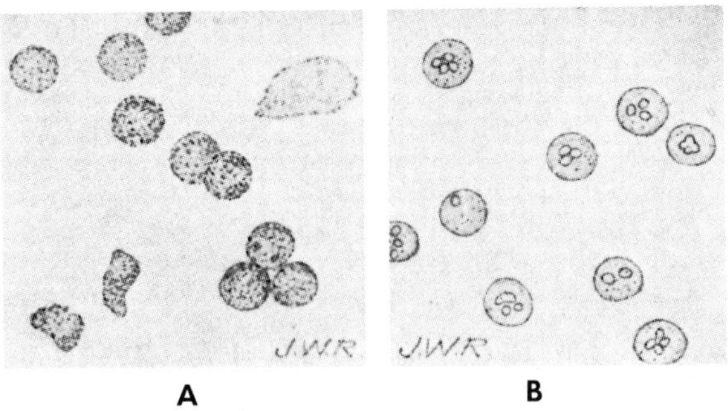

Figure 2–2. Neutrophilic leukocytes. A, Usual appearance. B, With acetic acid (×475).

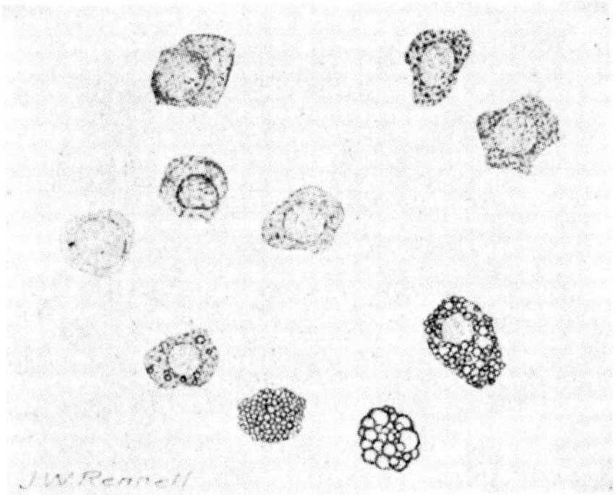

Figure 2–3. Renal epithelial cells. Lower four cells con tain fat (×475).

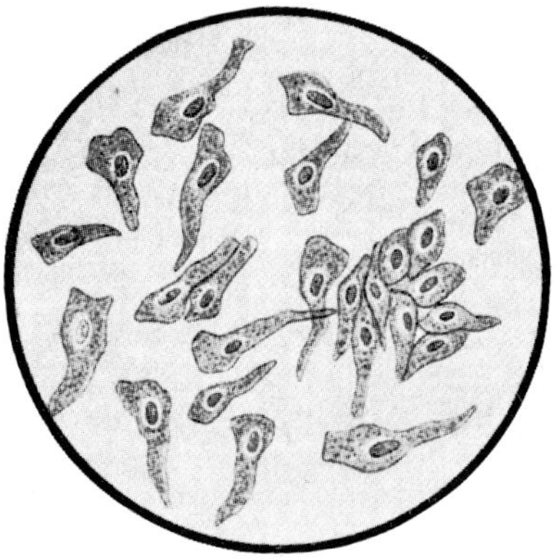

Figure 2–4. Caudate epithelial cells from renal pelvis (Jakob).

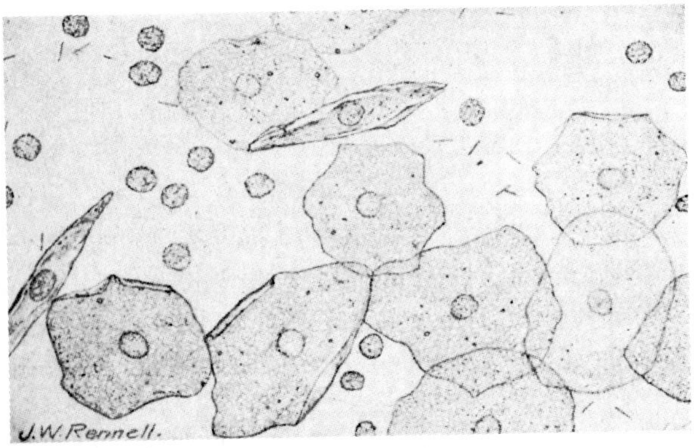

Figure 2–5. Squamous epithelial cells, leukocytes, and bacteria. Vaginal contamination (×300).

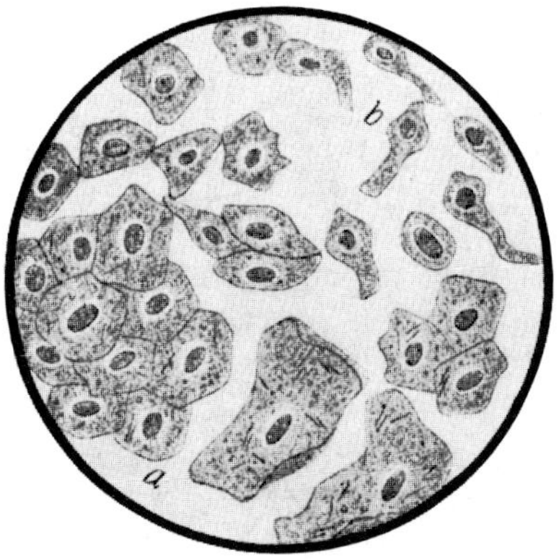

Figure 2–6. Transitional epithelial bladder cells. a, Flattened from superficial layer. b, Deeper cells (Jakob).

FIGURES 2–1 TO 2–6: CELLS IN THE URINARY SEDIMENT

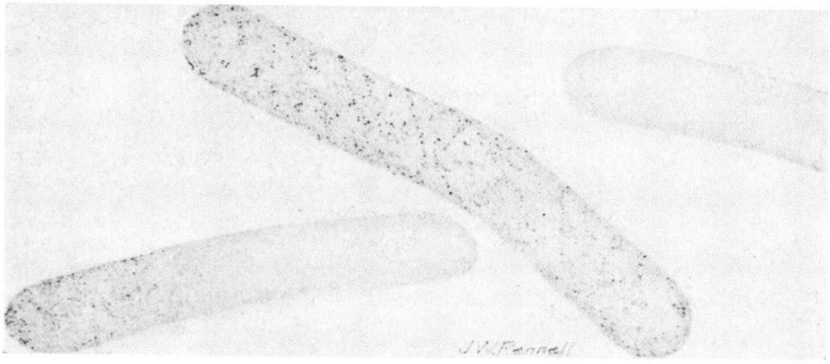

Figure 2-7. Finely granular casts (×350).

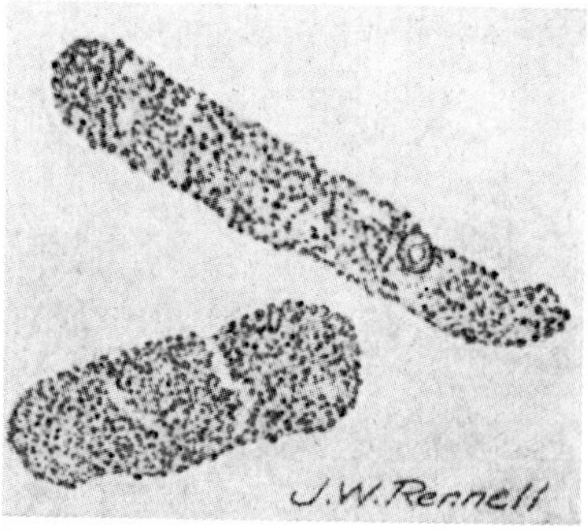

Figure 2-8. Coarsely granular casts (×350).

Figure 2-9. Convoluted hyaline and tapering hyaline casts (×350).

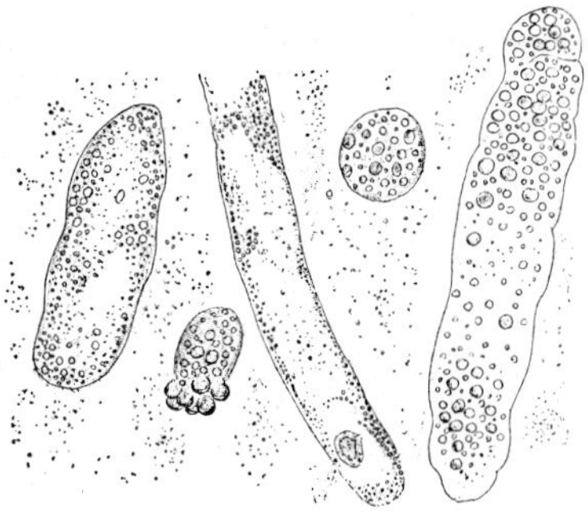

Figure 2-10. Granular and fatty casts and two fat bodies (×350).

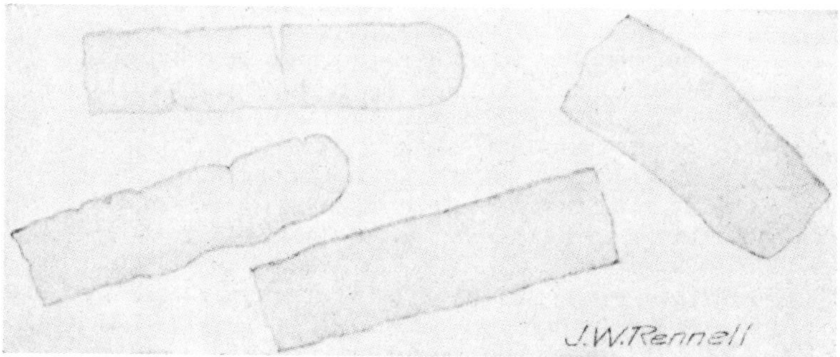

Figure 2-11. Waxy casts (×350).

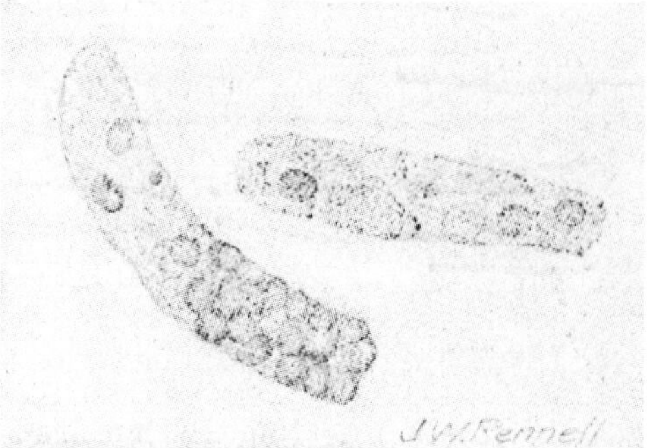

Figure 2-12. Leukocyte cell casts (×350).

FIGURES 2-7 TO 2-12: CASTS FOUND IN THE URINARY SEDIMENT

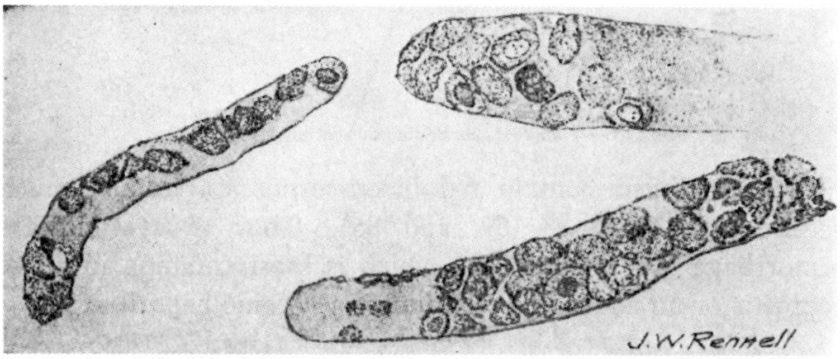

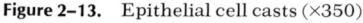

Figure 2–13. Epithelial cell casts (×350).

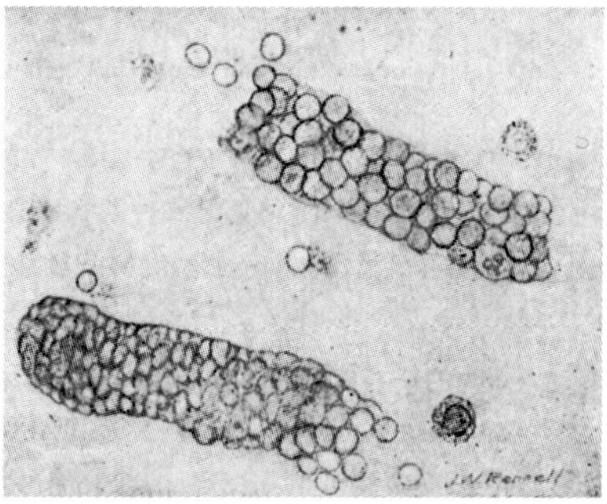

Figure 2–14. Red blood cell casts: two renal epithelial cells and six red blood cells (×300).

(Figs. 2–11 and 2–24). On staining, they are light to dark purple.

Bacterial casts are rarely seen; on staining, these show dark purple bacteria enmeshed in pale pink matrix.

Structures commonly confused with casts are mucous threads and squamous epithelial cells which have rolled into cigar shapes. Mucous threads are long, ribbon-like strands with poorly defined edges and pointed or split ends. Often they appear to have longitudinal striations. Fibers of plant or animal origin are longer and sharply defined. Scratches on the slide or coverslip may also cause confusion (see Figs. 2–30 and 2–34).

Fat. Free globules of fat are seen frequently in grape-like clusters. The globules vary in size more than yeast cells or red cells.

Crystals Found in Normal Acid Urine. See Figures 2–36, 2–44 and 2–46.

1. *Amorphous urates:* Yellow-red granules.
2. *Uric acid:* Yellow or red-brown, irregular but usually "whetstone" crystals or rhomboids.
3. *Calcium oxalate:* Refractile, octahedral "envelopes."

Crystals Found in Normal Alkaline Urine. See Figures 2–35, 2–45, and 2–47.

1. Amorphous phosphates, fine precipitate.
2. Triple phosphate, colorless, three- to six-sided prisms. Occasionally fern leaf.
3. Ammonium biurate, yellow brown spheres, "thorn apple."
4. Calcium phosphate, stellate prisms.
5. Calcium carbonate, colorless spheres or dumbbells, tiny.

Crystals Seen in Abnormal Urine. See Figures 2–37 to 2–43 and 2–48.

1. *Cystine:* Colorless, refractile, hexagonal plates.
2. *Tyrosine:* Fine needles arranged in sheaves or clumps, usually yellow, silky.
3. *Leucine:* Yellow, oily-appearing spheres with radial and concentric striations. Leucine and tyrosine crystals may occur together.
4. *Sulfonamide crystals (sulfadiazine):* Yellow-brown asymmetrical, striated sheaves and round forms with radial striations.

Significance of Urinary Crystals and Amorphous Deposits. A variety of crystals are found in the normal urine sediment. The type of crystal or amorphous deposit depends to some extent on the acidity of the urine. In *acid urine,* calcium oxalate, uric acid, and urate crystals may be seen; uric acid and urates redissolve on warming to 60° C. In *alkaline urine,* phosphate and carbonate crystals and amorphous phosphates are often seen; these will dissolve on acidifying the urine sample. Calcium oxalate and calcium hydrogen phosphate crystals are found in neutral urine (see Figs. 2–35 and 2–36).

One should be able to recognize commonly occurring crystals in order that unusual crystals (e.g., cystine or sulfonamides) may be distinguished. See Figures 2–37, 2–41, 2–43, and 2–48 and Table 2–5.

Cystine crystals are colorless hexagonal plates, which may be confused with uric acid. They occur in the urine in patients with a specific congenital defect of renal tubular reabsorption (see aminoaciduria, p. 47, chemical screening test, p. 49, and cystine calculi, p. 50). Tyrosine and leucine crystals are occasionally seen in the urine of patients with severe liver disease. Sulfonamide crystals are not often seen since the introduction of more soluble sulfonamide drugs. See page 76 for chemical test for sulfonamide in urine. Since the introduction of large parenteral doses of ampicillin, this antibiotic is occasionally seen as masses of long, thin, colorless crystals in acid urine. X-ray media, meglumine diatrizoate, appears as flat, four-sided plates or long, thin rectangles. The urine is cloudy and the specific gravity very high.

Abnormal Cells and Other Formed Elements

Tumor Cells. Rarely, tumor cells may be found in urine (Rofe, 1955). If clumps of cells from bladder tumors are found, they may be identified; neoplasms of the kidney cannot be diagnosed from a urine sediment. Epithelial

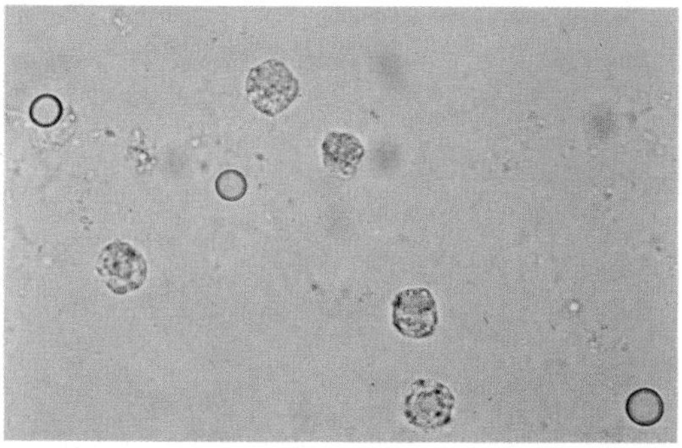

Figure 2–15. Two red blood cells and five polymorphonuclear leukocytes. Air bubble upper left. (×500).

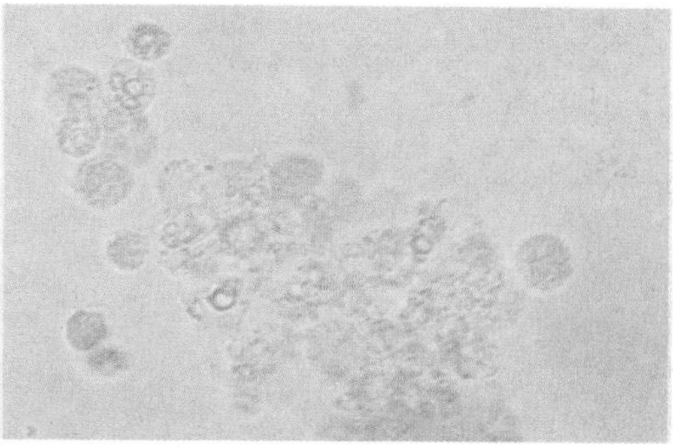

Figure 2–16. Clump of neutrophilic leukocytes showing granules and some nuclei (×500).

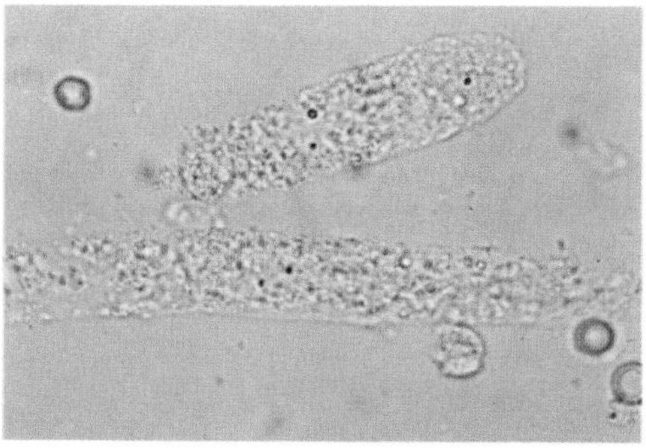

Figure 2–17. Granular casts, a leukocyte, and three red blood cells (×500).

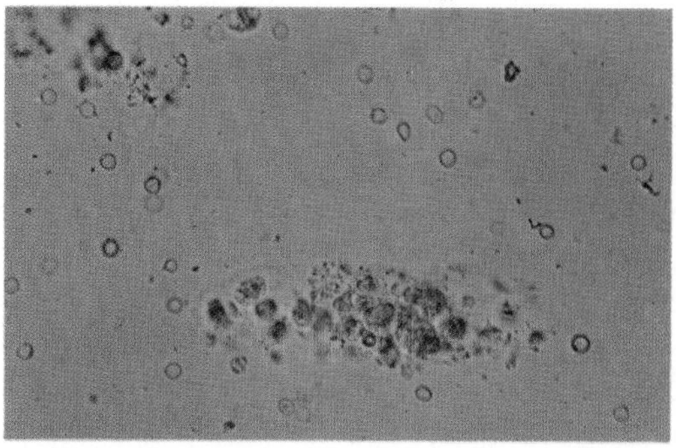

Figure 2–18. Mixed cellular cast and red blood cells (×400).

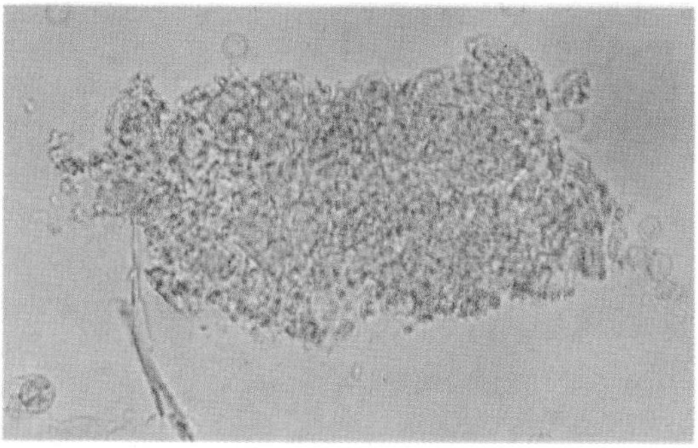

Figure 2–19. Broad blood cast (×400).

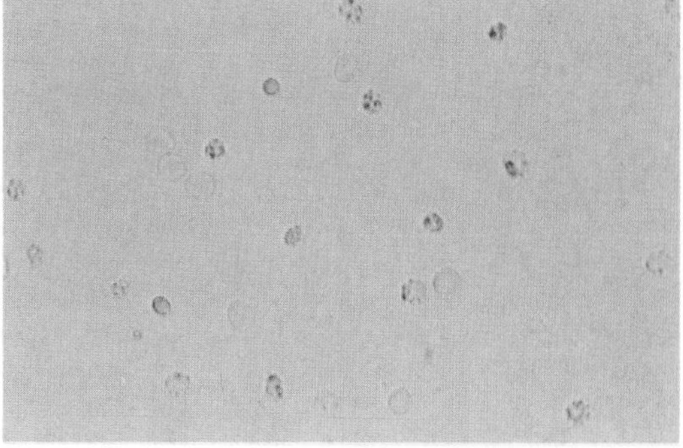

Figure 2–20. Red blood cell cast (×400).

Table 2–5. CHARACTERISTICS OF AMORPHOUS AND CRYSTALLINE URINARY SEDIMENTS

SUBSTANCE	DESCRIPTION	URINE pH WHERE FOUND			SOLUBILITY CHARACTERISTICS
		ACID	NEUTRAL	ALKALINE	
Bilirubin	Reddish-brown; amorphous needles, rhombic plates or cubes. May color uric acid crystals	+	−	−	Soluble in alkali, acid, acetone, chloroform
Cholesterol	Rare; flat, colorless plates with corner notch	+	+	−	Very soluble in chloroform, ether, hot alcohol
Calcium carbonate	Small, colorless dumbbells or spheres; rarely needles	−	+	+	Soluble in acetic acid with effervescence
Calcium oxalate	Small, colorless octahedron common; dumbbell, ring form	+	+	Slight	Soluble in dilute HCl
Cystine	Colorless, hexagonal, flat; rapidly destroyed by bacteria. May be confused with uric acid	+	−	−	Soluble in alkali, especially ammonia, and dilute hydrochloric acid. Insoluble in boiling water, acetic acid, alcohol, ether
Hematin	Small, biconvex whetstone seen with hemoglobinuria	+	−	−	
Hemosiderin	Clumps of golden brown granules	+	+	−	Blue with Prussian blue
Hippuric acid	Rare; colorless needles, rhombic plates, and four-sided prisms. Distinguish from phosphates	+	+	+	Soluble with hot water, alkali. Not soluble in acetic acid
Indigotin	Rare; amorphous blue or small crystals. Colors other crystals	+	+	+	Very soluble in chloroform. Soluble in ether. Insoluble in acetone
Leucine	Yellow spheroids with radial striations. Seen with tyrosine. Probably not pure	+	−	−	Soluble in hot alcohol, alkali. Slightly soluble in hot water. Crystallizes out as hexagonal plates in pure form
Phosphates					
Ammonium magnesium (triple phosphate)	Common form. Colorless, three- to six-sided prisms, "coffin lid." Sometimes fern leaf	−	+	+	Soluble in dilute acetic acid
Calcium hydrogen	Less common. Star-shaped or long, thin prisms; needles or occasional plates	Slight	+	+	Soluble in dilute acetic acid
Sulfonamides					
Sulfadiazine	Dense, greenish globules	+	+	−	Soluble in acetone
Acetylsulfadiazine	Wheat sheaves, eccentric binding	+	+	−	
Tyrosine	Colorless or yellow, fine silky needles in sheaves or rosettes	+	−	−	Soluble in alkali, dilute mineral acid, relatively heat soluble. Insoluble in alcohol, ether
Urates	Yellow, calcium, magnesium, and potassium, mostly amorphous	+	−	−	Soluble in alkali, soluble at 60°C.
	Ammonium – thorn apple, brown	−	+	+	Soluble at 60°C. with acetic acid; soluble strong alkali
	Potassium – small, spherical, brown Sodium acid urate – colorless, needles or amorphous	+	−	−	Soluble at 60°C.
Uric acid	Yellow, red-brown, large variety of crystals – rhombic, four sided plates, rosettes. Colorless, smaller crystals	+	−	−	Soluble in alkali. Insoluble in alcohol, acids
Xanthine	Rare, colorless, rhombic plates	+	+	−	Soluble in alkali, soluble with heat. Insoluble in acetic acid
X-ray Media (Diatrizoate)	Colorless, thin, rhombic, some with notch	+	−	−	Soluble in 10% NaOH. Insoluble in ether, chloroform.

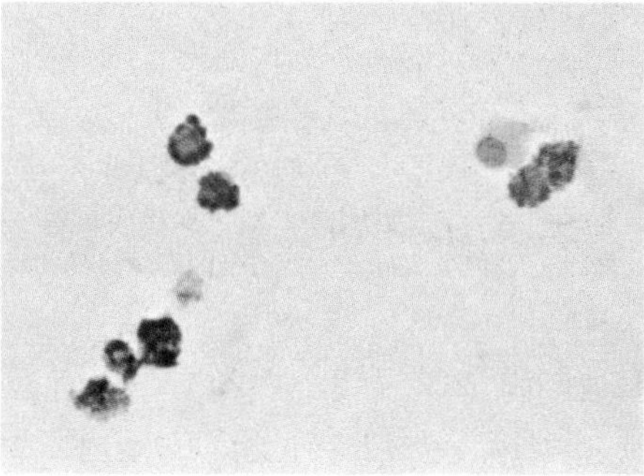

Figure 2–21. One renal epithelial cell (red) and several neutrophilic leukocytes (peroxidase stain; ×500).

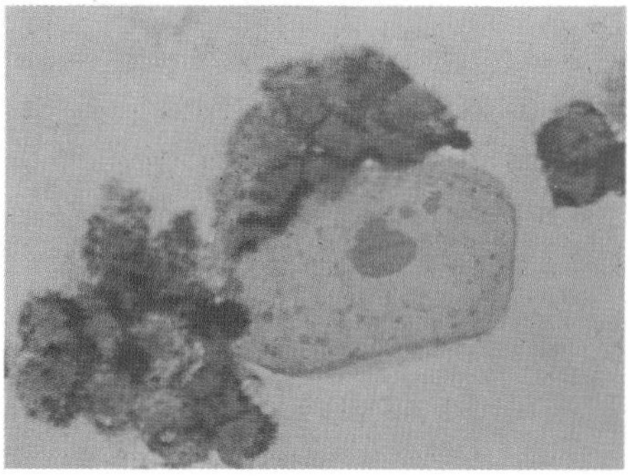

Figure 2–22. Clump of neutrophilic leukocytes and one squamous epithelial cell (peroxidase stain; ×500).

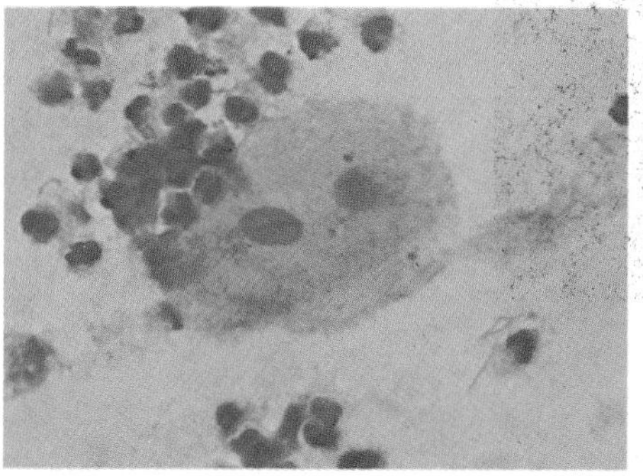

Figure 2–23. Clump of neutrophilic leukocytes and two squamous epithelial cells (crystal violet-safranine stain; ×500).

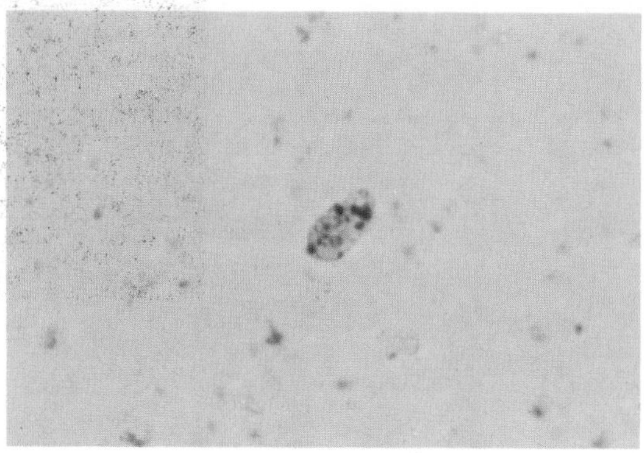

Figure 2–24. Waxy appearance; slightly granular, bilirubin-stained cast (×400).

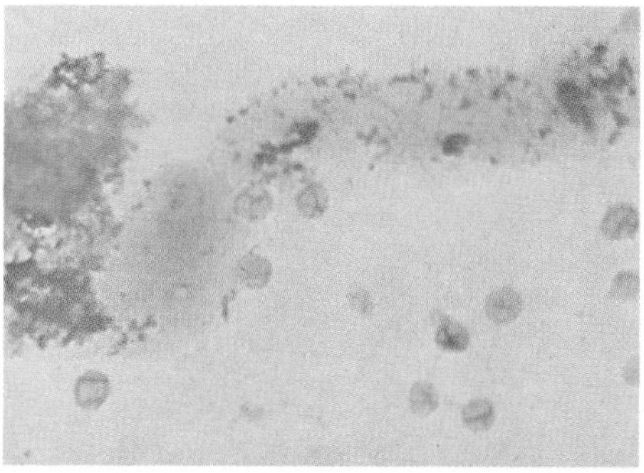

Figure 2–25. Convoluted cast with coarse granules (purple). Red blood cells (crystal violet-safranine stain; ×500).

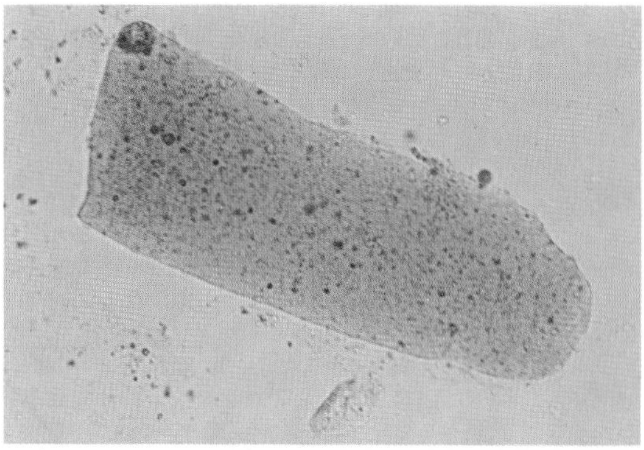

Figure 2–26. Hemosiderin in a cast. Prussian blue stain (×400).

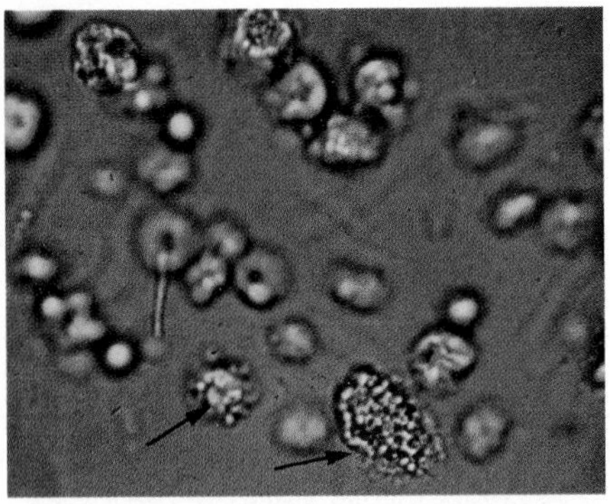

Figure 2–27. Renal epithelial cells containing refractile globules of fat. Oil immersion.

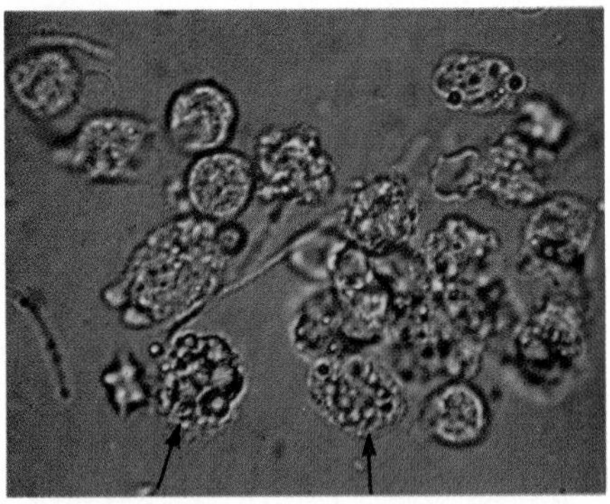

Figure 2–28. Renal epithelial cells containing fat. Stained orange with Sudan III. Oil immersion.

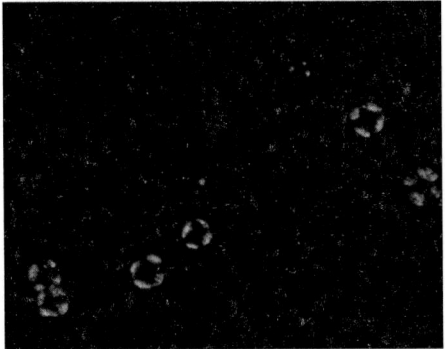

Figure 2–29. Anisotropic lipid in oval fat bodies (Maltese cross) seen with polarized light. Oil immersion.

cells with inclusion bodies may be found in the urine in viral diseases (Dewall, 1966). Occasionally syncytial giant cells containing nuclear inclusions are seen in the urine in measles. In children with cytomegalic inclusion disease (salivary gland virus disease) epithelial cells with nuclear inclusion bodies are found in the urine.

For cytologic study, the urine should be collected into an equal volume of 70 per cent alcohol. A dried film of centrifuged sediment may be stained with Papanicolaou stain or a special stain for inclusion bodies (Lippman, 1957).

Bacteria, Fungus, and Parasites. Bacteria may or may not be significant, depending on the method of urine collection and how soon after collection of the specimen the examination takes place. A dry film may be made by spreading a drop or two of the urine sediment on a glass slide. It may then be fixed and stained with Gram's stain. The uncentrifuged urine may be examined in the same manner. If bacteria are identified in the uncentrifuged specimen under an oil-immersion lens, it suggests that more than 100,000 organisms per ml. are present, i.e., significant bacteriuria. Most commonly, rod-shaped bacteria are seen, since the enteric organisms are most often found in urinary tract infection. If urinary tract infection is indeed present, usually many leukocytes also will be seen in the sediment.

Acid-fast staining of the urine sediment may reveal tubercle bacilli, but since smegma contains nonpathogenic acid-fast organisms, the presence of tubercle bacilli in urine must be substantiated by culture. An early morning catheterized specimen is preferred for culture purposes.

Yeast cells (Candida) may be found in urinary tract infection (e.g., in diabetes mellitus), but yeasts are also common contaminants from skin and air. They may be confused with red blood cells; budding is usually seen and helps to identify them as yeast cells. Pseudomycelial forms of Candida are occasionally found.

Parasites and parasitic ova may be seen in

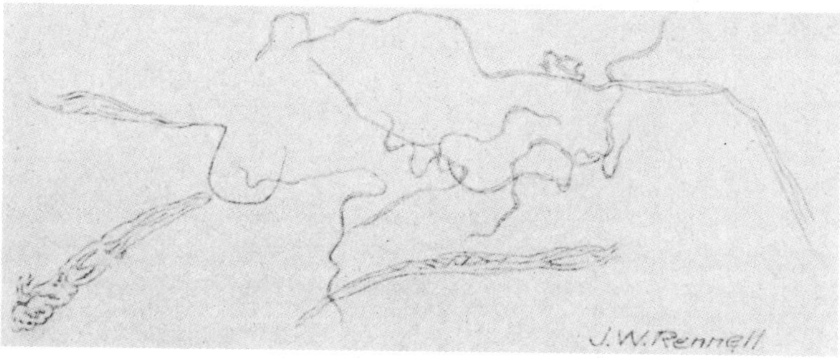

Figure 2–30. Mucous threads may be confused with casts (×350).

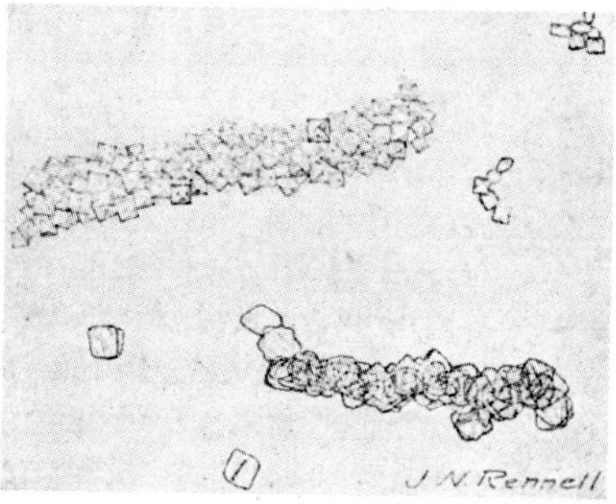

Figure 2–31. Crystals forming pseudocasts (×300).

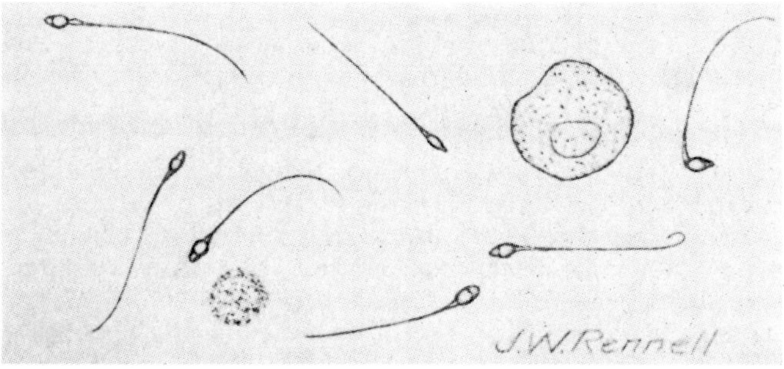

Figure 2–32. Spermatozoa, bladder epithelial cell, and leukocyte (small) (×475).

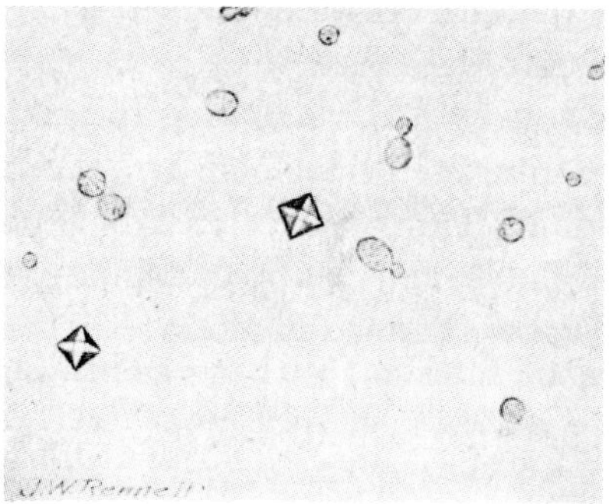

Figure 2–33. Yeast with buds and calcium oxalate crystals (×450).

Figure 2–34. Extraneous matter found in urine: *a*, flax fibers; *b*, cotton fibers; *c*, feathers; *d*, hair; *e*, potato-starch granules; *f*, rice-starch granules; *g*, wheat-starch granules; *h*, air bubbles; *i*, muscle fibers; *k*, plant cells; *l*, oil globules.

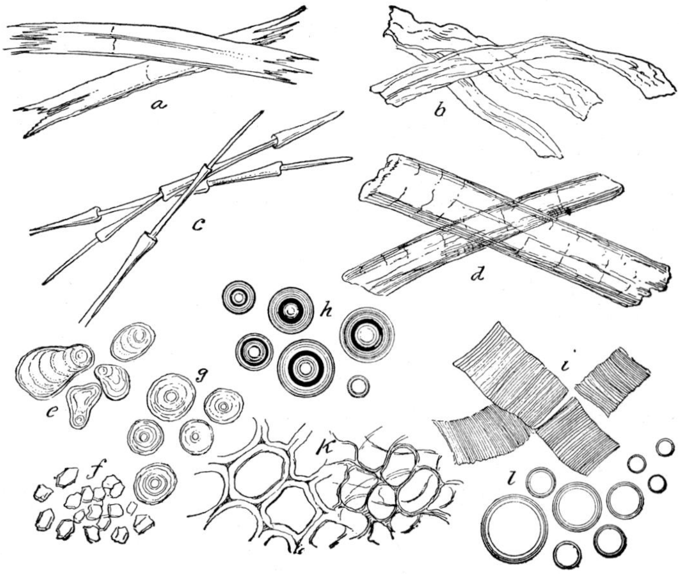

FIGURES 2–30 TO 2–34: URINARY SEDIMENT STRUCTURES WHICH MAY CAUSE CONFUSION

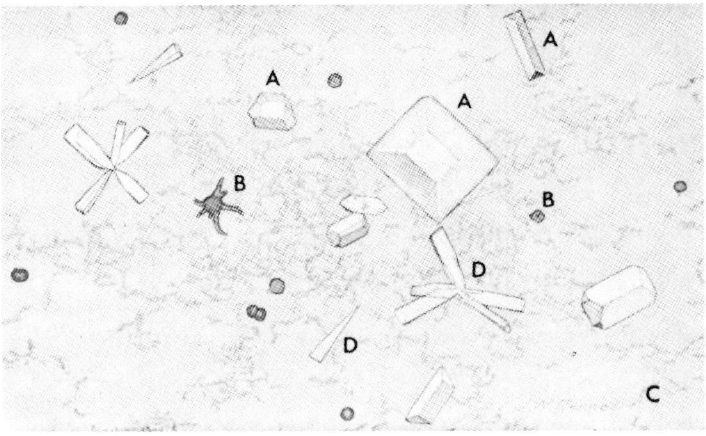

Figure 2–35. Alkaline urine. A, Ammonium magnesium phosphate (triple phosphate) crystals; B, ammonium urate (brown); C, amorphous phosphate; D, stellate calcium phosphate crystals (less common) (×150).

urine sediments as a result of fecal or vaginal contamination. When these are noted, the examination should be repeated on a fresh, clean-voided urine specimen. In patients with schistosomiasis due to *Schistosoma haematobium*, typical ova may be found in the urine accompanied by red blood cells from the urinary bladder. *Trichomonads* may be present in urine as a result of vaginal contamination. When urethral or bladder infection is suspected, the protozoa should be searched for immediately in a wet preparation of the sediment; the motility of the organism is helpful in making the appropriate identification. Ameba are rarely seen in the urine; these may reach the bladder from lymphatics or more likely from fecal contamination of the urethra. The pathogenic *Entamoeba histolytica* is usually accompanied by erythrocytes and leukocytes.

Contaminants and Artifacts. The vinegar eel, fly larvae, and other parasites may be found in urine as a result of dirty or contaminated containers. Partly digested muscle fibers or vegetable cells may be found when there is fecal contamination (Fig. 2–34).

Spermatozoa are generally present in the urine of men after nocturnal emissions. They are easily recognized (Fig. 2–32).

Cotton, hair, and other fibers may be seen and are easily identified. Wood fibers from applicator sticks may be found if sticks are used to mix the sediment. Oil droplets from lubricants may be confused with cells, especially red cells, but are structureless. Granules of starch appear bright and striated and should not be confused with cells.

CELLS AND CASTS IN THE URINE SEDIMENT

Interpretation of the sediment takes time, skill, and experience acquired through constant use of the procedure and correlation of the findings with the clinical status of the pa-

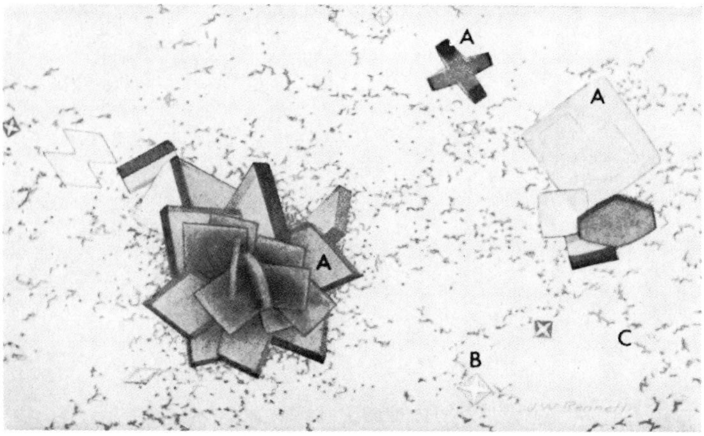

Figure 2–36. Acid urine. A, various forms of uric acid crystals (colored); B, calcium oxalate crystals (also seen in alkaline urine); C, amorphous urates (×150).

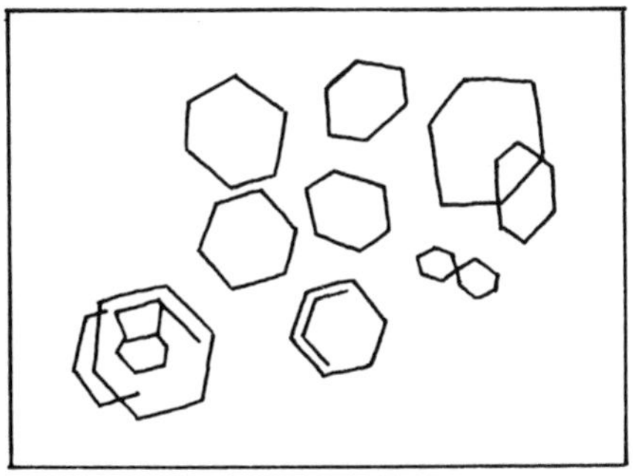

Figure 2–37. Cystine – colorless, hexagonal plate.

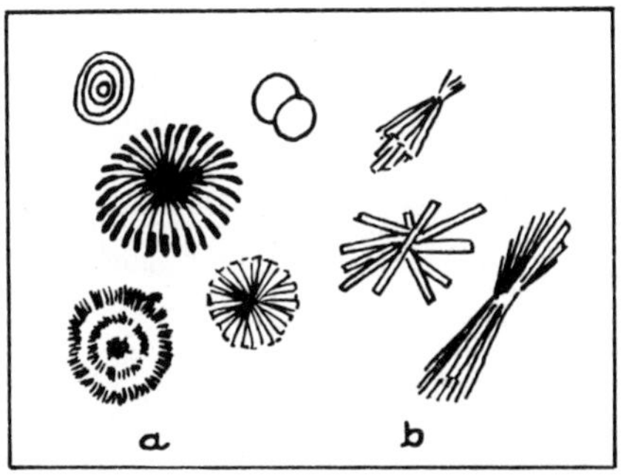

Figure 2–38. *a*, Leucine spheres; *b*, tyrosine needles.

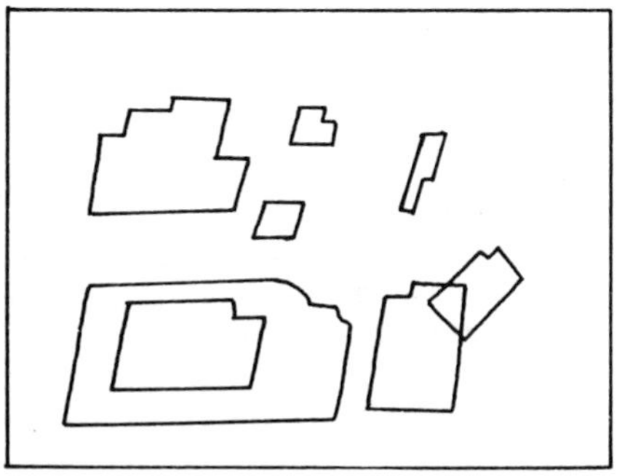

Figure 2–39. Cholesterol – flat, notched plates.

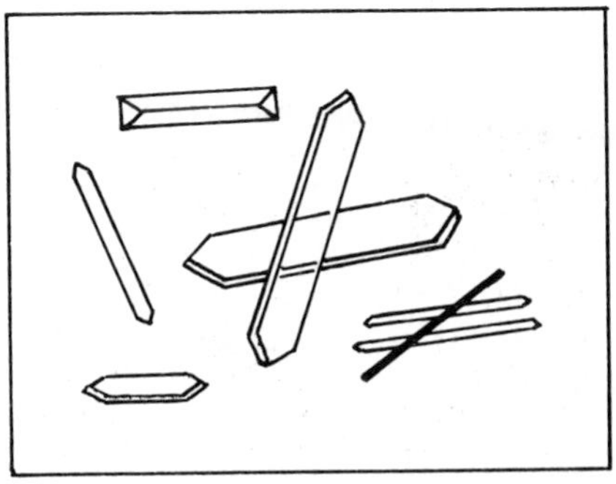

Figure 2–40. Hippuric acid prisms.

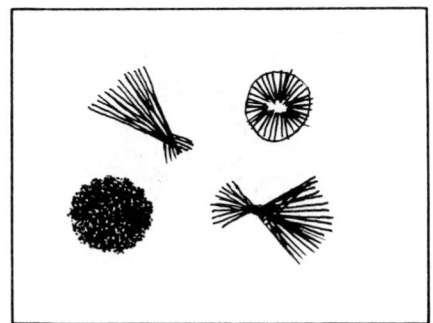

Figure 2–41. Sulfadiazine – (round) and acetyl sulfadiazine (sheaf).

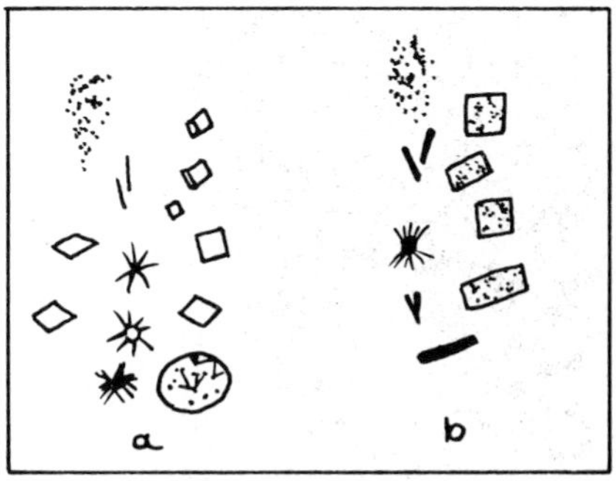

Figure 2–42. *a*, Bilirubin (brown, amorphous forms, needles, and four-sided plates, occasionally intracellular); *b*, indigotin (blue, amorphous forms, needles, and four-sided plates).

FIGURES 2–37 TO 2–42: CRYSTALS OCCASIONALLY SEEN IN THE URINARY SEDIMENT

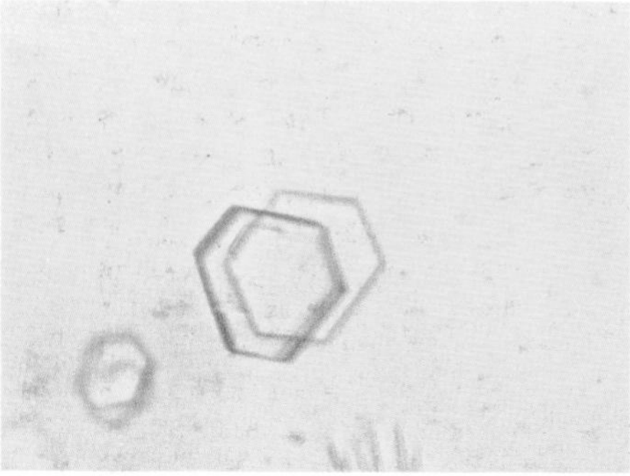

Figure 2–43. Two cystine crystals, six sided, with one small calcium oxalate crystal (×500).

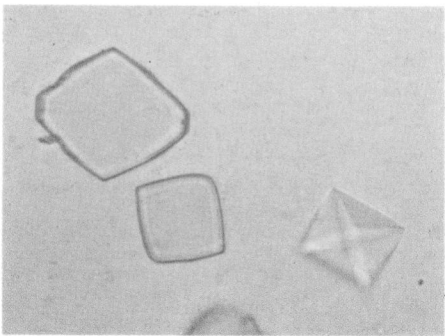

Figure 2–44. Two uric acid crystals, four sided, and one calcium oxalate crystal (×500).

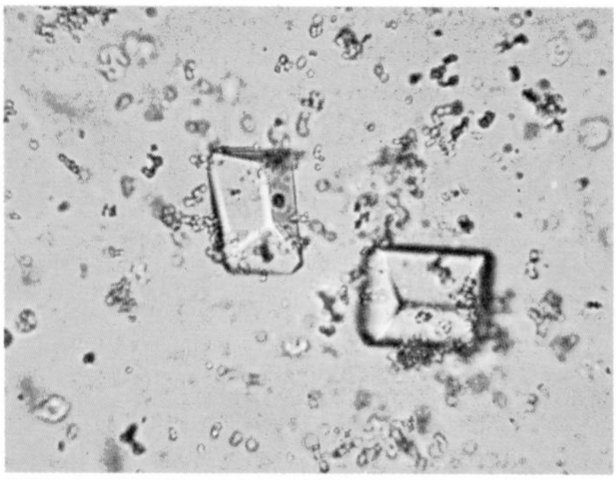

Figure 2–45. Two ammonium magnesium phosphate crystals, "triple phosphate" with amorphous phosphate granules (×500).

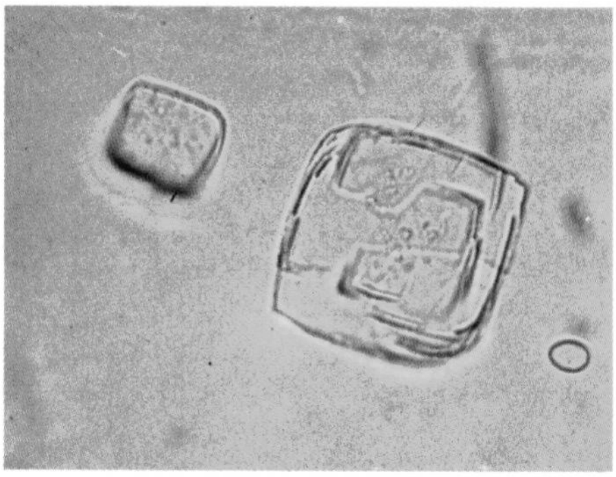

Figure 2–46. Two uric acid crystals, one large and multilayered (×500).

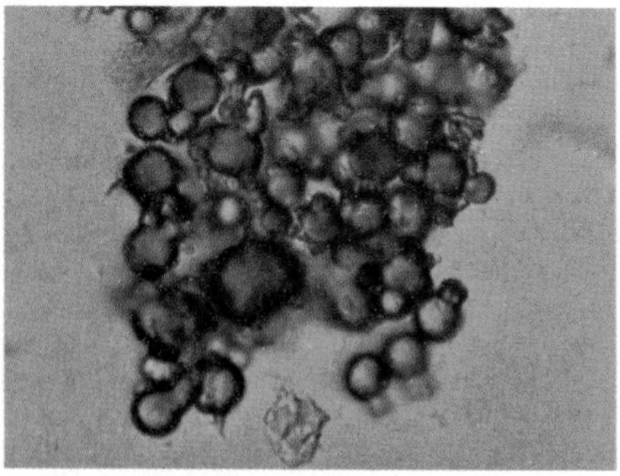

Figure 2–47. Many ammonium urate crystals, a few showing thorns (×500).

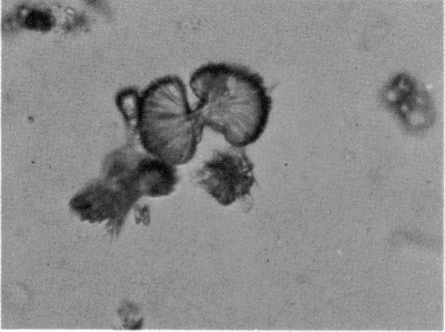

Figure 2–48. Sulfonamide crystal, sheaf form, with central binding (×500 .

tient. In the diagnosis of renal disease, cells and casts are the important structures to be sought; these are often referred to as the formed elements. Crystals and amorphous materials, commonly found in the urinary sediment, are generally of lesser importance but occasionally may provide information of key importance.

Formed Elements of Urine. Cells found in normal urine come from two sources—desquamation of the lining of the urinary tract and adjacent structures (epithelial cells) and cells of the circulating blood (leukocytes and red blood cells). Casts formed in the renal tubules and ducts are the other formed elements seen. (Other cellular structures, bacteria, and parasites which may be found are discussed above. "Normal" values for formed elements will vary from one laboratory to another. Because of the variation in the concentration of random urine specimens and different methods used for concentration of the sediment (1:10, 1:20, complete or none) at different centrifuge speeds, there are no valid qualitative normal values.

Epithelial Cells. The urinary tract is lined with a variety of epithelial cells. Cuboidal, squamous, and columnar cells are found in the nephron, and transitional epithelium is found in the ureter and bladder. In the female, the urethra is lined with columnar and stratified squamous epithelial cells, while the male genital tract and bulbourethral glands are lined with columnar cells. The number of epithelial cells seen in normal urine is small and apparently represents the normal sloughing off of aging cells. Stratified squamous epithelial cells are seen most frequently in urine from females, especially in noncatheterized specimens, and presumably come from the vagina and vulva. Increased numbers of epithelial cells are seen in urine after prostatic massage and after urethral catheterization. Other than squamous cells and some flattened transitional cells, epithelial cells from the kidney and urinary tract cannot usually be distinguished from each other in the urine. Usually epithelial cells of tubules and the urinary tract are not distinguished from the leukocytes of the blood, and a total count of nonsquamous white cells is reported, for example, in Addis counts. With a differential staining technique, which depends on the peroxidase reaction of polymorphonuclear leukocytes, epithelial cell counts have been made in normal subjects and found to be fairly constant in a given individual. The excretion rate of leukocytes, on the other hand, varies considerably from hour to hour in the same subject. Renal tubular epithelial cells are excreted in larger numbers than leukocytes in the normal newborn (Cruikshank and Edmond, 1967). (For normal values, see Table 2–2.)

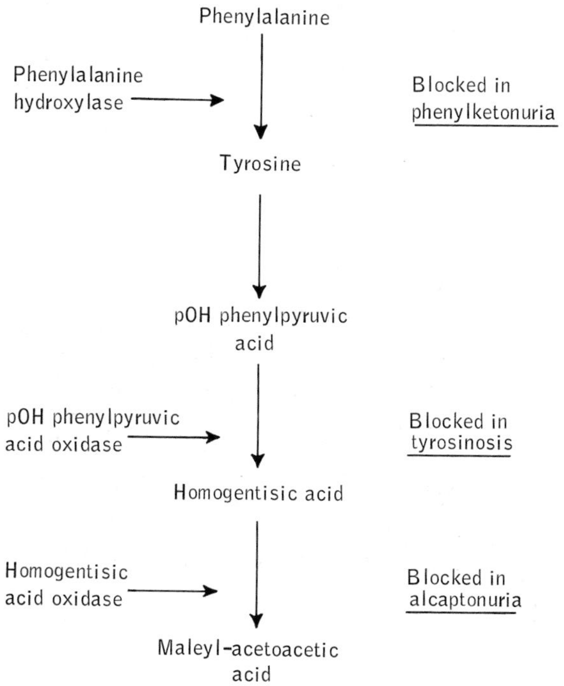

Figure 2–49. Outline showing points at which metabolic impairment occurs in phenylketonuria, tyrosinosis, and alcaptonuria.

EPITHELIAL CELLS IN RENAL DISEASE. Inflammatory changes may cause greater sloughing of renal epithelial cells. Tubular epithelial cells undergo fatty degeneration, especially when there is marked proteinuria, as in the nephrotic syndrome; and when these degenerated cells are found in the urine sediment, they are termed *oval fat bodies*. Probably, some "oval fat bodies" are macrophages. The source of the fatty material in tubular cells is thought to be the lipoprotein that passes through the damaged glomerulus in the nephrotic syndrome. The tubule cells may ingest the fat, which is then metabolized into cholesterol and appears as coarse fat droplets. The droplets may be anisotropic if cholesterol is present, and with polarized light are seen as a light cross against a dark background. Neutral fats, triglycerides, do not show this effect with polarized light. Free droplets of fatty material may accompany the oval fat bodies, and these along with cellular or granular casts containing fat are characteristic of the urinary sediment in the nephrotic syndrome (Zimmer *et al.*, 1961).

Excretion of large numbers of renal epithelial cells and casts containing renal epithelial cells suggests active degeneration of the tubules and may be seen in glomerulonephritis and active pyelonephritis. Clumps of epithelial cells may be seen in acute tubular necrosis and necrotizing papillitis.

Erythrocytes and Leukocytes. Erythrocytes and leukocytes are found in small numbers in normal urine. How these cells enter the urine is not known. The proportion of leukocytes to erythrocytes is much greater in urine than in blood; thus, diapedesis of leukocytes through the glomerular membrane or tubules may be postulated.

ERYTHROCYTES. In normal males and females, in most instances, no red cells will be seen on microscopic examination of sediment (Wright, 1959). In about 10 per cent of the patients in one study, one red cell in every two or three high-power fields was noted. The normal values for excretion of erythrocytes in 24 hours is shown in Table 2–2. Exercise, lordosis, and fever will increase the rate of excretion of erythrocytes (Goldring, 1931).

Increased numbers of red cells in the urine may originate in any part of the urinary tract. When increased red cells (hematuria) and red cell casts are seen together, it may be assumed that the source of hematuria is renal. Massive hematuria is most often associated with trauma to the kidney or urinary tract; in trauma to the kidneys (as, for example, renal biopsy), hematuria and red cell casts are characteristically seen. The presence of hematuria with no red cell casts and little or no proteinuria suggests that the bleeding is originating in the lower urinary tract.

Some causes of hematuria are as follows: *renal*—glomerulonephritis, lupus nephritis, calculus, tumor, acute infection, tuberculosis, infarction, renal vein thrombosis, trauma (including renal biopsy), hydronephrosis, polycystic kidney, and occasionally acute tubular necrosis and malignant nephrosclerosis; *lower urinary tract*—acute and chronic infection, calculus, tumor, and stricture; *extrarenal*—acute appendicitis, salpingitis, diverticulitis, and tumors of the colon, rectum, and pelvis.

Hematuria is also seen in acute febrile infections, malaria, subacute bacterial endocarditis, polyarteritis nodosa, malignant hypertension, blood dyscrasia, and scurvy and may be associated with toxic reactions to drugs, such as sulfonamides, salicylates, and methenamine, and with anticoagulant therapy. Hemorrhagic cystitis is associated with cyclophosphamide therapy.

LEUKOCYTES. The urinary sediment of most normal males will show on microscopic examination an occasional leukocyte or nonsquamous epithelial cell. In the normal female, the number may be higher. The number of leukocytes and nonsquamous epithelial cells (white cells) excreted per day and the number of neutrophil leukocytes excreted per hour in the normal adult is shown in Table 2–2 (see also Houghton and Pears, 1957, and Little, 1962). The rate of excretion of cells increases with exercise and with fever (Goldring, 1931).

Increased numbers of leukocytes in the urine, principally neutrophils, is seen in almost all renal diseases and in diseases of the urinary tract. When accompanied by leukocyte casts or mixed leukocyte-epithelial cell casts, the source of the increased leukocytes is considered to be the kidney.

The presence of many leukocytes (pyuria) and clumps of leukocytes in the sediment is usually indicative of acute infection and when found should lead to urine culture. In such instances, repeated sterile routine cultures may indicate tuberculosis or lupus nephritis. Rupture of a renal abscess or urinary tract abscess may result in gross pyuria.

Moderate numbers of leukocytes and mixed leukocyte casts are seen in the sediment in acute and subacute glomerulonephritis and in lupus nephritis. Leukocytes and leukocyte casts may be present in the urine in chronic pyelonephritis but are frequently absent. Renal or urethral calculi may give rise to increased numbers of leukocytes. Acute or chronic cystitis and bladder tumors also produce increased leukocytes in the urine, as does prostatitis, urethritis, and balanitis. Collection of the urine specimen in two containers may indicate whether urethritis is present as opposed to bladder or renal infection; in urethritis the leukocytes will be found predominantly in the first container. It should be noted that, in normal circumstances, some leukocytes are found in the secretions of the male and female genital tracts.

Leukocytes are rapidly lysed in hypotonic alkaline urines; approximately 50 per cent are lost in two to three hours at room temperature (Triger and Smith, 1966). This circumstance emphasizes the importance of prompt examination of the urine sediment. In dilute or hypotonic urine, leukocytes swell and the cytoplasm may exhibit Brownian movement. When stained with a crystal-violet safranine stain, these swollen cells are a paler blue than other leukocytes and are known as "glitter" cells. Glitter cells are found when the specific gravity of the urine is low (Berman, 1956).

Casts (Schreiner, 1957). Urinary casts are formed from gelled protein precipitated in the tubules and molded to the tubular lumen; pieces of casts are broken off and washed out with the urine. Casts are thought to form in two ways. The first is by precipitation and gelling of protein in the tubular fluid, a process accelerated by high protein concentration, low pH, and relatively high solute concentration. According to McQueen (1966), casts are composed of urinary mucoprotein secreted by the tubules. With fluorescent antibody technique, casts recovered from healthy volunteers after severe exercise were found to contain tangled masses of thread-like material, probably mucoprotein. Casts may also form by clumping of cells in the tubule in a matrix of protein. Such cells may be leukocytes, erythrocytes, or tubular epithelial cells. Normally the number of these cells present is too small to form cellular casts.

In the normal person, very few casts are seen. Those found are hyaline casts and usually contain no cells but may show a few fine granules. In very hypotonic urine, no casts are seen; they also dissolve in very alkaline urine. Casts are seen in increased numbers after exercise, in fever, and in postural proteinuria. The number of casts excreted per day in the normal person is shown in Table 2–2.

Increased numbers of casts in the urine is known as *cylindruria*. Cylindruria usually accompanies proteinuria. The presence of increased numbers of casts establishes the existence of renal disease rather than lower urinary tract disease, since they are formed in the nephron. They are, therefore, a valuable aid in the differential diagnosis of renal and urinary tract diseases.

Casts are thought to form in the lower parts of the nephron, and the width of the cast will depend on whether it forms in the distal tubule or the collecting ducts. Presumably the broader casts are formed in the collecting tubules or ducts. Since their presence in large numbers indicates widespread stasis in the nephron, they have been referred to as renal failure casts; for example, many are washed out in the diuretic phase following anuria. Frequently the broader casts have a homogeneous waxy appearance.

Classification of casts is based on morphologic appearance rather than chemical composition, about which little is known. Casts that are commonly seen are usually classified as hyaline, cellular (formed by the clumping of erythrocytes, leukocytes, tubular epithelial cells, or degenerating fatty tubular epithelial cells), or granular casts, which may be degenerated cellular casts. Coarsely granular casts containing aggregations of plasma proteins or fatty casts containing droplets of fatty debris are usually seen in association with oval fat bodies and heavy proteinuria; this triad is found in the nephrotic syndrome. Occasionally fatty casts are seen in other renal disorders associated with degeneration of tubular cells and in diabetic nephropathy. Leukocyte casts are indicative of interstitial nephritis, frequently pyelonephritis.

Pigment casts are seen as blood casts, that is, casts which contain degenerated red blood cells or hemoglobin casts, or myoglobin casts. Blood casts are commonly seen in active glomerulonephritis. Bile-stained casts are seen when there is renal excretion of bilirubin. In hemoglobinuria, hemochromatosis and microangiopathic anemias, epithelial cells or cell casts may contain hemosiderin.

Very rarely a uric acid crystal cast or pseudocast may occur.

Method for Examining Refractile Bodies in Urine. Lipid droplets containing cholesterol are anisotropic in polarized light, show up brightly against a dark field, and appear to be divided into four quadrants. This appearance resembles a Maltese cross. Visible evidence of anisotropy depends on the orientation of the crystal in the field; not all will be seen. Crystals, hair, and clothing fibers also show up brightly, but do not exhibit Maltese cross forms. Neutral fat, triglyceride, does not show anisotropy.

A polarizing microscope with rotating stage may be used in this examination. If one is not available, an ordinary light microscope can be easily made usable by the addition of suitable filters. Polaroid filters, consisting of an analyzer circle and a polarizer circle, are used. Install the analyzer disc in the ocular lens of a microscope by unscrewing the eye lens assembly. Insert the polarizer disc in the slotted opening under the substage condenser.

Sediment from a fresh urine sample is examined. Using high-power magnification and bright illumination, turn the polarizing filter in the eyepiece by turning the ocular itself until a maximum darkening of the field is produced. The refractile bodies will have the typical Maltese cross form. They may be counted by standard techniques for all counts previously described (see Fig. 2–29).

Method for Examining Fat Droplets in Urine

Reagent. Saturated solution of Sudan III in 70 per cent alcohol.

Procedure

1. Urine specimen must be collected in clean, fat-free container (glass, Pyrex, or polyethylene). Waxed cardboard containers are not suitable.

2. Centrifuge about 15 ml. of the urine in a clean centrifuge tube for 15 minutes.

3. With a clean medicine dropper, carefully take a drop of urine from the surface of the centrifuged specimen and transfer to a slide, making two deposits. Add a drop of Sudan III to one and coverslip. Coverslip the unstained deposit.

4. Look at unstained specimen for fat. Examine the stained deposit microscopically for round droplets of fat which are colored red-orange with Sudan III. Use the low-power objective with subdued light and then the high-powered objective. The staining reaction may take some minutes (see Figs. 2–27 and 2–28).

Leukocyte Peroxidase Stain (Kaplow, 1965). This is a stain for localizing perioxidase activity in which benzidine dihydrochloride is used as the indicator compound in a single, stable, reusable staining solution. The method is a rapid and highly sensitive one. The cells are fixed, thereby preserving cell morphology. A method for staining cells in the wet sediment has also been proposed (Prescott and Brodie, 1964). By this technique, renal epithelial cells and neutrophilic leukocytes are easily differentiated.

PROCEDURE

1. Use fresh smears of the urinary sediment. The urine should be at acid pH. Smears are made by placing a drop of the sediment on a glass slide and making a short smear with another slide edge as for peripheral blood smears. Dry the preparation by waving it rapidly in the air. Thicker smears are made by placing a drop or two of the sediment on a slide and tilting to spread. Allow these to dry in air. Satisfactory smears have been made from refrigerated sediments up to 24 hours old providing the pH of the specimen is acid. An adhesive is not needed.

2. After proper drying of the smear, fix slides for 60 seconds at room temperature in 10 per cent formol-ethanol (made by adding 10 ml. of 37 per cent formaldehyde to 90 ml. of absolute ethyl alcohol in a Coplin jar). Wash for 15 to 30 seconds under very gently running tap water. Shake off excess water.

3. Place *wet* slides in incubation mixture in a Coplin jar for 30 seconds at room temperature. The *incubation* mixture is made as follows:

30 per cent ethyl alcohol	100 ml.
Benzidine dihydrochloride	0.3 gm.
0.132 M (3.8 per cent w/v) $ZnSO_4 \cdot 7\ H_2O$	1.0 ml.
Sodium acetate ($NaC_2H_3O_2 \cdot 3\ H_2O$)	1.0 gm.
3 per cent hydrogen peroxide (must be fresh)	0.7 ml.
1.0 N sodium hydroxide	1.5 ml.
Safranine O	0.2 gm.

The reagents should be added in the order listed and be mixed well with each addition. The benzidine salt may contain a small amount of inert residue which will not go into solution. A precipitate forms upon addition of the zinc sulfate; this dissolves upon addition of the remaining reagents. The final pH is 6.00 ± .05. The solution should be filtered and stored in a capped Coplin jar or bottle at room temperature. The same solution has been used satisfactorily for as long as six months.

4. Wash briefly (5 to 10 seconds) in running tap water, dry, and examine.

5. If greater nuclear detail is desired, the stained preparations may be counterstained in 1 per cent aqueous cresyl violet acetate for 1 minute.

6. After drying, the slides may be rinsed with xylol and mounted with Permount and a coverslip. The stained preparation is stable for at least 12 months.

Peroxidase activity is represented by discrete dark blue granules in the cytoplasm of granulocytes and monocytes. The cytoplasm of neutrophils is filled with blue granules. Rarely, a neutrophil is observed that is weakly stained or unstained. Renal epithelial cells, squamous epithelial cells, and bacteria stain only with the safranine counterstain (see Figs. 2–21 and 2–22).

Hemosiderin in Urine (Rous, 1918). Hemosiderin appears in the urine sediment in diseases involving a true siderosis of kidney parenchyma (e.g., pernicious anemia, chronic hemolytic anemia, microangiopathic hemolytic anemia, multiple transfusions, paroxysmal nocturnal hemoglobinuria, and hemochromatosis). It may be found as yellow-brown granules that are free or in epithelial cells and occasionally in casts. The Prussian blue reaction is used to demonstrate hemosiderin (Fig. 2–26).

PROCEDURE

1. Centrifuge a complete morning specimen or random urine sample and pool the sediment. Examine several drops of sediment microscopically, searching for coarse brown granules, especially within epithelial cells.

2. If such granules are seen, suspend the rest of the sediment in a fresh mixture of 5 ml. of 2 per cent potassium ferrocyanide and 5 ml. of 1 per cent HCl and allow to stand for 10 minutes.

3. Centrifuge, and discard the supernatant. Examine the sediment microscopically. Coarse granules of hemosiderin appear blue in this preparation. If granules do not stain, reexamine after 30 minutes (occasionally, the reaction is delayed).

Metachromatic Staining of Urine Sediment in Metachromatic Leukoencephalopathy (Austin, 1957). Large quantities of metachromatic staining granules are accumulated free in tissues (liver, renal tubules) or within the glial cells of the brain in a demyelinating disease in young children known as metachromatic leukoencephalopathy. The material is a sulfuric acid ester of a cerebroside and results from deficiency of a sulfatase.

Metachromatic staining is seen when the tissue dye complex has an absorption spectrum different from the original dye. The change is caused by polymerization of the dye induced by the negative charge of the sulfatides.

PROCEDURE

A sample of fresh urine (10 ml.) is centrifuged for 5 minutes at 2000 r.p.m. Decant the supernatant. One drop of sediment is placed on a slide. Add 1 to 2 drops of 2 per cent toluidine blue solution to the remaining sediment and stir gently. Transfer one drop of the stained sediment to the slide, place coverslip over it, and examine microscopically.

The abnormal material stains golden brown and is found as free granules or in casts. A negative sediment will remain blue.

Addis Count. A method of quantitative enumeration of red blood cells, white cells, and casts in a 12-hour urine specimen is known as the Addis count (Addis, 1948). The chief value of the Addis count is in following the progress of known renal disease, e.g., acute glomerulonephritis. (For diagnostic purposes, careful examination of the sediment from a random fresh urine sample is usually sufficient.)

An accurately timed 12-hour urine specimen should be collected, with attention to the factors which contribute toward preservation of the formed elements, which are to be counted. A 6- to 9-hour specimen may be used. A concentrated specimen of low pH is desirable; this is most easily obtained by collection of the specimen overnight while the patient is not normally eating or drinking. Intake of fluids should be restricted during the collection period as the patient's condition permits. Particular attention should be paid to avoiding contamination of the specimen with vaginal discharge or feces.

Formalin is the preservative of choice for preservation of cells and casts; it also inhibits bacterial growth. Sufficient formalin is introduced by rinsing the collection bottle with a solution of 10 per cent formaldehyde in water and discarding the excess solution. It is advisable to keep the specimen at room temperature during and after collection in order to prevent precipitation of dissolved materials, for precipitation obscures the cells and casts and makes counting difficult. The specimen should be examined as soon as possible after collection.

PROCEDURE

1. Mix the specimen well and measure the volume carefully.

2. A preliminary microscopic examination of the urinary sediment should be performed with a 10:1 concentration of the sediment (see method, p. 21). From the results of this examination, the volume in which to resuspend the sediment in step 5 can be determined.

3. Transfer 10 ml. of urine to a special Addis graduated centrifuge tube and centrifuge for 5 minutes at 2000 r.p.m.

4. Pour off the supernatant urine and save for protein determination. Adjust the volume of the remainder to 1 ml. When the amount of sediment is large, adjust the volume to 2 to 5 ml. Alter the calculations appropriately.

5. Mix well to resuspend the sediment, and with a capillary pipette, mount the resuspended sediment on both sides of *two* Levy-Hausser counting chambers with improved Neubauer rulings.

6. Under low power, count the number of casts in the four ruled areas ($4 \times 9 = 36$ sq. mm.) on the two sides of the two counting chambers. Using the high-power objective, count the red blood cells and white blood cells and epithelial cells in 4 sq. mm. (usually 1 sq. mm. from each side of each chamber). Squamous epithelial cells are not counted.

The number of cells and casts excreted in 12 hours or 24 hours may be reported. This number is determined as follows:

Number counted per sq. mm. × 1/10 =
number/sq. mm. corrected for concentration of specimen.

Number/sq. mm. × 1 mm./0.1 mm. =
number/cu. mm.

Number/cu. mm. × 1000 = number/ml.

Number/ml. × 12 hr. vol. in ml. = number/12 hr.

INTERPRETATON. Normal values (see Table 2–2): *Red blood cells,* 0 to 500,000 per 12 hr. *Nonsquamous white cells,* 0 to 1,000,000 per 12 hr. *Casts,* 0 to 5000 hyaline casts per 12 hr.

In children the number of erythrocytes and leukocytes may be lower and the number of casts greater (Lyttle, 1933).

Addis (1948) has given the following average counts per 12 hours in cases of glomerulonephritis.

	CASTS	ERYTHROCYTES	WHITE CELLS
Acute	690,000	405,000,000	48,000,000
Chronic active	1,850,000	34,000,000	14,000,000
Chronic latent	48,000	16,000,000	2,400,000
Chronic terminal	398,000	26,400,000	10,000,000

Common Renal Diseases

In *acute glomerulonephritis* an acute, diffuse inflammation of the glomeruli of the kidneys occurs. The disease is more common in children than in adults and usually follows an infection with group A, beta hemolytic streptococci. Polymorphonuclear leukocytes infiltrate the swollen glomeruli, endothelial and epithelial cells proliferate, and red cells escape through the inflamed tissue.

The urine may show gross hematuria (often appearing as a smoky turbidity) or only microscopic hematuria. The finding of red cell casts confirms the renal origin of the red cells; mixed red cell and epithelial cell casts, hyaline and granular casts, and an increased number of leukocytes are usually found. Occasionally fatty casts and fat droplets appear late in the course of the disease (Addis, 1948).

Proteinuria, usually about 2 gm. per day, may range as high as 6 to 8 gm. per day. During recovery, casts disappear, and proteinuria may be reduced to a trace while microscopic hematuria is still present. Persistence of heavy proteinuria denotes a poor prognosis.

Coliform organisms are most often the cause of *acute pyelonephritis;* infections involving Proteus and Pseudomonas may follow catheterization. Quantitative urine cultures should always be undertaken to establish the significance of the bacteriuria. The disease is found in children, especially girls; it is also relatively common in pregnancy and also may be the result of obstructive lesions of the urinary tract (such as urinary calculi) and neurogenic bladder dysfunction. In patients with diabetes mellitus, a fulminating infection (necrotizing papillitis) may occur.

The urine often appears grossly cloudy and has a strong odor. Examination of urinary sediment reveals numerous leukocytes (many in clumps), bacteria, and occasional red blood cells and leukocyte casts. The presence of leukocytes in casts is an important finding differentiating pyelonephritis from infection lower in the urinary tract. Occasionally only a few white cell casts are present and may represent the only clue to a diagnosis of pyelonephritis.

The amount of proteinuria is usually less than 2 gm. per day. With response to treatment, bacteria and leukocytes disappear, but protein in trace amounts may persist.

The course of *chronic glomerulonephritis* and the findings in this disease may vary considerably. In general, there is inflammation and scarring of the glomeruli.

Gross hematuria and heavy proteinuria may occur in patients with rapidly progressive disease, culminating in oliguria and uremia. In terminal stages, granular and waxy casts appear in the urine.

Examination of the urinary sediment is not always helpful in diagnosis or prognosis. A few red cell casts, red cells, and leukocytes may be found intermittently in patients with moderate proteinuria of 2 to 3 gm. per day. With exacerbations of the disease, proteinuria and hematuria are increased. The presence of epithelial cell casts, red cell casts, and lipid droplets may help to distinguish this disease from primary nephrosclerosis and chronic pyelonephritis.

The diagnosis of *chronic pyelonephritis* is often not easily made, even at autopsy, although the patient will sometimes have a history of acute pyelonephritis. The urinary sediment may intermittently contain leukocytes, epithelial cell and white cell casts, and bacteria. Red blood cells and red blood cell casts are found infrequently. The finding of leukocyte casts is most important in making a diagnosis of chronic pyelonephritis. Glitter cells (large leukocytes) occur frequently in this disease when hypotonic urine is formed. Proteinuria of less than 2 gm. per day is usual, but the level may be higher. In most cases of chronic pyelonephritis, diagnosis can be made from the history, urinary findings, and radiographic findings, and by renal biopsy. Diagnostic difficulties occur when the patient presents with impairment of renal function or proteinuria in the absence of other findings.

The *nephrotic syndrome* may result from a variety of causes. It is commonly associated with proliferative glomerulonephritis, membranous glomerulonephritis, systemic lupus erythematosus, and diabetic glomerulosclerosis; it is also occasionally found in certain generalized disease processes such as amyloidosis and periarteritis, circulatory diseases such as constrictive pericarditis and renal vein thrombosis, infections such as malaria and subacute bacterial endocarditis, and toxic states such as those due to mercurial and gold therapy and other drugs (Schreiner, 1963).

The syndrome is characterized by edema, proteinuria, hypoalbuminemia, and hyperlipemia, with little or no impairment of renal function.

The urinary findings are similar regardless of cause. Proteinuria is marked, usually more than 4 to 5 gm. per day, and may be as high as 30 gm. per day. Albumin is the chief protein in the urine; alpha-1, beta, and gamma globulins are usually also present in significant quantities. During remissions, proteinuria is decreased or absent.

The urine sediment contains cellular or granular casts showing fatty degeneration, oval fat bodies, and droplets of fat. Red blood cells are usually absent.

For further details concerning the urinary sediment in these and other renal diseases, Lippman's monograph should be consulted (1957) and also Strauss and Welt (1971).

Physicochemical Tests

Possibly because an unwarranted amount of attention was given for many centuries to the appearance of the urine, and because the yield in terms of positive results is small, simple gross examination of the urine has been too often ignored by the physician and the medical student. There are certain characteristics of the gross urine specimen, however, which provide useful diagnostic information and should not be overlooked.

Appearance of Normal Urine. The amber-yellow color of urine is due largely to the pigment urochrome and to small amounts of urobilin and uroerythrin. Urochrome excretion is thought to be proportional to the metabolic rate and is increased during fever, thyrotoxicosis, and starvation. The pink pigment (uroerythrin) may be deposited on uric acid or urate crystals (brick dust deposit), and these should not be confused with blood. Pale urine in a normal person follows high fluid intake. Darker urines may be seen when fluids are withheld. Thus, the color roughly indicates the degree of concentration, but the latter, of course, should always be checked. For example, pale urine of high specific gravity may be found in diabetes mellitus.

Normal urine may show a sedimentary deposit if allowed to stand after cooling from body temperature. This deposit is usually a compact white crystalline precipitate composed largely of inorganic phosphate; in acid urine it may be due to orange urate crystals and amorphous urate material. Mucus from the urinary and genital tracts may appear in sediment as small, cloudy patches (nubeculae) in normal urine.

Appearance of the Urine in Abnormal States. When a patient's urine has an unusual color or appearance, a detailed history of dietary intake of food, candies and drugs should be obtained. Certain food and candy dyes will color urine, as will drugs used for investigation and therapy. The family history may be important in the investigation of the autosomal recessive inheritance of alcaptonuria, which is associated with black or brown urine. Red urine associated with ingestion of beets is seen in genetically susceptible persons.

Some of the more important changes in the gross appearance of the urine are described below. A comprehensive listing is given in Table 2–6.

Cloudy Urine. Cloudy urine is most often normal and due to *phosphate* precipitation (and occasionally carbonate) in alkaline urine; the phosphates and carbonates redissolve when acetic acid is added. *Urates* cause a white or pink cloud in acid urine and redissolve on warming to 60° C. *Leukocytes* may form a white cloud similar to that caused by phosphates, but in this case the cloud remains after the addition of dilute acetic acid; the presence of leukocytes is confirmed by microscopic examination of the sediment. *Bacterial growth* will cause a uniform opalescence which is not removed by acidification or by filtering through paper; the odor of these specimens is unpleasant and usually ammoniacal because of the splitting of urea by the bacterial organisms. When the turbid urine is examined microscopically, rod-shaped bacteria, sometimes motile, are most commonly seen, e.g., *E. coli* and Proteus. Enterococcus, a coccal form, is also common.

Turbidity or smokiness may be due to *red blood cells*—hematuria. This turbidity does not clear on acidification or warming, and the presence of erythrocytes may be confirmed microscopically. *Spermatozoa and prostatic fluid* may cause turbidity not cleared by acidification or heating. Prostatic fluid normally contains a few leukocytes and other formed elements. *Mucin* from the urinary passages may cause a fluffy, bulky deposit; this is increased in inflammatory states of the lower urinary tract or genital tract. Turbidity due to blood clots, menstrual discharge, and other particulate material such as pieces of tissue, small calculi, clumps of pus, and fecal material is sometimes seen. Turbidity due to fat droplets, *chyluria* (Pomerantz, 1966), may be the result of obstruction of intra-abdominal lymphatics (for example, in filariasis). Fat may be found floating on the top of the urine specimen in cases of fat embolism or phosphorus poisoning. Turbidity or milkiness due solely to fat can be removed by shaking the urine with ether. Contamination with powders or with antiseptics which become opaque with water (phenols) will also cause a turbid urine.

Red Urine. The most common abnormal color is red or red-brown. When seen in the female, contamination with menstrual flow should be considered. The urine in *hematuria* (presence of red blood cells) may appear cloudy, smoky, pink, red, or brown. The urine in *hemoglobinuria* may be clear red, clear red-brown, or dark brown. *Methemoglobin* has a dark brown color and may develop in bladder urine of acid pH or in acid urine on standing. Blood and blood pigments are easily detected by means of a reagent strip or tablet containing orthotolidine. The benzidine and guaiac tests may also be used. A positive test will indicate the presence of hemoglobin or myoglobin. In order to distinguish hematuria from hemoglobinuria, sediment from a fresh urine specimen should be examined microscopically for red blood cells. A markedly hypotonic urine may cause lysis of erythrocytes, and therefore the specific gravity of the specimen should also be checked. *Myoglobin* in urine has a red-brown color and will give a positive orthotolidine, benzidine, or guaiac test. In myoglobinuria brown pigment casts and an occasional red cell may be found. If myoglobin is present in sufficiently concentrated amounts, it may be recognized by its characteristic spectrum in the hand spectroscope (see method for differentiating myoglobin from hemoglobin, p. 61). For causes of myoglobinuria, see Table 2–7.

Table 2–6. APPEARANCE AND COLOR OF URINE

APPEARANCE	CAUSE	REMARKS
Colorless	Very dilute urine	Polyuria, diabetes insipidus
Cloudy	Phosphates, carbonates	Soluble in dilute acetic acid
	Urates, uric acid	Dissolve at 60°C.
	Leukocytes	Insoluble in dilute acetic acid
	Red cells ("smoky")	Lyse in dilute acetic acid
	Bacteria, yeasts	Insoluble in dilute acetic acid
	Spermatozoa	Insoluble in dilute acetic acid
	Prostatic fluid	
	Mucin, mucous threads	May be flocculent
	Calculi "gravel"	Phosphates, oxalates
	Clumps, pus, tissue	
	Fecal contamination	Rectovesical fistula
	X-ray media	In acid urine
Milky	Many PMN (pyuria)	Insoluble in dilute acetic acid
	Fat	
	Lipuria, opalescent	Nephrosis, crush injury – soluble in ether
	Chyluria, milky	Lymphatic obstruction – soluble in ether
Yellow	Acriflavine	Green fluorescence
	Mepacrine	
	Nitrofurantoin	Antibiotic
	Riboflavin	Large doses
Yellow-orange	Concentrated urine	Dehydration, fever
	Urobilin in excess	No yellow foam
	Bilirubin	Yellow foam
	Pyridium	Color increases with HCl
Yellow-green	Bilirubin-biliverdin	Yellow foam
Yellow-brown	Bilirubin-biliverdin	"Beer" brown, yellow foam
	Senna, rhubarb, cascara	In acid urine

APPEARANCE	CAUSE	REMARKS
Red	Hemoglobin	o-Tolidine pos.
	Red blood cells	o-Tolidine pos.
	Myoglobin	o-Tolidine pos.
	Porphyrin	o-Tolidine neg., may be colorless
	Phenindione	Anticoagulant
	Amidopyrine	
	Fuscin, aniline dye	Foods, candy
	Beets	Yellow alkaline, genetic
	Menstrual contamination	Clots, mucus
Red-pink	Phenolsulfonphthalein	In alkaline urine
	Phenolphthalein	In alkaline urine
	Sulfobromophthalein	In alkaline urine
	Santonin	In alkaline urine
	Rhubarb, senna, cascara	In alkaline urine
Red-purple	Porphyrin	May be colorless
Red-brown	Red blood cells	
	Hemoglobin on standing	
	Methemoglobin	
	Myoglobin	
Brown-black	Methemoglobin	
	Homogentisic acid	On standing, alkaline
		Alkaptonuria
	Melanin, methyldopa	On standing
	Phenols	Reduce Benedict's
Blue-green	Methylene blue	
	Indigo-carmine	Decolorize with alkali
	Indicans	Intestinal putrefaction
	Pseudomonas infection	
Dark brown	Levodopa	Large dose

Table 2–7. TYPES AND CAUSES OF MYOGLOBINURIA

Paroxysmal myoglobinuria:	Muscle cramps with myoglobinuria for 72 hours after attack.
"March" myoglobinuria:	Excessive unaccustomed exercise, anterior tibial syndrome.
Trauma:	Beating, bullet, crush injury.
Infection:	Acute polymyositis.
Toxin:	Fish poisoning (Haff's disease); sea snake bite.

Hemoglobinuria follows sudden transitory increases in the concentration of plasma hemoglobin, which usually results from intravascular hemolysis. Appearance of hemoglobin in the urine will depend upon the number of red cells destroyed; if more than a total of 3 gm. of hemoglobin (20 ml. of blood) is released rapidly, the hemoglobin-binding properties of haptoglobin will be saturated and free hemoglobin will appear in the urine. For causes of hemoglobinuria, see Table 2–8.

In the porphyrias the urine may be normal, red, or purple. It is usually red in congenital erythropoietic porphyria and the cutanea tarda form of porphyria. In acute intermittent hepatic porphyria, it is normal but darkens to red-brown on standing. In lead porphyrinuria, the urine color is normal. Tests for porphyria are given on page 66. Red urine also may be associated with the use of drugs and dyes in diagnostic tests; for example, phenolsulfonephthalein, which is used in testing renal function, will cause a red color in alkaline urine.

Yellow-brown or Green-brown Urine. Yellow-brown or green-brown urine is most often associated with bile pigments, chiefly bilirubin. Bilirubin becomes oxidized to green biliverdin on standing. In severe obstructive jaundice, the urine may be dark green. On shaking the urine specimen, a yellow foam may be seen which distinguishes bilirubin from a normal, dark, concentrated urine, which will have white foam. See tests for bilirubin on p. 65.

Orange-red or Orange-brown Urine. Urine containing large amounts of urobilin may resemble a dark, concentrated normal urine. Excreted urobilinogen is colorless but is converted in the presence of light and acid pH to urobilin which is dark yellow or orange. Urobilin will not color the foam on shaking a urine sample. See test for urobilinogen on page 62. Urinary analgesics (phenazopyridines) will cause an orange color and will color any foam present.

Dark Brown or Black Urine. An acid urine containing hemoglobin will darken on standing because of the formation of methemoglobin. Other rarer causes of dark brown urine are homogentisic acid (alcaptonuria) and melanin. In both cases the urine turns darker on standing; urine containing homogentisic acid will darken more rapidly when alkaline (see p. 47). In patients with extensive malignant melanoma, a colorless pigment called melanogen is excreted. The addition of a few drops of 10 per cent ferric chloride will produce a gray precipitate that darkens to black. Occasionally a colorless pigment, pyrocatechol, may be excreted; this is a breakdown product of melanin and will turn yellow with ferric chloride. Occasionally melanuria is seen in patients with Addison's disease and in highly pigmented persons with chronic intestinal obstruction. For tests for melanuria, see page 70. Dark brown urine is seen in the urine of some patients taking levodopa.

Odor. Normal urine has a faint, aromatic odor of undetermined source. Odor is chiefly important in the recognition of specimens that, due to bacterial contamination on standing, are ammoniacal, fetid, and unsuitable for laboratory examination.

Characteristic urine odors are produced after ingestion of asparagus or thymol. In maple syrup urine disease, a congenital metabolic disorder in amino acid metabolism, the urine smells like maple syrup. In phenolketonuria, a mousy odor has been noted. In Oasthouse disease, also a congenital metabolic disorder, the urine has a distinctive odor due to excessive alpha-hydroxybutyric acid.

The pH of Urine. The pH of urine is a reflection of the ability of the kidney to maintain normal hydrogen ion concentration in plasma and extracellular fluid. The metabolic activity of the body produces nonvolatile acids which cannot be extracted by the lungs – principally sulfuric, phosphoric, and hydrochloric acids, but also small amounts of pyruvic, lactic, and citric acids and some ketone bodies. These acids are excreted by the glomerulus with cations, chiefly sodium. The distal tubular

Table 2–8. TYPES AND CAUSES OF HEMOGLOBINURIA

Paroxysmal nocturnal hemoglobinuria:	Hemosiderinuria is present.
"March" hemoglobinuria:	Unaccustomed excess exercise and low renal threshold.
Glucose-6-phosphate dehydrogenase deficiency:	(1) Ingestion of fava beans; (2) drug ingestion, primaquin and probably phenothiazine, nitrofurantoin, and others.
Cold hemoglobinuria:	Donath-Landsteiner antibody.
Autoimmune hemolytic anemia:	(1) Cold antibody with lupus, lymphomas, and viral pneumonias; (2) warm antibody (rare) with lupus erythematosus.
Incompatible blood transfusion:	Severe intravascular hemolysis.
Infections:	(1) *Plasmodium falciparum,* especially on quinine therapy (black-water fever); (2) clostridial infections.
Drugs:	Sulfonamides, phenacetin, quinine, arsenic.

cells exchange hydrogen ions for sodium of the glomerular filtrate, and the urine becomes acid in reaction. For a discussion of this exchange process, see Chapter 3.

Normal pH. The average adult on a normal diet excretes urine about pH 6. In health, urine pH may vary from pH 4.6 to pH 8. When protein intake is high more phosphates and sulfates are produced; this results in more acid urine. On a predominantly vegetable diet, as in many nonwestern countries, the urine may have a pH higher than 6. The urine becomes less acid following a meal as a result of secretion of acid into the stomach (the so-called alkaline tide). At night, during the mild respiratory acidosis of sleep, a more acid urine may be formed.

Interpretation of Urine pH in Pathologic States. The capacity to exchange hydrogen ion for cation and the formation of ammonia is decreased when tubular function is impaired. In *renal tubular acidosis*, glomerular filtration is normal, but tubular ability to form ammonia and exchange hydrogen ions for cations is defective. The urine is relatively alkaline, and the pH cannot be lowered below pH of 6 to 6.5, even with the administration of an acid loading substance. Titratable acidity and the concentration of ammonium are decreased.

In metabolic acid-base disturbances, the pH of the urine may reflect attempts at compensation by the kidneys. In *metabolic acidosis* an acid urine is produced and titratable acidity and ammonium ion concentrations are increased. In *metabolic alkalosis* an alkaline urine is produced and ammonia production is decreased. In *respiratory acidosis* an acid urine is formed and the amount of ammonium excreted is increased; in *respiratory alkalosis* an alkaline urine is produced which is associated with increased excretion of bicarbonate. In *potassium depletion* such as in hypokalemic alkalosis of prolonged vomiting or in hypercorticism, there may be paradoxical aciduria with slightly acid urine in the presence of a metabolic alkalosis. Potassium and hydrogen ions are excreted and bicarbonate is reabsorbed.

Acid urine may be produced by a diet high in meat protein and in some fruits such as cranberries. Ammonium chloride, methionine, or methenamine mandelate is often used to produce an acid urine in treatment of calculi, such as phosphate and calcium carbonate, which are formed in an alkaline urine and in urinary tract infection.

Alkaline urine may be induced by use of a diet high in certain fruits and vegetables, especially citrus fruits. Sodium bicarbonate, potassium citrate, and acetazolamide may be used to induce alkaline urines in the treatment of calculi, since uric acid, calcium oxalate, and cystine precipitate in acid urine. They may also be used in some urinary tract infections, (the antibiotics neomycin, kanamycin, and streptomycin are more active in alkaline urine), in sulfonamide therapy in which sulfadiazine or sulfamerazine is used (sulfisoxizole is more soluble in the tubular lumina), and in the treatment of salicylate poisoning.

Measurement of Urine pH. Measurement of urine pH and acidity must always be made on freshly voided specimens. If precise measurements are required, the urine should be covered tightly and the container filled in order to minimize the amount of dead space. On standing, the pH tends to rise because of loss of carbon dioxide (the P_{CO_2} of freshly voided urine is approximately 40 mm. Hg that of normal plasma) and because bacterial growth produces ammonia from urea.

A rough estimate of the pH is usually sufficient and may be made with indicator paper. In patients with disturbances of acid-base balance, urinary pH may be accurately measured with a pH meter with a glass electrode. In measuring titratable acidity, the specimen should be fresh, or if a 24-hour urine collection is made, the pooled urine should be refrigerated from the onset of collection.

Determination of pH in Urine. Urinary pH may be measured by means of a closed glass electrode and read directly from the scale of a pH meter. Since the pH meter may tend to drift, it must be standardized with a buffer of known pH immediately prior to use. After standardization, spray the electrodes with distilled water, clean, and dry with tissue. Immerse the electrodes in the urine sample. Report the pH of urine at the temperature of measurement.

Titratable Acidity of Urine. The pH of the urine is largely dependent on the amount of mono- and dibasic phosphate present. Titratable acidity is measured by titrating a fresh or preserved (toluol) specimen of urine with 0.1 N NaOH with pH 7.4 as an endpoint. If phenolphthalein is used as an indicator, the endpoint is pH 8.3 (Palmer and Henderson, 1913). The test may be used together with urinary ammonia determination in patients with chronic acidosis of obscure origin.

PROCEDURE. To 25 ml. of urine in a flask, add 10 gm. of powdered potassium oxalate (to precipitate calcium). Mix well. Titrate to pH 7.4 using 0.1 N NaOH. If phenolphthalein is used as the indicator, titrate to a pale pink color (pH 8.3).

Titratable acidity is usually reported as number of milliliters of 0.1 N NaOH required to neutralize a 24-hour specimen.

$$= \frac{\text{ml. NaOH} \times \text{24-hour volume}}{25}$$

Normal titratable acidity is in the range of 200 to 500 ml. 0.1 N NaOH (or 6 ml. 0.1 N NaOH per kg. body weight).

Specific Gravity and Osmolality. The volume of excreted urine and its concentration of solute is varied by the kidney to maintain homeostasis of body fluid and electrolytes. In order to achieve this the kidneys produce a urine much more concentrated than the plasma from which it is derived. The solute concentration of the urine varies with water and solute ingestion, the state of the tubular cells and the influence of antidiuretic hormone (ADH) on water reabsorption in the distal tubules. Final concentration of urine takes place in the collecting system of the medulla. The inability to concentrate or dilute urine is an indication of renal disease or hormonal deficiency (ADH). See Chapter 3 for a discussion of the concentrating ability of the kidney.

Urines of low specific gravity are called *hyposthenuric*, the specific gravity being less than 1.007. Urines of fixed specific gravity of about 1.010 are known as *isosthenuric*. The specific gravity of the protein-free glomerular filtrate is about 1.007. Its osmolal concentration is about 285 mOsm., or the osmolality of protein-free plasma (the plasma protein makes little contribution to the total osmolality of the plasma, only about 2 mOsm.).

The measurement of specific gravity or osmolality should give an indication of the urinary total solute concentration. The measurement of osmolality of urine and plasma is preferred to the measurement of specific gravity, although it may be well to measure both properties. The reader should refer to Chapter 3 for a discussion of osmolality versus specific gravity of urine.

Specific Gravity. Useful clinical information can be obtained from the measurement of maximal specific gravity, although the usual methods are technically not as precise as the measurement of osmolality. Urea (20 per cent), chloride (25 per cent), and sulfate and phosphate (25 per cent) contribute most to the specific gravity of normal urine.

NORMAL VALUES. Normal adults with normal diets and normal fluid intake will produce urine of specific gravity 1.016 to 1.022 during a 24-hour period. If a random specimen of urine has a specific gravity of 1.023 or more, concentrating ability can be considered normal.

Urinary specific gravity after taking no fluids for 12 hours overnight should be about 1.022, and after 24 hours without fluid, 1.026. For values in children, see Table 2–1. After vasopressin (5 units) urinary specific gravity should reach at least 1.020.

Minimum specific gravity after a standard water load should be less than 1.003. For details of concentration and dilution tests, see Chapter 3.

MEASUREMENT OF SPECIFIC GRAVITY. In the measurement of specific gravity, the hydrometer (urinometer) is used. There are certain technical limitations in the method, but careful attention to detail will provide a reasonably accurate measurement. Measurements of concentrating ability are useless in the presence of diuresis, solute diuresis (glucose, urea), and radiographic dyes. Corrections should be made for protein and for glucose; however, since glucose produces a solute diuresis, it is debatable whether corrections for it are of value. If a high specific gravity is found in a pale urine, the presence of glucose should be suspected.

The *urinometer* is a hydrometer adapted to measure the specific gravity of urine at room temperature. It should be checked each day by measuring the specific gravity of distilled water, which has a specific gravity of 1.000. If the urinometer does not give a reading of 1.000, an appropriate correction must be applied to all readings taken with that urinometer.

Procedure. The urinometer vessel is filled three-fourths full with urine (minimum volume of urine required is about 15 ml.). The urinometer is inserted with a spinning motion to make sure that it is floating freely. (When reading the urinometer, be sure that it is not touching the sides or the bottom of the cylinder. Avoid surface bubbles which obscure the meniscus.) Read the bottom of the meniscus.

Because temperature influences the specific gravity, urines should be allowed to come to room temperature before a reading is made, or a correction of 0.001 should be made for each 3° C. above or below 20° C.; e.g., a reading of 1.018 at 17° C. would be corrected to 1.017.

For accurate determinations of specific gravity in concentration-dilution tests, correction must be made for protein or sugar present. Subtract 0.003 for every 1 gm. per 100 ml. of either glucose or protein.

The accuracy of a urinometer may be further checked in solutions of known specific gravity; e.g., a solution of potassium sulfate with a specific gravity of 1.015 may be prepared by diluting 20.29 gm. potassium sulfate to 1 liter with distilled water.

SPECIFIC GRAVITY OF SMALL VOLUMES. When only a small amount of urine is available, specific gravity may be measured by using a small volume urinometer, by weighing the urine, by a falling-drop technique in organic solvent solution, e.g., chloroform and benzene in a graded series of mixtures, or by measuring the refractive index. It should be mentioned that osmolality determination requires as little as 0.2 ml. of urine.

The *refractometer* requires only a few drops of urine; the method is easy and rapid, and it correlates well with urinometer readings. The method depends on the relationship between the refractive index of a solution and its content of dissolved solids. A temperature compensated hand model with a built-in scale showing specific gravities is available.

The Goldberg refractometer (American Optical Company) has been calibrated to read directly the specific gravity of urine. The instrument is temperature compensated between 60° and 100° F. It is damaged by heat above 150° F. and by immersion of the eyepiece and focusing ring in water. It should read zero with distilled water; the zero reading can be reset if necessary by breaking the seal over the setscrew, turning it with a small screwdriver, and resealing. To prevent dropping and lens damage, a stand is recommended to support the refractometer.

To make a specific gravity determination of urine, first clean the surfaces of the cover and prism with a drop of distilled water and a damp cloth and then dry. Close the cover. Apply a drop of urine at the notched bottom of the cover so that it flows over the prism surface by capillary action.

Point the instrument toward a light source at an angle that gives optimum contrast. Rotate the eyepiece until the scale is in focus. Read directly on the specific gravity scale the *sharp* dividing line between light and dark contrast.

The entire procedure should be repeated with a second drop of urine from the same sample.

Osmolality (Normal Values). The normal adult on a normal diet with a normal fluid intake will produce a urine of about 500 to 850 mOsm. per kg. water. The normal kidney is able to produce urine of osmolality in the range of 800 to 1400 mOsm. per kg. water in dehydration and a minimal osmolality of 40 to 80 mOsm. per kg. water during water diuresis. After a period of dehydration, the osmolality of the urine should be three to four times that of the plasma (e.g., with a normal plasma osmolality of 285 mOsm. per kg. water, the urine osmolality should be at least 855 mOsm. per kg. water).

METHODS FOR MEASURING OSMOLALITY. The freezing point depression method is commonly employed. A solution containing 1 osmol or 1000 mOsm. per kg. water depresses the freezing point 1.86° below that of water (take as 0° C.). For method, see Chapter 12.

Urine Volume. Measurement of the urine volume during timed intervals may be a valuable aid in clinical diagnosis. The average daily volume in the normal adult is 1200 to 1500 ml., the range of normal being from 600 to 2000 ml. The night urine is generally not in excess of 400 ml., which is to say that the ratio of day to night urine is better than 2:1 and often more than 3:1. Young children excrete about three to four times as much urine per kilogram of body weight as do adults. See Table 2–1.

A volume of more than 2000 ml. is termed *polyuria.* Any increase in urine volume, even though transitory, is called *diuresis.* By definition, *oliguria* is the excretion of less than 500 ml. of urine daily, and *anuria* is the complete suppression of urine formation. *Nocturia* is arbitrarily defined as the excretion by an adult of more than 500 ml. of urine with a specific gravity of less than 1.018 at night. This is characteristic of chronic glomerulonephritis and is due to the kidney's inability to concentrate the urine. It occurs also in other polyuric states. Under ordinary physiological conditions, the chief determinant of urine volume is the intake of water. Water is excreted extrarenally by the lungs, skin, and large bowel. These are not particularly sensitive to the body's needs either to conserve or excrete water. It thereby falls upon the kidney to control the body's state of hydration in the face of variations of water intake.

Increases in Urine Volume. Excessive intake of water (polydipsia), such as may occur occasionally in neurotic states, will result in a polyuria that may be confused with diabetes insipidus.

Certain pharmacologic preparations exert a diuretic effect. Among these are caffeine, alcohol, and mercurial diuretics. Intravenous saline or glucose solutions may increase the urine output.

The classic pathological states characterized by a continuous polyuria are diabetes insipidus and diabetes mellitus. In both these conditions polyuria is frequently so marked as to be quite noticeable to the patient; it results in excessive thirst and in excessive water intake. The mechanism of the polyuria in these two conditions, however, is quite different. In diabetes insipidus, it is the result of lack of antidiuretic hormone or, less often, insensitivity of the renal tubule to vasopressin, as in nephrogenic diabetes insipidus. The loss of this function is associated with a decreased reabsorption of water from the tubular urine, and urine has the specific gravity of an ultrafiltrate of plasma (1.010) or less. In diabetes mellitus the polyuria is related to an increase in renal solute load in the form of glucose, causing a solute diuresis.

In chronic progressive renal failure, functioning renal tissue is lost and the kidney gradually loses its ability to concentrate urine. In order to excrete the daily renal load, an increase in urine volume is inevitable. The normal urine day and night volume ratio is lost. Increased output of urine is observed in primary aldosteronism due to hyperplasia or tumor of the adrenal cortex and may occur in any condition in which prolonged and severe potassium depletion leads to renal tubular injury. In Addison's disease, secondary adrenal insufficiency, and adrenalectomy, deficiency of adrenocortical hormones is responsible for the relative inability of the kidneys to reabsorb sodium and therefore water. In a high percentage of cases, hyperparathyroidism is associated with polyuria.

Decreases in Urine Volume. Water deprivation will cause a decrease in urine volume even before signs of dehydration appear. Excessive loss of water by extrarenal routes has the same effect. This latter commonly occurs in hot weather when excessive sweating takes place.

Decreases in urine volume to oliguric levels occur also under pathologic circumstances such as the following:

1. *Dehydration.* In prolonged vomiting, diarrhea, or excessive sweating, such as may occur in febrile states, loss of body water without adequate replacement results in dehydration and hemoconcentration. Oliguria occurs, and there may even be retention of nitrogenous waste products due to a decrease in the glomerular filtration rate. Specific gravity is elevated to about 1.030.

2. *Renal ischemia.* In shock from any cause, with its characteristic low blood pressure and reduced blood volume, oliguria occurs even to the point of anuria. Anuria (or oliguria) also follows major hemolytic *transfusion reactions* and also accompanies the "crush" syndrome. Anuria in these conditions is thought to be related to loss of functioning renal mass. Renal ischemia is a likely etiologic factor.

3. Renal disease due to exposure to certain toxic agents, such as mercury bichloride, carbon tetrachloride, diethylene glycol, and the sulfonamides, may result in anuria due to acute tubular necrosis.

4. *Acute glomerulonephritis.* In acute glomerulonephritis, there is frequently oliguria, and there may be anuria. This is apparently due to blockage of glomerular capillary tufts, which results in decreased renal blood flow and decreased glomerular filtration. Decreased urine output is also seen in acute pyelonephritis and terminal chronic nephritis.

5. *Obstruction.* Bilateral hydronephrosis, resulting as it does from high-grade or long-standing obstruction of the urinary tract, may be associated with a marked decrease in urine flow and even anuria. The anuria associated with sulfonamide intoxication appears, at times, to be at least partially due to obstruction caused by the precipitation of crystals in the renal tubules or in the intramural portion of the ureter. Uric acid crystals and urates may precipitate after therapy with uricosuric agents or leukemia therapy. On the other hand, retention of urine in the bladder is not synonymous with oliguria or anuria, because there may be no decrease in urine formation by the kidney. Catheterization, of course, permits one to distinguish such retention from true oliguria.

AMINOACIDURIA

Aminoacidurias may be classified into two general types – overflow and renal.

Overflow Type. Abnormal metabolism of amino acids results in the abnormal accumulation of an amino acid or amino acids in plasma and their excretion in the urine. The kidney is normal, but the amount of amino acids excreted in the glomerular filtrate exceeds the threshold value for reabsorption. Examples of this type of aminoaciduria include phenylketonuria, tyrosinosis, alkaptonuria, maple syrup urine disease, and the generalized aminoaciduria of liver disease. In a few instances (e.g., homocystinuria) the substrate does not accumulate in the blood because there is no reabsorption in the kidney; therefore, blood levels are low, but urine levels are increased. This is known as the "no-threshold" type of aminoaciduria. See Tables 2–9 and 2–10.

Patients receiving protein hydrolysates show gross aminoaciduria, since the D-amino acids of the DL mixture are poorly metabolized and are excreted. Cachectic patients excrete excess beta-amino-isobutyric acid, as is also seen in starvation. In severe liver disease, such as massive hepatic necrosis, and in hepatic coma, breakdown of amino acids by the liver is reduced, and a generalized aminoaciduria is seen with cystine and methionine present. Leucine and tyrosine crystals are sometimes observed in the urine sediment. In hepatic coma, glutamine is often the dominant amino acid excreted. In acute hepatitis the patterns are normal if the disease is not severe, but in more severe cases, a generalized aminoaciduria with the appearance of cystine is seen.

Alkaptonuria is one of the better known abnormalities of amino acid metabolism. Homogentisic acid accumulates in the plasma because of the absence of homogentisic acid oxidase. The breakdown of phenylalanine and tyrosine is therefore arrested at the homogentisic acid stage, although there is no accumulation of amino acids in this disease. Homogentisic acid may be detected by qualitative tests, but chromatography of the urine is needed for confirmation. (See Fig. 2–49.)

Table 2–9. PRIMARY OVERFLOW AMINOACIDURIAS*

DISEASE	AMINO ACIDS INCREASED IN BLOOD AND URINE	ABNORMAL ENZYME
Phenylketonuria	Phenylalanine	Phenylalanine hydroxylase
Tyrosinosis	Tyrosine	p-Hydroxyphenylpyruvic acid oxidase
Histidinemia	Histidine	Histidase
Maple-syrup urine disease	Valine, leucine, and isoleucine	Branched chain keto acid decarboxylase
Hypervalinemia	Valine	Probably valine transaminase
Hyperglycinemia	Glycine (lysine on high protein diet)	Associated with CP synthetase deficiency and other disorders
Hyperprolinemia		
Type I	Proline	Proline oxidase
Type II		Δ^1pyrrolin-5-carboxylate dehydrogenase
Hydroxyprolinemia	Hydroxyproline	Hydroxyproline oxidase
Homocystinuria	Methionine, homocystine	Cystathionine synthetase
Hyperlysinemia	Lysine	Not known
Citrullinemia	Citrulline	Argininosuccinic acid synthetase
Alcaptonuria	Homogentisic acid (2:5 dihydroxyphenyl-acetic acid). No abnormal amino acid.	Homogentisic acid oxidase
Oasthouse urine disease	Methionine, phenylalanine, valine, leucine, isoleucine and tyrosine and also alpha-hydroxybutyric acid in urine.	Possibly methionine malabsorption syndrome

*From M. L. Efron: Aminoaciduria. New Eng. J. Med., *272*:1060, 1965.

In *phenylketonuria* the chromatogram shows a normal amino acid pattern with the addition of phenylalanine. The assay of plasma phenylalanine and chromatograms of the urine are used to diagnose and follow the treatment of phenylketonuria. After therapy with low-phenylalanine diet, the abnormal amino acid disappears in two to three weeks.

In maple syrup urine disease, so called because of the characteristic odor of the urine, there is excessive excretion of valine, leucine, and isoleucine and their keto acids and hydroxy acids in the urine. Whereas the ferric chloride test may be a useful screening test in cases of phenylketonuria, the dinitrophenylhydrazine test is somewhat more specific for high levels of keto acids in urine (Hsia, 1966). Diagnosis should be based on the characteristic urinary amino acid excretion pattern on chromatography.

Renal Type. A renal tubular defect is the cause of aminoaciduria. The plasma level of amino acids is normal. Examples are congenital disorders (e.g., the Fanconi syndrome, cystinosis, Hartnup disease, and cystine-lysinuria) and the secondary renal tubular disorders seen in Wilson's disease, galactosemia, rickets, scurvy, and occasionally the nephrotic syndrome. Heavy metal poisoning, oxalic acid poisoning, phenol poisoning, and

Table 2–10. NO-THRESHOLD AMINOACIDURIAS*

DISEASE	AMINO ACIDS IN URINE	ABNORMAL ENZYME
Argininosuccinic aciduria	Argininosuccinic acid (also citrulline)	Argininosuccinase
Cystathioninuria	Cystathionine	Cystathioninase
Homocystinuria	Homocystine	Cystathionine synthetase
Hypophosphatasia	Phosphoethanolamine	Serum alkaline phosphatase

*Modified from Efron, 1965.

Table 2–11. RENAL TRANSPORT AMINOACIDURIAS*

DISEASE	AMINO ACIDS IN URINE	ABNORMALITY
Cystinuria (cystine stones)	Cystine; lysine; arginine ornithine (basic amino acids)	Incomplete absorption of cystine, lysine, arginine and ornithine
Hartnup disease	Monoaminomonocarboxylic (neutral) amino acids (proline, glycine, hydroxyproline and methionine not increased)	Incomplete absorption of monoaminomonocarboxylic amino acids
Glycinuria – renal type Familial Iminoglycinuria	Glycine – proline, hydroxyproline	Membrane transport defect

*Modified from Efron, 1965.

occasionally burns may also produce renal tubular defects resulting in aminoaciduria. (See Tables 2–11 and 2–12.)

The aminoaciduria seen in the Fanconi syndrome, hepatolenticular degeneration (Wilson's), and infantile galactosemia is generalized; all amino acids appear in the urine in increased amounts. In cystinosis the aminoaciduria and other findings are similar to those of Fanconi syndrome, but cystine crystals accumulate in the tissues.

Cystinuria results from a defect of tubular reabsorption. The plasma amino acid concentrations are normal, but urinary amino acid chromatograms show increased amounts of cystine and lysine with variable amounts of ornithine and arginine present. The remaining amino acids are normal in amount. Cystine precipitates in the urinary tract and forms calculi. Patients with recurrence of urinary calculi should be screened for cystinuria. Cystinuria may be detected by screening tests (Brand, 1930), but this should be confirmed by amino acid chromatography.

For further discussion of aminoaciduria and its clinical manifestations, see Efron, 1965; Smith, 1960; and Stanbury *et al.*, 1972.

Normal Values. In the normal adult, urinary excretion of amino acids is fairly constant, averaging 200 mg. of alpha-amino nitrogen excreted in a 24-hour period. Although most amino acids found in normal humans have been detected in normal urine, usually not more than about 6 to 8 are detected by paper chromatography or column chromatography in more than trace amounts. In the normal urine amino acid chromatogram *glycine* is usually most prominent. This is followed by *alanine, serine,* and *glutamine* and then by *taurine, histidine,* and *methylhistidine.* With a high-protein (meat) diet, histidine and methylhistidine are excreted in larger amounts. Other amino acids which may be demonstrated in normal urine, depending on the technique used, are glutamic acid, threonine, tyrosine, and lysine and a trace of arginine; beta-amino-isobutyric acid may also be seen.

In infants the pattern may vary with feeding. The level of amino acid excretion is relatively higher in infants, and increased amounts of cystine, asparagine, glutamine, glutamic acid, and occasionally proline are seen. Relatively large amounts of taurine are present in the urine at birth, but adult levels are seen at six months of age. Children show the same pattern as adults (Smith, 1960).

Screening Tests for Aminoaciduria. The overflow aminoacidurias, including phenylketonuria, are probably best diagnosed by examining the amino acid composition of plasma. Examination of urine should also be performed, since in renal aminoaciduria of the no-thresh-

Table 2–12. SECONDARY AMINOACIDURIA*

PRIMARY DISORDER	AMINO ACIDS IN URINE	ABNORMAL ENZYME
Wilson's disease	Generalized (cystine and threonine often most prominent)	Ceruloplasmin
Galactosemia	Generalized aminoaciduria	Galactose-1-phosphate-uridyl-transferase
Cystinosis	All plasma amino acids (also loss of glucose, phosphate, potassium, water, and Fanconi syndrome)	Unknown

*Modified from Efron, 1965.

old type, where the mechanism of reabsorption of amino acids is abnormal, blood levels of amino acids will be normal or only slightly increased, but urine levels may greatly increase.

A bacterial inhibition assay with dried blood has been successfully used in screening programs for phenylketonuria (Efron, 1965; Guthrie, 1963). A simple chromatographic method with serum from whole blood collected in capillary tubes is also useful and will detect all the overflow types of aminoaciduria with raised plasma levels of amino acids (Culley *et al.*, 1962).

A number of simple screening tests have been described for the diagnosis of inborn errors of metabolism (Buist, 1968, Renuart, 1966) (Table 2–13). A laboratory using these tests should have the capability of further investigation or access to a central laboratory to provide confirmation.

The ferric chloride test for urine is nonspecific (see Table 2–14). It gives a color reaction with several amino acid disorders but may be useful in screening urine for phenylketonuria (see p. 52), maple syrup urine disease, alkaptonuria, histidinemia, tyrosinosis, and Oasthouse urine disease. In a newborn infant a positive urine ferric chloride test may be due to transient excretion of tyrosine rather than phenylketonuria. A positive test with ferric chloride should therefore be followed by chromatographic examination of blood and urine for amino acids.

Chromatographic Methods. For one- and two-dimensional paper chromatography of urinary amino acids, consult Smith, 1960, and Hsia and Inouye, 1966. Column chromatography (Spackman *et al.*, 1958) will give a quantitative answer for each of the amino acids excreted at a significant level as opposed to the semiquantitative result with paper chromatography.

Table 2–14. FERRIC CHLORIDE TEST IN URINE*

SUBSTANCE OR DISEASE	COLOR CHANGE
Acetoacetic acid	Red or red-brown
Bilirubin	Blue-green
Homogentisic acid	Blue or green; fades quickly
o-Hydroxyphenylacetic acid	Mauve
o-Hydroxyphenylpyruvic acid	Red-brown; turns to green or blue then fades to mauve
p-Hydroxyphenylpyruvic acid	Green; fades in seconds
Imidazolepyruvic acid	Green or blue-green
α-Ketobutyric acid	Purple; fades to red-brown
Maple-syrup urine disease	Blue
Melanin	Gray precipitate; turns black
Phenylpyruvic acid	Green or blue-green; fades to yellow
Pyruvic acid	Deep gold-yellow or green
Xanthurenic acid	Deep green; later brown
Drugs	
Aminosalicylic acid	Red-brown
Antipyrines and acetophenetidines	Red
Cyanates	Red
Phenol derivatives	Violet
Phenothiazine derivatives	Purple-pink
Salicylates	Stable purple

*Modified from Henry, 1964.

Table 2–13. URINARY SCREENING TESTS FOR INBORN ERRORS OF METABOLISM: AMINOACIDURIA

DISEASE	FERRIC CHLORIDE TEST	DNPH* TEST	NITROPRUSSIDE-CYANIDE TEST
Phenylketonuria	Green	+	−
Homocystinuria	−	−	+
Cystinuria	−	−	+
Maple syrup disease	Blue	+	−
Histidinemia	Olive	±	−
Tyrosinosis	Quick-fading green	+	−
Hyperglycinemia	−	+	±
Glycogen storage	−	+	−

*2,4-dinitrophenylhydrazine.

The combination of high-voltage paper electrophoresis and paper chromatography will give good separation (Rothman and Higa, 1962). Amino acids are first partially separated by paper electrophoresis (Fig. 2–50); the paper strip is then cut, and the group of amino acids well separated by electrophoresis are identified (Fig. 2–51). The remaining clustered amino acids are then separated by descending chromatography (Fig. 2–52). Urine collected for chromatography should be acidified with mineral acid to prevent destruction of amino acids. Either random samples or 24-hour specimens from which an aliquot is taken may be collected. When total daily excretion is required, total amino acid nitrogen should be determined. (See 14th edition, p. 54, for details of amino acid electrophoresis.)

Figure 2–50

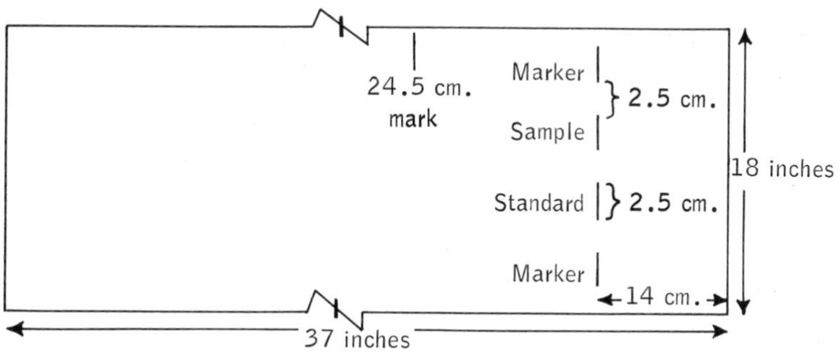

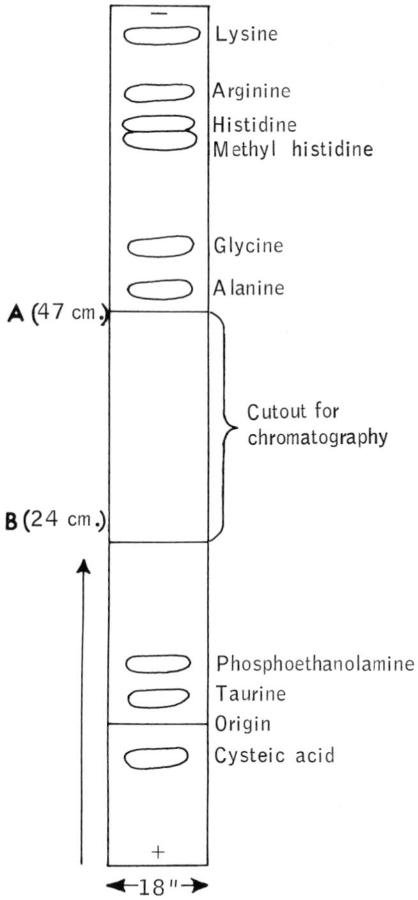

Figure 2–51

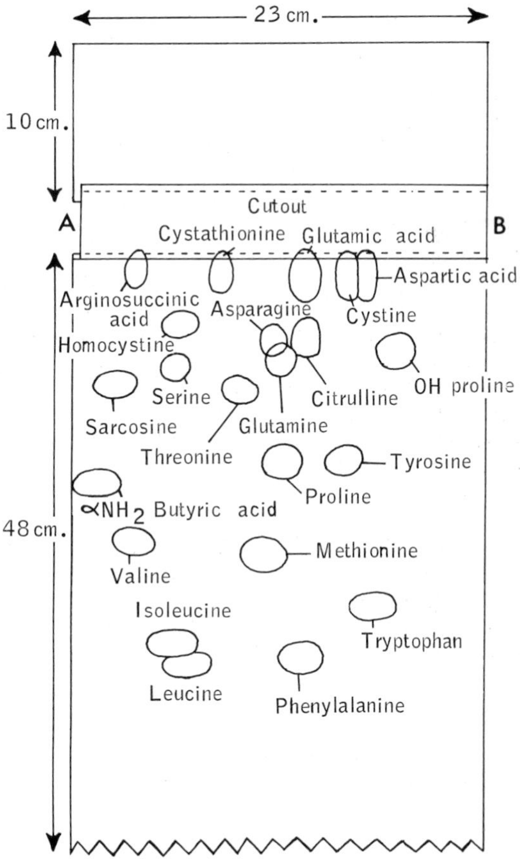

Figure 2–52

Figure 2–50. Illustration of Whatman 3MM paper for use in urinary amino acid electrophoresis showing positions of sample and marker application points.

Figure 2–51. Amino acids separated by high-voltage electrophoresis. The mixed amino acids present in section *AB* (24 to 47 cm.) are further separated by chromatography. *Note:* The diagram is not drawn to scale.

Figure 2–52. Separation of amino acids from strip *AB* after descending chromatography. *Note:* The diagram is not drawn to scale.

Qualitative Tests for Phenylpyruvic Acid in Urine

Principle. Phenylpyruvic acid reacts with ferric ions in an acid medium to form a blue-green color. Phosphate ions, which could cause a false negative result if present, are removed by precipitation as $MgNH_4PO_4$.

Ferric Chloride Test

REAGENTS

1. Magnesium reagent. Dilute 11 gm. $MgCl_2$, 14 gm. NH_4Cl, and 20.0 ml. concentrated NH_4OH to 1 liter with water.
2. HCl, 10 per cent in distilled water.
3. $FeCl_3$, 10 per cent in distilled water.

PROCEDURE

1. Add 1 ml. magnesium reagent to 4 ml. urine. Mix, let stand 5 minutes and filter.
2. Acidify filtrate with 2 drops 10 per cent HCl and add 2 drops 10 per cent $FeCl_3$. Observe color. A positive result is green.

Reagent Strip Test. Phenistix* reagent strips contain ferric ammonium sulfate, magnesium sulfate, and cyclohexylsulfamic acid. The cyclohexylsulfamic acid provides optimum acidity for the reaction.

PROCEDURE. Dip the reagent-impregnated portion of the strip into the urine and remove immediately or press it against a wet diaper. At 30 seconds compare the color of the dipped end of the strip with the color chart provided. A positive test is a gray to gray-green color. Report as positive or negative.

Sensitivity. For both methods, the sensitivity is 5 to 10 mg. per 100 ml.

Specificity. Beta-imidazolepyruvic acid is the only substance other than phenylpyruvic acid that gives the typical green color with ferric chloride or gray-green with reagent strip at 30 seconds. It is excreted in the urine in a rare disorder of children – deficiency of the enzyme histidine alpha-deaminase.

Ferric chloride reacts with p-hydroxyphenylpyruvate to produce a green color, but the color fades in seconds. Salicylates and metabolites of phenothiazine derivatives may cause a pink to purple color. High concentrations of bilirubin in the urine may alter the color reaction with phenylpyruvic acid.

Alkaline urines which are old and decomposed will interfere with the color reactions. Fresh or refrigerated specimens should be used. See Table 2-14 for ferric chloride color reactions.

Screening Test for Cystine in Urine. *Cystine* in urine may be detected by examination of the urine sediment; characteristic colorless hexagonal plates are seen (Figs. 2-37 and 2-43). A screening test in which the nitroprusside reaction for sulfhydryl groups is used shows a cherry-red color when cystine is present. The concentration of sulfhydryl in normal urine is too low to give a color reaction.

PROCEDURE. Add 2.5 ml. 5 per cent sodium cyanide solution to 5.0 ml. urine in a test tube. Allow to stand 10 minutes. Then add a few drops of a weak, freshly prepared sodium nitroprusside solution.

RESULT. A deep red color is seen if cystine is present. Normal urine may give a pale pink color if some cystine is present.

Note: A nitroprusside spot test may be useful if routine screening of urine from pediatric patients is undertaken (Fischl *et al.*, 1961).

Screening Tests for Homogentisic Acid in Urine

Homogentisic acid (alkaptonuria) causes urine to change color on standing, especially if it is alkaline. The urine becomes dark at the surface, and the color then spreads. (See Table 2-6 for other substances causing dark urine.) In many cases the dark color has not been observed by the patient, and the diagnosis is made in adult life with the onset of arthritis or because of positive findings in a routine urinalysis. Homogentisic acid reduces copper reagent (Benedict's) to form a yellow-orange precipitate which then darkens to a muddy orange because of the alkalinity of the solution. The glucose oxidase test and yeast fermentation test are negative. Ferric chloride will form a transient blue color with homogentisic acid (see p. 50). For a paper chromatographic method for homogentisic acid detection, consult Hsia and Inouye, 1966.

PROCEDURE

1. To 2 ml. urine in a test tube, add 10 per cent NaOH drop by drop. The urine will darken in alkaline solution if positive.
2. To 2 ml. urine in a test tube, add 10 per cent $FeCl_3$ drop by drop. A transient blue color will be seen if positive.
3. The alkaline urine from step 1 is dropped onto glossy photographic paper in daylight. The paper will turn black, as the homogentisic acid acts as a developer (Fischberg, 1942).
4. Benedict's qualitative test for reducing substances in urine will show a muddy orange color. It is also reduced in the cold.

Dinitrophenylhydrazine Test. This test indicates the presence of keto amino acids in the urine. A positive result is, therefore, likely in phenylketonuria (phenylpyruvic acid); histidinemia (imidazole pyruvic acid); methionine malabsorption (Oasthouse syndrome) (α-ketobutyric acid). The test is positive with acetone (hyperglycinemia, isovaleric acidemia, and glycogen storage diseases Type 1, 3, 5, and 6) and with ketonuria due to other causes. A preliminary screening test for ketonuria should be done.

*Ames Company, Elkhart, Indiana.

REAGENTS

1. 100 mg. of 2-4-dinitrophenylhydrazine in 100 ml. of 2 N HCl. The reagent should be stored in a brown bottle in the refrigerator.

PROCEDURE

1. Reagents should be at room temperature.
2. Add 10 drops of reagent to 1 ml. of clear urine.
3. After or within 10 minutes look for a yellow or chalky white precipitate to indicate a positive reaction.

Nitrosonaphthol Test for Tyrosine. An orange-red color is given within 3 to 5 minutes by tyrosine and its metabolites. It will be positive in tyrosine transaminase deficiency, tyrosinosis (tyrosinemia), and transient tyrosinosis of the newborn.

REAGENTS

1. 2.63 N nitric acid (1 volume of concentrated nitric acid in five volumes of water). Refrigerate.
2. 2.5 per cent sodium nitrite – 2.5 gm. in 100 ml. water. Store in the refrigerator.
3. 100 mg. of 1-nitrose-2-naphthol dissolved in 100 ml. of 95 per cent ethanol. Store refrigerated.

PROCEDURE

1. To 1 ml. of 2.63 N nitric acid add 1 drop of 2.5 per cent sodium nitrite and 10 drops of nitrosonaphthol reagent.
2. Mix.
3. Add 3 drops of urine and mix.
4. Observe color in 3 to 5 minutes.

CALCIUM IN URINE

The urinary output of calcium depends upon dietary intake of calcium, skeletal weight, and endocrine factors.

Estimation of calcium excretion may be useful if a 24-hour collection of urine is made and the dietary intake of calcium is known. The Albright-Reifenstein diet (1948), for example, contains about 130 mg. calcium per day. The patient is placed on the diet for three days before urine collections are started and continues on the diet for the next three days while urine is collected.

On a normal diet the daily output of calcium in urine in adults is 2.5 to 15 mEq. or 50 to 300 mg. With a dietary intake of less than 200 mg. per day the normal excretion is 13 to 180 mg. per day. With an intake of 200 to 600 mg. per day the normal output is 50 to 200 mg. per day. With an intake of about 1 gm. calcium per day the output of calcium in urine is less than 300 mg. per day.

High levels of calcium are seen in urine in hyperparathyroidism; hence, if more than 400 mg. per day is excreted on a normal diet, hyperparathyroidism should be suspected. In osteolytic bone diseases, in osteoporosis, especially after immobilization, and in hyperthyroidism, there is increased excretion of calcium. Hypercalciuria occurs in renal tubular acidosis when there is excessive loss of base and in vitamin D intoxication from increased intestinal absorption (Chap. 9).

Urinary calcium levels are low when serum calcium levels are low, except in renal disease; low serum levels occur in hypoparathyroidism due to defective mobilization of calcium from bone and with reduced calcium absorption, steatorrhea, or vitamin D deficiency (Chap. 9).

Methods for measuring calcium include ethylenediaminetetra-acetic acid (EDTA) titration, titration of oxalate precipitate, and by atomic absorption spectrophotometry, polarography, and glass electrodes sensitive to divalent cations (Henry, 1964).

Screening Test for Urinary Calcium (Barney, 1937). The normal serum calcium level is above the renal threshold for calcium, which is about 7 mg. per 100 ml. If the serum level is below this, no calcium is excreted. The test may be useful as a rapid screening test for hypoparathyroidism. See Ritter *et al.*, 1960, for criticisms of the test. Results will be affected by concentration of the urine and calcium intake (Albright and Reifenstein, 1948).

PRINCIPLE. Calcium is precipitated as calcium oxalate at a pH at which the calcium and magnesium phosphates are soluble. The degree of precipitation is noted visually.

REAGENTS

1. Glacial acetic acid.
2. Calcium solution, 25 mg. per 100 ml. Dissolve 69 mg. anhydrous $CaCl_2$ in water and dilute to 100 ml. with water.
3. Sulkowitch reagent:
   - 2.5 gm. oxalic acid.
   - 2.5 gm. ammonium oxalate.
   - 5.0 ml. glacial acetic acid.
   - 150.0 ml. distilled water.

PROCEDURE

1. Adjust the pH of the urine sample to 5 with acetic acid. If the urine specimen is cloudy, it may be centrifuged after the pH has been adjusted to 5. If the centrifugate is still cloudy, a blank should be made with 5 ml. of urine and 5 ml. of water. Compare to the test to see if turbidity has increased.
2. Pipette 5 ml. of urine into a test tube. Add 5 ml. of Sulkowitch reagent and mix by inversion. Also carry out the test on 5 ml. of solution containing 25 mg. per 100 ml. calcium.
3. Wait 2 minutes and observe the turbidity. Report as *decreased* (little or no precipitate) and serum calcium probably less than 8.5 mg. per cent (4.3 mEq./L.), *moderate* (turbidity seen but less than that produced by the 25 mg. per 100 ml. calcium solution), or *increased*

(turbidity equal to or greater than that produced by the 25 mg. per 100 ml. calcium solution) and serum calcium probably above 12 mg. per cent (6 mEq./L.).

GLUCOSE AND OTHER SUGARS

Glucose. Glucose in the glomerular filtrate is reabsorbed by the tubules. The tubular maximal reabsorptive capacity for glucose is usually about 160 mg. per 100 ml., ±20 mg. At blood concentrations above this value, glucose appears in the urine in concentrations high enough to be detected by the usual screening methods. This condition is known as glycosuria. In the normal adult an average of 130 mg. of glucose is excreted during a 24-hour period, with lesser amounts of other sugars (Date, 1958).

Glycosuria. Routine screening of urine samples for glucose, a part of the basic urine examination, has as its primary goal the detection of *diabetes mellitus.* Since there are other causes of glycosuria, notably recent ingestion of large amounts of carbohydrates and impaired renal tubular ability to reabsorb glucose, one is faced with the necessity of either confirming or excluding a diagnosis of diabetes mellitus when glucose is detected in a urine sample. As a general rule, if the reducing substance in the urine is glucose and a persistent glycosuria occurs, a diagnosis of diabetes mellitus should be considered. If there is no glucose in a urine specimen collected 2 hours after a meal, diabetes mellitus is probably not present, although high renal thresholds may occur in older diabetic patients with arteriosclerosis. The finding of an elevated fasting blood glucose level and an elevated postprandial (2-hour) blood glucose level on repeated occasions confirms the diagnosis. In doubtful cases a glucose tolerance test should be conducted (Wilkerson, 1964). See Editorial, 1966, and Chapter 9.

NONDIABETIC GLYCOSURIA. The glycosuria of diabetes mellitus is associated with an elevation of the blood glucose level, hyperglycemia. On the other hand, glycosuria without hyperglycemia occurs classically in a condition known as *renal glycosuria.* Here, the renal threshold for glucose is abnormally low, which allows glucose to appear in the urine at normal or rather low blood sugar levels. The differentiation between this condition and diabetes mellitus is an important one. The distinction is made by determining the fasting blood sugar and the glucose tolerance curve. These are both normal or low in renal glycosuria. In a small percentage of pregnant women, glycosuria occurs as a result of a lowering of the renal threshold for glucose.

ALIMENTARY GLYCOSURIA. Alimentary glycosuria is seen after gastrectomy and in some persons after ingestion of large amounts of glucose or sucrose. Alimentary glycosuria is also associated with thyrotoxicosis.

EPINEPHRINE. Epinephrine, whether injected or liberated from the adrenals as the result of excitement or pain, is capable of producing a marked hyperglycemia. This phenomenon is dependent upon the presence of stored carbohydrate in the liver, which can be mobilized. The oxidation of carbohydrates is not impaired. The effect is usually transient and occasional. Tumors of the adrenal medulla, notably *pheochromocytomas,* produce hyperglycemia and glycosuria by means of epinephrine discharges. The patient with pheochromocytoma may have clinical signs and symptoms and laboratory findings that closely resemble those of diabetes mellitus.

PANCREATITIS. Pancreatitis, in its acute stages, is often accompanied by disturbed carbohydrate utilization, with hyperglycemia and glycosuria. Chronic pancreatitis may be present with no disturbance in the function of the islets of Langerhans. However, in about one-third of advanced cases typical diabetes mellitus may ensue. Also, following total pancreatectomy, diabetes mellitus is seen though, interestingly enough, it is usually mild in terms of insulin requirement.

Other endocrinopathies, not involving primarily the islets, may also be associated with disturbed carbohydrate utilization.

HYPERTHYROIDISM. Hyperglycemia and glycosuria frequently occur in thyrotoxic states. In some cases they may result from an increased rate of glucose absorption from the gastrointestinal tract. On the other hand, fasting hyperglycemia may occur, and in these instances the disturbance in carbohydrate metabolism resembles that of diabetes mellitus. This diabetes may disappear after satisfactory treatment of the hyperthyroidism. It may persist, however, as true diabetes mellitus, but even in this case it will be markedly ameliorated on return to the euthyroid state.

ACROMEGALY. Nearly 25 per cent of patients with acromegaly demonstrate hyperglycemia and glycosuria in the active phase of the disease. The diabetogenic action of growth hormone is poorly understood but is thought to inhibit the peripheral action of insulin on carbohydrate metabolism.

CUSHING'S SYNDROME. Hyperglycemia, glycosuria, and impaired glucose tolerance result from either prolonged increased secretion of cortisol or *administration of cortisol* or its analogs. Cortisol increases hepatic gluconeogenesis and inhibits the condensation of pyruvic acid and coenzyme A to form acetyl coenzyme A, an intermediate in the tricarboxylic acid cycle.

GLUCAGON-SECRETING ALPHA CELL TUMOR OF THE ISLETS. Glucagon produces hyperglycemia in the same way as epinephrine. Stimulation of liver phosphorylase reactivation results in hepatic glycogenolysis. The rare alpha cell tumor of the islet tissue of the pancreas is believed to produce excessive amounts of glucagon.

STARVATION DIABETES. After an individual has fasted for several days, glucose tolerance may be so impaired that intake of food results in glycosuria. This effect may be marked and it has been referred to as starvation diabetes.

LIVER DAMAGE. When liver damage is present, a rather confusing picture is apt to occur. When glucose or foods that will yield it are ingested, glycosuria may occur because of the liver's inability to convert glucose to glycogen adequately. In fasting, however, because the blood sugar is normally maintained by contribution of glucose from the liver, low blood sugars are frequently seen, and the patient may exhibit hypoglycemic manifestations.

ASPHYXIA. In asphyxia, such as in carbon monoxide poisoning, hyperglycemia is frequently seen; it has also been noticed after *general anesthetics*, after morphine, and after strychnine administration.

INTRACRANIAL INJURY. In intracranial injury, glycosuria and hyperglycemia are frequently seen, especially in event of subarachnoid hemorrhage. These are generally attributed to injury in the region of the pons, the floor of the fourth ventricle, or the hypothalamus.

RENAL TUBULAR DISEASE. In renal tubular disease, the Fanconi syndrome, there is often lowered renal absorption of glucose.

Reducing Sugars Other Than Glucose. Consult Stanbury *et al.*, 1972, for detailed information.

Fructose. Fructose may appear in the urine in diabetes mellitus. Fructosuria occurs with a very rare inherited metabolic defect. It is accompanied by proteinuria and aminoaciduria (Froesch *et al.*, 1963).

Lactose. Lactose is found in the urine in late pregnancy and lactation. Lactosuria is often accompanied by glycosuria during pregnancy. Lactose intolerance with lactosuria is a rare metabolic disease (Lowe and Auerback, 1964).

Galactose. Galactose appears in the urine in rare cases of galactose intolerance and in the inherited disease galactosemia. Galactosuria, usually accompanied by glucosuria or fructosuria, is also present in severe hepatitis or biliary atresia in neonatal infants. *Galactosemia* in infancy, due to a deficiency in galactose-1-phosphate uridyl transferase, is accompanied by liver damage, mental retardation, and cataracts and may be prevented by dietary restrictions early in life (Lowe and Auerback, 1964). The finding of a positive copper reduction test (Benedict's) and a negative glucose oxidase test in an infant urine is highly significant, and the reducing substance should be identified by chromatography. In patients with galactosemia there are usually proteinuria and aminoaciduria. The enzyme deficiency should be confirmed by a red cell utilization test (Hsia and Inouye, 1966).

Pentose. The ingestion of fruits rich in pentoses, such as plums or cherries, may cause pentosuria. A rare familial disorder is characterized by the excretion of xylulose, a pentose (Freedberg *et al.*, 1959).

Reducing sugars are differentiated from each other and from glucose by use of paper or thin-layer chromatography (Fig. 2–53). See Table 2–15 for nonsugar reducing substances found in the urine.

Methods for Measuring Reducing Sugars in Urine. Qualitative and quantitative procedures are available. Two methods are used, one in which glucose reduces alkaline copper sulfate to cuprous sulfate (Benedict's test) and one in which glucose is oxidized to gluconic acid by glucose oxidase. The second method is specific for glucose, since, with the exception of ascorbic acid, nonglucose reducing agents do not interfere with it.

Qualitative Tests for Glucose in Urine. The simplest, most specific test is the *glucose oxidase paper strip* method (Free *et al.*, 1957a). It is more sensitive than copper reduction methods and will detect levels of 10 to 12 mg. per 100 ml. of urine glucose. It is not affected over a pH range of 5 to 9 or by the addition of significant amounts of uric acid (200 mg. per 100 ml.), creatinine (100 mg. per 100 ml.), or protein. Ascorbic acid, however, will completely inhibit the test for at least 2 minutes when the ascorbic acid level is about twice as great as the glucose level (Nakamura *et al.*, 1965). It is important to remember that ascorbic acid is added to many antibiotic preparations as a stabilizer. As a screening test, the glucose oxidase test will not detect increased levels of galactose or homogentisic acid in urine. It is therefore important that a copper reduction test such as Benedict's should be routinely used for pediatric patients.

Of the copper reduction tests used for screening purposes, the *qualitative Benedict's test* (1909) is more sensitive to reducing substances in urine than the single-tablet copper reduction test (Clinitest) (Cook *et al.*, 1953). Benedict's test becomes positive at levels of 50 to 80 mg. per 100 ml. of reducing substance (Henry, 1964). See Table 2–3 for a comparison of glucose test sensitivities. Urines containing nonglucose reducing substances may give positive results in healthy persons. Reducing substances normally excreted in the urine are creatinine and uric acid; abnormal reducing

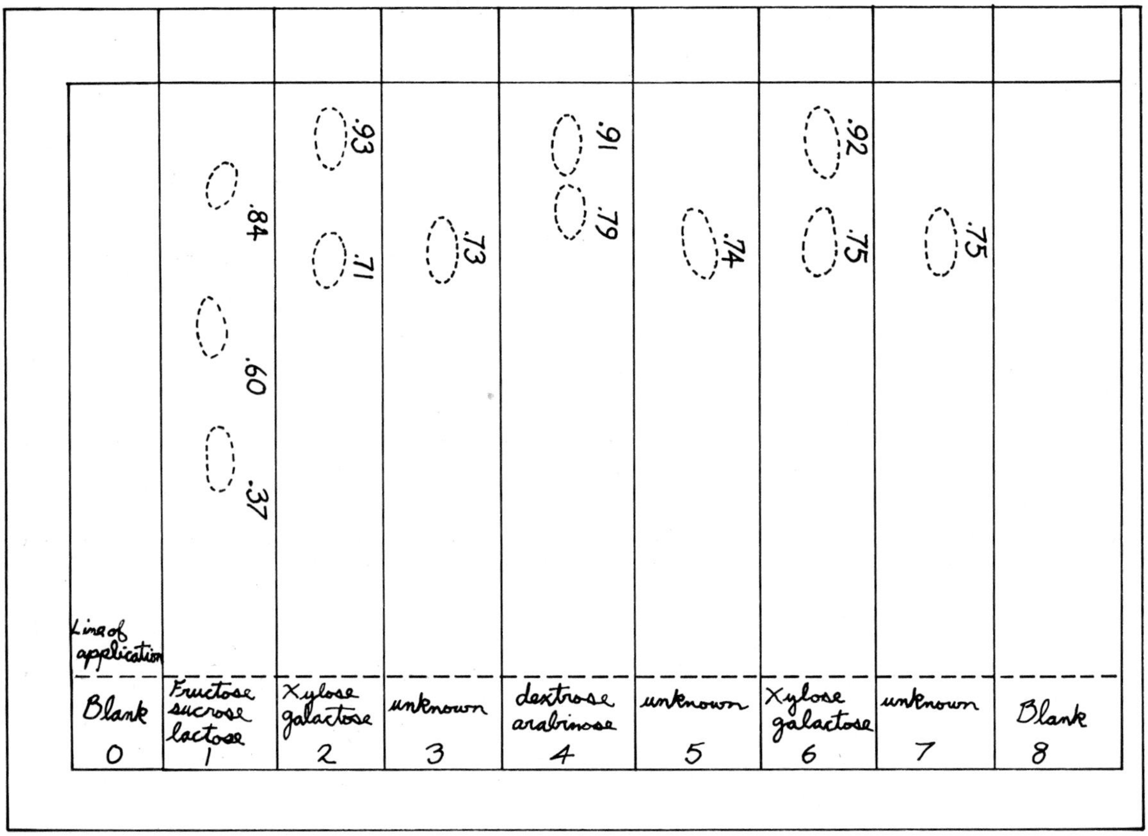

Figure 2–53. Xerox copy of thin-layer chromatographic plate showing Rf values of sugars. Unknown urine (columns 3 and 7) contained galactose (compare with columns 2 and 6).

Table 2–15. REACTIONS OF SUBSTANCES FOUND IN URINE TO TEST FOR GLUCOSURIA

CONSTITUENTS	GLUCOSE OXIDASE REAGENT STRIP	BENEDICT'S COPPER REDUCTION
Glucose	Positive	Positive
Sugars other than glucose		
Fructose		
Galactose		
Lactose	No effect	Positive
Maltose		
Pentose		
Urine constituents*		
Creatinine		
Homogentisic acid (alcaptonuria)	No effect	May cause false pos.
Uric acid		
Drug* or contaminants in urine		
Ascorbic acid (therapy or in antibiotic prep.)	Large quantities may delay color†	May cause false pos.
Hydrogen peroxide	False pos.	
Hypochlorite (bleach)	False pos.	

*Also amino acids, carinamide, cephalothin, chloral, chloroform, chloramphenicol, chlortetracycline, formaldehyde, hippuric acid, homogentisic acid, isoniazid, ketone bodies, nalidixic acid, oxalic acid, oxytetracycline, p-aminosalicylic acid, penicillin, phenols, protein, salicylates, streptomycin, and uronates may cause positive Benedict's test (Caraway, 1962; Wirth, 1965).

†Does not affect Diastix (Ames), but Ketones will.

Table 2–16. IDENTIFICATION OF URINARY SUGARS

SUGAR	COPPER REDUCTION	FERMENTABLE	CONFIRMATORY TEST
Glucose	+	+	Glucose oxidase
Lactose	+	−	Chromatography (Rubner's test)
Fructose	+	+	Chromatography (resorcinol test)
Galactose	+	−	Chromatography (red cell enzyme test)
Maltose	+	+	Chromatography
Mannose	+	+	Chromatography
Pentose	+	−	Chromatography
Sucrose	−	+	Chromatography

substances include homogentisic acid and many drugs. See Table 2–15 for a comprehensive listing.

The methods that follow include the glucose oxidase reagent strip technique for glucose and qualitative Benedict's test.

Identification of Sugars Other Than Glucose. Identification of sugars other than glucose is best accomplished by using thin-layer chromatography. The technique presented is simple and a specific result is obtained. The yeast fermentation test and qualitative tests for fructose and lactose are also presented. Qualitative tests for other urine sugars are generally nonspecific. Table 2–16 shows a comparison of results with yeast fermentation and copper reduction tests for sugars found in urine.

Qualitative Measurement of Glucose in Urine

Oxidase Method

PRINCIPLE. Glucose oxidase reacts with glucose in the urine to remove two hydrogen ions and forms gluconolactone, which is promptly hydrated to gluconic acid. The removed hydrogen ion is then combined with atmosphere oxygen to form hydrogen peroxide. The overall reaction is expressed as follows:

$$\text{Glucose} + O_2 \xrightarrow{\text{glucose oxidase}} \text{gluconic acid} + H_2O_2$$

The hydrogen peroxide, in the presence of peroxidase, oxidizes orthotolidine, which in its oxidized state turns blue.

$$H_2O + \text{orthotolidine} \xrightarrow{\text{peroxidase}} \text{oxidized orthotolidine (blue)} + H_2O$$

PROCEDURE. Using glucose oxidase test strips (Clinistix*), dip test end of strip briefly into urine or urine stream. Ten seconds later note color of test area.

*Ames Company, Elkhart, Indiana. Reagent strips showing different color results are also available from Eli Lilly Co. Ames Diastix give different color results.

INTERPRETATION

Negative: No purple color. Test area remains red. (Check both sides of reagent strip.) *To check for false negatives,* redip negative test strip in 1 per cent glucose solution. If a negative or delayed positive reaction is seen, the specimen should be checked with a copper reduction method.

Positive: Purple color is present in test area. Generally a light color corresponds to a small amount of glucose and a dark color to a larger amount, but quantitation is not accurate.

Reagent strips are more sensitive to glucose than copper reduction tests. Reagent strips will detect as little as 0.01 per cent glucose in urine under optimum conditions and under average conditions approximately 0.1 per cent (100 mg. of glucose per 100 ml. of urine) (Table 2–3). Of reducing substances occurring in urine, the reagent strips will react positively only with glucose. Contamination of urine with hydrogen peroxide or hypochlorite (bleach) will cause a false positive reaction. See section on routine screening urinalysis for storage of reagent strips (p. 21).

INHIBITORY SUBSTANCES IN URINE. With the glucose oxidase test, color development may be delayed because of interfering substances that may be present in the specimen. Ketones in large quantities will depress the color results on the Diastix form of reagent strip.

Ascorbic acid is the major interfering substance of clinical importance. The effect depends on the relative amounts of ascorbic acid and glucose present. Reagent strips may be satisfactory for use in the case of diabetic patients taking small daily doses of ascorbic acid. Any color developing after the usual 10-second waiting period should be considered positive, without reference to the color chart.

A lapse of 1 minute should be allowed for color development.

Qualitative Benedict's Method (1911)

PRINCIPLE. Glucose in urine reduces blue alkaline copper sulfate reagent (Benedict's reagent) to red cuprous oxide precipitate (see Fig. 2-54). A green, yellow, or orange color and precipitate is formed, depending upon the amount of glucose and other reducing substances present.

REAGENT

1. Dissolve 17.3 gm. $CuSo_4 \cdot 5H_2O$ in 100 ml. hot water in large beaker.

2. Dissolve 173 gm. sodium citrate and 100 gm. anhydrous sodium carbonate in 800 ml. water with heat. Cool and pour into first reagent and dilute to 1 liter with water.

PROCEDURE. Place 5 ml. of Benedict's qualitative reagent in a test tube. Add 0.5 ml. of urine (8 drops). Mix by shaking. Place rack into pan of boiling water for 5 minutes (or over flame for 2 minutes). Remove from boiling water and read immediately.

INTERPRETATION

REACTION	REPORT AS	APPROXIMATE GLUCOSE CONCENTRATION MG./100 ML.
Clear blue or green opacity, no precipitate	0 or trace	0 to 100
Green with yellow precipitate	1+	100 to 500
Yellow to green with yellow precipitate	2+	500 to 1400
Muddy orange with yellow precipitate	3+	1400 to 2000
Orange to red precipitate–clear supernatant	4+	2000 or more

The sensitivity of the test is approximately 50 to 80 mg. glucose per 100 ml. (Henry, 1964). According to Apthorp (1957), a negative Benedict's test corresponds to a blue, blue-green, or green color with gray precipitate and is usually equivalent to less than 50 mg. per 100 ml. of reducing sugar. The green-with-yellow precipitate is equivalent to 50 mg. per 100 ml. Specimens showing green-with-a-dull-yellow precipitate are "doubtful." Bickel (1961) found that green-yellow reactions were equivalent to 115 to 550 mg. per 100 ml. of reducing sugars, but specimens showing the opaque green reaction could contain from less than 50 mg. per 100 ml. to 290 mg. per 100 ml. of reducing sugars. The interpretation of the opaque green reaction is therefore difficult (Wright, 1956), and it is recommended that it be reported as trace.

The bulk of the precipitate is the index of positivity of the reaction according to Benedict (1909) and is associated with the presence of cuprous creatinine. A dilute urine with low creatinine levels of less than 0.03 mg. per 100 ml. may therefore appear negative, even when glucose is present (Samson, 1939). False negative reactions may be associated with inadequate heating (Cook *et al.*, 1953). False positive results may be due to prolonged boiling.

NORMAL VALUES. The urine of normal children and adults is negative. Normal neonatal infants during the first 10 to 14 days of life may excrete urine giving a positive reaction due to glucose, galactose, fructose, and lactose (Bickel, 1961). Normal pregnant and postpartum women may give positive reactions to tests for lactose.

Quantitative Urine Sugar

Quantitative Test for Glucose in Urine. The techniques commonly used measure reducing substances rather than glucose. Glucose oxidase methods may be applied to the urine if uric acid and other inhibitory substances are removed by charcoal used with Lloyd's reagent (Beach and Turner, 1958) or resin (Weatherburn and Logan, 1966). The urine specimen is stable for 24 hours if stored in a refrigerator; aliquots may be frozen. Thymol and sodium fluoride may be added as preservatives; inferior grades of thymol or old solutions of thymol should not be used, since some samples reduce copper (King *et al.*, 1941). The aliquot of measured urine should be tested for approximate glucose levels so that appropriate dilutions will be made for the quantitative method used for blood glucose.

INTERPRETATION. Normal values for copper *reducing substances* in urine are given as 0.5 to 1.5 gm. in 24 hours (Bradley, 1945). Normal values for total *sugars* in urine are given as 116 to 656 mg. in 24 hours, with a mean value of 254 mg. in 24 hours, with a chromatographic separation technique. Values for individual sugars are as follows: glucose, 57 to 542 mg./24 hr. (mean 130 mg.); lactose, 23 mg./24 hr.; galactose, 14 mg./24 hr.; xylose, 49 mg./24 hr.; arabinose, 38 mg./24 hr. mean values (Date, 1958).

YEAST FERMENTATION TEST. Fermentable sugars split into ethanol and carbon dioxide when exposed to yeast. This test is used in the further identification of reducing sugars found in urine but is not as helpful as thin-layer chromatography. Glucose and fructose are readily fermented by a suspension of fresh yeast. Galactose, lactose, and pentose are not fermented. See Table 2-16.

REAGENTS

1. Fresh cake of yeast (brewer's, baker's, or compressed).

2. 1 per cent glucose solution.

3. 1 per cent lactose solution.

PROCEDURE

1. Make a qualitative test for sugar on the

known specimen. Specimens showing a 3+ reaction should be diluted 1:2 before making the fermentation test. Specimens showing a 4+ reaction should be diluted 1:5 or 1:10.

2. To 10 ml. of boiled patient's urine or diluted urine add a piece of yeast about the size of a pea. Mix well to obtain an even emulsion. Fill the long arm of the Einhorn saccharometer and tip until the closed arm is full and free of bubbles. (A **U** tube closed at one end may be used.)

3. Set up two controls, one of glucose, to check the activity of the yeast, and one of lactose, to be sure the strain of yeast used will not ferment sugars considered nonfermentable. Use 5 ml. of the 1 per cent solution plus 5 ml. of normal boiled urine for each control. Add yeast and fill tube as for unknown.

4. Place all three tubes in an incubator (37.0° C.) for 2 hours. At the end of this time note the fermentation in each tube and repeat the qualitative sugar on the patient's fermented specimen and the controls.

The glucose control should show fermentation. The lactose control should show no fermentation. The unknown urine, if the reducing sugar was glucose or fructose, will show fermentation, and the qualitative sugar test will now be negative. If the reducing sugar was pentose, lactose, or galactose, the urine will show no fermentation, and the qualitative sugar will be as positive as before unless a dilution was used.

COMMENT. Since glucose may be identified by the glucose oxidase paper strip method, the fermentation test will help only to separate fructose from the nonfermenting lactose, galactose, and pentoses. Further identification requires the use of thin-layer chromatography.

Fructose in Urine

Resorcinol Test

PROCEDURE (Selivanoff, 1887). Boil 5 ml. of urine with 5 ml. of 25 per cent HCl. Add about 5 mg. resorcinol and boil for 10 seconds. Fructose will cause the formation of a heavy red precipitate. Separate the precipitate by filtration and dissolve it in ethanol. The precipitate should form a red solution in ethanol for the test to be positive.

Note: Fructose will form from glucose in an alkaline urine, so the specimen should be fresh. For an enzyme method for measuring fructose, see Hsia and Inouye, 1966.

Lactose in Urine

PROCEDURE (Rubner, 1884). To 15 ml. urine in a test tube, add 3 gm. lead acetate. Shake and filter. Boil filtrate, add 2 ml. concentrated NH_4OH, and boil. Lactose will cause the formation of a brick-red solution and then a red precipitate with clear supernatant. Glucose will cause a yellow solution and yellow precipitate.

Detection of Urine Sugars by Thin-layer Chromatography

PRINCIPLE. Thin-layer chromatography (TLC) is a micro method of chromatography on a thin layer of adsorbent. It is a supplement to older systems of paper, column, ion-exchange, and precipitation chromatography (see Stahl, 1965).

A glass plate is coated with a uniform, thin (e.g., 250 micra) layer of adsorbent containing a bonding medium, such as $CaSO_4$, to improve adhesion to the glass. Use of inorganic adsorbents, such as silica gel or kieselguhr, permits a wide range of chromogenic reactions for detection. The layer thickness is adjustable and when accurately controlled results in a high degree of reproducibility. The layer represents an open column. After the layer is dried, samples of a complex multicomponent system, such as steroids or proteins or drugs, are applied as solutions to one end of the plate. The plate is placed vertically in a tank containing a suitable solvent. Separation is achieved usually by the ascending technique of development and is produced either by preferential adsorption to the adsorbent (stationary phase) or by distribution between the solvent (mobile phase) and the water held in the adsorbent. Only short travel distances are required, so the time involved for separation is 30 minutes or less for most complex systems. The separation can be visualized by spraying with a suitable stain or by viewing under ultraviolet light. Identification is made by the position and color of the spot produced. The ratio of the distance between the point of application and the position of the spot to the total travel distance of the solvent is called Rf. Under controlled conditions, the Rf for each component of a system is quite a reproducible figure. If known standards are included on each plate, any changes in this reproducibility from batch to batch can be more easily evaluated.

Advantages of TLC over other chromatographic procedures are speed, sharper separations with less tailing of spots, and avoidance of fluorescent background substances by using inorganic adsorbent layers. These layers also allow the use of more corrosive visualization sprays. Other advantages are higher sensitivity and the small quantities of sample required.

EQUIPMENT

1. Thin-layer chromatography plates (8 by 8 inches) prepared with kieselguhr (MN) and calcium sulfate binder (Mann Research Laboratories Inc., New York, and other manufacturers).

2. Storage rack (Brinkmann Instruments, Des Plaines, Illinois).

3. Desiccator to store TLC plates.

4. Drying oven, 100° C.

5. Glass developing tank with cover; TLC Chromatank (Shandon), 9 by 12 by 6 inches, (Colab, Chicago).

6. Plastic labeling template (Brinkmann).

7. Microsyringe, 10 μliter with 2 inch fixed needle. (Hamilton Co. Inc., Whittier, California.)

8. Glass spray bottle (50 or 125 ml. size), preferably one which can be adjusted to produce a fine mist using compressed air.

Storage. Plates are stored in a rack in a desiccator, layer-side up. Plates are activated prior to use by setting up the rack (for 30 minutes) in an oven preheated at 105° to 120° C.

Procedure

Standards. Prepare solutions of the most commonly encountered sugars of urine in a concentration of 0.01 per cent in pyridine. Include fructose, sucrose, dextrose, lactose, xylose, galactose, and arabinose. These solutions may be stored indefinitely in a refrigerator in brown glass bottles. Mixtures of standards can be made and applied if greater speed is desired. The absolute values for Rf have been much more variable with sugars than with the barbiturates, for example, so the use of a full panel of standards with each batch is necessary.

Solvent. Mix 65 ml. of ethyl acetate, 24 ml. of isopropyl alcohol, and 12 ml. of distilled water. One batch is sufficient to develop one plate and should be made fresh for each run. It is especially important with sugars to have a chamber which is oversaturated with mixture vapors, so place the solvent in the developing tank 1 hour before the run is to begin. Filter papers may be placed along the sides of the tank to aid in saturation.

Spray. Mix 9 ml. of 95 per cent ethyl alcohol, 0.5 ml. of concentrated sulfuric acid, and 0.5 ml. of anisaldehyde. Prepare fresh for each run. It may be convenient to prepare a double quantity.

Unknown. There is no extraction of the urine. The specimen, which has a negative glucose oxidase test and a positive Benedict's test, may be stored frozen until used. A 1:10 solution of urine in pyridine is prepared (1 ml. of urine in a 10 ml. volumetric flask is suitable, but smaller volumes may be prepared). Two μliters of the unknown and standards are applied to the plate.

1. Apply the test substance and standards to the activated plate: Carefully scrape about 3 mm. of adsorbent from the bottom and sides of the plate to reduce the edging effect. However, if too much is removed from the bottom edge, the amount of solvent prescribed above will not be sufficient to reach the adsorbent layer.

Use the marking template to mark with a sharp pencil the 10 cm. distance that the solvent is to be allowed to travel. The template will straddle any plate up to 200 mm. wide in bridge form without coming in contact with the adsorbent layer. The template may be used to spot samples at fixed intervals by using the marking ruler on its edge as guide.

Apply samples at least 2 cm. from the edge of the plate or in such a way that the spots are not immersed in the solvent at the bottom of the developing tank. Rinse syringe in 95 per cent alcohol between each application.

Allow the spot to dry after application.

2. After the sample spot has dried, place the glass plate vertically in a developing tank in which the solvent mixture has been placed one-half to 1 hour before. (Ample time for saturation of the atmosphere inside the tank with mixture vapors is required.) Lean the plate against the wall of the tank in such a way that the layer side is not in contact with the wall.

3. After the solvent front has reached the 10 cm. line, remove the plate from the tank and let it dry. Approximately 30 to 45 minutes is required for the solvent to move 10 cm.

4. Place approximately 9 to 18 ml. of spray reagent in a spray bottle. Connect the bottle to compressed air and adjust the pressure until a fine mist is obtained. Spray the plate under a fume hood.

5. Outline the position and shape of each spot with a sharp pencil.

6. Measure Rf distance (i.e., distance spot has moved). If distance solvent has moved is 100 mm. and unknown 74 mm., its Rf is 0.74. (Measure to center of spot.) For a permanent record of the pattern, have the plate photocopied with the Xerox photocopier. Label this copy with respect to each component separated, its Rf, and the color achieved. (See Fig. 2–53.)

7. Obtain from patient's record a list of drugs given the patient or accessible to him. This information can be added to the photocopy.

Comments. It is important to remove the plate immediately when the 10 cm. travel distance line is reached because xylose and arabinose travel so close to the solvent front that they may be lost. The solvent cannot cross a space barrier such as a pencil line. If there is tailing of the spot, the urine may be diluted 1:50 or 1:100 and another test made.

When spraying with the stain, care must be taken not to overspray or the background will darken and the spots will be difficult to differentiate. The amount of spray required can only be determined with practice. After a light spray, it is necessary to heat the plate to from 90° to 120° C. for 5 to 10 minutes to bring out the blue color. Overheating will also intensify the background color.

Results. Dextrose, fructose, lactose, and sucrose will be blue; galactose will be gray; arabinose and xylose will be yellow.

Sensitivity. Optimal sensitivity is 0.5 μg. per spot; minimal sensitivity is 0.05 μg. per spot; maximal sensitivity 5.0 μg. per spot.

HEME PIGMENTS AND PYRROLES

Hemoglobin in Urine. The presence of an abnormal number of red blood cells in urine is known as *hematuria,* whereas the term *hemoglobinuria* indicates the presence of hemoglobin in solution in urine. See page 36 for causes of hematuria and Table 2–8 for causes of hemoglobinuria.

Because of the diagnostic importance of small amounts of hematuria, and because of the tendency of red blood cells to undergo lysis in urine, a screening test for hemoglobinuria is a useful adjunct to the microscopic examination of the sediment. Normal urine may contain an average of 1000 red blood cells per milliliter (Wright, 1959). Cook *et al.* (1956) found that the addition of about 66,000 red blood cells to 1 ml. of urine was the lowest amount clearly detectable as abnormal by microscopic examination. The combination of a positive test for hemoglobin and normal urinary sediment suggests that a fresh urine sample should be examined for red blood cells. The microscopic examination for red cells should not be omitted, because a few red cells that do not react to the usual screening test may occasionally be present; in a series of 1052 urine specimens, 65 sediments showed an occasional red blood cell, but 35 of these specimens had negative orthotolidine tests (Damron, 1963).

Screening Test for Hemoglobin in Urine. The orthotolidine and benzidine tests are sensitive to a hemoglobin level of about 0.0003 mg. per ml. equivalent to 10 million red blood cells per liter (10,000 per ml.). Because of the carcinogenic effect of benzidine, the orthotolidine test is recommended. Either a wet chemical test (Henry, 1964) or a reagent strip or tablet may be used. In this test, hemoglobin and other iron porphyrin derivatives including myoglobin catalyze the oxidation of orthotolidine to a blue product by oxygen release from hydrogen peroxide.

Procedure. Using an orthotolidine reagent strip (Hemostix, Ames), dip test end of strip into well-mixed urine or briefly pass through urine stream and observe at 1 minute. Do not use brown or discolored strips. See page 21 for precautions in using reagent strips.

Interpretation

Negative: No blue color is present at 1 minute.

Positive: Test end of strip turns blue within 1 minute. The color blocks indicate reactions that are obtained with small, moderate, and large amounts of excreted blood.

Specificity. The orthotolidine reagent strip is specific for red blood cells, hemoglobin, and myoglobin in urine. False positive results are not seen within the 1 minute reading time with specimens containing as much as 1000 mg. per 100 ml. of potassium iodide. Oxidizing agents may cause false positive reactions.

Sensitivity. The reagent strip is more reactive to urine specimens containing free hemoglobin than to specimens containing only intact red blood cells. Free hemoglobin, however, has been detected in over 90 per cent of urine specimens containing red blood cells. With urine specimens containing little or no free hemoglobin and only a small number of red blood cells, the reagent strips may or may not produce a color reaction.

Ascorbic acid, when present in large amounts in urine, may retard or inhibit the chemical reaction of hemoglobin with the peroxide-orthotolidine system. Therefore, the reagent strips should not be the only test procedure used when testing for occult blood in urines from patients taking large therapeutic dosages of ascorbic aid or parenteral antibiotics (tetracyclines) containing large amounts of ascorbic acid as a preservative. When there is a possibility of large amounts of ascorbic acid in the urine, microscopy is the procedure of choice.

Myoglobinuria and Differentiation from Hemoglobinuria. When there is rapid destruction of skeletal muscle, myoglobin and other muscle proteins are released into the blood and myoglobin appears in the urine. See Table 2–7 for causes of myoglobinuria. The urine becomes red or brown in color. This is similar to the color seen with hemoglobin and some other substances. Among these are nonprotein substances such as porphyrin, homogentisic acid, drugs, and dyes; these will all remain in the solution when proteins are precipitated with sulfosalicylic acid. Hemoglobin is precipitated from urine that is 80 per cent saturated with ammonium sulfate, but myoglobin is not.

Procedure (Blondheim *et al.,* 1958)

1. Use a fresh morning urine specimen or one voided after exercise. Observe the color of urine. Characteristically, urine with myoglobinuria is red when fresh and turns black on standing.

2. Mix 1 ml. of urine and 3 ml. of 3 per cent sulfosalicylic acid. Filter. If the pigment is precipitated, it is a protein. If the filtrate is a normal color, no abnormal nonprotein pigment is present. (*Note:* the heat + acetic acid test does not precipitate myoglobin or hemoglobin.)

3. To 5 ml. of urine in a test tube, add 2.8 gm.

of ammonium sulfate. Dissolve by mixing. The urine is now 80 per cent saturated with ammonium sulfate. This is optimum for precipitation of hemoglobin. Filter or centrifuge. If the supernatant shows a normal color, the precipitated pigment is hemoglobin. If the supernatant fluid is colored, this is presumptive evidence of myoglobin. The presumptive test should be confirmed spectrophotometrically and/or by paper electrophoresis (Henry, 1964; Whisnant *et al.*, 1959).

Urobilinogen in Urine. After bile is excreted into the intestine, conjugated bilirubin is reduced by bacterial action to mesobilirubin, stercobilinogen, and urobilinogen. Stercobilinogen and urobilinogen are colorless and are oxidized to the colored pigments urobilin and stercobilin.

The reduced products of bilirubin are normally reabsorbed into the portal circulation to be reexcreted by the liver. Part of the reabsorbed urobilinogen and stercobilinogen is excreted in the urine together with mesobilirubinogen. Urobilin, the oxidized form of urobilinogen, is also found in normal urine.

Normal adult urine contains from about 0.5 to 2.5 mg. of urobilinogen in a 24-hour collection; less than 1 Erhlich unit in 2 hours is excreted as measured by a semiquantitative method (Balikov, 1957). Urinary and fecal urobilinogen is increased when there is hemolysis of red cells, as in hemolytic anemia. Raised levels of urinary urobilinogen may also be present in liver disease because the liver cells may not be able to reabsorb or reexcrete circulating urobilinogen, thus causing more to appear in the urine. Urobilinogen may be absent from the urine (and decreased in feces) in patients with complete obstruction of the bile duct, as in carcinoma of the head of the pancreas.

Methods for Measuring Urobilinogen in Urine. Methods for measuring urobilinogen in urine measure the total chromogens in the urine. Ehrlich's reagent, p-dimethylaminobenzaldehyde in concentrated hydrochloric acid, reacts with urobilinogen and the other chromogens to form a colored urobilinogen-aldehyde. The acidity is then decreased by adding sodium acetate, which intensifies the red color of the aldehyde and inhibits color formation by skatoles and indoles. The reaction is not specific for urobilinogen; consequently, extractions with petroleum ether are employed to separate urobilinogen from other Ehrlich's reactive compounds. If the extraction is performed, the result may be reported in terms of mg. urobilinogen. If no extraction is made, the results are reported in Ehrlich units.

The oxidation product of urobilinogen, urobilin, is not detected by the Ehrlich reaction. A reduction of urobilin to urobilinogen with ferrous hydroxide is therefore necessary on 24-hour urine specimens. Neither an extraction nor a reduction step is included in the analysis of a 2-hour urine collection.

SCREENING TEST. A reagent strip containing paradimethylaminobenzaldehyde in an acid buffer* has correlated well with the qualitative test below. The color change is read at one minute. Blood and bilirubin do not interfere with the color, but pyridium dyes will produce a color change. Substances which interfere with the qualitative test below will also affect this test.

The qualitative test which follows may be used to indicate the presence of urobilinogen or porphobilinogen. The semiquantitative method is employed to measure the amount of urobilinogen excreted in a 2-hour period. The 2-hour test is usually made in the afternoon, when the level of urobilinogen excretion is thought to be highest. A quantitative method for 24-hour urine specimens is also presented (see Watson and Hawkinson, 1947; Schwartz *et al.*, 1944; and Henry *et al.*, 1961).

REAGENTS

1. Ehrlich's reagent: 0.7 gm. paradimethylaminobenzaldehyde, 150 ml. concentrated hydrochloric acid, 100 ml. deionized water.
2. *Saturated* sodium acetate in deionized water.
3. Chloroform.
4. Butanol.

For quantitative procedure:

5. Ferrous sulfate, 20 per cent solution in deionized water. Make this reagent just before use.
6. Sodium hydroxide, 10 per cent solution in deionized water.
7. Petroleum ether.

STANDARDIZATION. Standards of pure crystalline stercobilin hydrochloride are preferred for the calibration of spectrophotometers. Watson and coworkers proposed an alternate standard for the *Evelyn colorimeter, filter 565*, using a mixture of Pontacyl dyes that, in a stated combination and concentration, has an absorbency equivalent to certain concentrations of urobilinogen reacting with Ehrlich's reagent and sodium acetate. This calibration with Pontacyl dyes is described below.

Another artificial standard has been proposed which may be applicable to other colorimeters. It makes use of phenolsulfonphthalein (Balikov, 1957).

Pontacyl dye solution

1. *Stock:* 10 mg. per 100 ml.
   95 mg. Pontacyl violet 6R 150 per cent.†
   5 mg. Pontacyl carmine 2B.†

*Urobilistix, Ames.

†Pontacyl dye may be obtained from Dyestuffs Division, E. I. DuPont de Nemours Co., Wilmington, Delaware.

5 ml. glacial acetic acid.
Dilute to 1 liter.

2. *Working standard:* 2.04 mg. per 100 ml. Dilute 20.4 ml. of stock to 100 ml. with distilled water.
2.04 mg. per 100 ml. dye = 0.6 mg. per 100 ml. urobilinogen.

QUALITATIVE METHOD FOR UROBILINOGEN (AND PORPHOBILINOGEN) IN RANDOM URINE SPECIMENS

Procedure (Watson and Schwartz, 1941; see Fig. 2–55)

1. To one volume (approximately 5 ml.) of urine in a test tube add one volume of Ehrlich's reagent. Mix well by inversion.

2. Add two volumes of saturated sodium acetate to the tube and again mix. A pink or red color indicates that the specimen contains urobilinogen, porphobilinogen, or other Ehrlich's reactive compounds. If the test is positive, proceed.

3. Add a few milliliters of chloroform to a portion of the solution if a positive reaction results and observe whether the color is completely extracted into the chloroform layer (lower layer). Extract more than once, if necessary, to insure complete extraction. Color due to urobilinogen will be extracted into chloroform; that due to porphobilinogen will not be extracted.

4. If the chloroform does not extract the pink color, which suggests the presence of porphobilinogen, extract another portion of the colored mixture with a few milliliters of butanol. Butanol (top layer) will, like chloroform, extract color due to urobilinogen but will not extract color due to porphobilinogen. It may extract intermediate Ehrlich positive compounds.

5. Report as negative, positive for urobilinogen, positive for porphobilinogen, positive for Ehrlich's reactive compounds that are neither urobilinogen nor porphobilinogen, or, in rare cases, positive for both urobilinogen and porphobilinogen.

Comment. Sulfonamides, procaine, 5-hydroxy indoleacetic acid, and other compounds react with Ehrlich's reagent and may interfere (Henry *et al.*, 1961). Before testing, fresh urine should be cooled to room temperature, since normal urine contains a chromogen (probably indoxyl) which gives the "warm aldehyde" reaction with Ehrlich's reagent.

QUANTITATIVE 2-HOUR URINE UROBILINOGEN (Watson and Hawkinson, 1947)

Collection. A urine specimen is collected at 1 and 3 P.M. The patient voids at 1 P.M. and the urine is discarded. The patient voids again at 3 P.M. and the total specimen is collected and sent to the laboratory immediately. Because urobilinogen is rapidly oxidized to urobilin, the determination should be done within one-half hour of collection of the specimen.

Procedure

1. Measure and record the total 2-hour volume.

2. Into a colorimeter tube, pipette 3 ml. of urine.

3. To the tube add 3 ml. of Ehrlich's reagent, mix, and immediately add 6 ml. of saturated aqueous sodium acetate. Mix again.

4. To the second tube, which is to serve as a blank, the reagents are added in reverse order to prevent color development. First combine 6 ml. of saturated sodium acetate and 3 ml. of Ehrlich's reagent. Mix. Then add 3 ml. of urine. Mix again. The blank should be colorless.

5. The color development is not stable. Measure it immediately using the 565 filter in the spectrophotometer. Set the "blank" at 100 per cent T, remove the "blank" and record the center setting. Put the "test" in the colorimeter and record its per cent transmission.

6. If the concentration of urobilinogen is high, dilute *both* blank and test with water. Record the volumes in making these extra dilutions.

7. Using the calibration curve made with Pontacyl dyes or urobilinogen standards, determine the concentration in mg. per 100 ml. that corresponds to the per cent T of the "test."

$$\text{Ehrlich Units per 2 hr.} = \text{mg. per 100 ml. of colored solution (from graph)} \times \frac{1}{100}$$
$$\text{(to convert to mg. per ml. of colored solution)} \times 12 \text{ ml. (total volume of colored solution)} \times \frac{\text{total volume of specimen}}{3 \text{ ml.}}$$

Normal values. Less than 1 Ehrlich unit in 2 hours.

MEASUREMENT OF UROBILINOGEN IN 24-HOUR URINE COLLECTIONS (Schwartz *et al.*, 1944)

Collection. The 24-hour urine should be collected in a bottle containing 5 gm. of anhydrous sodium carbonate and kept refrigerated during the collection period.

Procedure

1. Measure and record the volume of urine.

2. Mix 50 ml. of urine with 25 ml. of 20 per cent ferrous sulfate and 25 ml. of 10 per cent sodium hydroxide in an Erlenmeyer flask. Cover and let stand in the dark for at least 1 hour.

3. Centrifuge or filter a portion of the mixture. The clear filtrate should be analyzed immediately.

4. In order to choose a suitable volume for analysis, add approximately 1 part filtrate and 1 part Ehrlich's reagent; mix; and add 2 parts saturated sodium acetate. If the color is in-

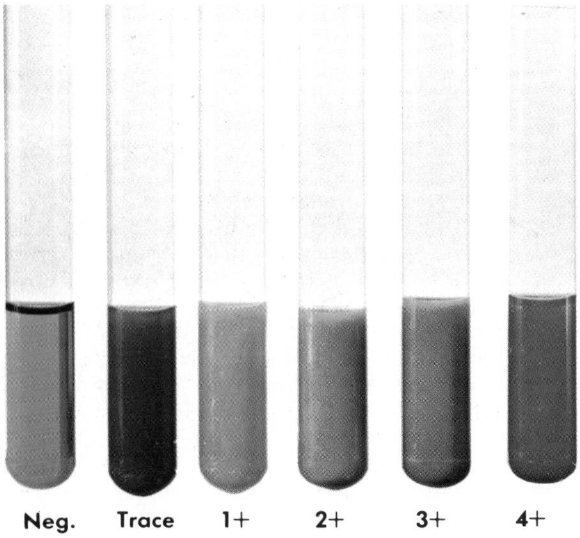

Figure 2–54. Benedict's qualitative test for reducing substances.

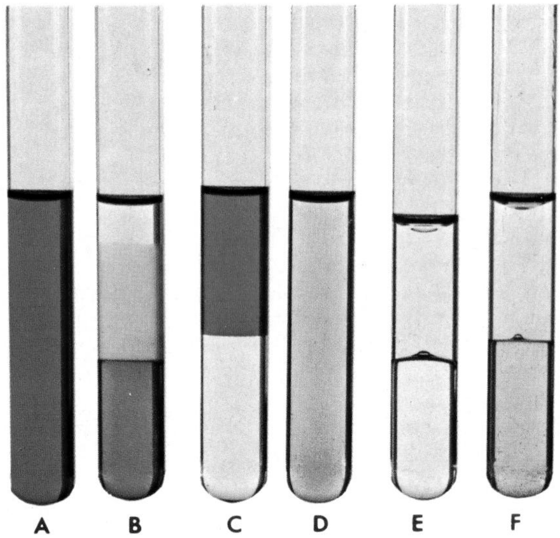

Figure 2–55. Test for porphobilinogen and urobilinogen. *A* and *D*, Ehrlich reaction. *B*, Chloroform extraction (lower layer, urobilinogen). *C*, Butanol extraction (top layer, urobilinogen). *E*, Chloroform extraction (aqueous top layer, porphobilinogen). *F*, Butanol extraction (aqueous lower layer, porphobilinogen; top layer, "intermediate Ehrlich compounds").

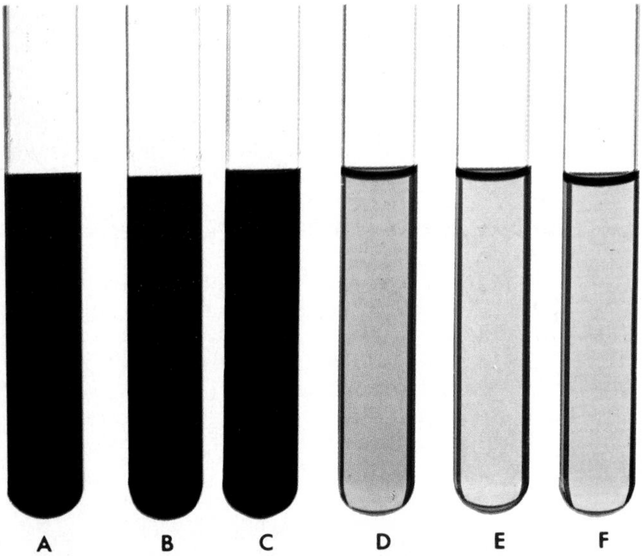

Figure 2–56. Ferric chloride test. *A*, Salicylate. *B*, Salicylate boiled. *C*, Acetoacetic acid. *D*, acetoacetic acid boiled. *E*, Phenothiazine. *F*, Phenylpyruvic acid.

tense, proceed with 5 ml. of filtrate; if pale red, use 10 ml.

5. Transfer the selected volume of filtrate to a separatory funnel. Add water to bring the volume to 49 ml.

6. Add 1 ml. of glacial acetic acid and mix.

7. Add 35 ml. of petroleum ether and shake vigorously for 7 minutes. After separation of the layers, discard the lower aqueous phase.

8. Wash the petroleum ether twice with approximately 25 ml. of water. Discard the wash water.

9. Shake the petroleum ether vigorously with 3 ml. of Ehrlich's reagent. Add 9 ml. of saturated sodium acetate. Shake. Transfer the colored aqueous solution to a graduate. Repeat the extraction with Ehrlich's reagent and sodium acetate until no further color is extracted. Combine the aqueous layers, mix, *record their volume*, and read in a colorimeter, filter setting 565, setting a reagent blank at 100 per cent T. Dilute a portion of the colored solution with water if the color is too intense.

Calculation

$$\text{Urobilinogen mg. per 24 hr.} = \text{mg. per 100 ml. of colored solution (from graph)} \times \frac{1}{100} \text{ ml.} \times \text{total volume colored solution} \times \frac{\text{total urine volume}}{50 \text{ ml.}} \times \frac{100 \text{ ml.}}{\text{ml. filtrate extracted}}$$

(total volume of reducing mixture).

Normal excretion of urobilinogen: 0.05 to 2.5 mg./24 hr.

Urinary Bile Pigments. Bilirubin is a breakdown product of hemoglobin formed in the reticuloendothelial cells of the spleen and bone marrow and carried in the blood by protein. Free or unconjugated bilirubin is not able to pass through the glomerular barrier of the kidney. When free bilirubin is conjugated in the liver with glucuronic acid, it becomes water soluble and is able to pass through the glomerulus of the kidney. Conjugated bilirubin is normally excreted in the bile. In patients with obstructive jaundice, bilirubin is found in the urine; urine with yellow foam may accompany pale acholic stools. Bilirubin is also found in the urine when intracanalicular pressure rises because of periportal inflammation or fibrosis and from swelling of liver cells. Bilirubin may, for example, appear in the urine in hepatitis before the appearance of jaundice. A positive test for urinary bilirubin with a negative test for urobilinogen in urine is indicative of intra- or extrahepatic biliary obstruction.

The normal adult urine contains about 0.02 mg. of bilirubin per 100 ml. (With, 1954).

A screening test for bilirubin in urine may be used to detect latent or unsuspected liver disease. It should be performed when the color of the urine indicates the possibility of bilirubin. The screening test is also of value in the differential diagnosis of jaundice, since bilirubinuria is not found with hemolytic jaundice, but accompanying obstructive and parenchymatous jaundice. It is helpful in diagnosis and in following the course of infectious hepatitis. In persons exposed to toxins and ingesting certain drugs, a positive test for bilirubinuria may be an early indication of liver damage.

CHEMICAL DISTINCTION OF THE PORPHYRIAS*

	URINE			FECES		
	PBG	URO	COPRO	PROTO	URO	COPRO
				μg./gm./dry weight		
NORMAL VALUES	<4 mg./day	<60 μg./day	<280 μg./day	<107	<32	<4.6
I. Erythropoietica						
A. Congenital	n	++++	+	n	+	++++
B. Protoporphyria	n	n	n	+++	n—+	n—+
II. Hepatica						
A. Acute intermittent	++++	++	+	n	n—+	n—+
B. Variegata† (South Africa)	n—++++	n—+	++—+++	++++	+—++	+++
C. Coproporphyria	n—++	n—+	++++	n	+	++++
D. Cutanea tarda	n	+++—++++	+	n	++	++

*Watson, C. J., 1972.
†Values rise with relapse.

PBG = Porphobilinogen.
URO = Uroporphyrin.
COPRO = Coproporphyrin.
PROTO = Protoporphyrin.

Two tests are commonly used: the diazo method, in which bilirubin is coupled to p-nitrobenzene diazonium p-toluene sulfonate to form a blue or purple color (this is in the form of a tablet) and one which employs a ferric chloride reagent to oxidize bilirubin to a green biliverdin. Both tests will detect levels of bilirubin in urine of 0.05 to 0.1 mg. per 100 ml. Since bilirubin is not stable in urine, especially in light, and is oxidized to biliverdin, the urine should be examined within 1 hour of collection. The diazo test may give a false negative reaction, while the oxidation test is positive due to biliverdin. In severe jaundice, biliverdin may be excreted in the urine. See Bryant and Flynn (1955).

Diazo Method (Free and Free, 1953)

REAGENTS. Tablets containing p-nitrobenzene diazonium p-toluene. The tablets also contain sulfosalicylic acid and sodium bicarbonate to provide an acid medium for the reaction and an effervescent mixture that will insure the solution of a portion of the tablet when water is added. (Ictotest kit including asbestos-cellulose mats and reagent tablets, available through Ames Co., Elkhart, Indiana.)

PROCEDURE

1. Place 5 drops of specimen on an asbestos-cellulose mat provided with the kit. Bilirubin, if present, will be adsorbed onto the mat surface.
2. Place a reagent tablet on the moistened area of the mat.
3. Allow 2 drops of water to flow over the tablet. If bilirubin is present, there will be a coupling of bilirubin with p-nitrobenzene diazonium p-toluene sulfonate from the tablet, as shown by the formation of a blue to purple color within 30 seconds. A pink or red color is negative.

SPECIFICITY. The diazo test reacts positively to bilirubin. There is no purple reaction with urobilin or other pigments or with any other known constituent of normal urine. High levels of urobilin or indican will give a red color; salicylates may give an orange to red color (Bryant and Flynn, 1955). Ascorbic acid may interfere with the test.

SENSITIVITY. The diazo test has a sensitivity ranging between 0.1 and 0.05 mg. of bilirubin per 100 ml. of urine (Giordano and Winstead, 1953).

STABILITY OF REAGENT. Ictotest reagent tablets are effervescent and are somewhat hygroscopic and, accordingly, they should be protected from moisture or high humidity. The tablets are packed in a brown bottle, since prolonged direct exposure to strong light results in decomposition of the stabilized diazonium compound. Prolonged exposure of several weeks to temperatures of 100° F. or more may also result in deterioration of the tablets.

*Reagent Strip:** The diazotized 2,4-dichloroaniline reacts with bilirubin to form azobilirubin. These are read after dipping at 20 seconds. The colors – yellow to brown – may be difficult to interpret. Sensitivity is about 0.2 mg. per cent. Pyridium may cause a color change.

Oxidation Method (Watson and Hawkinson, 1946)

REAGENTS

1. Thick filter paper (Schleicher & Schuell, No. 470) that has been soaked in saturated barium chloride, dried, and cut into small strips.
2. Fouchet's reagent. Dissolve 25 gm. trichloroacetic acid in 100 ml. distilled water. Add 10 ml. of 10 per cent $FeCl_3$ solution.

PROCEDURE

1. Hold the strip of $BaCl_2$ paper perpendicularly in the urine for a few seconds so that it is about one-half inch below the surface. Remove.
2. Drop 1 to 2 drops of Fouchet's reagent on the saturated area. A green color, usually deepening on standing because of the formation of biliverdin, represents a positive test.

High levels of urobilin or indican may cause a brown-purple color; salicylates give a purple color; high levels of urobilinogen may cause a red color over the green of biliverdin.

Porphyrinuria and Porphyria. Porphyrins are cyclic tetrapyrrole pigments that are precursors of the hemoglobins and cytochromes. Porphyrins found in the body exist in two isomeric forms, types I and III, principally coproporphyrin and uroporphyrin and possibly others.

Erythrocytes contain protoporphyrin. In the normal person, small amounts of the porphyrin precursors, delta-amino-levulinic acid and porphobilinogen, together with coproporphyrin and uroporphyrin are excreted in the urine. Coproporphyrin, normally the predominant urinary porphyrin, is also found in feces.

In the *porphyrias,* large amounts of porphyrin are excreted in the urine; in the *porphyrinurias,* moderate increases in porphyrin excretion (coproporphyrin) are seen. Porphyrinuria is associated with alcoholic cirrhosis of the liver, anemias, and chemical poisoning, such as lead poisoning. Lead interferes with porphyrin metabolism in several ways – by inhibiting the conversion of ALA to porphobilinogen, inhibiting the conversion of coproporphyrinogen III to protoporphyrin, and interfering with incorporation of iron into protoporphyrin (Stich, 1961; Brooks, 1951).

Delta-amino-levulinic acid (ALA) is synthesized from glycine and succinyl-coenzyme A. Urinary excretion of ALA is greatly in-

*Ictostix, Bililabstix, Ames.

creased in lead poisoning and in acute intermittent porphyria; it may be increased in carcinoma of the liver and in hepatitis. Normal urinary excretion is 1 to 7 mg. per day.

Porphobilinogen (PBG) is a monopyrrole formed by condensation of two molecules of delta-amino-levulinic acid. It is a precursor of the porphyrins. Porphobilinogen is colorless but converts to red porphobilin and uroporphyrin after excretion. Urinary excretion of porphobilinogen is greatly increased in acute intermittent porphyria, and may be increased in hepatitis and carcinomatosis.

Uroporphyrins are tetrapyrroles formed as a by-product during heme synthesis. Uroporphyrin excretion is greatly increased in the acute porphyrias and may be increased in lead poisoning, cirrhosis of the liver, and hemochromatosis.

The *coproporphyrins* are tetrapyrroles. Coproporphyrin I excretion is increased when there is increase in erythropoietic activity, also in infectious hepatitis and obstructive jaundice. Some increase in coproporphyrin III excretion is seen in infections, malignant disease, alcoholic cirrhosis, and following ingestion of many chemicals. In lead poisoning, coproporphyrin III urinary excretion is increased, and the level may be used for following the course of the disease.

The *porphyrias* may be classified as follows (Watson, 1960; Waldenström, 1957; Kark, 1955):

1. *Porphyria erythropoietica,* congenital type, is inherited as a recessive congenital disorder. Photosensitivity and anemia are present. Excess uroporphyrin I and coproporphyrin I are produced, probably in the bone marrow, and deposited in subcutaneous tissues and other organs. Urine is usually pink to dark burgundy. The protoporphyric type shows no increase in urinary porphyrins but an increased amount of protoporphyrin in the feces and red blood cells.

2. *Porphyria hepatica,* acute intermittent type, is the most common type and occurs more often in young adult females. Precursors of porphyrins are produced in excess by the liver. Symptoms include intermittent acute abdominal pain and neurologic manifestations. Urinary porphobilinogen and delta-amino-levulinic acid are increased in amount, although the findings may be intermittent. The urine may be normal in appearance and then darken on standing as the colorless porphobilinogen changes to porphobilin and uroporphyrin. There is increased excretion of coproporphyrin and uroporphyrin I.

Porphyria cutanea tarda clinically has some features of acute intermittent porphyria, but the onset occurs later in life. It is apparently due to a liver metabolic defect. The urine is red in color. Porphyrins are present in the urine in increased amounts, but porphobilinogen excretion is normal or rarely increased. Acquired porphyria cutanea tarda is an occasional complication of alcoholic cirrhosis. Uroporphyrins and coproporphyrins are both excreted in increased amounts in the urine.

For a discussion of methods for measuring porphobilinogen and delta-amino-levulinic acid in urine, see Henry (1964) and Patterson *et al.,* (1966).

The purple-red pigment is not always seen in urine, since porphyrins may be present in amounts of 500 μg. per liter without causing a color change (Henry, 1964). An orange-red fluorescence due to porphyrins is frequently seen if the specimen is placed near an ultraviolet light source.

Urine specimens should be protected from light, since porphobilinogen will convert slowly to uroporphyrin in the presence of light, and coproporphyrin will decrease in amount.

The screening test for porphobilinogen (Watson and Schwartz, 1941) is described with the tests for urobilinogen. (See test, p. 62.)

Screening Test for Uroporphyrins (Kark, 1955). Porphobilinogen is converted to fluorescing uroporphyrin by heat and acidification.

REAGENTS AND APPARATUS

1. Ultraviolet lamp with filter, 100 watts, passing light at 3660 Å.
2. Glacial acetic acid, C.P.
3. pH test paper.

PROCEDURE

1. Irradiate 10 ml. of urine in the dark with ultraviolet light. A red or orange-red fluorescence indicates the presence of uroporphyrins but may be masked or altered by the blue-green fluorescence of the urine. A normal urine may be compared as a control.
2. If the test is negative, acidify the urine with acetic acid to pH 4 (pHydrion paper), and heat for 15 minutes in a 100° C. bath.
3. Cool. Clean the outside of the test tube and again irradiate. Red or orange-red fluorescence is seen in the presence of uroporphyrin.

Screening Test for Coproporphyrin III (Brooks, 1951; Schwartz *et al.,* 1951)

REAGENTS AND APPARATUS

1. Ultraviolet lamp (as above).
2. Quartz test tube.
3. Glacial acetic acid.
4. Ethyl ether.
5. Hydrogen peroxide, 3 per cent.

PROCEDURE

1. To about 5 ml. of clear urine in a 16 by 150 mm. quartz test tube, add in this order 1 ml. glacial acetic acid, 5 ml. ethyl ether, 3 drops *fresh* 3 per cent hydrogen peroxide.
2. Close tube with clean rubber stopper and invert 12 times to mix and extract. Allow tube to stand 10 minutes. (If clear separation does not occur, centrifuge for 2 minutes to break the emulsion.)

3. Inspect tube in a dark room under ultraviolet *reflected* light, and estimate presence and approximate concentration of urinary coproporphyrin III as follows:

COLOR OF ETHER, TOP LAYER	INTERPRETATION
Pale blue, no pink cast	Negative or normal
Violet	1+
Pink	2+
Light rose	3+
Deep rose red	4+

Indican in Urine. Indole is produced by bacterial action on tryptophan in the intestine. Most is eliminated in the feces, the remainder is absorbed and detoxified to be excreted as *indican* in the urine.

$$\text{Indole} \xrightarrow{\text{oxidized}} \text{indoxyl} + H_2SO_4 \longrightarrow$$
$$\text{indoxyl sulfuric acid} \xrightarrow{+K} \text{indican}$$
(indoxyl potassium sulfate)

In normal urine the amount of indican excreted is small; it is increased with high-protein diets. It originates from putrefactive reactions and is increased with intestinal obstruction, gastric cancer and hypochlorhydria, and biliary obstruction. Positive results are obtained in Hartnup's disease.

Detection of indoxyl potassium sulfate depends upon its decomposition and subsequent oxidation of the indoxyl to indigo blue and its absorption by chloroform.

PROCEDURE. To 5 ml. of fresh urine in a test tube, add 5 ml. ferric chloride reagent (0.2 per cent in concentrated HCl). Mix. Add 2 ml. chloroform and invert several times. Allow the chloroform to settle and observe. When indican is present, the chloroform layer shows a deep violet to blue color. Normal urine may give a faint blue color. Report as positive or negative.

COMMENT. Indigo red may form occasionally because of slow oxidation. If iodides are present, iodine will be formed by oxidation and cause a violet color; thymol will also cause a violet color. These are removed by adding a crystal of sodium thiosulfate.

Bile pigments interfere with the reaction and should be removed by shaking the urine with barium chloride and filtering. Formalin will also interfere with the reaction.

Urine from cows and horses will usually give positive reactions and may be used for comparison.

Urinary 5-Hydroxy Indoleacetic Acid Screening Test. Serotonin (5-hydroxytryptamine) is produced by the argentaffin cells of the intestines from tryptophan and is carried in the blood by platelets.

Tryptophan→ 5-OH tryptophan→

$$\text{5-OH tryptamine} \xrightarrow[\text{monoamine oxidase}]{}$$
$$\text{5-OH indole acetaldehyde} \xrightarrow[\text{oxidase}]{}$$
5-OH indoleacetic acid.

Carcinoid tumors (argentaffinoma) arising from the argentaffin cells produce excessive amounts of serotonin, especially when metastatic. Serotonin causes intestinal disturbances, vasomotor disturbances, and bronchoconstriction. Edema, right-side valvular heart disease, and neurologic symptoms are seen. The screening test (Sjoerdsma *et al.*, 1955) is useful for the detection of the serotonin metabolite 5-hydroxy indoleacetic acid in the urine if it appears in fairly large amounts. The quantitative method is more sensitive, since it eliminates the interfering ketoacids and indoleacetic acid (Udenfriend *et al.*, 1955).

Normal excretion of 5-hydroxy indoleacetic acid in 24 hours is 1 to 5 mg. A random specimen of urine is usually sufficient for screening purposes; if a 24-hour collection is made, it should be acidified with HCl or acetic acid. Patients should not take any drugs for 72 hours before the test; phenothiazines or acetanilid drugs will interfere with this test.

The principle of the test is based on the development of a purple color specific for 5-hydroxy indoles with nitrous acid and 1-nitroso-2-naphthol. Ethylene dichloride is used to remove interfering chromogens.

REAGENTS. 1-nitroso-2-naphthol, 0.1 per cent in 95 per cent ethanol. Nitrous acid prepared fresh by adding 0.2 ml. of 2.5 per cent sodium nitrite solution to 5 ml. 2 N H_2SO_4. Ethylene dichloride.

PROCEDURE. Pipette into a test tube 0.2 ml. urine, 0.8 ml. distilled water, 0.5 ml. 1-nitroso-2-naphthol solution. Mix well. Add 0.5 ml. fresh nitrous acid and mix. Allow to stand at room temperature for 10 minutes. Shake with 5.0 ml. ethylene dichloride and allow the two layers to separate. A positive test shows a purple color in the upper aqueous layer.

INTERPRETATION. A purple color may appear with as little as 40 mg. 5-hydroxy indoleacetic acid in 24 hours. Patients with malignant carcinoid tumors may excrete up to 350 mg. 5-hydroxy indoleacetic acid per day and the test will show a black color. Positive findings should be checked with a quantitative method.

KETONES

Ketonuria. In ketonuria the three ketone bodies present in the urine are acetoacetic acid (20 per cent), acetone (2 per cent), and betahydroxybutyric acid (about 78 per cent) (Henry, 1964). Acetone is formed by nonreversible spontaneous decarboxylation from acetoacetic acid. Beta-hydroxybutyric acid forms reversibly from acetoacetic acid.

$$\text{Acetoacetic acid} \xrightarrow{-CO_2} \text{acetone}$$

$$\text{Acetoacetic acid} \underset{-2H}{\rightleftharpoons} \text{hydroxybutyric acid}$$

Ketone bodies are the products of incomplete fat metabolism, and their presence is indicative of acidosis. Ketonuria is commonly seen in uncontrolled diabetes mellitus.

Nondiabetic Ketonuria. In infants and children, ketonuria commonly occurs in a variety of conditions, such as acute febrile diseases and toxic states accompanied by vomiting or diarrhea (Riekers and Miale, 1958). Ketonuria is also present in vomiting of pregnancy, cachexia, and following anesthesia. In these cases, it is related most probably to increased tissue catabolism in the face of limited food intake. The use of the ketogenic diet in treatment of seizures in children will produce ketonuria. In glycogen storage disease (Gierke's), hypoglycemia and ketonuria are seen because of the limited availability of glucose. Occasionally ketonuria is seen following exposure to cold or severe exercise.

As a rule, examination of the urine for ketone bodies is not a part of the routine urine examination except in specimens from young children. However, in the presence of any of the above conditions, or whenever acidosis or ketosis is suspected clinically, the urine should be examined for ketones.

Diabetic Ketonuria. The presence of ketonuria indicates the presence of ketoacidosis (ketosis) and may provide a warning of impending coma. Up to 50 mg. per 100 ml. of acetoacetic acid may be present without clinical evidence of ketosis (Killander *et al.*, 1962). Diabetic children and young adults are more prone to episodes of ketosis, often associated with infection as well as other problems in management. It is the usual practice in the management of diabetes to test for ketonuria when the urine, on qualitative examination, displays more than a 2+ glycosuria. It is suggested that the urine of diabetic patients controlled with *oral* hypoglycemic agents should be tested regularly for ketone bodies as well as glucose, especially in the presence of infection, since insulin may then be required for control. Ketonuria should also be checked for when changes in diabetic therapy are prescribed.

Normal Values. Depending on the methods used, total ketone bodies (as acetone) range from 1.7 to 42 mg. per 100 ml. (Henry, 1964). According to Killander and associates (1962), up to 2 mg. per 100 ml. acetoacetic acid is normal.

Methods for Testing Ketonuria. Since it seems that the three ketone bodies have equal significance (Riekers, 1958), there is no need to attempt separation. The Gerhardt ferric chloride test has been used for many years as a test for acetoacetic acid (see Fig. 2–56); however, ferric chloride tests are not very specific and the sensitivity is low—about 25 to 50 mg. per 100 ml. Tests for acetone alone are unsatisfactory, and there are no practical tests for beta-hydroxybutyric acid.

The nitroprusside test of Rothera is sensitive to acetoacetic acid, about 1 to 5 mg. per 100 ml., and acetone with a sensitivity of 10 to 25 mg. per 100 ml. (Nash *et al.*, 1954). In the simplest form of the nitroprusside test reagent strips are used, impregnated with sodium nitroprusside and alkali. A tablet form of the same test is available with similar sensitivity. The blood level of ketone bodies may also be estimated by the nitroprusside test; this is especially helpful in determining the severity of ketosis in the treatment of diabetic acidosis. See Table 2–17 for approximate values of acetoacetic acid or acetone corresponding to qualitative nitroprusside test results.

GENERAL PRINCIPLE. Acetone and acetoacetic acid react with sodium nitroprusside in the presence of alkali to produce a purple colored complex.

REAGENT STRIP METHOD. A paper strip impregnated with sodium nitroprusside, glycine, and disodium hydrogen phosphate (Ketostix, Ames) is used.

Procedure. Dip test end of strip in urine, serum, or plasma or briefly pass through urine stream; 15 seconds after moistening, compare color developed with color chart.

Interpretation

Negative: No color develops within 15 seconds.

Positive: Within 15 seconds, the reagent strip develops a purple color, the intensity of

Table 2–17. COMPARISON OF QUALITATIVE NITROPRUSSIDE TEST RESULTS AND APPROXIMATE KETONE LEVELS

REAGENT STRIP RESULT	ROTHERA'S TEST	APPROXIMATE LEVELS OF KETONE BODIES, MG./100 ML.	
		ACETOACETIC ACID	ACETONE
±	Trace	5	20-40
"Small"	1+	10	100
"Moderate"	2+	20-100	250-500
"Large"	4+	100-300	800-4000

the color depending upon the amount of ketone bodies in the specimen. Color charts show three intensities of color, which represent three degrees of positivity.

ROTHERA'S TEST—URINE (1908)

Reagents

1. Pulverize and mix 7.5 gm. sodium nitroprusside and 200 gm. ammonium sulfate.

2. Concentrated ammonium hydroxide.

Procedure

1. To 5 ml. of urine in a test tube, add approximately 1 gm. of Rothera's reagent. Mix well.

2. Overlay with about 1 ml. of concentrated ammonium hydroxide. A positive test is the appearance of a reddish purple ring at the interface within 1 minute and 30 seconds. A brown ring is not a positive reaction.

3. Report as follows: *Negative*—No ring, or a brown ring. *Trace*—A faint pinkish purple ring appearing slowly 2+—Narrow dark purple ring. 4+—Wide dark purple ring appearing very rapidly.

ROTHERA'S TEST—SERUM OR PLASMA

Reagents. Same as for urine.

Procedure

1. In a small tube place enough of the sample so that it will be possible to observe a ring at the interface, above the curvature of the tube.

2. Reduce the amounts of all reagents so that they are present in the same ratios to each other and to the volume of specimen as the ratios described above for urine.

3. Carry out the test as described for urine.

SPECIFICITY. The reagents react with both acetoacetic acid and acetone in urine, plasma, or serum. They do not react with salicylates. Levodopa may cause a false positive result. Urine containing bromsulphalein and phenylketones will cause color reactions with the reagent similar to that produced by acetoacetic acid and acetone. Bromsulphalein reacts to the alkaline buffers of the reagent strips to form a colored complex. If the level of phenylketones is 100 mg. per 100 ml. or greater, a color may develop; however, such high levels of phenylketones are uncommon and are seldom present in patients with phenylketonuria.

SENSITIVITY. In urine, reagent strips react to 10 mg. of acetoacetic acid per 100 ml. and are less sensitive to acetone (Free and Free, 1958). When a patient is being followed with repeated determinations of acetone and diacetic acid in plasma, the concentrations of these compounds may start at a high level and fall but still give "large" results. Therefore, repeated reports of "large" would not reflect the change taking place. In such an instance, semiquantitative results can be obtained with either the reagent strip or Rothera's test by testing several different dilutions of each specimen. Report these analyses in a form such as this: undiluted "large," 1:2 dilution "large," 1:4 dilution "moderate," etc.

STABILITY OF KETONES. In urine, bacterial action will cause loss of acetoacetic acid. This may happen *in vivo* as well as *in vitro* (Free and Free, 1958). Acetone is lost at room temperature but not if kept in a closed container in a refrigerator. If a sample cannot be tested immediately, it should be refrigerated.

MELANIN IN URINE

Melanin is a pigment derived from tyrosine, which is normally present in hair and skin and in the eye.

Patients with widespread melanotic tumors excrete in the urine a colorless precursor, a conjugate of 5,6-dihydroxyindole, which polymerizes into a dark pigment after about 24 hours at room temperature.

Screening tests for melanin should be made on fresh specimens of urine. If a small amount of melanogen is present, it may be extracted by evaporation of the urine over a water bath followed by repeated washings until clear with absolute methyl alcohol. Melanin is left in the residue and is then extracted with acidified (2 drops concentrated HCl per 100 ml.) methyl alcohol. Melanin is then precipitated by ether and may be recovered after centrifugation.

Ferric Chloride Test for Melanin

PROCEDURE. To 5 ml. urine in a test tube, add 1 ml. 10 per cent $FeCl_3$ in 10 per cent HCl. A gray or black precipitate will form if positive. The HCl prevents phosphate precipitation. Melanogen is oxidized to melanin. Homogentisic acid, which also causes a dark color in urine, gives a transient blue-green color with ferric chloride (see Table 2–14).

Nitroprusside Test for Melanin

PROCEDURE. To 2 ml. urine in a test tube, add 3 to 4 drops fresh solution of sodium nitroprusside (shake a few crystals in 10 ml. water). Add 2 drops of 10 per cent NaOH to make the solution alkaline. Shake. A red color will develop if acetone, creatinine, or melanin is present. Acidify with 2 drops of glacial acetic acid. Small amounts of melanogen cause a green color; larger amounts cause blue, then black. Acetone causes a purple color and creatinine an amber color.

MUCOPOLYSACCHARIDES

Acid mucopolysaccharides are high molecular weight polymers of disaccharide units containing hexosamine with sulfate attached and uronic acid. They are normally present in the ground substance of connective tissue.

In the normal person, chondroitin sulfate A

is the principal mucopolysaccharide found in the urine; chondroitin sulfate B, now called dermatan sulfate, and heparin sulfate are also present. Normal excretion based on the measurement of uronic acid by the Dische carbazole reaction is 0 mg. per 100 ml. (Hsia, 1966), or 2.1 to 8.2 mg. in 24 hours as glucuronic acid (Kerby, 1954).

In Hurler's syndrome, an inherited generalized disorder of connective tissue, the urine contains large amounts of dermatan sulfate and heparin sulfate. Similar findings occur in Hunter's syndrome. In Sanfilippo urine heparin sulfate predominates (Dorfman and Matalon, 1972). In Morquio-Ullrich disease, keratosulfate is principally excreted. Smaller amounts of mucopolysaccharide are excreted in the urine of patients with collagen diseases such as systemic lupus erythematosus and rheumatoid arthritis.

Screening Test for Mucopolysaccharides (Berry and Spinlanger, 1960). The test is based on the metachromasia produced with the basic groups of the toluidine blue dye in the presence of large amounts of acid mucopolysaccharide. Further separation and identification of the mucopolysaccharide should be made by paper chromatography.

EQUIPMENT

1. Whatman filter paper No. 1. Micropipettes.
2. Control solution of chondroitin sulfate containing 0.1 mg. per ml. in distilled water.
3. Toluidine blue, 0.04 per cent in 1 M sodium acetate at pH 2. Use a certified buffer tablet.

PROCEDURE

1. 5, 10, and 25 μliters of urine are placed in separate spots on a piece of filter paper. Each spot should be allowed to dry before the next is made. A normal urine may be spotted for comparison.
2. 5 μliters of the standard chondroitin sulfate solution is applied separately and dried.
3. The dry paper is dipped into the toluidine blue solution for 1 minute.
4. Rinse the paper in 95 per cent alcohol 2 or 3 times. Dry, then examine.

RESULT. Urine from children with Hurler's syndrome will show a purple spot against a blue background, as will the standard chondroitin sulfate. Normal urine is blue.

COMMENT. The pH of 2 is important in achieving a good result. Control must be run for comparison. False positive results were obtained in most newborn infants, but after 2 weeks of age, only 0.2 per cent of the normal infants gave positive results (Berry, 1960). Heparin may give false positive results.

Test for Excessive Mucopolysaccharides

This test requires 5 ml. of fresh urine at room temperature (cold urine will give a positive test). One milliliter of 5 per cent cetyltrimethyl-ammonium bromide (CTAB) in 1 M citrate buffer at pH 6 is added to the urine and mixed well. A heavy flocculent precipitate at 30 minutes is positive for excess mucopolysaccharides. False positives may occur (Pennock *et al.*, 1970; Dorfman and Matalon, 1972).

PHENOTHIAZINE DRUGS IN URINE

Screening Test. Phenothiazine drugs are used in the treatment of psychiatric disorders. The average daily urinary excretion is about one-half of the daily intake; some continues to be excreted over a period of time after therapy has ceased. The screening test has been used to monitor the amount of drug ingested (or not ingested) by the patient. For identification of the drug, spectrophotometric methods are used. Refer to Chapter 10.

PROCEDURE (Forrest *et al.*, 1961). Mix 1 ml. urine in a test tube with 1 ml. of ferric chloride reagent (5 ml. $FeCl_3$ 5 per cent in water, 45 ml. perchloric acid 20 per cent, and 50 ml. nitric acid 50 per cent).

Read immediately. Disregard colors appearing after 10 seconds.

INTERPRETATION. Shades of pink to purple indicate dosage levels of 20 to 2000 mg. per day. False negative results of up to 25 per cent have been reported (Brownstein and Roberge, 1966). These may be due to low dose levels, overhydration, and the lack of sensitivity of some related drugs. Prochlorperazine, trifluoperazine, perphenazine, and thioridazine (Mellaril) are not as sensitive as chlorpromazine.

False positive results may be seen when high doses of para-aminosalicylic acid are ingested or with estrogens or phenylketonuria. Indican may cause a purple color. Aspirin does not produce false positive reactions. (Phenothiazine drugs may cause positive reactions in other urine tests—for urobilinogen, porphyrins, 5-hydroxy indoleacetic acid—and may interfere in the starch test for amylase. Lazerte and McMillin, 1964.)

PROTEIN IN URINE

Normal urine contains a small amount of protein, although the normal glomerulus for the most part bars the passage of albumin (M.W. 69,000) and larger plasma proteins from plasma to the glomerular filtrate. In general, detection of protein in urine is considered evidence of renal disease and, usually, of glomerular disease.

Normal Values. The concentration of protein in normal urine at normal flow rates is about 2 to 8 mg. per 100 ml. An upper limit of 150 mg. of protein excreted per day has been reported in normal adults (Relman and Levinsky, 1971). Normal newborn infants may have higher levels of protein in urine during the first three days of life (Rhodes *et al.*, 1962).

Urine albumin has the same immunologic and ultracentrifugal properties as plasma albumin (Webb *et al.*, 1958). Urine globulins comprise about one-half to two-thirds of the normal urine protein; the predominant globulins are alpha-1 and alpha-2, with smaller amounts of beta and gamma globulins present (Boyce *et al.*, 1954). Other proteins found in normal urine include prealbumin, products of fibrinogenolysis, transferrin, haptoglobin, ceruloplasmin (Berggard, 1961), and possibly, also, light chain fractions of immunoglobulin. Large lipoproteins are not found. A large mucoprotein (Tamm Horsfall protein) that is not found in plasma is present in normal urine in amounts up to 2.5 mg. per 100 ml.; it originates in the distal tubules and collecting ducts (Pollak and Arbel, 1969). Some protein found in normal urine comes from the lower urinary tract, the prostate, and seminal vesicles (Grant, 1959).

Proteinuria. Most commonly, an increase in protein in urine of more than 150 mg. per day is the result of increased glomerular filtration of protein caused by glomerular damage of some kind. In general, the rate of excretion of a plasma protein is related to its molecular size; for example, albumin and alpha-1-globulin have greater clearance in patients with proteinuria than gamma, beta, and alpha-2 globulins. In most kidney diseases involving proteinuria, albumin is the predominant protein (Wolvius and Verschure, 1957; Joachim *et al.*, 1964). In a few instances the globulins predominate, notably in multiple myeloma and in macroglobulinemia (Osserman and Lawlor, 1961). In some cases of pyelonephritis or renal tubular diseases, a "tubular" pattern of decreased albumin and increased globulin fractions appears (Manuel *et al.*, 1970).

The degree of proteinuria varies with the type of renal disease and with the severity of the disease process. Measurement of the amount of protein excreted may be helpful in diagnosis and in following the course of a disease. Continued proteinuria of any amount, even in an apparently healthy person, usually indicates minimal renal disease. Examples of how the degree of proteinuria may be related to the specific disease process are given in the following paragraphs. These examples are taken from a review by Relman and Levinsky (1971), and the reader is referred to this book for more details.

Heavy Proteinuria (> 4 gm. per day). Heavy proteinuria is characteristically seen with the nephrotic syndrome. It may also be found in acute and chronic glomerulonephritis, lupus nephritis, amyloid disease, and severe venous congestion of the kidney.

Moderate Proteinuria (0.5 to 4 gm. per day). Moderate proteinuria may be found in a large number of renal diseases, including those mentioned above and nephrosclerosis, pyelonephritis with hypertension, (also multiple myeloma, diabetic nephropathy, pre-eclampsia of pregnancy, and a variety of toxic nephropathies including radiation nephritis).

Minimal Proteinuria (< 0.5 gm. per day). Minimal proteinuria may be noted in chronic pyelonephritis, in which it may be intermittent, and in relatively inactive phases of glomerular diseases. It is also seen with polycystic kidney disease and in renal tubular diseases. Minimal proteinuria is present in "benign" postural proteinurias.

Proteinuria may be absent in phases of acute pyelonephritis, in chronic pyelonephritis, and in the presence of obstructive nephropathy, kidney stones, kidney tumors, and congenital malformations.

Postural Proteinuria. Postural proteinuria (orthostatic) occurs in 3 to 5 per cent of healthy young adults. In these persons, proteinuria is found during the day but not at night when a recumbent position is assumed. Persistent proteinuria may develop in some of these healthy subjects at a later date, and renal biopsies have shown abnormalities of the glomerulus in a few cases (Robinson *et al.*, 1961). Proteinuria is apparently related to an exaggerated lordotic position and may result from renal congestion or ischemia. The total daily excretion of protein rarely exceeds 1 gm. In most instances, no other evidence of renal disease develops.

To evaluate the possibility of postural proteinuria, the patient is instructed to empty his bladder upon going to bed in the evening and to discard the specimen. Immediately upon rising in the morning, the patient voids and saves this specimen. After 2 hours of standing and walking about, the patient voids again and saves the specimen. The two urine specimens are tested for protein. If the first is negative and the second positive, the patient may have postural proteinuria. Frequent examination of the patient should be made to reevaluate this condition.

Functional Proteinuria. Functional proteinuria may be associated with fever, exposure to cold, emotional stress, or severe and unaccustomed exercise. Proteinuria of this type is transient and apparently benign, although it may persist for up to three days after severe exercise.

Measurement of Proteinuria. Qualitative, semiquantitative, and quantitative methods are available for analysis of protein in urine. Since the positive result of a screening test may have grave significance, it is important to be able to confirm it, by a second different method.

Screening Tests for Proteinuria. Screening tests should not be too sensitive, as they are required to differentiate normal protein excretion from abnormal and therefore should not detect less than about 8 to 10 mg. per 100 ml. in a normal adult with a normal rate of urine flow. It should be noted that a very dilute random specimen of urine may have a falsely low protein value.

In the simplest screening test a reagent strip is used. This is a colorimetric test that employs the principle of protein error of a pH indicator: bromphenol blue is yellow at pH 3, but with protein present, the color becomes green-blue. The sensitivity of the test is about 20 to 30 mg. per 100 ml. of albumin (Free, 1957b), and the results are graded as trace and 1 through 4+. The test material is not as sensitive to globulins as albumin (Clough and Reah, 1964). Although not so sensitive as precipitation tests, this test has the advantage of avoiding false positive reactions with organic iodides as used in renal pyelography and tolbutamides or other drugs. See Table 2–18.

Most other qualitative screening tests rely on a protein precipitation, e.g., with heat and acetic acid, with nitric acid, and with sulfosalicylic acid and trichloroacetic acid. (For details, see Henry, 1964). Probably the best standard test for routine screening of proteinuria is the acetic acid test. This test is based on the heat coagulation properties of albumin and globulin at pH 4 to 5 in the presence of inorganic salt. Acetic acid is used to produce the required pH, and in Purdy's modification (Purdy, 1900), sodium chloride provides the ionic strength needed in dilute urines. This method will also precipitate globulins and proteoses and has a sensitivity of 5 to 10 mg. per 100 ml.

Sulfosalicylic acid and trichloroacetic acids are used to precipitate protein in the cold and may be used as satisfactory screening tests. The sensitivity may be as low as 0.25 mg. per 100 ml. depending on the techniques used. See sulfosalicylic acid method, page 74.

Pseudoproteinuria. All the acid precipitation tests will give false positive results when organic iodine x-ray media are present. Urinary excretion may persist for three days after the administration of the dye. With the heat and acetic acid method, if the turbidity is due to albumin or globulin, it will increase with heat. Uric acid, proteose, and Bence Jones protein will redissolve with heat. An excretion product of the drug tolbutamide, an oral hypoglycemic agent, will also cause turbidity with acidification of the urine. See Table 2–18.

Semiquantitative and Quantitative Methods. Often more useful information may be obtained by quantitatively analyzing the amount of protein excreted over a 24-hour period than is available from a random specimen of urine.

In 1874 Esbach developed a method of urinary protein precipitation in which picric acid was used and by which the amount of precipitated protein could be estimated by volume. The Esbach method, even with modifications, is much less precise and accurate than the turbidimetric methods (Lewis and Richards, 1961). It should be used only in a semiquanti-

Table 2–18. FALSE POSITIVE AND FALSE NEGATIVE REACTIONS IN TESTS FOR PROTEINURIA*

URINARY CONSTITUENTS	BROMPHENOL REAGENT STRIP	SULFOSALICYLIC ACID	HEAT AND ACETIC ACID
Urine turbidity	No effect	May confuse reading	May confuse reading
X-ray contrast media	No effect	May cause false pos.	May cause false pos.
Tolbutamide metabolites	No effect	May cause false pos.	May cause false pos.
Penicillin (massive doses)	No effect	May cause false pos.	May cause false pos.
Sulfisoxazole metabolites	No effect	May cause false pos. with Exton's reagent	No effect
Aminosalicylic acid in urine containing preservative agents	No effect	May cause false pos.	May cause false pos.
Highly buffered alkaline urine	May cause false pos.	May cause false neg.	May cause false neg.
Quaternary ammonium compounds	" "	No effect	No effect

*Modified from Kark *et al.*, 1963.

tative fashion to give an estimate of protein present; and even in this case, unless the urine is acidified before precipitation, results will often be erroneous.

Sulfosalicylic acid and trichloroacetic acid are commonly used as precipitants; the resultant turbidity is measured by a photometer or nephelometer, or by eye, and compared with known standards. With sulfosalicylic acid, the turbidity produced with albumin is 2.4 times that produced with globulin (Henry *et al.*, 1956). Polypeptides, proteoses, and Bence Jones proteins are also precipitated. Exton's reagent contains sulfosalicylic acid, sodium sulfate, and an indicator—bromphenol blue. This produces a yellow turbidity that is usually compared with a set of standard tubes and provides an estimate of the amount of protein present (Exton, 1925). Trichloroacetic acid is a protein precipitant that causes gamma globulin to be precipitated with greater turbidity than albumin. However, the difference is not marked (Henry *et al.*, 1956). More precise measurements especially suitable for small amounts of protein are available. In these tests the trichloroacetic acid precipitate is taken up in nitric acid and reacted with ammonium hydroxide to produce a yellow color which is measured photometrically. Alternately, the precipitate may be dissolved in sodium hydroxide and measured by use of the biuret reaction (Kibrick, 1958). The biuret test as used for serum proteins is not sensitive enough to use as a test for proteinuria.

In routine clinical practice, quantitative measurement of protein by the turbidimetric procedure with sulfosalicylic acid as the precipitant is satisfactory. See page 75.

Measurement of Protein in Urine

Heat Coagulation Method (Henry, 1964)

PRINCIPLE. Albumin and globulin are coagulated by heat at an acid pH. Acetic acid is used to provide optimum pH, and sodium acetate provides inorganic salt for protein flocculation as well as buffering capability.

REAGENT

1. Acetic acid, glacial, 23.7 ml.
2. Sodium acetate, anhydrous, 7.4 gm. (or sodium acetate $3H_2O$, 12.4 gm.).
3. Distilled water to 100 ml.

PROCEDURE

1. Centrifuge 10 ml. of urine to clarify. Usually the sediment is saved for microscopic examination.
2. Place 7.5 ml. of clear urine in a 5/8-inch test tube and add 3 drops of reagent. Mix by inversion. If mucus precipitates, remove by filtration or centrifugation.
3. Heat upper half of urine in flame to boiling point and then compare upper half with lower half in normal room light.

INTERPRETATION

No difference	Negative	
Barely visible turbidity	Trace	About 5 mg./100 ml.
Distinct turbidity with print visible through it	1+	10 to 30 mg./100 ml.
Moderate turbidity	2+	40 to 100 mg./100 ml.
Heavy turbidity	3+	200 to 500 mg./100 ml.
Heavy flocculation	4+	500 mg./100 ml. or more

SPECIFICITY. Positive with albumin, globulins, and proteoses.

SENSITIVITY. About 5 to 10 mg./100 ml.

Bromphenol Method

PRINCIPLE. This protein test is based on the phenomenon of a "protein error of indicators." At a fixed pH certain indicators will have one color in the presence of protein and another color in the absence of protein. The citrate buffer provides a hydrogen ion concentration of approximately pH 3. At this pH tetrabromphenol blue has a yellow color, whereas at this same pH in the presence of increasing amounts of protein the indicator will have a green to blue color.

REAGENT AND PROCEDURE. Using reagent strips (Albustix, Ames), dip the yellow end of strip in urine, or briefly pass it through the urine stream. Compare color of dipped end with color chart provided.

INTERPRETATION

Negative: No color change occurs.

Positive: If protein is present, the yellow end of the test strip changes immediately to a yellow-green to green to blue-green color, depending on the quantity of protein present. Report qualitatively as trace or 1+ to 4+.

SPECIFICITY. The reagent is unaffected by urine turbidity, other urine constituents, contrast media, preservatives, or metabolites of tolbutamide and other drugs. A decomposed urine, or a highly buffered alkaline urine which is protein-free, may give a false positive reaction.

SENSITIVITY. The reagent is sensitive to clinically significant proteinuria. Tests such as the heat and acetic, nitric acid ring, and sulfosalicylic acid carried out with maximum refinements are more sensitive. The first positive color on the color scale represents about 30 mg. per 100 ml. of albumin. The test is less sensitive to globulins than albumin.

Precautions: See page 21 for care of reagent strips.

Sulfosalicylic Acid Turbidity Method

PRINCIPLE. Sulfosalicylic acid precipitates protein in urine with a turbidity that is approximately proportional to the concentration of protein in a solution. The turbidity may be measured with a photometer.

REAGENTS

1. Sulfosalicylic acid solution 3 per cent w/v in distilled water.
2. 1.25 per cent HCl.

PROCEDURE

1. Centrifuge an aliquot of a measured 24-hour collection of urine, and use the supernatant for determination.
2. Pipette into Coleman cuvettes:

Unknown	*Blank* (for *each* patient)
2 ml. urine	2 ml. urine
8 ml. sulfosalicylic acid solution	8 ml. HCl

3. Mix by inversion and let stand 5 minutes before reading.
4. Read in Coleman Jr. photometer at 500 mμ, using the blank to set the transmittance at 100 per cent.
5. Read the values from a calibration chart. If greater than 140 mg. per 100 ml., repeat with 1:10 dilution with normal saline.

PREPARATION OF STANDARD CURVE. A standard solution with a known amount of protein (Versatol, 7 gm. per 100 ml. or a Bovine Albumin Standard) is used in several dilutions. A normal serum of known protein concentration may be used.

1. Add 5 ml. distilled water to a vial of protein standard and swirl gently until well mixed. Let stand 30 minutes, then dilute 1:50 with 0.85 per cent NaCl to make a solution containing 140 mg. per 100 ml.
2. Set up a series of test tubes numbered 1 through 7 and add the following:

TUBE NO.	PROTEIN SOLUTION	0.85% NaCl	PROTEIN MG./100 ML.
1	4.5 ml.	1.5 ml.	105
2	3.0 ml.	3.0 ml.	70
3	2.4 ml.	3.6 ml.	56
4	1.5 ml.	4.5 ml.	35
5	0.9 ml.	5.1 ml.	21
6	0.3 ml.	5.7 ml.	7
7	0.0 ml.	6.0 ml.	0

3. Read each tube as an unknown, using tube 7 as blank, and plot results on semilog paper.

INTERPRETATION. Report result as mg. per 100 ml. urine, or mg. or gm. per 24-hour volume of urine. Average normal excretion of protein is about 2 to 8 mg. per 100 ml., or up to 150 mg. in 24 hours. See page 72.

COMMENT. Each acidified urine is used as its own blank to offset the effects of urinary pigments. Sulfosalicylic acid precipitates urinary proteose, polypeptides, and Bence Jones protein in addition to albumin and globulin. See Pseudoproteïnuria, page 73.

Bence Jones Proteinuria (Bence Jones, 1848). The presence of Bence Jones globulin is indicated by a single sharp peak in the globulin region on paper electrophoresis. Bence Jones globulin represents the light chain of a high molecular weight immunoglobulin of the plasma. Bence Jones proteinuria is associated with multiple myeloma, macroglobulinemia, and malignant lymphomas (Creipell, 1970). The degree of Bence Jones proteinuria varies with the type of myeloma present. The heaviest proteinuria appears with the Bence Jones, gamma-D, and gamma-A types and the least proteinuria with gamma-G type. The amount of proteinuria may parallel the extent of the disease and the amount of renal damage (Hobbs *et al.*, 1966). The incidence of Bence Jones proteinuria in multiple myeloma has been estimated as 50 to 80 per cent; however, its demonstration depends greatly on the technique used.

Measurement of Bence Jones Protein. Many techniques have been proposed, most of them based on the unusual heat solubility properties of Bence Jones protein. This protein precipitates at temperatures between 40° and 60° C. and redissolves again near 100° C. Other tests depend on precipitation in the cold with salts, ammonium sulfate, and acids. More recently, electrophoretic and immunoelectrophoretic analysis of concentrated urine specimens has been used in detecting Bence Jones proteins (Osserman and Lawlor, 1961).

In the presence of marked Bence Jones proteinuria, most tests yield positive results. When only a small amount of Bence Jones protein is present, or when other globulins are also present, results may be doubtful. With proper pH control and salt concentration, precipitation may be achieved at levels of about 30 mg. per 100 ml. (Putnam *et al.*, 1959). False positive reactions are seen when other globulins are precipitated by acetic acid in the heat precipitation method or because of clearing due to acid hydrolysis in the sulfosalicylic acid heat test. A false negative reaction may occur if the Bence Jones protein is too concentrated and the precipitate does not redissolve on boiling (Naumann, 1965).

The best method for detection of Bence Jones protein in urine is by protein electrophoresis, when a homogeneous band in the globulin region will be seen on paper or cellulose acetate. For electrophoretic analysis, urine needs to be concentrated; this is usually accomplished by dialysis in cellophane tubing or by vacuum dialysis.

METHOD. The qualitative sulfosalicylic acid test for urine protein (Putnam *et al.*, 1959) is performed first; if negative, no detectable Bence Jones protein is present.

Sulfosalicylic acid test. Clear the urine by centrifugation, saving the sediment if needed for microscopic examination. Place 2.5 ml. clear urine in a test tube and add 7.5 ml. of an aqueous solution of sulfosalicylic acid (3 gm. per 100 ml.). Mix by inversion. Allow to stand for 10 minutes in a rack. Results are graded in a similar manner to the heat and acetic acid test: trace, barely visible turbidity; 1+, distinct turbidity; 2+, moderate turbidity; 3+, heavy turbidity; 4+, heavy and flocculent turbidity. Positive results are obtained with protein, proteoses, and Bence Jones protein (see Table 2–18 for false positive reactions with this test).

REAGENT. Acetate buffer, pH 4.9, 2 M. Place 17.5 gm. sodium acetate trihydrate in a 100 ml. volumetric flask, add 4.1 ml. glacial acetic acid, and add water to 100 ml.

PROCEDURE

1. Place 4 ml. clear urine in a test tube (centrifuge or filter urine if turbid). Add 1 ml. acetate buffer and mix. Final pH should be 4.9 ± 0.1.

2. Heat for 15 minutes in a 56° C. water bath. Any precipitation is indicative of Bence Jones protein.

3. If there is a turbidity or precipitate, heat the same tube in a boiling water bath for 3 minutes and observe for any *decrease* in the amount of precipitate or turbidity. Bence Jones protein will redissolve at 100° C.

4. An increase in turbidity or precipitate on boiling indicates the presence of albumin and globulin. This will mask any dissolving Bence Jones protein. Filter the contents of the tube taken directly from the boiling water, and observe the filtrate. If it is clear, becomes cloudy as it cools, and then becomes clear again at room temperature, the test is positive for Bence Jones protein.

COMMENT. A heavy precipitate of Bence Jones protein at 56° C. may not redissolve on boiling; the test should be repeated with diluted urine. The urine specimen should be fresh or refrigerated, since heat coagulable protein will denature or decompose if the urine is left at room temperature and give false positive reactions.

Concentration of Urine for Protein Electrophoresis. Because the amount of protein in urine is frequently too low for satisfactory electrophoresis (less than 0.5 to 1 gm. per 100 ml.), a method for concentration is needed that will not denature the proteins and is preferably simple and rapid. Urine may be concentrated by dialysis against powdered sucrose (McFarlane, 1964) or polyvinylpyrrolidone or dextran solutions. Rapid results are more easily achieved by using dialysis against a dextran solution under vacuum (Burrows, 1965). Two different methods are described.

EQUIPMENT. Cellophane dialysis tubing 22/100 (Visking Company, Chicago) and dextran of molecular weight of 59,000 or more (Pharmachem Corp.) or polyvinylpyrrolidone (Plasdone, General Aniline).

PROCEDURE. About 10 ml. of clear urine is placed in the dialysis sac and suspended in a glass container with stopper containing either a 30 per cent solution of dextran in normal saline or a 30 per cent solution of polyvinylpyrrolidone in water. Dialysis is carried out in a refrigerator; it is convenient to set this up in the evening in order to allow dialysis to proceed overnight. Dialyze until the urine is concentrated tenfold or more. The collapsed sac is removed and patted dry and the contents aspirated with a pipette.

EQUIPMENT (Method 2). Collodion bags (Membrane filter S13200, Sartorius Division, Brinkman Instruments, Inc.) and glass suction apparatus.

PROCEDURE. The collodion bag is filled with about 5 to 7 ml. of clear urine on which a total protein determination has been made. The suction vessel is filled with 10 per cent dextran in saline. A small vacuum pump is attached. The urine may be concentrated to 0.1 ml. in about 2 hours. The level is clearly visible and should be watched. More urine may be added at any time, since the inner glass tube with the collodion sac attached is open.

COMMENTS. The second procedure is preferable; it is simple and rapid and allows a large volume of urine to be concentrated, if necessary. The concentrated urine is more easily accessible. (The manufacturer's directions should be followed regarding the use and storage of the collodion bags.) Specimens may be lost with the use of the cellophane dialysis method because the procedure may go to dryness if not watched and because the concentrated urine is difficult to recover from the sac. It was thought that globulins might adsorb to the cellophane surface of the sac, but this has been discounted (Henry, 1964).

ELECTROPHORESIS OF URINE PROTEIN. Paper or cellulose acetate is suitable. If the protein concentration is low, the sample may be applied to cellulose acetate several times on the same spot to achieve better results. For further details consult Chapter 9.

Sulfonamide in Urine. Sulfonamides are conjugated in the body by acetylation. Both free and acetylated forms can be found in the blood and urine.

Newer sulfonamides, such as sulfisoxazole, are less likely to form crystals in the urine than the older sulfanilamide, sulfapyridine, or sulfathiazole. Acetylated sulfadiazine is more soluble in urine than free sulfadiazine.

The sulfonamides contain a sulfonamide group and a free amino group. The sulfonamide is diazotized with nitrous acid and coupled with N-(1-naphthyl)-ethylenediamine to produce a colored compound. Since acetylation blocks the amino group, the conjugated form cannot be diazotized. To measure total sulfonamide, the sample is first hydrolyzed with HCl. A protein-free specimen of urine is used.

PROCEDURE. See Bratton and Marshal, 1939; Gershenfeld, 1943.

REAGENTS

1. 15 per cent aqueous solution of trichloroacetic acid.

2. 0.1 per cent aqueous solution of sodium nitrate.

3. 0.5 per cent aqueous solution of ammonium sulfamate.

4. 0.4 N hydrochloric acid solution (dilute 3.8 ml. concentrated HCl with 100 ml.).

5. 0.1 per cent aqueous solution of N-(1-naphthyl)-ethylenediamine dihydrochloride (Eastman Organic Chemicals, Division of Eastman Kodak Co., Rochester, New York). Keep in a dark bottle in the refrigerator.

STANDARDS

Stock Standard. A 0.2 per cent aqueous solution of a sulfonamide. It is desirable to use as a standard the identical form of the sulfa drug that is administered. Keep in a dark bottle in the refrigerator. Stable for several weeks.

Dilute Standards. Into three 100 ml. flasks containing 18 ml. of the 15 per cent trichloroacetic acid solution, add the following amounts of the *stock standard* and dilute to the mark:

No. 1: 1.0 ml. (10 ml. contains 0.02 mg.).
No. 2: 2.5 ml. (10 ml. contains 0.05 mg.).
No. 3: 5.0 ml. (10 ml. contains 0.10 mg.).

TECHNIQUE

Free Sulfanilamide. Protein-free urine is diluted by mixing 1 ml. with sufficient distilled water to 250 ml.

If the urine contains proteins, mix 1 ml. of urine with 1 ml. of 15 per cent trichloroacetic acid, dilute to 10 ml. and filter. Dilute a portion of the filtrate 1 to 25.

To 5 ml. of either of the above final dilutions, add 5 ml. of 0.4 N HCl. To the 10 ml. of this mixture and to 10 ml. of each of the three dilute standards, add 1 ml. of the sodium nitrite solution, mix, and after allowing it to stand 3 minutes, add 1 ml. of the ammonium sulfamate solution. Allow to stand 2 minutes and add 1 ml. of the ethylenediamine reagent. Compare in a colorimeter with the dilute standard (which matches closest) within 1 hour.

Total Sulfanilamide. Five ml. of diluted protein-free urine (freed of protein if necessary and diluted as above) is mixed with 5 ml. 0.4 N HCl and kept for 1 hour in a boiling water-bath. Cool and adjust to 10 ml. to replace evaporated water. Proceed as above.

URINARY CALCULI

Analysis of the constituents of urinary calculi may be of help in the management of patients with calculous disease.

Calcium oxalate is the most commonly found constituent of urinary calculi. It precipitates out in both acid and alkaline urine and may form calculi in sterile urine. Calcium phosphate (hydroxy apatite $Ca_{10}(PO)_6(OH)_2$) forms calculi at the normal urinary pH of 6.0 to 6.5, whereas magnesium ammonium phosphate forms calculi in an alkaline urine probably associated with bacterial infection.

In Prien's series (1963), calcium oxalate or a mixture of oxalate and calcium phosphate were most often found in stones (80 to 84 per cent). Mixed calcium phosphate, magnesium ammonium phosphate, and uric acid were the next most common constituents (3 to 10 per cent each), and these were followed by cystine (1 to 2 per cent). Uric acid and cystine precipitate in acid urines at pH less than 6. Rarely, calculi containing sulfonamides are found, and silica calculi have been reported in patients ingesting silica gel over a long period of time (Lagergren, 1962). Carbonate, which is frequently detected in chemical analysis, probably results from adsorption of carbon dioxide to the calcium phosphate crystal. Supersaturation of the urine with oxalate, phosphate, uric acid, and calcium may lead to stone formation, depending on urinary pH. Calculi are commonly seen in hyperparathyroidism, since calcium excretion is high in this condition. Stasis in any part of the urinary tract will cause crystalline precipitation, usually phosphate.

The origin of oxalate in the urine is not entirely understood. When oxalates are ingested, they are eliminated, at least in part, unchanged in the urine. Common articles of diet which contain oxalate are asparagus, apples, cabbage, grapes, lettuce, rhubarb, spinach, and tomatoes, and these are probably the source of unmetabolized oxalic acid. Part of the oxalic acid of the body is formed, however, in the course of the metabolism of protein, fat, and carbohydrate, and increases have been noted in diabetes and in organic disease of the liver. The finding of clusters of calcium oxalate (or of uric acid) crystals in freshly voided urine suggests that conditions in the urinary passages are favorable for calculus formation but, of course, does not prove that calculi are present.

The passage of stones down the ureter produces renal colic, which is characterized by severe pain in the back radiating to the groin. Stones may also be passed through the urethra with great pain. Hematuria is a common urinary finding when symptoms of stone are present. If stones obstruct the pelvis of the kidney or ureter, hydronephrosis will result with pyelonephritis as a probable consequence.

Calculi may be of various sizes, commonly described as sand, gravel, and stone. Large round stones are characteristic of those found in the bladder. The physical characteristics of the various calculi rarely will suffice for their identification, but a few points are worth noting. Uric acid and urate stones are always colored yellow to brownish red and are moderately hard. Phosphate stones are usually pale and friable. Calcium oxalate stones are very hard, often of a dark color, and typically have a rough surface.

Several methods are available for the analysis of calculi, such as optical crystallography, x-ray diffraction, and infrared spectroscopy. A review of chemical methods is presented by Henry (1964).

Analysis of Urinary Calculi. The reagents needed for this method are available as a kit from C. W. Allan & Co., St. Louis, Missouri.

Gross Examination

1. Wash stone free from blood, mucus, preservative solution, etc., and dry in hot-air oven.
2. Measure stone's dimensions.
3. Describe briefly the color and texture of the stone's exterior surface.
4. Cut, saw, or break the stone so as to examine its interior. Look for a foreign body which may have acted as a nucleus for its formation. Describe the color and texture of the interior.
5. Reduce stone to a fine powder by pulverizing with a mortar and pestle.
6. If there is a very large stone, it may be advisable to make separate analyses of layers that appear to have different constituents.

Spot Plate Method. The spot plate method is suitable for screening purposes in most laboratories (see Feigl, 1946). For more detailed schemes, consult Henry (1964). A method for the examination of rare stones follows this discussion.

Place a small amount of powder in four spot depressions on a porcelain spot plate and a larger amount in the fifth spot. Add the following reagents, noting the reaction on each spot:

Rare Stones

SULFONAMIDES. To pulverized stone in test tube add 2 drops 10 per cent HCl (wait 30 seconds); then add 2 drops 0.1 per cent $NaNO_2$ (wait 30 to 60 seconds); then add 2 drops of 0.5 per cent NH_4–sulfamate and 2 to 3 drops 0.1 per cent N(1-naphthyl) ethylenediamine dihydrochloride in water. *Result:* Brownish pink to magenta color.

The presence of any sulfonamide derivative is determined by the diazotization of a free amino group. Excess $NaNO_2$ is destroyed by ammonium sulfamate and the purplish red azo dye is formed by the coupling of the diazotized sulfanilamide with N-(1-naphthyl) ethylenediamine dihydrochloride.

XANTHINE. To pulverized stone in evaporating dish add 2 drops concentrated HNO_3 and evaporate to complete dryness over steam bath. Cool slightly. Add 1 drop 20 per cent NaOH. Warm again. *Result:* Residue left after evaporation is yellow. After addition of NaOH, an orange color develops; this becomes red upon warming. *Xanthoproteic reaction:* This is due to the nitration of the phenyl rings present in tyrosine, phenylalanine, and tryptophan to give yellow nitro substitution products, which become orange-colored upon addition of alkali (salt formation).

In performing the qualitative test for xanthine, colored reactions will also be obtained from uric acid. While the dried residue after evaporation is lemon yellow with xanthine, it is orange with uric acid. After addition of NaOH, an orange color develops, becoming red with warming when xanthine is present; if uric acid is present, a cherry red to purple color develops immediately after addition of NaOH.

CHOLESTEROL. To approximately 0.5 ml. $CHCl_3$ extract in a test tube, add 3 drops acetic anhydride and 1 drop concentrated H_2SO_4. *Result:* Test solution becomes red, then blue, and finally blue-green in color.

REAGENT	REACTION
1. 1 drop sodium carbonate, 2 drops uric acid reagent.	Prompt *deep* blue color indicates uric acid and urates.
2. 3 drops HCl. Cool. Add pinch of magnesium dioxide.	Tiny bubbles of gas explosively released from bottom after MnO_2 is added indicate oxalates.
3. 5 drops ammonium molybdate. Warm over flame.	Distinct yellow precipitate indicates phosphates.
4. 1 drop ammonium hydroxide. 1 drop sodium cyanide. Wait 5 minutes. 3 drops sodium nitroprusside.	Beet-red color indicates cystine (see confirmatory tests, p. 52, and below).
5. Using the larger amount of powder in the fifth spot, add 10 drops HCl.	Foaming effervescence indicates carbonates.
Divide acid extract into 3 spots on plate and add:	
A. 3 drops NaOH. 3 drops of reagent "M."	Slow formation of blue precipitate indicates magnesium.
B. 3 drops NaOH. 3 drops Nessler's reagent.	Yellow to orange precipitate indicates ammonia.
C. 3 drops of sodium hydroxide.	Fine white precipitate indicates calcium oxalate. Dense precipitate indicates calcium phosphate.

Transient colors are probably due to halochromic salts of either the unsaturated sterol or a dehydrated product of it.

FIBRIN. To pulverized stone add approximately 1 to 2 ml. Millon's reagent. Heat. Note color. Add drop of concentrated HNO_3. Note color again. *Result:* A flesh pink color or yellow precipitate that dissolves in HNO_3 to form a pink or reddish solution.

A nitro compound is formed with phenol to produce the reddish color. The Millon test is especially recommended for para-substituted phenols, secondary proteoses, and peptones. It is not specific for proteins, but is given for phenols in general. The reaction depends upon the formation of a colored mercury compound with the hydroxyphenyl group.

CONFIRMATORY TESTS FOR CYSTINE

1. Burning test. *Result:* Blue flame causing a sharp, pungent odor.

2. Pulverized stone on small watchglass. Dissolve in a few drops of 10 per cent NH_4OH; (filter if necessary) and allow to evaporate spontaneously. *Result:* Cystine is recognized by the formation of typical hexagonal crystals. (Check under low power of microscope.)

3. Pulverized stone in test tube. Heat with 1 ml. 10 per cent NaOH. Add a few crystals of lead acetate; heat a little more. *Result:* A *heavy* black precipitate indicates the presence of cystine. Protein impurities that are incorporated with other ingredients of stones may yield a weakly positive test.

COLLECTION OF URINE

There are certain important considerations to be borne in mind relative to the collection of urine specimens for examination. If these are followed, one is less apt to commit serious errors in the interpretation of the results obtained.

Containers. Glass urine specimen bottles of about 6-oz. capacity are available. These should be washed with detergent and rinsed well with water and dried.

Disposable wax-coated paper specimen bottles and disposable plastic containers with lids are available in several sizes and are preferred by many for routine screening urinalysis. Conical containers are less likely to tip over.

A sterile kit for collection of urine for bacteriologic examination is available. It contains a disposable plastic bottle, detergent-impregnated pad, and dry pad. A sterile tray may be prepared for clean-voided specimens for hospital use. Sterile wrapped bedpans should always be available.

Pediatric urine collectors of clear pliable polyethylene are available for male and female infants. These are more comfortable than rigid tube containers. With these containers, an estimate of the volume excreted may be made. The bag may be folded and self-sealed for transportation. For a 24-hour collection, a tube is attached to the bag and can be connected to a collection bottle. Sterile and nonsterile plastic bags are available.

Large glass or plastic containers with wide mouths and screw caps are used for 24-hour collections, usually with added preservative or refrigeration between voidings. Bedpans used to collect voiding urine should be scrupulously clean.

Collection Procedure. The urine sample must be collected in a clean, dry container and should be examined when freshly voided. Red blood cells and leukocytes, which may be present, are affected adversely and will eventually be destroyed by hypotonicity of the urine. Casts, also, decompose in urine that has been allowed to stand for several hours. Bacterial contamination regularly occurs, resulting in alkalinization of the urine due to the conversion of urea to ammonia and loss of glucose. A rise in pH accelerates the loss of leukocytes and epithelial cells.

Collection of Urine for Quantitative Analysis. If it is necessary that the urine stand for more than 1 to 2 hours after it is voided, as in the collection of 24-hour urine specimens, a preservative should be added to it, or it should be refrigerated. Common preservatives for urine specimens are *formaldehyde, thymol, toluol, chloroform,* and *boric acid.* Preservative tablets are available that produce formaldehyde.* Formaldehyde is useful for preserving the cellular elements and casts. Thymol may be added as a 10 per cent solution in isopropanol, about 10 ml. per 24-hour collection. Boric acid, 0.8 per cent, is satisfactory. Of these, toluol and boric acid are the most satisfactory for general purposes. They do not interfere with the examinations for protein, sugar, or the ketone bodies. Sodium fluoride may be used to preserve glucose in urine. For many purposes, it is possible to keep the urine refrigerated without added preservatives. When analyses for total nitrogen, amino acids, and delta-amino-levulinic acid are to be made, the urine must be acidified with a strong mineral acid, e.g., HCl to pH 3.

For certain examinations, it is important to know the amount of time represented by the specimen. This is true of quantitative determinations for protein, sugar, and other urinary constituents. In this case, a 24-hour collection is most suitable. The patient is carefully in-

*Cargille Urinary Preservative Tablets. F. B. Kingsbury Formula, R. P. Cargille Laboratories, Inc., 117 Liberty Street, New York, N.Y.

structed to empty his bladder at 8:00 A.M. (this presumably being before breakfast) and discard this urine. He collects all subsequent urine up to and including that voided at 8:00 A.M. the following morning. The total volume of this sample is measured and recorded and the urine thoroughly mixed before a measured sample is withdrawn for analysis.

Collection of Urine for Screening Purposes. For *chemical* and *microscopic* examination, a voided specimen is usually suitable. If the specimen is likely to be contaminated by vaginal discharge or hemorrhage, a clean-voided specimen is collected. It may be necessary to pack the vagina or use a tampon in some cases, especially when examination of the urinary sediment is critical.

For most routine examinations, a fairly concentrated specimen is preferable to a dilute one. This is true of examinations for protein and also for the microscopic examination of the sediment. The concentration of solutes and formed elements in the urine varies throughout the patient's waking hours, depending upon his water intake. Ordinarily the first morning specimen of urine, voided on rising, is the most concentrated specimen, since the patient has not been drinking water during the hours of sleep. Therefore, this specimen is the best one to examine for protein and the contents of the sediment. (An ambulatory person will excrete larger amounts of protein, but for comparison the night specimens are probably better.) Valuable information may also be gained from determinations of the volume and specific gravity of this specimen. On the other hand, the first morning specimen is not the best one to examine for glucose.

In assessing the control of the blood sugar levels in diabetic patients, one is aided by examining urine specimens for glucose. Specimens are collected at the following hours: 6 A.M., 10 A.M., 4 P.M., and 8 P.M. The first of these specimens, that obtained in the fasting state on rising, is less likely to contain glucose than any of the others, which have been obtained from 2 to 3 hours after eating.

For *bacteriologic examination,* a clean-voided midstream specimen is desirable. Catheterization should be avoided because it is likely to cause urinary tract infections. When tubercle bacilli are sought, however, a catheterized early morning specimen is usually required in order to avoid contamination by smegma bacilli. Bacteriologic culture should be done immediately. When this is not possible, the urine should be refrigerated at 4° C. until cultured—for a period of not more than 12 hours as a rule, although specimens have been cultured without detriment after four days of adequate refrigeration (Ryan and Mills, 1963).

In the male the glans should be exposed adequately, thoroughly cleaned with a mild antiseptic solution, and dried. The midstream urine should be collected in a sterile container after the initial flow has been allowed to escape.

The female patient should be instructed to kneel or squat over a bedpan or to stand astride a toilet bowl. Using sterile gloves, the nurse should separate the labia minora widely to expose the urethral orifice and to keep the labia separated throughout the procedure. With sterile, soapy cotton balls, cleanse on each side of urinary meatus; then cleanse the meatus. Rinse the cleansed area with sterile, water-saturated cotton balls. Instruct the patient to void forcibly, and allow the initial stream of urine to drain into the bedpan or toilet, continuing to keep the labia separated. Catch the subsequent midstream specimen in a sterile container, and do not touch any portion of perineum with the container. About 30 to 100 ml. of urine should be collected. After obtaining the urine specimen, allow the labia to close. The patient then continues to void into the bedpan or toilet.

REFERENCES

Adams, F.: The Genuine Work of Hippocrates. New York, William Wood & Co., 1886.

Adams, R. D., Denny-Brown, D., and Pearson, C. M.: Diseases of Muscle. New York, Harper & Row, 1962.

Addis, T.: A clinical classification of Bright's diseases. J.A.M.A. *85*:163, 1925.

Addis, T.: The number of formed elements in the urinary sediment of normal individuals. J. Clin. Invest. 2:409, 1926.

Addis, T.: Glomerular Nephritis. New York, The Macmillan Company, 1948.

Albright, F., and Reifenstein, E. C., Jr.: The Parathyroid Glands and Metabolic Bone Diseases. Baltimore, The Williams & Wilkins Co., 1948.

Apthorp, G. H.: Investigation of the sugar content of urine from normal subjects and patients with renal and hepatic diseases by paper chromatography. J. Clin. Path. *10*:84, 1957.

Aukland, K.: Stop flow analysis of renal protein excretion in the dog. Scand. J. Clin. Lab. Invest. *12*:300, 1960.

Austin, J. H.: Metachromatic form of diffuse sclerosis; diagnosis during life by urine sediment examination. Neurology 7:415, 1957.

Balikov, B.: Urobilinogen excretion in normal adults, results of assays with notes on methodology. Clin. Chem. *3*:145, 1957.

Barney, J. D., and Sulkowitch, H. W.: Progress in the management of urinary calculi. J. Urol. 27:746, 1937.

Beach, E. F., and Turner, J. J.: An enzymatic method for glucose determination in body fluids. Clin. Chem. *4*:462, 1958.

Bence Jones, H.: On a new substance occurring in the urine of a patient with mollities ossium. Phil. Tr. Roy. Soc. (London) *138*:55, 1848.

Benedict, S. R.: A reagent for the detection of reducing sugars. J. Biol. Chem. 5:485, 1909.

Benedict, S. R.: Detection and estimation of glucose in urine: Reagent for quantitative use. J.A.M.A. 57:1193, 1911.

Berggard, I.: Studies on the plasma proteins in normal human urine. Clin. Chim. Acta 6:413, 1961.

Berman, L. B., Schreiver, G. E., and Feys, J. O.: Observations on the glitter-cell phenomenon. New Eng. J. Med. *255*: 989, 1956.
Berry, H. K., and Splinlanger, J.: A paper spot test useful in the study of Hurler's syndrome. J. Lab. Clin. Med. *55*: 136, 1960.
Bickel, H.: Mellituria, a paper chromatographic study. J. Pediat. *59*:641, 1961.
Blondheim, S. H., Margoliash, E., and Shafur, E.: A simple test for myohemaglobinuria (myoglobinuria). J.A.M.A. *167*:453, 1958.
Boyce, W. H., Garvey, F. K., and Norfleet, C. M., Jr.: Proteins and other biocolloids of urine in health and in calculous disease. J. Clin. Invest. *33*:1287, 1954.
Bradley, G. M.: Urinary screening tests in the infant and young child. Med. Clin. N. Amer. *55*:1457, 1971.
Bradley, S. E.: Laboratory findings in the blood and urine in health and disease. Med. Clin. N. Amer. *29*:1314, 1945.
Brand, E., Harris, M. M., and Biloon, S.: Cystinuria: The excretion of cystine complex which decomposes in the urine with the liberatum of free cystine. J. Biol. Chem. *86*:315, 1930.
Bratton, A. C., and Marshal, E. K., Jr.: A new coupling component for sulfanilamide determination. J. Biol. Chem. *128*:537, 1939.
Brooks, A. L.: An appraisal of a urinary porphyrin test in detection of lead absorption. Indust. Med. Surg. *20*:390, 1951.
Brownstein, H., and Roberge, A. R.: Detection of phenothiazine derivatives in urine. Clin. Chem. *12*:844, 1966.
Bryant, D., and Flynn, F. V.: An assessment of new tests for detecting bilirubin in urine. J. Clin. Path. *8*:163, 1955.
Buist, N. R. M.: Set of simple side room tests for detection of inborn errors of metabolism. Brit. Med. J. *2*:745, 1968.
Burrows, S.: Simple method for concentration of cerebrospinal fluid for protein electrophoresis. Clin. Chem. *11*: 1068, 1965.
Caraway, W. T.: Chemical and diagnostic specificity of laboratory tests. Am. J. Clin. Pathol. *37*:445, 1962.
Clough, G., and Reah, T. G.: A "protein error." Lancet *1*:1248, 1964.
Cook, M. H., Free, H. M., and Free, A. H.: The detection of blood in urine. Am. J. Med. Technol. *22*:218, 1956.
Cook, M. H., Free, A. H., and Giordano, A. S.: The accuracy of urine sugar tests. Am. J. Med. Technol. *19*:283, 1953.
Creipell, R.: *In* Manuel, Y., Revillard, J. P., and Betuel, H. (eds.): Proteins in Normal and Pathologic Urine. Baltimore, University Park Press, 1970.
Cruikshank, G., and Edmond, E.: "Clean catch" urine in the newborn – bacteriology and cell excretion patterns in the first week of life. Brit. Med. J. *4*:704, 1967.
Culley, W. J., Mertz, E. T., Luce, M. W., Calandro, J. M., and Jolly, D. H.: Paper chromatographic estimation of phenylalanine and tyrosine using fingertip blood; its application to phenylketonuria. Clin. Chem. *8*:266, 1962.
Damron, M.: Unpublished observations at University of Minnesota Medical Center, 1963.
Date, J. W.: Quantitative determination of some carbohydrates in normal urine. Scand. J. Clin. Lab. Invest. *10*: 155, 1958.
Dewall, C. P., Casazza, A. R., Grimley, P. M., Carbone, P. P., and Rowe, W. P.: Recovery of cytomegalovirus from adults with neoplastic disease. Ann. Intern. Med. *64*:531, 1966.
Dorfman, A., and Matalon, R.: *In* Stanbury, J. B., Wyngaarden, J. B., and Fredrikson, D. S.: Metabolic Basis of Inherited Disease. New York, McGraw-Hill Book company, 1972.
Editorial: Early diagnosis of diabetes. Brit. Med. J. *1*:497, 1966.
Efron, M. L.: Aminoaciduria. New Eng. J. Med. *272*:1058, 1965.
Esbach, G.: Dosage pratique de l'albumine: Tris méthodes. C. R. Soc. Biol. (Paris) *1*:33, 1874
Exton, W. G.: A simple and rapid quantitative test for albumin in urine. J. Lab. Clin. Med. *10*:722, 1925.
Farquhar, M. D., and Palade, G. E.: Segregation of ferritin in glomerular protein absorption droplets. J. Biophys. Biochem. Cytol. *7*:297, 1960.
Feigl, F.: Qualitative Analysis by Spot Tests. 3rd ed. Amsterdam, Elsevier Publishing Co., 1946.
Fischl, J., Sason, I., and Segal, S.: A rapid spot test for the determination of cysteinuria and aminoaciduria. Clin. Chem. *7*:674, 1961.
Fishberg, E. H.: The instantaneous diagnosis of alkaptonuria on a single drop of urine. J.A.M.A. *119*:882, 1942.
Folin, O., and McEllroy, W. S.: Copper-phosphate mixtures as sugar reagents. J. Biol. Chem. *33*:513, 1918.
Forrest, F. M., Forrest, I. S., and Mason, A. S.: Review of rapid urine tests for phenothiazine and related drugs. Am. J. Psychiat. *118*:300, 1961.
Foster, W. D.: A Short History of Clinical Pathology. London, E. & S. Livingstone, Ltd., 1961.
Free, A. H., and Free, H. M.: A simple test for urine bilirubin. Gastroenterology *24*:414, 1953.
Free, A. H., and Free, H. M.: Nature of nitroprusside reactive material in urine in ketosis. Amer. J. Path. *30*:7, 1958.
Free, A. H., Adams, E. C., Kercher, M. L., Free, H. M., and Cook, M. H.: Simple specific test for urine glucose. Clin. Chem. *3*:163, 1957a.
Free, A. H., Rupe, C. O., and Metzler, I.: Studies with a new colorimetric test for proteinuria. Clin. Chem. *3*:716, 1957b.
Freedberg, I. M., Feingold, D. S., and Hiatt, H. H.: Serum and urine L-xylulose in pentosuric and normal subjects and in individuals with pentosuria trait. Biochem. Biophys. Res. Com. *1*:328, 1959.
Froesch, E. R., Wolf, H. P., and Baitsch, H.: Hereditary fructose intolerance: An inborn defect of hepatic fructose-1-phosphate splitting enzyme. Am. J. Med. *34*:151, 1963.
Gershenfeld, L.: Urine and Urinalysis. 2nd ed. Philadelphia, Lea & Febiger, 1943.
Giordano, A. S., and Winstead, M.: A tablet test for bilirubin in urine. Am. J. Clin. Path. *23*:610, 1953.
Goldring, W.: Studies of the kidney in acute infection. J. Clin. Invest. *10*:355, 1931.
Gordon, B. L.: Medicine Throughout Antiquity. Philadelphia, F. A. Davis Co., 1949.
Grant, G. H.: The proteins of normal urine. II. From the urinary tract. J. Clin. Path. *12*:510, 1959.
Guthrie, R., and Susi, A.: Simple phenylalanine method for detecting phenylketonuria in large populations of newborn infants. Pediatrics *32*:338, 1963.
Henry, R. J.: Clinical Chemistry: Principles and Technics. New York, Harper & Row, 1964.
Henry, R. J., Jacobs, S. L., and Berkman, S.: Studies on the determination of bile pigments. III. Standardization of the determination of urobilinogen as urobilinogen-aldehyde. Clin. Chem. *7*:231, 1961.
Henry, R. J., Sobel, C., and Segalove, M.: Turbidometric determination of proteins with sulfosalicylic and trichloroacetic acids. Proc. Soc. Exp. Biol. Med. *92*:748, 1956.
Herdman, R. C., Michael, A. F., and Good, R. A.: Postural proteinuria. Ann. Intern. Med. *65*:286, 1966.
Hobbs, J. R., Slot, G. M. J., Campbell, C. H., Clein, G. P., Scott, J. T., Crowther, D., and Swan, H. T.: Six cases of gamma d. myelomatosis. Lancet *2*:614, 1966.
Hoffman, W. S.: The Biochemistry of Clinical Medicine. 4th ed. Chicago, Year Book Medical Publishers, Inc., 1970.
Houghton, B. J., and Pears, M. A.: Cell excretion in normal urine. Brit. Med. J. *1*:622, 1957.
Howell, T. H.: Urinary excretion after the age of ninety. J. Geront. *11*:61, 1956.
Hisa, D. Y., and Inouye, T.: Inborn Errors of Metabolism. Part 2. Laboratory Methods. Chicago, Year Book Medical Publishers, Inc., 1966.
Joachim, G. R., Cameron, J. S., Schwartz, M., and Becker, E. L.: Selectivity of protein excretion of patients with the nephrotic syndrome. J. Clin. Invest. *43*:2332, 1964.
Kaplow, L. S.: Simplified myeloperoxidase stain using benzidine dihydrochloride. Blood *26*:215, 1965.
Kark, R. M.: Clinical aspects of major porphyrinopathies. Med. Clin. N. Amer. *39*:11, 1955.
Kark, R. M., Lawrence, J. R., Pollak, V. E., Pirani, C. L., Muehrcke, R. C., and Silva, H.: A Primer of Urinalysis. 2nd ed. New York, Harper & Row, 1963.

Keele, K. D.: The Evolution of Clinical Methods in Medicine. Springfield, Illinois, Charles C Thomas, 1963.
Kerby, G. P.: The excretion of glucuronic acid and of acid mucopolysaccharides in normal human urine. J. Clin. Invest. *33*:1168, 1954.
Kibrick, A. C.: Extended use of the Kingsley biuret reagent. Clin. Chem. *4*:232, 1958.
Killander, J., Sjolin, S., and Zaar, B.: Rapid tests for ketonuria. Scand. J. Clin. Lab. Invest. *14*:311, 1962.
King, E. J., Pillai, S. S., and Beall, D.: Preservation of blood for sugar analysis. Lancet *1*:310, 1941.
Lagergren, C.: Development of silica calculi after oral administration of magnesium trisilicate. J. Urol. *87*:994, 1962.
Lange, C. F., Polos, A., and Dubin, A.: Chemical and physical characteristics of urinary proteoses associated with streptococcal glomerulonephritis. Clin. Chem. Acta *14*: 311, 1966.
Lazerte, G. D., and McMillin, T. J.: False positive urine tests due to drugs. Northwest Med. *63*:106, 1964.
Levine, J. M., Dubin, A., and Armstrong, S. H.: The finding of urinary proteose in certain renal diseases. Isolation and identification. J. Lab. Clin. Med. *53*:167, 1959.
Lewis, B., and Richards, P.: Measurement of urinary protein. Lancet *1*:1141, 1961.
Lippman, R. W.: Urine and the Urinary Sediment. 2nd ed. Springfield, Illinois, Charles C Thomas, 1957.
Little, P. J.: Urinary white-cell excretion. Lancet *1*:1149, 1962.
Lowe, C. U., and Auerback, V. H.: Inborn errors of metabolism. *In* Nelson, W. E. (ed.): Textbook of Pediatrics. 8th ed. Philadelphia, W. B. Saunders Company, 1964.
Lyttle, J. D.: The Addis sediment count in normal children. J. Clin. Invest. *12*:87, 1933.
Macfarlane, H.: A simple rapid method of concentrating urine for protein electrophoresis. Clin. Chem. Acta *9*: 376, 1964.
Major, R. H.: Classic Descriptions of Disease. Springfield, Illinois, Charles C Thomas, 1932.
Manuel, Y., Revillard, J. P., and Betuel, H. (eds.): Proteins in Normal and Pathologic Urine. Baltimore, University Park Press, 1970.
Maxwell, M. H., and Kleeman, C. R.: Clinical Disorders of Fluid and Electrolyte Metabolism. New York, McGraw-Hill Book Company, Blakiston Division, 1962.
McQueen, E. G.: Composition of urinary casts. Lancet *1*:397, 1966.
Nakamura, R. M., Reilly, E. B., Fujita, K., Brown, J., and Kunitake, G. M.: False negative reactions and sensitivity in the urine glucose oxidase test. Diabetes *14*:224, 1965.
Nash, J., Lister, J., and Vobes, D. H.: Clinical tests for ketonuria. Lancet *1*:801, 1954.
Naumann, H. N.: Differentiation of Bence Jones protein from uroglobulins. Am. J. Clin. Path. *44*:413, 1965.
Neubauer, K. T., and Vogel, J.: Analysis of the Urine. 4th ed. London, W. O. Markham, New Sydenham Society, 1863.
Osman, A. A.: Original Papers of Richard Bright on Renal Disease. London, Oxford University Press, 1937.
Osserman, E. F., and Lawlor, D.: Immunoelectrophoretic characterization of the serum and urinary proteins in plasma cell myeloma and Waldenström's macroglobulinemia. Ann. N.Y. Acad. Sci. *94*:93, 1961.
Palmer, W. W., and Henderson, L. J.: Clinical studies on acid base equilibrium and the nature of acidosis. Arch. Intern. Med. *12*:151, 1913.
Patterson, J. N., Catanzaro, C., and Dede, D. M.: The quantitative estimation of porphobilinogen and porphyrins in urine. *In* Manual for Workshop on the Porphyrins and the Porphyrias. Commission on Continuing Education. Council on Clinical Chemistry, American Society of Clinical Pathologists, Chicago, Illinois, 1966.
Pennock, C. A., Most, M. G., and Batstone, G. F.: Screening for mucopolysaccharidoses. Clin. Chim. Acta *27*:93, 1970.
Pollak, V. E., and Arbel, C.: The distribution of Tamm-Horsfall mucoprotein (uromucoid) in the human nephron. Nephron *6*:667, 1969.
Pomerantz, M., and Jones, W. R.: Chyluria with lymphographic abnormalities. J.A.M.A. *196*:452, 1966.
Prescott, L. F., and Brodie, D. G.: A simple differential stain for urinary sediment. Lancet *2*:940, 1964.
Prescott, L. F.: Urinary white cell excretion patterns. Lancet *2*:238, 1965.
Prien, E. L.: Crystallographic analysis of urinary calculi: A 23 year survey study. J. Urol. *89*:917, 1963.
Prout, W.: An Enquiry into the Nature and Treatment of Diabetes, Calculus and Other Affections of the Urinary Organs. Philadelphia, Towar and Hogan Company, 1826.
Purdy, C. W.: Practical Urinalysis and Urinary Diagnosis. Philadelphia, F. A. Davis Co., 1900.
Putnam, F. W., Easley, C. W., Lynn, L. T., Ritchie, A. E., and Phelps, R. A.: The heat precipitation of Bence Jones proteins. I. Optimum conditions. Arch. Biochem. Biophys. *83*:115, 1959.
Relman, A. S., and Levinsky, N. G.: Clinical examination of renal function. *In* Strauss, M. B., and Welt, L. G. (eds.): Diseases of the Kidney. Boston, Little, Brown and Company, 1971.
Renuart, A.: Screening for inborn errors of metabolism associated with mental deficiency or neurologic disorders or both. New Eng. J. Med. *274*:384, 1966.
Rhodes, P. G., Hammel, C. L., and Berman, L. B.: Urinary constituents of the newborn infant. J. Pediat. *60*:18, 1962.
Riekers, H., and Miale, J. B.: Ketonuria. An evaluation of tests and some clinical implications. Am. J. Clin. Path. *30*:530, 1958.
Ritter, S., Spencer, H., and Samachson, J.: The Sulkowich test and quantitative urinary calcium excretion. J. Lab. Clin. Med. *56*:314, 1960.
Robinson, R. R., Glover, S. N., Phillippi, P. J., Lecocq, F. R., and Langelier, P. R.: Fixed and reproducible orthostatic proteinuria. Am. J. Path. *39*:291, 1961.
Rofe, P.: The cells of normal human urine. J. Clin. Path. *8*:25, 1955.
Rothera, A. C. H.: Note on the sodium nitro-prusside reaction for acetone. J. Physiol. *37*:491, 1908.
Rothman, E., and Higa, A.: A new two-dimensional system for the separation of amino acids on paper. Anal. Biochem. *3*:173, 1962.
Rous, P.: Urinary siderosis. J. Exper. Med. *28*:645, 1918.
Rubin, M. I.: Urine and urination. *In* Nelson, W. E. (ed.): Textbook of Pediatrics. Philadelphia, W. B. Saunders Company, 1964.
Rubner, M.: Ueber die Einwirkung von Bleiacetat auf Trauben-und Milchzucker. Z. Biol. *20*:397, 1884.
Ryan, W. L., and Mills, R. D.: Bacterial multiplication in urine during refrigeration. Am. J. Med. Tech. *29*:175, 1963.
Samson, M.: The relation of cuprous creatinine to tests for sugar in urine. J. Am. Chem. Soc. *61*:2389, 1939.
Schreiner, G. E.: Identification and significance of casts. A.M.A. Arch. Intern. Med. *99*:356, 1957.
Schreiner, G. E.: The nephrotic syndrome. *In* Strauss, M. B., and Welt, L. G. (eds.): Diseases of the Kidney. Boston, Little, Brown and Company, 1963.
Schwartz, S., Sborov, V., and Watson, C. J.: Studies of urobilinogen. IV. Quantitative determination of urobilinogen by means of Evelyn photoelectric colorimeter. Am. J. Clin. Path *14*:598, 1944.
Schwartz, S., Zieve, L., and Watson, C. J.: An improved method for the determination of urinary coproporphyrin and an evaluation of factors influencing the analysis. J. Lab. Clin. Med. *37*:843, 1951.
Selivanoff, S.: Ber. d. deutch. chem. Gesellsch, *20*:181, 1887. *In* Silber, S., and Reiner, M.: Essential fructosuria. Report of three cases with metabolic studies. Arch. Intern. Med. *54*:412, 1934.
Sjoerdsma, A., Weissbach, H., and Udenfriend, S.: Simple test for diagnosis of metastatic carcinoid. J.A.M.A. *159*: 397, 1955.
Smith, I. (ed.): Chromatographic and Electrophoretic Techniques. Vols. I and II. New York, Interscience Publishers, Inc., 1960.
Somogyi, M.: Rapid estimation of urine sugar. J. Lab. Clin. Med. *26*:1220, 1941.
Spackman, D. H., Stein, W. H., and Moore, S.: Chromatography of amino acids on sulfonated polystyrene resins. An improved system. Anal. Chem. *30*:1190, 1958.

Stahle, E.: Thin Layer Chromatography. New York, Academic Press, 1965.
Stanbury, J. B., Wyngaarden, J. B., and Fredrikson, D. S.: Metabolic Basis of Inherited Disease. New York, McGraw-Hill Book Company, 1972.
Sternheimer, R., and Malbin, B.: Clinical recognition of pyelonephritis with a new stain for urinary sediments. Am. J. Med. *11*:312, 1951.
Stich, W.: γ-Aminolävulinacedurie. Ein neues biochemisches und diagnostisches Kriterium der Bleivergiftung. Klin. Wschr. *39*:338, 1961.
Strauss, M. B., and Welt, L. G., (eds.): Diseases of the Kidney. Vols. 1 and 2. Boston, Little, Brown and Company, 1971.
Sunderman, F. W., and Boerner, F.: Normal Values in Clinical Medicine. Philadelphia, W. B. Saunders Company, 1949.
Triger, D. R., and Smith, J. W. G.: Survival of urinary leucocytes. J. Clin. Path. *19*:443, 1966.
Udenfriend, S., Titus, E., and Weissbach, H.: The identification of 5-hydroxy-3-indoleacetic acid in normal urine and a method for its assay. J. Biol. Chem. *216*:499, 1955.
Waldenström, J.: The porphyrias as inborn errors of metabolism. Am. J. Med. 22:758, 1957.
Watson, C. J.: The problem of porphyria—some facts and questions. New Eng. J. Med. *263*:1205, 1960.
Watson, C. J.: Personal communication, 1972.
Watson, C. J., and Hawkinson, V.: Semiquantitative estimation of bilirubin in the urine by means of the barium strip modification of Harrison's test. J. Lab. Clin. Med. *31*:914, 1946.
Watson, C. J., and Hawkinson, V.: Studies on urobilinogen. VI. Further experiences with the simple quantitative Ehrlich reaction. Am. J. Clin. Path. *17*:108. 1947.
Watson, C. J., and Schwartz, S.: A simple test for urinary porphobilinogen. Proc. Soc. Exp. Biol. Med. *47*:393, 1941.
Weatherburn, M. W., and Logan, J. E.: A simplified quantitative enzymatic procedure for glucose in urine. Diabetes *15*:127, 1966.
Webb, T., Rose, G., and Sehon, A. H.: Biocolloids in normal human urine. II. Physicochemical and immuno-chemical characteristics. Canad. J. Biochem. Physiol. *36*:1167, 1958.
Whisnant, C. L., Jr., Owings, R. H., Cantrell, C. G., and Cooper, G. R.: Primary idiopathic myoglobinuria in a Negro female: Its implications and a new method of laboratory diagnosis. Ann. Intern. Med. *51*:140, 1959.
Wilkerson, H. L. C.: Diagnosis: Oral glucose tolerance tests. *In* Danowski, T. S. (ed.): Diabetes Mellitus: Diagnosis and Treatment. New York, American Diabetes Association, Inc., 1964.
Wirth, W. A., and Thompson, R. L.: The effect of various conditions and substances on the results of laboratory procedures. Am. J. Clin. Path. *43*:579, 1965.
With, T. K.: Biology of bile pigments, including a review of their chemistry and a discussion of analytical methods. Copenhagen, Arne Frost-Hansen, 1954.
Wolvius, D., and Verschure, J. C. M.: The diagnostic value of the protein excretion pattern in various types of proteinuria. J. Clin. Path. *10*:80, 1957.
Wright, W. T.: Significance of an opaque green Benedict reaction. New Eng. J. Med. *254*:570, 1956.
Wright, W. T.: Cell counts in urine. Arch. Intern. Med. *103*: 76, 1959.
Zimmer, J. G., Dewey, R., Waterhouse, C., and Terry, R.: The origin and nature of anisotropic urinary lipids in the nephrotic syndrome. Ann. Intern. Med. *54*:205, 1961.

Chapter 3

RENAL FUNCTION AND ITS EVALUATION

by S. THOMAS SHAW, JR., M.D., and ELLIS S. BENSON, M.D.

ELEMENTS OF RENAL PHYSIOLOGY

Renal Hemodynamics and Glomerular Filtration

The renal tissue of man, totaling only 0.4 per cent of body weight, receives 20 per cent or more of his cardiac output. This section describes briefly the physical distributions and chemical alterations of this continuous and profuse transfusion which allow the kidneys to function as prime regulators of body fluid. This description should provide a useful basis for the subsequent discussion of renal function tests.

Obviously the amount of blood flowing into the kidneys each minute is reduced by the volume of urine excreted into the two renal pelves in that time.* This is proportionately a small reduction, averaging about 1.0 ml. per min., but it can range with normal kidneys from about 0.3 ml. per min. in dehydration to more than 15 ml. per min. in excessive hydration. Such a range of urine flow allows for a flexible response by the excretory mechanism to various normal and abnormal states of fluid volume and dynamics in the body.

The extraction of fluid from the blood flowing into the renal vessels occurs first in the glomeruli of the renal cortex. Approximately one million glomeruli per kidney filter about 60 ml. of fluid from the blood into the proximal nephrons each minute. The average glomerular filtration rate (GFR) in a man with two normal kidneys, thus, is roughly 120 ml. per min.*

*This ignores the water that is metabolically formed or consumed in the kidneys each minute.

Because of the diffusion properties of the glomerular membrane, the filtered water contains all the solutes of molecular weight below about 50,000 that it had in the blood plasma. Only those solutes of molecular weight below about 5500, however, maintain the same concentration in filtered water as in plasma water. The fluid entering Bowman's space and the beginning of the proximal convoluted tubule, therefore, is commonly referred to as an ultrafiltrate of plasma.

Total renal blood flow (TRBF) is the volume of blood which passes each minute into the renal arteries (normally 1200 ml. per min. or greater). A small percentage of TRBF may circulate through nonfunctioning kidney tissue, such as renal pelvis, peripelvic fat, and the renal capsule. Essentially all the remaining blood flow is believed to circulate through the glomeruli and peritubular capillaries. The effective renal plasma flow (ERPF) measured by clearance methods probably represents the amount of blood plasma flowing through functional renal tissue each minute. ERPF averages about 660 ml. per min.

The volume of blood flowing out of the glomeruli via the efferent arterioles is reduced by about 120 ml. of glomerular ultrafiltrate per minute. The postglomerular blood then flows through the peritubular capillary network, which drains at various levels in the cortex and

*Unless otherwise stated, the values for biological data in this chapter represent mean values taken from various sources for the normal adult, generally corrected to 1.73 sq. m. of body surface area.

medulla into venules leading to the major venous channels of the kidney. Nearly all the 120 ml. per min. of plasma fluid extracted by the glomeruli is returned, after chemical alteration at various levels of the nephron, to the peritubular capillary system.

Tubular Function

The cells of the nephron* accomplish their regulating functions through both active transport and passive diffusion of ions and molecules between the luminal filtrate and the peritubular blood. Active transport requires metabolic activity by the cells, passive diffusion only specific structural arrangements. Both active transport and passive diffusion may occur in either direction; that is, from lumen to blood or vice versa. Flow in the former direction is referred to as tubular reabsorption; and, when active, the latter directed process is referred to as tubular secretion. Probably all solutes move in both directions, but the disparity of rates in the two directions is so great for most solutes that, in effect, their movement may be considered unidirectional. For some substances, however, the rates of reabsorption and secretion are more nearly equal.

Although reabsorption of some materials may be completed in the proximal convoluted tubule (most notably glucose), many others apparently may be reabsorbed along nearly the full length of the nephron (sodium, chloride, and bicarbonate are examples). Secretion of organic molecules apparently occurs only in the proximal convoluted tubule. On the other hand, hydrogen ions and ammonia may be secreted into the lumen filtrate along nearly the entire length of the nephron, although their largest increments of concentration are known to occur in the distal segments.

The kidneys vary the excretory rate of urine solutes either by varying the rates of reabsorption from the ultrafiltrate back to the blood or, in the case of some solutes, by varying the rates of secretion into the ultrafiltrate from the postglomerular capillary blood. The processes of solute and water transfer by the tubules and ducts are influenced by many factors, including renal blood flow and GFR, type and magnitude of solute load, acid-base status, the activities of endogenous and exogenous metabolic inhibitors, and the level of various hormones. At least two hormones, antidiuretic hormone (ADH) and aldosterone, apparently have as their primary action the control of transport processes in nephron cells.

*For the sake of simplicity, the term "nephron" refers throughout this chapter to collecting ducts as well as renal tubules and their glomeruli.

Flowing at 120 ml. per min., the plasma ultrafiltrate entering the renal tubules will be reduced to an average rate of 1 ml. per min. by the time it issues from the medullary collecting ducts into the renal pelves as urine. This reduction occurs by intricate processes, still not completely comprehended, that occur along segments of the nephron. Apparently luminal fluid is largely reabsorbed by passive diffusion secondary to active sodium transport from filtrate to interstitium and plasma. If a countercurrent multiplier-and-exchange mechanism is active in the kidney, as appears to be the case, fluid reabsorption would be greatly enhanced by the anatomic arrangement and structure of Henle's loops, their contiguous blood channels, and the collecting ducts in the renal medulla.

Along with the net transfer of water from the ultrafiltrate, shifts of various solutes back and forth between nephron lumen and plasma result in either the concentration or dilution of these solutes in the final urinary product as compared to the plasma. Most of this solute movement, as far as total transfer of molecules and ions is concerned, is from nephron lumen to renal interstitium and then to the blood of the peritubular capillaries. Thus, all but about 0.3 to 15.0 ml. (1.0 ml. as a normal average) of total blood volume entering the kidneys each minute is restored to the circulation before the blood leaves these organs, in spite of the initial glomerular extraction of 20 per cent of the ERPF. This small net extraction of modified fluid from the blood is sufficient to balance the volume and composition of body fluid under widely variable conditions because it is continuous for 1440 minutes every day and because the extracted fluid may become drastically altered in its solute composition as it is changed from postglomerular ultrafiltrate to urine. For instance, the urine of man can contain over four times as many milliosmols of total solute per liter as his blood plasma normally contains. With a urine flow of only 0.5 ml. per min., an amount of solute, measured in milliosmols, equivalent to all the solute in the total circulating plasma could be excreted within 24 hours if maximal urine concentration were maintained.

Principles of Renal Clearance

The concept of blood or plasma clearance developed in the 1920's has had important application in the study of renal function. Renal plasma clearance of any substance is expressed as the volume of plasma freed of that substance by renal activity per unit time (usually 1 minute). Depending on the type of substance, clearance may be achieved predominantly by glomerular filtration, by cellular transport at various locations in the nephron, or by a combination of glomerular filtration and cellular function of the nephron. Thus, renal clearance of specific solutes can be usefully related to these components of renal function.

Some typical clearance data in a normal man are the following: 0.2 ml. per min. for glucose, 12 ml. per min. for sulfate, 120 ml. per min. for creatinine, and 400 ml. per min. for phenolsulfonphthalein (PSP). Such clearance data tells nothing about *how* these substances are excreted. When the process of function involved in the excretion of a given solute is known, however, the renal clearance of that solute may then become a useful measurement of that function.

In order to clearly and simply depict the clearance concept, an artificial representation of plasma fluid containing a particular solute flowing through the kidneys is made in Figure 3–1. The example closely approximates the situation occurring in the renal plasma clearance of PSP. Box *a* represents the volume of plasma flowing into functional renal tissue each minute (this will be designated "entrance plasma"). The dots in the box represent the plasma solute.

Box *b* represents the volume of plasma leaving functional kidney tissue per minute (designated "exit plasma") where urine minute volume is 1.0 (urine is excreted at the rate of 1 ml. per min.). The dots are less concentrated in the exit plasma (box *b*) because of renal extraction of solute into the 1 ml. of urine formed each minute. Box *c* represents the same exit plasma volume and solute density as box *b*; however, in *c* the solute has been artificially gathered into a compartment having the same concentration as the entrance plasma (box *a*). This leaves a virtual volume (the cleared volume) which contains none of the solute. This is the volume expressed by the plasma clearance equation; it is the minute volume of plasma cleared of the solute under consideration. Although boxes *b* and *c* are equivalent, box *b* more nearly represents actual exit plasma in the body, while box *c* gives a clearer picture of the virtual volume defined by renal clearance.*

If U_x equals the urine concentration of substance X and V equals urine volume flowing per unit time (usually 1 minute is used), then (U_x) (V) is equivalent to the amount of substance X excreted per unit time. If P_x equals the plasma concentration of substance X and C_x equals the volume of plasma cleared of substance X per unit time, then the amount of X cleared from plasma per unit time is (P_X) (C_X). The amount of any substance excreted in the urine per unit time is equal to the amount cleared from the plasma by the kidneys in that same time; therefore, (P_X) (C_X) equals (U_X) (V).† From this equation, the well-known clearance formula $C_X = \frac{(U_X)\,(V)}{P_X}$ is derived.

In the example of Figure 3–1, the exit plasma has a concentration of 0.8 μg. per ml., whereas entrance plasma has a 2.0 μg. per ml. concentration (each dot represents 44 μg. of solute). Thus, 1.2 μg. of solute is removed from each milliliter of plasma flowing through functional renal tissue per minute, and 793 μg. is removed from 661 ml. of plasma each minute. Since 1 ml. of urine is formed per minute and the solute extracted from the plasma is concentrated in this volume, urine concentration (U_X) is 793 μg. per ml. The plasma concentration in peripheral venous blood usually approximates

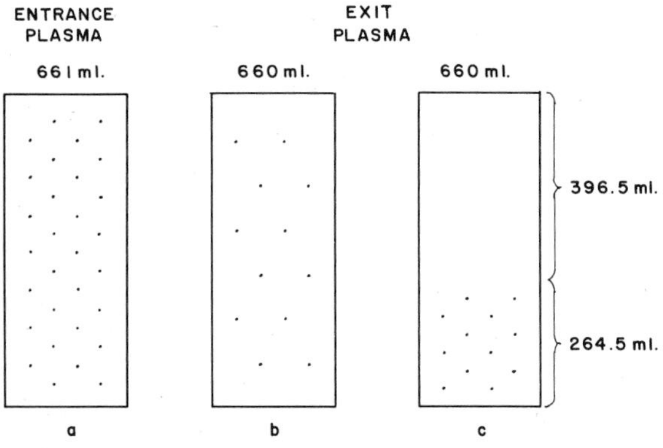

Figure 3–1. Boxes *a* and *b* represent plasma entering and leaving functional kidney tissue each minute. If each dot represents 44 μg. of solute, the concentration in the entrance plasma is 2.0 μg. per ml., while that in the exit plasma is 0.8 μg. per ml. (1.2 μg. per ml. being cleared). The 793 μg. cleared from the entrance plasma by the kidneys each minute (1.2 μg. per ml. solute cleared × 661 ml.) is excreted at a urine concentration (U) of 793 μg. per ml., since the urine output (V) is 1.0 ml. per min. Plasma clearance ($C = \frac{UV}{P}$) therefore equals 793 μg. per ml. (1.0 ml. per min.)/2.0 μg. per ml. = 396.5 ml. per min. Box *c* is an artificial representation of exit plasma and the virtual volume (396.5 ml.) of plasma freed of the solute under consideration. Note that the concentration in the virtual volume not cleared of the solute (264.5 ml.) is the same as that of the entrance plasma.

*Plasma clearance, in the strictest sense, defines the volume of arterial or entrance plasma cleared of the solute per unit of time (note that the cleared volume, 396.5 ml., and the uncleared volume, 264.5 ml., add up to 661 ml., the minute volume of the entrance plasma).

†Actually, with urine flows as high as 2 to 6 ml./min., a period of approximately 30 minutes is required for bladder urine to reach equilibrium with arterial plasma after a constant plasma concentration of any solute is reached (Smith, 1956). The equation (P_X) $(C_X) = (U_X)$ (V) therefore holds only during periods of constant arterial plasma concentration of sufficient length.

entrance plasma concentration. Its value is usually taken as P_X (given in Figure 3–1 as 2.0 μg. per ml.). Therefore, in the example just given, $C_X = \frac{(U_X)(V)}{P_X} = \frac{(793\ \mu g./ml.)\ (1.0\ ml./min.)}{2.0\ \mu g./ml.} =$ 396.5 ml./min.

Since renal clearance always expresses a plasma *volume* cleared of a given substance per unit of time, useful hemodynamic measurements can be acquired from clearance methods. For instance, the clearance of any substance that is excreted solely by glomerular filtration (is neither reabsorbed nor secreted by the nephron) will reflect GFR. Furthermore, if such a substance is completely filterable from the plasma (that is, if it is filtered from glomerular plasma into the ultrafiltrate at the same concentration as in plasma water), its clearance will *equal* the GFR. Several substances are suitable in this regard, but the clearance of inulin (a polymer of fructose) is considered ideal for estimation of GFR.

In addition to determining GFR, the clearance of any substance which is completely extracted from the plasma with each passage through functional kidney tissue will measure ERPF. The clearance of para-aminohippuric acid (C_{PAH}) is taken to represent ERPF because its renal extraction from plasma, at low plasma concentration, approaches 100 per cent in the normal man. Although part of the plasma PAH filters through the glomerular membrane, it is primarily the secretory function of the proximal convoluted tubule which extracts PAH from the peritubular blood and allows the complete (or nearly complete) clearance of plasma circulating through active renal tissue.

Methods of Clearance Measurement

Although inulin clearance (C_{In}) and p-aminohippuric acid clearance (C_{PAH}) are excellent measures of GFR and ERPF, respectively, tests utilizing the clearance of other substances have found more general use in clinical medicine as mirrors of these functions. Furthermore, clearance tests representing other activities of the nephron, such as water and osmol clearance, have received some clinical attention in recent years.

Techniques may be sorted into two categories: exogenous and endogenous clearance methods. In the exogenous type of measurement, clearance is assessed during a continuous infusion of the clearance substance. This infusion may augment the concentration of a material naturally present in plasma, or it may introduce a substance which is normally not present in plasma. In the endogenous method, the clearance of a substance at plasma concentrations which are naturally occurring in plasma is determined (urea and creatinine clearances are examples of such methods).

EXOGENOUS CLEARANCE METHOD

In classic constant-infusion methods of exogenous clearance, a substance is infused intravenously at a rate which provides a constant blood level after an initial loading dose and a period of equilibration in the fluid compartments of the body. For accurate and complete collections of timed urine specimens, the urinary bladder is generally catheterized. Urine flow is increased by oral or intravenous hydration to a high rate, preferably above 2 ml. per min. This helps to minimize errors in urine collection and avoids excessive lag between the time of glomerular filtration and the time of excretion into the collected specimen of each unit of the substance being measured. Three or more carefully timed urine collections, each of 15 to 30 minutes, are made. The bladder is rinsed at the end of each period (the rinse fluid being added to the specimen), and blood is collected at accurately measured intervals during the collection periods, usually at the midpoint of each period. A preinfusion blank sample of blood and of urine should also be taken.

If blood concentrations of the material fluctuate during the urine collection periods, clearance values may be falsely high or low. The plasma concentration of the blood specimen taken during each period must represent the average concentration for that period if the clearance calculation is to be accurate.

For one anticipating the performance of clearance determinations, consultation of the textbook by Smith (1956, pp. 196–202) is recommended.

Several modified exogenous clearance methods have been proposed to circumvent the complications and errors inherent in timed urine collections (Earle and Berliner, 1946; Sapirstein *et al.*, 1955; Blaufox *et al.*, 1963; Slapak and Hume, 1965). These methods utilize single intravenous injection of the clearance substance followed by multiple peripheral blood samplings to monitor the falling concentration curve of the substance injected. Being partly a function of renal clearance, the decay curve is used to calculate clearance. Urine samples are not used. At their present stages of development, however, these methods appear to have either theoretical (Newman *et al.*, 1944; Conn *et al.*, 1964) or practical drawbacks that prevent their general use for diagnostic purposes in humans.

ENDOGENOUS CLEARANCE METHOD

Measuring endogenous clearance offers several advantages over determinations with exogenous substances. Generally speaking, in both health and disease the concentration of many endogenous substances is quite constant from hour to hour. Even in renal disease, the change in concentration of many of these substances is so gradual that, for practical purposes, the concentration over a 24-hour period may be considered constant.* For this reason, urine collection periods can be much longer than 15 to 30 minutes. If such periods are of several hours' duration and the urine output is normal, the errors caused by imperfect timing of sample collection and incomplete bladder emptying are minimized. This means that the patient can void voluntarily, avoiding the discomfort and hazard of bladder catheterization, and one collection period may be sufficient. The patient may even collect the total sample himself at home. The plasma concentration of the substance being measured can be determined by a single blood collection, although more than one collection may be advisable.

CHEMICAL ASSAYS

For chemical assays of urea and creatinine, one may refer to Chapter 9, Clinical Chemistry. Inulin may be measured colorimetrically by hydrolysis to fructose followed by reaction with one of several types of reagents. These include anthrone, diphenylamine, resorcinol, and indolylacetic acid (Roe *et al.*, 1949; Schreiner, 1950; Smith, 1956; Heyrovsky, 1956). PAH may be assayed by the diazotization reaction used for sulfonamides (Bratton and Marshall, 1939; Smith *et al.*, 1945). These methods require protein-free filtrates of plasma. Several reports adapting these methods to automated analysis are now available (Dawborn, 1965; Wright and Gann, 1966; Wilson *et al.*, 1969; Looyé, 1970).

Urea, creatinine, inulin, and PAH may all be measured from the same plasma and urine samples. Several clearances may be simultaneously determined, therefore, in the same individual.

In exogenous clearance studies, analyses may be simplified by the use of radioactively labeled clearance substances, the concentrations of which in urine and plasma may be determined by appropriate counting techniques.

*Exceptions do occur and they should not be overlooked when clearances are being performed in such cases.

MEASUREMENTS OF RENAL FUNCTION

Glomerular Filtration Rate

In the foregoing paragraphs, the clearance of inulin (C_{In}) was described as an accurate measurement of the glomerular filtration rate. Clinical use of this measurement, however, is limited because of the difficulties inherent in any exogenous clearance technique. Other substances whose clearance accurately represents GFR include cyanocobalamin, carboxyl- and allyl-inulin and diatrizoate. These substances may be radioactively labeled, and measured by appropriate radioisotope techniques. In descending order of accuracy, other materials whose clearance approximates GFR are mannitol, other hexitols, creatinine, and urea. Since the latter two substances are endogenous solutes, their use offers the advantages of endogenous clearance determinations.

CREATININE CLEARANCE

The rate of excretion of creatinine is primarily a function of the GFR. The rate of creatinine production in an individual subject is quite constant. If renal excretion is also constant, plasma levels remain rather stable. Even with kidney disease, the rate of excretion usually falls so slowly that plasma levels change very slightly over a 24-hour period. For these reasons, endogenous creatinine clearance has been widely used as a clinical test of renal function. The popularity of this test undoubtedly results from its relative simplicity, as compared with exogenous methods, and also from its greater accuracy than endogenous urea clearance in estimating GFR. The method of creatinine clearance, however, has disadvantages relative to inulin clearance, and it is subject to errors in both method and interpretation.

At normal plasma concentrations a small amount of tubular secretion of creatinine occurs in man. When creatinine concentration in plasma rises above normal, this secretion by the tubules becomes proportionately larger. Because a variable proportion is cleared by tubular secretion in man, creatinine is not an ideal substance with which to estimate GFR. Practically speaking, however, endogenous creatinine clearance agrees fairly closely with inulin clearance in both health and early renal disease (Brod and Sirota, 1948; Doolan *et al.*, 1962). The reason for this agreement in the face of tubular secretion of creatinine may be explained by the "noncreatinine chromogens" of plasma which are measured by the Jaffé reaction (alkaline picrate method) commonly employed to quantitate creatinine. Most of these nonspecific chromogens do not appear in the urine to any significant extent. Their presence in the plasma and absence from the urine thus lower the apparent creatinine clearance to a level comparable to that of inulin. In other words, in the clearance ratio of U_{creat} V/P_{creat}, the value of U_{creat} of the numerator results from glomerular filtration augmented by creatinine secretion, while the value of P_{creat} of the denominator results from plasma creatinine augmented by noncreatinine chromogens in the plasma. Thus, the augmentation of the numerator by creatinine secretion tends to be offset by augmentation of the denominator by chemical inaccuracy, and the resultant value of the clearance ratio for creatinine is fortuitously close to that for inulin.

In advanced renal disease, however, as plasma creatinine levels elevate considerably, the proportion of secreted creatinine increases while the level of noncreatinine chromogens in the plasma remains relatively stable. The effect of this additional creatinine secretion by the tubules is not compensated, and discrepancies between C_{creat} and C_{In} develop.*

The normal concentration of creatinine in plasma is quite low (around 1 mg. per 100 ml.) and the precision of chemical estimation at this level is not good. Thus, precision of creatinine clearance determinations in the normal range is not ideal.

Another source of error for this method (applicable to all endogenous clearances) is inaccurate collection of timed urine samples. The long urine sample period still requires complete collection during a measured period of time. The patient or his attendant must be thoroughly instructed in the details of timing and the routine of collection. If a 24-hour collection is to be made from one morning to the next, the bladder must be emptied the first morning, the time carefully recorded, and all *subsequently* voided urine collected until precisely the same time the following morning, at which time the bladder must be emptied again and this volume included in the collection. If the voided sample prior to the collection period is included in the 24-hour sample, the clearance will be falsely high. If urine samples voided during the collection period are lost or discarded, the clearance will be falsely low. In the laboratory, all the 24-hour urine volume collected must be accurately measured and thoroughly mixed before an aliquot is taken for measurement of creatinine concentration.

Although error caused by incomplete bladder emptying is increased as the collection period is shortened, Doolan *et al.* (1962) found that properly supervised 1-hour collection periods can give acceptable results.

*Four separate studies of patients with renal disease, reviewed by Doolan *et al.* (1962), reported mean ratios of C_{creat}/C_{In} ranging from 1.02 to 1.29. Among individual patient determinations in these series, however, there were ratios as low as 0.49 and as high as 1.86. Although C_{creat} tends to be higher than C_{In} and true GFR by virtue of tubular secretion, some workers have found that normal infants (Brod and Sirota, 1948) and patients with cardiac failure (Baldwin *et al.*, 1950; Miller *et al.*, 1952) have creatinine clearances which are lower than C_{In}.

UREA CLEARANCE

Urea clearance was the first clearance method to be used clinically. Since urea is freely filtered by the glomeruli in the same way as inulin and creatinine, C_{urea} is a measure of GFR. Urea, however, also diffuses across the nephron epithelium; thus, much of this solute is reabsorbed from the ultrafiltrate, and its clearance volume is considerably less than the GFR. Although urea clearance data offer significant information when properly evaluated, creatinine clearances are more easily performed and provide more straightforward interpretation. The reader is referred to the discussion by Shaw and Benson (1969) for a more complete description of urea clearance.

Renal Blood Flow and Effective Renal Plasma Flow

The only means of estimating total renal blood flow (TRBF) is by direct measurement of flow at the renal artery or vein. Since an average of 91 per cent of TRBF perfuses functioning renal tissue (Smith, 1956), ERPF can be used as an index of renal blood flow. One can approximate TRBF rather closely with the following equation:

$$TRBF = ERPF\left(\frac{100}{100\text{–}Hct}\right)\left(\frac{100}{91}\right)$$

There are no known solutes natural to the circulation of man which are suitable for clearance estimation of ERPF. Therefore, such estimations require exogenous clearance methods. Several derivatives of hippuric acid are apparently ideal for measuring ERPF, since they seem to be completely cleared from the plasma which circulates through functioning renal tissue. PAH (p-aminohippuric acid) has been used extensively for clinical and research investigations. Other compounds, such as o-iodohippuric acid, may be synthesized with radioiodine, so their concentrations in plasma and urine are easily determined by radioactive count rate. A less suitable substance is PSP (phenolsulfonphthalein or phenol red), which is not completely cleared from the plasma during each pass through nephron tissue. C_{PSP} values are generally about 60 per cent of those for C_{PAH}. PSP can, however, be quantitated very simply (see later) and, probably for this reason, the substance has been used for a simple excretion test indicating the state of renal blood flow. (See PSP Excretion Test.)

ERPF and GFR may be determined simultaneously in the same subject by performing almost any combination of various exogenous and endogenous clearance tests simultaneously. For example, C_{PAH} and C_{In} can be done by chemical determinations of PAH and inulin on the same plasma and urine specimens. Should radioisotopic methods be desirable, clearances of o-iodohippuric acid (for measuring ERPF) and of diatrizoate (for measuring GFR) can be used. To differentiate these two compounds in the same sample, o-iodohippuric acid may be labeled with ^{131}I and diatrizoate with ^{125}I, or vice versa, and their respective concentrations determined by counting samples in a gamma ray spectrometer.

PSP EXCRETION TEST

The rate of PSP excretion has been one of the most widely used tests for clinical evaluation of renal function for many years. Since the maximum tubular transport mechanism for PSP is far from saturated in normal kidneys at the plasma levels achieved during this test, the rate of its excretion in the urine is proportional to RBF and not to tubular transport capacity (see discussion that follows).

In this test, in an adult, a single intravenous dose of 6 mg. of phenol red (PSP) is administered. One or several urine collections follow the injection. Although the 15-minute urine specimen is by far the most important one, specimens are often obtained precisely 15, 30, 60, and 120 minutes after the dye is given. The patient should be well hydrated so that the excreted PSP is rapidly passed into the bladder urine, and adequate samples can be accurately collected at the standard time intervals. About 600 ml. of water taken orally 30 minutes before the injection usually induces adequate urine flow, but supplementary fluid intake during the test may be necessary to facilitate voiding. An exact dose given in an accurate 1-ml. syringe is injected rapidly, and the exact time of injection is noted. The percentage of the injected dose excreted in each timed specimen is easily determined by the following procedure: Prepare a 100 per cent standard solution by injecting a 1-ml. dose (6 mg.) of phenol red into a 1000-ml. volumetric flask. To this add 5 ml. of 10 per cent sodium hydroxide to develop maximum red color; then dilute to 1000-ml. volume with water. Mix by inversion several times. Prepare 10, 20, 30, 40, and 50 per cent standard solutions by appropriate dilution of aliquots of the 100 per cent standard. Transfer each urine specimen into a separate graduated cylinder. If any specimen is less than 40 ml. in volume, results for that specimen will not be reliable. Add to each specimen 5 ml. of 10 per cent sodium hydroxide to develop color, and then dilute each with water until the color is equivalent to a standard. The per cent of PSP dose in each specimen may then be calculated by photometry or by visual comparison with the series of standards. The calculation is made by comparing the final diluted volume of a specimen to that of the standard having equivalent color intensity. For instance, if a specimen diluted to 1000 ml. compares closely with the 30 per cent standard, then the specimen contains approximately 30 per cent of the PSP dose. If a sample diluted to 500 ml. compares closely with the 30 per cent standard, the sample contains only approximately 15 per cent of the dose. Exact quantitation can be achieved using this principle by interpolation of specimen percentages from photometric readings and a standard curve. In the normal subject, no less than 25 per cent of the injected PSP dose should be excreted in the first 15 minutes. Seventy per cent is usually excreted by 2 hours.

Since the rate of excretion of PSP by the kidneys is proportional to the amount presented to these organs in the blood, this rate is greatest just after the dye is administered, and it falls as plasma concentration decreases with time. If sufficient time is allowed for repeated recirculations of the dye through the kidneys, even those organs with markedly diminished RBF may excrete a relatively normal amount in 1 or 2 hours (Relman and Levinsky, 1963). In this test, therefore, the rate of excretion during the first 15 minutes is the most sensitive measure of RBF. Many conditions impairing renal circulation will depress early PSP excretion. These include cardiac failure, primary vascular diseases, and most primary renal diseases. The test is worthless in evaluating renal function if voluntary voiding of timed urine specimens is used in patients with bladder retention, since excretion from the bladder will be delayed. Conversely, conditions associated with hypoalbuminemia can give falsely high excretion rates (Ochwadt and Pitts, 1956). The apparent reason for this artifact is that normally 80 per cent of the PSP is bound to albumin, from which it must dissociate in the peritubular blood before it is extracted into the urine by the tubular cells. With hypoalbuminemia, therefore, a larger proportion of PSP is not protein bound and can be cleared more rapidly by the tubules.

When proper regard is paid to technique and due caution is taken in interpretation of results, the PSP test may be useful in the detection of renal damage prior to azotemia (Chapman and Halsted, 1933; Relman and Levinsky, 1963). Because rapid hydration may be dangerous to the patient with highly restricted renal function, the test is not recommended in patients with azotemia (Relman and Levinsky, 1963).

Tubular Function Tests

Substances with plasma clearances less than GFR undergo positive net transfer from luminal filtrate to blood across the nephron cells (reabsorption). Conversely, substances with plasma clearances greater than GFR have positive net transfer in the opposite direction. Filtered glucose ($C_{glucose} = 0.2$ ml./min.) is thus almost completely reabsorbed; filtered sulfate ($C_{sulfate} = 12$ ml./min.) is 90 per cent reabsorbed; and filtered PSP ($C_{PSP} = 400$ ml./min.) is greatly augmented by tubular secretion.

The filtered load of a substance presented to the tubules is equal to the product of plasma concentration, glomerular filtration rate, and a constant (f) representing the filterable fraction of the substance in the plasma ($f \cdot P_X \cdot GFR$ or $f \cdot P_X \cdot C_{In}$). The constant (f) is equal to 1 for substances that are freely filtered through the glomerular membranes. Many substances, particularly those that are secreted by the renal tubules, are partially bound to plasma proteins. The average value of f for PAH at plasma levels between 30 and 50 mg. per 100 ml. in man is 0.78, whereas that for PSP at plasma levels between 20 and 40 mg. per 100 ml. is 0.25. The latter value indicates that in the concentration range of from 20 to 40 mg. per 100 ml. PSP is 75 per cent bound to plasma protein (albumin) and only 25 per cent of the dye entering the kidneys is filterable by the glomeruli.

Solute transfer from plasma to urine by tubular secretion is not as restricted by protein binding as is glomerular filtration. The reason for this may be illustrated by the example of PSP. As the unfiltered plasma leaves the glomerulus and begins to pass through the proximal peritubular capillaries, some of the diffusible PSP molecules not bound to protein pass out of the plasma into the interstitial fluid and are transported across the cell into the tubular fluid. This cellular extraction of dye molecules from the interstitium maintains a negative concentration gradient from the peritubular plasma to the interstitial fluid for PSP. As more free dye molecules leave the plasma, more protein-bound molecules dissociate to maintain equilibrium between bound and unbound PSP (75 per cent bound $\rightleftharpoons$ 25 per cent unbound). In the case of PAH, this process continues until all the molecules have dissociated from protein and the plasma has been cleared of its contained PAH before entering the venous circulation.

For a substance such as inulin, which is neither reabsorbed nor secreted by the nephron, the excretion rate is equal to the filtered load ($U_{In} \cdot V = f \cdot P_{In} \cdot GFR$). On the other hand, the excretion rate for a substance such as sulfate is less than the filtered load by the amount of net reabsorption (T_r) which takes place in the nephron ($U_{sulfate} \cdot V = f \cdot P_{sulfate} \cdot GFR - T_{r\ sulfate}$). Tubular reabsorption rate (T_r) thus can be calculated by measuring GFR (usually by C_{In} or C_{creat}) and excretion rate and calculated from $T_{r_X} = f \cdot P_X \cdot GFR - U_X \cdot V$.*

*Clinical use of such measurement is found in the tubular phosphate reabsorption test for parathyroid function. In this test the percentage of filtered phosphate reabsorbed by the tubules is represented by the formula $\%\ TRP = \frac{Tr_{phos}\ (100)}{GFR \cdot P_{phos}}$. With C_{creat} representing GFR, this formula is commonly expressed in the following form:

$$\%\ TRP = \left(1 - \frac{U_{phos} \cdot P_{creat}}{U_{creat} \cdot P_{phos}}\right)\ 100.$$

Excretion of a substance such as PSP is *more* than the filtered load by the amount of net secretion (T_S) that takes place in the nephron ($U_{PSP} \cdot V = f \cdot P_{PSP} \cdot GFR + T_{S_{PSP}}$). Secretory rate may therefore be determined by the same type of measurements used for tubular reabsorption by using the following equation: $T_{S_X} = U_X \cdot V - f \cdot P_X \cdot GFR$.

The clearance of PAH from plasma by normal tubules is related to the capacity of the proximal convoluted tubule to transport many organic compounds from the interstitium into the tubular lumen. A partial list of these compounds (taken from Weiner and Mudge, 1964) includes the following endogenous and exogenous substances: 5-hydroxy-indoleacetic acid, indolylacetic acid, pantothenic acid, oxalic acid, salicylic acid, nitrofurantoin, phenol red, sulfathiazole, probenecid, penicillin G, and chlorothiazide.

Most of the organic molecules secreted by the proximal nephron are not completely cleared from the adjacent blood stream as is PAH; but like PAH, they apparently share transport mechanisms with many other compounds, and all exhibit transport saturation. Thus, the excretion rate of both PSP and penicillin G can be reduced by concomitant administration of either probenecid (Benemid) or PAH; probenecid inhibits tubular secretion of PAH, and the latter inhibits probenecid transport (Weiner and Mudge, 1964). All secreted molecules will saturate their tubular transport mechanisms at a specific renal load (i.e., at a specific plasma level for a given ERPF). For PAH, the venous plasma draining tubular areas is essentially free of this material until the saturation concentration in the "entrance plasma" for a given plasma flow is approached. When this level is reached, further increments in renal load escape extraction from the postglomerular blood. The value for tubular secretion (T_s) at saturation concentration is called the tubular maximum (or tubular maximal secretory rate) and is designated T_m. The tubular maximum can be determined for substances which undergo net reabsorption in the nephron as well as for those which are secreted. For substances which are reabsorbed, T_m is the maximum value of T_r (tubular reabsorption rate) as renal load is increased.

The value of T_m for a given substance is considered to be highly reproducible in each normal individual (Smith, 1951), and a range of values for a population may be defined. Secretion or reabsorption T_m values for various substances (PAH, PSP, glucose) are probably the best quantitative measurements available of functioning tubular mass in the kidneys. In other words, when the T_m for a substance is one-half its normal value, the functioning parenchymal mass of the kidneys is probably reduced by about 50 per cent.

Simple measurements of excretory rate, as in the PSP test, do not properly assess nephron function, because the tubular cells are not necessarily working at saturation levels. With the standard PSP dose, for instance, the plasma level produced is probably no more than one-fifth the concentration which would normally produce a saturation load (Relman and Levinsky, 1963). For the excretion rate of PSP to be depressed at such a plasma concentration, the tubular transport capacity would have to be decreased about 80 per cent. Therefore, in a hypothetical patient with normal ERPF but with 70 per cent depression of $T_{m_{PSP}}$ (corresponding to marked tubular impairment), the PSP excretion rate could be normal. In a patient with 30 per cent reduction in ERPF but relatively normal $T_{m_{PSP}}$, decreased renal load (by virtue of decreased PSP delivery via plasma flow) can be expected to result in depressed excretion of the dye.

Decreased renal perfusion without impairment of tubular function is well known (Smith, 1951; Bradley, 1964); such a patient might have cardiac failure or renal vascular disease. The PSP excretion test thus may well detect depressed RBF in the face of normal tubular function. On the other hand, the combination of severe depression of general tubular function and normal RBF is an unlikely one. Marked impairment of general parenchymal function is usually accompanied or caused by decreased RBF. Abnormal 15-minute PSP excretion in a patient with renal disease may certainly mean that tubular function is impaired, but the direct cause for the poor excretion rate is decreased ERPF.

Although T_m determinations may represent the best quantitative measurements of functioning nephron mass, the complexity of such determinations prevents their general use in clinical medicine. They are performed during intravenous infusions calculated to produce saturation renal loads of the solute studied; they require concurrent determination of GFR by C_{In} or C_{creat}, preferably the former. Because of this, simpler tests of tubular function are necessary. To date, the so-called concentration tests have received the widest clinical attention.

CONCENTRATION TESTS

Urine solute concentration above that of the glomerular ultrafiltrate of plasma depends primarily on tubular ability to transport sodium from luminal filtrate in such a way that solute concentration in the renal medulla is higher than that of plasma. This process, in turn, depends on the anatomic integrity of the medulla, which enables the tubular and vascular loops to act, as they apparently do, as countercurrent multipliers and countercurrent exchangers, respectively. This mechanism accounts for the increasing osmotic pressure found in the kidney extending from the corticomedullary junction to the tip of the renal papillae. This high osmotic pressure probably acts effectively as a pump by which water may be drawn from the glomerular filtrate in the collecting duct in the final concentration process before the filtrate escapes into the renal pelvis as urine. Under hydrated conditions, when ADH secretion is inhibited and circulating levels are low, the collecting duct epithelium of normal kidneys is apparently quite impermeable to water. Little water can be drawn from the duct lumen. Urine flow is consequently high and the solute concentration low. During dehydration, however, ADH secretion is stimulated and circulating levels of this factor increase. With normal renal function, this results in decreased urine flow and high urinary solute concentration. A large part of the process of urine concentration during dehydration is believed to be due to an increased permeability of the collecting duct epithelium to water, resulting in osmotic flow of luminal water into the medullary interstitium and capillaries. The degree of permeability apparently depends on the level of circulating ADH.

The most common techniques used in concentration tests are those of measuring specific gravity, refractive index, or osmolality of the urine by the use of simple and convenient devices. A simple hydrometer (commonly referred to as a urinometer) may be used for specific gravity. A light refractometer is used for refractive index measurement (the measured refractive index is usually calibrated in terms of total urinary solids or specific gravity). Osmometers employing the principle of freezing-point depression have been the most popular instruments used in measuring osmolality.

Determinations of total solute concentration, as they are usually performed, do not give the same functional information as T_m determinations, but they have similar implications as far as renal disease is concerned. To enlarge on this point, it should be noted that the major solutes of the urine (sodium, potassium, chloride, and urea) undergo the largest increases in concentration in urine flowing through nephron segments located in the renal *medulla*. On the other hand, tubular disposition of such specific solutes as glucose and PAH, commonly used for T_m measurements, is primarily a function of *cortical* segments. Furthermore, the process of concentration of the major urinary solutes is extremely sensitive to such factors as postural hemodynamic changes, variation in solute load, ionic composition, and osmolality of body fluids and various hormones (notably ADH). Urine solute concentration can range in physiologic circumstances from below 100 to above 1000 mOsm. per kg. of urine water. T_m values are considerably less variable (Smith, 1951; Bradley, 1964).

Keeping in mind the limitations just discussed, inability to concentrate the urine may indicate tubular dysfunction. The use of a 12- to 24-hour period of strict fluid deprivation is the most frequently used method of invoking a stimulus to the concentrating ability of the tubules under controlled conditions. Of course, if normal concentrating ability is noted in a randomly collected urine sample, the use of a concentration test becomes needless.*

The Fishberg concentration test (Fishberg, 1954) is performed as follows: The patient has his usual breakfast, including fluids. After this he takes no more liquids until the test is completed. Lunch and dinner may be eaten, but all fluids are omitted. High protein intake is encouraged if the subject is not azotemic. All urine voided until the following morning may be discarded. On awakening in the morning, the patient voids and the specimen is saved. Remaining in bed after the first void, the patient voids again 1 hour later. He is then up and about for another hour before he passes the third specimen. The patient has by then had approximately 24 hours in which to concentrate his urine, generally with little inconvenience. The specific gravity of each of the three specimens is then measured. If renal tubular function is normal, the specific gravity of at least one of the specimens will exceed 1.022 and may be 1.032 or higher.

Fishberg (1954) points out that diuresis of edema fluid may produce low specific gravity after the dehydration period and thereby simulate renal impairment and that a spontaneous nocturnal diuresis is common in patients with hypertension and cardiac failure. In such cases, the third morning specimen may be more concentrated than the first.

A more comfortable test for the patient, and one which is adequate for routine testing (Relman and Levinsky, 1963), requires withholding fluids from the patient following dinner and throughout the night. The subject voids after awakening the following day, and the specific gravity of the specimen voided next is determined. The specific gravity of this specimen should be 1.026 or above in normals. If the specific gravity is lower, fluid restriction is continued another 6 hours and a new urine sample is tested.

When osmolality is measured, the normal individual is expected to concentrate urine to a value of 850 mOsm. per kg. or higher. This value is based on a study involving a 14-hour dehydration period (Jacobson *et al.*, 1962). Wolf (1962) gives a range for normal refractive index of urine in a renal concentration test as 1.3413 to 1.3462 at 22° C and a corresponding range of total solids of 5.4 to 8.5 gm. per 100 gm. urine.

In all concentration tests the subject should be on a normal diet and consuming normal quantities of water prior to the test. Certain dietary constituents enhance solute concentration, protein being very important in this regard. Chronic, excessive water intake prior to a concentration test may produce submaximal concentration by normal kidneys (Fishberg, 1954; Relman and Levinsky, 1963).

*The physician must be wary of interpreting a specific gravity measured on urine within a short period following a radiographic test in which intravenous radiopaque dye has been employed. High-density dye molecules can produce very high specific gravities in spite of impaired renal concentration. Whenever urine specific gravity is higher than 1.035 in any individual, radiocontrast dye or other abnormal solutes in the urine should be suspected.

Obviously the patient must not be taking diuretics. Glucosuria invalidates a concentration test by virtue of its diuretic effect. Proteinuria does not in itself cause a diuresis, however, and a valid test may be performed in the presence of this condition. For each 10 gm. of protein per liter of urine (1 per cent proteinuria), a value of 0.003 should be subtracted from the observed specific gravity because of the influence of heavy protein molecules on this measurement.

A few subjects who have normal kidney function in all other respects may not achieve maximal urinary concentration prior to 18 to 24 hours of dehydration (Fishberg, 1954). In addition, the dehydration period sometimes must be discontinued prematurely because of the patient's discomfort or indications of serious impairment of his clinical status. In these cases the concentration test may be replaced by a test in which ADH (vasopressin) is used. The ADH is then administered *without* fluid restriction; urine samples are collected and tested within a few hours of administration (Relman and Levinsky, 1963). If kidney function is normal, urine concentration values will reach or closely approach those in dehydration tests. ADH should not be given to patients with coronary artery disease, however, because of its vasopressor effects.

Technical points of importance for specific gravity tests are as follows: (1) The temperature of the urine at the time of measurement should be that at which the hydrometer has been calibrated; (2) proper and standardized technique in reading the urinometer must be carried out by those involved with this responsibility; otherwise, accuracy and reproducibility can be seriously jeopardized (Galambos *et al.*, 1964). For a discussion of these and other important considerations in the use of urinometers, the reader is referred to the textbook by Henry (1964) and to Chapter 2 of this text.

Additional discussion of refractive index and osmolality determinations are found in Chapters 2 and 12 of this text.

Conditions other than renal disease may account for impaired concentration of the urine. In diabetes insipidus, the posterior pituitary gland and hypothalamus may fail to respond to the stimulus of increasing osmolality of body fluid by secretion of ADH. Nephrogenic diabetes insipidus is a rare condition in which kidney function is normal except for an inability to respond to ADH. As mentioned above, diuresis can impair nephron capacity to concentrate solutes in normal kidneys. This diuresis results from osmotic or pharmacologic diuretic agents, or it may be caused by increased GFR associated with augmented cardiac output or improved renal circulation. Finally, abnormalities in body fluid composition (such as those accompanying hypercalcemia or hypokalemia) can result in reversibly depressed concentrating ability by the kidney tubules.

Like concentration, dilution of total urinary solutes is a nephron function and can be used as a test of renal performance.

A normal individual should dilute his urine to a

specific gravity of less than 1.003 during a 3-hour period following a 1-liter intake of water (Relman and Levinsky, 1963). The water is taken over a 30-minute period, and urine may be collected at intervals over the following 3 hours.

Dilution tests are a far less critical gauge of renal function than concentration tests. Their significance, relating to renal tubular function, is probably also dependent on different factors than those related to concentrating ability. Dilution tests employing rapid hydration should be avoided in azotemic patients.

Specific Gravity vs. Refractive Index vs. Osmolality

The specific gravity of urine depends primarily upon the density of the various kinds of solute molecules and their respective numbers in solution. The same osmolal or total solids concentration of two species of solute may produce solutions with considerably different specific gravities. The great advantages of gravimetric determinations, however, are the low cost of equipment and the simplicity and rapidity of the method.

The refractive index of a solution depends on the concentration of its dissolved solutes. In pure solutions this dependence is linear (or nearly linear) when the concentration is expressed in terms of solute weight per solution volume (w/v). Since there is a high correlation between the refractive index of urine specimens and the total concentration of their dissolved solutes (Rubini and Wolf, 1957), this method appears to be rather insensitive to differences in the type of urinary solutes. Some refractometers are calibrated in terms of specific gravity and/or per cent total solids (gm. per 100 ml.). For the specific gravity calibration to be completely valid, either each type of solute in urine must have the same density per unit concentration by weight or there must be constant ratios between the various solute concentrations in all urine specimens. Because neither condition truly exists, this calibration (specific gravity) is based on a normalized chemical constitution of urine. Measurement with a refractometer is simple and rapid and requires only a few drops of urine.

Osmolality depends entirely on the number of primary particles (both undissociated molecules and ions) effectively in solution. Mathematically this is expressed by $\varnothing \cdot N \cdot C$, in which C is the molality (or number of mols. of a given compound in each kilogram of water); N is the number of particles into which each molecule of the compound dissociates in solution; and $\varnothing$ is the osmotic coefficient of the respective molecules or ions. For single univalent ions, this coefficient is approximately 0.9 at urine concentrations and is generally less for bivalent and trivalent ions. With ideal nonelectrolyte molecules, the coefficient is 1. With modern instrumentation, osmolality can be accurately determined with small samples (down to 0.2 ml.). The method is relatively simple and rapid but not so much so as gravimetry or refractometry.

It is clear that these three methods commonly used to measure total solute concentration in urine do not give equivalent information, since the proportions of urinary constituents are variable. Thus, to raise the specific gravity 0.001 at 15° C., 3.595 gm. of urea or 1.473 gm. of sodium chloride must be added to a liter of urine.* The osmolality of the resulting urine solution would be raised 60 mOsm. per kg. by such an addition of urea or about 47 mOsm. per kg. by the sodium chloride. Not only are ratios of normal urinary substances variable within the normal as well as the diseased population, but abnormal solutes, such as glucose, protein, and ketones, *are* known to have markedly different *effects* on specific gravity, total solids, and osmolality.

The words "concentration" and "dilution" of urine are intended to describe the degree to which the nephron changes solute density above or below that of the plasma ultrafiltrate, respectively, before it is excreted as urine. Implicit in such a description is an assumed normal value of this ultrafiltrate. Plasma has a mean total solids concentration of 8 per cent and mean specific gravity of 1.025. The values for plasma ultrafiltrate would be considerably lower, however, by virtue of the large contribution of plasma proteins to both parameters (about 7 per cent to total solids and 0.018 to specific gravity). While the large, dense protein molecules in plasma have considerable effect on these measurements, they have relatively little effect on plasma osmolality. Sodium, chloride, and bicarbonate normally account for 90 per cent or more of plasma osmolality, the normal mean value being 285 mOsm. per kg. of plasma water. Approximately 2 mOsm. per kg. are contributed by protein. The osmolality of plasma ultrafiltrate, therefore, does not appreciably differ from that of plasma.

Although the solute concentration of the glomerular filtrate varies little from one patient to another, there are occasional cases in which the variation may be sufficiently great that a comparison of final urine concentration to that of the plasma ultrafiltrate is desirable. This is particularly true in patients in whom primary or secondary alteration of renal function seems likely (polyuric subjects who may have chronic pyelonephritis, diabetes insipidus, or hypokalemic nephropathy serve as examples). Since there is no practical method of measuring plasma ultrafiltrate directly, the simplest means of comparison is that of measuring plasma and urine osmolality. This comparison is valid from a practical standpoint because the osmolality of the glomerular filtrate is roughly 99 per cent of that for plasma. Neither refractive index nor specific gravity of urine can be conveniently compared to that of plasma because of the large and variable protein effect on such measurements in the latter fluid.

In one study (Jacobson *et al.*, 1962), 26 normal subjects had serum osmolalities ranging from 280 to 307 after a 14-hour fluid fast. Urine osmolalities ranged from 855 to 1335, while specific gravities ranged from 1.018 to 1.029 in these subjects, and the urine to plasma osmolal ratios (U_{osm}/P_{osm}) fell between 3.0 and 4.7. In the same study, serum osmolality values varied from 270 to 322 in 58 patients with chronic renal disease after the 14-hour dehydration period. Urine osmolality and specific gravity ranged from 255 to 1082 and from 1.005 to 1.027, respectively. The U_{osm}/P_{osm} ratio varied from 0.8 to 3.8 in this group. Only 11 of the 58 patients were able to

---

*Taken from the data of Albarran as presented by Fishberg (1954).

develop U_{osm}/P_{osm} values of 3.0 or more with urine osmolalities of 850 or higher.

The concentrating and diluting ability of the kidneys can be quantitatively expressed by use of osmol and free water clearance determinations. Such studies require only endogenous clearance techniques and simple measurement of urine and plasma osmolality.

Osmol clearance represents the volume of plasma water cleared of its solutes (or osmotic pressure) per unit time ($C_{osm} = \frac{U_{osm} \bullet V}{P_{osm}}$). Free water clearance (C_{H_2O}) is measured by subtracting osmol clearance per unit time from urine output per unit time ($C_{H_2O} = V - C_{osm}$). When its value is positive, C_{H_2O} represents the volume of solute-free water cleared from plasma per unit time. When its value is negative, C_{H_2O} is the volume of osmotically free water *added* to the plasma per unit time (or cleared from the tubular filtrate). Negative C_{H_2O} may be expressed positively as $T^{C}_{H_2O}$ (tubular reabsorption rate for osmotically free water). C_{H_2O} is positive when the urine is being diluted ($U_{osm}/P_{osm} < 1.0$), and it is negative when the urine is being concentrated ($U_{osm}/P_{osm} > 1.0$).

URINE pH AND TITRATABLE ACIDITY

Additional tubular function tests are urine pH and titratable acidity. The reaction of the urine varies ordinarily from pH 5.6 to 6.6, with extremes of pH 4.4 to 8.0 under nonphysiologic conditions (Milne, 1963). Hydrogen ion (H^+) is excreted in the urine in several forms. It may be bound to ammonia as ammonium ion; it may be buffered by certain anions, phosphate and organic anions predominating; or it may exist as free H^+. Although the latter form of hydrogen ion is almost a negligible fraction of the total excreted, it is the concentration of this form that accounts for the pH of the urine.

Titratable acidity of urine may be defined as the mEq. of H^+ neutralized by titrating the 24-hour output of urine with base to the pH of plasma (pH 7.4 at body temperature or pH 7.56 at 25° C). This titration neutralized free H^+ and most of the H^+ buffered by organic anions and monohydrogen phosphate. It does not neutralize ammonium ion hydrogen.

A normal individual on an average mixed diet excretes 30 to 50 mEq. of H^+ each day as ammonium ion and from 10 to 30 mEq. as titratable acid. An abnormal acid load to the kidneys can increase the excretion of both forms of H^+ five- to tenfold (Pitts, 1945).

In chronic renal failure, reduction of nephron mass results in a decreased ability to synthesize ammonia. Less H^+ can be excreted as a consequence, and systemic acidosis may develop even though the urine may continue to have a low pH. The ability to produce a high H^+ gradient between urine and plasma may be well preserved in uremia, although the daily excretion of ammonium ion and buffer anions is reduced. In addition, the ratio of urinary ammonia to titratable acid falls in chronic renal failure (Pitts, 1963).

In renal tubular acidosis the ability to produce the normal pH gradient between urine and plasma is lost. Renal tubular acidosis may be defined as an inability to acidify urine to a pH of 5.4 or lower under the stimulus of ammonium chloride ingestion (12 gm. daily for three days) or of spontaneous metabolic acidosis (Milne, 1963). Although the patient with tubular acidosis has a tendency to develop systemic acidosis, plasma pH and bicarbonate concentrations are usually within the normal range in nonazotemic cases.

For a discussion of causes and types of renal tubular acidosis, the reader is referred to the chapter by Milne (1963, pp. 826–831).

INTERPRETATION OF RESULTS

The aims of renal function testing in clinical medicine are the detection of renal impairment as early as possible in its course and the quantitative measure of change in function with time. Although function tests may detect kidney disease well before symptoms develop, and demonstrate large increments of damage prior to definite elevation of nitrogenous products in plasma, they are of little diagnostic value in determining the *etiology* of renal disease. Etiologic diagnosis is still largely based on patient history, physical findings, and examination of urinary sediment early in the course of renal disease. In addition, urine chemistry and culture, x-ray examination, renal biopsy, and other tests are often necessary to assess pathogenesis.

The most widely used renal function tests for clinical purposes at present are relatively simple ones, such as endogenous creatinine clearance, PSP excretion rate, and total solute concentration tests. The following discussion will be concerned with these tests and the physiologic changes which occur during the course of chronic progressive renal failure. Patterns of physiologic change will be generalized and, therefore, an approximation of those encountered in most chronic diseases. Discussion of acute, potentially reversible diseases of the kidneys has been omitted. It should be understood that such processes as acute tubular necrosis ("shock kidneys") and acute glomerulonephritis and pyelonephritis are accompanied by transient and sometimes severe depressions of function followed by complete or partial recovery if the patient survives the acute phase. Acute glomerulonephritis and pyelonephritis may occur also as recurrent episodes in a process of chronic progressive disease. In such cases, sudden and often marked disturbances of function occur that are superimposed on chronically impaired functional patterns.

Numerous pathologic mechanisms, both systemic and focal in origin, can produce chronic renal failure. The explanation of impaired kidney function, however, may be reduced to fairly simple terms. No matter if the process is located primarily in the glomeruli or tubules, vessels or interstitium, cortex or medulla, the affected kidneys may be considered to be composed of three types of nephrons. First, there are the destroyed nephrons, which no longer function. Second, there are those undergoing destruction and atrophy but having some degree of residual function. The third type of nephrons are those not yet significantly involved by the disease process. The following description of functional variation with renal tissue loss is based on the "intact nephron theory" of chronic renal failure, which assumes that residual function depends primarily on the number of residual, intact nephrons that have undergone varying degrees of "compensatory hypertrophy". Although the "intact nephron theory" may represent an oversimplification of the true circumstances, it is helpful in explaining functional data accompanying chronic renal failure.

Creatinine Clearance and Plasma Concentration

Plasma creatinine concentration (P_{creat}) does not adequately reflect early renal damage. Besides analytical imprecision in its estimation, its value in detecting early functional impairment may be obscured by compensatory increases in creatinine excretion.

Figure 3–2 illustrates the relationship between plasma concentration and clearance of creatinine and the number of functioning residual nephrons. It assumes a constant daily creatinine formation in the body of 1728 mg. (a value within the normal range arbitrarily chosen for convenience) and a creatinine clearance of 120 ml. per min., corresponding to a full complement of renal subunits (two million nephrons). Figure 3–2 *A* ignores the effect of nephron hypertrophy in order to conceptually isolate the first explanation for poor early sensitivity of P_{creat} to changed function. Before the onset of kidney damage, plasma creatinine concentration is 1.0 mg. per 100 ml. Daily creatinine excretion rate = daily plasma clearance rate × plasma concentration = 120 ml./min. × 1440 min./day × 0.01 mg./ml. = 1728 mg. = daily formation rate. Obviously, so long as excretion and formation rates are equal, plasma concentration remains constant.

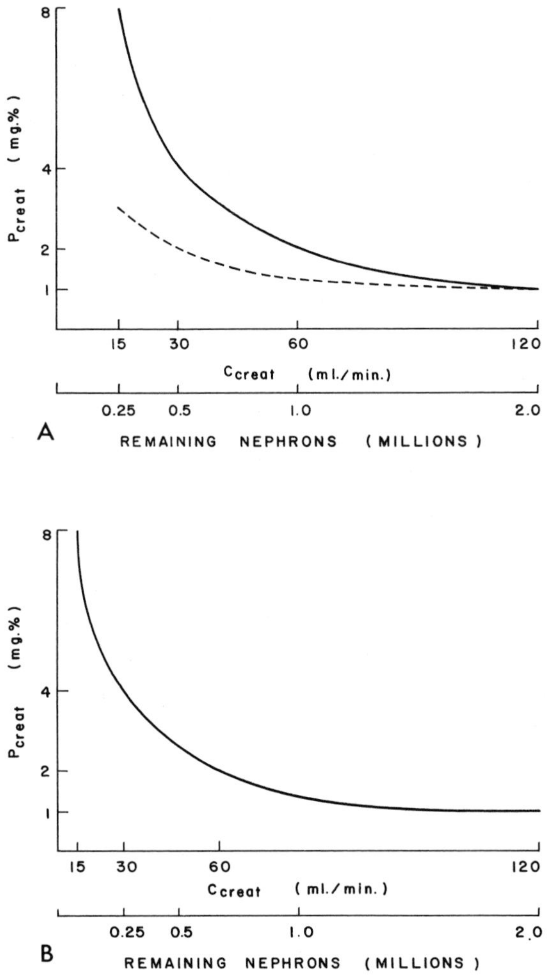

Figure 3–2. *A*, Plasma creatinine concentration (P_{creat}) as a function of creatinine clearance (C_{creat}) and number of residual nephrons. The graph does not allow for nephron hypertrophy (see text). *B*, Plasma creatinine concentration (P_{creat}) as a function of creatinine clearance (C_{creat}) and number of residual nephrons. Graph assumes progressive nephron hypertrophy with advancing disease (see text).

If, for example, one million nephrons are destroyed over a period of days, months, or years and one million intact nephrons remain, creatinine clearance (C_{creat}) will fall to 60 ml. per min. providing there is no hypertrophy of the remaining nephrons (following the solid line in Figure 3–2 *A*). P_{creat} will subsequently become elevated, eventually reaching or approaching a level at which the remaining renal subunits are able to excrete the 1728 mg. of creatinine formed each day.* At a P_{creat} of 2.0

*Formation rate for creatinine remains fairly constant until late in the course of renal disease (Relman and Levinsky, 1963).

mg. per 100 ml., excretion rate again equals formation rate if the clearance remains at 60 ml. per min. (60 ml. per min. × 1440 min. per day × 0.02 mg. per ml. = 1728 mg. per day). If the disease does not progress beyond this point (*only* one million nephrons are destroyed), P_{creat} will eventually reach the level of 2.0 mg. per 100 ml. and remain there. Each remaining nephron thus will excrete twice as much creatinine per unit volume of glomerular filtrate, on the average, as it did before the onset of the disease. A higher P_{creat} produces a larger creatinine load per nephron to bring formation and excretion into new equilibrium. If renal parenchyma is progressively destroyed, however, in rapid continuous or discontinuous steps, P_{creat} may only *approach* a concentration at which equilibrium between formation and excretion is again established (illustrated by broken line in Figure 3–2 *A*).

Consider Figure 3–2 *A* as representing the relationship between plasma creatinine and creatinine clearance found in a patient with progressive renal failure. The solid line would then connect several points found during the course of slow, steady destruction of nephrons; there is adequate time for the plasma level to rise and establish a balance between formation and excretion prior to the next decrement of nephrons. The broken line connects points found during a more rapid course of destruction in which P_{creat} can only approach a level at which new formation-excretion equilibrium is established.

Figure 3–2 *B* illustrates the effect of nephron hypertrophy on the relationship between plasma concentration and clearance and the extent of slowly progressive kidney damage. Although the scale for creatinine clearance values is different from that in Figure 3–2 *A*, the solid line relationship between P_{creat} and C_{creat} in the two figures is actually the same (e.g., P_{creat} of 2.0 mg. per 100 ml. at C_{creat} of 60 ml. per min., and so on). In Figure 3–2 *B*, however, a loss of one million nephrons produces a decrease in clearance to 75 ml. per min. rather than the expected 60 ml. per min. The change in clearance scale illustrates the effect of a 25 per cent functional hypertrophy of the remaining units.

At one-quarter million nephrons, there has been nearly 100 per cent hypertrophy in function per average nephron, since clearance is nearly 30 ml. per min. rather than 15 ml. per min. without hypertrophy (see Figure 3–2 *A* and *B*). The relationship between plasma concentration, clearance, and the remaining nephrons in this illustration applies to slow disease progression, in which intact nephrons have time to undergo steady increments of hypertrophy. The reader must understand that the dependency shown here between clearance and nephron numbers is based on estimation and not on actual measurements. The proper location of clearance values along the abscissa corresponding to given degrees of kidney destruction (as in Fig. 3–2 *B*) in an individual case of renal disease depends on the degree of hypertrophy occurring after progressive decrements in nephron number. This, in turn, probably depends on several factors, including the nature of the disease, its rate of progression, the metabolic and circulatory state of the patient, and other variables.

Values of plasma creatinine corresponding to given clearance levels must also be variable from one case to another. They will certainly depend on the rate of creatinine formation in a given individual. They will also depend on the accuracy and precision of the method used to measure creatinine. With rapidly progressive renal disease, they vary with the rate at which clearance is falling.

As a consequence of many factors, therefore, it is apparent that the kidneys may be severely damaged when, by current methods and definitions, the plasma creatinine level is still normal. This points out the importance of renal function tests, such as creatinine clearance, in the detection of early kidney impairment. Figure 3–2 illustrates that plasma creatinine is a reliable index only after advanced destruction (beyond 50 per cent tissue loss).

The type of hyperbolic relationship illustrated in Figure 3–2 between plasma or serum creatinine and renal function also is seen in the case of other nitrogenous products. Measurement of creatinine has an advantage over measurement of other nitrogenous compounds in that changes in concentration of creatinine are highly specific for alterations of renal function. Because rate of formation of creatinine depends almost exclusively on body muscle mass and its elimination almost entirely on the GFR, its circulating concentration is quite insensitive to factors such as hydration, diet, and metabolic status. This is not the case with urea, uric acid, or the concentration of total nonprotein nitrogen.

PSP Excretion

During the course of renal failure, if effective plasma flow is reduced in rough proportion to that of glomerular filtration rate, decreased PSP excretion rates should correlate well with decreased creatinine or urea clearances. Although data to substantiate this expectation are scarce, one study comparing urea clearance with 15-minute PSP excretion in 254 patients with renal disease supports this suggestion (Freyberg, 1935). Clinical experience also indicates, however, that each of these tests may at times give evidence of poor function when the other is normal. In some cases this disparity may result from variations in the relationship between glomerular filtration rate and renal plasma flow.

Because of susceptibility of the PSP test to technical errors, including failure to inject an exact amount of dye and collect the full volume of urine excreted in the first 15 minutes, the creatinine clearance test is probably a more reliable function test for clinical use.

Concentration Tests

Concentration tests generally reflect progressive inability of the kidneys to increase the osmotic pressure of urine above that of the glomerular filtrate in chronic renal failure. If residual function is primarily the result of intact nephrons, defective concentrating ability may be explained in two general ways. First, an increased load of solutes presented to the remaining functioning nephrons produces a constant osmotic diuresis. Secondly, although residual units may themselves be capable of optimum performance, nephron functions such as osmotic concentration of the urine are to some extent dependent on the anatomic relationships between segments of adjacent nephrons (particularly the loops of Henle, the collecting ducts, and the vascular loops in the renal medulla). When this relationship is disturbed by the loss of intervening nephrons and by interstitial cellular infiltrates and scarring, the countercurrent concentrating mechanism will also be disturbed.

Generally speaking, total loss of urinary concentrating ability with fixed specific gravity near 1.010 (or osmolality between 300 and 400 mOsm. per kg.) is not seen until very late in the course of renal disease – at about 10 to 20 per cent of normal urea clearance (Freyberg, 1935; Relman and Levinsky, 1963). Occasionally subnormal concentrating ability is seen when other function tests indicate little or no renal damage (Freyberg, 1935).

Tests for Renal Ischemia Producing Hypertension

Lowered arterial pressure in the kidney stimulates the release of renin from juxtaglomerular cells into the blood stream. Renin is an enzyme which, with other plasma factors, generates the octapeptide, angiotensin II. This peptide can produce an increase in systemic blood pressure through its vasoconstrictive effect and an increase in the secretion of aldosterone by the adrenal gland. When lowered renal arterial pressure is caused by a systemic hypotension, renin release may compensate for the hypotension by the vasoconstrictive action of angiotensin and the fluid retention effect of aldosterone. If, however, arterial pressure in the kidney is low owing to a local process (in the vascular tree or parenchyma of the kidney itself), high blood concentration of renin resulting from the ischemic kidney may cause systemic arterial hypertension. However, a direct causal relation between renin levels and hypertension or between normal control of blood pressure and the renin-angiotensin system has not been demonstrated. Hence, we encounter in the literature guarded statements such as elevated blood renin activity may be "associated with" rather than "cause" certain types of hypertension.

Non-nephrogenic, benign phase hypertension is ordinarily associated with mild depression, normal, or mild elevation of renin activity in the blood. The malignant or accelerated phase of any type of hypertension, however, is usually associated with very high renin levels. Renin activity is very low when hypertension is caused by primary aldosteronism.

Thus, renin assays may be very helpful in evaluating the cause of hypertension in patients with early disease. Distinctly high renin activity suggests a renal or renovascular lesion, although peripheral vein renin activity is not always elevated in renovascular hypertension. Normal to low activities suggest other mechanisms. When peripheral blood renin remains low in a subject following salt deprivation and ambulant posture for several hours, primary aldosteronism is suggested.

Often it is necessary to catheterize the inferior vena cava in order to collect renal vein samples for renin assays. In a patient with systemic hypertension and radiologic or other evidence to indicate unilateral renal ischemic atrophy, marked elevation of renin in the venous blood from the atrophic kidney over that of the opposite kidney is generally taken as an indication of operable renal hypertension. Oftentimes reconstructive surgery or unilateral nephrectomy will cure or greatly alleviate this hypertension. Maximum stimulation (e.g., low salt diet, upright position, possibly diuretics) should be employed for renal vein sampling to reduce the incidence of falsely negative renin results. (See Chapter 11.)

Many methods of measuring renin activity are available, including a commercial kit based on the radioimmunoassay of Haber *et al.* (1969). There is probably not yet available, however, a renin concentration assay which can be reliably performed in most clinical laboratories.

So-called split or differential renal function tests may be done to detect renal artery obstruction with ischemia. These tests may substitute for, or complement, renin assays. They are based on the finding that an ischemic kidney will retain sodium and water while greatly concentrating other urinary solutes. These tests are technically based on complete and separate collection of urine from each kidney. This requires ureteral catheterization. The volumes of urine collected over a period of time are measured exactly, and the urine samples from each side are analyzed for various solutes. The Howard Test (Connor *et al.,* 1960) is based on determination of sodium and creatinine concentration in the urines of each kidney. Other variations of split function tests include measurement of PSP, PAH, osmolality, urea-creatinine ratios, and so on. The criteria for the diagnosis of unilateral renal ischemia using the Howard Test are the following: (1) a 60 per cent reduction in urine volume, (2) a 15 per cent decrease in sodium concentration, and (3) a 50 per cent increase in creatinine concentration in the urine from the affected kidney as compared to the presumed normal kidney. A high percentage of patients with unilateral renal artery obstruction causing hypertension will exhibit positive split function results, whereas these tests are usually negative with parenchymal disease even when it is the apparent cause of hypertension (Dossetor *et al.,* 1970).

REFERENCES

Baldwin, D. S., Sirota, J. H., and Villareal, H.: Diurnal variations of renal function in congestive heart failure. Proc. Soc. Exp. Biol. Med. 74:578, 1950.

Blaufox, M. D., Frohmuller, H. G. W., Campbell, J. C., Tuz, D. C., Orvis, A. L., and Owen, C. A., Jr.: A simplified method of estimating renal function with iodohippurate-I^{131}. J. Surg. Res. *3*:122, 1963.

Blaufox, M. D., Sanderson, D. R., Tauxe, W. N., Wakim, K. G., Orvis, A. L., and Owen, C. A.: Plasmatic diatrizoate-I^{131} disappearance and glomerular filtration in the dog. Amer. J. Physiol. *204*:536, 1963.

Bradley, S. E.: Clearance studies of nephron dysfunction in shock. Fed. Proc. *23*:689, 1964.

Bratton, A. C., and Marshall, E. K., Jr.: A new coupling component for sulfanilamide determination. J. Biol. Chem. *128*:537, 1939.

Brod, J., and Sirota, J. H.: The renal clearance of endogenous "creatinine" in man. J. Clin. Invest. 27:645, 1948.

Chapman, E. M., and Halsted, J. A.: The fractional phenolsulphonphthalein test in Bright's disease. Amer. J. Med. Sci. *186*:223, 1933.

Conn, R. B., Sabo, A. J., Landes, D., and Ho, J. Y. L.: Inconstancy of renal clearance values with changing plasma concentrations. Nature (London) *203*:143, 1964.

Connor, T. B., Thomas, W. C., Jr., Haddock, L., and Howard, J. E.: Unilateral renal disease as a cause of hypertension: Its detection by ureteral catheterization studies. Ann. Intern. Med. 52:544, 1960.

Dawborn, J. K.: Application of Heyrovsky's inulin method to automatic analysis. Clin. Chim. Acta *12*:63, 1965.

Doolan, H. P., Alpen, E. L., and Thiel, G. B.: A clinical appraisal of the plasma concentration and endogenous clearance of creatinine. Amer. J. Med. *32*:65, 1962.

Dossetor, J. B., Fam, W., Gutelius, J. R., Turgeon-Knaack, C., and Morehouse, D. D.: Differential renal function studies in the diagnosis of renal hypertension. Canad. Med. Ass. J. *102*:500, 1970.

Earle, D. P., and Berliner, R. W.: A simplified clinical procedure for measurement of glomerular filtration rate and renal plasma flow. Proc. Soc. Exp. Biol. Med. 62:262, 1946.

Fishberg, A. M.: Hypertension and Nephritis. 5th edition. Philadelphia, Lea & Febiger, 1954.

Freyberg, R. H.: The choice and interpretation of tests of renal physiology. J.A.M.A. *105*:1575, 1935.

Galambos, T. T., Herndon, E. G., and Reynolds, G. H.: Specific gravity determination. Fact or fancy? New Eng. J. Med. *270*:506, 1964.

Haber, E., Koerner, T., Page, L. B., Kliman, B., and Purnode, A.: Application of a radioimmunoassay for angiotensin I to the physiologic measurements of plasma renin activity in normal human subjects. J. Clin. Endocr. *29*:1349, 1969.

Henry, R. J.: Clinical Chemistry: Principles and Techniques. New York, Paul B. Hoeber, Inc., 1964.

Heyrovsky, A.: A new method for the determination of inulin in plasma and urine. Clin. Chim. Acta *1*:470, 1956.

Jacobson, M. H., Levy, S. E., Kaufman, R. M., Gallinek, W. E., and Donnelly, O. W.: Urine osmolality. A definitive test of renal function. Arch. Intern. Med. *110*:83, 1962.

Looyé, A.: Automated simultaneous determination of p-acetylaminohippurate and inulin in serum. Clin. Chem. *16*:753, 1970.

Miller, B. J., Leaf, A., Mamby, A. R., and Miller, Z.: Validity of the endogenous creatinine clearance as a measure of glomerular filtration rate in the diseased human kidney. J. Clin. Invest. *31*:309, 1952.

Milne, M. D.: Renal tubular dysfunction. *In* Strauss, M. B., and Welt, L. G. (eds.): Diseases of the Kidney. Boston, Little, Brown and Company, 1963.

Newman, E. V., Bordley, J., and Winternitz, J.: The interrelationships of glomerular filtration rate (mannitol clearance), extracellular fluid volume, surface area of the body, and plasma concentration of mannitol. A definition of extracellular fluid clearance determined by following plasma concentration after a single injection of mannitol. Johns Hopkins Hosp. Bull. *75*:253, 1944.

Ochwadt, B. K., and Pitts, R. F.: Disparity between phenol red and Diodrast clearances in the dog. Amer. J. Physiol. *187*:318, 1956.

Pitts, R. F.: The renal regulation of acid-base balance with special reference to the mechanism for acidifying the urine. Science *102*:49, 1945.

Pitts, R. F.: Physiology of the Kidney and Body Fluids. Chicago, Year Book Medical Publishers, 1963.

Relman, A. S., and Levinsky, N. G.: Clinical examination of renal function. *In* Strauss, M. B., and Welt, L. G. (eds.): Diseases of the Kidney. Boston, Little, Brown and Company, 1963.

Roe, J. H., Epstein, J. H., and Goldstein, N. P.: A photometric method for the determination of inulin in plasma and urine. J. Biol. Chem. *178*:839, 1949.

Rubini, M. E., and Wolf, A. V.: Refractometric determination of total solids and water of serum and urine. J. Biol. Chem. *225*:869, 1957.

Sapirstein, L. A., Vidt, D. G., Mandel, M. J., and Hanusek, G.: Volumes of distribution and clearances of intravenously injected creatinine in the dog. Amer. J. Physiol. *181*:330, 1955.

Schreiner, G. E.: Determination of inulin by means of resorcinol. Proc. Soc. Exp. Biol. Med. *74*:117, 1950.

Shaw, S. T., Jr., and Benson, E. S.: Tests of renal function. *In* Davidsohn, I., and Henry, J. B. (eds.): Todd-Sanford Clinical Diagnosis By Laboratory Methods. 14th ed. Philadelphia, W. B. Saunders Company, 1969.

Slapak, M., and Hume, D. M.: A new method of estimating glomerular-filtration rate. Use of diminishing blood concentration of labelled vitamin B_{12}. Lancet *1*:1095, 1965.

Smith, H. W.: The Kidney. New York, Oxford University Press, 1951.

Smith, H. W.: Principles of Renal Physiology. New York, Oxford University Press, 1956.

Smith, H. W., Finkelstein, N., Aliminosa, L., Crawford, B., and Graber, M.: The renal clearances of substituted hippuric acid derivatives and other aromatic acids in dog and man. J. Clin. Invest. *24*:388, 1945.

Weiner, I. M., and Mudge, G. H.: Renal tubular mechanisms for excretion of organic acids and bases. Amer. J. Med. *36*:743, 1964.

Wilson, B. W., Thorburn, G. D., and Stacy, B. D.: Automated determination of inulin in the estimation of glomerular filtration rate. Aust. J. Exp. Biol. Med. Sci. *47*:113, 1969.

Wolf, A. V.: Urinary concentrative properties. Amer. J. Med. *32*:329, 1962.

Wright, H. K., and Gann, D. S.: An automatic anthrone method for the determination of inulin in plasma and urine. J. Lab. Clin. Med. 67:689, 1966.

Chapter 4

THE BLOOD

by ISRAEL DAVIDSOHN, M.D., and DOUGLAS A. NELSON, M.D.

METHODS USED IN THE STUDY OF BLOOD

PRELIMINARY CONSIDERATIONS

Certain observations of the formed elements of peripheral blood, their precursors and some of their products, form a separate branch of medical science called clinical hematology. Examinations of the blood derive their value in the care of patients only as they are correlated with the entire clinical condition.

The blood consists of a fluid of complicated and variable composition, the plasma, in which are suspended erythrocytes, leukocytes, and platelets. If coagulation is prevented, the formed elements can be separated from the pale, straw-colored plasma. When blood coagulates, the fluid that remains after separation of the clot is called serum. Serum differs from plasma mainly by loss of the protein fibrinogen, which is converted to insoluble fibrin strands in the process of coagulation. Serum and plasma are used for many important studies in clinical chemistry and immunology. The techniques of hematology are concerned chiefly with the cellular constituents of the blood, their number or concentration, the relative distribution of various types of cells, and the structural or biochemical abnormalities that promote disease.

Methods of Obtaining Blood

There are two sources of blood for laboratory tests: capillary or peripheral blood and venous blood. Both have their advocates, advantages, and disadvantages.

CAPILLARY OR PERIPHERAL BLOOD

It is claimed that what we call peripheral blood is more likely arteriolar than capillary.

For most clinical examinations, including cell counts and determination of the concentration of hemoglobin, blood is best obtained from a vein. However, for making differential blood counts and also for the enumeration of cellular elements, blood may be obtained from the lobe of an ear, the palmar surfaces of the tip of a finger, or, in the case of infants, the plantar surfaces of the great toe or the heel. In the case of the ear, the free margin of the lobe, not the side, should be punctured. Puncture can be made deliberately and slowly because there is almost no pain connected with it. The puncture should be about 3 mm. deep. It is possible to make 100 blood smears or to collect several milliliters of blood from a well-made puncture. If the patient is bedridden, the finger will be found more convenient because the approach is easier; otherwise the ear is preferable because it is less sensitive. An edematous or congested part should not be used. Free flow of blood is essential to obtain reproducible results comparable to those of venous blood. Cold and cyanotic skin is a source of errors. It is responsible for false high figures for red cell and white cell counts, but can be obviated by massage before the puncture until the skin is pink and warm. Vigorous squeezing after the puncture is another source of errors.

Equipment. Equipment consists of gauze pads, 70 per cent alcohol, and a lancet or scalpel blade. Several varieties of blood lancets are available. Disposable lancets or blades are recommended. If needles are to be reused, they must be sterilized by autoclaving before being used on different patients. Simple disinfectant solutions will not destroy the etiologic agent of hepatitis.

Technique of Puncture. The site is first rubbed well with a gauze pad moistened with 70 per cent alcohol to remove dirt and epithelial debris and to increase the amount of blood in the part. After the skin has dried and the circulation has returned, a puncture 2 to 3 mm. deep is made with a disposable blade or lancet. The puncture is practically painless if properly made with a sharp blade. It should be made with a firm quick stab, which, however, must not be made so quickly or from so great a distance that its site and depth are uncertain. A deep puncture is no more painful than a superficial one and makes it unnecessary to repeat the procedure.

The first drop of blood that appears is wiped away because it contains tissue juices; the second is used for examination. If the skin at the site of the puncture is not dry, the blood will not form a rounded drop as it exudes. The blood must not be pressed out, since this dilutes it with fluid from the tissues, but moderate pressure some distance above the puncture is allowable. After the needed blood has been obtained, a pad of sterile gauze is applied to the puncture and the patient instructed to apply slight pressure until bleeding has ceased. When the heel is used, it must be made warm, probably done most easily by immersion in warm water or by use of a hot-water compress. Otherwise, values significantly higher than in venous blood may be obtained, especially in the newborn. On the first day of life average differences as high as 2 gm. of hemoglobin per 100 ml. may be present.

After the newborn period, the values for hematocrit, red cells, hemoglobin, platelets, and osmotic fragility are the same in peripheral blood as in venous blood, provided the capillary blood is freely flowing.

VENOUS BLOOD

Veins have become important in the modern practice of medicine in two ways: as a source of blood for the many and constantly rising number of blood tests and as an avenue for introduction of various therapeutic agents, including blood itself.

Three factors are involved in a good venipuncture: the venipuncturist, the patient and his veins, and the equipment.

Venipuncturist. The venipuncture is in most instances a relatively simple procedure. The operator must be aware of the old phrase in ancient medicine that the doctor's main motto should be *primum non nocere*—"the first thing is not to inflict damage." The vein that one tries to enter should be preserved for innumerable future uses. Actually the life of the patient may sometimes depend on vein patency.

The hematomas displaying all the colors of the rainbow in antecubital fossae, around wrists, and other sundry places testify eloquently to the operator's lack of skill or lack of judgment. As a rule, the damage is only temporary, but it may be long lasting or even permanent. A venipuncture is an operation that is by no means trifling; it must be approached with due care and deliberation.

The Patient and His Veins. The patient should be reassured with a few words well chosen to fit the particular situation. Self-assurance and poise will do much to establish the proper rapport. The patient should be made comfortable, and the approach to his arm should be convenient for the operator. There is no need to add to the difficulties by trying to do the puncture in an inconvenient position. Ambulatory patients should be seated comfortably, preferably in a chair provided with an armrest or at a table on which the arm can be placed comfortably. The operator sits at the opposite side of the table.

The veins should be inspected and evaluated. When veins are deep and not felt distinctly, an attempt to enter them is bad practice because it amounts to blind probing. One can minimize this difficulty by using a tourniquet, which makes the veins more prominent and palpable for orientation. Such trial compression should be released and repeated again when one is ready for the actual puncture.

In patients who have had many punctures in the past and sequelae thereof, such a preliminary study of the veins is particularly important and may reveal more available veins than would seem apparent at first glance.

Equipment. The syringe should be of the proper size for the amount of blood to be drawn. Disposable plastic syringes are widely used. With reusable glass syringes, the fit of the plunger and barrel and the integrity of the syringe tip should be checked; following use, the syringe should be rinsed in cold water to remove the blood.

The needle is chosen as to gauge and length for the specific job. The gauge number expresses the thickness of the needle. The smaller the number, the thicker the needle. The length of the needle used depends upon the depth of the vein. The tip should be inspected carefully. A blunt or bent tip will damage the patient's vein and often leads to failure.

Method of Obtaining Blood from a Vein. It is best to have the patient lying down. If he is sitting, his arm should be firmly supported. Never have the patient standing or seated on a high stool. Although few patients faint as a result of venipuncture, this danger must always be kept in mind.

A rubber tourniquet is used to increase venous pressure and to make the veins more prominent and easier to enter, but to prevent hemoconcentration the pressure should not be maintained longer than necessary.

A soft rubber tube bound firmly around the upper part of the arm is a suitable form of tourniquet. The outer end should be tucked under the last round in such a manner that a slight pull will release the bandage. The cuff of a blood pressure apparatus answers admirably and has the advantage that it permits adjustment of the compression to a level sufficient to reduce the flow of venous blood without stopping arterial circulation. This is usually midway between the systolic and diastolic pressures. Also, reduction or release of pressure after the needle has entered the vein is facilitated. Occasionally it will be sufficient for an assistant or even the patient to grasp the upper arm firmly. If one uses a rubber tubing as tourniquet, he can apply the proper pressure by first compressing the arm so as to suppress the radial pulse and then releasing the pressure just enough to feel the radial pulse feebly. The patient is asked to open and close his fist several times. This causes the veins to become distended. Giving the patient an active role in the procedure helps to take his mind off the puncture. Even if not seen, veins can usually be felt beneath the skin. In fat persons, veins that show as blue streaks are usually too superficial and too small.

After all preliminary steps have been taken, the skin is cleansed with 70 per cent alcohol or another suitable disinfectant and allowed to dry. It is desirable to apply the tourniquet while the alcohol is drying. The next step is to fix the vein in position. This is done by supporting the patient's forearm with the operator's hand and compressing and pulling the soft tissues just below the intended puncture site with the operator's thumb. The syringe is held between the thumb and the last three fingers of the other hand. The back of these fingers are rested on the patient's arm. The free index finger rests against the hub of the needle and serves as a guide. A prominent vein may be entered with a single direct puncture of skin and vein. This one-step procedure is less painful.

When veins are difficult to find, a two-step procedure is used. First the skin is punctured in the vicinity of the vein and then the vein itself is punctured. Successful entrance into the vein is followed immediately by appearance of blood in the syringe. If that does not take place, the plunger is withdrawn slightly and in most instances blood appears. Next the tourniquet may be loosened if blood flows freely; otherwise, it may be left as put on originally until the desired amount of blood is obtained. At this point the patient is asked to open his fist, the tourniquet is released, a small additional amount of blood is permitted to enter the syringe, the needle is withdrawn, gentle pressure is applied to the site of the puncture with a pad of dry gauze or cotton, and the patient is instructed to take over pressing the pad and to raise the outstretched arm for a few minutes. This usually stops the bleeding and prevents formation of a hematoma. A small dressing (Band-Aid) may be applied, mainly to prevent a stain on the rolled-down sleeve. The operator must see that the patient's condition is satisfactory before he is dismissed. If there is any sign of continued discomfort, anxiety, bleeding, or shock, the patient should be kept lying down and seen by a physician.

It is usually easy to secure 5 to 15 ml. of blood, or even more, if required. If the needle is sharp and smooth, the procedure causes the patient surprisingly little inconvenience. There is rarely any difficulty in inserting a needle into a vein except in children and in patients in whom the arm is fat and the veins are small. If desired, one of the veins about the ankle can be used. In infants, blood may be secured from the femoral or the external jugular vein.

When the blood has been expelled, the plunger should be separated from the barrel of reusable syringes, and both washed in cold water. Otherwise the syringe may become "frozen" when the blood clots or dries.

Instead of a syringe, other devices for securing blood from a vein may be employed. One of these is the B-D Vacutainer. Vacutainer tubes are supplied with a measured amount of anticoagulant (or none) and sufficient vacuum to draw a predetermined volume of blood and are sealed with a rubber stopper. The disposable needle screws into the holder and the Vacutainer tube is placed in the holder so that the rubber stopper just reaches the guide line. The short needle is thereby embedded in the rubber stopper but does not penetrate through it to break the vacuum. After the needle is inserted into the arm vein as described above, the tube is pushed all the way into the holder, vacuum is broken, and the blood flows into the tube. After the flow ceases, the tube may be removed and another tube inserted into the holder, or if only one tube is needed, the whole unit is withdrawn as described above for the syringe. This convenient system eliminates the need for syringes and uses disposable needles and tubes.

Hemolysis interferes with many examinations. It can be minimized by using clean glassware and clean and not too thin needles, by drawing the blood slowly, not faster than the vein is filling, by avoiding admixture of air with resulting frothing, and, after the blood is drawn, by removing the needle and then emptying the blood again slowly and without force into the test tube.

Complications of Venipunctures and Suggestions for Their Prevention

Immediate Local Complications. Hemoconcentration is the result of prolonged application of the tourniquet. Even 60 seconds will produce measurable increases in the concentration of the blood cells.

Failure of blood to enter the syringe is the result of several factors. Excessive pull on plunger may collapse a small vein. This may be remedied by using a slight back-and-forth movement and reducing the force of aspiration. Piercing the outer coat of the vein without entering the lumen may also account for the failure of blood to enter the syringe. This may be remedied by withdrawing slightly and reentering the vein. This complication may occasionally be followed by hematoma formation. As soon as signs of beginning hematoma are noticed, the needle should be withdrawn, local pressure applied, and venipuncture attempted on the other arm. Transfixation of the vein also accounts for failure to obtain blood. This may be remedied by slight withdrawal followed by gentle aspiration to see whether blood appears. If this fails, the puncture may have to be repeated. This complication is frequently followed by formation of a hematoma, and the same remedy is followed as outlined above. Circulatory failure is another cause, and the situation is entirely beyond the control of the operator.

In the case of these or of any other complications, failure to draw blood after two attempts should be an indication not to make further attempts but to request another operator to try.

Another not infrequent immediate complication is syncope. This is best treated by having the patient lie down, if he is not already in this position. A physician should check the patient immediately.

Continued bleeding may occur in patients with a bleeding tendency, whatever the source. Local pressure, as a rule, solves the problem.

Late Local Complications. Thrombosis of the vein is sometimes due to trauma, especially following many venipunctures at the same site. Rarely, infection results in thrombophlebitis. These complications are rare if the precautions and recommendations discussed in this chapter are observed.

Late General Complications. Serum hepatitis may be caused by transmission of the virus by contaminated needle or syringe. The use of disposable needles has virtually eliminated this source of transmitted disease.

Venipuncture in Infants. In infants and children venipuncture presents special problems because of the small size of the veins and the difficulty of control. However, even here much can be achieved by the same approach that was outlined for procedures in adults.

Restraining the infant to reduce mobility, use of sharp needles of appropriate size, careful inspection of the veins, and making certain that the pressure applied with the tourniquet is not excessive (best checked by feeling pulsation of the radial artery) will contribute to a successful venipuncture when others may have failed. External jugular puncture may be tried in difficult cases and is frequently successful. Occasionally the internal jugular vein may have to be used. Puncture of the superior sagittal sinus is mentioned here only to discourage its use. Any complication that would be harmless in another area, for example, a hematoma, may have serious consequences.

For hematologic examination, blood obtained by venipuncture is delivered to bottles or tubes containing a suitable anticoagulant. This transfer must be made without delay. Mixing with the anticoagulant is accomplished by thorough but gentle rotation of the container. A drop of blood from the needle or syringe tip is placed on a slide and the smear is made directly.

To obtain serum, blood is kept at room temperature or in a 37° C. incubator until a clot has formed and begins to retract; then it is centrifuged and the serum pipetted off. To accelerate retraction the clot may be separated from the wall of the container with a platinum needle, a thin glass rod, or wooden applicator before it is placed in the refrigerator. To obtain serum more rapidly, the blood may be defibrinated with glass beads or a glass rod.

Anticoagulants. The four most popular are a mixture of ammonium and potassium oxalate, trisodium citrate, Versene (EDTA), and heparin. The first three prevent coagulation by removing calcium from the blood plasma by precipitation or binding in un-ionized form. Heparin inhibits thrombin and other stages of clotting factor activation.

Trisodium citrate is used to prevent coagulation of blood for transfusions. EDTA and heparin may be used for the same purpose, but not the toxic oxalate mixture.

The mixture of ammonium (six parts) and potassium oxalate (four parts), 2 mg. per 1 ml. of blood, does not affect the mean corpuscular volume and may be used for hemoglobin, hematocrit, and cell counts. Its usefulness for blood films is limited to the first few minutes. The reason: crenation of red cells, vacuolation in the cytoplasm of granulocytes, phagocytosis of oxalate crystals, artefact formation in the nuclei of lymphocytes and monocytes, and other malformations develop rapidly. *Warning:* Blood collected in this anticoagulant mixture cannot be used for chemical determinations of nitrogen or potassium.

Trisodium citrate is used in a mixture of one part of a 3.8 per cent aqueous solution and nine parts of blood in blood coagulation studies.

Versene (EDTA) is used in a concentration of 1 to 2 mg. per 1 ml. of blood. The dipotassium or disodium salt of ethylenediaminetetraacetic acid is probably the most widely used anticoagulant for blood cell counts. It must be mixed thoroughly with the blood. It equals oxalate for hematocrit studies and is superior for morphologic studies because it prevents formation of artefacts even on prolonged standing. Acceptable blood smears can be prepared after 2 to 3 hours and cell counts even up to 24 hours, if the blood is refrigerated. Also, platelet counting is still possible after several hours.

Heparin, 0.1 to 0.2 mg. per 1 ml. of blood, does not affect the corpuscular size and hematocrit. It is the best anticoagulant for prevention of hemolysis and for osmotic fragility tests. It is not satisfactory for leukocyte counts or when blood films are to be prepared; in the latter case it produces a troublesome blue background in Wright's-stained slides.

Sources of Error from the Use of Anticoagulants. Even with the use of the best anticoagulant, changes take place that may lead to errors unless suitable precautions are taken.

Blood films should be prepared immediately. If other determinations cannot be performed within 2 or 3 hours, the blood should be refrigerated at 4° C. If the blood is kept at room temperature, sometime between 6 and 24 hours swelling of erythrocytes raises the hematocrit and mean corpuscular volume (MCV) and lowers the mean corpuscular hemoglobin concentration (MCHC) and the erythrocyte sedimentation rate. At 24 hours, however, the white cell count (WBC), red cell count (RBC), hemoglobin, hematocrit, and the red cell indices are all unchanged if the blood has been anticoagulated with EDTA and stored at 4°C. (Brittin *et al.*, 1969); under these conditions this is true also for the reticulocyte count and the platelet count (Lampasso, 1968). According to Gambino *et al.* (1965), the sedimentation rate must be performed within 12 hours.

Before taking a sample from a tube of venous blood for a hematologic determination it is important to mix the blood thoroughly. This requires at least 60 inversions of the tube, which is easily accomplished in two minutes on a mechanical rotator; less than this leads to unacceptable deterioration in precision (Fairbanks, Fahey and Beutler, 1971, p. 178).

Macroscopic Examination

Important information may be obtained from the appearance of the blood. If the hematocrit is performed by centrifugation, inspection of the specimen after spinning may furnish valuable data. The relative heights of the red cell column, buffy coat, and plasma column should be noted.

Normally the buffy coat is a thin white layer at the line of separation between red cells and plasma. In the centrifuged hematocrit tube each 1 per cent buffy coat is roughly equivalent to 10,000 leukocytes per cu. mm. For example, a buffy coat of 1 per cent of the total volume in the tube indicates a leukocyte count in the range of 10,000 per cu. mm., if the platelets are not markedly elevated. If the leukocyte count is over 12,000 per cu. mm., a buffy coat of 1 per cent of the total volume represents a leukocyte count closer to 20,000 per cu. mm. than 10,000 because of greater packing (Wintrobe, 1967). The size of the cells will alter the estimate if they are much different from normal. These estimates apply best to the macrohematocrit; in the microhematocrit they underestimate the leukocyte count because of the greater packing. The estimates give only a crude idea of the count, but they are sometimes useful.

An orange or green color of the plasma suggests increased bilirubin, and pink or red suggests hemoglobinemia. It should be kept in mind that poor technique in collecting the blood specimen is the most frequent cause of hemolysis. If the specimens are not obtained within an hour or two after a fat-rich meal, cloudy plasma may point to nephrosis or certain abnormal hyperglobulinemias, especially cryoglobulinemia.

Hemoglobin

Hemoglobin, the main component of the red blood cell, is a conjugated protein that serves as the vehicle for the transportation of oxygen and CO_2. When fully saturated, each gram of hemoglobin holds approximately 1.34 ml. of oxygen. The red cell mass of the adult contains approximately 600 gm. of hemoglobin, capable of carrying 800 ml. of oxygen.

A molecule of hemoglobin consists of two pairs of polypeptide chains ("globin") and four prosthetic heme groups, each containing one atom of ferrous iron. Each heme group is precisely located in a pocket or fold of one of the polypeptide chains. Located near the surface of the molecule, the heme reversibly combines with one molecule of oxygen or carbon dioxide.

The main function of hemoglobin is to transport oxygen from the lungs, where oxygen tension is high, to the tissues where it is low. At an oxygen tension of 100 mm. Hg in the pulmonary capillaries, 95 to 98 per cent of the hemoglobin is combined with oxygen. In the tissues, where the oxygen tension may be as low as 20 mm. Hg, the oxygen readily dissociates from hemoglobin; in this instance, less than 30 per cent of the oxygen would remain combined with hemoglobin.

Reduced hemoglobin is hemoglobin with

iron unassociated with oxygen. When each heme group is associated with one molecule of oxygen, the hemoglobin is referred to as oxyhemoglobin. In both reduced hemoglobin and oxyhemoglobin, iron remains in the ferrous state. With iron oxidized to the ferric state, methemoglobin is formed, and the molecule loses its capacity to carry oxygen or carbon dioxide.

Hemoglobinometry is the measurement of the concentration of hemoglobin in the blood. Anemia, a decrease below normal of the hemoglobin concentration, erythrocyte count, or hematocrit, is a very common condition and frequently a complication of other diseases. Clinical diagnosis of anemia based on estimation of the color of skin and of visible mucous membranes is highly unreliable. To make matters even more complicated, anemia is frequently masked in many diseases by other manifestations. To a limited extent similar considerations apply to conditions with abnormally high hemoglobin. For all these reasons the correct estimation of hemoglobin is important and is one of the routine tests done on practically every patient.

DETERMINING THE CONCENTRATION OF HEMOGLOBIN

The concentration of hemoglobin is expressed in grams per 100 ml. of blood, or grams per deciliter (gm./dl.). The custom of recording hemoglobin as a percentage of some arbitrary normal is ambiguous and should not be used.

When one evaluates the relative merits of clinical laboratory tests, at least four desiderata are considered: the accuracy of a single determination as compared with a known standard; the reproducibility of a series of determinations when done by the same technician, by a group of technicians in the same laboratory, and by different laboratories; the speed from the point of view of availability in case of emergency; and the simplicity of the procedure from the point of view of economy.

The methods used in hemoglobinometry can be grouped into four main classes, depending on the basic technique employed, with variants within each class: colorimetric methods, gasometric methods, specific gravity methods, and chemical methods.

COLORIMETRIC METHODS

Principle. Hemoglobin (Hb) is measured as oxyhemoglobin or is first converted into a derivative, such as acid hematin, alkaline hematin, or cyanmethemoglobin. The measurement is done by comparing the unknown sample with a standard. The method of comparison may be visual or photoelectric. The latter is considerably more accurate.

Direct Matching Methods. Methods that are based on the direct matching of the red color of whole fresh blood with some color standard are not satisfactory.

Acid Hematin Methods. Also outmoded are methods that depend on converting hemoglobin into acid hematin with dilute hydrochloric acid and matching the brownish yellow

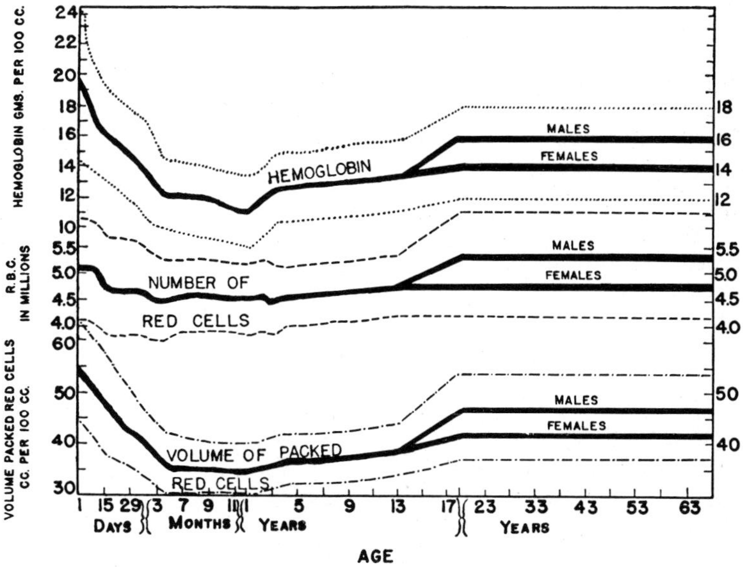

Figure 4–1. Normal curve for hemoglobin, red cells and volumes of packed red cells, from birth to old age. The mean values are heavily outlined. The range of variation is indicated by dotted lines for hemoglobin, interrupted lines for red cell count and dotted interrupted lines for volume of packed red cells. The scales for hemoglobin, red cell count and volume of packed red cells are similar and therefore the relative changes in these values are apparent on inspection. The scale for age, however, is progressively altered. (Derived from the data of Williamson, Appleton, Haden and Neff, Merritt and Davidson, Poncher, Guest, Osgood and Baker, Kato, Mugrage and Andresen, and Wintrobe. From Wintrobe, M. M.: Clinical Hematology. Philadelphia, Lea & Febiger, 1967.)

color of this solution with a standard in some sort of a colorimeter or comparator.

Nonhemoglobin substances (protein, lipids) in plasma and cell stroma influence the color of blood diluted with acid because the acid hematin is in colloidal suspension and not a true solution. This is also the reason why the acid hematin method is not satisfactory for photometry.

From 2 to 12 per cent of the total hemoglobin of the blood is in an inactive form, mainly as carboxyhemoglobin, methemoglobin, and sulfhemoglobin. In alkaline solutions these abnormal hemoglobins are converted to hematin, whereas acid has no such effect.

Alkali Hematin Method. Addition of an excess of alkali produces a true and relatively stable solution of hematin.

Since the blood of the newborn and the young infant contains alkali-resistant fetal hemoglobin, this method introduces a significant source of error in newborns. The method is no longer used in routine hemoglobinometry.

Oxyhemoglobin Method. No longer widely used, but still a satisfactory method is the determination of hemoglobin as oxyhemoglobin. In this procedure 0.02 ml. of blood measured with a Sahli-type hemoglobin pipette is washed into 5.0 ml. of approximately 0.007 N ammonium hydroxide solution prepared by adding 4 ml. of reagent grade NH_4OH to 1 liter of water and mixing. Rinse the pipette three times with diluting fluid. The water used in the preparation of ammonia solution must be glass distilled, because minute amounts of copper in distilled water or other diluents employed in oxyhemoglobin determinations may cause oxyhemoglobin to be converted to methemoglobin and lower the values. Shake well to insure mixing and oxygenation of hemoglobin. The solution is read in a photometer in which are used a green filter (540 nm.) and a 0.007 N ammonium hydroxide solution as blank. The test can be read within a few seconds or with a stoppered cuvette any time up to three days. The standard curve can be set up with one of the procedures to be listed later.

Cyanmethemoglobin Method. This method is the outcome of the long-felt need for improvement of standardization of hemoglobin determinations; it is now the method of choice.

In 1964 the Subcommittee on Hemoglobinometry of the International Committee for Standardization in Hematology proposed that hemoglobinometry be standardized by international agreement. The cyanmethemoglobin method was recommended, with a cyanmethemoglobin solution as a standard. Hemoglobin constants and the standard were defined. In the United States, the College of American Pathologists is entrusted with the certification of standards. Among the forms of hemoglobin well adapted to photometry, cyanmethemoglobin has outstanding advantages. All forms of hemoglobin likely to be found in blood – oxyhemoglobin, reduced hemoglobin, carboxyhemoglobin, and methemoglobin, but not sulfmethemoglobin – are quantitatively converted to cyanmethemoglobin upon the addition of a single reagent.

Solutions of cyanmethemoglobin are the most stable of the various hemoglobin pigments. It is certainly safe to say that solutions of cyanmethemoglobin are stable for at least six months when kept in the refrigerator. Another advantage of cyanmethemoglobin solutions is that they can be standardized accurately. The absorption band of cyanmethemoglobin in the region of 540 nm. is broad rather than sharp, and consequently its solutions can be used in filter-type photometers and in narrow-band spectrophotometers.

Photoelectric colorimeters or photometers make it possible to determine hemoglobin with an accuracy of from ±1 to 2 per cent in automated systems and ±2 to 5 per cent in standard manual techniques. However, this degree of accuracy, though possible, is not always achieved in practice. The main obstacle is the difficulty of standardizing the instrument, especially for hemoglobinometry. "Recalibration" by the manufacturer is rarely reliable and frequently creates a false sense of security. To be reliable, standardization has to be done under the conditions prevailing in the laboratory and must be checked frequently. Several photometers are available. Whichever is used, it must be used exactly according to the instructions provided by the manufacturer. Calibration of the instrument is the first step. The method differs with each make.

It is advisable to have an independent "photometric" standard in addition to the cyanmethemoglobin standards. This will help to check both the instrument and the cyanmethemoglobin standard if the photometric readings of the standard used in the test show excessive variations in duplicate readings.

Preparation of independent "photometric" standards:

Copper sulfate · $5H_2O$	1.5 gm.
2 M ammonium hydroxide	500.0 ml.

Store in tightly stoppered Pyrex flasks. Keeps for a year.

Preparation of 2 M ammonium hydroxide: Dilute 136 ml. of concentrated reagent grade ammonium hydroxide to 1 liter with distilled water.

Selection and Matching of Cuvettes

ROUND CUVETTES

1. Clean and dry several dozen cuvettes inside and out.

2. Examine each cuvette and select only those free of scratches or other flaws.

3. Add 0.2 ml. of whole blood to 50 ml. of

distilled water, mix well, and fill each cuvette with this solution.

4. Set the photometer at the 540 nm. band or insert the appropriate green filter.

5. Set a water blank at 100 on the transmittance scale (T) or at zero on the density scale (D). This setting should be checked frequently.

6. Insert a filled cuvette in the well. Set the galvanometer beam near the middle of the scale. Rotate the tube slowly, watching the movement of the beam. At the midpoint of the beam's swing, mark the cuvette with a diamond point pencil in relation to a stable mark on the housing of the well.

7. Repeat the same procedure with each cuvette and rotate it until the reading of the galvanometer corresponds with the reading of the first cuvette, marking each in relation to the same stable mark of the colorimeter.

8. All precautions should be taken to avoid scratching the cuvettes. For that reason wooden or coated wire test tube racks are preferable.

SQUARE CUVETTES. Steps 1 to 5 are identical.

6. Place each cuvette in the well. If inexpensive cuvettes are used, only those giving identical readings should be kept. If high-grade expensive cuvettes are used, a correction factor has to be determined for each and applied each time the cuvette is used.

Pipettes. The 0.02 ml. pipette (Sahli) that is used to measure the blood should be accurate to ±1 per cent. Several supply houses offer 0.02 ml. pipettes with a claimed accuracy of this order. However, it would appear advisable to calibrate a few such pipettes in order to verify the degree of accuracy. (For technique of calibration see p. 109.) The pipettes should be acid cleaned and thoroughly washed with water at least once a week. They should be washed and thoroughly dried between each measurement.

The transfer pipettes used to measure the diluent solution should be of a good order of accuracy and preferably within ±0.5 per cent. Some of the commercially available pipettes are well within these limits. (The Bureau of Standards tolerance on 5 ml. pipettes is ±0.2 per cent.) If a burette or automatic pipette is used for this purpose, it should be of the same order of accuracy. The task of matching cuvettes can be bypassed by using the flow-through cuvette with which most instruments are now supplied. After each reading, the solution is discarded by means of a valve in the bottom of the cuvette. Since all readings, both standards and unknowns, are taken through the same cuvette, errors due to imperfectly matched cuvettes are eliminated.

Standard

PRINCIPLE. Potassium ferricyanide–cyanide solution is used. Ferricyanide converts hemoglobin iron from the ferrous to the ferric state to form methemoglobin, which combines with potassium cyanide to produce the stable cyanmethemoglobin.

The stock standard, which has been certified by the College of American Pathologists, is available commercially from several firms. The exact concentration is within ±2 per cent of the value stated on the label. It is about 60 mg. of cyanmethemoglobin per 100 ml. The spectrophotometric characteristics of cyanmethemoglobin are such that D is directly proportional to the concentration. Three different concentrations of the reagent must be used for the preparation of a standard curve, the one purchased containing 60 mg. and two more with 40 and 20 mg. of cyanmethemoglobin per 100 ml. They are equivalent to 15, 10, and 5 gm. of hemoglobin per 100 ml. when blood is diluted 1:251.

DILUTION OF STANDARD

1. Transfer 5 ml. of the stock standard to each of three large clean test tubes, using a clean 5-ml. volumetric pipette. Allow the pipette to drain. Do not blow it out. Add a second 5-ml. volume of the standard to the second tube, using the same pipette.

2. Rinse pipette five times with Drabkin's diluent.

3. Add 5 ml. of the diluent to tube 2 and 10 ml. to tube 3.

4. Mix contents of tube 3 and of tube 2 in the order mentioned.

5. Beginning with tube 3 and continuing with tubes 2 and 1, transfer 5 ml. of contents of each tube into each of three matched cuvettes.

6. The concentration of cyanmethemoglobin in tube 1 is the same as stated on the label of the standard solution. The concentration in tube 2 is two-thirds and in tube 3, one-third of the standard.

7. The procedure is different if one uses the Evelyn photometer because the dilution of blood is 1:501. Therefore, 5 ml. of the stock standard is added to each of the three test tubes, followed by 5 ml. of the diluent to tube 1, 10 ml. to tube 2, and 20 ml. to tube 3. The resulting concentration of cyanmethemoglobin in tube 1 is one-half of the stock solution, one-third in tube 2, and one-fifth in tube 3.

DRABKIN'S DILUENT SOLUTION

Sodium bicarbonate ($NaHCO_3$)	1.0 gm.
Potassium cyanide (KCN)	0.05 gm.
Potassium ferricyanide ($K_3Fe(CN)_6$)	0.20 gm.
Distilled water to make	1000.0 ml.

This is a clear, pale yellow solution. It should be discarded if it turns turbid. It should be kept in a brown bottle and not more than a month's supply should be prepared. Reagent grade quality chemicals should be used.

Precautions in the Use of Cyanide. Salts and solutions of cyanide are poisonous, and care should be taken to avoid getting them into the mouth or inhaling their fumes. Most clinical laboratories use for the determination of uric acid a reagent containing 50 gm. of this salt per liter. In view of this, and of the fact that laboratories of clinical pathology are disciplined in the use of such dangerous materials as isotopes and virulent pathogens, it would seem that the handling of the proposed reagent constitutes a quite negligible hazard.

The concentration of cyanide in the stock standard and the diluent is 50 mg. per liter. The smallest dose of potassium cyanide that has been known to kill a human is 300 mg. Nonetheless, this is not a substance to be handled by irresponsible persons. Especially the salt itself must be handled with great circumspection. The following precautions have been recommended:

1. A suction bulb should be employed to fill pipettes.
2. Blood should be mixed with the cyanide solution by swirling.

If the standard or the diluent is prepared in the laboratory, special care must be taken in handling the chemical. If during weighing it is spilled accidentally on the bench or floor, the dry powder should be wiped up with a damp cloth. The cloth should be carefully discarded into a suitable closed container. The solution or powder should not be placed in a sink with acid. The solution may be discarded into a sink if the water is flowing freely. The solid potassium cyanide should be kept under lock and key.

It is common now for the diluent to be supplied from the manufacturer already prepared so that handling of the salt is avoided.

The standard solution is bacteriostatic and will remain free of bacterial growth if not contaminated in handling. It is recommended to place the standard in clean matched cuvettes and to seal them permanently. Stoppers are not recommended. It should be stored in a refrigerator in darkness together with the blank solution at about 5° C. but not frozen. Before use, the outside of the cuvettes should be wiped free of moisture, finger marks, and lint, and the standard should be permitted to reach room temperature to prevent condensation on the cuvettes and formation of bubbles when the cold solution is heated suddenly by the light source. Both events may be a source of error. The standard must be discarded every six months.

Calibration of Instrument with the Cyanmethemoglobin Standards

1. The readings are taken at the 540 nm. band. The filter appropriate for the instrument must be in place.
2. The current is turned on and the instrument allowed to warm up according to the instructions of the manufacturer.
3. Distilled water or the diluent solution is used as blank. The absorption of light by the diluent at 540 nm. is negligible.
4. The blank is set at 100 on the per cent transmittance (T) scale or at zero on the optical density (OD) scale.
5. The three standard tubes are placed in the cuvette well and the readings recorded beginning with the tube with the lowest concentration and proceeding with next higher concentration tubes. This standardization procedure takes about 5 minutes. It should be done by the beginner before each determination. Later, as experience grows and the instrument performs well and reliably, checking with the standards may be done at intervals to be determined by the operator's and supervisor's judgment.

Preparation of a Standard Curve and Table. The following formula is used:

$$\frac{S \times D}{1000} = \text{gm. hemoglobin per 100 ml.}$$

where S is concentration of cyanmethemoglobin standard and D is the dilution of the blood sample. For example, if the concentration of the cyanmethemoglobin standard is 60.4 mg. per 100 ml. and the dilution is 251, then

$$\frac{60.4 \times 251}{1000} = 15.16 \text{ gm. of hemoglobin per 100 ml.}$$

The procedure may be facilitated by preparing a curve from which the readings of the galvanometer can be readily translated into hemoglobin values.

If the galvanometer readings are in terms of per cent of transmission (T), the readings of the standards are entered on semilogarithmic graph paper. The abscissa (bottom axis) represents grams of hemoglobin, and the ordinate, the percentage of light transmittance. A line is drawn through the three points. It should pass through or very near T per cent = 100. This graph will show the value in grams of hemoglobin per 100 ml. corresponding to each reading. When many tests are done, it may be more convenient to construct a table of hemoglobin values for every possible per cent reading. Each photometer must be standardized individually against the standards and should be checked frequently.

If the meter readings are in terms of optical density (OD), the values are plotted on linear graph paper with the density values on the ordinate and the hemoglobin in grams per cent on the abscissa. A line connecting the three points should pass through or very near zero.

The readings for unknown can be translated into grams of hemoglobin.

Test

1. Exactly 5 ml. of Drabkin's solution is transferred into each of two matched cuvettes, using an accurate volumetric transfer pipette (meeting U.S. Bureau of Standards requirements of tolerance). A suction bulb, an automatic pipette, or a burette should be used, depending on the amount of work.

2. The blood sample may be taken from a freely bleeding capillary puncture or from a venous sample. The latter must be thoroughly mixed by gently tipping the tube end over end at least 60 times before blood is taken from it. Exactly 0.02 ml. of whole blood is transferred with an accurate standardized Sahli pipette into one of the two cuvettes. Great care must be exerted to fill the pipette exactly to the mark. If the excess is minimal (not more than 2 mm.), it may be removed by touching the point of the pipette with a cloth; otherwise the pipette has to be emptied, cleaned and dried, and the procedure repeated.

3. The blood and solution are mixed by swirling the cuvette. They are left standing for 10 minutes to permit formation of cyanmethemoglobin.

4. The second cuvette serves as a blank. (Instead of Drabkin's solution distilled water may be used.)

5. If a filter-type photometer is used, the filter appropriate for the make of the instrument is put in place. If the instrument is a spectrophotometer, the wavelength scale is adjusted to 540 nm. Then proceed for the blank and unknown as described previously (see p. 108). The hemoglobin values are read from the curve or table.

The details of procedure vary with each instrument. These include calibration of the instrument with cyanmethemoglobin standards, preparation of a standard curve and a standard table for hemoglobinometry, and hemoglobinometry by the cyanmethemoglobin method.

Sources of Error—Inaccuracy of the Pipette. In view of the fact that 0.02 ml. Sahli pipettes may be less accurate than claimed, it is desirable to reserve several carefully calibrated pipettes for hemoglobin tests. Calibration of blood diluting pipettes can be carried out by the following procedure recommended by Stevenson *et al.* (1951).

EQUIPMENT. Redistilled mercury; tuberculin syringe; single-hole, size 0 rubber stopper; mineral oil or stopcock grease; apparatus support stand; 50-ml. beaker; weighing bottles; thermometer; analytical balance.

CALIBRATION

1. 0.02 ml. pipettes are cleaned with concentrated nitric acid, washed, and dried.

2. The equipment is kept at room temperature. The mercury and pipettes are allowed to reach room temperature before calibration is started. The temperature of the mercury is recorded. Mercury is placed in the beaker. The weighing bottles are weighed and the weight recorded.

3. The plunger of the syringe is coated with mineral oil or grease and the syringe assembled. The tip of the syringe is inserted into the hole of the rubber stopper, which is then clamped vertically to a heavy apparatus support about 18 inches above the bench.

4. The proximal end of the pipette is inserted into the other end of the stopper.

5. The plunger of the syringe is slightly withdrawn. The tip of the pipette is immersed in the mercury. Slow withdrawal of the plunger fills the pipette with mercury. When the 0.02 mark is reached, the beaker is removed. If some mercury is lost in this procedure, the procedure must be repeated. The mercury is emptied into the weighing bottle. The determination should be done in duplicate. The weight of the mercury is established by subtracting the weight of the empty weighing bottle from the final weight with mercury.

6. The volume of the weighed mercury is established by dividing the weight by a temperature correction factor (the specific gravity of mercury in gm./ml.):

TEMPERATURE (°C.)	CORRECTION FACTOR
20	13.547
21	13.545
22	13.543
23	13.541
24	13.539
25	13.537
26	13.534
27	13.532
28	13.530
29	13.528
30	13.526

7. The actual volume of the pipette expressed in milliliters divided by the number of milliliters supposed to be measured by the pipette (0.02) gives a correction factor for the pipette, which should be scratched on the pipette with a diamond pencil.

Example

(1) Weight of weighing bottle = 39.8731 gm.

(2) Weight of weighing bottle plus mercury = 40.1311 gm.

Weight of the mercury = (2) − (1) = 0.2580 gm.

Volume of mercury delivered by pipette

$$\frac{W}{TCF} = \frac{0.2580}{13.528} \text{ at } 29^\circ \text{C.} = 0.0191 \text{ ml.}$$

where W is the weight of mercury and TCF is the correction factor for the temperature.

Correction factor for the pipette =

$$\frac{VM}{SVP} = \frac{0.0191}{0.0200} = 0.96, \text{ where VM is the}$$

volume of mercury delivered at prevailing temperature and SVP is the supposed volume measured by the pipette.

Other Sources of Error. Lipemic blood is a source of error. (This applies to all methods employing colorimetry.)

Occasionally hypochromic red cells will not be lysed by the Drabkin's solution, and the resulting dilution of unknown blood in diluent is turbid. In this case, exactly 5 ml. of distilled water added to the turbid fluid will lyse the cells and make it clear. The value determined for the hemoglobin from the calibration curve must then be corrected for the additional dilution by multiplying by 2.

According to Green and Teal (1959), false high hemoglobin values were seen in two patients with easily precipitable globulins, one with myeloma and the other with idiopathic macroglobulinemia. This was corrected by adding 0.1 gm. of K_2CO_3, which increased the alkalinity of the reagent; the globulin remained in solution. Otherwise the composition of the reagent remained identical.

Omission of the sodium bicarbonate from Drabkin's reagent and addition of 140 mg. of KH_4PO_4 and 0.5 ml. of Sterox SE (Hartman-Leddon Co., Philadelphia), a nonionic detergent, will also minimize turbidity due to protein precipitation. In addition, time for full color development is shortened to 3 minutes with this reagent compared to 20 minutes with Drabkin's (van Assendelft, 1972).

GASOMETRIC METHOD

Van Slyke's Oxygen Capacity Method. This is an indirect method, which estimates the amount of hemoglobin from the amount of oxygen it will absorb and utilizes the Van Slyke apparatus that is used for the estimation of carbon dioxide. It serves as an accurate method for standardizing the various hemoglobinometers but is too complicated for clinical work (R. J. Henry, 1964).

SPECIFIC GRAVITY METHOD

The specific gravity of the blood is the ratio of the weight of a volume of blood to the weight of the same volume of water at a temperature of 4° C. The normal specific gravity ranges from 1.048 to 1.066. The average for men is 1.057 and for women 1.053. Reflecting the normal diurnal variation in hemoglobin concentration of blood, there is a variation of about 0.003, the values in the afternoon and after meals being somewhat lower and those after exercise and at night, higher. The specific gravity of the serum is 1.026 to 1.031 and that of the erythrocytes, 1.092 to 1.095.

The copper sulfate method of measuring the specific gravity of the blood is a simple and rapid procedure requiring no precision equipment. Drops of blood are permitted to fall into a series of solutions of copper sulfate of known specific gravity, and one observes whether the drops sink or rise in the solutions. Upon immersion, the drops of blood become coated with a layer of copper proteinate, remain discrete for 15 to 20 seconds, and fall if their specific gravity is higher than that of the copper sulfate solution and vice versa. The accuracy of the method depends on the number of solutions used. If 16 are used with specific gravity intervals of 0.004, the gravities are accurate to 0.001. The solutions can be used repeatedly.

Test

REAGENT. Place 4 lb. of "fine crystals" of $CuSO_4 \cdot 5H_2O$ in a 4-liter bottle.

Add distilled water to 2500 ml. Stopper bottle and shake vigorously for 5 minutes. Measure the temperature of the solution. Pour off the supernatant and filter through cotton or dry filter paper into a clean 4-liter bottle. With the help of a table, in the original publication (Phillips *et al.*, 1950), a volume of the saturated solution, which varies with the temperature, is diluted with a volume of distilled water to make up a stock solution with a specific gravity of 1.100. From the stock, solutions of lower specific gravities of any other desired range are prepared.

METHOD. Venous blood is released into the solution from a height of about 1 cm. directly from the syringe and needle or from a medicine dropper from the tube with blood collected in an anticoagulant. The drop penetrates 2 to 3 cm. below the surface. In a few seconds the drop begins to rise or continues to fall. The specific gravity of the drop does not change for another 10 to 15 seconds. If the drop is of the same specific gravity as the test solution, it will become stationary for about 10 to 15 seconds and will then resume its downward course. If it is lighter, it will rise for a few seconds and then begin to sink. If it is heavier, it will continue to fall.

The method has found its main use in screening potential blood donors for anemia. The same method can be used for measuring plasma protein.

CHEMICAL METHODS

Hemoglobin may be measured by determining its iron content. Iron must first be

Nitrosobacilli (some)
Pneumococcus
Str. viridans
Benzene and derivatives
Dinitrobenzene
Nitrobenzene
Nitrosobenzene
Chlorates
Dimethylamine
Ferrocyanide
Ferrous sulfate
Formaldehyde
Hydrogen peroxide
Hydroquinone
Hydroxylacetanilide
Hydroxylamine
Iodine
Methylacetanilide
Nitrites
Amyl nitrite
Ethyl nitrite
Sodium nitrite
Nitroglycerin
Ozone
Para-aminopropriophenone
Permanganate
Phenacetin
Phenylenediamine
Phenylhydroxylamine
Pyrogallol
Sulfonal (sulfon-methanol)
Sulfonamides
Prontosil
Sulfanilamide
Sulfapyridine
Sulfathiazole
Toluenediamine
Tolylhydroxylamine
Trinitrotoluene

Methemoglobin is reduced back to Hb by the erythrocyte enzyme systems. It can also be reduced (slowly) by the administration of reducing agents, such as ascorbic acid or sulfhydryl compounds (glutathione, cysteine, BAL); these, as well as methylene blue, are of value in cases of hereditary NAD-methemoglobin reductase deficiency. In cases of acquired or toxic methemoglobinemia, methylene blue is of great value; its rapid action is not based on its own reduction capacity but on its acceleration of the normally slow NADP-methemoglobin reductase pathway.

Methemoglobin can combine reversibly with various chemicals (e.g., cyanides, sulfides, peroxides, fluorides, and azides). Because of its strong affinity for cyanide, the therapy of cyanide poisoning is to administer nitrites to form methemoglobin which then combines with the cyanide. Thus, the free cyanide (which is extremely poisonous to the cellular respiratory enzymes) becomes less toxic when changed to cyanmethemoglobin.

Sulfhemoglobin. *In vitro* and in the presence of oxygen, hemoglobin reacts with hydrogen sulfide to form a greenish derivative of hemoglobin called sulfhemoglobin. Since oxygen is necessary for the formation, it is assumed that oxyhemoglobin reacts directly with the H_2S. The role of sulfur or compounds containing sulfur in the *in vivo* production of sulfhemoglobin is unclear. Sulfhemoglobin implies an irreversible change in the polypeptide chains or globin part of the molecule. It may form in response to an oxidant stress; further change can result in denaturation and precipitation of hemoglobin as Heinz bodies.

Sulfhemoglobin cannot transport oxygen, but it can combine with CO to form carboxysulfhemoglobin. Unlike methemoglobin, sulfhemoglobin cannot be reduced back to hemoglobin, and it remains in the cells until they break down.

Sulfhemoglobin has been reported in patients receiving treatment with sulfonamides, aromatic amine drugs (phenacetin, acetanilid), and sulfur as well as in those with severe constipation, in cases of bacteremia due to *Clostridium welchii,* and in a condition known as enterogenous cyanosis. The concentration of sulfhemoglobin *in vivo* is within the range of a few percentage points, as a rule, and seldom exceeds 10 per cent.

Carbon Monoxide Hemoglobin (Carboxyhemoglobin, HbCO). Hemoglobin has the capacity to combine with carbon monoxide in the same proportion as with oxygen. However, the affinity of the hemoglobin molecule for carbon monoxide is 210 times greater. This means that carbon monoxide will bind with hemoglobin even if its concentration in the air is extremely low (e.g., 0.02 to 0.04 per cent). In those cases, HbCO will build up until typical symptoms of poisoning appear.

HbCO cannot bind oxygen and therefore is not available as an oxygen carrier. Furthermore, the HbO_2-HbCO mixture does not release oxygen so readily as in normal blood, thus adding to the anoxia. If a patient poisoned with carbon monoxide receives pure oxygen, the conversion of HbCO to HbO_2 is greatly enhanced. HbCO is light sensitive and has a typical, brilliant, cherry red color.

Acute carbon monoxide poisoning has long been well known. Chronic poisoning, due to prolonged exposure to small amounts of carbon monoxide, is less well known but is assuming increasing importance. The chief sources of the gas are gasoline motors, illuminating gas, gas heaters, and defective stoves and furnaces. Exposure to carbon monoxide is thus one of the hazards of modern civilization. The gas has even been found in the air of busy streets of large cities in sufficient concentration to cause mild symptoms in persons such as traffic policemen who are exposed to it over long periods of time.

Healthy persons exposed to various concentrations of the gas for an hour do not experience definite symptoms (headache, dizziness, muscular weakness, and nausea) unless the concentration of the gas in the blood reaches 26 or 30 per cent of saturation; however, it appears that in chronic poisoning, especially in children, serious symptoms may occur with lower concentrations. The figures reported for cases of clinical poisoning are often misleading, since the carbon monoxide largely or wholly disappears from the blood after the patient has breathed pure air for a few hours, although the symptoms may continue for a long time.

Tests for Abnormal Hemoglobin Pigments. Some information can be obtained by naked eye examination of the blood specimen. Normal appearance of the serum or plasma identifies the red cells as the site of the pigment. Shaking of normal whole blood in the air for 15 minutes imparts to it a bright red color as the reduced hemoglobin is converted to oxyhemoglobin. The blood is cherry red when the pigment is carboxyhemoglobin in carbon monoxide poisoning. The color is chocolate brown in methemoglobinemia and mauve-lavender in sulfhemoglobinemia.

The specimen must be obtained carefully to avoid hemolysis and promptly analyzed, because certain abnormal pigments disappear on institution of therapy. If carbon monoxide is suspected, dry sodium citrate in small well-stoppered tubes should be used. If methemoglobin is to be tested for, heparin is the anticoagulant of choice, because oxalate tends to elevate the pH and favors conversion of neutral to alkaline methemoglobin. For all other tests, dry oxalate anticoagulant is preferable. Plasma containing hemoglobin is pink or red; it is brown in the presence of methemoglobin or methemalbumin. The red cells and the plasma or serum must be examined.

Identification of Hemoglobin Pigments with the Hand Spectroscope. Whole blood or washed red cells are added to distilled water in a ratio of 1 to 10 or 1 to 100, depending on the concentration of the abnormal pigment. A few milliliters of the hemolyzed blood are placed in each of two test tubes. In the case of methemoglobin and methemalbumin a dark band is seen in the spectroscope between 620 and 630 nm. in the red portion of the spectrum between the Frauenhofer lines C and D. Sulfhemoglobin produces a similar band at 618 nm. To distinguish the pigments, 2 to 3 drops of a 5 per cent solution of potassium cyanide are added (with a dropper, not a pipette) to the second tube with blood. The band will disappear if the pigment is methemoglobin, and the color of the specimen will change from brown or black to dark red, but not if it is sulfhemoglobin or methemalbumin. Three per cent hydrogen peroxide causes the bands of sulfhemoglobin and methemoglobin to disappear. Carboxyhemoglobin and oxyhemoglobin are difficult to distinguish with the spectroscope. Both produce bands at approximately the same location (576 nm.).

Other Tests. Naked eye examination of diluted blood (one drop in 5 ml. of water) shows a yellowish red color of oxyhemoglobin and pinkish or bluish red color of carboxyhemoglobin.

ALKALI TEST. Two drops each of normal blood and of the patient's blood are placed on a spot plate. Two drops of 25 per cent sodium hydroxide are added to each. Carboxyhemoglobin remains unchanged. The normal control turns brown.

A simple qualitative test may be useful in an emergency and will be described.

KATAYAMA'S TEST (1888). This simple test for carbon monoxide hemoglobin will detect as little as 10 per cent of saturation. Place about 10 ml. of water in each of two test tubes. To one tube, add 5 drops of the suspected blood and to the other add 5 drops of normal blood to serve as a control. To each tube, add 5 drops of fresh orange-colored ammonium sulfide. Mix gently and make faintly acid with acetic acid. The color of blood containing carbon monoxide hemoglobin becomes more or less rose red, depending on the concentration of the gas; normal blood becomes a dirty greenish brown.

SPECTROPHOTOMETRIC IDENTIFICATION OF HEMOGLOBINS. The various hemoglobins have characteristic absorption spectra, which can be determined easily with a spectrophotometer. Hemoglobin, for instance, has an absorption maximum at 565 nm. The maxima for oxyhemoglobin are at 514, 544.8, 576.9, and 640.2 nm. Carboxyhemoglobin is characterized by an absorption peak of 535 and 570.9 nm. Methemoglobin has maxima at 500, 540, 578, and 634 nm. and cyanmethemoglobin has its maxima at 414 and 540 nm.

The identification of different forms of hemoglobins by determining the absorption spectrum can be carried out in a very simple way. Approximately one-half of a drop of blood is put into a test tube and diluted with approximately 20 ml. of de-ionized or double-distilled water. The actual dilution of the hemoglobin depends on the concentration of the hemoglobin (e.g., if extremely low, one might have to add less water; if the hemoglobin content is high, one might have to dilute the specimen more). For maximal accuracy, the peak of absorption should be somewhere between 60 and 40 per cent transmittance. After the blood has been diluted with water, samples are read in a spectrophotometer with water as the blank. A recording spectrophotometer is especially

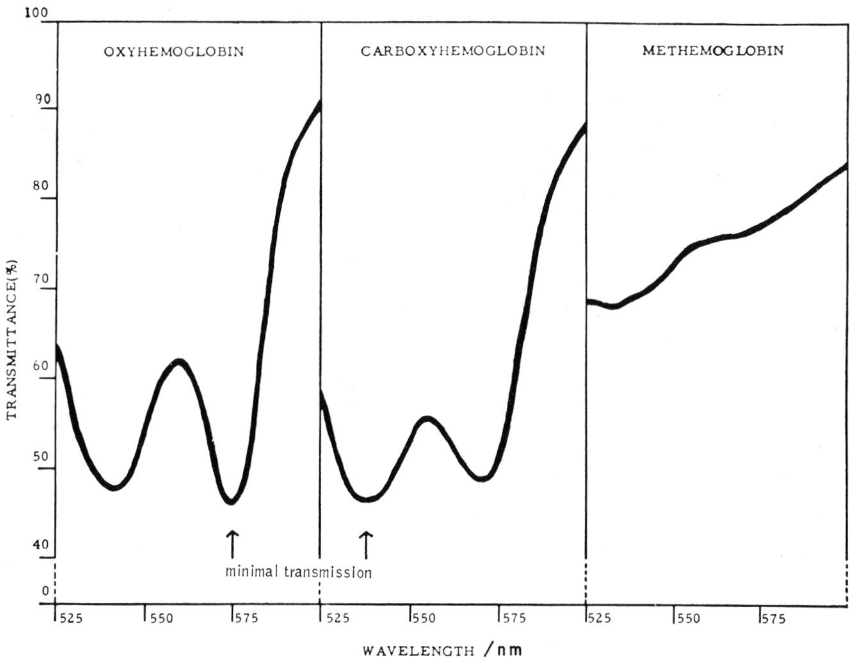

Figure 4–2. Spectrophotometric identification of hemoglobins.

convenient for this determination. Otherwise, the absorption is read at intervals of 5 nm. between 620 and 500 nm. (Fig. 4–2).

In the differentiation between oxyhemoglobin and carbon monoxide hemoglobin, one can take advantage not only of the different absorption spectra but also of the following characteristic: In the case of pure oxyhemoglobin, the absorption at 576.5 nm. will be greater than that at 544.8 nm. In the case of carboxyhemoglobin, however, the absorption at 570.5 nm. will be less than that at 535 nm. (Fig. 4–2).

Hematocrit (Packed Cell Volume)

Definition. Hematocrit is the volume of erythrocytes expressed as a percentage of the volume of whole blood in a sample. The venous hematocrit agrees closely with the hematocrit obtained from a skin puncture; both are greater than the total body hematocrit. Dried heparin, balanced oxalate, or EDTA is satisfactory as an anticoagulant.

Macromethod of Wintrobe

EQUIPMENT. The Wintrobe hematocrit tube is a thick-walled glass tube with a uniform internal bore and a flattened bottom. It is graduated in millimeters from 0 to 105 and has a rubber cap to prevent evaporation during the long period of centrifugation.

Of the various forms of filling pipettes available, a disposable capillary (Pasteur) pipette with a rubber bulb is the most convenient.

The essential requirement of a centrifuge is that it generate a centrifugal field of not less than 2500 G. at the bottom of the cup.

PROCEDURE. After adequate mixing of the sample, the hematocrit tube is filled. The tip of the pipette is introduced to the bottom of the tube. As filling proceeds, the tip of the pipette is raised, but it remains under the rising blood meniscus in order to avoid foaming. The level of the blood should be noted and the tubes capped to avoid evaporation during the required centrifugation for 30 minutes at 2500 G.

Reading is done without disturbing the specimen. The result is calculated from the formula:

$$\text{Hematocrit (per cent)} = \frac{100\ L_1}{L_2}$$

where L_1 is the height of the red cell column in mm. and L_2 is the height of the whole blood specimen (red cells and plasma). The gray-white layer of leukocytes and platelets above the erythrocytes is not included in L_1.

Micromethod

EQUIPMENT. A capillary hematocrit tube about 7 cm. long with a uniform bore of about 1 mm. is recommended. The capillaries are filled with a 1 to 1000 dilution of heparin, dried at 56 or 37° C., and stored. Special centrifuges are available, producing centrifugal fields ranging from 5000 to 10,000 G. This permits shortening of centrifugation to 5 minutes for the latter and 10 minutes for the former.

PROCEDURE. The microhematocrit (capillary) tube is filled by capillary attraction, either from a free-flowing puncture wound or a well-mixed venous sample. The capillary tubes should be at least half full. The empty end is sealed in a small flame of a microburner or plugged with modeling clay, e.g., Plasticine. The filled tubes are placed in the radial grooves of the microhematocrit centrifuge head with the sealed end away from the center.

The air at the outermost end of the capillary will be displaced in the course of centrifugation and the air gap will disappear. Leakage, especially if modeling clay was used for sealing, can be prevented by using a rubber gasket at the periphery of the hematocrit head to act as a cushion. Place the bottom of the tube against the rubber gasket to prevent breakage. Centrifugation for 5 minutes at 10,000 to 12,000 G. is satisfactory unless the hematocrit exceeds 50 per cent; in this case an additional 5 minutes' centrifugation should be employed in order to ensure that plasma trapping has been minimized.

The capillary tubes are not graduated. The length of the whole column, including the plasma, and of the red cell column alone must be measured in each case with a millimeter rule and a magnifying lens or with one of several commercially available automatic or semiautomatic devices. The instructions of the manufacturer must be followed.

INTERPRETATION OF RESULTS. The normal hematocrit for males is 47.0 ± 7, for females 42.0 ± 5. A value below an individual's normal or below the normal range for age and sex indicates anemia, and a higher value, polycythemia. The hematocrit reflects the concentration of red cells, not the total red cell mass. The hematocrit is low in hydremia of pregnancy but the total number of circulating red cells is not reduced. The hematocrit may be normal or even high in shock accompanied by hemoconcentration, though the total red cell mass may be considerably decreased owing to blood loss.

SOURCES OF ERROR

Centrifugation. Adequate duration and speed of centrifugation are essential for a correct hematocrit. The red cells must be packed so that additional centrifugation does not further reduce the packed cell volume. In general, the higher the hematocrit, the more powerful the centrifugal force required.

In the course of centrifugation, a small proportion of the leukocytes, platelets, and plasma are trapped between the red cells. The error resulting from the former is, as a rule, quite insignificant. The increment of the hematocrit due to trapped plasma is somewhat greater than that due to leukocytes and platelets, but this too is of little practical consequence. The lower the relative centrifugal force, the larger the amount of trapped plasma; therefore, the amount of trapped plasma is larger in high hematocrits than in low hematocrits, and is larger with the macromethod than the micromethod. With the macromethod, the trapped plasma accounts for 3 to 4 per cent of the red cell column at normal hematocrits compared with less than 1.5 per cent of the micromethod (Dacie and Lewis, 1968). Because less time is necessary for centrifugation, and because there is less error due to trapping of plasma, the micromethod is preferred over the macromethod.

Sample. Prolonged stasis caused by constriction with a tourniquet for one minute or longer may result in a falsely high hematocrit of from 2.5 to 5 per cent (Mollison, 1967, p. 124). This error will also apply to hemoglobin and cell counts. Unique to the hematocrit is the error due to excess EDTA (inadequate blood for a fixed amount of EDTA): the hematocrit will be falsely low due to cell shrinkage, but the hemoglobin and cell counts will not be affected.

A free flow of blood from a skin puncture for microhematocrit is essential. The hematocrit is unreliable as an estimate of total red cell mass immediately after a loss of blood, even if moderate, and immediately following transfusions.

Other Errors. Technical errors include failure to mix the blood adequately before sampling, improper reading of the level of cells and plasma, and inclusion of the buffy coat as part of the erythrocyte volume. Irregularity of the inside diameter of the tubes will also lead to inaccurate hematocrits.

With good technique the precision of the hematocrit, expressed as ±2 C.V. (coefficient of variation), is ±1 per cent.

Blood Cell Counting

Quantitative studies of the formed elements of the blood – red cells, white cells, and platelets – are concerned with the concentration of each in a microliter (cubic millimeter) of blood. The unit of volume for cell counts traditionally has been expressed as cubic millimeters ($mm.^3$) because the method of measuring that volume is in terms of the linear dimensions of the hemacytometer chamber. However, the International Committee for Standardization in Hematology has now recommended that all units of volume be expressed in liters. Since 1 $mm.^3$ = 1.00003 μl., an insignificant difference, the *microliter* will be used as equivalent to and in preference to the *cubic millimeter* in this chapter.

Except for platelet counts, the hemacytometer is no longer used for routine blood cell counting in any but the smallest of laboratories. Yet it is still necessary for the technologist to be able to use this method effectively and to know its limitations.

Any cell counting procedure includes three steps: dilution of the blood, sampling the diluted suspension into a measured volume, and counting the cells in that volume.

HEMACYTOMETER METHOD (RBC)

Counting Chamber. The type of hemacytometer or counting chamber most widely used (Fig. 4–3) consists of a heavy, colorless glass slide, on the middle third of which are fixed three parallel platforms extending across the slide. In the "double counting chamber," the central platform is subdivided by a transverse groove into two halves, each wider than the two lateral platforms and separated from them and from each other by moats. The central platforms or "floor pieces" are exactly 0.1 mm. lower than the lateral platforms. Each of the central platforms has a so-called improved Neubauer ruling (Fig. 4–3), which consists of a square measuring 3 by 3 mm. (9 sq. mm.) subdivided into nine secondary squares, each 1 by 1 mm. (1 sq. mm.). The four corner squares, labeled A, B, C, D in this figure, are used for the white cell count and are subdivided into 16 tertiary squares.

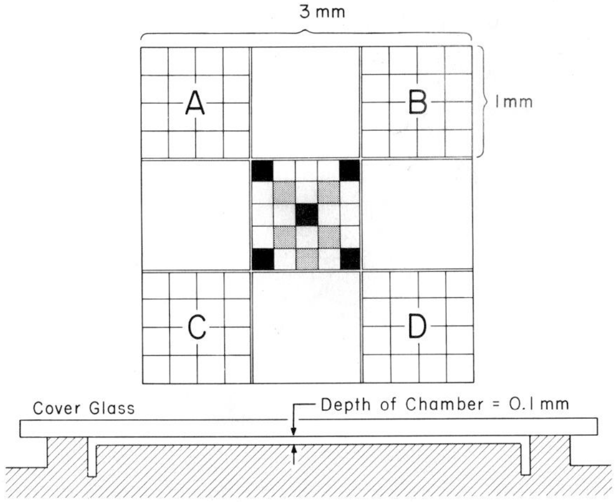

Figure 4–3. The upper figure is a diagram of the improved Neubauer ruling; this is etched on the surface of each side of the hemacytometer. The large corner squares, A, B, C, and D, are used for leukocyte counts. The five black squares in the center (colored only for purposes of illustration) are used for red cell counts or for platelet counts, and the 10 black plus checked squares for platelet counts. Actually, each of the 25 squares within the central sq. mm. has within it 16 smaller squares for convenience in counting.

The lower figure is a side view of the chamber with the coverglass in place.

The central square millimeter is divided into 25 tertiary squares, each of which measures 0.2 by 0.2 mm. Each of these is further subdivided into 16 smaller squares. The total number of the smallest squares in the central square is 400. As a rule, five of the tertiary squares, amounting to 80 of the smallest squares, are used for red cell counts.

A thick coverglass, ground to a perfect plane, accompanies the counting chamber. Ordinary coverglasses have uneven surfaces and should not be used. When the coverglass is in place on the platform of the counting chamber (Fig. 4–3), there is a space exactly 0.1 mm. thick between it and the ruled platform; therefore, each square millimeter of the ruling forms the base of a space holding exactly 0.1 cu. mm.

Counting chambers and coverglasses should be rinsed immediately after use in lukewarm water, never in hot water. The water may be wiped off with a clean lint-free cloth. The counting chamber and coverglass may be allowed to dry in the air. The surfaces must not be touched with gauze or linen, because they may scratch the ruled areas. A scratch across the chamber or coverglass ruins it. The chamber and coverglass should not be touched because fingerprints are difficult to remove and may be responsible for errors. Before use, the surfaces must be absolutely clean, dry, and free from lint and water marks. After they have been cleaned they must not be touched except at the edges.

Red Cell Counting Pipette. The Thoma glass pipettes (Fig. 4–4) consist of a graduated capillary tube, divided into 10 parts and marked 0.5 at the fifth mark and 1.0 at the tenth, a mixing bulb above it containing a glass bead, and above the bulb, another short capillary tube with an engraved mark 11 on the white and 101 on the red cell pipette. The red cell pipette has a red bead in the mixing bulb and the white cell pipette a white bead. The graduations on the pipettes are arbitrary. The volume of the red cell pipette is made up of one-half part at the level of the 0.5 mark, one part at the level of the 1.0 mark, and 100 parts in the bulb. When the blood is drawn to the 0.5 mark and the diluting fluid to the 101 mark, all the blood cells are washed into the bulb and the resulting dilution in the bulb is 1 to 200. The capillary portion of the pipette contains no blood but only diluting fluid; therefore, it is not included in the total volume, and its contents must be expelled before the red cell suspension is introduced into the chamber.

In the white cell diluting pipette, the marks on the capillary tube are the same as in the red pipette, but the bulb is smaller, with an

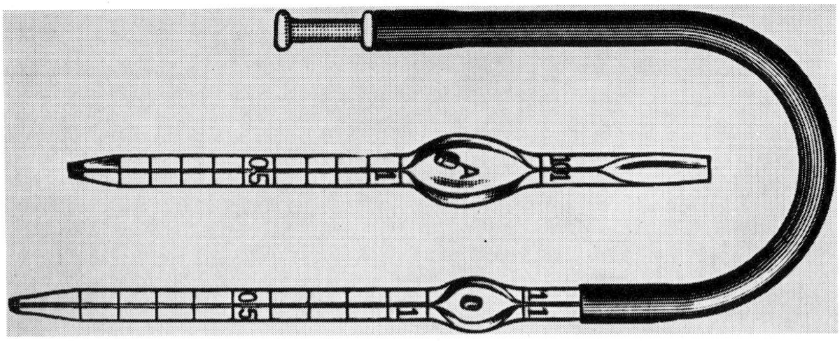

Figure 4–4. Thoma red and white cell diluting pipettes.

engraved mark 11 above it. When the blood is drawn to the 0.5 mark and diluted to the 11 mark, the dilution is 1 to 20. Again the cell-free fluid in the capillary is not included in the total volume.

Pipettes should have a guaranteed error of no more than ± 1.0 per cent. Inferior pipettes should not be used. Alternatively it is perfectly acceptable to make the 1:200 dilution of blood with a 20 μl. hemoglobin or Sahli pipette of ± 1.0 per cent accuracy into an ordinary test tube containing exactly 4 ml. of red cell diluting fluid.

The rubber tubing that is attached to the pipette should be sufficiently heavy walled to resist collapse during suction and should be long enough (at least 10 inches) to permit easy reading of the graduation marks.

After use, pipettes should be rinsed with tap water and then three times with distilled water, filling the bulb through the capillary end, shaking, and emptying through the large-bore end. This is followed by similar treatment with acetone or 95 per cent alcohol and finally with ether, using a water suction pump. The interior of the pipettes should then be dried with a current of dry air. The bulb is dry if the bead rolls freely. If the lumen of the capillary pipette contains coagulated blood or other debris, it can be cleaned with a horsehair or with a special, delicate, commercially available wire. If the pipette contains impurities, it should be filled with cleaning solution and allowed to stand overnight. Washing devices are available that permit cleansing and drying many pipettes simultaneously. If cleansing or at least thorough rinsing cannot be done immediately after use, the pipettes should be placed upright in a container with water. Utmost care must be exerted to prevent damage to the delicate point of the pipette, for even the slightest damage that affects the bore makes the pipette useless because it leads to inaccuracy in the dilution.

Red Cell Diluting Fluid. The diluting fluid must be isotonic to prevent lysis and crenation of red cells. It should contain a fixative to preserve the shape of the cells and to prevent agglutination and autolysis if the count cannot be performed within an hour. Gower's solution (sodium sulfate, 12.5 gm.; glacial acetic acid, 33.3 ml.; distilled water, 200 ml.) meets these requirements; it should be filtered before use. It is even simpler to use Isoton* or its equivalent, which is likely to be readily available if an electronic flow-through counter is in the laboratory.

Counting Procedure

1. Venous or capillary blood is suitable. If capillary blood is used, it must be flowing freely. If venous blood is used, it must be thoroughly mixed by inversion at least 60 times.

2. The tip of the pipette is placed beneath the surface of the blood which is then quickly aspirated just to the 0.5 mark on the red cell pipette. No air bubbles can be in the column of blood. If the blood rises slightly above the mark, it can be drawn back to the mark by touching the tip of the pipette to the finger. If a large excess of blood has been drawn up, the pipette should be cleaned and the procedure repeated, because even though it is withdrawn, enough will remain adhering to the inside of the pipette to introduce a significant error. Painstakingly accurate technique in this part of the procedure is important, because any error is magnified 200 times by the subsequent dilution.

3. The blood adhering to the tip is wiped off quickly, the tip is plunged into the diluting fluid, and the fluid is sucked up to the mark 101, while rotating the pipette. It is best to hold the pipette nearly horizontally in order to avoid aspiration of air bubbles in the bulb, but when the bulb is almost full the pipette should be raised to the vertical position. At this stage the blood sample has been diluted 1 to 200 or 1 to 100, depending on the amount of blood

*Coulter Diagnostics, Hialeah, Fla.

taken. Except in cases of severe anemia, a dilution of 1 to 200 is preferable.

4. The ends of the pipette are now closed with the thumb and middle finger, and the pipette is shaken for about 30 seconds to facilitate the initial mixing. The bead contained in the bulb should move freely. The shaking should be done at a 90 degree angle to the long axis of the pipette. If capillary blood is used, all these steps must be carried out rapidly to prevent coagulation before blood is mixed with the diluting fluid.

When it is not convenient to count the erythrocytes at once, a heavy rubber band is placed around the pipette to close both ends.

5. When the counting chamber and the coverglass have been cleaned, the coverglass is adjusted in place. The pipette is held between the thumb and middle finger or in a special shaking machine and shaken for 2 to 3 minutes at right angles to the long axis of the pipette.

6. The first 3 to 4 drops are blown off to eliminate the cell-free fluid from the capillary tube. The pipette is held at an angle of about 35 degrees while the tip is touched to the angle between the edge of the coverglass and one of the projecting ends of the floor piece. The fluid will run under the coverglass by capillary attraction. The fluid is allowed to enter in a controlled manner by pressure from the index finger on the open end of the pipette or from the pressure of the tongue on the mouthpiece of the pipette. Care must be exercised to permit just enough fluid to fill the space beneath the coverglass. This is especially important when the chamber lacks clamps, since an excess of fluid will tend to raise the coverglass appreciably and erroneously increase the erythrocyte count. A small excess remaining at the mouth of the counting chamber can be removed by touching the drop gently with the finger but not with gauze or a towel.

The characteristics of a properly filled counting chamber are that the fluid fills the space beneath the coverglass entirely or almost entirely, none of the fluid has run over into the moat, and there are no bubbles. If any of these conditions are not met, the count will not be reliable and the chamber has to be cleaned, dried, and recharged.

7. The cells in the chamber are permitted to settle for several minutes. Then the ruled area is surveyed with the low-power objective to see whether they are evenly distributed. If they are not, the procedure has to be repeated. If the chamber is filled and the cells not counted promptly, the fluid should be protected against evaporation by placing the chamber under a Petri dish containing a moistened piece of filter paper, which is applied to the top inner surface.

8. Counting. The square millimeter with the 400 small squares in the center of the ruled area lies under a volume of 1/10 μl. In this volume, one usually counts the red cells in 80 small squares (5 of the 25 tertiary squares, see Fig. 4–3); in other words, the cells in one-fifth of this volume of 1/10 μl. of the diluted cell suspension. Since the dilution is 1 to 200, one is counting the number of red cells in $1/5 \times 1/10 \times 1/200 = 1/10{,}000$ μl. of blood. This means that the red cell count in 1 μl. of blood is the number of cells counted $\times$ 10,000.

9. In counting the 5 tertiary squares, each with 16 small squares, the following rule is suggested to avoid confusion in counting cells that lie on borderlines: Erythrocytes that touch any one of the three lines or the single line on the left and the top borders of the small square should be counted as though they were within the squares, but those that touch any of the lines on the right and the bottom borders of the small squares should not be counted. In this way no cell is counted twice. The cells are counted in each small square, first from left to right, beginning with the top of four small squares, and then from right to left for the next row, and so on. The number of cells for each of the five groups of 16 squares is recorded separately and the results are added.

Sources of Error. Numerous possibilities for error exist in all cell counts using the hemacytometer. Errors that can be minimized by careful technique are errors due to the nature of the sample, to the operator's faulty technique, and to inaccurate equipment. Errors that are inherent in the distribution of cells in the counting volume are called "field" errors and can be minimized only by counting more cells.

Errors due to the Nature of the Sample. Partial coagulation in either capillary or venous blood introduces errors by changes in the distribution of the cells or decrease of their number. Drawing a drop of blood from pale, cold, or cyanotic skin is another serious source of error, as is excessive massage to improve the flow of blood.

With venous blood, stasis due to prolonged application of the tourniquet produces hemoconcentration. The distribution of the cells in the plasma changes rapidly due to sedimentation. Failure to mix the blood thoroughly and immediately before drawing the sample into the pipette is bound to introduce an error, which is directly proportionate to the degree of sedimentation during the interval since the blood was mixed. This is accentuated in a variety of diseases in which the sedimentation is significantly accelerated. The fact that the specimen is a suspension and that the cells have to be in a uniform suspension in order to be counted correctly opens the door to other possible errors. Currents of all kinds may alter the uniformity of the suspension. Yeast cells growing in contaminated diluting fluid may be mistaken for erythrocytes.

Operator's Errors. These include errors due to faulty technique, such as may occur when blood and the diluting fluid are drawn into the pipette (use of an unclean or wet pipette or failure to wipe off the pipette tip), and errors introduced when the chamber is loaded and when the cells are counted. A frequent source of trouble is faulty application of the coverglass, especially when it is raised by introduction of an excess of diluted blood, or movement of the coverglass after the counting chamber has been filled. Overflowing of the suspension into the moat is another example. This may reduce the count by as much as 1,000,000. The number of technical errors of this kind is legion but can be reduced to a minimum in the hands of an experienced technologist.

Errors due to Equipment. Inaccuracies in the graduations of the pipettes and of the ruled areas and depth of the counting chambers are frequent sources of error. They can be diminished by using pipettes and hemacytometers certified by the U.S. Bureau of Standards.

Inherent or Field Error. Even in a perfectly mixed sample, variation occurs in the number of suspended cells that are distributed in a given volume (i.e., come to rest over a given square).

According to Poisson's law of distribution, the variation among the different squares in the chamber is given by the formula S.D. = $\sqrt{m}$, where m is the mean number of erythrocytes per unit area and S.D. is the standard deviation of the counts in these areas. *Example:* The mean count per 80 squares is 500 (as for a count of 5,000,000 per μl.). The S.D. of counts of different sets of 80 squares in the chamber will be $\sqrt{500}$ or 22.4. Expressed relatively as a per cent, this is $\frac{22.4}{500} \times 100 = 4.5$ per cent. This expression of the standard deviation as a percentage of the mean $\left(\frac{\text{S.D.}}{\text{mean}} \times 100\right)$ is known as the coefficient of variation (C.V.).

Since ±2 S.D. is generally accepted as a significant limit, the error of a count of 5,000,000 per cu. mm. made in the hemacytometer chamber owing merely to the variation in the field of observation is $\pm 2 \times 4.5 = \pm 9$ per cent. This "error of the field" measured as S.D. = $\sqrt{m}$ is the minimal error, but is not the only one to which the hemacytometer count is subject. Separate fillings of different standard chambers with the same blood will result in different total counts per measured unit volume in the different chambers owing to variations in calibration, variations in the filling technique, and variations in pressure of the coverglass. This may be referred to as the *"error of the chamber."*

Similarly, separate fillings of different standard pipettes with the same blood will result in different total counts per measured unit volume in the different pipettes. This may be referred to as the *"error of the pipette."* Berkson *et al.* (1940) have determined the S.D. of the pipette error as 4.7 per cent of the mean count. For the total error, they gave for a count of 5,000,000 $\sqrt{4.1^2 + 4.6^2 + 4.7^2} = 7.7$* or about 8 per cent. Since twice the S.D. is the usually accepted limit of significance, the error of a single estimate of the erythrocyte count was given by them as ±16 per cent. This, of course, is a minimal error under the best of circumstances. Counting twice as many cells (two pipettes and two chambers) is preferable and can reduce the error somewhat, but not into the range of clinical usefulness.

DILUTORS

The method previously described for diluting the blood for hemoglobin or for cell counts can be performed more rapidly and accurately both manually and semiautomatically (Bull, 1971).

Semiautomated and Automated Methods. Several instruments are now available for precise and convenient diluting, which both aspirate the sample and wash it out with the diluent. In some instruments the volumes are adjustable; in others, one or both volumes are fixed. In either case the dilutor should perform a 1:250 or 1:500 dilution with a coefficient of variation of less than 1 per cent.

A semiautomatic dilutor, the Hem-Aliquanter (Bull *et al.*, 1968), dispenses the diluent and the sample separately. The sample is dispensed simultaneously for several tests with errors of less than 1 per cent. This dilutor should be considered for the laboratory without a multichannel instrument.

Manual. For capillary sampling, manual methods are still necessary. Accurate disposable pipettes are now available; some are similar to the classic Sahli pipette. More convenient and reliable are microcapillary pipettes that fill by capillarity and cannot overfill;† when added to the diluent in an appropriate-sized test tube they empty satisfactorily, with

*The total error is given as the square root of the sum of the squares of the constituent errors. The 4.1 per cent for the error of the field is a slight modification found by Berkson *et al.* (1940) of what is given by the Poisson distribution (for a normal red cell count) as 4.5 per cent. The 4.6 per cent is the error of the chamber.

†Drummond Hemocaps, Drummond Scientific Company, Broomall, Pa.

sufficient washout of sample by diluent. These pipettes are available with an accuracy of ±0.25 per cent, which is suitable for calibration. Less expensive pipettes with an accuracy of ±1 per cent are usually used for routine work.

Combining a microcapillary tube with a plastic vial containing a premeasured volume of diluent, the Unopette* is a valuable system for manual dilutions. After the capillary is filled, it is pushed into the container and the sample is washed out by squeezing the soft plastic vial. This system is especially convenient for finger-puncture sampling. Unopettes are available with diluents for red cell counts, white cell counts, platelet counts, and hemoglobin determinations.

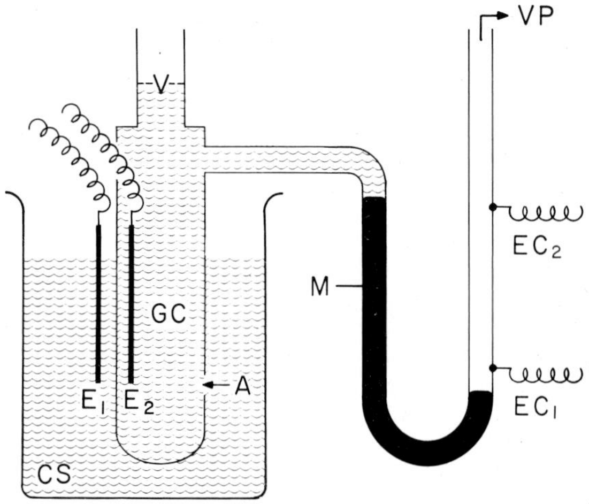

Figure 4–5. Schematic diagram of particle counter in which changes in electrical resistance are counted as voltage pulses. CS = cell suspension, GC = glass cylinder, A = aperture, E_1 and E_2 = platinum electrodes, V = valve, M = mercury column, EC_1 and EC_2 = electrical contacts, VP = vacuum pump. (Diagram adapted from Ackermann, 1972.)

ELECTRONIC COUNTING OF RED CELLS

(Brittin and Brecher, 1971; Bull, 1971; Ackermann, 1972)

The most widely used methods of cell counting today are electronic, employing one of two principles:

1. Cells passing through an aperture cause changes in electrical resistance which are counted as voltage pulses. This principle is used in the Coulter Counter† and in the Celloscope.‡

2. Cells passing through a flow cell cause deflections in a beam of light which are converted to electric pulses by a photomultiplier tube. This principle is used in the Technicon Autoanalyzer§ and the Fisher Autocytometer.**

Counting Voltage Pulses

PRINCIPLE. Cells passing through an aperture through which a current is flowing cause changes in electrical resistance which are counted as voltage pulses. This principle, used in the Coulter Counter and in the Celloscope, is illustrated in Figure 4–5. An accurately diluted suspension of blood (CS) is made in 0.85 per cent saline or, preferably, in an isotonic conductive solution (such as Isoton†) which preserves the cell shape. The instrument has a glass cylinder (GC) that can be filled with the conducting fluid and has within it an electrode (E_2) and an aperture (A) of 100 μm. diameter in its wall. Just outside the glass cylinder is another electrode (E_1). The cylinder is connected to a U-shaped glass tube which is partly filled with mercury (M) and which has two electrical contacts (EC_1 and EC_2). The glass cylinder is immersed in the suspension of cells to be counted (CS) and is filled with conductive solution and closed by a valve (V). A current now flows through the aperture between E_1 and E_2. Then, as a vacuum pump (VP) draws the mercury up the tube, the cell suspension flows through the aperture into the cylinder. Each cell that passes through the aperture displaces an equal volume of conductive fluid, increasing the electrical resistance and creating a voltage pulse, because its resistance is much greater than that of the conductive solution. The pulses, which are proportional in height to the volume of the cells, are counted.

The counting mechanism is started when the mercury contacts EC_1 and stopped when it contacts EC_2; during this time the cells are counted in a volume of suspension exactly equal to the volume of the glass tubing between contact wires EC_1 and EC_2.

If two or more cells enter the aperture simultaneously, they will be counted as one pulse; this produces a coincidence error for which a correction must be made. The size of the coincidence error can be diminished by decreasing the concentration of cells and decreasing the size of the aperture. However, decreasing the cell concentration increases the effect of errors in dilution, increases the inherent counting error, and makes more critical the error due to the background "noise" of contaminating particles. With decreased aperture size, partial or complete plugging of the aperture with debris becomes a problem. Therefore, a balance is struck, and for a given count above a critical number, a coincidence correction is made by referring to a chart supplied by the manufacturer.

*Becton-Dickinson, Rutherford, N.J.
†Coulter Diagnostics, Hialeah, Fla.
‡Lars Ljungberg & Co., Stockholm, Sweden.
§Technicon Co., Ardsley, N.Y.
**Fisher Scientific Co., Pittsburgh, Pa.

A threshold setting or pulse discriminator allows the exclusion of pulses below an adjustable height on the Coulter Counter Models A and F.

Note: On the Models B and Z a second threshold also excludes the counting of pulses *above* a certain height. One therefore counts only the cells in the "window" between the two settings. By systematically changing each threshold by given increments, one can determine a frequency distribution of relative cell volumes. Such cell size distributions can now be automatically plotted by attachments available for the Coulter Counter Models B or Z (Channelyzer) and may be valuable in the study of red cells or platelets when two or more changing populations of cells are present.

Instruments that handle the data from the changes in electrical resistance digitally (e.g., the Coulter Counter) are stable and infrequently require calibration. Therefore, they can be relied upon as primary reference machines to give a correct red cell count if the specimens are properly mixed and diluted (Brittin and Brecher, 1971; Bull, 1971).

Before counting, the adjustment of the threshold is checked by counting the diluted suspension of red cells at successively increasing increments. To ensure that smaller particles (background "noise") are excluded from the count, the adjustment should be in the middle of the plateau. Larger foreign particles in the diluent are quantitated in a background or blank count which may be subtracted from the cell count. However, if the blank count is too high, the accuracy of the cell count will be impaired. The final cell dilution should allow a particle count of at least 5000, which should be at least 20 times the blank count. Specific directions for operation of the instruments are given by the manufacturer.

In the Coulter Counter, the dilution for the red cell count is 1:50,000, usually made in two steps: first, 20 μl. of blood in 10 ml. (1:500), followed by 100 μl. of the first dilution in 10 ml. of diluent (1:100). Since 0.5 ml. of the cell suspension is counted, 50,000 cells (after correction for coincidence) will be counted for a normal red cell count of $5 \times 10^6/\mu$l.

For a normal red cell count, therefore, the Poisson error will be about 0.5 per cent $\left(\text{C.V.} = \frac{\sqrt{n}}{n}\right)$ and for a very low count, closer to 1 per cent. The actual precision of red cell counting is about twice this, or 1 to 2 per cent (C.V.), and errors of dilution bring the precision achieved in practice to 2 to 4 per cent (Brittin and Brecher, 1971).

The Celloscope 401 operates on the same principle as the Coulter Counter, but deals with the problem of coincidence in a different way. Instead of counting all the pulses and correcting for coincidence, the Celloscope 401 counts every 64th pulse and no coincidence correction is necessary. The precision of red cell counting is comparable to that of the Coulter Counter; Lappin *et al.* (1972) found the mean coefficient of variation to be 1.2 per cent.

Counting Light-Scattering Events. In electron-optical counters (Fig. 4–6) a photomultiplier tube detects light scattering either from external reflections from the surface of cells, from transmitted and refracted light passing through the cells, or from diffracted light which has passed tangential to cell surfaces (Mansberg, 1970). In the Technicon cell counter, the intensity of the diffraction events provides the highest signal-to-noise ratio (about 100:1) in the small scattering angle that is necessary for adequate depth of focus. Because of a uniform pulse amplitude, the high signal-to-noise ratio, and the forward-angle scattering character of the system, there is a broad threshold curve which is the same for leukocytes and erythrocytes. A small sensing volume is defined by illumination (44×10^3 fl.) in the flow cell and allows a lesser dilution (1:10,000) than the voltage pulse counter, resulting in minimal coincidence. The characteristics described yield an accuracy and precision in cell counting that is limited only by the qualities of the pumping system.

The Technicon cell counter consists basically of the following modules: sampler, proportion-

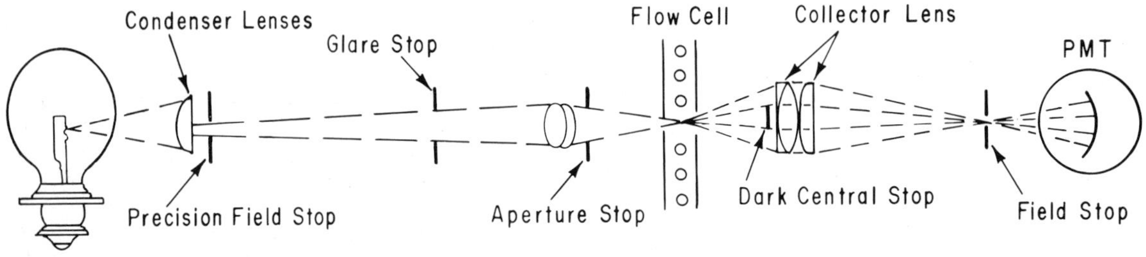

Figure 4–6. Schematic diagram of the electron-optical cell counter. Light is focused on the flow cell. Only light scattered by a cell reaches the photomultiplier tube (PMT), which converts it to an electrical pulse. (From Mansberg, H. P.: Advanc. Automated Anal. *1*:213, 1970.)

ing pump with manifolds having plastic tubing, glass helical mixing and phasing coils, a cell counter, and a single pen recorder. Anticoagulated blood in a tube or sample cup is mixed by two paddles (one minute each) before being sampled during a third minute. (The capacity is 60 samples/hour.) The continuous flow system incorporates dilution with diluent and mixing before the diluted cell suspension reaches the flow cell for counting. The output of the photomultiplier tube is recorded by the pen on moving preprinted paper. The instrument must be calibrated with a known blood or particle suspension at the beginning of each series of counts; since this takes a relatively large volume of known or reference standard blood, it is not practical to run small numbers of samples.

The Technicon red cell counter is now almost always used as part of a multichannel instrument, the SMA 4A or SMA 7A or the Hemalog. The coefficient of variation of the red cell count on these instruments is between 1.5 and 3.5 per cent (Nelson, 1969).

Red Cell Corpuscular Values; Red Cell Indices

Wintrobe introduced procedures for the study of anemia which have substituted objective quantitative standards for subjective impressions: Mean corpuscular volume (MCV), mean corpuscular hemoglobin (MCH), and mean corpuscular hemoglobin concentration (MCHC). Three accurately determined basic values are needed: red cell count, hemoglobin, and hematocrit. Venous blood is used with heparin, balanced oxalate (ammonium and potassium oxalate), or EDTA added.

MCV. The MCV is the average volume of the individual red cells in cubic microns (μ^3) or femtoliters (fl.). One fl. $= 10^{-15}$ liters $= 1\ \mu^3$.

CALCULATION

$$\text{MCV} = \frac{\text{hematocrit (per cent)} \times 10}{\text{red cell count (millions per } \mu\text{l.)}}$$

Normal (N) $= 90 \pm 8$ femtoliters per cell.

EXAMPLES

Hematocrit = 20; red cell count = 1,500,000

$$\text{MCV} = \frac{20 \times 10}{1.5} = 133 \text{ fl. (macrocytic anemia)}$$

Hematocrit = 20; red cell count = 3,000,000

$$\text{MCV} = \frac{20 \times 10}{3} = 67 \text{ fl. (microcytic hypochromic anemia)}$$

MCH. The MCH is the content (weight) of hemoglobin of the average individual red cell in micromicrograms ($\mu\mu$g.) or picograms (pg.).

CALCULATION

$$\text{MCH} = \frac{\text{hemoglobin (gm./dl.)} \times 10}{\text{red cell count (millions per } \mu\text{l.)}}$$

$$N = 30 \pm 3 \text{ pg.}$$

In most anemias, changes in the average size of the red cells (MCV) parallel similar changes in the weight of hemoglobin in the red cells (MCH). Consequently, the MCV and MCH show similar variations.

EXAMPLES

Hemoglobin = 6 gm./dl.; red cell count = 1,200,000

$$\text{MCH} = \frac{6 \times 10}{1.2} = 50 \text{ pg. (macrocytic anemia)}$$

Hemoglobin = 5 gm./dl.; red cell count = 2,400,000

$$\text{MCH} = \frac{5 \times 10}{2.4} = 21 \text{ pg. (microcytic hypochromic anemia)}$$

MCHC. The MCHC is the average hemoglobin concentration per 100 ml. of packed red cells in per cent.

CALCULATION

$$\text{MCHC} = \frac{\text{hemoglobin (gm./dl.)} \times 100}{\text{hematocrit (per cent)}}$$

$N = 34 \pm 2$ per cent (increased only in spherocytosis)

EXAMPLES

Hemoglobin=7 gm./dl.; hematocrit=20 per cent

$$\text{MCHC} = \frac{7 \times 100}{20} = 35 \text{ per cent (normochromic anemia)}$$

Hemoglobin=6 gm./dl.; hematocrit=21 per cent

$$\text{MCHC} = \frac{6 \times 100}{21} = 29 \text{ per cent (hypochromic anemia)}$$

Discussion. The red cell indices are used to determine the morphologic type of anemia, which is helpful in outlining a diagnostic approach to the patient with anemia. The appearance of the erythrocytes on the blood film should always be compared with the values obtained for the indices in order to check on their accuracy and to detect variations in size and shape within the red cell population. It must be remembered that the indices give only an average value.

Red cell indices are useful only if they are reasonably accurate, and this depends upon the accuracy of the measurements from which they are calculated. When only the hemacytometer is available for red cell counts, the MCV and MCH have too great an inherent variability and the MCHC is the most useful of the indices. But even a small laboratory that does 10 to 15 white cell counts per day can justify an electronic cell counter. When the latter is used for red cell counts, all three of the indices can have useful accuracy.

When the workload is over 100 (certainly over 150) blood cell counts per day, an automated multichannel instrument can be justified.

Leukocyte Count (White Cell Count)

In the total leukocyte count, no distinction is made among the five normal cell types (neutrophils, lymphocytes, monocytes, eosinophils, and basophils, in order of decreasing numbers). Each cell type has its own particular function in defending the body against foreign threats. How they are distinguished from one another is considered later; here we are concerned with the total leukocyte concentration in the blood. The normal range for adults is 4500–11,000/μl.

Sample. Heparin is unsatisfactory as an anticoagulant; EDTA or double oxalate should be used.

Hemacytometer Method. Though this method is rarely used in routine leukocyte counting any longer, the technologist should be able to perform it (1) as a check on the validity of electronic methods for calibration purposes and in cases with profound leukopenia; and (2) as a back-up method.

EQUIPMENT. The white cell pipette has a stem and a mixing chamber (Fig. 4–4). The stem is divided into 10 parts, which measure the volume of the blood sample. The fifth and tenth graduations are marked as 0.5 and 1.0, respectively. The mixing chamber extends from the mark 1.0 to 11.0. It contains a white bead, which aids in the mixing. The volume of the mixing chamber is 20 times the volume of the stem at the mark 0.5 and 10 times the volume at the mark 1.0. When blood is drawn to the 0.5 mark (1 volume) and the diluting fluid to the 11.0 mark (11 volumes), the dilution of the blood sample is 1 to 20 and the dilution factor is 20. When blood is drawn to the 1.0 mark and the diluting fluid to 11.0, the dilution factor is 10.

The counting chamber with the improved Neubauer ruling is used.

DILUTING FLUID. The diluting fluid should lyse the erythrocytes so that they will not obscure the leukocytes. The simplest diluting fluid is a 2 per cent solution of acetic acid. More satisfactory is the following:

Glacial acetic acid	2 ml.
1 per cent aqueous solution of gentian violet	1 ml.
Distilled water	100 ml.

The fluid must be filtered frequently to remove yeasts and molds.

TECHNIQUE. All recommendations made previously relating to the erythrocytes apply also to leukocytes and will not be repeated here.

1. The blood is drawn carefully to the 0.5 mark and the diluting fluid to the mark 11. This gives a dilution of 1 to 20.

2. The outside of the tip of the pipette is wiped off with cotton to remove any blood that may be adhering to it and the diluting fluid is drawn to fill the mixing chamber to the mark 11.

3. Mixing the pipette for 3 minutes, discharging the first few drops of diluting fluid from the stem, and loading the two counting chambers are performed as described for the red cell count.

4. The condenser diaphragm of the microscope is partially closed to make the leukocytes stand out clearly under a low-power (10×) objective lens. The diluting fluid lyses the red cells but not the leukocytes. If the distribution of the latter in the four corner squares is uneven, the procedure thus far must be repeated with clean hemacytometer and pipette.

5. The leukocytes are counted in each of the four large (1 sq. mm.) corner squares (A, B, C and D in Fig. 4–3), each of which is divided into 16 smaller squares for convenience. Eight large squares in two chambers are counted.

6. Each large square encloses a volume of 1/10 mm.^{3} and the dilution is 1 to 20. Therefore, in the volume in the chamber over one large square, one is counting the number of leukocytes in $1/10 \times 1/20 = 1/200$ mm.^{3} of blood. This means that the leukocyte count is the average number of cells in each large square (N) multiplied by 200. A general formula is:

$$\text{leukocyte count (cells/mm.}^3) = \frac{\text{cc}}{\text{lsc}} \times \text{d} \times 10$$

where cc is the total number of cells counted, d is the dilution factor, 10 is the factor transforming the surface area of the square millimeter to the volume in mm.^{3}, and lsc is the number of large squares counted.

In leukopenia, with a total count below 2500, the blood is drawn to the 1.0 mark and the dilution factor is 10.

Example: 120 cells counted in eight squares.

$$\text{Number of leukocytes per mm.}^3 = \frac{120 \times 10 \times 10}{8} = 1500.$$

In leukocytosis with high counts, red cell pipettes are used, and the dilution may be 1 to 100 or even 1 to 200.

SOURCES OF ERROR. The errors are caused by the same factors as in counting red cells (q.v.). The largest element is the small number of cells counted and the field error contributed by the Poisson distribution. If the leukocyte count is 5000/μl., 200 cells will be counted in all 8 squares. The C.V. $= \frac{\sqrt{200}}{200} = 0.07$ or 7 per cent, and the 95 per cent confidence limits (based on this error alone) would be 4650–5350 cells/μl. Errors of pipette and counting chamber add another 2 to 3 per cent; for blood with a true count of 5000/μl., therefore, the 95 per cent confidence limits would be $\pm$20 per cent, or 4000–6000/μl. Though this is a larger percentage error than the hemacytometer red cell counts, it is of less practical consequence because of the greater physiologic variation of the leukocyte count.

Nucleated red cells will be counted and cannot be distinguished from leukocytes with the magnification used. If their number is high as seen on the stained smear, a correction should be made according to the following formula:

$$\text{True leukocyte count} = \frac{\text{total count} \times 100}{100 + \text{No. of NRBC}}$$

where the No. of NRBC = the number of nucleated red cells which are counted in the differentiated count per 100 leukocytes.

EXAMPLE. The blood smear shows 25 nucleated red cells per 100 leukocytes. The total white cell count is 10,000.

$$\text{True leukocyte count} = \frac{10{,}000 \times 100}{125}$$

$$= 8000/\mu\text{l.}$$

Electronic Counting of Leukocytes. (Gagon *et al.*, 1966; Brittin and Brecher, 1971). The principle is the same as that for red cells, except that in either electro-optical or voltage pulse counting, the red cells are lysed before counting. Discussion here will be confined to voltage pulse counting since this is the most widely used of the methods.

DILUENT SOLUTION

1. Physiological saline, Isoton,* or one of the other commercially available diluting fluids is used, 10 ml. for 20 μl. of blood.
   a. To this are added two drops of a 3 per cent saponin solution* for lysis of the red cells. Five minutes are required to ensure complete stromatolysis.
   b. Alternatively, one can use Coulter's Zaponin* or Zap-oglobin.* The latter has the advantage of both selectively lysing red cells and converting the hemoglobin to cyanmethemoglobin so that the hemoglobin concentration may be determined from the same dilution.

2. Cetrimide-citrate-saline has advantages over saponin in that stromatolysis and dilution occur with one procedure and the leukocytes are stable for several hours (Cartwright, 1968). A 1:500 dilution is made by diluting 20 μl. of blood directly in 10 ml. of cetrimide-citrate-saline.

THRESHOLD (PULSE DISCRIMINATOR) SETTING. Prior to counting with any new instrument, diluent, or lysing agent, it is necessary to construct a threshold curve. This is done by performing multiple leukocyte counts on a normal blood sample at threshold settings differing by small increments from zero to a point at which the cells are no longer being counted. They may have to be done at different aperture current settings in order to select one that yields a good plateau. The threshold setting is selected so that baseline noise and small particles are not included in the count. The height of the plateau should be checked by several replicate hemacytometer leukocyte counts.

TECHNIQUE. Details of operation and coincidence correction charts are supplied by the instrument manufacturer. Background counts greater than 100 should be corrected for coincidence and subtracted from the corrected leukocyte count; if less than 100, background counts can be ignored.

SOURCES OF ERROR. With the Coulter counter, 0.5 ml. of the 1 to 500 dilution of blood is counted, so that 10,000 cells are actually counted for a white cell count of 10,000 per μl. If two counts are made from one dilution and averaged, the error ($\pm$2 C.V.) is approximately $\pm$10 per cent in the normal range. If two dilutions of blood are made with an automatic dilutor and triplicate counts are done on each and averaged, the error ($\pm$2 C.V.) is $\pm$4.6 per cent in the normal range. Gagon *et al.* (1966) showed that the leukocyte concentration in blood anticoagulated with EDTA is stable for 24 hours at 8° C. or 25° C. and, in blood anticoagulated with double oxalate, for 24 hours at 8° C. and 6 hours at 25° C. Counts with heparinized blood were often higher than those with other anticoagulants and were not reproducible.

The speed of performance, the elimination of visual fatigue of the technician, and the improved precision are decisive advantages of the electronic cell counter over the hemacytometer.

Platelet Count

Normally 2 to 4 μm. in diameter, the platelets are the smallest formed elements in the blood. They function in hemostasis and in maintaining vascular integrity in addition to participating in the process of blood coagulation. The normal range is 150,000–400,000/μl.

Platelets are difficult to count, because they are small and must be distinguished from debris. Another source of difficulty is their

*Coulter Diagnostics, Hialeah, Fla.

tendency to adhere to glass, to any foreign body, and particularly to each other. It is often possible to recognize a significant decrease in the number of platelets by a careful inspection of stained films. With capillary blood, films must be made evenly and very quickly after the blood is obtained in order to avoid clumping and to minimize the decrease due to adhesion of platelets to the margins of the injured vessels. A better estimate is possible by examining stained films made from venous blood anticoagulated with EDTA, in which platelets are evenly distributed and where clumping and loss due to the hemostatic process do not occur. Therefore, a remark regarding platelets should be a part of the report on the differential count in the form of a reference to their abnormal shape and inadequacy in numbers, if noted.

The visual method of choice employs the phase contrast microscope. This is the reference method. Laboratories performing over 20 platelet counts per day can justify electronic platelet counting; both the voltage pulse counting and the electro-optical counting systems are satisfactory.

Hemacytometer Method. Phase Contrast Microscope (Brecher and Cronkite, 1964).

Equipment. Flat bottom counting chamber and a No. 1 or 1½ coverslip. "Long working distance" phase condenser with 43 × annulus and matching 43 × phase objective and 10 × eyepiece. For American Optical Company equipment, "medium dark contrast" should be specified.

Diluent Solution. One per cent ammonium oxalate in distilled water. Stock bottle is kept in refrigerator. The amount needed for the day is filtered before use and the unused portion discarded at end of day.

Procedure

1. Though blood collected in plastic or siliconized syringes and test tubes is theoretically preferable, glass tubes in the Vacutainer system have proved satisfactory. Platelet clumping must be avoided by a good venipuncture and prompt anticoagulation. EDTA is the anticoagulant of choice. Although less desirable, blood from a skin puncture wound may be used if only the first few drops are used and the blood is flowing freely.

2. Two red cell pipettes (Fig. 4–4) are used. Each is filled rapidly with blood exactly to the 1 mark, carefully wiped, then filled with ammonium oxalate to the 101 mark, and rotated in a mechanical pipette rotor. The Bryant-Garrey rotors have been found satisfactory. Rotation for as long as 8 hours does not affect the counts.

3. The hemacytometer is filled in the usual fashion, using a separate pipette for each side.

4. The chamber is covered by a Petri dish for 15 minutes to allow settling of the platelets in one optical plane. A piece of wet cotton or filter paper is left beneath the dish to prevent evaporation.

5. The platelets appear round or oval and frequently have one or more dendritic processes. Their internal granular structure and a purple sheen allow the platelets to be distinguished from debris, which is often refractile. Ghosts of the red cells which have been lysed by the ammonium oxalate are seen in the background.

6. Platelets are counted in 10 small squares (as for red cell counts, the black squares in Figure 4–3), 5 on each side of the chamber. If the total number of platelets counted is less than 100, more small squares are counted until at least 100 platelets have been recorded; 10 squares per side (black plus checked squares, Figure 4–3) or all 25 squares in the large central square on each side of the hemacytometer, if necessary. If the total number of platelets in all 50 of these small squares is less than 50, the count should be repeated with 1:20 dilutions of blood in white cell pipettes.

Calculation. Since each of the 25 small squares defines a volume of 1/250 μl. (1/25 mm.² area × 1/10 mm. depth), the platelet count (per μl.) $= \frac{\text{no. cells counted}}{\text{no. squares counted}} \times$ dilution × 250.

By adjusting the number of squares so that at least 100 platelets are counted, the field error (the statistical error due to counting a limited number of platelets in the chamber) can be kept in the same range for low platelet counts as for high platelet counts. It has been shown that the coefficient of variation (C.V.) due to combined field, pipette, and chamber errors is about 11 per cent when at least 100 platelets are counted, 15 per cent when 40 platelets are counted, and 30 per cent when only 10 platelets are counted. With this method the range of values in 95 per cent of healthy controls is from 140,000 to 440,000.

Sources of Error. Most of the sources of error are the same as those discussed previously for the red cell and white cell counts. Blood in EDTA is satisfactory for 5 hours after collection at 20° C. and 24 hours at 4° C, provided no difficulty was encountered in collection. Platelet clumps present in the chamber imply a maldistribution and negate the reliability of the count; a new sample of blood must be collected. The causes of platelet clumping are likely to be initiation of platelet aggregation and clotting before the blood reaches the anticoagulant, imperfect venipuncture, delay in the anticoagulant contacting the blood, or, in skin puncture technique, delay in sampling. Capillary blood gives similar values, but errors are about twice those with venous blood, probably because the platelet level varies in successive drops of blood from the skin puncture wound.

ELECTRONIC COUNTING

Voltage Pulse Counting

SAMPLE. In order to use the Coulter counter or Celloscope for platelet counts, the red cells must first be removed from the blood sample by one of three methods:

1. Bull *et al.* (1965) devised a sedimentation method in which a short length of plastic tubing (sealed at one end) is filled with blood and placed at an angle in a rack to speed sedimentation, which provides sufficient separation of red cells from platelet-rich plasma in 10 to 50 minutes.

2. Fry and Hoak (1969) showed that closely controlled centrifugal force (300 g. for 5 minutes) can provide reproducible separation of red cells without significant loss of platelets from the plasma.

3. Vertically held test tubes in a modified table top centrifuge (Serufuge, Clay-Adams, New York) can be spun 40 G. for 25 seconds to produce rouleaux, which then rapidly sediment to yield platelet-rich plasma in 2 minutes (Bull, 1970).

EQUIPMENT. The Coulter Counter Model B or Model Z is more convenient than the Model A or F because it has two thresholds; the lower one excludes particles smaller than platelets, and the upper one excludes red cells or white cells larger than platelets. With the Coulter Counter Model A or F or the Celloscope 401, two counts must be taken at different thresholds and the platelets determined by subtraction. A 70-μm. aperture is used with the Coulter counters. The procedure for setting the amplification and aperture current controls and thresholds is given by Bull *et al.* (1965).

PROCEDURE. A 1:3000 dilution of platelet-rich plasma is made in Isoton* or saline using a 3-μl. capillary pipette in 9 ml. of diluent or 3.33 μl. in 10 ml. The background count should not exceed 300; if over 150, it should be corrected for coincidence and subtracted from the corrected platelet count before calculation. Two or three counts are made and the results averaged. For platelet counts of less than 25,000/μl., a 1:300 dilution is made by adding 20 μl. of plasma to 6 ml. of diluent.

CALCULATION. Since the number of platelets is expressed per μl. of whole blood, a correction must be made for the hematocrit. In addition, platelet-free plasma is trapped by red cells during sedimentation, giving an excess of platelets in the supernatant plasma. For this, an experimentally derived correction also dependent on the hematocrit is applied and is available in a table (Bull *et al.*, 1965). These corrections have been combined with that for coincidence into a circular slide rule (commercially available); from the uncorrected plasma platelet count and the hematocrit one can read the whole blood platelet count (Bull, 1970).

The coefficient of variation of this method is about 4 per cent, which compares favorably with the hemacytometer-phase contrast method of 11 to 16 per cent. The normal values are the same.

SOURCES OF ERROR. Careful technique is especially important at all steps in platelet counting: collection of blood, having a particle-free diluent, obtaining platelet-rich plasma without losing platelets or having too many red cells remain, microtechnique in diluting, and cleanliness in glassware and the aperture of the counter.

Excessive numbers of red cells in the plasma will give falsely low counts, because platelets entering the aperture at the same time as red cells will not be detected. High leukocyte counts will also produce a falsely low platelet count, because white cells erratically filter out platelets when aspirating into the microcapillary tube. Platelets as large as red cells will be screened out by the upper threshold, also giving a falsely low count. On the other hand, if the sample is hemolyzed, or if red cell fragments are present in the blood, the platelet count is apt to be falsely high.

Always in platelet counting the blood film must be examined before reporting the count, both for concordance of the apparent numbers on the film with that from the machine, and to detect abnormalities such as those just mentioned that are prone to produce erroneous counts.

Electro-optical Counting (Brittin *et al.*, 1971; Simmons *et al.*, 1971). A semiautomatic instrument for counting platelets, the Autocounter* utilizes the darkfield optical microscope system (Fig. 4–6) described previously for red cell counts. Whole blood is sampled automatically from test tubes or plastic cups, diluted approximately 1:1500 in 2 M urea which lyses the red cells. Platelets and leukocytes are counted. For a platelet count of 350,000/μl., about 10,000 light-scattering events are counted in a small optically determined sensing volume (44,000 fl.) in the flow cell; this gives a linear response with no significant coincidence. The results are recorded on a moving pen recorder. The instrument is calibrated with a stable standard of fixed platelets* before each batch of samples. For each sample, the leukocyte count is separately determined and subtracted from the total count.

This instrument counts platelets with a greater precision than the voltage pulse

*Coulter Diagnostics, Hialeah, Fla.

*Technicon Corporation, Tarrytown, N.Y.

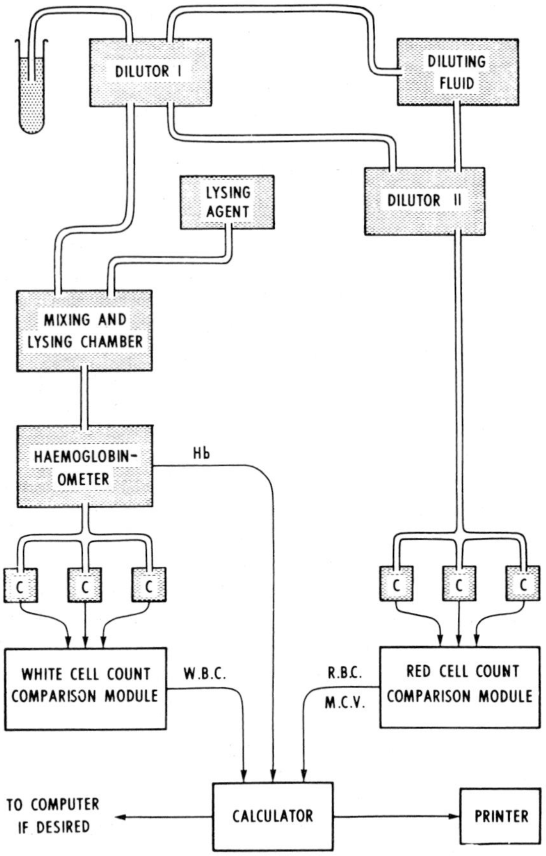

Figure 4–7. Flow diagram of the Coulter Model S. The blood sample is presented manually to the instrument as indicated by the tube, upper left. (From Pinkerton, P. H., *et al.*: J. Clin. Path. 23:68, 1970.)

counters in most hands (C.V. = 1 to 3 per cent versus 4 to 6 per cent for the Coulter method) and at least equal precision in others (C.V. = 2.0 to 2.5 per cent).

The Autocounter has the advantage of using whole blood and automatic mixing, diluting, and counting. Consequently it is easier to use and more reliable, since it is less prone to technical errors in handling samples. In addition, it is readily used for skin-puncture sampling using prediluted whole blood taken with the Unopette system.*

No matter which method is used for platelet counting, the blood film (prepared from EDTA-blood) must be checked to corroborate the height of the count, to detect platelet clumping which may invalidate the count, and to detect abnormalities in platelets or other blood elements that may give a false value. One must always confirm abnormal results with a newly drawn sample.

*Becton-Dickinson, Rutherford, N.J.

Multichannel Instruments

Coulter Counter Model S

DESCRIPTION. The Coulter Counter Model S produces seven simultaneous measurements (leukocyte count, red cell count, hemoglobin, hematocrit, and the red cell indices) in 40 seconds' time, employing the principles of voltage pulse counting and size analysis together with a photosensitive device for measuring hemoglobin concentration. A power supply provides a negative pressure which aspirates the blood and moves the diluting fluids and dilutions through the system. The instrument can accept a new sample every 20 seconds, as it counts one sample while diluting the next. The analysis may be performed on whole blood, of which the machine aspirates about 1.3 ml.; most is used for flushing, then 44.7 μl. is diluted 1:224 with Isoton* (Fig. 4–7). From this (Dilutor I) a second dilution of 1:224 is made, and from the resulting 1:50,000 dilution the red cell count and the MCV are determined by each of three Coulter counters (C). From Dilutor I, also, the original dilution is brought to a mixing chamber where a lysing agent is added to lyse the red cells and convert the hemoglobin to cyanmethemoglobin, and the dilution from 1:224 to 1:250. After the hemoglobin concentration is measured, the suspension of white cells (in dilute cyanmethemoglobin solution) is brought to three counters (C). The red cells and white cells are counted simultaneously, in triplicate, and each group is averaged. This result is printed out unless one result disagrees with the other two by more than 3 standard deviations from the mean, in which case the discordant result is discarded and the mean of the other two is printed out. If all three results disagree by more than 3 standard deviations, none is accepted and the print-out reads zero. After each sample the hemoglobinometer is automatically zeroed. The MCV is determined directly from voltage pulse heights, and the hematocrit is calculated from the MCV and the red cell count. The other indices are calculated and the seven results appear in digital print-out form on a special card which has been inserted in the printer to receive the data. Simultaneously, the results can pass to a computer.

Capillary blood from skin-puncture sampling can be easily handled by diluting 44.7 μl. of blood in 10 ml. of Isoton. This prediluted

*Coulter Diagnostics, Hialeah, Fla.

sample can then bypass the first dilution step by means of a separate aspirator. The instrument is not fully automatic, in that the technologist must hold the tube of blood up to the aspirator. This is not entirely disadvantageous in that it allows interruption for the rapid processing of urgent specimens with minimal trouble. Also, the operator is continually watching the oscilloscope screen, the diluting chambers and other working parts, which helps in early detection of malfunction.

The Coulter Model S has been thoroughly evaluated and found to correlate well with the results from the routine laboratory methods (Brittin *et al.*, 1969a; Pinkerton *et al.*, 1970). It is currently the most widely used multichannel instrument in hematology. The precision in all the red cell measurements, actual and calculated, has proved to be in the vicinity of 1 per cent (C.V.); the white count slightly higher, 2 to 3 per cent. These values for the coefficient of variation are superior to the routine methods discussed, even when automatic pipettes are used. The reason for this appears to lie in the automatic diluting system which itself has excellent precision.

CALIBRATION. No certified standard cell suspensions are available, though several stabilized suspensions are commercially available. We prefer to calibrate the instrument with normal fresh blood in EDTA, which is analyzed by conventional methods as described by Brittin *et al.*, 1969a. Hemoglobin is determined by the cyanmethemoglobin method, using a certified standard and the Coleman Jr. spectrophotometer. Hematocrit is measured by the microhematocrit technique. Red cell counts and white cell counts are performed with the Coulter Counter Model F. For the former, the 1:50,000 dilution is made in a single step to reduce error. A 2 μl. ± 0.25 per cent Microcap* is used to deliver the blood into 100 ml. (±0.08) of Isoton† in a volumetric flask. The blood for white cell count is diluted 1:500, again with a Microcap, 20 μl. ± 0.25 per cent. Each of the above is performed on the normal blood in five to 10 replicate determinations, except that only two separate dilutions are made for the red cell count. The values are averaged and the red cell indices calculated. The white cell count is checked by performing duplicate hemacytometer counts. Using this normal blood, the Model S is primed several times and the average values set in. Now that the initial calibration is made, it is desirable to carry out final calibration over a period of several days to get the benefit of a larger number of determinations and to minimize any day-to-day variation in the less precise conventional methods. It is important that this calibration not be changed until a "drift" away from these values has been demonstrated on a statistical basis by quality control procedures. At that time, after any necessary maintenance work has been done, the instrument is recalibrated in the same fashion. The calibration settings must not be changed on the basis of a single determination of a control suspension of cells. The Model S has been found to be quite stable; recalibration is usually unnecessary oftener than every two or three weeks.

The method of calibration described gives values for red cell indices from the Model S comparable to those calculated from conventional methods. It has been proposed that the calibration for the hematocrit be set at 1.5 per cent less than the microhematocrit value in order to eliminate the error in the conventional hematocrit (and MCV) due to trapped plasma (England *et al.*, 1972). This proposal has merit, but would change the normal ranges. It is clear that in conditions in which trapped plasma is considerably increased due to rigidity or shape of red cells, such as iron deficiency anemia and sickle-cell disease, the hematocrit and MCV are lower and the MCHC slightly higher with the Model S than with conventional methods. It appears quite likely that the Model S gives the more correct values.

QUALITY CONTROL. A commercially available cell control blood may be used and charted every morning and at intervals during the day, but this is quite expensive and not entirely satisfactory. Brittin and Brecher (1971) have discussed this problem in their excellent review of instrumentation, and Brittin *et al.* (1969b) presented a useful method for using patient blood samples in quality control. They demonstrated that all seven values are stable in blood collected in EDTA for at least 24 hours at 4° C. At least five and preferably 10 specimens with hematologic values in the normal range are selected on Day 1, kept in the refrigerator, and re-analyzed on Day 2. A significant change in any channel between the two days can be detected statistically using the Student-t test for paired samples:

$$t_n = \frac{\bar{d}}{S_d}\sqrt{n}, \text{ with } n-1 \text{ degrees of freedom}$$

n = number of pairs of observations

$\bar{d}$ = mean of the differences (from day to day)

S_d = standard deviation of the differences

$$= \sqrt{\frac{\sum(d^2) - \frac{(\Sigma d)^2}{n}}{n-1}}$$

*Drummond Scientific Co., Broomall, Pa.
†Coulter Diagnostics, Hialeah, Fla.

The t value is calculated for each channel. If the calculated t value exceeds that critical value for the 95 per cent limits found in a statistical table of t-values, the difference is significant at the 5 per cent level. For $n = 5$, the critical t value is 2.78. For example, if the t score calculated from the five pairs of white cell counts exceeds 2.78, we can be 95 per cent confident that there is a significant difference between the two days, and we must look for trouble in the white cell channel. Often it is possible to ascertain from simple inspection of the values whether the mean difference from one day to the next differs significantly from zero. The calculations can be easily programmed for a desk top computer, and it is helpful to chart the t values for each channel.

It would be theoretically desirable to continuously monitor the tendency for drift throughout the day, and this would be feasible with an on-line computer of sufficient size. However, the Model S has proved sufficiently stable so as to make the method described quite satisfactory.

Sources of Error. Carry-over is a problem, especially on low white cell counts, since it amounts to about 2 to 3 per cent. If the ratio of successive counts exceeds 3.3:1, the second count will be in error by 5 per cent (Brittin and Brecher, 1971). It is therefore necessary to repeat any low white count (following a normal or high one) and to use the second value; this should also be done with very low red cell counts.

Increased white cell counts, over 25,000/μl., usually produce a slight but significant false elevation of the hemoglobin as a result of turbidity. A very high white count can also elevate the hematocrit and the MCV because the white cells are counted and sized with the red cells.

Cold agglutinins in high titer tend to give spurious macrocytosis and low red cell counts with impossibly high MCHCs (Hattersley *et al.*, 1971). Warming the blood or the diluent eliminates this problem.

In some patients with leukemia the white cells appear to be fragile and escape being counted, giving a falsely low count. Erroneously low white counts may also be found in uremia or in some patients receiving immunosuppressive drugs (Luke *et al.*, 1971). Hemacytometer counts should be used to check the white counts of such patients.

The following instruments have been discussed by Brittin and Brecher (1971), to which the reader should turn for a critical analysis.

Technicon SMA–4A/7A. The SMA-4A uses the electro-optical principle to count red cells and white cells, uses a colorimetric cyanmethemoglobin determination, and measures the hematocrit by the conductivity of the blood. This method has a serious limitation of giving erroneous hematocrits when there are severe electrolyte or serum protein abnormalities. The SMA-7A is the same as the SMA-4A but adds the calculated values for the red cell indices.

Technicon Hemalog. This is a newer development which has not yet been thoroughly evaluated. It adds to the SMA-7A system a centrifuged hematocrit, a platelet count (Autocounter), prothrombin time, and partial thromboplastin time. It also calculates the ratio of the spun hematocrit/conductivity hematocrit, for the purpose of detecting discrepancies which indicate abnormal plasma conductivity.

Fisher Hem-Alyzer. The white cell count and red cell count are performed by the electro-optical principle, and the hemoglobin is determined as oxyhemoglobin. The instrument has been found reliable, but suffers from the lack of the hematocrit and, because of this, it cannot calculate the MCV and MCHC, which are the most useful of the indices in analyzing anemia.

Volume of Blood and Plasma

Many methods have been devised for determining the total volume of blood.

There are two basic indirect methods: One may inject intravenously Evans blue dye, which binds firmly to albumin. The dilution of the dye after equilibrium is reached allows calculation of total plasma volume. Hematocrit permits calculation of total blood volume. More widely used are ^{125}I- or ^{131}I-tagged human serum albumin for plasma volume and ^{51}Cr-tagged red cells for red cell volume. (For details see Chapter 7, p. 474.)

Clinical Applications. Surgical patients with anemia and hemoconcentration may have a normal red cell count and hematocrit. Administration of fluid postoperatively and transfusion therapy are best guided by tests for total blood volume, plasma volume, and red cell mass. Patients may need packed red cells but not saline or plasma, or, vice versa, patients may need only plasma and not whole blood. Prior to transfusion therapy, the hematocrit may be misleading. Volume studies may help to decide if whole blood or only plasma is needed.

Fragility Tests

Erythrocyte Osmotic Fragility Test. The osmotic fragility test provides an indication of the change of shape (surface/volume ratio) of the red cell from the normal biconcave disc. Its chief value is in establishing a diagnosis of hereditary spherocytosis.

PRINCIPLE. Red cells suspended in hypotonic solution of sodium chloride take up water, swell, become spheroidal and, after reaching the critical volume, eventually burst. The cell that is thicker than normal (spheroidal as in hereditary spherocytosis) has a decreased surface/volume ratio, and its capacity to expand is limited. Consequently it bursts upon intake of small amounts of water in relatively high concentrations of the salt. Its osmotic fragility is increased and its osmotic resistance is decreased. On the other hand, the thin or flat cell in hypochromic anemia can take up considerable amounts of water and reaches the critical volume for lysis at lower concentrations of sodium chloride. Its osmotic fragility is decreased; its resistance is increased.

The osmotic fragility test measures how nearly spherical red cells are, but it does not measure the fragility of the red cells. Increased osmotic fragility or decreased resistance means spherocytosis. The degree of the latter parallels the degree of the former.

Increased fragility is found in hereditary spherocytosis and in those idiopathic and symptomatic acquired hemolytic anemias in which a tendency to spherocytosis is present. Contrariwise, diminished osmotic fragility or increased resistance means excessive flatness of red cells; it is seen in the presence of obstructive jaundice, in iron deficiency anemias, in thalassemia, in sickle cell anemia, after splenectomy, and in a variety of anemias in which target cells are found. In thalassemia a portion of red cells may remain unlysed in 0.03 per cent saline and even in distilled water. In tests for osmotic fragility, identical amounts of blood are added to decreasing concentrations of sodium chloride solution. After a period of incubation, the highest concentration of sodium chloride with minimum hemolysis determines beginning hemolysis; the highest concentration in which hemolysis is complete expresses the complete hemolysis.

Incipient hemolysis in higher concentrations of sodium chloride is an indicator of increased osmotic fragility of red cells. In other words, osmotic fragility of red cells is increased if hemolysis occurs in concentrations greater than 0.5 per cent sodium chloride. On the other hand, osmotic fragility is decreased if hemolysis is incomplete in 0.3 per cent sodium chloride.

Two tests of osmotic fragility of varying degrees of simplicity will be described.

Screening Test

REAGENTS

1. Stock solution of sodium chloride. A 1 per cent solution of sodium chloride is prepared by dissolving 1.0 gm. of C.P. sodium chloride in 100 ml. of distilled water. The salt must be first dried in a desiccator.

2. Dilute solutions. The 0.85 per cent solution is prepared by placing 8.5 ml. of the stock solution in a test tube and adding 1.5 ml. of distilled water. Similarly, the 0.5 per cent solution is prepared by mixing 5.0 ml. amounts of the stock solution and of distilled water.

PROCEDURE. One milliliter of each of the two solutions is placed in one of two tubes. One-tenth milliliter of venous blood is added. To a similar set of two tubes, blood of a normal person is added and serves as a control. The control blood must be obtained approximately at the same time as the patient's. The tubes are shaken gently, and if the tube with the 0.5 per cent sodium chloride solution shows hemolysis and the one with 0.85 per cent is not hemolyzed, the osmotic fragility of the red cells is probably increased and a quantitative test is indicated.

Quantitative Method—Unincubated

EQUIPMENT

1. Test tube rack containing two rows of 13 matched, chemically clean, and dry colorimeter tubes.

2. Ten-milliliter serologic pipettes.

3. Pipettes calibrated to contain or deliver 0.05 ml.

Sahli pipettes delivering 20 μl. have been recommended for transfer of blood.

REAGENTS

1. Stock solution of 10 per cent NaCl (pH 7.4).

NaCl	180.00 gm.
Na_2HPO_4	27.31 gm.
$NaH_2PO_4 \cdot 2H_2O$	4.86 gm.

Dissolve in distilled H_2O and dilute to 2 liters. Keeps well at room temperature in a tightly stoppered bottle.

2. Starting with a 1 per cent solution prepared from the 10 per cent solution, 50 ml. of the following solutions are made: 0.85, 0.75, 0.65, 0.60, 0.55, 0.50, 0.45, 0.40, 0.35, 0.30, 0.20, 0.10, and 0.00 per cent NaCl.

The solutions can be prepared in 50 ml. volumetric flasks as follows: To each flask the following volumes of the 1 per cent solution are added: 42.5, 37.5, 32.5, 30.0, 27.5, 25.0, 22.5, 20.0, 17.5, 15.0, 10.0, and 5.0 ml. The solutions are made up to volume (50 ml.) with distilled water. A 1.2 per cent solution of sodium chloride is prepared by diluting 6 ml. of the 10 per cent solution to 50 ml. The solutions keep well at 4° C. for weeks. They should be discarded if molds develop.

3. Freshly obtained heparinized or defibrinated blood is preferable to oxalated or citrated blood. To defibrinate, 10 to 15 ml. of aseptically drawn venous blood is placed in a sterile flask containing one glass bead (3 to 4 mm. in diameter) for each milliliter of blood. The flask should be rotated gently until the beads become coated with fibrin. The control blood should be obtained at approximately the same time.

Procedure. Five milliliters of each of the dilutions of sodium chloride are added to the 13 test tubes of each row. The second row of tubes is set up as a control. Five one-hundredths ml. of the patient's blood is added to each tube of the first row, and the same amount of the normal control blood is added to the second row. After each transfer of blood, the pipettes should be rinsed thoroughly with saline and blown out vigorously. The tubes are immediately mixed well. They are allowed to stand at room temperature for 20 minutes, remixed, and centrifuged at 2000 r.p.m. for 5 minutes. In a photoelectric colorimeter provided with a 540 nm. filter, the degree of hemolysis in the supernatant (diluted 1 to 2 or 1 to 5) is measured by comparing with 100 per cent hemolysis in the tube with no saline and using the supernatant of the 0.85 per cent sodium chloride as a blank. The dilutions are made so that the optical density readings fall between 0.2 and 0.8. The per cent hemolysis in each of the tubes is calculated by dividing the hemoglobin value by the value in the tube containing no saline. A good colorimeter permits recognition of as little as 1 per cent hemolysis.

Range of osmotic fragility in normal blood:

Per Cent NaCl	*Per Cent Hemolysis*
0.30	97–100
0.40	50–90
0.45	5–45
0.50	0–5
0.55	0

Each laboratory should determine its own normal values.

Recording of Results. Beginning hemolysis or minimum resistance is expressed by the percentage concentration of sodium chloride in the tube in which the first trace of lysis is visible. Complete hemolysis or maximum resistance is expressed accordingly. A more accurate picture is obtained by plotting on graph paper the percentage of hemolysis in each tube against the corresponding concentration of sodium chloride (Fig. 4–8). Another way of expressing the results is the median corpuscular fragility (MCF), which is the concentration of NaCl at which 50 per cent of the cells have lysed. Before incubation, the normal range for the MCF is 0.40 to 0.445 per cent NaCl.

Interpretation of Results. Although osmotic fragility is essentially a measure of spherocytosis, it provides a more objective measurement than inspection of a blood smear. A difference of more than one tube between the patient and the control is significant.

Sources of Error

1. Chemical purity of sodium chloride is essential. Even minute impurities may act as hemolytic agents.

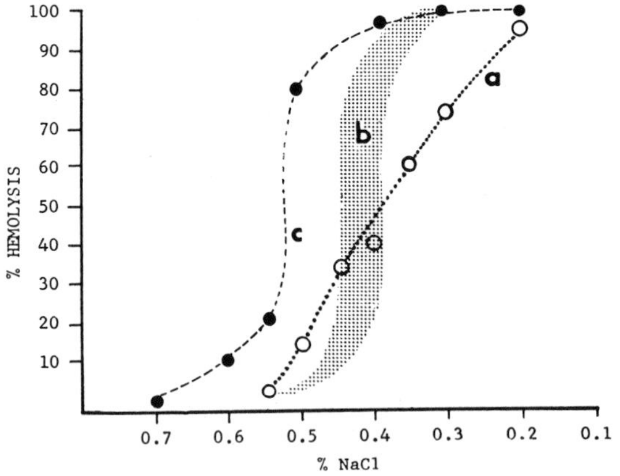

Figure 4–8. Red cell osmotic fragility; *a* indicates thalassemia; *b*, normal zone; and *c*, hereditary spherocytosis.

2. Accuracy of the sodium chloride solution.

3. The relative volumes of blood and saline. A 1 to 100 dilution is recommended, because the degree of hemolysis can be read directly in most colorimeters without further dilution, and the minimal amount of plasma does not affect the tonicity of the solution. Because of differences between arterial and venous blood, the latter should be mixed until bright red.

4. A change of pH by 0.1 equals the change of tonicity by 0.01 per cent; specifically, a lowering of pH increases fragility.

5. A temperature rise increases fragility; a rise of 5° C. is equivalent to a change of tonicity of about 0.01 per cent. Room temperature is generally sufficiently constant.

Quantitative Method after Incubation.

Procedure. Duplicate 2-ml. volumes of sterile, defibrinated blood in stoppered test tubes are incubated at 37° C. for 24 hours. The second test tube is included to have a spare in case of contamination. The test is set up similarly to the way described for the quantitative fragility test, but with the addition of a tube containing a 1.2 per cent solution of sodium chloride to serve as a blank in case of increased hemolysis.

Recording of Results. As above, the per cent hemolysis is plotted against sodium chloride concentration on graph paper for both patient and control. The MCF after incubation normally is 0.465 to 0.590 per cent NaCl.

Interpretation. Incubation at 37° C. for 24 hours increases the fragility of normal erythrocytes (Fig. 4–9 [1A]). The increase is even more marked for red cells of hereditary spherocytosis and of congenital hemolytic anemia due to pyruvate kinase deficiency; hemolysis may begin between 0.70 and 0.65 per cent sodium chloride and may be complete at about 0.40 per cent (Fig. 4–9 [2A]). The test permits recognition of low-grade hereditary

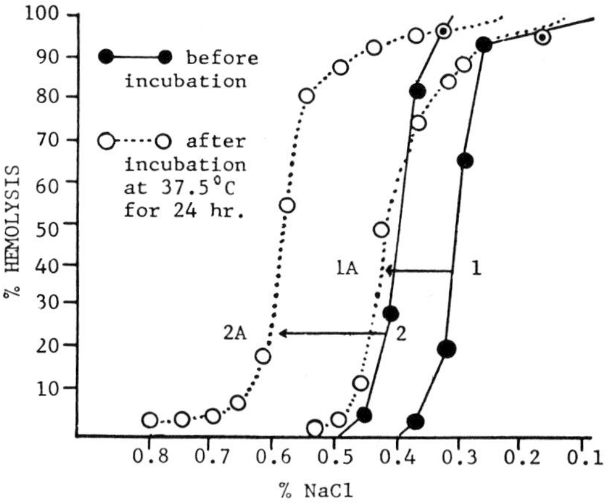

Figure 4–9. The effect of incubation on red cell osmotic fragility.

spherocytosis in which the unincubated osmotic fragility may be normal.

SOURCES OF ERROR. In addition to those mentioned for the unincubated test, bacterial contamination may occur and increase the degree of hemolysis.

INDICATIONS FOR THE INCUBATED OSMOTIC FRAGILITY TEST. Only when hereditary spherocytosis is suspected, i.e., unexplained hemolytic anemia with splenomegaly, is the incubated osmotic fragility test indicated. Since the unincubated osmotic fragility test may be normal in mild hereditary spherocytosis, an abnormal incubated test may be decisive in establishing the diagnosis.

Mechanical Fragility. Red cells with increased osmotic fragility also show an increased mechanical fragility, but the latter may be abnormally increased when the former is normal. Sickled cells and agglutinated cells have an increased mechanical fragility. The mechanical fragility of red cells of newborn infants is about twice that of older children and adults. The procedure does not offer enough additional information to justify its inclusion here. Details are given by Dacie and Lewis (1968).

Erythrocyte Sedimentation Rate (ESR)

An increased tendency toward sedimentation of erythrocytes in shed blood in certain pathologic conditions, particularly inflammation, has long been recognized. Following the work of Fahraeus and other investigators with blood rendered noncoagulable by heparin, citrate, or oxalate, the rate of sedimentation has been actively studied and applied clinically.

It has been found that the erythrocytes settle more rapidly in the blood of women than of men and very much more rapidly after the third or fourth month of pregnancy. In pregnancy, acceleration begins with the tenth to twelfth week, increasing moderately and progressively. Normal rates return about one month post partum. Increased speed of sedimentation is also observed in tuberculosis and other chronic infectious diseases, in which it increases with the activity of the disease; in cancer, in which it more or less closely parallels the extent of the malignant process; in various so-called connective tissue diseases, such as rheumatic fever and rheumatoid arthritis; in localized acute inflammation, in which the rate appears to increase with the leukocyte count; and in dysproteinemias, such as multiple myeloma.

Various factors have been demonstrated to play a role.

Plasma Factors. An accelerated ESR (erythrocyte sedimentation rate) is favored by elevated levels of fibrinogen and, to a lesser extent, of globulin. These plasma components cause increased formation of rouleaux, which sediment more rapidly because of their increased weight as compared with single cells. Removal of fibrinogen by defibrination lowers the ESR, except when plasma globulin is markedly elevated.

The effect of globulin on acceleration of the ESR is less pronounced than that of fibrinogen, except in liver disease, in which close correlation between the two has been noted in the presence of low fibrinogen levels. That fibrinogen and globulin are not the only responsible factors is shown by the fact that ESR may be accelerated in the presence of normal levels and in patients with anemia. There is no absolute correlation between the ESR and any of the plasma protein fractions. Alpha and beta globulins are more effective than gamma globulin. Albumin retards sedimentation.

Extreme increase in plasma viscosity slows down the ESR by counteracting the accelerating effect of blood proteins on rouleaux formation. Cholesterol accelerates and lecithin retards the ESR.

Red Cell Factors. Anemia is responsible for accelerated ESR. The change in the erythrocyte-plasma ratio favors rouleaux formation.

Microcytes sediment significantly more slowly and macrocytes somewhat more rapidly than normocytes. The larger the cells, the smaller the surface in relation to the volume. The sedimentation rate is directly proportionate to the weight of the cell aggregate and inversely proportionate to the surface area. Rouleaux formation is an aggregation of erythrocytes into units of larger size and proportionately decreased surface area, which is smaller in relation to the volume of the aggregate than the combined surface area of the individual cells. The result is acceleration of the ESR. If the red cells have an abnormal or irregular shape which does not allow rouleaux formation, the ESR will be low; sickle cell disease and spherocytosis are cases in point.

Anticoagulants. Sodium citrate or EDTA does not affect the rate of sedimentation, but oxalates and heparin may.

Stages in the ESR. Three stages can be observed: (1) The initial period of aggregation. During this phase the rouleaux are formed and the sedimentation is relatively slow. It lasts about 10 minutes of the 1-hour observation period. (2) The period of fast settling. During this period the settling rate is constant. It lasts about 40 minutes. (3) The final period of packing continues for the balance of the hour and for a longer time afterwards.

METHODS FOR DETERMINING THE SEDIMENTATION RATE

Westergren Method. Because of its simplicity the Westergren method is widely used. The National Committee for Clinical Laboratory Standards has recommended it as the basis for an acceptable standard method.

EQUIPMENT. The Westergren tube is a straight pipette 30 cm. long and 2.5 mm. in internal diameter. It is calibrated in millimeters from 0 to 200. It holds about 1 ml. The Westergren rack is also used.

REAGENT

A 0.105 molar solution of sodium citrate is used as the anticoagulant-diluent solution (31 gm. of $Na_3C_6H_5O_7 \cdot H_2O$ added to 1 liter of distilled water in a sterile glass bottle). This is filtered and kept without preservatives.

TECHNIQUE

1. Exactly 1.0 ml. of the sodium citrate is transferred with a graduated pipette to a tube with a mark at the 5-ml. level.

2. Five milliliters of venous blood is withdrawn in a dry syringe, and 4 ml. of it is placed in the tube containing the anticoagulant. The tube, now filled to the 5-ml. mark, is inverted two or three times to mix thoroughly the anticoagulant with the blood. This blood-citrate mixture should be used within 2 hours if kept at 20° C. or within 12 hours if kept at 4° C.

3. A Westergren pipette is filled exactly to the 0 mark and placed in the rack. The bottom of the tube must be pressed firmly against the rubber stopper in the base of the rack before removing the finger from the top of the tube. The tube must be held firmly by the clip at the top of the rack in an *exactly vertical* position. The rack is constructed to hold 12 or more tubes.

4. The room temperature must be constant and the tube cannot be exposed to direct sunlight. The tube must not be disturbed, either by moving it or by vibrations of the bench.

After exactly 60 minutes, the distance from the bottom of the surface meniscus to the top of the column of red cells is recorded in millimeters as the ESR value. If the demarcation between plasma and red cell column is hazy, the level is taken where the full density is first apparent.

Modified Westergren Method. A modification of the Westergren method employs blood anticoagulated with EDTA rather than citrate. This is more convenient, since it allows the ESR to be performed from the same tube of blood as is used for other hematologic studies. Two milliliters of well-mixed EDTA anticoagulated blood is diluted either with 0.5 ml. of 3.8 per cent sodium citrate (Dawson, 1960) or with 0.5 ml. of 0.85 per cent sodium chloride (Gambino *et al.*, 1965), which yields the same degree of dilution as is used in the classic Westergren method. Results are reproducible and are almost identical with those obtained by the classic Westergren method. The blood must be diluted, since undiluted blood anticoagulated with EDTA or double oxalate gives inaccurate and poorly reproducible results. Blood anticoagulated with EDTA may be kept for 12 hours at 4° C. without affecting the ESR.

The ESR is higher in women than in men and gradually increases with age. Westergren's original upper limits of normal (10 mm. per hour for men and 20 mm. per hour for women) appear to be too low. After studying a large number of healthy working people, Böttiger and Svedberg (1967) recommended that the upper limit of normal should be 15 mm. per hour for men and 20 mm. per hour for women below the age of 50 and 20 mm. per hour for men and 30 mm. per hour for women over the age of 50. The work of others (e.g., Boyd and Hoffbrand, 1966) indicates that in some individuals over the age of 65 the ESR may be as high as 40 mm. per hour without obvious cause.

Sources of Error

1. The anticoagulant. The exact concentration is important. If it is higher than recommended, the ESR may be slowed down.

2. Hemolysis may modify the sedimentation.

3. The cleanliness of the tube is important, and all traces of alcohol and ether must be removed.

4. Effect of the acceleration by tilting. The red cells aggregate along the lower side while the plasma rises along the upper side. Consequently the retarding influence of the rising plasma is less effective. An angle of even 3 degrees from the vertical may accelerate the ESR by as much as 30 per cent.

5. The filling of the tube. Bubbles affect sedimentation.

6. Temperature. Constant at 20° C. Little variation from 22° to 27° C. Otherwise a correction must be made for the temperature or the tube should be placed in a constant tempera-

ture bath at 20° C. If the blood has been kept in a refrigerator, it should be permitted to reach room temperature before the test is set up.

7. Time. The test should be set up within 2 hours after the blood sample is obtained (or 12 hours if EDTA is used as the anticoagulant and the blood is kept at 4° C.); otherwise, the ESR may be lowered. On standing, erythrocytes tend to become spherical and less inclined to form rouleaux; hence, retarded ESR.

8. Anemia. A decrease in the number of erythrocytes accelerates the ESR; an increase as in polycythemia retards it. This was the reason for the attempts to make a correction for the anemia, but as stated elsewhere in this chapter, the present tendency is to recognize that the value of the ESR is extremely limited in the presence of anemia and that a correction for the anemia is hardly worth the effort and may be actually misleading.

9. Anisocytosis may interfere with rouleaux formation. Pronounced poikilocytosis, for example, sickling, may inhibit sedimentation.

10. Factors favoring slowing of the ESR: defibrination, partial clotting with resulting defibrination, low temperature, excess of dry anticoagulant, and diameter of tube less than 2 mm.

Interpretation. Many aspects of the ESR have not been settled. The rate has been shown to be higher in females than in males and becomes higher with increasing age. This does not appear to be related to lower red cell levels or, at least in males, to changes in plasma proteins.

According to the current interpretation, the accelerated ESR is a nonspecific response to tissue damage. It is only an indication of the presence of disease and does not precisely reflect severity. Its value is greatest when used as one evidence of subsidence of an inflammatory process.

It may help in differentiating certain conditions, e.g., myocardial infarction from angina pectoris, rheumatoid arthritis from osteoarthritis, and advanced cancer of the stomach from peptic ulcer.

It may also be elevated without apparent inflammation or necrosis, mainly in so-called dysproteinemias.

On the other hand, it may be within normal limits in the presence of tissue destruction, for example, in some cases of acute myocardial infarction and acute rheumatic fever and in the presence of congestive heart failure.

The test must be used with great caution. It is most valuable in following the course of certain inflammatory processes, e.g., tuberculosis and rheumatic fever.

The Zeta Sedimentation Ratio. Recently a centrifugal device (the Zetafuge*) has been introduced which spins capillary tubes in a vertical position in four 45-second cycles (Bull and Brailsford, 1972). This results in controlled compaction and dispersion of erythrocytes, allowing rouleaux to form and sediment in this 3-minute period of time. The capillary tube is then read as if it were a standard hematocrit tube, giving a value referred to as a zetacrit. The true hematocrit is divided by the zetacrit, and the result, expressed as a percentage, is the zeta sedimentation ratio (ZSR). With the ZSR, the normal values (51 per cent or less) are the same for men and women. It is not affected by anemia, which should make it easier to interpret. Its sensitivity to elevation of the ESR by fibrinogen is the same as the Westergren method. This ZSR requires only a 100-μl. sample and is considerably faster (Bull and Brailsford, 1972).

Although clinical trials with this instrument have not yet been published, it seems to have sufficient advantages to merit consideration as an alternative to the ESR.

*Coulter Diagnostics, Hialeah, Fla.

Examination of Stained Blood

MAKING AND STAINING BLOOD FILMS

The information gathered from the examination of the blood smear is extremely important. It may furnish the diagnosis as does a histologic section; it may serve as a guide to therapy and as indicator of harmful effects of chemotherapy and radiotherapy. The reliability of the information obtained depends to a considerable extent on the quality of the smears. Properly spread films are essential to accurate work. They more than compensate for the time spent in learning to make them.

The slides and coverglasses must be *perfectly clean* and free of grease. Commercially available precleaned slides are usually quite satisfactory. Otherwise, one of the following procedures may be used.

1. Wash the slides with soap and water, then with abundant clean hot water (the water should not be permitted to cool before all the soap has been removed), followed by distilled water, and then dry and polish with a clean, lint-free cloth. From then on they must be handled by touching only their edges. Washed slides and coverglasses may be stored in 95 per cent alcohol. Dry coverglasses may also be stored in a clean, dry Petri dish.

2. Slides and coverglasses may be cleaned in advance with acid cleaning solution, which is prepared as follows: Twenty-five grams of

powdered potassium dichromate is dissolved in a Pyrex beaker in 25 ml. of water with the aid of heat. Let it cool and add slowly 1 liter of technical grade concentrated sulfuric acid. This step must be done cautiously because intense heat develops.

The slides and coverglasses are dropped individually into the cleaning solution and left in it for from 4 to 24 hours. The cleaning solution is poured off and the slides washed with multiple changes of tap water. The removal of the acid may be accelerated by heating. The complete removal of the acid is established when the tap water is negative with litmus paper. They should then be rinsed in distilled water. The slides and coverslips are then stored as described previously.

The drop of blood must *not be too large*.

The work must be done *quickly*, before coagulation begins. The blood is obtained from the fingertip or the lobe of the ear, as for a blood count. Only a very small drop is required, usually about twice the size of a pinhead. The size of the drop largely determines the thickness of the film. The proper thickness depends on the purpose for which the film is made. For a study of the structure of blood corpuscles and examination for malarial parasites, it should be so thin that, throughout the greater part of the film, the erythrocytes lie in a single layer, close together but not overlapping. For routine differential counting of leukocytes, a film in which the erythrocytes are piled up somewhat is best because the leukocytes are more evenly distributed, the number of leukocytes in a given area is greatly increased, and the tedium of counting is correspondingly lessened. The film must not, on the other hand, be so thick that identification of the various leukocytes becomes difficult. In some cases of severe anemia, it is very difficult to make good films because of the large proportion of plasma, which leads to slow drying with consequent distortion of the erythrocytes and the appearance of artefacts. To overcome this, the films should be made very thin and dried quickly.

The Two-slide Method. The coverglass method has the advantage of more even distribution of leukocytes. In every other respect the slide method is preferable. Slides are easier to handle and to label and are less fragile.

Take a small drop of blood on a chemically clean and dust-free slide about ¾ inch from the end, using care that the slide does not touch the skin. Place the slide on a table or flat surface. (At the bedside it may be more convenient to hold the end of the slide away from the drop by the thumb and forefinger of the left hand and to support the other end with the small finger.) With the thumb and forefinger of the right hand hold the end of a second slide against the surface of the first at an angle of 30 to 40 degrees (the free edge of the spreader slide will then be about an inch above the table) and draw it back against the drop of blood until contact is established. The drop will immediately run across the end, filling the angle between the two slides. Push the "spreader slide" at a moderate speed forward so that the blood spreads evenly on the other slide behind the edge of the spreader, keeping contact between the two until all the blood has been spread into a moderately thin film.

The slides are rapidly air dried; rapid drying is aided by waving the slide in the air or by using an electric fan. If the drop of blood was of appropriate size, the thin portion of the film is about 3 cm. long. The thickness of the film can be regulated by changing the angle at which the spreader slide is held, by varying the pressure and the speed of spreading, and by using a smaller or larger drop of blood. At a given speed, increasing the angle at which the spreader slide is held will increase the thickness of the film. At a given angle, increasing the speed with which the spreader slide is pushed will increase the thickness of the film. The film should not cover the entire surface of the slide. In a good film there is a thick portion and a thin portion and a gradual transition from one to the other. The film should have a smooth, even appearance and be free from ridges, waves, or holes. The edge of the spreader must be absolutely smooth. If it is rough, the film has ragged tails containing many leukocytes. A "margin-free" blood spreader prepared by cutting off the corners of a regular slide is preferred in some laboratories. This makes the smear narrower than the slide.

The speed of spreading the film is a factor in the quality of the preparation. The faster it is spread, the more even and the thicker it is. In films of optimum thickness there is some overlap of red cells in much of the film but even distribution and separation of red cells toward the thin tail. However, in a good smear the leukocytes should not be crowded. The faster the film is air dried, the better the spreading of the individual cells on the slide. Slow drying (in humid weather, for example) results in contraction artefacts of the cells.

It is very easy by this method to make large numbers of thin, even films.

The slide may be labeled by writing the identification with a lead pencil directly on the thicker end of the blood film.

Two-coverglass Method. This method is widely recommended, but considerable practice is required to get good results. No. 0 or No. 1 coverglasses ⅞ inch square are recommended. No. 2 coverglasses are too thick for oil immersion.

Touch a coverglass (22 by 22 mm. square) to the top of a small drop of blood (about 2 to 3 mm. in size) without touching the skin and place it, blood side down, crosswise on another coverglass so that the corners appear as an eight-pointed star. If the drop is not too large and if the coverglasses are perfectly clean, the blood will spread out evenly and quickly in a thin layer between the two surfaces. Just as it stops spreading and before it begins to coagulate, pull the coverglasses quickly but firmly apart on a plane parallel to their surfaces. They should not be separated by lifting. They should be placed smear side up on clean paper and allowed to dry in the air, or they may be placed back to back cornerwise in slits made in a cardboard box.

Films from venous blood may be prepared similarly by touching the tip of a hypodermic needle to a coverslip, placing on it a drop 1 to 2 mm. in size, and proceeding as described. It has also been recommended to empty the syringe quickly into the container with anticoagulant except for the last few drops, to hold it in vertical position with the tip up, and to apply gentle pressure on the plunger until a small drop of blood appears on the tip. The drop is then touched with the coverglass. Venous blood with an anticoagulant is less suitable for the study of white cells. Oxalate is especially poor because of the presence of vacuoles and other degenerative changes and phagocytized crystals of oxalate. EDTA is perhaps the most satisfactory anticoagulant for examining the morphology of blood cells because vacuoles and other degenerative changes appear more slowly than with other anticoagulants; only minimal changes occur within 2 or 3 hours of collection. Blood with other anticoagulants and defibrinated blood are less satisfactory for the study of leukocytes.

Separation of the coverglasses must be done just at the right moment to get good results. If it is done too soon, the smear will be too thick. If it is done too late, the blood will clot and it may be difficult to pull the coverglasses apart.

The coverglass method is especially recommended for accurate differential counts, since all the leukocytes in the drop will be found on the two coverglasses and thus the error due to unequal distribution can be excluded by counting all the leukocytes. The blood usually is much more evenly spread on one of the coverglasses than it is on the other.

Fixation. In general, films must be "fixed" before they are stained. Stains that are dissolved in methyl alcohol, e.g., Wright's stain, combine fixation with the staining process. Fixation takes place during the first minute when the undiluted stain is applied. With aqueous stains, chemicals or heat must be used prior to application of the stain.

Chemical Fixation. Soak the film 1 to 2 minutes in pure methyl alcohol or absolute ethyl alcohol, or 15 minutes or longer in equal parts of absolute alcohol and ether. One minute in a 1 per cent solution of mercuric chloride or in a 1 per cent solution of formalin in alcohol is preferred by some workers. The film must be well washed in water after fixation with mercuric chloride. Chemical fixation may precede staining with hematoxylin and eosin and with other simple stains.

Fixation with Heat. This may precede any of the methods that do not combine fixation with a staining process. The best method is to place the film in an oven, raise the temperature to 150° C., and allow to cool slowly. Without an oven, the proper degree of fixation is difficult to attain.

BLOOD STAINS

The aniline dyes, which are extensively used in blood work, are of two general classes: basic dyes, such as methylene blue, and acid dyes, such as eosin. Nuclei and certain other structures in the blood are stained by the basic dyes and, hence, are called basophilic. Certain structures take up only acid dyes and are called acidophilic, oxyphilic, or eosinophilic. Certain other structures are stained by a combination of the two and are called neutrophilic. Recognition of these staining properties marked the beginning of modern hematology.

Polychrome Methylene Blue and Eosin Stains. These stains, which are the outgrowth of the original time-consuming Romanowsky method, have largely displaced other blood stains for routine laboratory use. They stain differentially most normal and abnormal structures in the blood. Most of them are dissolved in methyl alcohol and combine the fixing with the staining process. Numerous methods of preparing and applying these stains have been devised, among the best known being Giemsa's and Wright's.

Wright's Stain. This is called a polychromatic stain because it produces a variety of colors. It is a methyl alcoholic solution of an acid and a basic dye. It is one of the best and is the most widely used stain. Wright's stain certified by the Commission of Staining is commercially available. It is satisfactory and ready for use. One can also purchase the powder certified by the Commission on Staining.*

PREPARATION. The solution is prepared by dissolving 0.1 gm. of powder per 60 ml. of chemically pure absolute methyl alcohol (C.P., acetone-free). The powder (0.1 gm.) is ground in a mortar adding a few milliliters

*H. J. Conn and M. S. Darrow: Staining Procedures Used by the Biological Stain Commission. 2nd ed. Baltimore, The Williams & Wilkins Co., 1960.

of the alcohol at a time until 60 ml. have been added and the entire stain has gone into solution. This requires 20 to 30 minutes. The stain should then be left standing for a day or two and filtered before use. The stock dye is filtered when prepared and each time when samples are taken from the stock. The dye is sensitive to contamination with water in reagents or glassware. The reagent bottle must be tightly stoppered at all times to prevent entry of water vapor. Exposure to acid or alkaline fumes must also be avoided.

Buffer for dilution of Wright's stain (pH 6.4): primary (monobasic) potassium phosphate (KH_2PO_4), anhydrous 6.63 gm.; secondary (dibasic) sodium phosphate (Na_2HPO_4), anhydrous 2.56 gm.; and distilled water to make 1 liter. A more alkaline buffer (pH 6.7) may be prepared by using 5.13 gm. of the potassium salt and 4.12 gm. of the sodium salt.

STAINING THE FILM

1. For best results the films should be stained as soon as they have been dried in the air but in any case not later than after a few hours. If they must be kept longer without staining, they must be fixed. In smears left unfixed for a day or more, the dried plasma stains and produces a background of pale blue. Uniform staining is difficult to achieve, because smears tend to vary in thickness except when exceptionally good technique is used in their preparation.

2. Place the slide with the air-dried film side up on a stain rack over a pan; the coverslip is placed best on a support, i.e., a cork attached to the bottom of a pan with paraffin.

3. Without previous fixation, cover the film with a noted quantity of the staining fluid with a medicine dropper. There must be plenty of stain in order to avoid too great an evaporation and consequent precipitation. This step fixes the smear. When slides are used, the stain may be confined to the desired area by two heavy wax-pencil marks.

4. After 2 minutes, add to the staining fluid on the film an equal quantity of the buffer solution with a second medicine dropper. In some parts of the country tap water may be used with equally good results. To mix the stain with the diluent, blow gently on the diluted stain on several portions of the slide to set up gentle currents and to make an even distribution. The quantity of the fluid on the preparation must not be so large that some of it runs off. Allow the mixture to remain for 3 to 4 minutes. Look for a greenish metallic scum to appear. The margins should show a reddish tint. A longer period of staining may produce a precipitate. The time of optimum staining with the undiluted stains has to be established for each batch. Eosinophilic granules are best brought out by a short period of staining. The optimum time for the most effective combination of stain and diluent varies from batch to batch.

5. Float off the stain with a stream of water (preferably distilled), first slowly and then more vigorously, preferably from an overhead water bottle, until all traces of excessive stain have disappeared. During the entire procedure the slide must remain horizontal. The washing takes 5 to 30 seconds until the thinner portions of the film become yellowish or pink in color. The preparation should be flooded with water while the stain is still on it. If the stain is poured off before rinsing, the scum tends to settle on the blood film, where it clings in spite of subsequent washing. If the color is too dark, the excessive blue can be removed by further washing. The stain remaining on the back of the slide is removed with gauze moistened in alcohol.

6. The washing completed, the excessive water is drained by tilting the slide and touching a blotter with the lower edge.

7. The slide may be dried by evaporation by leaving it in the tilted position, or by blotting gently with filter paper.

8. The coverslide, film side down, is mounted on a side with neutral Canada balsam. Coverglass films may be mounted temporarily by placing them, blood slide down, on a glass slide on which a drop of immersion oil has been placed. Using a drop of isobutyl methacrylate dissolved in xylol or toluol at an approximately neutral pH will give permanent mounts.

Films stained well with Wright's stain have a pink color when viewed with the naked eye and give the following picture on microscopic examination (see Fig. 4–10): When inspected under low-power magnification of the microscope, the cells should be evenly distributed and separated from each other. The red cells are pink, not lemon yellow or red; they are lying flat without overlapping or forming rouleaux. At least eight satisfactory low-power fields on a slide are present in a good preparation. There should be only a minimum of precipitate. The areas between the cells are clear. The color of the film should be uniform without pale or dark green areas indicative of excessive staining of thick portions of film. The blood cells should be free from artefacts, such as vacuoles. The nuclei of leukocytes are purplish blue, the basi- and oxychromatin (chromatin and parachromatin) clearly differentiated, and the cytoplasmic neutrophilic granules lilac or violet pink. The eosinophilic granules are red-orange and each distinctly discernible, so that one may count the individual granules.

The basophil has dark bluish purple granules. Platelets have dark lilac granules. Bacteria are blue. The cytoplasm of lymphocytes is generally robin's-egg blue; that of the monocytes

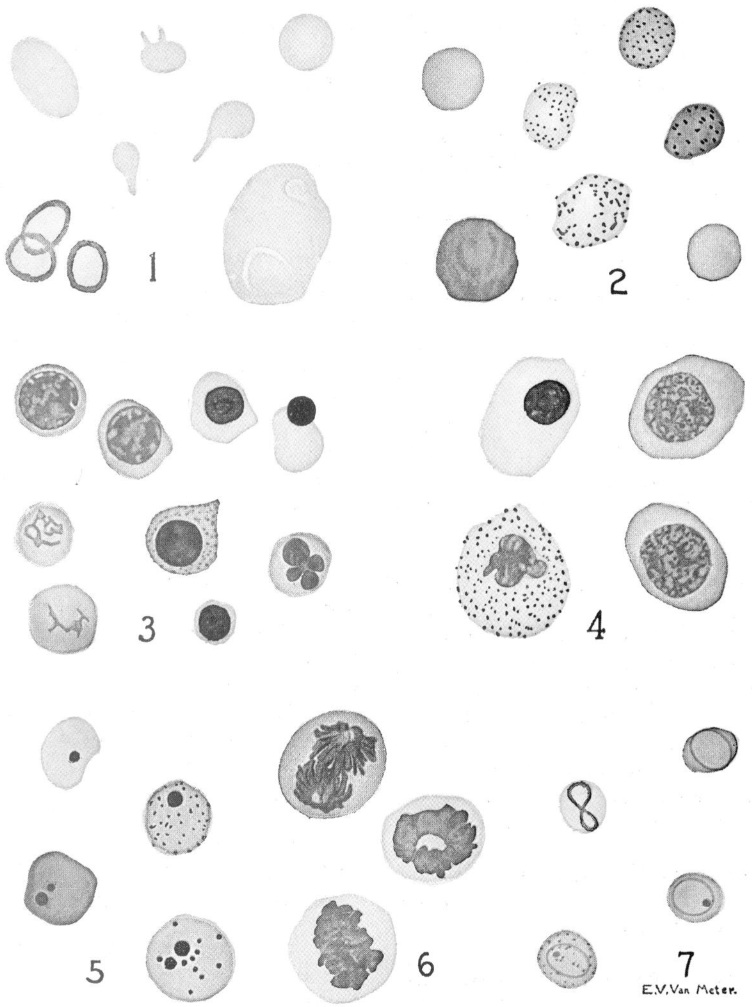

Figure 4–10. Abnormal erythrocytes. All drawn from actual specimens and all stained with Wright's stain except where noted (× 1000) (1 mm. = 1 μm.). *1,* Variations in size, shape, and hemoglobin content; from cases of pernicious anemia and iron deficiency anemia. *2,* Polychromatophilia and basophilic stippling in cases of lead poisoning and pernicious anemia. *3,* Normoblasts, reticulated erythrocytes, and one microblast; the top row represents stages in the development of the normoblast. The two reticulated erythrocytes are stained with brilliant cresyl blue. *4,* Megaloblasts in pernicious anemia. Two show polychromatophilia and fairly typical nuclei, two have condensed nuclei, and one of these has basophilic cytoplasmic granules. *5,* Nuclear particles or Howell-Jolly bodies. One cell also shows basophilic stippling. *6,* Mitotic figures. *7,* Cabot's ring bodies. Two cells also contain nuclear particles and one shows basophilic stippling (Leishman's stain). (E. V. Van Meter, pinx.)

has a faint bluish tinge. Malarial parasites stain characteristically: the cytoplasm, sky blue; the chromatin, purplish red. These colors are not invariable; two films stained from the same bottle sometimes differ greatly. In general, a preparation is satisfactory when both the nuclei and the neutrophilic granules are distinct, regardless of their color, and when the film is free from precipitated dye. The colors are prone to fade if the preparation is mounted in a poor quality of balsam or if it is exposed to the light.

Failure to get satisfactory results with the polychrome methylene-blue-eosin stains, when they are properly used, may be due to imperfect polychroming of the powder but is most frequently due to incorrect reaction of the staining fluid. When the solution is too acid (pH too low), the erythrocytes stain bright red and the nuclei of the leukocytes are pale sky blue or even colorless. When the reaction is too alkaline (pH too high), the erythrocytes stain deep slate blue and there is little differentiation of colors. The reaction of the solution is determined partly by that of the powder when, as is the case with Wright's stain, its reaction is not accurately adjusted, but it depends to a still greater degree on the methyl alcohol, which is prone to develop formic acid as a result of oxidation on standing. A given powder may afford perfect results when dissolved in methyl alcohol from a freshly opened bottle but may produce poor results when dissolved in the same lot of alcohol after it has stood for some months exposed to the air. Deterioration of old solutions is largely due to the same cause. Pathologic blood may stain poorly with solutions that are correct for normal blood.

SOME CAUSES OF BAD RESULTS

Causes of Excessively Blue Stain. Thick films, overstaining, inadequate washing, or too high an alkalinity of stain or diluent. In such smears the erythrocytes appear blue or green, the nuclear chromatin is deep blue to black, and the granules of the neutrophilic granulocytes are deeply overstained and appear large and prominent. The granules of the eosinophils are blue or gray. Such stain can be corrected by staining for a shorter time with the stain itself and for a longer time with the diluent, or by using less stain and more diluent. If these steps are ineffective, the buffer may be too alkaline and a new one with a lower pH should be prepared.

Causes of Excessively Pink Stain. Insufficient staining; too long a washing; mounting the coverslips before they are dry; or too high an acidity of the stain, buffer, or water. In such smears the erythrocytes are bright red or orange and not pink, the nuclear chromatin is pale blue, and the granules of the eosinophils are sparkling brilliant red. One of the causes of the increased acidity is exposure of the stain or buffer to acid fumes. The situation may be corrected by a new batch of stain or buffer. If the local tap water is alkaline, using it in place of distilled water may improve the stain.

Causes of Pale, Inadequately Stained Red Cells, Nuclei, or Eosinophilic Granules. Understaining or excessive washing. Prolonging the staining or reducing the washing may solve the problem.

Causes of Precipitate on the Film. Unclean slides, drying during the period of staining, inadequate washing of the stain at the end of the staining period, especially failure to hold the slide horizontally during washing or inadequate filtration of the stain, and permitting dust to settle on the slide or smear.

Other Useful Blood Stains. Although Wright's stain suffices for most clinical work and is to be recommended if only one blood stain is to be used, certain other stains demand brief mention.

GIEMSA'S STAIN. This widely used stain is probably the best modification of Romanowsky's stain for demonstrating blood parasites and other protozoa, and it is also highly satisfactory as a routine blood stain. Its composition is as follows:

Azur II-eosin	3.0 gm.
Azur II	0.8 gm.
Glycerin (Merck, C.P.)	250.0 ml.
Methyl alcohol (Kahlbaum I or Merck's reagent)	250.0 ml.

The solution is troublesome to make and is best purchased already prepared. Blood films are fixed in methyl alcohol and are then immersed for 20 minutes or longer in a freshly prepared mixture of 1 ml. of stain and 10 ml. of distilled water. In order to prevent precipitate from forming on them, the slides or coverglass should be placed on edge in the stain. Satisfactory results may also be obtained by placing about 30 drops of distilled water on the fixed film, adding 3 drops of Giemsa's stain, mixing, and allowing it to act for 15 or 20 minutes.

PAPPENHEIM'S PANOPTIC METHOD. In order to combine the advantages of the several stains, Pappenheim recommended the following procedure: Stain for 1 minute with the May-Grünwald stain; add an equal quantity of water; after 1 minute, pour off the fluid and stain 15 minutes with the diluted Giemsa solution. The May-Grünwald stain is the same as Jenner's stain. Wright's stain, diluted with an equal quantity of water, may be substituted for Giemsa's stain, but the time of staining should then not exceed 5 minutes.

JENNER'S STAIN OR THE MAY-GRÜNWALD STAIN. Jenner's eosinate of methylene blue, dissolved in methyl alcohol, brings out leukocytic granules well and is therefore especially useful for differential counting. It stains nuclei poorly and is much inferior to Wright's stain for the detection of malarial parasites, since it does not produce the so-called Romanowsky staining.

It may be purchased in solution, in the form of tablets, or as a powder, 0.5 gm. of which should be dissolved in 100 ml. of neutral absolute methyl alcohol. The unfixed blood film is covered with the staining solution and after 3 to 5 minutes is rinsed with water, dried in the air, and mounted.

CARBOLTHIONIN BLUE. Carbolthionin blue is especially useful for the study of basophilic granular degeneration (basophilic stippling) of the erythrocytes. Nuclei, malarial parasites, and basophilic granules are brought out sharply. Polychromatophilia is also evident. The films can be fixed with an alcoholic solution of formalin or saturated solution of mercuric chloride.

PAPPENHEIM'S METHYL GREEN PYRONINE. Pappenheim's methyl green pyronine can be used as a blood stain and is very satisfactory for study of the erythrocytes and lymphocytes and for demonstration of Döhle's inclusion bodies. At the appropriate pH (4.7 or 4.8), methyl green stains DNA blue-green and pyronine stains RNA red. All nuclei are blue to reddish purple; basophilic granules, cytoplasm of lymphocytes, and Döhle bodies are red. Polychromatophilia is well demonstrated, the affected cells taking more or less of the red color. Heat fixation is probably best.

STUDY OF STAINED BLOOD FILMS

It has been said with much truth that an intelligent study of the stained film, together with an estimation of the concentration of hemoglobin, will yield 90 per cent of all the diagnostic information obtainable by hematologic examination. The stained films furnish the best means of studying the morphology of the blood and blood parasites, and, to an experienced person, they give a fair idea of the amount of hemoglobin and of the number of erythrocytes and leukocytes. An oil-immersion objective is required.

Erythrocytes. In a healthy person the erythrocytes, when not crowded together, appear as circular, homogeneous discs of nearly uniform size, ranging from 6 to 8 μm. in diameter (Fig. 4–11). However, even in normal blood there may be individual cells as small as 5.5 μm. and as large as 9.5 μm. The center of each is somewhat paler than the periphery. Erythrocytes are liable to be crenated when the film has dried too slowly. In disease, erythrocytes vary in their hemoglobin content, size, shape, staining properties, and structure.

Variation in Color

Hemoglobin Content. The depth of staining furnishes a rough guide to the amount of hemoglobin in red cells, and the terms normochromic, hypochromic, and hyperchromic are used to describe this feature of red cells. *Normochromic* refers to normal intensity of staining (Fig. 4–11). When the amount of hemoglobin is diminished, the central pale area becomes larger and paler. This is known as *hypochromia.* The MCH and MCHC are usually decreased (Fig. 4–13). In megaloblastic anemia, because the red cells are larger and hence thicker, many stain deeply and have less central pallor (Figs. 4–14 and 4–16). These cells are *hyperchromic* because they have an increased hemoglobin content (MCH), but the hemoglobin concentration (MCHC) is normal. In hereditary spherocytosis the cells are also hyperchromic; though the hemoglobin content (MCH) is normal, the hemoglobin concentration (MCHC) is increased because of a reduced surface/volume ratio.

The presence of hypochromic cells and normochromic cells in the same film is called *anisochromia* or, sometimes, a dimorphic anemia (Fig. 4–18). This is characteristic of sideroblastic anemias, but also is found some weeks after iron therapy for iron deficiency anemia or in a hypochromic anemia after transfusion with normal cells.

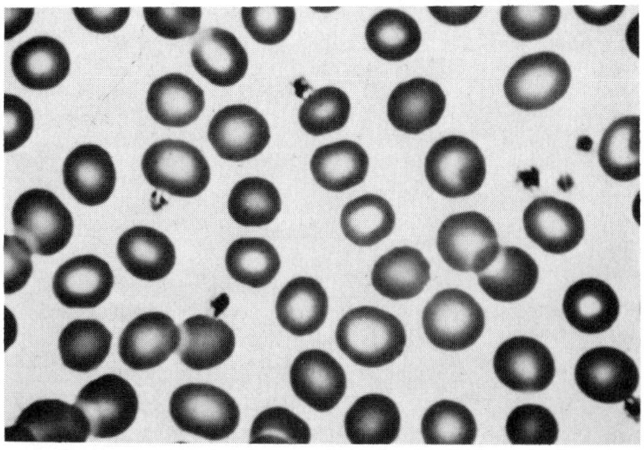

Figure 4–12. This blood film shows a small number of slightly hypochromic red cells; most are normochromic. Cell diameters are normal. MCV and MCHC were normal. The irregular bodies 2 to 3 μm. in diameter are normal blood platelets. (× 875.)

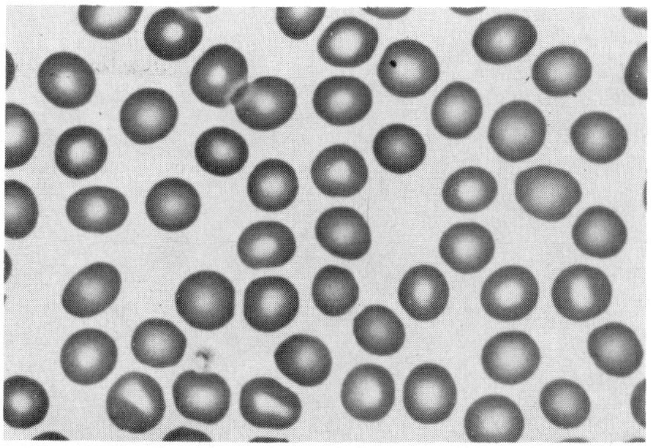

Figure 4–11. Normal blood film. (× 875.)

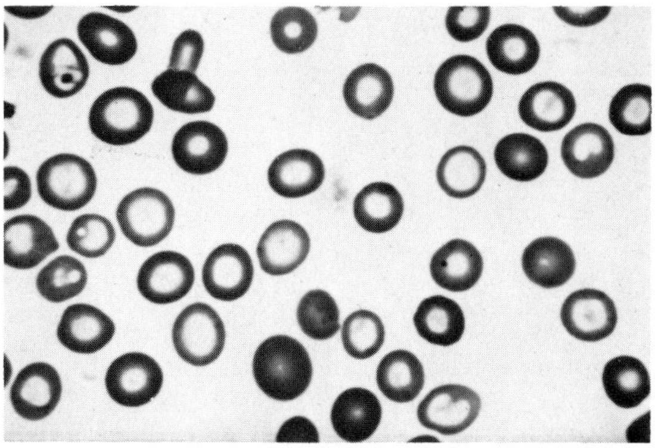

Figure 4–13. Iron deficiency anemia. Most of the cells are hypochromic and microcytic. Note elliptical cells. Anisocytosis is slight in degree. (× 875.)

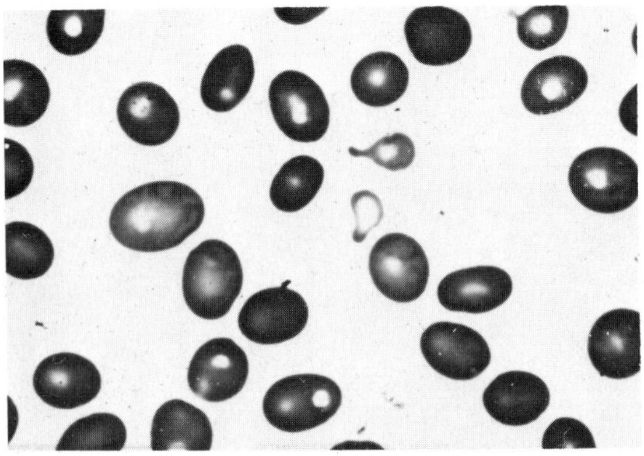

Figure 4–14. Megaloblastic anemia. Macrocytosis. Marked anisocytosis. Note elliptical cells and teardrop-shaped cells. (× 875.)

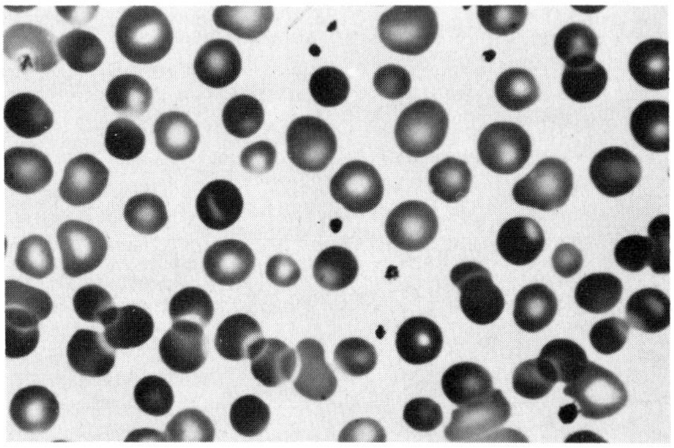

Figure 4–15. Hereditary spherocytosis. The denser cells are more spherocytic. Note that they have minimal and eccentric pallor, moderate anisocytosis. Though the cell diameter is reduced, the MCV is within the normal range. (× 875.)

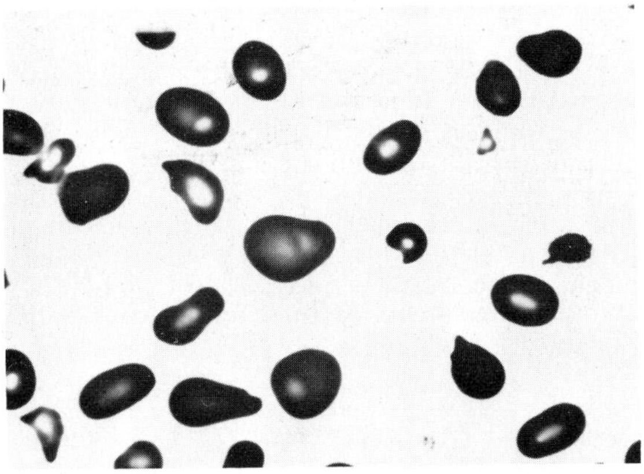

Figure 4–16. Megaloblastic anemia, macrocytosis, marked anisocytosis. (× 875.)

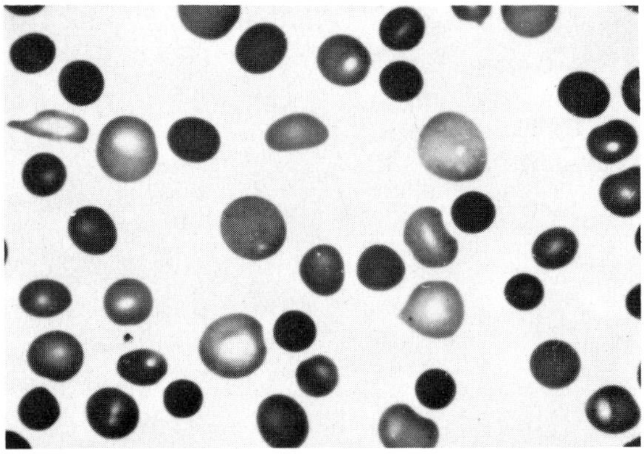

Figure 4–17. Autoimmune hemolytic anemia. The paler, large cells are polychromatic macrocytes (i.e., young reticulocytes.) The small, dense cells are spherocytes. Moderate anisocytosis. (× 875.)

Polychromatophilia. A blue-gray tint to the red cells (polychromatophilia or polychromasia) is a combination of the affinity of hemoglobin for acid stains and the affinity of RNA for basic stains. The presence of residual RNA in the red cell indicates that it is a young red cell which has been in the blood one to two days. These polychromatic red cells are larger than the mature red cells and may lack the central pallor. Young cells with residual RNA are polychromatophilic red cells on air-dried films stained with Wright's stain, but are reticulocytes when stained supravitally with brilliant cresyl blue. Therefore, increased polychromasia implies reticulocytosis; it is most marked in hemolysis and in acute blood loss.

Variation in Size. The red cells may be abnormally small or *microcytes* (Figs. 4–13, 4–16, and 4–19), abnormally large or *macrocytes* (Figs. 4–14, 4–16, and 4–18), or show abnormal variation in size (*anisocytosis*) (Figs. 4–13 through 4–19). Anisocytosis of varying degree is a feature of most anemias; when it is marked in degree, both macrocytes and microcytes are usually present (Figs. 4–14 and 4–16). In analyzing causes of anemia, the terms *microcytic* and *macrocytic* have most meaning when considered as cell volume rather than cell diameter. The mean cell volume, of course, is measured directly on the Coulter Counter Model S, or is calculated from the spun hematocrit and the red cell count. The diameter we perceive directly from the blood film, and infer from it (and the hemoglobin content) the volume. Thus, the red cells in Figure 4–13 are microcytic; since they are hypochromic they are thinner than normal and the diameter is not decreased proportionately to the volume. Also, the mean cell volume in the blood of the patient with spherocytosis (Fig. 4–15) is in the normal range; though many of the cells have a small diameter, their volume is not decreased because they are thicker than normal.

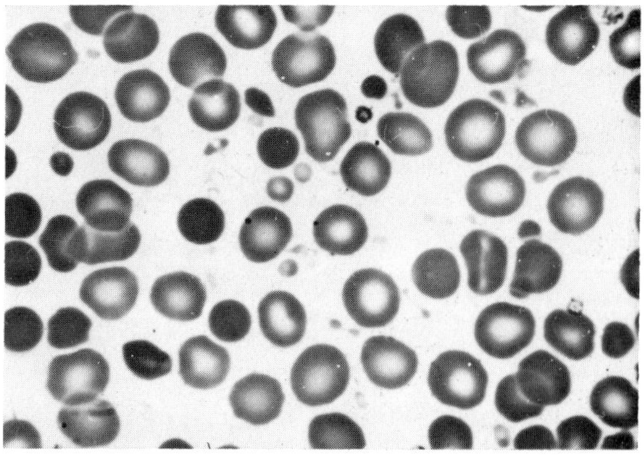

Figure 4–19. Blood film from a patient who has just suffered extensive body burns. Note the many tiny red cell fragments that have budded off the red cells as a result of the heat, leaving spherocytes. Marked anisocytosis. (× 875.)

Variation in Shape. Variation in shape is called *poikilocytosis*. Any abnormally shaped cell is a poikilocyte. Oval, pear-shaped, tear drop-shaped, saddle-shaped, helmet-shaped and irregularly shaped cells may be seen in a single case of anemia such as megaloblastic anemia (Figs. 4–14 and 4–16).

Elliptocytes are most abundant in hereditary elliptocytosis (Fig. 4–20), in which the majority of the cells are elliptical; this is a dominant condition that is only occasionally associated with hemolytic anemia. Elliptocytes are seen in normal persons' blood, but number less than 10 per cent of the cells. They are more common, however, in iron deficiency anemia, myelofibrosis with myeloid metaplasia (Figs. 4–21 and 4–22), megaloblastic anemias (Figs. 4–14 and 4–16), and sickle cell anemia.

Spherocytes are nearly spherical erythrocytes in contradistinction to normal biconcave

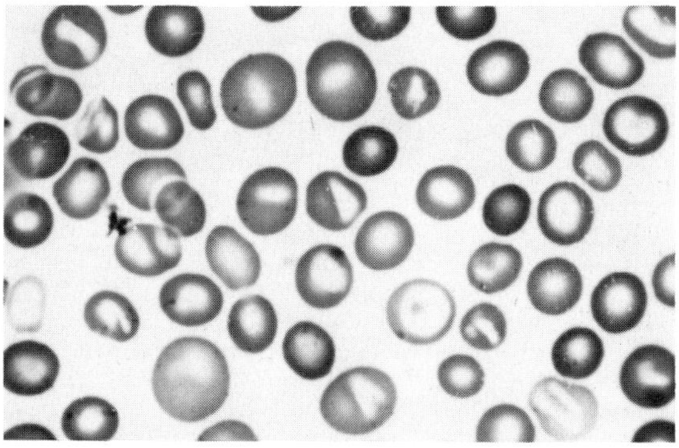

Figure 4–18. Sideroblastic anemia. Dimorphic populations of hypochromic cells and normochromic cells, some of which are macrocytic. Moderate anisocytosis. (× 875.)

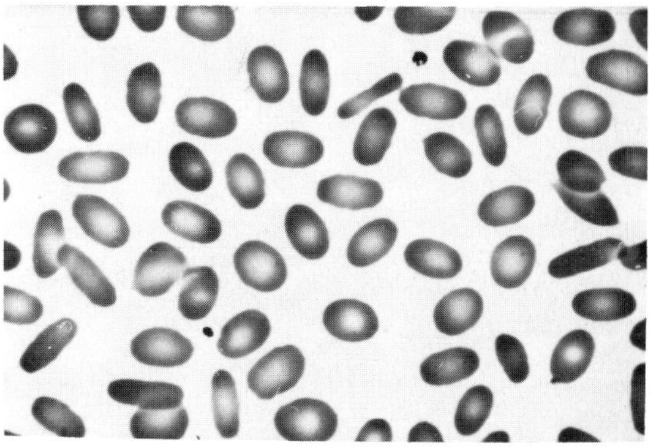

Figure 4–20. Hereditary elliptocytosis. Incidental finding, no anemia. (× 875.)

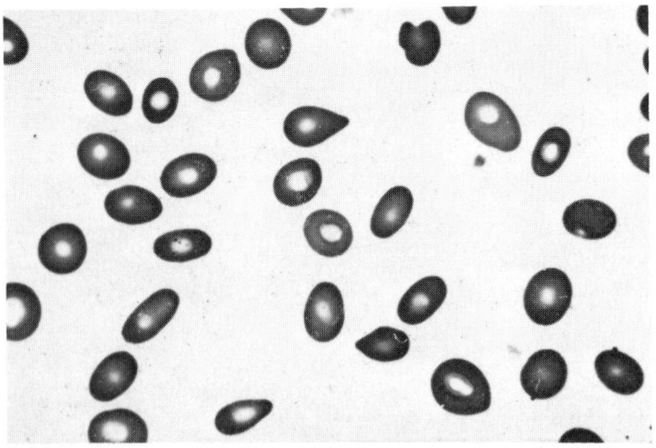

Figure 4–21. Blood film from patient with myelofibrosis with myeloid metaplasia. Numerous elliptocytes. Teardrop-shaped cells. (× 875.)

discs. Their diameter is smaller than normal. They lack the central pale area or have a smaller, often eccentric, pale area (because the cell is thicker and can come to rest somewhat tilted instead of perfectly flattened on the slide). They show increased fragility in hypotonic salt solutions and are found in hereditary spherocytosis (HS, Fig. 4–15), in some cases of acquired hemolytic anemia (AHA, Fig. 4–17), and in some conditions in which there has been a direct physical or chemical injury to the cells, such as heat (Fig. 4–19). In each of these three instances tiny bits of membrane (in excess of hemoglobin) are removed from the adult red cells, leaving the cell with a decreased surface/volume ratio. In HS and AHA this occurs in the reticuloendothelial system; in other instances (e.g., the patient with body burns), this may occur intravascularly.

Target cells are erythrocytes that are thinner than normal (leptocytes) and when stained show a peripheral rim of hemoglobin with a dark, central, hemoglobin-containing area. The two are separated by a pale unstained ring, which contains less hemoglobin. These cells, as well as other hypochromic cells, seem to be more resistant to hypotonic salt solution than are normal erythrocytes. They are found in obstructive jaundice (e.g., Fig. 4–23), in which there appears to be an augmentation of the cell surface membrane; in the postsplenectomy state, in which there is a lack of normal reduction of surface membrane as the cell ages; in any hypochromic anemia, especially thalassemia; and in hemoglobin C disease.

Schistocytes (cell fragments) indicate the presence of hemolysis, whether in megaloblastic anemia (Fig. 4–16), severe burns (Fig. 4–19), or microangiopathic hemolytic anemia (Fig. 4–24). The latter process is associated with either small blood vessel disease or fibrin in small blood vessels and results in intravascular fragmentation; particularly characteristic are helmet cells and triangularly shaped cells. Burr cells are irregularly contracted red cells with prominent spicules and are seen in the same process; however, this term is used differently by different hematologists, and therefore leads to confusion.

Acanthocytes are spiculated red cells in which the ends of the spicules are bulbous and rounded (Fig. 4–25); they are seen in abetalipoproteinemia, hereditary or acquired, and certain cases of liver disease. *Crenated cells* or echinocytes (Fig. 4–26) are regularly contracted cells which may commonly occur as an artefact during preparation of films, or may be due to hyperosmolarity, or to the discocyte-echinocyte transformation. *In vivo* the latter may be associated with decreased red cell ATP due to any of several causes (Brecher and Bessis, 1972).

Artefacts resembling crenated cells consisting of tiny pits or bubbles indenting the red cells (Fig. 4–27) may be caused by a small amount of water contaminating the Wright's

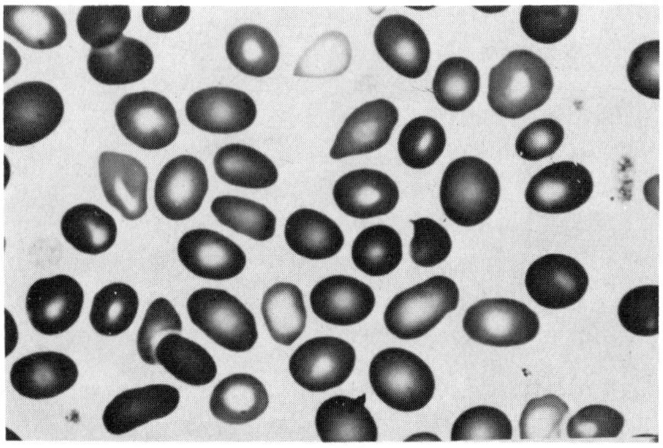

Figure 4–22. Same as Figure 4–21. A few hypochromic microcytic cells are present also. (× 875.)

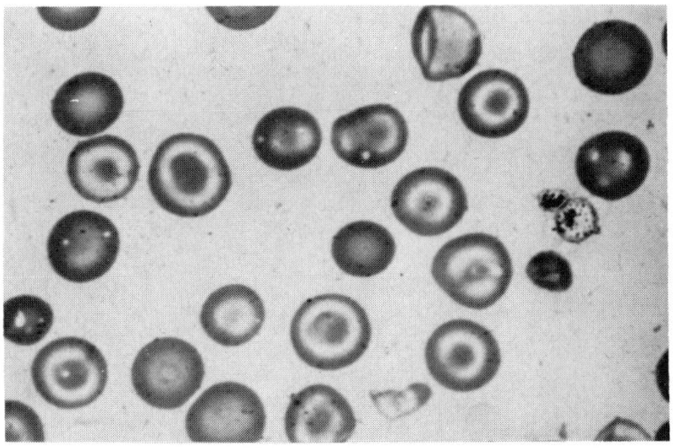

Figure 4–23. Target cells that have an increased cell diameter. Blood film from a patient with obstructive jaundice. (× 875.)

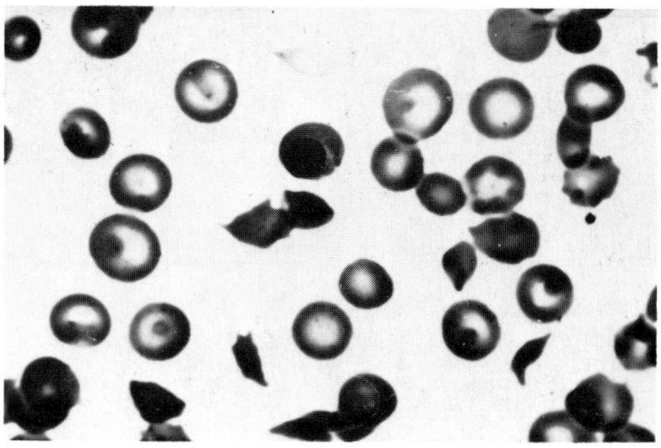

Figure 4–24. Microangiopathic hemolytic anemia; hemolytic-uremic syndrome. Note irregularly contracted cells, schistocytes, a few crenated cells. One nucleated red cell. (× 875.)

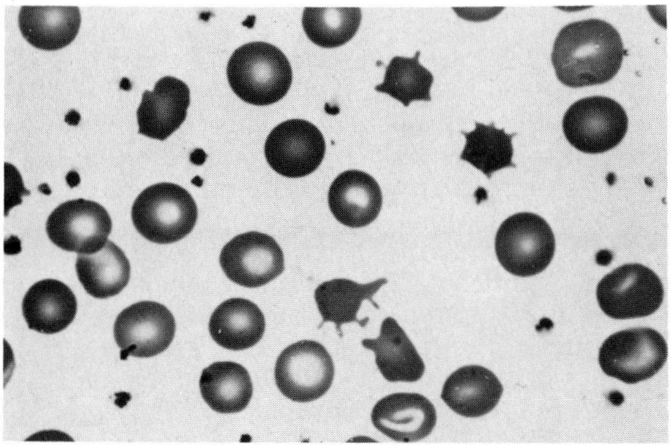

Figure 4–25. Acanthocytes. Note the long spicules, which tend to have bulbous ends (× 875.)

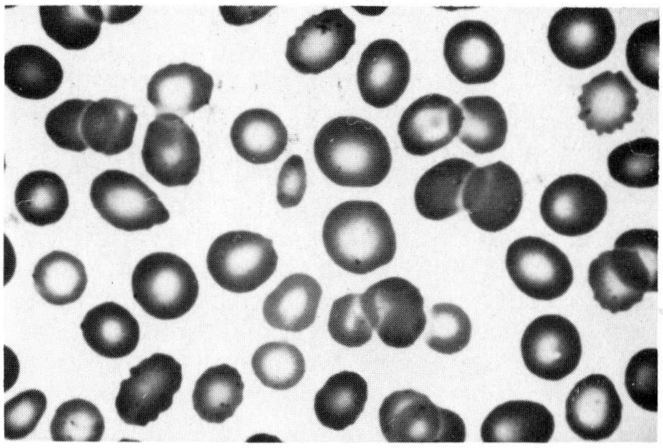

Figure 4–26. Megaloblastic anemia. A few crenated cells are present. (× 875.)

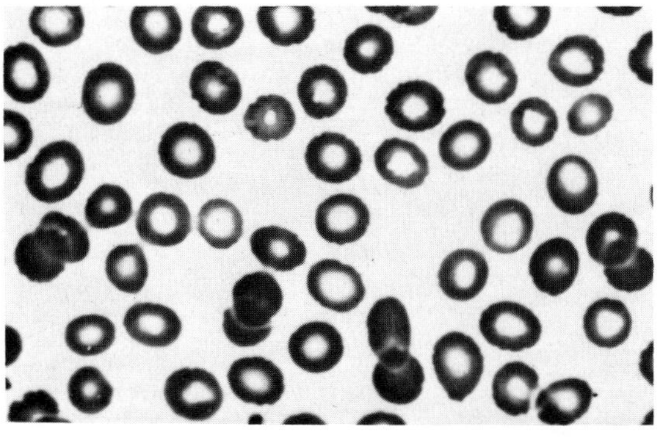

Figure 4–27. Artefact due to water in the methyl alcohol fixative. If bubbles are small in size (as here) they cause an indented appearance which may be confused with crenation. (× 875.)

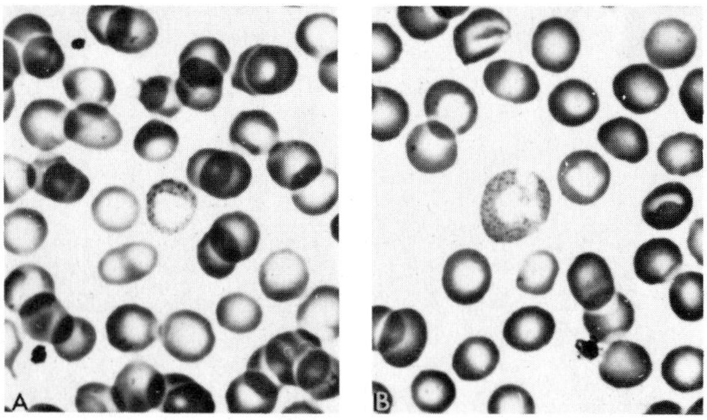

Figure 4–28. Basophilic stippling. One stippled red cell in the center of each field. *A*, thalassemia minor; *B*, lead poisoning (× 875.)

stain (or absolute methanol, if this is used first as a fixative).

Variations in Structure

BASOPHILIC STIPPLING (BASOPHILIC GRANULAR DEGENERATION; PUNCTATE BASOPHILIA). This is characterized by the presence, within the erythrocyte, of irregular basophilic granules, which vary in size from scarcely visible dots to granules nearly as large as azurophil granules of promyelocytes (Fig. 4–28). The number of these granules present in an erythrocyte commonly varies in inverse ratio to their size. They stain deep blue with carbolthionin blue or Wright's stain. The erythrocyte containing them may stain normally in other respects or it may exhibit polychromatophilia. Fine stippling is commonly seen when there is increased polychromatophilia, and, therefore, with increased production of red cells. Coarse stippling may be seen in lead poisoning or other diseases with impaired hemoglobin synthesis, in megaloblastic anemia, and in other forms of severe anemia; it is attributed to an abnormal instability of the RNA in the young cell.

Red cells with inorganic iron-containing granules (as demonstrated by stains for iron) are called *siderocytes*. Sometimes these granules stain with Wright's stain; if so, they are called *Pappenheimer bodies*. In contrast to basophilic stippling, Pappenheimer bodies are few in number in a given red cell and are rarely seen in the peripheral blood except after splenectomy.

HOWELL-JOLLY BODIES. These particles are smooth, round remnants of nuclear chromatin. Single Howell-Jolly bodies may be seen in megaloblastic anemia, hemolytic anemia, and after splenectomy. Multiple Howell-Jolly bodies in a single cell (Fig. 4–29) usually indicate megaloblastic anemia or some other form of abnormal erythropoiesis.

CABOT RINGS. These are ring-shaped, figure-of-eight, or loop-shaped structures (Fig. 4–10). Occasionally they are formed by double or several concentric lines. They have been observed rarely in erythrocytes in pernicious anemia, lead poisoning, and certain other disorders of erythropoiesis. They stain red or reddish purple with Wright's stain and have no internal structure (on close examination they are seen to consist of fine granules). In addition to Cabot's rings, erythrocytes may occasionally contain basophilic granules, nuclear fragments, or even complete nuclei. The rings have been thought to be the remains of a nuclear membrane or denatured protein or lipoprotein resulting from cellular degeneration. They are interpreted as evidence of abnormal erythropoiesis.

MALARIAL STIPPLING. This term has been applied to the finely granular appearance of erythrocytes that harbor the parasites of tertian malaria. It was formerly classed with basophilic stippling but is undoubtedly different. Not all stains show it. With Wright's stain it can be brought out by staining longer and washing less than when ordinary blood is examined. The minute granules, "Schüffner's granules," stain purplish red. They are sometimes so numerous

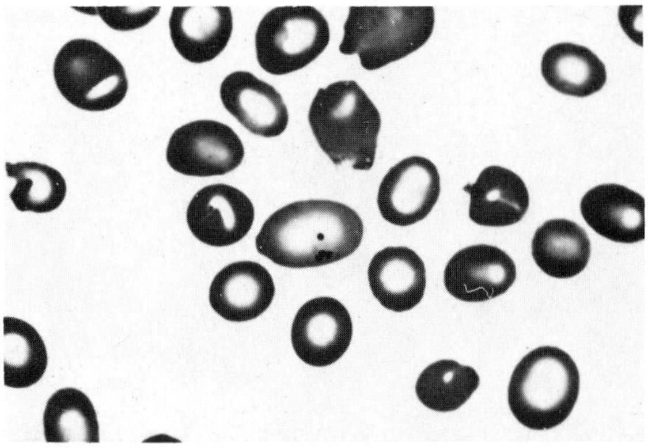

Figure 4–29. Megaloblastic anemia. The central oval macrocyte has four Howell-Jolly bodies; the lower three are touching one another. (× 875.)

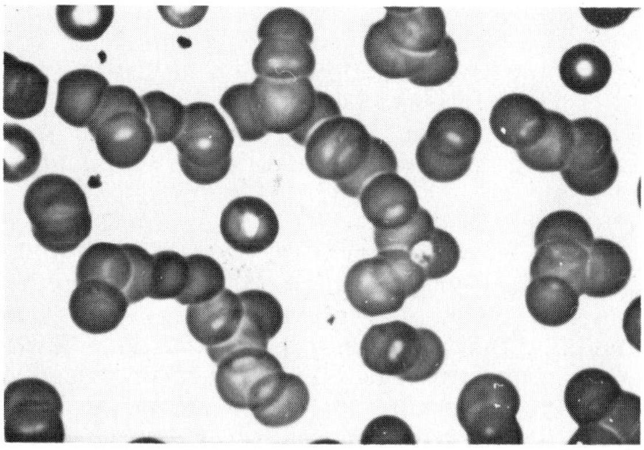

Figure 4–30. Rouleaux in a blood film from a patient with multiple myeloma. (× 875.)

that they almost hide the parasites. These red cells are, as a rule, larger than normal.

ROULEAU FORMATION. This is the alignment of red cells one upon another so that they resemble stacks of coins in wet preparations. On air-dried films, rouleaux appear as in Figure 4–30; the red cells are not evenly distributed. Elevated plasma fibrinogen or globulins cause rouleaux to form and, because of this, also promote an increase in the erythrocyte sedimentation rate. Rouleau formation is especially marked in paraproteinemia (monoclonal gammopathy). *Agglutination* or clumping of red cells is more surely separated from rouleaux in wet preparations, but on air-dried films (Fig. 4–31) tends to show more irregular and round clumps than the linear rouleaux. Cold agglutinins are responsible for this appearance.

Nucleated Red Cells. In contrast to erythrocytes of lower vertebrates and to other cells of the body, a unique characteristic of the mammalian erythrocyte is the absence of a nucleus. Nucleated red cells (*normoblasts*) are normally present only in the bone marrow in the human (Fig. 4–32, 4–59 and 4–60). *Pronormoblasts* are the largest, with a large nucleus, prominent nucleolus, rather fine but distinct chromatin, and abundant blue cytoplasm. The *basophilic normoblast* (prorubricyte) is somewhat smaller, with coarser chromatin, and distinct open spaces (parachromatin). The openings are arranged at the periphery and, with the chromatin bars between them, suggest a wheel with broad spokes. The cytoplasm is deep blue and evidence of hemoglobin is not yet visible. Pronormoblasts and basophilic normoblasts are rarely seen in peripheral blood.

With increased production of hemoglobin the blue color of the cytoplasm is progressively replaced by red, which results in various shades of gray (*polychromatophilic normoblast;* rubricyte). When the nucleus becomes smaller and dense (pyknotic) and the cytoplasm gains more hemoglobin, the *orthochromatic normoblast* (metarubricyte) stage is reached; usually some cytoplasmic polychromatophilia remains. Older normoblasts are smaller and the nuclei are very densely staining. In the peripheral blood film, their nuclei stain more deeply than any other cell type; therefore, normoblasts can be recognized under the low power (10 ×) objective lens. Sometimes the nuclei of normoblasts may be irregular in shape and clover-leaf forms may be found.

The megaloblast (Fig. 4–33) is a distinct cell, not merely a larger normoblast. It is present in pernicious anemia and in other megaloblastic anemias. The cells of this series are not found in the normal marrow. They are all larger than the corresponding cells of the normal series. Deficiency of vitamin B_{12} or folic acid is responsible. The result is abnormal DNA synthesis resulting in defective nuclear matura-

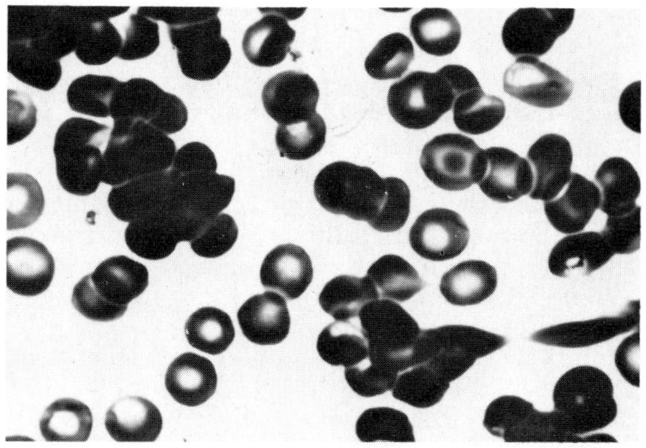

Figure 4–31. Blood film from a patient with a high titer of cold agglutinins. Red cells aggregate in clumps. Separation of cells during making the film may distort the cells (lower right). (× 875.)

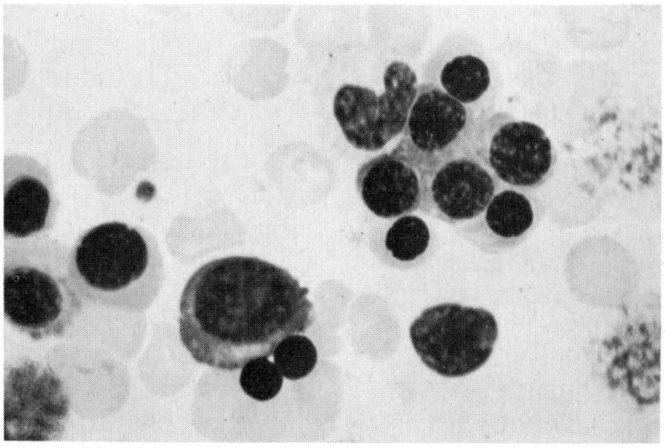

Figure 4–32. Normoblasts in the marrow from a patient with hemolytic anemia. Largest cell is a basophilic normoblast. (× 875.)

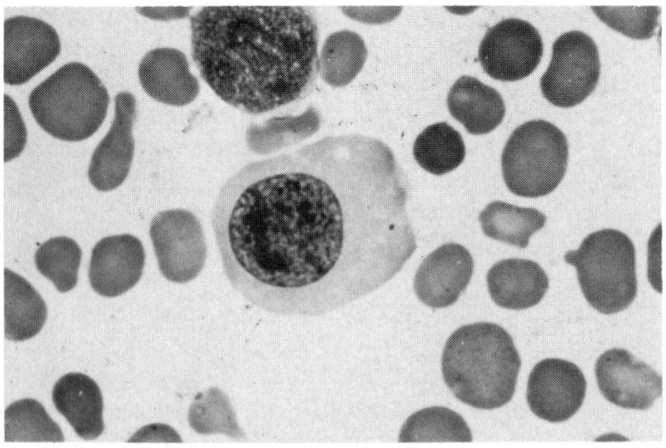

Figure 4–33. Polychromatic megaloblast. Above: "smudge cell" (damaged nucleus; no cytoplasm). (× 875.)

tion; cytoplasmic development continues as cell division is delayed. Hemoglobin synthesis is, as a rule, essentially normal. The result of the discrepancy in the growth of the nucleus and cytoplasm is the formation of abnormally large cells with an increased amount of hemoglobin in the cytoplasm and an immature nuclear chromatin pattern.

The megaloblastic series is illustrated in Figures 4–64, 4–65 and 4–71. In the typical megaloblast the nucleus is characteristic. The youngest cell of the series usually has nucleoli. It is large, round, or oval. The cytoplasm stains deeply blue with a light juxtanuclear zone. It has a more delicate chromatin network with larger and more numerous openings than has the nucleus of the normoblast at the corresponding stage of development (Figs. 4–32 and 4–33). Sometimes it appears as if it were composed of coarse granules.

As the megaloblast grows older and goes through the stages from promegaloblast (the mother cell of this series) through basophilic megaloblast and polychromatophilic megaloblast to orthochromatic megaloblast, the nucleus becomes smaller and the chromatin denser, coarser, and more solidly stained. Nuclei of megaloblasts at the end stages of development may show degenerative changes (pyknosis, karyorrhexis, and multiple Howell-Jolly bodies). The end stage is a megalocyte, a larger anuclear cell without the central pale zone of the normocyte and, as a rule, with abundant hemoglobin. At the same time the cytoplasm shows less tendency to polychromatophilia. The recognition of megaloblasts is important, but is not always easy unless the nucleus is typical.

In general, young nucleated erythrocytes are prone to exhibit polychromatophilia. In some nucleated erythrocytes, the cytoplasm is so blue and shows so little of its characteristic smooth texture that it is difficult to recognize the cell as an erythrocyte except by the character of the nucleus. Such erythroid cells are often mistaken for lymphocytes or for Türk's irritation leukocytes, an error that careful observation of the nucleus will usually prevent.

Significance of Nucleated Erythrocytes. Normoblasts are present normally only in the blood of the fetus and of very young infants. In the healthy adult they are confined to the bone marrow and appear in the circulating blood only in disease, in which their presence usually denotes an excessive demand made on the blood-forming organs to regenerate erythrocytes. In response to this demand, immature and imperfectly formed cells are thrown into the circulation. Their number, therefore, is usually regarded as an indication of the extent to which the bone marrow reacts rather than of the severity of the disease. A contributing factor may be a "lowered bone marrow threshold," which allows immature cells to pass into the circulation more readily at some times than at others.

In general, normoblasts appear when regeneration of blood takes place in a normal manner, although with excessive activity as in severe hemolytic anemia. In erythroblastosis fetalis, there are abnormally large numbers of normoblasts. This disease of the newborn is characterized by splenomegaly, an enlarged liver, jaundice, and a macrocytic anemia if the disease is caused by Rh blood factor incompatibility. If the disease is caused by AB blood factor incompatibility, varying numbers of spherocytes are present, but macrocytes are less common. In thalassemia major, circulating normoblasts may be extremely numerous, an observation which led to an older name for this condition, "erythroblastic anemia."

The presence of normoblasts and immature cells of the neutrophilic series in the blood is known as a *"leukoerythroblastotic reaction."* This may be found in any of the conditions already mentioned, but in addition is often indicative of space-occupying disturbances of the marrow, such as myelofibrosis with myeloid metaplasia, metastatic carcinoma, leukemias, multiple myeloma, Gaucher's disease, and others. When leukoerythroblastotic reactions occur in these conditions, the number of normoblasts is usually out of proportion to both the degree of the anemia and the amount of polychromasia (the amount of effective production of red cells) present.

The presence of megaloblasts indicates a change in the type of blood formation. This is seen most characteristically in pernicious anemia and other megaloblastic anemias. It indicates the presence of megaloblasts in the marrow and is therefore important in the diagnosis of this disease.

Leukocytes. The total white blood cell count is determined as previously described (p. 124). The percentage distribution of the different types of leukocytes and the qualitative study are done on a stained smear. Such studies are called differential counts and often yield more helpful information than any other single procedure used in examination of the blood.

Wright's stain is widely used. A thin blood film is best for the study of details and identification of the cells. One should first glance over the preparation to note the general staining of leukocytes. Two films stained side by side will sometimes show differences in the color reactions of the leukocytes due to variations in staining technique.

To make the differential count, the film is examined carefully with an oil-immersion objective and a mechanical stage. Each leukocyte seen is classified and the percentage of each cell type is calculated. For accuracy, 500 to 1000 leukocytes should be counted, but for practical reasons, a smaller number is classified. It is imperative to count leukocytes in all parts of the film, since the different varieties may be unevenly distributed. A record of the count may be kept by placing a mark for each leukocyte in its appropriate column, ruled on paper. It is more convenient to use one of several commercially available recording tabulators. They have a separate key for each type of blood corpuscle, and the percentages can be read directly as the instrument automatically indicates when 100 corpuscles have been counted. Leukocytes that cannot be classified should be placed together in an unidentified group. In some conditions, notably leukemia, there may be many of these unidentified leukocytes.

The actual number of each variety of leukocyte in a microliter (or $mm.^3$) is easily calculated from these percentages and the total leukocyte count. It should form part of the record if this is to be complete. An increase in actual number is an *absolute increase;* an increase in percentage only is a *relative increase.* It is evident that an absolute increase of any variety may be accompanied by a relative decrease if the total white cell count is high.

One should always make it a rule, before making a differential count, to attempt to estimate the total leukocyte count from the number of leukocytes seen in a field with the low-power objective. After some practice this can be done with a considerable degree of accuracy. Similarly, the platelets should be examined and a note made of whether they are normal, increased, or decreased in number; morphologic abnormalities should also be recorded.

plt

One should remember, in addition, that the examination of the blood smear provides an excellent opportunity to study and to note the morphology of the red cells. The number of nucleated erythrocytes seen while making the count should also be noted in the record as the number per 100 leukocytes.

If blood films are poorly made, the white cells will be irregularly distributed. If the spreader has a rough edge, or if the film is too thin, a disproportionately large number of the white cells end up at the feather (thin) end of the film. Even in well-made films, there is a tendency for lymphocytes to stay in the middle of the film and larger cells (neutrophils, monocytes) to be at the sides and the feather end. On well-made films this tendency is slight enough to allow worthwhile differential counts to be made. In the crenellation technique of counting, the field of view is moved from side to side across the whole width of the slide in the "counting area," just behind the feather edge, where the red cells are separated from one another and free of artefacts. Another technique is to count all the cells as the field of view is moved from the thick end to the feather end, which encompasses all the cells in one part of the original drop of blood. The disadvantage of this latter method is the difficulty in identifying contracted, heavily stained cells in the thicker part of the film.

In a poorly made film there is no use performing a differential count, as the number will be misleading.

Sources of Error in the Differential Leukocyte Count. Even in the most perfectly made blood films, the differential count is subject to the same errors of random distribution as are other cell counts. For interpretation of day-to-day or slide-to-slide differences in the same patient, it is helpful to see how much of the variation is ascribable to chance alone. Table 4–1 gives 95 per cent confidence limits for different percentages of cells in differential counts performed, classifying a total of 100 to 1000 leukocytes. In comparing the percentages from two separate counts, if one number lies outside the confidence limits of the other, one can be 95 per cent certain that the difference is significant (i.e., not due to chance). Thus, on the basis of a 100-cell differential count, if the monocytes were 5 per cent one day and 10 per cent the next, it is quite probable that the difference is due solely to sampling error. Although the difference *could be* real, one cannot be confident that it *is* real, because of the small number of cells counted. If, on the other hand, the differential count totaled 500 cells, the difference between 5 per cent and 10 per cent is significant; one can be reasonably certain (with a 5 per cent chance of being wrong) that the difference is a real one and not due to chance alone. Of course, this is a minimal

Table 4–1. NINETY-FIVE PER CENT CONFIDENCE LIMITS FOR THE PERCENTAGE OF CELLS WITH A PARTICULAR CHARACTERISTIC, GIVEN THAT *a* PER CENT OF CELLS WITH THIS CHARACTERISTIC ARE FOUND IN A STUDY OF *n* CELLS*

	n							
a	100		200		500		1000	
0	0	4	0	2	0	1	0	1
1	0	6	0	4	0	3	0	2
2	0	8	0	6	0	4	1	4
3	0	9	1	7	1	5	2	5
4	1	10	1	8	2	7	2	6
5	1	12	2	10	3	8	3	7
6	2	13	3	11	4	9	4	8
7	2	14	3	12	4	10	5	9
8	3	16	4	13	5	11	6	10
9	4	17	5	14	6	12	7	11
10	4	18	6	16	7	13	8	13
15	8	24	10	21	12	19	12	18
20	12	30	14	27	16	24	17	23
25	16	35	19	32	21	30	22	28
30	21	40	23	37	26	35	27	33
35	25	46	28	43	30	40	32	39
40	30	51	33	48	35	45	36	44
45	35	56	38	53	40	50	41	49
50	39	61	42	58	45	55	46	54

*For $n = 100$, the confidence limits were calculated exactly; for n over 100, with $a \times n$ over 2000, the normal approximation was applied; and for n over 100 with $a \times n$ under 2000, Poisson's approximation was used.

For x over 50, obtain confidence limits by reading limits for $100 - x$ in the table and subtracting them from 100. For example, the confidence limits for 75 per cent in a sample of $n = 100$ are 65 and 84.

From C. L. Rümke: Variability of results in differential counts on blood smears. Triangle, the Sandoz Journal of Medical Science, *4*:156, 1960.

estimate of the error involved in differential counts, since it does not include mechanical errors (due to variations in collecting the blood samples, inadequate mixing, irregularities in distribution depending on the type and quality of the blood films, and poor staining) or errors in cell identification, which depend upon the judgment and experience of the observer. Meticulous technique and accurate and consistent cell classification are therefore demanded of the technician. The physician who interprets the results must be aware of the possible sources of error, especially the minimal error due to chance in the distribution of cells.

Table 4–2 shows the distribution of the various types of leukocytes in the blood of normal persons. Absolute concentrations are given, as these have considerably greater significance than percentages alone. It has been shown in several studies that there is a lower normal limit for neutrophils in the black population than in the white; other cell types have the same normal ranges. In the adult, age and sex differences are insignificant.

The student should thoroughly familiarize himself with the five types of leukocytes found in normal blood and with the cells that most commonly enter the blood in disease: neutrophil precursors, myeloblasts, atypical lymphocytes, and lymphoblasts.

Leukocytes Normally Present in Peripheral Blood

LYMPHOCYTE

Description. Lymphocytes are mononuclear cells without specific cytoplasmic granules. Small lymphocytes are about the size of an erythrocyte or slightly larger (6 to 10 μm.), although their diameter is influenced by the thickness of the film, being greatest in very thin films in which the leukocytes are much flattened (Fig. 4–34 *A*). The typical lymphocyte has a single, sharply defined nucleus containing heavy blocks of chromatin. The chromatin stains dark blue with Wright's stain, while the parachromatin stands out as lighter stained streaks; at the periphery of the nucleus, the chromatin is condensed. The characteristic feature of the nucleus is that there is a gradual transition between the chromatin and the parachromatin so that it is practically impossible to tell where chromatin ends and parachromatin begins. The nucleus is generally round but is sometimes indented at one side. The cytoplasm stains pale blue except for a clear perinuclear zone.

Larger lymphocytes, 12 to 15 μm. in diameter, with less densely staining nuclei and more abundant cytoplasm, are frequently found, especially in the blood of children, and may be difficult to distinguish from monocytes. The misshapen, indented cytoplasmic margins of lymphocytes are due to pressure of neighboring cells. In the cytoplasm of about one-third of the large lymphocytes a few round, red-purple granules are present. They are larger than the granules of neutrophilic leukocytes (Fig. 4–34 *B*). It appears that there is a continuous spectrum of sizes between small and large lymphocytes and, indeed, there can be a transition from small to large to blast forms as well as the reverse. It does not appear to be meaningful to classify small lymphocytes and large lymphocytes separately in differential counting. The presence of blast forms (nonleukemic lymphoblasts; reticular lymphocytes) must be noted, however, as this indicates transformation of lymphoid cells as a response to antigenic stimulation.

Production and Function. According to current concepts (Craddock *et al.*, 1971), during fetal life lymphocyte precursors originate in the bone marrow and are influenced or pro-

Table 4-2. ABSOLUTE LEUKOCYTE CONCENTRATION IN NORMAL ADULTS*

		95% RANGE	MEDIAN
Total leukocytes	White subjects	4500–10,100	7100
	Black subjects	3600–10,200	6300
Band neutrophils	White subjects	200–2100	600
	Black subjects	60–1600	300
Segmented neutrophils	White subjects	1500–6000	3000
	Black subjects	1100–6700	2700
Total neutrophils	White subjects	2000–6800	3700
	Black subjects	1300–7400	3400
Eosinophils		30–800	150
Basophils		0–160	30
Lymphocytes		1500–4000	2400
Monocytes		200–1000	460

*Data from Orfanakis, *et al.*: 1971 (Salt Lake City, Utah). Absolute concentrations derived from electronic leukocyte count and 200 cell differential counts (total leukocyte count × percentage of each cell type).

grammed to perform a certain function by one of the primary lymphoid organs, either the thymus gland or the "bursal equivalent" (a distinct organ, the bursa of Fabricius, is found in birds; the bursal equivalent is postulated to exist in man and other mammals, but the anatomic site is unknown). Those lymphocytes influenced by the thymus (thymus-dependent lymphocytes or T-cells) and their progeny function in cell-mediated immunity, which includes delayed hypersensitivity, graft rejection, graft-versus-host reactions, defense against intracellular organisms (such as tubercle bacillus and brucella), and probably defense against neoplasms. The lymphocytes influenced by the bursal equivalent (bursa-dependent lymphocytes or B-cells) and their progeny perform in humoral immunity, or the production of antibodies, either as a lymphocyte or after transformation into a plasma cell.

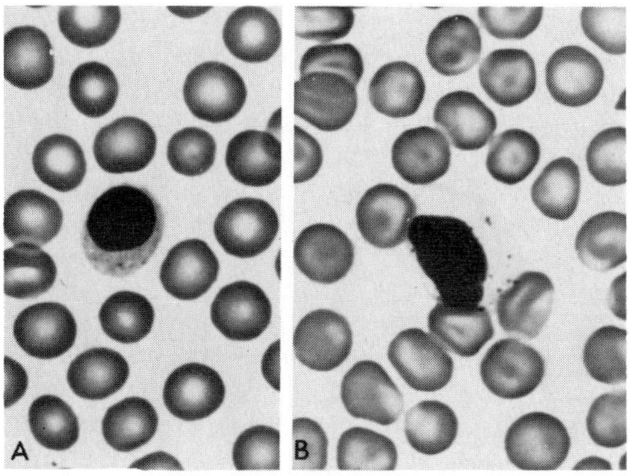

Figure 4-34. *A*, Small lymphocyte. *B*, Larger lymphocyte with granules; note that many of the red cells are target cells. (× 875.)

In late fetal and postnatal life, lymphocytes are produced in the lymphoid tissue: spleen, lymph nodes, and intestine-associated-lymphoid tissue. B-cells and T-cells tend to localize in anatomically distinct parts of the lymphoid tissue where proliferation can take place. In the blood, B-cells and T-cells comprise most of the circulating lymphocytes (other types are probably also present) but cannot be distinguished by size or by Wright's stain; special techniques are required. The majority of the circulating lymphocytes are T-cells, which have a life span of months to years. The B-cells are a minor population (10 to 30 per cent of the lymphocytes), probably have a short life span measured in days, and are distinguished by the presence of considerable immunoglobulin on their surface membrane.

Lymphocytes, especially T-cells, recirculate from blood to lymph; in the postcapillary venule in lymphoid tissue the lymphocyte travels from the blood through the endothelium and into the lymphoid tissue where it may stay or percolate through and return to the blood via the thoracic duct lymph. After antigenic stimulation, small lymphocytes (B-cells or T-cells, depending on the nature of the antigen) become activated and undergo blast transformation. On Wright's stained films, these blasts are large cells (15 to 25 μm.) with abundant rather deep blue cytoplasm, a large reticular nucleus with uniform chromatin, and prominent nucleoli. This is the cell which is called the reticular lymphocyte (nonleukemic lymphoblast; "immunoblast"). If the blasts are derived from B-cells, the new lymphocytes function in the production of antibodies (B-cells, plasma cells); or, if the blasts are derived from T-cells, the progeny act in the cellular immune response. The latter is mediated by several soluble factors produced by the activated T-cell, including: transfer factor, which can transfer the capacity for delayed hypersensitivity to another cell; lymphotoxin, which is directly toxic to cells; and migratory inhibition factor, which promotes adherence of macrophages and keeps them at the site.

Plasma cells have abundant blue cytoplasm, often with light streaks or vacuoles, an eccentric round nucleus, and a well-defined clear (Golgi) zone adjacent to the nucleus. The nucleus of the plasma cell has heavily clumped chromatin, which is sharply defined from the parachromatin, and often arranged in a radial or "wheel-like" pattern.

Lymphocytes constitute about 20 to 40 per cent of all leukocytes; 1500 to 4000 are present in each microliter of blood. They are more abundant in the blood of children, averaging about 60 per cent of all leukocytes in the first year of life and decreasing to about 36 per cent in the tenth, with immature cells being more numerous than in adults. Lymphocytes constitute about 5 to 15 per cent of the nucleated cells in the marrow.

The lymphocytes and their derivatives, the plasma cells, operate in the immune defenses of the body. Lymphocytosis is discussed beginning on page 256, plasmacytosis on p. 267.

MONOCYTE

Description. The monocyte is the largest cell of normal blood (Fig. 4–35). It generally is about two to three times the diameter of an erythrocyte (14 to 20 μm.), although smaller monocytes sometimes are encountered. It contains a single nucleus, which is lobulated, deeply indented, or horseshoe-shaped. Occasionally the nucleus of a monocyte may appear round or oval. Careful inspection and adjustment of the oil-immersion lens to observe the nucleus at several levels often reveals that even in those cases there is an indentation of the nucleus, which is obscured by the position of the cell.

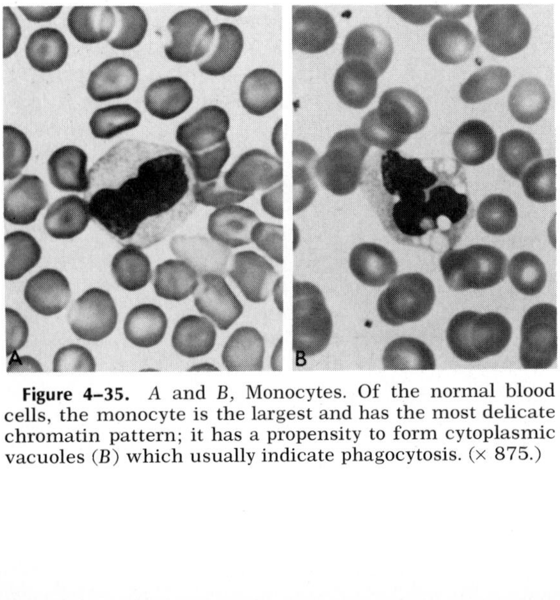

Figure 4–35. *A* and *B*, Monocytes. Of the normal blood cells, the monocyte is the largest and has the most delicate chromatin pattern; it has a propensity to form cytoplasmic vacuoles (*B*) which usually indicate phagocytosis. (× 875.)

The cytoplasm is abundant. With Wright's stain the characteristic feature of the nucleus is for the chromatin to be in strands. There is also a relatively sharp distinction between the chromatin and the parachromatin, which reresults in a less densely stained nucleus than that seen in the lymphocyte. The cytoplasm is slate colored, ground glass, or "muddy" in appearance and sometimes appears dusted, uniformly or in patches, with fine reddish granules which are less distinct than the granules of neutrophilic leukocytes. Occasionally bluish granules may be seen.

When the monocyte transforms into a macrophage it becomes larger (20 to 40 μm.); the nucleus may become oval and the chromatin more reticular or dispersed so that nucleoli may be visible. A perinuclear clear zone (Golgi) may be evident. The fine red or azurophil granules are variable in number or may have disappeared. The more abundant cytoplasm tends to be irregular at the cell margins and to contain vacuoles. These are phagocytic vacuoles which may contain ingested red cells, debris, pigment, or bacteria. Evidence of phagocytosis in monocytes or the presence of macrophages in directly made films of capillary blood is pathologic and often indicates the presence of active infection.

The size of the cell, the width of the zone of cytoplasm, its bluish gray color, evidences of phagocytosis, and the depth of color and the folds and indentations of the nucleus, usually with the absence of peripheral condensation of nuclear chromatin and of a clear perinuclear zone, are the points to be considered in distinguishing monocytes that have a round nucleus from lymphocytes. For comparison, condensation of nuclear chromatin in clumps and at the nuclear margin, a perinuclear clear zone in the cytoplasm, and a homogeneous agranular cytoplasm are characteristic for lymphocytes. It must be borne in mind that the thickness of the film has a great influence on the apparent size of all leukocytes. They are larger and paler when flattened out in the thin part of the film.

Production and Function. The monocyte is produced largely if not entirely in the marrow from monoblasts (which may be identical with myeloblasts) and promonocytes. The promonocyte is a somewhat larger cell; an oval or indented large nucleus has fine uniform chromatin and two to five nucleoli. The cytoplasm is more basophilic than the monocyte, the Golgi zone may be conspicuous, and there are variable numbers of dust-like red or azurophilic granules which are smaller than the azurophilic granules of neutrophil precursors.

These cells in the marrow form a rapidly dividing precursor pool for the blood monocytes (van Furth, 1970). The process of maturation continues in the blood, where it is common (especially in infection) to find immature stages, including the presence of nucleoli. After spending one to three days in the blood, the monocyte moves into the tissues where it transforms into a macrophage and may live for weeks to months unless it is called to duty in an inflammatory reaction.

The azurophil granules of monocytes are lysosomes containing acid hydrolases and peroxidase, similar to the azurophil granules of neutrophils and the specific granules of eosinophils. However, as the monocyte transforms into a macrophage, its azurophil granules disappear (as they are utilized in the digestive process) and new lysosomal enzymes are formed in large quantities and packaged in a second form of granule which is not visible by light microscopy (Nichols *et al.*, 1971). It has been shown that lysosomal granules fuse with the phagocytic vacuole in the process of digestion of phagocytized material.

The monocyte, then, is formed in the marrow, is transported by the blood, and migrates into the tissues where it functions as a macrophage. This appears to be the origin of tissue macrophages, including at least some of the fixed reticuloendothelial cells (e.g., Kupffer cells of the liver, pulmonary alveolar macrophages). Macrophages ingest and destroy particles or cells (including bacteria) coated with IgG immunoglobulin or complement and, hence, participate as effector cells in humoral immunity. They act also as phagocytes in cell-mediated immunity, being stimulated by soluble factors from activated T-lymphocytes. There is evidence also that macrophages are important in initiating immune responses by processing antigens.

Recently it has been shown that monocytes are the source of a soluble factor that stimulates growth and differentiation of granulocytes and monocytes *in vitro*, implying that this cell type may be involved in regulation of granulocytopoiesis (Chervenick and LoBuglio, 1972). Monocytes constitute about 2 to 10 per cent of the total number of leukocytes in the peripheral blood – 200 to 1000 per microliter of blood. Monocytosis will be discussed on page 266.

SEGMENTED NEUTROPHILIC GRANULOCYTE (POLYMORPHONUCLEAR NEUTROPHILIC LEUKOCYTE; NEUTROPHIL)

Description. Neutrophils average 12 μm. in diameter; they are smaller than monocytes and eosinophils and slightly larger than

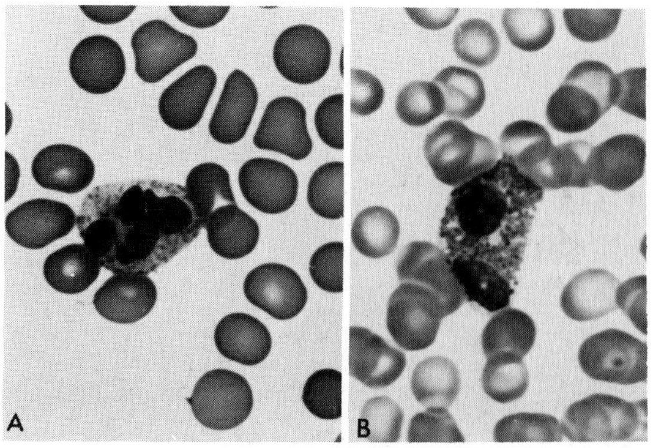

Figure 4–36. *A*, Neutrophil. The cytoplasm is filled with tiny granules, some of which stain more deeply than others (toxic granulation). Note that most of the red cells lack central pallor, an artefact seen near the feather edge of the film. *B*, Eosinophil. Typically this cell has fewer nuclear lobes and larger cytoplasmic granules than the neutrophil. (× 875.)

basophils. The nucleus stains deeply; it is irregular and often assumes shapes comparable to such letters as E, Z, and S. Frequently there appear to be several separate nuclei, hence, the widely used name "polynuclear leukocyte." On careful inspection, however, delicate filaments connecting the segments can usually be seen.

A filament has length but no breadth as one focuses up and down. A segmented or mature neutrophil has at least two of its lobes separated by such a filament. The number of lobes in normal neutrophils ranges from two to five, with a median of three. The nuclear lobes have coarse blocks of chromatin with rather sharply defined parachromatin spaces. The cytoplasm, itself colorless, is packed full of tiny granules (0.2 to 0.3 μm.) which stain tan to pink with Wright's stain (Fig. 4–36). About two-thirds of these are specific granules and one-third azurophil granules; the latter's intensity of staining has diminished from that in the immature cell.

Production and Function. Neutrophils are produced in the marrow (Figs. 4–38 and 4–61). The stem cell (common to erythroid, megakaryocytic, and granulocytic cells) gives rise to the *myeloblast,* a cell 15 μm. in diameter with a large oval nucleus, very fine, uniform chromatin pattern, delicate nuclear membrane, and two to five nucleoli. The cytoplasm is pale, clear blue. The appearance of azurophil granules (~0.5 μm. diameter) heralds the earliest promyelocyte and indicates that the cell is to be a granulocyte. The *promyelocyte* stage encompasses the entire period of production of azurophil granules. The promyelocyte is slightly larger than the myeloblast. The nuclear chromatin begins to condense a bit and the

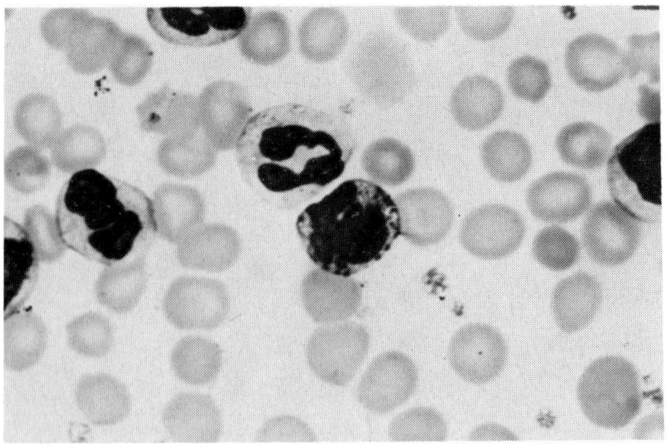

Figure 4-37. Neutrophil (above) and basophil (below). The basophil is smaller, has large deeply basophilic granules which often can be partially washed out, leaving vacuoles. (× 875.)

nucleoli are less obvious. The cytoplasm is basophilic and is filled by more and more azurophil granules. The *neutrophil myelocyte* stage begins with the appearance of specific neutrophil granules, at first only in the Golgi region; as more specific granules develop they spread throughout the cytoplasm. With successive mitoses the number of azurophil granules (which have ceased production at the end of the promyelocyte stage) are diminished. The early neutrophil myelocyte, therefore, has a rather fine, dispersed nuclear chromatin pattern, many azurophil granules, and few specific granules. The late neutrophil myelocyte has a somewhat more condensed chromatin pattern, a cytoplasm well filled with specific granules, and rather few azurophil granules. The myelocyte is the latest stage capable of cell division. No cytoplasmic granules are formed and no cell division occurs in later stages. Next is the *neutrophil metamyelocyte,* distinguished by an indented, kidney-shaped nucleus with more condensed chromatin. From this stage on, changes in the cytoplasm are insignificant. In the *band neutrophil* (stab form) the nucleus has more condensed chromatin and a rather uniform elongated shape. Partial constriction of the nucleus is included in the band stage, until a fine filament (length but no breadth) is formed between two of the lobes, at which point the cell is classified as a *segmented neutrophil.*

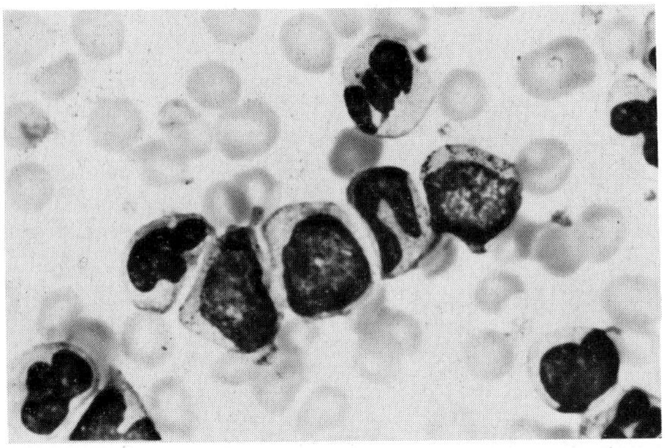

Figure 4-38. Neutrophil precursors. The five touching each other are, left to right, a band, metamyelocyte, myelocyte, band, and myelocyte. (× 875.)

Two well-defined granule types are present in the human neutrophil (Bainton *et al.*, 1971). The *azurophil granules*, formed in the promyelocyte stage, contain lysosomal enzymes (acid hydrolases: acid phosphatase, β-glucuronidase, and so forth), peroxidase, one-third of the muramidase, and cationic antibacterial proteins. The *specific neutrophil granules,* formed in the myelocyte stage, contain alkaline phosphatase, two-thirds of the muramidase, lactoferrin, and collagenase. The mature human neutrophil has twice as many specific as nonspecific (azurophil) granules. It has the capacity for both glycolytic and respiratory energy production.

The distribution of this cell series in the body is summarized in Table 4-3. For each neutrophil in the blood vessels, about 20 precursors are present in the marrow. From the time of differentiation into a promyelocyte until the time the progeny of that cell reach the blood is nine days, the last five of which have been in the maturation and storage pool. When a neutrophil enters the blood, it moves readily between a circulating granulocyte pool (CGP), which is sampled in the leukocyte count, and a marginal granulocyte pool (MGP), which is not, but is either marginated along vessel walls or sequestered in capillary beds. In less than a day after it arrives, the neutrophil emigrates from the circulation in a random manner and enters the tissues. From there, if not utilized in an inflammatory exudate, neutrophils leave the body via secretions in bronchi, saliva, gastrointestinal tract, urine, or they are destroyed by the R.E. system.

Neutrophils are able to move in a zigzag manner, but their motion changes to a straight line path if a chemotactic attractant (e.g., a bacterium coated with certain components of complement) is within a certain distance. Neutrophils have receptors for complement and bind and phagocytize the coated particle. Phagocytosis occurs, with the formation of a phagocytic vacuole that contains the ingested particle; accompanying this process is an increase in metabolic activity and energy production. Specific granules, followed shortly by azurophil granules, empty their contents into the phagocytic vacuoles, a process known as degranulation. Bactericidal activity occurs within the vacuole, mediated by H_2O_2, peroxi-

Table 4–3. DISTRIBUTION OF NEUTROPHILS*

	COMPARTMENT OR POOL	CELL TYPES	TIME IN COMPARTMENT (days)	SIZE OF COMPARTMENT (Cells × 10^9/kg.)
Marrow	Mitotic pool	Myeloblast Promyelocyte N. myelocytes ↓	4	3.8
	Maturation and storage pool	N. metamyelocyte N. band Neutrophil ↓	5	7.6
Blood	Circulating pool	Neutrophil ⇅	< 1	0.39
	Marginal pool	Neutrophil ↓		0.31
Tissues		Neutrophil	up to 5 days	

*Data from Craddock, C. G.: *In* Williams, W. J., Beutler, E., Erslev, A. J., and Rundles, R. W. (eds.): Hematology. New York, McGraw-Hill Book Co., Inc., 1972, Chapter 71.

dase, and a halide ion generating the free halogen, or by other enzymatic activity.

Neutrophils thus are important in defense against infectious disease. If their enzymes are activated and released outside the cell, neutrophils can cause tissue necrosis, as occurs in the Arthus or Shwartzman reaction. Neutrophils, which are active in inflammation, release an endogenous pyrogen that produces fever by acting on the hypothalamus to set the body's thermostat at a higher level.

Segmented neutrophils constitute 50 to 70 per cent of the circulating leukocytes; 1500–6000/μl. are present in white subjects, and 1100–6700/μl. in blacks. Band neutrophils, defined as lack of a nuclear filament, are normally present, up to 2000/μl. Neutrophils are the only leukocytes that have a significantly different range between races. Children generally have a lower number of neutrophils than adults.

Normally about 35 per cent of the segmented neutrophils have two lobes, 41 per cent have three lobes, 17 per cent four, and no more than 3 per cent have five lobes. A "shift to the left" occurs when there are increased bands and less mature neutrophils in the blood, as well as a lower average number of lobes in segmented cells.

Neutrophilic leukocytosis (neutrophilia) is discussed on page 246.

The segmented granulocytes of pernicious anemia and other megaloblastic anemias are called "macropolycytes" (Fig. 4–39). They are about 50 per cent larger by measurement of their diameters than are normal segmented granulocytes. They have more nuclear segments than do normal granulocytes. They may be present before the other signs of megaloblastic anemia are present.

Eosinophilic Granulocyte (Eosinophil)

Description. The structure of these cells is similar to that of the polymorphonuclear neutrophils, with the striking difference that, instead of the neutrophilic granules, their cytoplasm contains larger round or oval granules having a strong affinity for acid stains (Fig. 4–36 *B*). They are easily recognized by the size and color of the granules, which stain bright red with stains containing eosin. In well-stained preparations a distinct highlight can be seen on each granule. Their cytoplasm is colorless or has a faint sky-blue tinge. The nucleus stains somewhat less deeply than that

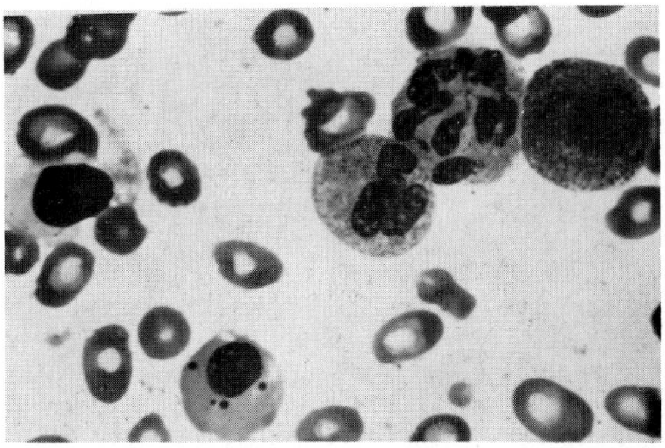

Figure 4–39. Megaloblastic anemia. Below, orthochromatic megaloblast with four Howell-Jolly bodies. Above, right, two giant neutrophils (one of which has nine nuclear lobes and could be called a macropolycyte) and an eosinophil with poor nuclear maturation (× 875.)

of the polymorphonuclear neutrophils and usually has two connected segments, rarely more than three. Eosinophils average 13 μm in diameter.

Production and Function. Eosinophils are formed in the bone marrow (Fig. 4–61). In contrast to neutrophils, only one type of granule appears in eosinophils. In the early myelocyte stage the eosinophilic granules are dark staining, but as the cell matures (in a similar fashion to the neutrophil in other respects) the granules assume the bright staining reaction. The eosinophil granules are lysosomes and contain acid hydrolases and, in addition, peroxidase and histamine. Less is known of the kinetics of this system than of the neutrophils, but they are probably similar. The ratio of blood to tissue eosinophils in man is about 1/100; tissue eosinophils are located primarily in skin, lung, and gastrointestinal tract, i.e., the epithelial barriers to the outside world.

Less is known also about the function of the eosinophils than of the neutrophils. Eosinophils carry about one-third of the blood histamine. The eosinophil is capable of locomotion and phagocytosis, though less actively than the neutrophil. Its granules release their contents into phagocytic vacuoles. Eosinophils respond, usually together with plasma cells, late in inflammation. They are attracted to and ingest antigen-antibody complexes.

The normal number of eosinophils varies from 50 to 250 for each microliter of blood and they comprise 1 to 4 per cent of the leukocytes. However, recent series indicate that in apparently normal people the eosinophil count may be as high as 800/μl. An increase is called eosinophilia, which is discussed on page 255.

BASOPHILIC GRANULOCYTE (BASOPHIL)

Description. In general, basophilic granulocytes resemble polymorphonuclear neutrophils, except that the nucleus is less irregular (usually merely indented or slightly lobulated) and granules are larger and have a strong affinity for basic stains (Fig. 4–37). They are easily recognized. In some basophils, most of the granules may be missing because they are readily soluble in water, leaving clean-cut openings in the cytoplasm. The granules then are a mauve color. In a well-prepared smear stained with Wright's stain, the granules are deep purple, while the nucleus is somewhat paler and is often nearly or completely hidden by the granules so that its form is difficult to distinguish.

Unevenly stained granules of basophils may be ring shaped and resemble *Histoplasma capsulatum* or protozoa.

Production and Function. Basophils originate in the bone marrow from basophilic myelocytes in a manner similar to that of eosinophils (Fig. 4–61). No nonspecific granules appear to be present in the developing basophil. Basophil granules contain heparin or heparin-like substance and histamine, as well as 5-hydroxytryptamine. Acid mucopolysaccharide is responsible for the metachromatic staining property of basophil granules. In contrast to those of other granulocytes, basophil granules are not lysosomes.

Despite their small number, basophils carry about one-half of the blood histamine. Basophils appear to react in allergic states, especially atopy. They have been shown to take up IgE (reaginic) antibodies from sera of atopic individuals (Wilson *et al.*, 1971). Basophils from atopic individuals degranulate when treated with specific allergens.

Basophils are the least numerous of the leukocytes in normal blood and rarely comprise more than 0.5 per cent of the total leukocytes. The normal range is 0 to 160 per microliter.

Basophilic leukocytosis is discussed on page 256.

DEGENERATED FORMS. Degenerated forms of leukocytes are frequently encountered but have no significance unless they are present in large numbers. They include vacuolated leukocytes and bare nuclei from ruptured cells. The latter vary from fairly well-preserved nuclei without cytoplasm to mere strands of palely stained nuclear substance arranged in a coarse network—the so-called basket cells (Fig. 4–40).

Occasionally, in acute leukemia or in chronic lymphocytic leukemia, frayed-out nuclei without cytoplasm exceed the usual lymphocytes in number. Such nuclei may represent fragile lymphocytes that have been broken in making the film.

Automated Methods for the Differential Leukocyte Count.

COMPUTER IMAGE PROCESSING. A uniformly made and stained blood film is scanned automatically with a microscope, and the optical

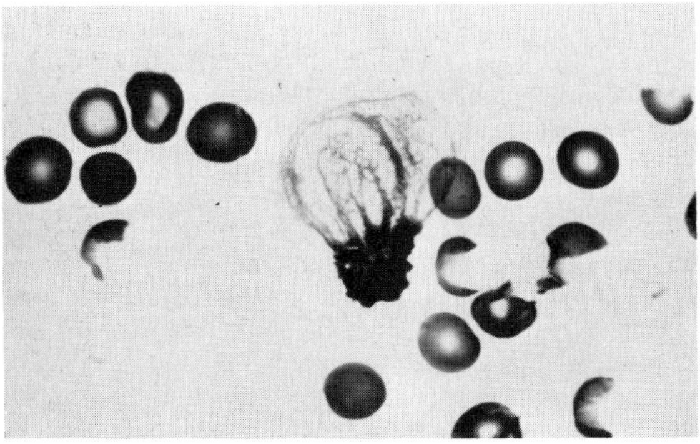

Figure 4–40. Basket cell. This is a nuclear remnant from a damaged or broken cell. (× 875.)

images are converted to digital form by a computer. Up to eight blood cell types can be recognized and classified in this manner (Bacus and Gose, 1972). This system has recently been introduced (LARC: Leukocyte Automatic Recognition Computer*), but evaluations have not yet been published. Unclassified cells can be automatically relocated and identified by a technologist. At present, one to two minutes are required for a 100-cell differential count.

CYTOCHEMICAL DIFFERENTIAL COUNTING. The Hemalog-D† is a continuous flow instrument which samples 1.5 ml. of whole blood, lyses the red cells, separates the sample containing leukocytes into different channels, fixes them in formalin, and introduces reagents for cytochemical reactions (Ansley and Ornstein, 1970). In the current phase of development (Saunders *et al.*, 1972) the *peroxidase* channel counts band neutrophils, neutrophils, and eosinophils, all of which contain peroxidase. A pH of 3.8 is used; eosinophils stain more deeply than neutrophils and are discriminated from them by degree of absorption. Juvenile neutrophils have a somewhat greater peroxidase activity than mature neutrophils. Light scattering measurements are also made in this channel. Large unstained cells give a large signal; the densely stained eosinophil gives a smaller scatter signal than a neutrophil despite its slightly larger size. When light scattering and absorption measurements are combined, the "juvenile" neutrophils (including band neutrophils, metamyelocytes, myelocytes, and promyelocytes) stain intensely and give a large scatter signal; neutrophils stain less intensely and give a smaller scatter signal; eosinophils stain intensely and give a small scatter signal; lymphocytes do not stain and give a small scatter signal. In addition, this channel has a cell counter that provides a total white cell count. In the *lipase* channel, monocytes are stained for lipase activity; the substrate α-naphthyl butyrate is used. In a third channel, basophils are measured by the reaction of their granules with *toluidine blue*. Large unstained cells are also counted. Ten thousand cells are counted for each channel, and the results are expressed in both percentage and absolute numbers.

The Hemalog-D has had encouraging trials. Its advantages are the enhanced precision from the large number of cells counted; cytochemical staining should give improved cell recognition and offer information not currently available by the visual pattern and color recognition techniques which have dominated hematology.

---

*Corning Scientific Instruments, Medfield, Mass.
†Technicon Corp., Tarrytown, N.Y.

Platelets

Description. Platelets are round or oval, 2 to 4 μm. in diameter and separated from one another in films made from blood anticoagulated with EDTA. In blood films taken from skin puncture wounds, they may have sharp projections or be elongated and tend to clump together in proportion to the time after the wound is made. Considerably larger platelets can be seen when platelet production is increased or after splenectomy. In Wright stained smears, the center (the granulomere), about one-third to one-half of the platelet, is filled with fine purplish red granules. It is surrounded by homogeneous pale blue cytoplasm (the hyalomere). The separation into a "granulomere" and "hyalomere" is probably due to the circumferential band of microtubules discernible with the electron microscope. (See p. 347.)

Physiologic variations in number of platelets are considerable. The newborn, especially during the first two days of life, have fewer platelets (150,000 to 250,000) than older infants. The number of platelets decreases progressively before menstruation, even more precipitously during the first day of menstruation. They begin to rise on the third day. Violent exercise is followed by a rise, possibly caused by a change in distribution. The number increases as one ascends to a higher altitude, and is higher in winter than in summer. There are unexplained variations from day to day; hence, a single abnormal count should not be taken to indicate a pathologic condition.

Production. Platelets originate in the marrow from cells of the megakaryocyte series, which are the largest of all hematopoietic cells and arise from the same stem cell as granulocytes and erythroid cells.

The *megakaryoblast* is the earliest cell in this series; it is 20 to 30 μm. in diameter and has basophilic cytoplasm and an oval to irregularly lobulated nucleus. The chromatin pattern is reticular and somewhat densely staining; nucleoli are small. Megakaryoblasts engage in DNA synthesis and division of the nucleus several times, without cytoplasmic division, a process known as endomitosis. The ploidy varies from 4 N to 32 N. Separate nuclear lobes are connected by strands of nuclear material. Cytoplasmic size increases coincident with nuclear division. Only after DNA synthesis ceases do fine, red cytoplasmic granules begin to appear in the *promegakaryocyte.* During this stage, as granules increase in number, nuclear lobulation becomes more pronounced. In the *megakaryocyte,* cytoplasmic basophilia has disappeared. The granules, at first diffuse, later become clustered into small aggregates (separated by demarcation channels as visualized in the electron microscope). The nuclear chromatin is densely staining, but small nucleoli are often visible. One of the helpful morphologic features is that nucleoli of megakaryocytes are always small. Platelets are shed as cytoplasmic fragments (probably by fusion of the demarcation membranes that separate them) from the mature megakaryocyte. The time from megakaryoblast to platelet formation is 4 to 5 days in man (Aster, 1972).

Distribution, Life Span, Function. At any instant about one-third of the platelets in the vascular system are in slow transit through the spleen because of the anatomic characteristics of the red pulp. This means that two-thirds are in the rest of the circulation. If the spleen enlarges significantly, more of the platelets are located within it at any one time. In marked splenomegaly up to 80 to 90 per cent of the platelets may be within the spleen, resulting in thrombocytopenia based on this distributional change.

Platelets live for 8 to 11 days in the vascular system. Some platelets probably are used up in maintaining vascular integrity and in plugging vascular injuries. Others appear to be removed by the reticuloendothelial system when they become senescent.

Platelets normally function in supporting the endothelium of blood vessels by plugging gaps between them; in severe thrombocytopenia tiny hemorrhages (petechiae) occur spontaneously from vascular leaks.

Another major function of platelets is their primary role in hemostasis. When a blood vessel is damaged, platelets adhere to collagen, aggregate with one another, and form a plug in an attempt to stop the blood from leaving the vessel. In the process they make available platelet factor 3, a phospholipid, which promotes the intrinsic coagulation mechanism.

Hematopoiesis

An approximation of how blood cells are formed is shown in Figure 4–41; however, the story remains incomplete, and modification will undoubtedly be necessary. The uncommitted stem cell is morphologically undefined. That a myeloid stem cell is a common precursor to the series indicated is supported, for example, by the fact that in chronic granulocytic leukemia a common chromosomal abnormality (Ph^1) is found in erythroid, granulocytic, and megakaryocytic cells but not in lymphocytes. Committed stem cells are assumed to exist for each cell line, that is, they have limited potential for differentiation and respond to specific controlling factors. Regulation of cell production is best worked out for erythropoiesis; a hormone, erythropoietin, induces differentiation of a committed stem cell into erythroid precursors without affecting other cell lines. Evidence for hormones of factors controlling platelet production (thrombopoietin) and granulocyte production (leukopoietin) exists but is less complete. Recent work indicates that the monocyte produces a colony-stimulating factor (CSF) that can induce a morphologically undefined colony-forming cell (CFC) to differentiate *in vitro* into granulocytes and macrophages (Stohlman and Quesenberry, 1972; Chervenick and LoBuglio, 1972). It is likely that our understanding of the control of granulocytopoiesis will be clarified in the near future.

PRODUCTION AND DESTRUCTION OF ERYTHROCYTES*

The erythrocyte is a vehicle for the transport of hemoglobin, which is produced in precursor cells of the erythrocytes, the normoblasts. The function of hemoglobin is the transport of oxygen and carbon dioxide. The erythrocyte is also metabolically capable of keeping hemoglobin in a functional state.

In the adult, all erythropoiesis occurs in the marrow. The nutrient arteries give rise to distributing arterioles, from which arise the sinusoidal beds of the marrow. The sinusoids are lined by a single layer of flattened reticulum cells, which can take up dye supravitally. This cell lining is discontinuous and relatively unstable. If a reticulum cell differentiates into another cell type, it may leave in its place a gap in the lining. The reticulum cells are associated with a ground substance but no basement membrane, unless the reticulum cell is adjacent to a fat cell. Hematopoiesis takes place outside the sinusoids in the stroma of the marrow. Reticulocytes and other blood cells enter the sinusoids via diapedesis.

The committed stem cell differentiates into the earliest recognizable precursor of the erythrocyte, the pronormoblast. When the stem cell divides, one daughter cell goes into the specific maturation sequence and the other remains undifferentiated to maintain the pool of marrow stem cells.

During differentiation a definite sequence of events occurs. The bulk of the iron is transferred from the plasma transferrin into the cells of the pronormoblast and basophilic normoblast stages. These cells have the highest content of RNA, which begins to decline in the polychromatic normoblasts (an intermediary stage between basophilic and orthochromatic normoblast) as hemoglobin increases in amount. Synthesis of RNA gradually decreases in each stage through the orthochromatic nor-

*See Harris and Kellermeyer (1970) and Finch (1969).

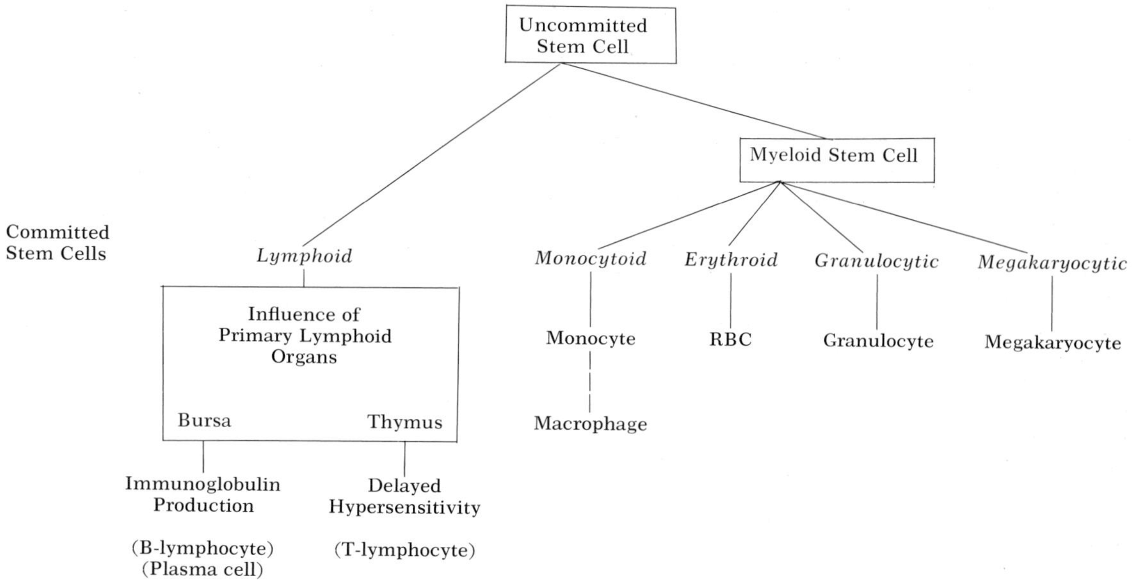

Figure 4–41. Possible relationships among hematopoietic stem cells. (Modified from Nowell and Wilson, 1971.)

moblasts. Of course, when the nucleus is no longer present (that is, when it is ejected and the cell becomes a reticulocyte) RNA synthesis ceases, yet the RNA already present remains for a few days, and protein and heme synthesis continue in the reticulocyte. Hemoglobin can be recognized in the basophilic normoblast spectrophotometrically but is not visually evident until the stage of the polychromatic normoblast. Hemoglobin synthesis continues until the reticulocyte loses its mitochondria and RNA.

During this differentiation process, approximately three mitotic divisions occur from the pronormoblast stage to the orthochromatic normoblast. This takes about two to three days. In the orthochromatic stage the nucleus becomes condensed and is incapable of further mitosis. In another day or two the nucleus is extruded along with a small part of the cytoplasm and the cell now assumes the anucleate stage of the reticulocyte. This sequence provides a basis for the picture we see in the distribution of erythropoietic cells in the bone marrow: most are orthochromatic and polychromatic normoblasts, fewer are basophilic normoblasts, and fewer still pronormoblasts. A small proportion of cells mature directly without dividing, but most have undergone three mitoses in four days.

Reticulocytes are larger than mature red cells and are sticky. It may be because of this that they remain in the marrow for one to two days before they are released into the blood, where they continue their maturation and hemoglobin synthesis for about a day before their synthetic ability is lost.

The reticulocytes in the marrow remain in the stroma and are about equal in number to the nucleated erythrocytes in the marrow and slightly more in number than the reticulocytes in the circulating blood. If sufficiently severe hypoxia is present, this marrow pool of reticulocytes can be released. This approximately doubles the number of circulating reticulocytes.

The mature erythrocytes circulate for about 120 days. During this time they gradually age, certain enzymatic activities diminish, and they are finally destroyed within phagocytic cells of the reticuloendothelial system.

Regulation of Erythrocyte Production. Normally the level of erythrocytes in the blood is determined by the rate of production of cells. The rate of erythrocyte destruction does not vary appreciably in normal individuals. The evidence indicates that increased production of erythrocytes occurs when oxygen transport to the tissues is impaired as in anemia, poor delivery of oxygen to the tissues in cardiovascular disorders, and low oxygen environment, as in high altitudes. On the other hand, production of erythrocytes is decreased when an individual is hypertransfused or exposed to high oxygen pressures.

In general, the hemoglobin level correlates

(Text continued on page 165.)

Figure 4–42. Development of blood cells. This illustration comprises a survey of all blood cells. The horizontal double line separates the cells that are found in the marrow and in lymphoid tissue from the mature cells below the line seen normally in the peripheral blood. The first of the two vertical double lines separates the cells produced exclusively in the marrow from the cells of the monocytic series. The second vertical double line in the upper part of the illustration separates the two types of immature cells of extramedullary origin, lymphoblasts and plasmoblasts.

1. The cells near the top of the illustration have a characteristically basophilic cytoplasm, are free from granules, and have large, round, or slightly oval nuclei with a delicate chromatin structure (with the exception of the nucleus of the plasma cell in the left upper corner, which will be discussed in more detail later). As presented, the primitive erythrocyte, the pronormoblast, the primitive granulocyte, the myeloblast, and the young megakaryocyte, the megakaryoblast, originate directly from the primitive reticulum cell. This is an assumption and not at all certain, since the morphologic characteristics of the uncommitted stem cell are not known. Blue nucleoli are seen in the nuclei of the pronormoblast, myeloblast, and lymphoblast.

Certain changes take place with progressive maturation of all blood cells. Some are common to all of them; some are different and specific for each type.

As one descends along the line of development from the top of the illustration to the bottom, one sees:

The size of the whole cell and of the nucleus decreases in the erythroid, the granulocytic, and the lymphocytic series. The chromatin of the nucleus progressively loses its delicate granular structure and becomes more dense, more coarse, and clumped. The basophilia of the cytoplasm disappears completely in the cells originating in the marrow. The cells of extramedullary origin behave differently. Their cytoplasm remains basophilic but becomes less deep in the lymphocyte; it actually becomes more intense in the plasma cells.

Lymphoid cells probably have a different stem cell from the other series; it is shown here as the lymphocytic reticulum cell. Not shown here is the common myeloid stem cell known to exist for erythroid, granulocytic, megakaryocytic, and probably for the monocytic cell lines. Then each line has a "committed" stem cell that is responsive to regulation by humoral factors (Fig. 4–41). The morphologic identity of each of these stem cells is not certain.

2. *The erythrocyte.* The pronormoblast is the most primitive recognizable erythroid cell. A second stage (not illustrated), the basophilic normoblast, has an even more intensely blue cytoplasm, the nuclear chromatin is more clumped, and nucleoli are less distinct. As the deep blue of the cytoplasm fades, orange to gray patches of forming hemoglobin appear in the cytoplasm: the polychromatic normoblast. As the amount of hemoglobin increases, so does the pink of the cytoplasm: the orthochromatic normoblast.

As all this goes on in the cytoplasm, the nucleus shrinks and its chromatin contracts into a small, round, black clump and eventually is thrown out of the cell; the erythrocyte has arrived. The cell still contains a vestige of cytoplasmic RNA, the reticulum, invisible in smears stained with any of the usual Romanowsky stains but recognizable by the larger size and the faint purplish gray color of the polychromatophilic erythrocyte. In a smear vitally stained with cresyl blue, for example, the residual RNA appears as a delicate blue network of fibrillae and dots, the reticulocyte. At this stage the cell enters peripheral blood; the reticulum disappears progressively until the fully functional mature erythrocyte has evolved.

3. *The granulocyte.* Again from the primitive reticulum cells, via the stem cell, the myeloblast has evolved.

All these transitions are rapid and distinct when measured in days. Actually they take place slowly when observed from minute to minute. As we see them during this progressive evolution, we cannot always discern the differences, no more than we can set apart a two-year-old child from one who is two and one-half years old, but we can as a rule distinguish between a two- and a four-year-old. And so it is in the case of the five different blast cells. At first we cannot tell them apart, even as we cannot note any differences in the stem cells. In early stages of their embryonal life we have to resort to "judging a cell by the company it keeps."

Now let us go back to the changes taking place in the granulocyte. A most characteristic innovation has taken place. Granules appear in the cytoplasm, at first coarse and of indefinite color. This together with the coarsening of the nuclear chromatin and the disappearance of the nucleoli results in the promyelocyte. According to the illustration, a promyelocyte is not classified as eosinophilic, neutrophilic, or basophilic. However, some hematologists designate later promyelocytes as eosinophilic, neutrophilic, or basophilic when just a few specific granules are recognized, though most of the granules are azurophilic (nonspecific) and the cytoplasm is largely blue. When the differentiation into the three colors – the red, the deep blue, or the black and the in-between, the neutral – becomes clear cut, the next phase has developed: the myelocyte – the eosinophilic, the basophilic, and the neutrophilic cell. The abundance of granules is frequently so great that the structure and even the outlines of the nucleus are hazy, but its round or oval shape and the progressive coarsening of its chromatin can be made out. The brilliant dazzling red of the discrete eosinophilic granules stands out and is maintained during the remainder of this cell's functional life. Occasionally, in poorly stained smears, the granules of the neutrophilic cell appear coarse and deeper red than they should. The inexperienced may fall into this trap and report eosinophilia where it does not exist. Paying attention to the brilliancy and discreteness of true eosinophils protects against this mistake.

The basophilic myelocyte is just as distinct in its appearance as is the eosinophilic. In this case the tendency to obscure the nucleus is even greater. The granules in the basophilic cells are water soluble, and when exposed to water, the pigment disappears, leaving a bunch of grape-like vacuoles.

The changes in the cytoplasm of granulocytes reach their peak in the myelocyte. Nothing of importance happens in the cytoplasm during the subsequent transformations. It is the nucleus that changes. It becomes indented and kidney shaped, and the metamyelocyte has developed. The metamyelocyte is the first cell of the series to break through the marrow-blood barrier normally and then only as an occasional cell. In the next phase, the band form, the shape of the nucleus is just what the name implies. Finally, as the cell ages, the band subdivides into segments connected with thin filaments – first two segments, then three, and so on until the usual maximum of five segments is reached. Presence of more than five segments is a sign of advanced age: polysegmentation, a shift to the right. This progressive segmentation is characteristic for the segmented neutrophilic granulocyte. The eosinophilic and basophilic segmented granulocytes have fewer segments than the neutrophil, as a rule only two segments, rarely more. Eventually, as the cell reaches the end of its useful life, it disintegrates. It swells, its outlines become vague and its cytoplasm loose, its granularity appears structureless, the segments of the nucleus fall apart, and their chromatin congeals, as shown at the bottom of the illustration. If it reaches this stage before it has emigrated from the blood, the senescent cell is destroyed in the reticuloendothelial system.

4. The story of the *megakaryocyte* is less dramatic. The megakaryoblast at the top in the third major vertical column is a giant of a cell with a restless nucleus and a homogeneous basophilic cytoplasm, which very soon begins to show a fine granularity as the cell becomes the functioning megakaryocyte. This cell is probably the largest normal cell of the body. Its octopus-like, multilobed, gigantic nucleus looks threatening. The cytoplasm spreads out like the web of a spider. Interestingly, this restless giant of a cell gives birth to the smallest formed particle of the body, the platelet or thrombocyte.

5. The next series, the *monocytic* in the fourth vertical column, is represented merely by one cell and that one only as it is seen in the peripheral blood. Where the blast form of this series should have been, a question mark fills the void because

(Legend continued on page 165.)

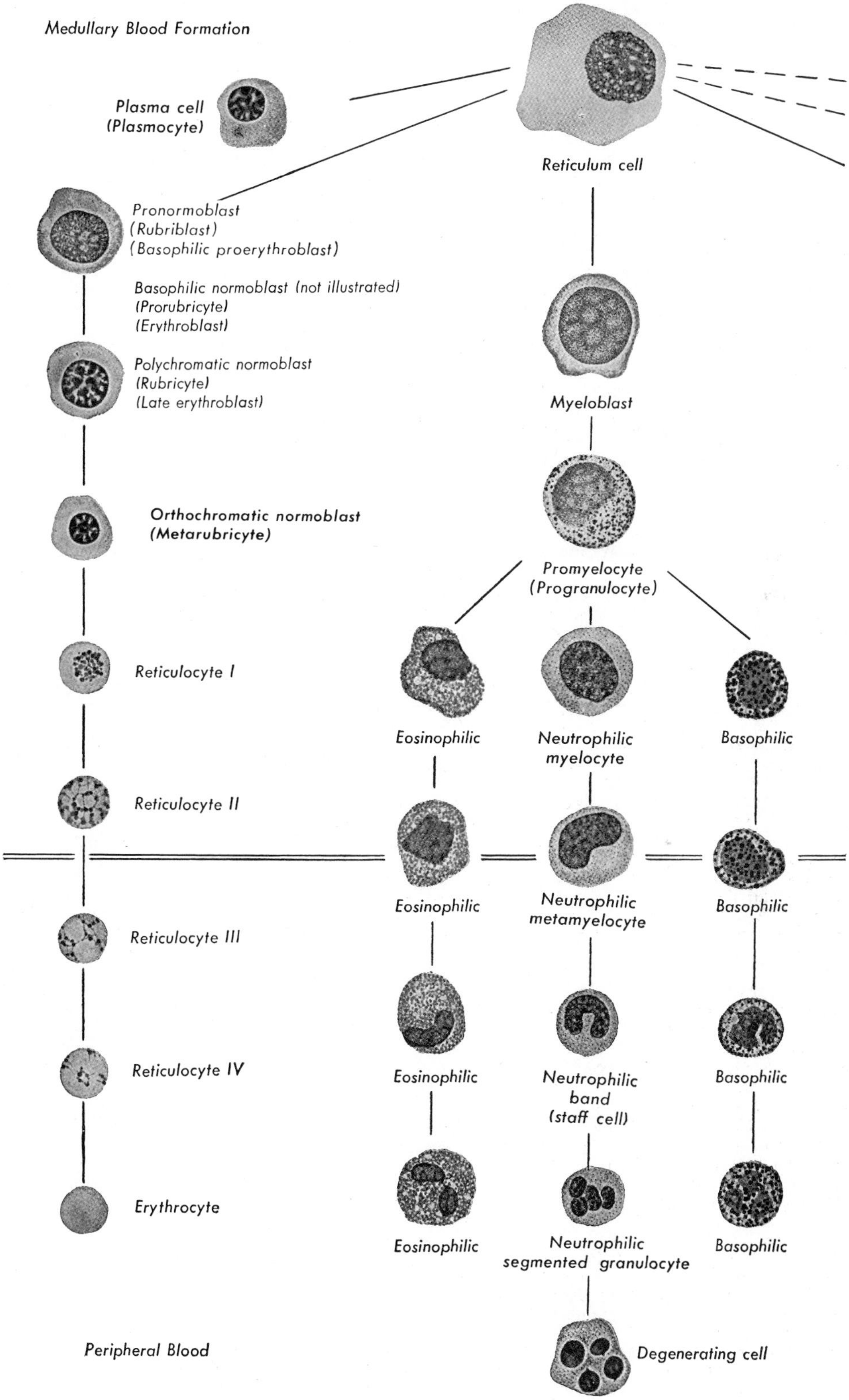
Medullary Blood Formation
Plasma cell
(Plasmocyte)
Reticulum cell
Pronormoblast
(Rubriblast)
(Basophilic proerythroblast)
Basophilic normoblast (not illustrated)
(Prorubricyte)
(Erythroblast)
Polychromatic normoblast
(Rubricyte)
(Late erythroblast)
Myeloblast
Orthochromatic normoblast
(Metarubricyte)
Promyelocyte
(Progranulocyte)
Reticulocyte I
Eosinophilic
Neutrophilic
myelocyte
Basophilic
Reticulocyte II
Eosinophilic
Neutrophilic
metamyelocyte
Basophilic
Reticulocyte III
Reticulocyte IV
Eosinophilic
Neutrophilic
band
(staff cell)
Basophilic
Erythrocyte
Eosinophilic
Neutrophilic
segmented granulocyte
Basophilic
Peripheral Blood
Degenerating cell

Fig. 4–42.

(Figure 4–42 continued on following page.)

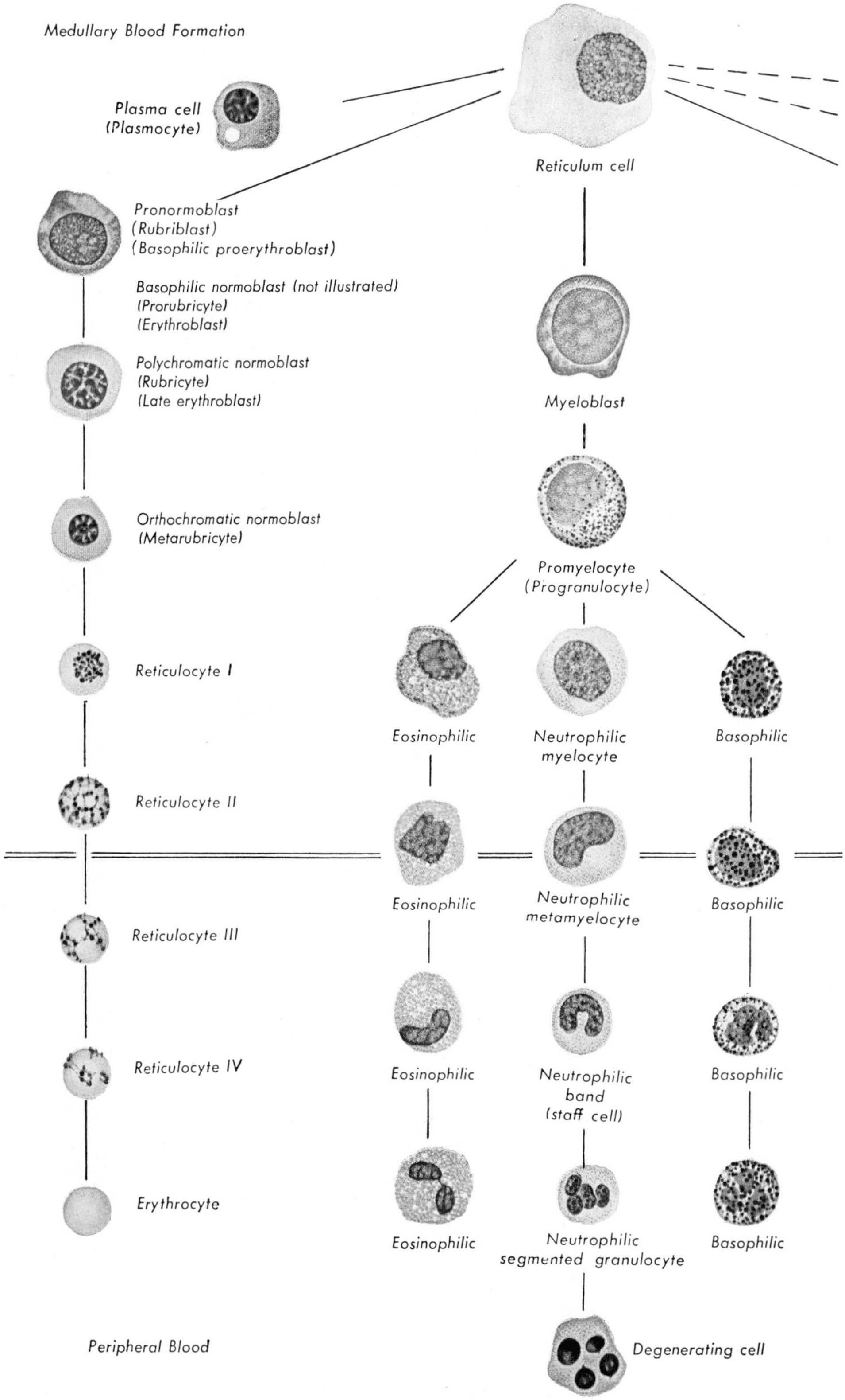

Figure 4–42. *Continued.*

(*Figure 4–42 continued on opposite page.*)

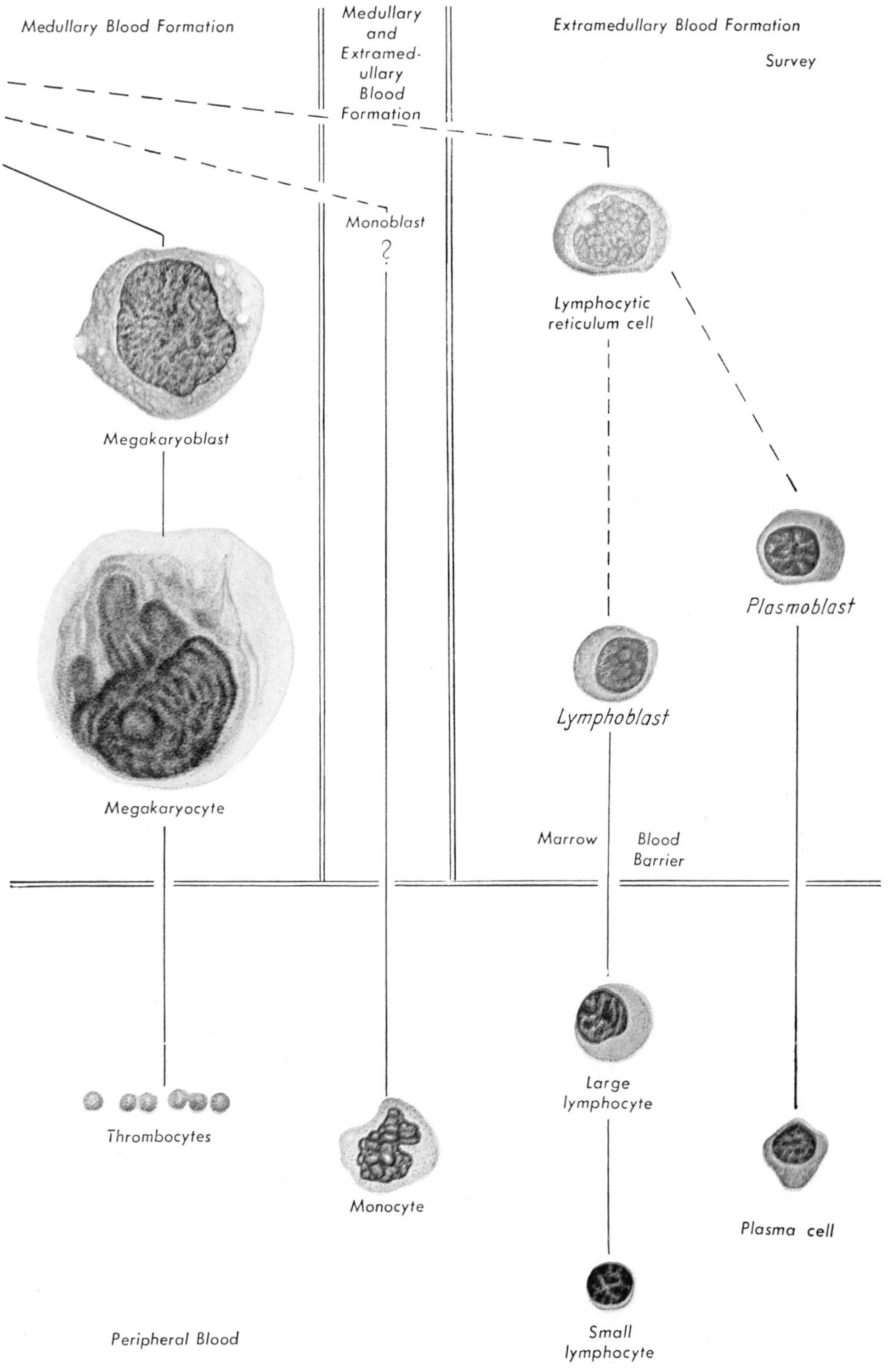

Figure 4–42. *Continued.*

(*Figure 4–42 continued on following page.*)

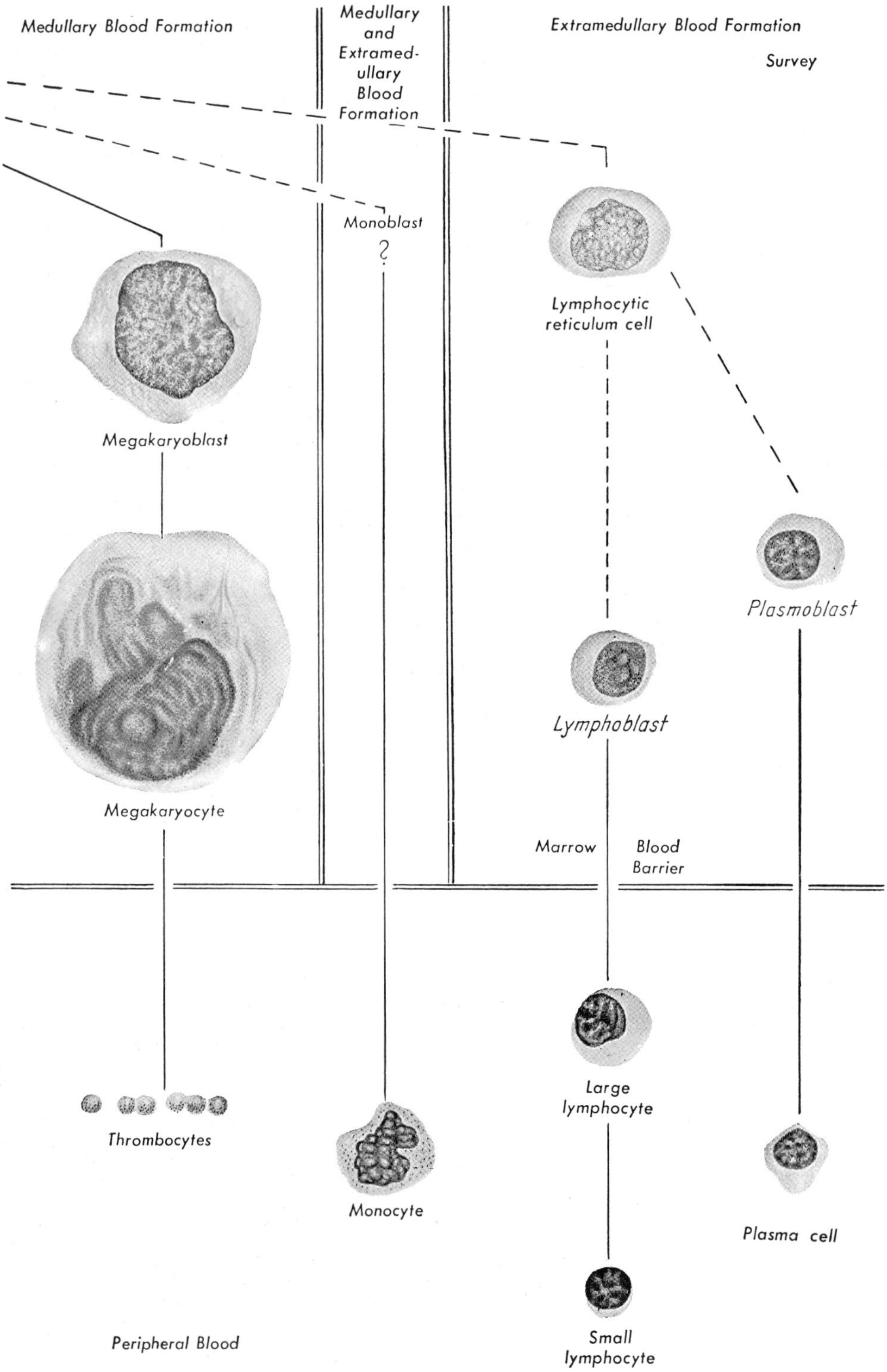
Medullary Blood Formation
Medullary and Extramed- ullary Blood Formation
Extramedullary Blood Formation
Survey
Monoblast
?
Megakaryoblast
Lymphocytic reticulum cell
Plasmoblast
Megakaryocyte
Lymphoblast
Marrow
Blood Barrier
Large lymphocyte
Thrombocytes
Monocyte
Plasma cell
Small lymphocyte
Peripheral Blood

Figure 4–42. *Continued.*

with the delivery of oxygen to the tissues, but this is modified by variation in the oxygen affinity of hemoglobin, which is modulated by the concentration of certain phosphates in the red cell. Intracellular phosphates, in particular 2,3-diphosphoglycerate (2,3-DPG), combine with reduced hemoglobin and diminish its affinity for oxygen. In areas of tissue hypoxia, as oxygen moves from hemoglobin into the tissues, the amount of reduced hemoglobin in the red cells increases, binding more 2,3-DPG, depleting free 2,3-DPG in the cell, leading to increased glycolysis with the production of more 2,3-DPG. In turn, the latter is bound by hemoglobin, further reducing its oxygen affinity so that more oxygen can be delivered to the tissues (Erslev, 1971).

Tissue hypoxia induces formation of a factor or hormone that travels in the plasma to the marrow where it effects the production of more red cells. This erythropoietic factor is known as erythropoietin. It is found in the mucoglycoprotein fraction of the plasma and migrates electrophoretically in the alpha-2-globulin range. It is relatively heat stable and is inactivated by proteolytic enzymes. Erythropoietin (or an enzyme which produces erythropoietin from a substrate in the plasma) is produced mainly in the kidney. Erythropoietin appears to act by inducing the committed stem cell of the marrow to differentiate into erythropoietic cells. The rate of cell division is also increased, and the release of reticulocytes from the marrow is promoted. When we sample a marrow which is producing more erythrocytes than normal, we see increased numbers of normoblasts but in a normal ratio of cell types, a condition we speak of as normoblastic hyperplasia.

Measurement of erythropoietin at present requires a bioassay procedure. The patient's plasma or urine is injected into the polycythemic mouse. The mouse is made polycythemic by transfusions or hyperoxia in order to depress its own erythropoietin production and to make it more sensitive to any injected activity. The response of the mouse is measured by the incorporation of radioactive iron into circulating erythrocytes. Increased amounts of erythropoietin can be detected in the plasma of patients with certain types of anemia, but in plasma, normal or decreased levels cannot be detected. Methods for concentrating the urine have been devised, and well-defined levels of erythropoietic activity can be measured in normal urine (Adamson *et al.*, 1966). Elevated levels are detected in patients with erythroid hyperplasia and in aplastic anemia. Decreased levels below the normal range are found in normal individuals after transfusion and in polycythemia vera.

Synthesis of Hemoglobin

Heme Synthesis. Heme synthesis occurs in most cells of the body, except the mature erythrocytes, but most abundantly in the erythroid precursors. Succinyl-coenzyme A condenses with glycine to form the unstable intermediate alpha-amino-beta-keto-adipic acid, which is readily decarboxylated to delta-amino-levulinic acid (ALA) (Fig. 4–43). This

---

Figure 4–42. Continued. Development of blood cells.
the beginning of the monocyte is shrouded in mystery. It is supposed to originate predominantly within the marrow, and there is no question that there is such a cell in the circulation as it is depicted at the bottom of the column. As the picture shows, it is the largest white cell in the peripheral blood. Its nucleus is irregularly lobated. It cannot be reduced to a pattern. Its chromatin structure is the most delicate and the least clearly outlined of all the white cells in the peripheral blood. Its structural haziness is made even more indefinite by the fine granulation of the abundant cytoplasm, which is described as of "ground glass" appearance.

6. The mother cell of the *lymphocyte*, as shown in the illustration, stems from the embryonal reticulum cell by way of the lymphatic reticulum cell, which proceeds to the lymphoblast (reticular lymphocyte) and then to the lymphocytes of the peripheral blood, the large and the small lymphocyte. It must be remembered that the small lymphocyte is not an end cell, as might be assumed from this figure. Under antigenic stimulation, the small lymphocyte can transform back into the lymphoblast (reticular lymphocyte) or the lymphocytic reticulum cell, divide again, and become a plasma cell or another lymphocyte. It is worth repeating that in this series the basophilia of the cytoplasm of the embryonal precursors does not disappear with maturity. It assumes a lighter hue. Small numbers of deep red granules appear, but only in some lymphocytes – the azurophilic granules. The mature small lymphocyte is an unassuming cell with a bare rim of cytoplasm, which is sometimes lost and leaves exposed the dense, almost structureless nucleus. In the large lymphocyte, the cytoplasm is abundant – frequently a beautiful transparent blue; the nuclear chromatin is much more loosely patterned.

7. In the *plasma cell* series, in the last right-hand vertical column, the plasmoblast is shown branching away from the lymphatic reticulum cell, a blast cell, outside the marrow in the lymphoid tissue. Another view, that small lymphocytes undergo transformation into blast-like cells which can divide and form plasma cells, is not shown.

The top cell in the left upper corner of the illustration shows a plasma cell originating directly from the primordial reticulum cell of the marrow, which is in keeping with the well-known presence of plasma cells in the marrow in health and their increase there in various conditions.

The characteristic eccentric location of the nucleus, the arrangement of the chromatin clumps, and their separation by the colorless parachromatin with the resulting resemblance to the spokes of a wheel are well shown. (From L. Heilmeyer and H. Begemann: Atlas der Klinischen Hämatologie und Cytologie. Springer, 1955.)

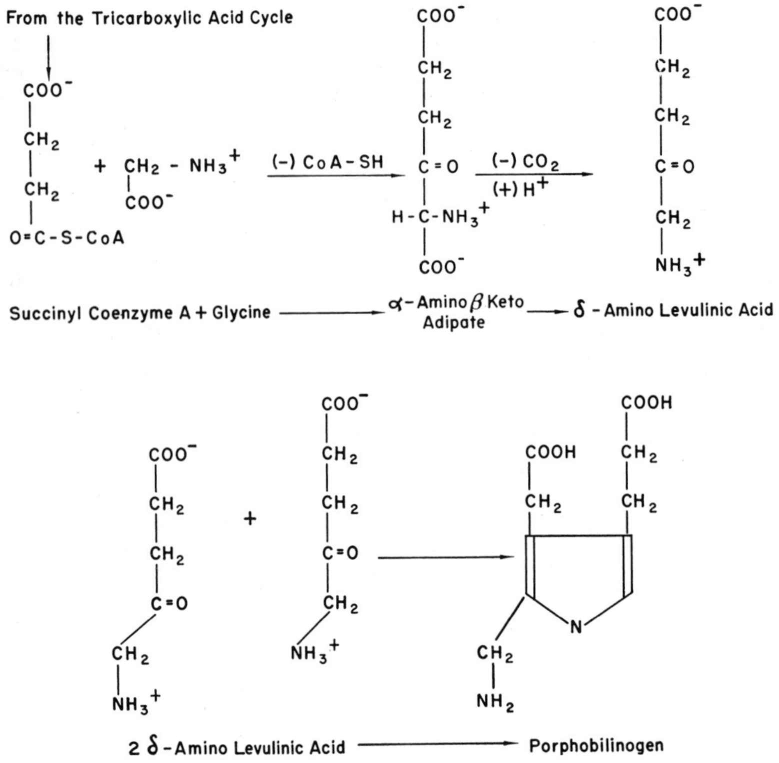

Figure 4–43. Formation of porphobilinogen from succinyl-coenzyme A and glycine. (From B. S. Leavell and O. A. Thorup: *Fundamentals of Clinical Hematology*. 3rd ed. 1971.)

condensation requires pyridoxal phosphate (vitamin B_6) and must take place in intact mitochondria.

ALA is excreted normally in small amounts in the urine; in certain abnormalities of heme synthesis (for example, lead poisoning) excretion is increased. Two molecules of ALA condense to form the monopyrrole, porphobilinogen, catalyzed by the enzyme ALA-dehydrase. Porphobilinogen is also normally excreted in small amounts in the urine. Markedly elevated amounts appear in the urine in acute intermittent porphyria, easily detected by a color reaction with Ehrlich's aldehyde reagent.

Four molecules of porphobilinogen react to form uroporphyrinogen III or I (Fig. 4–44). It is the type III isomer that is converted, by way of coproporphyrinogen III and protoporphyrinogen, to protoporphyrin. In certain diseases when this pathway is partially blocked, the type I isomers of uroporphyrinogen and coproporphyrinogen are formed and their oxidized excretion products, uroporphyrin I and coproporphyrin I, are increased in amount.

Protoporphyrin is normally found in mature erythrocytes. In abnormalities of heme synthesis, levels of free erythrocyte protoporphyrin may be increased.

Iron is inserted into protoporphyrin by the mitochondrial enzyme iron chetalase to form the finished heme moiety.

Globin Synthesis. Globin synthesis occurs in the cytoplasm of the erythroblast and reticulocyte. According to the prevailing doctrine of protein synthesis, the polypeptide chains (which constitute the protein part of hemoglobin) are manufactured on the ribosomes, which are located mainly in the cytoplasm of the young erythroid cell. Specific small sRNA (soluble RNA) molecules attach to each amino acid and determine the placement of that amino acid according to the code in the mRNA (messenger RNA). Progressive growth of the polypeptide chain begins at the amino end. This process of protein synthesis occurs on ribosomes which are aggregated as polysomes. The polysomes are probably held together by the messenger RNA strand. Since the reticulocyte can synthesize hemoglobin for at least two days after loss of its nucleus, it appears that the messenger RNA for hemoglobin is stable. It is probable that the globin polypeptide chains formed on the polysome are folded into their three-dimensional configurations spontaneously.

Control of hemoglobin synthesis is not entirely elucidated, but it has been shown that hemin inhibits heme synthesis and either hemin or iron increases globin synthesis.

Structure of Hemoglobin. In each hemoglobin molecule, one heme group is inserted into a hydrophobic pocket of one folded polypeptide chain. Normal adult hemoglobin A consists of four heme groups and four polypeptide chains (two alpha chains and two beta chains) which form a roughly globular hemoglobin molecule. The ferrous iron atoms have six coordination bonds, four to the pyrrole nitrogens of heme, one to the imidazole nitrogen of histidine of the globin chain (87 alpha or 92 beta), and one that is reversibly bound to oxygen. As the oxygen partial pressure increases, the four heme groups sequentially bind one molecule of oxygen each. In the process, a change in the overall configuration of the hemoglobin molecule occurs, and this altered configuration appears to favor the heme-heme interaction in the binding of oxygen.

The sigmoid-shaped oxygen dissociation curve of hemoglobin reflects this affinity for oxygen with increasing partial pressure of oxygen, such as occurs in the lungs. With the conditions prevailing in the tissues with decreasing pH and increasing temperature produced by metabolic events, the curve shifts downward and to the right, favoring the release of oxygen. Rapidly metabolizing tissue will extract more oxygen from hemoglobin than will metabolically inactive tissue.

Carbon dioxide is also transported in the blood by hemoglobin. The enzyme carbonic anhydrase catalyzes the transformation of carbon dioxide to bicarbonate in the red cell while in the tissue capillary bed and catalyzes the reverse reaction (the release of carbon dioxide from bicarbonate) in the erythrocyte when it is in the capillary bed of the lungs.

Destruction of Erythrocytes and Degradation of Hemoglobin. From the time an erythrocyte enters the circulation and loses its RNA, it gradually undergoes metabolic changes over the course of its 120-day life span. At this time, the less viable senescent cell is removed from the circulation. We know that certain glycolytic enzymes diminish in activity as the cell ages. It is probable that changes in the cell surface, possibly indirectly related, render the cell more liable to phagocytosis. Fragmentation of the red cell, without hemolysis, can occur with the formation of schistocytes or cell fragments. These particles are then readily removed by the reticuloendothelial system. Some people believe that this process of fragmentation prior to removal by phagocytosis plays an important role in eliminating senescent erythrocytes from the circulation. This explanation has been used to account for the fact that there is little or no morphologic evidence of erythrophagocytosis in the reticuloendothelial system of the normal individual, despite the removal of three million erythrocytes per second from the blood. The other possibility is phagocytosis of the

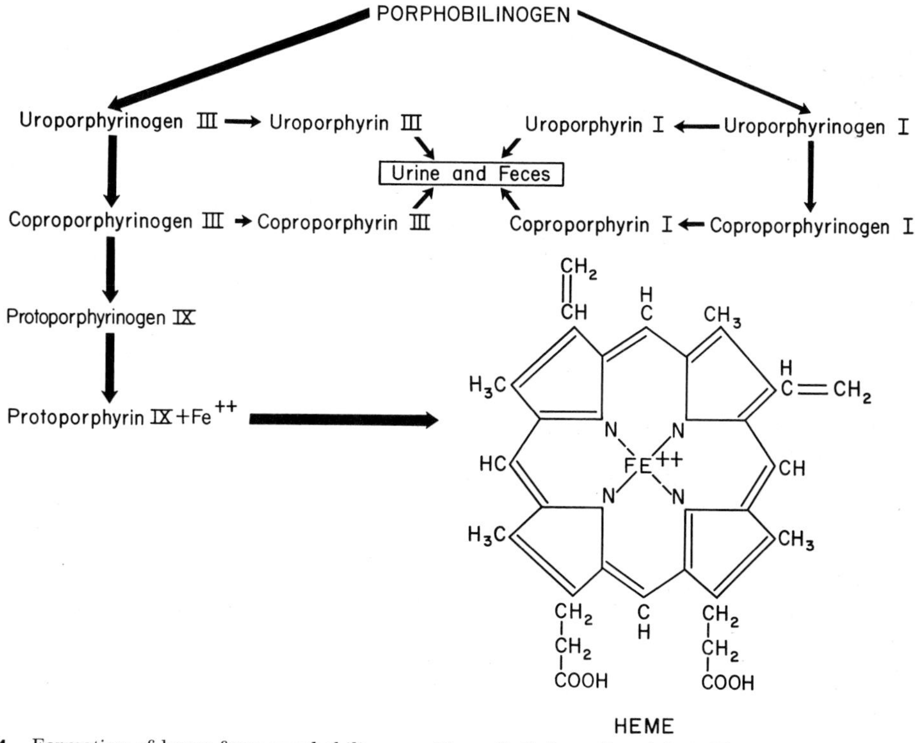

Figure 4–44. Formation of heme from porphobilinogen. (From B. S. Leavell and O. A. Thorup: Fundamentals of Clinical Hematology. 3rd ed. 1971.)

intact aged erythrocytes and rapid breakdown within the phagocytes.

Whether one process predominates or both coexist, we know that the cells are removed by the macrophages or phagocytic cells of the reticuloendothelial system.

Under normal conditions in man, the major part of erythrophagocytosis appears to occur in the bone marrow. In pathological states when the erythrocyte is damaged and the red cell survival is shortened, the site of destruction depends upon the extent to which the erythrocyte is damaged. If the damage is small, the erythrocytes are removed primarily by the spleen. If the damage is great, the cells are removed mainly by the liver.

Degradation of Hemoglobin. After removal of the red cell from the circulation, hemoglobin is broken down within the cells of the reticuloendothelial system into its three constituents—iron, protoporphyrin, and globin. The iron goes into storage and may be completely reutilized. The polypeptide chains of globin are probably degraded and returned to the amino acid pool of the body. In contrast, the protoporphyrin ring is split, converted to bilirubin, and excreted from the body.

The cleavage of the protoporphyrin ring occurs only at the alpha-methene bridge. The carbon atom at this point is oxidized to carbon monoxide. This appears in the blood as carboxyhemoglobin. It has been shown that the concentration of carboxyhemoglobin within the blood can be used as a measure of the amount of hemoglobin destruction.

In conditions associated with intravascular hemolysis, hematin (the oxidized form of heme) may be detected in the plasma bound to albumin (methemalbumin). Normally, hematin cannot be found in the blood, since hemoglobin catabolism occurs within the reticuloendothelial cell.

The formation of bilirubin from hemoglobin proceeds rapidly in the reticuloendothelial cells. In rats, the time of appearance of bilirubin in the bile after administration of labeled hemoglobin is 3 hours. The bilirubin is then transported to the liver, firmly bound to plasma albumin. It is removed from the plasma by the liver cell, conjugated mainly with glucuronide and excreted in the bile. In the intestine, reduction by bacteria occurs, and bilirubin is transformed into urobilinogen, mesobilirubinogen, and stercobilinogen, compounds which are collectively designated urobilinogens.

Estimation of fecal urobilinogen is a measure of hemoglobin breakdown. When production of red cells is diminished and the level of circulating hemoglobin is low, as in aplastic anemia, pigment excretion is reduced. When destruction of erythrocytes is increased, as in hemolytic anemia, excretion of urobilinogen is increased in amount.

In normal man about 80 to 90 per cent of the excreted bile pigment measured as fecal urobilinogen is derived from breakdown of senescent erythrocytes which have lived 100 to 120 days. However, about 10 to 20 per cent of the pigment is excreted within the first few days. This early labeled bile pigment could not be derived from erythrocytes destroyed at the end of their normal life span. There is evidence now that, though a small amount of this comes from nonhemoglobin heme formed in the liver, most of this early labeled pigment comes from the breakdown of newly formed hemoglobin in the bone marrow. Much of it may represent hemoglobin from the nucleus and pieces of cytoplasm of the orthochromatic normoblast that are lost during the process of nuclear extrusion.

In certain hematologic diseases, notably thalassemia, pernicious anemia, refractory normoblastic anemia, and erythropoietic porphyria, this early labeled bile pigment fraction may be markedly increased. This excessive intramedullary destruction of hemoglobin, which never appears in circulating erythrocytes, is known as ineffective erythropoiesis.

SITES OF BLOOD FORMATION

Undifferentiated cells of the mesenchyma and endothelial cells of the primitive blood spaces give rise to blood cells in the embryo. Later, in due course, production of blood cells becomes organoid and the liver and spleen become the main sites. Eventually the bone marrow takes over. At birth, the marrow is active and red and contains only minimal amounts of fat. Later in childhood, only the proximal portions of the long bones and the flat bones (the skull, vertebrae, thoracic cage, shoulder, and pelvis) are the sites of blood formation. The rest of the marrow space is occupied by fat, which can be replaced by hematopoietic cells when the need arises. As the individual ages, the proportion of marrow space occupied by fat increases slightly, probably due to expansion of the marrow cavity.

Examination of Marrow

Marrow aspiration biopsy, introduced by Arinkin in 1929, was considered at first a formidable and highly specialized procedure. It is now widely used in the diagnosis of hematologic diseases and many conditions not primarily affecting the blood system. A number of techniques have been devised by which a suitable specimen of marrow can be obtained with little discomfort to the patient. The simple aspiration type of biopsy can be carried out as an office procedure on ambulatory patients. The risks involved are minimal. They compare favorably with ordinary venipuncture and are decidedly less traumatizing than a lumbar puncture. As for any other special procedure, however, the indications for marrow examination should be clear. In each instance the physician should have in mind some reasonable prediction of its result and consequent benefit to the patient. Without exception, the peripheral blood should be examined carefully first. It is a relatively uncommon circumstance to find hematologic disease in the bone marrow either earlier or more certainly than it can be discovered in the peripheral blood. If an examiner is not able to find at least suggestive evidence of abnormality referable to the marrow from the clinical data or the study of the peripheral blood, he is not likely to do better with the marrow.

It is estimated that the weight of the marrow in man varies from 1300 to 1500 gm. The unique feature of this organ is its extreme lability. It can undergo complete transformation in a few days and occasionally even in a few hours. As a rule, this rapid transformation involves the whole organ, as evidenced by the fact that a small sample represented by a biopsy or aspiration is usually fairly representative of the whole marrow. This conclusion is in accord with results of studies of biopsy samples simultaneously removed from several sites. According to these observations, the various sites chosen for removal of marrow for studies are in most instances equally good. Consequently, the difficulty of access, the risks involved, and the discomfort of the patient are the main reasons for selection of a site in the particular patient. Occasionally the failure to obtain quantitatively or qualitatively adequate material in one site may be followed by success in another location. Also the need for repeated aspirations or biopsies may indicate the use of several different sites. The iliac bone and the vertebral spinous processes are less traumatic to the patient and seem to be more promising as sources of marrow for demonstration of cancer cells. We regard the posterior iliac crest as the preferred site. The large marrow space allows both aspiration and biopsy to be performed with ease at one time.

TECHNIQUE OF MARROW ASPIRATION BIOPSY

In the adult patient, the sternum, the spinous processes of the vertebrae, and the anterior or posterior iliac crest are readily accessible areas from which bone marrow material can be obtained. In infants and young children the upper end of the tibia is frequently used to obtain marrow. The various methods of obtaining and handling material are essentially identical in principle so that comparable results are achieved by workers of equal skill and experience.

Surgical biopsy of the marrow, in which intact fragments of tissue are obtained by incision or by trephining, at one time had many advocates. These procedures have now been largely replaced by aspiration and needle biopsy techniques which have the advantages of simplicity and less discomfort to the patient. Stained sections are not as suitable for accurate differentiation of cell types as the smeared preparations. In addition to aspiration, needle biopsy should be used when it is important to see the cells in their anatomic relation to one another and to the inactive fat or connective tissue stroma (as in aplastic anemia and myelofibrosis) or in diseases that produce focal rather than diffuse changes (Hodgkin's disease, multiple myeloma, malignant lymphoma, metastatic tumors, granulomatous diseases, and so forth). Another method of histologic examination uses aspirated marrow particles (fragments of marrow tissue) clotted together with thrombin and plasma, placed in fixative, and sections made. Histologic sections of needle biopsy and of aspirated particles will usually yield sufficient information in the situations mentioned above so that surgical biopsy will be unnecessary.

The technique for handling aspirated marrow outlined here is known to yield good films and to show reasonably smooth distribution of cells, and it can be carried out with a minimum of technical complexity.

Equipment. The needle must be of short, stout construction, properly molded for a firm grasp, with a short bevel and well-fitted stylet. The lumen needs to be rather large, not less than about 14 gauge. Several varieties of needles are available. A widely used needle is the University of Illinois sternal needle* (Fig. 4–45). It has an adjustable guard, which, when properly set, will prevent perforation of the inner plate of the sternum. With each complete turn the guard moves 1 mm. The stylet can be fixed firmly. A small needle of same construction is available for infants and children.

The Jamshidi bone marrow biopsy needle† (Fig. 4–46) is preferred for biopsies of adequate size and free of crushing artefact (Jamshidi and Swaim, 1971). The tapered distal end of

*V. Mueller & Co., Chicago, Ill.

†Kor Med Corporation, Minneapolis, Minn.

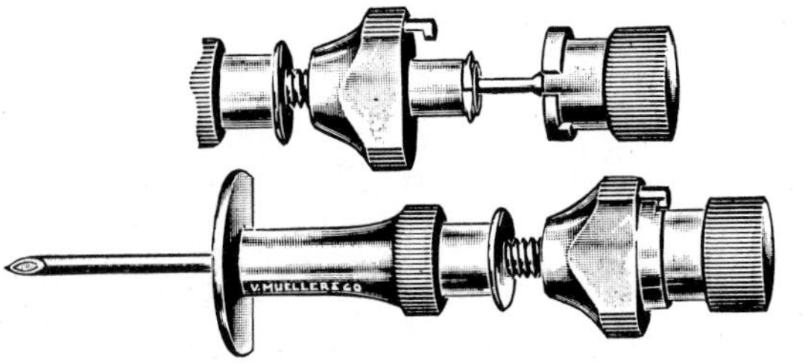

Figure 4–45. University of Illinois sternal needle with adjustable guard, special locking device for the stylet, and Luer-Lok hub set into the needle. (Courtesy of V. Mueller and Co., Chicago.)

the biopsy needle makes loss of the sample less probable. Biopsies 1 to 3 cm. long and 2 mm. in diameter are easily obtained.

Other biopsy needles, such as the Westerman-Jensen and the stout Vim-Silverman needles, are also satisfactory.

Clean glass slides, coverslips, test tubes, and watch glasses should be available.

Ten- or 20-ml. syringes are better than smaller sizes because they have a stronger pull. Syringes with metal tips are preferable. An extra syringe and a *separate* small syringe for the anesthetic should be available.

Sterile equipment to be used by the operator should be ready on a marrow puncture tray. It should contain the following: towels, emesis basin, cotton sponges, hemostat, two 10-ml. syringes preferably with metal tips, one 5-ml. syringe, one 24-gauge hypodermic needle, one 22-gauge needle, and a marrow needle (University of Illinois type) wrapped and sterilized. In addition: several pairs of sterile rubber gloves, procaine, alcohol, iodine, or another local antiseptic (e.g., Zephiran), clean and preferably new glass slides, Band-Aids, and collodion.

EDTA is the preferred anticoagulant for preservation of cellular detail.

Iliac Crest Aspiration and Biopsy. Occasionally a mild, rapidly acting sedative may be useful, though for most patients it will be unnecessary.

The patient should be informed and reassured concerning the nature of the procedure to put him in the proper frame of mind. The next step is to put him at ease physically by having him lie comfortably on his side with his back flexed and knees drawn toward his chest.

The site for the puncture is selected. The posterior superior iliac spine is located and marked. With the use of sterile technique, the

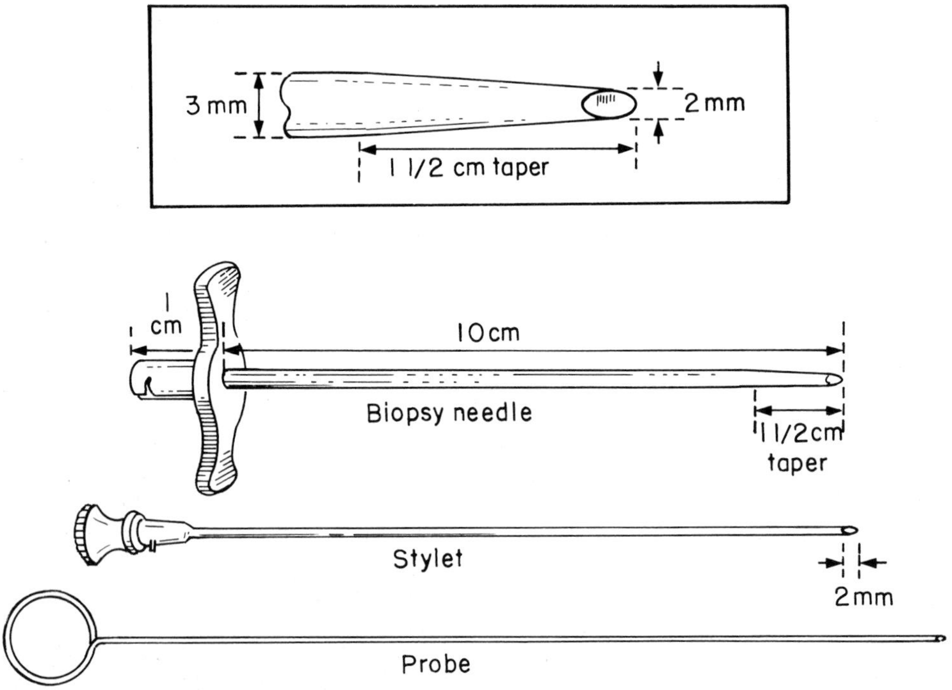

Figure 4–46. Biopsy needle. The biopsy device has a uniform, external cylindrical configuration with a core of substantially constant internal diameter except for the tapered distal portion. The distal tip is beveled and has a sharp cutting edge. The interior diameter of the distal portion is tapered radially toward the cutting tip. This provides space within the interior of the instrument which has a larger diameter than the cutting tip, avoids compression of the tissue, and allows one to obtain specimens without plugging the lumen of the needle. The proximal end is calibrated for syringe attachment and has finger grips. The stylet is designed to interlock, to fit the tapered internal core, and projects 1 to 2 mm. beyond the tip in order to protect the cutting edge and provide a means of entering the marrow. (From Jamshidi, K., and Swaim, W. R.: J. Lab. Clin. Med. 77:335, 1971.)

skin is prepared with an antiseptic solution over the entire posterior iliac crest and several centimeters around it. The field surrounding the puncture site is protected with a sterile drape or sterile towels. Sterile gloves are worn. Aseptic technique should be used during the operation.

Using a solution of 1 per cent procaine or lidocaine (Xylocaine), raise a skin wheal just over the posterior iliac spine. Change to the 22-gauge needle and infiltrate the subcutaneous tissue and the periosteum over a few square centimeter area of the iliac crest.

One must make sure that the patient is not sensitive to the particular anesthetic; if sensitivity is known or demonstrated, another should be chosen. Another recommended precaution is to withdraw the needle slightly at the start of the injection to make certain that the local anesthetic is not being injected intravenously.

A one-eighth inch stab wound in the skin avoids the possibility of pushing a plug of skin into the marrow cavity. With its stylet in place and locked in position, the University of Illinois needle is grasped firmly and introduced vertically through the anesthetized area until its point impinges upon the outer table of the bone. The guard is screwed down until it touches the skin. It is then screwed back about four turns. Now, with steady pressure and a slight clockwise-counterclockwise rotation of the needle, push the needle firmly into the bone. A sudden loss of resistance may be felt as the needle enters the marrow cavity.

When the point of the needle is in the marrow, the stylet is removed and a 10- or 20-ml. syringe is attached. Using sharp, firm aspiration, quickly withdraw not more than 0.2 to 0.3 ml. of material. The small amount is more suitable for cytologic studies. When greater volumes are aspirated, only additional peripheral blood is drawn into the syringe, and the results may be completely vitiated by dilution. A slightly larger amount may be drawn if the specimen is to be concentrated by centrifugation. Many patients experience pain or distress when marrow is being aspirated. Prepare the patients for the pain by warning them just before aspirating; it does not come as a surprise and is tolerated better. If material is not obtained at once, the stylet can be replaced and the needle advanced further after rotating back the guard.

The syringe and needle are removed and handed to an assistant who proceeds to make the slides. If a biopsy is not to be done, the operator places a sterile compress over the wound and holds it firmly in place for a few minutes. Then a sterile gauze or cotton bandage is taped over the wound, after making certain that its edges are approximated.

A biopsy can easily be performed through the same incision used for the aspiration. With the stylet in place, the operator now takes the Jamshidi biopsy needle and advances it through the incision to the periosteum a centimeter or two superior to the previous site on the iliac crest. The needle is pointed toward the anterior iliac spine (in a slight superior and lateral direction) as it is firmly pushed through the bony cortex. When decreased resistance indicates that the marrow cavity has been entered, the stylet is removed and the biopsy needle is slowly and smoothly advanced while rotating it in a clockwise-counterclockwise manner. After 2 to 3 cm. of further advance, the biopsy needle is rotated completely several times and then slowly removed while continuing a slight rotational motion. The wound is treated as described above. The probe is inserted through the distal cutting end to push the marrow core out of the biopsy needle.

The biopsy specimen, if handled gently, can be used for smears or imprints before being fixed in Zenker's acetic solution for 18 to 24 hours.

Sternal Aspiration. The same basic technique for preparation, anesthesia, and aspiration is used; of course, biopsy must not be performed in the sternum because of the danger of penetrating the inner cortex and piercing the heart or great vessels beneath.

The patient lies on his back with arms at his sides. Find the sternomanubrial prominence (angle of Louis) and, using a skin pencil, mark this with a horizontal line. Locate the jugular notch of the manubrium and mark the midline of the sternum in its long axis. The site of puncture in the body of the sternum will lie in the midline or slightly to one side of the midline, 1 to 2 cm. below the angle of Louis, opposite the second interspace. This location is recommended because it contains marrow and is rarely deformed. The outer table in that region varies from 0.2 to 3 mm. in thickness and the marrow cavity from 5 to 15 mm. in depth. The area between the costal insertions should not be used; it may be cartilaginous. The manubrium itself should be avoided because it is often more fatty than the rest of the sternum.

The University of Illinois needle is especially recommended for sternal puncture. With the stylet in place, the needle is advanced vertically, at right angles to the sternum in the midline opposite the second interspace and placed firmly on the periosteum. The guard is rotated down until it is tightly flush with the skin, then rotated back three turns. Firm pushing with only slight rotation of the needle will advance the needle into the marrow cavity; the guard will prevent its going through the inner cortex (because it allows only a 3 mm. advance from the outside of the outer cortex). (Fig. 4–45).

Aspiration is performed as described previously. Sternal aspiration should not be used in children before adolescence.

Anterior Iliac Crest Aspiration. The patient lies on his back. The puncture site is about 1 cm. below the crest posterior to the anterior iliac spine. The needle is directed slightly cephalad.

Vertebral Spinous Process Aspiration. This site has the psychologic advantage that the patient cannot see the operation. The patient sits leaning forward or lies on his side or with his face down. The lower thoracic or lumbar vertebral spinous process is punctured. More pressure is needed than for sternal puncture. The needle should be inserted slightly to the side of the middle at right angle to the skin surface.

Obtaining Marrow from Infants and Children

Tibia. This site is frequently used in infants and young children up to about two years of age. The preferable site for the puncture is the superior medial surface of the tibia, inferior to the medial condyle and medial to the tibial tuberosity.

Posterior Iliac Crest. The procedure is essentially the same as for the adult, except that a smaller needle is used. This is the most useful site for children of any age as well as adults.

PREPARATION OF THE ASPIRATE FOR EXAMINATION

Many procedures are in use and each has its advocates. The three most frequently used are: marrow films, gross quantitative study, and histologic sections.

Marrow Films. Delay, no matter how brief, is undesirable. To avoid delay in handling aspirated bone marrow, it is well to have an assistant on hand to prepare the smears. When small amounts of material are taken as suggested previously, films can be made in a similar manner as for ordinary blood counts. Gray particles of marrow are usually seen with the naked eye. They are the best material for the preparation of good films and serve as landmarks for the microscopic examination of stained smears.

Direct Films. Drops of marrow are placed on a slide a short distance away from one end. Most of the blood is sucked off with a capillary pipette, leaving the particles behind. A smear 3 to 5 cm. long is made with a spreader, not wider than 2 cm., dragging the particles behind but not *squashing* them. A trail of cells is left behind. Criteria of a good preparation: particles and free marrow cells are present.

Imprints. Marrow particles can also be used for preparation of imprints. One or more visible particles are picked up with a capillary pipette, the broken end of a wooden applicator, or a toothpick and transferred immediately to a slide and made to stick to it by a gentle smearing motion. The slide is air dried rapidly by waving and then is stained.

Crush Preparations. Marrow particles in a small drop of aspirate may be placed on a slide near one end. Another slide is carefully placed over the first. Slight pressure is exerted to crush the particles, and the slides are separated by pulling them apart in a direction parallel to their surfaces.

All smears should be dried rapidly by whipping them through the air or by exposing them to a fan.

A careful cytologic study is a good index of the composition of the marrow. Qualitative changes detected by examination of well-prepared smears of adequate marrow aspirates are, as a rule, more significant diagnostically than any amount of quantitative data. As the marrow is being spread, the appearance of fat as irregular holes in the films gives assurance that the desired material (not peripheral blood) has been obtained.

Gross Quantitative Study. This method is usually combined with the study of smears or of histologic sections. The aspirate is transferred to a Wintrobe hematocrit tube with a capillary pipette. Some or all of the visible particles are included, depending on their use for preparation of direct smears. The tube is centrifuged at high speed (2500 r.p.m.) for 10 minutes. Four layers can be distinguished in the centrifugate: fat, plasma, myeloid-erythroid (M:E) portion, and erythrocytes. Their height is recorded in percentages by reading on the scale of the tube. Normally the fat layer is 1 to 3 per cent of the total volume and the M:E layer, 5 to 8 per cent. The volumes of the plasma and erythrocyte layers vary considerably. The erythrocyte volume is generally more than the hematocrit because of shorter centrifugation. The admixture of sinusoidal blood, not an uncommon occurrence in marrow aspiration, may alter the proportions of the different fractions more or less significantly. Smears of the M:E layer may be made by aspirating this complete layer with an equal volume of plasma, mixing in a watch glass, and preparing films.

Interpretation of Quantitative Findings. High myeloid-erythroid and low fat values, in the absence of a significant peripheral leukocytosis, suggest marrow hyperplasia. Low myeloid-erythroid and high fat values suggest hypoplasia, at least of the aspirated sample. If the myeloid-erythroid layer is less than 2 per cent and fat is absent, the sample is mainly sinusoidal blood. Examination of histologic sections is an essential check on the quantitative data. Concentration by centrifugation is particularly valuable in group studies, but in the study of individual patients the use of particles and of histologic preparations is more advantageous. Dilution with sinusoidal blood may amount to 40 to 100 per cent in aspirates as small as 0.25 to 0.5 ml.

Histologic Sections. The needle biopsy and the clotted marrow particles (fragments) are fixed in Zenker's fluid, run through in one of several ways, and embedded in paraffin or celloidin. Sections provide the best estimate of cellularity and a picture of marrow architecture, but are somewhat inferior for the study of cytologic details. Another disadvantage is that particles adequate for histologic sections are not always obtained, especially in conditions in which the diagnosis depends on marrow evidence, e.g., myelofibrosis or metastatic cancer.

Berman (1953) recommended the following technique: The aspirated marrow is deposited in a paraffin-coated vial. A small amount of powdered topical thrombin is placed on a clean glass slide, dissolved in a drop of water, and allowed to dry. The marrow particles in the aspirate tend to stick to the paraffin coating. They are transferred with the broken end of a wooden applicator and placed close to each other on the thrombin-coated area on the slide. A few drops of plasma from the centrifuged aspirate are added. The plasma clots by action of thrombin. The marrow particles are included in the clot, which is transferred to a suitable fixative. The latter is changed repeatedly until it remains water clear and then run through, embedded, sectioned, and stained.

Staining of Marrow Preparations. Good fixation is essential. In some stains the fixative is included; otherwise, fixation has to be done separately.

Wright's Stain. The stain as it is used for blood smears is diluted with an equal quantity of absolute methyl alcohol. The slide is covered with a measured number of drops of the stain for 2 minutes, followed by an equal amount of buffered distilled water for 4 to 8 minutes. A longer staining time may be necessary in marrows with greater cellularity. The stain is rinsed as recommended for blood smears.

May-Grünwald-Giemsa Stain. The slide is covered with a measured number of drops of May-Grünwald stain for 2 minutes. An equal amount of buffered distilled water is added, the slide agitated for two minutes, the mixture poured off, and the slide covered with double-strength Giemsa's stain (2 drops of stock to 1 ml. buffered distilled water) for 10 to 12 minutes. The slide is rinsed in neutral distilled water until the water is clear. The slide is placed vertically and air dried.

Wright-Giemsa Stain. The technique is the same as the preceding, except that Wright's stain is substituted for May-Grünwald.

EXAMINATION OF MARROW FILMS

The ability to interpret marrow cytology can be attained only by experience. It must be regarded more as a qualitative examination than as a quantitative test. For this reason, the examiner should be informed of the clinical nature of the patient's disease.

In general, there are two ways in which a marrow film can be examined: First, by scanning several slides under low, then high dry, and finally under oil-immersion magnification; and on the basis of previous experience, one can arrive at impressions concerning the number and distribution of cells in very much the same manner as the pathologist reads his sections of tissue. Second, one can actually make a differential count of large numbers of cells (300 to 1000) and calculate the percentage of each type of cell. Finally, a combination of both methods can be used.

The second of these methods, painstaking differential counting, is an essential part of training in this work without which accuracy in the first method may be difficult to achieve. The differential count also affords an objective record from which future changes may be measured. The recognition of cell types, and particularly recognition of the maturation phase within any given series, tends to vary rather widely from one laboratory to another despite a great many efforts to standardize nomenclature with descriptions, photographs, and drawings. No average normals, or even ranges of normal, can be accepted as universal. The most valid baseline is that determined in each individual laboratory, and even then, unless "group training" is used, there may be significant variations from one examiner to another. Fortunately these limitations of the method are serious only when they are not recognized. By practice and experience laboratory workers are able to obtain gratifying practical results and establish a high degree of reproducibility in their marrow differential counts. The following procedure for the studies of marrow preparations can be recommended:

1. Naked eye inspection of the slides to select the smear-containing particles.
2. Low-power (16 mm.) survey of the particles to form a preliminary opinion whether the marrow is normoplastic, hypoplastic, or hyperplastic.
3. Selection of a cellular area, usually in the tail portion of the film around the particles, is followed by high-power and oil-immersion study of cytologic details.

The following points are particularly significant:

Cellularity. The degree of cellularity or whether the marrow is generally hyperplastic or hypoplastic is a difficult point to determine by examination of aspirated material. When this issue is crucial, we can be certain only by the study of histologic sections of aspirated particles or of material obtained by needle biopsy or surgical biopsy. If aspiration is carried out in a uniform manner, and if minimal amounts of material are withdrawn, it is possible to make useful, although rather crude, estimates of cellularity.

The cellularity (expressed as the ratio of the volume of hematopoietic cells in the marrow to the total volume of cells plus fat) normally varies with the age of the subject and the marrow site. For example, at age 50 years average cellularity in the vertebrae is 75 per cent; sternum, 60 per cent; iliac crest, 50 per cent; and rib, 30 per cent. Normal cellularity of the iliac bone at different ages has been well defined by Hartsock *et al.* (1965) (Fig. 4–47).

The report should include references to the following: description of the general cellularity, type of erythropoiesis, general maturity of the erythropoietic and leukopoietic cells, and an estimate of the M:E ratio based on a count of 500 to 1000 cells.

A differential count is useful, especially in selected cases, for example, in leukemia to follow up the effect of therapy. Examination of more slides in the time that would otherwise be spent for differential counts is usually more fruitful.

Myeloid-Erythroid (M:E) Ratio. In the normal adult the M:E ratio is about 3 or 4 to 1. This widely used term refers to differential counts from which mature granulocytes have not been excluded.

The M:E ratio at birth is 1.85 to 1. It rises rapidly soon afterward, and during the first two weeks of life it reaches the highest normal level of 11 to 1. It then gradually drops to the 1 to 20-year average of 3 to 1.

Interpretation. An *increased* M:E ratio, e.g., 6 to 1, may mean a reaction to an infection or may mean leukemia, a leukemoid reaction, or erythroid hypoplasia. A *decreased* M:E ratio, i.e., less than 2 to 1, may mean a depression of leukopoiesis or a hyperplasia of erythropoiesis. Normoblastic erythroid hyperplasia may be the result of one of the many forms of anemia or of liver diseases or polycythemia. Megaloblastic erythroid hyperplasia may be caused by a deficiency of folic acid, or vitamin B_{12}, as in pernicious anemia. A normal M:E ratio does not necessarily mean normal marrow.

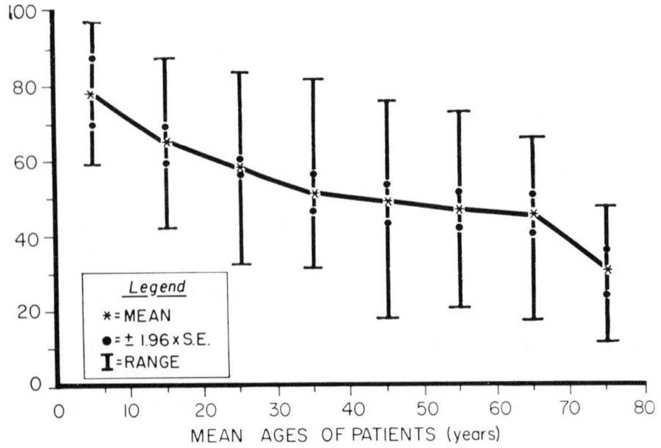

Figure 4–47. Variation in marrow cellularity with age, anterior iliac crest. Per cent cellularity on the ordinate versus age, grouped by decade, on the abscissa. (From Hartsock *et al.*: Amer. J. Clin. Path. *43*:326, 1965.)

Because of the irregular distribution of the various cell types, differential counts of nucleated marrow cells are not more than approximations. The irregularity is caused partly by the tendency of normoblasts and mature neutrophilic granulocytes and platelets to aggregate. A low-power survey of the entire smear may give the experienced examiner a more accurate picture of the relative proportions of the cells than a differential count. An estimate expressed as increased, normal, or reduced cellularity is all that is necessary for practical purposes.

One soon learns to note with some accuracy the expected 20 to 25 per cent of nucleated cells in the erythrocytic series without the necessity of making actual counts. A diminished proportion of nucleated red cells usually signifies bone marrow suppression or displacement by leukemic or other malignant cells. An increased number of nucleated red cells, usually seen in a generally hyperplastic marrow, characterizes the hemolytic anemias in which normoblasts predominate and the macrocytic anemias in which erythroblasts or megaloblasts predominate.

Marrow Differential. The data available in the literature for so-called "normal" marrow cell counts vary from investigator to investigator. One misses the generally accepted normals for the peripheral blood. The various "normal" differentials reflect the particular investigator's technique of counting and manner of interpretation. Therefore, it is best to establish one's own normals. Our own collected observations are recorded in our table of normals (Table 4–4).

Interpretation of Cytologic Findings

1. Cells normally present may be increased in numbers. This includes arrest of maturation and presence of younger cells in abnormally large numbers.
2. Eosinophil counts above 5 per cent, lymphocyte counts above 20, and plasma cell counts above 5 may be significant.
3. Cells normally absent: neoplastic cells, metastatic (cancer) or primary (multiple myeloma) cells, cells seen in storage diseases (Gaucher's disease).
4. Granulomatous lesions: tuberculosis, Hodgkin's, and sarcoidosis.
5. Parasites: malaria, histoplasmosis.

Table 4–4. MYELOGRAM

FOUND	NORMAL AVERAGE	NORMAL RANGE
Undifferentiated cells	0.0	0 – 2.0
Myeloblasts	1.6	0.4 – 5.0
Promyelocytes	4.0	1.0 – 8.0
Myelocytes:		
Neutrophilic	12.0	5.0 –19.0
Eosinophilic	1.5	0.5 – 3.0
Basophilic	0.3	0.0 – 0.3
Metamyelocytes:		
Neutrophilic	26.4	13.0 –32.0
Eosinophilic	2.0	0.5 – 3.0
Basophilic	0.3	0 – 0.3
Segmented granulocytes:		
Neutrophilic	15.4	7.0 –30.0
Eosinophilic	2.0	0.6 – 4.0
Basophilic	0.3	0 – 0.4
Pronormoblasts	0.6	0.2 – 4.0
Basophilic normoblasts	2.4	1.5 – 5.8
Polychromatic normoblasts	10.6	5.0 –20.0
Orthochromatic normoblasts	6.6	3.0 –20.0
Promegaloblasts	0	0
Basophilic megaloblasts	0	0
Polychromatic megaloblasts	0	0
Orthochromatic megaloblasts	0	0
Megakaryocytes	0.4	0.04– 2.0
Monocytes	2.0	0.4 – 4.0
Prolymphocytes / Lymphocytes	10.0	3.0 –17.0
Reticulum cells	1.0	0.2 – 3.0
Plasma cells	0.6	0 – 2.0
M:E ratio	3–4:1	
No. of cells classified		

Megakaryocytes. Because of their large size and unique appearance, these cells are readily recognized under low magnification. Since they tend to accumulate at the edges or thick end of the smear, it is best to look for them first at low magnification before proceeding to a more detailed study under the oil-immersion lens. Attempts at actual counting of megakaryocytes are usually disappointing, and even after examining several films one is usually satisfied to state that megakaryocytes appear to be present in normal numbers or that they are increased, decreased, or absent. In direct smears made from marrow aspirate of dubious quality, the distribution of megakaryocytes is so unpredictable that their decrease or absence should excite little concern unless associated with thrombocytopenic purpura, in which case more material must be obtained. Smears of selected marrow fragments are more reliable for this observation. In idiopathic thrombocytopenic purpura, megakaryocytes are usually present in normal or even in increased numbers. Qualitative changes in their appearance should be noted, although they are difficult to evaluate. It has been recommended that not less than 25 megakaryocytes be examined for such a study. Morphologic evidence of immaturity, increased size, diminished or absent cytoplasmic granulation, vacuolization or hyalinization of the cytoplasm, and absence of peripheral fragmentation or "platelet budding" have been noted by various observers in the study of thrombocytopenic disorders.

Distribution of Cell Types. In overt disease of the blood system, an abnormal distribution of cells is often immediately evident upon scanning the marrow smear. This may be true in the aleukemic leukemias, when the diagnosis is difficult or impossible by examination of peripheral blood, so that this group of diseases constitutes one of the more important indications for bone marrow aspiration. The cell pattern in pernicious anemia and other megaloblastic anemias is often helpful in diagnosis or in noting response to therapy. Other valuable uses of marrow biopsy will be discussed in relation to the various blood diseases.

Presence of Malignant Cells. In spite of the focal nature of its lesions, multiple myeloma is often diagnosed by marrow aspiration. It is less frequent, but not rare, to find other types of malignant tissue including carcinomas metastasizing to bone.

INDICATIONS FOR MARROW ASPIRATION

In the differential diagnosis of macrocytic anemia, there are some cases in which the changes in the blood are minimal, yet the marrow is megaloblastic. This is more apt to occur in folate deficiency than in untreated pernicious anemia. In these instances, of megaloblastic anemia especially, examination of the marrow may assist in recognizing the true nature of the condition.

In a variety of conditions, such as hemolytic, aplastic, and regenerative anemias, leukopenia, thrombocytopenic purpura, multiple myeloma, metastatic carcinoma, lipid storage diseases, myeloproliferative disease, splenomegaly, lymph node enlargements, in various skin lesions and in other situations, marrow examination may help to make the correct diagnosis or may exclude a primary disease of the blood.

In obscure fevers and suspected infections in which blood cultures were negative, culture of marrow aspirate may show growth of the infectious agent.

Examination of marrow is essential for correct diagnosis of *pancytopenia*. It may help to diagnose or rule out leukemia.

Examination of histologic sections prepared from particles of marrow or needle biopsy may be helpful in the recognition and diagnosis of neoplastic and granulomatous lesions of marrow, such as malignant lymphoma, metastatic carcinoma, multiple myeloma, sarcoidosis, tuberculosis, brucellosis, and histoplasmosis, and of storage diseases, e.g., Gaucher's. This method also permits one to study the architecture of marrow that is essential for the diagnosis of aplastic anemia and myelofibrosis and may not be demonstrated with the smear method. It is in most of the conditions listed in this paragraph that "dry taps" are common. In such cases needle biopsy or surgical biopsy may furnish suitable material. In experienced hands a "dry tap" or a film showing only peripheral blood is a significant finding and should arouse suspicion of bone marrow aplasia, replacement by malignant tissue, myelofibrosis, or a similar condition.

Contraindications are hemophilia and other major disturbances of coagulation.

Interpretation of the marrow may be difficult if the patient has had specific therapy (iron, liver, vitamin B_{12}, folic acid); if he has been transfused within the preceding few weeks, the diagnosis may be obscured. Bone marrow should be obtained for examination before any therapy that might alter it is given.

HAZARDS OF MARROW ASPIRATION

Complications may occur during aspiration. One should be prepared to administer intravenously a short-acting barbiturate from ready-to-use sterile ampules if the patient develops convulsions.

Death has been reported from puncture of the heart and tamponade after an overaggressive sternal puncture. Caution is essential. Indications for the procedure should be observed. Neophytes should be carefully trained and closely supervised, especially with sternal marrow puncture.

SURGICAL BIOPSY

If the marrow cannot be aspirated, needle biopsy should be performed. With proper technique, needle biopsy as described above is almost always successful except, perhaps, in osteosclerosis.

Only when needle biopsy fails will open surgical biopsy be necessary.

STUDY OF MARROW OBTAINED AT AUTOPSY

Samples of marrow should be obtained at every autopsy, but to secure useful material for imprints or smears it has to be removed within 2 hours after death. Tissue from the following sites should be obtained: a segment of a rib and sternum, a wedge of a lumbar vertebral body, and a segment of marrow removed from the midfemur. The femoral marrow is particularly useful as an indicator of response of the marrow to hematopoietic stimuli, whereas the rib, sternum, and vertebra, which contain red marrow at all ages, are sensitive indicators of damage of various kinds.

SPECIAL DIAGNOSTIC STAIN

Prussian Blue Reaction for Iron. Iron stain is useful for differentiation of anemias due to iron deficiency from anemia of thalassemia and other disorders in which iron accumulates because it cannot be utilized for hemoglobin synthesis.

PROCEDURE

1. Use only marrow smears which contain particles. A slide known to contain iron should be included as a positive control.
2. Fix slides for 10 minutes in a Coplin jar containing a filter paper moistened with two drops of 10 per cent formalin.
3. Prepare staining solution just before use by mixing 12 ml. of 2 per cent potassium ferrocyanide with 36 ml. of 1 per cent hydrochloric acid (HCl).
4. Remove filter paper and add staining solution to Coplin jar.
5. Stain for 10 minutes.
6. Rinse slides with distilled water and allow to dry.
7. Counterstain one slide with Nuclear Fast Red for 10 minutes.
8. Rinse counterstained slide with tap water and allow to dry.
9. Coverslip.

RESULT. The slide without the counterstain is most easily read for storage iron, and the slide counterstained with Nuclear Fast Red for sideroblasts (see later).

Hemosiderin and ferritin are blue; iron in hemoglobin is not stained. Report as negative or 1+ to 5+. Storage iron, which is contained in macrophages, can be evaluated only in the marrow particles on the smear. In adults, 2+ is normal, 3+ slightly increased, 4+ moderately increased, and 5+ markedly increased. Marrow hemosiderin is comparable to hemosiderin in the rest of the body.

INTERPRETATION. Storage iron in the marrow is located in macrophages. Normally a small number of blue granules are seen. None or extremely rare hemosiderin granules are seen in iron deficiency states. Storage iron is increased in infections, pernicious anemia, hemolytic anemia, hemochromatosis, hemosiderosis, hepatic cirrhosis, uremia, and cancer, and after repeated transfusions.

Sideroblasts. It is sometimes informative to determine the amount of stainable iron in normoblasts. This is performed simply by doing an iron stain on slides previously stained with Wright's stain (Sundberg and Broman, 1955) or, preferably, by counterstaining the iron stain with Nuclear Fast Red. A normoblast with stainable iron (green-blue particles) is a sideroblast. Normally with this method, about 30 to 50 per cent of the normoblasts are sideroblasts. The percentage of sideroblasts is decreased in iron deficiency anemia (where storage iron is decreased) and also in the common anemias associated with infection, rheumatoid arthritis, and neoplastic disease (where storage iron is normal or increased). The number of sideroblasts is increased when erythropoiesis is impaired for other reasons; it is roughly proportional to the degree of saturation of transferrin (Bainton and Finch, 1964).

Vital Staining

ERYTHROCYTES

Reticulocytes. In vital stains, using new methylene blue or brilliant cresyl blue dyes, the blue granules or filaments represent precipitated RNA in the reticulocyte; when air-dried films are stained with Wright's stain, staining of the RNA results in diffuse basophilia in the young red cell, and the same cell type is known as a polychromatic cell. Reticulation is a characteristic of very young erythrocytes, and the number of reticulocytes in the circulating blood is probably the best easily available index of effective erythropoiesis. An increase may be interpreted as indicating both an excessive demand for new erythrocytes and a competent bone marrow; when the demand lessens or the bone marrow fails to function, the number of reticulated erythrocytes decreases.

REAGENT. Brilliant cresyl blue or new methylene blue, 1.0 gm., is dissolved in 100 ml. of citrate saline (one part of 3 per cent sodium citrate plus four parts of 0.9 per cent sodium chloride).

PROCEDURE. Place three drops of dye solution in a small test tube, add three drops of blood, and mix. Incubate for 15 minutes at 20° C. Mix the suspension well, make two films on glass slides, and allow them to dry in air.

Viewed with the oil-immersion lens without further staining, reticulocytes have the appearance shown in Figure 4–48. The precipitated RNA is reticular or granular and stains deep blue; the red cells themselves stain paler blue or blue-green.

The proportion of erythrocytes containing reticulum or granules is calculated. As a basis for calculation, at least 1000 erythrocytes (preferably 3000) should be examined for reticulation. These should be examined on several different portions of the slide. To obviate the difficulty of examining large fields that contain a confusing number of erythrocytes, the field of vision may be made smaller by placing a metal or paper diaphragm in the oculars to show about 25 cells per field.

The Miller ocular is a convenient device which aids in the rapid counting of large numbers of red cells and, hence, the reticulocytes among them (Brecher and Schneiderman, 1950). It is a glass insert that fits into the eyepiece of the microscope and imposes a large square onto the field of view. In the corner of the large square is a smaller square equal to one-tenth the area of the large square. Traversing the slide, one counts the reticulocytes in the large square and the red cells in the small square in successive fields. At least 300 red cells should be counted in the small square, providing an estimate of reticulocytes among 3000 red cells. The calculation is:

$$\text{Reticulocytes (\%)} = \frac{\text{No. reticulocytes in large square}}{\text{No. red cells in small square} \times 10} \times 100$$

After the reticulocyte percentage has been calculated, the absolute reticulocyte count should be determined by multiplying the percentage by the red cell count.

NORMAL VALUES. Normal adults have a reticulocyte count of 0.5 to 1.5 per cent or 24,000 to 84,000 reticulocytes per microliter. In newborn infants the percentage is 2.5 to 6.5 per cent; this falls to the adult range by the end of the second week of life.

Interpretation of the reticulocyte count is discussed on p. 184.

SOURCES OF VARIATION. Because such a small number of actual reticulocytes are counted, the sampling error in the reticulocyte count is relatively large. According to Cartwright (1968), the 95 per cent confidence limits may be expressed as $R \pm 2\sqrt{\frac{R\,(100 - R)}{N}}$ where R is the reticulocyte count in per cent and N is the number of erythrocytes examined. This means that if 1000 erythrocytes are evaluated, the error expressed as ± 2 C.V. for a 1 per cent reticulocyte count is 60 per cent and, for a 10 per cent count, 19 per cent. In practical terms, this is less disturbing than it seems, since the 95 per cent confidence limits for a 1 per cent count are 0.4 to 1.6 per cent; for a 5 per cent count, 3.6 to 6.4 per cent; and for a 10 per cent count, 8.1 to 11.9 per cent. Other values may be calculated from the formula. It is important that this unavoidable sampling

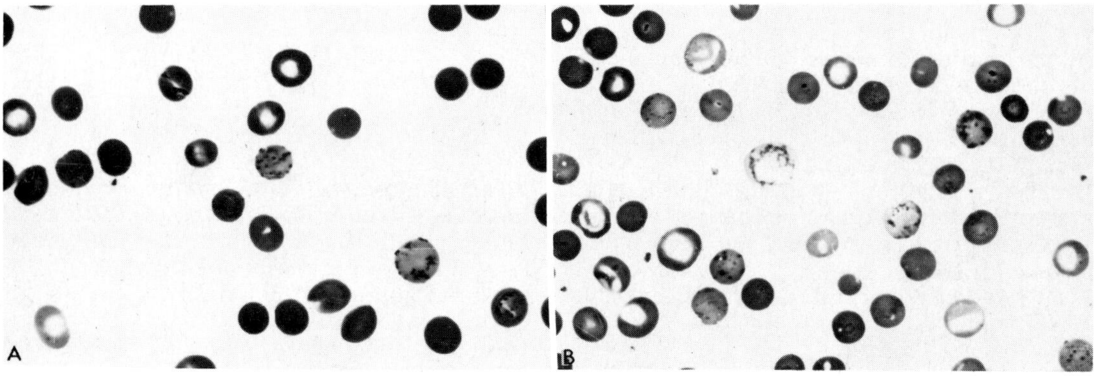

Figure 4–48. Reticulocytes; on air-dried film made after vital staining of blood with new methylene blue dye. RNA precipitates with the dye and appears as blue granules, which are sometimes connected into a network or reticulum.

variation be kept in mind when one evaluates the significance of day-to-day changes in the reticulocyte count.

In preparations made as just described, the leukocytes and thrombocytes are stained blue and the erythrocytes are blue-green. The reticulated erythrocytes often are decidedly larger than the other erythrocytes. The network and granules are stained deep blue and stand out distinctly (Fig. 4–48). The only serious source of error will be particles of stain adhering to the surface of the corpuscles. The preparations retain their color well if kept away from light.

The films also may be stained with Wright's stain, which, combined with brilliant cresyl blue, produces beautiful preparations that are very satisfactory.

Heinz Bodies. Heinz bodies are precipitates of denatured hemoglobin which characteristically attach themselves to the red cell membrane. Normally red blood cells do not contain Heinz bodies. Their presence usually means that one of the following three situations exists: (1) A drug such as phenylhydrazine, chlorate, or an aromatic nitro or amino compound has been administered in an appropriate dose to the subject (or to the red cells *in vitro*), resulting in the oxidative denaturation of hemoglobin and the formation of Heinz bodies. (2) A drug such as primaquine or one of the above drugs in a lower dosage (insufficient to affect normal red cells) has been administered to a subject who has glucose-6-phosphate dehydrogenase deficiency (or some other red cell defect resulting in a deficiency of reduced glutathione) so that the hemoglobin cannot be protected from oxidative denaturation (p. 202). (3) The subject has a hereditary defect, a hemolytic anemia associated with an unstable hemoglobin (p. 213).

Heinz bodies cannot usually be detected in Wright's stained films but can be seen with phase microscopy or with the following method:

Reagent. Methyl violet, 0.5 gm., or crystal violet, 2.0 gm., is dissolved in 100 ml. of saline and filtered.

Procedure. One volume of whole blood plus four volumes of the dye solution are incubated for 10 minutes in a small test tube. Films are then made, air dried, and examined without further staining. Alternatively, the incubation may be carried out between a slide and coverslip and examined as a wet preparation.

Result. Heinz bodies stain deep purple and vary from 1 to 4 μm. in diameter. They tend to be attached to the red cell membrane (Fig. 4–49). Reticulocytes do not stain with this dye.

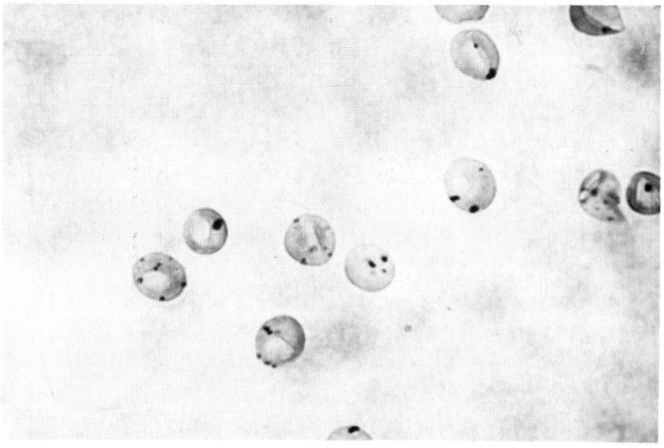

Figure 4–49. Heinz bodies. After supravital staining with methyl violet, denatured hemoglobin precipitates and tends to adhere to the cell membrane. In this instance, normal blood was incubated with acetyl-phenylhydrazine.

Hemoglobin H. Hemoglobin H is an abnormal, unstable hemoglobin composed of four beta chains (β_4). It is found in alpha-thalassemia trait in very small amounts and in hemoglobin H disease in larger amounts (Gabuzda, 1966; Weatherall and Clegg, 1972).

Reagent. Brilliant cresyl blue, 1.0 gm., in 100 ml. of citrate-saline. (See reticulocyte count, above.)

Procedure. Equal volumes of the dye solution and whole blood are placed in a small test tube, mixed, and incubated at 37° C. Films are made and air dried at 10 min., 1 hour, and 24 hours; they are examined without counterstaining.

Result. Hemoglobin H inclusions are multiple, small, pale blue, round bodies. They must be distinguished from: (1) the granules and reticular networks in reticulocytes, which are darker blue in color; and (2) Heinz bodies, which are darker blue (with this stain), larger, and often attached to the membrane.

The 10-minute sample is the control by which to gauge the number of reticulocytes. Hemoglobin H inclusions should be present at 1 hour in over half the cells in hemoglobin H disease and in a very rare cell in alpha-thalassemia trait. Heinz bodies due to unstable hemoglobins are likely to appear only later (Atwater and Schwartz, 1972).

VITAL STAINING OF LEUKOCYTES

Florence Sabin introduced a simple method for studying the leukocytes in the living condition. This method opened a fertile field for research but has not become a widely used clinical procedure.

Technique

1. Carefully clean slides and coverglasses in the following manner: Soak them in bichromate cleaning fluid three or four days, place in running water for 2 or 3 hours, separate occasionally, rinse in three or four changes of distilled water, soak overnight, and store in

80 per cent alcohol. Before use, wipe them with a clean towel and polish the slides with jeweler's rouge applied on a piece of silk.

2. Flame the slides and flood with a very dilute solution of the selected dye in absolute alcohol; drain off excess dye and place the slides upright until dry. The film must be very thin and evenly spread. Prepared slides may be stored until needed but must be kept away from dust. Many stains will serve. Sabin preferred neutral red (specify for vital staining), because it is relatively nontoxic and is also an indicator, showing the chemical reaction of the parts of the cell that take the stain. The very dilute solution that is applied to the slides is prepared by mixing 0.4 ml. of a 1 per cent solution of neutral red in absolute alcohol with 10 ml. of absolute alcohol. When it is also desired to bring out the mitochondria of the cells, 3 drops of saturated solution of Janus green in absolute alcohol may be added to each 2 ml. of the diluted solution of neutral red.

3. Receive a very small drop of blood from a puncture on a perfectly clean coverglass. Invert the coverglass on the prepared slide and immediately seal with petrolatum of high melting point or with a mixture of petrolatum and paraffin. The slide must not be cold but need not be warmed.

4. Within 10 minutes place the slide on a warm stage or preferably in a microslide incubator. Examine at once with the oil-immersion objective. Normally the corpuscles remain alive for at least an hour, sometimes for 3 or 4 hours.

Each lot of cleaned slides and each new bottle of diluted stain should be tested with normal blood to insure uniform conditions. Leukocytes are very sensitive to the least trace of acid that may be left on the slides and to an excess of the dye. Any coloring of the nucleus indicates injury to the cell.

APPEARANCE OF LEUKOCYTES. Polymorphonuclear neutrophilic leukocytes are constantly moving about because of their characteristic ameboid motion and are readily seen. Their cytoplasmic granules, which are numerous, of small size and pale red, are constantly streaming through the cytoplasm. As the leukocytes move about, the nucleus, with its several lobes, is usually in the rear part. In addition to the granules, the cytoplasm of most of these leukocytes contains one or more rounded bodies, which take the stain slowly. These are larger than the granules and are presumably digestive vacuoles, indicating phagocytic activity. They vary in color, depending on the chemical reaction of their contents. Certain leukocytes are rounded and motionless, the nucleus is structureless and nearly fills the cell, and the granules, although distinctly visible, do not take the stain. These are interpreted as dead or dying neutrophils. Their number varies at different hours; it usually is greater near the middle of the day. The number may be greatly increased by faulty technique (excessive heat, pressure of the coverglass, and so forth).

The cytoplasmic granules of *eosinophils* and *basophils* stain with the neutral red. The basophilic granules are somewhat smaller than the eosinophilic granules and differ among themselves in size and depth of staining. Digestive vacuoles are apparently absent from both cells. Eosinophils are actively motile; basophils are slightly so.

The younger *monocytes*, with oval nuclei, are rounded and practically nonmotile. Their cytoplasm contains very fine salmon-colored granules, which are grouped around a clear spot, the centrosphere. With these fine granules are a variable number of larger red bodies, apparently digestive vacuoles. The older cells, with lobulated or saddle-shaped nuclei, are more irregular in shape, usually elongated, and are sluggishly motile. The red vacuoles are usually numerous and may displace or at least obscure the fine granules.

The cytoplasm of *lymphocytes* is clear except for a few small vacuoles that take the red stain. When Janus green is added, a clump of blue mitochondria may be seen opposite the nucleus. The nucleus is oval or indented, seldom round. The large and small lymphocytes show no locomotion. Those of intermediate size move very slowly, and the nucleus is then at the front end and its shape changes.

HEMATOLOGIC CHANGES IN DISEASE

The results of hematologic examinations, forming what we call the "blood picture," are an essential part of the clinical description of practically every disease. A normal number and distribution of cells and a normal hemoglobin concentration in the blood are so important as physiologic constants that the absence of disease can scarcely be asserted until these observations have been made. That certain diseases do not produce significant changes in the blood is often a valuable point in differential diagnosis. Most hematologic changes are the result of pathologic processes not primarily affecting the blood or blood-forming tissues. The granulocytosis of acute suppurative diseases, the anemia of bleeding peptic ulcer, the lymphocytosis of whooping cough, and many other "blood pictures" constitute important diagnostic information, in each instance forming an essential part of the clinical description of the particular disease. It is evident, therefore, that clinical hematology is almost coextensive with the entire field of medical diagnosis.

By far less common are some of the so-called true blood diseases in which the first and most obvious deviations from normal are noted in the blood or blood-forming tissues. The leukemias, multiple myeloma, and some of the anemias are representative of this group. We also recognize a group of diseases which, although not primarily involving the blood system, present such conspicuous changes in the blood picture that this feature becomes the key to diagnosis and treatment. Toxic or allergic agranulocytosis, nutritional anemia, and certain forms of aplastic anemia are suitable examples of this group. In addition, the field of clinical hematology is generally defined to include the hemorrhagic diseases or those conditions in which there is disturbance of the blood-clotting mechanism. All these divisions are arbitrary and not sharply outlined. Their consideration may serve, however, to give some general notion as to the scope and meaning of clinical hematology.

Types of Hematologic Examination

Some hazard is involved in adopting a routine or set of routines for laboratory orders, since the problem of each patient must be given individual consideration. However, certain tests are used so frequently that time and effort can be saved by putting them into groups as indicated in the following paragraphs.

Routine or Screening Examinations. It is generally considered a wise policy to include a few hematologic procedures in the examination of every patient without relation to any known or suspected diagnosis. The procedures are selected with reference to the most common diseases and abnormalities. Their chief purpose is to indicate whether or not more detailed examinations are needed. Since these tests must be done on large numbers of patients and often, it is also important that they be simple and economical and consume as little time as possible. In small hospitals, an accurate hemoglobin or hematocrit, a total leukocyte count, and a differential leukocyte count with evaluation of the stained smear are usually accepted as an adequate hematologic routine. In large hospitals, the hemoglobin, hematocrit, red cell count, white cell count, and red cell indices are performed on one automated instrument and are available on every patient. The differential white cell count and evaluation of the blood film should also be performed.

Special Hematologic Procedures. Almost any of the examinations on blood may be included in the routine or ordered from time to time, depending on the type of practice being conducted and the needs of the individual patient. For example, a sedimentation rate may be used in the routine of clinics in gynecology, tuberculosis, or rheumatology where the presence or absence of systemic reactions to inflammatory processes is a very common differential point. Likewise, it may be well to perform screening tests for sickle cell hemoglobin on all black patients whether or not there are clinical suggestions of sickle cell disease. Single procedures, or groups of procedures, will be indicated by the nature and course of the patient's illness.

Complete Hematologic Examination or Consultation. If it is evident that hematologic changes are the primary or principal component of the patient's illness, or if the presence of such changes must be ruled out, the physician should seek a complete hematologic examination. In order to get the most immediate and effective study of the patient it may be necessary to ask for consultation with the clinical pathologist or hematologist. In any event, the purpose of this examination is to get the maximal amount of information concerning the blood system with as little discomfort to the patient and as little loss of time as possible. It is a matter of common experience that both the technical accuracy and diagnostic value of blood studies are improved when several observations are made at one time and, so far as possible, with a single sample of blood. There will, of course, be some selection of procedures, depending on the clinical findings, but the risk of making a few extra observations in this type of work is much less than the hazard involved in trying to piece together bits of information obtained at different times on separate samples of blood.

The Anemias

DEFINITION

Anemia is a disorder characterized by a reduction of the O_2-carrying substance in a certain volume of blood due to reduction below normal in the number of red blood cells per microliter, in hemoglobin concentration, and in hematocrit. Normal range varies with age and sex (Fig. 4–1). For practical purposes, 12 gm./dl. of hemoglobin may be accepted as the dividing line for adult females and 13.5 gm./dl. for adult males. Values below these indicate anemia.

The loss of hemoglobin and consequent

Table 4–5. MORPHOLOGIC, ETIOLOGIC, AND CLINICAL CLASSIFICATION OF ANEMIA*

TYPE OF ANEMIA	MEAN CORPUSCULAR VOLUME (fl.)	MEAN CORPUSCULAR HEMOGLOBIN CONCENTRATION (%)	CAUSE	CLINICAL SYNDROME
I. Macrocytic	>99†	>30	Deficiency of vitamin B_{12} or folic acid (megaloblastic macrocytic anemias)	Pernicious anemia Sprue Idiopathic steatorrhea Some cases of intestinal stricture or resection, gastrocolic fistula, celiac disease
			Faulty absorption	Other forms of chronic diarrhea "Tropical" nutritional macrocytic anemia Less frequently, dietary deficiency in temperate zones Rare cases of carcinoma of the stomach Following total gastrectomy
			Need outstrips supply	Macrocytic anemia of pregnancy Megaloblastic anemia of infancy *Diphyllobothrium latum* infestation "Refractory megaloblastic" and "achrestic" anemia
			Overactivity of marrow(?) (nonmegaloblastic macrocytic anemias)	Conditions usually associated with normocytic anemia, especially: Sickle cell anemia Macrocytic hemolytic anemias of obscure etiology Chronic and extensive liver disease Macrocytic anemia of hypothyroidism
			Chronic radiation effect	"Internal radiation"
II. Normocytic	83–99	>30	Sudden loss of blood	Acute posthemorrhagic anemia, including scurvy, hemophilia, and purpura
			Excessive destruction of blood (for details see Table 4–6)	Hemolytic anemia due to: Infectious, chemical, physical, vegetable, and animal agents
Spherocytes may be present			Extracorpuscular causes	Immune reactions Nonimmune reactions
The intrinsic structural abnormality may be morphologically apparent as: Spherocytosis Elliptocytosis Sickling Targeting			Corpuscular causes (intrinsic structural abnormality)	Hereditary spherocytosis
			Abnormal hemoglobin molecule	Sickle cell anemia and other hereditary hemoglobinopathies Paroxysmal nocturnal hemoglobinuria
			Specific enzyme defects	Hereditary nonspherocytic and other hemolytic anemias
			Defective blood formation	Aplastic or hypoplastic anemia, induced by: Agents that regularly produce marrow hypoplasia (ionizing radiation, mustards, antimetabolites) Agents occasionally associated with hypoplasia (antimicrobials, anticonvulsants) Unknown causes

(Table 4–5 continued on the opposite page.)

reduction in the oxygen-carrying capacity of the blood is the most conspicuous feature of anemia and is the pathologic basis for most of the associated signs and symptoms, such as dyspnea, tachycardia, weakness, and so on. Anemia, without the addition of a qualifying or descriptive term, is not a satisfactory diagnosis or a valid basis for treatment. In most instances anemia occurs as a sign or complication of disease, often remote from the blood system itself. When anemia is encountered, a careful reevaluation of the patient's condition and a search for the underlying cause are demanded (Table 4–5).

Table 4–5. MORPHOLOGIC, ETIOLOGIC, AND CLINICAL CLASSIFICATION OF ANEMIA* *(Continued)*

TYPE OF ANEMIA	MEAN CORPUSCULAR VOLUME (fl.)	MEAN CORPUSCULAR HEMOGLOBIN CONCENTRATION (%)	CAUSE	CLINICAL SYNDROME
				Chronic anemia associated with various inflammatory and noninflammatory diseases, especially renal disease, malignant disease, and chronic infections
				"Myelophthisic" anemia due to metastatic carcinoma in bone marrow, Hodgkin's disease, leukemia, multiple myeloma, myelosclerosis, and marble bone disease
				Pure red cell anemia
				Congenital pancytopenia (Fanconi)
				Congenital hypoplastic anemia (Diamond-Blackfan)
			Hydremia (?)	"Physiologic" anemia of pregnancy
III. Simple microcytic	<83‡	>30	"Imperfect" formation of blood	Subacute and chronic inflammatory diseases and chronic noninflammatory conditions
IV. Hypochromic microcytic	<83	<30	Deficiency of iron through:	
			Deficient diet	Diet deficient in foods containing iron, especially in infants
			Defective absorption	In association with achlorhydria
				Following gastrectomy (total or partial)
				Sprue, idiopathic steatorrhea, celiac disease, chronic diarrhea
			Continued loss of blood	Chronic alimentary or genitourinary tract bleeding
				Multiple hereditary telangiectasia
			Excessive demands for iron	Requirements for growth
				Repeated pregnancies
			Above causes in various degrees and combinations	Chlorosis
				Chronic hypochromic anemia of women
			Deficient antenatal storage or postnatal supply	Hypochromic anemia of infants
Target cells			Genetic anomaly	Thalassemia
				Hereditary sex-linked anemia
				Sideroblastic anemias, including pyridoxine-responsive anemia

*Modified from Wintrobe: Clinical Hematology. 6th edition. 1967. Used by permission of the author.
†The sign > indicates "greater than."
‡The sign < indicates "less than."

ERYTHROKINETICS

The balance between delivery of erythrocytes to the blood and removal of erythrocytes from the blood is maintained tenaciously and results in a relatively constant hemoglobin mass in the circulation. Anemia results when the removal of erythrocytes from the blood is increased and cannot be compensated for by increased production or when the delivery of erythrocytes or hemoglobin to the blood is decreased or when both processes exist together.

When anemia develops, the resultant tissue hypoxia leads to elevated levels of erythropoietin in the plasma. Resultant normoblastic hyperplasia produces more erythrocytes for delivery to the circulation. The marrow in a normal individual is capable of six to eight times the normal output of erythrocytes with extreme stimulation. This capacity must be compared with the output actually attained when one is evaluating the marrow response of a given patient.

Measurements that attempt to assess effective erythropoiesis (production and delivery of erythrocytes to the circulation), ineffective erythropoiesis, and destruction of erythrocytes are often necessary to determine the mechanism and the cause of anemia (Harris and Kellermeyer, 1970).

Measurements of Total Production of Erythrocytes or Hemoglobin. The *total mass of erythropoietic cells* in the body cannot be easily measured. An estimate is made by examining a sample of bone marrow from a normally active site and determining the cellularity (ratio of the volume of hematopoietic cells to the volume of fat plus hematopoietic cells compared with the normal) and the percentage of total nucleated cells that are erythropoietic (see section on bone marrow, p. 168). When marrow activity increases, usually the additional hematopoietic cells replace the fat in the red marrow sites before extension occurs into the yellow marrow of the long bones. One assumes that the sample is representative of the total marrow picture, an assumption that usually holds, but one sometimes finds exceptions.

The *plasma iron turnover* is calculated from the serum iron level and the rate of removal of injected radioactive iron from the plasma. About 25 to 30 per cent of the iron is not used in erythropoiesis and is probably taken up by the liver. The remaining 70 to 75 per cent is taken up by erythropoietic cells and is therefore a measure of total erythropoiesis, both effective and ineffective.

Measurement of Total Destruction of Erythrocytes or Hemoglobin. Determination of *fecal urobilinogen* is an estimate of the total excretion of bile pigments—the breakdown products of heme. This measurement includes pigment derived from hemoglobin formed and destroyed in the marrow without ever reaching the circulation, as well as that from the destruction of circulating erythrocytes. Limitations include diminished conversion of bilirubin to urobilinogen because of oral administration of broad-spectrum antibiotics and failure of pigment to reach the intestine in obstructive jaundice. In severe liver disease less reabsorbed urobilinogen is excreted in the bile and more is excreted in the urine. The urine urobilinogen is not so good a measure of urobilinogen excretion for two reasons: Removal by the kidney is usually a minor component of the total excretion, and with a normally functioning liver, clearance of reabsorbed urobilinogen in the plasma is so effective that considerable increases in the circulating blood may result in little or no elevation of the urine urobilinogen.

Measurement of Effective Production of Erythrocytes

Reticulocyte Count. Since the RNA of the reticulocyte disappears about a day after its entry into the blood, enumeration of reticulocytes will be a measure of the number of cells being delivered by the marrow to the blood, that is, a measure of effective erythropoiesis. The normal absolute reticulocyte count is approximately 50,000 per microliter, or 1 per cent of the circulating erythrocytes. If the erythrocyte count is determined, one can calculate the absolute reticulocyte count by multiplying the reticulocyte percentage by the erythrocyte count. To give a meaningful expression of erythropoiesis, the absolute reticulocyte count, or some estimate of it, and not simply the percentage must be used (Hillman and Finch, 1967; 1969).

A second consideration is an increased maturation time of reticulocytes in the blood due to accelerated release from the marrow, an effect of erythropoietin. The need for this is recognized by the presence of large, polychromatic cells or nucleated red cells in the blood film, indicating a shift of excessively immature reticulocytes from the marrow into the blood. An approximate correction is to assume that the reticulocyte life span has doubled.

If a patient has a Hct. = 26 per cent, red count = 2.89 million/μl., and a reticulocyte count = 7 per cent, he will have an absolute reticulocyte count = 202,000/μl. Therefore, he has $\frac{202{,}000/\mu l.}{50{,}000/\mu l.}$, or four times as many reticulocytes as normal. However, this must be corrected for the increased maturation time (shift): $4 \times 1/2 = 2$. Therefore, two times as many reticulocytes are entering his blood per day as in a normal individual; that is, his red cell production is two times normal.

If only the hematocrit is available, this same correction can be made as follows:

Correction for hematocrit:

$$\text{“absolute percentage”} = \text{reticulocyte count } (7\%) \times \frac{\text{Patient's Hct. } (26\%)}{\text{Normal Hct. } (45\%)} = 4\%$$

Correction for shift:

$$\text{Corrected reticulocyte count} = \frac{\text{Absolute reticulocyte percentage } (4\%)}{\text{Maturation time } (2 \text{ days})} = 2$$

Corrections are necessary in order to assess the degree of red cell production in response to anemia.

A normal individual with a normal supply of iron can increase red cell production by two times normal within a week if the hematocrit drops to 35 per cent, or to three times normal if the hematocrit drops to 25 per cent. Only if there is a parenteral supply of iron (such as in hemolysis) can the maximal red cell production of six to eight times normal be achieved (Hillman and Finch, 1969).

If an appropriate marrow response to anemia has not been reached in one to two weeks, we can infer that some impairment of red cell production exists.

The *erythrocyte utilization of iron* is a measure of the amount of an injected dose of iron which appears in the hemoglobin of circulating erythrocytes. It is derived from the plasma iron turnover and the percentage of radioactive iron which has been injected and which appears in the circulating erythrocytes after two weeks, assuming that none of the newly formed cells have been destroyed in that time interval. This, too, is a measure of effective erythropoiesis.

Measurement of Effective Duration of Erythrocytes in the Blood. The *erythrocyte survival* can be determined by removing a sample of blood, labeling the erythrocytes with ^{51}Cr, inactivating the excess ^{51}Cr remaining in the plasma and reinjecting the labeled erythrocytes into the patient. The ^{51}Cr is bound to the beta chain of the hemoglobin molecule and for the most part is not released until the red cell is removed from the circulation and the hemoglobin is degraded. Measurements of radioactivity in the red cells are made at 2 hours or 24 hours (the zero time, or 100 per cent level) and at 1- to 3-day intervals until over 50 per cent of the activity has disappeared. The results are usually expressed as the ^{51}Cr half survival time. The normal range is 28 to 38 days. (The reason it is not 60 days is that ^{51}Cr is eluted from the hemoglobin at the rate of about 1 per cent per day.) If the production of erythrocytes equals destruction (i.e., if a steady state exists), the erythrocyte survival is also a measure of effective production of erythrocytes.

Summary. Total erythropoiesis refers to the total production of hemoglobin or red cells; effective erythropoiesis refers to production of hemoglobin or red cells that reach the circulation; and ineffective erythropoiesis refers to production of hemoglobin or red cells that never reach the circulating blood. These concepts of the *erythrokinetic* approach to the study of anemia are useful, especially in situations that defy easy classification.

CLINICAL SIGNS OF ANEMIA

Certain clinical signs and symptoms are directly associated with anemia *per se* and are more or less independent of the particular cause. For the most part these signs and symptoms result from the diminished oxygen-carrying capacity of the blood and, therefore, are roughly proportionate to the hemoglobin concentration. It is not possible to state a critical level beyond which the vital processes are deranged, since there are always a number of factors operating at one time. Consideration must be given to the underlying disease process and its complications other than anemia, the metabolic requirements of the tissues as conditioned by the illness, the nutritional state and other factors, and the rate at which the anemia develops. When anemia develops slowly in a patient who is not otherwise severely ill, erythrocyte counts below 2,000,000 per microliter, or hemoglobin concentrations as low as 6 gm./dl. may develop without producing any discomfort or physical signs as long as the patient is at rest.

In general, the anemic patient complains of easy fatigability and dyspnea on exertion. He may complain also of faintness, vertigo, and palpitation. Headache is a common symptom. Tinnitus is occasionally mentioned. Dysphagia, ulcers on the buccal mucous membrane, and glossitis have a somewhat more specific relation to the type of anemia. The more common physical findings are pallor, a rapid pulse, low blood pressure, slight fever, some dependent edema, and systolic murmurs. In addition to these general signs and symptoms there are many clinical findings characteristic of the specific type of anemia. It is not our present purpose to discuss these in full, but the point to be emphasized is that the anemias are not laboratory diseases but are conditions in which the clinical record has both specific and differential diagnostic value.

ACUTE POSTHEMORRHAGIC ANEMIA

Definition. This anemia is due to a sudden loss of blood of whatever cause.

Blood. An increased platelet count and a shortened coagulation time are the earliest manifestations and may be demonstrable in less than an hour. The next development is a moderate leukocytosis from 10,000 to 35,000 and a shift to the left reaching the peak in 2 to 5 hours. Twenty-four to 48 hours later an outpouring of reticulocytes begins and becomes maximal four to seven days after the hemorrhage. There is a progressive decrease in serum iron. The red cell count, hemoglobin, and hematocrit are elevated immediately following hemorrhage owing to vasoconstriction and changes in blood distribution. This is followed by a drop, which persists even though the loss of blood has stopped. Dilution by tissue fluids, which compensate for the lost blood volume, is responsible for the progressive fall in hematocrit which may not reveal the full extent of the red cell loss for two days. As a rule, the anemia is normocytic and normochromic, with a normal MCV and MCH. The morphologic characteristics are only minimal anisocytosis, poikilocytosis, and achromia regardless of the severity of the anemia. Following severe hemorrhage young basophilic erythrocytes (polychromatophilia) and normoblasts appear. This may give rise to transient macrocytosis.

Regeneration following acute blood loss is progressive. The red cells return to normal levels in about four to six weeks; the hemoglobin takes about two more weeks to come back. It takes about two weeks after the blood loss for the morphologic changes to disappear and two to four days for the leukocyte count to return to normal. A persistent high reticulocyte count and leukocytosis indicate continued bleeding if an infection has been excluded.

CHRONIC POSTHEMORRHAGIC ANEMIA

When blood is lost slowly or in small quantities, the reactive mechanisms of the body are not excited; hence, both the clinical and hematologic features that characterize acute posthemorrhagic anemia are lacking. Instead of being stimulated, the hematopoietic tissues are likely to be suppressed once iron is depleted. The leukocyte count is low, the percentage of granulocytes is decreased, reticulocytes and other evidence of red cell immaturity do not appear, the serum bilirubin is normal or diminished, and there is no increase in the urobilinogen. Over a period of time the anemia of chronic blood loss becomes a chronic iron deficiency anemia. Acute episodes of hemorrhage may occur during the course of chronic blood loss, in which event certain features of the hematologic picture described in the previous section may be noted. The presence of microcytic red cells containing less than the normal complement of hemoglobin is evidence of chronic blood loss, even in the presence of signs characteristic of acute posthemorrhagic anemia. In any instance, the source and cause of the blood loss must be found if possible, since it is toward these that definitive treatment must be directed.

IMPAIRED FORMATION OF ERYTHROCYTES DUE TO DEFICIENCY OF ESSENTIAL NUTRIENTS

Iron Deficiency Anemia. When iron loss exceeds iron intake for a time long enough to deplete the body's iron stores, insufficient iron is available for the normal rate of hemoglobin production. When well developed, iron deficiency anemia is characterized by a decrease of hemoglobin and, to a lesser degree, of the hematocrit, both more marked than the decrease in the number of red cells: a hypochromic microcytic anemia.

Iron Metabolism. Iron is an essential component of hemoglobin and of other body cells. The average diet contains 5 to 15 mg. per day. The normal adult has 4 gm. of iron in the body. Over 60 per cent of the body's iron is in the hemoglobin of circulating red cells. About 1 mg. of iron is contained in each milliliter of red cells. About 3 to 4 per cent of the body's iron is present in enzymes and in myoglobin, and the rest is stored as ferritin, submicroscopic particles of iron in tissues, and as hemosiderin, larger particles of iron demonstrable microscopically. Very little iron is excreted from the body. Only a few milligrams of iron can be absorbed daily from the food, even in the presence of an iron deficiency anemia. *Transferrin*, a serum iron-binding protein, a beta globulin, transports absorbed iron. The body's iron is used again and again practically without any loss. Twenty to 25 mg. of iron are returned to the body's iron stores each day from degraded red cells and the same amount reutilized in the formation of new red cells. Less than 1 mg. of iron is lost daily in the urine, bile, and other secretions. Consequently iron deficiency results only when there is an increased need for iron (e.g., during rapid growth in infancy and childhood or during pregnancy) or when excessive loss of blood has reduced the body's reserves of iron, as following repeated hemorrhages, excessive menstruation, and multiple pregnancies. For these reasons the highest incidence of iron deficiency anemia is in women during the reproductive period of life.

In infancy and childhood, iron deficiency is probably the most common cause of anemia, especially between the ages of six and 24 months. It is caused by an amount of dietary iron insufficient to meet the needs of rapid growth. After the first four to six months of life, the iron stores of the normal infant present from birth have been exhausted, and he depends on his diet for iron. If the infant is maintained on milk and carbohydrates without supplements of iron-containing foods, he is likely to develop an iron deficiency anemia, the so called milk anemia of infancy. Defective absorption of iron and eventual iron deficiency anemia occur in most patients after total gastrectomy and in nearly half the patients after subtotal gastrectomy (Fairbanks *et al.*, 1971). Except for the sprue syndrome, other causes of malabsorption of iron are extremely rare.

The adult male has no increased physiologic demands for iron. If he had absolutely no iron intake or absorption (which would be extremely rare), his body iron stores of 1000 mg. would last for three to four years before he would even begin to become iron deficient. Therefore, almost all cases of iron deficiency anemia in adult males are due to chronic blood loss.

An understanding of the sequence of events in the development of iron deficiency anemia is helpful in interpreting intermediate stages (Harris and Kellermeyer, 1970). When iron loss exceeds absorption, absorption increases. If the negative balance continues, iron is mobilized from body stores until they become depleted. At this point *iron depletion* exists. Then iron-binding capacity (transferrin) increases and plasma-iron concentration falls. Particulate iron is no longer seen in the cytoplasm of normoblasts in the marrow, i.e., sideroblasts are absent. This is the stage of *iron deficiency without anemia.* Only then does impairment of hemoglobin formation occur, resulting in increased erythrocyte protoporphyrin and anemia. At first, this is a normocytic normochromic anemia—perhaps for several months before the marrow puts out smaller cells (microcytic normochromic anemia). Later the anemia becomes microcytic and hypochromic.

Laboratory Findings

BLOOD. In early iron deficiency anemia, the stained blood film often shows normochromic normocytic erythrocytes (Fairbanks, 1971). In later stages the picture is one of microcytosis, anisocytosis, poikilocytosis (including elliptical and elongated cells), and varying degrees of hypochromia (see p. 141). Reticulocytes are usually decreased in absolute numbers except following iron therapy. The number of red cells is rarely as low as in pernicious anemia. The hemoglobin and hematocrit may be extremely low. Osmotic fragility may be decreased because the red cells are thinner than normal (Fig. 4–13).

Chemical examination shows decreased serum iron, increased serum iron-binding capacity, and increased serum copper and erythrocyte protoporphyrin. Increases of the latter comparable to those seen in iron deficiency anemia have been reported in anemia due to heavy metal intoxication and somewhat less elevated levels in anemia of chronic infection. The white blood cell count is normal or slightly lowered. Granulocytopenia, relative lymphocytosis, and a small number of hypersegmented neutrophils may be present. Platelets may be increased, whether the iron lack is due to blood loss or dietary deficiency, but tend to be decreased in severe anemia. Achlorhydria is common.

MARROW. Normoblastic hyperplasia occurs early, but in later stages the limiting effect of severe iron deficiency restricts erythropoiesis to the basal level. The normoblasts are smaller than normal, deficient, and irregular in shape with frayed margins. Smears stained for iron show sideroblasts and storage iron to be absent.

Laboratory Diagnosis. In many cases, the diagnosis of iron deficiency in a patient with hypochromic microcytic anemia is readily made on clinical grounds. When the diagnosis is not clear, differentiation must be made from other hypochromic microcytic anemias.

SERUM IRON. The normal range is from 75 to 150 μg. of iron per 100 ml. of serum. Lower levels are presented in iron deficiency but may be seen also in chronic infections and a number of other chronic diseases.

SERUM IRON-BINDING CAPACITY. This determination helps to distinguish iron deficiency from the other conditions with low serum iron. In iron deficiency anemia, the serum iron-binding capacity is increased. It is decreased in the other conditions with low serum iron. If, however, chronic infection coexists with chronic blood loss, the serum iron-binding capacity may not be increased, even though the patient is iron deficient. The normal total serum iron-binding capacity is 250 to 400 μg. per 100 ml.

STORAGE IRON IN MARROW. Hemosiderin in marrow is a sensitive indicator of iron deficiency. The diagnosis is established if no stainable iron is found in good preparations stained for the Prussian blue reaction.

THERAPEUTIC TRIAL. A reticulocyte response to oral or parenteral administration of iron occurs in iron deficiency and is proportional to the severity of the anemia. The degree of reticulocytosis is less in iron deficiency anemia responding to iron therapy than it is in megaloblastic anemia responding to specific therapy.

DIFFERENTIAL DIAGNOSIS. Thalassemia is distinguished by normal or elevated serum iron, normal serum iron-binding capacity, increased storage iron in the marrow, increase in hemoglobin A_2 or F, and the presence of the condition in family members.

Simple chronic anemia (in chronic infection, rheumatoid arthritis, or neoplastic disease) may be hypochromic and microcytic and shows low serum iron, normal or low serum iron-binding capacity, and decreased sideroblasts but increased storage iron in the marrow.

Sideroblastic anemia may be hypochromic and microcytic, but usually is dimorphic, with a second population of normocytic or macrocytic cells. Serum iron is elevated and there is a striking increase of sideroblasts and storage iron in the marrow. Some sideroblastic anemias are responsive to pyridoxine; these may show abnormal tryptophan derivatives in the urine.

Hypochromic anemia in chronic plumbism is caused by the injurious effect of lead on heme synthesis. Basophilic stippling is evident. Pronounced increase of aminolevulinic acid and coproporphyrin III in the urine is characteristic of lead poisoning, but increased levels of lead in urine and blood are required for definitive diagnosis.

Macrocytic and Megaloblastic Anemia. Macrocytic anemias which are not megaloblastic may be due to early release of erythrocytes from the marrow, as in response to acute blood loss or hemolysis; this is a "shift" macrocytosis since it results from a premature release of reticulocytes from the marrow (Finch, 1969). Macrocytosis without reticulocytosis may also be seen in liver disease, some aplastic or refractory anemias, or hypothyroidism.

Macrocytic anemias associated with megaloblastic changes in the bone marrow have certain morphologic differences from nonmegaloblastic macrocytic anemias in the peripheral blood (Chanarin, 1969; Hoffbrand, 1971). The finding of macro-ovalocytes and giant hypersegmented neutrophils is distinctive of megaloblastic anemia.

Megaloblastic anemia is characterized by enlargement of all rapidly proliferating cells of the body. Both nucleus and cytoplasm are enlarged, but the increase is more pronounced in the cytoplasm. The major cellular abnormality appears to be the diminished capacity of the cells to synthesize DNA.

The cells have both a prolonged intermitotic resting phase and a block early in mitosis. The number of mitotic figures is increased. RNA synthesis is less impeded than is DNA synthesis; hence, cytoplasmic maturation and growth continue, accounting for enlargement of the cells. In the bone marrow, hemoglobin appears at an unusually early stage in the erythroid cells, as judged by nuclear maturation. The delicate, finely reticulated chromatin and the prominent parachromatin result in a distinctly more "open" chromatin pattern than is seen in the normoblastic series. The nuclei undergo karyorrhexis readily, and multiple Howell-Jolly bodies may be present. Basophilic stippling is frequently seen. There are relatively more cells analogous to the pronormoblast and basophilic normoblast (i.e., the promegaloblast and basophilic megaloblast) than are seen in normal erythropoiesis. This has sometimes been termed "maturation arrest," or nuclear cytoplasmic asynchrony. Giant polychromatic megaloblasts are especially distinctive. The same general features are seen in the other cell lines. In the granulocytic series, the cells are larger, with retarded nuclear maturation and large cytoplasmic mass; often the specific granules themselves are distinctly larger. The chromatin pattern is less condensed (more "open") and, as a result, the nucleus appears to stain poorly. Abnormally contorted nuclear configurations are common. The giant metamyelocyte is the most characteristic of the abnormal granulocytes. Megakaryocytes, too, are large and have abnormally pronounced nuclear segmentation and often fragmentation.

All these features characterize the *morphologic entity* of megaloblastic anemia.

The *etiology* of megaloblastic anemia is almost always vitamin B_{12} or folic acid deficiency.

Classification of Megaloblastic Anemia

VITAMIN B_{12} DEFICIENCY. Vitamin B_{12} (cyanocobalamin) has a molecular weight of 1355 gm. per mole. The molecule's two major parts are (1) a "planar group" (the corrin nucleus), a ring structure surrounding a cobalt atom, and (2) a "nucleotide" group, which consists of the base, 5,6-dimethylbenzimidazole, and a phosphorylated ribose esterified with 1-amino, 2-propanol. A cyanide group is in coordinate linkage with the trivalent cobalt. Different forms of vitamin B_{12} result from replacement of the cyanide by hydroxy, aquo, or nitro groups.

Vitamin B_{12} is unique in that it is the only vitamin exclusively synthesized by microorganisms. It is found in practically all animal tissues. It is stored primarily in the liver. The human liver contains approximately 1 to 2 μg. per gm. of liver. Vitamin B_{12}, in its coenzyme form, is released by digestion of proteins of animal origin and then is bound by gastric intrinsic factor (I.F.), which is essential for absorption. This vitamin B_{12}-I.F. complex then adheres to specific receptor sites on the epithelial cells of the ileum, at which site the vitamin B_{12} is absorbed. The daily requirement is in the range of 2 μg. per day. Since the liver contains 1 to 2 μg. per gm. of tissue, the body's vitamin B_{12} stores will last for from three to six years if intake is cut off, as is the case if total gastrectomy is performed.

Vitamin B_{12} deficiency is produced by any of several mechanisms.

Inadequate Intake. A dietary deficiency is an *extremely rare* cause of megaloblastic anemia and is seen only in persons who completely abstain from animal food, including milk and eggs. For example, strict vegetarians are known to develop this form of vitamin B_{12} deficiency.

Defective Production of Intrinsic Factor. This is the most common cause of vitamin B_{12} deficiency.

PERNICIOUS ANEMIA (PA). Pernicious anemia is a "conditioned" nutritional deficiency of vitamin B_{12} which is caused by a failure of the gastric mucosa to secrete intrinsic factor. This abnormality is genetically determined but usually is not manifested until late in life.

Clinical Features. The disorder is equally common in males and females. Anorexia, malaise, weakness, shortness of breath, and the combination of skin pallor and jaundice giving a lemon-yellow appearance of the skin are often present. The tongue may be sore, smooth, and pale (atrophic glossitis) or red and raw (acute glossitis). Three systems are commonly involved: *Gastrointestinal symptoms* may be prominent and include episodic abdominal pain, constipation, and diarrhea. Diffuse and irregular degeneration of the white matter of the *central nervous system* characteristically involves the posterior and lateral columns of the spinal cord (subacute combined degeneration) and sometimes other sites. Symmetrical sensations of "pins and needles" of the distal extremities, numbness and tingling, loss of position sensation (difficulty with balance and gait), and loss of vibratory sensation (perhaps the most constant sign) are indicative of posterior column lesions. Lateral column involvement gives rise to weakness, spasticity, and increased deep tendon reflexes. Sometimes, in advanced cases, the brain may be affected, and the patient shows irritability, emotional instability, or a change in personality; the term "megaloblastic madness" has sometimes been applied to the latter.

Peripheral Blood. The *hematopoietic* is the third system involved. Pancytopenia (a decrease in all the formed elements of the blood) is the rule. The anemia is macrocytic with an elevated MCV and is characterized by macro-ovalocytes and often extreme degrees of anisocytosis and poikilocytosis. Microcytes and teardrop forms are common. Basophilic stippling, multiple Howell-Jolly bodies, nucleated red cells with karyorrhexis, and even megaloblasts may be seen. Leukopenia is present. Giant macropolycytes, or PA neutrophils, have increased numbers of lobes, presumably a result of abnormal nuclear maturation and large neutrophilic granules. Thrombocytopenia is usually encountered and on rare occasions is sufficiently severe to be responsible for bleeding. It is worth noting that significant morphologic changes may occur in the blood in the absence of anemia and also that neurologic symptoms may be present in the absence of anemia (Figs. 4–14, 4–16, 4–26, 4–29, 4–33, 4–39, 4–63, 4–64, and 4–65).

Bone Marrow. The bone marrow is hyperplastic. The fat is replaced, and red marrow extends into the long bones. The number of erythroid precursors (megaloblasts) is increased. Instead of the normal myeloid-erythroid ratio of 3 to 1, the ratio is more likely to approach 1 to 1. The cytologic changes have been described. If the megaloblastic process is incompletely developed, or if the patient has been inadequately treated, the findings may be only partial. Since they persist longer, the granulocytic alterations are especially helpful in assessing partially treated megaloblastic anemia. The marrow findings are due to the effects of the vitamin B_{12} deficiency on nucleic acid synthesis (DNA synthesis impeded more than RNA synthesis) and to hypoxic stress, giving rise to increased numbers of erythroid cells. If the patient is transfused with packed red cells, the number of erythroid precursors diminishes but the cytologic abnormalities persist.

Stomach. The chief cells of the stomach secrete pepsinogen. In man both intrinsic factor and HCl are secreted by parietal cells. Gastric atrophy involving all coats of the wall (a paper-thin stomach) is found in approximately 40 per cent of cases; the remainder show varying degrees of atrophic gastritis. It is generally held that these are successive stages of the same process. Except for the few patients with juvenile pernicious anemia who have free acid secretion but no intrinsic factor, adult patients with pernicious anemia have histamine-refractory achylia and achlorhydria—a decreased volume of gastric juice and a total lack of acid secretion. It must be remembered here that a small proportion of hematologically normal persons over the age of 60 have histamine-fast achlorhydria but usually not achylia.

Historical Observations. Addison's name has been linked with pernicious anemia because of his clinical description of the disease in 1855. The term pernicious anemia reflected the inevitable fatal outcome. Gastric atrophy was later noted on autopsy of these patients.

Whipple's observations that liver was a particularly effective food to induce hemoglobin production in dogs led Minot and Murphy to feed raw liver in huge amounts to patients with pernicious anemia. Their success and their recognition of the importance of the gastric lesion won them a Nobel prize and led Castle to his classic experiments, which defined the extrinsic factor and the intrinsic factor.

Castle used the daily reticulocyte count to assess the effectiveness of his therapeutic efforts. For 10 days he gave beef and normal human gastric juice, 12 hours apart, and got no reticulocytosis. Then, for a succeeding 10-day period, he gave the beef and normal human gastric juice together and achieved a reticulocyte response. He reasoned that for effective erythropoietic activity the interaction of an extrinsic factor (beef) and an intrinsic factor (in normal gastric juice) was essential.

Later, vitamin B_{12} was crystallized (1948), and after enormous effort its structure was determined (1955). Vitamin B_{12} experimentally was shown to be identical to Castle's extrinsic factor. Intrinsic factor is a mucoprotein secreted by the parietal cells of the stomach. It binds vitamin B_{12} and facilitates its absorption in the ileum.

Erythrokinetics in Pernicious Anemia. As previously noted, the mass of erythroid tissue in the marrow is increased. The plasma iron turnover is very rapid, with uptake in the marrow. From the marrow the iron does not move into the circulating red cells but to the liver instead. Fecal urobilinogen is usually increased. Thus, measures of total erythropoiesis indicate an *increase* of up to three times normal.

In untreated pernicious anemia, in addition to poor RBC utilization of iron, the reticulocyte count is low and the survival of circulating erythrocytes is shortened. The effective erythropoiesis is below normal. Since total erythropoiesis is increased, this implies that a great deal of the erythropoietic activity is *ineffective*. This has also been directly shown with glycine-^{15}N studies.

Diagnosis of Pernicious Anemia. The symptoms are nonspecific, except that evidence of CNS involvement is highly suggestive of the diagnosis.

Laboratory Findings.

1. Blood and marrow evidence of megaloblastosis.
2. Histamine-fast achlorhydria and achylia (gastric juice).
3. Evidence of vitamin B_{12} deficiency.

Microbiological assay of serum vitamin B_{12} employs the organism *Euglena gracilis,* which requires vitamin B_{12} for growth (Anderson, 1964).

A radioisotope dilution technique gives more rapid results, which are comparable to the Euglena assay. One uses $^{57}CoB_{12}$, a standardized intrinsic factor preparation, and albumin-coated charcoal (Lau *et al.,* 1965). By either method, the normal serum B_{12} level is 200 to 900 pg. per ml.

Measurement of urinary methylmalonic acid: Since a vitamin B_{12} coenzyme is essential for the isomerization of methylmalonate, excretion of increased amounts of methylmalonate in the urine is found in vitamin B_{12} deficiency. This is a sensitive test, provided the inborn error of metabolism, methylmalonic aciduria, is not present. Thin-layer chromatography, gas chromatography, or colorimetric methods are available (Hoffbrand, 1971).

Demonstration of a typical reticulocyte response and clinical response with administration of physiologic doses of vitamin B_{12} (parenteral, 1 μg. per day): The reticulocytes begin to rise on about the fourth day and reach a peak somewhere between the seventh and tenth days, at which time the hemoglobin and number of red blood cells have begun to rise on their way back to normal levels. This shows that vitamin B_{12} deficiency was responsible for the anemia.

4. Demonstration that the patient lacks intrinsic factor.

Several methods have been used for the *in vitro* assay of intrinsic factor activity in the gastric juice (Yamaguchi and Glass, 1967). These remain research procedures and are not available in most laboratories.

In vivo determination of the ability of the patient to absorb an oral dose of radioactive vitamin B_{12} has become standard practice in the diagnosis of pernicious anemia. This can be done in several ways—measuring fecal excretion, hepatic uptake, urinary excretion, plasma uptake, or even whole body counting. The most convenient is the Schilling test, the measurement of radioactivity in a 24-hour sample of urine (See p. 480). Two hours after oral administration of 0.5 to 2.0 μg. of radioactive vitamin B_{12}, a large "flushing" dose of nonlabeled vitamin B_{12} is given parenterally. Normal individuals will excrete somewhere between 5 and 40 per cent of a 1μg. dose of ingested vitamin B_{12} in the urine in 24 hours, whereas patients lacking intrinsic factor excrete less than 3 per cent. The crucial and integral part of this test is repetition, using oral vitamin B_{12} plus intrinsic factor and showing that this brings the patient's absorption of vitamin B_{12} into the normal range. The validity of the results depends upon good renal function and an accurate urine collection. The determination of whether the patient has intrinsic factor activity in his gastric juice is the one finding that is demonstrable both in remission and relapse.

5. Serum antibody studies (Hoffbrand, 1971).

Two types of autoantibodies have been found in the serum of patients with pernicious anemia. One reacts with gastric parietal cells and is present in 80 to 90 per cent of patients who have been tested. This parietal cell antibody is also present in patients with chronic gastritis, such as that associated with iron deficiency, in some patients with thyroiditis and myxedema, and it may be present in healthy controls, especially in older age groups. This is a nonspecific finding that probably indicates the presence of gastritis. The other autoantibodies are directed against intrinsic factor. Sixty per cent of patients with pernicious anemia have in their serum anti-intrinsic factor antibodies of the "blocking" type (which block the binding of intrinsic factor to B_{12}) with or without the "binding" type (which inhibit the binding of intrinsic factor to the ileal mucosa). Intrinsic factor antibodies in the absence of PA have not been found, except in hyperthyroidism (Graves' disease), where the incidence is 3 to 6 per cent, and in a similar percentage of insulin-dependent diabetics. There appears to be an immunologic relationship of some kind between stomach and thyroid.

Family studies in patients with pernicious anemia have shown an increased incidence of the disease in relatives, and many relatives have achlorhydria and partial defects of vitamin B_{12} absorption. Relatives of patients with pernicious anemia also have a higher incidence of gastric parietal cell antibodies and of thyroid antibodies than normal.

Studies such as these have led to the suggestion that adult pernicious anemia may be a genetically determined autoimmune gastritis. This hypothesis is supported by the fact that in some adult patients, in relapse, administration of prednisolone has resulted in return of chief cells and parietal cells in gastric mucosa, return of intrinsic factor and HCl production, improvement in vitamin B_{12} absorption, a hematologic response, and some decrease in the level of antibody to intrinsic factor.

Therapy of Pernicious Anemia. Parenteral injection of vitamin B_{12} at regular intervals is the therapy of choice. The maximal reticulocyte response occurs in seven to 10 days. Within 4 to 6 hours after the initial injection, the bone marrow shows a decrease in the number of early megaloblasts and the appearance of normal pronormoblasts. Progressive change toward normal occurs so that by two to four days the marrow is predominantly normoblastic. Of help to the hematologist in partially treated patients is the fact that the cytologic abnormalities in the granulocytes return to normal more slowly than do those in the erythroid cells. Patients with pernicious anemia can be kept in complete remission with monthly parenteral injections of vitamin B_{12}.

It is extremely important to recognize that treatment with large doses of folic acid (pharmacologic doses of 5 to 15 mg. per day) will provide a hematologic response in patients with vitamin B_{12} deficiency while failing to effect any improvement in the neurologic lesions. This is important because failure to recognize that a patient has pernicious anemia may be due to masking of the diagnosis by folic acid therapy; this allows the neurologic complications to progress to an irreversible stage.

Let us return to our classification of vitamin B_{12} deficiency.

Defective Production of Intrinsic Factor

GASTRECTOMY. Surgical removal of the stomach (total or even subtotal occasionally) will remove the source of intrinsic factor. This will lead to clinical and laboratory findings almost identical with those of PA after the body's stores of vitamin B_{12} have been exhausted, in three to six years.

Defective Absorption of Vitamin B_{12}

MALABSORPTION SYNDROMES. Celiac disease, tropical sprue, resection of small bowel, or inflammatory disease of the small bowel may be associated with multiple defects of absorption, including other vitamins. Folic acid deficiency (absorbed principally in the upper small bowel) is more commonly seen than vitamin B_{12} deficiency (absorbed principally in the lower small bowel) in diseases leading to malabsorption. The reason for this is probably the lesser time necessary for depletion of body stores of folic acid.

Extremely rare cases have been reported in which there is specific intestinal failure of absorption of vitamin B_{12} in the presence of normal intrinsic factor.

LACK OF AVAILABILITY OF VITAMIN B_{12}. In certain countries infestation with the fish tapeworm (*Diphyllobothrium latum*) is common enough so that vitamin B_{12} deficiency may occur occasionally when it is present. The worm successfully competes with the host for the ingested vitamin B_{12}. Most common in Finland, it is rarely seen in the United States.

Bacteria in a blind-loop of intestine may also preferentially utilize ingested vitamin B_{12} to the detriment of the host.

In all these latter conditions, due to malabsorption or lack of availability of vitamin B_{12}, the Schilling test will show lack of absorption of vitamin B_{12} which is not corrected by intrinsic factor.

FOLIC ACID DEFICIENCY (Hoffbrand, 1971; Streiff, 1970). Folic acid deficiency may also be produced by any of several mechanisms. Folic acid is present in a wide variety of foods, such as eggs, milk, leafy vegetables, yeast, liver, and fruits, and also is formed by bacteria in the intestines. It is almost impossible to achieve a diet deficient in folic acid. The daily requirement is about 50 μg. in adults. Dietary folic acid deficiency produced in normal man (Herbert, 1962) has elucidated the sequence of events in the onset of folate-deficient megaloblastic anemia. After initiating the folate-deficient diet, the various abnormalities were established as follows: 3 weeks, low serum folate; 11 weeks, hypersegmentation of neutrophils; 13 weeks, high excretion of formiminoglutamic acid (FIGLU) in urine; 17 weeks, low erythrocyte folate; 18 weeks, macro-ovalocytosis of erythrocytes; 19 weeks, megaloblastic bone marrow; 19 to 20 weeks, anemia.

At this time, changes in the intestinal epithelium had not yet appeared. Therefore, in man, with no dietary intake of folic acid, anemia will appear in three to six months. The peripheral blood and bone marrow features of megaloblastic anemia due to folic acid deficiency are similar to those of vitamin B_{12} deficiency; however, leukopenia and thrombocytopenia are less constant. Folic acid deficiency has usually been found in association with some complicating factor.

Classification of Folic Acid Deficiency

INADEQUATE INTAKE OF FOLIC ACID

Megaloblastic Anemia of Infancy. Megaloblastic anemia of infancy is rare in the U.S.A. because it is associated with general malnutrition. It occurs more readily when infections or diarrhea increases the folate requirements.

Megaloblastic Anemia in Pregnancy. Megaloblastic anemia in pregnancy is not uncommon, because of the fetal requirements for folate. The mother's plasma folate level gradually falls during pregnancy, and at birth the plasma level in the newborn averages five times that of the mother. Megaloblastic anemia is more frequent in multiparae, may be precipitated by infection, and is usually due to folate deficiency rather than B_{12} deficiency. A legitimate case can be made for prophylactic supplementation of the diet during pregnancy with oral folic acid.

Nutritional Megaloblastic Anemia. Nutritional megaloblastic anemia is found particularly in the tropics and in India, and even there it is usually associated with increased demand for folate as in pregnancy, rapid growth in infancy, infection, or hemolytic anemia. Elderly persons on inadequate diets in this country have developed folate-deficient megaloblastic anemia, a fact increasingly recognized in recent years.

Liver Disease. Liver disease associated with alcoholism may lead to folate-deficient megaloblastic anemia because of the grossly inadequate diet of the alcoholic. With an adequate dietary folic acid intake, however, the anemia that is found with liver disease is macrocytic and normoblastic, not megaloblastic.

DEFECTIVE ABSORPTION OF FOLIC ACID. Defective absorption of folic acid occurs in association with malabsorption syndromes discussed above and in the blind-loop syndrome, in which bacteria preferentially utilize folate.

INCREASED REQUIREMENTS FOR FOLIC ACID. The increased need in pregnancy and in infants (multiple birth) has been mentioned. The increased cell turnover that occurs in neoplasia or in the markedly stimulated hematopoiesis of hemolytic anemias may result in megaloblastic erythropoiesis. The basis for this is increased need and a marginal supply of folate.

INADEQUATE UTILIZATION OF FOLIC ACID. Inadequate utilization of folic acid is relatively rare but applies in certain cases.

Folic acid antagonists, such as methotrexate, block folic acid metabolism and because of this are used in therapy of some malignant neoplasms. In addition to inhibiting the growth of the tumor, they will also induce megaloblastic erythropoiesis.

Some anticonvulsants (e.g., diphenylhydantoin and pyrimethamine, which is used in the therapy of malaria) have antifolate effects.

In addition to the previously mentioned nutritional problem in alcoholics, *alcohol* may exert a direct effect in suppressing hematopoiesis by blocking metabolism of folate.

Diagnosis of Folic Acid Deficiency. Folic acid deficiency or vitamin B_{12} deficiency is suspected when the blood and bone marrow show findings characteristic of megaloblastic anemia; usually tests of serum folate and B_{12} levels are then performed.

SERUM AND RED CELL FOLATE. A microbiologic assay for folic acid activity employing *Lactobacillus casei* has been most widely used, but a radioisotopic assay has become available (Waxman *et al.*, 1971). Low serum folate levels precede the development of low red cell levels in the development of folate deficiency. The normal serum level is in the range of 7 to 16 ng. per ml. The level is decreased in folate deficiency and normal in vitamin B_{12} deficiency.

URINARY FORMIMINOGLUTAMIC ACID (FIGLU). Folic acid coenzymes are required for the conversion of FIGLU to glutamic acid in the catabolism of histidine. When oral histidine is given, FIGLU will appear in increased amounts in the urine if folate deficiency is present. However, its value in discriminating between vitamin B_{12} and folate deficiency is lessened by the fact that many patients (50 per cent) with pernicious anemia who are not deficient in folic acid have increased FIGLU excretion.

THERAPEUTIC TRIAL. The therapeutic trial remains an excellent way to discriminate between folic acid and vitamin B_{12} deficiency. Physiologic doses of folic acid (parenteral, 50 to 200 μg. per day) will allow an adequate reticulocyte response in patients with folic acid deficiency, but not in vitamin B_{12} deficiency. Physiologic daily doses of vitamin B_{12} (parenteral, 1 to 5 μg. per day) will lead to hematologic response in patients with vitamin B_{12} deficiency and not folic acid deficiency.

On the other hand, the usual therapeutic doses of folic acid (5 to 15 mg. per day) or larger doses of vitamin B_{12} (500 to 1000 μg.) may induce a partial response in any patient with megaloblastic anemia.

The therapy of pernicious anemia with folic acid sufficient to lead to a hematologic response (5 to 15 mg. per day) must be condemned because of the danger of allowing subacute combined degeneration of the cord to progress.

OTHER DEFECTS OF NUCLEOPROTEIN SYNTHESIS. Other defects of nucleoprotein synthesis may very rarely lead to megaloblastic anemias which do not respond to vitamin B_{12} or folic acid.

Congenital Defects. Oroticaciduria is a very rare autosomal recessive condition in which certain enzymes required for pyrimidine synthesis are absent. The findings are excessive urinary excretion of orotic acid, failure of normal growth and development, and megaloblastic anemia which is refractory to vitamin B_{12} and folate but which responds to uridine.

Synthetic Inhibitors. Synthetic inhibitors of purine metabolism (6-mercaptopurine, thioguanine) or of pyrimidine metabolism (5-fluorouracil) are used in chemotherapy for neoplasia and may concomitantly produce megaloblastosis.

IMPAIRED FORMATION OF ERYTHROCYTES NOT DUE TO DEFICIENCY OF ESSENTIAL NUTRIENTS

Anemia of Chronic Disorders. The anemia most commonly seen in chronic infections and chronic systemic disease is usually mild and is overshadowed by the basic disease. Occasionally the basic disease may be obscured by the anemia. This mild "simple chronic anemia" associated with chronic infections, rheumatoid arthritis, and neoplastic disease does not progress in severity and has characteristic morphologic, biochemical and kinetic disturbances (Cartwright, 1966; Cartwright and Lee, 1971).

Blood. The erythrocytes are usually normocytic and normochromic, but they are often normocytic and hypochromic and occasionally microcytic and hypochromic. As the anemia develops, hypochromia usually precedes the development of microcytosis; this is in contrast to iron deficiency anemia, in which the reverse is true. Anisocytosis and poikilocytosis are slight. The reticulocyte count is usually not elevated. Leukocytes and platelets are not distinctively altered, except by the causative disease.

Marrow. The marrow is normocellular or minimally hypocellular or hypercellular, and the cell distribution is not greatly disturbed. The normoblasts may have frayed hypochromic cytoplasm and the appearance of hemoglobin in the cells may be delayed (as in iron deficiency anemia). Sideroblasts are decreased, but storage iron is normal or increased.

Biochemical Features. The serum iron is characteristically decreased, the total iron-binding capacity (TIBC) is decreased or normal (in contrast to iron deficiency anemia where the TIBC is elevated), and the per cent saturation is somewhat decreased. Erythrocyte protoporphyrin is elevated.

Erythrokinetics. Red cell production, though normal or even slightly increased, is insufficient to compensate for a moderately decreased red cell survival. In these patients, erythropoietin can be produced with other types of stimulation (e.g., cobalt), and the marrow is capable of responding to erythropoietin; but for unknown reasons, this anemia fails to induce erythropoietin production.

The defect in iron metabolism is principally a block in the movement of iron from the storage sites in the reticuloendothelial cells to the erythroid marrow; this results in the low serum iron and in an iron-deficient type of erythropoiesis, despite the presence of adequate storage iron. The anemia usually fails to respond to therapy with iron or other measures; spontaneous improvement will occur when the underlying disorder is corrected.

The abnormalities are characteristic of a large number of anemias secondary to systemic disease. Cartwright (1966) has proposed the term "sideropenic anemia with reticuloendothelial siderosis" as more descriptive than "simple chronic anemia" for a condition that is not simple and that is not always chronic.

Anemia of Renal Insufficiency. A direct correlation between the severity of the anemia and the degree of elevation of the blood urea nitrogen has been described but does not always hold.

Several factors are often involved in the anemia of chronic renal failure (Erslev, 1972). Decreased production of erythropoietin by the damaged kidney is probably a factor in most cases in which the blood urea nitrogen exceeds 100 mg./dl. Even with complete loss of kidney function (e.g., bilateral nephrectomy) there is a basal level of erythropoiesis; it is not known whether this is the result of extrarenal erythropoietin production. Both ineffective erythropoiesis and impaired ability of the marrow to respond to erythropoietin appear to be present in some degree.

Hemolysis is a significant feature in many cases of chronic renal failure. There appears to be an extracorpuscular factor in uremic plasma which has a detrimental effect on red cell metabolism and results in morphologically deformed cells (irregularly contracted and spiculated red cells, the so-called burr cells). Numerous irregularly contracted and fragmented cells are seen in malignant hypertension as a result of traumatic damage incurred by the red cells in traversing the damaged small blood vessels (Brain *et al.*, 1962).

In addition, bleeding is a common problem in chronic renal disease, probably due either to thrombocytopenia, in some patients, or to platelet functional defects, which are present in most patients. Anemia due to iron deficiency from blood loss should always be suspected. Folic acid deficiency may be a problem in patients in a dialysis program, since folic acid is readily moved into the dialysis bath.

Anemia of Liver Disease. Chronic posthemorrhagic anemia, folate-deficient megaloblastic anemia due to poor nutrition in chronic liver disease, and acquired hemolytic anemias associated either with Coombs' positive red cells, congestive splenomegaly, or lipid disturbances (Zieve's syndrome) may occur in liver disease. In addition to these, there is an anemia associated with liver disease which is characterized by increased red cell destruction and relatively inadequate red cell production. It is exaggerated by an increased blood volume. The red cells are normocytic or macrocytic (thin macrocytes). Frequently target cells are present, especially in obstructive jaundice. (See p. 144.) Reticulocytes may be slightly increased, and platelets are low normal or decreased. The bone marrow may be slightly hypercellular and erythropoiesis is macronormoblastic rather than megaloblastic. Changes in leukocytes, such as are present in megaloblastic anemias, are not seen, and this type of anemia does not respond to vitamin B_{12} or folic acid. The anemia is of unknown origin.

A few patients with severe cirrhosis have a hemolytic anemia associated with "spur cells," which are red cells with thorny projections similar to acanthocytes. As with target cells, the spur cells are secondary to lipid abnormalities in the plasma and have increased surface membrane with increased cholesterol in the membrane. Why the excess membrane leads to spur cells and not target cells, however, is not known. These irregular rigid cells tend to be trapped in the spleen and destroyed.

Anemia Associated with Bone Marrow Infiltration (Myelophthisic Anemia). This anemia is associated with marrow replacement by (or involvement with) metastatic carcinoma, multiple myeloma, leukemia, lymphoma, lipidoses or storage disease, and certain other conditions.

The characteristic finding in the blood is the presence of varying numbers of normoblasts and immature neutrophils; these are responsible for the descriptive terms *leukoerythroblastotic reaction, leukoerythroblastic anemia* and *leukoerythroblastosis.*

Normochromic and normocytic (occasionally macrocytic) anemia of varying severity is present. Reticulocytes are often increased, and the number of normoblasts is usually out of proportion to the severity of the anemia. The leukocyte count is normal or reduced (occasionally elevated), and immature neutrophils and even myeloblasts may be found. Platelets are normal or decreased, and bizarre, atypical platelets can sometimes be seen.

Examination of the marrow will usually reveal the condition responsible for this reaction. Mechanical crowding out of the hematopoietic tissue by the pathologic process has been assumed but not proved and probably is not the usual cause. Often the amount of erythropoietic tissue in the marrow as determined by morphologic and kinetic studies is normal or increased. The mechanism described in the section on anemia of chronic disorders (p. 193) may often play a role, but the reason for the outpouring of immature cells into the blood is not clear.

In addition to myelophthisic anemias, circulating normoblasts and immature neutrophils can also be seen in severe anemias due to other causes, severe infections, and congestive heart failure, but usually the normoblasts are not so numerous.

The *leukoerythroblastotic reaction* associated with myelophthisic anemias cannot always be distinguished from the blood picture of myelosclerosis with myeloid metaplasia (MMM), which is usually regarded as one of the myeloproliferative disorders. In MMM, enlargement of the spleen and liver is almost always found. In the blood film, more severe red cell abnormalities, leukocytosis, myeloblasts and immature granulocytes of all varieties (not just neutrophils), increased basophils, more atypical platelets, more numerous megakaryocyte fragments, and dwarf megakaryocytes are all findings more characteristic of MMM than of a leukoerythroblastotic reaction of some other cause. Examination of the bone marrow by a needle biopsy or surgical biopsy may be necessary to differentiate MMM from other myelophthisic anemias.

Aplastic and Refractory Anemias. The term aplastic anemia usually refers to pancytopenia associated with hypocellularity of the bone marrow—that is, a severe reduction in the amount of hematopoietic tissue which results in deficient production of blood cells. The marrow, though hypocellular, may have patchy areas of normocellularity or even hypercellularity.

The clinical course may be acute and fulminating, with profound pancytopenia and a rapid progression to death, or the disorder may have an insidious onset and a chronic course. The symptoms and signs are related to the degree of the deficiencies: bleeding may be caused by thrombocytopenia; infection may be the result of neutropenia; and other signs and symptoms are those of anemia. As a rule, splenomegaly and lymphadenopathy are absent.

Aplastic anemias are of diverse etiology. In approximately half the cases, the marrow has apparently been injured by ionizing radiation, drugs, or chemicals; and in the remainder, no antecedent cause of exposure to an injurious agent can be found (Lewis, 1965).

Aplastic Anemia Associated with Chemical or Physical Agents

TOXIC APLASTIC ANEMIAS. Toxic aplastic anemias are caused by a number of physical and chemical agents that produce marrow damage in all humans and animals exposed to a sufficient dose. Here belong ionizing radiation, mustard compounds, benzene, and antineoplastic agents, such as busulfan, urethane, and antimetabolites.

Benzene Poisoning. The changes in the blood frequently include anemia, either alone or in combination with leukopenia and thrombocytopenia, Occasional changes are eosinophilia, leukocytosis, and leukemoid reactions. The marrow may vary from acellular to hypocellular to hypercellular. Occasionally extramedullary hematopoiesis and splenomegaly may be present.

Organic Arsenicals. There is no apparent relationship between the size of the dose, the frequency or duration of exposure, and the injury to the blood. The various compounds differ in their effectiveness.

Ionizing Radiation. The effects on blood cells depend on the radiosensitivity of the cells, the capacity of the cells to regenerate, and the survival rate of the cells in the peripheral blood. The erythroid cells are most sensitive, granulocytes have intermediate sensitivity, and the megakaryocytes are the least sensitive of the three. Reticulum cells and connective tissue cells are relatively insensitive.

After acute exposure to radiation, the reticulocyte count falls, but the red cells decline very slowly because of their long survival. Within the first few hours there is a neutrophilic leukocytosis due to a shift from marginal and probably marrow storage pools. A fall in lymphocytes occurs after the first day and is responsible for the early leukopenia. After five days or so, granulocytes begin to fall. The last cells to decrease are usually the platelets; these are often the last to return to normal in the recovery phase.

The effects of massive exposure depend on the dose and sensitivity. In the acute radiation syndrome, systemic effects (prostration, fever), leukopenia, and infection may lead rapidly to death. Or thrombocytopenia and purpura may develop. This form may lead to diarrhea, dehydration, infection, aplastic anemia, hemorrhage, and death in weeks. The effect of radioactive isotopes is more gradual, more persistent, and longer lasting. Late effects of ionizing radiation include increased susceptibility to leukemia.

Blood counts at regular intervals for persons exposed occupationally to ionizing radiation have been recommended, but this practice has little to recommend it. The use of film badges is more practical.

HYPERSENSITIVE APLASTIC ANEMIAS. There is a long, constantly increasing number of drugs that produce marrow damage in some individuals after single or repeated exposures. These drugs are not capable of damaging the marrow of animals, as are the chemicals in the first group. They include antimicrobial drugs (salvarsan, chloramphenicol, sulfonamides, chlortetracycline, streptomycin), anticonvulsants (Mesantoin, Tridione), analgesics (phenylbutazone), antithyroid drugs (carbimazole), antihistaminics (Pyribenzamine), insecticides (DDT), and other chemicals—some known (gold compounds, Atabrine, chlorpromazine, hair dyes, bismuth, mercury) and others to come.

Chloramphenicol is a drug in this category that appears important in the causation of aplastic anemia. Reactions of the marrow to chloramphenicol are of two types which are possibly unrelated (Yunis and Bloomberg, 1964; Wintrobe, 1967).

In about half the patients who receive chloramphenicol, a reversible increase in serum iron, reticulocytopenia with anemia, neutropenia, and thrombocytopenia occur. The marrow may show decreased erythroid cells and vacuolization of primitive erythroid and granulocyte precursors. These changes are dose and time dependent and reversible.

In a very small proportion of persons receiving chloramphenicol, an irreversible aplastic anemia develops which may be fatal. No relationship has been established between the reversible erythropoietic lesion and the development of aplastic anemia; it may be that individual susceptibility is responsible for the latter. For this reason it is essential that restraint be employed in using the drug, because monitoring its administration with blood cell counts is unlikely to be an effective preventative measure (Wintrobe, 1967).

Aplastic Anemia Associated with Other Disease

INFECTION. Marrow aplasia has been described as an infrequent sequel to infectious hepatitis, occurring a few months after onset when the hepatitis is resolving. These patients are usually males and under age 20; the prognosis is usually grave (Rosner, 1970). Other viral infections can cause hematopoietic depression and rarely are followed by aplastic anemia.

PAROXYSMAL NOCTURNAL HEMOGLOBINURIA (PNH). This rare hemolytic process (see p. 220) may be followed by aplastic anemia. Usually in PNH a variable degree of marrow hypofunction coexists. Curiously, in some patients who present with aplastic anemia, the red cell defect of PNH may be present or may appear during the course of the disease. According to Lewis and Dacie (1967), about 15 per cent of patients with aplastic anemia have a demonstrable PNH red cell defect, with or without clinical hemolysis.

Idiopathic Aplastic Anemia. In patients with pancytopenia and a hypocellular bone marrow, search should be made for evidence of significant exposure to radiation, drugs, and chemicals of known or possible propensity to injure the marrow so that further exposure can be eliminated. Nevertheless, in approximately half the cases of aplastic anemia, no suspected causal relationship to toxic agents can be found, and it is these that are designated as idiopathic.

The symptoms and signs do not differ, but the onset is more commonly insidious than in toxic or hypersensitive aplastic anemias.

BLOOD. The red cells are usually normal in size and shape, though in some cases there may be varying degrees of anisocytosis and poikilocytosis or macrocytosis. Polychromasia, stippling, and normoblasts are most often conspicuously absent. Leukopenia with marked decrease in granulocytes and a relative lymphocytosis are observed. In severe leukopenia there is often also an absolute lymphocytopenia. Neutrophil granules may be larger than normal and may stain dark red (unlike the "toxic" granules found in infections), and the leukocyte alkaline phosphatase may be elevated (Lewis, 1962). Thrombocytopenia is part of the picture. The finding of immature leukocytes or normoblasts is not characteristic and should occasion the search for other causes of pancytopenia. The serum iron is usually increased.

BONE MARROW. In most cases the aspirate consists of red cells, lymphocytes, some plasma cells, and fatty particles. Marrow sections will show fatty tissue with inconspicuous fibrosis and islands of lymphocytes and plasma cells. Though focal areas of normocellularity or hypercellularity may sometimes be present, the overall cellularity is decreased.

ERYTHROKINETIC STUDIES. The increased serum iron is a valuable early sign of erythroid hypoplasia and reflects the decreased plasma iron turnover. In addition, the erythrocyte utilization of iron is decreased. Both effective and total erythropoiesis, therefore, are decreased in aplastic anemia.

Familial Hypoplastic Anemia (Fanconi's Anemia; Congenital Pancytopenia). Pancytopenia becomes obvious after infancy and usually by the eighth year of life. Often more than one member of a family is affected. The anemia is usually normochromic and may be macrocytic; the marrow is generally hypocellular. Developmental anomalies are present and include short stature, hypogonadism, malformations of the extremities (e.g., aplasia of the radius and abnormalities of the thumbs), and malformations of other organs (e.g., heart and kidneys). Chromosomal defects have been described (Fanconi, 1967).

A small proportion of patients with aplastic anemia and a hypocellular bone marrow have, after a time, developed leukemia. This has been described after roentgen irradiation, benzene intoxication, phenylbutazone or chloramphenicol administration, and in some cases of idiopathic aplastic anemia, including Fanconi's anemia. An attractive hypothesis is that aplastic anemia and leukemia are expressions of a similar fundamental injury or disturbance at the level of the stem cell.

Refractory Anemia with Hypercellular Bone Marrow. Anemia or pancytopenia of unknown cause is sometimes associated with a hypercellular bone marrow showing erythroid hyperplasia and low or inadequate levels of reticulocytes in the blood. Red cell life span may be somewhat shortened, but hemolysis is not a major problem. Plasma iron turnover is increased, but the erythrocyte utilization of iron is decreased. Characteristically, therefore, ineffective erythropoiesis is increased. These anemias have been reviewed by Vilter and his associates (1967).

Sideroblastic Anemia. This is characterized by hypochromic, often microcytic, red cells in the blood, with or without leukopenia and thrombocytopenia. The serum iron is increased, and the per cent saturation of the iron-binding protein is greatly elevated. The marrow shows markedly increased storage iron, erythroid hyperplasia with evidence of defective hemoglobinization, and increased numbers of sideroblasts. In addition to increased numbers of normoblasts with Prussian blue-positive granules in the cytoplasm, there are increased numbers of granules per normoblast and at least a few "ring" sideroblasts (Fig. 4–50). In the latter, the granules line up around the nucleus and the iron can be shown to be located within mitochondria. These findings reflect defective heme synthesis, which may be due to any of several possible enzyme defects; in most instances the exact defect is unknown (Dacie and Mollin, 1966). Occasionally, megaloblast-

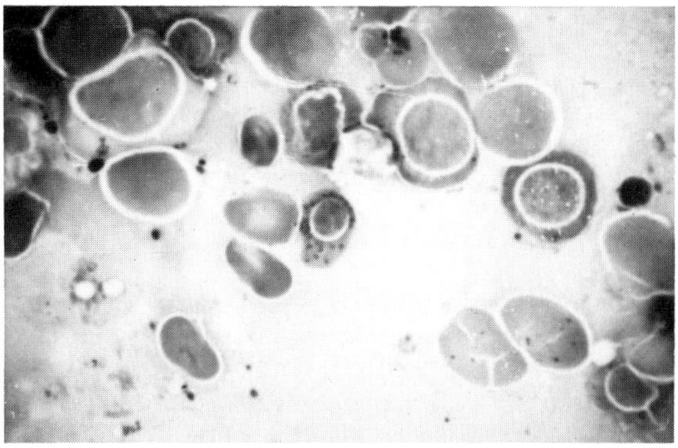

Figure 4–50. Nucleated red cells from the marrow of a patient with sideroblastic anemia. The Prussian blue reaction stains nonhemoglobin iron as blue granules (here shown as dark granules) in the cytoplasm. The perinuclear space is artefactually widened. In the center is a late normoblast with multiple granules of iron, hence, a sideroblast; it is a ring sideroblast, since the granules almost completely surround the nucleus. In the lower right are two siderocytes, i.e., non-nucleated red cells containing stainable iron granules. (× 875.)

like changes are seen in the erythroid cells, but changes typical of vitamin B_{12} or folate deficiency are not seen in granulocytes unless folate deficiency coexists. The following classification is that of Hines and Grasso (1970):

Refractory Sideroblastic Anemia

HEREDITARY SEX-LINKED SIDEROBLASTIC ANEMIA. This occurs in males and may not appear until adolescence. It is rare, but a few well-documented family studies exist.

ACQUIRED REFRACTORY SIDEROBLASTIC ANEMIA

Primary acquired sideroblastic anemia is more common and has its onset in later adult life and in either sex. This is usually a dimorphic anemia with a mixed population of hypochromic and normochromic red cells. In addition to the marrow findings described previously, tissue mast cells are usually increased in number. About one-third of these patients have either folic acid deficiency or an abnormality in pyridoxine metabolism, or both, and show partial improvement when treated with these agents.

Secondary acquired sideroblastic anemia is associated with another disease (which may or may not be hematologic) and usually shows less of the ring sideroblasts than the primary form. Hines and Grasso (1970) state that about half the patients in this group show a hematologic response to folic acid, or pyridoxine, or both.

Reversible Sideroblastic Anemia. This is due to some agent which interferes with heme synthesis; recognition is important because hematologic improvement occurs if the agent is removed.

The *antituberculosis drugs* isoniazid, cycloserine, and pyrazinamide cause sideroblastic abnormalities in some patients on long-term therapy.

Lead poisoning is an important member of this group because environmental exposure to lead is usually unrecognized and needs to be detected. Lead interferes with heme synthesis by blocking the enzymes ALA synthetase, ALA dehydrase, and heme synthetase. These blocks are only partial and of different degree, because in lead poisoning, aminolevulinic acid and coproporphyrin are increased in the urine.

Alcoholism is perhaps the most common of the reversible sideroblastic anemias. Folate deficiency, hypomagnesemia, and hypokalemia are concomitant findings. After withdrawal of alcohol intake, the abnormal sideroblasts usually disappear within a few days.

Pyridoxine-responsive Anemia. Individuals who partially respond to pyridoxine have been included in other categories above. Those in whom anemia is completely corrected form a smaller group. They are young or middle-aged males with a severe microcytic and hypochromic anemia and are dependent upon extraordinary amounts of dietary pyridoxine to maintain a normal hemoglobin level.

REFRACTORY ANEMIA WITH DYSHEMATOPOIESIS. Included here is a group of ill-defined refractory anemias with hypercellular marrow, macrocytic or normocytic anemia, usually with neutropenia and thrombocytopenia. The marrow shows bizarre megaloblastoid erythropoiesis but is without all the characteristic morphologic alterations seen in typical megaloblastic anemia of vitamin B_{12} and folate deficiency, and the process does not respond to these agents. Sideroblasts are not so prominent here, and the erythroblasts may have PAS-positive cytoplasm. Abnormalities in the granulocytes may be present, and the leukocyte alkaline phosphatase is sometimes very high or very low. Abnormalities in megakaryocytes are common and include bizarre giant forms, complete separation of nuclear lobes, or small fragmented forms with one or two apparently diploid nuclei. Myeloblasts may be increased up to about 20 per cent for long periods of time, accounting for the designation "refractory anemia with partial myeloblastosis." Among the refractory anemias with a hypercellular marrow, this group may be particularly likely to eventuate in acute myelogenous leukemia or erythroleukemia, and some authors believe it belongs in the myeloproliferative syndrome (Vilter *et al.*, 1967; Dameshek and Gunz, 1964).

CONGENITAL DYSERYTHROPOIETIC ANEMIA (CDA). Several forms of hereditary anemias characterized by abnormal erythropoiesis with ineffective erythropoiesis and splenomegaly have recently been collected. They appear to have an autosomal recessive mode of inheritance. In general, they tend to be more benign than β-thalassemia major, which forms another group of hereditary anemias with ineffective erythropoiesis.

At least four types have thus far been separated on the basis of marrow and serologic findings. CDA-I has megaloblastic changes with some binuclearity, internuclear chromatin bridges, and a macrocytic anemia (Heimpel *et al.,* 1971). CDA-II is normoblastic and has multinuclearity of normoblasts with much karyorrhexis. The anemia is normocytic. CDA-II is distinguished from the others because it has a positive acidified serum test (with some, but not all normal sera) and a negative sucrose hemolysis test, indicating a red cell membrane abnormality (Crookston *et al.,* 1969). CDA-III, described first by Björkman in 1965, has more pronounced multinuclearity, with giant erythroid precursors and a macrocytic anemia. CDA-IV is similar to CDA-II but lacks the serologic abnormality.

Pure Red Cell Aplasia

Transitory Arrest of Erythropoiesis. This may occur during the course of a hemolytic anemia (often preceded by an infection), and the combination of aplasia and hemolysis becomes a threatening situation (Bauman and Swisher, 1967). Red cell production may occasionally cease during rather minor infections in normal children or adults, at which time the marrow will show absence of all but a few of the most immature erythroid precursors. Since a temporary arrest in production, e.g., a week or two, may not result in enough fall in hemoglobin to become symptomatic, it is quite possible that such events are considerably more common than we realize. If the arrest in erythropoiesis persists, anemia will result (Chanarin *et al.,* 1964).

Congenital (Erythroid) Hypoplastic Anemia (Erythrogenesis Imperfecta; the Anemia of Blackfan and Diamond). This is a rare pure red cell aplasia which usually becomes obvious during the first few months of life. The severe anemia is normochromic and normocytic; reticulocytes are low; leukocytes and platelets are normal; and the marrow shows a marked reduction in all developing erythroid cells but normal granulocytic and megakaryocytic cell lines (Diamond *et al.,* 1961).

Acquired Pure Red Cell Anemia. In adults this anemia is also rare. The marrow is cellular but with virtual absence of erythroid precursors. In about half the cases, this condition is associated with a thymoma, a relationship that must be more than accidental (Havard, 1965). In some patients with thymoma, pancytopenia, hypoplasia of the marrow, and myasthenia gravis were present. In the cases without thymoma, about 10 per cent terminated in leukemia (Schmid *et al.,* 1963).

HEMOLYTIC ANEMIAS

Hemolytic anemias are caused by excessive destruction of red cells manifested by a shortening of the red cell survival (Table 4–6).

Red Cell Survival Studies. A shortened red cell survival constitutes the definition of hemolysis. If the hemolytic process is severe, other laboratory measurements will suffice to demonstrate that hemolysis is in fact present. If the hemolytic process is mild or obscure, it may be necessary to perform red cell survival studies.

Differential Agglutination Method of Ashby (1919)

Principle. Compatible blood possessing a blood group factor that the recipient does not possess is transferred to the recipient, e.g., O cells to recipients A or B or AB and ON cells to M or MN recipients. After the transfusion, serums with potent agglutinins for the red cells of the recipient are added to samples of the recipient's blood and the unagglutinated red cells are counted.

Test. A sample of the recipient's blood obtained prior to the transfusion is tested first to serve as a control and for the selection of a serum reacting strongly with the cells of the recipient.

After the transfusion, 0.1 ml. of the recipient's blood is added to 4.9 ml. of 3 per cent sodium citrate. To 0.25 ml. of this suspension, 0.25 ml. of a potent agglutinating serum is added.

The optimum dilution of the agglutinating serum is determined with pretransfusion blood. The optimum dilution is one with which less than 10,000 unagglutinated red cells are found when the tested blood sample contains 5,000,000 red cells. The blood serum mixture is left at room temperature for at least 2 hours and then centrifuged at about 1500 r.p.m. (300 G.) for 1 minute. The tube is shaken vigorously to break up the large clumps into small ones. The specimen is permitted to settle for not more than 1 minute, and the upper three-fourths of the suspension is transferred with a pipette to another test tube, which is then recentrifuged for 1 minute. The sediment is mixed with the supernatant according to a standard procedure, i.e., 50 inversions at an angle of about 90 degrees at the rate of one per second. A counting chamber is filled with the upper layer of the cell suspension. The cells are permitted to settle for not less than 2 minutes. Only the free cells are counted. The

Table 4–6. ETIOLOGIC CLASSIFICATION OF HEMOLYTIC ANEMIAS*

Corpuscular Defects

- *Hereditary*
  - Membrane abnormalities
    - Hereditary spherocytosis
    - Hereditary elliptocytosis
  - Metabolic abnormalities
    - Glucose-6-phosphate dehydrogenase deficiency
    - Pyruvate kinase deficiency
    - Other enzyme deficiencies
  - Hemoglobin abnormalities
    - Structural
      - Homozygous – S, C, D, E
      - Heterozygous –
        - Altered oxygen affinity
        - Unstable
    - Rate of synthesis
      - Thalassemia
    - Double heterozygotes – thalassemia and structural hemoglobin abnormality
- *Acquired*
  - Paroxysmal nocturnal hemoglobinuria

Extracorpuscular Defects (Acquired)

- *Chemical*
  - Hemolytic to normal cells
    - Acetanilid
    - Allyl-propyl-disulfide
    - Anilin
    - Arsine
    - Benzene
    - Colloidal silver
    - Dinitrobenzene
    - Lead
    - Lecithin
    - Methyl chloride
    - Naphthalene (moth balls)
    - Nitrobenzene
    - Phenacetin
    - Phenylhydrazine
    - Promin
    - Saponin
    - Toluene
    - Trinitrotoluene
    - Water

Extracorpuscular Defects (Acquired) (***Continued***)

- Hemolytic to G-6-PD deficient cells (hereditary element)
  - above, plus
  - Benzedrine
  - Diphenylsulfone
  - Mesantoin
  - Neoarsphenamine
  - Nitrofurans
  - Pamaquine (Plasmochin)
  - p-Aminosalicylic acid (PAS)
  - Paraphenylenediamine (in hair dyes)
  - Phenacetin
  - Primaquine
  - Probenecid
  - Quinine
  - Sulfonamides
- *Physical agents*
  - Heat and severe thermal burns
  - Red cell fragmentation syndrome
- *Vegetable and animal poisons*
  - Vegetable poisons
    - Fava bean (favism) – (hereditary element)
    - Baghdad spring anemia
    - Castor bean
  - Animal poisons
    - Snake venoms
    - Endogenous agents
- *Infectious agents*
  - Protozoal parasites: malaria
  - Nonprotozoal blood parasites: bartonella (Oroya fever)
  - Bacteria: *Cl. welchii, V. cholerae*
- *Immune reactions*
  - Isoimmune reactions
    - Hemolytic transfusion reactions
    - Hemolytic disease of the newborn due to blood group incompatibility
  - Autoimmune reactions
    - Idiopathic hemolytic anemia
    - Symptomatic hemolytic anemia
- *Idiopathic nonimmume hemolytic anemia*
- *Symptomatic nonimmune hemolytic anemia*
- *Paroxysmal cold hemoglobinuria*

*Modified from Wintrobe, 1967. Used with permission of the author.

number of the unagglutinated cells is expressed in absolute numbers per microliter or as a percentage of the number present after the transfusion. Full details are given by Mollison (1967).

Limitations. The differential agglutination method of Ashby is important historically but has been virtually supplanted by the radiochromium method. Disadvantages are that one is limited to suitably "matched" donors and recipients; the survival of the patient's cells in his own circulation cannot be studied; and it is necessary to transfuse large volumes of donor blood.

Radiochromium Method (^{51}Cr). Blood cells tagged with sodium chromate containing a small amount of ^{51}Cr are transferred to the recipient. The survival of the tagged cells is determined in samples removed at intervals.

A sample of the patient's own or donor's blood is removed, labeled and injected into the patient (for details of the technique see p. 477).

The classification of hemolytic anemias is based on red cell survival studies. When erythrocytes from a patient with a hemolytic anemia are injected into a normal individual, and their survival is still *shortened,* it is concluded that the abnormality responsible for the anemia is located in the patient's red cells. These are called *intracorpuscular* defects and are usually (but not always) hereditary. On the other hand, when the patient's erythrocytes are found to have a *normal* survival in the blood stream of a normal person, it is concluded that the abnormality is located somewhere outside the patient's red cells. These defects are called *extracorpuscular* and are usually acquired.

Normal red cells survive normally in a patient with an intracorpuscular defect, but have a shortened survival if the patient's defect is extracorpuscular.

Laboratory Findings in Hemolytic Anemia. Laboratory findings differ, depending on the site of blood destruction, the amount of destroyed blood, and the rate of destruction. If the destruction is *intravascular* and the quantity of destroyed blood is large, free hemoglobin and methemalbumin will be present in the plasma (hemoglobinemia and methemalbuminemia). The urine may contain free hemoglobin and may also show hemosiderin.

Free hemoglobin readily dissociates into $\alpha\beta$ dimers ($\alpha_2\beta_2 \rightarrow 2\alpha\beta$). These are bound to haptoglobin, an α_2-globulin, and the hemoglobin-haptoglobin complex is rapidly removed from the circulation and catabolized by the reticuloendothelial system. This process prevents hemoglobin from appearing in the urine. However, when the plasma hemoglobin level exceeds 50–200 mg./dl. (i.e., when the plasma haptoglobin has been complexed with hemoglobin and removed), the free $\alpha\beta$ dimers of hemoglobin readily pass through the glomerulus of the kidney. Part of the hemoglobin is then absorbed by the proximal tubular cells where the hemoglobin iron is converted to hemosiderin. When these tubular cells are later shed into the urine, *hemosiderinuria* results. If the amount of hemoglobin in the tubular lumen exceeds the capacity of the tubular cell to absorb it, it reaches the urine (*hemoglobinuria*). In the process, it may be oxidized to methemoglobin. The normal plasma hemoglobin level is 2 to 3 mg./dl. A rise to 5 to 10 mg. imparts to the plasma a yellow to orange color. With further increase the color becomes pink. Levels up to 25 to 30 mg./dl. are common in hemolytic anemia. Higher levels are usually indicative of intravascular hemolysis and are seen in hemolytic transfusion reactions and in paroxysmal cold and nocturnal hemoglobinurias.

Plasma Hemoglobin. Careful technique to avoid adding to the hemolysis is essential for correct interpretation of all tests for plasma hemoglobin. In small amounts, hemoglobin is measured by its catalytic action on the oxidation of benzidine by H_2O_2. The test is described in Dacie and Lewis (1968). The benzidine method does not distinguish between hemoglobin, sulfhemoglobin, and methemalbumin.

Methemalbumin. The Schumm test is a qualitative test for methemalbumin. Nine volumes of plasma or serum are overlaid with a layer of ether in a large test tube. One volume of saturated solution of ammonium sulfide is added with a pipette. After thorough mixing, the contents is poured into a hand spectroscope. An absorption band at 558 nm. indicates a positive test for methemalbumin. An ammonium hemochromogen formed from methemalbumin gives a more intense color at this wavelength than methemalbumin itself.

Serum Haptoglobin. A semiquantitative method is based on simple serum electrophoresis. The haptoglobin-hemoglobin complex migrates faster than free hemoglobin and slower than methemalbumin. Known amounts of hemoglobin are added to the patient's (and a control's) serum. If hemoglobin is added in an amount less than the binding capacity of the haptoglobin present, only one band of hemoglobin will be seen on the unstained electrophoretic strip; this is the haptoglobin-hemoglobin complex which migrates as an α_2-globulin. If more hemoglobin is added than can be bound by haptoglobin, a second band of hemoglobin is seen, that of free hemoglobin which migrates with the β-globulins. Thus, if increasing amounts of hemoglobin are added to several samples of the patient's serum, the quantity of haptoglobin can be estimated. Absence of hemoglobin in the α_2-globulin region indicates absent haptoglobin. Hemoglobin migrating in the albumin band is methemalbumin, which indicates intravascular hemolysis; usually in this case the haptoglobin band is missing. Details of the method may be found in Brus and Lewis (1959) or Dacie and Lewis (1968).

Another type of haptoglobin measurement is made by combining the available haptoglobin in plasma with methemoglobin and measuring the peroxidase activity, which is much greater than that of free methemoglobin (Owen *et al.*, 1960). The measurement is spectrophotometric and is more convenient than the electrophoretic method when large numbers of samples must be investigated.

Decreased or absent haptoglobin, as mentioned above, indicates hemolysis, either intravascular or extravascular, but also may occur in infectious mononucleosis, severe liver disease, and congenital ahaptoglobinemia.

Increased serum haptoglobin may occur in any inflammatory disease or during steroid therapy; in such situations the presence of hemolysis cannot be ruled out if the haptoglobin concentration is normal.

If hemolysis is primarily *extravascular*, no hemoglobinemia, hemoglobinuria, or hemosiderinuria is present. Hemolysis is detected by measuring an increase in one of the products of heme catabolism (see also p. 168):

1. An increase in CO expired; currently this is a research technique and not generally available.

2. An increase in indirect-reacting serum bilirubin; since this is bound to albumin, it will not appear in the urine.

3. An increase in urine urobilinogen or, more consistently, in fecal urobilinogen.

The normal urobilinogen in a 24-hour specimen is 0 to 3.5 mg. in urine and 40 to 280 mg. in the stool. Following excessive hemolysis it may increase to 5 to 200 mg. in the urine and to 300 to 4000 mg. in the stool. The examination of feces is more dependable than examination of the urine because it may show an increase when the urine shows none. It may show an increase even when the serum bilirubin is not raised. The latter finding is explained by the fact that the normal liver has the capacity to remove large amounts of free (indirectly reacting) bilirubin from the blood.

Hemolytic anemia is characterized also by increased red cell production. Because of the availability of maximal amounts of iron for hemoglobin formation, red cell production reaches the maximal degree possible (about eight times normal) in severe chronic hemolytic anemia, if complicating factors such as folate deficiency do not intervene. If the red cell destruction exceeds the capacity of the marrow to replace red cells at the same rate, hemolytic anemia occurs. With less severe hemolysis, the marrow may be able to produce enough red cells so that anemia does not occur; this is called compensated hemolysis.

Blood Smear. The anemia is normocytic, as a rule. It may be macrocytic. Macrocytosis is an expression of the presence of immature red cells, which are larger than normocytes. What one sees in the blood smear is an expression of the capacity of the marrow to compensate for the lost blood. Present are anisocytosis and poikilocytosis (usually more of the former than of the latter), reticulocytosis (much larger number of reticulocytes in massive acute hemolysis than in chronic), polychromatophilia (i.e., reticulocytes without the benefit of vital stain), and normoblasts.

When in response to excessive blood destruction the call for increased production reaches the marrow, it releases excessive numbers and younger forms of leukocytes and platelets together with erythrocytes. The result is leukocytosis with a "shift to the left" and thrombocytosis with both normal and giant platelets. Examples of other red cell abnormalities are: spherocytes in hereditary and acquired hemolytic anemia (Figs. 4–15 and 4–17); schistocytes (fragmented red cells) in traumatic hemolysis (Fig. 4–24); and erythrophagocytosis in immune hemolysis.

The laboratory consequences of spherocytosis are defective rouleaux formation, which may exert a retarding influence on the sedimentation rate of erythrocytes, and a "shift to the left" of the osmotic fragility curve.

Bone Marrow. Normoblastic hyperplasia is the rule, and may be striking in degree (Fig. 4–59). Storage iron is usually increased and sideroblasts are normal or increased in number, reflecting the abundance of available iron for hemoglobin synthesis.

Sudden worsening of the degree of anemia may occur in chronic hemolytic anemias and be due to either of two basic mechanisms. Occasionally episodes of bone marrow failure characterized by erythroid hypoplasia and reticulocytopenia may upset the equilibrium between production and destruction of red cells. In most instances these "aplastic crises" are thought to be precipitated by infection (Bauman and Swisher, 1967). On the other hand, a sudden increase in the rate of red cell destruction may occur accompanied by an increased reticulocytosis in an insufficient attempt to compensate. This is called a "hemolytic crisis."

Hemolytic Anemias Due to Intrinsic Abnormalities

Membrane Defects

HEREDITARY SPHEROCYTOSIS. Hereditary spherocytosis is characterized by spherocytic red cells which are intrinsically defective, splenomegaly, and familial occurrence (probably autosomal dominant). The hemolytic process is variable in severity and is corrected by splenectomy, though the spherocytosis remains.

The osmotic fragility of freshly drawn blood is usually increased but may be normal in mildly affected patients; that of blood incubated at 37° C. for 24 hours is uniformly increased (p. 130). The increased osmotic fragility is characteristic, but not specific; it may occur in some acquired hemolytic anemias.

The laboratory findings are those of a chronic extravascular hemolytic process: evidence of increased pigment catabolism, erythroid hyperplasia, and reticulocytosis. The Coombs' test is negative, spherocytes are present, and osmotic fragility is increased. Spherocytes are more intensely stained than normal erythrocytes and lack the central pallor (Fig. 4–15). The MCHC is often increased, reflecting a decrease in cell surface.

Since the diagnosis is established by familial occurrence, siblings and the parents should be studied. In a few cases, neither parent may be affected.

The erythrocytes are abnormally permeable to sodium, and there is no defect in energy metabolism, which is, in fact, increased. The increased metabolic activity has been explained as an attempt to compensate for a membrane defect which leaks cations, with degenerative changes and the loss of cell surface accelerated by the metabolic and physical stress of passage through the spleen (Jandl, 1968). The primary defect appears to be in the erythrocyte membrane, possibly an abnormal structural protein (Jacob *et al.*, 1971).

HEREDITARY OVALOCYTOSIS (HEREDITARY ELLIPTOCYTOSIS). This autosomal dominant condition probably includes more than one genetic variant. Nonhypochromic ovalocytes (elongated erythrocytes) are abundant in the blood smear (Fig. 4–20). The deformity is increased in sealed, moist preparations. Most persons with this cellular abnormality are asymptomatic; about 10 to 15 per cent develop a mild hemolytic anemia. No specific biochemical lesion has been identified.

Metabolic Defects. Disorders characterized by a relative lack of spherocytes, normal hemoglobin structure, normal osmotic fragility, and failure of splenectomy to correct the anemia were in the past called hereditary nonspherocytic hemolytic anemias.

AUTOHEMOLYSIS TEST (Dacie and Lewis, 1968)

Principle. When sterile defibrinated blood is incubated at 37° C. normal red cells undergo a complex series of changes with slow hemolysis. Cells with membrane or metabolic defects hemolyze to a greater extent than normal.

Test. Sterile defibrinated blood is used. The patient's blood and a normal control blood are tested in parallel. One-milliliter samples are delivered into four sterile screw-capped test tubes, and 0.05 ml. of sterile 10 per cent glucose is added to two of the tubes. The tubes are incubated at 37° C. for 24 hours, then gently mixed by inversion and incubated for another 24 hours.

After the 48-hour incubation, the blood in each pair of tubes is pooled and well mixed (10 minutes on a rotary mixer at 15 revolutions/min.). A small sample is removed for microhematocrit and another for hemoglobin concentration (1:200 dilution) in Drabkin's solution. The remainder of each sample is centrifuged and the serum is placed in a clean test tube. A 1:10 dilution of the incubated serum is made in Drabkin's solution (a higher dilution is made if hemolysis is severe); the blank for the hemoglobin determination is a preincubation serum sample.

Normal Range

Without added glucose	0.2 to 2.0 per cent
With added glucose	0 to 0.9 per cent

Interpretation. In hereditary spherocytosis, lysis is almost always increased; with glucose, the lysis is diminished to a variable extent. In hereditary nonspherocytic anemias, Selwyn and Dacie found two patterns: Type I cases had slightly to moderately increased lysis without glucose; when glucose was added, some reduction in lysis occurred, but less than with normal blood. Type II cases had increased lysis but no improvement with added glucose.

It later was shown that glucose-6-phosphate dehydrogenase (G6PD) deficiency gave a Type I pattern and pyruvate kinase deficiency gave a Type II pattern of autohemolysis.

ERYTHROCYTE METABOLISM. The mature red cell lacks mitochondria and therefore oxidative phosphorylation and Krebs' cycle activity. Energy production is mainly glycolytic, 90 per cent of which occurs through the Embden-Meyerhof pathway, as glucose goes to lactic acid with the net production of two moles of ATP (Fig. 4–51). ATP is needed for the energy-requiring reactions in the cell: for active cation transport across the membrane; for maintaining membrane deformability; and for preserving the cell's biconcave shape. The pentose phosphate pathway (hexose monophosphate shunt) generates NADPH in the first two steps, through the enzymes G6PD and 6-phosphogluconate. NADPH production is linked to glutathione reduction and, through this mechanism, to preservation of vital enzymes and hemoglobin. Small amounts of oxidized hemoglobin (methemoglobin) are reduced by GSH (glutathione). Activity of the pentose phosphate pathway increases when the cell is exposed to an oxidant drug. If an enzyme in this pathway is lacking in activity, GSH cannot be produced and hemoglobin will be oxidized by the oxidant stress. The result is denatured hemoglobin in the form of Heinz bodies which adhere to the membrane, inducing rigidity and a tendency to lysis. Moderate enzyme deficiencies in this pathway (e.g., G6PD) may not be associated with anemia; however, if the cells are challenged by an oxidizing drug an acute hemolytic episode occurs.

Deficiencies in the Embden-Myerhof path-

Calculation

$$\text{Lysis } (\%) = \frac{R_t \times \left(\dfrac{100 - \text{Hct}_t}{100}\right) \times 100}{R_o \times \dfrac{\text{Dilution of whole blood}}{\text{Dilution of serum}}} = \frac{R_t\,(100 - \text{Hct}_t)}{R_o \times \dfrac{200}{10}}$$

R_o = optical density of diluted whole blood.
R_t = optical density of diluted serum at 48 hours.
Hct_t = hematocrit at 48 hours.

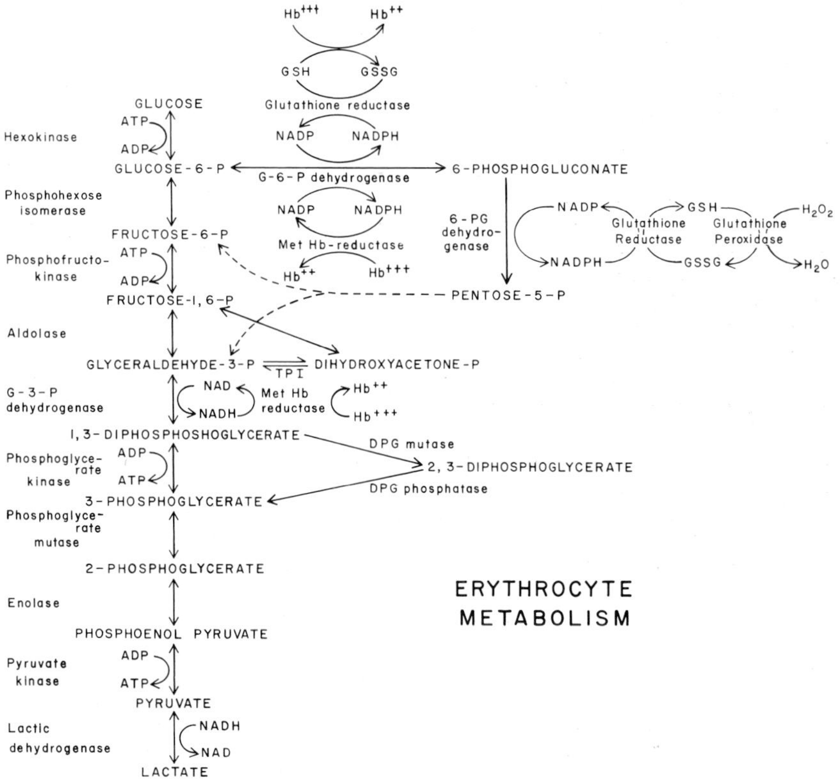

Figure 4–51. Erythrocyte metabolism is discussed in the text. Some of the points where linked systems operate (e.g., glutathione, methemoglobin reduction) are indicated. Normally most methemoglobin is reduced by NAD-linked methemoglobin reductase. NADP-linked methemoglobin reductase requires methylene blue for activation and is more effective in drug-induced methemoglobinemia than the normal cell mechanism.

way result in impaired ATP generation and a chronic hemolytic anemia. The mechanism of the red cell destruction here is less clear. Heinz bodies are not formed. It appears that lack of cell deformability and impaired cation pumping may be important in the hemolytic process (LaCelle and Weed, 1971).

Another shunt, the Rapoport-Luebering shunt, provides for the conversion of 1,3-diphosphoglycerate (1,3-DPG) to 2,3-diphosphoglycerate (2,3-DPG) instead of directly to 3-phosphoglycerate (3-PG) (Fig. 4–51). If this shunt is operating, generation of two moles of ATP (per mole of glucose) is bypassed; the result is no net energy production in glycolysis. However, 2,3-DPG combines with the β-chain of hemoglobin and decreases the affinity of hemoglobin for oxygen. At a given partial pressure of oxygen, therefore, increased 2,3-DPG allows more oxygen to leave hemoglobin and go to the tissues; the oxygen dissociation curve is shifted to the right (Chapter 12). Increased activity of this shunt is apparently stimulated by hypoxia.

Glucose-6-phosphate Dehydrogenase (G6PD) Deficiency (Beutler, 1971; Carson and Frischer, 1966). About 10 per cent of male American blacks who were given 30 mg. of primaquine a day developed a self-limited, acute hemolytic anemia. Only the older red cells were destroyed, and it was found that the deficiency in the susceptible red cells was in G6PD.

It has since been found that G6PD deficiency is widespread throughout the world. Among Caucasians, the highest incidence is in Mediterranean people; the deficiency is also found in blacks and in Orientals.

Since G6PD is determined by a gene on the X-chromosome, full expression of the deficiency is found in the male hemizygote. Partial expression may be found in the heterozygous female who has two populations of red cells, one normal and one deficient. The deficiency of G6PD results in a limitation of the regeneration of NADPH, which renders the cell vulnerable to oxidative denaturation of hemoglobin. Since, normally, G6PD is highest in young cells and decreases as the cell ages, in persons with G6PD deficiency the older cells are preferentially destroyed.

Hemolytic susceptibility in affected persons can increase greatly during intercurrent illness or upon exposure to various drugs (e.g., primaquine, sulfonamides, nitrofurans, and aminoquinolones) which have oxidant properties.

The genetic heterogeneity is great and is expressed in different groups as variation in the electrophoretic and catalytic properties of the enzymes, in the degree of deficiency, in the types of cells in the body affected, in the types of drugs which will produce hemolysis, and in the susceptibility to chronic hemolysis or to neonatal jaundice (Oski and Naiman, 1972). Blacks have a milder deficiency than Caucasians, have fewer cell types of the body affected and, as a rule, do not have chronic hemolytic anemias. The rarer forms of G6PD deficiency that result in chronic hemolytic anemias are more common in people of northern European extraction. In some but not all Caucasians with G6PD deficiency, exposure to fava beans results in a severe and sometimes fatal hemolytic reaction (favism) in which serum factors are also involved.

The laboratory findings during active hemolysis are those of hemolytic anemia in general. In the blood film, poikilocytes, irregularly contracted cells, and occasional spherocytes may be found. After supravital staining with methyl violet, Heinz bodies may be present early in an acute hemolytic episode (p. 179).

Screening Tests for G6PD Deficiency. Several types of tests may be used; they vary in their specificity, sensitivity to the heterozygous state, and the amount and freshness of blood required. For positive results in nonspecific screening tests or for equivocal results in specific tests, the diagnosis must be confirmed by a quantitative assay.

HEINZ BODY TEST FOR G6PD-DEFICIENT CELLS (Beutler *et al.*, 1955)

Principle. Acetylphenylhydrazine, an oxidant drug, is added to the patient's and to control blood. After 2- and 4-hour incubation at 37° C., samples from each are examined for Heinz bodies.

Reagents

1. Acetylphenylhydrazine, 100 mg., is dissolved in 100 ml. of 0.066 M phosphate buffer at pH = 7.6. To this is added 200 mg. glucose.
2. Methyl violet, 0.5 gm./100 ml. saline, or crystal violet, 2 gm./100 ml. saline.
3. Blood sample: EDTA, double oxalate, or heparin may be used as anticoagulant, or defibrinated blood may be used.

Procedure. To 2 ml. of acetylphenylhydrazine solution in a test tube add 0.1 ml. blood, mix well, and place in a 37° C. water bath. At 2 hours place a small drop of the mixture on a coverslip which is then inverted over a large drop of methyl violet or crystal violet on a slide. After 10 minutes examine slides from patient and control for Heinz bodies. This is repeated at 4 hours, if necessary.

Result. The percentage of cells with 5 or more Heinz bodies is determined for control and patient. Control values should be 0 to 30 per cent. Values for persons with G6PD deficiency (or defects in the glutathione system or unstable hemoglobins) will be greater, usually over 45 per cent.

DYE REDUCTION TEST OF MOTULSKY (Dacie and Lewis, 1968). This test is conveniently performed using commercially available kits* which include detailed instructions. In principle, a mixture of glucose-6-phosphate, NADP, and brilliant cresyl blue dye in tris buffer is incubated with hemolysate. If G6PD is present, the NADP will be reduced to NADPH (Fig. 4–51) which, in turn, will reduce the blue dye to its colorless form. The time needed for this reduction to take place is noted for the patient's blood and for that of a normal control with an identical hemoglobin concentration (adjusted if necessary). This time is inversely proportional to the amount of G6PD present and is prolonged in G6PD deficient subjects.

The dye reduction test is quite specific and can be performed on stored blood. It has the advantage that it can be performed on microsamples, but is likely to give false negative results in heterozygotes and black males with G6PD deficiency during a hemolytic episode (Fairbanks and Fernandez, 1969).

ASCORBATE CYANIDE TEST (Jacob and Jandl, 1966).

Principle. Blood is incubated with a solution of sodium cyanide and sodium ascorbate. Hydrogen peroxide is generated from the coupled oxidation of ascorbate and hemoglobin. Since cyanide inhibits catalase, the hemoglobin is oxidized by the hydrogen peroxide and the brown color of methemoglobin is discernible. This occurs more rapidly in G6PD-deficient cells than in normal cells.

Reagents

1. Sodium ascorbate, 10 mg., and glucose, 5 mg., are added to test tubes which are stoppered and may be stored indefinitely at −20° C.
2. Sodium cyanide, 500 mg., dissolved in 50 ml. distilled water plus 20 ml. of isotonic phosphate buffer, pH 7.4. The solution is neutralized to pH 7.0 with HCl, and the volume is made up to 100 ml. with distilled water. This solution is stable indefinitely at room temperature.
3. Blood: EDTA, ACD, or heparin but not oxalate may be used as anticoagulant (hexose monophosphate shunt activity is inhibited by oxalate). Storage of blood at 4° C. for 14 days in ACD does not alter the results of the test.

Procedure. Aerate the blood to a bright red color before adding 2 ml. to the ascorbate and glucose mixture. Add 2 drops of the sodium

*G6PD kit, Dade, Miami, Fla.

cyanide solution and incubate the unstoppered blood suspension in a water bath at 37° C., preferably with agitation. Again mix the suspensions at 2 hours and at 3 or 4 hours, noting the color each time.

Result. G6PD-deficient blood appears brown after thorough mixing at a time normal blood remains red. For either hemizygote or heterozygote, this occurs at 1 to 2 hours when EDTA is the anticoagulant and at 2 to 4 hours when heparin or ACD is used. Normal blood changes color slowly over a period of several hours.

Interpretation. The ascorbate cyanide test is not specific, in that pyruvate kinase deficiency, paroxysmal nocturnal hemoglobinuria, and unstable hemoglobins will give a positive result. It is the most sensitive of the screening tests, in that it uses intact cells and will detect the deficiency in black males during hemolytic episodes and in heterozygotes (Fairbanks and Fernandez, 1969).

FLUORESCENCE OF NADPH (Beutler, 1971b)

Principle. Whole blood is added to a mixture of glucose-6-phosphate, NADP, saponin, and buffer, and a spot of this mixture is placed on filter paper and observed for fluorescence with ultraviolet light. If G6PD is present, NADP is converted to NADPH. Since phosphogluconate dehydrogenase is present in most hemolysates, further NADP is converted to NADPH (Fig. 4–51). NADPH fluoresces but NADP does not; therefore, lack of fluorescence indicates G6PD deficiency. By reoxidizing any small amounts of NADPH formed, oxidized glutathione (GSSG) enhances the ability of the test to detect mild G6PD deficiency.

Reagents

1. A screening mixture is made up with the following composition: G6P, 0.01 M, 1 part; NADP, 7.5 mmol., 1 part; saponin (Sigma) 1 per cent, 2 parts; tris-HCl buffer, 750 mmol., pH 7.8, 3 parts; GSSG, 8 mmol., 1 part; and water, 2 parts. This mixture is stable in the frozen state for several months, but is available in lyophilized form from Hyland Laboratories, Costa Mesa, California.

2. Whatman No. 1 filter paper (nonfluorescing).

3. Blood in heparin, ACD, or EDTA, which may be several weeks old. Spots of dried blood on filter paper are also satisfactory.

Procedure. Add 10 μl. of blood to 100 μl. of the screening mixture and make a spot on the filter paper. After incubating the mixture at room temperature for 5 to 10 minutes, make a second spot. Examine spots under long-wave ultraviolet light.

Interpretation. With the normal control sample, the first spot may fluoresce slightly and the second spot will fluoresce brightly. In G6PD deficiency, neither spot will show fluorescence.

QUANTITATIVE ASSAY OF G6PD (AND OTHER RED CELL ENZYMES). Methods currently in use are presented by Beutler (1971b). For G6PD, most assays are based on the rate of reduction of NADP to NADPH, measured spectrometrically at 340 nm., when a hemolysate is incubated with G6P. Often an assay for 6-PGD activity is done simultaneously, using appropriate steps, because NADPH is formed in the first two reactions of the hexose monophosphate shunt.

In heterozygotes or in acute hemolysis in black subjects with G6PD deficiency, the diagnosis may be obscured even with the assay because of the increased level of G6PD in reticulocytes and younger erythrocytes. Usually, however, the ascorbate cyanide screening test will be positive in these instances.

PYRUVATE KINASE (PK) DEFICIENCY (Tanaka *et al.*, 1962; Tanaka and Paglia, 1971). Though G6PD deficiency is the most common red cell enzyme abnormality, it does not usually produce a chronic hemolytic anemia. Deficiency of the glycolytic enzyme *pyruvate kinase* is probably the most common cause of hereditary nonspherocytic hemolytic anemia. The type II pattern of autohemolysis is usually seen, though it is not established that all type II patterns are due to PK deficiency. It is inherited as an autosomal recessive characteristic. Heterozygotes are asymptomatic and have normal hemograms, but most can be detected by enzyme assay. The disease may appear in infancy. Irregularly contracted erythrocytes and crenated cells may be prominent on the blood film in some cases. Reticulocyte counts are often very high.

Heinz bodies are not found. The diagnosis is established by a specific screening test or by enzyme assay.

Screening Test for PK Deficiency (Beutler, 1971b)

PRINCIPLE. Pyruvate kinase catalyzes the phosphorylation of ADP to ATP by phosphoenolypyruvate (PEP) with the formation of pyruvate. Pyruvate then reduces any NADH present to NAD with the formation of lactate. Loss of fluorescence of NADH under ultraviolet light is observed as evidence of the presence of PK.

Leukocytes must be removed from the sample because normally they contain about 300 times as much PK as do red cells, and in PK deficiency the red cells but not the leukocytes are deficient. Removing the buffy coat removes most of the leukocytes; lysing the red cells by hypotonicity allows the rest to remain intact, keeping the PK from the leukocytes out of the reaction.

Reagents

1. Mixture No. 1: In each milliliter are the

following: phosphoenolypyruvate (PEP) cyclohexyl ammonium salt, 0.15 M (neut.), 30 μl.; ADP, 30 mmol. (neut.), 100 μl.; $MgCl_2$, 80 mmol., 100 μl.; KPO_4 buffer, 0.25 M, pH 7.4, 50 μl.;* water, 720 μl. This mixture is stable indefinitely when frozen.

2. Dry NADH vial, 0.5 mg. (Sigma).

3. Mixture No. 2: Add 0.5 ml. of mixture No. 1 to a 0.5-mg. NADH vial just before using.

4. Whatman No. 1 filter paper (nonfluorescing).

5. Blood may be collected in EDTA, ACD, or heparin.

PROCEDURE. After centrifuging the blood, carefully remove the buffy coat and plasma with a capillary pipette, and add 0.9 per cent NaCl to the red cells to make a 20 per cent suspension. Add 10 μl. of the red cell suspension to 100 μl. of mixture No. 2 screening mixture. Make one spot of this mixture on filter paper immediately and a second spot after 30 minutes' incubation at 37° C. After the spots are dry, examine them under long-wave ultraviolet light.

INTERPRETATION. With a normal control blood, the first spot should fluoresce brightly, but the second should have no fluorescence. Blood from a pyruvate kinase-deficient patient will show fluorescence in both spots.

Quantitative Assay of PK. The same principle is employed as in the screening test, but the rate of decrease of O.D. at 340 nm. is measured. A negative screening test or a normal PK assay (using the standard high substrate [PEP] concentrations) does not rule out PK-deficient hemolytic anemia. It has been clearly shown that hemolytic anemia may be associated with mutant PK enzymes which have normal activity at high substrate concentration but decreased activity at a lower substrate concentration which prevails in the cell. Performing the PK assay at different substrate concentrations is therefore recommended (Beutler, 1971b).

DEFICIENCY OF OTHER RED CELL ENZYMES

Embden-Meyerhof Pathway Enzymes. Hemolytic anemia has been described in deficiencies of hexokinase, glucose phosphate isomerase, triose phosphate isomerase, diphosphoglyceromutase, and phosphoglycerate kinase. These are rare entities (Valentine, 1971).

Nonglycolytic Enzymes. Glutathione peroxidase deficiency and glutathione reductase (GR) deficiency have been described in association with chronic hemolytic anemia. However, mild to moderate deficiency of GR may be found in many disorders (probably due to riboflavin deficiency) and does not appear to play a measurable role in red cell destruction (Beutler, 1971b). Deficiency of glutathione has been described in mild chronic hemolytic anemia due to deficiency of either one of two enzymes involved in the synthesis of glutathione (Konrad *et al.*, 1972).

In general, the deficiencies of the glutathione system that result in hemolytic anemia are rare; patients with these deficiencies show autosomal recessive inheritance, have increased susceptibility to oxidant drugs, and may be expected to show Heinz bodies during episodes of acute hemolysis (Figs. 4–49 and 4–51).

Hemoglobinopathies and Thalassemia

In 1949 Pauling and his associates described specific properties of a hemoglobin type in patients with sickle cell anemia. Their studies initiated the concept of molecular disease; that is, a molecular variation in a single protein can be responsible for the entire spectrum of clinical, laboratory, and pathologic manifestations that characterize a disease. The subsequent finding that the abnormality was due to the substitution of a single amino acid in a polypeptide chain of hemoglobin has rapidly developed into the exciting field of biochemical genetics.

At present, over 200 different hemoglobins have been described, about three-fourths of which have been characterized as a single amino acid substitution; undoubtedly the end has not been reached.

NORMAL HEMOGLOBINS

The heme group is identical in all variants of human hemoglobin. The protein part of the molecule (globin) consists of four polypeptide chains. At least three distinct hemoglobin types are found in normal individuals, and the structure of each has been determined.

HbA ($\alpha_2\beta_2$). Hemoglobin A is the major normal adult hemoglobin. The polypeptide chains of the globin part of the molecules are of two types: two identical alpha chains, each with 141 amino acids, and two identical beta chains, with 146 amino acids each. Each chain is linked with one heme group. The molecule is ellipsoidal, with the four heme groups at the surface of the molecule, where they function by combining reversibly with oxygen or carbon dioxide (Fig. 4–52).

HbF ($\alpha_2\gamma_2$). Hemoglobin F is the major hemoglobin of the fetus and the newborn infant. The increased affinity for oxygen of fetal blood over adult blood is not due to the hemo-

*KPO_4 buffer, 0.25 M, pH 7.4, is made up by mixing 8.25 ml. of a stock solution of 1 M K_2HPO_4 with 1.75 ml. of 1 M KH_2PO_4 and 30 ml. of distilled water (Beutler, 1971b, p. 23).

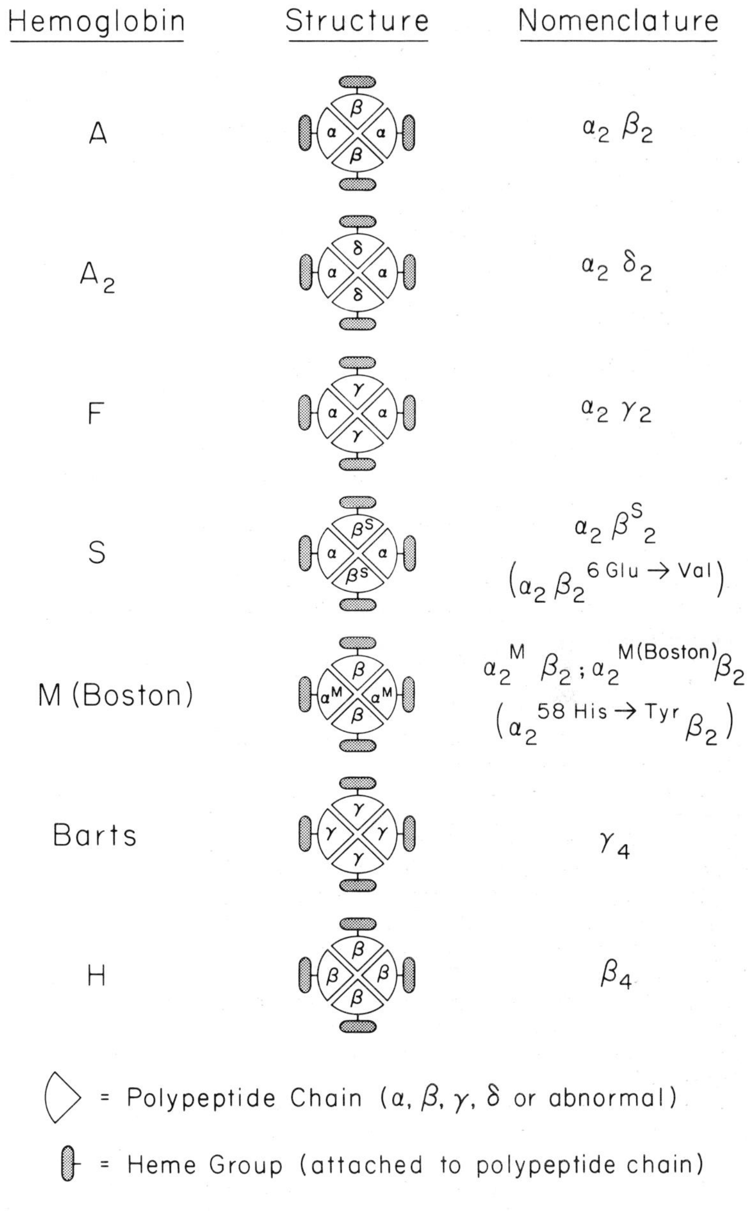

Figure 4–52. Configuration and nomenclature of normal and abnormal hemoglobins. Each triangle represents one folded polypeptide chain; the bar attached to its external surface represents a heme group. The drawing is schematic. Each heme group is near the surface of the molecule, located in a pocket formed by folds of its polypeptide chain and attached to that chain by an imidazole group. In most hemoglobinopathies (e.g., Hb S, Hb $G_{Philadelphia}$), the affected polypeptide chain differs from normal in only one amino acid. In Hb S, the designation could also be written $\alpha_2\beta_2^{6\ Val}$, and in Hb $G_{Philadelphia}$, $\alpha_2^{68\ Lys}\beta_2$, indicating the site of the substitution and the amino acid which replaces the one usually present (After Krieg and Henry, 1967).

globin itself, but probably to the environment in the red cell. The two alpha chains are identical to those of HbA, and two gamma chains, with 146 amino acid residues, differ from beta chains. During fetal life, HbF predominates, as alpha chain production and gamma chain production are high (Fig. 4–53). Beta chain production begins before the twentieth week of prenatal life, so that HbA is 10 per cent of the total between 20 and 35 weeks and 15 to 40 per cent at the time of birth. After birth, smaller amounts of HbF are produced; at four months HbA is 90 to 95 per cent of the total. Only traces of HbF (<0.5 per cent) are found in adults. The mechanism of "switching" from gamma to beta chain production is unknown. If for some reason beta chain production is impaired during this time of switching, gamma chain production may continue in considerable degree into adult life, so that high levels of HbF often indicate an anemia of early onset (e.g., thalassemia major).

HbA_2 ($\alpha_2\delta_2$). Hemoglobin A_2 accounts for 1.5 to 3.5 per cent of normal adult hemoglobin. Its two alpha chains are the same as in HbA and HbF; its two delta chains differ from beta chains in only eight of their 146 amino acids.

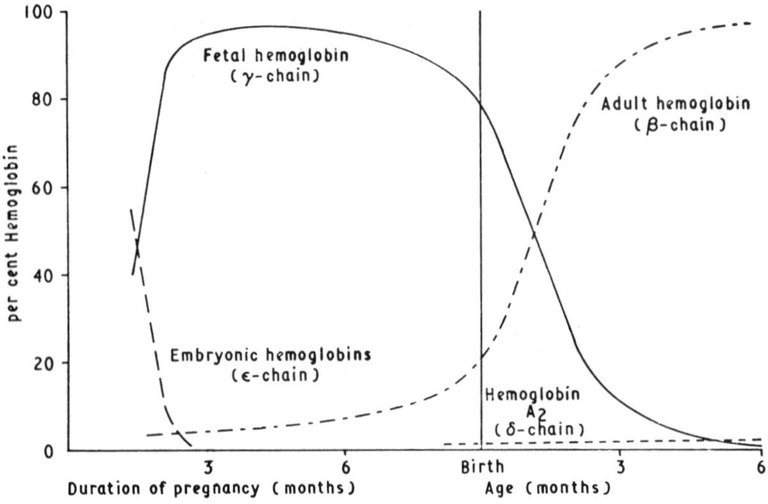

Figure 4–53. The developmental changes in human hemoglobins. (After Huehns and Shooter, 1965.)

Quantitation has become important, for HbA_2 is increased in certain types of thalassemia.

Embryonic Hemoglobins: Hb-Gower-1 (ϵ_4) **and Hb-Gower-2** ($\alpha_2\epsilon_2$). Two different hemoglobins have been found in normal human fetuses with a gestational age of less than three months; both contain a polypeptide chain (ϵ) distinct from the α, β, γ and δ chains. After the γ-chain production has become maximal early in fetal life, ϵ-chain production ceases (Fig. 4–53).

Investigations of hemoglobin structure and inheritance of abnormal hemoglobins have resulted in the concept of four genetic loci on chromosomes, which govern the structure of the alpha, beta, gamma, and delta polypeptide chains. Available evidence indicates that beta and delta loci are closely linked. The alpha locus is either farther removed or on a different chromosome.

ABNORMAL HEMOGLOBINS AND NOMENCLATURE

Most abnormal hemoglobins are the result of the substitution of a single amino acid for another on one of the polypeptide chains. Normal adult hemoglobin was designated HbA; fetal hemoglobin, HbF; and that found in sickle cell anemia, HbS. Thereafter, as hemoglobin variants were discovered, they were given sequential letters of the alphabet according to their electrophoretic mobility. When more than one hemoglobin was found with the same electrophoretic mobility, it was designated with the subscript indicating the geographical location in which it was found; there are several variants of HbD, G, J, and M, for example. If it is known on which polypeptide chain the abnormality is present, this can be indicated as a superscript; e.g., HbS = $\alpha_2^A\ \beta_2^S$; HbI = $\alpha_2^I\ \beta_2^A$ (Fig. 4–52). Further, once the site of the amino acid substitution is known, this is designated by the number of the amino acid residue in the superscript along with the substitution; e.g., HbS = $\alpha_2\beta_2^{6Val}$; HbI = $\alpha_2^{16Asp}\beta_2$. Amino acid substitutions in some of the known hemoglobin variants are listed and classified by functional characteristics in Table 4–7.

ABNORMAL HEMOGLOBIN SYNDROMES

In *hemoglobinopathies* the structure of one of the four types of polypeptide chains formed is abnormal; this is usually due to substitution of a single amino acid. A larger number of hemoglobin variants which do not cause disease have been discovered in surveys. In clinically significant disease, either the beta chain or the alpha chain is affected; involvement of the gamma chain and delta chain occurs, but this is rare. Depending on the type of amino acid and the site involved, the hemoglobin may be functionally abnormal and have altered chemical and physical properties.

In *thalassemias,* globin chains of normal structure are formed, but the rate of production of one type of polypeptide chain is diminished. Beta thalassemia refers to decreased production of beta chains and HbF ($\alpha_2\gamma_2$) or HbA_2 ($\alpha_2\delta_2$) would be expected to be increased. More rarely, alpha chain production is affected (alpha thalassemia).

In *homozygous beta hemoglobinopathies,* both allelic genes for the abnormal beta chains are present, so that no normal beta

Table 4–7. FUNCTIONAL CLASSIFICATION OF HEMOGLOBIN VARIANTS

I. Homozygous: Hemoglobin variants causing hemolytic anemia in the homozygous state; asymptomatic in the heterozygous state.

Hb S	$\alpha_2\beta_2^{6\,Val}$	Sickling
Hb C	$\alpha_2\beta_2^{6\,Lys}$	Three different Hb Cs exist; two of which sickle
Hb D Punjab	$\alpha_2\beta_2^{121\,Gln}$	Several different Hb Ds exist
Hb E	$\alpha_2\beta_2^{26\,Lys}$	

II. Heterozygous: Hemoglobin variants causing functional aberrations or hemolytic anemia in the heterozygous state.

A. Hemoglobins associated with methemoglobinemia and cyanosis.

1. Hb M Boston $\alpha_2^{58\,Tyr}\beta_2$
2. Hb M Iwate $\alpha_2^{87\,Tyr}\beta_2$
3. Hb M Saskatoon $\alpha_2\beta_2^{63\,Tyr}$
4. Hb M Milwaukee $\alpha_2\beta_2^{67\,Glu}$
5. Hb M Hyde Park $\alpha_2\beta_2^{92\,Tyr}$

B. Hemoglobins associated with altered oxygen affinity.

1. Increased affinity and polycythemia.

a. Hb Chesapeake	$\alpha_2^{92\,Leu}\beta_2$
b. Hb J Capetown	$\alpha_2^{92\,Gln}\beta_2$
c. Hb Malmo	$\alpha_2\beta_2^{97\,Gln}$
d. Hb Yakima	$\alpha_2\beta_2^{99\,His}$
e. Hb Kemp	$\alpha_2\beta_2^{99\,Asn}$
f. Hb Ypsi (Ypsilanti)	$\alpha_2\beta_2^{99\,Tyrl}$
g. Hb Hiroshima	$\alpha_2\beta_2^{143\,Asp}$
h. Hb Rainier	$\alpha_2\beta_2^{145}$
i. Hb Bethesda	$\alpha_2\beta_2^{145\,His}$

2. Decreased affinity—"anemia" (low hemoglobin concentration with few symptoms of anemia) and cyanosis.

a. Hb Kansas	$\alpha_2^{102\,Thr}\beta_2$
b. Hb Seattle	$\alpha_2^{76\,Glu}\beta_2$
c. Hb Bristol	$\alpha_2\beta_2^{67\,Asp}$
d. Hb Yoshizuka	$\alpha_2\beta_2^{108\,Asp}$

C. Unstable Hemoglobins

1. Hemoglobins which may precipitate as Heinz bodies after splenectomy: "Congenital Heinz body hemolytic anemia."

a. α-chain abnormalities

Hb Torino	$\alpha_2^{42\,Val}\beta_2$
Hb L-Ferrara	$\alpha_2^{47\,Gly}\beta_2$
Hb Hasharon	$\alpha_2^{47\,His}\beta_2$
Hb Ann Arbor	$\alpha_2^{80\,Arg}\beta_2$
Hb Etobicoke	$\alpha_2^{84\,Arg}\beta_2$
Hb Dakar	$\alpha_2^{112\,Glu}\beta_2$
Hb Bibba	$\alpha_2^{136\,Pro}\beta_2$

b. β-chain abnormalities

Hb Leiden	$\alpha_2\beta_2^{6\text{ or }7}$	(Glu deleted)
Hb Sogn	$\alpha_2\beta_2^{14\,Arg}$	
Hb Freiburg	$\alpha_2\beta_2^{23}$	(Val deleted)
Hb Riverdale Bronx	$\alpha_2\beta_2^{24\,Arg}$	
Hb Genova	$\alpha_2\beta_2^{28\,Pro}$	
Hb Tacoma	$\alpha_2\beta_2^{30\,Ser}$	
Hb Philly	$\alpha_2\beta_2^{35\,Phe}$	
Hb Louisville	$\alpha_2\beta_2^{42\,Leu}$	
Hb Hammersmith	$\alpha_2\beta_2^{42\,Ser}$	
Hb Zurich	$\alpha_2\beta_2^{63\,Arg}$	
Hb Toulouse	$\alpha_2\beta_2^{66\,Glu}$	
Hb Bristol	$\alpha_2\beta_2^{67\,Asp}$	
Hb Sydney	$\alpha_2\beta_2^{67\,Ala}$	
Hb Shepherd's Bush	$\alpha_2\beta_2^{74\,Asp}$	
Hb Seattle	$\alpha_2\beta_2^{76\,Glu}$	
Hb Boras	$\alpha_2\beta_2^{88\,Arg}$	
Hb Santa Ana	$\alpha_2\beta_2^{88\,Pro}$	
Hb Gun Hill	$\alpha_2\beta_2^{91-97}$	(5 a.a. deleted)
Hb Sabine	$\alpha_2\beta_2^{91\,Pro}$	
Hb Köln	$\alpha_2\beta_2^{98\,Met}$	
Hb Kansas	$\alpha_2\beta^{102\,Thr}$	
Hb Wein	$\alpha_2\beta_2^{130\,Asp}$	
Hb Olmsted	$\alpha_2\beta_2^{141\,Arg}$	

2. Tetramers of normal chains; appear in thalassemias.

Hb Barts	γ_4
Hb H	β_4
Hb α_4^A	α_4

chains (hence, no HbA) are produced. Examples are sickle cell disease (HbS) and hemoglobin C disease (HbC). Since alpha, gamma, and delta genes (and chain production) are normal, the HbF and HbA_2 formed are structurally normal, though they may be increased in amount.

Homozygous alpha hemoglobinopathies have not been described.

In *heterozygous beta hemoglobinopathies,* the abnormal hemoglobin is present in addition to HbA; HbF and HbA_2 again are structurally normal, since only a portion of the beta chains are abnormal. Examples are sickle cell trait (HbA + HbS); hemoglobin C trait (HbA + HbC). The normal HbA quantitatively exceeds the abnormal hemoglobin present because of either slower production of abnormal beta chains than normal beta chains or selective early destruction of the red cells with higher concentrations of the abnormal hemoglobin (see Fig. 4–54).

In *heterozygous alpha hemoglobinopathies,* the abnormality in the alpha chain will affect all three hemoglobin types. Therefore, six different hemoglobin types are found—the three normal hemoglobins and the three abnormal forms. Examples are $HbD_{Baltimore}$, Hb Ann Arbor and HbM_{Boston}.

Combinations of abnormalities exist. *Double heterozygotes for two beta chain abnormalities* produce two different abnormal beta chains; therefore, there are two abnormal hemoglobins and no hemoglobin A. An example of this is HbS-C disease. Double heterozygotes for beta and delta chain abnormalities and for alpha and beta chain abnormalities are rare but have provided important information.

Double heterozygotes for beta hemoglobinopathy and beta thalassemia are well known. Here, the quantity of abnormal hemoglobin exceeds the normal hemoglobin, in contrast to the heterozygous beta hemoglobinopathies, in which the reverse is true. Examples are HbS thalassemias and HbE thalassemia (see Fig. 4–54).

Beta Hemoglobinopathies. The only known disorders that are homozygous for a structural hemoglobin abnormality involve the beta chain.

Sickle Cell Disease. Homozygous HbS disease is a serious chronic hemolytic anemia, first manifest in early childhood and often fatal before the age of 30 years. With modern medical care, however, many patients live longer. Hemoglobin S is found almost exclusively in the black population; 0.2 per cent of the blacks born in the United States have sickle cell anemia.

In Hemoglobin S the amino acid glutamic acid in the sixth position on the beta chain is replaced by valine. This substitution is on the surface of the molecule and changes its charge and, hence, its electrophoretic mobility. Hemoglobin S is freely soluble when fully oxygenated; when oxygen is removed from HbS, polymerization of the abnormal hemoglobin occurs, forming tactoids (fluid crystals) which are rigid and deform the cell into the shape which gave the cell its name. In homozygous HbS disease, sickling occurs at physiologic oxygen tensions and the rigidity of the red cells is responsible for the hemolysis as well as for most of the complications. The rigid cells are more vulnerable to trauma and are readily trapped by the reticuloendothelial system, especially the spleen, accounting for the hemolysis. As a result of the hemolysis, severe continued marrow hyperplasia during childhood produces bone changes: expansion

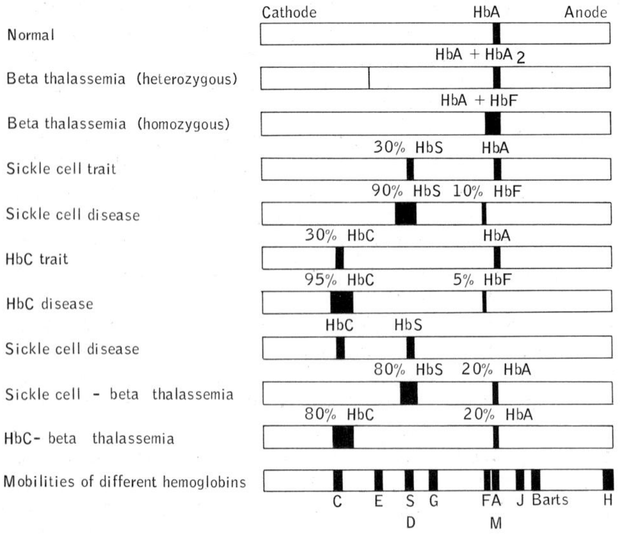

Figure 4–54. Hemoglobin electrophoresis in different clinical conditions. The mobilities are representative of those obtained on zone electrophoresis at an alkaline pH. Special techniques required to separate and measure HbA_2 and HbF. (Krieg and Henry, 1967.)

of the marrow space, thinning of the cortex, and radial striations seen in the skull on x-ray. Leg ulcers are common.

COMPLICATIONS. In early childhood, bilateral painful swelling of the dorsa of the hands or feet is known as the *hand-foot syndrome* or sickle cell dactylitis. It lasts about two weeks, is accompanied by changes of periostitis as observed by x-ray, and does not occur after the age of three.

The spleen is central to three complications: A *sequestration crisis* refers to sudden pooling of blood and rapid enlargement of the spleen, resulting in hypovolemic shock. This may occur in early childhood when splenomegaly is present. *Functional asplenia* (Pearson *et al.*, 1969) consists of inadequate antibody responses under some conditions and an impaired ability of the reticuloendothelial system to clear bacteria from the blood, probably due to reticuloendothelial blockade. This may partly explain the increased risk of infection in children with the disease. Salmonella and pneumococcal infections are unusually prevalent in children with sickle cell anemia. *Autosplenectomy* is the result of vaso-occlusive episodes, resulting in progressive infarction, fibrosis, and contraction of the spleen. Though splenomegaly is present in childhood, a small fibrotic remnant is the rule in the adult.

From early childhood, patients cannot produce a concentrated urine, apparently as a result of anoxic damage to the vasa recta in the medullae of the kidneys.

Vaso-occlusive crises are debilitating episodes of abdominal and bone or joint pain, accompanied by fever, which are probably due to plugging of small blood vessels by masses of sickled cells.

Aplastic crises can occasionally afflict any patient with chronic hemolytic anemia. A temporary failure of red cell production which would not be noticed in a person with a normal red cell life span will cause a serious fall in hemoglobin concentration in hemolytic anemia. This may be a result of infection, exposure to toxic drugs, or folic acid deficiency; sometimes no cause can be found.

BLOOD. The anemia is normochromic and normocytic; polychromasia is increased; normoblasts are present. Target cells are numerous (up to 30 per cent) and Howell-Jolly bodies are regularly seen in older children and adults, as a result of asplenia. Sickle cells are often found in the stained smear (Fig. 4–55). Osmotic fragility is usually decreased, and mechanical fragility is increased. Neutrophilia and thrombocytosis are usual. Sickle cell preparations are rapidly positive. The marrow shows normoblastic hyperplasia and increased storage iron.

ELECTROPHORESIS. If the patient has not been recently transfused, no HbA, 60 to 99 per cent HbS, 1 to 40 per cent HbF, and normal concentration of HbA_2 are present. The fetal hemoglobin is distributed unevenly among the red cells. HbS, HbD and several unstable hemoglobins have the same electrophoretic mobility but, of these, only HbS gives a positive sickle cell test.

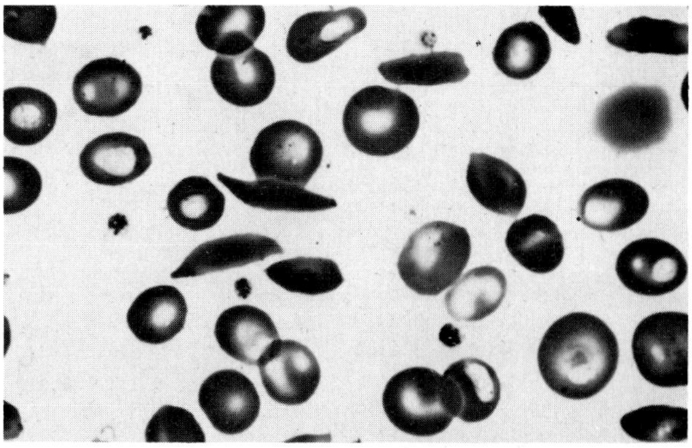

Figure 4–55. Sickle cell anemia. Note that the elongated, pointed cells have greater density in the center than near the edges, in contrast to elliptocytes. Linked molecules of reduced Hb S, forming tactoids, distort the cells. (× 875.)

Sickle Cell Trait. Sickle cell trait is probably the most common hemoglobinopathy in the United States. This heterozygous condition (HbA + HbS) is present in about 10 per cent of American blacks. Under normal circumstances no clinical signs of disease or hematologic abnormalities are present. However, acidosis or hypoxia due to aircraft flight, respiratory infection, anesthesia, or congestive heart failure may cause sickling and vascular complications with visceral infarcts. Impaired ability to concentrate urine is found in adults with the trait. Hematuria, particularly on the left side, may occur. Sickle cell trait confers protection on the individual from the lethal effects of falciparum malaria, which may account for the major distribution of HbS in central Africa. The stained film appears normal, except perhaps for a few target cells. The sickle cell preparation is positive, and almost all the red cells eventually sickle.

ELECTROPHORESIS. HbA, 60 to 80 per cent; HbS, 20 to 40 per cent; HbF, normal.

Hemoglobin C Disease. Homozygous hemoglobin C disease is a mild hemolytic anemia with splenomegaly which is often asymptomatic but occasionally results in jaundice and abdominal discomfort.

BLOOD. Slight normochromic normocytic anemia with an admixture of microcytes and spherocytes, minimal increase in reticulocytes, and numerous target cells (40 to 90 per cent) are seen in the blood. Osmotic fragility is biphasic, with both increased and decreased fragility. Hexagonal or rod-shaped crystals may be seen in erythrocytes in the stained smear, especially after splenectomy or after slow drying of the smear (Fig. 4–56). If red cells are incubated in 3 per cent saline, crystal-like inclusions appear in almost every cell. This tendency of the hemoglobin to form rod-shaped inclusions apparently increases the rigidity of the cells and increases their likelihood of being trapped and destroyed in the spleen (Conley and Charache, 1967).

ELECTROPHORESIS. No HbA; almost 100 per cent HbC; less than 7 per cent HbF.

Hemoglobin C Trait. Hemoglobin C is found in West Africans and in about 2 to 3 per cent of American blacks. The heterozygous state is asymptomatic, without anemia, and generally without any abnormality of the blood smear (Lehmann and Huntsman, 1966), though some authors state that mild hypochromia and target cells (up to 40 per cent) may be present (Chernoff, 1955).

ELECTROPHORESIS. HbC, 20 to 40 per cent; HbA, 60 to 80 per cent.

Hemoglobin D Disease and Trait. Hemoglobin D is found in India and in approximately 0.4 per cent of American blacks. The trait is asymptomatic, with no anemia and a normal blood smear. Homozygous HbD disease is very rare, with virtually no symptoms and a mild hemolytic anemia. The blood film is very similar to homozygous HbC disease, with numerous target cells, but rod-like inclusions do not form. Several variants with identical electrophoretic mobility have been identified.

ELECTROPHORESIS. HbD has a mobility on alkaline electrophoresis identical to that of HbS but is easily distinguished by the absence of the sickling phenomenon. In the trait, HbD accounts for less than half of the total hemoglobin.

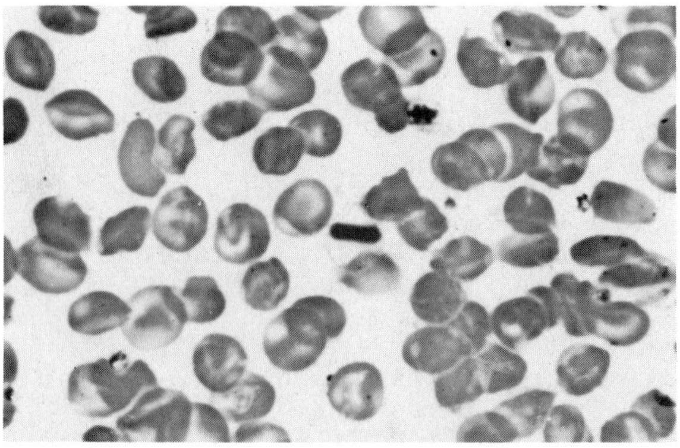

Figure 4–56. Hemoglobin C disease, postsplenectomy. Prior to splenectomy the only morphologic abnormality was the presence of target cells. After splenectomy Howell-Jolly bodies and hemoglobin crystals, such as that in the center, were present. Note that almost all the hemoglobin in this particular cell is in the dark bar, and the membrane is still visible. Some such crystals are distinctly hexagonal. (×875.)

Hemoglobin E Disease and Trait. Hemoglobin E is found chiefly in Southeast Asia. The trait is asymptomatic, with a normal blood smear and no anemia. In HbE disease, the clinical findings and the blood film are very similar to those of HbD.

Doubly Heterozygous States (Two Beta Hemoglobinopathies). A different abnormal beta chain inherited from each parent may result in interaction of HbC, D, or E with HbS to produce hemolytic anemia of variable severity.

Sickle Cell–Hemoglobin C Disease (SC Disease). Severity is intermediate between sickle cell trait and sickle cell disease, with almost all the manifestations of sickle cell anemia appearing but with less frequency. The onset is usually early in childhood, but real difficulties do not occur until the teens or later. Fatigue, dyspnea on effort, frequent upper respiratory infections, attacks of mild jaundice, and arthralgias are seen. Crises are usually rare and mild. Painful crisis occurs more often in joints and muscles than in the abdomen. Constant hip and low back pain may be present with aseptic necrosis of the head of the femur on x-ray. Hematuria and splenic infarcts have been described. Leg ulcers occur only occasionally. In pregnancy there is a tendency toward increased frequency of crises—both clinical and hematologic. Painful crises are related to infarction, and sudden death may occur following childbirth. In contrast to sickle cell anemia, splenomegaly is usually present. The body habitus is normal or stocky in contrast to the asthenic features in sickle cell anemia.

BLOOD. Mild chronic normochromic slightly microcytic anemia is seen in some cases but is compensated for during remissions. The anemia is more severe in other cases. Anisocytosis and poikilocytosis are mild to severe, and target cells are numerous—up to 85 per cent of the erythrocytes. The sickle cell test is positive.

ELECTROPHORESIS. HbC and HbS occur in about equal amounts. HbF ranges from normal to 7 per cent. Because no normal beta chains can be produced, HbA is absent.

Sickle Cell–Hemoglobin D Disease (SD Disease). SD disease simulates but is less severe than sickle cell anemia, and thus may also resemble SC disease. The sickle cell test is positive.

ELECTROPHORESIS. The pattern is indistinguishable from sickle cell anemia because HbS and HbD cannot be separated on routine (alkaline) electrophoresis. Agar-gel electrophoresis at pH 6.2 will separate HbS and HbD; solubility studies (HbD is more soluble than HbS) and family studies will help to reveal the true nature of the condition. One parent is likely to have a negative sickle cell test and an abnormal hemoglobin with the mobility of HbS.

Other doubly heterozygous beta hemoglobinopathies are known but are even less common.

Heterozygous Hemoglobinopathies. A number of amino acid substitutions occur in the heme pocket where they either increase the stability of the methemoglobin form (HbM) or alter the affinity of the heme for oxygen; the latter usually alters the stability of the molecule as well.

Other substitutions affect the $\alpha\beta$ contact sites; these also can change stability and oxygen affinity of the molecule (Perutz and Lehmann, 1968; Lehmann and Carrell, 1969).

These functionally significant hemoglobinopathies are heterozygous; in all, the concentration of the abnormal hemoglobin is less than 50 per cent.

Hemoglobins Associated with Methemoglobinemia and Cyanosis

HEMOGLOBIN M.* Several abnormal hemoglobins are associated with clinical methemoglobinemia and cyanosis which do not respond to methylene blue (Table 4–7). Some are alpha chain abnormalities (e.g., HbM_{Boston} and HbM_{Iwate}); others are beta chain abnormalities (e.g., $HbM_{Saskatoon}$ and $HbM_{Hyde\ Park}$). The common feature is that all have an amino acid substitution at or near the heme group so that a stable complex is formed with heme in the oxidized state; reduction to ferrous heme and hence reversible binding of oxygen is prevented.

Cyanosis from birth is seen in hemoglobin M disease with alpha chain abnormalities, but does not appear for two to four months if the abnormality is in the beta chain—that is, until beta chain production reaches adult levels. The cyanosis is, of course, not associated with enzyme abnormalities in the red cell, toxic drugs, or cyanotic heart disease, conditions which must be considered in the differential diagnosis.

All HbM disorders thus far discovered are heterozygotes. Some types of HbM will not separate from HbA on alkaline electrophoresis. If the hemolysate is first converted to methemoglobin, the HbM will migrate differently from normal methemoglobin at pH 7.1. Then absorption spectra of the eluted HbM, which may be distinctive, can be compared with that of normal methemoglobin. Further analysis will be necessary to identify an example of HbM—rate of reaction with cyanide, absorption spectrum of the cyanmethemoglobin, and amino acid analysis of the globin.

*See Gerald and Scott, 1966, and Lehmann and Huntsman, 1966.

Hemoglobins Associated with Altered Oxygen Affinity

INCREASED AFFINITY AND POLYCYTHEMIA. Several alpha and beta chain abnormalities have been described (Table 4–7). The oxygen dissociation curve is shifted to the left. Since the hemoglobin has high affinity for oxygen, the tissues are relatively hypoxic at any given Po_2, resulting in increased erythropoietin and polycythemia. Since the amino acid substitution is inside the molecule, usually the abnormal hemoglobin is indistinguishable from HbA on electrophoresis (Stamatoyannopoulos *et al.*, 1971).

Hemoglobin Chesapeake. An alpha chain abnormality associated with mild asymptomatic polycythemia in a Caucasian family was the first described (Charache *et al.*, 1966). The features were similar to those of benign familial polycythemia. The abnormal hemoglobin, accounting for about 30 per cent of the total, had an increased affinity for oxygen which resulted in significantly elevated hematocrit levels. The abnormal hemoglobin could be detected by starch block or starch gel electrophoresis.

DECREASED AFFINITY AND CYANOSIS. In all known instances, those hemoglobins which have decreased oxygen affinity (and a shift of the oxygen dissociation curve to the right) are also unstable to some degree.

Hemoglobin Kansas. This hemoglobin, described in a Caucasian boy, had just the opposite property from Hb Chesapeake, an abnormally low affinity for oxygen. The clinical features were cyanosis since infancy, normal arterial oxygen tension, and reduced oxygen saturation. Electrophoresis after conversion to methemoglobin allowed separation from HbA (Reissman *et al.*, 1961).

Unstable Hemoglobins (White and Dacie, 1971). Over 30 variants have been described in which the hemoglobin precipitates within the red cell as Heinz bodies (Tables 4–7 and 4–8). Some of these unstable hemoglobins have been defined as the cause of what were originally called "congenital Heinz body hemolytic anemias."

All patients have been heterozygous. The clinical features have shown considerable variation, from severe hemolytic anemia in the first year of life (e.g., Hb Hammersmith, Hb Bristol) to a very mild chronic hemolytic anemia (e.g., Hb Louisville, Hb Hasharon) which may be exacerbated by drugs (e.g., Hb Zurich). A few unstable hemoglobins have been discovered incidentally in clinically normal individuals (e.g., Hb Toulouse, Hb Sogn).

Jaundice and splenomegaly are common, as in other hemolytic anemias. More distinctive in some cases are the excretion of darkly pig-

Table 4–8. SOME UNSTABLE HEMOGLOBINS*

	DEFECT	SEVERITY OF DISEASE	% ABNORMAL HEMOGLOBIN	ELECTROPHORETIC MOBILITY†	OXYGEN AFFINITY
β-chain					
Hb Toulouse	$\alpha_2\beta_2^{66\,\mathrm{Gln}}$	none	40	like Hb I	normal
Hb Gun Hill	$\alpha_2\beta_2^{91-97}$ (5 a.a. deleted)	mild	30	like Hb C	high
Hb Louisville	$\alpha_2\beta_2^{42\,\mathrm{Leu}}$	mild	30–35	like Hb A	low
Hb Seattle	$\alpha_2\beta_2^{76\,\mathrm{Glu}}$	mild	43	like Hb J	low
Hb Freiburg	$\alpha_2\beta_2^{23}$ (deleted)	mild	30	like Hb F	high
Hb Zürich	$\alpha_2\beta_2^{63\,\mathrm{Arg}}$	mild	25	like Hb S	
Hb Köln	$\alpha_2\beta_2^{98\,\mathrm{Met}}$	mild-mod.	10–15	like Hb S; free chains; heme depleted bands	high
Hb Genova	$\alpha_2\beta_2^{28\,\mathrm{Pro}}$	mod-severe	25	like Hb A; also small bands like S; free chains	–
Hb Hammersmith	$\alpha_2\beta_2^{42\,\mathrm{Ser}}$	severe	30	like Hb A	low
Hb Bristol	$\alpha_2\beta_2^{67\,\mathrm{Asp}}$	severe	35	like Hb A	low
α-chain					
Hb Hasharon	$\alpha_2^{47\,\mathrm{His}}\beta_2$	mild	14–19	like Hb S	normal
Hb Torino	$\alpha_2^{42\,\mathrm{Val}}\beta_2$	mod-severe	8	like Hb A	low
Hb Etobicoke	$\alpha_2^{84\,\mathrm{Arg}}\beta_2$	mild	15	like Hb S	high

*Data from White and Dacie, 1971; Keeling *et al.* 1971.

†The mobilities are given as reported in the literature; several buffer systems and media were used. For references see White and Dacie, 1971.

mented urine (only during hemolytic crises in mild variants) and cyanosis in the more severe cases. The urine pigment appears to be a dipyrrole, probably a breakdown product of denatured hemoglobin. The cyanosis is due in part to met- and sulfhemoglobinemia and in part to low oxygen affinity.

The anemia is normocytic and normochromic to hypochromic, the latter because of the loss of hemoglobin from the cells (in the form of Heinz bodies) in the reticuloendothelial organs. Patients with relatively high hemoglobin concentrations in the steady state usually have hemoglobin variants with a high oxygen affinity and an unexpectedly high reticulocyte count (e.g., Hb Köln, Hb Gun Hill). On the other hand, patients with rather low hemoglobin concentrations may be relatively asymptomatic if their hemoglobin has a low oxygen affinity; their reticulocyte counts are unexpectedly low for the hemoglobin concentration (e.g., Hb Hammersmith). Heinz bodies are rarely seen in circulating red cells before splenectomy, though sometimes they may be generated by incubating the red cells with brilliant cresyl blue or new methylene blue. After splenectomy, Heinz bodies are readily demonstrable in a large proportion of cells; blood film shows irregularly contracted cells and basophilic stippling which may be pronounced.

In splenectomized patients, the Heinz bodies interfere with hemoglobin determinations and with electronic platelet and white cell counts. Before reading the O.D. of the hemolysate it should be centrifuged to remove the Heinz bodies. Platelet and leukocyte counts should be performed by visual methods.

The key laboratory estimation is the heat denaturation test (p. 219); unstable hemoglobins precipitate at a temperature at which normal hemoglobin does not. It should be noted that hemoglobin electrophoresis may be either normal or show the mobility of another abnormal hemoglobin (Table 4–8).

THALASSEMIAS

Thalassemias comprise a group of hereditary diseases of hemoglobin synthesis in persons of Mediterranean, African, and Asian ancestry.

According to current concepts, the common characteristic of this group of diseases is impaired production of one of the polypeptide chains of hemoglobin; that is, the *rate* of synthesis is diminished in varying degree, but the chain formed is structurally normal. Most common are the beta thalassemias, in which beta chain production is impaired. Other disorders are alpha thalassemia, delta thalassemia, and beta-delta thalassemia, with decreased synthesis of their respective polypeptide chains. These various conditions are the "thalassemia syndromes" (Weatherall, 1969, 1972). Nathan (1972) and Bank and Marks (1973) have summarized evidence for the hypothesis that the primary genetic defect in beta thalassemia is either an unstable messenger RNA (mRNA) or, more probably, a deficient production of normal mRNA responsible for directing beta chain synthesis.

Beta Thalassemia

Thalassemia Major (Homozygous Thalassemia; Cooley's Anemia). Clinical findings in thalassemia major are as follows: Severe hemolytic anemia with jaundice and splenomegaly become evident early in childhood. Prominent facial bones and slanting eyes give rise to a mongoloid appearance. These changes and the roentgenographic findings of thinned cortex of the long and flat bones and thickening of the skull with osteoporosis ("hair-on-end" appearance) reflect the extreme bone marrow hyperplasia in response to the hemolytic process.

BLOOD. Unlike most hemolytic diseases, the anemia is hypochromic and microcytic. This is probably due to a defect in heme metabolism, which is felt to be secondary to the major problem of globin synthesis. Reticulocytosis, extreme poikilocytosis with bizarre shapes, target cells, ovalocytosis, Cabot rings, Howell-Jolly bodies, nuclear fragments, siderocytes, anisochromia, anisocytosis, and often extreme normoblastosis are present. Poikilocytosis is more striking in patients with intact spleens; normoblastosis is more severe after splenectomy. Osmotic resistance of the red cells, serum iron, and indirect-reacting bilirubin are increased.

MARROW. Marked normoblastic hyperplasia is present. Many late normoblasts show inclusion bodies which stain like hemoglobin but are best seen after vital staining with methyl violet. Fessas (1963) proposed that these inclusions were aggregates of excess, denatured alpha chains. Intramedullary destruction of hemoglobin (ineffective erythropoiesis) is markedly increased in thalassemia major. Storage iron and sideroblasts are increased.

ELECTROPHORESIS AND ALKALI DENATURATION. Almost all cases of thalassemia major fall into the group of the homozygous *high A_2 beta thalassemias* (true β-thalassemia). HbF is increased, usually 40 to 60 per cent, and may be as high as 90 per cent. HbA has even been undetectable in some individuals. HbA_2 is elevated only in some cases, but the ratio of A_2 to A is always increased.

Thalassemia Minor (Heterozygous Thalassemia Minima; Cooley's Trait). Clinical findings are as follows: The features in heterozygous beta thalassemia vary from moderately severe anemia (thalassemia intermedia) to completely normal clinical findings. The severe intermediate forms of heterozygous thalassemia are rare and are found in Mediterranean individuals but not in blacks; in the latter, heterozygous thalassemia is uniformly mild. In many persons, there is a mild hypochromic, microcytic anemia with slightly hemolytic jaundice and splenomegaly. Most individuals with thalassemia minor, however, have no symptoms or abnormal physical signs.

BLOOD. Usually there is no anemia. Most characteristically, the red cell count is elevated and the hemoglobin and hematocrit are reduced. The MCH is almost always low, the MCV is usually low, and the MCHC is sometimes low but often normal. On stained film, the cells have a moderate degree of microcytosis and poikilocytosis; target cells and basophilic stippling are present. The serum iron is normal or high.

MARROW. Normoblastic hyperplasia and elevated storage iron are characteristic.

ELECTROPHORESIS AND ALKALI DENATURATION. Most common is heterozygous *high A_2 beta thalassemia* (true beta thalassemia). HbF is slightly elevated in 50 per cent of cases in the 2 to 6 per cent range. HbA_2 is elevated in the 3.5 to 7 per cent range. The remainder is HbA.

High HbF Beta Thalassemia (beta-delta thalassemia). HbF is elevated in the range of 5 to 20 per cent; HbA_2 is normal or slightly decreased. This variant is much less common than the high A_2 beta thalassemia; only eight homozygous cases have been discovered. High HbF beta thalassemia may be distinguished from a nonthalassemic condition, *hereditary persistence of HbF*, by the fact that in the latter the HbF is uniformly distributed among the red cells. In thalassemias, HbF is unevenly distributed in the red cell population, as shown by the acid elution staining technique (Shepard *et al.*, 1962). Other forms of beta thalassemia exist but are less common, and description in some is incomplete. It is evident that no single finding is diagnostic and that family studies are of great importance.

Beta Thalassemia in Association with Beta Hemoglobinopathies (Doubly Heterozygous States). Study of these conditions has yielded much information about the behavior of thalassemia genes. The beta thalassemia gene selectively depresses synthesis of the normal beta chains of HbA. For example, patients doubly heterozygous for beta thalassemia and HbS have levels of HbA which are *less* than the level of HbS. In the simple sickle cell trait, the level of HbA always exceeds that of HbS.

Sickle Cell–Thalassemia Disease. Although anemia may be slight, a moderately severe hemolytic anemia is more typical with manifestations similar to those of sickle cell anemia.

BLOOD. Pronounced microcytosis, variable hypochromia, and many target cells are present. Sickled cells are uncommon.

ELECTROPHORESIS. HbS is 60 to 90 per cent;

HbA is less than 35 per cent; increased levels of HbA_2 are present; and HbF varies from normal levels to 25 per cent. Some patients have very high levels of HbS and no HbA, the remainder being HbF and HbA_2, which gives a pattern apparently identical to homozygous HbS disease. These cases are severe clinically.

Hemoglobin C Thalassemia. This occurs mainly in blacks, in whom it tends to result in little disability. Patients of Mediterranean extraction usually have moderately severe hemolytic anemia.

BLOOD. The MCH and MCV are reduced. On the blood film are hypochromic target cells, fragmented red cells, and microspherocytes, many of which have a folded appearance.

ELECTROPHORESIS. HbC, 65 to 95 per cent; HbF, variable; HbA, about 20 per cent. HbA_2 levels cannot be studied when HbC is present, as there are no satisfactory methods for separating the two.

Hemoglobin E Thalassemia. In this Southeast Asian disorder, a clinical and hematologic picture similar to thalassemia major is usual.

ELECTROPHORESIS. HbE, 15 to 95 per cent; HbF, 5 to 85 per cent. It is of interest that HbA is nearly always absent. This emphasizes the fact that absence of HbA cannot be taken as proof of homozygosity; it must be supported by family studies.

Alpha Thalassemias. The thalassemias characterized by decreased synthesis of alpha chains are rare and the diagnosis is difficult to establish.

The *homozygous state* is probably incompatible with fetal survival. Stillborn infants with hydrops fetalis in the absence of ABO or Rh blood group incompatibility have been described, mainly in Orientals. Their blood has contained large quantities of Hb Barts (γ_4), small amounts of HbH (β_4), some HbA, but no HbF. Both Hb Barts and HbH move faster on alkaline electrophoresis than does HbA. It is felt that, in a great lack of alpha chains, excess beta chains and gamma chains aggregate; the alpha chains that are available appear to bind with beta chains (HbA) in preference to gamma chains (HbF).

The *heterozygous state* is diagnosed with certainty in neonatal infants, in whom it is recognized by increased levels of Hb Barts in cord blood. (It has been shown that normal cord blood contains trace amounts of Hb Barts.) In adults, mild hypochromia and target cells and decreased osmotic fragility may be found. Hb Barts is usually absent, and HbH may be present in only small amounts if at all. HbH is an unstable hemoglobin and forms intracellular inclusion bodies similar to Heinz bodies upon vital staining with brilliant cresyl blue (p. 179).

Hemoglobin H Disease. Persons with a thalassemia-like disorder similar to thalassemia minor, with 5 to 30 per cent HbH, have been described in almost all racial groups and especially in Southeast Asia, Greece, and parts of the Middle East. Clinically the disease resembles thalassemia intermedia. The MCH is low and the red cells are markedly hypochromic. The bone marrow has marked normoblastic hyperplasia. The disease is detected by finding the rapidly migrating hemoglobin on electrophoresis and inclusion bodies of the unstable HbH using vital staining with brilliant cresyl blue (p. 179). The genetics are not completely worked out, but a current hypothesis suggests double heterozygosity for two different alpha thalassemia genes (Weatherall and Clegg, 1972).

Hereditary Persistence of Hemoglobin F. Continuation of HbF synthesis in adult life without any hematologic abnormalities has been described in blacks (0.1 per cent of American blacks) and persons of Mediterranean extraction; these may be separate entities. Levels of HbF range from 10 to 30 per cent and the feature that distinguishes this from other causes of increased HbF (as in thalassemias) is that HbF is uniformly distributed among the red cells as demonstrated with the acid elution technique.

LABORATORY STUDIES IN HEMOGLOBINOPATHIES AND THALASSEMIAS

Careful history, with emphasis on anemic disorders, jaundice in the family, and ethnic background, and physical examination are necessary.

Routine hematologic studies will include red cell indices, reticulocyte count, and examination of a well-made blood smear.

If the red cells are hypochromic, iron deficiency anemia is first considered because of its frequency. Serum iron and iron-binding capacity and Prussian blue reaction of the marrow for sideroblasts and storage iron will effectively determine whether the patient has iron deficiency.

Demonstration that the patient is hemolyzing may require serum bilirubin, urine or fecal urobilinogen, serum haptoglobin, or red cell survival studies.

Osmotic Fragility (see p. 130) may be helpful. Unless some cells show increased resistance to hypotonic saline, a hemoglobinopathy is unlikely. If osmotic fragility is increased, the hemolytic process is not likely to be due to a hemoglobinopathy (Lehmann and Huntsman, 1966).

Tests for Sickling

Metabisulfite Microscopic Test

PRINCIPLE. Deoxygenated cells containing HbS sickle. The process of deoxygenation is

Table 4–9. HEMOGLOBIN DISEASES*

DISEASE	Hb TYPES	HbF (PER CENT)	CLINICAL SEVERITY	CRISES	SPLENO-MEGALY	SEVERITY OF ANEMIA	RED CELL CONSTANTS	TARGET CELLS (PER CENT)	ANISOCYTOSIS AND POIKILOCYTOSIS	SICKLING
Homozygous										
Sickle cell anemia	S + S	2-25	+++	++++	−	+++	Normocytic normochromic	5-30	Minimal	+
HbC disease	C + C	<7	+	−	++	±	Slightly microcytic normochromic	40-90	Minimal	−
HbD disease	D + D	2	−	−	−	−	Microcytic normochromic	40-80	Minimal	−
HbE disease	E + E	<7	+	−	±	±	Microcytic normochromic	25-60	Minimal	−
Mixed Heterozygous										
Sickle cell-HbC disease	C + S(F†)	<7	− to +++	− to +++	± to +++	− to +++	Slightly microcytic, slightly hypochromic to normochromic	20-85	Minimal	+
Sickle cell-HbD disease	D + S(F†)		++	+	− to +++	+++	?	Infrequent	Marked	+
Thalassemia Syndrome										
Thalassemia major	A + F		++++		++++	++++	Microcytic hypochromic	10-35	+++	−
Thalassemia-HbS disease	S + F + A		+ to ++++		+ to +++	++ to ++++	Microcytic hypochromic	20-40	+++	+
Thalassemia-HbC disease	A + C(F†)		+ to ++		?	− to ++	Microcytic hypochromic	10-30	++	−
Thalassemia-HbE disease	E + F		+ to ++++		+ to ++++	+ to ++++	Microcytic hypochromic	10-40	+++	−

*Modified from Chernoff (1958).
†F may be present.

enhanced by adding a reducing substance to the preparation.

METHOD. One drop of blood is added to 2 drops of freshly prepared 2 per cent sodium metabisulfite (conveniently available as 200-mg. capsules ready to add to 10 ml. of distilled water). A coverslip is placed on the slide and may be sealed with petrolatum, or the slide may be kept in a moist chamber, preferably at 37° C. A similar preparation, but with saline instead of the reducing agent, is set up as a control. The slides are examined under the microscope immediately with the high dry objective and again at 30 minutes. It is advisable to reexamine at 2 hours before concluding that the test is negative. Sickling is best seen near the edge of the coverslip. Partially sickled cells have a "holly-leaf" shape (Fig. 4–57).

INTERPRETATION. The test does not differentiate sickle cell anemia from sickle cell trait or other HbS syndromes; all the cells will sickle since the HbS is distributed homogeneously among the cells. Certain other abnormal hemoglobins ($HbC_{Georgetown}$, HbC_{Harlem}, or HbI) will also sickle.

SOURCES OF ERROR. Deterioration of the reducing agent will give false negative results. False negative tests may also occur when the amount of HbS is too small for detection, from admixture with alcohol (from skin preparation), from trapped air under the coverslip, or from inadequate sealing. Distortion of cells caused by ovalocytosis, extreme poikilocytosis, and crenation may be distinguished from sickle cells by comparison with the saline control.

Microscopic Test Without Reducing Agent. If a reducing solution is not available, a drop of blood may be placed on a slide, and a coverslip

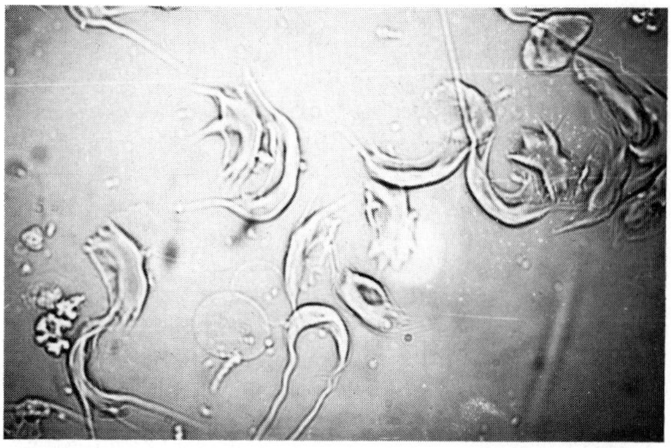

Figure 4–57. Positive sickle cell preparation. Sodium metabisulfite, after 24 hours. Note holly-leaf forms and sickled forms. After long incubation, unusually long crystals sometimes develop.

applied over it and sealed. Sickling will occur after several hours in sickle cell anemia; it will take longer in sickle cell trait. Placing a rubber band around the finger to deoxygenate the blood *in vivo* before sampling by finger stick will shorten the times involved.

Dithionite Tube Test

PRINCIPLE. HbS is reduced by dithionite and is insoluble in concentrated inorganic buffers. The polymers of reduced HbS obstruct light rays from passing through the solution. This test is particularly useful for screening large numbers of people for HbS. Positive results must be confirmed.

REAGENTS. Sickledex (Ortho Diagnostics, Raritan, N.J.) is a commercially available kit which provides all the reagents (Diggs and Walker, 1971). Alternatively, these may be made up as follows at a considerable saving in cost per test (Greenberg *et al.*, 1972):

1. Phosphate buffer, 2.36 M. Dissolve 236.7 gm. of potassium hydrophosphate and 135.9 gm. of potassium dihydrophosphate in distilled water and adjust the final volume to one liter. The pH should be about 7.0.
2. Precipitating reagent: Add 2 ml. of 5 per cent saponin and 2 ml. of 20 per cent sodium dithionite ($Na_2S_2O_4$) to 100 ml. of the phosphate buffer. Fresh dithionite must be used each day, as it deteriorates readily.
3. Blood may be fresh or anticoagulated. Hemolysates may be used.

PROCEDURE. Patients and normal control blood are tested.

Place 0.02 ml. of blood in a test tube 12 mm. in diameter. Add 2 ml. of the precipitating reagent. Invert the tube three times to mix. After three minutes' incubation at room temperature, examine the tube for opacity or transparency. Opacity is present when black newsprint cannot be seen through the solution in good light at a distance of 2.5 cm. from the tube.

INTERPRETATION. Opacity indicates an insoluble hemoglobin which is almost always hemoglobin S (or a non-HbS sickling hemoglobin), whether in homozygous, or heterozygous, or mixed heterozygous state. Normal blood or other abnormal hemoglobins result in transparency. Positive or doubtful tests are confirmed with the metabisulfite test and electrophoresis.

SOURCES OF ERROR

False positive reactions may occur:

1. In unstable hemoglobin disorders after splenectomy, when large numbers of Heinz bodies are present.

2. In blood protein disorders, such as multiple myeloma, due to precipitation of plasma proteins.

3. If the tube is held too far from the newsprint.

4. If there is too much blood for the quantity of reagent.

False negative reactions may occur if:

1. The patient is severely anemic. It is advisable to double the quantity of blood if the hematocrit is less than 30 per cent.

2. The dithionite has deteriorated, in which case the characteristic color (purple to red) may have changed to orange.

3. The saponin has deteriorated.

4. The tube is held too close to the newsprint.

Inclusion Bodies (Hemoglobin H and Heinz Bodies). See p. 179.

Alkali Denaturation Test for HbF (Singer et al., 1951). Fetal hemoglobin resists alkali denaturation; adult hemoglobin does not. A hemolysate is alkalinized and then neutralized, and the denatured adult hemoglobin is precipitated by ammonium sulfate. A filtrate will then contain only alkali-resistant hemoglobin, which is measured and expressed as a percentage of the total.

REAGENTS. N/12 KOH or NaOH, kept in refrigerator in plastic- or paraffin-lined containers (alkaline reagent). Fifty per cent saturated $(NH_4)_2SO_4$ is prepared by adding 500 ml. saturated $(NH_4)_2SO_4$ to 500 ml. distilled water; to this, 2.5 ml. concentrated (11 N) HCl is added (precipitating solution).

PROCEDURE. A hemolysate is prepared by washing blood once with 0.85 per cent saline, centrifuging, discarding the supernatant, and adding 1.5 volumes of distilled water to the volume of cells plus 0.4 volume of toluene. Shake vigorously for 5 minutes. Centrifuge at 3000 r.p.m. for 10 minutes. Discard the upper two layers. Adjust the concentration of the hemolysate to about 10 gm. hemoglobin per 100 ml. with distilled water. Determine the hemoglobin concentration (H_1). Add 0.1 ml. of the H_1 hemolysate to 1.6 ml. of the alkaline reagent. To mix, rinse the pipette five to six times while shaking the tube.

After exactly 1 minute, add 3.4 ml. precipitating reagent to stop the reaction and precipitate the nonresistant hemoglobin. Invert the tube three to four times and filter immediately. The filtrate (H_2) is a 1 to 50 dilution of the original hemoglobin solution (H_1). It is convenient to measure the optical density of H_2 directly and of a dilution of 0.02 ml. of H_1 in 4 ml. of distilled water (H_3) at 540 nm. The percentage of alkali-resistant hemoglobin is:

$$\frac{\frac{1}{4}\text{ optical density of } H_2}{\text{optical density of } H_3} \times 100.$$

INTERPRETATION. The filtrate (H_2) from normal adult blood is colorless and is less than 2 per cent of the total hemoglobin. Filtrates from blood with over 2 per cent HbF are brown to red. The alkali denaturation method is insensitive to less than 2 per cent HbF, so all figures below that level are considered to be normal.

Distribution of HbF on Stained Films. If the alkali-resistant hemoglobin is in the range of 10 to 30 per cent in a person with clinical features of thalassemia minor, the distribution of HbF in stained blood films should be examined. The modification of the original method of Kleihauer and Betke by Shepard *et al.* (1962) is useful.

PRINCIPLE. Hemoglobins other than HbF are eluted from the red cells on an air-dried blood film by a citric acid–phosphate buffer (pH 3.3). Only HbF remains in the fixed red cells, and the distribution can be determined after staining.

INTERPRETATION. If the high HbF is caused by the high F gene for hereditary persistence of HbF, all the red cells will contain the same amount of HbF. If the cause is thalassemia or a hemoglobinopathy, some red cells will contain little HbF or none (ghosts), and others will contain considerable amounts.

Heat Labile Hemoglobin. Most unstable hemoglobins will precipitate within 3 hours if incubated at 50° C. (Dacie and Lewis, 1968). The original test has been modified; more rapid precipitation of unstable hemoglobin occurs with nonphosphate buffers (Schneiderman *et al.*, 1970).

REAGENTS

Buffer a. Tris-(hydroxymethyl) aminomethane (Tris), 0.1 M, pH = 7.4,
or b. Sodium barbital, 0.1 M, pH = 7.4.

PROCEDURE. Wash 1 ml. of fresh blood (in any anticoagulant) twice in 0.9 per cent NaCl. Lyse the packed red cells by adding 5 ml. distilled water and mixing gently. Add 5 ml. of buffer and centrifuge at 1500 g for 10 minutes. Place 2 ml. of the clear supernatant in a clean test tube and incubate at 50° C. in a waterbath. Examine the solution at 1, 2, and 3 hours for a precipitate.

If there is a precipitate, determine the amount of unstable hemoglobin present. Centrifuge the solution at 1200 G for 10 minutes. Dilute both the clear supernatant and the original hemolysate 1:20 with Drabkin's reagent. Read the optical density at 540 nm.

$$\%\ \text{Unstable hemoglobin} = \frac{(\text{OD unheated sample} - \text{OD heated sample})}{\text{OD unheated sample}} \times 100$$

INTERPRETATION. Normally no precipitate occurs at one hour and only a trace at three hours at 50° C. Greater amounts of precipitates, from 10 to 40 per cent of the total, are found in hemoglobinopathies owing to unstable hemoglobins.

Electrophoresis of Hemoglobin. Hemoglobin molecules in an alkaline solution have a net negative charge and move toward the anode in an electrophoretic system at a speed proportional to the strength of their charge. Those with an electrophoretic mobility greater than that of HbA at pH 8.6 in barbital buffer are known as the "fast hemoglobins"; these include Hb Barts and the two fastest, HbH and HbI. HbC is the slowest of the common hemoglobins. A few of those with increasing mobility (in order) are HbA_2, HbE, HbO, HbD = HbS, HbL, HbG, HbA (Fig. 4–58). HbF can be separated from HbA on agar gel, but not on paper or cellulose acetate.

Different types of apparatus are commercially available or can be devised for Hb electrophoresis. The hemolysate is applied to a suspending medium (e.g., filter paper, cellulose acetate, starch gel, agar gel, or starch block) between chambers containing buffer solution, and a constant voltage is applied. Different media and different buffers vary in efficiency of separation. None is both practical and adequate for *all* separations and for screening purposes (Lehmann and Huntsman, 1966).

Filter paper electrophoresis with barbital

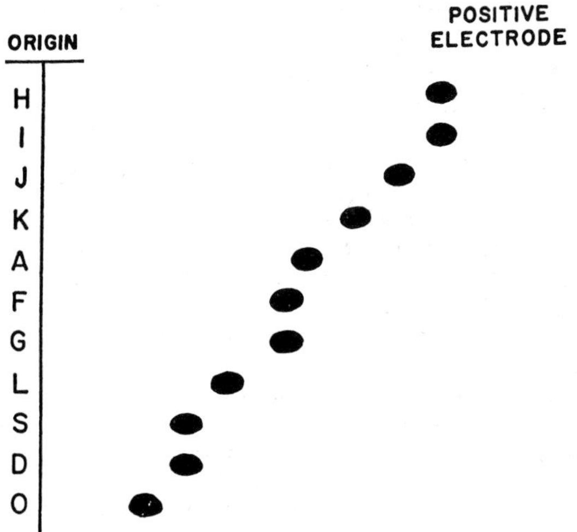

Figure 4–58. Relative migrations of the human hemoglobins after electrophoresis on filter paper in 0.05 M barbital buffer at pH 8.6. Hemoglobins H and I may be separated by filter paper electrophoresis at pH 6.5 (phosphate buffer). Hemoglobins S and D may be differentiated by virtue of their different solubilities in phosphate buffer under standard conditions. Hemoglobins F and G may be differentiated from each other by the resistance of the former to denaturation by alkali. (From Page and Culver: *A Syllabus of Laboratory Examinations in Clinical Diagnosis: Critical Evaluation of Laboratory Procedures in the Study of the Patient.* Revised edition. Cambridge, Harvard University Press, 1960.)

buffer is simple and satisfactory for routine use and gives separations indicated above but will not show HbA_2. Tris buffer will allow the demonstration of small Hb fractions, including HbA_2, but is less satisfactory for separating S and C or S and E.

Cellulose acetate electrophoresis requires less hemolysate, is more rapid, and allows essentially similar separations. Starch-gel and starch-block electrophoresis provide more distinct separations and are particularly valuable for the best quantitation of HbA_2 (the bands can be cut out, eluted, and the optical density measured), but they are more troublesome to employ. Agar gel appears to be best for electrophoretic separation of HbF.

For quantitation of HbA_2, the starch-block method of Kunkel *et al.* (1957) is probably most consistently reliable. Examples of other methods that can be used somewhat more readily in a routine clinical laboratory are cellulose acetate (Marengo-Rowe, 1965), DEAE cellulose chromatography (Huisman and Dozy, 1961), starch gel (Aksoy and Erdem, 1965), and agar gel (Yakulis *et al.*, 1960).

Final characterization of abnormal hemoglobins is beyond the scope of the usual routine laboratory. It consists of purification of the abnormal hemoglobin with starch-block electrophoresis, hybridization experiments to determine whether the abnormality lies in the alpha or beta chain, and "fingerprinting." In the latter procedure, the polypeptide chains are split by enzymatic digestion into peptides that are separated by performing horizontal paper electrophoresis and vertical chromatography in sequence. This peptide map, or "fingerprint," is compared with that prepared from normal hemoglobin, and the peptide in which the abnormality occurs can be located. The abnormal peptide is then eluted and its amino acid content determined.

PAROXYSMAL NOCTURNAL HEMOGLOBINURIA (PNH)

PNH is characterized by chronic intravascular hemolysis and hemoglobinuria which are more marked during and after sleep and may be related to the increased susceptibility of the red cells to an acid pH. Hemoglobinuria may be intermittent, but hemosiderinuria is more consistently present. The disease shows spontaneous remissions and exacerbations and is refractory to therapy.

The blood shows a normochromic anemia with a reticulocytosis which is often less than expected for the degree of anemia. Pancytopenia is common. Red cell acetylcholinesterase and leukocyte alkaline phosphatase are decreased. Osmotic fragility is not increased. The direct Coombs' test is negative.

The marrow may be hypercellular with normoblastic hyperplasia, or it may be hypocellular. It is becoming clear that in some patients marrow failure may occur during the course of PNH, and that in others, aplastic anemia is the initial diagnosis, with signs of PNH later manifesting themselves. Possibly an abnormal line of cells develops in an aplastic or regenerating marrow (Lewis and Dacie, 1967).

PNH is an acquired intrinsic defect of erythrocytes which renders them sensitive to complement. The nature of the red cell defect is unknown, but it allows the cell to lyse in the presence of complement, without the apparent necessity for antibody.

The diagnosis of PNH requires a positive acidified serum test (Ham test). Screening tests are the sucrose hemolysis test and the cold antibody lysis test. All three depend upon the unusual susceptibility of the PNH cells to lysis by complement.

Sucrose Hemolysis Tests (Hartmann *et al.*, 1970)

Whole Blood Screening Test

PRINCIPLE. In both screening and confirmatory tests, red cells adsorb complement when exposed to oxalated or citrated plasma in a medium of low ionic strength, whether antibody is present or not. PNH red cells have increased sensitivity to complement-mediated lysis.

REAGENT. "Sugar water." Dissolve 10 ml. of table sugar in distilled water to make a final volume of 100 ml. This reagent is prepared freshly each day.

PROCEDURE. Add one part citrated or oxalated blood to nine parts of sugar water solution. Mix at once, then incubate for 30 minutes at room temperature. Centrifuge to sediment the red cells and note any hemolysis in the supernate.

INTERPRETATION. Lack of hemolysis is evidence against PNH. Presence of hemolysis means that the confirmatory sucrose hemolysis test must be performed. A normal control blood sample must give a negative result.

Confirmatory Sucrose Hemolysis Test

REAGENT

1. Isotonic sucrose solution: Dissolve 92.4 gm. reagent grade sucrose in 91 ml. of 50 mM. NaH_2PO_4 and 9 ml. of 50 mM. Na_2HPO_4 and adjust the pH to 6.1 with HCl or NaOH. Add distilled water to a volume of 1000 ml. This solution may be kept for two weeks at 4° C. Fresh sugar water solution (above) can be used as an alternative.

2. Fresh ABO type compatible serum from a normal individual (not from the patient). Serum stored at −70° C. or less is satisfactory for at least one year.

3. Red cells from patient and from a normal person are washed three times and 50 per cent suspensions prepared in 0.9 per cent NaCl.

4. Ammonium hydroxide (NH_4OH), 0.04 per cent.

PROCEDURE. Prepare two tubes by adding 0.05 ml. of ABO type compatible serum to 0.85 ml. sucrose solution and mixing. Add 0.1 ml. of 50 per cent suspension of patient's red cells to one tube and 0.1 ml. of 50 per cent suspension of normal red cells to the other and mix promptly. Incubate the tubes at room temperature for 30 minutes. Centrifuge and note any hemolysis in the supernate. If hemolysis is present, determine percentage. Use as a blank the serum-sucrose mixture and as a standard 0.1 ml. of the suspension of patient's red cells plus 0.9 ml. of 0.04 per cent NH_4OH; read at 540 nm.

INTERPRETATION. Five per cent hemolysis or less is a negative result. A number of other hematologic diseases may cause this degree of hemolysis. Five to 10 per cent is doubtful and over 10 per cent is positive and virtually diagnostic for PNH.

SOURCES OF ERROR. False positive results may occur: (1) if defibrinated blood is used; (2) if the patient's own serum is used, in cases of immune hemolytic anemia; (3) in the whole blood screening test, if the patient is severely anemic (this is not a problem in the confirmatory sucrose hemolysis test); or (4) if sucrose or sugar water solutions are stored for long periods of time before use. False negative results occur if the serum has been stored improperly, i.e., has lost its complement activity.

Acidified Serum Test (Ham Test) (Dacie and Lewis, 1968)

PRINCIPLE. The red cells in PNH are sensitive to lysis by complement, which is adsorbed to the red cell in acidified serum in the absence of antibody. A positive acidified serum test is required for the diagnosis of PNH, by definition.

REAGENTS

1. Red cells from patient and ABO compatible normal control, as above.
2. Fresh (or properly stored, at −70° C. or less) serum from patient and normal control.
3. Heat inactivated normal serum is prepared by heating at 56° C. for 30 minutes.
4. 0.2 N HCl.

PROCEDURE. Set up seven tubes. Add 0.5 ml. of normal serum to the four tubes indicated in Table 4–10, then add the other sera and acid as indicated and mix. After adding the red cell suspensions to the tubes, mix, and incubate in a waterbath at 37° C. After one hour centrifuge and examine supernatant serum for lysis.

The hemolysis is measured by pipetting 0.3 ml. of the supernatant sera into 5.0 ml. of 0.04 per cent NH_4OH and measuring the O.D. at 540 nm. As a blank use 0.5 ml. of serum, and as a 100 per cent standard use 0.05 ml. red cells + 0.55 ml. saline; both are diluted in the same manner as the supernatant sera.

INTERPRETATION. Lysis of PNH cells occurs with acidified normal serum and acidified patient serum (often to a lesser degree). If lysis also occurs with heat inactivated normal acidified serum the test is not positive, as markedly spherocytic cells will react in this way. Normal cells should not lyse in any of the three tubes. Lysis of PNH cells is always partial, usually between 10 and 50 per cent.

A positive acidified serum test defines the PNH abnormality, whether in typical PNH or in aplastic anemia. It has also been found in a rare condition, congenital dyserythropoietic anemia, type II (p. 197). In the latter, however, lysis never occurs with the patient's own serum, only with normal sera.

Hemolytic Anemias Due to Extracorpuscular Factors

Chemical Agents

Agents Hemolytic to Normal Cells. The action of chemical agents depends on the dose and on other factors, many of which are known only vaguely. They range from simple substances, such as water, to some that are highly complex.

When it was used as irrigating fluid, distilled

Table 4–10. ACIDIFIED-SERUM TEST*

	1	2	3	4	5	6	7
Fresh normal serum	0.5	0.5			0.5	0.5	
Patient's serum			0.5				
Heat inactivated normal serum				0.5			0.5
0.2 N HCl		0.05	0.05	0.05		0.05	0.05
50% Patient's red cells	0.05	0.05	0.05	0.05			
50% Normal red cells					0.05	0.05	0.05
Pattern of lysis in positive test	Trace	+++	+	−	−	−	−

*Modified from Dacie, J. V., and Lewis, S. M.: Practical Haematology. 4th ed. New York, Grune & Stratton, Inc., 1968.

water was found responsible for acute hemolytic anemia as a result of entry into venous channels during transurethral resection. In addition to anemia some of these chemicals produce methemoglobinemia, and some are responsible for cyanosis (toluene, trinitrotoluene, nitrobenzene, acetanilid, and phenacetin). Some may lead to aplastic anemia (toluene and trinitrotoluene). Promin, a sulfone derivative, makes blood turn chocolate brown. Lead administered therapeutically may produce progressive anemia, with basophilic stippling, reticulocytosis, normoblastemia, Cabot's rings, Howell-Jolly bodies, and leukocytosis. Lead not only causes damage to the red cell and hemolysis, but also produces defects in the heme synthetic pathway. In cases of chronic exposure to lead, basophilic stippling, more in the marrow than in the peripheral blood, and coproporphyrinuria are the characteristic findings. These changes produce defective erythrocytes, which are removed by the spleen.

Agents Hemolytic to Defective Cells (Hereditary Element). Certain drugs and chemicals which have oxidizing activity (e.g., nitrobenzene, aniline, phenylhydrazine, trinitrotoluene, sulfonamides, and primaquine) may produce hemolytic anemia in only a few of the many persons who are exposed to them. It is now clear that some biochemical defects of the red cell prevent it from keeping hemoglobin in the reduced state under the stress of these oxidant drugs; as a result, methemoglobinemia is present, and denatured hemoglobin (in the form of Heinz bodies) can be found. These biochemical defects have been mentioned in the section on metabolic defects of the cell or hereditary nonspherocytic hemolytic anemias (p. 203) and include glucose-6-phosphate dehydrogenase (G6PD) deficiency, glutathione deficiency, and glutathione reductase deficiency. In addition, unstable hemoglobins such as Hb Zürich have a propensity for drug-induced hemolytic anemia. Premature infants, although they have high levels of G6PD, have glutathione instability and low levels of glutathione and may develop hemolytic anemia when given large doses of synthetic water-soluble analogues of vitamin K.

It must be remembered that, if the exposure to these oxidant substances is great enough, acute hemolytic anemia may be produced in normal individuals; persons with biochemical abnormalities are sensitive to lower doses.

During the acute hemolytic episode, Heinz bodies can frequently be demonstrated by direct vital staining of blood with methyl violet (p. 179). Red cells with Heinz bodies are removed from the circulation by the spleen, or the Heinz bodies are extracted from the red cells by splenic action. Therefore, Heinz bodies will no longer be found in the blood once the acute hemolytic process has abated.

Tests for G6PD deficiency, the most common underlying cause for drug-sensitive hemolytic anemia, are described on p. 204.

Physical Agents. Extensive third degree burns produce hemolytic anemia, probably because of direct damage to red cells. The blood film may show remarkable morphologic abnormalities of the red cells, including numerous schistocytes (fragments) and irregularly contracted cells. The most severe abnormalities are often found immediately after extensive burns before a reticulocyte response has had time to develop (Fig. 4–19). The badly damaged cells are rapidly removed from the circulation.

Hemolytic anemia characterized by striking morphologic abnormalities of the red cells and occurring in certain other conditions has been attributed to physical trauma to the red cells. The red cell abnormalities are present in varying degree and include fragments (schistocytes) and irregularly contracted cells (burr cells, triangular cells, helmet cells) (Fig. 4–24). The basis of the hemolytic process has been thought to be physical damage to the red cells in their contact with loose fibrin meshworks (intravascular coagulation) or with pathologic vascular lesions. Fragmentation of the cells results with or without intravascular lysis. Two general categories are recognized in this group of disorders, aptly termed the "red cell fragmentation syndrome."

Cardiac Valvular Disease and Prostheses. Chronic intravascular hemolysis associated with low serum haptoglobin, hemosiderinuria, reticulocytosis, and red cell abnormalities (e.g., schistocytes and irregularly contracted cells) may occur after surgical replacement of a diseased heart valve with a prosthesis or after surgical repair of a septal defect with a plastic patch (Marsh and Lewis, 1969). This has been attributed to mechanical damage of red cells in the turbulent environment of a leaky valve or of a roughened surface uncovered by endothelial cells. Repair of the valve or coverage of the patch by endothelium has improved the hemolytic process. Other studies have shown that some patients with cardiac valvular disease have a hemolytic process which may be altered by surgery.

Microangiopathic Hemolytic Anemia. Hemolytic anemia with red cell abnormalities (e.g., schistocytes and irregularly contracted cells) has been described in malignant hypertension, thrombotic thrombocytopenic purpura, and disseminated carcinoma, in which a common factor was the presence of pathologic lesions involving small blood vessels. The hypothesis was advanced that the hemolytic anemia in these conditions may be an expression of mechanical or perhaps chemical effects of the vascular lesions on the red cells, and the process was designated "microangiopathic"

isoantibodies. They are of two types: In one, the isoantibody (made by the patient himself) is already present in his serum, and the disease is due to introduction of the corresponding isoantigen (not normally present in the patient's cells or tissues). An example of this is the hemolytic transfusion reaction that results when Group O individuals are transfused with red cells of groups A, B, or AB (p. 397). Anemia, strictly speaking, is not a part of this clinical syndrome (although the patient may have been anemic to begin with!), since the patient's own cells are not destroyed.

In the second type of isoimmune hemolytic disease, isoantibody made by another individual is introduced into the patient's blood stream. For example, if Group O plasma (containing isoagglutinins anti-A and anti-B) is transfused into a person of Group A, a hemolytic anemia may result if the plasma contains high titers of isoantibodies.

HEMOLYTIC DISEASE OF THE NEWBORN. Erythroblastosis fetalis is an isoimmune disease of this type. Antibody is made by the mother against antigen present on fetal cells, but not on her own cells. This occurs when fetal cells bearing this antigen are introduced into the mother's circulation. The antibody, if then able to cross the placenta, attaches to the fetal red cells and results in shortened survival.

Blood Findings in Hemolytic Disease of the Newborn. Early examination of the blood usually reveals an increase of immature nucleated erythrocytes (pronormoblasts and normoblasts). On the other hand, although this finding gave the disease its name, erythroblastemia is not always present, especially if the examination is not done immediately after birth.

Up to 2000 nucleated red cells/μl. in term infants and up to 5000/μl. in premature infants are commonly seen; normally, nucleated red cells average 500/μl. in term infants and 1000–1500/μl. in premature infants. Blood from the umbilical vein for early examination is more reliable than peripheral (capillary) blood because the erythrocyte count and the hemoglobin may be significantly altered between birth and ligation of the cord.

Generally there is a macrocytic anemia of varying severity and an increase in reticulocytes. In fetal erythroblastosis caused by ABO incompatibility, spherocytes are conspicuous. Occasionally anemia may appear suddenly on the second or third day or even later. The platelet count is frequently below the lower normal value of 150,000 per microliter. The leukocyte count is frequently elevated, with many immature leukocytes including myelocytes and even blasts (Fig. 4–59). There is pronounced normoblastic hyperplasia of the marrow (Fig. 4–60).

Figure 4–59. Hemolytic disease of the newborn (fetal erythroblastosis), peripheral blood. The erythrocytes are predominantly macrocytic and show considerable aniso- and poikilocytosis. This finding alone suggests Rh incompatibility as the cause of the erythroblastosis. In erythroblastosis caused by ABO incompatibility, spherocytes are frequent.

The predominant nucleated cells in this preparation are orthochromatic normoblasts with dense, compact, and coarse nuclei, many of them deformed and lobated. At 3 o'clock the arrow points at a polychromatophilic normoblast. Its large nucleus with its chromatin subdivided by the lighter parachromatin testifies to its younger age when compared with the more mature, almost orthochromatic normoblast just touching it toward the center. The signs of advancing age of the latter cell are its small compact nucleus and more hemoglobin and the consequent lighter blue of its cytoplasm. A polychromatophilic normoblast with a misshaped nucleus having three finger-like projections is at 7 o'clock, another almost orthochromatic normoblast with a single knob on its nucleus is at 8 o'clock, followed clockwise by a polychromatophilic, larger, and somewhat younger normoblast. The arrow at 10 o'clock points at a neutrophilic myelocyte. Sharply at 12 o'clock is a neutrophilic metamyelocyte surrounded clockwise by an orthochromatic normoblast, a proerythroblast, the youngest cell in the preparation, and by another orthochromatic normoblast. (From L. Heilmeyer and H. Begemann: Atlas der Klinischen Hämatologie und Cytologie, Springer, 1955.)

Figure 4–60. Hemolytic anemia, marrow. The illustration shows the characteristic findings of a reactive, predominantly normoblastic hyperplasia. We will start just a little to the right of the very top of the circle, at 1 o'clock, where, conveniently located for orientation, is the familiar segmented granulocyte. What seems to be a separate nucleus on the left in this cell is actually connected with a fine filament that cannot be seen here. To the right of the granulocyte, touching it and slightly deformed by it, is probably a basophilic normoblast. As we travel down the circle, we find at 2 o'clock two polychromatophilic normoblasts of which there are many in the preparation. These cells are somewhat younger than a number of almost orthochromatic normoblasts with their small dense pyknotic nuclei. One of them is impinging on or, more correctly, is being impinged upon by the second of two polychromatophilic normoblasts which we have just described. At 4 o'clock we find in a colony of eleven cells three varieties of erythroid cells. The one at which the arrow is pointing is a proerythroblast. Its chromatin is loosely knitted, and it has three distinct nucleoli and a deeply basophilic cytoplasm. Touching it toward the center of the field is a normoblast that differs from the proerythroblast just described by the coarsening of its nucleus and the almost polychromatophilic color of its cytoplasm owing to advancing hemoglobinization. This cell, which is best labeled as a polychromatophilic normoblast, is just slightly younger than the two fully ripened polychromatophilic normoblasts just above and the six just below the proerythroblast. The large cell toward the center of the field bordering on the six polychromatophilic normoblasts just described is another proerythroblast.

At 7 o'clock the arrow points at a neutrophilic myelocyte. Covering it toward the center are two polychromatophilic normoblasts, followed in the same direction by a promyelocyte. Note the difference between the fewer and coarser granules of the promyelocyte and the abundant and finer granules of the myelocyte. At 8 o'clock the arrow points to another proerythroblast distinctly younger than the one at 4 o'clock. The large nucleus and the looser structure of the chromatin testify to its younger age. Roughly at 11 o'clock we see what looks like the cytoplasmic body of a neutrophilic myelocyte cut in half with the nucleus left outside. The amputated cell is surrounded by two basophilic normoblasts. (From L. Heilmeyer and H. Begemann: Atlas der Klinischen Hämatologie und Cytologie. Springer, 1955.)

Autoimmune Diseases. The antigen is an autoantigen (a modified part of the patient's own body). The antibody is an autoantibody (also a modified part of the patient's own body). Examples are idiopathic and symptomatic autoimmune hemolytic anemia, autoimmune leukopenia, and paroxysmal cold hemoglobinuria.

Knowledge of autoimmune diseases goes back to the end of the 19th century but was pushed into the background by the authority of Paul Ehrlich, who coined the phrase "horror autotoxicus," with which he expressed his conviction that antibodies could not be formed in the body against its own tissues, because this would not be compatible with life. There were occasional breakthroughs, such as Donath and Landsteiner's test for cold paroxysmal hemoglobinuria and studies on hemolytic anemia by the French hematologists of the beginning of the century.

The recent great advances have been made possible by the progress in our knowledge and understanding of antibodies, which vary widely in their properties and behavior. Some do not react in saline but need plasma, albumin, macromolecular substances in general, or proteolytic enzymes. These are *incomplete antibodies* as compared with *complete antibodies,* which react well in saline. Much of this new knowledge came as a by-product of studies on the Rh factor.

Some antibodies react only at warm (body) temperatures and others at cold temperatures, with optimums at a particular degree of temperature. Some react only at a certain pH. Some agglutinate only but do not hemolyze directly. The agglutinated red cells become subject to destructive forces in the reticuloendothelial system. Some are hemolysins, lysis taking place at only one temperature, warm or cold (monothermal). Some are hemolysins but require two temperature levels, first cold and then warm (bithermal).

In recent years, some of these phenomena have been explained by the modern theory of antibody (i.e., immunoglobulin) structure (p. 572) and by more detailed analysis of the factors involved in red cell agglutination and lysis. Normal red cells suspended in saline carry a net negative surface charge, which causes them to repel each other and remain separated. The large, bulky IgM antibodies are able to bridge this electrostatic "gap" and thus can agglutinate red cells in saline. This is the definition of a "complete" antibody. IgG antibodies, because of their smaller size, are usually unable to agglutinate cells in saline and so are called "incomplete" antibodies. They will, however, cause agglutination in albumin (which neutralizes some of the negative charge), or when the cells are subsequently exposed to antiglobulin serum (p. 359).

The lytic behavior of various antibodies can best be explained in terms of variation in their ability to fix complement. Since one IgM molecule is sufficient to bind a molecule of C′1, it is frequently found that IgM antibodies are potent hemolysins. But some of the most powerfully lytic antibodies known, such as the Donath-Landsteiner antibody, are IgG antibodies; this may reflect both antigen-site density and the varying efficiency of complement fixation among the different IgG subclasses (IgG_1, IgG_2, and so forth).

Finally, most warm-reacting antibodies are IgG, and most cold antibodies are IgM. The physicochemical basis for this variation in thermal behavior is still unknown.

Because knowledge is still incomplete, the terms "warm" and "cold," "complete" and "incomplete" will be used in the discussion that follows. Although they may be retained for convenience and historical interest, there is little doubt that these empiric terms will eventually be supplanted by more precise biochemical ones.

Incomplete Warm Autohemoantibodies

DEFINITION. These are IgG antibodies that combine with red cells at 37° C. Demonstrable reactions, e.g., agglutination, do not occur in saline except when the red cells are treated with proteolytic enzymes, but reactions can be demonstrated in macromolecular mediums, such as serum albumin and plasma, and with antiglobulin serum.

ELUTION OF AUTOANTIBODIES. Incomplete autoantibodies can be separated from the red cells by suspending the latter in small amounts of saline of suitable temperature and centrifuging at the same temperature. The supernatant contains the antibodies. Maximum elution of warm antibodies takes place at 56° C. In the body, red cells coated with these antibodies are rapidly destroyed. Warm antibodies are responsible for idiopathic and symptomatic acquired hemolytic anemia.

Warm autohemolysins occasionally are present together with warm autoagglutinins and react best at 37° C.

Cold Agglutinins. Cold agglutinins are antibodies that agglutinate the patient's own and almost all other human erythrocytes. Once thought to be nonspecific, these antibodies are now known to be specific for an antigen called I. This is present on the red cells of almost all adult humans, the only exceptions being a very few individuals who have instead an antigen called i. Newborn infants have the i antigen but lose it and develop the I antigen during infancy. Reaction temperature ranges from 0 to 20° C. At 0 to 10° C. cold agglutinins are almost universal. Antibodies reacting only at such low temperatures have no pathologic significance. They are the so-called physiologic cold agglutinins.

Pathologic agglutinins also exert maximal effect at 0° C. but have a wider thermal amplitude. The highest temperature at which they react is, as a rule, 30° C.

The range of titers of physiologic cold agglutinins at 0° C. is 0 to 128. The most frequent titer is around 1 to 8. In chronic cold agglutinin disease the range is 4000 to 512,000. Erythrocytes coated with cold agglutinins have increased mechanical fragility.

Hemolysins. *Natural isohemolysins* are rare. They have been reported in some of the blood group systems, e.g., Lewis.

Immune isohemolysins are seen following injection of incompatible blood or so-called purified specific blood group substances.

Bithermal autohemolysins are seen in paroxysmal cold hemoglobinuria.

Bithermal cold autohemolysins are abnormal serum globulin capable of hemolyzing the patient's own and other persons' red cells.

They combine with erythrocytes (sensitization of erythrocytes) at temperature below 20° C. They do not combine with red cells at temperature higher than 20° C. When temperature rises to 25° C., hemolysis begins. The optimum temperature for hemolysis is 40° C. The titers are low: 2 to 16; the highest recorded was 64, and even then it was transient.

Monothermal cold autohemolysins, having a thermal range of 15 to 30° C. (optimum: 22° C.), occur simultaneously with high-titer cold agglutinins. They are the cause of excessive destruction of red cells and of hemolytic anemia. They react best at slightly acid pH (acid hemolysins); the optimum pH is 6.3 and the range, pH 6 to 7. The serum is acidified by adding 10 volumes per cent of 0.4 N HCl. The range of titers of cold monothermal autohemolysins is 320 to 2048; the highest reported titer was 8000.

Collection of Blood and Serum. For the study of cold autoantibodies it is best to collect the blood with a prewarmed syringe in a prewarmed test tube (both at 37° C.) and to place the tube immediately into a container with water maintained at 37° C. until it is transferred into an incubator. There it remains until it clots and the clot is retracted. Centrifugation must also be carried out at the same temperature. The serum is then removed with a capillary pipette. If cells are mixed with the serum, the specimen must be recentrifuged at 37° C. The procedure may be simplified somewhat by using a prewarmed Vacutainer tube.

Red cells can be obtained from the same specimen by breaking up the warm clot, transferring them to a test tube with warm (37° C.) saline, washing with warm saline, and centrifuging at the same temperature. They can also be obtained with an anticoagulant, e.g., acid citrate-dextrose (ACD) or oxalate, but again maintaining 37° C. is essential.

For shipping by mail, the serum should be obtained as described and whole blood collected in ACD solution. Upon arrival at the destination the whole blood will have to be placed in an incubator before the cells are washed. Serum should be stored frozen in 1- to 2-ml. vials at −20° C. or less. Red cells will keep for two to three weeks in ACD or in another suitable solution. They can be kept for considerably longer periods at −20° C. in glycerin. Once washed and suspended in saline, they must be used within a few hours.

RED CELL SUSPENSION. For agglutination tests a 2 per cent suspension is used, and for hemolysin tests a 4 to 5 per cent is used.

Testing for Autoantibodies. The direct antiglobulin (Coombs') test detects antibodies attached to red cells (see p. 371). The indirect antiglobulin (Coombs') test (ICT) detects free autoantibodies in the serum. Warm autoantibodies are detectable more readily with enzyme-treated red cells than with the ICT test (for technical details see p. 372). On the other hand, cold autoantibodies are readily detected with the indirect antiglobulin test. Successful use of the ICT depends on meticulous technique and attention to sources of error. The following outline is based on the recommendations of Dacie (1960–1967).

TEMPERATURE. The temperature recommended for incubation must be adhered to strictly. Carrying out the test at 37° C. means carrying out the entire procedure at that temperature from the moment one obtains the blood specimen until the reading of the results. Tests at 4° C. are less informative than those at 20° C., because normal incomplete cold antibodies may interfere.

pH. For detection of incomplete cold hemolysins, acidification of the test serum with 10 per cent by volume of 0.25 N HCl is essential before the red cells are added.

COMPLEMENT. Inactivation of the test serum at 56° C. for as little as 5 minutes destroys its reactivity in the ICT. To use such inactivated serum one has to add one or more volumes of fresh normal serum but only after normal incomplete cold antibody has been absorbed from it. The same applies to serum that has lost its complement activity on prolonged standing.

On the other hand, the warm autoantibody of the gamma globulin type does not require complement and can be used after inactivation.

TEST CELLS. Some warm autoantibodies are specific, especially for certain types in the Rh system. Hence, cells of known Rh genotypes should be used, i.e., Rh_1Rh_1(CDe/CDe), Rh_2Rh_2(cDE/cDE), and rh (cde/cde), and not just Rh-(D)-positive and -negative cells. For screening purposes, ORh_1Rh_2(CDe/cDE) cells should be used.

ANTIGLOBULIN SERUM. At least two dilutions

Figure 4–61.

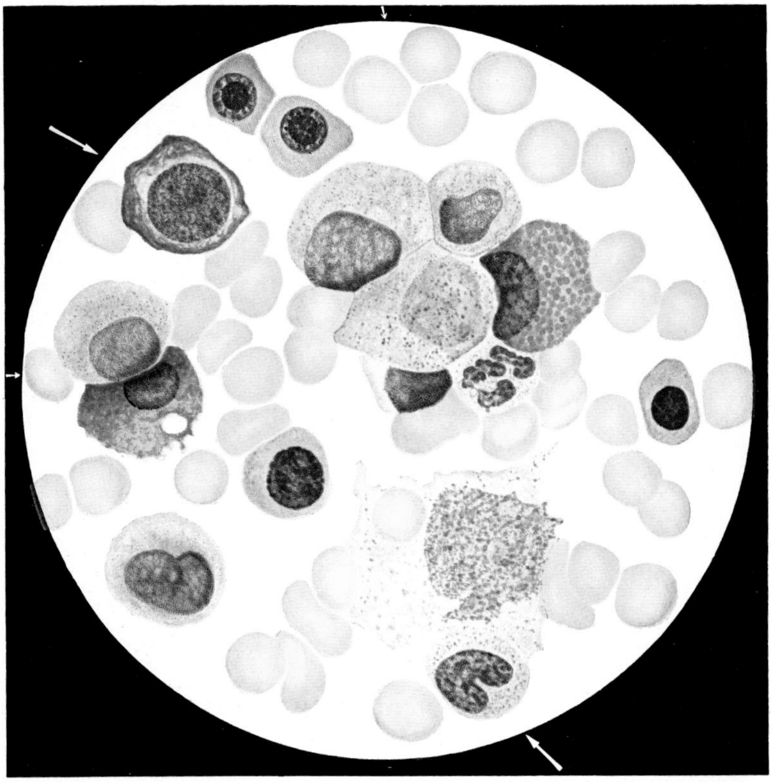

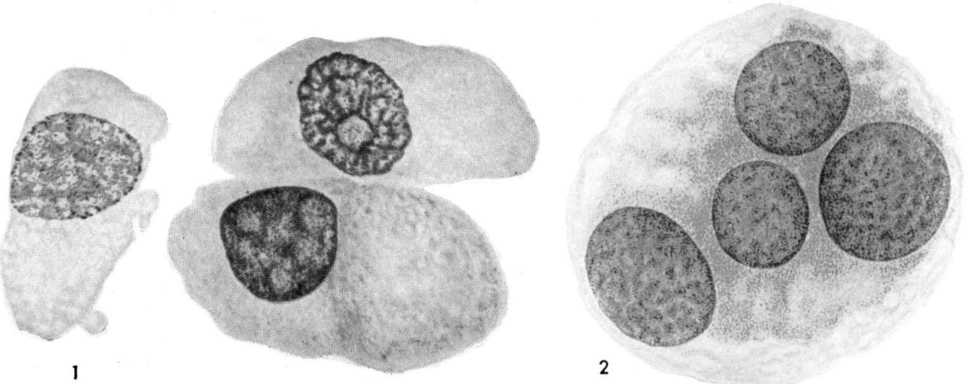

Figure 4–62.

Figure 4–61. Normal marrow. At the 12 o'clock position the arrow points to an island of six cells. Two at the top are neutrophilic myelocytes lying next to each other. The next two toward the center are a promyelocyte on the left and an eosinophilic myelocyte on its right. The visible portion of a cell partly covered by the promyelocyte is probably a normoblast. Next to it on the right is a neutrophilic segmented granulocyte.

At the bottom of the circle the arrow is directed at a metamyelocyte. Just above it is a reticulum cell, somewhat deformed and crowded by the adjacent red cells.

At 7 o'clock there is a metamyelocyte.

At 9 o'clock there is a myelocyte and next to it and below, a plasma cell.

At 10 o'clock a proerythroblast is seen, and just a short distance away clockwise are two orthochromatic normoblasts.

There is a superficial resemblance between the proerythroblast and the plasma cells. The main difference is in the size and structure of the nucleus. In the proerythroblast the nucleus is larger and the chromatin is delicately reticulated and granular. In the plasma cell it is more compact and clumped. In this reproduction of the plasma cell the separation into chromatin and parachromatin masses is not apparent. The presence of hemoglobin in the cytoplasm of the proerythroblast, even

(*Legend continued on opposite page.*)

have to be used: 1 to 4 and 1 to 64. The former is more likely to detect cold autoantibodies and the latter, the warm autoantibodies.

PROCEDURE. Fourteen test tubes are set up, seven in each of two racks.

RACK 1 (FOR INCUBATION AT 37° C.)	RACK 2 (FOR 20° C.)
Tube 1: To 0.25 ml. (5 drops) of serum add 0.05 ml. (1 drop) of 20 to 30 per cent suspension of ORh_1Rh_2 (CDe-cDE) cells.	same set-up
Tube 2: As tube 1, but serum acidified with 1/10 volume of 0.25 N HCl is used.	same
Tube 3: As tube 1, but an equal volume of fresh normal serum is added to the patient's serum.	same
Tube 4: As tube 3, but both the patient's and normal serum are acidified with 1/10 volume of 0.25 N HCl.	same
Tube 5: As tube 2, but patient's serum is inactivated at 56° C. for 30 minutes.	same
Tube 6: As tube 1, but with normal serum instead of patient's serum.	same
Tube 7: As tube 2 with normal serum instead of patient's serum.	same

The racks are shaken gently at intervals. After a 2-hour incubation the test tubes are inspected for agglutination or hemolysis and so recorded. The cells are washed at least three times in saline and the indirect antiglobulin test carried out.

INTERPRETATION OF RESULTS. Tube 1 determines the presence of warm autoantibodies at 37° C. Tube 6 is a negative serum control, and if positive, it invalidates a positive result in tube 1.

Tube 2 determines the presence of acid type of autoantibodies if the result is positive in it but negative in tube 1. Tube 7 is a negative serum control, and if positive it invalidates a positive result in tube 2.

A positive result in tube 3 establishes the role of complement in the reaction if tube 1 is negative. This is confirmed by a negative result in tube 5.

Tube 4 is a positive control for tubes 2 and 3.

The results in rack 2 show the presence and thermal reactivity of the antibodies at room temperature.

This is a qualitative test. If positive, the titer of the antibody and its specificity remain to be determined.

Gamma Globulin Neutralization Test (Dacie). Described by Dacie in 1951, this test involves the addition of gamma globulin to antiglobulin serum, which permits distinction of two types of antiglobulin reactions in autoimmune hemolytic anemia: (1) The reaction is inhibited by gamma globulin. This is the gamma globulin type which includes the majority of autoimmune hemolytic anemias due to warm autoantibodies. (2) The reaction is not inhibited by gamma globulin.

This test is now obsolete because of the availability of specific antiglobulin sera, i.e., anti-IgG, anti-IgM, anti-IgA, and also anticomplement sera. If these are unavailable, an anti-non-gamma antiglobulin serum can be made by adding an appropriate amount of IgG to a broad spectrum antiglobulin serum (Dacie and Lewis, 1968).

It is now known that the "gamma" antiglobulin reaction indicates the presence of antibody on the cells, particularly IgG. A positive "non-gamma" reaction, on the other hand, indicates that the globulin on the cell is not antibody but some other protein. This non-gamma globulin is actually one or more of the complement components. In the cold antibody type of immune hemolytic anemia, it is usually impossible to detect more than small amounts of antibody on the red cells, because the IgM antibody efficiently fixes complement; therefore, it is the rule for the non-gamma antiglobulin reaction to be positive.

Classification of Autoimmune Hemolytic Anemias (AIHA)

1. Acquired hemolytic anemias caused by incomplete warm autoantibodies.

A. *Chronic idiopathic AIHA.* Slow to start, insidious, not related to another disease. The immune nature of the hemolytic process is more frequently demonstrable in this form of anemia than in the symptomatic.

---

if only traces of it are present, may sometimes be another differential point. (From L. Heilmeyer and H. Begemann: Atlas der Klinischen Hämatologie und Cytologie. Springer, 1955.)

Figure 4–62. Osteoblasts and osteoclasts.

1. The three oval-shaped cells on the left are osteoblasts. They measure about 30 microns in their longest diameter. The nucleus is somewhat eccentrically located. Its chromatin structure is coarse. It contains one or more deeply blue nucleoli. The cytoplasm is purplish blue. Within it, some distance away from the nucleus, in the part of the cell with more abundant cytoplasm, is an indefinitely outlined, light colored area, the archoplasm.

Familiarity with this marrow cell is important, because otherwise it may be mistaken for a plasma cell, and if such cells are present in sheets, they may be mistaken for cancer cells.

2. The multinucleated cell on the right is an osteoclast. It has four nuclei with a finely reticulated chromatin structure and a distinct margin. The cytoplasm is reddish purple and finely granular. It may contain coarse inclusions, which are interpreted as phagocytosed osseous debris. These cells are seen frequently in children and in osteitis fibrosa. They may have as many as 100 nuclei. Familiarity with them is essential because they also are easily mistaken for cancer cells. (From L. Heilmeyer and H. Begemann: Atlas der Klinischen Hämatologie und Cytologie. Springer, 1955.)

Figure 4–63.

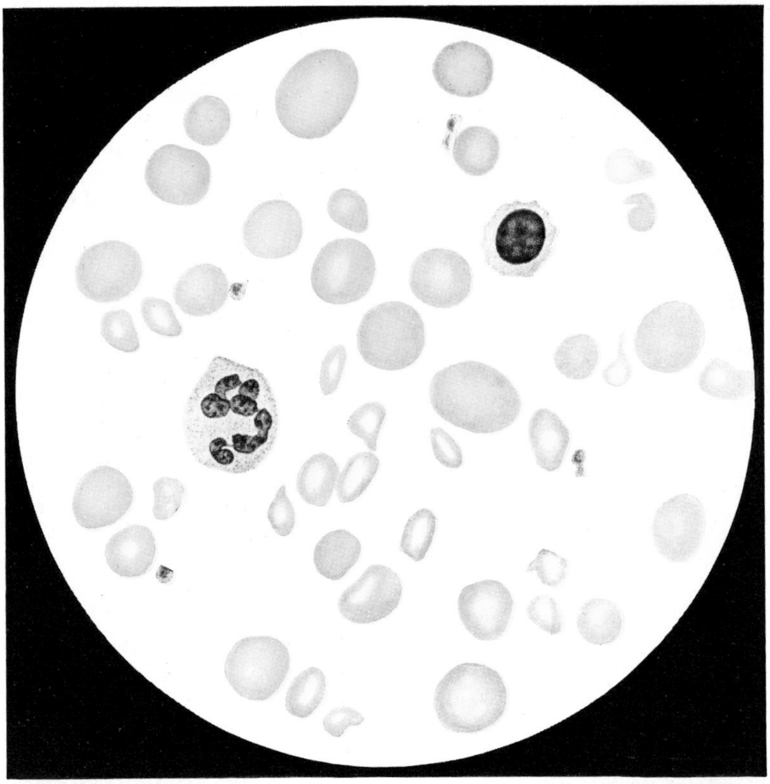

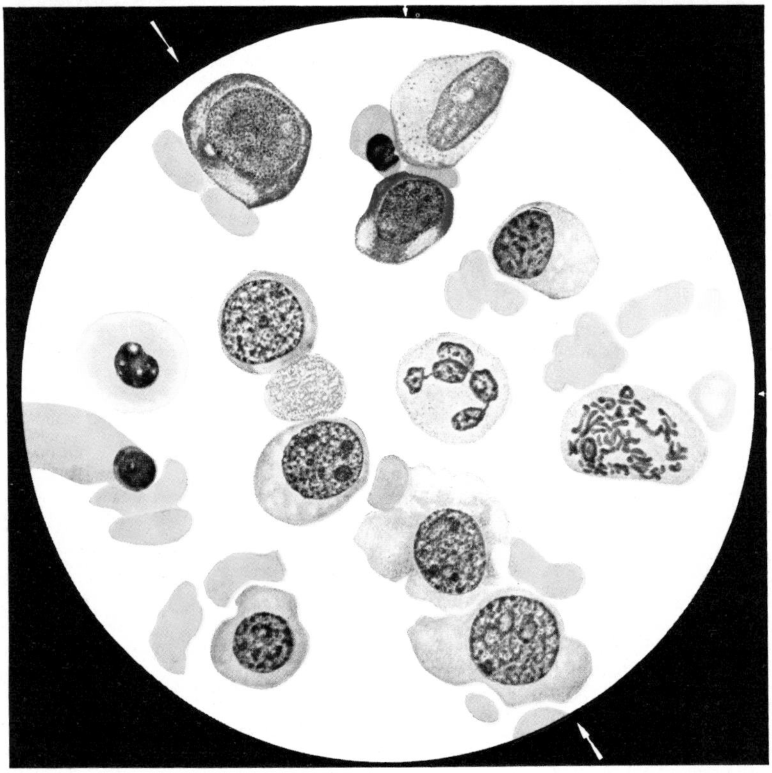

Figure 4–64.

(See opposite page for legends.)

B. *Secondary or Symptomatic AIHA.* Accompanies chronic inflammatory, reticuloendothelial, and neoplastic diseases.

C. *Acute idiopathic AIHA.* Sudden onset; dramatic blood destruction. Usually occurs in second week after a clinically clear-cut, seemingly insignificant infection.

2. Acquired hemolytic anemias caused by cold autoantibodies, mainly agglutinins.

A. Chronic.

B. Acute, transient.

3. Paroxysmal cold hemoglobinuria (PCH) caused by bithermal autohemolysins.

A. Chronic (syphilitic).

B. Transient (nonsyphilitic).

4. Atypical autoimmune hemolytic anemia.

Acquired Hemolytic Anemias Caused by Incomplete Warm Autoantibodies

CHRONIC IDIOPATHIC AUTOIMMUNE HEMOLYTIC ANEMIA

Pathogenesis. Red cell survival is shortened. Most antibodies are IgG and do not fix complement. The red cells are preferentially sequestered in the spleen, except when heavily coated by antibody and when hepatic exceeds splenic sequestration. Mechanisms of hemolysis involve: (1) adherence of red cells to specific IgG receptors on the membrane of macrophages with either erythrophagocytosis or phagocytosis of small pieces of membrane from the red cells, resulting in production of spherocytes; (2) red cells coated with antibody and spherocytes less deformable than normal red cells, resulting in trapping in splenic cords and further damage; and (3) agglutinated red cells, which are also more prone to be trapped in narrow blood vessels or splenic cords.

Clinical Findings. Pallor, slight jaundice, tachycardia, cardiac murmur, and slight to moderate splenomegaly may be found.

Laboratory Findings. The MCV is normal or increased and the MCH is normal. On the blood film there is considerable anisocytosis. The large cells are polychromatophilic, indicating that any macrocytosis is due to reticulocytosis. Spherocytes are usually prominent, and schistocytes and normoblasts may be present. The reticulocyte production index is usually over three and may be as high as six to eight times normal.

The marrow shows normoblastic hyperplasia. Urine urobilinogen and serum bilirubin and lactic dehydrogenase are usually increased. The direct Coombs' test is positive, and this is usually an anti-gamma globulin reaction (reacts with IgG). Rarely this may be IgM, or IgA along with IgG, or IgM alone (Dacie, 1970).

Complications. Marrow hypoplasia, megaloblastosis (folic acid deficiency may be responsible), thrombocytopenia and purpura, thromboembolism, and neurologic complications with spinal cord involvement. Blood transfusion problems: difficulty of correct typing and donor selections with sensitization and its dangers resulting.

Anatomic Pathology. Spleno- and hepatomegaly, moderate; marrow hyperplastic. Extramedullary hematopoiesis in 20 per cent of the patients; hemosiderosis and erythrophagocytosis in spleen and liver.

SECONDARY OR SYMPTOMATIC AUTOIMMUNE HEMOLYTIC ANEMIA

Definition. Hemolytic anemia with autoantibodies and associated with another disease.

The clinical picture of the disease is the result of two entities: the *basic* lesion (neoplasm, lymphoma, chronic infection) and *anemia*. The anemia is frequently the minor manifestation but may be in the foreground. As a rule, the anemia disappears when the basic ailment is treated successfully. There is no fundamental difference from the idiopathic

---

Figure 4–63. Pernicious anemia, peripheral blood. Several oval-shaped megalocytes, one of them at 11 o'clock, many macrocytes well filled with hemoglobin and without a trace of polychromatophilia, pronounced anisocytosis and extreme poikilocytosis, and the oversized polysegmented neutrophilic granulocyte add up to the characteristic picture of a macrocytic anemia of pernicious anemia type. The normoblast adds to the findings but is not essential for the diagnosis. A study of the marrow and the other laboratory tests described elsewhere in this chapter are essential. (From L. Heilmeyer and H. Begemann: Atlas der Klinischen Hämatologie und Cytologie. Springer, 1955.)

Figure 4–64. Pernicious anemia, marrow. The youngest cell in this preparation is at 11 o'clock. It is large, its cytoplasm is deeply basophilic, and its nucleus has a fine filigreed, dispersed chromatin with several blue nucleoli barely visible through the cloud of the granular chromatin. This is a promegaloblast. Just opposite, at 5 o'clock, is a more mature polychromatic megaloblast with its more advanced condensation, which still retains its delicate structure of chromatin and has clearly visible nucleoli. Bordering on this cell toward the center of the field is a basophilic megaloblast. Then, almost in linear sequence, are another polychromatophilic megaloblast, a giant platelet, and a third polychromatophilic, smaller megaloblast. At 3 o'clock is a polychromatophilic megaloblast in mitosis.

At 12 o'clock is a neutrophilic myelocyte; touching it on its left is a ripe orthochromatic normoblast, and toward the center of the field is a promegaloblast. (From L. Heilmeyer and H. Begemann: Atlas der Klinischen Hämatologie und Cytologie. Springer, 1955.)

variety. Here, too, incomplete antibodies are responsible for the shortened survival of red cells.

Diseases in Which Symptomatic Autoimmune Hemolytic Anemia Occurs. Chronic lymphocytic leukemia, lymphoma (lymphosarcoma), Hodgkin's disease, myeloma, macroglobulinemias, myelofibrosis, myeloproliferative disorders, cancer (stomach, pancreas, cervix, marrow metastases), and ovarian cysts and teratomas.

Diseases in Which Hypersensitivity May Play a Part. Tuberculosis, Boeck's sarcoid, lupus erythematosus, acute rheumatic fever, rheumatoid arthritis, periarteritis nodosa, scleroderma, and dermatomyositis.

Clinical and Serologic Findings. Essentially the same as in idiopathic.

Relation of Hemolytic Anemia to Basic Disease. Basic disease may be hidden. Anemia may be presenting first and may be mistakenly interpreted as idiopathic.

The autoimmune nature of the anemia is established by the antiglobulin test.

The nonimmune variety of idiopathic and symptomatic hemolytic anemia differs little from the immune in clinical manifestations. Autoimmune hemolytic anemia is more likely to respond to steroid therapy. On the other hand, selection of donors for blood transfusions may be difficult in autoimmune anemia because autoantibodies are only rarely isospecific and react frequently with blood of all groups.

ACUTE IDIOPATHIC AUTOIMMUNE HEMOLYTIC ANEMIA

Onset is dramatic, with high fever. More frequent in the young. Anemia usually noticed after early manifestations subside. Patients much more sick than in the chronic disease. Leukocytosis with shift to left.

Blood Smear. Microspherocytes, normoblasts, erythrophagocytosis.

Therapy. Transfusion may be urgent. Corticosteroids. Recovery usually spontaneous, more often than in chronic, with less tendency to relapses. Fatal outcome is rare.

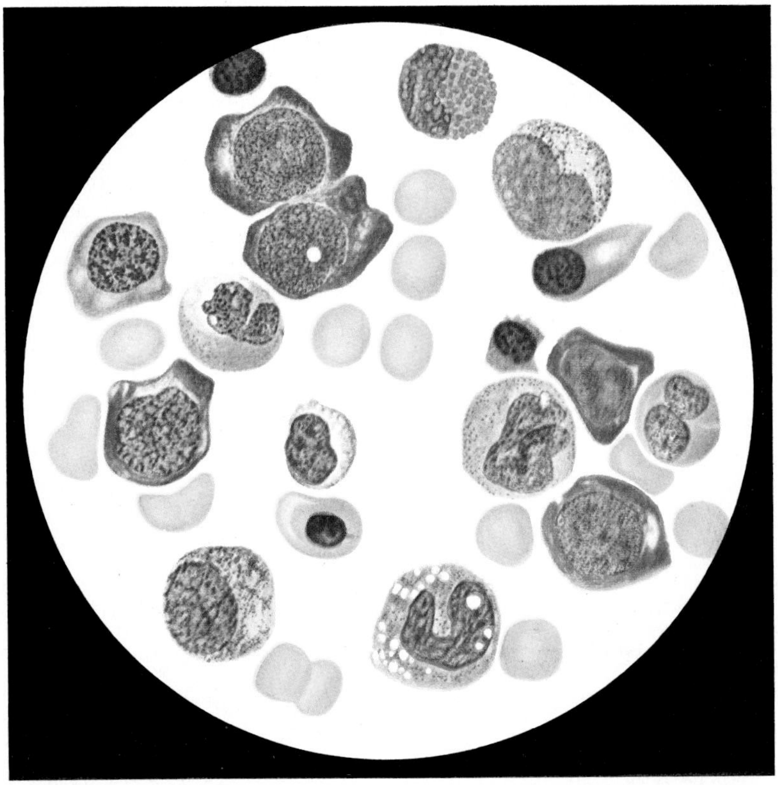

Figure 4–65. Pernicious anemia marrow. The cells are identified by the key. The giant band cell at 6 o'clock may be pointed out as an illustration of the fact that granulocytes in pernicious anemia tend to be excessively large as do erythroid cells – and possibly for the same reason, i.e., deficiency of vitamin B_{12} or folic acid. (From L. Heilmeyer and H. Begemann: Atlas der Klinischen Hämatologie und Cytologie. Springer, 1955.)

(Fig. 4–65 continued on opposite page.)

Acquired Hemolytic Anemias Caused by Cold Autoantibodies

CHRONIC COLD AGGLUTININ DISEASE

Synonyms. Acquired hemolytic anemia of cold agglutinin type, cryoagglutinemia, cold hemagglutinin disease, cold agglutinin syndrome, hemopathic acrocyanosis.

Clinical Findings. Long-lasting (years and decades). No known therapy. Increased red cell destruction, occasionally with hemoglobinuria. Disturbance of blood circulation in skin, especially in exposed areas, due to intravascular autohemagglutination (acrocyanosis) and hemolytic anemia. Onset usually in winter. General well-being not affected. Sensation of pinpricks but no severe pain. Another diagnostic finding is that all fingers are cyanotic; after warming the hand, if one finger is dipped in cold water, only this finger becomes cyanotic.

Pathogenesis. Cold agglutinin is inactive at inner body temperature, but in exposed areas of skin, temperature may drop to below 30° C.

In order to produce cold agglutinin disease, the antibody must be active in the range of 28 to 32° C. Agglutination occurs in areas of the body which reach this temperature and may produce acrocyanosis and Raynaud's phenomenon. The intensity of these symptoms is not necessarily well correlated with the degree of hemolysis, which depends largely upon the binding of complement by the antibody. The agglutinates are reversible when the blood is rewarmed, but the complement remains on the cell and may produce hemolysis either by: (1) completion of the lytic sequence, resulting in intravascular hemolysis; or (2) interaction of complement on the membrane with receptors for complement on macrophages of the reticuloendothelial system. The latter process results in either erythrophagocytosis or phagocytosis of small fragments from the surface of red cells, producing spherocytes which have enhanced susceptibility to splenic trapping and lysis (Dacie, 1972b).

Laboratory Findings. Autoagglutination of

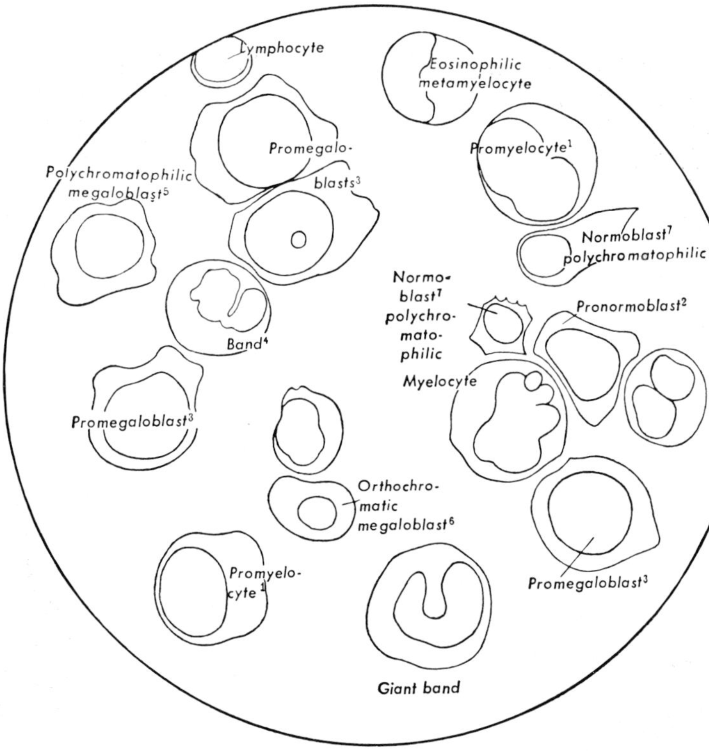

Synonyms

1. Progranulocyte
2. Rubriblast (Pernicious anemia—P.A. type) Basophilic proerythroblast
3. Rubriblasts (P.A. type)
4. Staff cell
5. Rubricyte (P.A. type)
6. Orthochromatic metarubricyte (P.A. type)
7. Metarubricyte

Figure 4–65. *Continued.*

blood samples at room temperature, difficulty in doing blood count, slight normocytic, normochromic anemia, shortened survival of erythrocytes, both patient's own and transfused, with Ashby's method and with ^{51}Cr. Hemoglobinuria and hemosiderinuria associated with exposure to cold may be found at one time or another in most patients; occasionally they cannot be demonstrated.

Serologic Tests

1. Cold agglutinin titers from 8000 to 64,000. Optimal conditions for cold monothermal hemolysis: pH 6.5, 22° C.

2. Test for cold monothermal hemolysins: 0.1 ml. of patient's serum, 0.1 ml. of normal fresh serum of same blood group (complement), 0.02 ml. of 0.25 N HCl, and 0.02 ml. of 50 per cent red cells of group O or patient's own. Centrifuge. Supernatant is red in many patients.

3. Positive direct Coombs' test if a potent broad spectrum antiglobulin serum (or an anti-non-gamma serum or anticomplement serum) is used. Complement is invariably fixed and remains on the cells.

4. Positive indirect Coombs' test with the patient's serum at 10° C.

5. The antibody, eluted from the red cells or present in the serum, can usually be shown to have anti-I specificity (p. 364), occasionally anti-i. In most patients with anti-I, the light chains of the IgM antibody are of a single type (usually kappa), indicating that this is probably a monoclonal blood protein disorder (Dacie and Worlledge, 1969).

Differential Diagnosis

Acute Transient Cold Agglutinin Disease. Short duration. Preceding pneumonia.

Raynaud's Syndrome. Vascular lesion (vasomotor nerves), mainly in extremities. Not all fingers uniformly involved. Cold temperature is not only factor. Reversibility by warm temperature is not so impressive. May be very painful. Serologic findings negative.

ACUTE TRANSIENT HEMOLYTIC ANEMIA CAUSED BY COLD AGGLUTININS AFTER MYCOPLASMA OR VIRUS INFECTION

Mycoplasma Infection. During the recovery phase of *Mycoplasma pneumoniae* infection (primary atypical pneumonia) a transient episode of hemolysis may occur.

Clinical Findings. The disease starts as an acute pneumonia with characteristic physical and radiologic findings. Just as recovery begins, usually in the second or third week, the patient becomes ill again, with pallor and jaundice. The spleen may become palpable. The attack of hemolytic anemia lasts only a few days or weeks.

Laboratory Findings. Autoagglutination, neutrophilic leukocytosis, reticulocytosis, and spherocytosis are usual.

Serologic Findings. Cold agglutinins in titers of 2000 to 64,000. Monothermal cold hemolysins are demonstrable, reacting even at 30° C. The direct Coombs' test (DCT) is positive with anti-non-gamma serum; this is due to complement on the cells. The IgM cold agglutinin usually does not remain on the cells at 37° C. The IgM usually has anti-I specificity in mycoplasma infections, and both kappa and lambda type light chains are usually present in contrast to chronic cold agglutinin disease.

Virus Infection. Although this acute transient hemolysis due to cold agglutinins is most common with mycoplasma infections, a similar process may occur rarely in association with some viral diseases.

In infectious mononucleosis the serologic findings are similar, but the IgM antibodies usually have anti-i specificity. In a large proportion of patients these cold antibodies are present in low titer; rarely, however, are they in sufficient amount and with the thermal amplitude to cause hemolysis.

PAROXYSMAL COLD HEMOGLOBINURIA CAUSED BY BITHERMAL HEMOLYSINS

Paroxysmal cold hemoglobinuria (PCH) is a syndrome characterized by: (1) attacks of acute intravascular hemolysis brought on by exposure to cold, and (2) the presence of a cold-acting antibody which binds to the red cell in the cold and causes hemolysis when the blood is warmed, if complement is present.

Etiology. Congenital or late *syphilis* was the cause in most cases of PCH in the older literature. More recently, most cases are nonluetic.

Nonluetic PCH may occur in an acute transient form associated with acute viral infections. More rarely it may be chronic and have no demonstrable cause.

Clinical Findings. The signs and symptoms related to the hemolytic episode are in addition to those of the underlying disease, if present. Beginning about 10 minutes after exposure to cold, the patient has a sudden attack of malaise, headache, nausea, vomiting, chills and high fever, and urticaria on the exposed skin. The first urine passed is red brown; the urine has cleared within 24 hours.

Laboratory Findings. Spherocytosis may accompany the attack; reticulocytosis occurs a few days after the hemolytic episode. Leukopenia occurs abruptly, during and after the cooling. Erythrophagocytosis may be observed. Minor attacks may occur with hemoglobinemia but without hemoglobinuria.

Serologic Findings. The direct Coombs' test (DCT) may be positive with an anti-gamma globulin (IgG) serum if the cells are washed at a low temperature so the antibody is not eluted, but is negative if the cells are washed at 37° C. The DCT should be positive in either case with a broad spectrum anti-globulin or an anti-non-gamma serum, which will detect complement on the cells. The indirect Coombs' test is positive.

Demonstration of a bithermal hemolysin with the Donath-Landsteiner test is essential for the diagnosis. This bithermal antibody is an IgG which binds to the red cell only in the cold (often only below 15° C.) and fixes complement. Lysis occurs owing to completion of complement activation when the blood is warmed. IgG antibodies with these bithermal characteristics are known as Donath-Landsteiner antibodies and have been shown to have anti-P specificity by Levine and his colleagues (Dacie and Worlledge, 1969).

The Donath-Landsteiner (D-L) Test for Paroxysmal Cold Hemoglobinuria

Qualitative Test. One blood sample is collected in a previously warmed (37° C.) test tube and incubated at 37° C. until it clots. The other is placed in melting ice for 30 minutes and then transferred without shaking to a water bath at 37° C. Both specimens are inspected after an hour or two when the clots have retracted. In paroxysmal cold hemoglobinuria the chilled and then warmed specimen will show hemolysis of the serum. The specimen kept at 37° C. will not show hemolysis.

Indirect Test. Serum is obtained from a specimen that has been permitted to clot at 37° C. One volume of a 50 per cent suspension of washed normal O cells is added. The suspension is placed in melting ice for 30 minutes, followed by incubation in a water bath at 37° C. for 60 minutes and centrifugation. Hemolysis is seen in the centrifuged specimen.

In another tube, a volume of fresh normal serum is added to the patient's serum as a source of complement to compensate for a possible complement deficiency.

A control test tube is set up as for the patient's serum but is kept at 37° C. and should show no hemolysis.

Drug-induced Immune Hemolytic Anemias

Mechanisms. There are four varieties of immune hemolytic anemias mediated by drugs or chemicals.

1. The drug binds tightly to red cells; antibody (usually IgG) attaches to the drug-coated erythrocytes, and the sensitized cell is destroyed prematurely by the RE system. The drug most frequently implicated in this type is penicillin.

In the laboratory the characteristic finding is a positive direct antiglobulin test, with a negative indirect antiglobulin test. In addition, eluates prepared from the patient's red cells fail to react with any of a panel of normal red cells. However, if drug-coated cells are used (Spath *et al.*, 1971), both the eluate and the indirect antiglobulin test will be positive.

2. The drug and antibody combine in the plasma, and the antigen-antibody complex binds nonspecifically to the red cells (or, even more frequently, to platelets). The complement sequence is then activated, and the complement-coated cells are either lysed intravascularly or destroyed in the RE system. Quinidine, stibophen, and chlorpropamide are among the drugs associated with this mechanism.

In the laboratory, if the direct antiglobulin test is positive, it is of the non-gamma or complement type. Frequently, it is only possible to demonstrate the phenomenon if drug, patient's serum, and cells are incubated together. It is, in fact, not necessary to use the patient's cells at all. PNH cells, which are particularly susceptible to complement-mediated hemolysis, may be used as the "indicator" cell (Logue *et al.*, 1970); so may normal platelets (Deykin and Hellerstein, 1972).

3. The drug alters the red cell membrane so that it takes up proteins, including antibody and complement, from the plasma in a nonspecific fashion. The coated cells may have a shortened survival. Cephalothin is the best example of this process.

A positive direct antiglobulin test, when present, may be either gamma, non-gamma, or both. In addition, albumin, fibrinogen, and other globulins may be detected on these cells (Spath *et al.*, 1971).

4. Alpha-methyl dopa (Aldomet) and levodopa have been associated in a significant number of cases with a positive direct antiglobulin test, and in a few cases with hemolytic anemia. Fifteen per cent of patients receiving Aldomet develop a positive DCT and 1 per cent develop hemolytic anemia. In contrast to the three other types, eluates prepared from these patients' cells do agglutinate normal red cells and, in fact, often show Rh specificity. This, therefore, appears to be an autoimmune hemolytic anemia. The pathogenesis of this phenomenon is, as yet, still unknown.

Summary of Immunohematologic Tests for the Diagnosis of Autoimmune Hemolytic Anemia

Available methods permit a step-by-step analysis of acquired autoimmune hemolytic anemia. The direct antiglobulin test detects cell-bound antibodies. The quantitative antiglobulin test and the gamma globulin neutralization test answer the question as to the thermal range of the autoantibodies. The specificity of the autoantibodies can be determined with the antiglobulin test, with enzyme-treated red cells, with the elution technique, and by typing and genotyping the patient's red cells. The free autoantibodies in the circulating blood can be studied with agglutination and indirect antiglobulin tests at various temperatures and with the Donath-Landsteiner test. The hemolytic autoantibody can be studied with acidified serum and with enzyme-treated red cells. The role of the complement can also be studied with appropriate set-ups.

ANEMIA IN PREGNANCY

Normal Hematologic Values

Plasma volume begins to increase in the second trimester and becomes pronounced (40 to 50 per cent above normal) during the third. It returns to normal promptly after childbirth.

Red cell mass shows a moderate decrease during the first two months, followed by a slight increase during the remainder of the pregnancy to a level 25 to 30 per cent above normal in the third trimester. It returns to normal post partum but more slowly than the plasma volume.

Because the plasma volume normally increases more than the red cell volume during pregnancy, the hemoglobin concentration gradually falls. Lowenstein *et al.* (1966) have suggested that the lower limit of normal during pregnancy should be 11.6 gm./dl. in the first 16 weeks, 11.0 gm./dl. between 17 and 24 weeks, and 10.4 gm./dl. after the 25th week. The lowest levels are reached at the 32nd week, after which the hemoglobin concentration increases slightly.

Erythrocyte sedimentation rate is increased beginning with the third month. It returns to normal beginning with the third postpartum week.

Leukocytes (mainly granulocytes) may show a slight increase in the third trimester. The increase is more pronounced in primiparas. The leukocyte count rises frequently to 15,000 to 20,000 immediately post partum.

Platelets may be slightly decreased during the third trimester. An increase occurs during labor.

The marrow shows a slight normoblastic hyperplasia during the final weeks of the pregnancy.

Iron-binding capacity may be slightly increased during the second trimester and is frequently and significantly increased during the third trimester even if iron stores are not depleted.

Plasma proteins drop progressively. They return to normal rapidly after childbirth.

IRON DEFICIENCY ANEMIA

If no iron supplementation is given during pregnancy, nearly 100 per cent of women will have iron depletion or iron deficiency and 30 per cent will have iron deficiency anemia (Fairbanks *et al.*, 1971); therefore, it is almost a universal practice to give supplemental iron therapy during pregnancy. A variety of factors contribute to this situation. Primiparas may enter their child-bearing career with an iron deficiency brought on by periodic blood losses in menstruation, which may be aggravated by dieting and faulty food habits. In multiparous women the deficiency is increased by further loss of iron in each successive pregnancy and lactation. The iron requirements during a pregnancy amount to about 725 mg. This requires correction for the amount of iron that would have been lost with each menstruation. The fetus derives its initial iron stores from the mother.

MEGALOBLASTIC ANEMIA

The cause of megaloblastic anemia of pregnancy is almost always folic acid deficiency. It has been shown that healthy pregnant women need, in addition to folate available in the diet, another 100 μg. per day to maintain normal red cell folate levels (Chanarin, 1969). Indeed, about 25 per cent of pregnant women will develop a megaloblastic bone marrow with normal dietary folate intake. It is now recommended that supplemental folate be given to all pregnant women.

The incidence of this form shows striking geographic differences. It is seen frequently in India and in the tropics, especially in advanced pregnancy and early after childbirth, more often in multiparas, and in women with poor dietary habits.

The peripheral blood picture is similar to but not identical to that seen in true pernicious anemia. Aniso- and poikilocytosis are less pronounced. Leukopenia is present less regularly. Bone marrow examination is necessary if anemia in pregnancy does not respond to iron therapy. In the presence of low MCH values and without macrocytosis, megaloblastic anemia may coexist with iron deficiency. Frequently in a combined deficiency the megaloblastosis does not become obvious until the iron deficiency is corrected. The marrow resembles addisonian pernicious anemia closely, except that normoblastic hyperplasia may be present simultaneously with the megaloblastic.

LABORATORY DIAGNOSIS OF ANEMIA

This section is based on the useful approach given by Wheby (1966). The diagnosis and study of anemia require the proper use and interpretation of laboratory measurements. Prerequisite for the efficient use of the laboratory are a careful history and physical examination, both of which lead to the initial laboratory measurements and provide important guidance in determining the nature of the anemia.

The first question to be answered is whether the patient is anemic (or polycythemic) and can be ascertained by determining whether his hemoglobin, hematocrit, or erythrocyte count lies outside the normal range for his age and sex. The second task is to define the underlying cause or mechanism for the anemia.

Usually the CBC (WBC, RBC, Hb, Hct, MCV, MCH, MCHC) and examination of a Wright's stained smear are parts of the routine examination of the blood. It is possible that all these values could be normal in the presence of a mild macrocytic anemia, in which the RBC does not fall below the normal range, and the macrocytes present (and detectable on the blood film) do not elevate the MCV above the normal range.

Once anemia is discovered, the basic examination of the blood should include the following: (1) hemoglobin, hematocrit, and RBC count, for calculation of *indices* (if not already available with multichannel instrument); (2) blood film examination; (3) leukocyte count; (4) platelet count (if apparently abnormal on examination of the film or if suspected to be abnormal on clinical grounds); and (5) reticulocyte count.

With the Coulter Counter Model S, all red cell values and the indices have comparable precision. It must be remembered that indices are *mean* values, and will not detect different populations of cells which balance each other. For example, combined deficiencies of folate and iron may give rise to populations of macrocytic and hypochromic microcytic cells, which could yield normal indices. This emphasizes the need for careful examination of the blood film. Determination of erythrocyte indices and examination of the blood film are not substitutes for one another but are complementary.

Examination of the blood film will determine the *morphologic type* of anemia. In addition, certain changes or combinations of findings will suggest the mechanism involved.

Increased numbers of *polychromatic* macrocytes, with or without normoblasts, suggest increased erythropoiesis, and in the untreated patient this is usually due to hemorrhage or hemolysis. Here, the history (of blood loss) or physical examination (jaundice or splenomegaly) may help.

Findings suggestive of hemolysis are *poikilocytes* (abnormally shaped cells), *sickle cells*, *irregularly contracted forms* (including red cell fragments or schistocytes), and *spherocytes*. Sometimes it is difficult to detect spherocytes in hereditary spherocytosis because of minimal anisocytosis. The two findings in the red cells that are helpful here are the presence of a low MCD (mean cell diameter) between 6.0 and 6.5 μm (normal = 7.0 to 7.4) and spheroidocytes. Spheroidocytes are cup-shaped forms, spheroids, or flattened spheres as seen on the blood film or in a wet preparation.

Target cells may be found in hemoglobinopathies, especially in homozygous states for HbC, HbD, and HbE, and in thalassemia. They may be present in any *hypochromic* anemia, though usually in smaller numbers. Target cells without microcytosis are also found in liver disease and in the absence of a spleen.

Fine *basophilic stippling* (which is due to precipitation of RNA) can be found in polychromatic red cells associated with a significant increase in the generation of erythrocytes, as in response to hemorrhage or hemolysis. Coarse basophilic stippling suggests an abnormality in hemoglobin synthesis. It is found in megaloblastic anemias, thalassemias, refractory anemias, and lead poisoning. In particular, hypochromasia or microcytosis with stippling is against the diagnosis of iron deficiency anemia and more suggestive of thalassemia or lead poisoning.

The combination of *oval macrocytes* and *hypersegmented neutrophils* indicates the very likely existence of megaloblastic anemia. In some laboratories the *lobe average* is used. This is computed on the basis of counting and averaging the number of nuclear lobes in one hundred neutrophils. In the normal individual this is about three. The presence of megaloblastic anemia is strongly suggested by oval macrocytes, an increased lobe average (especially with giant PA neutrophils), and pancytopenia.

Finally, examination of the blood film allows the evaluation of *qualitative abnormalities in leukocytes and platelets* as well as an estimate of their numbers. Blood diseases that may be first suspected or detected in this manner are many, and include chronic lymphocytic leukemia, compensated hemolytic anemia, early megaloblastic anemia, and anomalies of red cells, such as hereditary elliptocytosis, or of leukocytes, such as the Pelger-Huët anomaly.

After the routine studies just mentioned the choice of further procedures depends upon the morphologic type of the anemia as determined by the indices and the blood smear.

Macrocytic Anemia (MCV Greater than 99 fl.). These anemias are normochromic, as determined by appearance on the smear and by the MCHC. The first step is to ascertain whether the anemia is megaloblastic. The clues from the smear have been mentioned. A *bone marrow aspiration* should be done to confirm the presence of megaloblastosis.

Megaloblastic Marrow. If the marrow is *megaloblastic,* with characteristic changes in both red cell and white cell precursors, the anemia in all likelihood is due to folate or vitamin B_{12} deficiency. We now have two questions: "Which type is it?" and "What is the *cause* of the deficiency?"

DIRECT METHODS OF DETERMINING WHETHER LACK OF VITAMIN B_{12} OR FOLATE IS RESPONSIBLE. Serum and red cell assay for folic acid are low in folate deficiency and normal in vitamin B_{12} deficiency.

Serum assay for vitamin B_{12} is low in vitamin B_{12} deficiency and normal in folate deficiency.

INDIRECT METHOD OF DETECTING DEFICIENCY OF VITAMIN B_{12}. Urinary MMA (methylmalonic acid) is increased in vitamin B_{12} deficiency, and normal in folate deficiency.

If the above measurements indicate a deficiency, the cause of the deficiency must still be found, and in vitamin B_{12} deficiency, this will include an assessment of gastric function, as indicated below. If the measurements described above are not available, a perfectly satisfactory alternative exists in the following.

GASTRIC ANALYSIS. The presence of free HCl provides valuable information, since it virtually excludes pernicious anemia in adults. The character and volume of the gastric juice should also be noted. In pernicious anemia the volume of gastric juice is small and the fluid is viscid, whereas with normal juice or with lack of free acid seen in many older people, the fluid is watery and of nearly normal volume.

Intrinsic factor assay, if possible, is helpful, for the gastric juice in pernicious anemia lacks intrinsic factor. This assay is not widely available.

TESTS OF VITAMIN B_{12} ABSORPTION. The Schilling test is most widely used and is discussed elsewhere (p. 480). It should be considered in two stages. If the initial absorption of vitamin B_{12}-^{60}Co is low, it indicates impaired absorption but does not distinguish between lack of intrinsic factor or defective absorption due to intestinal disease; therefore, the second stage must be performed—giving B_{12}-^{60}Co + intrinsic factor, which will correct impaired absorption caused by lack of intrinsic factor.

It is imperative that the Schilling test be delayed until bone marrow examination has been completed.

THERAPEUTIC TRIAL. If free acid is present in the gastric analysis, or if folic acid deficiency appears more likely than pernicious anemia, a therapeutic trial with 50 to 200 μg. of folic acid (intramuscularly) per day would be a logical approach. Reticulocyte count and hematocrit are performed daily. A good response indicates folate deficiency. If there is no response, either a Schilling test or a similar therapeutic trial with 1 μg. of vitamin B_{12} per day (intramuscularly) can then be performed.

Once the actual deficiency is established, the *cause* of it is ascertained by considering the various disorders discussed earlier (see pp. 189 and 192).

Nonmegaloblastic Marrow. If the marrow is *not megaloblastic,* conditions which can be associated with macrocytosis should be investigated. These include liver disease, hemolytic anemias, hypothyroidism, and refractory or hypoplastic anemia. But anemias associated with these disorders, though they *may* be macrocytic, are more usually normocytic and thus are considered with the normocytic anemias.

Microcytic and Hypochromic Anemias (MCV <83 fl.; MCHC <32 Per Cent). If the counts are performed on a Coulter Counter Model S, the MCHC is likely to still be in the normal range, with slight to moderate degrees of hypochromia (see p. 141). Consequently the MCV has assumed the leading role in the detection of microcytic hypochromic anemias.

These anemias reflect a quantitative defect in hemoglobin synthesis.

1. *Iron deficiency anemias* are due to increased requirement or blood loss not balanced by intake.

2. *Anemia of chronic disorders,* otherwise known as sideropenic anemia associated with reticuloendothelial siderosis, or simple chronic anemia, is associated with infection, neoplasia, or collagen disease. This anemia may be normochromic and normocytic or hypochromic and normocytic but is sometimes hypochromic and microcytic.

3. *Thalassemia* is a genetically determined impairment in the rate of globin synthesis.

4. *Sideroblastic anemia* is that group of refractory anemias with erythroid hyperplasia of the marrow in which a defect in hemoglobin synthesis predominates. A few of these respond to pyridoxine and are called pyridoxine-responsive anemias.

Since *iron deficiency* is the most common, the first step is to determine whether the body lacks iron.

When blood loss cannot be documented, serum iron and iron-binding capacity and bone marrow study for iron should be performed. These will usually discriminate between the two most common anemias in this category, iron deficiency and simple chronic anemia associated with some other disease–frequently chronic infection or cancer. In both, the serum iron is low, but in iron deficiency the total iron-binding capacity is elevated, whereas in simple chronic anemia it is normal or decreased. Storage iron in the marrow is depleted in iron deficiency but is normal or elevated in simple chronic anemia. Iron deficiency anemia in an adult male almost always means chronic blood loss; the source must be found and corrected, if necessary.

Hypochromic anemias with basophilic stippling and increased serum iron are most likely *thalassemias,* and the next examinations to perform are hemoglobin electrophoresis and determinations of HbA_2 and HbF (see pp. 218 and 220). Investigation of other members of the patient's family is often essential in order to establish a diagnosis of thalassemia.

Least common in this group are the *sideroblastic anemias.* In addition to refractory sideroblastic anemia already discussed, a very similar picture may occur after therapy with certain drugs (e.g., isoniazid) and in chronic lead poisoning. Basophilic stippling is common in this group of anemias.

Table 4–11 summarizes the laboratory distinctions in hypochromic anemias.

Normocytic and Normochromic Anemias (MCV 83–99 fl.). This large group of anemias has many causes. A useful approach is evaluation of the erythrokinetics in a given patient (Hillman and Finch, 1967). Often a reticulocyte production index (RPI) or absolute reticulocyte count and evaluation of a bone marrow aspirate will suffice. The reticulocyte count is the simplest measure of effective erythropoiesis.

Normochromic Anemias with an Optimal Bone Marrow Response; Reticulocyte Production Index over Two Times Normal. If the output of reticulocytes has reached between three and six times normal, as determined by the absolute reticulocyte count or RPI, it can be assumed that the marrow has reached an optimal response. The cause for the anemia is then either *acute blood loss* or *hemolysis.* If blood loss cannot be proved, evidence that hemolysis is in fact present must be sought.

Erythroid hyperplasia of the marrow, serum bilirubin, urine or fecal urobilinogen will indicate whether erythropoietic activity and destruction are increased. Red cell survival determination may be needed to prove hemolysis in some cases. Low serum haptoglobin points to hemolysis, but a normal level does not exclude it. None of these measurements will specify whether hemolysis is intravascular or extravascular, but elevated plasma hemoglobin, hemoglobinuria, and hemosiderinuria indicate intravascular hemolysis.

Once it is determined that excessive hemolysis is occurring, the type of hemolytic mechanism must be ascertained.

The *direct antiglobulin (Coombs') test* is a useful guide to further study.

If the direct antiglobulin (Coombs') test is *positive,* tests to determine the type and specificity of the antibody should be undertaken. If the antibody is nonspecific, tests such as cold agglutinins, the Donath-Landsteiner test, and serum protein electrophoresis may help to define the process.

If the direct antiglobulin (Coombs') test is *negative,* what examinations are performed next will depend upon the clinical findings and the results of the measurements already made.

If hereditary spherocytosis is suspected, osmotic fragility before and after 24-hour incubation at 37° C. and family studies will be necessary.

If a nonspherocytic congenital hemolytic anemia is suspected, an autohemolysis test, screening for glucose-6-phosphate dehydrogenase deficiency, hemoglobin electrophoresis, and a sickle cell test will be helpful.

If thalassemia seems likely, determinations of HbA_2 and HbF are appropriate. Thalassemia is unique in that it is both hypochromic and hemolytic. Again, family studies are often helpful.

If drug-induced hemolysis is suspected, a test for Heinz bodies, screening test for glucose-6-phosphate dehydrogenase and, if possible, tests for a drug-dependent autoantibody are indicated.

If the nature of the hemolytic anemia is obscure, a sugar-water test for paroxysmal nocturnal hemoglobinuria should be performed.

Normochromic Anemias Without an Adequate Marrow Response; Reticulocyte Production Index Under Two. The mechanism of the anemia may be ineffective erythropoiesis. Conditions with the greatest degree of ineffective erythropoiesis appear in other categories (e.g., megaloblastic anemia and thalassemia), but some idiopathic refractory anemias have a hyperplastic bone marrow and impaired delivery of the cells to the blood. In some of these, abnormalities in erythroid precursors suggestive of megaloblastic change may be present, but the granulocytic and megakaryocytic changes usually seen in megaloblastic anemia are lacking.

A low reticulocyte count may indicate decreased production caused by inadequate stimulation of the marrow. Chronic renal disease may result in impaired production of erythropoietin. Certain endocrinopathies, such

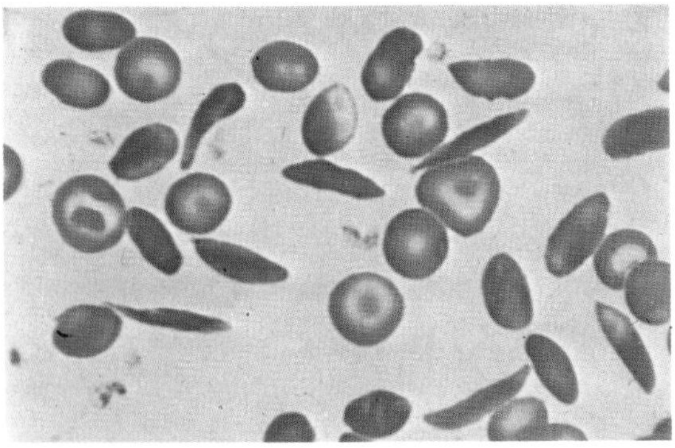

Figure 4–66.

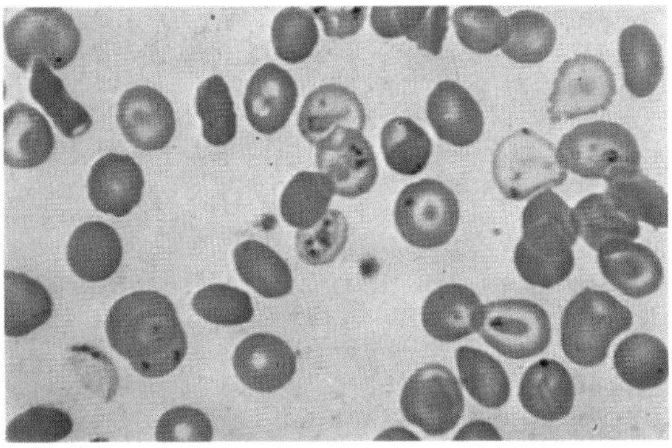

Figure 4–67.

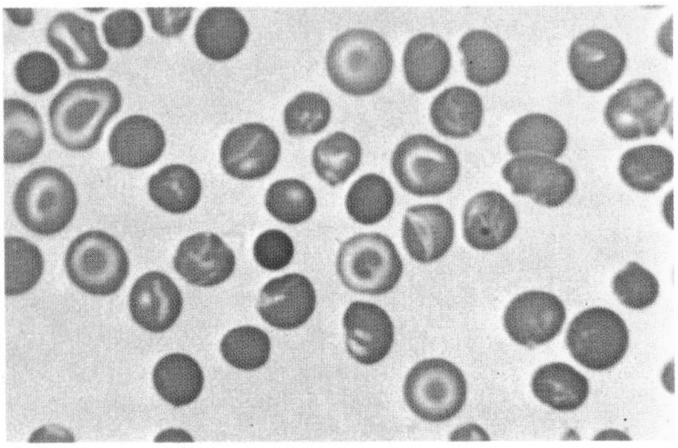

Figure 4–68.

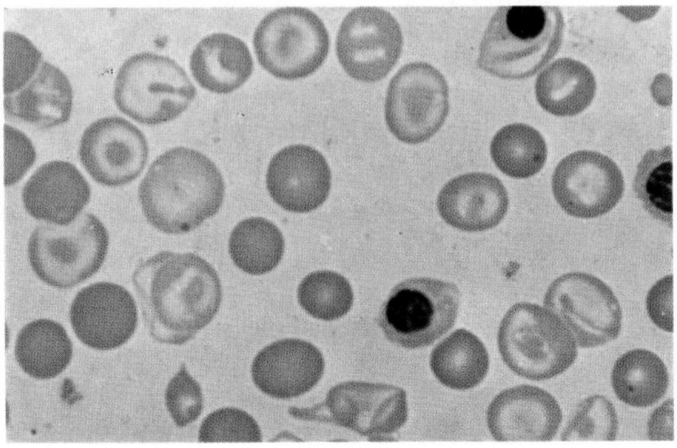

Figure 4–69.

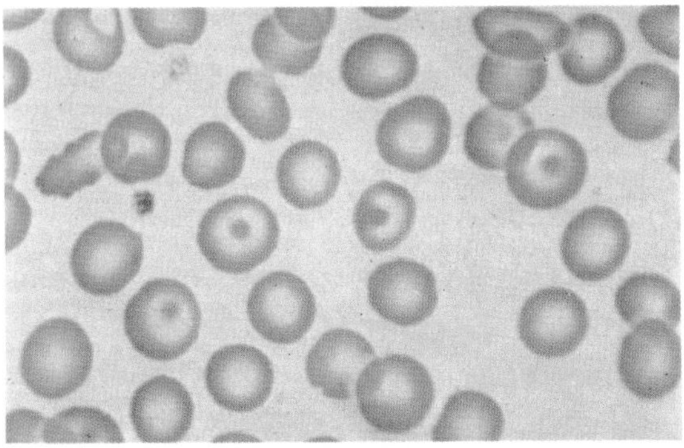

Figure 4–70.

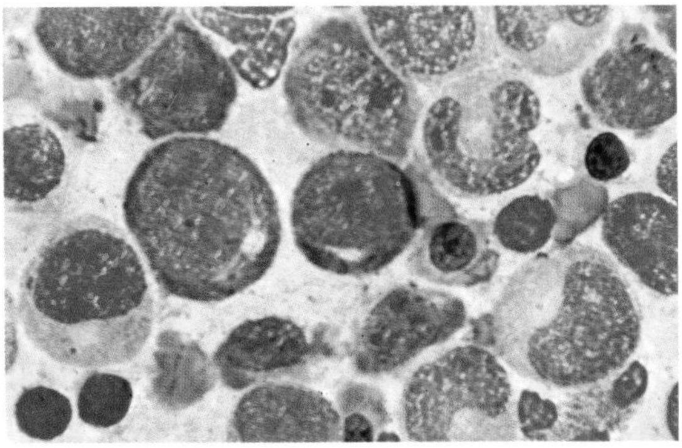

Figure 4–71.

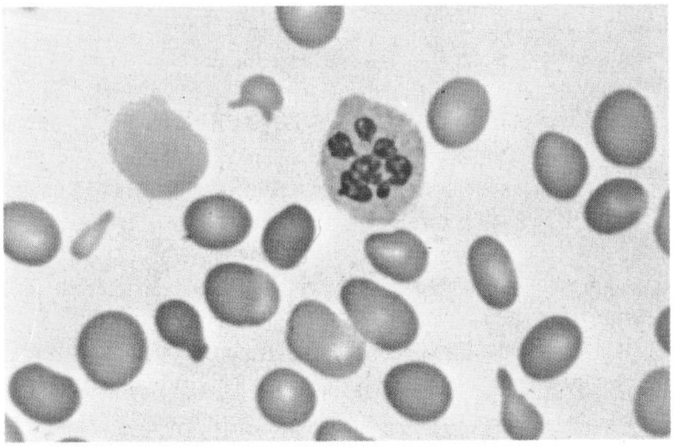

Figure 4–72.

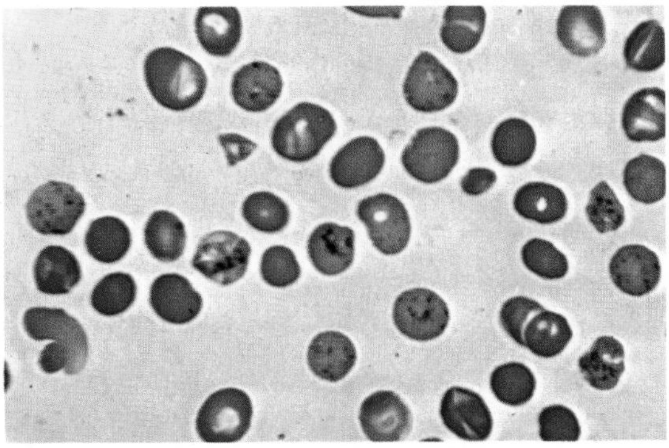

Figure 4–73.

(See opposite page for legends.)

Table 4–11. LABORATORY FINDINGS IN HYPOCHROMIC ANEMIAS*

	SERUM IRON	TIBC†	SATURATION OF TIBC†	MARROW		HEMOGLOBIN	
	75-150 μg./ 100 ml.	250-400 μg./ 100 ml.	35-40 PER CENT	IRON STORES	SIDEROBLASTS	A_2	F
Iron lack	↓	↑	↓	Absent	↓	N	N
Simple chronic anemia (some are normochromic)	↓	↓ or N	↓	N or ↑	↓	N	N
Thalassemia major	↑	↓	↑	↑	N or ↑	N	↑
Thalassemia minor	N or ↑	N	N or ↑	N or ↑	N	↑	N or ↑
Sideroblastic	↑	↓ or N	↑	↑	↑	N	N

*Adapted from Wheby, 1966.
†Total iron-binding capacity.

as hypopituitarism or hypothyroidism, may result in regulation of hemoglobin production at a lower level due to decreased tissue need for oxygen.

A large group of normochromic anemias associated with various chronic diseases form a heterogeneous group characterized by failure of the marrow to meet the need of a slightly decreased red cell survival. Some of these are simple chronic anemias associated with infection, cancer, or rheumatoid arthritis and have the defect in iron metabolism noted above under the hypochromic microcytic anemias. The reasons for inadequate stimulation or response of the marrow are not well understood.

Inability of the marrow to respond to erythropoietin may be due to damage to the marrow by drugs or toxic chemicals, to unknown causes, or to infiltration of the marrow by neoplastic cells or fibrous tissue.

In these conditions with low reticulocyte counts in which the marrow is not effectively producing erythrocytes, it is usually helpful to examine the bone marrow. Other studies to determine the underlying disease process can then proceed according to the marrow picture, the assessment of erythrokinetics, and the clinical findings.

POLYCYTHEMIA

Polycythemia is an increased concentration of erythrocytes in the blood that is above the normal for age and sex. Usually, but not always, the hematocrit and hemoglobin are also elevated.

Absolute polycythemia refers to an increase in the total red cell mass in the body; in *relative polycythemia,* the total red cell mass is normal, but the hematocrit is elevated because the plasma volume is decreased. Polycythemia may be classified as follows:

Relative polycythemia

Diminished plasma volume: dehydration; burns; shock; and so forth.

Absolute polycythemia

1. Autonomous cell production (panmyelosis): polycythemia vera.
2. Hypoxia:
    a. Arterial oxygen unsaturation: high altitude, pulmonary disease, cyanotic heart disease, methemoglobinemia, HbM.
    b. High affinity hemoglobinopathy.

Figure 4–66. Hb-S disease. Peripheral blood of a 14-year-old girl. Severe anemia, reticulocytosis, and poikilocytosis. Many typical sickles and occasional target cells.

Figure 4–67. Hb-S disease in a 22-year-old woman. Severe anemia, reticulocytosis, and poikilocytosis. Target cells. Siderocytes. Howell-Jolly bodies. Peripheral blood (May-Grünwald-Giemsa stain).

Figure 4–68. Hb-C disease in a 19-year-old black man. Hb, 12 gm. per 100 ml. Moderate reticulocytosis. Many target cells. Spherocytes.

Figure 4–69. Thalassemia major following splenectomy in a five-year-old Italian girl. Hb, 5.2 gm. per 100 ml.; Hct, 21. HbF, 71 per cent. Normoblastemia. Many target cells.

Figure 4–70. Thalassemia minor. Moderate number of target cells.

Figure 4–71. Megaloblastic anemia, marrow in a 66-year-old woman. Anemia, leukopenia, and thrombocytopenia. Megaloblasts with characteristic chromatin structure of nuclei and deeply basophilic cytoplasm in the center and upper half of the field. Next to them, on the left, a giant band cell, and below three giant metamyelocytes.

Figure 4–72. Megaloblastic anemia. Same patient as in Figure 4-71. Peripheral blood. Oval macrocytes, anisocytosis, and poikilocytosis; a characteristic polysegmented neutrophilic granulocyte.

Figure 4–73. Megaloblastic anemia. Same patient as in Figure 4-71, after therapy was started. Reticulocytosis. Vital stain and Wright's stain.

3. Autonomous ESF (erythrocyte stimulating factor) production:
   a. Neoplasm or growth: hypernephroma, cerebellar hemangioma, and so forth.
   b. Hereditary: recessive familial erythrocytosis.
4. Benign familial polycythemia.

Relative Polycythemia

Relative polycythemia refers to an increase in hematocrit or red cell count due to decreased plasma volume; total red cell mass is not increased. This occurs in acute dehydration, e.g., in severe diarrhea or burns.

In cases of burns there is marked hemoconcentration as the fluid portion of the blood leaks into the tissues. The concentration of hemoglobin has been found to be reduced after hemorrhage and increased during shock. In shock there is reduction in the plasma volume, which results in hemoconcentration. In anaphylactic shock the same hemoconcentration as is found in surgical shock has been noted by some investigators. Hemoconcentration occurs several hours before blood pressure sinks to critical levels. Studies of blood concentration made early may show a rising curve that acts as a warning signal of the more serious circulatory failure that will follow unless active treatment is immediately carried out.

Stress polycythemia and probably some instances of Gaisböck's syndrome are also examples of relative polycythemia.

Absolute Polycythemia

POLYCYTHEMIA VERA
(Erythremia, Vaquez-Osler Disease, Osler's Disease, Primary Polycythemia)

Polycythemia vera is one of the myeloproliferative disorders characterized by panmyelosis (excessive proliferation of erythroid, granulocytic, and megakaryocytic elements in the marrow and also in extramedullary sites) and reflected in the blood predominantly in an absolute increase in the red cell mass but also by leukocytosis and thrombocytosis. Erythropoietin excretion in the urine is decreased. The production of red cells appears to be autonomous, but it does respond to erythropoietin when the patient has become anemic through blood loss. The cause of this panmyelosis and pancytosis is unknown.

Clinical Findings. The disease is more frequent in men than in women. It begins in middle age and its prevalence is highest after 50. Affected patients exhibit a peculiar and striking ruddy cyanosis. Splenomegaly is present in two-thirds of patients. Thrombotic or hemorrhagic phenomena occur in about one-half of patients. Myocardial infarction, cerebral thrombosis, splenic infarction, pulmonary infarcts, and thrombophlebitis account for the most frequent thrombotic episodes; upper gastrointestinal bleeding, often from peptic ulcer, is the most common bleeding problem (Wasserman and Gilbert, 1966). Pruritus, especially after bathing, is common. Polycythemia occurring with hypertension but without splenomegaly has been referred to as Gaisböck's syndrome; polycythemia in combination with hepatic cirrhosis is known as Mosse's syndrome.

Blood. The erythrocytes number 6 to 12 million per microliter and the hemoglobin is 18 to 24 gm. per deciliter. The MCV, MCH, and MCHC are normal or low. The red cells are hypochromic and microcytic if chronic blood loss has occurred. Macrocytes, microcytes, polychromatic cells, and normoblasts may be found but are not a prominent feature of the disease. Red cell production is increased. Red cell destruction is normal during the period of erythrocytosis; later in the disease, as splenomegaly develops, the red cell survival diminishes. The total blood volume is increased, primarily because of the increased red cell mass, though the plasma volume may also be elevated to a lesser degree. Blood viscosity is high, and it may be difficult to prepare good smears. The ESR is reduced. The platelet count is increased in about two-thirds of patients, often to levels exceeding 1 million per microliter.

High platelet counts have been associated with increased likelihood of thrombosis and hemorrhage, and very high counts have been shown to exert an anticoagulant effect. No consistent clotting defect has been found in polycythemia vera. Clotting and clot retraction occur rapidly; the clot retracts to a small size and, frequently, large numbers of red cells fall out of the clot, which thus becomes very small. This may result in a false assumption of fibrinolysis, but the whole blood clot lysis and euglobulin clot lysis times are usually normal (Wasserman and Gilbert, 1964). Moderate neutrophilic leukocytosis in the range of 10,000 to 30,000 per microliter is the rule. Immature granulocytes are seen in about one-half of cases and basophils are often absolutely increased. The leukocyte alkaline phosphatase is almost always markedly elevated.

The arterial oxygen saturation is normal. Hyperuricemia appears in many patients with polycythemia vera due to the increased nucleic acid metabolism, and in some patients, secondary gout or renal uric acid stones occur.

Marrow. The marrow is characteristically hypercellular, with all the elements (erythroid, granulocytic, and megakaryocytic) sharing the hyperplasia; fat is decreased. Increased reticulin is present and correlated positively with the cellularity. Storage iron is decreased or absent. In the few patients with polycythemia vera who do not show leukocytosis or thrombocytosis, the marrow may not be helpful.

If doubt remains about the diagnosis of polycythemia vera, a search for other causes of polycythemia should be made. This especially should include an intravenous pyelogram (see below).

Course. Polycythemia vera is a chronic disease; patients usually live 10 to 20 years under good control. Phlebotomy, busulfan, and ^{32}P have been used to control the manifestations of the disease. Because of the high incidence of complications in untreated cases, surgery should not be undertaken unless the hematocrit has been reduced to normal levels (Wasserman and Gilbert, 1964).

In about 10 to 20 per cent of patients, progressive anemia, gradual splenic enlargement, and further elevation of the leukocyte count, with more immature granulocytes and more circulating nucleated red cells, may occur. Many red cells become oval, tear drop-shaped cells become prominent, and poikilocytic red cells increase in number (Figs. 4–21 and 4–22). Bone marrow aspiration becomes impossible because of myelofibrosis, and splenomegaly is due to increasing extramedullary hematopoiesis. The manifestations at this stage of the disease are indistinguishable from myelofibrosis with myeloid metaplasia (Fig. 4–76). The latter, therefore, is not uncommonly a sequel of polycythemia vera (Dameshek and Gunz, 1964).

Another late complication of polycythemia vera is acute blastic leukemia. It is still not clear whether this is etiologically related to prior therapy with radiomimetic drugs, x-ray or ^{32}P. In the study of Modan and Lilienfeld (1965), about 10 per cent of American patients with polycythemia vera who received ^{32}P or x-ray developed acute leukemia. In a British series, however, no cases of acute leukemia were found in equivalent numbers of patients treated with or without radiation (Halnan and Russell, 1965). No conclusions can be drawn since these were retrospective, nonrandomized studies. A prospective study is now in progress to settle this issue (Wasserman, 1971).

HYPOXIA

Arterial Oxygen Unsaturation. Lack of oxygen reaching the blood for one reason or another results in arterial unsaturation, impaired oxygen delivery to the tissues, increased production of erythropoietin, erythroid hyperplasia in the marrow, and resultant erythrocytosis. The red cell mass is increased. As a response to the hypoxia, the red cell 2,3-DPG and the P_{50} are increased. In contrast to polycythemia vera, there is usually no leukocytosis or thrombocytosis, and the leukocyte alkaline phosphatase is normal. Arterial oxygen unsaturation may be the cause of polycythemia in persons living at high altitudes; in patients with chronic pulmonary disease and a block in diffusion of oxygen into the blood; in cyanotic heart disease in which there is right to left shunt; and in methemoglobinemia whether due to enzyme deficiency, chronic drug effect, or a structurally abnormal hemoglobin (HbM).

High Affinity Hemoglobinopathy. Another cause of tissue hypoxia is the presence of a structurally abnormal hemoglobin which has a high affinity for oxygen. As in other functional hemoglobinopathies, the disorder occurs in the heterozygote (Table 4–7, p. 209). The abnormal hemoglobin releases less oxygen to the tissues than does normal hemoglobin at the Po_2; the oxygen dissociation curve is shifted to the left and the P_{50} is decreased. The red cell 2,3-DPG is not increased. As in arterial oxygen unsaturation there is increased erythropoietin production and erythrocytosis. It must be emphasized that routine hemoglobin electrophoresis usually does not detect these hemoglobin variants because the amino acid substitution is at one of the $\alpha\beta$ contact sites or near the heme pocket. A low P_{50} therefore is presumptive evidence for a hemoglobinopathy. The heat lability test for unstable hemoglobin should be done, since some hemoglobins with high affinity and polycythemia are unstable.

AUTONOMOUS ERYTHROPOIETIN (ESF) PRODUCTION

Neoplasms or growths may be associated with absolute polycythemia, which is corrected when the tumor is removed. Some of these neoplasms have been shown to contain, and presumably produce, ESF (e.g., cerebellar hemangioma, hypernephroma, some hepatomas). In other neoplasms or growths (e.g., renal cysts, hydronephrosis, ovarian carcinoma, some hepatomas) it appears that the mass impinging on the kidney induces increased renal production of ESF due to increased pressure or local hypoxia within the kidney.

Recessive familial erythrocytosis has recently been ascribed to increased ESF production which is unresponsive to changes in hemoglobin concentration or oxygen carrying capacity of the blood induced by phlebotomy (Adamson *et al.*, 1973). Red cell 2,3-DPG and P_{50} were normal in the polycythemic patients as well as the unaffected family members. The physiologic basis for this unregulated (autonomous) ESF production remains to be explained.

BENIGN FAMILIAL POLYCYTHEMIA

Also known as primary erythrocytosis of childhood, benign familial erythrocytosis is a rare disorder. Originally this was described as a pure erythrocytosis without splenomegaly, and with normal leukocyte and platelet counts, occurring in one or more siblings and sometimes a parent (Abildgard *et al.*, 1963). It now seems clear that at least some of the patients in families with autosomal dominant hereditary patterns in this group have high oxygen affinity hemoglobinopathies, and at least some with autosomal recessive hereditary patterns have autonomous ESF production (see above). What is not clear at the present time is whether different pathophysiologic mechanisms may be operative in other patients with "benign familial erythrocytosis," since most of the patients reported have not been studied with currently available techniques.

Differentiation of polycythemia vera from other forms of absolute polycythemia is alluded to in the above discussion. To be emphasized in the latter are the lack of leukocytosis and thrombocytosis, the normal leukocyte alkaline phosphatase, and the marrow, which shows only erythroid hyperplasia and not panmyelosis.

HEMATOPOIESIS IN THE NEWBORN AND INFANT

Erythrocytes

In the seven- to ten-week-old (18 to 38 mm. long) embryo, about 25 per cent of the circulating cells are nucleated. At the intrauterine age of four or five months (length 160 to 250 mm.), the number of nucleated red cells is reduced to less than 1 per cent. The number of erythrocytes increases with the progression of pregnancy by about 500,000 every four weeks from 1 million per microliter at eight weeks of intrauterine life. In addition to age, other factors, prenatal and postnatal, influence the blood picture.

One such factor is size. In single ovum twins with common placental circulation, differences in body weight are reflected in corresponding differences in the numbers of erythrocytes and levels of hemoglobin, for example, 25 gm. of hemoglobin and 7,500,000 erythrocytes in the larger twin and 3.7 gm. and 1,800,000 erythrocytes in the smaller.

Bleeding from the fetal into the maternal circulation is evidenced by the presence of elevated amounts of fetal hemoglobin in the maternal circulation.

At the time of clamping the cord, as much as 100 to 125 ml. of placental blood may be added to the newborn if tying of the cord is postponed until the pulsation of the cord ceases. In a study of newborns whose cords had been clamped late, the average capillary red cell counts were 400,000 higher 1 hour after and 800,000 higher 24 hours after birth as compared with newborns whose cord had been clamped early.

Capillary blood (obtained by skin prick) gives higher red cell and hemoglobin values than venous blood (cord, sinus). The differences may amount to about 500,000 red cells per microliter for the former and about 3.0 gm. per 100 ml. for the latter. The slowing of capillary circulation and the resulting loss of fluid may be the responsible factor. Examination of venous blood furnishes more consistent results than examination of capillary blood.

Dramatic changes take place in the blood and marrow during the first few days and even during the early hours after birth. These are reflected in the values of all formed elements and in the rapid fluctuations. The number of erythrocytes tends to reach a peak during the first 24 hours, remains the same for about two weeks, and then declines slowly.

The calculated average of 480 erythrocyte counts in capillary blood was reported as 5,640,000, with a range of 3,500,000 to 8,230,000. The calculated average of 249 counts in venous blood was 4,820,000, with a range of 3,100,000 to 6,850,000. Both compilations were based on examinations done during the first postnatal day. It is apparent that the high counts are seen mainly in capillary blood, whereas values obtained in venous blood are not significantly different from what one finds in healthy older children.

In the full term infant, nucleated red cells are most numerous at birth with about 500/μl. The normoblast count declines to about 200/μl. at 24 hr., 25/μl. at 48 hr. and less than 5/μl. at 72 hr. By four days it is rare to find circulating normoblasts (Oski and Naiman, 1972).

The normal reticulocyte count at birth ranges from 3 to 7 per cent during the first 48 hours, during which time it rises slightly. After the second day it falls rather rapidly to 1 to 3 per cent on the third day and reaches 1 per cent by the seventh day of life.

Hemoglobin concentration in capillary blood

during the first day of life averages 19.0 gm./dl., with 95 per cent of normal values falling between 14.6 and 23.4 gm./dl. In cord blood the average is 16.8 gm./dl., with 95 per cent of normals between 13.5 and 20.1 gm./dl. (Oski and Naiman, 1972). There is frequently an initial increase in the hemoglobin level of venous blood at the end of 24 hours as compared with that of cord blood. At the end of the first week, the level is about the same as in cord blood and it does not begin to fall until after the second week. During the first two weeks the lower limit of normal is 14.5 gm./dl. for capillary blood and 13.0 gm./dl. for venous blood.

The hematocrit in capillary blood on the first day of life averages 61 per cent, with 95 per cent of normal values between 46 and 76 per cent. In cord blood, the average is 53 per cent. The changes during the first few weeks parallel the hemoglobin concentration.

The normal MCV at birth ranges from 104 to 118 fl., macrocytic when compared to the normal adult range of 83 to 99 fl. The MCV gradually falls to reach about 83 fl. by age 6 months. The MCH parallels the MCV. The average MCHC is about 32 per cent at birth, and after the second week, rises slightly during the first few months to about 34 per cent.

The high erythrocytic values at birth are explained by the stimulating effect on the marrow of the partial anoxia *in utero,* which becomes more progressive with the growth of the fetus. With the change in the environment and improved oxygenation after birth, the stimulus to blood production ceases abruptly, with resulting lowering of all the erythrocytic values and later a more gradual development of a "physiologic" anemia. The role of hypoxia is illustrated by reports of continued high erythrocyte values in the neonatal period in infants with congenital heart disease. These infants do not develop "physiologic" anemia.

Another factor that contributes to the lowered values is the shortened survival of neonatal erythrocytes.

There are conflicting reports in the literature regarding osmotic resistance of fetal erythrocytes, but the consensus is that they are significantly more resistant than adult cells.

Leukocytes

The total white cell count at birth and during the first 24 hours varies within wide limits. The numbers range from 4000 to 40,000, granulocytes being the predominant cell and a large proportion of them being nonsegmented with occasional myelocytes and without evidence of disease. According to most opinions there are increases of the total number and of the granulocytes during the first 24 hours. The count begins to drop progressively at the beginning of the second day, mainly owing to a decrease of granulocytes. According to a careful study by Forkner, during the first day the average was a total white cell count of 25,000, with 69 per cent neutrophilic granulocytes, 2 per cent eosinophils, 7 per cent monocytes, 18 per cent lymphocytes, and 4 per cent myelocytes. Ten days later the corresponding figures were 13,000, 29 per cent, 3 per cent, 17 per cent, 49 per cent, and 0.2 per cent.

In premature infants examined on the first day, the total white cell count is usually lower (average: about 7500). The number of immature white cells in the differential count is higher, and the replacement of granulocytes by lymphocytes takes place somewhat later than in term infants.

The dramatic variations in the total white cell count and in the differential count suggest caution in correlating such findings with clinical manifestations of disease.

Platelets

The platelet count is in the lower normal adult range at birth and during the first week and then rises rapidly to adult levels.

DISORDERS INVOLVING LEUKOCYTES

The examination of leukocytes includes two technical phases. In the quantitative phase, one determines the number of all the white cells, the total white blood count (WBC), and the relative and absolute numbers of the various forms of white cells. The term *leukocytosis* refers to an increase in the total WBC above the upper limit of normal for age and sex. *Leukopenia* is a total WBC below normal. Although all leukocytes act in defending the body in one way or another, their functions are somewhat different and it is best to regard them as separate systems. An increase or decrease in the absolute number of cells in each series is termed: *neutrophilia* (neutrophilic leukocytosis) and *neutropenia; eosinophilia* (eosinophilic leukocytosis) and *eosinopenia; basophilia* (basophilic leukocytosis) and *basopenia; lymphocytosis* and *lymphocytopenia; monocytosis* and *monocytopenia,* though the latter is not clearly defined. In the qualitative phase, one determines structural abnormalities in cytoplasm and nucleus and also, to an increasing extent, functional abnormalities as well. Examination also includes two anatomic phases: examination of peripheral blood (capillary or venous) and examination of marrow (obtained from sternum, tibia, iliac, or spinous process).

The purpose of the study of leukocytes is, first, to help in establishing a diagnosis. Occasionally the examination alone may furnish a positive specific diagnosis, for example, in leukemia. More frequently it may be diagnostically helpful together with other clinical or laboratory data, for example, in acute appendicitis or infectious mononucleosis. Another purpose is to help in establishing a prognosis. For example, a low white blood count in acute appendicitis or pneumonia is considered prognostically unfavorable.

Finally, study of the leukocytes is helpful in following the course of disease. For example, toxic effects of radiotherapy and chemotherapy may be recognized early by examination of leukocytes.

Examination of leukocytes may also reveal the existence of an entirely unsuspected disease. For example, leukemia may be found in a patient with the clinical picture of an acute infection, or infectious mononucleosis may be found in patients whose disease clinically resembles leukemia.

For this and other reasons the white blood count is one of the routine tests, which, according to recommendations of organizations supervising hospitals must be done on every patient admitted to the hospital regardless of disease.

In contrast to the red cells and platelets which function within the blood, the different white blood cells use the blood stream only for transportation; they perform their tasks in the tissues after leaving the blood (Boggs and Winkelstein, 1971). We have discussed the morphology, production, distribution within the body, life span, and function for each of the white cells in an earlier section, beginning on page 150. This background is assumed in the following sections, dealing with changes in number or function of the different cell types.

Neutrophilia

Neutrophilic leukocytosis or neutrophilia refers to an absolute concentration of neutro-

Table 4–12. THE NORMAL DIFFERENTIAL COUNT (95 PER CENT VALUES)*

	RELATIVE VALUES		ABSOLUTE VALUES	
	Average (per cent)	Range (per cent)	Average per cu. mm.	Range per cu. mm.
Segmented neutrophilic granulocytes				
Newborn – 1st day	60		9000	
Newborn – 2nd day			6000	
5 days to 14 years	38	16-60		
8 to 14 years			3250	
15 to 19 years	48	25-70		
Adolescents	48	25-70	4000	1500-7500
Adults	60	50-70	4500 (3000)	2500-7000 (1500-7000)
Band cells				
Newborn – 1st day	25			
1st year	17			
Adults	3	0-5	(600)	0-500 (200-2100)
Eosinophils				
Under 14 years	2.8	0-8		0-600
Over 14 years	3.0	1-5	200 (150)	50-500 (30-800)
Basophils	0.5	0-1	40 (30)	0-100 (0-160)
Lymphocytes				
Newborn – 1st day	30			
Newborn – 4th day	45			
4 to 7 years	48	20-70	5000	1500-8500
8 to 14 years	48	20-70	4000	1500-6500
15 to 19 years	42	22-62	3250	1500-5000
Adults	30	20-40	3000 (2400)	1000-4000 (1500-4000)
Monocytes				
All age groups			375	285-500
Birth to 4 years	5	0-12		
4 to 14 years	3	0-7		
14 years and over	4	1-6	300 (460)	50-600 (200-1000)
Disintegrating cells	5	0-12	400	0-1200

*For comparison with earlier data, the figures cited in parentheses are from Orfanakis *et al.*: Amer. J. Clin. Path. 53:647, 1970.

Table 4–13. PATHOLOGIC LEUKOCYTOSIS

CAUSE	CELL TYPE
Allergy	Eosinophil
Brucellosis	Lymphocyte, monocyte
Convulsions	Neutrophil or lymphocyte
Drugs and poisons	
ACTH	Neutrophil
Adrenalin	
Camphor	Neutrophil and eosinophil
Copper sulfate, phosphorus, carpine	Eosinophil
Tetrachlorethane, Adrenalin	Monocyte, neutrophil, and lymphocyte
Other (acetanilid, arsenicals, benzene, CO, digitalis, lead, phenacetin, turpentine, venoms)	Neutrophil
Hemolysis	Neutrophil
Hemorrhage	Neutrophil
Hodgkin's disease	Neutrophil, eosinophil and monocyte
Infectious lymphocytosis	Lymphocyte
Infectious mononucleosis	Lymphocyte, atypical changes
Leukemia	Granulocyte, lymphocyte, or monocyte
Loeffler's syndrome, periarteritis nodosa, pernicious anemia	Eosinophil
Polycythemia vera	Neutrophil, eosinophil, basophil
Toxemias:	
diabetic acidosis, eclampsia, gout, uremia	Neutrophil
Tuberculosis	Neutrophil, eosinophil, lymphocyte, monocyte
Tumors involving	
marrow and serous cavities	Neutrophil and eosinophil
ovarian tumor	Eosinophil
GI tract and liver	Neutrophil
Typhoid fever	Lymphocyte

phils in the blood above normal for age. Normal values for different ages are given in Table 4–12.

Mechanisms (Boggs and Winkelstein, 1971; Finch, 1972). The primary factors influencing the neutrophil count are: (1) the rate of inflow of cells from the bone marrow; (2) the proportion of neutrophils in the marginal granulocyte pool (MGP) and the circulating granulocyte pool (CGP); and (3) the rate of outflow of neutrophils from the blood (see p. 154).

Physiologic leukocytosis is an increased WBC produced by factors or situations that do not involve tissue damage. Severe exercise, hypoxia, or stress, or the injection of epinephrine will result in a decrease in the MGP and a corresponding increase in the CGP, resulting in a pseudoneutrophilia. This is a simple redistribution of cells between the CGP and MGP.

Stress of greater severity or injection of endotoxin, corticosteroids, or etiocholanolone results in an increased inflow of cells to the blood from the marrow storage pool. As a result, the maturation and storage pool in the marrow is diminished, and both MGP and CGP are enlarged. A greater neutrophilia is possible here because of the much larger size of the storage pool than the CPG and MGP. Band neutrophils and metamyelocytes are likely to be present.

In both of the above an acute neutrophilia occurs as a result of redistribution of cells, without input from increased production. Chronic neutrophilia may be produced by corticosteroids, which decrease the egress of neutrophils from the blood and result in increased CGP and MGP without necessarily increasing the production of neutrophils.

In contrast to the above, *pathologic leukocytosis* is an increased WBC which occurs as a result of disease, and usually is a response to tissue damage (Table 4–13). This leukocytosis is most often a neutrophilia.

In addition to the random loss of neutrophils from the circulation in various body secretions, neutrophils leave the blood by ameboid movement when attracted to a focus of inflammation in tissues, presumably by chemotactic substances. It is from the marginal granulocyte pool (MGP) that the neutrophils leave the blood, pass between capillary endothelial cells, and reach the tissues.

In acute infection, increased margination of neutrophils and outflow from blood to tissues would lead to neutropenia were they not

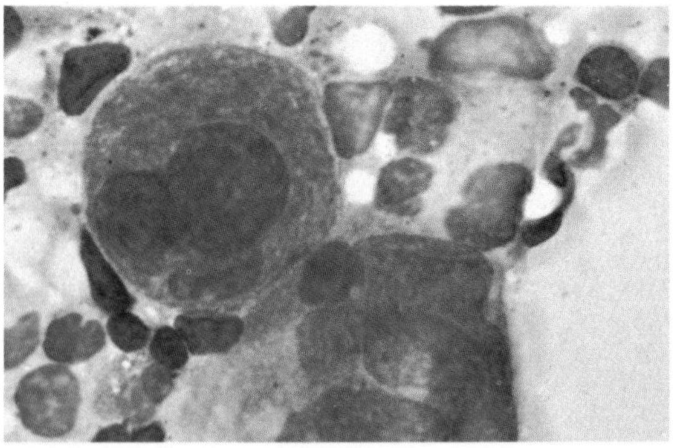

Figure 4–74.

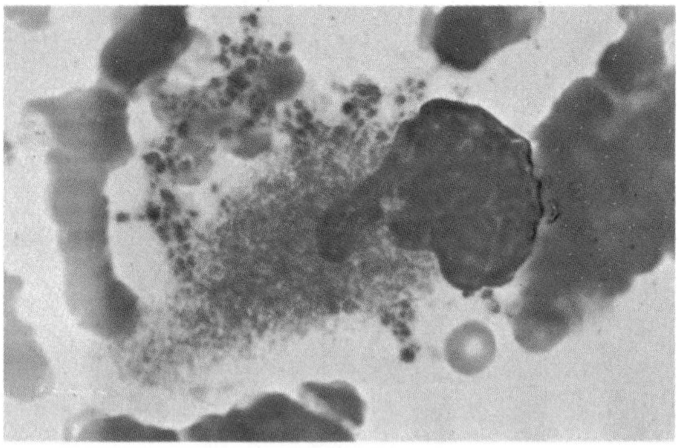

Figure 4–75.

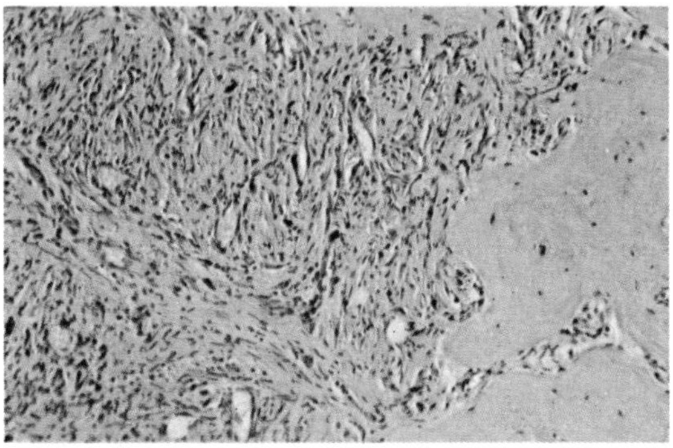

Figure 4–76.

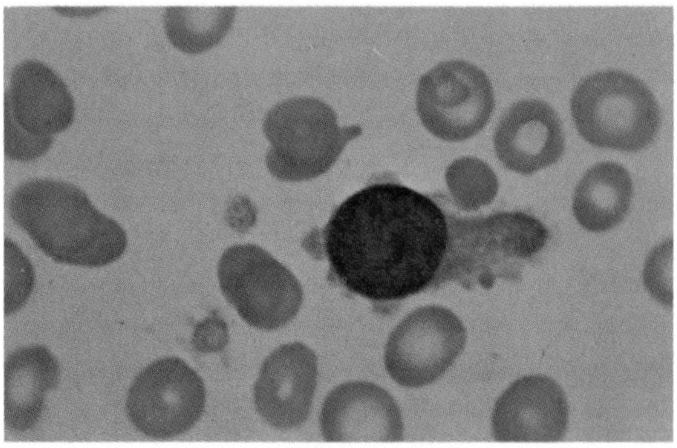

Figure 4–77.

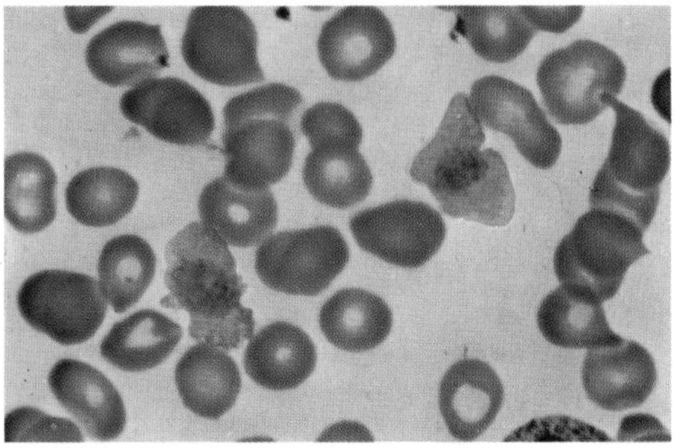

Figure 4–78.

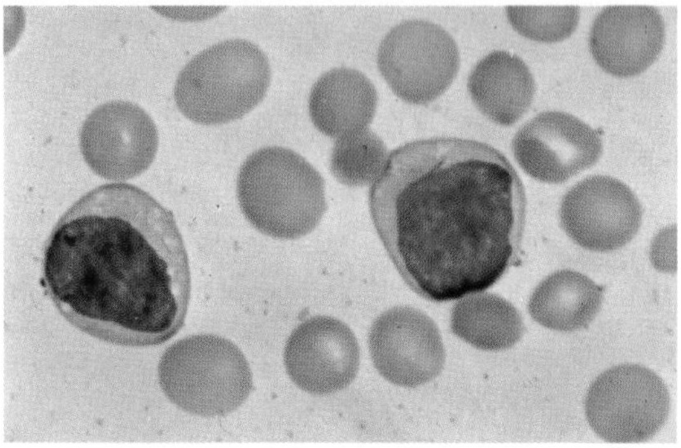

Figure 4–79.

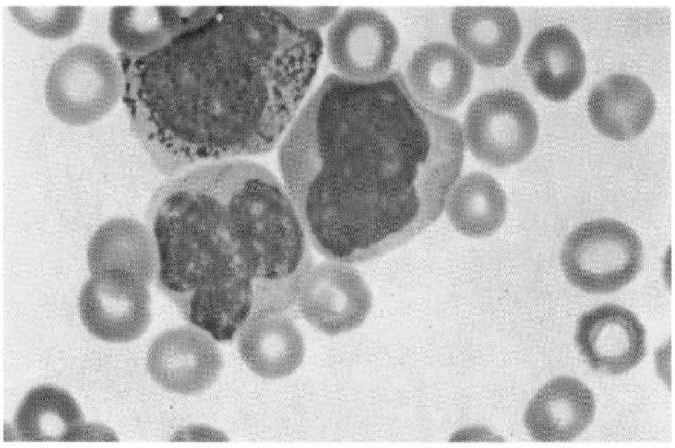

Figure 4–80.

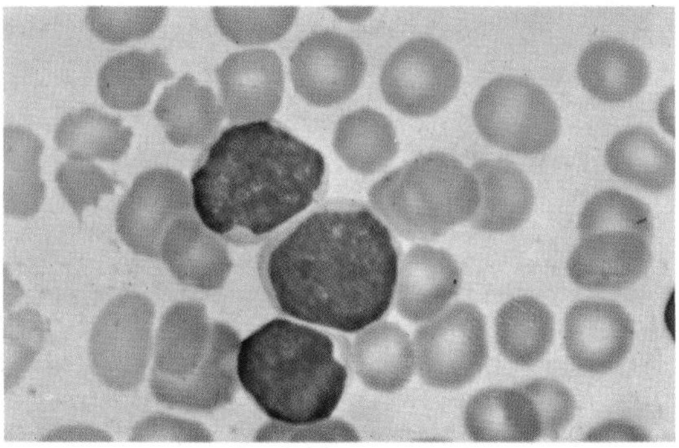

Figure 4–81.

(See opposite page for legends.)

quickly followed by a flow of neutrophils from the marrow storage compartment into the blood. Since the latter overcompensates, the result is a neutrophilia. Usually production and storage compartments then increase in the marrow and are able to sustain the increased CGP (i.e., neutrophilia) and MGP in the face of the increased flow of neutrophils from the blood into the inflammatory site. In these instances, the marrow will show granulocytic hyperplasia (decreased E/G ratio and increased cellularity), with maturation evidently intact.

If the demand for neutrophils is extremely great, as in severe infection, there may be depletion of the marrow storage pool and a decreased CGP (i.e., neutropenia) and MGP, because the supply of cells is insufficient for the demand. In these instances, the marrow will show increased numbers of early neutrophil precursors, through the myelocyte stage, but decreased numbers of metamyelocytes, bands, and neutrophils.

Causes

Infection. Systemic infections due to various bacteria, fungi, spirochetes, and viruses may cause neutrophilia. In some, this may be preceded by a transient neutropenia, especially if the infection is severe. Some bacterial infections result in persistent neutropenia, such as typhoid fever, paratyphoid fever, and brucellosis. Whether this is due to the mechanism cited above for severe infection, or to a toxic depression of the marrow, or to a combination, is not clear.

Appendicitis, salpingitis, otitis media, and other localized infections caused by pyogenic organisms usually result in neutrophilia.

A characteristic pattern of response to infection includes: progressive neutrophilic leukocytosis, increase of young forms (shift to the left), and fall in eosinophils. When the infection begins to subside and the fever drops, a gradual transformation in the blood picture occurs: the total number of leukocytes goes down, and the number of monocytes increases. This monocytic phase is gradually replaced by a relative or slight absolute lymphocytosis and eosinophilia as recovery proceeds.

Other disorders associated with neutrophilia are listed below. In some of them, one or more of the mechanisms described above are operating; in others, the mechanism is unclear.

Toxic

METABOLIC. Uremia, eclampsia, gout, diabetic acidosis.

DRUGS AND CHEMICALS. Lead, mercury, potassium chlorate, digitalis, epinephrine, corticosteroids, turpentine, ethylene glycol, benzene.

Physical and Emotional Stimuli. Heat, cold, muscular activity, anoxia, pain, fear, anger.

Tissue Destruction or Necrosis. Myocardial infarction; burns; surgical operations; crush injuries; fractures; neoplastic disease, especially with extensive necrosis.

Hemorrhage. Especially if bleeding has occurred within a serous cavity (peritoneal, pleural, joint, subdural).

Hemolysis. Especially with rapid hemolysis, as in hemolytic crises or hemolytic transfusion reactions.

Hematologic Disorders. Myeloproliferative disorders; granulocytic leukemia; postsplenectomy state.

Determinants. Certain host factors modify the degree of neutrophilic response. Children respond more intensely than adults. The degree of neutrophilia produced may be impaired by the same factors that impair erythrocyte production (iron lack, folate or vitamin B_{12} deficiency) or by marrow failure due to other causes. Imperfectly defined factors which enable the body to localize an infection may play a role: the more localized the process, the more pronounced the neutrophilia.

Other factors modifying the neutrophilic response are due more to the microorganism than the host. Pyogenic bacteria, especially, induce neutrophilia. Within limits the more virulent the agent, the higher the neutrophil count. When the infection is overwhelming, however, there is apt to be a neutropenia and greater shift to the left due to the mechanism described above.

It is claimed, and it is probably correct within wide limits, that the height of leukocytosis

---

Figure 4–74. Normal megakaryocytes. The cell at the bottom center is younger; it has completed nuclear division and has relatively few cytoplasmic granules. The cell above and to the left has more granules, which are clustering together in preparation for separation in platelets.

Figure 4–75. Megakaryocyte (broken in smear) showing separation of platelets from the cytoplasmic mass.

Figure 4–76. Myelofibrosis. Marrow is diffusely replaced by fibroblasts and cellular connective tissue.

Figure 4–77. Myelofibrosis. Dwarf megakaryocyte and two atypical platelets.

Figure 4–78. Myelofibrosis. Peripheral blood. Atypical platelets.

Figure 4–79. Acute granulocytic leukemia. Peripheral blood. Myeloblasts. Delicate reticular structure of chromatin. Indistinct Auer body in the right cell.

Figure 4–80. Acute granulocytic leukemia. Peripheral blood. An Auer body in a myeloblast and another in a cell with more differentiated nucleus. The third cell is a promyelocyte.

Figure 4–81. Acute lymphocytic leukemia. Peripheral blood. The two upper lymphoblasts resemble closely the myeloblasts in the preceding two slides. The cell at the bottom has a somewhat more differentiated nucleus.

is an indicator of the resistance of the individual and that the degree of the shift to the left is an indicator of the severity of the infection. In keeping with this conception, a simultaneous fall of the former and a rise of the latter are prognostically unfavorable.

The following are hematologic signs of recovery from infectious diseases:

1. Drop of the total leukocyte count and of the number of neutrophils.
2. Disappearance of shift to the left.
3. Transient increase in number of monocytes.
4. Increase of eosinophils when they were decreased or absent during the height of the disease.
5. Increase in number of lymphocytes.
6. Disappearance of toxic granulation.

Therefore, the following are unfavorable hematologic signs:

1. A moderate or slight rise in the total number of leukocytes associated with a marked shift to the left during the height of the disease.
2. Failure of eosinophils to reappear in the end stages of an infectious disease when they were absent before.
3. Absolute reduction of lymphocytes.
4. Excessive number of cells with toxic granulation.

Therapy of infections with antibiotic agents may modify the leukocytic response to infection. Steroid therapy, though causing neutrophilia, tends to impair the host response to infection, probably because of diminished movement of neutrophils into the tissues and increased lysosomal stability.

MORPHOLOGIC ALTERATIONS IN NEUTROPHILS

In addition to quantitative changes, qualitative morphologic alterations also occur in neutrophils. Some of these, such as toxic granules or cytoplasmic vacuoles, are acquired and disappear after the stimulus which provoked them is gone. Others are hereditary and persist through life, with or without functional impairment. These are well illustrated and reviewed by Brunning (1970).

It should be noted that disorders of leukocyte function may exist without any structural abnormality detectable with the usual modes of morphologic examination. These are briefly discussed on page 254.

Toxic Granulation. Toxic granules are dark blue to purple cytoplasmic granules in the metamyelocyte, band, or neutrophil stage. They are peroxidase positive and may be numerous or few in number; often, there is less peroxidase activity in toxic than in normal neutrophils. Toxic granulation is found in severe infections or other toxic conditions (Fig. 4–98 a).

Normally neutrophil granules are tan to pink in color in neutrophil metamyelocytes, bands, and mature forms. Even the nonspecific or azurophil granules which are dark blue on the promyelocyte stage normally lose their basophilia in the mature neutrophil, where they comprise about one-third of the granules in the human. It is probable that the toxic condition results in lack of maturation of the azurophil granules and persistence of their basophilic staining properties, accounting for the dark staining granules in mature cells. Possibly skipped divisions during the development of the neutrophil may result in a greater proportion of the granules being of the azurophil type. In some cells the presence of few granules implies prior utilization and senescence. Toxic granulation may be simulated by artefacts caused by imperfect staining; one must consider this and eliminate the possibility.

Irregular basophilia of the cytoplasm is also common in toxic conditions and appears to reflect impaired cytoplasmic maturation. If discrete, this focal basophilia is known as a Döhle inclusion body (v.i.).

Cytoplasmic vacuoles are also signs of toxic change if the possibility of degeneration artefacts can be eliminated by making films from fresh blood free of anticoagulant. Vacuoles imply that phagocytosis has occurred. One may also see irregular depletion of granules.

Another toxic change in the neutrophil is the occasional appearance of several sharp or blunt spicules extending out from the nucleus.

Döhle Inclusion Bodies. These are inclusions in the cytoplasm of polymorphonuclear neutrophils, which stain pale blue with Wright's stain. They are remnants of cytoplasmic RNA from an earlier stage of development. The typical inclusion bodies are about the size of micrococci or a little larger; some of them are pear shaped; others appear as short rods or cocci lying in pairs. Smaller, discrete, punctiform granules are sometimes seen but do not have the same significance. Originally Döhle bodies were described as being especially prominent in scarlet fever, but they are seen in many other infectious diseases, in burns, in aplastic anemia, and following administration of toxic agents. Therefore, they frequently accompany toxic granulation in the neutrophil. Döhle bodies are also present in the May-Hegglin anomaly.

The inclusion bodies appear blue in preparations stained with Wright's stain, but long staining with methyl green pyronine is preferable (see p. 140). When stained with the latter stain, nuclei are purplish and the bodies bright red.

May-Hegglin Anomaly. This is a rare autosomal dominant condition characterized by the presence of Döhle bodies in neutrophils, giant platelets, and, in some persons, thrombocytopenia (Oski *et al.*, 1962). The Döhle bodies are larger and more prominent than those usually found in infections (Fig. 4–98*B*); and they have been described in eosinophils, basophils, and monocytes as well as in neutrophils (Brunning, 1970).

Alder-Reilly Anomaly. A dense azurophilic granulation in all white blood cells was described by Alder in 1939 (Fig. 4–99A). In neutrophils it may resemble toxic granulation but is unrelated to infection and is not transient. In 1940 Reilly described similar granulocytes in some but not all patients with gargoylism (the Hurler syndrome or, more generally, the genetic mucopolysaccharidoses). Other observations have shown that the heavy granulation in neutrophils can occur either as a feature of the genetic mucopolysaccharidoses or independently in otherwise healthy persons (Brunning, 1970). In the former, other cells are usually involved. Occurring more often than the Alder-Reilly anomaly in the genetic mucopolysaccharidoses is a metachromatic inclusion in the lymphocytes surrounded by a clear space (Fig. 4–99B). This group of disorders is inherited and is characterized by abnormal deposition and excretion of mucopolysaccharides (Groover *et al.*, 1972).

Pelger-Huët Anomaly. This hereditary, autosomal dominant condition involves failure of normal segmentation of granulocytic nuclei. Most nuclei are band shaped or have two segments but no more (Fig. 4–100). The chromatin is quite coarse, and these are not normal young band forms. When a large number of band neutrophils appear in the differential count in a patient without infection or other cause, careful analysis of the smear of the patient and of family members will occasionally establish the presence of the Pelger-Huët anomaly.

A similar appearing, acquired disorder of nuclear segmentation in granulocytes may occasionally be found in cases of granulocytic leukemia, myeloproliferative disorders, some infections, and after exposure to certain drugs (Brunning, 1970); this is sometimes called the pseudo-Pelger anomaly. In addition to the band forms and neutrophils with only two segments, mature cells with round nonsegmented nuclei and coarse chromatin are common, in contrast to the congenital Pelger-Huët anomaly.

Chediak-Higashi Syndrome. This rare, autosomal recessive disorder is characterized by partial albinism, photophobia, abnormally large granules in leukocytes and other granule-containing cells, and frequent pyogenic infections. An accelerated lymphoma-like phase occurs, with lymphadenopathy, hepatosplenomegaly, and pancytopenia; lymphoid infiltrates are widespread and death ensues at an early age. (Blume and Wolff, 1972). Granulocytes, monocytes, and lymphocytes contain giant granules (Fig. 4–101), which appear to be abnormal lysosomes (White, 1967; Rozenszajn and Radnay, 1970).

Neutropenia

Neutropenia is a reduction of the absolute neutrophil count below 2000 per μl. for whites and below 1300 per μl. for blacks. The term *agranulocytosis* has been used for severe neutropenia; this is almost always associated with depletion of eosinophils and basophils as well. If the neutrophil count is less than 1000 per μl., the risk of infection is considerably increased over normal, and if there are less than 500 neutrophils per μl., the risk of infection is great.

Agranulocytic angina and malignant neutropenia are older terms that describe the common symptoms and rapidly fatal course that may be associated with infection and very severe neutropenia. Following a period of malaise comes the sudden onset of high fever and ulcerative lesions of the mouth, throat, and other mucous membranes. Death from sepsis occurs in a few days if effective antibiotic therapy cannot be achieved.

The mechanisms by which neutropenia occur include: (1) decreased flow of neutrophils from marrow into blood due to either lack of production or ineffective production; (2) increased removal of neutrophils from the blood; (3) altered distribution between circulating granulocyte pool (CGP) and marginal granulocyte pool (MGP); or (4) combinations of these. Neutropenias are not so neatly classified as anemias. In recent years, however, a sound approach has been made, using data from radioisotopic measurements of proliferative activity, maturation time, survival in the circulation, and measurement of MGP and CGP in addition to the usual bone marrow and peripheral blood studied (Kauder and Mauer, 1966; Finch, 1972). A classification according to Finch is given in Table 4–14, though some of the entries are uncertain and may need to be changed when more information becomes available. It should be noted that drugs induce neutropenia through several mechanisms and are a very important consideration in any differential diagnosis of leukopenia.

Myeloid Hypoplasia. Kostman's infantile genetic agranulocytosis is a rare, autosomal recessive condition appearing in early infancy. The marrow usually shows increased early granulocytes but few maturing forms, and the neutrophil survival is normal. A soluble factor

Table 4–14. CLASSIFICATION OF NEUTROPENIA*

I. *Myeloid hypoplasia*
  A. Infantile genetic agranulocytosis (Kostman); familial neutropenia; cyclic neutropenia; chronic (hypoplastic) neutropenia; myelophthisic neutropenia.
  B. Drug induced:
    1. Cytolytic:
      a. Alkylating agents (nitrogen mustard, cyclophosphamide, chlorambucil, busulfan).
      b. Ionizing radiation.
      c. Mitosis inhibitors (colchicine, vinblastine, vincristine).
      d. DNA depolymerization (procarbazine).
    2. Metabolic interference with DNA synthesis:
      a. Purine and pyrimidine antagonists (cytosine arabinoside,† methotrexate,† 6-mercaptopurine, azathioprine, hydroxyurea).
      b. Phenothiazine type (phenothiazines, dibenzazepine compounds, antithyroid compounds,† sulfonamides,† antibiotics, anticonvulsants).
      c. Others (chloramphenicol,† benzene†).
    3. Idiosyncratic:
      a. Acute, days to weeks (quinine, quinidine, indomethacin, procainamide, thiazides, sulfonamides,† phenylbutazone,† antithyroids†).
      b. Chronic, months to years (chloramphenicol,† phenylbutazone,† benzene,† gold salts†).

II. *Marrow hyperplasia with ineffective granulocytopoiesis*
  A. Chediak-Higashi syndrome; megaloblastic anemia; myeloproliferative disorders (these may belong in IV).
  B. Drug induced:
    1. Impaired nucleic acid synthesis (cytosine arabinoside,† methotrexate,† diphenylhydantoin).
    2. Others (alcohol, chloramphenicol†).

III. *Decreased survival in circulation* due to increased utilization or increased destruction.
  A. Bacterial infections; viral infections; protozoal infections; chronic benign neutropenia of childhood; chronic idiopathic neutropenia in adults; splenic neutropenia; neonatal isoimmunization neutropenia; acquired immunoneutropenia.
  B. Drug induced (immunologic mechanism):
    Aminopyrine, amidopyrine, phenylbutazone,† sulfapyridine.†

IV. Combination of impaired production (I or II) and decreased survival (III).
  A. Megaloblastic anemia; severe bacterial infections; mycobacterial infections; chronic idiopathic myelokathexis.
  B. Drug induced (very likely):
    Alcohol, purine and pyrimidine inhibitors, aminopyrine.

V. Pseudoneutropenia (shift from CGP to MGP).
  A. Endotoxin.
  B. Drug induced: (?) anesthetic agents, ether, pentobarbital.

*Adapted from Finch, S. C.: *In* Williams, W. J., Beutler, E., Erslev, A. J., and Rundles, R. W. (eds.): Hematology. New York, McGraw-Hill Book Co., Inc., 1972.

†Drugs cited for more than one mechanism.

necessary for granulocyte maturation appears to be lacking (Barak *et al.*, 1971).

Chronic familial neutropenia and cyclic neutropenia appear to be autosomal dominant conditions. The latter usually has a period of about 21 days, and appears to be due to periodic marrow failure. Other congenital and familial neutropenias have been described.

Isolated neutropenia or agranulocytosis is uncommon in adults. When the marrow is damaged, by a myelophthisic process such as metastatic carcinoma or Gaucher's disease replacing the marrow, or by drugs, usually the damage is not limited to granulopoiesis but affects normoblasts and megakaryocytes as well. Because of the short life span of granulocytes, however, neutropenia is the earliest recognizable effect in the blood. It takes weeks before damage to the erythropoietic tissue becomes manifest because of the long life span of erythrocytes. Platelets have a rather short life span but, on the other hand, megakaryocytes are more resistant to damage.

Drugs are an important cause of neutropenia, and, as outlined in Table 4–14, may act in different ways. Drugs that have the effect of destroying or interfering with mitosis of the proliferating cells are frequently used in the therapy of malignant disease. Important and limiting side effects of such chemotherapy are the results of marrow hypoplasia: severe neutropenia with its risk of infection, and severe thrombocytopenia with risk of bleeding; anemia is more readily controlled with transfusion. Of drugs used for therapy of other diseases, the phenothiazine group is responsible for most of the drug-related neutropenias at the present time.

Idiosyncratic drug effects refer to those in which host susceptibility factors predominate;

that is, there is little relationship with dose and duration of drug therapy.

Ineffective Granulocytopoiesis. Neutropenia due to increased ineffective granulocytopoiesis occurs in megaloblastic anemias as a result of drugs that have an antifolate effect. Of course, anemia is usually present if therapy is prolonged, and often thrombocytopenia as well. The marrow is usually hyperplastic. In addition to increased destruction of cells in the marrow there is some evidence that circulating neutrophils have a shortened survival. Indirect evidence for increased granulocyte turnover in this group of neutropenias with hypercellular marrow is an increased serum muramidase (lysozyme) (Catovsky *et al.*, 1971b).

Decreased Survival in Circulation. Transient neutropenia may occur early in some infections, followed by leukocytosis once the marrow production catches up with the demand. As previously noted, in severe, extensive bacterial infection, neutropenia with a shift to the left may be due to inability of marrow production to keep up with the peripheral utilization. Some bacterial infections, notably brucellosis and Salmonella infections, are prone to be associated with neutropenia; they may have some depressing effect on the marrow as well. Viral infections such as measles and rubella have neutropenia for several days after appearance of the rash; this is probably due in part to increased utilization. Lymphocytosis is present and persists after the neutropenia subsides.

The neutropenia of hypersplenism has been attributed to selective removal of neutrophils by the spleen. Described by Wiseman and Doan, it is associated with neutrophilic hyperplasia of the marrow and is corrected by splenectomy. Splenomegaly due to many causes may have shortened neutrophil survival and neutropenia; these include congestive splenomegaly, Felty's syndrome, Gaucher's disease, and lymphoma. In some cases, such as Felty's syndrome (neutropenia and splenomegaly in rheumatoid arthritis), there may be a leukocyte agglutinin involved.

Evidence has been accumulating that there are antibodies capable of clumping leukocytes of all varieties under proper experimental conditions (leukoagglutinins). The data thus far gathered permit a few general statements. The substance in the serum responsible for the agglutination of leukocytes has the characteristics of an antibody. It is present in the gamma globulin fraction. Both group-specific and nonspecific leukoagglutinins have been described. In most instances leukoagglutinins were found in persons with leukopenia, which suggests that they are an autoantibody. Leukopenia in the newborn may be produced by leukoagglutinins coming from the mother.

Drug-induced neutropenia due to immune mechanisms has been well described for aminopyrine since the first report in 1934 by Madison and Squier. In about 1 per cent of persons, seven to 10 days after first taking the drug, chills, headache, fever, and neutropenia with a shift to the left occur. Slight granulocytic hyperplasia is noted in the marrow. If the drug is continued, mucosal ulceration and sepsis may occur, and granulocytic precursors may disappear from the marrow. If, on the other hand, the drug is discontinued, the neutrophil count returns to normal levels in a week. An antibody develops in these patients which, in the presence of the drug, causes enhanced destruction of neutrophils. Of the possible mechanisms involved, a drug-plasma protein complex is probably the antigen; the antigen-antibody complex nonspecifically adsorbs on the cells and leads to their destruction (Finch, 1972).

Combinations. As indicated, some of the conditions discussed above are probably combinations of increased destruction and impaired effective production. As more detailed studies are done, some of the entries in this classification will be clarified and probably changed.

Pseudoneutropenia. Small doses of endotoxin will cause a shift of neutrophils into the MGP from the CGP, giving an apparent neutropenia, prior to causing a leukocytosis. In animals, anesthetic agents such as ether will cause the same kind of pseudoneutropenia (Boggs and Winklestein, 1971).

Laboratory Studies in Neutropenia. Absolute neutrophil counts should be calculated from the differential count and total WBC, and frequent counts should be charted to determine the possible periodicity and chronicity of the neutropenia. One should look carefully for immature neutrophils and normoblasts in blood films. Of course, one must determine whether anemia and thrombocytopenia are present. In patients with chronic disorders it may be fruitful to find out if other family members are leukopenic. Bone marrow examination of both smears and sections is done to check cellularity, E/G ratio, and numbers of neutrophils in different stages of maturation.

It has been proposed that the serum vitamin B_{12} binding capacity correlates well with the total blood granulocyte pool (MGP and CGP), and the serum muramidase (lysozyme) correlates with the granulocyte turnover; measurement of both and the ratio between them will help to determine the balance between these components of neutrophil behavior (Catovsky *et al.*, 1971). Monocytes contribute significantly to the serum muramidase, so monocytosis will negate its value in neutrophil studies. Spleen size determination is worthwhile, as it has been shown to correlate well with shortened survival of neutrophils (Bishop *et al.*, 1971). Though usually a research procedure only, granulocyte survival using $DF^{32}P$ (Diisopropyl fluorophosphate) is very useful in the kinetic classification of neutropenias (Finch, 1972).

Obviously the extent of the studies done will depend in part upon the severity of the neutropenia. Any drugs that the patient is using that might be responsible should be stopped.

Disorders of Neutrophil Function

In 1957 a condition was described in which increased susceptibility to infection was associated with normal-appearing neutrophils which lacked the ability to kill certain kinds of bacteria, a condition now known as chronic granulomatous disease of childhood. Since then, other disorders have been discovered which involve different stages of neutrophil function: random motility; chemotaxis (directed motility); opsonization; phagocytosis (including ingestion and degranulation); and bacterial killing (Nathan and Baehner, 1971; Douglas, 1971).

Defects in neutrophil motility, both random and directed (chemotaxis), have been described (Edelson *et al.*, 1973). Chemotaxis also may be abnormal because of defects outside the neutrophil, as in disorders of complement metabolism. Defects in opsonization are not primary in the neutrophil but may occur in some immunoglobulin or complement component deficiencies.

The most extensively studied disorder involving phagocytosis is *chronic granulomatous disease* (CGD) of childhood. Frequent suppurative infections occur with bacteria not ordinarily pathogenic; the pathologic response is granulomatous. Eczema, lymphadenopathy, and hepatosplenomegaly are common. Ingestion of organisms by the neutrophil and degranulation into the phagocytic vacuole appear normal, but bacteria are not killed. In normal neutrophils, two main bactericidal systems are present: (1) H_2O_2 (generated by the bacteria or by the neutrophil) plus peroxidase (from the azurophil granule) plus a halide ion generate a halogen that is toxic to the bacteria; and (2) lysosomal enzyme systems. In the CGD neutrophils and monocytes there is a failure to generate H_2O_2; the exact enzyme defect is not yet clear. The result is that catalase-positive bacteria are not killed, but catalase-negative bacteria which generate their own H_2O_2 are killed by this peroxidase system. CGD appears to be inherited as a sex-linked or autosomal recessive condition. It may be detected by the nitroblue tetrazolium (NBT) test during stimulation of phagocytic activity either morphologically (v.i.) or spectrophotometrically. Bactericidal assays are used with various organisms to characterize the disease.

Another neutrophil functional defect associated with certain infections is myeloperoxidase deficiency.

Though much new information has been developed in the past few years concerning the leukocyte functional disorders, in most instances the specific nature of the defects remains to be defined. In addition to the congenital disorders mentioned above, acquired defects at some stages in this complex defensive system are also being described, both in association with drug therapy and with other diseases (Douglas, 1971).

NITROBLUE TETRAZOLIUM TEST (NBT TEST)

Principle. When incubated with neutrophils, a colorless soluble dye, *nitroblue tetrazolium*, is reduced and produces a blue-black formazan precipitate. The proportion of neutrophils which reduce the dye can be quantitated by counting the cells on a slide, or by spectrophotometric means. Though the exact mechanism of this dye reduction is unclear, this process appears to be associated with stimulation of hexose monophosphate shunt activity and NADH-oxidase activity during phagocytosis.

Method (Park *et al.*, 1968; Matula and Paterson, 1971). Venous blood is anticoagulated with heparin (75–100 units/ml. of blood). Approximately 0.1 ml. of heparinized blood is placed in a siliconized concave microslide (Clay-Adams, New York); with this is mixed an equal volume of NBT solution (a 1:1 mixture of 0.2 per cent nitroblue tetrazolium in 0.85 per cent NaCl and 0.15 M phosphate buffered saline at $pH = 7.2$). The slide is placed in a Petri dish humidified by wet gauze, incubated at 37° C. for 15 minutes and then kept at room temperature for 15 minutes. After mixing again with a capillary pipette, coverslip smears are made carefully (trying to avoid damage to the leukocytes), air dried, and counterstained with Wright's stain.

Under oil immersion, 100 neutrophils are counted, scoring as *NBT positive* those with either a single large blue-black deposit or multiple smaller similar deposits (still larger than neutrophil granules). Monocytes or platelets that may contain formazan deposits are ignored. The result is recorded as percentage of NBT-positive neutrophils.

Interpretation. Normal individuals have less than 10 per cent NBT-positive neutrophils, as do patients with leukocytosis of nonbacterial origin (e.g., rheumatoid arthritis, lupus erythematosus), postsurgical states, and viral infections. In persons with localized bacterial infections the NBT test is also normal.

Elevated NBT-positive neutrophil percentages (11 per cent or greater) are characteristic of systemic bacterial infections and are also present in disseminated tuberculosis, systemic fungal infections, and malaria, and in newborn infants. This test, therefore, may be of value in helping to distinguish between systemic bacterial infection and nonbacterial infection or disease in febrile patients before definitive bacterial cultures are available.

The NBT test is also useful in detecting congenital defects of neutrophil function, such as chronic granulomatous disease (CGD). In this disorder the NBT-positive neutrophils are absent, or nearly so. More decisive is the stimulated NBT test (Windhorst *et al.*, 1967): in CGD there is a lack of increase in positive neutrophils (<10 per cent) when the cells are actively phagocytizing latex particles, whereas normal neutrophils show a dramatic increase (80 to 100 per cent positive neutrophils). The carrier females in the X-linked form of CGD show intermediate values.

Eosinophilia

Eosinophilia is an increase of eosinophilic granulocytes above the highest normal of 500 per μl. counted just like white blood cells with a special diluent.

The close association of eosinophilic leukocytes with allergy, broadly conceived, is impressive. One could easily correlate practically all eosinophilias with one form of allergy or another. An individual host factor has to be assumed to explain variations in eosinophil response. The eosinophils in the blood come from the marrow; those in the tissues come from the blood.

Allergic Diseases. Allergic diseases such as bronchial asthma, hay fever, angioneurotic edema, urticaria, and erythema multiforme are characterized by eosinophilia. Eosinophils are found in the peripheral blood, marrow, sputum (in bronchial asthma), nasal and conjunctival discharges (in hay fever), and urticarial skin lesions and vesicles. Blood eosinophilia is usually only mild or moderate.

The exact role of eosinophils in the allergic immunologic reaction has not been determined. Antigen-antibody complexes or histamine, which are involved in such reactions, may attract eosinophils chemotactically.

Skin Disorders. In some skin disorders the allergic background is apparent, for example, allergic eczema and dermatitis venenata; in others it may be surmised. There is frequently a clear-cut direct relation between the degree of eosinophilia and extent of cutaneous involvement.

Parasitic Infestations. Eosinophilia is more pronounced if tissues are invaded (for example, trichinosis) than when parasites are inhabiting the lumen of a viscus (for example, tapeworm). The role of free exchange of tissue fluids (metabolic continuity) is evident by disappearance of eosinophilia in some forms of infestation when encystment occurs (for example, cysticercosis).

In trichinosis eosinophils begin to rise in the blood within days after infection. The peak of the eosinophilia, from 40 to 60 per cent, is during the third or fourth weeks.

Leukocytosis and eosinophilia extending over months are seen in visceral larva migrans (dog and cat round worm) infestation. In this condition pulmonary lesions (Loeffler's syndrome) may be present. In Loeffler's eosinophilic pneumonitis, the fleeting pulmonary infiltrates are thought to be caused by passage of the parasites from the blood into the alveoli of the lung. (Regarding local tissue eosinophilia in Loeffler's syndrome, see below.)

Another parasitic infestation with eosinophilia is creeping eruption caused by larvae of the dog or cat hookworm.

Eosinophilia may be absent in severe infestations with trichinae. The prognosis in such cases seems aggravated.

Infectious Diseases. Eosinophilia of various degrees is seen in many infectious diseases. Some of them (for example, scarlet fever) have cutaneous rashes, probably of allergic nature; some (like brucellosis) have granulomatous lesions with obvious allergic overtones. It is possible that the blood and tissue eosinophilia of Hodgkin's disease is of a similar nature.

Neutrophilia depresses eosinophilia although it is not entirely clear how much of the latter effect is on the basis of enhanced corticosteroid secretion in disease. This is well shown in the disappearance of eosinophilia when a lesion that is responsible for eosinophilia (for example, echinococcus cyst) becomes infected, suppurates, and is followed by neutrophilia. The same phenomenon is also observed in acute infections (for example, pneumococcus pneumonia).

It is in infectious diseases that the depression of eosinophilia is particularly noticeable.

Chorea may show eosinophilia, although other forms of rheumatic fever do not.

Blood Diseases. In chronic granulocytic leukemia, general marrow hyperplasia may be responsible for the eosinophilia as well as for the basophilia. Eosinophilia may be seen in pernicious anemia to be replaced by eosinopenia in late stages. Marrow eosinophilia may be present in thrombocytopenic purpura. Eosinophilic leukemia is discussed with other leukemias.

Other Conditions. Splenectomy is frequently

followed by eosinophilia and lymphocytosis. Neutrophilia, if previously present, recedes. This may last for several months.

There is no satisfactory explanation for occasional instances of moderate and even severe eosinophilia, general or local, in patients with various neoplasms and a variety of other conditions (for example, ovarian cysts). Eosinophilia is seen more frequently in neoplasms involving serous surfaces and bone and in those with excessive necrosis.

Various drugs have been reported to be responsible for eosinophilia: pilocarpine, physostigmine, digitalis, phosphorus, benzene, parenterally administered liver extracts, and insulin. On the other hand, atropine is supposed to depress the eosinophils.

Local tissue eosinophilia with or without blood eosinophilia includes eosinophilic granuloma, polyps of the nose, intestinal eosinophilia, chronically inflamed pleura, and Loeffler's syndrome.

Familial eosinophilia is linked by some with a genetically determined allergic condition and by others with the effect of a common parasitic infection.

Eosinopenia

Eosinopenia is a decrease below the lowest normal of 50 per microliter. It is seen most frequently in the presence of infectious neutrophilia in severe infections. In Cushing's syndrome the count ranges from 0 to 30 per μl. It results from hyperactivity of the adrenal cortex. After major surgical operations there is a drop within 4 to 6 hours in the presence of adequate adrenal function. In postoperative shock not associated with massive hemorrhage, a normal or high eosinophil count indicates adrenal insufficiency.

Eosinopenia is seen after electric shock therapy, in eclampsia, and in labor.

The eosinopenia following parenteral administration of certain adrenocortical hormones and of substances (ACTH and epinephrine) that increase the output of these hormones is the basis for a test for adrenal function. Thorn *et al.* (1948) recommended a test for evaluation of adrenocortical function based on the development of eosinopenia following the injection of ACTH (adrenocorticotropic hormone). Absence of a significant drop of eosinophils is interpreted as evidence of adrenocortical insufficiency. At the present time, the value of the test is limited.

Technique of Absolute Eosinophil Count. Regular or special (Fuchs-Rosenthal) counting chamber and a special staining fluid are used. The technique of counting white blood cells described on page 124 applies to counting of eosinophils; see Dacie and Lewis (1968) for details.

Basophilia

Basophilia is an increase of basophilic granulocytes in the peripheral blood above 160 per microliter.

Basophilia is seen most frequently in allergic reactions, chronic granulocytic leukemia, myeloid metaplasia (extramedullary myelopoiesis), and polycythemia vera. Relative basophilia may be transient following irradiation. Basophilia may be present in chronic hemolytic anemia and following splenectomy. In some infections basophils disappear at the same time as eosinophils, and then both reappear when recovery sets in. Tissue basophils, mast cells, are different from basophilic granulocytes.

Basopenia

In view of the rarity of these cells in normal persons, a decrease cannot be readily detected. In acute infections, however, basophils disappear at first together with the eosinophils and reappear later with the lowering of the neutrophilia. ACTH or corticosteroids produce a decrease in basophils.

Lymphocytosis

Lymphocytosis is an increase in the number of lymphocytes in the peripheral blood above the normal range of 1500 to 4000 per microliter in the adult and 1500 to 8500 in the child.

Relative lymphocytosis is present in various conditions in which there is a neutropenia. True lymphocytosis is present in various infections but mainly late in the disease and during recovery. It is common in exanthems (for example, German measles) and also has been reported in brucellosis and secondary and congenital syphilis. It is considered a good omen in tuberculosis. In thyrotoxicosis, lymphocytosis is frequently present. In some of these patients there is also splenomegaly. In pertussis, lymphocytosis may be high early in the catarrhal stage and persist all through the entire course and late into convalescence.

INFECTIOUS LYMPHOCYTOSIS

This infectious and contagious disease of unknown etiology, described by C. H. Smith (1941), is characterized by lymphocytosis and occurs mainly in children. The incubation period is 12 to 21 days. The disease usually occurs without systemic manifestations, but sometimes with vomiting, fever, abdominal discomfort, signs suggesting involvement of the nervous system, cutaneous rashes, upper respiratory infections, and diarrhea. Usually the high white count (20,000 to 50,000, sometimes over 100,000 per μl.) precedes the clinical manifestations. From 60 to 95 per cent of the cells in the differential count are mature, adult, small lymphocytes, not like those seen in infectious mononucleosis. There is usually an eosinophilia. The lymphocytosis usually lasts three to five weeks, sometimes longer. There are no other blood changes. The marrow is not characteristic. Increase of lymphocytes has been observed but is probably due to admixture of peripheral blood. Lymph node enlargement is rare and minimal when present. The spleen and liver are rarely if ever enlarged. Lymph node biopsy may show reactive follicular hyperplasia but no characteristic changes.

The presumptive and differential tests for infectious mononucleosis are both negative. (For details regarding tests for infectious mononucleosis see p. 262.) In some cases there has been an increase of white cells in the cerebrospinal fluid, with about 40 per cent lymphocytes. The disease is distinctly infectious and contagious. The course is benign.

There is another form of infectious lymphocytosis, chronic in its course, with a leukocytosis of 10,000 to 25,000, with 60 to 80 per cent lymphocytes of normal appearance, and with a slight increase of eosinophils, monocytes, and plasma cells. As a rule, the children have enlarged tonsils, lymph nodes, and spleen and a history of recurrent upper respiratory infections. The marrow shows no abnormalities.

INFECTIOUS MONONUCLEOSIS

Infectious mononucleosis is an acute self-limited infectious disease of the reticuloendothelial tissues, especially of the lymphatic tissues, with characteristic clinical, hematologic, pathologic, and specific serologic changes.

The main reason for clinical interest in infectious mononucleosis is that it imitates many diseases, some of them serious, some inviting surgical intervention, and some with serious prognostic implications.

Clinical Features

Onset. The onset is vague, indefinite, and similar to the onset of other infectious diseases.

Duration. The disease proper lasts, as a rule, from 7 to 21 days.

Clinical Picture. Fever varies from mild to moderate, occasionally up to 106° F. Chills, sweats, headache, dizziness, malaise, pharyngitis, tonsillitis, retro-orbital aching, irritability, prostration, and asthenia may be seen, all of varying severity.

Lymph Nodes. Nodal enlargement is usually moderate in degree, but may vary from slight to marked. The enlargement may be simultaneous with the onset of fever or may follow or even precede it.

As a rule, cervical lymph nodes are the first to be enlarged, first on one side and then on the other, and then other regions are affected, including mediastinal and inguinal. The enlargement has usually regressed by three weeks.

Spleen. There is frequent splenomegaly of varying degrees. Occasionally the spleen may be enlarged without noticeable lymph node enlargement. It is frequently tender and the enlargement sometimes persists for a long time.

Liver. The liver is less frequently enlarged than the spleen and occasionally tender.

The various *complications*, the anatomic

Table 4–15. DISEASES SIMULATED BY INFECTIOUS MONONUCLEOSIS

DIAGNOSES MADE IN OUR SERIES (106 CASES) PRIOR TO BLOOD COUNT AND SEROLOGIC TESTS	NO. CASES	ADDITIONAL DIAGNOSES RECORDED IN THE LITERATURE
Agranulocytosis	1	Angioneurotic edema
Appendicitis	1	Asthma
Brucellosis	2	Bacterial endocarditis,
Diphtheria	4	subacute
Duodenal ulcer	1	Chickenpox
Gastroenteritis	1	Encephalitis
Hodgkin's disease	2	Erysipelas
Infectious hepatitis	3	Erythema multiforme
Influenza	7	Erythema nodosum
Leukemia	4	Glottis edema
Measles	1	Hyperthyroidism with
Meningitis	1	lymphocytosis
Nephritis	1	Infectious lympho-
		cytosis
Pharyngitis	7	Myocarditis (abnor-
Pharyngitis, ulcerative	2	mal ECG)
Pneumonia	1	Mumps
Pneumonia, virus	4	Obstructive jaundice
Purpura	2	Poliomyelitis
Scarlet fever	1	Rheumatic fever, acute
Serum disease	2	Scarlet fever
Sinusitis, frontal	1	Stomatitis, herpetic
Streptococcus sore throat	5	Syphilitic cervical
Tonsillitis, acute follicular	3	adenitis
Tonsillitis, acute		Syphilis, secondary
ulcerative	1	Thrombocytopenic
Tuberculous		purpura
lymphadenitis	1	Trichinosis
Vincent's angina	4	Tuberculosis, miliary
	63	

Table 4–16. CLINICAL FINDINGS IN 106 CASES OF INFECTIOUS MONONUCLEOSIS

	NO. CASES	PER CENT		NO. CASES	PER CENT
Lymphadenopathy	101	95.3	Epistaxis	3	2.8
Fever	93	87.7	Icterus	3	2.8
Pharyngitis	64	60.4	Loss of weight	2	1.9
without membrane	50	47.2	Diarrhea	2	1.9
with membrane	14	13.2	Arthritic pains	2	1.9
Splenomegaly	51	48.1	Purpura	2	1.9
Headache	26	24.5	Gingivitis	2	1.9
Hepatomegaly	24	22.6	Convulsions	1	0.9
Prostration	11	10.4	Toothache	1	0.9
Emesis	10	9.4			
Pain in abdomen	8	7.6	Albuminuria	14	13.2
upper abdomen	6	5.7	Positive test for syphilis	3	2.8
lower abdomen	2	1.9			
Stiffness or pain in neck	6	5.7	Relapses (17 days to 2 months)	7	6.5
Skin rash	5	4.7	Recurrence (1 year)	1	0.9

lesions underlying them, and the resemblance to various diseases are shown in Tables 4–15, 4–16, and 4–17.

Relapses. Relapses are not uncommon. Occasionally there may be several, and some may be more severe than the original attack.

Recurrences. Recurrences are rare, but they do occur sometimes after intervals of months or even years.

Age. The disease has been observed in patients from three months to 70 years of age, but the disease occurs rarely above college age. Most epidemics have been in adolescents and children.

Table 4–17. SOME DIFFERENTIAL DIAGNOSTIC PROBLEMS IN INFECTIOUS MONONUCLEOSIS

SIGNS AND SYMPTOMS	ANATOMIC LESIONS	RESEMBLANCE TO
Sore throat	Ulcerative or membranous pharyngitis	Diphtheria
Painful and stiff neck; occasionally convulsions and coma	Rapidly enlarged retrocervical lymph nodes. Acute hyperplastic lymphadenitis. Pleocytosis in cerebrospinal fluid may be present	Meningitis (serous meningitis may be present)
Generalized lymphadenopathy	Acute hyperplastic lymphadenitis	Leukemia
Abdominal pain and tenderness	Rapidly enlarged abdominal lymph nodes	
right lower quadrant		Acute appendicitis
left upper quadrant	Acute splenomegaly. Acute diffuse hyperplasia	Acute pleuritis; perinephritic abscess
acute tenderness and pain in right upper quadrant	Acute diffuse hepatitis; periportal infiltrations; enlarged lymph nodes around common bile duct	Acute hepatitis, especially if jaundice present
acute general abdominal pain, followed by shock	Ruptured spleen	Acute abdominal emergency
Cough (resembling whooping cough)	Enlarged mediastinal lymph nodes	Pertussis; Hodgkin's disease; tuberculosis
Cutaneous rashes		Exanthematous disease (measles); scarlet fever especially if angina is present; secondary syphilis, especially if enlarged inguinal lymph nodes and positive test for syphilis are present
Puffiness around eyes	Swelling of retrobulbar tissues	Trichinosis
Toothache	Acutely swollen submandibular lymph nodes	Pulpitis
Hematuria	Specific infiltration of renal parenchyma or purpuric renal hemorrhage	Acute glomerulonephritis

Differential Diagnosis. The diagnostic difficulties in infectious mononucleosis are illustrated in Tables 4–15 and 4–17.

The clinical picture of *acquired toxoplasmosis* may resemble infectious mononucleosis, especially in a form of the disease characterized by enlarged lymph nodes (Siim, 1960). The similarity may be even more pronounced since, in some of the cases reported, lymphocytes resembling those seen in infectious mononucleosis have been found.

A syndrome very similar to infectious mononucleosis consisting of fever, splenomegaly, abnormal liver function tests, and atypical lymphocytes may occur in adults with *cytomegalovirus (CMV) infections.* This was first recognized a few days to weeks after open heart surgery (Lang and Hanshaw, 1969). The heterophile antibody test is negative. Antibodies to CMV are detected in the serum and CMV may sometimes be found in the circulating white cells or in the urine.

Complications

Respiratory System. Extreme dyspnea may occur in the presence of severe inflammatory and ulcerative lesions of the pharynx and in laryngeal edema. Tracheostomy may have to be resorted to as a lifesaving operation. Fatal cases have been reported.

Hemolytic Anemia. Of the rare anemias associated with infectious mononucleosis, hemolytic anemia is the most common, occurring in 1 to 3 per cent of cases. The cause now appears to be related to the anti-i antibody produced frequently in this disease (Carter and Penman, 1969a).

Purpura. Mild thrombocytopenia occurs in about half the cases, but the platelet count is not often less than 100,000 per μl. Thrombocytopenic purpura with hemorrhagic complications is exceedingly rare (Carter and Penman, 1969b).

Spleen. Rupture of the spleen may occur in the acute stage of the disease. Prompt recognition and immediate surgical intervention may be lifesaving.

Liver. Involvement of the liver demonstrable by biopsy is common in infectious mononucleosis. Abnormal liver function tests indicative of hepatitis occur in 85 to 100 per cent of patients. Mild hyperbilirubinemia (up to 3 mg./dl.) has been noted in 30 to 50 per cent of patients (Carter and Penman, 1969c). Clinical jaundice is rare, but cases have been reported in which jaundice and acute pharyngitis were the only clinical manifestations of infectious mononucleosis, with positive hematologic and serologic findings.

The jaundice is, as a rule, hepatocellular, with both conjugated and nonconjugated bilirubin fractions in the serum and bilirubin and elevated urobilinogen in the urine.

Infections. Those due to pyogenic bacteria (sinusitis, otitis, bronchopneumonia) can be readily controlled, but staphylococcus infection may be serious or even fatal. Virus infection may be difficult to control. A fatality due to measles complicating infectious mononucleosis has been reported.

Other Complications. These include nasopharyngeal hemorrhage, hematuria, myositis or myalgia, hemoptysis, and uterine bleeding.

For additional information two monographs on infectious mononucleosis are recommended. One is the fruit of lifelong study of the disease in all its aspects (Hoagland, 1967). The other is a thorough review of the disease by several authors (Carter and Penman, 1969).

Blood Findings. There are no changes in the red blood cells and in platelets except in rare cases of complicating hemolytic anemia and the rather common mild thrombocytopenia. There is an increase of white blood cells ranging from 12,000 to 25,000 and sometimes higher. The highest counts in adults that have been observed were 40,000, but counts as high as 80,000 have been seen in children. The leukocytosis is usually brief. The total white count, as a rule, returns to normal within three weeks.

The increase is due to a rise in lymphocytes. These cells show characteristic changes, which can be summed up as follows:

1. Hyperplasia or an increase in their number.

2. Hypertrophy or an increase in size of the individual cells.

3. Nuclear changes are characterized by an increased density of the chromatin and by changes in shape. They show deep indentations and many are lobated, resembling in general outlines nuclei of monocytes ("leukocytoid lymphocytes," Downey type I) (Fig. 4–86). The cytoplasm shows basophilia, an increase of azurophilic granules, and frequently marked vacuolar degeneration. Some cells resemble plasma cells; some have nucleoli. Some cells resemble monocytes (monocytoid deviation). Cells which have a relatively smooth but still mature nucleus and abundant smooth cytoplasm with patchy peripheral and radial basophilia have been called "stress" lymphocytes or Downey type II (Figs. 4–82 to 4–85). They are often the most numerous. Occasionally lymphocytes have transformed or dedifferentiated into blasts in response to the viral stimulation. In general, the small percentage of immature lymphocytes present in infectious mononucleosis are the large reticular lymphocytes (nonleukemic lymphoblasts) with a coarsely reticular nucleus and abundant deeply basophilic cytoplasm (Downey type III) (Figs. 4–84 and 4–88). In contrast, the lymphoblasts of acute lymphocytic leukemia are usually smaller, with a very fine chromatin

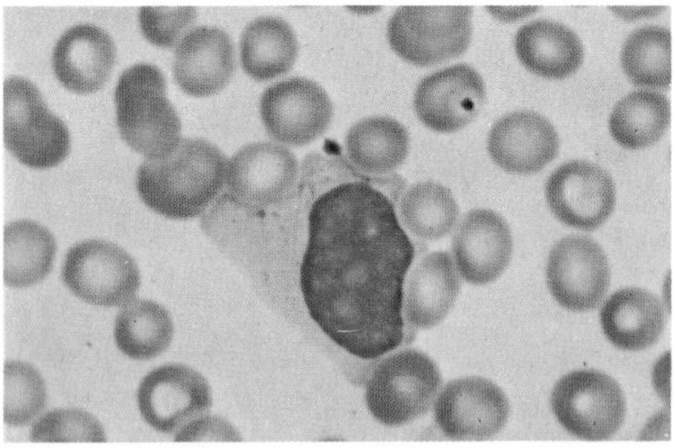

Figure 4–82.

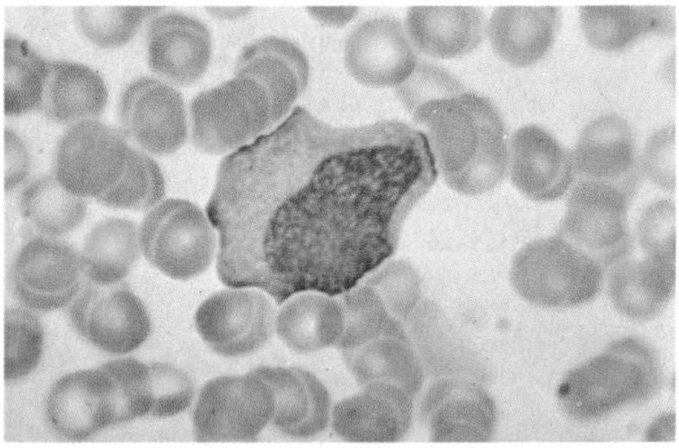

Figure 4–83.

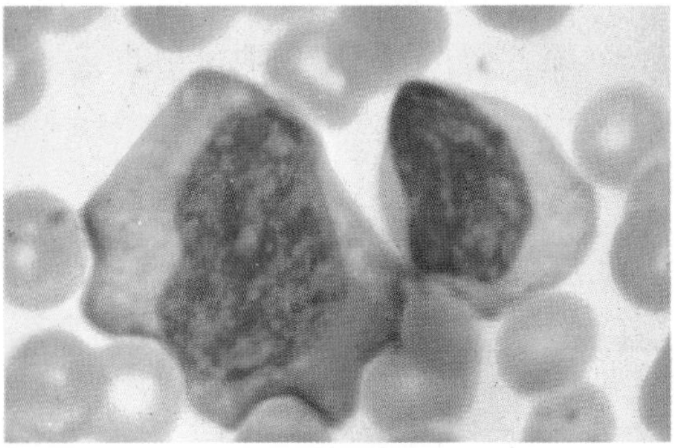

Figure 4–84.

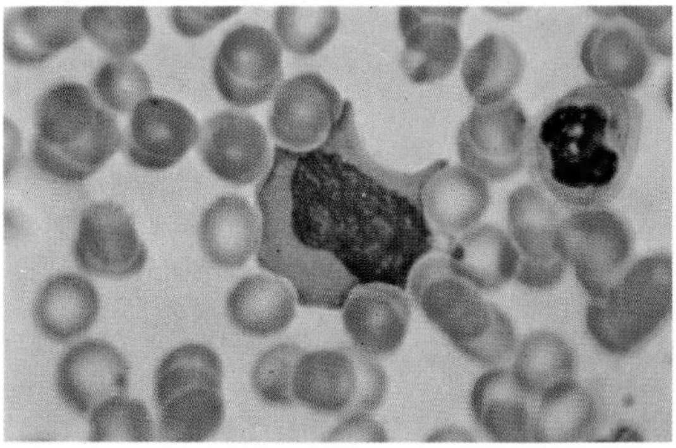

Figure 4–85.

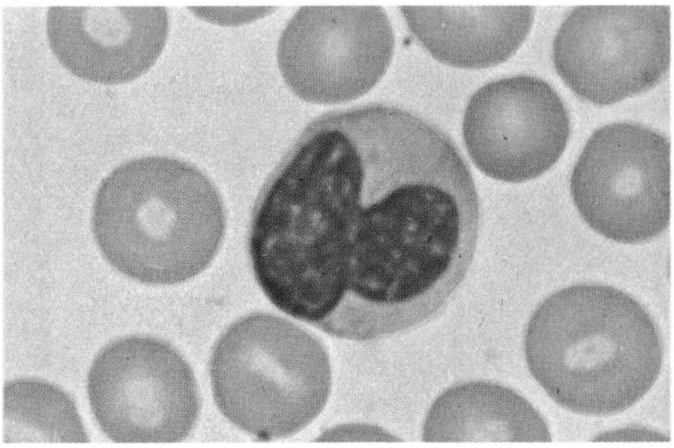

Figure 4–86.

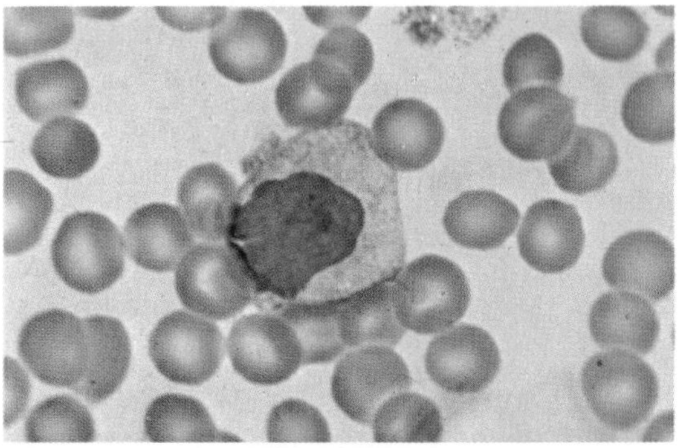

Figure 4–87.

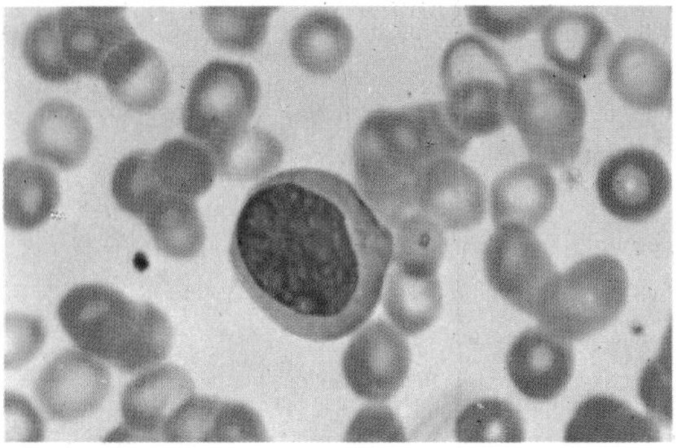

Figure 4–88.

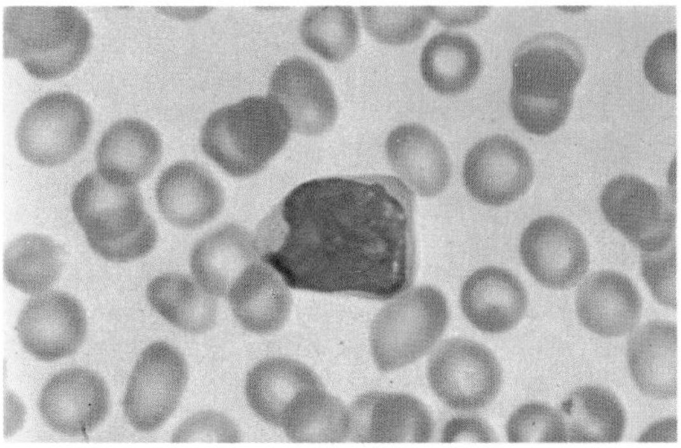

Figure 4–89.

(See opposite page for legends.)

pattern and very little cytoplasm (Figs. 4–81 and 4–89) (Downey and McKinlay, 1923).

The polymorphism of the lymphocytes is the striking feature of the differential blood picture. Collectively, the altered lymphocytes are often called atypical lymphocytes.

Not infrequently there are rapid and, as a rule, transient rises in the number of monocytes. The term mononucleosis refers to an increase of lymphocytes and not of monocytes. From 60 to 90 per cent of the cells in the differential white count are lymphocytes. Usually the lymphocytosis remains for two to three weeks but occasionally may persist longer.

The neutrophils are relatively and absolutely decreased in most cases. Early in the disease there may be a transient shift to the left, with an increase of band cells and metamyelocytes. Toxic granules and Döhle bodies may be seen. The eosinophils are within normal limits.

The cytologic changes are by no means pathognomonic of infectious mononucleosis. Similar cells in similar numbers may be found in other diseases, especially in upper respiratory infections in children, in liver diseases, and especially in viral infections, e.g., infectious hepatitis, viral pneumonia, varicella, mumps, and exanthemas of children.

Cerebrospinal Fluid. Pressure is slightly increased. There is frequently pleocytosis – as a rule, only moderate – but cell counts as high as 1000 per μl. have been seen. All, or almost all, the cells in the cerebrospinal fluid are mononuclear. The globulin is increased.

Other Laboratory Findings

Serologic Tests for Syphilis. Occasional positive results have been observed, usually only transient and becoming negative after a few days or weeks. Transient false positive Kahn tests in the blood serum and in the cerebrospinal fluid have been reported.

Urine. Traces of protein may be found in the urine.

Pathology. In addition to the previously mentioned gross changes in lymph nodes, spleen, and liver, studies have shown extensive microscopic changes, not only in lymph nodes but also in the spleen, liver, and other tissues. In the lymph nodes germinal centers are prominent and, in addition, there is crowding of the interfollicular cortex by lymphocytes, blast cells, and histiocytes. The blasts are pyroninophilic and, on lymph node imprint and in section, resemble the reticular lymphocytes (nonleukemic lymphoblasts) seen in small numbers in the blood. Atypical blast forms are seen, and multinucleated cells acceptable as Reed-Sternberg cells may be found occasionally (Lukes *et al.*, 1969).

In the spleen, which is large and extremely soft, similar changes are present. The follicles are small and compressed by the proliferating cells. The capsule and trabeculae are thinned out and eaten away by the proliferation. This explains the ease with which the spleen ruptures on slight trauma or increase of intra-abdominal pressure. In many places there are subintimal infiltrations in the trabecular veins,

---

Figure 4–82. Infectious mononucleosis. All the photographs of the lymphocytes of infectious mononucleosis are from patients with characteristic clinical findings and with positive differential tests. The lymphocyte is larger than any normal so-called large lymphocyte. The cytoplasm is abundant, clear, and moderately basophilic, especially close to the edges of the cell; red azure granules are accumulated along the upper periphery. The cytoplasm is delicate, the surrounding red cells leave an indentation in the cytoplasm, giving it a scalloped appearance. The plasticity of cytoplasm is not limited to infectious mononucleosis, but is characteristically frequent. The nucleus is oval, the chromatin is delicate and less dense than in normal large lymphocytes. Three nucleoli are seen clearly. The two red cells adjacent on the right made indentations, even in the nucleus, suggesting that it is plastic. There is a light perinuclear zone. The characteristic I.M. lymphocytes are called atypical lymphocytes or virocytes.

Figure 4–83. Infectious mononucleosis lymphocyte. The cytoplasm is deeply basophilic.

Figure 4–84. Infectious mononucleosis. High magnification emphasizes the delicate chromatin structure and variation in size.

Figure 4–85. Infectious mononucleosis. Contrast between the infectious mononucleosis lymphocyte, with its indented nucleus, and the normal small lymphocyte.

Figure 4–86. Infectious mononucleosis. Here the contrast between the infectious mononucleosis cells and segmented granulocyte is emphasized.

Figure 4–87. Normal monocyte.

Figure 4–88. Infectious mononucleosis; reticular lymphocyte (nonleukemic lymphoblast). The cytoplasm is homogeneous and deeply basophilic. The nuclear chromatin is uniform and granular (or reticular). Nucleoli are conspicuous. Note the difference between this cell and the blast cell of acute leukemia (Fig. 4–89).

Figure 4–89. Blast cell of acute leukemia.

and one can see masses of cells pouring out from the infiltration into the lumen of the blood vessels.

In the liver, infiltration is present in the periportal spaces, consisting of large cells resembling those seen in the spleen, lymph nodes, and the peripheral blood. Sometimes there is also infiltration within the sinusoids.

In cases with pulmonary lesions that are seen sometimes, there are massive peribronchial infiltrations, which explain some of the changes seen in the x-ray. Infiltrations have also been seen in the kidneys, in various parts of the central nervous system, and in peripheral nerves.

Serologic Tests. There are several tests for infectious mononucleosis.

Presumptive Test. This test is based on an increase of antisheep and antihorse agglutinins. Such agglutinins are present, in low titers, in the blood of most people. Their normal titer is, as a rule, less than 112. The titer is elevated in serum disease, sometimes to high levels, and in a variety of infections, especially those of the upper respiratory system. Another cause of the elevated titer of antisheep agglutinins is transfusion of blood to which blood group-specific substances have been added to neutralize the isoagglutinins. The test is nonspecific. If positive in a titer of 224 or more, it may be considered as confirming the diagnosis of infectious mononucleosis if the clinical and hematologic findings are characteristic for the disease (Paul and Bunnell, 1932). Details regarding the presumptive test are summarized in Tables 4–18 and 4–19.

Differential Test. The principle of the differ-

Table 4–18. THE PRESUMPTIVE TEST FOR INFECTIOUS MONONUCLEOSIS

Principle: The test is based on the agglutination of sheep red cells by the serum of patients with infectious mononucleosis.

Technique:

The physician: Obtain 5 to 10 ml. of blood under aseptic precautions. Send to the laboratory.

The laboratory:

Reagents:

Serum inactivated for 30 minutes at 56° C. 2 per cent suspension of sheep red cells.

Procedure:

Set up 13 tubes in a rack. Place 0.4 ml. of 0.85 per cent saline in the first tube and 0.25 ml. in each of the remaining tubes.

Add 0.1 ml. of the inactivated serum to the first tube, mix and transfer 0.25 ml. to the second tube, and so on until the twelfth tube is reached. Discard 0.25 ml. from the twelfth tube (Table 4–19). The serum dilutions are 1:5, 1:10, and so on.

Add 0.1 ml. of the 2 per cent suspension of sheep cells to each tube, including the thirteenth, which is the control. The final dilutions are 1:7, 1:14, and so on. Shake each tube.

Reading of results:

Let stand at room temperature. When speed is indicated, reading may be done after 15 minutes. If the result is positive (agglutination in dilutions 1:224 or higher), the test may be considered completed except that the final titer will be higher after a 2-hour incubation. If negative (titer less than 224), repeat reading at intervals as frequent as convenient. Final negative result (titer less than 56) should *not* be recorded until after a 2-hour incubation. If speed is not a factor, the results may be read only once, at the end of 2 hours.

Results are read after shaking the test tubes to resuspend the sediment. Check with the naked eye. If no clumping is visible, place the tube horizontally on the stage of the microscope and read with a low-power objective (scanning lens, e.g., 25 mm. or 35 mm.), permitting viewing of a test tube.

The titer is the reciprocal value of the highest serum dilution still showing agglutination.

Table 4–19. TECHNIQUE OF PRESUMPTIVE TEST FOR INFECTIOUS MONONUCLEOSIS

TUBES	SALINE ml.	SERUM ml.	SERUM DILUTIONS	2 PER CENT SHEEP CELLS ml.	FINAL DILUTIONS OF SERUM
1	.4	.1	1:5	.1	1:7
2	0.25	0.25 of 1:5	1:10	.1	1:14
3	0.25	0.25 of 1:10	1:20	.1	1:28
4	0.25	0.25 of 1:20	1:40	.1	1:56
5	0.25	0.25 of 1:40	1:80	.1	1:112
6	0.25	0.25 of 1:80	1:160	.1	1:224
7	0.25	0.25 of 1:160	1:320	.1	1:448
8	0.25	0.25 of 1:320	1:640	.1	1:896
9	0.25	0.25 of 1:640	1:1280	.1	1:1792
10	0.25	0.25 of 1:1280	1:2560	.1	1:3584
11	0.25	0.25 of 1:2560	1:5120	.1	1:7168
12	0.25	0.25 of 1:5120	1:10,240*	.1	1:14,336
Control 13	0.25	—	—	.1	

* Discard 0.25 ml. from last tube.

ential test is that absorption of serum with a suspension of a Forssman antigen (guinea pig or horse kidney) removes antisheep agglutinins in the serum of patients with serum disease and various other infections but not in the serum of patients with infectious mononucleosis. Here a substantial part of the antibodies remains after absorption. On the other hand, absorption with a suspension of beef cells removes the antisheep agglutinins in infectious mononucleosis but leaves them in some of the other bloods. It is this combination of no, or incomplete, removal of antibodies with Forssman antigen and complete removal with beef cells that is characteristic for infectious mononucleosis (Tables 4–20, 4–21, and 4–22).

SPECIFICITY OF THE DIFFERENTIAL TEST. In only two cases in our experience with the test, extending over 33 years, has it been positive in patients without a history or evidence of the disease. One patient had rheumatoid arthritis; the other was a young man with Hodgkin's disease. There were no clinical or blood changes suggestive of infectious mononucleosis. The diagnosis of Hodgkin's disease was made on a lymph node and confirmed by autopsy. Other cases of Hodgkin's disease and of serologically established infectious mononucleosis present simultaneously have been reported previously.

With these two exceptions, among the many hundreds of cases studied, the differential test was positive only in infectious mononucleosis and was negative in all other diseases. The differential test is a specific and qualitative test. The height of the titer is not important.

As a rule, the test is positive when the patient presents symptoms of the disease or when he is first examined. The test may be negative early in the disease and may remain negative as long as three weeks. Therefore, if the first test is negative and if clinical and hematologic findings still suggest the disease until at least the third week from onset, it is necessary to repeat the test. The test remains positive for weeks and sometimes months after the clinical symptoms have disappeared.

Table 4–20. THE DIFFERENTIAL TEST

PRINCIPLE

Antisheep agglutinins in *infectious mononucleosis* are *not* absorbed by Forssman antigen (guinea pig or horse kidney); they are *not* of the Forssman type.

Antisheep agglutinins in *serum disease* and in *normal persons* are readily absorbed by Forssman antigen; they are of the Forssman type.

Antisheep agglutinins in *infectious mononucleosis* are readily absorbed by beef cells.

Antisheep agglutinins in *conditions other than infectious mononucleosis* may or may not be absorbed by beef cells.

MATERIALS	PREPARATION OF ANTIGENS
1. Test tubes (a) for absorption: 85 × 13 mm. (inside diameter) rounded bottom and no lips. (b) for agglutination: 75 × 10 mm. (inside diameter) 2. Blood serum (0.5 ml. will suffice) inactivated for 30 minutes at 56° C. 3. Two per cent suspensions of sheep erythrocytes 4. Capillary pipettes 5. Physiologic salt solution	1. Guinea pig kidney Organs are stored frozen until needed and then thawed and washed with physiologic saline until washings are free of blood. They are now mashed into fine pulp and made into a 20 per cent suspension in physiologic saline. The suspension is boiled 1 hour on water bath, and loss by evaporation is made up with distilled water. 2. Horse kidney A 2 per cent suspension in physiologic saline is prepared. Otherwise the procedure is the same as for guinea pig kidney. 3. Beef red cells They are washed three times with physiologic saline and packed by centrifuging. One volume of packed cells is suspended in four volumes of saline, and the suspension is boiled on water bath for 1 hour. Loss by evaporation is made up with distilled water. To all antigens, phenol is added to make a 0.5 per cent solution. Can be kept in icebox for many months.

Table 4–21. DIFFERENTIAL TEST

PROCEDURE
1. Place in test tube (85 × 13 mm.) 1 ml. of thoroughly shaken Forssman antigen suspension.
2. Add 0.2 ml. of serum.
3. Shake and let stand at room temperature for 3 minutes.
4. Centrifuge at 1500 r.p.m. for 10 minutes or longer till supernatant is perfectly clear.
5. Remove the supernatant fluid with a capillary pipette, making sure not to take particles along.
6. Set up as many tubes (75 × 10 mm.) as needed, according to the titer of the presumptive test. Add 0.25 ml. of physiologic saline to each tube except the first.
7. Add 0.25 ml. of the absorbed serum to the first and second tubes.
8. Mix the second tube and transfer 0.25 ml. to the third tube, and so on. Discard 0.25 ml. from the last tube. The serum dilutions are 1:5, 1:10, 1:20, and so on.
9. Add 0.1 ml. of the 2 per cent suspension of sheep cells. Shake well. Final dilutions of serum are 1:7, 1:14, and so on.
10. Absorption with boiled beef cells. Follow the same procedure as above, using 1.0 ml. of the thoroughly mixed 20 per cent suspension of beef cells.
11. Let stand at room temperature. When speed is indicated reading may be done after 15 minutes. If test is positive, which means: (a) in test tubes containing serum treated with Forssman antigen, agglutination in the same dilution as the presumptive test or in not more than three dilutions or tubes below that of the titer of the presumptive test, and (b) no agglutination in test tubes containing serum treated with beef cell antigen, then the test can be reported as positive for infectious mononucleosis. If the result is negative, which means: more than three tubes' difference in the agglutination as compared with the titer of the presumptive test (or agglutination remaining after absorption with beef cell antigen), repeat readings at intervals as frequent as convenient. Final negative results should *not* be recorded until after two hours incubation. If speed is not a factor, results may be read only once, at the end of 2 hours.

In some of the other reported cases of alleged infectious mononucleosis, the presumptive test alone was used and not the complete differential test; in others the recommended technique was not followed, e.g., centrifugation was used to accelerate the incubation period, or the tests were kept in the refrigerator overnight. The latter modification brings into play cold agglutinins, which may increase the titer considerably, but not specifically, with resulting false positive readings.

Details regarding the differential test are summarized in Tables 4–20, 4–21, and 4–22.

Rapid Tests. Attempts to simplify tests for infectious mononucleosis began soon after Paul and Bunnell's original publication and have continued since. They have included the use of the microscope, slide, centrifugation, capillary tubes, of horse instead of sheep red cells, formalin-treated and enzyme-treated red cells, and a host of other modifications.

The spot test of Lee *et al.* (1967; 1968) is based on the following principles: (1) Horse erythrocytes are more sensitive than sheep erythrocytes in the test for infectious mononucleosis, and thus are especially valuable for low-titer sera found often early in the disease; (2) unwashed preserved horse erythrocytes remain usable for at least three months and give stronger and quicker agglutination with infectious mononucleosis sera than do formalinized horse erythrocytes; (3) some noninfectious mononucleosis sera also have high horse agglutinin titers, and, therefore, serologic diagnosis cannot depend on titers alone; and (4) fine suspensions of guinea pig kidney and of beef erythrocyte stromata result in satisfactory instant absorption of antibodies and a clear-cut differentiation between in-

TUBE	1	2	3	4	5	6	7	8	9*	10*	11*	12*
Saline (ml.)	1.9	1.0	1.0	1.0	1.0	1.0	1.0	1.0	1.0	1.45	0.95	
Positive control serum (ml.)											0.05	
Test serum (ml.)	0.1									0.05		
Beef cells, 1.1% (ml.)	0.5	0.5	0.5	0.5	0.5	0.5	0.5	0.5	0.5	0.5	0.5	0.25
Mix. Let stand 10 minutes at room temperature.												
Complement, 1:40 (ml.)	0.5	0.5	0.5	0.5	0.5	0.5	0.5	0.5	0.5		0.5	
Water (ml.)												1.75
Reciprocal of dilution	40	80	160	320	640	1280	2560					

*Controls	complement	serum	positive	50 per cent hemolysis standard
tube No.	9	10	11	12

Table 4–22. THE DIFFERENTIAL TEST: INTERPRETATION OF RESULTS

In serum of patients with infectious mononucleosis, absorption with Forssman antigen will result in a partial removal of the agglutinin for sheep red cells, but, as a rule, not less than one-fourth of the original titer will still be present in the serum after absorption. For example, an original titer of 112 may be reduced to 28 after absorption with Forssman antigen.

If all or almost all (more than 90 per cent) of the sheep agglutinins have been removed by absorption with Forssman antigen, this speaks against infectious mononucleosis.

On the other hand, so far no other condition has been found, except infectious mononucleosis, in which Forssman antigen fails to remove sheep agglutinins from the serum.

The absorption with beef red cells is a confirmatory procedure in infectious mononucleosis, since absorption with beef cells removes all or almost all (more than 90 per cent) of the sheep agglutinins from the serum. Failure of beef cells to remove sheep agglutinins speaks against infectious mononucleosis.

It may be preferable to do the absorption with Forssman antigen and with beef cell antigen in *every* case. The absorption with beef cells is essential in patients with elevated titers of antisheep agglutinins if no clinical or hematologic findings are present suggestive of infectious mononucleosis. In most of these instances the antisheep agglutinins will be completely removed by Forssman antigen, but, in rare instances, the absorption may be incomplete. The use of the beef cell antigen will then be decisive.

EXAMPLES

	TITER OF			
	PRESUMPTIVE TEST	DIFFERENTIAL TEST AFTER ABSORPTION WITH FORSSMAN ANTIGEN	DIFFERENTIAL TEST AFTER ABSORPTION WITH BEEF RED CELLS	RESULT
(a)	224	112	0	*Positive* for infectious mononucleosis
	224	0	112	*Negative* for infectious mononucleosis
	224	56	0	*Positive* for infectious mononucleosis
	224	56	56	*Negative* for infectious mononucleosis
	224	28	0	*Positive* for infectious mononucleosis
	224	14	0	*Negative* for infectious mononucleosis
	224	7	0	*Negative* for infectious mononucleosis
(b)	56	56	0	*Positive* for infectious mononucleosis
	56	56	28	*Negative* for infectious mononucleosis
	56	28	0	*Positive* for infectious mononucleosis
	56	14	0	*Positive* for infectious mononucleosis
	56	7	0	*Positive* for infectious mononucleosis
(c)	28	28	0	*Positive* for infectious mononucleosis
	28	14	0	*Positive* for infectious mononucleosis
	28	7	0	*Positive* for infectious mononucleosis

fectious mononucleosis and noninfectious mononucleosis sera (See Figure 4–102.)

The test is done on a slide. Serum is mixed thoroughly with guinea pig kidney on one spot of the slide and with beef erythrocyte stromata on another, and unwashed preserved horse erythrocytes are added immediately to each spot.*

In a series of 200 infectious mononucleosis sera, all showed agglutination within 2 minutes when absorbed with guinea pig kidney suspension, 76 per cent of them within 5 seconds, and 98 per cent within 1 minute. When absorbed with beef erythrocyte stromata, only 30 per cent of the sera showed agglutination, which appeared later and/or was weaker than in the corresponding sera absorbed with guinea pig kidney suspension (Fig. 4–102).

Ninety per cent of 300 noninfectious mononucleosis sera showed no agglutination on both spots within 2 minutes. Of the remaining sera, 7 per cent showed earlier and/or stronger agglutination after absorption with beef erythrocyte stromata than with guinea pig kidney suspension and 3 per cent showed agglutination only after absorption with beef erythrocyte stromata (Fig. 4–102).

Forty-five sera with sheep agglutinin titers of 56 or lower were examined with the spot test. The results were in complete agreement with the original diagnosis established by clinical, hematologic, and serologic findings, the latter with the differential test.

In our laboratory, the spot test has proved to be simple, rapid, highly specific, and sensitive.

*The reagents are available from Ortho Diagnostics, Raritan, New Jersey.

Laboratory Diagnosis of Infectious Mononucleosis*

Doubtful or Ambiguous Results. Although some of the widely used immunologic tests are known to be highly specific for infectious mononucleosis, none is 100 per cent reliable. False positive and false negative results have been reported in every known and well-studied test. Adequate and proper controls are always imperative as the only dependable method of detecting sources of technical errors and suggesting ways to prevent them. When the results are not clear cut, in spite of controls, it is important to repeat the tests and to conduct additional dependable serologic tests. Fortunately, several such tests are available. Repeat tests at a later date may be helpful.

Which Serologic Test? Our experience has been as follows:

The sheep agglutinin differential test is by far the most thoroughly investigated and the best reference test available at the present time. In cases with sheep agglutinin titers of 28 or below in the presumptive test, horse cells are recommended.

Of the rapid tests, the spot test is, in our experience, more dependable both as to sensitivity and specificity than other simplified tests.

Hematologic Findings. White blood cell and differential counts are essential and simple laboratory tests in the laboratory diagnosis of infectious mononucleosis. Lymphocytosis and the presence of adequate numbers of the characteristic lymphocytes, known as atypical lymphocytes, virocytes, or infectious mononucleosis lymphocytes, are just as important for the diagnosis as is the serologic test. Actually the absence of atypical lymphocytes during the active stage of disease speaks against the diagnosis of infectious mononucleosis. The hematologic findings alone are by no means diagnostic, but together with a positive serologic test they provide the most reliable laboratory aid for the diagnosis of the disease.

Etiology. It is claimed that strong serologic and epidemiologic evidence now exists to implicate the Epstein-Barr virus (EBV) as the cause of infectious mononucleosis (IM) (Stites and Leikola, 1971). The EBV was originally found in cell cultures of Burkitt's lymphoma. High titers of antibody to EBV are found in the serum of patients with Burkitt's lymphoma and carcinoma of the postnasal space. The relationship of EBV to IM is as follows: Antibody to EBV is consistently present in heterophile positive IM. In a study of 268 college students, who originally had no serum EBV antibody, 15 per cent developed typical IM during college and all 15 per cent also developed antibody to EBV in their sera. Of 94 students who originally had a low titer of antibody to EBV, none developed IM. About 10 per cent of adults and even more pediatric patients with IM have no heterophile antibody, but most have antibody to EBV (Henle and Henle, 1973). EBV has now been isolated from the throats of patients with IM (Miller *et al.*, 1973).

Epidemiology. The peaks of morbidity in a military academy occurred in February and August, exactly on the forty-fifth day following vacations. According to Hoagland (1967) the disease may be transmitted by kissing, for which the vacation period offers greater opportunities. The incubation in 71 to 73 patients was 42 to 49 days following intimate oral contact in one series. In 68 per cent of another series the incubation was 31 to 60 days. Other epidemiologic observations indicate that kissing is by no means the only means of transmission.

Epidemiologic evidence has suggested that there are carriers of the disease who are free of clinical manifestations. Recently it has been shown that EBV is present in the oropharynx up to 16 months after onset of infectious mononucleosis, long after the disappearance of clinical symptoms (Miller *et al.*, 1973).

Lymphocytopenia

Lymphocytopenia is an absolute lymphocyte count below 1500 per μl. in adults and below 3000 per μl. in children. A number of immunologic deficiency disorders which are genetically determined have lymphocytopenia along with various other immunologic defects of either humoral or cell-mediated immunity (Hoyer *et al.*, 1968). Increased levels of adrenocortical hormones, the administration of chemotherapeutic drugs, or irradiation will result in lymphocytopenia. Impaired drainage of the intestinal lymphatics with loss of lymphocytes into the intestines due to a number of causes has been implicated as a mechanism for lymphocytopenia. Though decreased cell-mediated immunity may be evident early in the course of Hodgkin's disease, lymphocytopenia occurs late, in advanced disease (Cassileth, 1972; Zacharski and Linman, 1971).

Monocytosis

Monocytosis is an increase of monocytes above the upper limit of normal; this is usually given as 500 or 800 per μl. Some normal per-

*See Lee and Davidsohn, 1967.

sons may have as many as 1000 per μl. (Table 4–2), so it is probably safest to regard counts exceeding this as monocytosis.

Monocytosis is present during the recovery stage from acute infections and is usually considered a favorable sign except in tuberculosis. An increase of monocytes in tuberculosis is a poor prognostic sign.

Monocytosis may be present in subacute bacterial endocarditis. In this condition monocytes may show phagocytosis of other blood cells, red blood cells, and leukocytes. It may be present in mycotic, rickettsial, protozoal, and viral infections.

Infectious disease, however, is an uncommon cause of monocytosis in current medical practice. Maldonado and Hanlon (1965) reviewed 160 successive cases of absolute monocytosis at the Mayo Clinic. Over half (85) were associated with *hematologic disease:* 20 had monocytic or granulocytic leukemia; 20 had lymphoma (Hodgkin's disease was most frequent); 7 had multiple myeloma; 6 had myeloproliferative disorders; and, in 18, the cause was indeterminate. *Malignant disease* accounted for 13 cases; *connective tissue disorders,* 16; *infectious disease,* 9; fever of unknown origin, 7; ulcerative colitis, 4; regional enteritis, 4; nontropical sprue, 2; and cirrhosis, 3 cases. Miscellaneous and indeterminate causes made up the remaining 17 cases. Among hematopoietic dysplasias, an unexplained monocytosis occasionally seems to precede the development of leukemia by months or years.

Plasmacytosis

Plasma cells are not normally present in circulating blood. They are increased in a variety of chronic infections, in allergic states, in the presence of neoplasms, and in other conditions in which the serum gamma globulin is elevated. They are moderately increased in cutaneous exanthemas, infectious mononucleosis, syphilis, subacute bacterial endocarditis, sarcoidosis, and collagen diseases. Their increase is usually linked with an increase in lymphocytes, monocytes, and eosinophils. These four cells form the antigen-antibody quartet.

In the marrow, normally less than 1 per cent of plasma cells are present. An increase beyond 2 per cent is significant. Increases up to 20 per cent of plasma cells may be found in a variety of conditions other than multiple myeloma, including metastatic carcinoma, chronic granulomatous infections, conditions linked with hypersensitivity, and following administration of cytotoxic drugs. They are often increased in aplastic anemia, but this is probably just a relative increase. On the other hand, they are decreased or absent in agammaglobulinemia.

PROLIFERATIVE DISORDERS OF BLOOD-PRODUCING TISSUES; BLOOD AND MARROW FINDINGS

Leukemia

Leukemia is a generalized neoplastic proliferation or accumulation of leukopoietic cells with or without involvement of the peripheral blood. Leukocytosis, abnormal circulating cells, and infiltration of nonhematopoietic tissues are frequently but not invariably present.

If no abnormal cells are present in the blood the leukemia is described as *aleukemic*; if abnormal cells are present but the total leukocyte count is not elevated, the term *subleukemic* leukemia is used.

The *acute leukemias,* if no remission is induced, usually are fatal within three months. The bone marrow is usually packed with primitive cells of the series involved with very little evidence of differentiation.

Subacute leukemias are often categorized with the acute leukemias, but when the term is used it implies a longer natural history of three to 12 months and cells of intermediate differentiation. Patients with *chronic leukemias* usually survive more than one year after the onset of symptoms if no remission occurs. The cell type is more differentiated (Woodliff and Dougan, 1972).

CLASSIFICATION

1. *Chronologic* (based on natural history)
   a. Acute.
   b. Subacute.
   c. Chronic.
2. *Cytologic* (based on predominant cell type)
   a. Undifferentiated blast cell leukemia (hematopoietic reticulum cell; stem cell), rare.
   b. Granulocytic leukemia: acute (myeloblast); chronic (myelocyte).
   c. Lymphocytic leukemia: acute (lymphoblast); chronic (lymphocyte).
   d. Monocytic leukemia: acute (monoblast), chronic (monocyte).
   e. Plasma cell leukemia.
   f. "Lymphosarcoma cell" leukemia.
3. *Functional capacity of release mechanism*
   a. Leukemic.
   b. Subleukemic.
   c. Aleukemic.

4. *Localized proliferation of cells of same type*
   a. Chloroma (myeloblast).
   b. Myeloma (plasma cell).
   c. Lymphoma (lymphoblast or lymphocyte).

ETIOLOGIC FACTORS

The etiology of human leukemias remains unknown. Leukemia is an abnormal, uncontrolled proliferation or accumulation of one cell type at some level of maturation. It is probable that the initial event in the development of leukemia is a mutation in one cell, and that this event occurs as a result of one or more environmental determinants acting at a particular moment in a susceptible individual.

Marrow Damage. Irradiation may result in an increased incidence of leukemia. In physicians the incidence is 1.7 times that in the general population, and in radiologists it is eight to 10 times that in other physicians. Following the dropping of the atomic bomb in 1945, an increased incidence of leukemia appeared in those of the Japanese population who were exposed to radiation. Treatment of ankylosing spondylitis with radiation has also been followed by an increased occurrence of leukemia. Generally, following radiation, when leukemia occurs it is acute or chronic granulocytic or acute lymphocytic.

Marrow damage due to *chemical agents* such as chloramphenicol, phenylbutazone, or benzene has been followed in a few cases by acute granulocytic leukemia. *Aplastic anemia* of unknown cause and *paroxysmal nocturnal hemoglobinuria* are other examples of marrow injuries that are associated with a small but increased incidence of leukemia.

Immunologic Function. In patients with hereditary defects of the immune system, an increased frequency of lymphocytic leukemia and lymphoma has been noted. It may be that survival of malignant cells requires some defect in immune surveillance. Also, persons with a long-term proliferation of the lymphoid system, as in autoimmune hemolytic anemia, may eventually develop a lymphoma.

Genetic Factors. Multiple occurrences of leukemia have been described in the same family, more in chronic lymphocytic than in chronic granulocytic leukemia. Monozygotic twins are much more likely to both have leukemia than are dizygotic twins.

Chromosome number 22 has shown an apparent deletion of one of the long arms in the myeloid cells of about 90 per cent of patients with chronic granulocytic leukemia. This abnormal chromosome is called the Philadelphia chromosome (Ph^1). Also, in children with an extra chromosome number 21 and mongolism there is an increased incidence of both acute granulocytic leukemia and an unusual myeloid dysplasia that resembles leukemia but eventually regresses.

Viruses. In some animal leukemias, viruses have been proved to be the etiologic agent, and they are suspected to be so in human leukemia.

INCIDENCE

Expected deaths from leukemia in the United States in 1973 are estimated to be 15,300, or about 7 per 100,000 population. The death rate increased from 3.9 per 100,000 in 1940 to 6.5 per 100,000 in 1954.

Estimated new cases of leukemia in the U.S. in 1973 are 19,000 (American Cancer Society, 1973).

Acute leukemias account for about 60 per cent of all leukemias; chronic granulocytic leukemia and chronic lymphocytic leukemia are each about 20 per cent of the total. Overall, males with leukemia outnumber females about 1.3 to 1; this ratio is larger in chronic lymphocytic leukemia.

Peaks in the age distribution for acute leukemia are at 3 to 4 years of age, and at 15 to 20 years of age. Acute lymphocytic leukemia accounts for most of the former and acute granulocytic for most of the latter. Most cases of chronic granulocytic leukemia occur between the ages of 20 and 50 years, and chronic lymphocytic leukemia, above 50. Monocytic leukemia, which is usually acute, favors middle age and is rare before age 30.

ACUTE LEUKEMIAS

Clinical Features. The onset of the disease is sudden and differs strikingly from the insidious onset of chronic leukemia. The disease resembles an acute infectious or even a septic condition. Other changes include fever, rapidly developing anemia, and signs of granulocytic insufficiency, with ulcerations of mucous membranes, especially of the mouth and throat, and purpura. Enlargement of lymph nodes, spleen, and liver is not very pronounced. Rheumatoid pains, sometimes resembling acute rheumatic fever, are frequent. Marked prostration and general malaise may be present. The course is rapidly progressive. Acute leukemia may imitate a variety of diseases.

Lymph node enlargement is conspicuous only in acute monocytic leukemia, especially cervical. Moderate generalized lymph node enlargement is more frequent in acute lymphocytic leukemia. In monocytic leukemia cervical lymph nodes are also tender.

The spleen is only slightly enlarged, except

in acute lymphocytic leukemia, in which it may be moderately or even greatly enlarged.

Lesions in the mouth, with swelling, ulceration, and hemorrhages in the gums, are especially frequent in monocytic leukemia but may also occur in other forms. Mucosal ulcerations may also be present in other parts of the gastrointestinal tract. Also, these lesions are more frequent in monocytic leukemia.

In addition to rheumatoid pains previously referred to, there may also be tenderness of bones and swelling and tenderness of joints. The responsible pathologic lesion is the presence of subperiosteal leukemic infiltrations.

Signs of central nervous system (CNS) involvement are seen primarily in acute lymphocytic leukemia (ALL). CNS symptoms appear in about one-third of children with ALL who live longer than one year. Usually due to meningeal infiltration with leukemic cells, the symptoms are related to increased pressure or to focal lesions. Other CNS problems are the result of high circulating blast counts leading to leukostatic thrombi and intracerebral hemorrhage, or to severe thrombocytopenia, which may result in subarachnoid hemorrhage.

Blood Findings. Anemia is present almost without exception—certainly in any case with fully developed clinical manifestations. It is usually normocytic. Frequently young nucleated red cells are present. Thrombocytopenia of moderate to marked degree is the rule. Prolonged bleeding time, poor clot retraction and positive tourniquet test are present. The leukocyte count is occasionally very high (over 100,000 per μl.), often is slightly elevated, but is perhaps most frequently normal or decreased. A combination of anemia, thrombocytopenia, and leukopenia is a common finding in acute leukemia.

The predominant cell is an immature blast cell, most frequently a myeloblast in the adult and a lymphoblast in the child (Figs. 4–79 through 4–81).

Marrow Findings. By the time the patient is symptomatic, the hematopoietic cells and fat are usually replaced by diffuse infiltration of blasts. The bony trabeculae and cortex may be thin.

Chromosomal Abnormalities in Blood-Forming Cells. In almost half of patients with acute leukemia, the karyotype is normal. In the remainder, no consistent abnormality of the karyotype is found in any one form of acute leukemia. Most patients apparently have a normal (diploid) mode, but some have abnormal karyotypes, which are usually consistent for the individual but not for the type of leukemia. Sandberg *et al.* (1964) found that in the patients with acute granulocytic leukemia who had an abnormal karyotype, the aneuploidy was hypodiploid except for those with a bimodal, unstable cell population. In acute lymphocytic leukemia, the aneuploidy in the patients with abnormal karyotypes was hyperdiploid.

Cytochemistry. Hayhoe *et al.* (1964) analyzed 140 cases of acute leukemia using standard Romanowsky staining characteristics and four cytochemical reactions: Sudan black B, peroxidase, neutrophil alkaline phosphatase, and periodic acid-Schiff (PAS). Virtually all cases could be classified into one of four groups: lymphoblastic, myeloblastic, myelomonocytic, and erythremic myelosis. Lymphoblastic was quite clearly separable, but there was some overlap among the other three groups. In a recent review, Hayhoe and Cawley (1972) have included data from cytochemical esterase reactions which have added some discriminatory power. The usefulness of these cytochemical characteristics is described in the following sections, the methods are given beginning page 273, and some of the reactions are illustrated in Figures 4–90 through 4–97.

Acute Lymphocytic Leukemia

Morphology. The cell type is the lymphoblast. The nuclear-cytoplasmic ratio is high. The nuclei may have deep clefts (known as Rieder cells) but are not indented or twisted. The chromatin pattern is fine and uniform. Usually only one or two nucleoli are present. The cytoplasm is scanty in amount, pale blue, and homogeneous, without granules (Figs. 4–81, 4–89, 4–108, and 4–109).

Normoblasts are not usually found in the blood, nor are they predominant in the marrow. Auer rods, agranular neutrophils, or the acquired pseudo-Pelger anomaly are not found.

Cytochemistry. The blasts are negative for Sudan black B, peroxidase, and naphthol AS-D chloroacetate esterase; Hayhoe and Cawley (1972) state that no more than 5 per cent of the cells can be positive (Fig. 4–93). The PAS stain usually shows coarse blocks of material in at least some lymphoblasts. The neutrophil alkaline phosphatase score is normal or high.

Acute Granulocytic Leukemia. Acute granulocytic leukemia, myelomonocytic leukemia, and erythroleukemia share certain features. The latter two are usually considered variants of the former. This commonality suggests a common stem cell for granulocytes, monocytes, erythroid cells, and probably also megakaryocytes, since the latter are frequently abnormal when erythroid cells are involved (Hayhoe and Cawley, 1972).

Morphology. The cell type is the myeloblast, which is usually slightly larger than the lymphoblast (Figs. 4–79, 4–80, and 4–107). The nuclear-cytoplasmic ratio is not high. The nucleus is round to oval. The chromatin is very fine, delicate, and uniform, without condensation. The nuclear membrane is indistinct. Three to five nucleoli are usually evident. The

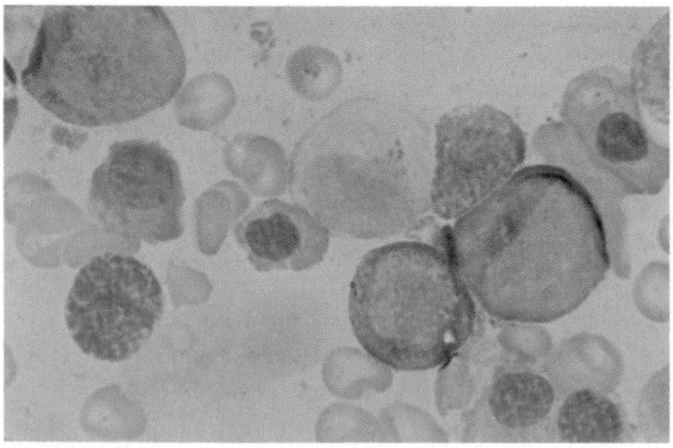

Figure 4–90.

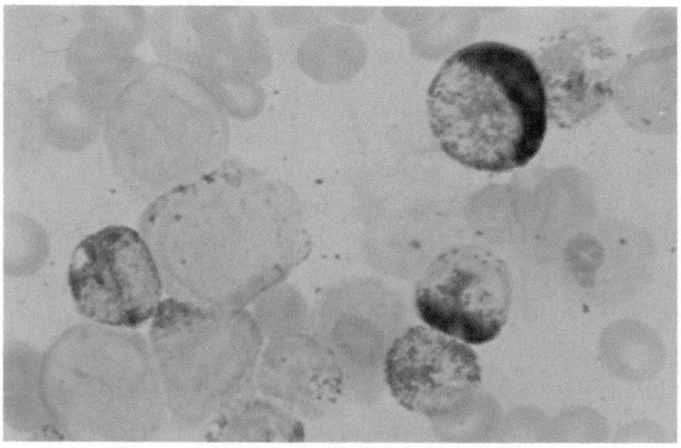

Figure 4–91.

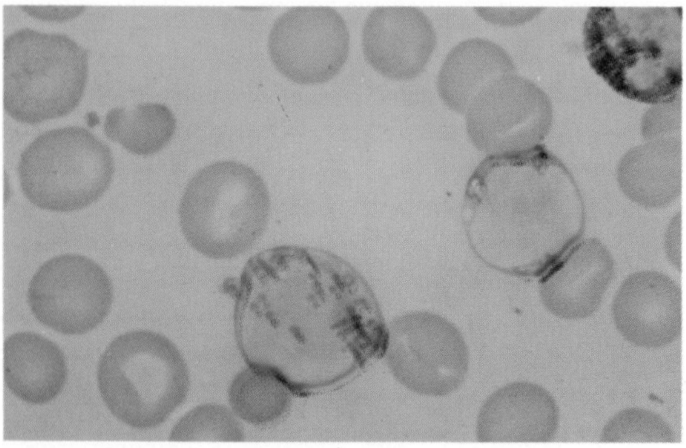

Figure 4–92.

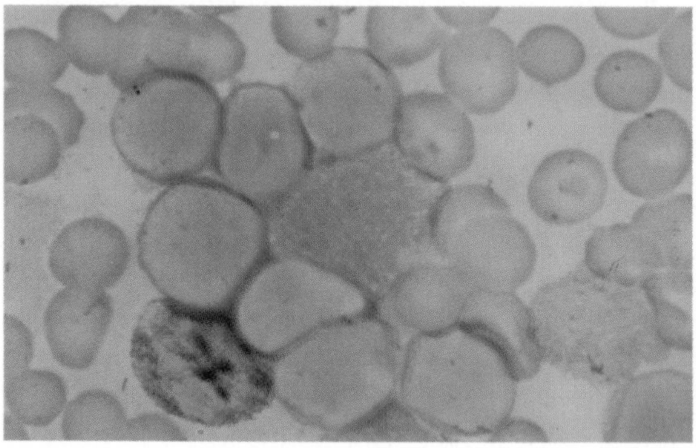

Figure 4–93.

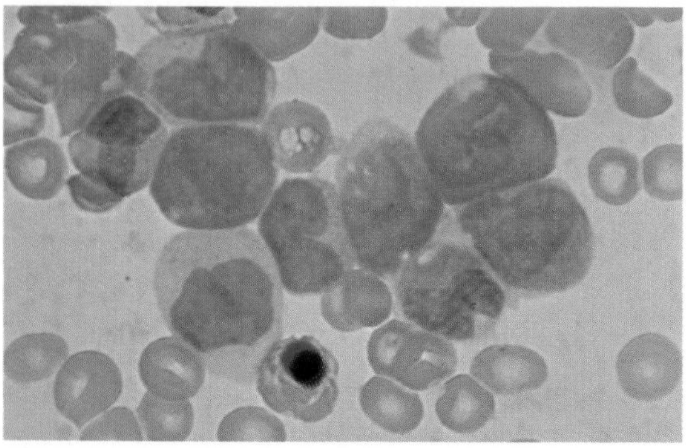

Figure 4–94.

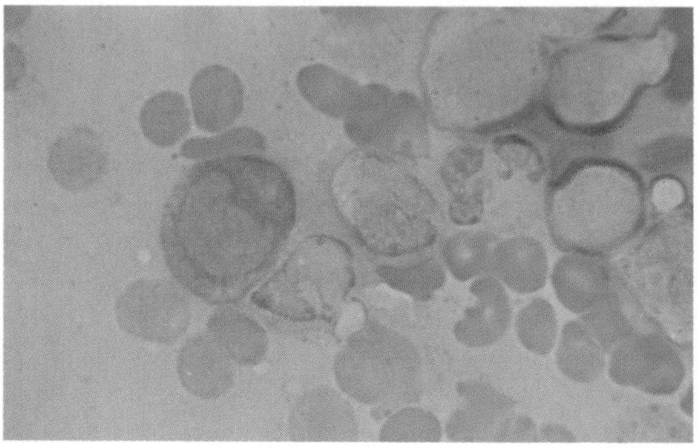

Figure 4–95.

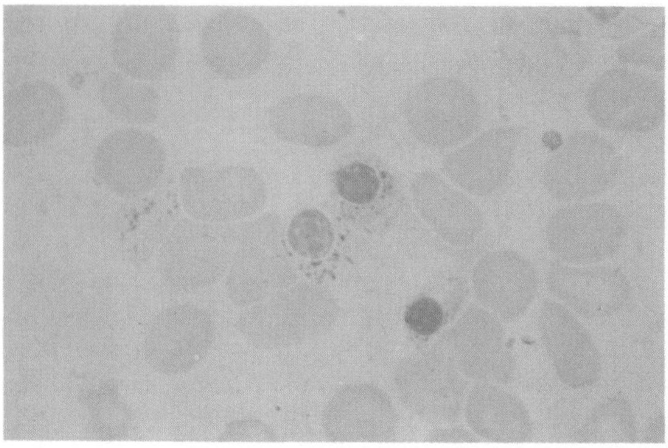

Figure 4–96.

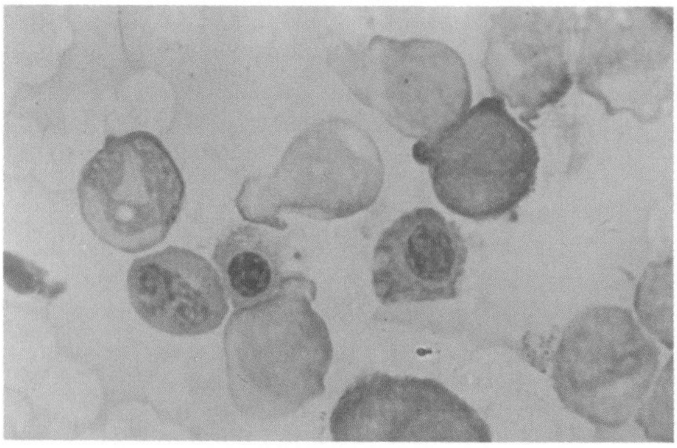

Figure 4–97.

(*See opposite page for legends.*)

cytoplasm is homogeneous, without granules or with a very few azurophilic granules.

Less than 1 per cent of blood leukocytes are monocytes, and normoblasts do not predominate in the marrow. Promyelocytes are usually present, but intermediate cells between the blasts and mature neutrophils are not numerous. This lack of maturing cells is known as a *leukemic hiatus* and is characteristic of acute granulocytic leukemia. If many myelocytes and metamyelocytes or increased basophils are present, it suggests that the picture may be one of a blast transformation of chronic granulocytic leukemia rather than *de novo* acute granulocytic leukemia.

Deficient granulation in mature neutrophils or hyposegmentation of the nuclei (pseudo-Pelger anomaly) may be present.

With Wright's stain, *Auer rods* are characteristic rod-shaped red to purple staining inclusions in the cytoplasm of myeloblasts or promyelocytes in acute granulocytic leukemia (Figs. 4–79, 4–80, and 4–107). Less commonly they may be seen in more mature neutrophils. Auer rods are derivatives of azurophilic granules and stain positively for Sudan black B, peroxidase, and naphthol AS-D chloroacetate esterase. Auer rods are found in the majority of cases of acute granulocytic leukemia, and almost never in any other condition except for myelomonocytic leukemia and erythroleukemia.

Acute promyelocytic leukemia is a variant of acute granulocytic leukemia in which promyelocytes predominate instead of myeloblasts. The azurophil granules tend to be abundant and darkly staining. This disorder usually has a fulminant course, punctuated by bleeding which is more severe than would be expected from the degree of thrombocytopenia. This is due to intravascular coagulation that in some way apparently is initiated by the procoagulant material from the granules of the abnormal cells.

Cytochemistry. According to the defining criteria of Hayhoe and Cawley (1972), over 5 per cent of the cells (and usually more than 85 per cent) have strong positive staining of granules with Sudan black B (Figure 4-92). More than 5 per cent of the cells are also peroxidase positive (Figs. 4–91 and 4–107). Staining of the late myeloblasts or early promyelocytes is the important criterion; occasionally the blasts fail to show these reactions if they have failed to show any development of azurophilic granules; on the other hand, sometimes no granules can be seen with Wright's stain, and yet the blasts are peroxidase and Sudan black B positive. Almost always these two stains react in parallel. Auer rods are positive with these staining reactions. Naphthol AS-D chloroacetate esterase is positive in developing granulocytes also, but alpha-naphthol acetate esterase is negative (Fig. 4–94). The PAS stain shows faint diffuse or granular staining in some blasts or early promyelocytes.

The neutrophil alkaline phosphatase score is usually low, suggesting that these neutrophils are derived from the leukemic blasts.

Acute Myelomonocytic Leukemia. In the past, two forms of monocytic leukemia have been recognized. In the *Naegeli type*, myeloblasts are numerous and abnormal proliferation is evident in developing granulocytes as well as monocytes; this has been considered a variant of acute granulocytic leukemia, with monocytes being derived from myeloblasts. The *Schilling type* of monocytic leukemia has been considered a "pure" monocytic leukemia, with monocytes derived from the reticuloendothelial

---

Figure 4–90. Sudan black B stain. Three myelocytes, a band neutrophil, and a mature neutrophil contain many Sudan-positive granules. Erythroid precursors (which are slightly megaloblastic) are negative. From a case of erythroleukemia.

Figure 4–91. Peroxidase reaction. Large cell near center with few granules is an early promyelocyte. Most darkly staining cell, upper right, is a neutrophilic myelocyte. Note that here the more mature neutrophils have fewer peroxidase-positive granules than the myelocyte. Same case as Figure 4–90.

Figure 4–92. Acute granulocytic leukemia, Sudan black B stain. The two cells near the center are early promyelocytes; they have a few positive granules (brown-black), and the lower cell has an Auer rod which is positive. In the upper right corner is a neutrophil.

Figure 4–93. Acute lymphocytic leukemia, Sudan black B stain. Seven lymphoblasts; none contains any positive granules. The neutrophil, with its many Sudan black-positive granules, serves as a positive control.

Figure 4–94. Naphthol AS-D chloroacetate esterase reaction. Neutrophil myelocytes, metamyelocytes, and band forms have many positive granules (red), but the two monocytes and the normoblast are negative. The metamyelocytes are large with rather poorly condensed chromatin, and might otherwise be mistaken for monocytes. Same case as Figure 4–90.

Figure 4–95. Alpha-naphthyl acetate esterase reaction. The monocyte contains positively staining granules (orange), but the neutrophil bands and the mature neutrophil do not. Same case as Figure 4–90.

Figure 4–96. Sideroblastic anemia, Prussian blue reaction. Three abnormal sideroblasts with multiple iron-containing granules (green). The cell at the lower right has many granules circling the nucleus; if the granules, lying close together, encompass at least three-fourths of the circumference of the nucleus, the cell is designated a ring sideroblast. In this cell it was obvious when the focal plane was moved up and down. In normal erythropoiesis only about one-third of the normoblasts contain granules, and these are one to two in number and very small.

Figure 4–97. Erythroleukemia, periodic acid-Schiff stain. Neutrophil bands at left contain PAS-positive material (red). The three erythroid precursors at the right contain abundant PAS-positive material. Two myeloblasts near the center are negative or very faintly positive. Same case as Figure 4–90.

system, and with no evidence of abnormality in granulocyte development; the Schilling type is considerably less common.

It seems now, however, less likely that monocytes have a dual origin. It now appears that monocytes originate in the bone marrow from a stem cell common to granulocytes, erythroid cells, and megakaryocytes. In the monocytic leukemias there is a spectrum, from cases with slight monocytic and strong myeloblastic components to those that are almost purely monocytic. The Naegeli and Schilling types are classified as variants, then, of myelomonocytic leukemia (Hayhoe *et al.*, 1964; Hayhoe and Cawley, 1972).

Morphology. The nucleus has delicate reticular chromatin and several (3 to 5) nucleoli. The nucleus is folded, indented, and frequently twisted or even coarsely segmented. There is usually abundant cytoplasm (the nuclear-cytoplasmic ratio is not high) and often many fine azurophilic granules. Phagocytosis of red cells or cell debris may be seen. Auer rods may be present in the abnormal monocytes as well as in the blasts; neutrophils may have diminished granules; the pseudo-Pelger anomaly may be present; and eosinophils may be abnormal.

Monocytes comprise over 1 per cent of the circulating leukocytes. Normoblasts are not usually found in the blood, nor do they predominate in the marrow. Megakaryocytes are less likely to be depleted in the marrow in this form of acute leukemia, and thrombocytopenia is less frequent.

Cytochemistry. Sudan black B positivity is present in the monocytes and is finer than that seen in granulocyte precursors. The peroxidase reaction also tends to be less strong, and usually is negative in the younger cells. The alpha-naphthol acetate esterase reaction is positive in the monocytes (Fig. 4–95), and the naphthol AS-D chloroacetate esterase is negative, the reverse of the findings in the granulocyte precursors in acute granulocytic leukemia. This makes these esterase reactions particularly valuable in the diagnosis of myelomonocytic leukemia. The PAS reaction may be negative or show diffuse cytoplasmic staining of fine granules.

Muramidase. Patients with myelomonocytic leukemia characteristically have markedly increased levels of muramidase (lysozyme) in the serum and urine (Osserman and Lawlor, 1966). Muramidase is an enzyme capable of lysing bacteria; it is present in normal neutrophils and monocytes. The source of the normal serum lysozyme is probably the neutrophil, and its concentration appears to correlate with neutrophil turnover. In myeloproliferative disorders the serum muramidase is also increased, and this correlation appears to hold (Catovsky *et al.*, 1971 a and b). The highest levels, however, occur in myelomonocytic leukemia, and here the muramidase level reflects the proliferation of monocytes. It appears probable that the muramidase is produced and secreted from the monocyte during its life, but that the muramidase is not released from the neutrophil until its death. If the cells are poorly differentiated or significantly abnormal morphologically they may not produce muramidase (Catovsky *et al.*, 1971b). Muramidase may be estimated by a turbidometric method, observing the decrease in optical density (Δ O.D.) produced in a suspension of *Micrococcus lysodeikticus* when exposed to serum or urine, compared to the Δ O.D. produced by a known concentration of egg-white lysozyme (Parry *et al.*, 1965). It may also be measured utilizing an agar plate diffusion method in which the bacterial cells are present in the agar (Osserman and Lawlor, 1966).

DiGuglielmo Syndrome. Another variant of acute granulocytic leukemia is erythroleukemia, which refers to an abnormal proliferation of both erythroid precursors and granulocytic precursors. Morphologic abnormalities are usually pronounced.

Very rarely there is virtually no granulocytic involvement in the neoplastic process, in which case the condition is called *erythremic myelosis*. This disease has a rapid course resembling acute leukemia.

Usually there is a mixture of variable proportions of erythroid precursors and myeloblasts, *erythroleukemia*, which may include megakaryocytic and monocytic abnormal proliferations in addition. This also usually has a rapid course, but is more variable and sometimes may be subacute or even chronic.

When the abnormal erythroid proliferation is minimal and the myeloblastic proliferation predominates, the picture of *acute granulocytic leukemia* is seen.

Although each disorder may be seen *de novo*, occasionally one sees progression from an initial erythremic myelosis to erythroleukemia to a final termination in acute granulocytic (myeloblastic) leukemia in a single patient. This group of disorders has been designated the *Di Guglielmo syndrome* (Dameshek and Gunz, 1964).

Morphology. Erythroid precursors, though abnormal, usually are easily recognized. They predominate in the hyperplastic marrow and are usually present in the blood. They are irregular in outline, often with pseudopods. The nuclear:cytoplasmic ratio is not high. Nuclear shape is often bizarre, with atypical megaloblastic features. Nucleoli tend to be large. Mitoses and multinucleated giant forms are numerous. Vacuolation of cytoplasm in pro- and basophilic erythroblasts is often present.

In erythremic myelosis and the more acute forms of erythroleukemia, there is an apparent arrest of maturation and fewer polychromatic and orthochromatic forms are present. In chronic forms of erythroleukemia, later normoblasts are present in larger numbers. Myeloblasts are increased in erythroleukemia, and Auer rods may be found in them or in promyelocytes. Abnormalities in neutrophils and eosinophils may be seen. Monocytic proliferation may be a part of the process. Abnormal megakaryocytes are often prominent and include giant forms with bizarre nuclear fragmentation and small fragmented megakaryocytes with one or two apparently diploid nuclei. Atypical platelets may be found in the blood (Figs. 4–77 and 4–78).

Cytochemistry. Some of the erythroid precursors at all stages of maturation show strong cytoplasmic PAS positivity. This is granular in early erythroid precursors and diffuse in later stages (Fig. 4–97). Erythroid precursors are normally PAS negative, and they are negative in most diseases, including nutritional megaloblastic anemia. They are sometimes positive, however, in iron deficiency anemia and thalassemia and in refractory sideroblastic anemia or refractory anemia with dyshematopoiesis (Hayhoe *et al.*, 1964). The latter disorders are part of a heterogeneous group which have been regarded as chronic forms of the Di Guglielmo syndrome (Dameshek and Gunz, 1964).

In erythroleukemia increased numbers of primitive cells showing Sudan black and peroxidase positivity are found. Abnormal neoplastic erythroid precursors are positive for the alpha-naphthol acetate esterase reaction (Hayhoe and Cawley, 1972).

Cytochemistry: Methods

Neutrophil Alkaline Phosphatase (Kaplow, 1963)

PRINCIPLE. The enzyme, located in the neutrophil-specific granules, is exposed to the substrate (a naphthol phosphate) in the presence of a diazonium salt (fast blue or fast violet) at an alkaline pH, 9.5. The substrate is hydrolyzed by the enzyme, releasing a phosphate and an aryl naphthol amide. The latter is immediately coupled to the diazonium salt, forming an insoluble azo dye.

REAGENTS

1. Fixative: 10 per cent formalin in absolute methanol. (To 10 ml. 37 per cent formaldehyde add 90 ml. absolute methanol. Store at –10 to –20° C.)
2. Buffer: *Stock:* 0.2 M propanediol.* Dissolve 21 gm. of 2-amino-2-methyl-1,3-propanediol in distilled water and dilute to 1000 ml. Store at 4° C.

   Working: 0.05 M propanediol pH 9.4-9.6. Add 70 ml. 0.1 N HCl to 250 ml. of stock buffer and dilute to 1000 ml. with distilled water. Store at 4° C.
3. Substrate mixture: Dissolve 5 mg. of naphthol AS-BI phosphate* (or naphthol AS-MX phosphate or naphthol AS phosphate) in 0.2 to 0.3 ml. dimethyl formamide in a dry flask and add 60 ml. of 0.05 M propanediol buffer and 40 mg. of Fast Blue Salt RR, BB, or BBN* (or Fast Red Violet Salt LB). Shake well, filter into a Coplin jar, and use immediately.
4. Counterstain: Mayer's hematoxylin. Add 1 gm. hematoxylin to 500 ml. distilled water. Heat just to boiling and add another 500 ml. distilled water. Add 0.2 gm. sodium iodate and 50 gm. aluminum potassium sulfate; shake well, filter, and store in brown bottle at room temperature.

*Eastman Kodak, Rochester, N.Y.

PROCEDURE. Use freshly made blood films. If venous blood is used, heparin should be the anticoagulant, as the enzyme activity diminishes rapidly in EDTA.

Fix air-dried blood films in 10 per cent formol-methanol for exactly 30 seconds at 0 to –10° C.

Wash in gently running tap water for 30 to 60 seconds.

Air dry slides, then place them in substrate mixture for exactly 10 min. Wash in gently running tap water again for 30 to 60 seconds.

Counterstain for 6 to 8 minutes in filtered Mayer's hematoxylin.

Wash in running tap water for 2 minutes. Air dry.

Positive controls are run with each batch of slides. Women in the last trimester of pregnancy are good controls, because their scores are high normal or somewhat increased.

Scoring Procedure. Examine 100 mature neutrophils in the thin part of the film, where red cells barely touch one another, and score each as follows:

Unstained cells	0
Cells stained faintly, diffusely, or a few discrete granules	1
Cells with moderate number of granules	2
Cells with granules filling the cell	3
Cells staining deeply, almost obscuring the nucleus	4

Adding the scores for the 100 neutrophils will give a total score with a possible range of 0 to 400.

Normal Range. Each laboratory must establish its own normal range. Only a portion (0 to 60 per cent) of the neutrophils normally stain under these conditions. The normal range with this method is about 20 to 100.

*Sigma Chemical Co., St. Louis, Mo.

INTERPRETATION. Increased activity is seen in infections with leukocytosis, polycythemia vera, some cases of myelofibrosis with myeloid metaplasia, and in Hodgkin's disease. Decreased activity is seen in chronic granulocytic leukemia, acute granulocytic leukemia, paroxysmal nocturnal hemoglobinuria, hereditary hypophosphatasia, and in some viral infections.

SOURCES OF VARIATION. It is preferable to perform the reaction immediately or to fix the films and store in the freezer, in which case they will lose only 10 per cent activity in 2 to 3 weeks. At room temperature, unfixed air-dried films tend to have a small decrease in activity in the first 2 hours, then increasing to an average of 9 per cent above the original value at 4 to 6 hours, then declining gradually to 20 per cent below the original value at 24 hours and 35 per cent below at 48 hours (Kaplow, 1963).

Sudan Black B Stain (Sheehan and Storey, 1947)

PRINCIPLE. Sudan black B stains phospholipids and other lipids. It appears to stain both azurophilic and specific granules in neutrophils, whereas the peroxidase is found only in azurophilic granules. In early forms, late myeloblasts, and early promyelocytes, the Sudan black B reaction is therefore parallel to the peroxidase in its utility in separating acute lymphocytic from acute granulocytic leukemia.

REAGENTS

Stock Stain Solution. Dissolve 0.3 gm. of Sudan black B powder in 100 ml. ethyl alcohol.

Buffer Solution. Dissolve 16 gm. crystalline phenol in 30 ml. ethyl alcohol. Add this to a solution of 0.3 gm. hydrated disodium hydrogen phosphate ($Na_2HPO_4 \cdot 12H_2O$) dissolved in 100 ml. distilled water.

Working Stain Solution. Add 40 ml. buffer solution to 60 ml. stock stain solution. Filter, using suction. This solution is stable for approximately two months.

PROCEDURE

1. Fix air-dried films in formalin vapor for 10 minutes. Slides need not be freshly made.
2. Wash slides in running tap water for 10 minutes.
3. Place slides in working stain solution (in Coplin jar) for 60 minutes.
4. Wash slides with 70 per cent ethyl alcohol for 2 to 3 minutes to remove excess dye.
5. Wash slides in tap water for 2 minutes.
6. Allow slides to dry. Counterstain slides with Wright's stain or hematoxylin.

INTERPRETATION. Cytoplasmic granules stain faintly in neutrophil precursors and strongly in mature neutrophils with a brown-black color. Eosinophilic granules are brown, but often show a central pallor. Monocytes have scattered fine brown-black granules. Lymphocytes and lymphoblasts are negative, but at least some myeloblasts contain Sudan black-positive granules (Figs. 4–90, 4–92, 4–93).

The peroxidase and Sudan black B reactions show roughly similar patterns in the various cell types (Hayhoe *et al.,* 1964). These techniques are most useful in distinguishing myeloblasts from lymphoblasts when large numbers of primitive blast forms are present in acute leukemias.

Peroxidase (Myeloperoxidase) (Kaplow, 1965)

PRINCIPLE. In the presence of hydrogen peroxide, peroxidase in leukocyte granules oxidizes benzidine from a colorless form to a blue or brown derivative which is localized at the site of the enzyme.

REAGENTS

Fixative: Mix 10 ml. of 37 per cent formaldehyde with 90 ml. of absolute ethanol.

Incubation mixture:

Ethanol, 30 per cent (v./v.) in water	100 ml.
Benzidine dihydrochloride*	0.3 gm.
$ZnSO_4 \cdot 7\ H_2O$, 0.132 M (3.8 per cent, w./v.)	1.0 ml.
Sodium acetate ($NaC_2H_3O_2 \cdot 3\ H_2O$)	1.0 gm.
Hydrogen peroxide, 3 per cent	0.7 ml.
Sodium hydroxide, 1.0 N	1.5 ml.
Safranin O†	0.2 gm.

Reagents are mixed in the stated order. A precipitate forms after adding the zinc sulfate, but dissolves after other reagents are added. The pH is not critical between 5.8 and 6.5. The mixture is filtered and may be kept in a closed container and reused for a period of several months.

PROCEDURE

1. Freshly made films or imprints are used. Peroxidase is unstable in the light, but unfixed films are satisfactory for as long as 3 weeks if kept in the dark. Heparin, oxalate, or EDTA does not interfere with the reaction.
2. Place slides in fixative for 60 seconds at room temperature. Wash in gently running tap water.
3. Place slide in incubation mixture for 30 seconds at room temperature. Wash slides again in running tap water for 30 to 60 seconds.
4. Allow slides to dry, and examine under the microscope.
5. The slides may be counterstained with Wright's stain or with 1 per cent aqueous cresyl violet if greater nuclear detail is desired.

INTERPRETATION. Peroxidase activity is indicated by blue granules in the cytoplasm. The nucleus and background cytoplasm stain red.

---

*Harleco, Philadelphia, Pa.

†National Biological Stains and Reagents, Division of Allied Chemical Co., Morristown, N.J.

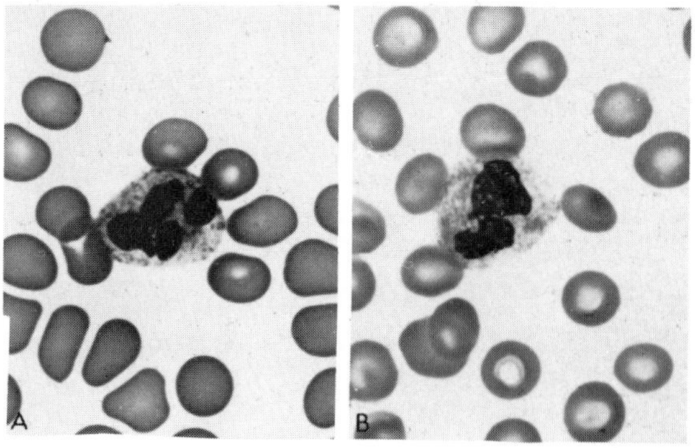

Figure 4–98. *A*, Neutrophil with small proportion of toxic granules. Infection. (× 875). *B*, Neutrophil with large Döhle bodies. Dark areas in the cytoplasm stain pale blue with Wright's stain. May-Hegglin anomaly. In infection, Döhle bodies tend to be single and smaller in size. (× 875.)

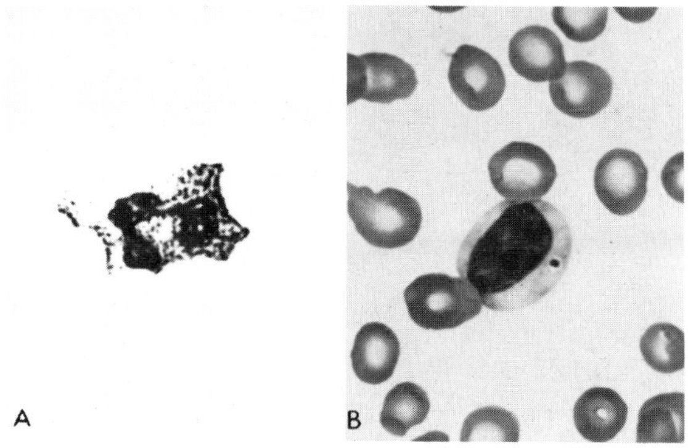

Figure 4–99. Hurler syndrome (genetic mucopolysaccharidosis, Type I). *A*, Neutrophil with Alder-Reilly granules. Entire cytoplasm was filled with dark, purple granules, almost obscuring the nucleus. This high contrast photograph shows only part of the granulation. *B*, Lymphocyte with large purple granule surrounded by "halo." (× 875.)

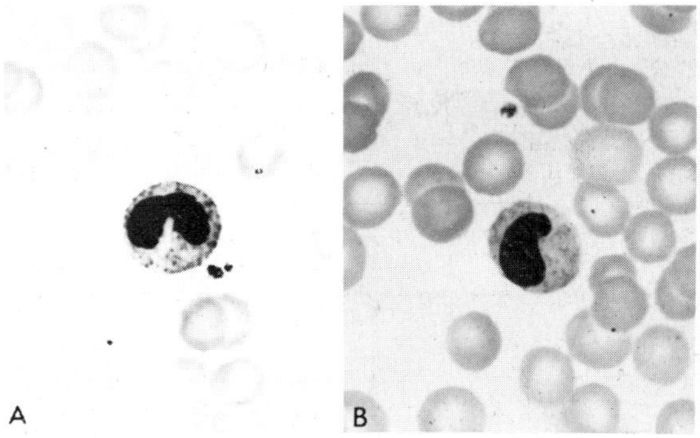

Figure 4–100. Pelger-Huët anomaly. In 50 to 90 per cent of the neutrophils the nucleus is band-shaped or has only two segments. Usually the chromatin is coarse and open; this is not shown here. (× 875.)

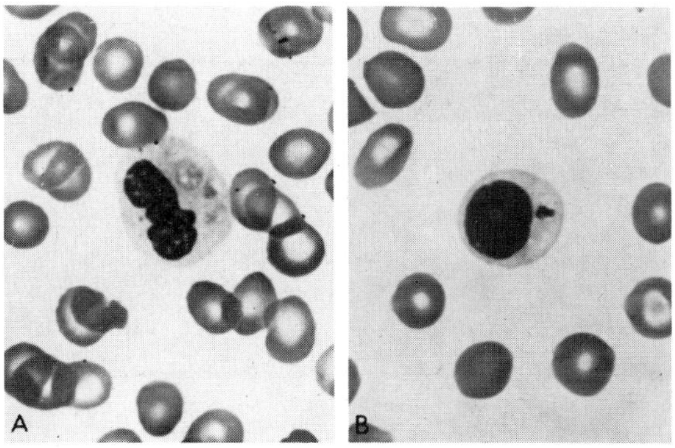

Figure 4–101. Chediak-Higashi syndrome. *A*, Neutrophil with three very large, unevenly staining granules to the right of the nucleus. With Wright's stain they are slate gray to olive green. *B*, Lymphocyte with large red-purple inclusion. (× 875.)

In the neutrophil series the peroxidase occurs in the azurophilic (nonspecific) granules (Figs. 4–91 and 4–107). Therefore, granules may appear first in late myeloblasts; they increase in number in the promyelocytic stage; and with subsequent cell division one would expect them to become fewer in number in the mature neutrophils. However, there appears to be increased activity in the mature cell for reasons that are not clear. In eosinophils the specific granules contain peroxidase. Basophils, lymphocytes, and erythroid cells do not stain. Monocytes stain less intensely than do neutrophils, and the granules are smaller.

This peroxidase reaction finds its greatest usefulness in distinguishing between acute granulocytic and acute lymphocytic leukemia (Fig. 4–107). It parallels the Sudan black B reaction; Auer rods are positive with both. Peroxidase appears earlier in cell development than the naphthol AS-D chloroacetate esterase activity.

Peroxidase activity may be absent in some toxic neutrophils in infection, in some neutrophils in acute granulocytic or myelomonocytic leukemia, and in the rare congenital myeloperoxidase deficiency.

Nonspecific Esterases. Nonspecific esterases are found in many tissues. There appear to be different enzymes which act on different substrates. Their usefulness in hematology depends upon their ability to provide distinguishing reactions between different cell types, both normal and leukemic. The two esterases presented here are particularly useful in distinguishing neutrophil precursors from monocytes in acute granulocytic and acute myelomonocytic leukemias.

Naphthol AS-D Chloroacetate Esterase (Daniel *et al.*, 1971)

REAGENTS

1. Fixative: Mix 10 ml. of 37 per cent formaldehyde with 90 ml. of absolute methanol.
2. Buffer: Michaelis veronal acetate buffer, pH 7.4.

Stock Solution A:	Sodium acetate, anhydrous, 11.704 gm.
	Sodium diethylbarbiturate (Barbital) 29.428 gm.
	Distilled water, CO_2 free, to make 1000 ml.
Stock Solution B:	HCl, concentrated, 8.4 ml.
	Distilled water, to make 1000 ml.

Mix 5.0 ml. of Stock Solution A, 5.0 ml. of Stock Solution B, and 13.0 ml. of CO_2-free distilled water.

3. Incubation mixture: Add in the following order:

Distilled water	20 ml.
Buffer	20 ml.
Propylene glycol	1 ml.

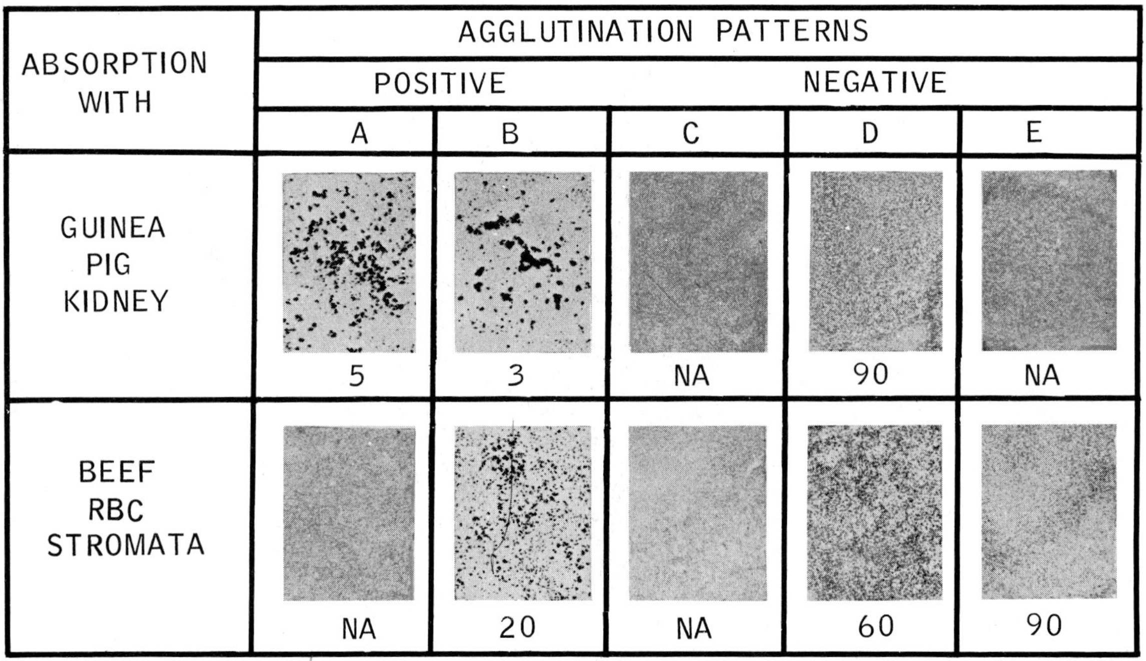
ABSORPTION WITH
AGGLUTINATION PATTERNS
POSITIVE
NEGATIVE
A
B
C
D
E
GUINEA PIG KIDNEY
5
3
NA
90
NA
BEEF RBC STROMATA
NA
20
NA
60
90

Figure 4–102. Agglutination patterns in spot test for infectious mononucleosis. (Numbers indicate time in seconds when aggregates appeared; NA indicates no agglutination within 2 minutes.)

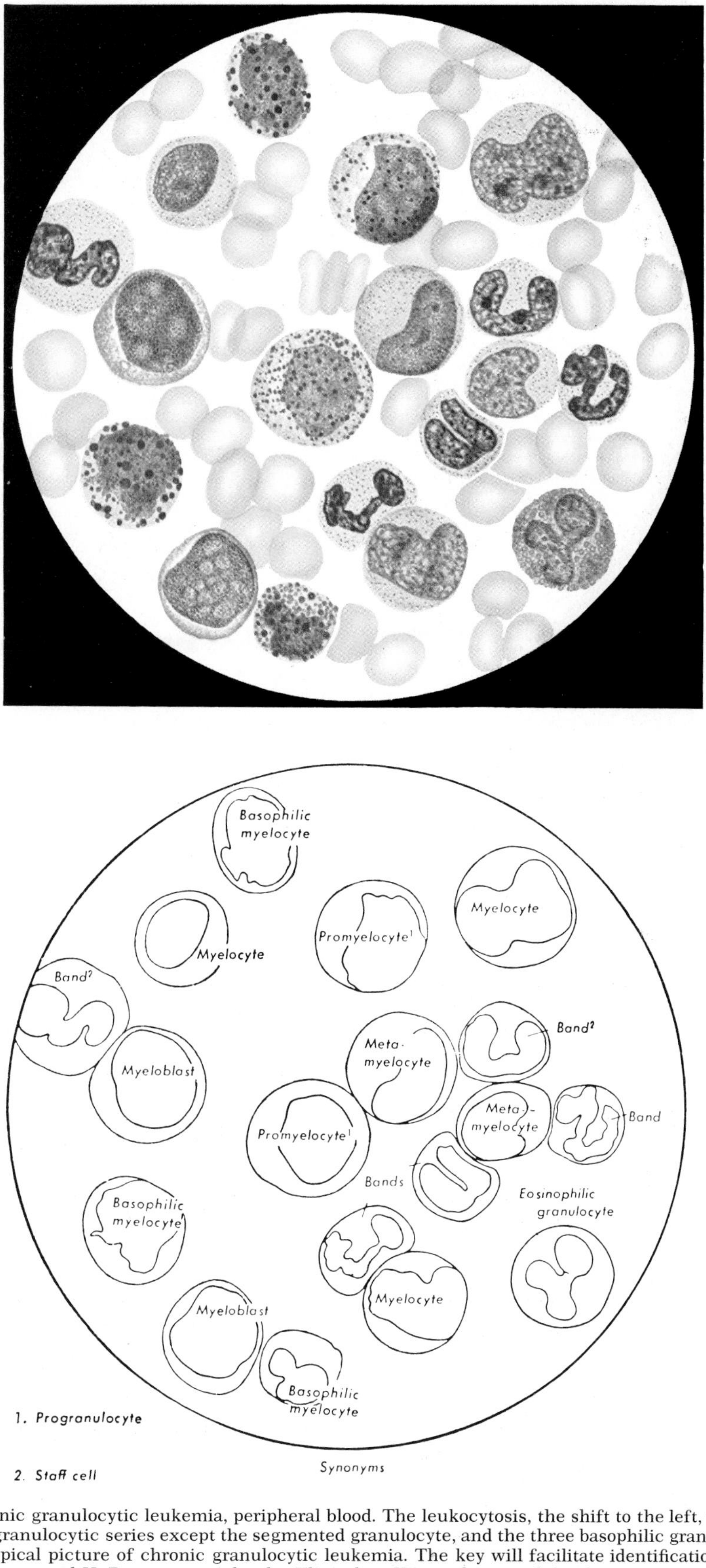

Figure 4–103. Chronic granulocytic leukemia, peripheral blood. The leukocytosis, the shift to the left, the presence of the whole gamut of the granulocytic series except the segmented granulocyte, and the three basophilic granulocytes in a single field add up to the typical picture of chronic granulocytic leukemia. The key will facilitate identification of the individual cells. (From L. Heilmeyer and H. Begemann: Atlas der Klinischen Hämatologie und Cytologie. Springer, 1955.)

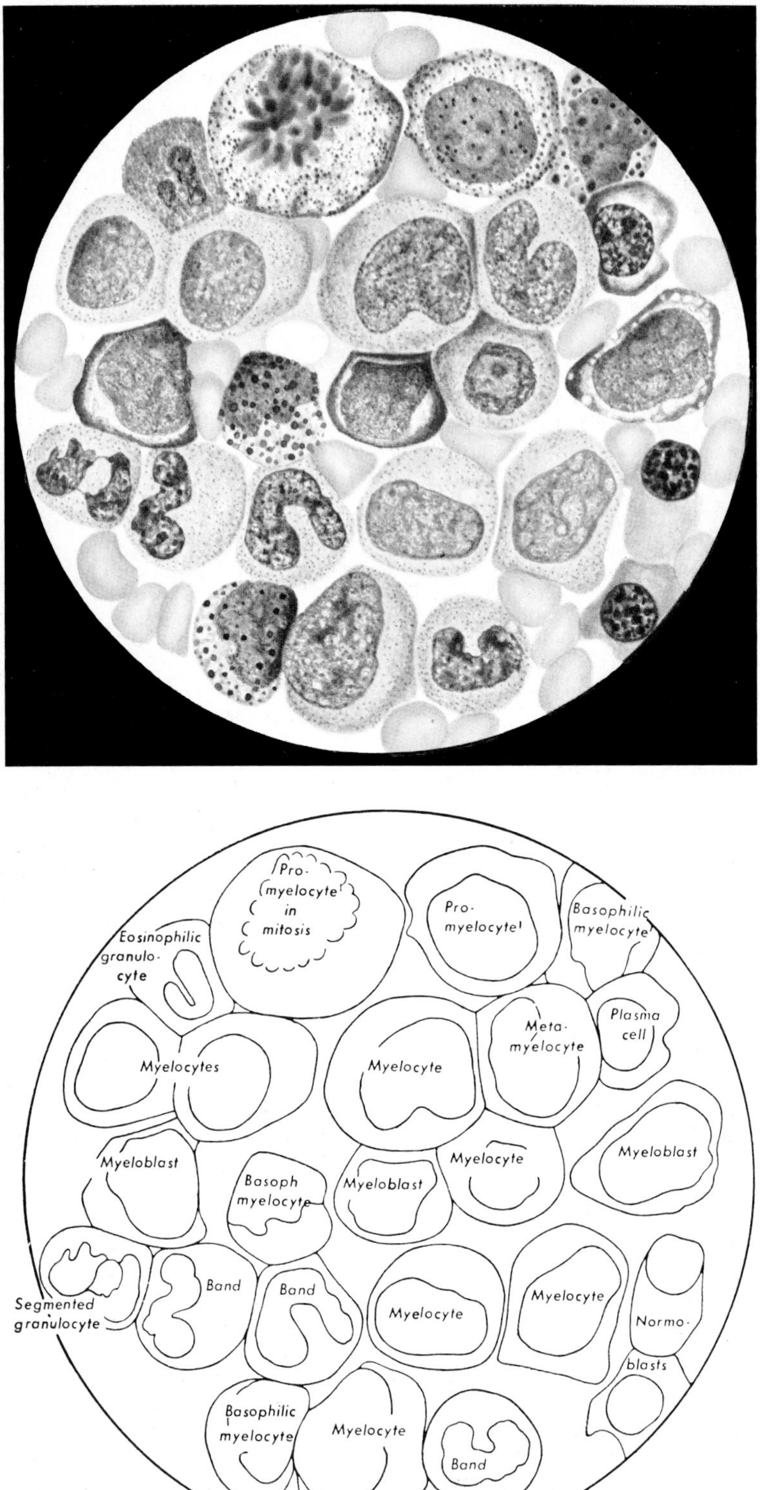

Synonyms

1. Progranulocyte

Figure 4–104. Chronic granulocytic leukemia, marrow. Here, as in the peripheral blood smear, all stages of development of granulocytes from the myeloblast through promyelocyte, myelocyte, metamyelocyte, band form, and segmented cell are present. The basophilic granulocytes are equally prominent. (From L. Heilmeyer and H. Begemann: Atlas der Klinischen Hämatologie und Cytologie. Springer, 1955.)

Naphthol AS-D chloroacetate,*
(20 mg. dissolved in 1.6 ml.
acetone) 20 mg.
Fast Garnet GBC† 40 mg.
Filter mixture through Seitz filter.
4. Harris hematoxylin

PROCEDURE

1. Place air-dried blood or marrow films in fixative for 30 seconds at 4° C. The films can be stored unfixed at room temperature for 2 weeks without significant loss of activity. Wash in running tap water.

2. Place in incubation mixture for 30 minutes. Wash in running tap water.

3. Counterstain with hematoxylin for 10 minutes.

INTERPRETATION. In neutrophils the naphthol AS-D chloroacetate esterase reaction parallels the peroxidase activity and is found in azurophilic granules (Fig. 4–94). In some cases blasts may be peroxidase positive and naphthol AS-D chloroacetate esterase negative, indicating that peroxidase appears earlier in development. The chloroacetate esterase activity is weak or negative in monocytes and negative in lymphocytes.

Alpha-Naphthol Acetate Esterase (Yam *et al.*, 1971)

REAGENTS

1. Fixative: Buffered formalin and acetone: Formaldehyde, 37 per cent, 25 ml.; Na_2HPO_4, 20 mg.; KH_2PO_4, 100 mg.; distilled water, 30 ml.; acetone, 45 ml.

2. Buffer: Sorenson's phosphate buffer (M/15, pH = 7.6).

3. Incubation mixture: Add in the following order:

Buffer	44.5 ml.
Hexazotized pararosanilin (1.5 ml. Parasanilin‡ hydrochloride plus 1.5 ml. fresh 4 per cent sodium nitrite)	3.0 ml.
Alpha-naphthol acetate,§ 50 mg. dissolved in 2.5 ml. ethylene glycol monomethyl ether	

Filter mixture through Seitz filter.
4. Harris hematoxylin

PROCEDURE

1. Place air-dried blood or marrow films in fixative for 30 seconds at 4° C. Wash in running tap water.

2. Place slides in incubation mixture for 60 minutes. Wash in running water.

3. Counterstain with Harris hematoxylin for 10 minutes.

INTERPRETATION. Alpha-naphthol acetate esterase activity is found in monocytes but not in neutrophils or neutrophil precursors, other granulocytes, or lymphocytes (Fig. 4–95). It may be found, however, in activated or atypical lymphocytes, in lymphocytes in imprints of active lymphoid tissue, and probably in the poorly differentiated lymphocytes of some lymphomas.

Periodic Acid-Schiff (PAS) Reaction (Hayhoe *et al.*, 1964)

PRINCIPLE. Periodic acid (HIO_4) is an oxidizing agent that converts hydroxy groups on adjacent carbon atoms to aldehydes. The resulting dialdehydes are combined with Schiff's reagent to give a red-colored product. A positive reaction is therefore seen with polysaccharides, mucopolysaccharides, and glycoproteins.

REAGENTS

1. Fixative: Mix 10 ml. of 37 per cent formaldehyde with 90 ml. of absolute ethanol.

2. Periodic acid, 5 gm., is dissolved in 500 ml. of distilled water. Stored in a dark bottle, the solution is good for three months.

3. Schiff's reagent: Dissolve 5 gm. of basic fuchsin in 500 ml. of hot distilled water, and filter after it has cooked. Saturate with sulfur dioxide gas by bubbling for 1 hour. Extract the solution with 2 gm. of activated charcoal for a few seconds in a hood and immediately filter through Whatman No. 1 filter paper into a dark bottle. The solution keeps for 2 to 3 months.

4. Harris hematoxylin

PROCEDURE

1. Place air-dried blood and marrow films or imprints in fixative for 10 minutes. Wash briefly with tap water.

2. Control slides are exposed to digestion with saliva (salivary amylase) for 30 minutes. Place slides in periodic acid for 10 minutes. Wash briefly with tap water and blot dry.

3. Immerse slides in Schiff's reagent for 30 minutes.

4. Rinse slides in several changes of sulfur dioxide water for 20 to 30 minutes.

5. Wash for 5 to 10 minutes in tap water and counterstain with Harris hematoxylin for 10 minutes.

INTERPRETATION. In blood cells a positive PAS reaction usually indicates the presence of glycogen. This is demonstrated by digestion with amylase and consequent loss of staining. Neutrophils react at all stages of development, the most strongly in the mature stage. The same is true of eosinophils. The glycogen is not in the granules, but in background cytoplasm. Myeloblasts contain a few small PAS-positive granules. Monocytes have a faint staining reaction in the form of fine granules. Lymphocytes may contain a few small or large granules. Normoblasts are normally PAS negative.

*Nutritional Biochemicals Corp., Cleveland, Ohio.
†Sigma Chemical Co., St. Louis, Mo.
‡National Biological Stains and Reagents, Division of Allied Chemical Co., Morristown, N.J.
§Sigma Chemical Co., St. Louis, Mo.

Figure 4–105

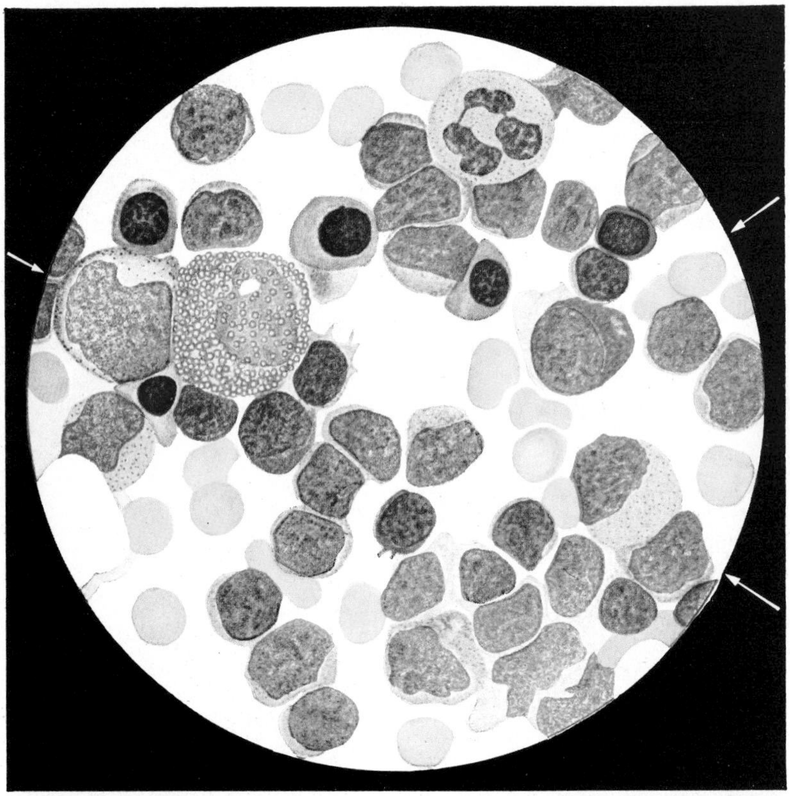

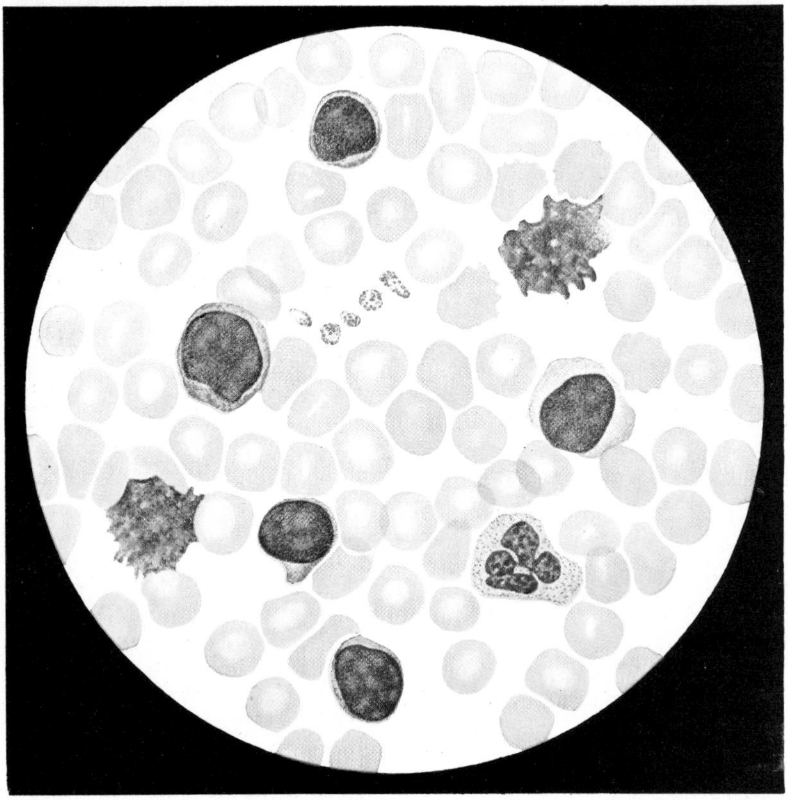

Figure 4–106

(*See opposite page for legends.*)

In erythroleukemia (Fig. 4–97) and in thalassemia some of the erythroid precursors are PAS positive. This is true to a lesser extent in iron-deficiency anemia and sideroblastic anemias. In acute lymphocytic leukemia the lymphoblasts often contain large coarse clumps of PAS-positive material. In chronic lymphocytic leukemia and lymphomas as well as in infectious mononucleosis the lymphocytes may have increased numbers of PAS-positive granules.

CHRONIC GRANULOCYTIC LEUKEMIA (CGL)

Clinical Findings. CGL occurs primarily in young and middle-aged adults. The onset is insidious and the disorder may be discovered accidentally on a routine blood test. The patient may have symptoms of anemia, or he simply may complain of malaise. The spleen enlarges progressively, and the patient begins to lose weight and have fever and night sweats associated with the increased metabolism due to increased granulocyte turnover. The discomfort associated with an enlarged spleen may bring the patient to the doctor. Infarcts in the spleen may produce left upper quadrant pain. Excessive bleeding or bruising may occur in the later stages of the disease. Lymphadenopathy is not usually present.

Laboratory Findings

Blood. The leukocyte count is usually over 50,000 per μl. and may exceed 300,000 per μl. The differential count is characteristic. There is a complete spectrum of granulocytic cells, from a few myeloblasts down to mature neutrophils. Myeloblasts are less than 10 per cent of the cells. Two peaks are present: myelocytes and neutrophils both exceed the other cell types. This is a feature that helps to exclude other myeloproliferative disorders (Galton and Spiers, 1971). Eosinophil precursors and eosinophils may be increased. Increased basophils are a prominent feature of the disease. Monocytes may be increased in an occasional patient.

Early, no anemia is present, but it appears during the course of the disease as a result of decreased RBC production. Erythrocytes are normochromic and normocytic. A few normoblasts may be present.

Thrombocytosis occurs in early stages of the disease in some patients. As the marrow is replaced by granulocytic proliferation, the megakaryocytes are crowded out and thrombocytopenia supervenes. Another factor in producing thrombocytopenia is the large pool of platelets in the spleen.

Marrow. The marrow is markedly hypercellular due primarily to granulocytic proliferation, with all stages represented. Eosinophil and basophil precursors are often increased. Normoblasts tend to be decreased. Frequently the marrow cannot be aspirated because of increased reticulin in the marrow, which can be demonstrated on marrow biopsy.

It is well to remember that even a typical bone marrow is not diagnostic of CGL. On the other hand, the diagnosis can be made from the peripheral blood film alone.

Neutrophil Alkaline Phosphatase (p. 273). The neutrophil alkaline phosphatase (NAP) is greatly reduced or absent in most patients with chronic granulocytic leukemia. It is greatly elevated in polycythemia vera; elevated, normal, or low in myelofibrosis with myeloid metaplasia; and normal or elevated in leukemoid reactions (Dameshek and Gunz, 1964). Although a low NAP is characteristic of chronic granulocytic leukemia, it is not specific, for low values may be found in paroxysmal nocturnal hemoglobinuria and in some cases of pernicious anemia, infectious mononucleosis, and aplastic anemia; these conditions do not, however, lead to diagnostic confusion. During remissions of chronic granulocytic leukemia with a normal appearing blood picture, in some cases, the NAP continues to be low; in others, the NAP returns to normal and may increase in response to infection as it does in normal individuals.

Chromosomal Abnormalities. In direct bone marrow preparations and in metaphases of cultured peripheral blood, most patients with

Figure 4–105. Chronic lymphocytic leukemia, marrow. A monotonous picture. The predominant cell is the lymphocyte. It has replaced the native marrow cell to a considerable degree. The arrow at 2 o'clock points to a plasma cell with its eccentrically located nucleus. At 4 o'clock is a neutrophilic myelocyte. At 9 o'clock there is a promyelocyte, above and below it are normoblasts, and to its right is an eosinophilic myelocyte. (From L. Heilmeyer and H. Begemann: Atlas der Klinischen Hämatologie und Cytologie. Springer, 1955.)

Figure 4–106. Chronic lymphocytic leukemia, peripheral blood. The five lymphocytes have a somewhat less dense chromatin. This is the only deviation from the normal, and even that is not impressive. The two degenerating cells are commonly seen in this disease. (From L. Heilmeyer and H. Begemann: Atlas der Klinischen Hämatologie und Cytologie. Springer, 1955.)

Figure 4–107

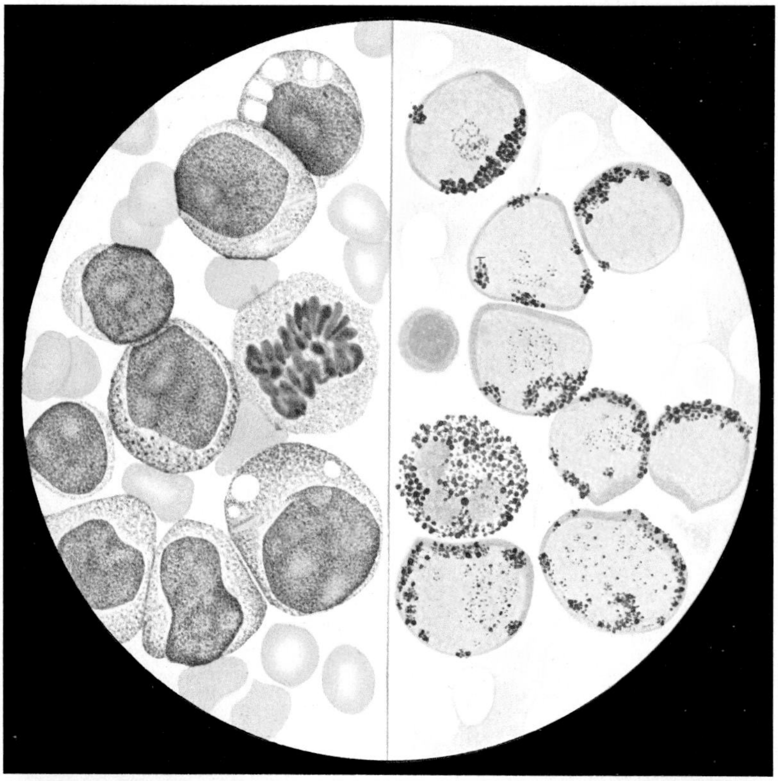

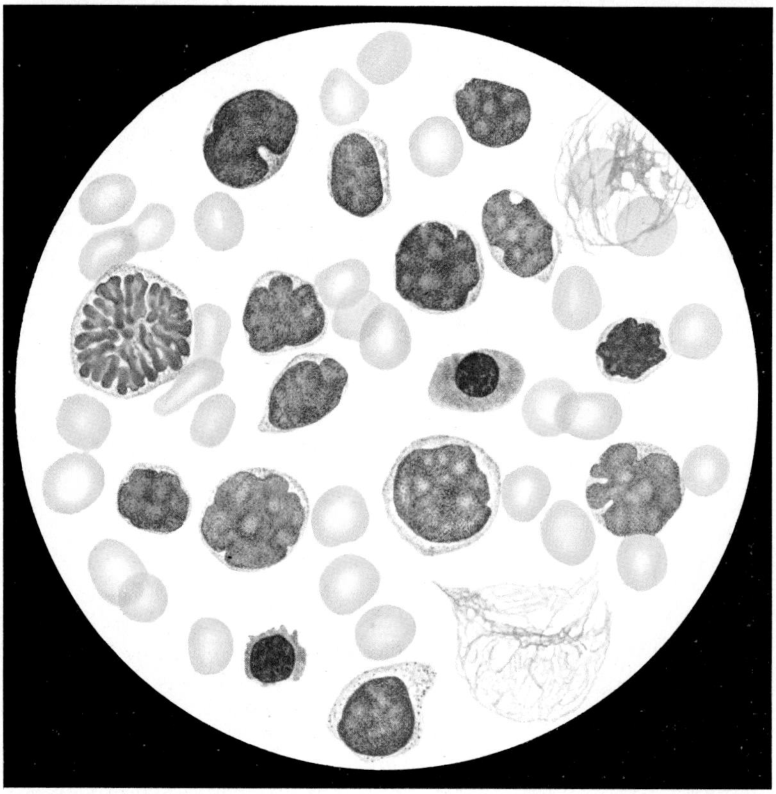

Figure 4–108

(*See opposite page for legends.*)

chronic granulocytic leukemia have a unique abnormality: an abnormally small acrocentric chromosome in the 21-22 group. In most cases, it appears to be chromosome number 22. This was first described in 1960 by Nowell and Hungerford and is called the Philadelphia (Ph^1) chromosome. The Ph^1 chromosome is present in blood and marrow cells during relapse and can be found in the marrow but not the blood during remission. It appears that the Ph^1 chromosome is present in precursors of granulocytes, in erythroblasts, and in megakaryocytes, but not in lymphocytes or skin cells.

The small proportion of patients with chronic granulocytic leukemia who lack the Ph^1 chromosome are characteristic in most other respects: average age, spleen size, marrow and blood picture, and NAP values. On the average, however, the patients in this Ph^1-negative group have less elevated white blood cell counts, have lower platelet counts, include a larger proportion of children, respond less well to therapy, and have a shorter survival (Tjio *et al.*, 1966).

Other Findings. Serum vitamin B_{12} and vitamin B_{12}-binding proteins are sometimes greatly increased. These are thought to reflect the total blood granulocyte pool. The serum muramidase is also increased.

Course. Treatment with busulfan or radiation usually yields one or more remissions. Yet, in most patients, the disease transforms into a more aggressive phase after two to three years. This may be in the form of a "blast transformation," with the rapid appearance of large numbers of myeloblasts and promyelocytes, an appearance resembling acute granulocytic leukemia. (Incidentally, Auer rods are rarely found in the blastic phase of CGL). Increasing numbers of basophils or of bizarre monocytes may also be the morphologic indicator of a transformation. If cytogenetic studies are done, other chromosomal abnormalities in addition to the Ph^1 may appear. The NAP tends to go up in the terminal phase of CGL.

CHRONIC LYMPHOCYTIC LEUKEMIA (CLL)

Clinical Findings. CLL is rare under the age of 40; most cases occur over the age of 60. It is more common in men. The onset is insidious and the disease is commonly discovered by chance during the investigation of another problem. Lymphadenopathy, asymptomatic or associated with symptoms such as weakness, fatigue, anorexia, and weight loss, may cause the patient to come to the physician. Enlarged lymph nodes are usually evident, and frequently hepatosplenomegaly is also found, though splenomegaly is of lesser degree than that seen in CGL or myelofibrosis with myeloid metaplasia (MMM). Skin lesions, gastrointestinal infiltration and symptoms, and bone pain or tenderness are rather common.

Blood. The leukocyte count is usually between 30,000 and 200,000 per μl., and 80 to 90 per cent of these are small lymphocytes. Damaged or smudged cells are common on the film, probably indicating fragile cells. Occasionally the leukocyte count by electronic counter will be significantly lower than a hemacytometer count because of the more fragile cells. It is advisable to check the electronic count by hemacytometer on new cases, and thereafter to check the appearance of the blood film with the count from the machine, keeping this problem in mind.

The lymphocytes are monotonously similar in appearance and usually look normal. Nuclear chromatin may be coarsely condensed and more sharply separated by parachromatin than in normal lymphocytes or, in some cases, the chromatin is less condensed than normal. Sometimes nucleoli are evident in many of the lymphocytes. Size variation is minimal. Cytoplasm is of small to moderate amount. In a minority of patients a small proportion of the lymphocytes are immature. Usually these are prolymphocytes or reticular lymphocytes (transformed lymphocytes).

Figure 4–107. Acute granulocytic leukemia, peripheral blood. The large myeloblasts with the immature granular and reticulated chromatin and the somewhat indistinct nucleoli are characteristic. The cytoplasm shows no granules in some of the cells and varying numbers of different distinctness in the others. The peroxidase stain in the right half of the smear shows varying numbers of oxidase-positive granules in all the cells. That all cells have the peroxidase-positive granules, whereas granules are seen in only a few of those stained with the regular stain, indicates that the granules demonstrated by the two stains are not identical. The Auer bodies in three of the cells on the left side are characteristic for this type of leukemia. (From L. Heilmeyer and H. Begemann: Atlas der Klinischen Hämatologie und Cytologie. Springer, 1955.)

Figure 4–108. Acute lymphocytic leukemia, marrow. The lymphoblasts have immature nuclei, many of which are indented. The chromatin pattern is delicate. Usually only one or two nucleoli are present in lymphoblasts; all the light staining areas in the nuclei do not represent nucleoli. Two degenerating cells, two normoblasts, and one cell in mitosis are present. (From L. Heilmeyer and H. Begemann: Atlas der Klinischen Hämatologie und Cytologie. Springer, 1955.)

Figure 4–109

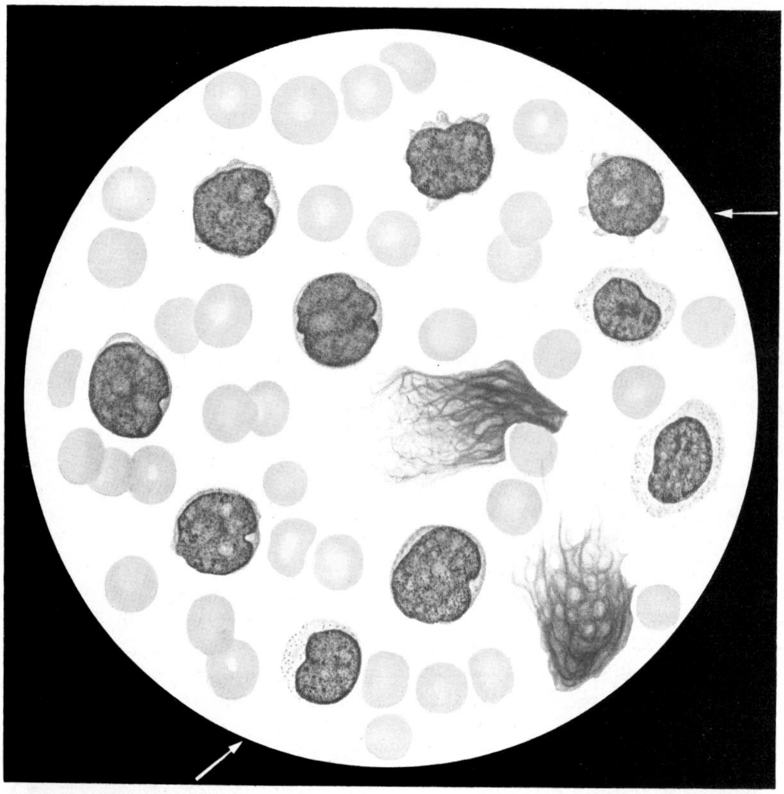

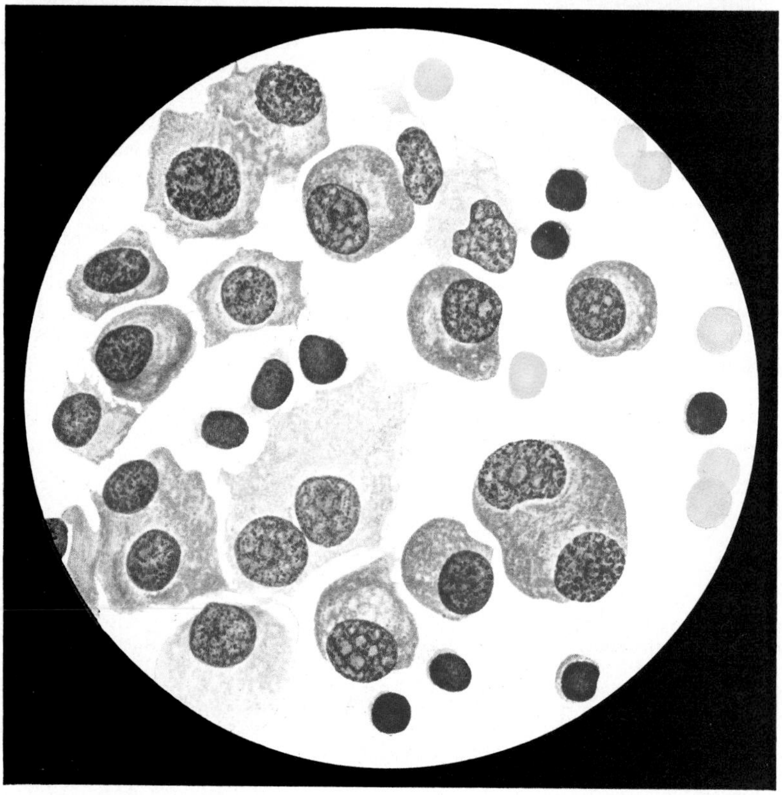

Figure 4–110

(*See opposite page for legends.*)

Often there is neither anemia nor thrombocytopenia at the time of diagnosis. Anemia due to impaired production does develop as the marrow is replaced by leukemic cells. Autoimmune hemolytic anemia develops in about 10 per cent of patients with advanced disease; among the leukemias, it has the greatest frequency in CLL. Thrombocytopenia is often slight and occasionally becomes severe as the disease progresses, so that hemorrhagic manifestations appear.

Marrow. Very early in the disease marrow involvement may be lacking. The usual early finding, however, is the presence of slight to moderate lymphocytosis. Since the lymphocytes are morphologically normal, examination of marrow smears may be equivocal. Histologic sections of aspirated particles or biopsy material may then be very helpful. Small to medium-sized areas of lymphocytes are present and have indistinct margins; lymphocytes are infiltrating into adjacent hematopoietic tissue. If an autoimmune hemolytic anemia is present, erythropoiesis becomes prominent. Later in the disease, lymphocytes overrun the marrow, largely replacing hematopoietic tissue.

Differential Diagnosis. Persistent lymphocytosis in excess of 15,000 lymphocytes per μl. over a period of several weeks or months in an adult over 40 years of age is good evidence for CLL. Marrow examination, especially histologic sections, should confirm this diagnosis. In children lymphocyte counts in excess of 100,000 per μl., morphologically mimicking CLL, may be found transiently in infectious lymphocytosis or pertussis.

In contrast to CLL with normal-appearing lymphocytes is a somewhat less common variety, *lymphosarcoma cell leukemia*. In the latter the cells have variably condensed chromatin, usually less than in CLL, and notched nuclei. Deep clefts in the nuclei are characteristic. This type of lymphocytic leukemia is associated with poorly differentiated lymphocytic lymphoma, which is almost always nodular in its histologic pattern. In CLL, on the other hand, the histologic pattern of the involved lymph node is a well-differentiated lymphocytic lymphoma that is diffuse.

Other Findings. Most patients with CLL have no detectable chromosomal abnormalities.

Hypogammaglobulinemia develops in many patients with CLL; all classes of immunoglobulins may be affected. Along with neutropenia, this defect in humoral immunity accounts for an increased likelihood of infectious complications. In about 5 per cent of patients there is a monoclonal immunoglobulin elevation; usually this is IgM.

In studies thus far, virtually all patients with CLL have had surface immunoglobulins on most of the leukemic cells, indicating that they are probably B-lymphocytes (Aisenberg and Bloch, 1972). It appears that the surface immunoglobulin is usually restricted to IgM and to a single light chain, supporting the clonal origin of the leukemic cells. The fact that most of the lymphocytes are B-cells would explain their lack of responsiveness to phytohemagglutinin, which is considered to be a T-cell characteristic. Lymphosarcoma cells (cells from poorly differentiated lymphocytic lymphoma) have been found to have greater concentrations of immunoglobulin, again mainly IgM, on their surfaces.

Course. As the disease becomes extensive, problems with anemia (myelophthisic or hemolytic), thrombocytopenia with bleeding, or infection tend to prevail. The duration of life from diagnosis is quite variable, the median survival being between three and four years, but many patients live much longer than the median. Very rarely (in contrast to CGL) does a blastic phase supervene in CLL; in those rare cases the blasts morphologically resemble reticular lymphocytes ("transformed" lymphocytes) or hematopoietic reticulum cells.

OTHER FORMS OF LEUKEMIA

Leukemic Reticuloendotheliosis (Histiocytic Leukemia; "Hairy Cell" Leukemia) (Bouroncle *et al.*, 1958). This rare disorder is clinically variable in its manifestations. It has an insidious onset and is characterized by reticuloendothelial (RE) cell proliferation in the RE organs and blood. Splenomegaly is the predominant physical finding.

Figure 4–109. Acute lymphocytic leukemia, peripheral blood. This preparation is from the same adult patient as in Figure 5–99. The lymphocytes at 3 o'clock (just below the arrow) and at 4 and 7 o'clock are more mature as indicated by the presence of azurophilic granules in their cytoplasm and, in the case of the lymphocyte at 4 o'clock, also by the more compact structure of the chromatin. (From L. Heilmeyer and H. Begemann: Atlas der Klinischen Hämatologie und Cytologie. Springer, 1955.)

Figure 4–110. Multiple myeloma, marrow. The abnormal plasma cells, like normal plasma cells, have a paranuclear *Hof* and an eccentric nucleus. Multinucleated plasma cells, though seen occasionally in reactive plasmacytosis, are not so common as in myeloma. Abnormal here is the lack of chromatin condensation and prominence of the nucleoli (i.e., immaturity of the nucleus) compared with the degree of cytoplasmic development and with the lesser immaturity usually seen in reactive plasmacytosis. (From L. Heilmeyer and H. Begemann: Atlas der Klinischen Hämatologie und Cytologie. Springer, 1955.)

Pancytopenia is the usual finding, with variable numbers of RE cells. In the majority of cases bone marrow aspiration is difficult. Marrow biopsy shows a marrow that varies in cellularity, often having both hypocellular and hypercellular areas. RE cells are considerably increased in number.

Morphologically the cells are medium sized (10 to 20 μm. diameter), with round to oval nuclei, though many are notched or dumbbell shaped. The chromatin pattern is usually uniformly reticular, and nucleoli are small and inconspicuous. In some cells chromatin is more condensed, resembling that of a lymphocyte. The cytoplasm is moderate in amount, often has numerous hair-like projections and frayed borders, and stains gray with Wright's stain.

Cytochemically these cells contain acid phosphatase which is resistant to inhibition by tartrate; this is in contrast to the isozymes of acid phosphatase present in other hemic cells (Yam *et al.,* 1971b). This reaction separates these cases from lymphoma and lymphocytic and monocytic leukemias.

Functionally it appears that some cells with these characteristics may be lymphocytic in character, i.e., synthesis of IgG, lack of adherence to nylon, lack of phagocytic properties (Rubin *et al.,* 1969). The clinical course is usually chronic, but may be acute or subacute.

Stem Cell Leukemia. This is a variety of acute leukemia in which the predominant cells are primitive undifferentiated leukocytes that cannot be classified as one of the three blast forms. Using cytochemical methods in classifying acute leukemia, Hayhoe *et al.* (1964) were able to classify all cases of acute leukemia in other previously described categories, virtually eliminating the category of stem cell leukemia. We believe that it occurs, but is very rare.

Plasma Cell Leukemia. Often in multiple myeloma a few plasma cells are found in the peripheral blood. Only in the rare instances of myeloma in which large numbers of plasma cells circulate is the term plasma cell leukemia used.

Chloroma. Rarely in acute myeloblastic leukemia there is formation of tumors originating from periosteum, especially of skull, orbits, nasal sinuses, ribs, and vertebrae. Exophthalmus with disturbances of vision may occur. The sectioned surface of the tumor shows a green color, and the tumor contains large amounts of verdoperoxidase and protoporphyrin. It fades on exposure and can be restored with hydrogen peroxide and preserved by glycerin. There are aleukemic and leukemic forms, the latter with myeloblasts in the blood. Clinically the latter cases are identical with acute granulocytic leukemia.

Myeloblastoma. This localized tumor of myeloblasts differs from chloroma only by absence of pigment. Like chloroma it is exceedingly rare, since the tissue involvement in the acute granulocytic leukemia is a diffuse infiltrative process.

Eosinophilic Leukemia. This occurs but is extremely rare. Acute and chronic forms have been described, with tissue changes similar in every way to those in other forms of granulocytic leukemia, except that most of the cells in the tissues as well as in the circulating blood have been eosinophilic granulocytes of varying stages of differentiation. It is generally regarded to be a variant of acute or chronic granulocytic leukemia, as the case may be, since other myeloid elements are usually involved, but to a lesser degree. It may be difficult or impossible to differentiate this lesion from reactive hyperplastic changes, especially early in the disease. Leukocytosis and eosinophilia, no matter how high, are not sufficient to establish the diagnosis of leukemia; both can be seen in parasitic infestation. But the diagnosis can be made when there are, in addition, excessive immaturity of the cells, enlargement of spleen and lymph nodes, progressive anemia, thrombocytopenia, and normoblastemia.

Basophilic Leukemia. Extremely high basophil counts overshadowing other myeloid involvement are seen rarely in granulocytic leukemia. Both chronic and acute cases have been described. A basophilic phase of CGL is sometimes seen as part of a terminal metamorphosis in the type of proliferating cell. It should be kept in mind that mast cells that resemble basophilic granulocytes are present in large numbers in the skin and marrow in urticaria pigmentosa.

Neutrophilic Leukemia. This is similar to eosinophilic and basophilic leukemia, but the cell type is the segmented granulocyte with very few immature forms. It is extremely rare.

Lymphosarcoma Cell Leukemia. This is discussed in the following section.

Malignant Lymphoma

Malignant lymphoma is a neoplastic proliferation of one of the cell types of the lymphopoietic-reticular tissue. Stem cells, lymphocytes, or histiocytes are the cells involved. If a mixture of more than one cell type appears to be present, it probably represents a variation in the size, configuration, or degree of differentiation of one cell type, rather than separate cell lines (Lukes, 1971).

Usually lymphoma begins in and involves lymph nodes predominantly, though other sites such as the spleen and the gastrointestinal tract are frequent areas of origin as well.

As the disease progresses, proliferation spreads to lymphoid tissue beyond the site of origin. In advanced disease, infiltrations of neoplastic cells are found in many organs throughout the body. When lymphoma originates in extranodal tissue, e.g., the stomach or lung, the course is likely to be more benign than otherwise.

NON-HODGKIN'S LYMPHOMAS

Classification. A widely used classification is given in the left column of Table 4–23 for non-Hodgkin's lymphomas. Classification is based upon the cell type involved and the pattern of histologic involvement, whether nodular or diffuse. The common criteria for diagnosis are obliteration of normal lymph node architecture (including germinal centers) by the proliferating cells, infiltration of the capsule of the lymph node, and cellular atypia. Lukes (1971) has pointed out, however, that all these criteria can be fulfilled in some severe reactive processes, and he has emphasized the importance of positive identification of the specific cell type.

In addition to morphologic criteria for cell identification, newer techniques are beginning to allow more precise cellular identification in lymphoma and leukemia.

B-Lymphocytes are identified by the presence of surface immunoglobulin, and of receptors for C_3 on the membrane of the cells as determined by immunofluorescence technique. T-Lymphocytes are identified by their ability to bind sheep red blood cells in rosettes, and to undergo blast transformation in response to phytohemagglutinin (PHA). It seems clear that the current understanding and, hence, the classification of lymphomas and related lymphoid disorders will be modified and refined by using these and other techniques (Preud'homme and Seligmann, 1972).

Lymphocytic Lymphoma, Well Differentiated. The cell type is the small lymphocyte, with clumped chromatin indistinguishable from the normal lymphocyte. Mitoses are rarely seen. The pattern of node and marrow involvement is more often diffuse than nodular. Though it may begin in lymph nodes, the accumulative process involves the bone marrow quite early in its course, and the blood lymphocyte count is then elevated. The usual diagnosis, therefore, is chronic lymphatic leukemia rather than well differentiated lymphocytic lymphoma. It is essentially the same disease. CLL appears to be a B-cell disease since in most patients studied the lymphocytes have surface immunoglobulins (see p. 285).

This is a disorder of late adult life. Hypogammaglobulinemia is frequent, and autoimmune hemolytic anemia occurs in 10 to 20 per cent of patients.

Lymphocytic Lymphoma, Poorly Differentiated. The proliferating cell is a lymphocyte with a nucleus which has less condensation of chromatin than the normal circulating lymphocyte, irregular, cleft, or indented nuclear shape, and small inconspicuous nucleoli. The cytoplasm is scant in amount. It is similar to the cell in the germinal centers of normal lymph nodes. The pattern of node involvement is usually nodular, especially in adults. Spread to the marrow and other organs tends to be in nodular or discrete masses rather diffuse. A few poorly differentiated lymphocytes occasionally enter the circulation. Late in the course of the disease in about 20 per cent of patients the marrow becomes more heavily involved, and larger numbers of these cleft or notched immature lymphocytes are found in the blood. The terms *"lymphosarcoma cell leukemia"* and "leukosarcoma" have been used to designate this manifestation of the disease. These terms, however, are better reserved for the small proportion of cases in which the leukemic process is found early in the course of the disease, at the time of diagnosis (Sheehan, 1971). In this case the tissue and marrow involvement tends to be diffuse rather than nodular. The cells vary from the cleft or notched nucleus to a larger cell with

Table 4–23. CLASSIFICATION OF THE NON-HODGKIN'S LYMPHOMAS*

LYMPHOMA (NODULAR OR DIFFUSE)	CELL TYPE INVOLVED	LEUKEMIC VARIANT
Lymphocytic, well differentiated	Differentiated lymphocyte	Chronic lymphocytic leukemia
Lymphocytic, poorly differentiated	Poorly differentiated lymphocyte Lymphoblast	Lymphosarcoma cell leukemia Acute lymphocytic leukemia
Stem cell (undifferentiated)	Stem cell	Stem cell leukemia (rare)
Histiocytic	Histiocyte	

*Classification is from Lukes, R. J.: *In* Ultmann, J. E., Griem, M. L., Kirsten, W. H., and Wissler, R. W. (eds.): Current Concepts in the Management of Lymphoma and Leukemia, New York, Springer-Verlag, Inc., 1971, p. 6.

more abundant basophilic cytoplasm, a reticular chromatin pattern and one or more large nucleoli.

Poorly differentiated lymphocytic lymphoma is a disease of adults more often than children. In contrast to adults, the involvement in children is usually diffuse and leukemic rather than nodular and aleukemic; in other words, notched cells of this type may be found instead of (sometimes in addition to) lymphoblasts as a variant of acute lymphocytic leukemia of childhood.

Stem Cell Lymphoma. The cell type is a medium-sized blast with round to oval nucleus, reticular chromatin, small nucleoli, and a moderate amount of cytoplasm. The cell resembles a hemocytoblast or some of the primitive cells in a normal germinal center. In tissue sections the cells appear to grow as a syncytium; macrophages with abundant pale cytoplasm interspersed among the tumor cells give the "starry-sky" histologic appearance.

This lymphoma is rarely leukemic, even with marrow involvement. It is seen in children in this country and has a high incidence in children in Central Africa, where it is known as Burkitt's lymphoma.

Histiocytic Lymphoma. Formerly called reticulum cell sarcoma, this variety is characterized by a variable cell type. A large cell with an oval nucleus, reticular chromatin, a large prominent nucleolus, and abundant cytoplasm forms one cell type. When pleomorphic, this form has multiple nuclei, which may resemble the Sternberg-Reed cells of Hodgkin's disease. Another variant has a smaller nucleus and nucleolus and more abundant cytoplasm, which occasionally may show evidence of phagocytosis. As with stem cell lymphoma, histiocytic lymphoma is rarely leukemic, though a few cells may appear in the blood late in the course of the disease.

Generally in lymphomas, depression of other hematopoietic cell lines (the red cells, platelets, and granulocytes) occurs either chronically, as a result of marrow involvement by the tumor late in the disease, or acutely, as a result of chemotherapy or radiation treatment.

HODGKIN'S DISEASE

The right side of Table 4–24 shows the current classification of Hodgkin's disease, which was proposed at the Rye conference (Lukes *et al.*, 1966b). This is generally regarded as a malignant lymphoma, but has different histology in that the cells reacting to the neoplasm usually predominate rather than the neoplastic cells themselves. The hallmark of Hodgkin's disease is the Sternberg-Reed cell, which is a large binucleated or multinucleated cell with each nucleus bearing a very large nucleolus.

Hodgkin's disease may occur from early childhood to old age. Increased frequency is noted between 15 and 35 years and after age 50. Males predominate, especially in childhood; disease in females under age 30 is usually of nodular sclerosis in type.

The *lymphocytic predominance* group histologically shows a variable degree of histiocytic proliferation without necrosis or fibrosis and few Sternberg-Reed cells. Prognosis is best in this group, which tends to be localized to the cervical nodes and occurs most frequently in young males.

Nodular sclerosis is characterized by broad bands of collagen separating nodules of lymphoid tissue and the presence of "lacunar cells," which are large atypical histiocytes

Table 4–24. CLASSIFICATIONS OF HODGKIN'S DISEASE*

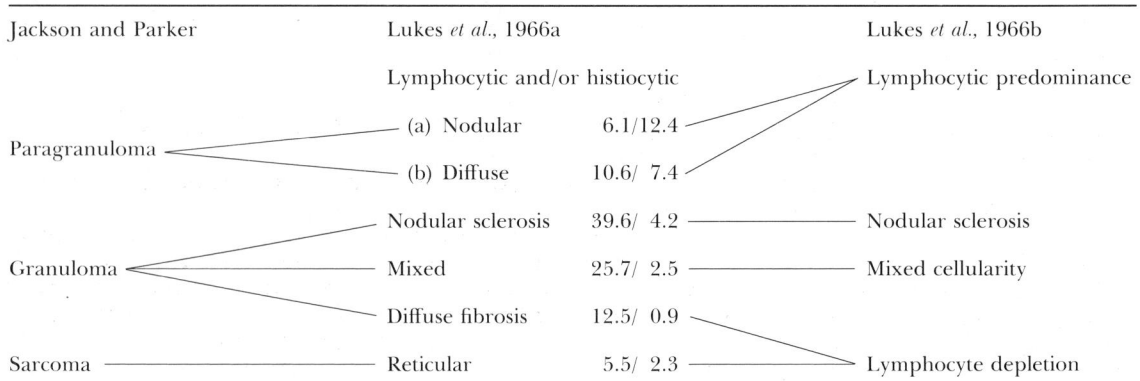

Jackson and Parker	Lukes *et al.*, 1966a		Lukes *et al.*, 1966b
	Lymphocytic and/or histiocytic		Lymphocytic predominance
Paragranuloma	(a) Nodular	6.1/12.4	
	(b) Diffuse	10.6/ 7.4	
Granuloma	Nodular sclerosis	39.6/ 4.2	Nodular sclerosis
	Mixed	25.7/ 2.5	Mixed cellularity
	Diffuse fibrosis	12.5/ 0.9	
Sarcoma	Reticular	5.5/ 2.3	Lymphocyte depletion

*The figures in the left column represent the per cent of cases of that type and the figures in the right column represent the median survival in years for all clinical stages of that type from the series reported by Lukes, R. J., Butler, J. J., and Hicks, E. B.: Cancer *19*:317, 1966.

with abundant pale cytoplasm. Sternberg-Reed cells are difficult to find. This variety of Hodgkin's disease is common and often is first discovered as a mediastinal mass in a young woman.

The *mixed type* has a variety of cell types: lymphocytes, plasma cells, eosinophils, histiocytes, and Sternberg-Reed cells, which are often quite numerous. Necrosis and disorderly fibrosis may be present.

The rare *lymphocyte depletion* type is more often diffuse fibrosis than reticular and is an acute febrile illness without lymphadenopathy associated with pancytopenia and lymphocytopenia. The lack of leukocytosis and thrombocytosis and more frequent involvement of the bone marrow contrast with other forms of Hodgkin's disease (Neiman *et al.,* 1973).

Clinical staging is currently employed to determine the extent of the disease at the time of diagnosis. Besides history and physical examination, extensive radiographic studies, radioisotope scans, CBC, platelet count, erythrocyte sedimentation rate, leukocyte alkaline phosphatase, bone marrow biopsy, liver function studies, urinalysis, and skin tests for delayed hypersensitivity are performed. Stage I disease is limited to lymph nodes in one anatomic region or two contiguous regions on one side of the diaphragm. Stage II disease involves more than two contiguous regions or two noncontiguous regions on one side of the diaphragm. Stage III disease is present on both sides of the diaphragm but confined to lymphoid tissue. Stage IV disease involves bone marrow or any other organ, in addition to lymphoid tissue. All stages are additionally classified as A if systemic symptoms are absent, B if they are present. This extensive diagnostic approach is to define areas of involvement and facilitate radiation therapy, which is combined with chemotherapy. It is part of the current aggressive approach to the management of Hodgkin's disease, which is resulting in longer survival and even apparent cure in some patients.

Hodgkin's disease is the lymphoma which has thus far been most studied immunologically. Cell-mediated immunity is defective when extensive disease is present; Hodgkin's disease is considered a disorder of T-lymphocyte function (Aisenberg, 1973).

Blood Findings. Normocytic, sometimes severe, anemia is seen in about 50 per cent of cases.

The leukocyte count may be elevated, normal, or reduced (leukopenic). The differential count shows neutrophilia, lymphocytopenia, monocytosis, and eosinophilia. Either all or any combination of these may be present.

Neutrophilic leukocytosis is seen, especially when lymph nodes are involved, and neutropenia, when bone marrow is involved. The blood changes seem to depend on the stage of the disease and on some individual, as yet unknown, factors. The neutrophil alkaline phosphatase is elevated during activity of the disease; it returns to normal during remissions.

The most frequent finding is a moderate leukocytosis, with white cell counts ranging from 12,000 to 25,000 per μl. and a relative and even absolute lymphopenia. In the differential count the lymphocytes may decrease below 10 per cent. A slight shift to the left may be present in the neutrophils. As a rule, lymphopenia is prognostically a poor omen.

Monocytosis is frequent, with values of 10 per cent or higher. Eosinophilia has been described in about 20 per cent of patients and may be extreme. The platelet count may be increased, normal, or decreased, the latter especially with marrow involvement.

Both the histologic changes noted above and the blood and marrow findings appear to be manifestations of different host responses to the disease.

Marrow Findings. Frequently there is a granulocytic hyperplasia with a shift to the left, slight monocytosis, and eosinophilia. As a rule, findings are not characteristic. Amyloid degeneration of various grades is sometimes present in various organs and with it plasma cell hyperplasia in the marrow.

If marrow biopsy is performed in patients with systemic symptoms or with clinical Stage III or Stage IV disease, it will be positive in about 10 per cent of patients (Rosenberg, 1971). Positive biopsy is interpreted as: (1) the presence of Sternberg-Reed cells in an appropriate pleomorphic cellular stroma; or, less commonly (2) abnormal infiltration of lymphocytes, histiocytes, and fibrosis without classic Sternberg-Reed cells, but with documented Hodgkin's disease in other sites.

In the rare lymphocyte depletion type of Hodgkin's disease, dissemination is widespread and bone marrow is involved in most cases.

Blood Protein Disorders

Immunoglobulins are discussed in Chapter 9, page 571 ff.

Polyclonal gammopathy refers to an increase in the serum of several different immunoglobulins which are the products of many different clones of plasma cells. This is usually a response to antigenic stimulation.

Monoclonal gammopathy refers to an increase in the serum of one specific class, subclass, and type of immunoglobulin molecule (or fragment thereof); this is the product of plasma cells or lymphocytes which originated from a single cell or clone. Monoclonal gammopathy is found in multiple myeloma, some lymphomas (including Waldenström's macroglobulinemia and heavy chain diseases), some patients with primary amyloidosis, a few patients with carcinoma, and some individuals with no known underlying disease. The latter group may comprise up to one-third of all monoclonal gammopathies (Ritzmann *et al.*, 1972); it includes primarily elderly individuals who have a lower concentration of the homogeneous immunoglobulin (less than 2 gm./dl.) which does not change for long periods of time.

MULTIPLE MYELOMA

This is a neoplastic proliferation of plasma cells or morphologically abnormal plasma cells (myeloma cells), primarily occurring in the bone marrow either in nodules or diffusely. Though plasma cells also proliferate in lymph nodes and spleen, these organs are rarely enlarged.

Multiple myeloma is rare under age 40. Bone pain is the commonest symptom, and pathologic fractures are frequent. Neurologic symptoms may be prominent from encroachment of tumor which has broken through the bony cortex on spinal nerves or spinal cord. Bone destruction leads to calcium mobilization, with increase of calcium in the serum and metastatic calcification. The growth of myeloma cells in the marrow produces multiple tumors, which appear on x-ray as multiple punched-out osteoporotic lesions; occasionally the growth is diffuse and appears as diffuse osteoporosis. An unusual propensity to infection is common because of impaired production of antibodies.

Blood. There is usually a normochromic normocytic anemia; normoblasts may be present in the blood. The leukocyte count is slightly decreased, normal, or slightly increased. Occasionally young neutrophils or even myeloblasts may be found. Usually myeloma cells can be located if careful search of the blood smears or buffy coat smears is made; on occasion, myeloma cells may be extremely numerous (plasma cell leukemia). The platelet count is usually normal, but may be decreased. The most striking feature of the blood smear is the marked degree of rouleaux formation, which may make cell counting difficult (Fig. 4–30).

Marrow. The bone marrow shows the presence of plasma cells or myeloma cells, varying from less than 1 per cent to over 90 per cent, depending upon the degree of involvement in the site of marrow aspirated. Cytologically the cells may be indistinguishable from normal plasma cells, but they usually show abnormalities, such as less clumping of nuclear chromatin, large nucleoli, lack of a perinuclear clear zone, lighter blue cytoplasm, or varying degrees of anaplasia (Fig. 4–110 shown on page 284.)

Immunoglobulins. Serum globulin is usually increased, often strikingly so. This increase is responsible for the tendency toward rouleaux formation and an elevated erythrocyte sedimentation rate (ESR). Serum protein electrophoresis usually shows an M-spot, a homogeneous band in the gamma or beta region; less commonly there is hypogammaglobulinemia (when only light chains are produced by the neoplastic plasma cells). Immunoelectrophoresis indicates that the monoclonal protein is IgG in over half the cases of multiple myeloma, IgA in about one-fifth, IgD in less than 1 per cent, and IgE very rarely. In each of these groups of myeloma, some patients secrete Bence Jones protein (light chains, kappa *or* lambda) in addition to the whole immunoglobulin molecule. In about one-quarter of patients with multiple myeloma, only light chains (Bence Jones protein) are produced by the abnormal plasma cells. Hypogammaglobulinemia is found in the latter group because light chains are filtered through the renal glomerulus, leaving little or none in the serum, in addition to the fact that immunoglobulin production by the nonmalignant plasma cells is greatly reduced in all patients with multiple myeloma.

Roughly 5 per cent of myeloma proteins are cryoglobulins, that is, proteins which precipitate from cooled serum and redissolve on warming.

Proteinuria is frequently present in multiple myeloma. In somewhat over 50 per cent of patients Bence Jones protein is present. This may be detected by its property of precipitating from acidified urine heated to 50° C. and redissolving when the urine is boiled, or by electrophoresis of a concentrate of urine on which it migrates as a narrow band in the gamma globulin region. If renal damage has occurred, albumin and whole immunoglobulin molecules are also found in the urine. Excretion of Bence Jones protein often results in obstruction and elimination of nephrons, and the so-called myeloma kidney. Renal insufficiency is common and is the presenting feature of multiple myeloma in some cases.

Amyloidosis, which is present in about 10 to 15 per cent of cases of multiple myeloma, may be a factor in the renal failure. Amyloid fibrils in cases of myeloma appear to have as the major protein component of their fibrils the light chains of immunoglobulin molecules (Glenner *et al.*, 1973).

The diagnosis of multiple myeloma is secure if the marrow contains large numbers of morphologically bizarre, malignant-appearing plasma cells. If large numbers of normal-appearing plasma cells and plasma-cell precursors are present in the marrow, the diagnosis is not established unless punched-out, lytic bone lesions are demonstrated by x-ray, or Bence Jones proteinuria or a monoclonal gammopathy is also present (Rapaport, 1971).

WALDENSTRÖM'S MACROGLOBULINEMIA

Macroglobulins (IgM immunoglobulins) comprise 3 to 10 per cent of serum proteins. They have a high molecular weight (1,000,000), a sedimentation constant of 18 to 20 Svedberg units, and a high carbohydrate content and are characterized by a mu heavy chain and either kappa or lambda light chains. Increases of serum macroglobulins which are polyclonal may be seen in chronic infections or in collagen diseases. Monoclonal macroglobulinemia is found in a few individuals without detectable disease; in some cases of malignant lymphoma, chronic lymphocytic leukemia, and carcinoma; and in a syndrome known as Waldenström's macroglobulinemia. Though many have regarded the latter as primary macroglobulinemia and the others as secondary, MacKenzie and Fudenberg (1972) state that this distinction cannot be maintained. They view monoclonal macroglobulinemia as a spectrum of disorders.

Waldenström's macroglobulinemia is found in individuals over the age of 40, with a peak incidence between ages 60 and 70. It is characterized by a general proliferation of lymphocytes (and plasma cells) and the presence of at least 1 gm. per dl. of monoclonal IgM in the serum, amounting to at least 15 per cent of the total serum protein.

The clinical features of the disease are effects of the increased serum macroglobulins, which commonly cause symptoms due to increased viscosity, and the cell proliferation itself, which accounts for hepatosplenomegaly and some degree of lymphadenopathy. In contrast to multiple myeloma, bone pain and osteolytic lesions on x-ray are rare. Hyperviscosity and sludging of blood may lead to visual disturbances, neurologic symptoms, impaired kidney function, and right-sided congestive heart failure. Hemorrhagic phenomena may be caused by the macroglobulins adhering to platelets, which interferes with their function, and forming complexes with plasma clotting factors, which impairs their activity. Cryoglobulinemia occurs somewhat more frequently than with myeloma and may be responsible for sensitivity to cold and Raynaud's phenomenon.

Blood. Normochromic, normocytic anemia is sometimes associated with thrombocytopenia or pancytopenia. Relative or slight absolute lymphocytosis is usually found. Marked rouleaux formation is present on the blood smear, and the sedimentation rate is usually extremely rapid, although it may be low if macrocryoglobulins are present and the test is carried out at a lower temperature. The anemia is occasionally hemolytic with a positive Coombs' test.

Marrow. Often the marrow cannot be aspirated readily. Lymphoid cells are increased in number. These usually resemble normal small lymphocytes, but sometimes plasmacytoid cells are present and plasma cells may be increased in number. PAS-positive inclusions are often seen in the cytoplasm and nucleus of the lymphoid cells. Tissue mast cells are increased in number.

Immunoglobulins. Serum globulin is usually markedly increased.

The *relative serum viscosity* may be simply measured using an Ostwald viscometer. The average time for descent of the serum at room temperature is expressed as a ratio to that of distilled water. The normal range is 1.4 to 1.8. It is considerably elevated in most patients with macroglobulinemia. Symptoms of hyperviscosity appear in most patients when the relative serum viscosity is between 6 and 8, though the threshold varies among patients (MacKenzie and Fudenberg, 1972).

The *Sia water test* is performed by allowing a drop of serum to fall into a tube of distilled water. Normally the drop disappears, leaving a faint haze. In macroglobulinemia a distinct precipitate forms, does not disappear, and falls to the bottom of the tube. The test is mentioned only because of its simplicity. It has the disadvantage of giving many false negative results, and it may be positive in polyclonal increases of IgM, such as rheumatoid arthritis.

Zone electrophoresis of serum proteins on paper or cellulose acetate reveals a homogeneous band between the beta and gamma areas, which suggests a monoclonal gammopathy. If a disulfide reducing agent which splits the IgM into its component subunits (such as mercaptoethanol) is added to serum before electrophoresis, the single band will separate into two or more bands; this does not occur with nonaggregating immunoglobulins such as IgG.

Ultracentrifugal study shows the molecular size to be large, with a sedimentation constant of 19S.

Final identification is achieved by *immunoelectrophoresis*, which is required for definitive characterization of the protein; together with the mu heavy chains is only one type of light chain. The total monoclonal IgM exceeds 10 mg./ml. (1 gm./dl.).

Bence Jones proteinuria occurs in about 10 per cent of patients.

Several studies have shown that in almost all cases of chronic lymphocytic leukemia (CLL), the lymphocytes are B-cells; the surface immunoglobulin is monoclonal and, in most cases, is IgM. In about a third of cases of CLL, there is also a small amount of monoclonal serum immunoglobulin as well. In Waldenström's macroglobulinemia, lymphoid cells and plasma cells of the marrow and many of the circulating lymphocytes have a surface IgM with the same light chain type as the serum IgM. It appears that Waldenström's macroglobulinemia is a variant of CLL (or well-differentiated lymphocytic lymphoma) in which there is a greater degree of maturation of the B-lymphocytes into plasma cells (Preud'homme and Seligmann, 1972).

HEAVY CHAIN DISEASE

A small number of patients have been discovered to produce and excrete heavy chain fragments without associated light chains. Some of these proteins show structural mutations (Frangione and Franklin, 1973).

Gamma Heavy Chain Disease (γ-HCD). This disorder clinically resembles malignant lymphoma rather than myeloma, with lymphadenopathy, hepatosplenomegaly, fever, and propensity to infections. Anemia is constantly present, often with leukopenia and thrombocytopenia. Atypical lymphocytes or plasma cells are frequently present in the blood, and two cases have terminated in plasma cell leukemia. The marrow is usually abnormal, with increased plasma cells and lymphocytes and eosinophils, but is not diagnostic. Usually, but not always, the histology of lymphoid tissue indicates a malignant lymphoproliferative disease. A rather broad serum protein "spike" has been found in the beta-gamma region in most patients, accompanied by hypogammaglobulinemia. The diagnosis is made by showing that the protein reacts on immunoelectrophoresis with antisera to γ-chains but not to light chains. The protein is also found in the urine in varying amounts, though concentration techniques may be necessary to demonstrate it.

Alpha Heavy Chain Disease (α-HCD). This disorder appears to be more common than γ-HCD, and involves a younger age group. The uniform clinical pattern in most patients is malabsorption and diarrhea due to a histiocytic lymphoma of the intestine, though in two patients the respiratory tract has been involved instead. Bone marrow and other lymphoid organs have not been involved. Usually routine protein electrophoresis is negative, but small amounts of alpha chain may be detected in the serum and sometimes in the urine with immunoelectrophoresis.

Mu Heavy Chain Disease (μ-HCD). The three patients who have been described have had chronic lymphocytic leukemia with vacuolated plasma cells in the marrow. Routine serum electrophoresis showed only hypogammaglobulinemia. The μ heavy chain was detected by serum immunoelectrophoresis; it was not found in the urine. In two patients, however, the urine contained Bence Jones protein.

Myeloproliferative Syndromes

The hypothesis of the myeloproliferative syndromes is based on the conception of the functional unity of the marrow, not only horizontally as it functions after birth, but vertically by including the periods which precede the participation of marrow in blood production in fetal life. The tissues involved in fetal production of blood may regain their capacity to produce blood cells in response to certain stimuli.

This concept is based on the well-known participation of megakaryocytes in the hyperplasia of chronic granulocytic leukemia and of granulocytes and megakaryocytes in polycythemia, on the frequent observation of polycythemia as a precursor of myelofibrosis with myeloid metaplasia, and on many other similar situations. In an effort to clarify these relationships among polycythemia vera, chronic myelogenous leukemia, myelofibrosis with myeloid metaplasia, thrombocythemia, megakaryocytic leukemia, and the Di Guglielmo syndrome, Dameshek in 1951 grouped them together as "myeloproliferative disorders."

Acute forms of myeloproliferative disorders are regarded by Dameshek and his collaborators (1964) as the Di Guglielmo syndrome (erythremic myelosis, erythroleukemia), acute granulocytic leukemia, and acute myelosclerosis with myeloid metaplasia.

A somewhat contrasting view is taken by Ward and Block (1971) in their extensive study of myelofibrosis with myeloid metaplasia. They separate chronic and acute granulocytic leukemia and erythroleukemia into a *myeloleukemia* group characterized by a neoplastic proliferation that invades and destroys both myeloid and nonmyeloid organs. On the other hand, myelofibrosis with myeloid metaplasia, polycythemia vera, and thrombocythemia form a *myeloproliferative* group, characterized by benign proliferation of the three myeloid (erythroid, granulocytic, and megakaryocytic) cell types in organs that were once hematopoietic in fetal life.

These groupings do not imply similar causation or similar expressions of a common underlying disorder; they only imply a common site of origin (the bone marrow) and a proliferative disorder of unknown etiology. Self-limited reactions of the marrow to known stimuli are not considered here to be among the myeloproliferative disorders.

Because of overlapping manifestations, and because of the occurrence of cases that are difficult if not impossible to classify in one category or the other, it is convenient to consider them together. Polycythemia vera, chronic granulocytic leukemia, and the Di Guglielmo syndrome have already been discussed.

The participation of the various cellular elements in the myeloproliferative disorders is shown in Table 4–25.

MYELOFIBROSIS WITH MYELOID METAPLASIA

Synonyms for what is probably the same basic disease process include myelosclerosis with myeloid metaplasia, myeloid megakaryocytic hepatosplenomegaly, aleukemic myelosis, agnogenic myeloid metaplasia, and many others (see Miale, 1972).

Definition. This is a chronic, progressive panmyelosis characterized by a triad of findings: varying degrees of fibrosis of the marrow, massive splenomegaly due to extramedullary hematopoiesis, and a leukoerythroblastic anemia with marked red cell abnormalities, circulating normoblasts, immature granulocytes, and atypical platelets (Dameshek and Gunz, 1964; Ward and Block, 1971).

Clinical Findings. The disorder occurs typically in persons over the age of 50 and has an insidious onset, with weight loss, signs and symptoms of anemia, and abdominal discomfort due to the large spleen. Often the liver is enlarged as well, and the patient may be slightly jaundiced. On x-ray, diffuse or patchy osteosclerosis may appear in one-third to one-half of patients; osteoporosis may be seen also.

Blood. A moderate normochromic, normocytic anemia (frequently with some hypochromic cells and basophilic stippling), moderate anisocytosis, and marked poikilocytosis, including prominent teardrop forms and elongated red cells, are characteristic (Figs. 4–21, 4–22). Normoblasts are often present in numbers out of proportion to the degree of anemia, and a slight reticulocytosis is frequently found. The anemia may have a complicated origin, with components of marrow failure, ineffective erythropoiesis, and hemolysis. The leukocyte count is normal or, more commonly, moderately increased; immature neutrophils and occasionally even myeloblasts are present. The neutrophil alkaline phosphatase is often elevated, but may be normal and is rarely decreased. Chromosomal studies have not shown the presence of the Philadelphia (Ph^1) chromosome, which is so characteristic of chronic granulocytic leukemia. Basophils are often increased in number. Platelets are normal or decreased in number (rarely increased) and often are atypical, with distinct "zones": a clear hyaloplasm and a central pale chromomere which lacks the usual concentration of azurophilic granules (Fig. 4–78). Small megakaryocytic fragments the size of lymphocytes with both nucleus and cytoplasm (dwarf megakaryocytes) or small megakaryoblasts may usually be found if searched for; on rare occasions, they are present in considerable numbers (Fig. 4–77).

Marrow. It is usually impossible to aspirate marrow, and a needle biopsy or a surgical biopsy is necessary for adequate study of the

Table 4–25. MYELOPROLIFERATIVE DISORDERS—CLASSIFIED AS TO DEGREE OF CELLULAR PROLIFERATION*

	RBC	WBC	MEGA-PLATELET	RETICULUM CELL	POTENTIAL (META-PLASTIC) BONE MARROW
Polycythemia vera	+++	++	++ (+)	+	+
Myelosclerosis-Myeloid metaplasia	–	+ (+)	++ (+)	+++	+++
Chronic granulocytic leukemia	+	+++	++	±	+
Thrombocythemia	±	±	+++	+	+
Di Guglielmo syndrome	++ (+)	++ (+)	+ (–)	–	–
Acute granulocytic leukemia	–	+++	–	–	–

*From Dameshek, W., and Gunz, F.: Leukemia. 2nd edition. New York, Grune & Stratton, Inc., 1964. By permission of the publisher.

marrow; this is especially true later in the course of the disease. If examined early in the disease, the marrow may be hypercellular, with panmyelosis and prominently increased megakaryocytes which are frequently abnormal. On histologic sections there is a diffuse increase in reticulin fibers which is demonstrable with silver stains (Rappaport, 1966); patchy fibrosis may be present.

Later the marrow becomes more fibrotic, with residual islands of atypical megakaryocytes, erythroid, and granulocytic precursors. The fibrosis is of loose connective tissue with scanty collagen, but reticulin fibers are abundant. Foci of osteoid may be found, and the bony trabeculae are sometimes irregularly thickened (myelosclerosis). The marrow may show a mixture of hyperplasia and fibrosis in one sample, or may differ in different sites of the body (Fig. 4–76).

Course. A significant proportion of cases of myelofibrosis with myeloid metaplasia are a late stage, after many years' progression, of typical polycythemia vera. The usual course is one of progressive anemia and enlargement of the spleen; hemolysis frequently becomes an increasing element in the anemia. Infections may be a serious problem. The average survival is slightly longer than that of chronic granulocytic leukemia, but considerably less than that of polycythemia vera; however, patients may occasionally live as long as 10 to 15 years. In patients with longer survival, frequently the terminal event is an acute blastic leukemia.

THROMBOCYTHEMIA

As distinguished from *thrombocytosis*, the term *thrombocythemia* should probably be confined to situations in which the platelet count is persistently elevated to levels at least three times normal (Dameshek and Gunz, 1964). It will be evident that thrombocythemia, thus defined, will usually be part of the general picture of other myeloproliferative disorders: polycythemia vera, chronic granulocytic leukemia and, rarely, myelofibrosis with myeloid metaplasia.

Occasionally, however, thrombocythemia may be the predominant feature of the hematologic picture, and in these cases it is commonly associated with bleeding problems. After reviewing most of the reported cases, Gunz (1960) regards them as constituting a clinical syndrome of *hemorrhagic thrombocythemia*.

Clinical Findings. Characteristic are recurrent, spontaneous hemorrhages, which are most commonly gastrointestinal. Hemorrhages are occasionally preceded or accompanied by thrombosis in superficial or deep veins. Purpura has not been described. Slight splenomegaly is the rule.

Blood. The most striking feature is the marked increase in platelets (maximum values: 0.9 to 14.0 million per μl.), often with abnormal and giant forms and usually accompanied by fragments of megakaryocytes. Neutrophilic leukocytosis is almost always present, and the neutrophil alkaline phosphatase has been elevated in most cases in which it has been examined. Hypochromic microcytic anemia due to chronic blood loss is present in many cases; at other times, polycythemia may be evident.

Marrow. The marrow shows a panmyelosis with increased megakaryocytes. Splenic extramedullary hematopoiesis may be present.

Gunz (1960) regards hemorrhagic thrombocythemia as a clinical syndrome; the pathologic features cannot be separated from those of the other myeloproliferative disorders. It is probably most closely related to polycythemia vera.

Leukemoid Reactions

A leukemoid reaction is an excessive leukocytic response to a stimulus that normally results in a lesser degree of leukocytosis or immaturity in the circulating cells. Here belongs leukocytosis of 50,000 per μl. or higher with a shift to the left, or lower counts, even below normal, but with considerable numbers of immature granulocytes or similar quantitative or qualitative changes in lymphocytes or monocytes. Depending on the predominant cell, leukemoid reactions may be neutrophilic, eosinophilic, lymphocytic, or monocytic.

CLASSIFICATION

Neutrophilic Leukemoid Reactions

1. Hemolytic crisis in hemolytic anemia. Normoblasts are commonly present in the peripheral blood.
2. Hemorrhage (WBC from 50,000 to 100,000).
3. Hodgkin's disease. Occasional counts over 100,000 with many eosinophils.
4. Various infections.
   A. Tuberculosis (lymphocytic leukemoid reactions also possible).
   B. Pneumococcus, meningococcus, and streptococcus infections; gas gangrene; diphtheria; leptospirosis; malaria.
   C. Congenital syphilis (lymphocytic leukemoid reaction also possible).

5. Burns.
6. Eclampsia.
7. Mustard gas poisoning.
8. Vascular thrombosis and infarction, e.g., mesenteric thrombosis, tissue necrosis.
9. Marrow replacement by tumors, including multiple myeloma and myelosclerosis (also eosinophilic, and lymphocytic leukemoid reactions possible). Normoblasts are characteristically present in the peripheral blood.
10. Myeloid metaplasia in the various myeloproliferative diseases.

Eosinophilic Leukemoid Reactions. High leukocytosis with total cell count in leukemic ranges and a high percentage of eosinophils but with few or no immature cells. Usually occur in children and may present differential diagnostic problems. As a rule, are not leukemias. The further course, with subsidence of the eosinophilia, solves the problem. A parasitic infestation is usually the cause.

Erythroblastosis. Normoblasts in peripheral blood in patients with or without anemia, frequently with a neutrophilic leukemoid blood picture. The finding of a moderate anemia with normoblasts in the peripheral blood is fairly common in metastatic carcinoma involving bone marrow.

Lymphocytic Leukemoid Reactions. These reactions occur in infectious lymphocytosis, infectious mononucleosis, pertussis, and varicella.

A leukemoid blood picture may be seen in a variety of infections for which various infectious agents are responsible. The reaction is irregular, even with the same infectious agent. The same microorganisms in most cases do not produce this kind of leukemoid blood picture. Hence, the conclusion is drawn that leukemoid blood pictures are frequently determined by the host reaction.

Myeloblastic leukemia-like pictures with severe anemia, fever, and splenomegaly have been seen, especially in tuberculosis with involvement of lymph nodes and spleen.

The differential diagnosis from leukemia is not always easy. Most important is the marrow examination, which is more helpful in the differentiation of lymphocytic leukemia than of granulocytic.

The increase of eosinophilic and basophilic granulocytes characteristically present in granulocytic leukemia is absent in the leukemoid blood picture. The leukemic hiatus of acute leukemia is absent.

The alkaline phosphatase cytochemical test in neutrophils is weak or negative in granulocytic leukemia and positive in nonleukemic cells. The reaction is particularly strong in leukemoid reactions. The values are also high in polycythemia and usually in myeloid metaplasia.

Hypersplenism

Hypersplenism is a condition characterized by exaggeration of some of the normal functions of the spleen, such as sequestration of blood cells, phagocytosis, and destruction of sequestered, over-aged, or abnormal blood cells, and humoral, possibly hormonal, control of certain marrow functions, specifically cytogenesis or release of marrow cells. Broadly speaking, hypersplenism may be described as a cytopenia involving any one or all of the formed elements of the blood and associated with splenomegaly and marrow hyperplasia. Correction of the cytopenia by splenectomy is possible.

Entities such as hereditary spherocytosis, thrombocytopenic purpura, and certain instances of agranulocytosis are included in this category by some, though others restrict the use of the term hypersplenism to conditions in which the cytopenia is secondary to the exaggeration of splenic function (due to whatever cause). Thus restricted, the diagnosis of hypersplenism is difficult and is often a matter of exclusion or clinical speculation. One expects to find in the bone marrow a compensatory hyperplasia of the element or elements being destroyed by splenic action. Injection of adrenaline, by producing contraction of the spleen, may increase the appearance in the peripheral blood of cells previously reduced below their normal number. This phenomenon is rejected by many observers as a valid test of hypersplenism; at best the results are irregular.

Hypersplenism is not a nosologic or gross anatomic or histopathologic entity. Perhaps the only accepted criterion of diagnosis is the prompt and permanent restoration of normal hematocytology after removal of the spleen.

Clinical Findings. Splenomegaly of varying degrees. Occasionally the clinical syndrome may be present without demonstrable splenomegaly.

Laboratory Findings. Pancytopenia, reticulocytosis and polychromatophilia, slightly increased RBC fragility, and normal or hyperplastic marrow.

Mechanisms (Jandl, 1967; Jacob, 1972). The red cells normally undergo a conditioning in their passage through the splenic cords, during which they are packed together and lack a normal plasma environment and are deprived of glucose, exposed to increasing acidity, and exposed intimately to macrophages. This conditioning process will normally cause the destruction of only limited numbers of cells but may impose a greater loss and a severe hemolytic process if the red cells are themselves defective. In splenomegaly the red cells are exposed to this stressful process to a considerably greater degree, and more are likely to be removed or damaged; especially in combination with any congenital or acquired red cell defect, this may result in a hemolytic anemia.

Leukopenia is less frequent than anemia in splenomegaly; it usually is attributed to splenic sequestration and probably increased destruction, and is more likely to occur in patients with the larger spleens.

Thrombocytopenia in patients with splenomegaly may often be due to displacement of platelets into a large splenic pool rather than to a shortening of their survival (Aster, 1966). This is in contrast to idiopathic thrombocytopenic purpura, in which the platelet survival is shortened on an immunologic basis and the spleen is not greatly enlarged.

Conditions Associated with Hypersplenism. Hypersplenism may be primary (idiopathic), without demonstrable cause or the result of various diseases, all of them producing stasis in, or hyperplasia of, splenic pulp and eventually splenomegaly (secondary hypersplenism).

Here belong portal hypertension following cirrhosis of the liver or thrombosis of the splenic vein (Banti's syndrome), congestive splenomegaly in chronic cardiac failure, rheumatoid arthritis (Felty's syndrome), chronic infectious diseases (e.g., malaria, syphilis, tuberculosis), kala-azar, Gaucher's disease and other lipid and nonlipid histiocytoses, and Hodgkin's disease. All these diseases have in common blood stasis or hyperplasia of histiocytes, monocytes, or lymphocytes.

In autoimmune acquired hemolytic anemia and idiopathic thrombocytopenic purpura, the spleen takes part in the process by producing autoantibodies, which attack the autologous antigen.

In certain chronic hypoplastic anemias the role of the spleen in the control of blood destruction is apparent from the fact that splenectomy reduces the requirement for blood transfusions.

In all these conditions anemia, leukopenia, and thrombocytopenia have been seen and have been, in some cases, relieved by splenectomy.

The LE (Lupus Erythematosus) Cell Test

Hargraves *et al.* described the LE cell in 1948; an interesting account of this discovery has been given (Hargraves, 1969).

Principle. A substance present in the gamma globulin fraction of the plasma or serum of patients with disseminated lupus erythematosus, the *LE factor* reacts with the nucleoprotein of white cell nuclei. The LE factor appears to be an antibody. The transformed nucleoprotein acquires chemotactic properties and attracts phagocytes, usually segmented neutrophilic granulocytes and occasionally monocytes. Rarely other leukocytes may act as phagocytes. The phagocytes with the ingested nuclear material are the LE cells. The phenomenon for LE cell formation requires the presence in the serum of the LE factor, damaged leukocytes, and normal active leukocytes.

Morphology. The LE cell contains two nuclei. The nucleus of the phagocyte is flattened out at the periphery of the cell. Its chromatin structure is well preserved. The bulk of the cytoplasmic portion of the cell is occupied by the ingested transformed nuclear mass. The cytoplasm forms a narrow margin at the periphery. In the fully developed LE cell, the normal chromatin structure of the ingested nucleus is absent and is replaced by a purplish, homogeneous, amorphous, round mass, which varies in size but is usually larger than the erythrocytes in the same preparation (Fig. 4–111). A phagocyte may engulf more than one nucleus. It is possible that in some cases the multiple nuclei are segments of a granulocyte that have not yet merged. The transformation of the nucleus is a progressive process. The stages can be followed step by step. The early chemotactic action of the transforming or transformed nucleus may attract several neutrophilic granulocytes, which surround it and form a so-called "rosette." This finding is not diagnostic.

Nucleophagocytosis is a fairly common finding and is fundamentally different from the LE cell phenomenon. In such cases, the phagocyte is more frequently a monocyte but may be a granulocyte. The phagocytized nucleus retains the intact chromatin pattern. It may show degenerative changes, mainly pyknosis that is diffuse or appears along the margins, and nuclear vacuoles. The inclusion is frequently smaller than in a true LE cell. These are the so-called "tart cells" (Fig. 4–112).

Several tests and modifications have been recommended.

Test No. 1 (Zimmer and Hargraves, 1952)

1. About 8 ml. of venous blood is collected in a sterile, dry, chemically clean test tube, allowed to clot, and left at room temperature for about 2 hours or at 37° C. for 30 minutes.

2. The clot is fragmented with several wooden applicators. What remains of the clot is removed from the bloody serum. The serum-cell mixture remaining after the removal of the clots is centrifuged for 5 minutes at 2000 r.p.m.

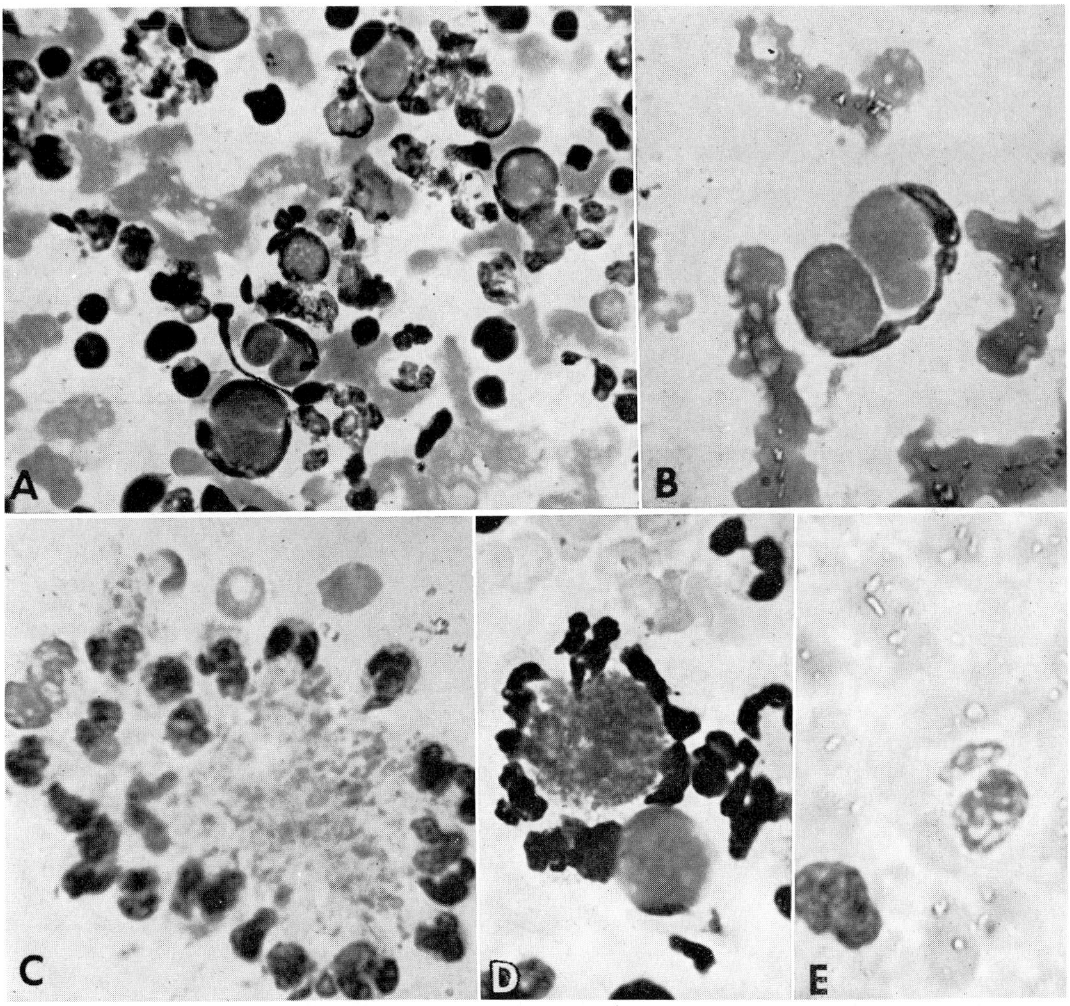

Figure 4–111. *A*, Many typical LE cells. In some of the phagocytes two nuclei are present. *B*, LE cell. The phagocyte is embracing two nuclei. The one to the right with the more uniform structure is the more typical. A deep indentation appears along the outer periphery of the one closer to the nucleus of the segmented phagocyte. The indentation may mean that the ingested nucleus was also from a segmented granulocyte or that the phagocyte has ingested three nuclei. The nucleus to the left still has vestiges of its chromatin structure. *C*, A so-called rosette. *D*, LE cell and a rosette. At the bottom is a typical LE cell. Just above is the rosette. *E*, In the center of the field is a vague outline of a cell containing two nuclei. The one at the top is the nucleus of a segmented granulocyte. The nucleus below it is less readily identified. Both are in relatively good stages of preservation. This is an example of phagocytosis but not an LE cell.

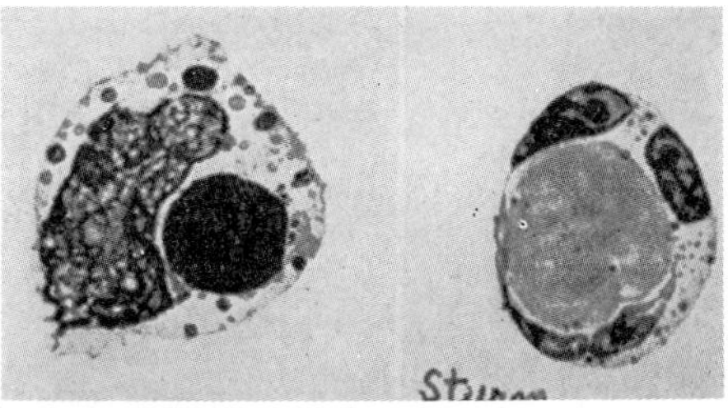

Figure 4–112. On the left is a monocyte with a phagocytized pyknotic nucleus (to be differentiated from lupus erythematosus cells). On the right is a neutrophil with a felt-like, purple staining mass in the cytoplasm; this is not quite typical of an LE cell in that the mass is not homogeneous. Typical LE cells should be found on the same slide. (Permission for reproduction from *The Morphology of Blood Cells*, by L. W. Diggs, was obtained from Abbott Laboratories.)

3. Most of the supernatant serum is removed with a pipette, leaving a column of about 1 cm. This together with the visible gray buffy coat layer is transferred to several Wintrobe hematocrit tubes.

4. The tubes are centrifuged for about 5 minutes at 1500 to 2000 r.p.m. or until three distinct layers (serum, buffy coat, and red cells) have formed.

5. The serum is discarded carefully with a pipette, leaving a layer of 1 or 2 mm. above the buffy coat and the buffy coat layer. The latter is transferred drop by drop to slides on which it is mixed. Smears are made and stained with Wright's stain.

6. The slide is surveyed with the low and high power of the microscope to locate areas suggestive of the presence of LE cells. These areas are then examined with the oil-immersion objective.

In our laboratory the following modification of the method used in the preparation of smears has been found satisfactory.

1. From each hematocrit tube most of the serum is removed, leaving a column of serum measuring about 5 mm. above the packed cells.

2. A pipette is now inserted 2 mm. below the lower level of the serum to remove the concentrated leukocytes together with the serum (Fig. 4–113 *A*). In this way the leukocytes are diluted mainly with serum, resulting in a mixture containing relatively few erythrocytes.

3. The serum-cell mixture from one Wintrobe tube is then placed on a slide (Fig. 4–113 *B*). Additional preparations can be made from each of the other Wintrobe tubes.

4. A second slide is placed diagonally upon the serum-cell mixture on slide 1 (Fig. 4–113 *C*). The mixture is allowed to spread. When fibrin is abundant, some pressure should be applied in order to separate the leukocytes from the fibrin threads. The top slide is then raised abruptly vertically from the bottom slide, but the slides should not be pulled apart horizontally. The bottom slide is held in slanting position (Fig. 4–113 *D*). The erythrocytes and serum flow toward the edge, while the leukocytes and fibrin threads (if any) remain in the center.

5. The smaller particles are removed with the short edge of a new clean slide and are used for the preparation of the final smear as follows: The short edge of the slide to which the material adheres is placed parallel to the long edge of a second slide, pushed forward at an angle of approximately 5 degrees almost to the edge of the horizontal slide (Fig. 4–113 *E*), and then lowered in such a manner that the surfaces of the two slides come into complete contact (Fig. 4–113 *F*). Finally the slides are pulled apart, with the two surfaces maintaining contact until separation is completed. When preparing the smears, the smaller particles rather than the larger ones are selected in order to insure more homogeneous preparation.

With this technique we have been able to observe, in positive cases, more intact LE cells than with the other methods previously employed. This has been particularly true in patients with leukopenia.

Report. The number of the characteristic cells is recorded until 1000 granulocytes have been counted. The report should make reference to this quantitative relation.

The presence of not yet fully transformed inclusions (questionable or pre-LE cells) and of rosettes should be noted, although they are not diagnostic. They indicate the need for examining more than 1000 leukocytes.

Phagocytosis of nuclei with preserved chromatin structure ("tart" cells) need not be reported.

This technique is one of several direct methods. In indirect methods the serum comes from the patient, and the leukocytes come from another person.

Test No. 2 (Magath and Winkle, 1952)

1. Prepare the blood sample as for test 1.

2. The clot is removed and passed through a copper wire screen of 30-mesh per inch, by use of the bottom of a test tube or a pestle. A special sieve and pestle are commercially available (Scientific Products Company). The effect of this procedure is twofold: the fibrin remains on the sieve, and some of the leukocytes are damaged.

3. The filtrate is transferred to several Wintrobe hematocrit tubes.

Continue with steps 4, 5, and 6 as in Test 1.

Test No. 3 (Zinkham and Conley, 1956)

1. Ten milliliters of venous blood is placed in a tube containing 3 drops of a 1 per cent aqueous solution of heparin (delivered with a

21-gauge needle) and 10 glass beads, 4 mm. in diameter. It has been shown that excess heparin will decrease the number of positive tests (Dubois and Freeman, 1957).

2. Let stand at room temperature for 90 minutes.

3. Rotate in a Shen type rotator set at 30 r.p.m. for 30 minutes. Transfer to one or more Wintrobe hematocrit tubes. Continue with steps 4, 5, and 6 as in Test 1.

Test No. 4 (Defibrination and Rotation)

1. Ten milliliters of venous blood is placed in an Erlenmeyer flask containing 10 glass beads, and the flask is rotated and swirled on a flat surface until defibrination has occurred.

2. Remove the clot, pour the defibrinated blood into a test tube containing five clean glass beads, and rotate at 30 r.p.m. for 30 minutes.

3. Incubate the tube at 37° C. for 15 minutes.

4. Transfer to Wintrobe hematocrit tubes and continue with steps 4, 5, and 6 as in Test 1.

Test No. 5 (Slide Test of Snapper and Nathan, 1955). This is an indirect method.

1. A substrate of leukocytes is prepared by placing a few drops of normal blood on a glass slide within a rubber ring about 0.8 cm. in diameter and 0.2 cm. high. Two such preparations are made on each slide. The slides are placed in a Petri dish, the bottom of which has been covered by moistened filter paper. After incubating at room temperature for 1 hour, the clot and ring are removed by pushing them off (without lifting) and the slide is washed with

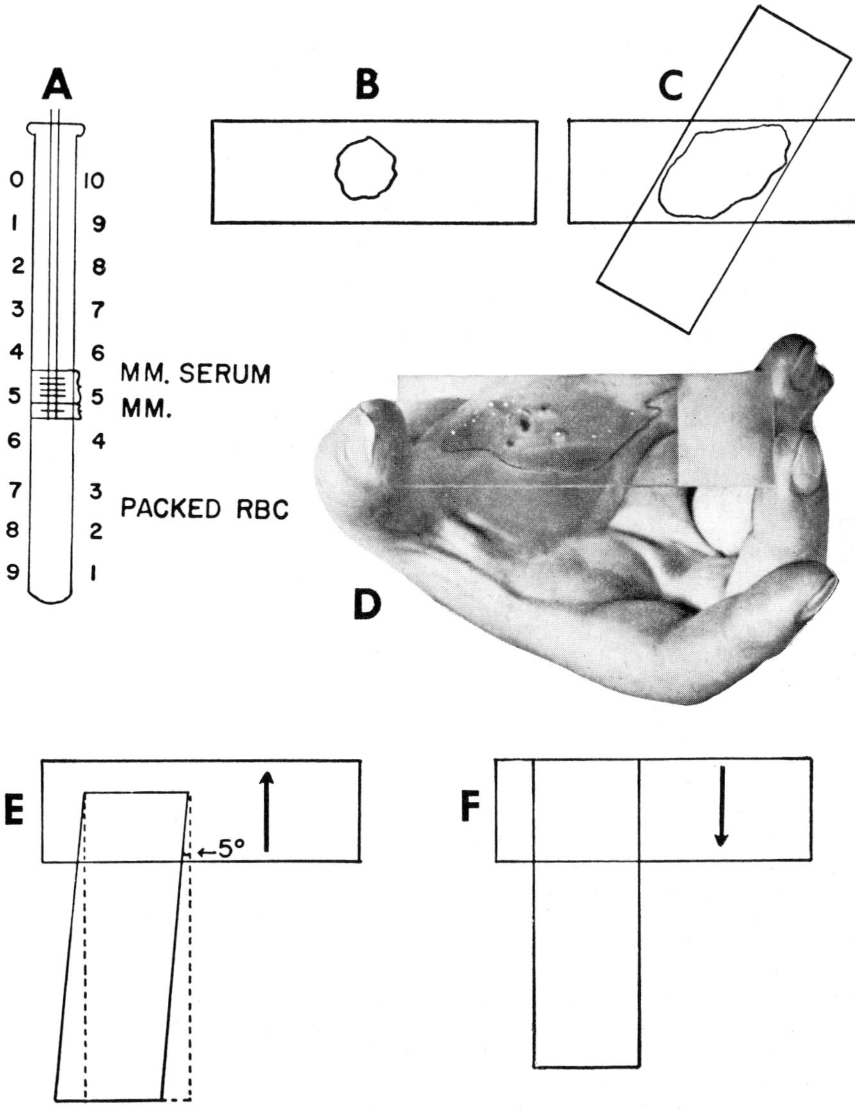

Figure 4–113. Preparation of LE slide. See text for explanation.

serum to remove the excessive free red cells. (The use of saline as a wash would distort the leukocytes.) The slides are then dried. They have been kept at room temperature as long as five weeks without losing their potency.

2. In order to test the blood of a suspected patient, a small piece of a No. 2 coverslip is placed on either side of the substrate area as a pillar. Then a large drop of finger blood is put on a square, 22-mm. wide coverslip and inverted over the substrate area, resting on the glass pillars.

3. The preparation is incubated at room temperature for 2 hours in a Petri dish, the bottom of which has been covered by a piece of moistened filter paper.

4. The coverslip is removed by pushing it off the glass slide. The substrate is washed to remove excessive red cells with either the patient's serum, if it is available, or normal serum. This step is not always necessary. Saline should not be used as a wash, because it distorts the leukocytes and causes poor staining.

5. The slides are stained with Wright's stain in the usual manner.

Test No. 6 (Capillary LE Cell Test; Mudrik et al., 1961)

1. Collect blood from finger or ear lobe puncture in four or more 1.5 × 75 mm. heparinized capillary tubes (used in microhematocrit determination). Fill at least three-fourths of each tube.

2. Seal the red end of each tube with Critoseal. Critocaps (both used in microhematocrit determination), or children's modeling clay.

3. Centrifuge in an International Hematocrit Centrifuge (8000 × G.) for 1 minute or in an International Clinical Centrifuge (700 × G.) for 5 minutes. Any other horizontal centrifuge may be used, provided a rubber cushion is used to avoid the breakage of capillary tubes.

4. Insert a wire stylet into capillary tube and mix plasma and buffy coat thoroughly by rotating either the stylet or the tube 15 times. The stylet is from a 20-gauge, three-inch hypodermic needle, and its tip is slightly bent. This step is important because it brings the plasma LE factor and leukocytes into close contact and, at the same time, traumatizes the leukocytes, a process that has proved to be an important factor in the formation of LE cells.

5. Incubate tubes at room temperature for 2 hours or at 37° C. for 30 minutes. Prolonged incubation does not increase the yield of LE cells.

6. Centrifuge again as in step 3.

7. Break tubes about 2 mm. below the buffy coat level with the aid of an ampule file. The 2-mm. erythrocyte column serves to prevent the loss of buffy coat during the following operation.

8. Deliver the buffy coat layer to a glass slide with a smallpox vaccination bulb. Care should be taken that no excess plasma is delivered to the slide.

9. Make the smear by placing another slide on top of the buffy coat, compressing gently, and pulling slides away from each other at parallel planes. Our experience has shown that this procedure distributes the cells on the LE smears more evenly than the conventional method used in making blood smears.

10. Stain with Wright or Giemsa stain as usual.

11. If previously drawn venous blood of the patient is already available, either clotted or unclotted, the buffy coat is concentrated by means of centrifugation, transferred to capillary tubes, and treated as outlined in steps 2 to 10.

12. If only serum or plasma of the patient is available, mix 1 drop of either with buffy coats from two to three capillary hematocrit tubes of a normal person, incubate the mixture in a capillary tube, and proceed as outlined in steps 5 to 10. Buffy coat of bone marrow may also be used but is less satisfactory.

The two alternate methods outlined in steps 11 and 12 make it unnecessary to again puncture the patient, but otherwise the regular procedure (steps 1 to 10) is preferable.

The capillary test has several advantages: (1) It does not require special equipment, such as rotating machine or sieve. (2) All reagents involved in the test come from the patient. (3) About 40 μl. of patient's blood is needed. (4) It can be done in the same capillary tubes that are used for routine microhematocrit determination, and actually the hematocrit test can be done with the same specimen. (5) The plasma LE factor is incubated chiefly with leukocytes rather than with a mixture consisting of considerably larger numbers of erythrocytes than leukocytes, as is the case in the other tests. The erythrocytes take no part in the reaction; therefore, reducing their number creates a more favorable medium for the leukocyte plasma reaction. (6) The incubation is performed in a minimum of space (less than 10 μl.), which facilitates phagocytosis. (7) After the capillary tube is broken, practically all the formed and concentrated LE cells are delivered onto a small area of a glass slide.

The capillary test has been shown to be highly sensitive in our laboratory.

The LE Battery. If the LE test employed is suspicious but not definitely positive, or if the diagnosis of SLE is strongly suspected, a group or battery of three types of LE cell tests should be performed. Dubois and Freeman (1957) showed that a battery produced more positives than any one single test. The rotary method (Test No. 3) was superior to the sieved clot method (Test No. 2) and the slide test (Test No. 5). We prefer the defibrination and rotation method (Test No. 4) and use this in lieu of the slide test (Test No. 5) in our LE battery.

PROPERTIES OF THE LE FACTOR

It is stable in the frozen state and resists repeated freezing and thawing. It passes the Seitz filter. It is destroyed by heating at 65° C. for 30 minutes but resists 60° C. for 15 minutes. It is inhibited by heparin in concentrations higher than 0.75 mg. per 10 ml. and by alcohol and phenol. The LE phenomenon is inhibited by EDTA.

It has been found also in the urine and pleural fluid and in the cord blood of children of mothers with the disease.

The LE factor is not limited in its activity to leukocytes. It reacts with nuclei of hepatic, splenic, and renal cells; with cancer cells; and with nuclei of cells of various animal species.

The nature of the chemical change involved in the transformation of the nucleus has been widely discussed. Various hypotheses have been suggested, such as depolymerization of DNA, alteration of the cell membrane, and others, but agreement has not been reached, except for the obvious fact that the LE factor reacts in some direct fashion with the nucleus.

ANTINUCLEAR ANTIBODIES AND THE DIAGNOSIS OF SYSTEMIC LUPUS ERYTHEMATOSUS

Tests for antinuclear antibodies, in addition to the LE cell test, include immunofluorescent techniques, complement fixation, antiglobulin consumption, precipitin tests, and agglutination of coated, inert particles such as latex fixation or bentonite flocculation. The detection of a particular antibody appears to depend upon the antigen employed rather than the particular immunologic method. Details of the more useful methods have been provided by Friou (1967b), and antinuclear antibodies have recently been discussed by Peltier and Estes (1972).

In systemic lupus erythematosus (SLE), the most characteristic antinuclear antibody is an antinucleoprotein (anti-DNP), which is the one that produces the LE cell phenomenon. This is almost always present in patients with untreated SLE and may be demonstrated by serologic tests even in the 25 per cent of patients with SLE who have negative LE cell tests. A low titer of the antibody or a failure of phagocytosis for some reason may be responsible for negative LE cell tests. Anti-DNP is also present in about 15 per cent of patients with rheumatoid arthritis who may have positive LE cell tests. Lower titers of the antibody may be found in some patients with chronic hepatitis, periarteritis nodosa, dermatomyositis, scleroderma, acute drug hypersensitivity (mainly hydralazine and procainamide), atypical pneumonia, tuberculosis, and anaplastic carcinoma or lymphoma. It is usually in such patients that positive LE cell tests have occasionally been reported; these have rarely been strongly positive.

A second important antibody in SLE reacts with DNA which is not linked to protein (anti-DNA). This antibody occurs in about two-thirds of patients with SLE. Absence, therefore, does not rule out SLE. Because anti-DNA is rarely found in any other condition, its presence is strong evidence in favor of SLE. Anti-DNA is usually found in the acute phase of the disease.

A third antinuclear antibody also present in SLE reacts with a nuclear antigen which is extractable in buffer solutions and does not contain DNA. This antibody is nonspecific in that it is present in many conditions other than SLE. Tests for this buffer-extractable, antinuclear antibody are, therefore, of little value. A positive test for total antinuclear antibody (which includes anti-DNP, anti-DNA, and the extractable antibody) will not be decisive; a negative test for total antinuclear antibody, however, is strong evidence against the diagnosis of SLE.

Variations of Blood Platelets in Disease

THROMBOCYTOSIS

An increase in the concentration of platelets above 400,000 per μl. is called thrombocytosis. It usually appears to be due to an increase in the production of platelets in situations such as iron deficiency, acute hemorrhage, hemolysis, inflammatory diseases, and malignancies. Myeloproliferative diseases are also frequently associated with an increased production of platelets, in extramedullary sites as well as marrow; these autonomous increases in platelets are usually referred to as thrombocythemia.

A change in distribution of platelets may also cause thrombocytosis. Loss of splenic function or splenectomy removes a site where normally one-third of platelets reside (p. 158) and results in thrombocytosis. Administration of epinephrine will result in thrombocytosis if the spleen is intact (Aster, 1966).

THROMBOCYTOPENIA

Mechanisms. Decreased production, altered distribution, and increased destruction or removal are causes of thrombocytopenia, which, when severe, is clinically important as a cause of bleeding (Harker and Finch, 1969).

Decreased production occurs either alone or more often in conjunction with other cytopenias in aplastic anemias (idiopathic or due to toxic agents), and in myelophthisic processes. Ineffective production appears to be a cause in megaloblastic anemia and in some myeloproliferative disorders.

An *altered distribution* of platelets results in thrombocytopenia in splenomegaly of various causes. In these instances there appears to be an increased pooling of platelets in the spleen, with a normal platelet survival (Aster, 1966).

Increased platelet destruction may be the cause of thrombocytopenia when consumption occurs at a rate exceeding an attempted compensatory increase in production. Consumption is usually the result of the utilization of the platelets in the process of disseminated intravascular coagulation. Daily platelet counts are helpful in monitoring the severity of the process.

Another important mechanism leading to increased destruction of platelets is immune, mediated by antibodies directed against platelet antigens. Immune thrombocytopenia is suspected when the low platelet count is accompanied by increased megakaryocytes in the bone marrow, assuming that disseminated coagulation can be ruled out. Large platelets in the blood film indicate increased production (Karpatkin, 1972); these are usually found in immune thrombocytopenia. Platelet antibodies may sometimes be demonstrated.

Immune thrombocytopenias include drug-induced thrombocytopenia, due usually to quinine, quinidine, barbiturates, or sulfa drugs. An antibody produced in response to a drug-protein complex reacts with the drug, and the drug-antibody complex nonspecifically coats platelets and promotes their destruction. *In vitro*, the drug plus patient's serum will inhibit the clot retraction of normal blood.

Idiopathic thrombocytopenic purpura (ITP) is a disorder due to increased platelet destruction in which an antibody appears to be responsible in most cases. An underlying disease or an etiologic agent cannot be identified, and the antibody is regarded as an autoantibody (Baldini, 1966). Acute, transient ITP occurs at any age, but is especially common in children and often follows a viral infection. Chronic ITP is similar to autoimmune hemolytic anemia; it occurs most commonly in young adults, with a greater frequency in women than in men.

Thrombocytopenia may be found in newborn infants due to isoantibodies formed in the mother to antigens on fetal platelets; the antibodies cross the placenta and destroy the infant's platelets. Isoantibodies against platelets are frequently formed in recipients of multiple whole blood or platelet transfusions; these antibodies limit the survival of further transfused platelets and also the patient's own platelets.

Laboratory Investigation of Thrombocytopenia (Rapaport, 1971). Examination of the blood film and the bone marrow is necessary to properly evaluate thrombocytopenia. Beyond these, the clinical history and physical examination will frequently provide a major clue to the etiology, and therefore determine which other tests will be employed.

Blood. The presence of thrombocytopenia is first suspected by examining the stained blood film and is quantitatively documented by platelet counts. Evidence suggesting the cause may be found in the CBC and in a careful examination of the blood film.

Impaired production of platelets is suggested by certain findings on the blood film. Marked anisocytosis and poikilocytosis of red cells or a leukoerythroblastotic reaction suggests a myelophthisic disorder of the marrow. Marked rouleaux formation suggests a blood protein disorder such as multiple myeloma. Pancytopenia without the presence of immature granulocytes or normoblasts is the typical finding in aplastic anemia. Careful search for blasts will usually be rewarding if the cause of the thrombocytopenia is acute leukemia. Oval macrocytes and hypersegmented neutrophils are presumptive evidence for megaloblastic anemia, which usually is accompanied by thrombocytopenia.

If the marrow is normally functional, increased destruction of platelets leads to increased production; this is accompanied by large platelets on the blood film. Evidence of hemolysis, with fragmented red cells, triangularly shaped cells, and helmet cells, should suggest the possibility of disseminated intravascular coagulation or thrombotic thrombocytopenic purpura. Evidence of hemolysis with spherocytic red cells suggests that there is an autoantibody against both red cells and platelets, as may occur in systemic lupus erythematosus. In the absence of an underlying disease, this combination of autoimmune hemolytic anemia and thrombocytopenia is known as Evans' syndrome.

Bone Marrow. Examination of marrow is necessary to ascertain the status of platelet production. A paucity of megakaryocytes indicates decreased production. When platelet production is increased, the megakaryocytes are increased in number, they tend to be larger and have more nuclear segments, and there is commonly a shift to the left in maturity and very few platelets surrounding or budding from them. Signs of increased production indicate that increased platelet destruction is the mechanism for the thrombocytopenia.

The other important reason for examining the marrow is to determine whether a myelophthisic process is responsible for the thrombocytopenia. Metastatic carcinoma, myelofibrosis, multiple myeloma, malignant lymphoma, and leukemia are among the diseases that are frequently associated with thrombocytopenia and which may be detected in the marrow biopsy or films.

Other Examinations. The clinical setting will suggest which other laboratory procedures are necessary. A diagnosis of ITP should not be made without performing a direct antiglobulin test, antinuclear antibody test, an LE cell test, and serum protein electrophoresis because of the frequency of thrombocytopenia in disorders of immune function, such as SLE, blood protein disorders, and malignant lymphoma.

Bleeding and Platelets. In general, with thrombocytopenia below 50,000 per μl., the risk of abnormal bleeding is enhanced, yet the functional effectiveness as well as the number of platelets is important in hemostasis. The bleeding time is a test of both platelet numbers and function. Using a standardized template bleeding time, Harker and Slichter (1972) showed that in patients with platelet counts between 100,000 and 10,000 per μl., the bleeding time becomes progressively and predictably longer as the count diminishes, if the platelets have normal function. If the patient's platelets are younger (and larger) and more hemostatically effective, as in ITP, the bleeding time is shorter than would be predicted for the level of the platelet count. If, on the other hand, the patient has a functional platelet defect, the bleeding time is longer than would be predicted from the platelet count.

Abnormalities of Platelet Function. Though adequate in numbers, qualitatively defective platelets may give rise to a bleeding disorder. The latter may be detected by a prolonged bleeding time and either diminished clot retraction or a defective release reaction (release of ADP with subsequent aggregation) and impaired ability to make platelet factor 3 available. Qualitative or platelet functional defects may be hereditary or acquired, and are considered briefly in Chapter 6, p. 418.

REFERENCES

Abildgard, C. F., Cornet, J. A., and Schulman, I.: Primary erythrocytosis. J. Pediat. *63*:1072, 1963.

Ackermann, P. G.: Electronic Instrumentation in the Clinical Laboratory. Boston, Little, Brown and Company, 1972.

Adamson, J. W., Alexanian, R., Martinez, C., and Finch, C. A.: Erythropoietin excretion in normal man. Blood *28*:354, 1966.

Adamson, J. W., Stamatoyannopoulos, G., Kontras, S., Lascari, A., and Detter, J.: Recessive familial erythrocytosis: Aspects of marrow regulation in two families. Blood *41*:641, 1973.

Aisenberg, A. C.: Malignant lymphoma. New Eng. J. Med. *288*:883; 935, 1973.

Aisenberg, A. C., and Bloch, K. J.: Immunoglobulins on the surface of neoplastic lymphocytes. New Eng. J. Med. *287*:272, 1972.

Aksoy, M., and Erdem, S.: A simple method for the quantitation of haemoglobin-A_2 by starch gel electrophoresis. Clin. Chim. Acta *12*:696, 1965.

Albritton, E. C.: Standard Values in Blood. Philadelphia, W. B. Saunders Company, 1952.

Anderson, B. B.: Investigations into the *Euglena* method for the assay of the vitamin B_{12} in serum. J. Clin. Path. *17*:14, 1964.

Ansley, H., and Ornstein, L.: Enzyme histochemistry and differential white cell counts on the Technicon Hemalog D. *In* Advances in Automated Analysis, Technicon International Congress. Miami, Thurman Associates, 1970, p. 437.

Ashby, W.: The determination of the life of the transfused blood corpuscles in man. J. Exper. Med. *29*:267, 1919.

Aster, R. H.: Pooling of platelets in the spleen: Role in the pathogenesis of "hypersplenic" thrombocytopenia. J. Clin. Invest. *45*:645, 1966.

Aster, R. H.: Production of platelets. *In* Williams, W. J., Beutler, E., Erslev, A. J., and Rundles, R. W. (eds.): Hematology. New York, McGraw Hill Book Co., Inc., 1972, p. 1042.

Atwater, J., and Schwartz, E.: Tests for hemoglobin H and other unstable hemoglobins. *In* Williams, W. J., Beutler, E., Erslev, A. J., and Rundles, R. W. (eds.): Hematology. New York, McGraw Hill Book Co., Inc., 1972, p. 1361.

Bacus, J. W., and Gose, E. E.: Leukocyte pattern recognition. I.E.E.F. Transaction on Systems, Man and Cybernetics, Vol. SMC-2, 513, 1972.

Bainton, D. F.: Origin, content, and fate of PMN granules. *In* Williams, R. C., Jr., and Fudenberg, H. H. (eds.): Phagocytic mechanisms in health and disease. New York, Intercontinental Medical Book Corp., 1972, p. 123.

Bainton, D. F., and Finch, C. A.: The diagnosis of iron deficiency anemia. Amer. J. Med. *37*:62, 1964.

Bainton, D. F., Ullyot, J. L., and Farquhar, M. G.: The development of neutrophilic polymorphonuclear leukocytes in human bone marrow. J. Exper. Med. *134*:907, 1971.

Baldini, M.: Idiopathic thrombocytopenic purpura. New Eng. J. Med. *274*:1245, 1966.

Bank, A., and Marks, P. A.: The thalassemia syndromes and the intracellular regulation of globin synthesis. Med. Clin. N. Amer. *57*:305, 1973.

Barak, Y., Paran, M., Levin, S., and Sachs, L.: In vitro induction of myeloid proliferation and maturation in infantile genetic agranulocytosis. Blood *38*:74, 1971.

Bauman, A. W., and Swisher, S. N.: Hyporegenerative processes in hemolytic anemia. Semin. Hematol. *4*:265, 1967.

Beck, W. S. (ed.): Hematology. Harvard Pathophysiology Series, Volume 1. Cambridge, The MIT Press, 1973.

Berkson, J., Magath, T. B., and Hurn, M.: Laboratory standards in relation to chance fluctuations of the erythrocyte count as estimated with the hemocytometer. J. Amer. Statist. A. *30*:414, 1935.

Berkson, J., Magath, T. B., and Hurn, M.: The error or estimate of the blood cell count as made with the hemocytometer. Amer. J. Physiol. *128*:309, 1940.

Berlin, N. I., Hennessy, T. G., and Gartland, J.: Sternal marrow puncture: The dilution with peripheral blood as determined by P^{32} labelled red cells. J. Lab. Clin. Med. *36*:23, 1950.

Berman, L.: A review of methods for aspiration and biopsy of bone marrow. Amer. J. Clin. Path. *23*:385, 1953.

Berman, L., Axelrod, A. R., Goodman, H. L., and McClaughry, R. I.: So-called "lupus erythematosus inclusion phenomenon" of bone marrow and blood: Morphologic and serologic studies. Amer. J. Clin. Path. *20*:403, 1950.

Beutler, E.: Abnormalities of the hexose monophosphate shunt. Semin. Hematol. *8*:311, 1971a.
Beutler, E.: Red Cell Metabolism: A Manual of Biochemical Methods. New York, Grune & Stratton, 1971b.
Beutler, E., Dern, R. J., and Alving, A. S.: The hemolytic effect of primaquine: VI. An in vitro test for sensitivity of erythrocytes to primaquine. J. Lab. Clin. Med. *45*:40, 1955.
Bishop, C. R., Rothstein, G., Ashenbrucker, H. E., and Athens, J. W.: Leukokinetic studies XIV. Blood neutrophil kinetics in chronic steady-state neutropenia. J. Clin. Invest. *50*:1678, 1971.
Björkman, S. E. (ed.): Haemoglobin and red cell production and destruction. Series Haematologica 2, 1965.
Block, M., Smaller, V., and Brown, J.: An adaptation of the Maximow technique for preparation of sections of hemopoietic tissues. J. Lab. Clin. Med. *42*:145, 1953.
Blume, R. S., and Wolff, S. M.: The Chediak-Higashi syndrome: Studies in four patients and a review of the literature. Medicine *51*:247, 1972.
Boggs, D. R., and Winkelstein, A.: White Cell Manual. Seattle, University of Washington Press, 1971.
Böttiger, L. E., and Svedberg, C. A.: Normal erythrocyte sedimentation rate and age. Brit. Med. J. *1*:85, 1967.
Bouroncle, B. A., Wiseman, B. K., and Doan, C. A.: Leukemic reticuloendotheliosis. Blood *13*:609, 1958.
Boyd, R. V., and Hoffbrand, B. I.: Erythrocyte sedimentation rate in elderly hospital in-patients. Brit. Med. J. *1*:901, 1966.
Brain, M. C.: Microangiopathic hemolytic anemia. Ann. Rev. Med. *21*:133, 1970.
Brain, M. C.: Microangiopathic haemolytic anaemia (MHA). Brit. J. Haematol. 23(Suppl):45, 1972.
Brain, M. C., Dacie, J. V., and Hourihane, D. O'B.: Microangiopathic haemolytic anaemia; the possible role of vascular lesions in pathogenesis. Brit. J. Haematol. *8*:358, 1962.
Brecher, G., and Bessis, M.: Present status of spiculated red cells and their relationship to the discocyte-echinocyte transformation: A critical review. Blood *40*:333, 1972.
Brecher, G., and Cronkite, E. P.: Estimation of the number of platelets by phase microscopy. *In* Tocantins, L. M., and Kazal, L. A.: Blood Coagulation, Hemorrhage and Thrombosis. New York, Grune & Stratton, Inc., 1964.
Brecher, G., and Schneiderman, M.: A time-saving device for the counting of reticulocytes. Amer. J. Clin. Path. *20*:1079, 1950.
Brecher, G., Schneiderman, M., and Cronkite, E. P.: The reproducibility and constancy of the platelet count. Amer. J. Clin. Path. *23*:15, 1953.
Brecher, G., Schneiderman, M., and Williams, G. Z.: Evaluation of electronic red blood cell counter. Amer. J. Clin. Path. *26*:1439, 1956.
Brittin, G. M., and Brecher, G.: Instrumentation and automation in clinical hematology. Prog. Hematol. 7:299, 1971.
Brittin, G. M., Brecher, G., and Johnson, C. A.: Evaluation of the Coulter Counter Model S. Amer. J. Clin. Path. 52:579, 1969a.
Brittin, G. M., Brecher, G., Johnson, C. A., and Elashoff, R. M.: Stability of blood in commonly used anticoagulants. Use of refrigerated blood for quality control of the Coulter Counter Model S. Amer. J. Clin. Path. 52:690, 1969b.
Brittin, G. M., Dew, S. A., and Fewell, E. K.: Automated optical counting of blood platelets. Blood *38*:422, 1971.
Brunning, R. D.: Morphologic alterations in nucleated blood and marrow cells in genetic disorders. Human Path. *1*:99, 1970.
Brus, I., and Lewis, S. M.: The haptoglobin content of serum in haemolytic anaemia. Brit. J. Haemat. 5:348, 1959.
Bull, B. S.: Aids to electronic platelet counting. Amer. J. Clin. Path. *54*:707, 1970.
Bull, B. S.: Automation in Haematology. *In* Goldberg, A., and Brain, M. C. (eds.): Recent Advances in Haematology. Edinburgh, Churchill-Livingstone, 1971, p. 357.
Bull, B. S., and Brailsford, J. D.: The Zeta sedimentation ratio. Blood *40*:550, 1972.
Bull, B. S., Dutcher, T. F., and Siggard-Andersen, O.: The Hem-Aliquanter: A dispenser-dilutor for hematology. Amer. J. Clin. Path. *49*:295, 1968.
Bull, B. S., Schneiderman, M. A., and Brecher, G.: Platelet counts with the Coulter Counter. Amer. J. Clin. Path. *44*:678, 1965.
Carson, P. E., and Frischer, H.: Glucose-6-phosphate dehydrogenase deficiency and related disorders of the pentose phosphate pathway. Amer. J. Med. *41*:744, 1966.
Carter, R. L., and Penman, H. G. (eds.): Infectious Mononucleosis. Oxford, Blackwell Scientific Publications, 1969: a, p. 82; b, p. 99; c, p. 55.
Cartwright, G. E.: The anemia of chronic disorders. Semin. Hematol. *3*:351, 1966.
Cartwright, G. E.: Diagnostic Laboratory Hematology. 4th edition. New York, Grune & Stratton, Inc., 1968.
Cartwright, G. E., and Lee, G. R.: The anemia of chronic disorders. Brit. J. Haematol. *21*:147, 1971.
Cassileth, P.: Lymphocytopenia. *In* Williams, W. J., Beutler, E., Erslev, A. J., and Rundles, R. W. (eds.): Hematology. New York, McGraw Hill Book Co., Inc., 1972.
Castle, W. B.: Development of knowledge concerning the gastric intrinsic factor and its relation to pernicious anemia. New Eng. J. Med. *249*:603, 1953.
Castle, W. B.: Disorders of the blood. *In* Sodeman, W. A. and Sodeman, W. A., Jr. (eds.): Pathologic Physiology: Mechanisms of Disease. 4th edition. Philadelphia, W. B. Saunders Company, 1967.
Catovsky, D., Galton, D. A. G., Griffin, C., Hoffbrand, A. V., and Szur, L.: Serum lysozyme and vitamin B_{12} binding capacity in myeloproliferative disorders. Brit. J. Haematol. *21*:661, 1971a.
Catovsky, D., Galton, D. A. G., and Griffin, C.: Significance of lysozyme estimations in acute myeloid and chronic monocytic leukemia. Brit. J. Haematol. *21*:565, 1971b.
Chalmers, J. N. M., and Boheimer, K.: Pure red-cell anaemia in patients with thymic tumors. Brit. Med. J. 2:1514, 1954.
Chanarin, I.: The Megaloblastic Anaemias. Oxford, Blackwell Scientific Publications, 1969.
Chanarin, I., Barkhan, P., Peacock, M., and Stamp, T. C. B.: Acute arrest of haemopoiesis. Brit. J. Haematol. *10*:43, 1964.
Charache, S., Weatherall, D. J., and Clegg, J. B.: Polycythemia associated with a hemoglobinopathy. J. Clin. Invest. *45*:813, 1966.
Chernoff, A. I.: The human hemoglobins in health and disease. New Eng. J. Med. *253*:322, 365, 416, 1955.
Chernoff, A. I., and Singer, K.: Studies on abnormal hemoglobins. IV. Persistence of fetal hemoglobin in erythrocytes of normal children. Pediatrics *9*:469, 1952.
Chervenick, P. A., and LoBuglio, A. F.: Human blood monocytes: Stimulators of granulocyte and mononuclear colony formation in vitro. Science *178*:164, 1972.
Cohen, R. J., Sachs, J. R., Wicker, D. J., and Conrad, M. E.: Methemoglobinemia provoked by malarial chemoprophylaxis in Vietnam. New Eng. J. Med. *279*:1127, 1968.
Conley, C. L., and Charache, S.: Mechanisms by which some abnormal hemoglobins produce clinical manifestations. Semin. Hematol. *4*:53, 1967.
Craddock, C. G.: Granulocyte kinetics. *In* Williams, W. J., Beutler, E., Erslev, A. J., and Rundles, R. W. (eds.): Hematology. New York, McGraw Hill Book Co., Inc., 1972, Chapter 71.
Craddock, C. G., Longmire, R., and McMillan, R.: Lymphocytes and the immune response. New Eng. J. Med. *285*: 324, and 378, 1971.
Crookston, J. H., Crookston, M. C., Burnie, K. L., Francombe, W. H., Dacie, J. V., Davis, J. A., and Lewis, S. M.: Hereditary erythroblastic multinuclearity with a positive acid serum test: A type of congenital dyserythropoietic anemia. Brit. J. Haematol. *17*:11, 1969.
Crosby, W. H., and Furth, F. W.: A modification of the benzidine method for measurement of hemoglobin in plasma and urine. Blood *11*:380, 1956.
Dacie, J. V.: Haemolytic Anaemias. Parts I, II, III, and IV. 2nd ed. New York, Grune & Stratton, Inc., 1960, 1963, 1967, and 1967.

Dacie, J. V.: Autoimmune haemolytic anaemias. Brit. Med. J. *2*:381, 1970.

Dacie, J. V.: Paroxysmal nocturnal haemoglobinuria. The Scientific Basis of Medicine: Annual Reviews. London, The Athlone Press, 1972a.

Dacie, J. V.: Mechanism of haemolysis in auto-immune haemolytic anaemias. Nouv. Rev. Franc. d'Hem. *12*:371, 1972b.

Dacie, J. V., Grimes, A. J., Meisler, A., Steingold, L., Hemsted, E. H., Beaven, G. H., and White, J. C.: Hereditary Heinz-body anaemia. A report of studies on five patients with mild anaemia. Brit. J. Haematol. *10*:388, 1964.

Dacie, J. V., and Lewis, S. M.: Practical Haematology. 4th ed. New York, Grune & Stratton, Inc., 1968.

Dacie, J. V., and Mollin, D. L.: Siderocytes, sideroblasts and sideroblastic anaemia. Acta Med. Scand. (suppl.) *445*:237, 1966.

Dacie, J. V., and Worlledge, S. M.: Auto-immune haemolytic anaemias. Progr. Hematol. 7:82, 1969.

Daland, G. A.: Color Atlas of Morphologic Hematology with a Guide to Clinical Interpretation. Cambridge, Harvard University Press, 1951.

Daland, G. A., and Castle, W. B.: A simple and rapid method for demonstrating sickling of the red blood cells; The use of reducing agents. J. Lab. Clin. Med. *33*:1082, 1948.

Dameshek, W., and Gunz, F.: Leukemia. 2nd edition. New York, Grune & Stratton, Inc., 1964.

Daniel, M-Th., Flandrin, G., Lejeune, F., Liso, P., and Lortholary, P.: Les estérases spécifiques monocytaires. Utilisation dans la classification des leucémies aigues. Nouv. Rev. Franc. d'Hematol. *11*:233, 1971.

Davidsohn, I.: Infectious mononucleosis. Amer. J. Dis. Child. *49*:1222, 1935.

Davidsohn, I.: Serologic diagnosis of infectious mononucleosis. J.A.M.A. *108*:289, 1937.

Davidsohn, I.: Test for infectious mononucleosis. Amer. J. Clin. Path. 8:56, 1938.

Davidsohn, I.: Immunohematology, a new branch of clinical pathology. Amer. J. Clin. Path. *24*:1333, 1954.

Davidsohn, I., and Lee, C. L.: Serologic diagnosis of infectious mononucleosis. Amer. J. Clin. Path. *41*:115, 1964.

Dawson, J. B.: The E. S. R. in a new dress. Brit. Med. J. *1*:1697, 1960.

DeGruchy, G. C.: Clinical Haematology in Medical Practice. 3rd ed. Oxford, Blackwell Scientific Publications, 1970.

Denst, J., and Mulligan, R. M.: The distribution of bone marrow in the human sternum. Amer. J. Clin. Path. *20*: 610, 1950.

Deykin, D., and Hellerstein, L. J.: The assessment of drug-dependent and isoimmune antiplatelet antibodies by the use of platelet aggregometry. J. Clin. Invest. *51*:3142, 1972.

Diamond, L. K., Allen, D. M., and Magill, F. B.: Congenital (erythroid) hypoplastic anemia: A 25-year study. Amer. J. Dis. Child. *102*:149, 1961.

Diggs, L. W.: The blood picture in sickle cell anemia. South. Med. J. *25*:615, 1932.

Diggs, L. W., and Walker, R.: Technical points in the detection of sickle cell hemoglobin by the tube test. Amer. J. Med. Technol. *37*:33, 1971.

Di Guglielmo, G.: Les maladies erythrémiques. Rev. Hémat. *1*:355, 1946.

Doan, C. A.: Clinical implications of experimental hematology. Medicine *10*:323, 1931.

Donohue, D. M., Motulsky, A. G., Giblett, E. R., Pirzio-Biroli, G., Viranuvatti, V., and Finch, C. A.: The use of chromium as a red-cell tag. Brit. J. Haematol. *1*:249, 1955.

Dougherty, T. F., Berliner, M. L., Schneebeli, G. L., and Berliner, D. L.: Hormonal control of lymphatic structure and function. Ann. N.Y. Acad. Sci. *113*:825, 1964.

Douglas, S. D.: Disorders of neutrophil and monocyte function. Brit. J. Haematol. *21*:493, 1971.

Downey, H.: Handbook of Hematology. New York, Paul B. Hoeber, Inc., 1938.

Downey, H., and McKinlay, C. A.: Acute lymphadenosis compared with acute lymphatic leukemia. Arch. Intern. Med. *32*:82, 1923.

Downey, H., and Stasney, J.: Infectious mononucleosis. II. Hematologic studies. J.A.M.A. *105*:764, 1935.

Dubois, E. L., and Freeman, V.: A comparative evaluation of the sensitivity of the L.E. cell test performed simultaneously by different methods. Blood *12*:656, 1957.

Ebaugh, F. G., Jr., Emerson, C. P., and Ross, J. F.: The use of radioactive chromium-51 as an erythrocyte agent for the determination of red cell survival in vivo. J. Clin. Invest. *32*:1260, 1953.

Edelson, P. J., Stites, D. P., Gold, S., and Fudenberg, H. H.: Disorders of neutrophil function. Defects in the early stages of the process. Clin. Exp. Immunol. *13*:21, 1973.

Emerson, C. P., Jr., Shen, S. C., Ham, T. H., and Castle, W. B.: The mechanism of blood destruction in congenital hemolytic jaundice. J. Clin. Invest. *26*:1180, 1947.

England, J. M., Walford, D. M., and Waters, D. A. W.: Reassessment of the reliability of the haematocrit. Brit. J. Haematol. *23*:247, 1972.

Erslev, A. J.: Feedback circuits in the control of stem cell differentiation. Amer. J. Path. *65*:629, 1971.

Erslev, A. J.: Anemia of chronic renal failure. *In* Williams, W. J., Beutler, E., Erslev, A. J., and Rundles, R. W. (eds.): Hematology. New York, McGraw Hill Book Co., Inc., 1972, Chapter 23.

Fairbanks, V. F.: Is the peripheral blood film reliable for the diagnosis of iron deficiency anemia? Amer. J. Clin. Path. *55*:447, 1971.

Fairbanks, V. F., Fahey, J. L., and Beutler, E.: Clinical Disorders of Iron Metabolism. 2nd ed. New York, Grune & Stratton, 1971.

Fairbanks, V. F., and Fernandez, M. N.: The identification of metabolic errors associated with hemolytic anemia. J.A.M.A. *208*:316, 1969.

Fanconi, G.: Familial constitutional panmyelocytopathy, Fanconi's anemia (F.A.). I. Clinical aspects. Semin. Hematol. *4*:233, 1967.

Fessas, P.: Inclusions of hemoglobin in erythroblasts and erythrocytes of thalassemia. Blood *21*:21, 1963.

Finch, C. A.: Red Cell Manual. Seattle, University of Washington Press, 1969.

Finch, S. C.: Granulocytopenia, (Chapter 75) and Granulocytosis (Chapter 76). *In* Williams, W. J., Beutler, E., Erslev, A. J., and Rundles, R. W. (eds.): Hematology. New York, McGraw Hill Book Co., Inc., 1972.

Finland, M., Peterson, O. L., Allen, H. E., Samper, B. A., and Barnes, M. W.: Cold agglutinins. J. Clin. Invest. *24*:451, 1945. (A series of six papers.)

Frangione, B., and Franklin, E. C.: Heavy chain diseases: Clinical features and molecular significance of the disordered immunoglobulin structure. Semin. Hematol. *10*:53, 1973.

Friou, G. J.: Antinuclear antibodies: Diagnostic significance and methods. Arthritis Rheum. *10*:151, 1967a.

Friou, G. J.: The LE cell factor and antinuclear antibodies. *In* Cohen, A. S. (ed.): Laboratory Methods in Rheumatic Diseases. Boston, Little, Brown and Company, 1967b.

Fry, G. L., and Hoak, J. C.: Improved method for electronic counting of platelets. J. Lab. Clin. Med. *74*:536, 1969.

Gabuzda, T. G.: Hemoglobin H and the red cell. Blood *27*:568, 1966.

Gagon, T. E., Athens, J. W., Boggs, D. R., and Cartwright, G. E.: An evaluation of the variance of leukocyte counts as performed with the hemocytometer, Coulter, and Fisher instruments. Amer. J. Clin. Path. *46*:684, 1966.

Galton, D. A. G., and Spiers, A. S. D.: Progress in the leukemias. Progr. Hematol. 7:343, 1971.

Gambino, S. R., DiRe, J. J., Monteleone, M., and Budd, D. C.: The Westergren sedimentation rate, using K_3EDTA. Amer. J. Clin. Path. *43*:173, 1965.

Garrey, W. E., and Bryan, W. R.: Variations in white blood cell count. Physiol. Rev. *15*:597, 1935.

Gerald, P. S., and Diamond, L. K.: The diagnosis of thalassemia trait by starch block electrophoresis of the hemoglobin. Blood *13*:61, 1958.

Gerald, P. S., and Scott, E. M.: The hereditary methemoglobinemias. *In* Stanbury, J. B., Wyngaarden, J. B., and Fredrickson, D. S.: The Metabolic Basis of Inherited Disease. 2nd edition. New York, McGraw-Hill Book Company, 1966.

Giorgio, A. J., and Plaut, G. W. E.: A method for the colorimetric determination of urinary methylmalonic acid in pernicious anemia. J. Lab. Clin. Med. *66*:667, 1965.

Glade, P. R. (ed.): Infectious Mononucleosis. Philadelphia, J. B. Lippincott Company, 1973.

Glenner, G. G., Terry, W. D., and Isersky, C.: Amyloidosis: Its nature and pathogenesis. Semin. Hematol. *10*:65, 1973.

Godman, G. C., Deitch, A. D., and Klemperer, P.: The composition of the L.E. and hematoxylin bodies of systemic lupus erythematosus. Amer. J. Path. *34*:1, 1958.

Goodman, L., and Gilman, A.: The Pharmacological Basis of Therapeutics. 3rd edition. New York, The Macmillan Company, 1965.

Green, P., and Teal, C. F. J.: Modification of hemoglobin in order to avoid precipitation of globulins. Amer. J. Clin. Path. *32*:216, 1959.

Greenberg, M. S., Harvey, H. A., and Morgan, C.: A simple and inexpensive screening test for sickle hemoglobin. New Eng. J. Med. *286*:1143, 1972.

Groover, R. V., Burke, E. C., Gordon, H., and Berdon, W. E.: The genetic mucopolysaccharidoses. Semin. Hematol. *9*:371, 1972.

Gunz, F. W.: Hemorrhagic thrombocythemia: A critical review. Blood *15*:706, 1960.

Halnan, K. E., and Russell, M. H.: Polycythaemia vera. Comparison of survival and causes of death in patients managed with and without radiotherapy. Lancet *2*:760, 1965.

Ham, T. H.: Studies in destruction of red blood cells. I. Chronic hemolytic anemia with paroxysmal nocturnal hemoglobinuria: An investigation of the mechanism of hemolysis with observations on five cases. Arch. Intern. Med. *64*:1271, 1939.

Ham, T. H., Gardner, F. H., and Wagley, P. F.: Studies on the metabolism of hemolytic anemia and hemoglobinuria occurring in patients with high concentrations of cold agglutinins. J. Clin. Invest. *27*:538, 1948a.

Ham, T. H., Shen, S. C., Fleming, E. M., and Castle, W. B.: Studies on the destruction of red blood cells. IV. Thermal injury. Blood *3*:373, 1948b.

Hargraves, M. M.: Discovery of the LE cell and its morphology. Mayo Clin. Proc. *44*:579, 1969.

Hargraves, M. M., Richmond, H., and Morton, R.: Presentation of two bone marrow elements: The "tart" cell and the "L.E." cell. Proc. Staff Meet. Mayo Clin. *23*:25, 1948.

Harker, L.: Hemostasis Manual. Seattle, University of Washington Press, 1969.

Harker, L. A., and Finch, C. A.: Thrombokinetics in man. J. Clin. Invest. *48*:963, 1969.

Harker, L. A., and Slichter, S. J.: The bleeding time as a screening test for evaluation of platelet function. New Eng. J. Med. *287*:155, 1972.

Harris, J. W.: Studies on destruction of red blood cells. VIII. Molecular orientation of sickle cell hemoglobin solutions. Proc. Soc. Exper. Biol. Med. *75*:197, 1950.

Harris, J. W., and Kellermeyer, R. W.: The Red Cell: Production, Metabolism, Destruction: Normal and Abnormal. Rev. ed. Cambridge, Harvard University Press, 1970.

Hartmann, R. C., Jenkins, D. E., Jr., and Arnold, A. B.: Diagnostic specificity of sucrose hemolysis test for paroxysmal nocturnal hemoglobinuria. Blood *35*:462, 1970.

Hartsock, R. J., Smith, E. B., and Petty, C. S.: Normal variations with aging of the amount of hematopoietic tissue in bone marrow from the anterior iliac crest. Amer. J. Clin. Path. *43*:326, 1965.

Haserick, J. R., and Lewis, L. A.: Blood factor in acute disseminated lupus erythematosus. II. Induction of specific antibodies against L.E. factor. Blood *5*:718, 1950.

Hattersley, P. G., Gerard, P. W., Caggiano, V., and Nash, D. R.: Erroneous values on the Model S Coulter due to high titer cold agglutinins. Amer. J. Clin. Path. *55*:442, 1971.

Havard, C. W. H.: Thymic tumours and refractory anemia. Series Haematologica *5*:18, 1965.

Hayhoe, F. G. J., and Cawley, J. C.: Acute leukaemia: Cellular morphology, cytochemistry and fine structure. Clin. Haemat. *1*:49, 1972.

Hayhoe, F. G. J., Quaglino, D., and Doll, R.: The Cytology and Cytochemistry of Acute Leukaemias. London. Her Majesty's Stationery Office, 1964.

Heilmeyer, L., and Begemann, H.: Atlas der klinischen Haematologie und Cytologie. Berlin, Springer-Verlag, 1955.

Heimpel, H., Forteza-Villa, J., Queisser, W., and Spiertz, E.: Electron and light microscopic study of the erythroblasts of patients with congenital dyserythropoietic anemia. Blood *37*:299, 1971.

Heller, P.: Hemoglobinopathic dysfunction of the red cell. Amer. J. Med. *41*:799, 1966.

Henle, W., and Henle, G.: Epstein-Barr virus and infectious mononucleosis. New Eng. J. Med. *288*:263, 1973.

Henry, R. J.: Clinical Chemistry: Principles and Technics. New York, Harper & Row, 1964: a, p. 423; b, p. 744.

Herbert, V.: Experimental nutritional folate deficiency in man. Trans. Assoc. Amer. Phys. *75*:307, 1962.

Herrick, J. B.: Peculiar elongated and sickle-shaped red blood corpuscles in a case of severe anemia. Arch Intern. Med. *6*:517, 1910.

Hillman, R. S., and Finch, C. A.: Erythropoiesis: Normal and abnormal. Semin. Hematol. *4*:327, 1967.

Hillman, R. S., and Finch, C. A.: The misused reticulocyte. Brit. J. Haematol. *17*:313, 1969.

Hoagland, R. J.: Infectious Mononucleosis. New York, Grune & Stratton, Inc., 1967.

Hoffbrand, A. V.: The megaloblastic anaemias. *In* Goldberg, A., and Brain, M. C. (eds.): Recent Advances in Haematology. Edinburgh, Churchill-Livingstone, 1971, p. 357.

Hoyer, J. R., Cooper, M. D., Gabrielsen, A. E., and Good, R. A.: Lymphopenic forms of congenital immunologic deficiency diseases. Medicine *47*:201, 1968.

Huehns, E. R., and Shooter, E. M.: Human haemoglobins. J. Med. Genet. *2*:48, 1965.

Huisman, T. H. J., and Dozy, A. M.: Quantitative determination of the minor hemoglobin component Hb-A_2 by DEAE-cellulose chromatography. Anal. Biochem. *2*:400, 1961.

Huisman, T. H. J., and Prins, H. K.: Chromatographic estimation of four different kinds of human hemoglobin. J. Lab. Clin. Med. *46*:255, 1955.

Itano, H. A., and Neel, J. V.: New inherited abnormality of human hemoglobin. Proc. Nat. Acad. Sci. *36*:613, 1950.

Ivy, A. C., Nelson, D., and Bucher, G.: The standardization of certain factors in the cutaneous "venostasis" bleeding time technique. J. Lab. Clin. Med. *26*:1812, 1941.

Jackson, J., Jr.: The protean character of the leukemias and of the leukemoid states. New Eng. J. Med. *220*:175, 1939.

Jacob, H. S.: Hypersplenism. *In* Williams, W. J., Beutler, E., Erslev, A. J., and Rundles, R. D. (eds.): Hematology. New York, McGraw Hill Book Co., 1972, Chapter 61.

Jacob, H. S., and Jandl, J. H.: A simple visual screening test for glucose-6-phosphate dehydrogenase deficiency employing ascorbate and cyanide. New Eng. J. Med. *274*:1162, 1966.

Jacob, H. S., Ruby, A., Overland, E. S., and Mazia, D.: Abnormal membrane protein of red blood cells in hereditary spherocytosis. J. Clin. Invest. *50*:1800, 1971.

Jacobson, L. O., Marks, E. K., and Lorenz, E.: The hematological effects of ionizing radiations. Radiology *53*:371, 1949.

Jaffé, E. R.: Hereditary methemoglobinemias associated with abnormalities in the metabolism of erythrocytes. Amer. J. Med. *41*:786, 1966.

Jamshidi, K., and Swaim, W. R.: Bone marrow biopsy with unaltered architecture: A new biopsy device. J. Lab. Clin. Med. *77*:335, 1971.

Jandl, J. H.: The spleen and reticuloendothelial system. *In* Sodeman, W. A., and Sodeman, W. A., Jr. (eds.): Pathologic Physiology: Mechanisms of Disease. Philadelphia, W. B. Saunders Company, 1967.

Jandl, J. H.: Hereditary spherocytosis. *In* Beutler, E. (ed.): Hereditary Disorders of Erythrocyte Metabolism. New York, Grune & Stratton, 1968.

Jandl, J. H., Jones, A. R., and Castle, W. B.: The destruction of red cells by antibodies in man. I. Observations on the sequestration and lysis of red cells altered by immune mechanisms. J. Clin. Invest. *36*:1428, 1957.

Kaplow, L. S.: Cytochemistry of leukocyte alkaline phosphatase. Amer. J. Clin. Path. *39*:439, 1963.

Kaplow, L. S.: Simplified myeloperoxidase stain using benzidine dihydrochloride. Blood *26*:215, 1965.

Karpatkin, S.: Human platelet senescence. Ann. Rev. Med. *23*:101, 1972.

Katayama, K.: Über eine neue Blutprobe bei der Kohlenoxydvergiftung. Virchows Arch. Path. Anat. *114*:53, 1888.

Kauder, E., and Mauer, A. M.: Neutropenias of childhood. J. Pediat. *69*:147, 1966.

Keeling, M. M., Ogden, L. L., Wrightstone, R. N., Wilson, J. B., Reynolds, C. A., Kitchens, J. L., and Huisman, T. H. J.: Hemoglobin Louisville (β 42(CDI) Phe $\rightarrow$ Leu): An unstable variant causing mild hemolytic anemia. J. Clin. Invest. *50*:2395, 1971.

Konrad, P. N., Richards, F. R., Valentine, W. N., and Paglia, D. E.: γ-Glutamyl-cysteine synthetase deficiency. A cause of hereditary hemolytic anemia. New Eng. J. Med. *286*: 558, 1972.

Kreig, A. F., and Henry, J. B.: Hemoglobin electrophoresis. Clinical pathology correlations of hemoglobinopathies and thalassemias. New York State J. Med. *67*:1275, 1967.

Kunkel, H. G., Ceppellini, R., Müller-Eberhard, U., and Wolf, J.: Observations on the minor basic hemoglobin component in blood of normal individuals and patients with thalassemia. J. Clin. Invest. *36*:1615, 1957.

LaCelle, P. L., and Weed, R. I.: The contribution of normal and pathologic erythrocytes to blood rheology. Progr. Hematol. *7*:1, 1971.

Lampasso, J. A.: Changes in hematologic values induced by storage of ethylene diaminetetraacetate human blood for varying periods of time. Amer. J. Clin. Path. *49*:443, 1968.

Lang, D. J., and Hanshaw, J. B.: Cytomegalovirus infection and the post-perfusion syndrome. New Eng. J. Med. *280*:1145, 1969.

Lappin, T. R. J., Lamont, A., and Nelson, M. G.: An evaluation of the Celloscope 401 electronic blood cell counter. J. Clin. Path. *25*:539, 1972.

Lau, K. S., Gottlieb, C., Wasserman, L. R., and Herbert, V.: Measurement of serum vitamin B_{12} level using radioisotope dilution and coated charcoal. Blood *26*:202, 1965.

Leake, C. D., Kohl, M., and Stebbins, G.: Diurnal variations in the blood specific gravity and erythrocyte count in healthy human adults. Amer. J. Physiol. *81*:493, 1927.

Lear, A. A., Harris, J. W., Castle, W. B., and Fleming, E. M.: The serum vitamin B_{12} concentration in pernicious anemia. J. Lab. Clin. Med. *44*:715, 1954.

Lee, C. L., and Davidsohn, I.: Workshop Manual on Serologic Tests for Infectious Mononucleosis. American Society of Clinical Pathologists, Commission on Continuing Education, 1967.

Lee, C. L., Davidsohn, I., and Panczyszyn, O.: Horse agglutinins in infectious mononucleosis. II. The spot test. Amer. J. Clin. Path. *49*:12, 1968.

Leeksma, C. H. W., and Cohen, J. A.: Determination of the life of human blood platelets using labelled di-isopropylfluorophosphate. Nature (London) *175*:552, 1955.

Lehmann, H., and Carrell, R. W.: Variations in the structure of human haemoglobin. Brit. Med. Bull. *25*:14, 1969.

Lehmann, H., and Huntsman, R. G.: Man's Haemoglobins. Philadelphia, J. B. Lippincott Co., 1966.

Leibowitz, S.: Infectious Mononucleosis. New York, Grune & Stratton, Inc., 1953.

Leitner, S. J., Britton, C. J. C., and Neumark, E.: Bone Marrow Biopsy. New York, Grune & Stratton, Inc., 1949.

Lewis, S. M.: Red cell abnormalities and haemolysis in aplastic anaemia. Brit. J. Haematol. *8*:322, 1962.

Lewis, S. M.: Course and prognosis in aplastic anemia. Brit. Med. J. *1*:1027, 1965.

Lewis, S. M., and Dacie, J. V.: The aplastic anaemia-paroxysmal nocturnal haemoglobinuria syndrome. Brit. J. Haematol. *13*:236, 1967.

Logue, G. L., Boyd, A. E., and Rosse, W. F.: Chlorpropamide-induced immune hemolytic anemia. New Eng. J. Med. *283*:900, 1970.

London, I. M.: The biosynthesis of hemoglobin and its control in relation to some hypochromic anemias in man. Series Haematologica 2:1, 1965.

Lowenstein, L., Brunton, L., and Hsieh, Y.-S.: Nutritional anemia and megaloblastosis in pregnancy. Canad. Med. Ass. J. *94*:636, 1966.

Luke, R. G., Koepke, J. A., and Siegel, R. R.: The effects of immunosuppressive drugs and uremia on automated leukocyte counts. Amer. J. Clin. Path. *56*:503, 1971.

Lukes, R. J.: Malignant lymphoma: Histologic considerations. *In* Ultmann, J. E., Griem, M. L., Kirsten, W. H., and Wissler, R. W. (eds.): Current Concepts in the Management of Lymphoma and Leukemia. New York, Springer-Verlag, Inc., 1971, p. 6.

Lukes, R. J., Butler, J. J., and Hicks, E. B.: The natural history of Hodgkin's disease as related to its pathologic picture. Cancer *19*:317, 1966a.

Lukes, R. J., Craver, L. L., Hall, T. C., Rappaport, H., and Rubin, P.: Hodgkin's disease, report of Nomenclature Committee. Cancer Res. *26*:1311, 1966b.

Lukes, R. J., Tindle, B. H., and Parker, J. W.: Reed-Sternberg-like cells in infectious mononucleosis. Lancet 2:1003, 1969.

MacKenzie, M. R., and Fudenberg, H. H.: Macroglobulinemia: An analysis of forty patients. Blood *39*:874, 1972.

Madison, F. W., and Squier, T. L.: Etiology of primary granulocytopenia (agranulocytic angina). J.A.M.A. *102*:755, 1934; J. Allergy 6:9, 1934.

Magath, T. B., Berkson, J., and Hurn, M.: Error of determination of erythrocyte count. Amer. J. Clin. Path. *6*:568, 1936.

Magath, T. B., and Winkle, V.: Technic for demonstrating "L.E." (lupus erythematosus) cells in blood. Amer. J. Clin. Path. *22*:586, 1952.

Maldonado, J. E., and Hanlon, D. G.: Monocytosis: A current appraisal. Mayo Clin. Proc. *40*:248, 1965.

Mansberg, H. P.: Optical techniques of particle counting. Advances in Automated Analysis. Technicon International Congress, 1969. *1*:213, 1970.

Marcus, A. J., and Zucker, M. B.: The Physiology of Blood Platelets. New York, Grune & Stratton, Inc., 1965.

Marengo-Rowe, A. J.: Rapid electrophoresis and quantitation of haemoglobins on cellulose acetate. J. Clin. Path. *18*:790, 1965.

Marsh, G. W., and Lewis, S. M.: Cardiac haemolytic anaemia. Semin. Hematol. *6*:133, 1969.

Matula, G., and Paterson, P. Y.: Spontaneous in vitro reduction of nitroblue tetrazolium by neutrophils of adult patients with bacterial infection. New Eng. J. Med. *285*:311, 1971.

Miale, J. B.: Laboratory Medicine: Hematology. 4th edition. St. Louis, The C. V. Mosby Co., 1972.

Miescher, P., and Strässle, R.: New serologic methods for the detection of the L.E. factor. Vox Sang. 2:283, 1957.

Miller, G., Niederman, J. C., and Andrews, L.-L.: Prolonged oropharyngeal excretion of Epstein-Barr virus after infectious mononucleosis. New Eng. J. Med. *288*:229, 1973.

Mitus, E. J., Mednicoff, I. B., and Dameshek, W.: Alkaline phosphatase of mature neutrophils in various polycythemias. New Eng. J. Med. *260*:1131, 1959.

Modan, B., and Lilienfeld, A. M.: Polycythemia vera and leukemia – the role of radiation treatment. A study of 1222 patients. Medicine *44*:305, 1965.

Mollin, D. L.: Sideroblasts and sideroblastic anaemia. Brit. J. Haematol. *11*:41, 1965.

Mollison, P. L.: Blood Transfusion in Clinical Medicine. 4th edition. Philadelphia, F. A. Davis Co., 1967.

Moloney, W. C., and Kastenbaum, M. A.: Leukemogenic effects of ionizing radiation on atomic bomb survivors in Hiroshima City. Science *121*:308, 1955.

Mudrik, P., Lee, C. L., and Davidsohn, I.: A capillary test for "L.E." cells. Amer. J. Clin. Path. *35*:516, 1961.

Muschel, L. H., and Piper, D. R.: Enzyme-treated red blood cells of sheep in the test for infectious mononucleosis. Amer. J. Clin. Path. *32*:240, 1959.

Nathan, D. G.: Thalassemia. New Eng. J. Med. *286*:586, 1972.

Nathan, D. G., and Baehner, R. L.: Disorders of phagocytic cell function. Progr. Hematol. 7:235, 1971.

Nathan, D. J., and Snapper, I.: On the interaction of dead leukocytic nuclei, L.E. factor and living leukocytes in the L.E. cell phenomenon. Blood *13*:883, 1958.

Neiman, R. S., Rosen, P. J., and Lukes, R. J.: Lymphocyte-depletion Hodgkin's disease. New Eng. J. Med. *288*:751, 1973.

Nelson, M. G.: Multichannel continuous flow analysis on the SMA-4/-7A. J. Clin. Path. 22(suppl. 3):20, 1969.

Nichols, B. A., Bainton, D. F., and Farquhar, M. G.: Differentiation of monocytes. Origin, nature and fate of their azurophil granules. J. Cell Biol. *50*:498, 1971.

Nowell, P. C., and Hungerford, D. A.: Chromosome studies on normal and leukemic human leukocytes. J. Nat. Cancer Inst. *25*:85, 1960.

Nowell, P. C., and Wilson, D. B.: Lymphocytes and hemic stem cells. Amer. J. Path. *65*:641, 1971.

Orfanakis, N. G., Ostlund, R. E., Bishop, C. R., and Athens, J. W.: Normal blood leukocyte concentration values. Amer. J. Clin. Path. *53*:647, 1970.

Osgood, E. E., and Seaman, A. J.: The cellular composition of normal bone marrow as obtained by sternal puncture. Physiol. Rev. *24*:46, 1944.

Oski, F. A., and Naiman, J. L.: Hematologic Problems in the Newborn. 2nd ed. Philadelphia, W. B. Saunders Co., 1972.

Oski, F. A., Naiman, J. L., Allen, D. M., and Diamond, L. K.: Leukocyte inclusions—Döhle bodies—associated with platelet abnormality (the May-Hegglin anomaly). Report of a family and review of the literature. Blood *20*:657, 1962.

Osserman, E. F., and Lawlor, D. P.: Serum and urinary lysozyme (muramidase) in monocytic and monomyelocytic leukemia. J. Exp. Med. *124*:921, 1966.

Owen, C. A., Jr.: The diagnostic use of radioactive isotopes. Postgrad. Med. *24*:449, 669, 1958; *25*:83, 196, 1959.

Owen, J. A., Better, F. C., and Hoban, J.: A simple method for the determination of serum haptoglobins. J. Clin. Path. *13*:163, 1960.

Page, L. B., and Culver, P. J.: A Syllabus of Laboratory Examinations in Clinical Diagnosis: Critical Evaluation of Laboratory Procedures in the Study of the Patient. Revised edition. Cambridge, Mass., Harvard University Press, 1966.

Park, B. H., Fikrig, S. M., and Smithwick, E. M.: Infection and nitroblue-tetrazolium reduction of neutrophils. Lancet 2:532, 1968.

Parry, R. M., Chandan, R. C., and Shahani, K. M.: A rapid and sensitive assay of muramidase. Proc. Soc. Exp. Biol. Med. *119*:384, 1965.

Paul, J. R., and Bunnell, W. W.: Presence of heterophilic antibodies in infectious mononucleosis. Amer. J. Med. Sci. *183*:90, 1932.

Pauling, L., Itano, H. A., Singer, S. J., and Wells, I. C.: Sickle cell anemia, a molecular disease. Science *110*:543, 1949.

Pearson, H. A., Spencer, R. P., and Cornelius, E. A.: Functional asplenia in sickle cell anemia. New Eng. J. Med. *281*:923, 1969.

Pease, G. L.: Granulomatous lesions in bone marrow. Blood *11*:720, 1956.

Peltier, A. P., and Estes, D.: Antinuclear antibodies. *In* Ioachim, H. L. (ed.): Pathobiology Annual 2:77. New York, Appleton-Century Crofts, Inc., 1972.

Perutz, M. F., and Lehmann, H.: Molecular pathology of human hemoglobin. Nature (London) *219*:902, 1968.

Phillips, R. A., Van Slyke, D. D., Hamilton, P. B., Dole, V. P., Emmerson, K., and Archibald, R. M.: Measurement of specific gravities of whole blood and plasma by standard copper sulfate solutions. J. Biol. Chem. *183*:305, 1950.

Piel, C. F., and Phibbs, R. H.: The hemolytic-uremic syndrome. Pediat. Clin. N. Amer. *13*:295, 1966.

Pinkerton, P. H., Spence, I., Ogilvie, J. C., Ronald, W. A., Marchant, P., and Ray, P. K.: An assessment of the Coulter counter model. S. J. Clin. Path. *23*:68, 1970.

Pizzolato, P., and Stasney, J.: Quantitative cytologic study of multiple sternal marrow samples taken simultaneously. J. Lab. Clin. Med. *32*:741, 1947.

Preud'homme, J. L., and Seligmann, M.: Surface bound immunoglobulins as a cell marker in human lymphoproliferative diseases. Blood *40*:777, 1972.

Proposal for adoption of an international method and standard solution for hemoglobinometry, specifications for preparation of the standard solution, and notification of availability of a reference standard solution. Blood *26*: 104, 1965.

Raman, K.: A method of sectioning aspirated bone marrow. J. Clin. Path. *8*:265, 1955.

Rapaport, S. I.: Introduction to Hematology. New York, Harper & Row, 1971.

Rappaport, H.: Tumors of the Hematopoietic System. Atlas of Tumor Pathology, Section III, Fascicle 8. Washington, D.C., Armed Forces Institute of Pathology, 1966.

Rath, C. E., and Finch, C. A.: Sternal marrow hemosiderin. J. Lab. Clin. Med. *33*:81, 1948.

Reimann, H. A., and de Berardinis, C. T.: Periodic (cyclic) neutropenia, an entity. Blood *4*:1109, 1949.

Reissman, K. R., Ruth, W. E., and Nomura, T. A.: A human hemoglobin with lowered oxygen affinity and impaired heme-heme interactions. J. Clin. Invest. *40*:1826, 1961.

Ritzmann, S. E., Daniels, J. C., Lawrence, M. C., Beathard, G. A., and Levin, W. C.: Monoclonal gammopathies, present status. Texas Med. *68*:91, 1972.

Rohr, K.: Das menschliche Knochenmark. 3rd edition. Stuttgart, Georg Thieme, 1960.

Rosenberg, S. A.: Hodgkin's disease of the bone marrow. Cancer Res. *31*:1733, 1971.

Rosner, F.: Aplastic anemia and viral hepatitis. (Letter.) Lancet 2:1080, 1970.

Rozenszajn, L. A., and Radnay, J.: The lysosomal nature of the anomalous granules and chromosome aberrations in cultures of peripheral blood in Chediak-Higashi syndrome. Brit. J. Haematol. *18*:683, 1970.

Rubin, A. D., Douglas, S. D., Chessin, L. N., Glade, P. R., and Dameshek, W.: Chronic reticulolymphocytic leukemia. Reclassification of "leukemic reticuloendotheliosis" through functional characterization of the circulating mononuclear cells. Amer. J. Med. *47*:149, 1969.

Rümke, C. L.: Variability of results of differential cell counts on blood smears. Triangle *4*:154, 1960.

Sandberg, A. A., Ishihara, T., Kikuchi, Y., and Crosswhite, L. H.: Chromosomal differences among the acute leukemias. Ann. N.Y. Acad. Sci. *113*:663, 1964.

Sandoz: Atlas of Hematology. Basel, Switzerland, Sandoz Ltd. 1952.

Sanford, A. H., and Sheard, C.: The determination of hemoglobin with the photoelectrometer. J. Lab. Clin. Med. *15*:483, 1930.

Saunders, A. M.: Hemalog D system—recent developments. Advances in Automated Analysis *3*:27, 1972. (Tarrytown, N.Y., Mediad, Inc., 1973.)

Schilling, R. F.: The effect of gastric juice on the urinary excretion of radio-activity after the oral administration of radioactive vitamin B_{12}. J. Lab. Clin. Med. *42*:860, 1953; *45*:926, 1955.

Schleicher, E. M.: A new apparatus for isolation and preparation of aspirated bone marrow particles. Amer. J. Clin. Path. *20*:476, 1950.

Schmid, J. R., Kiely, J. M., Pease, G. L., and Hargraves, M. M.: Acquired pure red cell agenesis. Report of 16 cases and review of the literature. Acta Haematol. *30*:255, 1963.

Schneiderman, L. J., Junga, I. G., and Fawley, D. E.: Effects of phosphate and nonphosphate buffers on thermolability of unstable hemoglobins. Nature (London) *225*:1041, 1970.

Seligson, D. (ed.): Standard Methods of Clinical Chemistry. Vol. II. New York, Academic Press Inc., 1958.

Selwyn, J. G., and Dacie, J. V.: Autohemolysis and other changes resulting from the incubation in vitro of red cells from patients with congenital hemolytic anemia. Blood *9*:414, 1954.

Shackman, N. H., Swiller, A. I., and Morrison, M.: Syndrome

simulating acute disseminated lupus erythematosus. Appearance after hydralazine (Apresoline) therapy. J.A.M.A. *155*:1492, 1954.

Sheehan, H. L., and Storey, G. W.: An improved method of staining leucocyte granules with Sudan black B. J. Path. Bact. *59*:336, 1947.

Sheehan, W. W.: The relationship between lymphocytic leukemias and lymphomas. *In* Ultmann, J. E., Griem, M. L., Kirsten, W. H., and Wissler, R. D. (eds.): Current Concepts in the Management of Lymphoma and Leukemia. New York, Springer-Verlag, Inc., 1971, p. 24.

Shepard, M. K., Weatherall, D. J., and Conley, C. L.: Semiquantitative estimation of the distribution of fetal hemoglobin in red cell populations. Bull. Johns Hopkins Hosp. *110*:293, 1962.

Siim, J. C.: Clinical and Diagnostic Aspects of Human Acquired Toxoplasmosis. *In* Human Toxoplasmosis. Copenhagen, Einar Munksgaard Forlag, 1960.

Simmons, A., Schwabbauer, M. L., and Earhart, C. A.: Automated platelet counting with the Autoanalyzers. J. Lab. Clin. Med. *77*:656, 1971.

Singer, K., Chernoff, A. I., and Singer, L.: Studies on abnormal hemoglobins. I. Their demonstration in sickle cell anemia and other hematologic disorders by means of alkali denaturation. Blood *6*:413, 1951.

Smiley, R. K., Cartwright, G. E., and Wintrobe, M. M.: Fatal aplastic anemia following chloramphenicol (Chloromycetin) administration. J.A.M.A. *149*:914, 1952.

Smith, C. H.: Infectious lymphocytosis. Amer. J. Dis. Child. *62*:231, 1941.

Smith, E. B., and Custer, R. P.: Rupture of the spleen in infectious mononucleosis. Blood *1*:317, 1946.

Snapper, I., and Nathan, D. J.: The mechanics of the L.E. cell phenomenon studied with a simplified test. Blood *10*:718, 1955.

Spath, P., Garratty, G., and Petz, L.: Studies on the immune response to penicillin and cephalothin in humans. I. Optimal conditions for titration of hemagglutinating penicillin and cephalothin antibodies. J. Immunol. *107*: 854, 1971.

Stamatoyannopoulos, G., Bellingham, A. J., Lenfant, C., and Finch, C. A.: Abnormal hemoglobins with high and low oxygen affinity. Ann. Rev. Med. *22*:221, 1971.

Stein, H., Lennert, K., and Parwaresch, M. R.: Malignant lymphomas of the B-cell type. Lancet *2*:855, 1972.

Stevenson, G. F., Smetters, G. W., and Cooper, J. A. D.: A gravimetric method for the calibration of hemoglobin micropipets. Amer. J. Clin. Path. *21*:489, 1951.

Stites, D. P., and Leikola, J.: Infectious mononucleosis. Semin. Hematol. *8*:243, 1971.

Stohlman, F., Jr., and Quesenberry, P. J.: Colony-stimulating factor and myelopoiesis. Blood *39*:727, 1972.

Streiff, R. R.: Folic acid deficiency anemia. Semin. Hematol. *7*:23, 1970.

Sundberg, R. D.: Sternal aspiration. Staff Meet. Bull. Hosp. Univ. Minnesota, *17*:389, 1946.

Sundberg, R. D.: Lymphocytogenesis in human lymph nodes. J. Lab. Clin. Med. *32*:777, 1947.

Sundberg, R. D., and Broman, H.: The application of the Prussian blue stain to previously stained films of blood and marrow. Blood *10*:160, 1955.

Sundberg, R. D., and Lick, N. B.: "L.E." cells in the blood in acute disseminated lupus erythematosus. J. Invest. Dermat. *12*:83, 1949.

Sunderman, F. W., MacFate, R. P., MacFadyen, D. A., Stevenson, G. F., and Copeland, B. E.: Symposium on clinical hemoglobinometry. Amer. J. Clin. Path. *23*:519, 1953.

Tanaka, K. R., and Paglia, D. E.: Pyruvate kinase deficiency. Semin. Hematol. *8*:367, 1971.

Tanaka, K. R., Valentine, W. N., and Miwa, S.: Pyruvate kinase (PK) deficiency hereditary non-spherocytic hemolytic anemia. Blood *19*:267, 1962.

Thorn, G. W., Forsham, P. H., Prunty, F. T. G., and Hills, A. G.: The response to pituitary adrenocorticotropic hormone as a test for adrenal cortical insufficiency. J.A.M.A. *137*:1005, 1948.

Timmes, J. J., Averill, H. H., and Metcalfe, J.: Splenic rupture in infectious mononucleosis. New Eng. J. Med. *239*: 173, 1948.

Tjio, J. H., Carbone, P. P., Whang, J., and Frei, E.: The Philadelphia chromosome and chronic myelogenous leukemia. J. Nat. Cancer Inst. *36*:567, 1966.

Turnbull, E. P. N., and Walker, J.: Haemoglobin and red cells in the human foetus. II. The red cells. Arch. Dis. Child. *30*:102, 1955.

Valentine, W. N.: Deficiencies associated with Embden-Meyerhof pathway and other metabolic pathways. Semin. Hematol. *8*:348, 1971.

Van Assendelft, O. W.: The measurement of hemoglobin. *In* Izak, G., and Lewis, S. M. (eds.): Modern Concepts in Hematology, New York, Academic Press, 1972, p. 14.

Van Furth, R.: Origin and kinetics of monocytes and macrophages. Semin. Hematol. *7*:125, 1970.

Van Loghem, J. J., and Van der Hart, M.: Varieties of specific autoantibodies in acquired hemolytic anemia (II). Vox Sang. *4*:129, 1954.

Vaughan, S. L., and Brockmyre, F.: Normal bone marrow as obtained by sternal puncture. Blood, Special Issue No. 1, p. 54, 1947.

Vilter, R. W., *et al.*: Refractory anemia with hyperplastic bone marrow. Blood, *15*:1, 1960. Semin. Hematol. *4*:175, 1967.

Waitman, W. B.: Effects of room temperature on sedimentation rate of red blood cells of man. Amer. J. Med. Sci. *212*:207, 1946.

Waldenström, J.: Incipient myelomatosis or essential hyperglobulinemia with fibrinogenopenia—a new syndrome? Acta Med. Scand. *117*:216, 1944.

Walsh, J. R., and Zimmerman, H. J.: The demonstration of the "L.E." phenomenon in patients with penicillin hypersensitivity. Blood *8*:65, 1953.

Ward, H. P., and Block, M. H.: The natural history of agnogenic myeloid metaplasia (AMM) and a critical evaluation of its relationship with the myeloproliferative syndrome. Medicine *50*:357, 1971.

Wasserman, L. R.: The management of polycythaemia vera. Brit. J. Haematol. *21*:371, 1971.

Wasserman, L. R., and Gilbert, H. S.: Surgical bleeding in polycythemia vera. Ann. N. Y. Acad. Sci. *115*:122, 1964.

Wasserman, L. R., and Gilbert, H. S.: Complications of polycythemia vera. Semin. Hematol. *3*:199, 1966.

Waxman, S., Schreiber, C., and Herbert, V.: Radioisotopic assay for measurement of serum folate levels. Blood *38*: 219, 1971.

Weatherall, D. J.: The genetics of the thalassaemias. Brit. Med. Bull. *25*:24, 1969.

Weatherall, D. J., and Clegg, J. B.: The Thalassaemia Syndromes. 2nd ed. Oxford, Blackwell Scientific Publications, 1972.

Weatherall, D. J., Gilles, H. M., Clegg, J. B., Blankson, J. A., Mustafa, D., Boi-Doku, F/S., and Chaudhury, D. S.: Preliminary surveys for the prevalence of the thalassaemia genes in some African populations. Ann. Trop. Med. Parasitol. *65*:253, 1971.

Weiner, W.: Eluting red-cell antibodies: A method and its application. Brit. J. Haematol. *3*:276, 1957.

Wheby, M. S.: Using a clinical laboratory in the diagnosis of anemia. Med. Clin. N. Amer. *50*:1689, 1966.

White, J. G.: The Chediak-Higashi syndrome: Cytoplasmic sequestration in circulating leukocytes. Blood *29*:435, 1967.

White, J. M., and Dacie, J. V.: The unstable hemoglobins—molecular and clinical features. Progr. Hematol. *7*:69, 1971.

Williams, W. J., Beutler, E., Erslev, A. J., and Rundles, R. W. (eds.): Hematology. New York, McGraw Hill Book Co., Inc., 1972.

Williamson, C. S.: Influence of age and sex on hemoglobin. Arch. Intern. Med. *85*:505, 1916.

Wilson, A. B., Marchand, R. M., and Coombs, R. R. A.: Passive allergisation in vitro of human basophils with serum containing IgE reaginic antibodies to castor allergen, demonstrated by rosette formation. Lancet *1*:1325, 1971.

Windhorst, D. B., Holmes, B., and Good, R. A.: A newly de-

fined X-linked trait in man with demonstration of the Lyon effect in carrier females. Lancet *1*:737, 1967.
Wintrobe, M. M.: Clinical Hematology. 5th and 6th editions. Philadelphia, Lea & Febiger, 1961, 1967.
Wintrobe, M. M.: The size and hemoglobin content of the erythrocyte; methods of determination and clinical application. J. Lab. Clin. Med. *17*:899, 1932.
Wong, S. Y.: Colorimetric determination of iron and hemoglobin in blood. II. J. Biol. Chem. 77:409, 1928.
Woodliff, H. J., and Dougan, L.: Leukaemia and allied disorders. I. Concepts, definitions and classifications. Med. J. Aust. *1*:1359, 1972.
Wright, J. H.: The histogenesis of the blood platelets. J. Morphol. *21*:263, 1910.
Wybran, J., Chantler, S., and Fudenberg, H. H.: Isolation of normal T-cells in chronic lymphatic leukemia. Lancet *1*: 126, 1973.
Yakulis, V. J., Heller, P., Josephson, A. M., and Singer, L.: Rapid demonstration of hemoglobin A_2 by means of agar gel electrophoresis. Amer. J. Clin. Path. *34*:28, 1960.
Yam, L. T., Li, C. Y., and Crosby, W. H.: Cytochemical identification of monocytes and granulocytes. Amer. J. Clin. Path. 55:283, 1971a.
Yam, L. T., Li, C. Y., and Lam, K. W.: Tartrate-resistant acid phosphatase isoenzyme in the reticulum cells of leukemic reticuloendotheliosis. New Eng. J. Med. *284*:357, 1971b.
Yamaguchi, N., and Glass, G. B. J.: The determination of intrinsic factor in gastric secretory analysis. Ann. N. Y. Acad. Sci. *140*:924, 1967.
Yunis, A. A., and Bloomberg, G. R.: Chloramphenicol toxicity: clinical features and pathogenesis. Progr. Hematol. *4*:138, 1964.
Zacharski, L. R., and Linman, J. W.: Lymphocytopenia: Its causes and significance. Mayo Clin. Proc. *46*:168, 1971.
Zimmer, F. E., and Hargraves, M. M.: The effect of blood coagulation on lupus erythematosus cell phenomenon. Proc. Staff Meet. Mayo Clin. 27:424, 1952.
Zinkham, W. H., and Conley, C. L.: Some factors influencing the formation of L.E. cells. Bull. Johns Hopkins Hosp. *98*:102, 1956.

Chapter 4—Addendum

ULTRASTRUCTURE OF THE BLOOD CELLS AND THEIR PRECURSORS

by RAOUL FRESCO, M.D., Ph.D.

In the past few years the electron microscope has graduated from a strictly research instrument to a useful diagnostic tool. Its use in renal pathology and in the differential diagnosis of soft tissue and endocrine neoplasms in particular has become firmly established. In other fields, and hematology is one of these, the electron microscope has so far been of only limited clinical value. However, it has been of considerable help in gaining a better insight into the morphology and pathogenetic mechanisms of the structures involved, and it is with this in mind that I have prepared this short appendix on the ultrastructure of some of the normal and abnormal cells found in the blood and bone marrow. Naturally, restrictions of space have made it necessary to select only a limited number of pathologic entities. For the reader wishing to obtain a more complete picture of the contributions of the electron microscope to hematology. I recommend the excellent recently published book by Tanaka and Goodman (1972).

The illustrations in this section are all of normal and pathologic human material. The specimens were fixed directly in 1 per cent osmium tetroxide, or first fixed in paraformaldehyde or glutaraldehyde followed by osmium. They were dehydrated and embedded in Epon according to the method of Luft (1961) and sectioned with glass knives. Thin sections were stained with uranyl acetate and lead citrate and photographed with an RCA-3G electron microscope.

Figures 1A to 5A:
LIFE CYCLE OF THE NORMAL ERYTHROCYTE

To the light microscopist, and particularly to the hematologist who has come to rely so much on the various colors and hues of the Romanowsky stains, the drab black and white electron micrographs may at first be somewhat disconcerting. He will soon appreciate the significance of the various organelles revealed by the increased resolution and magnification offered by the electron microscope and learn to interpret them in the light of the knowledge he has gained by examining stained specimens. This will become apparent by examining the first two pages of electron micrographs, which illustrate the life cycle of the normal erythrocyte.

Five normoblasts from a bone marrow spicule are seen in Figure 1A (× 6600). They are at various stages of maturation. The younger cells, basophilic normoblasts (BN), are larger, and their nuclei have coarse, partially clumped or condensed chromatin; nucleoli, which are present at this stage, are not included in this plane of section. The basophilia of the cytoplasm as seen by light microscopy is due to the presence of numerous clusters of five or six ribosomes, grouped because they are joined together by a thread of mRNA. These polyribosomes (arrows), better seen at higher magnification in the insert (× 34,000) synthesize the polypeptide chains of hemoglobin. Mitochondria (M) are also present and play an important role in the formation of hemoglobin by providing the enzymatic machinery for the synthesis of the heme ring.

As the cells mature they become smaller, their nuclei decreasing more rapidly in size, with the chromatin becoming progressively denser. In the polychromatophilic normoblast (PN) the cytoplasm shows a decrease in the number of polyribosomes and mitochondria and becomes darker as a result of the accumulation of electron-dense hemoglobin. This corresponds to the decreased basophilia and increased acidophilia seen by light microscopy.

In the acidophilic normoblast (Fig. 2A – × 7700), only a few ribosomes and mitochondria remain. The small pyknotic nucleus (N) becomes eccentric and bulges out on one side of the cell.

In the process of extrusion (Fig. 3A – × 8800), the nucleus (N) becomes surrounded by a very narrow, barely visible rim of cytoplasm. The plasma membrane (arrow) constricts about the neck formed between the nucleus and the main portion of the cytoplasm. Mitochondria (M) aggregate in the region of the constriction, presumably providing energy for the synthesis of the new plasma membrane and for the eventual complete separation of the nucleus from the young reticulocyte. The expelled nucleus, with its thin rim of hemoglobin-rich cytoplasm (Fig. 4A – × 10,500), is soon phagocytized by a macrophage and digested (Fig. 5A – × 8000). The hemoglobin which is lost with the nucleus comprises much of the ineffective hemoglobin production (or ineffective erythropoiesis) in normal people, i.e., the 10 to 15 per cent of hemoglobin produced that never reaches the circulating blood.

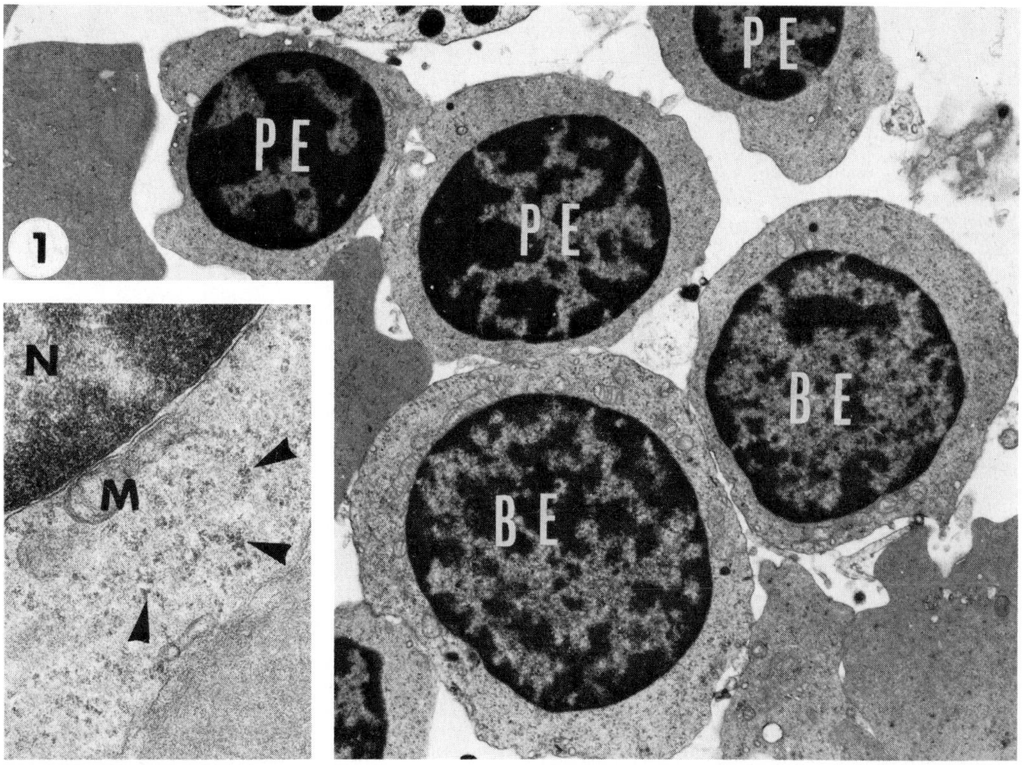
1
PE
PE
PE
BE
BE
N
M

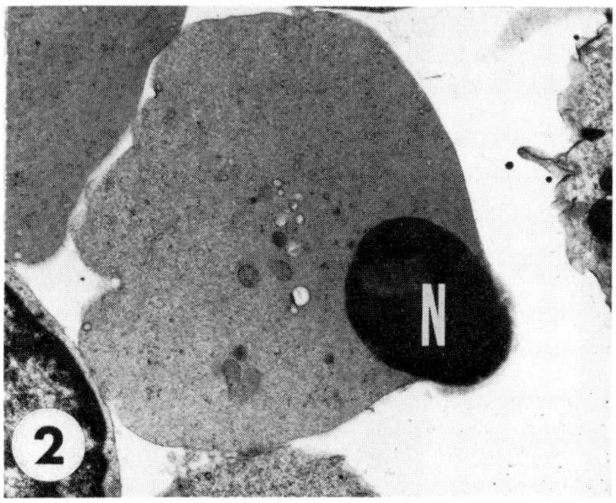
2
N

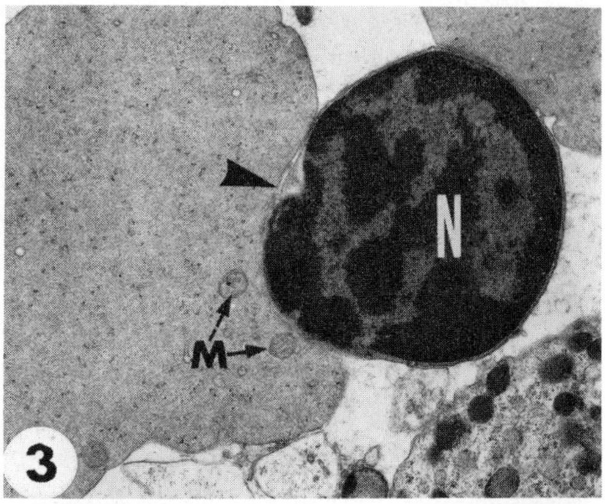
3
N
M

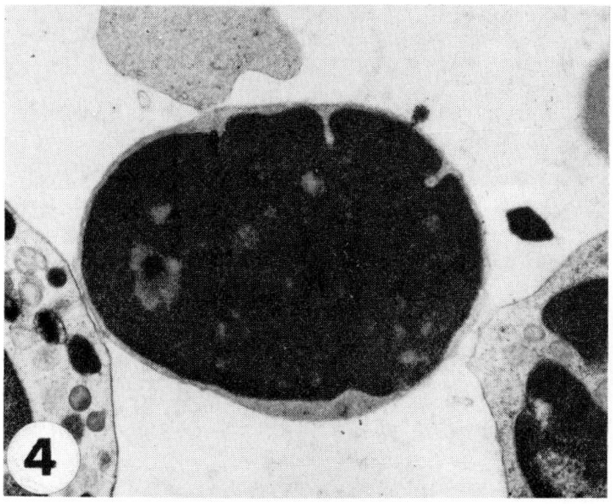
4

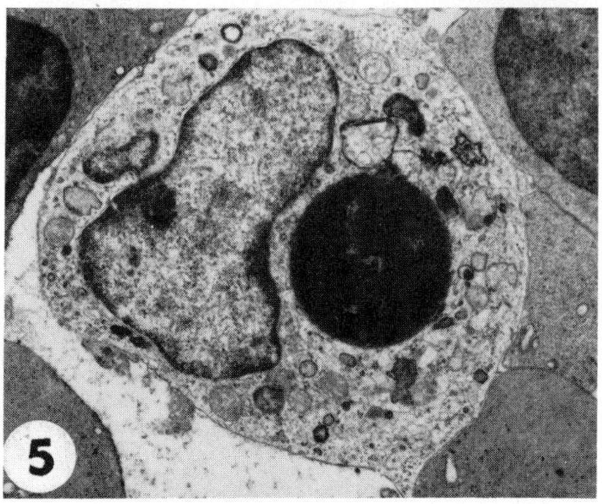
5

Figures 6A to 9A:
LIFE CYCLE OF THE NORMAL ERYTHROCYTE (continued)

The young reticulocyte (Fig. 6A – × 52,000) still often shows portions of plasma membrane clefts (arrow) at the site of nuclear expulsion as well as a few mitochondria (M) and ribosomes (R), which continue to synthesize small amounts of hemoglobin for about one to two days, at which time all the cytoplasmic organelles have disappeared. The mature erythrocyte can be seen as the familiar biconcave disk bound by a plasma membrane and rich in electron-dense hemoglobin (Fig. 7A – × 8800).

After from 80 to 120 days, the aged erythrocytes are phagocytized in turn by the reticulum cells of the bone marrow (Fig. 8A – × 4000) and some appear within the cytoplasm as whole cells, fragments, or "ghosts" (*). The hemoglobin is broken down and its iron is released and stored in the form of ferritin.

At higher magnification (Fig. 9A – × 100,000 – unstained), it can be demonstrated that ferritin can move between the red cell precursors and the reticulum cells of the bone marrow. It can be seen on the surface of these cells and in pinocytotic vesicles (PV). It was originally suggested by Bessis and Breton-Gorius (1957) that this ferritin is taken up by maturing erythroblasts surrounding the reticulum cell (erythroblastic island) to be resynthesized into new hemoglobin, but several workers have questioned the validity of this interpretation and have suggested a movement of ferritin in the opposite direction, namely, that the iron not immediately required for hemoglobin synthesis in red cell precursors is incorporated into ferritin and returned to the reticulum cell. In either case, an intimate relationship between normoblasts and macrophages in the marrow exists and is recognized morphologically as "the erythroblastic island" (Fig. 8A). To some extent normally, and to a greater extent in some abnormal circumstances, the spleen and liver are also involved in destroying erythrocytes.

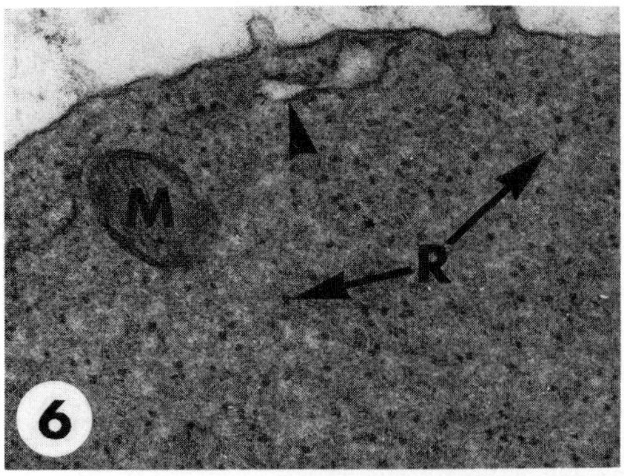
M
R
6

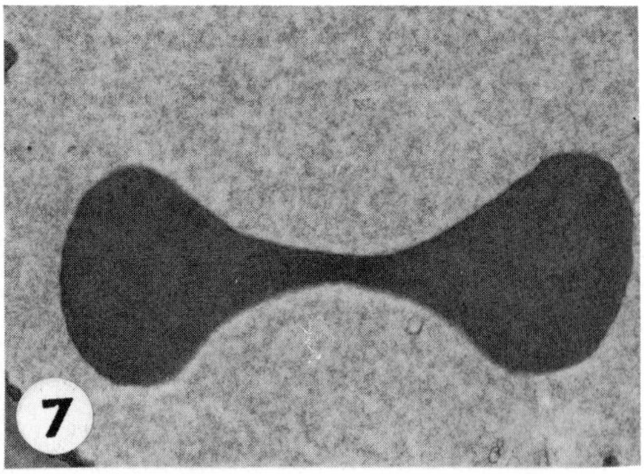
7

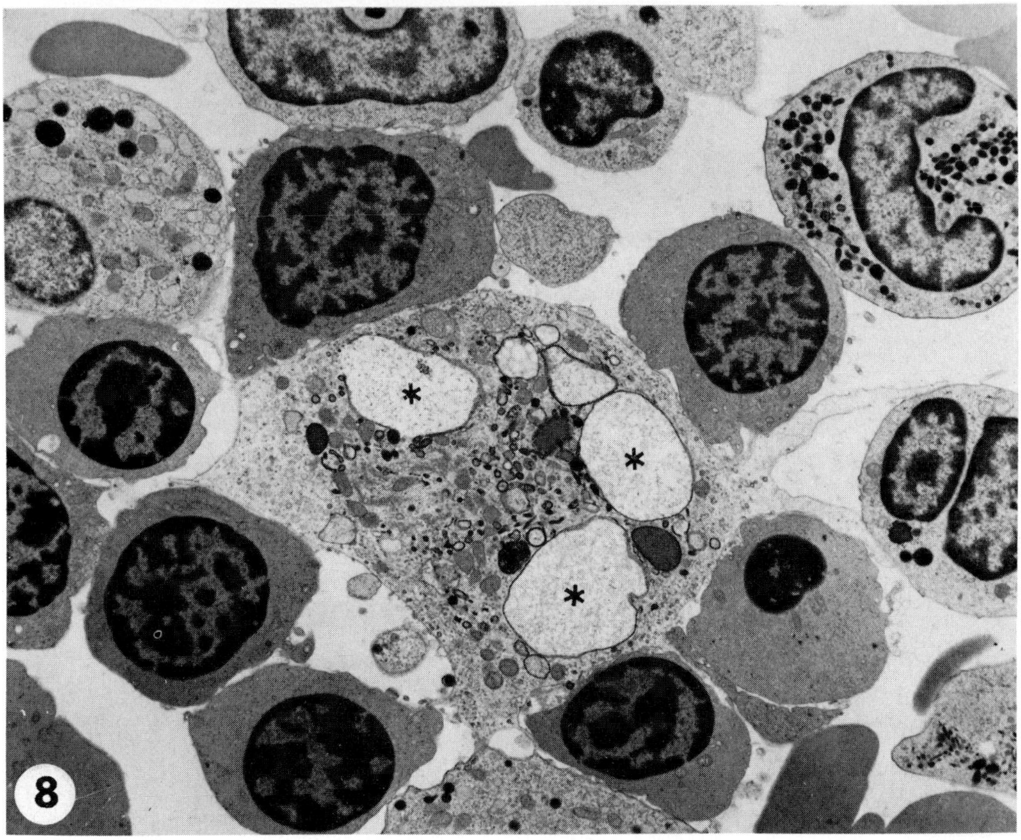
*
*
*
8

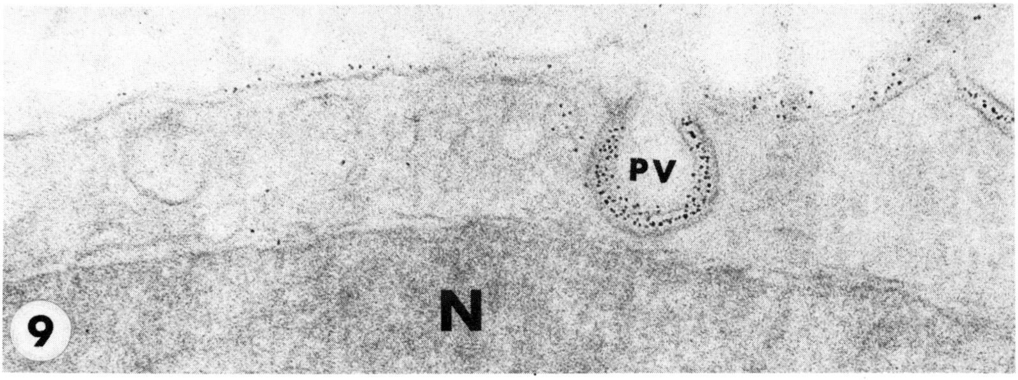
PV
N
9

Figures 10A to 15A:
GAUCHER'S DISEASE

A metabolic abnormality of the cells of the reticuloendothelial system responsible for the destruction of erythrocytes (see Figure 8A) is now known to be the cause of Gaucher's disease, a disorder in which these cells accumulate excessive quantities of glucocerebroside. The typical fibrillar appearance of the cytoplasm of the Gaucher cell seen by light microscopy is shown by electron microscopy (Fig. 10A – × 6600) to be due to the presence of many irregular spindle-shaped bodies, Gaucher bodies (GB), bound by a single limiting membrane and containing numerous elongated tubular elements (Fig. 11A – × 52,000). The tubules are roughly parallel to one another and variable in length; their diameters vary from 10 to 40 nm. (Fig. 13A – × 87,000). Numerous ferritin particles are present throughout the cytoplasm. Ultrastructural enzyme histochemistry has revealed high acid phosphatase activity in the Gaucher cytoplasmic bodies, suggesting that they are phagolysosomes, with the tubules representing residual structures from the partial digestion of membrane lipids. It has now been established that this incomplete digestion is due to a familial defect, the deficiency of a beta-glucosidase enzyme that catalyzes the cleavage of glucose from glucocerebroside. Various blood elements have been suggested as the source of the undigested glycolipid, including erythrocytes, leukocytes, and platelets. The common finding of phagocytized erythrocytes (E) in Gaucher cells (Fig. 12A – × 1700), the large number of ferritin particles in the cytoplasm of these cells, and their localization in the bone marrow, spleen, and liver, all sites of red cell destruction, favors the erythrocyte membrane as the main origin of the stored glycolipid. The cytoplasmic tubules present in Gaucher's disease have been isolated by density gradient centrifugation (Lee, 1968) and shown to contain more than 90 per cent glucocerebroside. The isolated tubules can be examined with the electron microscope after negative staining with phosphotungstic acid (Fig. 14A – × 125,000) or shadow casting with platinum-palladium (Fig. 15A – × 125,000). As described by Lee, each tubule appears to be made up of 10 to 12 fibrils gently twisted about the long axis, forming a spiral in a right-handed screw sense.

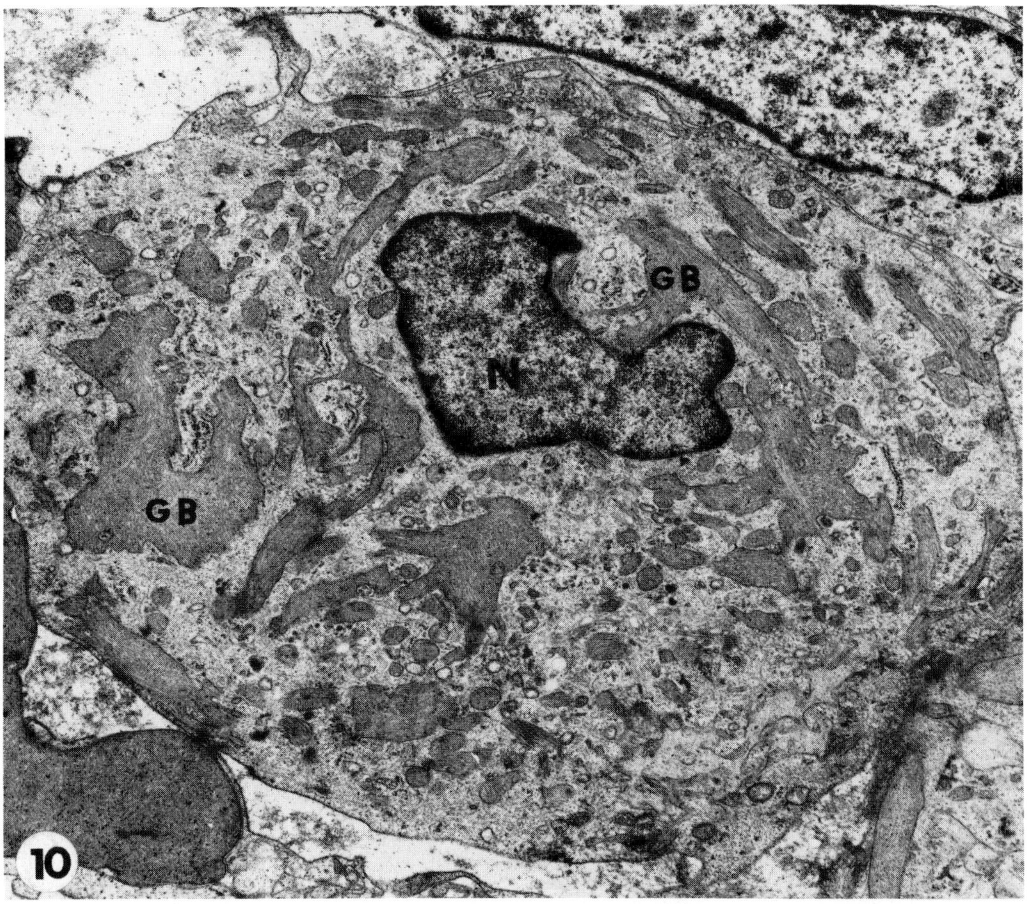
GB
N
GB
10

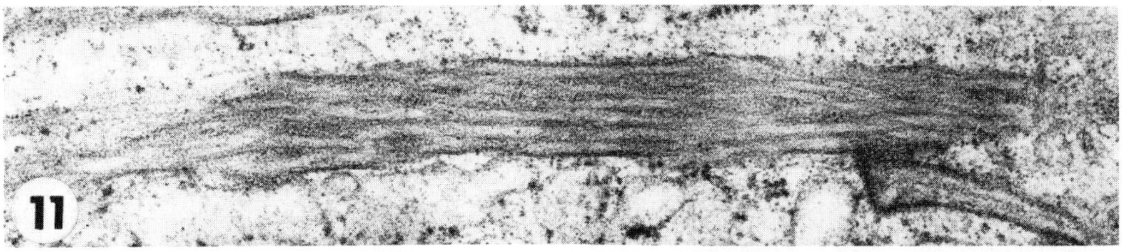
11

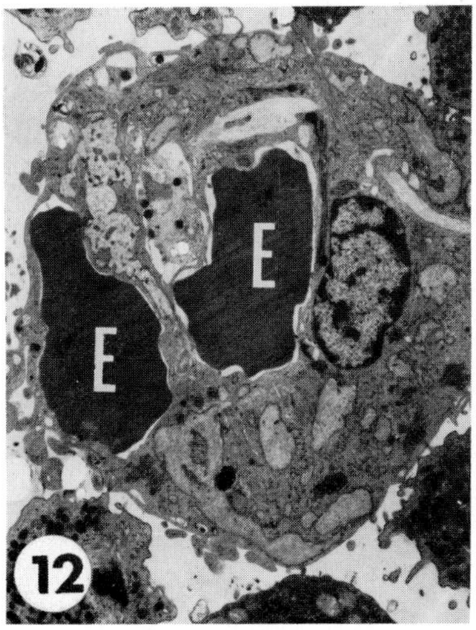
E
E
12

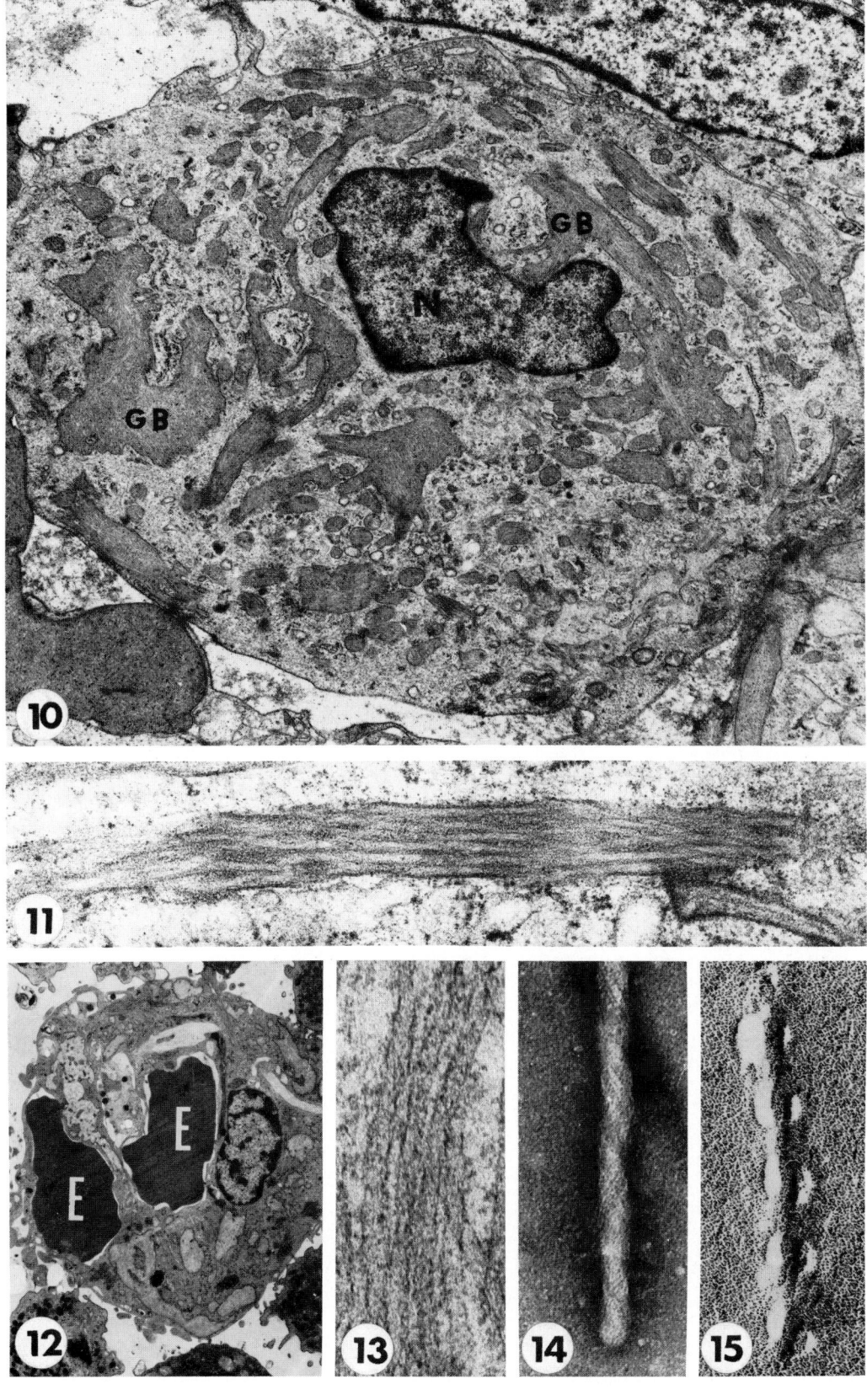
13

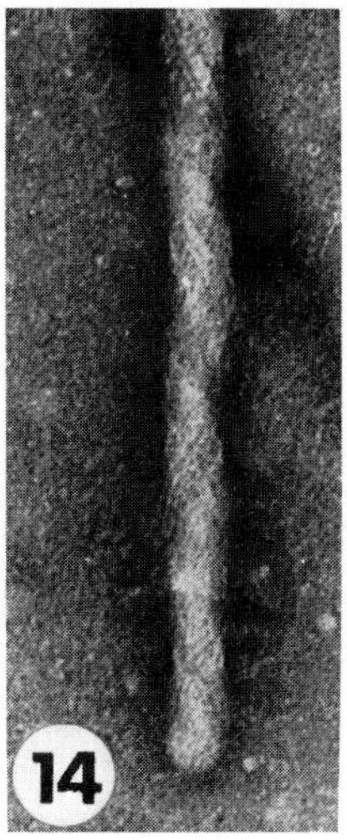
14

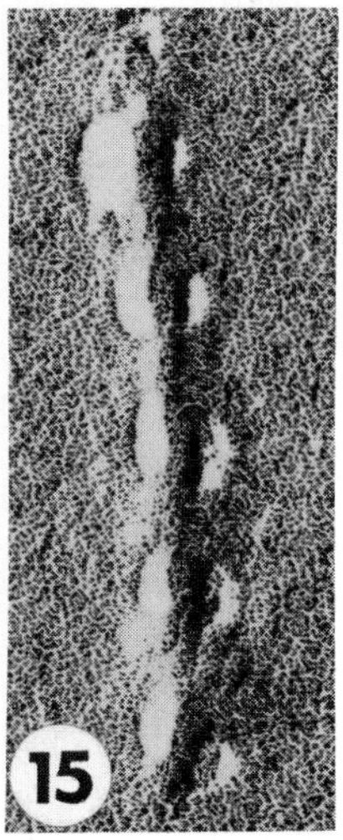
15

Figures 16A and 17A: SICKLE CELL ANEMIA

Electron microscopic examination of sickled erythrocytes (Fig. 16A–× 11,000) reveals the presence of numerous long, slender, parallel rods, representing polymerized reduced hemoglobin S, along the long axis of the deformed erythrocyte. At higher magnification (Fig. 17A *a*–× 150,000), as described by Stetson (1966), the rods can be seen to have a diameter of about 15 nm., and on cross-section (Fig. 17A *b*–× 150,000) show a tubular configuration with electron-dense borders. This structure conforms with the molecular model of reduced hemoglobin S proposed by Murayama (1966).

Figure 18A: SIDEROBLASTIC ANEMIA

Heme synthesis occurs within mitochondria, at least in part. In a number of hereditary and acquired refractory anemias with erythroid hyperplasia, there appears to be a defect in the mitochondrial enzymes involved in heme synthesis, and iron-laden mitochondria can be seen in the cells of the erythrocytic series in both the bone marrow and the peripheral blood. Figure 18A *a* (× 11,000) shows numerous iron-laden mitochondria surrounding the nucleus of a normoblast, the so-called ringed sideroblast. At higher magnifications the electron-dense iron is seen to accumulate in the matrix between the mitochondrial cristae (Fig. 18A *b*–× 76,500).

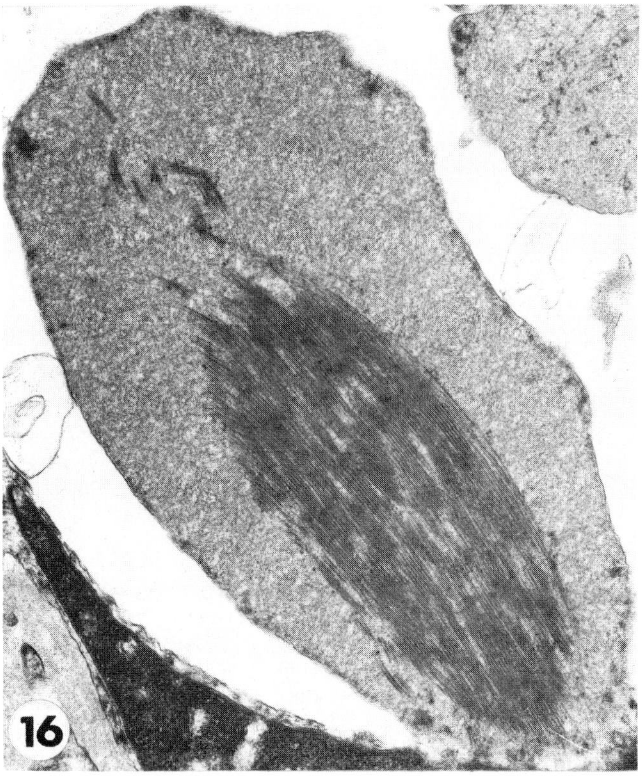
16

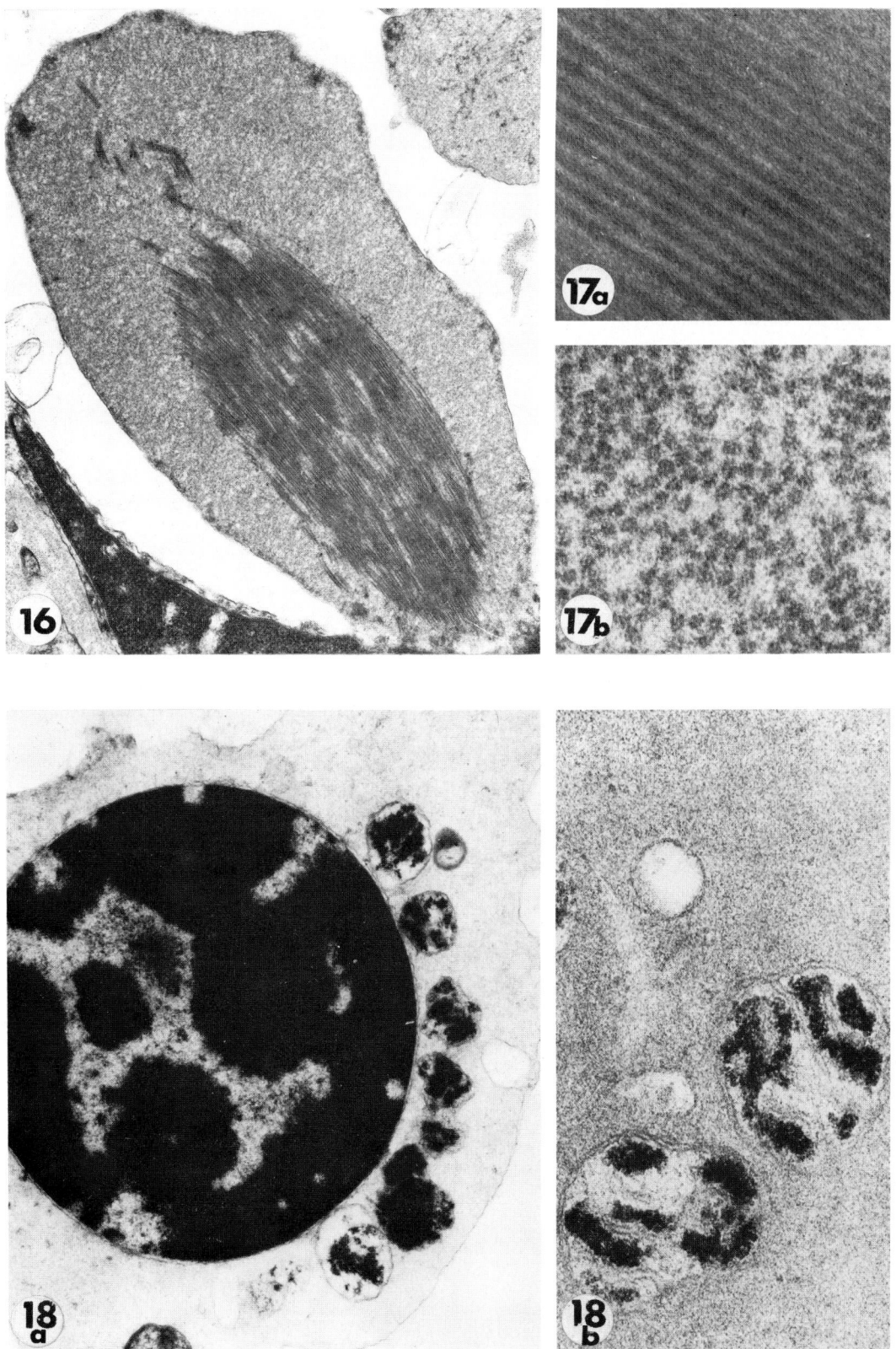
17a

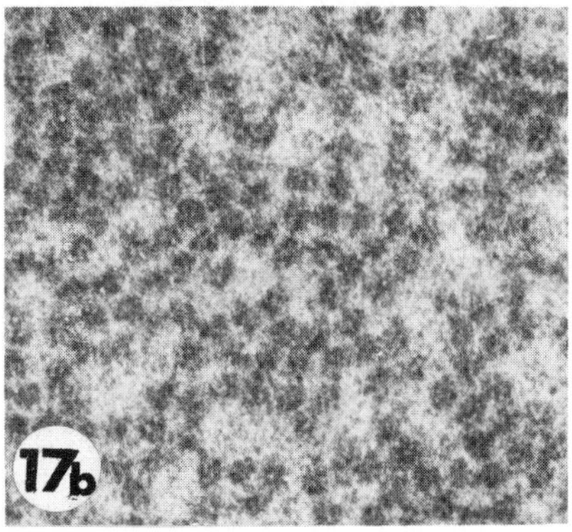
17b

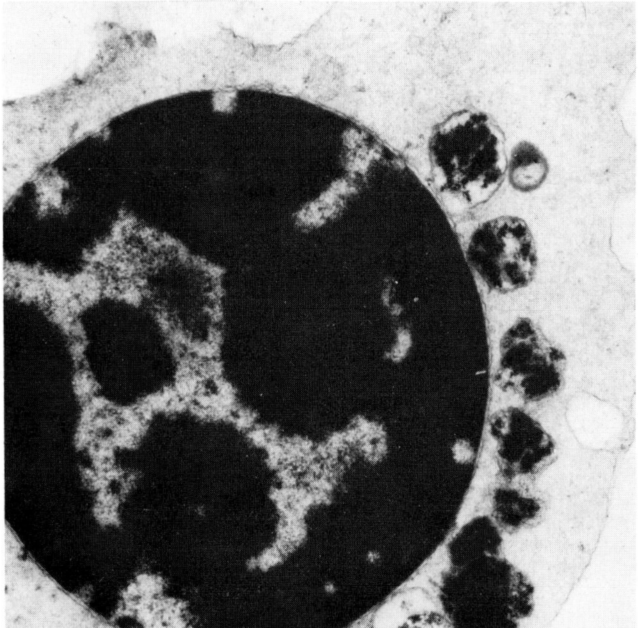
18a

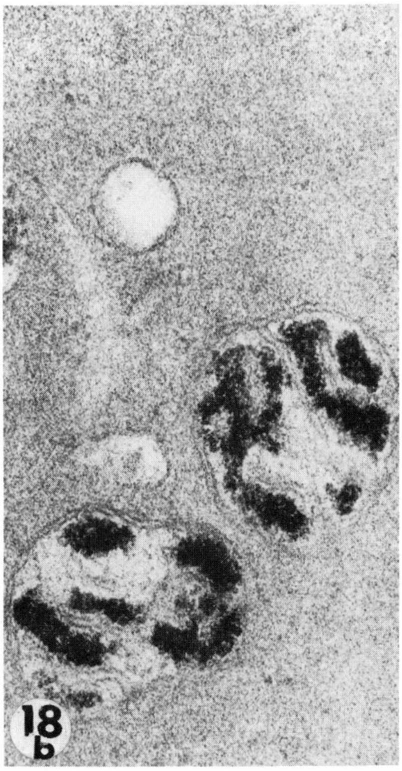
18b

Figure 19A
MATURATION OF GRANULOCYTES

The sequence of ultrastructural changes seen in the course of the maturation of granulocytes is illustrated in Figures 19A *a* to *d*.

The *myeloblast* (Fig. 19A *a*—× 13,200) is the most immature form of all three types of granulocytes (neutrophils, eosinophils, and basophils). The nucleus (N) is spherical to slightly angular, with finely granular evenly distributed chromatin, except for some clumps adjacent to the nuclear envelope. One or more nucleoli (n) are present near the center of the nucleus. The cytoplasm is relatively abundant, with numerous large mitochondria (M), a well-developed Golgi complex (G) often showing a few small dense granules associated with it, numerous polyribosomes (R) which are responsible for the marked cytoplasmic basophilia seen by light microscopy, and a few profiles of rough-surfaced endoplasmic reticulum.

The *promyelocyte* (Fig. 19A *b*—× 13,200) is the next stage in the maturation of the granulocytes. It is characterized by the presence of numerous profiles of rough-surfaced endoplasmic reticulum (RER) and numerous round or elongated primary (azurophil) granules scattered throughout the cytoplasm. The Golgi complex (G) is prominent, and a moderate number of mitochondria and free ribosomes are seen. The nucleus (N) is usually oval and shows increased condensation of its chromatin. A nucleolus (n) is still present at this stage.

Bainton and Farquhar (1966) have shown that the azurophil granules are formed only during the promyelocyte stage and arise from the proximal or concave face of the Golgi complex by budding and subsequent aggregation of vacuoles with a dense core.

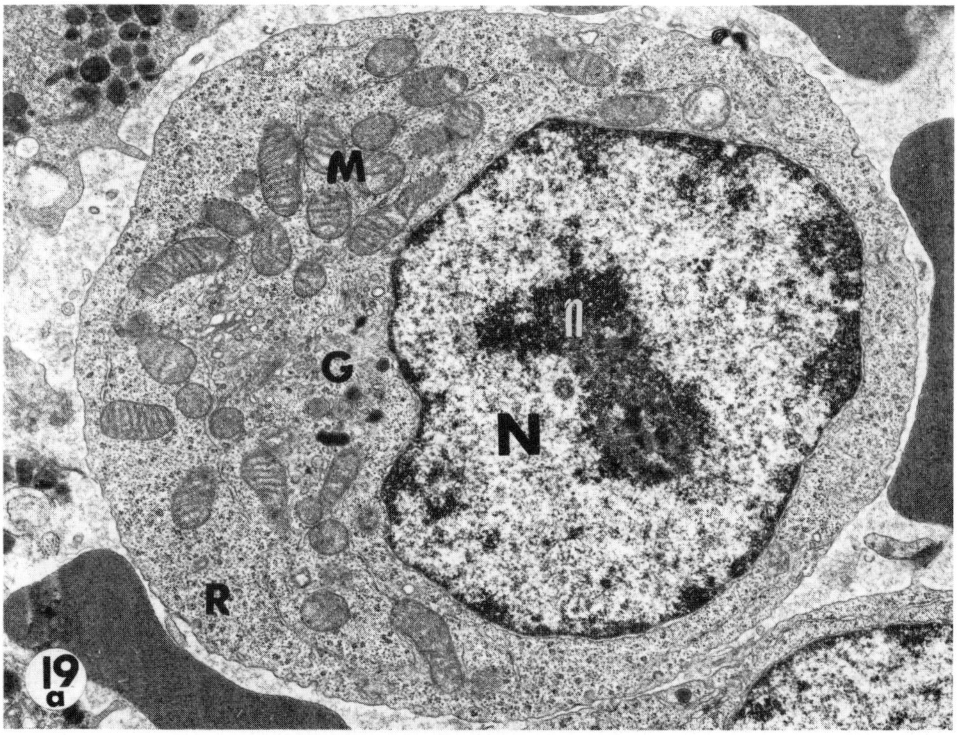
M
G
N
n
R
19
a

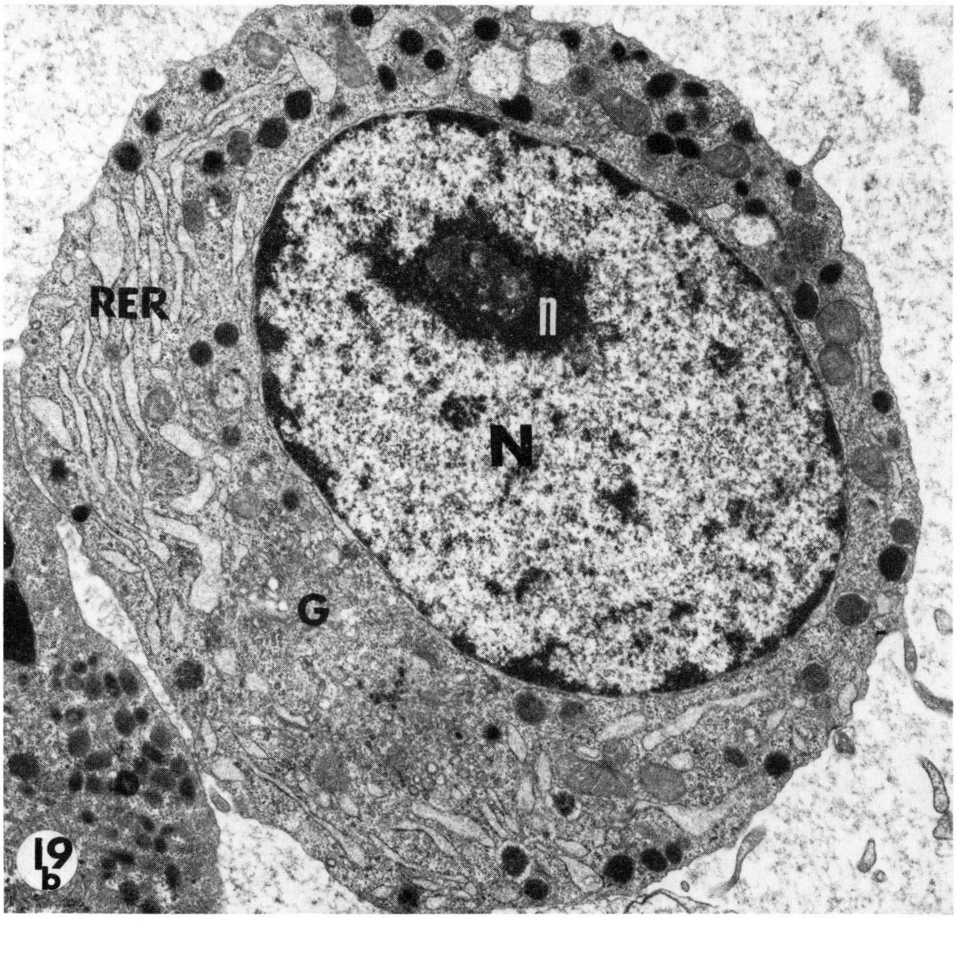
RER
n
N
G
19
b

Figure 19A
MATURATION OF GRANULOCYTES (continued)

A *neutrophil myelocyte* is illustrated in Fig. 19A *c* (× 13,200). At this stage of development the primary (azurophil) granule formation has ceased and has been replaced by the production of secondary (specific) granules. Depending on the type of specific granules produced, the myelocytes are classified as neutrophil, eosinophil, or basophil. The neutrophil granules are smaller and less dense than the azurophil granules and arise from the distal or convex face of the Golgi complexes by pinching-off and confluence of vesicles which have a finely granular content (Bainton and Farquhar, 1966).

The Golgi complex in the myelocyte continues to diminish in size and complexity. There is a depletion of rough endoplasmic reticulum and a decrease in the number of polysomes, free ribosomes, and mitochondria. The cytoplasmic matrix becomes denser and contains increasing amounts of particulate glycogen. The nucleus (N) begins to show an indentation. The nuclear chromatin is more condensed and the nucleoli disappear (Ackerman, 1971b).

The *neutrophil metamyelocyte* (Fig. 19A *d*–× 13,200) is a further step in the maturation process leading to the multilobed neutrophil granulocyte found in the peripheral blood. During this stage the cytoplasmic characteristics become those of the mature neutrophil, with a finely granular, more opaque matrix, few ribosomes and polysomes, and abundant particulate glycogen. Only a few strands of rough endoplasmic reticulum and relatively few small mitochondria are present. Specific granules predominate, forming about 80 per cent, with about 20 per cent azurophil granules. These two types of granules are quite difficult to distinguish morphologically at this stage without the use of selective peroxidase staining, which is positive only in the azurophil granules.

The nucleus (N) of the metamyelocyte is markedly indented or horseshoe shaped with coarsely clumped, peripherally condensed chromatin. The cell has lost the capacity for cell division, and further maturation consists predominantly of segmentation of the nucleus (Ackerman, 1971b).

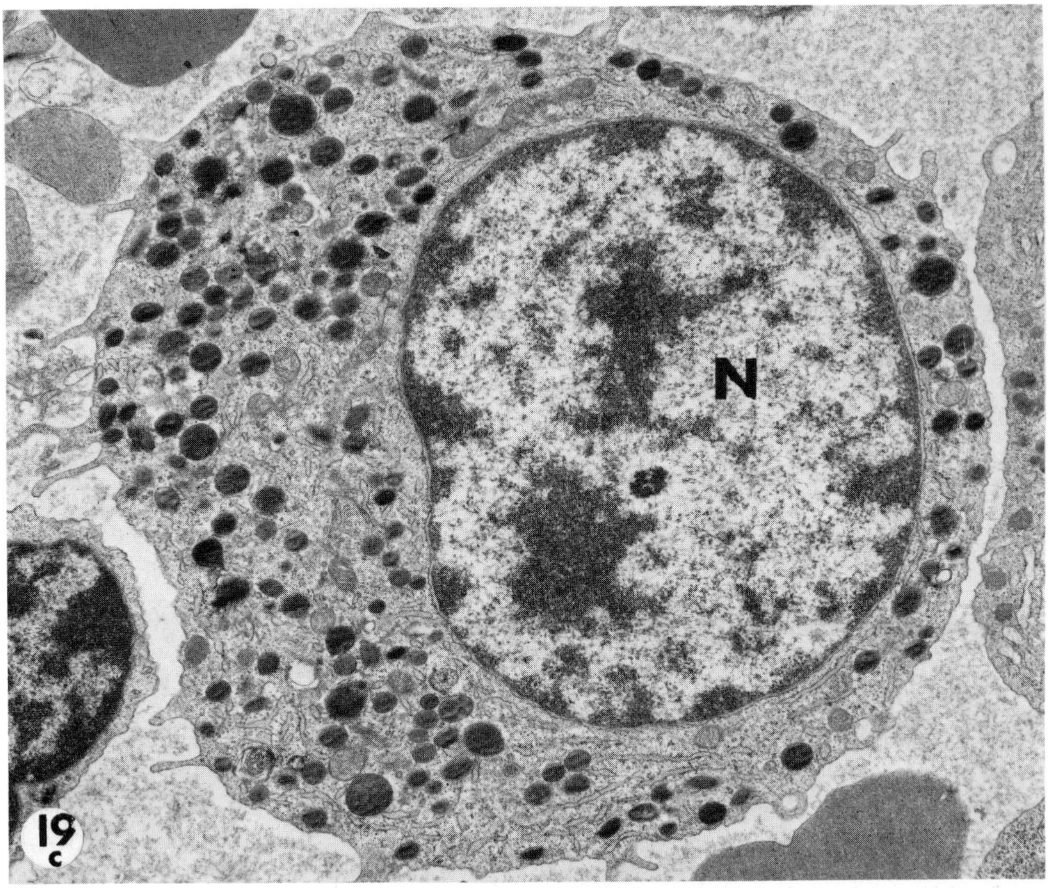
N
19c

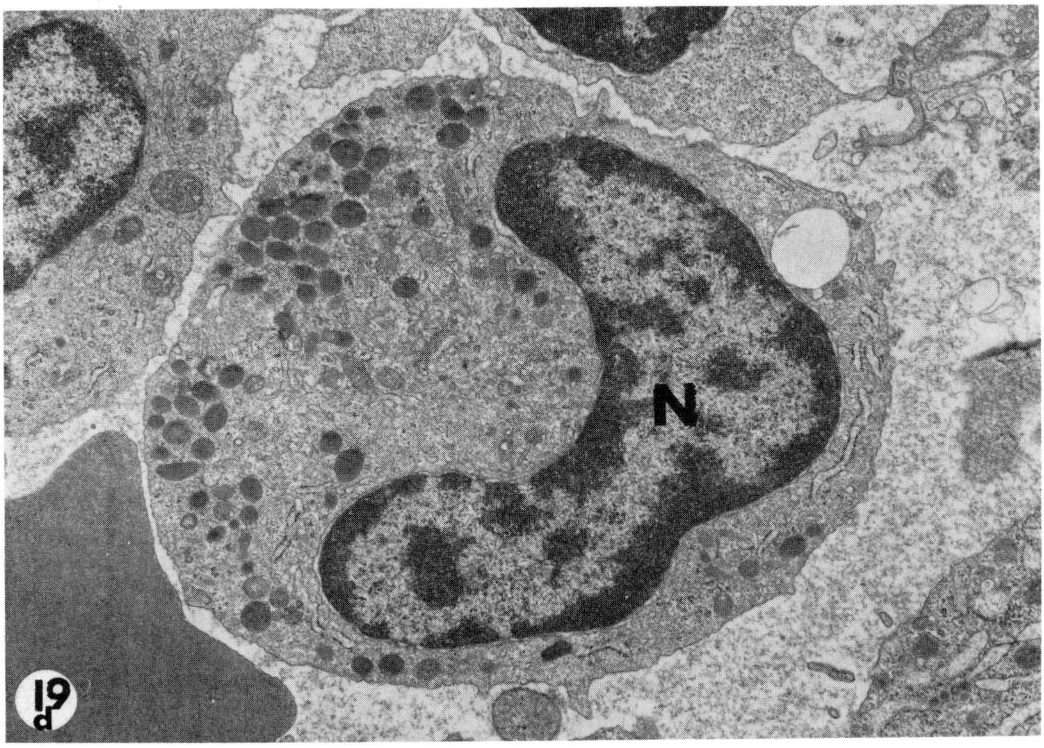
N
19d

Figure 20A:

NEUTROPHILIC GRANULOCYTE

Figure 20A *a* (× 12,400) is an electron micrograph of a mature neutrophilic granulocyte. There are three nuclear lobes (N) connected by thin filamentous strands not seen in this plane of section. The nuclear chromatin is condensed, particularly close to the nuclear membrane. A centriole (Ce) is situated close to the center of the cell, and the lamellae and cisternae of the Golgi complex (G) lie below and to the left of it. There are relatively few mitochondria. Ribosomes and glycogen granules are evenly distributed throughout the cytoplasm, as are numerous round or elongated specific granules (Sp G) and denser azurophil granules (Az). The heterogeneous appearance of the specific granules is better seen at higher magnification in Figure 20A *b* (× 52,000), which reveals a variety of sizes, shapes, and densities. Occasionally the granules (Fig. 20A *c* –× 170,000) have an internal crystalloid organization, in the form of regularly arranged electron-dense particles. The azurophil granules contain peroxidase and lysosomal hydrolytic enzymes; these constitute a minority of the granules of mature human neutrophils. Most are specific granules which contain alkaline phosphatase.

Figure 21A:

EOSINOPHILIC GRANULOCYTE

Figure 21A *a* (× 12,400) is an electron micrograph of an eosinophilic granulocyte. Its nucleus (N) is bilobed, showing chromatin condensation. A Golgi complex (G) occupies the center of the cell. The distinctive ultrastructural feature of the eosinophil is the presence of large round or oval membrane-bound specific granules with dense internal crystalloid structures (Cr) of various shapes. These structures are best seen at higher magnification (Fig. 21A *b*–×52,000) (Miller, de Harven and Palade, 1966).

Like the azurophil granules of the neutrophil, the eosinophil granules are lysosomes, containing several hydrolytic enzymes, including acid phosphatases, ATPase, cathepsin, ribonuclease, arylsulphatase, and beta-glucuronidase. They are particularly rich in peroxidases. Eosinophils have also been shown to contain profibrinolysin and may thus play an important function in the breakdown of fibrin in pathologic states.

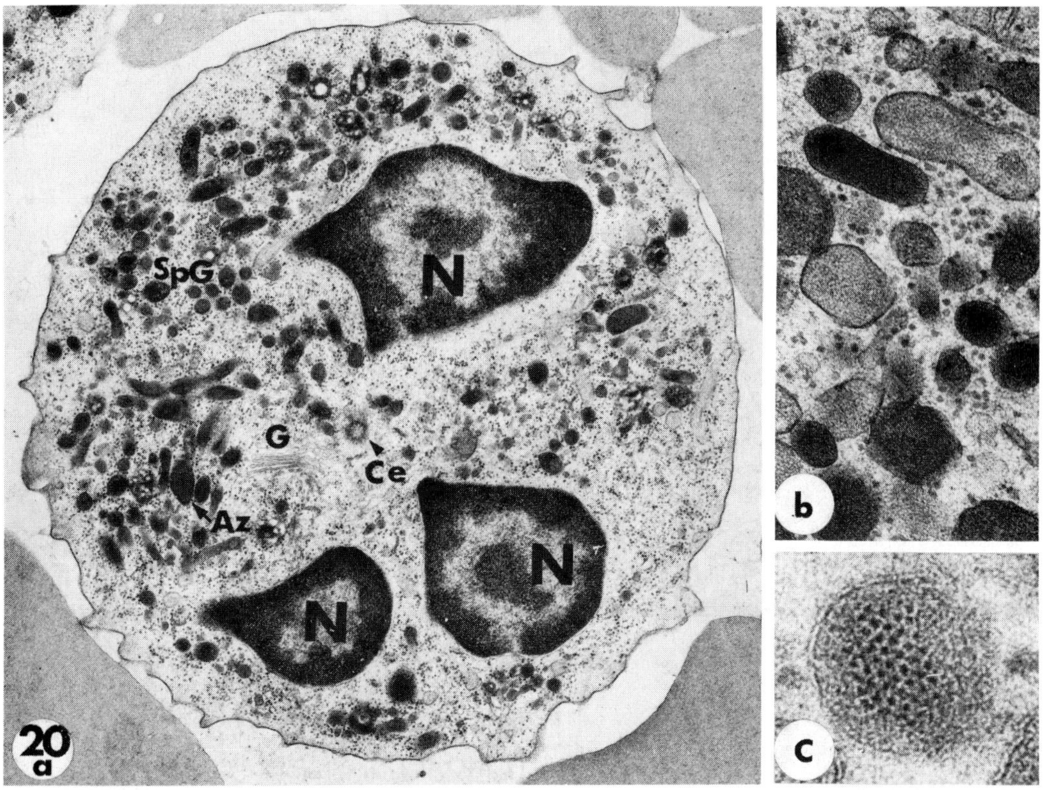
SpG
N
G
Ce
Az
N
N
20
a
b
c

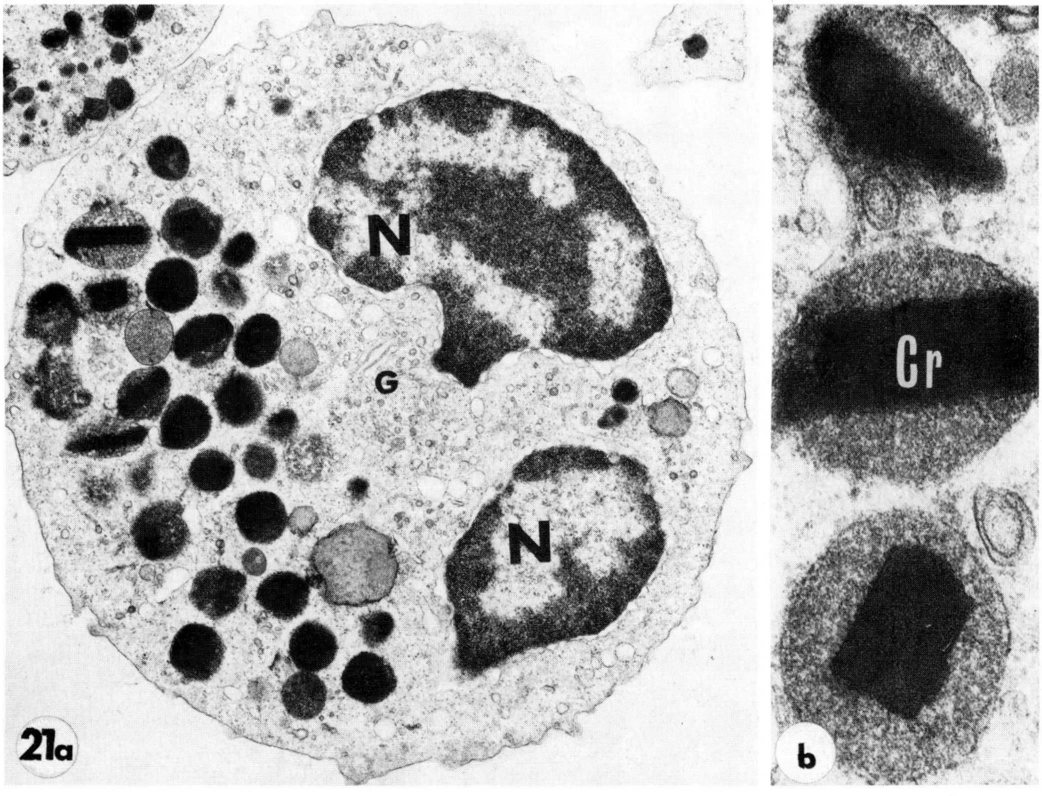
N
G
N
21a
Cr
b

Figure 22A:
BASOPHILIC GRANULOCYTE

Figure 22A (× 13,200). Basophilic granulocyte from peripheral blood showing a bilobed nucleus (N). The cytoplasm contains rare small mitochondria, a few profiles of rough endoplasmic reticulum, some free ribosomes and glycogen particles, and several specific granules. Some of these have lost their contents, leaving clear vacuoles lying close to the periphery of the cell. Myelin figures (My) are present in close association with the ruptured granules. One of the intact specific granules (arrow) is shown at higher magnification in the insert at the lower left-hand corner. It is bound by a "unit membrane" and is filled with uniform-sized particles, some of which are arranged in rows along and concentric with the unit membrane (× 52,000) (Zucker-Franklin, 1967). The granules are thought to contain histamine and heparin and have been shown to exhibit peroxidase activity (Ackerman and Clark, 1971).

Figure 23A:
MAST CELL

Though they bear a close functional relationship with the blood basophils and show similarities in the chemical composition and tinctorial qualities of their granules, the tissue mast cells (Fig. 23A – × 18,000) show distinctive ultrastructural features. There is a single, rounded or oval nucleus. Several mitochondria are present in the cytoplasm, as well as a few profiles of rough endoplasmic reticulum and ribosomal clusters. A Golgi complex (G) is found in the upper left, close to the nucleus. Most of the cytoplasm is filled with large electron-dense granules showing a complex internal organization. This is demonstrated by the granule indicated by the arrow, which is seen at higher magnification in the insert at the lower left-hand corner. Bound by a unit membrane, it contains structures which, when cut longitudinally, appear as parallel lines, and when seen in cross section have a spiral configuration. These have been called scroll forms but could also be described as resembling locks of hair in curlers(!) (× 75,000). The fine structure and cytochemical composition of mast cell granules vary considerably in different species. The scroll-like lamellae appear to be characteristic of human mast cells (Kobayasi, Midtgard and Asboe-Hansen, 1968) but their composition is as yet unknown. Like basophils, mast cell granules are rich in heparin and histamine, and in some species, but not in man, also contain serotonin.

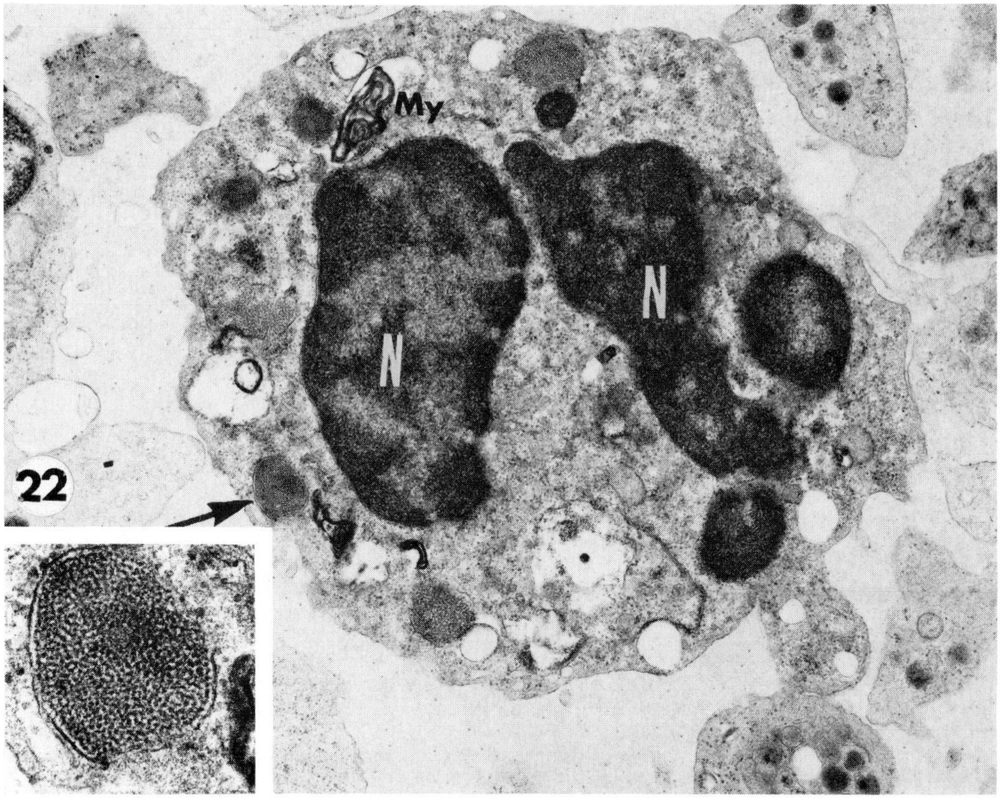
My
N
N
22

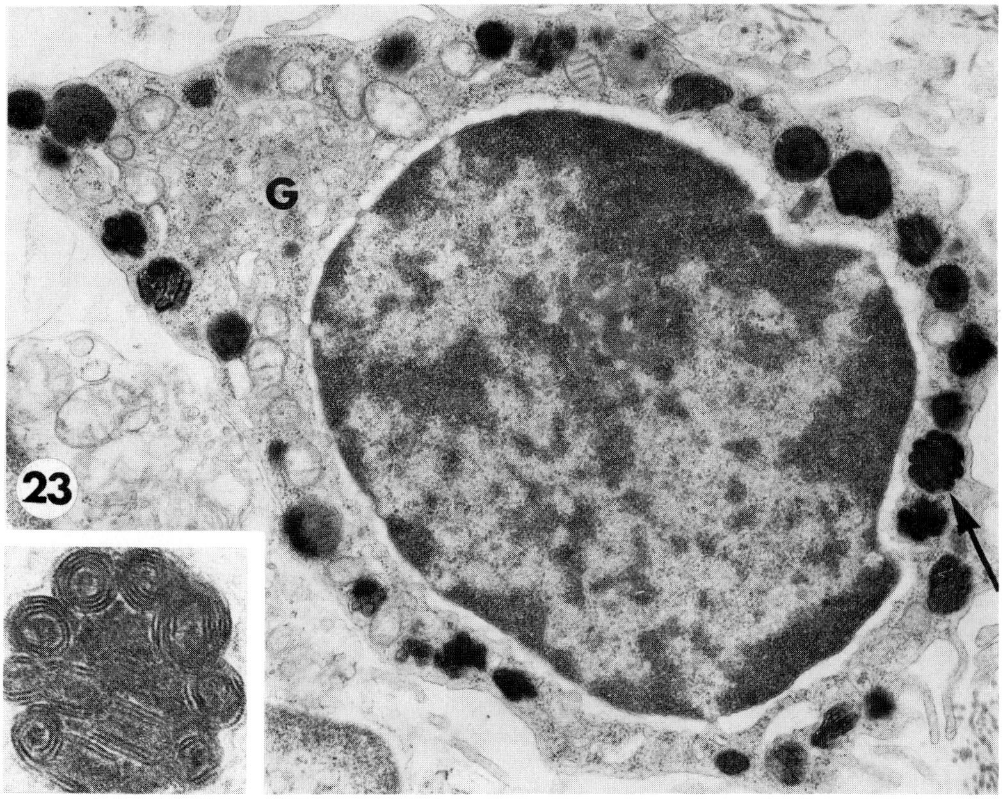
G
23

Figure 24A:
ACUTE GRANULOCYTIC LEUKEMIA

Considerable difficulty may arise in the differentiation of the various types of acute leukemia if diagnosis is based exclusively on the appearance of the leukemic cells stained by the Romanowsky method. This has given rise to the "lumping" of many of these cases in the category of undifferentiated or stem cell leukemia. Some progress has been achieved in the classification of acute leukemias through the help of cytochemical methods, particularly by Hayhoe and his co-workers (1964). Early hopes that the electron microscope would permit an easy differentiation between the neoplastic myeloblasts and lymphoblasts proved disappointing, because even at the ultrastructural level, these two primitive cell types are frequently indistinguishable. Figure 24A (× 11,000) is an electron micrograph of a myeloblast from a case of acute granulocytic leukemia. The nucleus (N) shows a deep indentation and poorly condensed chromatin. The cytoplasm contains a large number of free ribosomes, several mitochondria, and a number of electron-dense azurophilic granules. One structure probably derived from the azurophilic granules, and which when present is of great help in excluding the diagnosis of acute lymphocytic leukemia, is the Auer body (AuB). At higher magnification (Fig. 24A *b*– × 50,000), the Auer body is a rod-like structure surrounded by a single unit membrane and containing several electron-dense bars with a longitudinal lamellar substructure.

Figure 25A:
CHRONIC GRANULOCYTIC LEUKEMIA

In chronic granulocytic leukemia, the peripheral blood shows a large number of granulocytes in various stages of maturation, predominantly myelocytes and metamyelocytes. These demonstrate no ultrastructural features that would distinguish them from cells of the same type found in the normal bone marrow or in the blood of "reactive" granulocytosis, yet, in contrast to the latter, the specific granules in chronic granulocytic leukemia rather consistently contain very low levels of demonstrable alkaline phosphatase activity (× 4400).

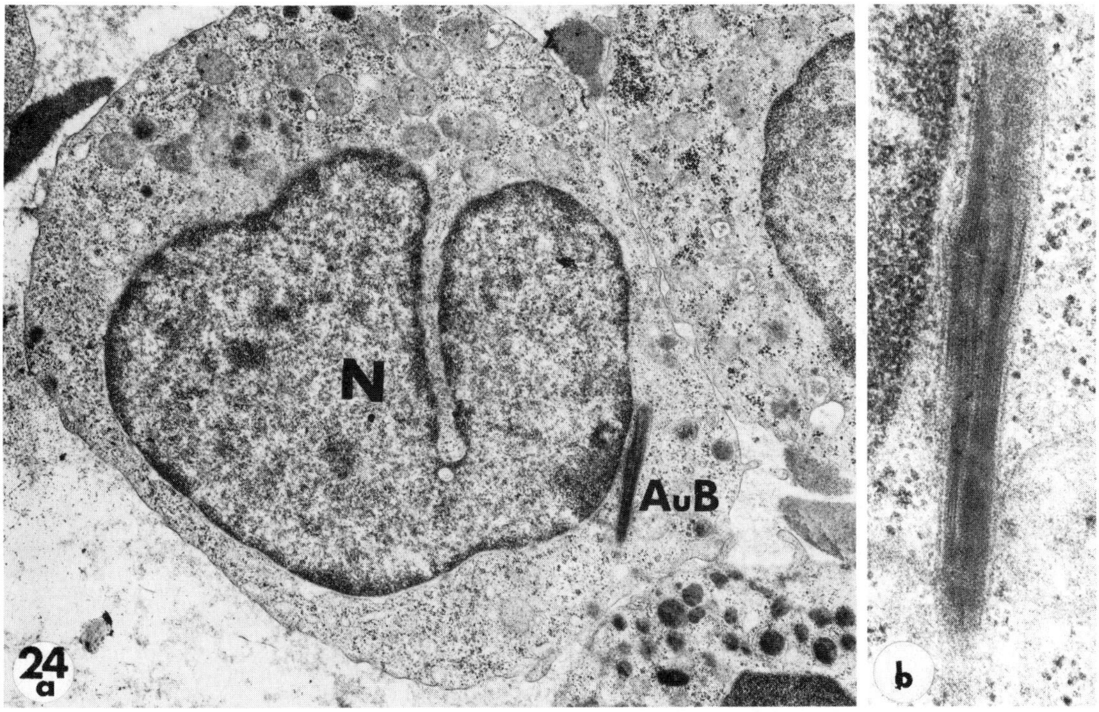
N
AuB
24
a
b

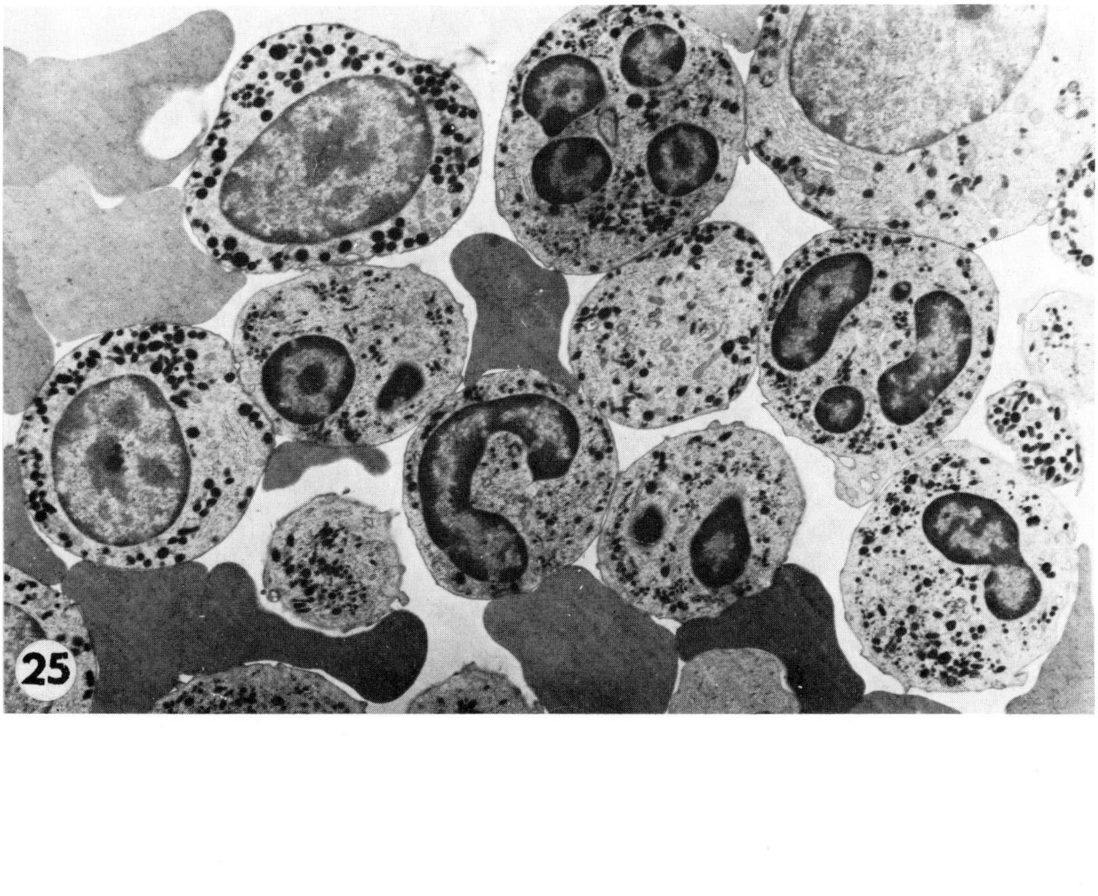
25

Figure 26A: LYMPHOCYTE

The lymphocyte has a round, or as in this case slightly indented, nucleus (N) with highly condensed chromatin. It is this dense chromatin which obscures the nucleolus (n) in conventionally stained blood smears, but which is often seen in thin sections and in electron micrographs. Thus, the mere presence of a nucleolus does not denote cell immaturity. A relatively scanty cytoplasm surrounds the nucleus. A poorly developed Golgi complex (G) and a pair of centrioles (Ce) arranged at right angles to one another are seen close to the nuclear indentation. Free ribosomes are distributed throughout the cytoplasm, and a few mitochondria (M) are present. Several small pseudopods (Ps) project from the surface (× 15,000).

Figure 27A: MONOCYTE

The monocyte has a horseshoe-shaped nucleus (N), with clumped chromatin occurring predominantly adjacent to the nuclear membrane. A nucleolus (n) is present. The cytoplasm is more abundant than in the lymphocyte, shows a better developed Golgi complex (G), several mitochondria (M), scattered free ribosomes, numerous vesicles of various sizes, as well as lysosomal (Ly) and denser azurophilic (Az) granules. The abundance of these various organelles is responsible for the "ground glass" appearance of the cytoplasm as seen by the light microscope. A large pseudopod (Ps) extends in the right upper corner (× 12,400).

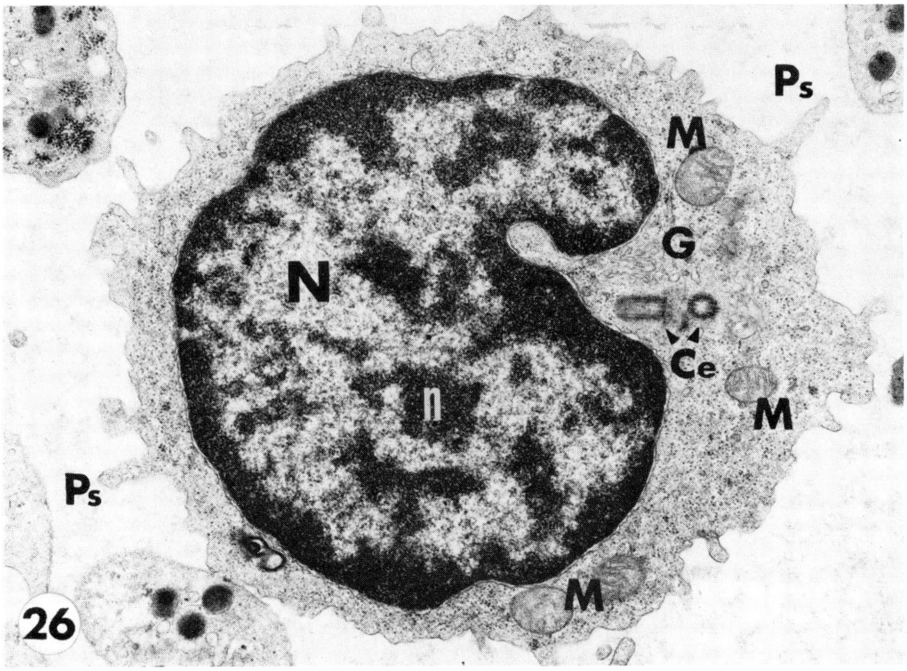
Ps
M
G
N
Ce
n
M
Ps
M
26

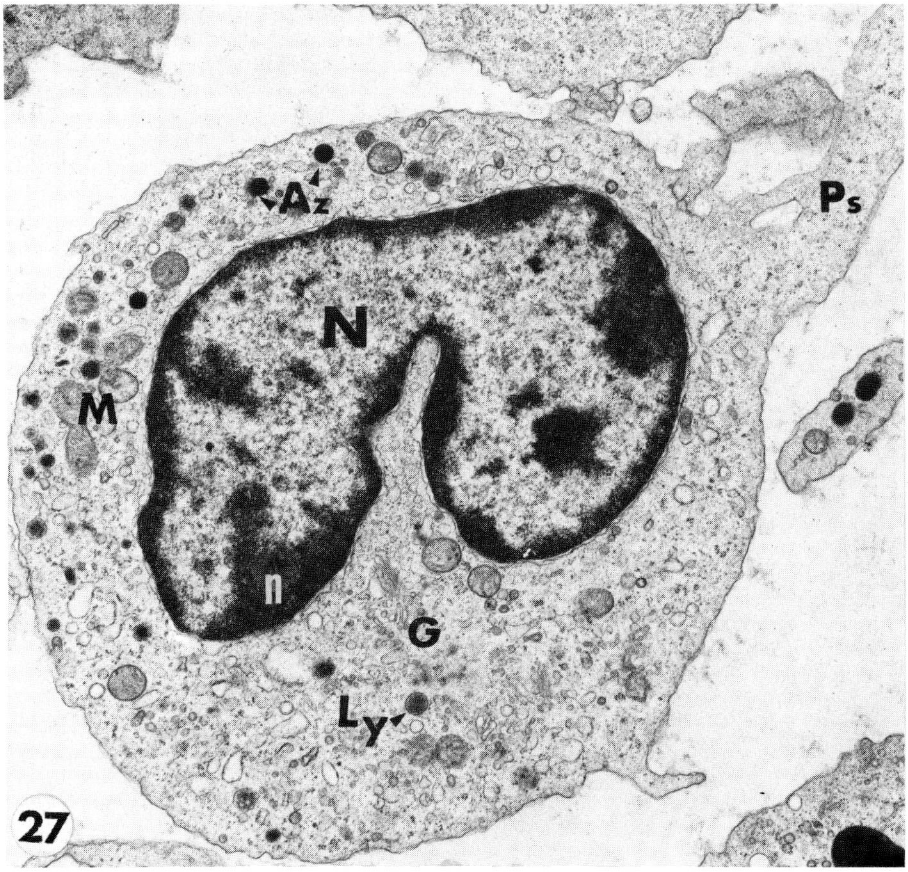
Az
Ps
N
M
n
G
Ly
27

Figures 28A and 29A: INFECTIOUS MONONUCLEOSIS

The atypical lymphocytes of infectious mononucleosis show an even greater degree of polymorphism at the ultrastructural level than they do with the light microscope. While maintaining many of the characteristics of lymphocytes as illustrated in Figure 26A, the atypical lymphocytes of infectious mononucleosis are generally larger in size, owing mostly to more abundant cytoplasm. This is shown in Figures 28A and 29A, which are electron micrographs of cells from the buffy coat of a patient with typical clinical and serologic manifestations of infectious mononucleosis. In Figure 28A all the cells are lymphocytoid. The nuclei have clumped chromatin and show one or more prominent nucleoli. There is an increase in the number of ribosomal aggregates, vesicular structures, and electron-dense lysosomal granules. Another area from the buffy coat of the same patient, in Figure 29A, shows more pronounced polymorphism. The cell at the lower left appears to be a typical lymphocyte, while the one just above it has plasmocytoid features, with prominent concentric lamellae of rough endoplasmic reticulum. The large cell at the right also has plasmocytoid features, the rough endoplasmic reticulum in this case being in the form of dilated cisternae. Portions of other atypical lymphocytes are also seen, with the characteristic increase of ribosomal aggregates (polysomes) (× 6600). (Douglas *et al.*, 1969).

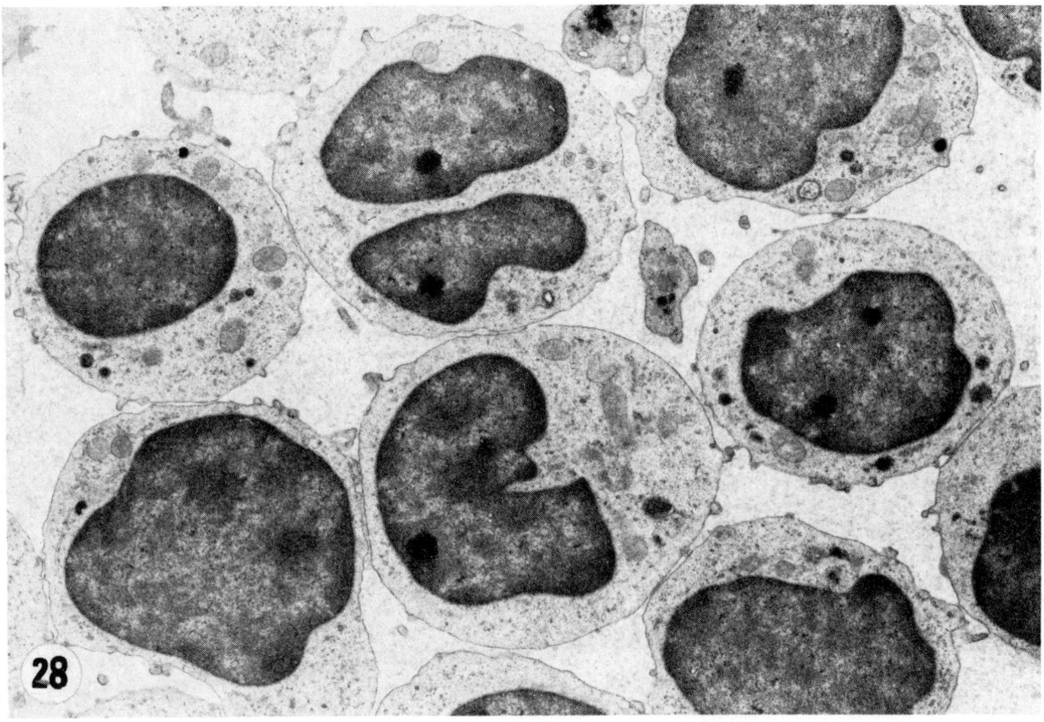
28

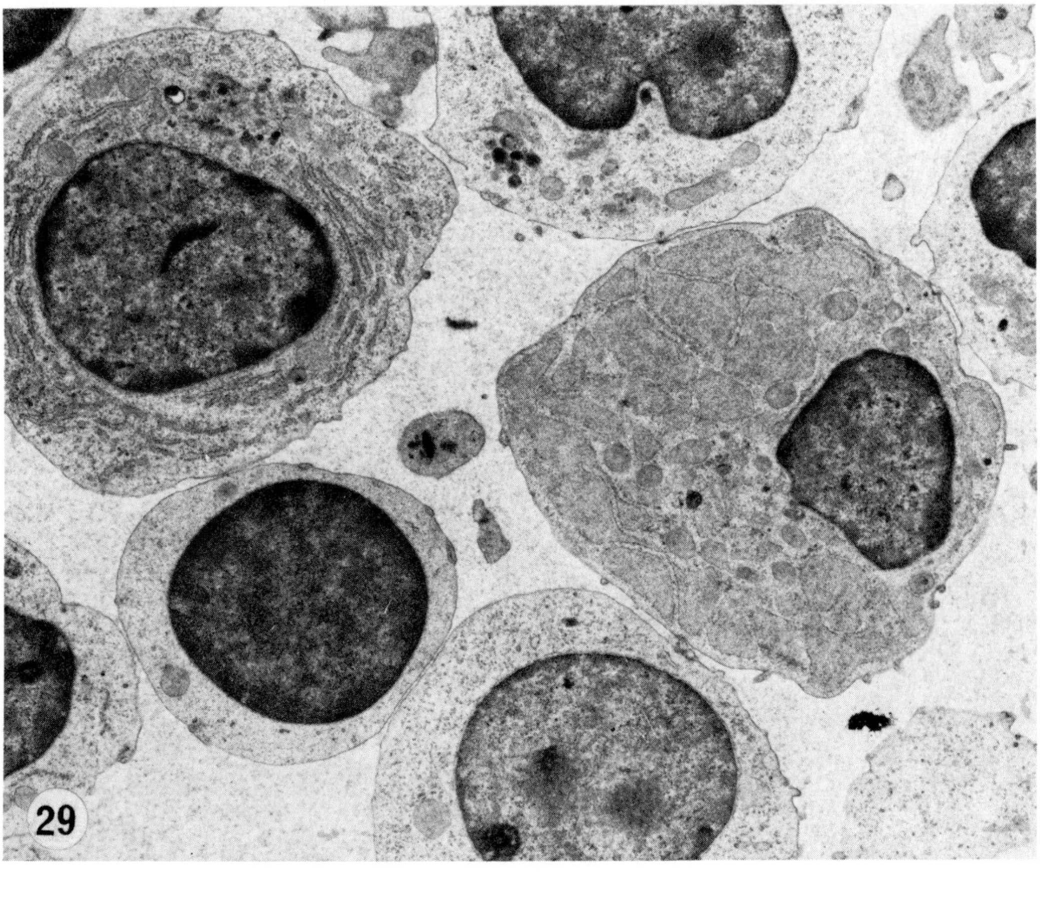
29

Figure 30A:
CHRONIC LYMPHOCYTIC LEUKEMIA

The cells in chronic lymphocytic leukemia most commonly have the appearance of mature small lymphocytes. They have round to oval nuclei, with occasional shallow indentations and scant cytoplasm with few organelles. Some of the cells show a prominent nucleolus (× 6600).

Figure 31A:
MONOCYTIC LEUKEMIA

A considerable degree of confusion has arisen in the classification and diagnosis of the monocytic leukemias, due in great part to the difficulty of distinguishing neoplastic monocytes and their precursors from immature cells of the granulocytic series, and the possible common origin of these two cell lines. Downey in 1938 separated monocytic leukemia into two types, a pure monocytic leukemia, the so-called Schilling type, and a mixed myelomonocytic, called the Naegeli type. The diagnosis of monocytic leukemia is based on the presence of large numbers of monocytoid and related blast precursors. In the pure form these comprise over 60 per cent of the leukocytes in the peripheral blood. As in the case of the acute blastic or stem cell leukemias, cytochemical methods have been of help in distinguishing pure monocytic from the myelomonocytic leukemias.

Occasional difficulties still occur in differentiating the Schilling from the Naegeli types of monocytic leukemia. However, in a recent publication, Freeman and Journey (1971) have studied the fine structure of seven cases of acute monocytic leukemia, and they believe that ultrastructural analysis can be of value in separating the two types of monocytic leukemia. In the Naegeli type, two distinct cell lines, a myeloid and a monocytic, were distinguished by their ultrastructure, while in the Schilling type, of which Figure 31A is an example, only one line of cells with distinctive ultrastructural configuration is found. These cells exhibit nuclear folding and irregularity with deep indentations, and there is scant condensation of the chromatin. One or more nucleoli are frequently present. The cytoplasm shows numerous mitochondria, prominent Golgi zones associated with numerous vesicles and granules and occasional larger vacuoles (× 6600).

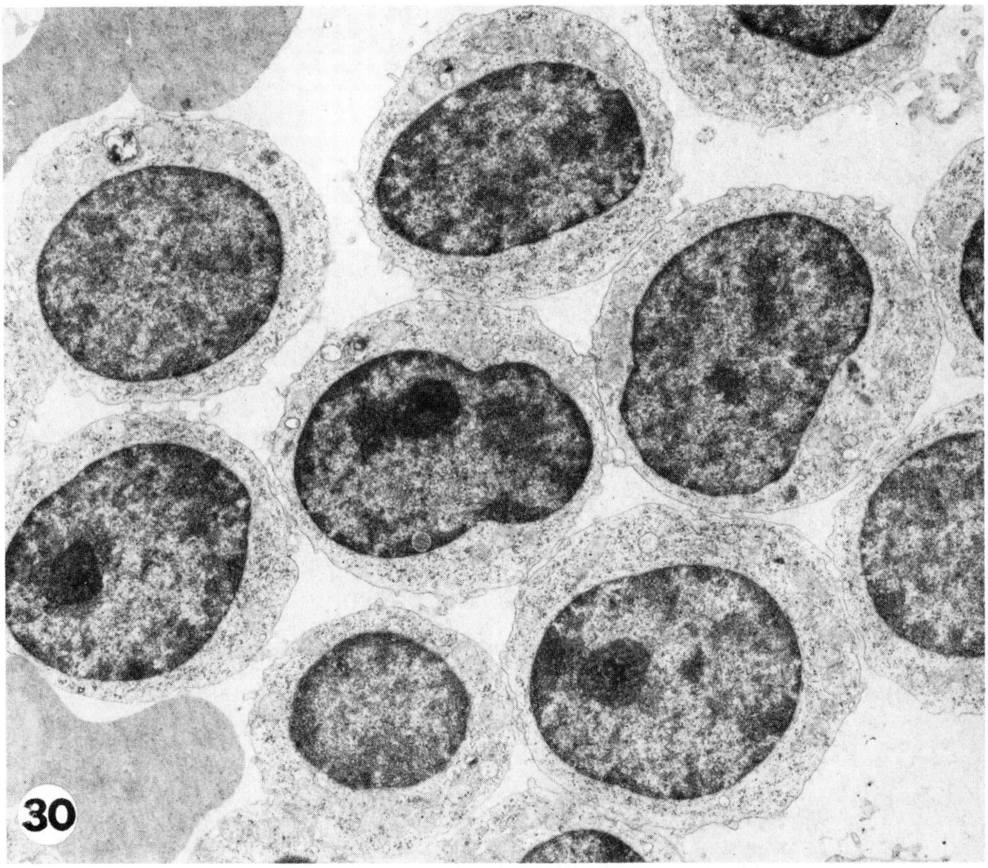
30

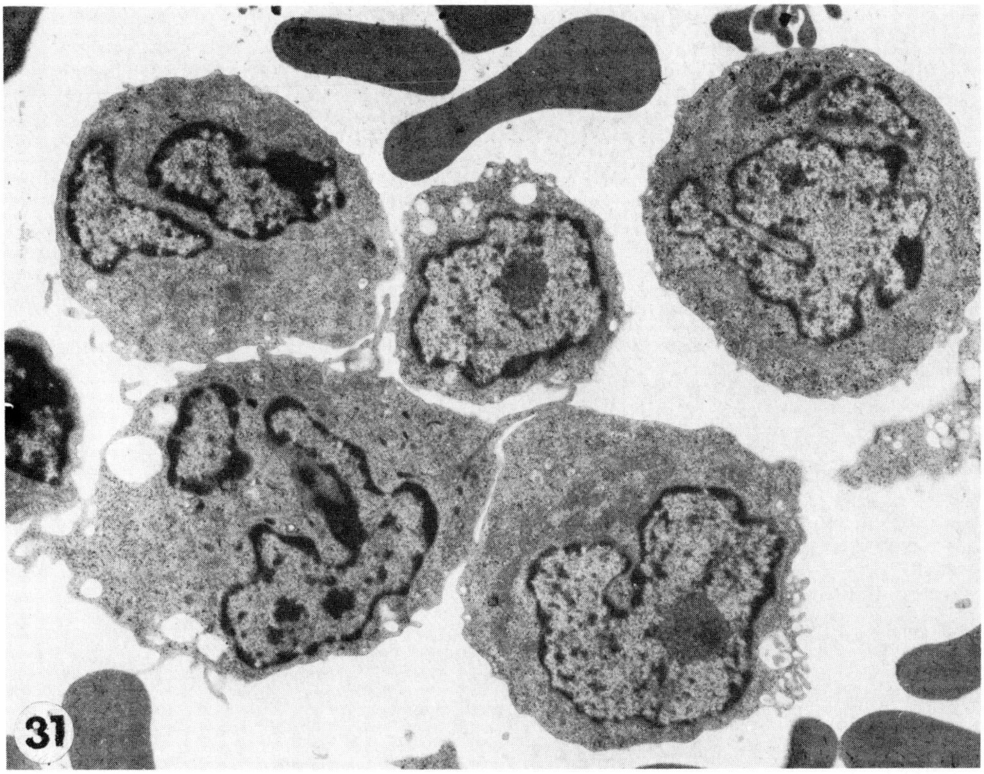
31

Figure 32A:
LYMPHOSARCOMA CELL LEUKEMIA

Lymphosarcoma cell leukemia is characterized by the presence in the peripheral blood of cells of the lymphoid series with highly atypical nuclei. These nuclei have deep thin indentations which, in certain planes of section, appear to divide the nuclei into two and sometimes three lobes. The chromatin shows peripheral condensation. Prominent electron-dense nucleoli (n) are present. The cytoplasm contains round or slightly elongated mitochondria, occasional electron-dense granules, rare strands of rough endoplasmic reticulum, and numerous free ribosomes. The Golgi complexes are poorly developed (× 5500).

Figure 33A:
RETICULUM CELL SARCOMA

The nuclei of these large neoplastic cells from the bone marrow of a patient with reticulum cell sarcoma range in shape from round or oval (upper left) to irregular and slightly notched (center) and multilobulated (lower right). The chromatin is generally finely dispersed, with minimal peripheral condensation. One or more large prominent nucleoli (n) are present in each cell. There is abundant cytoplasm, with numerous round or elongated mitochondria, many free ribosomes and several vacuoles (v). Many of the cells have prominent annulate lamellae (arrow), indicating rapidly growing and dividing cells (× 5500).

A stack of paranuclear annulate lamellae is seen at higher magnification in the insert at the lower left (× 26,000).

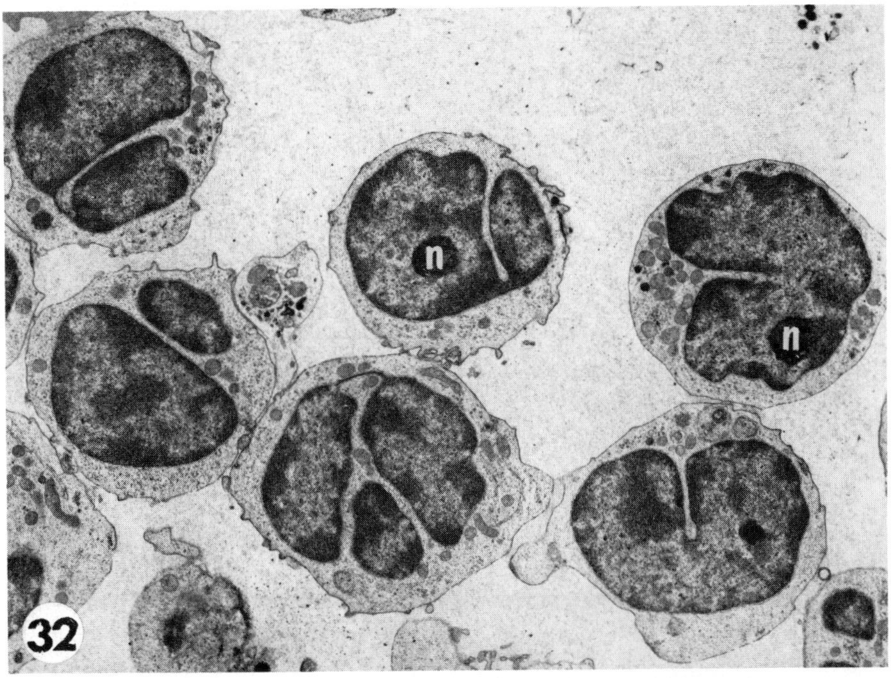
n
n
32

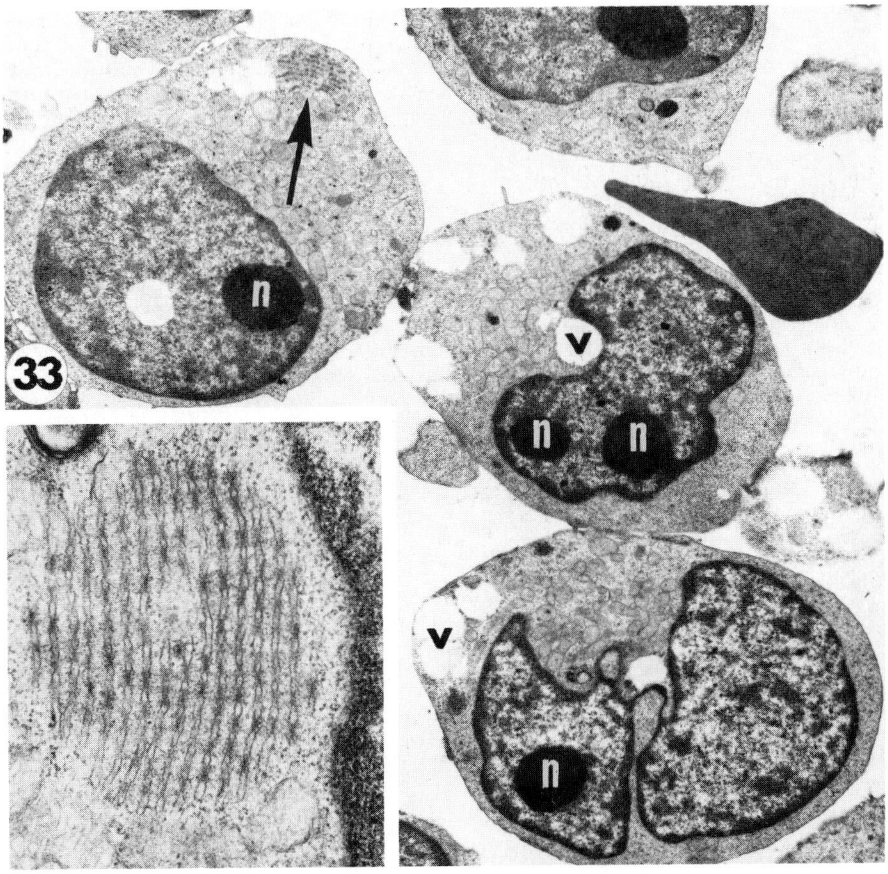
n
v
n
n
33
v
n

Figures 34A to 37A:
PLASMA CELL

Figure 34A (× 132,000) is an electron micrograph of a mature plasma cell from the bone marrow. It has a round eccentric nucleus (N) with clumped chromatin occurring mostly at the periphery, a distribution responsible for the wheel-like appearance seen by light microscopy. The most salient ultrastructural feature of the plasma cell is the presence of abundant arrays of well-packed rough endoplasmic reticulum (RER) throughout most of the cytoplasm. The cell also displays a prominent Golgi complex (G) composed of stacks of flattened sacs and vesicles, lined by smooth membranes. Several of the peripheral vesicles (V) are dilated, some containing a fluffy material. Several mitochondria (M) are present, mostly at the periphery of the Golgi complex. It is the rough endoplasmic reticulum that is responsible for the basophilia of the cytoplasm seen in the light microscope, and the paranuclear clear zone or "Hof" of the German authors is due to the Golgi and adjacent mitochondria.

The rough endoplasmic reticulum is seen at higher magnification (Fig. 35A–× 68,000) to consist of flattened membranous sacs containing finely granular material and lined on the outer surfaces by electron-dense ribosomes. These ribosomes are the sites of antibody formation. The newly synthesized immunoglobulins accumulate in the cisternae. Sometimes the cisternae become distended by the globulin (γ) as is seen in Figure 36A, forming what has been called a "flame cell." The lack of demonstrable membranes in this cell is due to aldehyde fixation without postosmication (× 6600). Occasionally plasma cells show localized, dense, rounded accumulations of protein, known as Russell bodies (Ru B) (Figure 37A–× 5500).

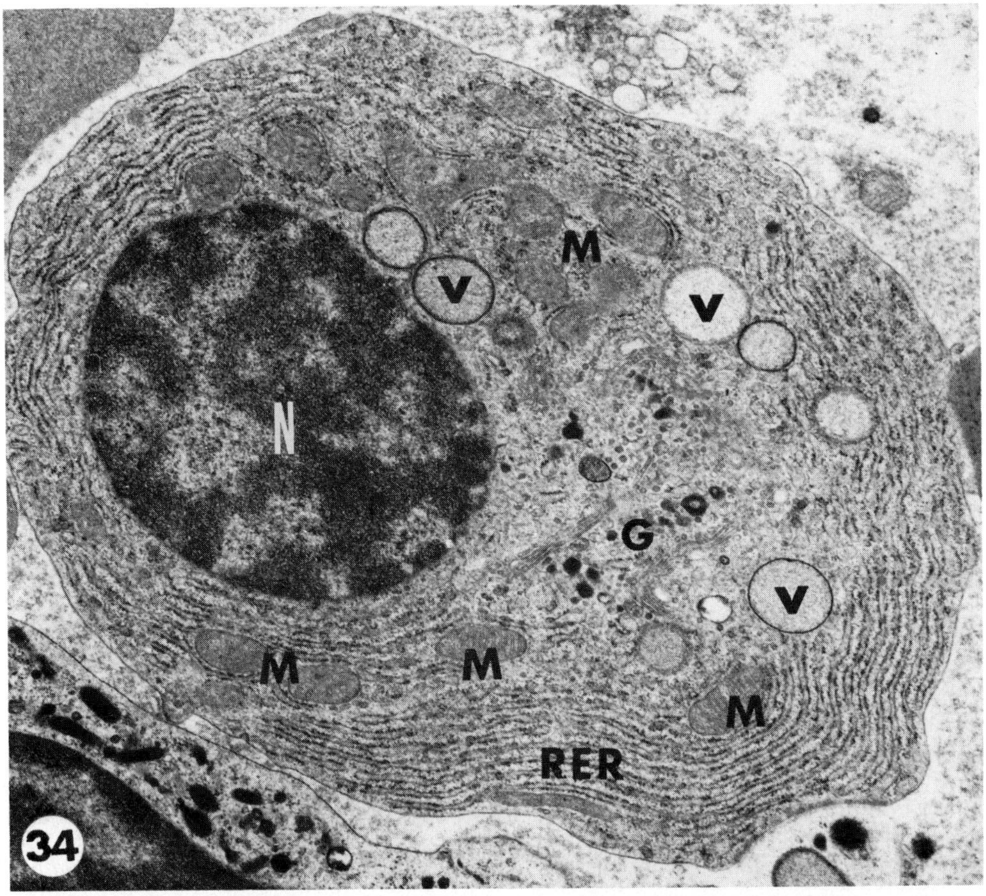
M
V
V
N
G
V
M
M
M
RER
34

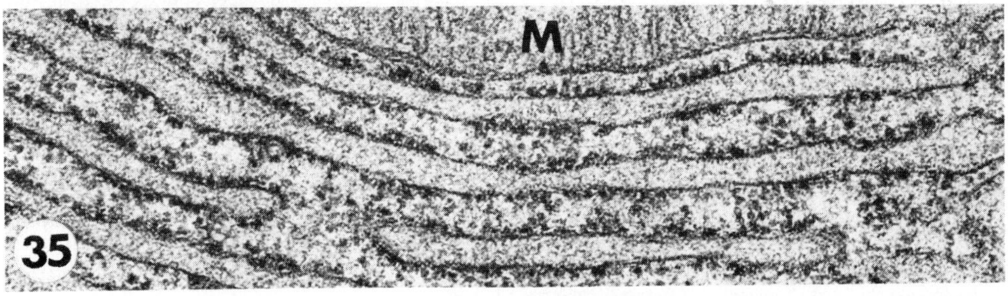
M
35

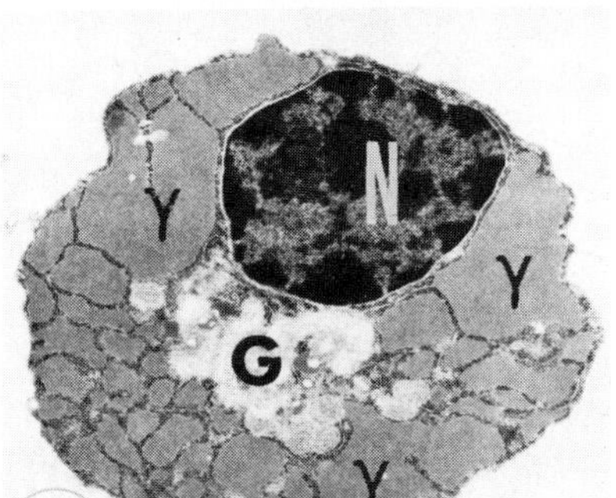
Y
N
Y
G
Y
36

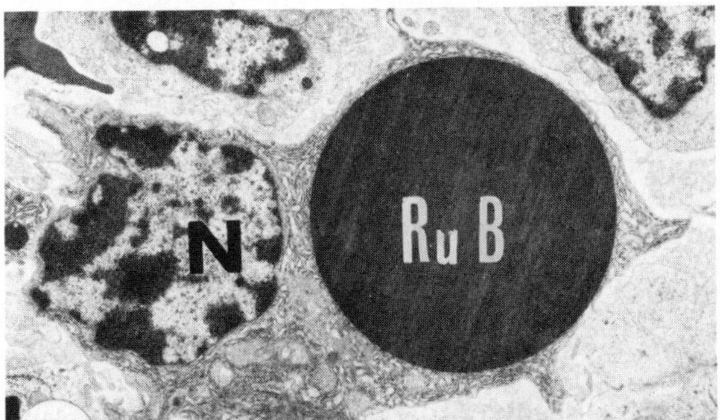
N
Ru B
37

Figures 38A and 39A:

MULTIPLE MYELOMA

Ultrastructural observations of the neoplastic plasma cells seen in the bone marrow of patients with multiple myeloma reveal a wide range of pleomorphism, ranging from cells which often cannot be distinguished morphologically from their normal counterpart (see Figure 34A) to highly atypical plasma cells as seen in Figures 38A and 39A. The atypical features of the two plasma cells in Figure 38A (× 6600) are the presence of nuclei having fine chromatin with minimal margination, the large prominent nucleoli (n), and the relatively small amount of cytoplasm showing large Golgi complexes (G). At higher magnification (Figure 39A—× 26,000) the cytoplasm shows an unusually large number of mitochondria (M) and relatively scant rough endoplasmic reticulum (RER).

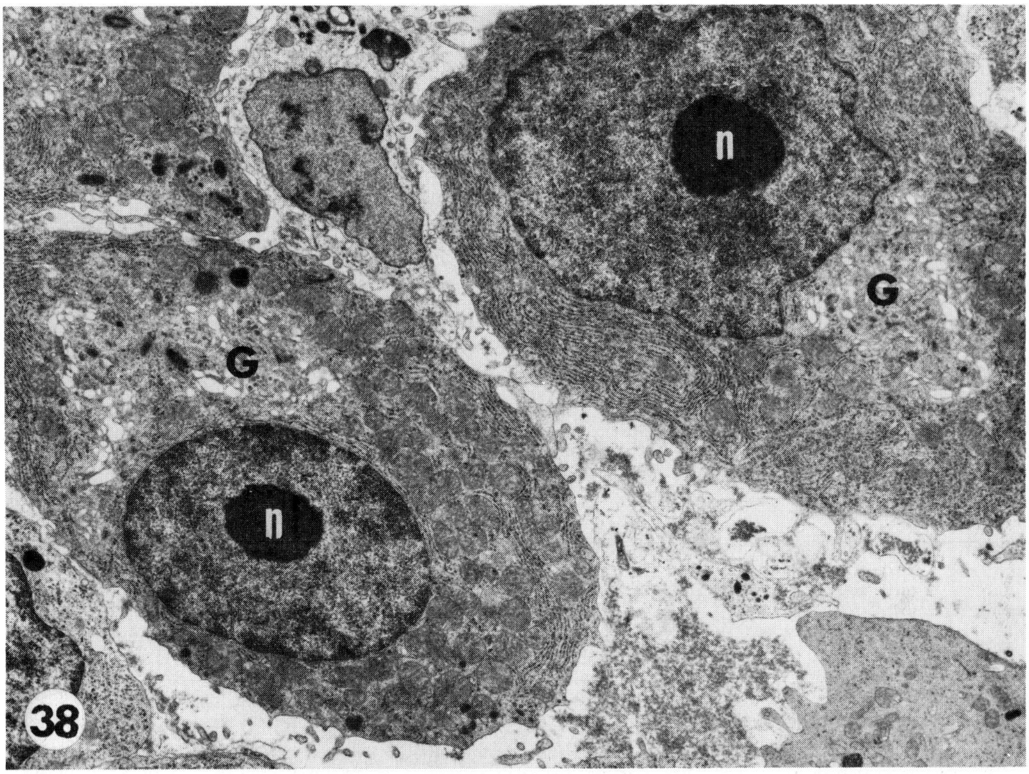
n
n
G
G
38

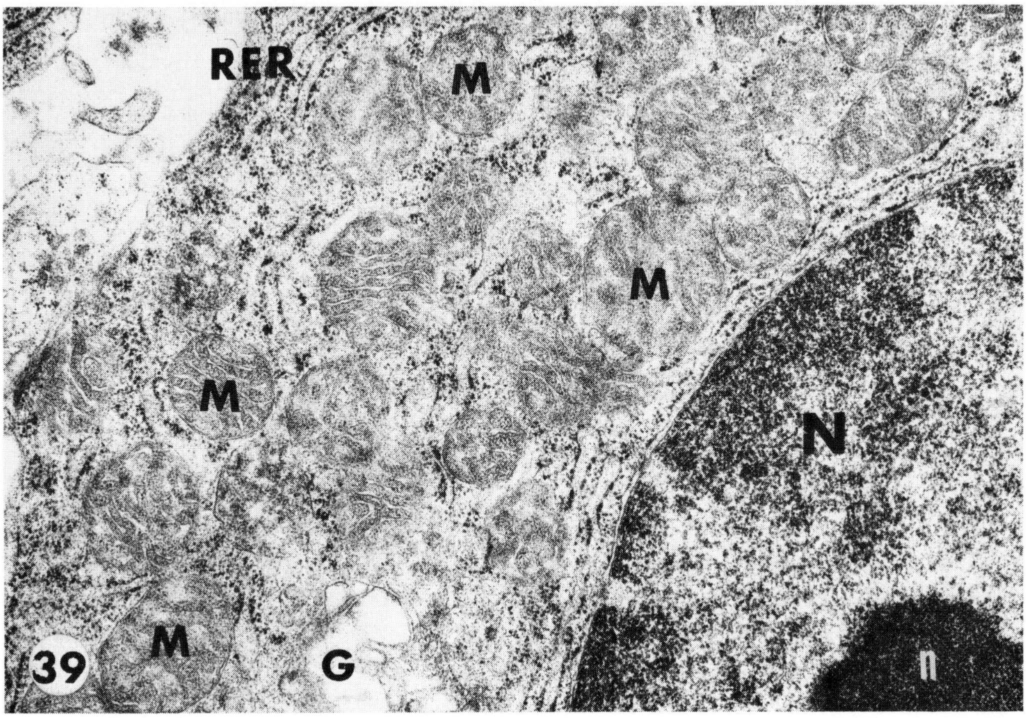
RER
M
M
M
N
M
G
n
39

Figures 40A and 41A:
MULTIPLE MYELOMA (continued)

The plasma cells in Figures 40A (× 6600) and 41A (× 13,200) are from the bone marrow of a patient with IgA myeloma. The outstanding ultrastructural feature in this case is the marked dilatation of all the cisternae of the rough endoplasmic reticulum, which are filled with a rather dense, granular, or flocculent material. The Golgi complex (G) is relatively inconspicuous, and only rare mitochondria (M) are seen. The nuclei (N) show marked clumping of the chromatin, and occasional binucleated cells are seen (cell at left in Figure 40A). Many cells show empty vacuoles at the periphery, which appear to be the result of rupture to the outside of the peripherally situated cisternae of the rough endoplasmic reticulum (Fig. 41A, arrow). This type of cell, the flame cell or thesaurocyte, is found predominantly but not exclusively in IgA myelomas.

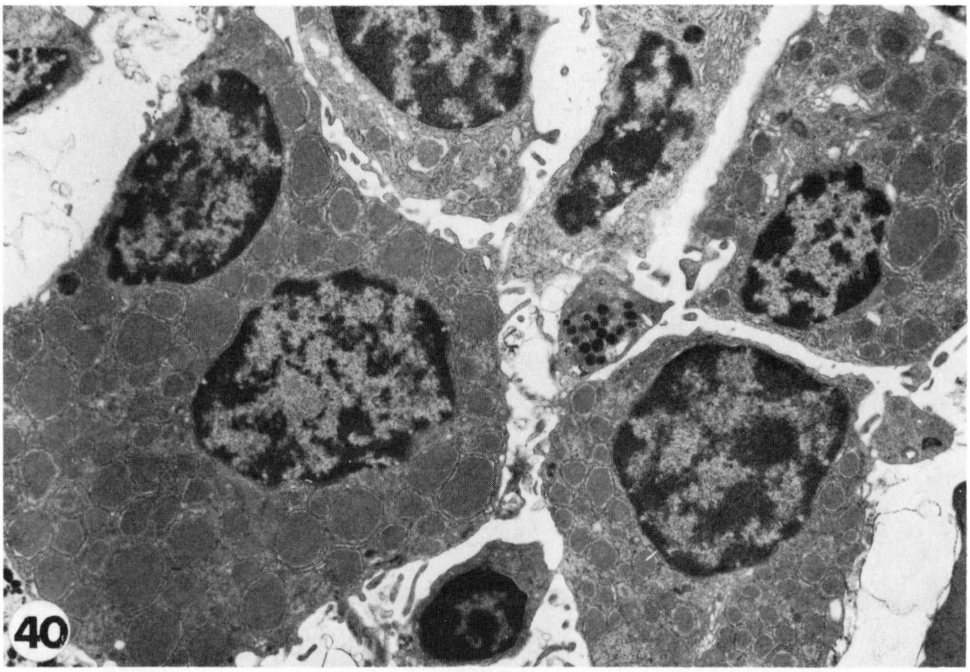
40

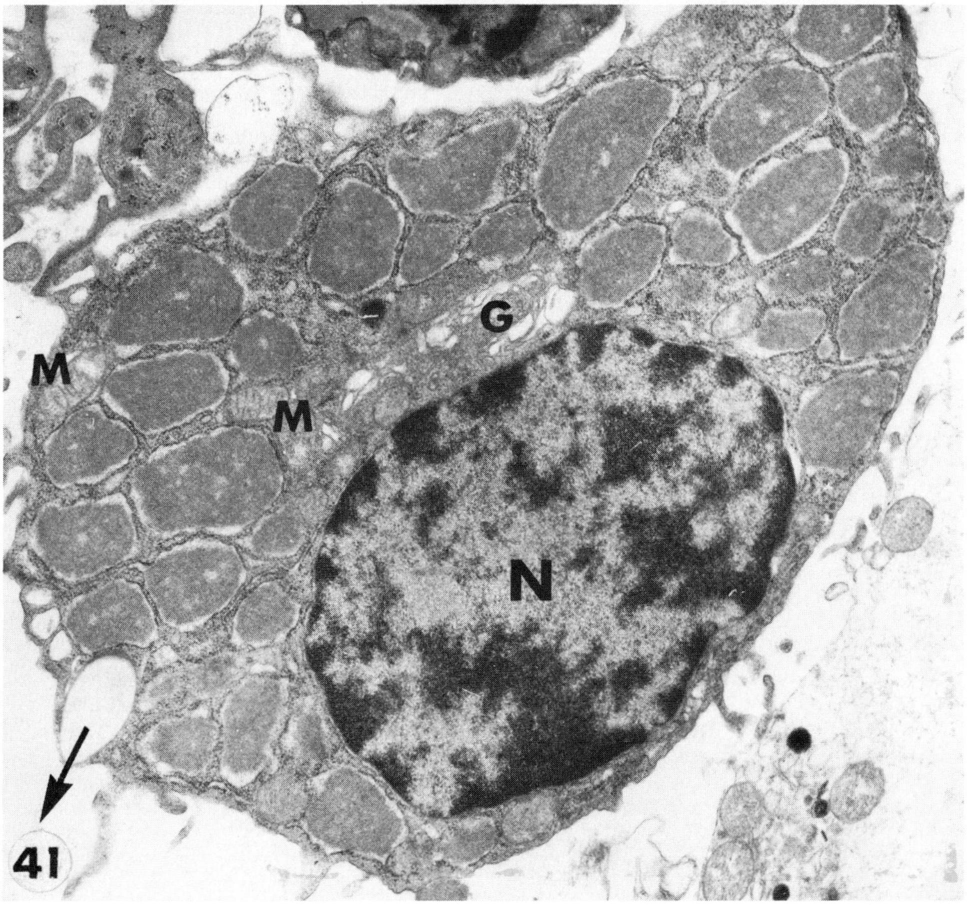
G
M
M
N
41

Figures 42A and 43A:
MEGAKARYOCYTES

The megakaryocytes are the largest cells found in the normal bone marrow, sometimes measuring up to 150 μm. in diameter. They have large multilobed nuclei. Figure 42A (× 6000) is an electron micrograph of a developing megakaryocyte showing three nuclear lobes (N) with irregular borders, the lobe on the left showing a nucleolus. The abundant cytoplasm contains numerous electron-dense granules, small Golgi complexes, and small round mitochondria, as well as numerous vesicles. These vesicles elongate, coalesce, and become continuous with the cell surface, thus segregating fragments of cytoplasm from the cell proper. These fragments are then released into the circulation as platelets. Occasionally the platelets may be released only from the surface of the megakaryocyte by the formation of blebs at the periphery, but most commonly the entire cytoplasm disintegrates (Figure 43A – × 4400).

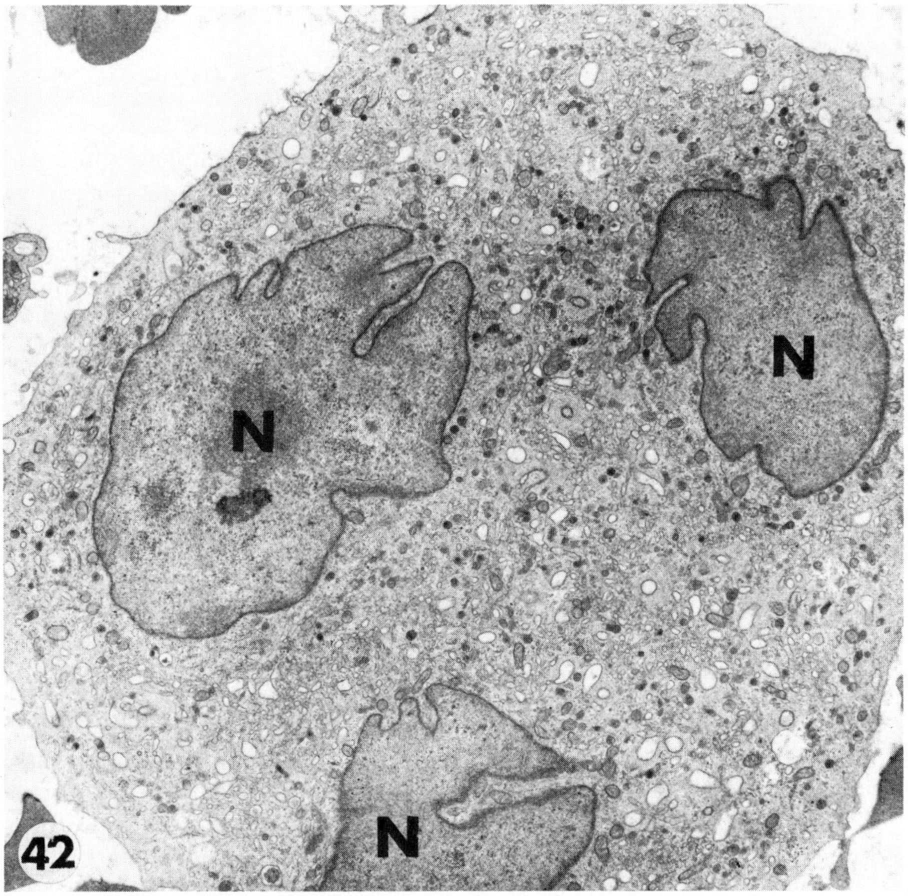
N
N
N
42

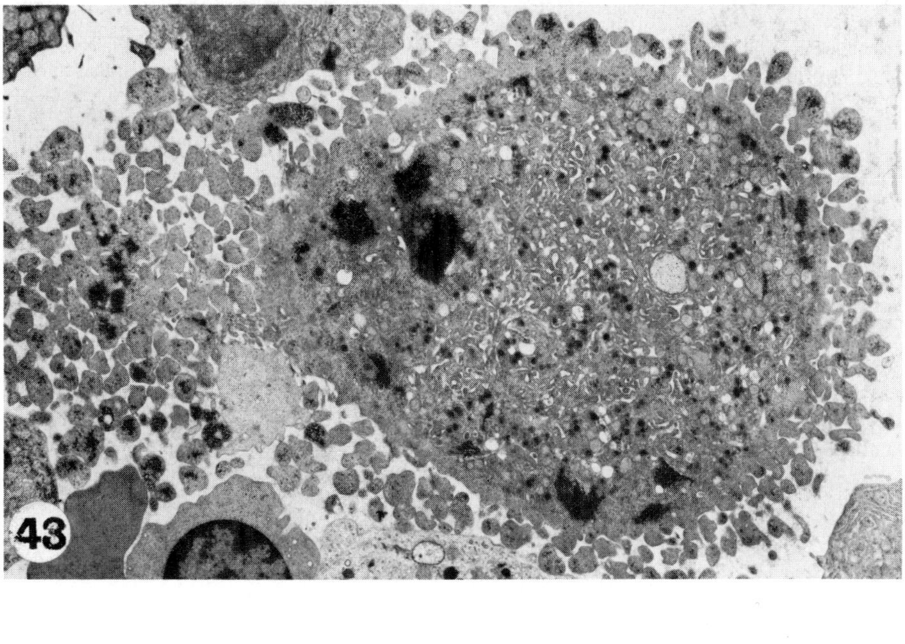
43

Figures 44A to 46A:

PLATELETS AND FIBRIN

As seen in Figure 43A, the platelets are fragments of the megakaryocyte cytoplasm and, as such, have no nucleus and rarely show structures such as Golgi complexes and endoplasmic reticulum, but retain organelles or inclusions such as vesicles, mitochondria, electron-dense granules, and glycogen particles from the mother cell. The circulating human platelets are disc-shaped structures with an average diameter of 2 μm. but can easily acquire irregular shapes during processing for electron microscopy through the action of anticoagulants, centrifugation, cold fixatives and, in fact, almost any stimulus (Figure 44A—× 13,200). When fixed in warm glutaraldehyde, as seen in Figure 45A (× 42,500), platelets reveal a marginal bundle of microtubules (arrows) beneath and parallel to the plasma membrane. It is these microtubules that are responsible for maintaining the discoid shape of the circulating platelets. In the central portions of the cytoplasm, but not in the pseudopods, are several round electron-dense granules, the alpha granules, surrounded by a unit membrane and often containing two zones of differing density.

The alpha granules are known to disintegrate during platelet aggregation and clot formation. Their nature and chemical composition is still a subject of debate. It is generally recognized that they are storage organelles, some of which, at least, are lysosomes, and they have been associated with platelet factors 3, 4, and fibrinogen. Other smaller and denser platelet granules are believed to contain serotonin, adenosine triphosphate, and histamine. For an extensive review of platelet morphology, the reader should consult White's publication (1971).

In the final phases of blood coagulation, in which the platelets play such an important role, thrombin converts fibrinogen to fibrin monomer, which spontaneously polymerizes and is transformed by the formation of cross-links into stable fibrin strands which have a characteristic ultrastructural appearance, showing an axial periodicity of 25 nm. (Figure 46A—× 100,000).

REFERENCES

1. Ackerman, G. A.: The human neutrophil promyelocyte. Z. Zellforsch. Mikrosk. Anat. *118*:467, 1971a.
2. Ackerman, G. A.: The human neutrophil myelocyte. Z. Zellforsch. Mikrosk. Anat. *121*:153, 1971b.
3. Ackerman, G. A., and Clark, M. A.: Ultrastructural localization of peroxidase activity in human basophil leukocytes. Acta Haematol. *45*:280, 1971.
4. Bainton, D. F., and Farquhar, M. G.: Origin of granules in polymorphonuclear leukocytes. J. Cell Biol. *28*:277, 1966.
5. Bessis, M. C., and Breton-Gorius, J.: Iron particles in normal erythroblasts and normal and pathological erythrocytes. J. Biophys. Biochem. Cytol. *3*:503, 1957.
6. Douglas, S. D., Fudenberg, H. H., Glade, P. R., Chessin, L. N., and Moses, H. L.: Fine structure of leukocytes in infectious mononucleosis: In vivo and in vitro studies. Blood *34*:42, 1969.
7. Freeman, A. I., and Journey, L. J.: Ultrastructural studies on monocytic leukaemia. Brit. J. Haematol. *20*:225, 1971.
8. Hayhoe, G. F. J., Quaglino, D., and Doll, R.: The Cytology and Cytochemistry of Acute Leukaemias. A Study of 140 Cases. M.R.C. Special Report Series, No. 304, London, Her Majesty's Stationery Office, 1964.
9. Kobayasi, T., Midtgard, K., and Asboe-Hansen, G.: Ultrastructure of human mast-cell granules. J. Ultrastruct. Res. *23*:153, 1968.
10. Lee, R. E.: The fine structure of the cerebroside occurring in Gaucher's disease. Proc. Nat. Acad. Sci. *61*:484, 1968.
11. Luft, J. H.: Improvements in epoxy resin embedding methods. J. Biophys. Biochem. Cytol. *9*:409, 1961.
12. Miller, F., de Harven, E., and Palade, G. E.: The structure of eosinophil leukocyte granules in rodents and in man. J. Cell Biol. *31*:349, 1966.
13. Murayama, M.: Molecular mechanism of red cell "sickling." Science *153*:145, 1966.
14. Stetson, C. A., Jr.: The state of hemoglobin in sickled erythrocytes. J. Exp. Med. *123*:341, 1966.
15. Tanaka, Y., and Goodman, J. R.: Electron Microscopy of Human Blood Cell. New York, Harper & Row, Inc., 1972.
16. White, J. G.: Platelet morphology. In Johnson, S. G. (ed.): The Circulating Platelet. New York, Academic Press, Inc., 1971, p. 45.
17. Zucker-Franklin, D.: Electron microscopic study of human basophils. Blood *29*:878, 1967.

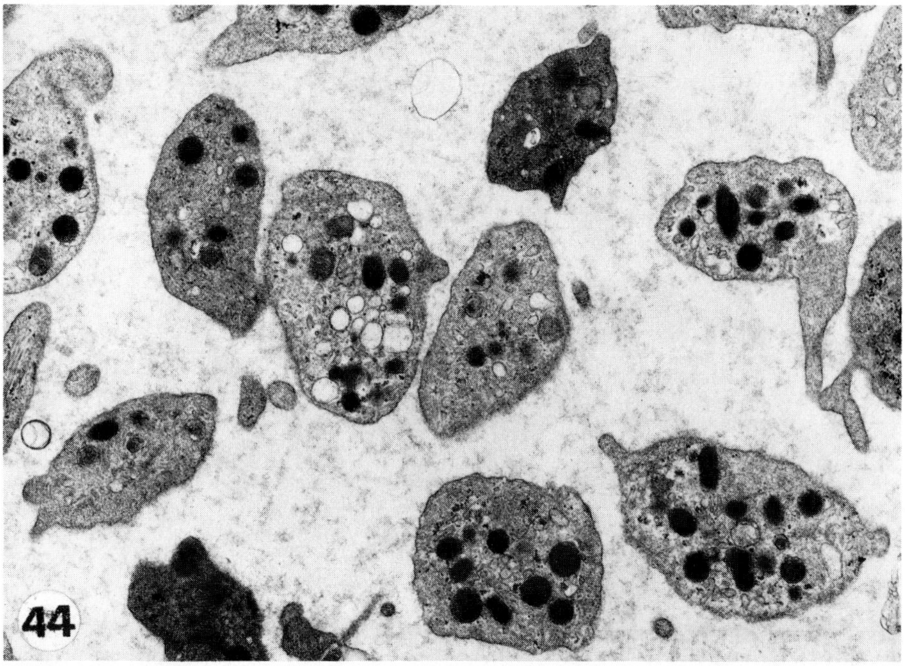
44

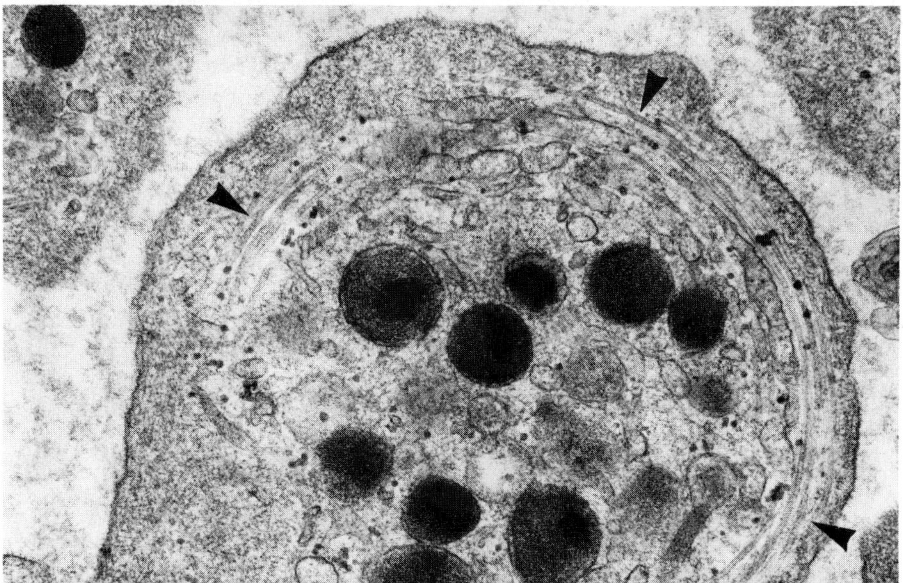
45

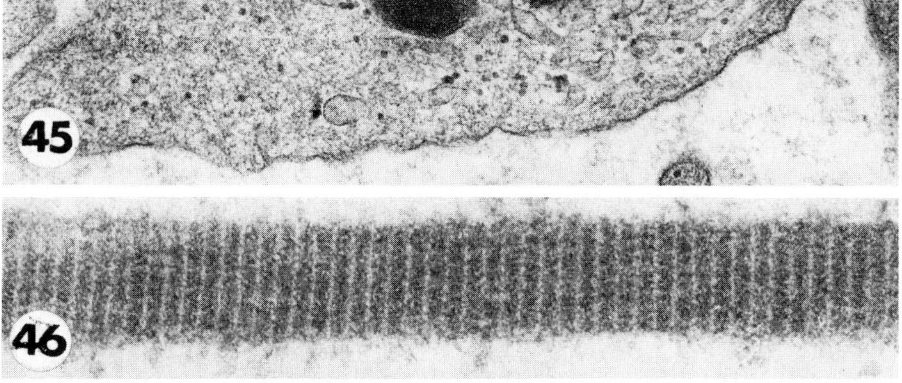
46

Chapter 5

BLOOD GROUPS AND THEIR APPLICATION

by KURT STERN, M.D., CHANG-LING LEE, M.D., and ISRAEL DAVIDSOHN, M.D.

IMMUNOHEMATOLOGY OF RED CELLS

Red cell antigens are chemical structures imparting specific properties to the surface of the red cell and are at present detectable only by the reactivity of red cells with antibodies corresponding to the antigens (homologous antibodies). Most of these antigen-antibody reactions involve clumping or *agglutination* of the red cells. Therefore, the antibodies are called *hemagglutinins* and the antigens, *hemagglutinogens.*

Isoagglutinogens and *isoagglutinins* are the antigens and antibodies, respectively, which differentiate red cells of some individuals from those of others belonging to the same species. *Heteroagglutinins* are antibodies that react with red cell antigens of different species. It is customary to differentiate between "natural" and "immune" agglutinins, the former term applying to agglutinins occurring without any known cause, such as transfusion or injection of blood or other antigenic substances eliciting antibody formation. On the other hand, immune isoagglutinins result from deliberate or unintentional immunization *(isoimmunization)*, such as may occur from injection or transfusion of blood or from the entry of fetal red cells into the maternal circulation. Some hemoantibodies, in the presence of complement, hemolyze red cells; hence, they are called *hemolysins.* In most instances, hemolysins develop after known immunization with hemoantigens.

The genetic background of morphologic and chemical variants of red cells is discussed elsewhere; the most significant polymorphism of red cells depends on immunohematologic ("serologic") characteristics. They are predicated on the presence or absence of surface chemical properties of red cells and they permit their differentiation and classification into a large number of well-defined blood group systems as determined by their reactions with specific hemagglutinins. They exhibit three important features: they are detectable on the basis of specific reactivity with corresponding antibodies producing agglutination or lysis; they are inherited according to Mendelian laws; and they appear at certain stages of fetal development and are fully formed either at birth or in early postnatal development and persist throughout life.

At present at least 13 independent and well-defined blood group systems are known. They are made up of at least 50 identifiable blood factors of practical significance, in addition to many more as yet unassigned. If red cells were to be tested for the presence of all these factors, several million different phenotypes could be differentiated (Race and Sanger, 1968). This imparts to blood from different persons an individuality suggesting that some time in the future each person's blood may be identifiable by its blood factors.

Is individuality a unique attribute of the human red blood cell or do other body cells show a similar degree of extreme differentiation? Actually, conclusive evidence is already available for complex systems of isoantigens differentiating leukocytes and platelets (see p. 409). In addition, the experience with skin and organ transplantations indicates that individuality is not limited to red blood cells; however, better methods are available for the dem-

Table 5-1. THE BLOOD GROUP SYSTEMS

BLOOD GROUP SYSTEM	ORIGINAL DISCOVERY	
	YEAR	AUTHORS
ABO	1900	Landsteiner
MNS	1927	Landsteiner and Levine
P	1927	Landsteiner and Levine
Rh-Hr	1937	Landsteiner and Wiener
Kell	1946	Coombs, Mourant, and Race
Lewis	1946	Mourant
Lutheran	1946	Callender and Race
Duffy	1950	Cutbush, Mollison, and Parker
Kidd	1951	Allen, Diamond, and Niedziela
Diego	1954	Levine, Koch, McGee, and Hill
I	1956	Wiener, Unger, Cohen, and Feldman
Xg	1962	Mann, Cahan, Gelb, Fisher, Hamper, Tippett, Sanger, and Race
Dombrock	1965	Swanson, Polesky, Tippett, and Sanger
Unclassified factors with very high or very low frequency	1952-1971	Several workers

onstration of differences in red cells of different individuals than for demonstration of tissue differences.

As can be seen from Table 5-1, immunologic definition of red blood cells has advanced especially rapidly during the last 30 years. This has been due to a large extent to development of new sensitive and specific techniques for demonstration of antigen-antibody reactions. Some of the factors responsible for the continuing progress in this branch of immunohematology are the increased use of blood transfusions, the relative ease in procuring material for study, the fact that the hemagglutination technique is a convenient and highly sensitive method that permits the study of the whole cell without destroying or even damaging its identity, and the consideration that results of this work have not only proved of great clinical value but have also contributed to our knowledge in such basic sciences as immunology, genetics, and anthropology.

Theory of Blood Group Systems

The ABO System. It is no coincidence that the ABO system was the first to be discovered. This is the only blood group system in which plasma and serum regularly contain agglutinins reacting with blood factors present in the red cells of other persons. Such random interactions of serums and red cell suspensions actually were the method by means of which Landsteiner demonstrated the presence of ABO blood groups in 1900. In addition to the "natural" occurrence of the isoagglutinins, two other factors aided the detection of isoagglutination in the ABO system: it occurs over a wide thermal range, including so-called room temperature (20 to 25° C.); and isoagglutinins responsible for agglutination in the ABO system are of the so-called complete type (IgM), which means that attachment of the antibody to the red cell possessing the homologous blood factor is followed automatically by agglutination (see p. 349).

Initially Landsteiner differentiated three types of blood: (1) Red cells of one group were not agglutinated by the serum of any other person; because of the apparent absence of agglutinogens from these red cells, this group was called *O.* (2) Red cells that were agglutinated by serums of some other persons were designated as group *A.* (3) Red cells that were agglutinated by serums of group A were called group *B.* Subsequently a rarer type of blood was found to have red cells which were agglutinated by serums of group A as well as of group B, i.e., group *AB.* The antibodies found in the serum are designated as anti-A and anti-B (Table 5-2).

It is apparent that two "laws" can be easily formulated: the serum of a person does not contain isoagglutinins capable of agglutinating his own red cells, and the serum of a person does contain the isoagglutinin(s) that react with the isoagglutinogen(s) absent from his red cells.

There are considerable variations in the reactivity of the blood factors. For example, a serum containing anti-B, when tested against a series of specimens of group B, may produce agglutinations differing considerably in strength from one specimen to the next. Technical factors, which also affect rapidity, in-

Table 5-2. ISOAGGLUTINOGENS AND ISOAGGLUTININS IN THE ABO SYSTEM

BLOOD GROUP	ISOAGGLUTINOGEN(S) IN RED CELLS	ISOAGGLUTININ(S) IN PLASMA OR SERUM	APPROX. FREQUENCY IN U.S. WHITES PER CENT
O	None	anti-A, anti-B	45
A	A	anti-B	41
B	B	anti-A	10
AB	A,B	none	4

tensity, and titer of agglutination, will be dealt with later.

Subgroups of A. In addition to the variable agglutinability of all blood factors, certain blood specimens of groups A and AB are consistently less agglutinable than others.

It was shown by means of absorption tests that certain weakly agglutinable cells of group A are not able to absorb completely anti-A, whereas complete absorption is accomplished by using comparable quantities of red cells with strong agglutinability. These observations have been generally accepted as proof of a qualitative difference between the A blood factor in strongly and weakly agglutinable red cells. Recent immunochemical studies disclosed absence from weakly reactive A red cells of antigenic determinants (oligosaccharides) present in strongly reactive A red cells. Most group A cells belong to subgroup A_1 (strongly agglutinable), whereas the weakly agglutinable specimens are designated as subgroup A_2. Similarly, red cells of group AB are subdivided into subgroups A_1B and A_2B. Table 5–3 lists the relative incidence of subgroups of A, including rarer subgroups designated as A_3, A_4, A_x, and A_m.

The main importance of the subgroups of A lies in the lesser agglutinability of red cells not belonging to subgroups A_1 and A_1B. This may lead to misidentification of blood as group O instead of group A or as group B instead of group AB. Such errors may be compounded by the presence in some blood specimens of isoagglutinins reacting specifically with subgroups of group A, e.g., the serum of a person of subgroup A_2 or A_2B may have anti-A_1, agglutinating A_1 and A_1B cells. In contrast to anti-A and anti-B, which are present regularly according to Landsteiner's laws (see Table 5–2), these antibodies are found only infrequently and therefore are called "irregular isoagglutinins." They are usually of low titer and can best be detected when the agglutination is performed at temperatures around 4° C. At room temperature and especially at body temperature (37° C.), agglutinations by these antibodies are weak or absent. Certain special features are found in three rare subgroups: when red cells of subgroup A_3 are exposed

Table 5–3. SUBGROUPS OF A AND AB

			REACTION OF RED CELLS WITH*				ISOAGGLUTININS IN SERUM	
GROUP	SUBGROUP	APPROXIMATE FREQUENCY OF SUBGROUP (PER CENT OF GROUP) IN U.S. WHITES	Anti-A (Present in Serum of Group B)	Anti-A_1 (Absorbed Serum of Group B)	Anti-A_1 Lectin	Anti-A (Present in Serum of Group O)	Regular	Irregular
A	A_1	78	+	+	+	+	anti-B	anti-H (very rare)
	A_2	22	+	–	–	+	anti-B	anti-A_1 (in 1–2% of A_2 persons)
	A_3	rare	+w (see text)	–	–	+w (see text)	anti-B	anti-A_1
	A_x	very rare	–	–	–	+	anti-B	anti-A_1 (commonly)
	A_m	extremely rare	–	–	–	–	anti-B	anti-H
AB	A_1B	70	+	+	+	+***	none	anti-H
	A_2B	30	+	–	–	+***	none	anti-A_1 (in 30% of A_2B persons)
	A_3B etc.**	extremely rare	+w or –	–	–	+***	none	anti-A_1 (commonly)

*+ Agglutination
+w Weak agglutination
– No agglutination

**Combinations of B with other subgroups of A
***Reflects also agglutination of factor B by anti-B

to anti-A serum, only a small number of red cells are agglutinated, as can be seen especially well on microscopic examination (mixed field agglutination). A_x red cells are clumped in most instances by anti-A in serum of group O but only rarely by anti-A present in group B. This phenomenon is not dependent on the titer of the isoagglutinins. Saliva of A_m but not of A_x persons contains A substance. Both contain H substance. Reference to the rare "Bombay" ABO types will be made on page 353.

General Properties of Isoagglutinogens A and B. By suitable methods the isoagglutinogens A and B can be demonstrated as early as the second month of fetal life. However, as a rule, they are not completely developed at birth. Specifically, red cells of group A or AB of newborn infants react in most instances as if they would belong to subgroup A_2 or A_2B. By the age of one year isoagglutinogens have reached full strength.

Although they were originally discovered in the red cells, the term "blood factors" A and B is to a certain extent a misnomer, since A and B antigens are present in some tissues other than blood. Within the blood itself they are probably present also in leukocytes and platelets. They are found abundantly in exocrine glands, such as the salivary glands, pancreas, and in the gastric mucosa. Demonstration of the antigens in tissues is not feasible by agglutination tests but may be accomplished by specific absorption of added antibody or by fluorescent antibody applied to tissue sections or by mixed cell agglutination. Davidsohn applied the specific red cell adherence (SRCA) test, a modification of the Coombs mixed cell agglutination reaction (Coombs *et al.*, 1945) to the demonstration of A, B, and H antigens in paraffin and frozen sections. This highly sensitive and specific technique is based on the sandwich principle. The unknown antigen in the tissue section is in the bottom layer. It is covered by a few drops of an appropriate antiserum or a similarly functioning reagent (a lectin) (middle layer). The top layer is a suspension of erythrocytes of the blood group that is suspected in the tissue of the bottom layer. If the erythrocytes remain attached, the presence of the blood group antigen in the bottom layer is established. The antigen is absent if the indicator red cells of the top layer have been washed away (Davidsohn, 1972). A and B antigens also occur in other species and even in bacteria. It is conceivable that introduction of such antigenic material into the body may induce formation of isoagglutinins early during life (Springer, 1967).

Highly purified preparations with A and B blood group activity have been obtained from various sources, including human meconium. Witebsky and Klendshoj (1941), Morgan and King (1943), Kabat (1956) and Watkins (1966) have made outstanding contributions to the elucidation of the chemistry of A and B blood group substances. They are complex mucopolysaccharides containing glucosamine and galactosamine, immunologic specificity depending on relatively small terminal portions of these macromolecules. Commercially available, purified, protein-free preparations of group-specific substance A are derived from porcine gastric mucosa and those of group-specific substance B from equine gastric mucosa. Such material has several useful applications. First, it can be safely injected into suitable persons in order to elevate titers of isoagglutinins anti-A or anti-B for preparation of diagnostic antiserums. Second, when added to blood containing the corresponding isoagglutinins, A and B substances at least partially neutralize these antibodies, and this was expected to increase the safety of group O blood for use as "universal donor." That this purpose is often not accomplished will be discussed later (p. 393). Third, group-specific substances A and B are of considerable usefulness in various laboratory techniques to be outlined later (pp. 381, 383).

Landsteiner's assignment of red cells possessing neither A nor B agglutinogens to group "O" (equivalent to "zero") was meant to indicate merely absence of these antigens. Subsequently, however, it was established that red cells of group O contain a specific polysaccharide distinguishable immunochemically from A and B. This agglutinogen is now designated as H. Anti-H antibodies occur only rarely in man (cf. Table 5-3 and p. 353). Not only red cells of group O, but also those of other groups contain H antigen, with A_1B red cells showing the poorest reactivity with anti-H.

Secretors of A, B, and H. In addition to the previously mentioned wide distribution of A and B substances throughout the human body, the corresponding blood group specific substance(s) are also found in glandular secretions, such as saliva and gastric juice, of roughly 80 per cent of persons of group A or B, respectively. Such persons are called "secretors." In the remaining 20 per cent, called "nonsecretors," blood group specific substances in tissues are present only as alcohol-soluble compounds, probably in the form of lipopolysaccharides, and this prevents their appearance in the aqueous secretions. On the other hand, in tissues of secretors, blood group specific substances occur in alcohol-soluble as well as in water-soluble forms. The property of being a secretor is transmitted genetically and depends on the presence of at least one of a pair of allelic genes designated as "*Se*." Persons who are nonsecretors are homozygous for the gene *se* (*sese*). Meconium of fetuses and infants who are secretors contains large amounts of blood group specific substance, reflecting concentration of material secreted during fetal life. Saliva and other secretions of secretors also contain H substance, which neutralizes anti-H reagents, e.g., anti-H lectin (see p. 385).

Isoagglutinins. As inferred from the "laws of Landsteiner," isoagglutinins anti-A or anti-B are regularly present in persons lacking the corresponding agglutinogen(s) in their red cells. In Table 5-3 reference was made to the irregular isoagglutinins anti-A_1 and anti-H. The latter shows the strongest reactivity with O and A_2 and the weakest with A_1 and A_1B red cells. Antibodies with similar reactivity are present in the serum of some animals, e.g., eels, and in certain plant extracts (lectins). It has been established that isoagglutinins develop postnatally. Isoagglutinins present in the newborn, as demonstrable in cord blood specimens, represent without exception maternal isoagglutinins transmitted transplacentally. Such passively transferred antibodies disappear gradually and, as a rule, the infant begins to produce his own isoagglutinins some time between the third and sixth months of postnatal life. This strongly suggests that the isoagglutinins are the result of some subtle antigenic stimulation, possibly through microorganisms or food, which inevitably occurs postnatally. In addition, earlier absence and subsequent appearance of isoagglutinins may also be attributed to the phenomenon of "immunologic maturation" postulated by Hirszfeld (1928). Absence of isoagglutinins corresponding to an isoagglutinogen present in the same person fits in well with the concept of immunologic tolerance to antigens present in, or introduced into, the fetus or neonate, a phenomenon which insures the inability of the normal host to form antibodies for his own antigens.

Although on the basis of this concept the term "natural" isoagglutinins may appear to be a misnomer, since they also result from some form of antigenic stimulation, practical considerations make it desirable to differentiate isoagglutinins developing in the "natural" course of events from those resulting from specific antigenic stimulation. Such antigenic stimulation includes transfusion of incompatible blood, entry into maternal circulation of red cells of a fetus with incompatible ABO group (e.g., a pregnant woman of group O with fetus A or B), and administration of group-specific substances including antigens closely related to A or B, such as those present in some bacterial vaccines (tetanus) or horse serum or those that may result from infections (*Escherichia coli*). In these instances it can be demonstrated that, in addition to increase in quantity, anti-A and anti-B antibodies have acquired certain properties that characterize IgG antibodies, to be described later (p. 359). Two specific properties of anti-A or anti-B isoagglutinins of considerable practical importance are mentioned now. First, they frequently possess not only the capacity to agglutinate but also to hemolyze red cells containing the corresponding isoagglutinogen. Since this hemolysis is dependent on presence of complement, it is apparent only with use of fresh serum or after addition of complement. Inactivation at 56° C. for 30 minutes destroys complement and prevents hemolysis while the corresponding agglutinin activity remains unaffected. Second, although the group-specific substances A and B are well capable of neutralizing IgM anti-A and anti-B isoagglutinin, the corresponding IgG antibodies are much less readily neutralized. Detailed procedures for demonstration of this property and its practical application are given on pages 381 to 383.

As are most antibodies, isoagglutinins anti-A and anti-B are found in the gamma globulin fraction. This has acquired a certain clinical significance in the disturbances of plasma proteins, namely, acquired and congenital hypogammaglobulinemia and agammaglobulinemia. As a rule, in such conditions isoagglutinins normally expected on the basis of the person's ABO group are either absent or present in unusually low titers. Hence, the absence during routine blood grouping tests of an expected isoagglutinin in the adult should arouse suspicion of lack or decrease in the serum gamma globulin fraction. Rarely, isoagglutinins are present only as IgG antibodies that are not detectable unless appropriate techniques are used (pp. 382–383). The physiologic absence of isoagglutinins in the serum of the newborn up to the age of three to six months has already been referred to.

In recent years plant extracts have been prepared containing proteins that specifically agglutinate red cells of certain human blood groups. In accord with the recommendation of Boyd (1954) these plant substances are called lectins. Lectins capable of differentiating between subgroups of A are especially useful, inasmuch as they agglutinate only A_1 and A_1B cells but not red cells A_2, A_2B, A_3, and so on. Anti-H lectins reacting strongly with group O red cells are particularly useful in testing for the presence of H antigen in secretions (p. 385).

Inheritance of ABO Groups. The fundamental principle of genetic transmission of the ABO characters is based on the fact that each of one autosomal chromosome pair (one derived from the father, the other from the mother) carries one locus on which one of the three alleles – A, B, or O – must be present (Fig. 5-1). Table 5-4 lists the resulting phenotypes and genotypes and their relative frequency in the U.S. white population. Three facts deducible

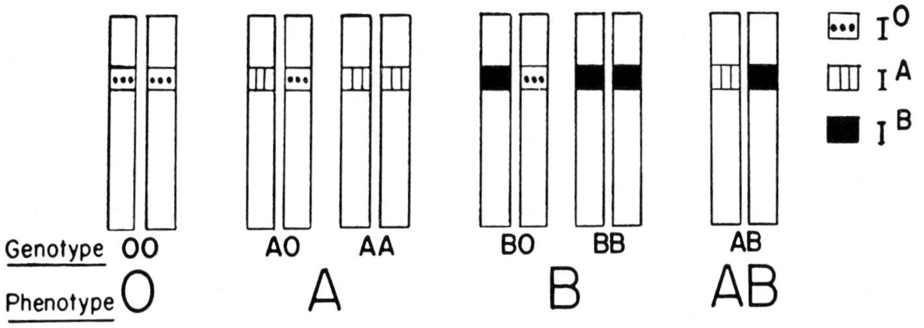

Figure 5–1. Diagrammatic representation of locus (I) containing genes of ABO factors.

from the table are worthy of mention: persons of group O are always homozygous; persons of group AB are always heterozygous; and persons of groups A and B may be either homozygous or heterozygous. Their genotypes are at present not susceptible to determination by laboratory tests. In other words, there is no reliable reagent available for determination of zygosity of phenotype A and B. Table 5–4 also presents information concerning inheritance of phenotypes of subgroups of A and AB. A_1, when present together with A_2, imparts to blood the phenotypic property A_1. Thus, one cannot differentiate between the homozygote A_1A_1 and the heterozygotes A_1A_2 or A_1O. By the same token, persons of group A_2 may have either genotype A_2A_2 or A_2O. In all these instances proof for zygosity of persons of group A_1, A_2, or B can be established reliably only by means of family studies; that is, heterozygosity can be proved by finding that one of the parents or children of the person in question belongs to group O.

New aspects of the mechanism of inheritance of ABO groups have been disclosed by investigations of exceptional blood specimens, first discovered in Bombay and therefore called "Bombay" types. Persons with this phenotype, designated as O_h, exhibit the following features: (1) the red cells are not agglutinated by anti-A, anti-B, or anti-H reagents; (2) the serum contains not only anti-A and anti-B, but also anti-H; (3) although the red cells possess neither A nor B agglutinogen, family studies may disclose presence of genes *A* or *B*: i.e., children of an $O_h \times O$ mating may be group A or B. In order to explain these anomalies, a gene pair *H-h*, inherited independently from the ABO antigens, has been postulated. Presence of at least one *H* gene is required in order to transform a precursor substance into a polysaccharide representing the antigen H which, in the presence of genes *A* and/or *B*, is converted into the corresponding antigens. This second step cannot occur in the rare homozygote *hh* ("Bombay type") since no H substance has been formed. This hypothesis is strongly supported by recent chemical studies, according to which antigens of the ABO and Lewis systems (p. 363) are products of sequential actions of transferases which modify a common precursor substance. Another significant deviation from the normal inheritance of ABO groups is the presence of both *A* and *B* genes on the same chromosome (*cis* arrangement). This rare phenomenon has been documented in a number of family studies and is associated with a weakly reacting B antigen. These observations and interpretations have made significant contributions to the understanding of genetic mechanisms. They are also important in connection with medicolegal applications of ABO inheritance, such as exclusion of parentage (p. 405).

Table 5–4. ABO PHENOTYPES AND GENOTYPES IN U.S. WHITE POPULATION

BLOOD GROUP PHENOTYPE	GENOTYPE	INCIDENCE (PER CENT)		
O	*OO*			45
A_1	A_1O	25	32	41
	A_1A_1	4		
	A_1A_2	3		
A_2	A_2O	8.5	9	
	A_2A_2	0.5		
B	*BO*	9.3		10
	BB	0.7		
A_1B	A_1B	2.8		4
A_2B	A_2B	1.2		

The MNS System. By contrast with the circumstances relating to the discovery of A and B agglutinogens, knowledge of M and N blood factors was derived from immunologic studies of Landsteiner and Levine (1927) in which animals of another species—rabbits—were injected with human blood. In addition to the expected species-specific hemoantibodies, serums of rabbits immunized with human red cells of one person also contained antibodies that discriminated between two classes of human red cells. After such serum was suitably absorbed with red cells belonging to one class, the remaining antibody agglutinated approximately 80 per cent of all blood specimens; the blood factor present in such blood was called "M." Blood specimens not containing the M factor and some of the M blood were found to be agglutinated by another antibody present in rabbits injected with human red cells free of the M factor. This second factor was called "N." As shown in Table 5–5, there are three possible combinations of M and N; namely, either of them may occur alone or combined with the other. When only one is present, they are homozygotes—MM or NN, respectively—whereas MN obviously is a heterozygote. It is apparent that, by contrast with the findings in the ABO system, no red cell can be devoid of both M-N factors. In other words in the MN system there is nothing corresponding to group O in the ABO system. Analyses of large series of specimens typed for M and N showed that incidence of the three types—M, N, and MN—was identical in persons of the four ABO groups. Thus, ABO and MN groups were proved to be independent of each other. Two differences between the MN and ABO systems are worthy of mention. M and N factors are present only in red cells and certain tissues but not in body fluids and secretions, and isoagglutinins anti-M and anti-N are not only of rare "natural" occurrence but are also hardly ever produced as a result of isoimmunization. In such rare exceptions anti-M isoagglutinins are encountered somewhat more frequently than anti-N. Human anti-M and anti-N react best at pH of 5 to 6; low levels of these antibodies may not be detectable at higher pH. Only a few cases have been recorded in the literature in which clinical manifestations, such as transfusion reactions or hemolytic disease of the newborn, could be traced to anti-M or anti-N. Hence, no consideration need be given to M and N factors in clinical medicine and specifically in pretransfusion tests. They are used in medicolegal and anthropologic studies. M and N are fully developed in red cells at birth and are apparently formed at an earlier stage of fetal development than A and B antigens.

Table 5–5. THE MN SYSTEM

PHENOTYPE	GENOTYPE	APPROXIMATE FREQUENCY (U.S. WHITES) PER CENT
M	*MM*	28
N	*NN*	22
MN	*MN*	50

As has been found subsequently in other blood group systems, the original simplicity of the MN system underwent numerous modifications after new data and facts became available. Weakly reacting forms of M and N have been encountered on rare occasions and designated as "M_2" and "N_2." Similar to weakly reacting subgroups of A, they may be missed because of poor agglutinability and thus give rise to erroneous interpretations. An extremely rare third allele of M and N has been described and called "M^g" (Allen *et al.*, 1958), the presence of which is important in connection with exclusion of parentage.

Several agglutinogens discovered during the last decade have been found to belong to the MN system. Two allelic factors, called "S" and "s," are regularly associated with M and N. In other words, each M or N agglutinogen is accompanied by and inherited with either the S or s agglutinogen. A rare antibody, discovered by Wiener *et al.* (1953) in a black patient and designated by them as anti-U, was subsequently shown to react with all red cells containing factors S or s. Thus, persons capable of forming this antibody lack both S and s and presumably are homozygous for a third allele, called S^u. This rare blood type occurs almost exclusively in blacks. Additional agglutinogens less regularly encountered include He and Hu, first described in African blacks. Also, two blood factors originally assumed to occur only in a few families and called Mi^a and Vw have been shown to be part of the MNS system.

The P System. Simultaneously with the discovery of M and N, Landsteiner and Levine (1927) established by means of antihuman red cell rabbit serums that human red cells contained a factor that they called "P," more recently referred to as P_1. This agglutinogen was found to be present in roughly 75 per cent of U. S. white adults. A much higher incidence of P_1-positive blood—over 95 per cent—was found in blacks. Presence of P_1 is independent of ABO, MN, and other blood group systems. There are considerable genetically determined differences in agglutinability of P_1-positive blood cells. Although P_1 is a poor isoantigen, low-titered anti-P_1 is found frequently in human serum, reacting best at low temperatures. A relationship of the P_1 antigen to Echinococcus has been demonstrated: some patients with this disease were found to have high-titered anti-P_1, and injection of echinococcal antigen into rabbits resulted in specific immune serum. Normal serums of some pigs, horses, and rabbits may also contain anti-P_1 agglutinin. Clinical implication of P_1 in transfusion reactions or other manifestations of isoimmunization is rare.

Modifications of the P system and its genetic background resulted from the discovery by Levine *et al.* (1951) of a "universal blood factor," designated by them as Tj^a (see p. 364). Absence from the red cells of this factor was responsible for serious difficulties in finding compatible blood for a particular patient whose serum agglutinated all blood specimens of the same ABO group tested as her own but did not agglutinate her own and her sister's red cells. The patient was said to be "Tj^a-negative" with anti-Tj^a antibody, i.e., to have antibodies for and lack in her red cells a blood factor which is present in practically all other individuals. Subsequently this rare property was found in approximately 20 other persons of 10 families living in different parts of the world. Sanger (1955) noted that all Tj^a-negative persons were also P_1 negative and proved the association of Tj^a with the P system serologically. When the antibody present in the serum of Tj^a-negative persons was absorbed with P_1-negative red cells, the residual antibody agglutinated specifically P_1-positive red cells. These observations led to the following reclassification of the antigens and genes of the P system: the antigen present in P_1-positive red cells is called P_1 and that in P_1-negative red cells, P_2. In addition to genes P_1 and P_2 determining the corresponding antigens, a third extremely rare gene, *p*, is assumed to exist and in its homozygous state, viz., *pp*, to be responsible for the blood type originally designated as Tj^a-negative. Additional family studies (Stern and Busch, 1963; Catino *et al.*, 1965) revealed several persons with this rare phenotype in a kinship with multiple consanguineous marriages. Most persons of type pp (Tj^a-negative) studied to date, had anti-Tj^a in the serum, even though there was no known preceding antigenic stimulation. On the basis of its serologic behavior, this antibody is to be designated as anti-$P + P_1$. In the presence of complement, it acts in most instances as hemolysin. Recently the hemolysin found in patients with paroxysmal cold hemoglobinuria (p. 234) has been shown to have the specificity of anti-$P + P_1$, i.e., it fails to react with pp red cells.

The Rh System. The Rh factor, like the MN and P blood factors, was discovered during animal experimentation. Landsteiner and Wiener (1940) injected rabbits and guinea pigs with red cells of the Rhesus monkey (*Macaca rhesus*) to study immunologic relationships between man and primates. In addition to expected hemoantibodies for Rhesus red cells the serum of rabbits so treated agglutinated approximately 85 per cent of human red cells. The significance of this discovery soon exceeded by far that of the M, N, and P factors when by fortunate coincidence and by ingenious reasoning Levine and Stetson (1939) and Levine, Burnham, Katzin, and Vogel (1941) demonstrated a clinical significance of the Rh factor that neither before nor since then has been possessed by any other blood groups except the ABO system. Specifically, previously unexplained hemolytic transfusion reactions, as well as the cause of hemolytic disease of the newborn (erythroblastosis fetalis), were shown to be the result of incompatibility in the Rh system as expressed in formation of Rh antibodies in the serum of persons whose red cells lack the Rh antigen.

The Rh system differs both from the ABO system and the MN system. In the Rh system there are no "natural" antibodies for agglutinogens absent from the red cells, but Rh antibodies develop frequently in persons who receive blood containing Rh antigen which they lack.

Extensive investigations were carried out soon after the discovery of the Rh factor, with outstanding contributions by Wiener, Levine, Diamond, Witebsky, and others in this country and Race and Sanger in England as well as numerous other workers throughout the world. Two different systems of terminology have developed from this work: one was originally proposed by Wiener, while a different set of notations elaborated by Race and Fisher in England was generally accepted in England and most parts of Europe and is also widely used in this country. It is not intended to discuss the relative merits of the two nomenclatures and to present specifically the serious objections based on principles of immunogenetics raised by Wiener against the Fisher-Race terminology, but the fact remains that both nomenclatures have today become firmly established. For this reason anybody working in the field must be familiar with both of them. In this presentation the recommendations by a committee appointed by the National Institutes of Health in 1949 have been followed, i.e., to use the notations of Wiener with the Fisher-Race notations added in parentheses. Table 5–6 contains a parallel listing of the most important notations expressed in both terminologies. A third notation has been proposed by Rosenfield, Allen, Swisher, and Kochwa (1962) which codes the various Rh types by assigning numbers to each antigenic determinant, e.g., Rh_0 = Rh1, rh′ = Rh2, rh″ = Rh3, hr′ = Rh4; hr″ = Rh5.

The Rh-Hr Factors. On the basis of the early work the conclusion was justified that the population could be divided into two main groups: one with red cells that were agglutinated by Rh antibodies and called Rh-positive,

Table 5–6. THE FIVE MAIN Rh FACTORS

DESIGNATION BY WIENER	DESIGNATION BY FISHER-RACE	PRESENT IN Rh-POSITIVE BLOOD	PRESENT IN Rh-NEGATIVE BLOOD
Rh_0	D	always	never
rh′	C	frequently	rarely
rh″	E	frequently	rarely
hr′	c	frequently	almost always
hr″	e	frequently	almost always

and another with red cells that were not agglutinated and called Rh-negative. However, further work soon disclosed the presence of at least two other Rh factors. This situation is similar to the one previously discussed for the association of S and s with M and N blood factors. The most important Rh factor was designated as Rh_0 by Wiener and as D by Fisher and Race. The two factors frequently associated with Rh_0 (D) were named rh′ (C) and rh″ (E). When suitable tests are done for these three factors, it is possible to differentiate eight different types as shown in Table 5–7: (1) If none of them is present, the blood is called Rh-negative, rh (cde); (2), (3), and (4) are rather rare types in which only rh′ (C), rh″ (E), or both are present; (5) Rh_0 (cDe) may occur by itself; or (6) it may be combined with rh′ (C), in which event it is called Rh_1 (CDe); or (7) in combination with rh″ (E), in which event it is called Rh_2 (cDE); (8) finally, all three factors may be present and yield the type Rh_1Rh_2 or Rh_z (CDE). Since for practical purposes, such as blood transfusions and prenatal tests, the Rh_0 (D) factor is most important, the first four types lacking this factor are designated as Rh-negative and the last four possessing it, Rh-positive.

Table 5–7. THE EIGHT MAIN Rh TYPES

	Rh FACTORS Rh_0 (D)	rh′ (C)	rh″ (E)	Rh TYPE** W.	F.R.	GENERAL DESIGNATION
1.	−	−	−	rh	cde	Rh-negative
2.	−	+	−	rh′	Cde	
3.	−	−	+	rh″	cdE	
4.	−	+	+	rh′rh″ or rh_y	CdE	
5.	+	−	−	Rh_0	cDe	Rh-positive
6.	+	+	−	Rh_1	CDe	
7.	+	−	+	Rh_2	cDE	
8.	+	+	+	Rh_1Rh_2 or Rh_z	CDE	

*+present
−absent
**W. = Wiener notations
F. R. = Fisher-Race notations

The subsequent developments in the Rh system almost invariably were connected with discoveries of "new" isoantibodies in pregnant women or recipients of blood transfusions. By means of statistical analysis these antibodies could be shown to react specifically with blood factors distributed irregularly in persons of different Rh types; e.g., they were more frequently found in Rh_0-(D)-positive than in Rh_0-(D)-negative individuals. Hence, they presumably belonged to the Rh system. An important advance was the recognition that absence of factors rh′(C) and rh″(E) was regularly associated with presence of a reciprocal blood factor detectable by some of these isoantibodies. In Wiener's system the blood factor determined by absence of rh′ was called hr′; the reversal of the letters Rh to Hr is intended to indicate the reciprocal relationship between Rh and Hr factors. In the Fisher-Race system small letters are used, such as *c* for hr′ in juxtaposition to C(rh′). Table 5–8 shows the reaction of the Hr antibodies with red cells of different Rh types and also indicates the relative frequencies of the corresponding phenotypes and genotypes. In addition to the significance of the Hr factors as occasional causes of incompatibility in blood transfusions or of maternal isoimmunization, they frequently make it possible to establish the probability of a person's having a certain Rh genotype. This, in turn, is important in prognosis of future pregnancies of Rh-immunized women. Having some information regarding the husband's genotype, one is able to state at least that there may be a 50 per cent chance for birth of an Rh-negative child (see p. 405). It must be stressed that to date no antibody has been detected reacting specifically with an antigen reciprocal to Rh_0 (D). In other words, anti-hr_0(d) has never been convincingly demonstrated.

In addition to the five well-established and readily determined Rh-Hr factors (Table 5–6), some additional isoantibodies of rare occurrence have been described that permit recognition of the following Rh factors: $rh^w(C^w)$ is a third allele of the rh′(C) factor. Since most but not all anti-rh′ (anti-C) serums also contain anti-C^w, one may suspect the presence of the C^w factor in a blood specimen that is agglutinated by some anti-rh′(C) serums and not by others. This suspicion may be confirmed by the reaction with "pure" anti-C^w antibody. Much rarer, and hence hardly ever of clinical significance, are other alleles of rh′(C), such as C^x and C^u, and of rh″ (E), designated as E^w and E^u. In blacks, variants of rh′(C), designated as rh'^N and variants of hr″ (e), called hr^S, may be present. In view of the irregular reactivity with standard antiserums for rh′ (C) and hr″ (e) of

Table 5–8. THE Rh-Hr PHENOTYPES AND GENOTYPES

Rh TYPE	REACTIONS* WITH ANTISERUMS FOR hr′ (c)	hr″ (e)	PHENOTYPES** W.	F.R.	POSSIBLE GENOTYPES** W.	F.R.	APPROXIMATE FREQUENCY IN U.S. WHITE POPULATION***
rh	+	+	rh	cde	*rr*	*cde/cde*	14.0
rh′	+	+	rh′rh	Ccde	$r'r$	*Cde/cde*	1.1
	−	+	rh′rh′	CCde	$r'r'$	*Cde/Cde*	Rare
rh″	+	+	rh″rh	cdEe	$r''r$	*cdE/cde*	0.4
	+	−	rh″rh″	cdEE	$r''r''$	*cdE/cdE*	Rare
rh′rh″ (rh_y)	+	+	$rh_y rh$	CcdEe	$r'r''$	*Cde/cdE*	Rare
					$r^y r$	*CdE/cde*	Rare
	−	+	$rh_y rh'$	CCdEe	$r^y r'$	*CdE/Cde*	Rare
	+	−	$rh_y rh''$	CcdEE	$r^y r''$	*CdE/cdE*	Rare
	−	−	$rh_y rh_y$	CCdEE	$r^y r^y$	*CdE/CdE*	Rare
Rh_o	+	+	Rh_o	cDe	$R^o r$	*cDe/cde*	2.4
					$R^o R^o$	*cDe/cDe*	0.1
Rh_1	+	+	$Rh_1 rh$	CcDe	$R^1 r$	*CDe/cde*	30.6
					$R^1 R^o$	*CDe/cDe*	2.6
					$R^o r'$	*cDe/Cde*	Rare
	−	+	$Rh_1 Rh_1$	CCDe	$R^1 R^1$	*CDe/CDe*	16.9
					$R^1 r'$	*CDe/Cde*	1.1
Rh_2	+	+	$Rh_2 rh$	cDEe	$R^2 r$	*cDE/cde*	12.5
					$R^2 R^o$	*cDE/cDe*	0.2
					$R^o r''$	*cDe/cdE*	Rare
	+	−	$Rh_2 Rh_2$	cDEE	$R^2 R^2$	*cDE/cDE*	2.7
					$R^2 r''$	*cDE/cdE*	0.2
$Rh_1 Rh_2$ (Rh_z)	+	+	$Rh_Z Rh_o$	CcDEe	$R^1 R^2$	*CDe/cDE*	12.9
					$R^1 r''$	*CDe/cdE*	Rare
					$R^2 r'$	*cDE/Cde*	Rare
					$R^Z r$	*CDE/cde*	0.2
					$R^Z R^o$	*CDE/cDe*	Rare
					$R^o r^y$	*cDe/CdE*	Rare
	−	+	$Rh_Z Rh_1$	CCDEe	$R^Z R^1$	*CDE/CDe*	0.2
					$R^Z r'$	*CDE/Cde*	Rare
					$R^1 r^y$	*CDe/CdE*	Rare
	+	−	$Rh_Z Rh_2$	CcDEE	$R^Z R^2$	*CDE/cDE*	Rare
					$R^Z r''$	*CDE/cdE*	Rare
					$R^2 r^y$	*cDE/CdE*	Rare
	−	−	$Rh_Z Rh_Z$	CCDEE	$R^Z R^Z$	*CDE/CDE*	Rare
					$R^Z r^y$	*CDE/CdE*	Rare

*+ present
− absent

**W = Wiener notations
F.R. = Fisher-Race notations

***Rare = frequency of 0.1% or less

blood specimens with these variants, results of such tests must be interpreted with caution, particularly when used for determination of genotypes or exclusion of parentage.

Red cells with factors rh′(C) and/or Rh_0 (D) share an antigen called rh^G(G), which, on rare occasions, may occur by itself, i.e., in red cells that appear to be Rh-negative. Introduction of such blood by transfusion or pregnancy into a person lacking Rh_0 (D) and rh′(C) may lead to formation of anti-rh^G (anti-G). Some Rh antibodies react with "compound antigens," that is, specific combinations of Rh factors. Thus, anti-hr (anti-f) reacts with red cells of persons carrying genes for hr′ (c) and hr″ (e) on the same chromosome. Anti-rh_i (anti-Ce) reacts with red cells of persons carrying genes for rh′(C) and hr″(e) on the same chromosome. An antigen V, found in about 20 per cent of blacks, but only rarely in whites, is associated with the gene complex *r* (*ce*). Antibodies of these specificities are rare, and some of their reactions are still imperfectly understood; hence, their use should be restricted to immunogenetic and anthropologic research.

Variants of Rh_0 Factor. Considerable practical importance must be assigned to Rh_0 (D) variants, which can be recognized by their atypical behavior in laboratory tests commonly employed for Rh typing (see p. 369). When such blood specimens were tested with a battery of serums containing Rh antibodies, it was noted that agglutination was produced by some but not by other serums. Furthermore, saline agglutinating Rh antibodies (see p. 370) were not capable of clumping these red cells. On the other hand, when more sensitive methods were used, e.g., the antiglobulin technique (see p. 370), it was always possible to demonstrate union of Rh antibody with Rh_0(D) antigen present in these specimens. These weakly reacting variants of the Rh_0(D) factor, commonly designated as D^u, require special methods for their detection *in vitro.* At the same time—and this is important—*in vivo* D^u blood behaves similarly to "regular" Rh_0-positive blood as far as isoimmunization by means of blood transfusions or pregnancy is concerned; hence, identification of D^u blood should be done routinely.

The strength of D^u antigens varies greatly from one specimen to the next—from strong antigens almost approaching the reactivity of the regular Rh_0(D) factor to weak D^u specimens that are most difficult to detect *in vitro.*

The D^u factor does not appear to be an antigen distinct from the Rh_0(D) factor, since it is neither possible to produce an antibody specific for D^u nor to separate by absorptions the portion of an anti-Rh_0(D) serum that reacts with the regular Rh_0(D) factor from that reacting with the D^u factor.

In addition to D^u factors, which are transmitted genetically, another form of weakly reacting Rh_0(D) factor has been encountered that results from a "gene interaction"; i.e., presence of rh′(C) depresses the reactivity of the Rh_0(D) antigen. This is important in connection with exclusion of parentage, since seemingly Rh-negative parents may give rise to an offspring found to be Rh-positive.

Variants of the D^u type are much more common among blacks than whites. Furthermore, in line with the greater frequency of the Rh type Rh_0(cDe) among blacks, D^u is found frequently without simultaneous presence of the rh′(C) and rh″(E) factors, whereas this is only rarely the case in whites.

A behavior opposite to that of D^u, namely, unusually strong reactivity of Rh_0(D), has been found in exceedingly rare blood specimens in which it is not possible to demonstrate presence of any of the other Rh or Hr factors. The Rh type thus produced has been called -D-$\bar{R}h_0$; according to Race and Sanger (1968), it may reflect a gene deletion and has been found to be inherited. Red cells with this factor, even when present in heterozygous form, have the unusual property of being agglutinated even in saline suspensions by IgG anti-Rh serums (see p. 359). The practical significance of -D- is predicated on serious difficulties encountered in transfusing persons with this Rh type, because they are capable of developing, and frequently do, antibodies reacting with rh′(C), hr′(c), rh″(E), and hr″(e); therefore, blood donors used for them must have the same rare Rh type as they. Implications of the -D- factor for exclusion of parentage will be discussed later (see p. 405). An even more exceptional Rh type, Rh_{null}, has been discovered in which red cells appear to lack all Rh factors (Vos *et al.,* 1961; Levine *et al.,* 1965). Most probably, such persons are negative for a gene, *LW,* which is almost universally present and initiates formation of a precursor antigen, LW, upon which *Rh* genes act in order to express the respective Rh factors of red cells. In some instances the property of Rh_{null} was associated with abnormal products of genes *M-N-S-s* and chronic hemolytic anemia, findings thought to reflect a complex genetic defect of red cell membranes.

Discoveries by Unger and Wiener (1957) have acquainted us with additional complications of the Rh system. Several observations were reported of apparently Rh_0-(D)-positive persons who formed antibodies reacting specifically with all other Rh_0-(D)positive cells except their own. This has been explained by attributing a mosaic nature to the Rh_0(D) factor. Very rarely Rh_0-positive blood specimens may occur in which one small part of this mosaic is missing. Such blood specimens have been designated as Rh^a, Rh^b, and Rh^c, and their possessors are thus capable of forming antibodies against the A, B, or C portion of Rh_0, such antibodies agglutinating "regular" Rh-positive blood specimens carrying these segments of the "mosaic."

Antigenicity of Rh Factors. In medicine the significance of blood factors is based on their capacity to immunize in transfusions or pregnancies. The Rh_0(D) factor is by far the most antigenic, and the other Rh factors are much less likely to produce isoimmunization. Antibodies for rh′(C) are frequently found together with anti-Rh_0(D) antibodies in the Rh-negative pregnant woman whose fetus or child was type Rh_1 and, hence, possessed both antigens. In many such instances, actually anti-rh^G (anti-G) is responsible for the reactivity with rh′(C). The combination of anti-Rh_0(D) and anti-rh″(E) antibodies occurs less frequently in women subjected to antigenic stimulation by a fetus with type Rh_2(cDE).

Rarely, factors other than $Rh_0(D)$ induce formation of antibodies in Rh-positive persons, their antigenicity decreasing in the following order: hr′(c), rh″(E), rh′(C), and hr″(e). By contrast with A and B factors, Rh factors have not been unequivocally demonstrated outside of blood cells, which therefore are the only agents capable of bringing about Rh immunization. In addition to pregnancy and blood transfusions, intramuscular injection of blood may be responsible for development of Rh antibodies.

Rh Antibodies. Three features differentiate Rh antibodies from hemagglutinins in the ABO blood group system: absence of regular "natural" antibodies, optimal temperature of reactivity and class of immunoglobulins. With exceedingly rare exceptions Rh antibodies do not occur without preceding antigenic stimulation, such as pregnancy, blood transfusion, or deliberate immunization consisting most commonly of intravenous injections.

Anti-A and anti-B antibodies react optimally when tested at 4° C., although their range may extend to and above 22° C. ("room temperature"). Such antibodies are called "cold agglutinins." By contrast, Rh antibodies are most readily, or only, detectable when tested at 37° C.; hence, they are designated "warm agglutinins."

Finally, unlike anti-A and anti-B, Rh antibodies are much more frequently present in the IgG than IgM classes of immunoglobulins. While chemical and physicochemical characteristics of immunoglobulins are discussed in another context (p. 571), the following considerations are essential for understanding differences in the hemagglutinating activities of IgM and IgG antibodies and the techniques best suited for their detection. Hemagglutination consists of two sequential events. The first is attachment of antibody molecules to the specific antigenic sites on the red cell surface. Antibody molecules possess at least two combining sites, making them bivalent. Thus, after attachment of antibody molecules to the antigenic sites, they may also initiate the second event, viz., formation of molecular bridges between red cells, expressed as visible agglutination. In order to facilitate physical contact between two or more red cells, antibody molecules must be capable of overcoming the repellent force resulting from the negative electric charge of red cells (zeta potential) which keeps them apart. The large, elongated and polyvalent IgM molecules possess this ability and, therefore, their attachment to antigenic sites on red cell surfaces is followed by visible agglutination, even when red cells are suspended in the highly ionized medium of saline solution. On the other hand, IgG hemagglutinins, although attached to antigenic sites, cannot overcome the mutual repulsion of red cells. Special techniques are required in order to bring about visible agglutination by IgG antibodies. Development of these techniques was not only essential for detection of Rh antibodies, but they also have made possible the rapid progress in several other blood group systems and in related areas of immunology.

In order to facilitate understanding of older literature, the following synonymous terms are mentioned: for IgM—complete, saline, thermolabile, 19S antibodies; for IgG—incomplete, blocking, serum albumin, thermostable, 7S antibodies.

One of the first methods for detecting the presence of IgG antibodies was based on the principle that IgG antibodies are unable to agglutinate but capable of preventing red blood cells from being agglutinated by specific IgM antibodies.

A second, more sensitive method for demonstration of IgG antibodies, frequently used for practical work (p. 375), consists of replacement of the saline medium by macromolecular substances, such as human serum or plasma, serum proteins, especially serum albumin, as well as other colloidal solutions, such as gelatin, gum acacia, or polyvinylpyrrolidone (PVP). In other words, when Rh-positive red cells suspended in albumin are added to a serum containing IgG Rh antibodies, agglutination occurs after suitable periods of incubation or other procedures (centrifugation, warming on slide). The effectiveness of these techniques is based on reducing the electric surface charges of erythrocytes in media with low ion concentrations and, thus, facilitating agglutination by IgG antibodies that had combined with red cell antigens. Many practical applications, such as Rh typing (see p. 370), make use of this property of IgG antibodies.

A third method with a wide range of practical applications in immunohematology and immunology is the antiglobulin test developed by Coombs (Coombs *et al.*, 1945).

Antiglobulin (Coombs) Test. There are two basic premises for the correct understanding, performance, and application of antiglobulin tests. First, human isohemoantibodies are globulins, in most instances gamma globulin. Second, addition of antiglobulin antibody to human red cells coated with isoantibody (i.e., globulin) results in agglutination of the coated red cells. For practical purposes such antiserums (antihuman globulin serum) may be produced by injection of human globulin into animals of a variety of species; rabbits and goats are most commonly employed. Figure 5–2 represents schematically the sequence of events in the antiglobulin test: in the first step (I) IgG antibodies unite with, or "coat," the red cells; this may occur *in vivo* or *in vitro.* The second step (II), addition of the antiglobulin reagent, is followed by the final event (III), agglutination of the globulin-coated red cells.

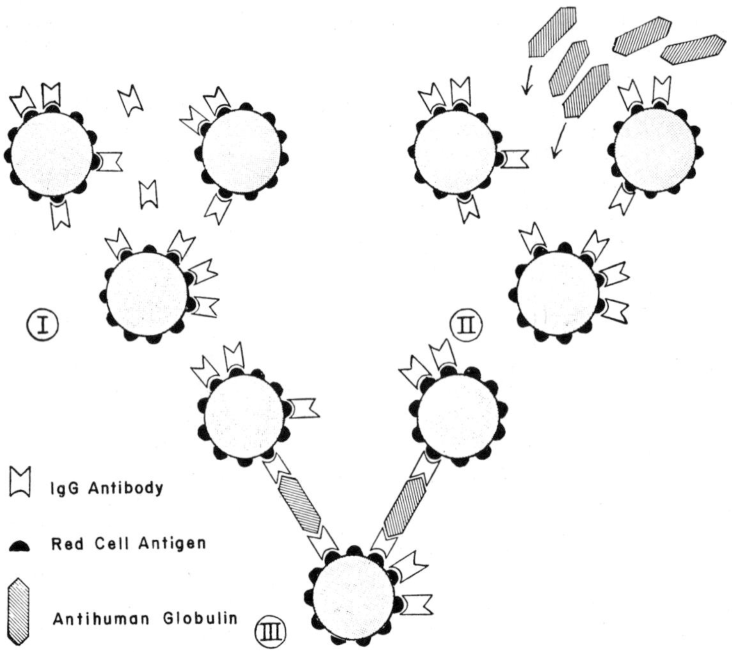

Figure 5–2. Schematic presentation of antiglobulin test.

There are two main applications of the antiglobulin test: (1) The direct antiglobulin test is designed for demonstration of *in vivo* coating of red cells. Basically a positive test shows agglutination of the suitably prepared red cell suspension after addition of the antiglobulin serum. The main indications for this test are diagnoses of hemolytic disease of the newborn (p. 402) and of autoimmune hemolytic anemia (p. 403), and investigation of hemolytic transfusion reactions (p. 397). (2) In the indirect antiglobulin test IgG antibodies are permitted to react *in vitro* with red cells containing the corresponding agglutinogen; after suitable periods and conditions of incubation of the red cell serum mixtures, antiglobulin serum is added to the suitably prepared red cells. The main applications of the indirect antiglobulin test are as follows:

1. Detection of IgG antibodies, e.g., IgG anti-Rh_0(D) by means of incubation of Rh_0(D)-positive red cells with the serum to be tested. Analogous procedures may be used for IgG antibodies of other specificities, including anti-A and anti-B.

2. Detection in red cells of blood factors for which IgG antibodies are available either exclusively or prevalently, e.g., Kell and Duffy (p. 362). This method is also used for demonstration of weakly reacting Rh_0 variants (D^u, see p. 358).

3. Demonstration of autoantibodies in the serum of patients with autoimmune hemolytic anemia.

4. Antiglobulin reactions also may be used for demonstration of other antigen-antibody reactions involving white cells, platelets, and tissue cells.

5. Since addition of gamma globulin neutralizes antiglobulin antibody and thus prevents the agglutinating activity of antiglobulin for coated red cells, the test has also been adapted to demonstrate the presence of hypogammaglobulinemia and agammaglobulinemia.

Enzyme Treatment of Red Cells. These techniques modify the red cell surface and thus reduce its electric charge. Consequently treatment with proteolytic enzymes, such as trypsin, papain, ficin, bromelin, or with neuraminidase makes saline-suspended red cells as agglutinable by IgG as by IgM antibodies. The enzyme techniques are fairly simple; their results are easier to read than those in some of the other methods for detection of incomplete antibodies; and they exceed them also in sensitivity as far as detection of Rh antibodies is concerned. On the other hand, some antigenic sites of other blood factors are destroyed or markedly weakened in reactivity after enzyme treatment and, hence, this technique cannot be employed for detection of antibodies for M, N, Duffy, and some other blood factors. Thus it is often necessary to utilize several of the techniques for detection of IgG antibodies for Rh and other blood factors, referred to in the preceding discussion.

Recently it has been shown that hemagglutination by IgG antibodies can be facilitated by addition of polyanions. Synthetic polymers such as polybrene, by virtue of their positive charge, overcome the repulsive force imparted to red cells by their negative charge, thus forming nonspecific red cell aggregates. If IgG antibodies of appropriate specificity are added to the mixture of red cells and polybrene, the aggregates are converted into true agglutinates. On the other hand, in absence of specific hemagglutinins, exposure to hypertonic salt solutions breaks up the nonspecific aggregates. Application of this method to automated hemagglutination procedures is detailed on page 383.

Specificity of Rh Antibodies. Depending on the antigenic compositions of the injected red cells and of the red cells of the recipient, antibodies with specificity for one or more Rh factors may be present in the same serum. The following general conditions must be met in isoimmunization to Rh factors or, for that matter, to any other antigen: the blood factor must be absent in the immunized person; the blood factor must be present in the immunizing blood; and the blood factor must be of sufficient antigenic strength. Other factors are the number of separate antigenic stimulations, the amount of blood involved in each stimulation, the time intervals between stimulations, and the individual variations in ability to produce antibodies. In line with the preceding statements about relative antigenicity, anti-Rh_0(D) antibodies are most commonly encountered. Rh-negative women bearing fetuses with type Rh_1(CDe) have also an opportunity to form antibodies to rh′(C) and/or rh^G(G), an event occurring in a majority of such pregnancies. If, on the other hand, a woman happens to be rh′(Cde) herself, pregnancy with an Rh_1(CDe) fetus makes possible only formation of anti-Rh_0(D). Such examples could be multiplied and apply equally to immunization by blood transfusions. Knowledge of exact specificity of isoantibodies is important for two reasons: for selection of blood transfusions for isoimmunized recipients, including treatment of erythroblastotic babies, and for proper utilization in laboratory tests of antiserums which may contain more than one antibody. Another important consideration concerns the possibility that antibodies with different specificity may also have different reactivity, as defined in the preceding section; e.g., a serum may contain anti-Rh_0(D) as IgG and anti-rh′(C) as IgM. Hence, the selection of techniques used for detection of such antibodies is of critical importance. As will be discussed in connection with antibody identification, testing for specificity of Rh antibodies requires availability of red cell panels, which, on the basis of their antigenic composition, permit discrimination between antibodies of different specificity.

Inheritance of Rh Factors. In general, the inheritance of Rh factors follows the same principles as those discussed in connection with the ABO and MN factors. Rh factors present in any one individual must have been inherited from one or both of his parents. If, for example, a person inherits the rh′(C) factor from both parents, he is homozygous: *r′r′ (Cde/Cde)*. On the other hand, a person heterozygous for rh′(C) has only one parent of type rh′(Cde), while the other may be Rh-negative (cde); his genotype is *r′r (Cde/cde)*. Table 5–8 lists the genotype and gene notations according to the Wiener and Fisher-Race nomenclatures.

Three facts must be stressed in connection with Rh genotypes. First, laboratory tests are limited to determination of genotypes for factors rh′(C) and rh″(E), and they cannot establish homozygosity or heterozygosity for factor Rh_0(D). Second, even when homozygosity or heterozygosity for one of the Rh factors has been established, there is frequently uncertainty as to location of the genes on the two chromosomes; e.g., a person found to be Rh_1Rh_2 (CcDEe) may belong to one of six genotypes (Table 5–8). Third, the most reliable evidence for presence of a specific Rh genotype is derived from knowledge of Rh types of parents and offspring of the person under test. In most other situations one can only refer to the most probable genotype on the basis of statistical information relating phenotypes to genotypes in populations of known ethnic background. In Table 5–9 the probability for association of the most common phenotypes of Rh-positive persons with heterozygosity has been estimated on the basis of the distribution of Rh types in the U.S. white population.

Information on the genotype is of prognostic value in cases of husbands of women immunized to one of the Rh factors. Knowledge of inheritance of Rh factors is indispensable for interpretation of Rh types in connection with exclusion of parentage as discussed subsequently (p. 405).

The Kell, Duffy, and Kidd Blood Group Systems. Instances of hemolytic disease of the newborn or hemolytic transfusion reactions have furnished the opportunity for discovery of a "new" antibody and permitted definition of the corresponding blood factor. The basic information concerning the incidence of Kell, Duffy, and Kidd blood factors in the U.S. white population is contained in Table 5–10. For practical purposes one should be aware of the following characteristic features of these three systems:

1. Among these blood factors Kell (K) is most and Kidd (Jk^a,Jk^b) is least antigenic. Actually, the immunogenicity of K may be exceeded only by that of Rh_0(D). That anti-Kell antibodies are not found more frequently as a result of isoimmunization by transfusion or pregnancy is explained by the low incidence of

Table 5–9. EVALUATION OF ZYGOSITY FOR Rh TYPE*

PHENOTYPE		REACTIONS** ANTI-hr′ (ANTI-c)	WITH ANTI-hr″ (ANTI-e)	MOST PROBABLE GENOTYPE		CHANCES % FOR GENOTYPE BEING HETEROZYGOUS Rh_0-POSITIVE
Rh_1	CDe	+	(+)	R^1r	*CDe/cde*	88
Rh_1	CDe	–	(+)	R^1R^1	*CDe/CDe*	6
Rh_2	cDE	(+)	+	R^2r	*cDE/cde*	98
Rh_2	cDE	(+)	–	R^2R^2	*cDE/cDE*	9
Rh_0	cDe	(+)	(+)	R^0r	*cDe/cde*	96
Rh_1Rh_2	CDE	+	+	R^1R^2	*CDe/cDE*	10

*Applied to U. S. white population.
**Results listed in parentheses can be anticipated on the basis of phenotype; hence the tests need not be done.

Kell in the general population. Since as a rule at least two antigenic stimulations are necessary for development of antibodies, chances for a Kell-negative person to be immunized (e.g., by two blood transfusions with Kell-positive blood) are less than one in 100.

2. Immunization to the k factor occurs extremely rarely because roughly only one out of 1000 persons is susceptible to such immunization by virtue of being homozygous for the Kell factor (KK).

3. The Duffy factor, Fy^a, is only weakly antigenic and, hence, corresponding antibodies are encountered only infrequently. This holds true to an even greater extent for the allele, Fy^b, and antibodies for Jk^a and Jk^b.

4. As a rule, antibodies for Kell, Duffy, and Kidd factors are best, or exclusively, detectable by the indirect antiglobulin technique. This is important in connection with crossmatching tests, which may fail to reveal incompatibility caused by such antibodies if this technique is not employed. Some examples of Kidd antibodies react best with enzyme-treated red cells subjected to the antiglobulin technique. On the other hand, the Duffy agglutinogens are readily destroyed by proteolytic enzymes, such as trypsin, papain, bromelin, and ficin, and hence such techniques are unsuitable for detection of Duffy factors and anti-Duffy antibodies.

5. The Kell system has become more complex with the discovery of additional alleles designated as Kp^a and Kp^b, which are associated with K and k in a similar fashion as are rh′(C) and rh″(E) with Rh_0(D). The "Sutter" blood factor, Js^a (Giblett, 1958), was initially thought to represent an independent blood group system. Subsequently, convincing proof for its association with the Kell system has become available. Js^a occurs in approximately 20 per cent of blacks but is exceedingly rare in persons of other races. Antibodies identifying the allelic factor, Js^b, have also been described. The rarity of immunization to these factors obviates the need for considering them in everyday laboratory work.

6. Fy^a and Fy^b appear to have a common antigenic determinant, possibly a precursor, as inferred from the observation of an antibody, anti-Fy3, which reacts with all red cells possessing Fy^a and/or Fy^b, but which fails to

Table 5–10. THE KELL, DUFFY, KIDD BLOOD GROUP SYSTEMS

BLOOD GROUP SYSTEM	PHENOTYPE	GENOTYPE	COMMON DESIGNATION	APPROXIMATE FREQUENCY (%) IN U.S. WHITE POPULATION
Kell	K	*Kk*	Kell-positive	6.9
		KK		0.1
		kk	Kell-negative	93
Duffy	Fy^a	Fy^aFy^b	Duffy-positive	48
		Fy^aFy^a		17
	Fy^b	Fy^bFy^b	Duffy-negative	35
Kidd	Jk^a	Jk^aJk^b	Kidd-positive	50
		Jk^aJk^a		23
	Jk^b	Jk^bJk^b	Kidd-negative	27

agglutinate the rare type lacking both antigens. A third allele, Fy4, has been described in the Duffy system. It is present in all red cells negative for Fy^a as well as for Fy^b. This red cell type is more common in blacks than in whites.

7. Considerable racial variations have been established for Kell, Duffy, and Kidd factors. For example, in U.S. blacks the incidence of Kell-positive persons is much lower – 2 per cent – than among U.S. whites (Table 5–10). The frequency of the Jk^a factor is greater in the U.S. black (over 90 per cent) than in the U.S. white population.

8. Family studies have shown Kell, Duffy, and Kidd factors to be inherited according to Mendelian genetics and to be independent of the other blood group systems.

The Lewis Blood Group System. In contradistinction to the other blood group systems of man, Lewis factors are primarily mucopolysaccharides present in body fluids, including plasma, and secretions, such as saliva. Secondarily these antigens are adsorbed to the red cells, which by means of suitable antiserums can be tested for presence of two factors – Le^a and Le^b. According to results of these tests, three phenotypes of red cells are recognized: Le(a+b–), Le(a–b+), Le(a–b–). Significantly, all persons found to have Le^a-positive red cells, are nonsecretors of blood group substances A, B, and H (p. 351). This behavior is best explained by assuming that ABH and Lewis antigens are derived from a common precursor compound for which secretor and Lewis genes compete. Thus, nonsecretors with the Lewis (*Le*) gene form large amounts of Lewis antigen which impart to red cells the property of Le^a. On the other hand, secretors with *Le* gene cannot produce Lewis antigen in amounts sufficient to make red cells Le^a-positive. The Le^b factor demonstrable in red cells of these persons may be a "hybrid antigen" resulting from interaction of *Le* and *H* genes. Finally, body fluids and red cells of persons without *Le* gene are devoid of any Lewis antigen, i.e., they are Le(a–b–). The latter phenotype is found in only 5 per cent of whites, but it exists in over 20 per cent of blacks.

Another distinctive feature of Lewis antigens is their postnatal development; cord blood specimens fail to react with anti-Lewis serums, although the antigens are present in saliva and serum. During the first year of life, reactivity of red cells with anti-Le^a rises to approximately 80 per cent. When children have reached the age of two years, their blood exhibits the adult reactivity. The cause of this variability is as yet unknown.

Anti-Lewis antibodies occur not uncommonly in persons of group Le(a–b–) as "natural" antibodies of low titer. In fresh serum they may have hemolytic activity, especially when tested with enzyme-treated red cells. Occasionally high-titered anti-Lewis antibodies may cause difficulties in selection of compatible blood or may be responsible for hemolytic transfusion reactions. In order to increase the reliability of tests required in such situations, Wiener (1965) has recommended supplementary determination of the Lewis group of red cells with tests for Lewis antigens in saliva.

The Lutheran Blood Group System. The factor Lu^a occurs in approximately 8 per cent of whites. Its allelomorphic factor, Lu^b is present in all Lu^a-negative and in the majority of Lu^a-positive individuals. Antibodies for Lu^a and Lu^b occur rarely, but occasionally they may have clinical significance. Anti-Lu^a is commonly an IgM antibody. Some examples of anti-Lu^b were found to react better with enzyme methods than with the antiglobulin technique. The Lu antigens may be subject to gene suppression, as shown in a family whose children expressed a Lu antigen in their red cells, although it was not detectable in the red cells of the parents. Evidence for linkage of Lutheran genes to secretor genes has been presented.

The Xg Blood Group System. Difficulties in finding compatible blood for a multitransfused patient led to the discovery of this unique blood group. Extensive testing showed the "new" antibody to be unrelated to previously known blood factors and blood group systems. Surprisingly, however, there was a significant sex-dependent variation in the reactivity of the antibody with random blood specimens; positive results were obtained with almost 90 per cent of the blood specimens taken from women, but with only roughly 60 per cent of those taken from men. These observations pointed to localization on the X chromosome of the gene determining the "new" antigen, because females with two X chromosomes are expected to possess X-linked genes more frequently than males with only one X chromosome. The new blood factor, designated as Xg^a, has been the subject of several interesting studies. Anti-Xg^a reacts exclusively with the antiglobulin technique, and because of its rare occurrence has only little clinical significance. The most important implications of Xg^a relate to genetics, since it is the first instance of assignment of a blood group gene to a specific chromosome. Its localization on the X chromosome made possible predictions inherent in X-linked inheritance: (1) daughters and mothers of Xg^a-positive men must be Xg^a-positive; (2) sons and fathers of Xg^a-negative women must be Xg^a-negative. With rare exception these expectations were corroborated by family studies. Violations of these rules can be anticipated in persons whose karyotypes have abnormal sex chromosomes, e.g., men with the Klinefelter syndrome (XXY) or women with Turner syndrome (XO). In such instances Xg^a determinations may disclose whether the supernumerary or missing X chromosome was of paternal or maternal origin. Other studies have utilized *Xg* as a "marker gene" in relation to other X-linked traits, such as hemophilia, color blindness, and glucose-6-phosphate dehydrogenase deficiency, in order to investigate gene linkage as the first step toward "chromosome mapping." The incidence of Xg^a in a population varies with racial origin, with its frequency decreasing in whites, blacks, and Chinese in the order of enumeration.

Other Blood Factors. In addition to the 13 blood group systems summarized in Table 5–1, a number of other blood factors discovered in recent years require more studies before their final classification. Some of these factors were originally found only in members of one family—"private" or "family" factors. The opposite behavior, namely, almost universal occurrence, has been reported for other blood factors that were absent in only one or a few individuals; familial distribution of the absence of such factors was observed and indicates a genetic mechanism.

In the course of further studies one of three developments may eventually take place with the "new" blood factors: they may turn out to belong to one of the other known blood group systems; they may be found to represent new, independent blood group systems, the main factor showing much greater frequency in some ethnic groups than in others; or they may remain "family factors," possibly attributable to rare mutations.

Examples of the first eventuality—assignment to "old" blood group systems of blood factors originally considered to be "family factors"—are Mi^a and Vw, which have been recognized as belonging to the MNS system. The integration of the "universal blood factor," Tj^a, into the P system has been described (p. 355). Other factors of universal distribution are Vel, Yt^a, and Ge.

The I factor, present in red cells of practically all adult persons, has some unusual properties. Wiener, Unger, Cohen, and Feldman (1956) showed that high-titered, cold autoagglutinins, sometimes responsible for autoimmune hemolytic anemia, have the specificity of anti-I and do not react with some exceedingly rare blood specimens that do not have the factor I but have the allelic factor i. Red cells of newborn and young infants regularly lack the I antigen, which gradually develops during the first years of life. The strength of the I antigen varies considerably from person to person.

In connection with universal blood factors, it should be noted that serums of persons possessing antibodies for the blood factors U (MNS system), Cellano (k), Lu^b, and hr''(e) will be found to agglutinate more than 98 per cent of random blood specimens tested and thus may at first glance arouse the suspicion that they are antibodies for one of the universal blood factors. Obviously such findings pose serious difficulties in connection with blood transfusions, and their solution requires cooperation of many blood banks. In such situations the "rare blood donor file," established by the American Association of Blood Banks, may prove valuable.

The second trend—development of a new blood group system—is exemplified by the Diego factor (Di^a), which was originally discovered in one single family but subsequently was shown to occur with frequencies of up to 10 to 45 per cent in certain populations, such as among certain South and North American Indians, and in Mongoloid populations (China, Japan).

Additional "family blood factors" have been reported. Their clinical importance is based on their etiologic role in isolated instances of hemolytic disease of the newborn and complications of blood transfusions.

Blood Groups and Disease. Progress made during the last decade in genetics probably has brought closer the time when blood group genes can serve as chromosome markers. Two approaches may prove useful for reaching this goal. On the one hand, family studies may disclose linkage between a particular blood group gene and a gene responsible for a hereditary disease. A few linkages of this type have been demonstrated, e.g., between *ABO* genes and the nail-patella syndrome or between Rh genes and some forms of elliptocytosis. Many more linkages have been suspected and are under scrutiny (Race and Sanger, 1968). On the other hand, the rapid advances in cytogenetics have permitted recognition of characteristic quantitative and qualitative chromosomal abnormalities and their association with disease. As exemplified by the gene for blood factor Xg^a, localized on the X chromosome, karyotypes with supernumerary or missing X chromosomes may be accompanied by deviations from the expected transmission of the *Xg* gene. By analogy, family studies of persons whose karyotypes exhibit autosomal trisomy, partial deletion, or translocation of an autosomal chromosome may lead to the discovery of abnormal transmission of one or the other blood group gene. Actually, within the last years combined cytogenetic and immunohematologic studies have made possible assignment of the genes for the Duffy blood group system to chromosome No. 1, and *MNSs* genes appear to be localized on either chromosome No. 2 or No. 4. Other pertinent studies have provided findings on the basis of which a particular chromosome or part thereof can be excluded from consideration as being the site of certain blood group genes.

Mutations, deletions, and other postnatal chromosomal changes that are associated with disease could also be expressed in changes of blood group phenotypes. This is probably the case in the rare but well-documented instances of leukemia in which the patient's red cells appear to have lost reactivity for blood factors A or B. Of considerable significance is the observation that in man and animals ionizing radiation may bring about decrease in antigenic strength or loss of reactivity of some blood factors.

A nongenetic mechanism seems to be responsible for what has been called "acquired B antigen" of red cells. Unexpected agglutinability of red cells by anti-B serum has been found in some patients with severe gastrointestinal disease, including carcinoma of colon and ulcerative colitis. Since family studies of these persons precluded presence of the *B* gene and their serums contained anti-B, it has been suspected that bacterial lipopolysaccharides, liberated in and penetrating the diseased gastrointestinal tract, became attached to the red cells and imparted to them B reactivity.

On the basis of statistical studies it has been stated that persons with certain diseases belong to one or the other blood group more frequently than expected. It has been claimed that this indicates an increased susceptibility of carriers of this blood group to the particular disease. Thus, an association between blood group O and duodenal ulcer and between blood group A and cancer of the stomach has been proposed. Since the validity of the data has been questioned and to date no biologic mechanism can be considered to fit with the alleged deviations of statistical surveys, it does not appear justified to accept these associations as proven.

A, B, and O (H) isoantigens are present in various secretions and tissues (p. 351). The effect of cancer on tissue isoantigens, especially A, B, and O (H), has been the subject of several investigations.

In carcinomas arising in tissues that normally contain isoantigens A, B, and H, the latter cannot be demonstrated when examined with the specific red cell adherence (SRCA) test. They are present in the normal tissue adjacent to the carcinoma. The loss of antigen in the carcinoma is parallel to the degree of anaplasia. It is interpreted as immunologic dedifferentiation in the course of cancerous transformation analogous to the morphologic dedifferentiation of anaplasia (Davidsohn *et al.*, 1966, 1968, 1972, 1973).

Specific blood group phenotypes carry health hazards which have an immunologic basis. Immunization, including that to blood group antigens, is predicated on the absence in the immunized individual of the particular antigen. Therefore, when a blood factor has two allelomorphs, e.g., S and s in the MNS system (p. 354), the homozygote SS is susceptible to immunization to s antigen and the homozygote *ss*, to S antigen, while the heterozygote *Ss* cannot be immunized to either antigen. The opposite holds true for the rare genotype, S^uS^u, in which red cells possess neither S nor s antigens; immunization to both S and s can and does take place. The absence of commonly encountered allelomorphs has been designated as "minus minus phenotype" (Allen, 1961; Race and Sanger, 1968). It is obvious that individuals with such phenotypes carry an exceptionally high risk of isoimmunization induced by transfusion or pregnancy. "Minus minus" phenotypes have been described in most blood group systems. Their frequency varies with racial origin. Probably more than one genetic mechanism is responsible for different phenotypes. In some instances the "silent" gene may be an *amorph,* i.e., fail to lead to a demonstrable gene product. Suppressor or modifier genes may prevent the expression of a gene, as it has been made likely for the Bombay types in the ABO system (p. 353). Gene deletions have been proposed to account for the phenotype -D- (Race and Sanger, 1968).

Admittedly the phenomena just described are rare and imperfectly understood. Nevertheless, in such instances the ability to provide compatible blood for a specific patient or to manage unusual problems associated with pregnancy will depend on awareness and adequate interpretation of exceptional immunohematologic findings. Moreover, new knowledge that may be acquired from investigation of these puzzling observations may have far-reaching impact on the understanding of inheritance in man and the pathogenesis and diagnosis of disease.

HEMAGGLUTINATION TECHNIQUES

General Principles

Specimen. Clotted blood is preferable, since it permits testing both for blood factors in red cell suspensions prepared from the clot and for antibodies in the serum. As soon as possible after clotting, the blood specimen should be placed in the refrigerator unless further work proceeds immediately. Refrigeration of blood specimens at 4° C. for several hours causes small amounts of cold agglutinins, frequently found in normal persons, to be absorbed into the clot and thus eliminates sources of error introduced by the presence of cold agglutinins in the serum (cf. p. 229). On the other hand, if tests for presence of cold agglutinins (cf. p. 229) are to be done, the serum should be separated from the clot before refrigeration. As a rule, blood grouping tests can be reliably carried out on properly preserved clotted specimens for periods up to five days, although the preservation of the reactivity of blood factors varies greatly with different blood group systems as well as with individual specimens. Tests for antibodies in the serum can be performed for several weeks with refrigerated (and for up to two years with properly frozen) specimens. Testing for blood factors on red cells from oxalated or citrated blood should be done within 24 hours; plasma is poorly suited for antibody tests. Blood from skin punctures may be directly transferred into physiologic saline and used for blood group tests.

Preparation of Red Cell Suspensions. Depending on the specific technique employed, 2, 5, 10, or 50 per cent red cell suspensions are required. These can be prepared by transferring freshly obtained blood from a skin puncture into saline or by suspending in saline the packed red cells obtained from citrated or oxalated blood. Preservative anticoagulant solutions are also available that permit preservation of red cells for one month or longer. This is most useful for controls and panel cells of known antigenic composition (reagent red cells). Most frequently, suspensions are made by gently breaking up blood clots with an applicator stick and transferring the red cell aggregates into saline or other suspending media.

In order to acquire skill in preparing red cell suspensions of specific concentrations, the following technique should be followed:

1. To about 5 ml. of physiologic saline add several drops of whole blood (fresh, citrated, oxalated, or fragments of clots).
2. Centrifuge for sufficient length of time in order to pack the red cells.
3. Withdraw the supernatant fluid as completely as possible.
4. Add 0.1 ml. of the packed red cells to a test tube containing 4.9 ml. of physiologic saline and mix well. Remove any small clots that may be present. This represents a 2 per cent suspension of red cells in saline. After one has acquired sufficient practice, one need not measure the amounts of red cells and suspending media but can estimate the density of the suspension by its appearance. Analogous procedures are used for preparation of red cell suspensions of different concentrations and in various media (e.g., serum, bovine albumin). All red cell suspensions must be refrigerated when not in use. They are unsuitable if they show hemolysis and should be used within 12 hours after preparation.

EQUIPMENT

1. Test tubes: for collection of blood (100 mm. long, 13 mm. wide) and for hemagglutination tests (75 mm. long, 10 mm. wide).
2. Test tube racks.
3. Centrifuge.
4. Waterbaths.
5. Miscellaneous: wooden applicators, capillary pipettes, rubber bulbs, slides, coverslips and so forth.

REAGENTS

Blood grouping serums and reagent red cells distributed commercially must meet specific minimum requirements established by the Division on Biological Standards, Food and Drug Administration.

1. Physiologic saline solution.
2. Blood grouping serums. A good typing serum must have the following properties:

   A. It should have a titer of recommended potency.

   B. It should be free of cold agglutinins.

   C. It should be free of so-called irregular agglutinins.

   D. It should not form rouleaux when mixed with red cells.

   E. It should be clear, of normal color (except when a dye is added for identification), and free of cells or any other particles, not hemolyzed, icteric, or chylous.

   F. It should be free of complement.

   Anti-A serum (minimum titer with A_1 cells 256).*

   Anti-B serum (minimum titer 256).*

   Anti-A,B serum (serum of group O) (minimum titer 256 with A_1 and B cells).

   Anti-A_1 reagent (absorbed anti-A serum; plant lectins).

   Anti-Rh_0(D) serum (minimum titer 32).

   Anti-rh′(C) serum (minimum titer 32).

   Anti-rh″(E) serum (minimum titer 32).

   Anti-hr′(c) serum (minimum titer 32).

   Anti-human globulin serum.

   Miscellaneous antiserums for other blood factors, such as hr″(e), K (Kell), and Fy^a, as required.
3. Bovine or human albumin (22 per cent or 30 per cent).
4. Reagent red blood cells: Suspensions of red cells in which presence or absence of significant blood group antigens has been determined may either be collected periodically from suitable donors or be purchased commercially.

Media for collection and preservation of reagent red cells include: (1) Modified Alsever's solution – 2.05 gm. dextrose, 0.8 gm. sodium citrate, 0.05 gm. citric acid, and 0.45 gm. sodium chloride are dissolved in 100 ml.

*In order to minimize errors, blue dye is added to commercial anti-A serum and yellow dye to anti-B serum.

distilled water; pH is expected to be 6.1. (2) Serum-lactose solution – 10 gm. lactose, 1.53 gm. dextrose, 1.38 gm. sodium citrate, and 0.5 gm. citric acid are dissolved in 100 ml. distilled water and mixed with 100 ml. of serum from a person of group AB (serum must be free of irregular and cold agglutinins).

5. Enzymes: Bromelin, ficin, papain, trypsin.

Antiserums must be refrigerated when not in use. Reagents and blood specimens for hemagglutination tests must be handled aseptically, since bacterial contamination may cause both falsely negative and falsely positive results (Davidsohn and Toharsky, 1942).

Positive and negative controls must be run daily with all antiserums.

The following specific techniques for the most commonly employed hemagglutination tests have been shown to give reliable results. Numerous variations of these methods are available and may be equally successful in the hands of properly trained and experienced persons. One must also keep in mind that the commercial antiserums commonly used have been standardized to give optimal results with certain techniques; hence, the instructions accompanying such antiserums must be closely followed.

ABO Grouping

Six-tube Technique

1. Separate the serum from red cells or clot of unknown specimen.

2. Prepare a 2 per cent suspension in saline of the red cells of the unknown specimen.

3. For each specimen six test tubes are labeled, showing in addition to proper identification of the unknown specimen the following information: Tube 1, anti-A; tube 2, anti-B; tube 3, anti-A,B; tube 4, A; tube 5, B; tube 6, O.

4. Place 1 drop of the anti-A serum into tube 1, 1 drop of the anti-B serum into tube 2, and 1 drop of the anti-A,B serum into tube 3.

5. Add 2 drops each of the serum of the unknown specimen to tubes 4, 5, and 6.

6. Add 1 drop each of the 2 per cent red cell suspension in saline of the unknown specimen to tubes 1, 2, and 3.

7. To tube 4 add 1 drop of a 2 per cent red cell suspension in saline of group A cells; to tube 5 add 1 drop of a 2 per cent red cell suspension in saline of group B cells; and to tube 6 add 1 drop of a 2 per cent suspension of red cells in saline of group O cells.

8. Mix the contents of all tubes by shaking the test tube rack.

9. Depending on the speed necessary for completing the test, one of two alternatives may be chosen: The test tubes may be left at room temperature (20 to 25° C.) for at least 2 hours, or after 2 to 3 minutes, the tubes may be centrifuged (1 minute at 1500 r.p.m. in clinical centrifuge or one-half to 1 minute in Serofuge or Hemofuge).

10. After incubation or centrifugation the red cell suspensions are redispersed by tapping the tubes. Presence of agglutination is checked with the naked eye, with the scanning lens of a microscope, and, if results are doubtful or negative, microscopically (16 mm. objective) after placing a drop on a slide.

11. All results are immediately entered in the proper work record, preferably with "plus" signs for agglutination and "minus" signs for absence of agglutination.

INTERPRETATION

1. The results of an ABO grouping test can be accepted as valid only if the findings obtained in the first three test tubes with known antiserums agree with those obtained in the second three test tubes with known red cell suspensions; this second part of the test is called "confirmation," "check," or "reverse" grouping. Figure 5–3 schematically compares the results in the four main ABO groups in such tests when both the unknown red cells and the unknown serum are tested. If at all possible, it is desirable that two different persons perform ABO groupings, one testing with known antiserums and the other with known cells. After they have completed the tests and recorded their readings independently, the results should be compared for final interpretation.

2. Absent or weak agglutination with the unknown serum may be simulated by hemolysis of the known red cells; this suggests the presence of hemolytic anti-A or anti-B antibody. It is important to record such findings (using the letter "H" for hemolysin), since they affect significantly the selection of blood to be used as "universal donor" or for transfusion of "universal recipients." The assumption that hemolysis is due to anti-A or anti-B must be confirmed by repeating the test with the serum after its inactivation in a water bath at 56° C. for 30 minutes; use of the inactivated serum is expected to result in agglutination instead of hemolysis.

3. If discrepancies in the two parts of ABO grouping are observed, the test should be repeated in order to rule out some mistake in the previous test. If a second test reveals the same discrepancy, the following possibilities are to be considered:

A. Cold agglutinins may cause agglutination of the known cells by the unknown serum regardless of its ABO group. This must be confirmed by testing the unknown serum with its own red cells at 4° C. for 1 to 2 hours. Under these conditions cold agglutinins produce agglutination, which disappears after transfer of the specimen to a water bath at 37° C. for 5 to 10 minutes. (For further tests for cold agglutinins, see pp. 229–234 and 404.)

B. Agglutination of the unknown red cells by known antiserums that conflict with the

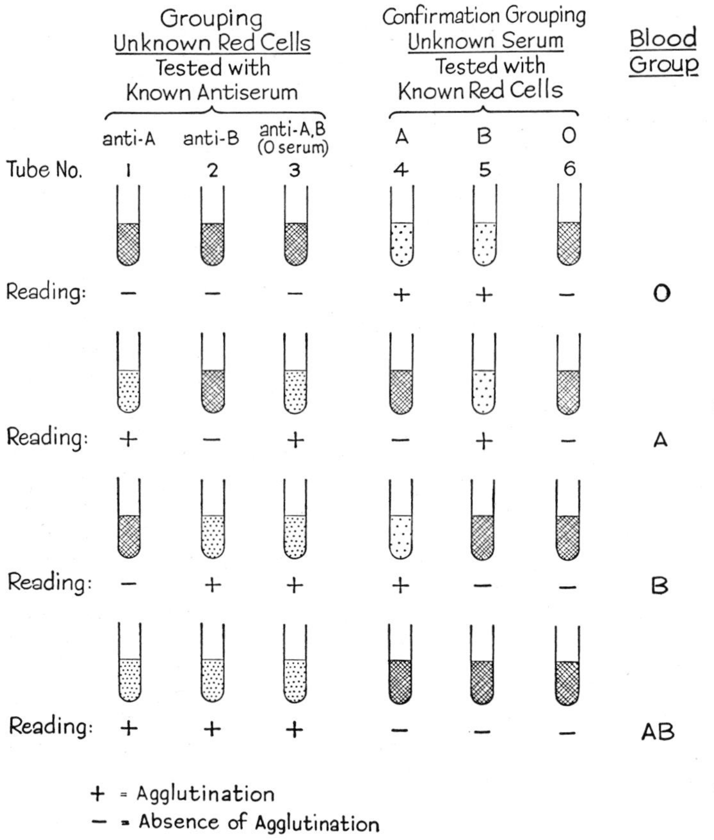

Figure 5–3. Schematic outline of ABO grouping test.

results obtained in the confirmation grouping may be due to coating of the red cells by *autoantibodies*. Confirmation of this phenomenon is obtained by performing on the unknown red cells the direct antiglobulin test and obtaining positive results. In order to obtain in such cases a reliable ABO grouping, the red cells should be washed several times with large amounts of physiologic saline solution, following which they are more likely to give adequate results.

C. Unexpected agglutination obtained with the unknown serum may reflect presence of *irregular agglutinins*, such as Rh antibodies, which react with the corresponding blood factor in the suspensions of the known red cells. This must be verified by demonstration of such irregular antibodies (see antibody identification, p. 376).

D. Discrepancies between the two parts of ABO grouping tests may be found in specimens of subgroups of A and AB. Most commonly these are specimens of group A_2 or A_2B containing anti-A_1 in their serums; thus, agglutination of the unknown red cells with anti-A serum may be associated with agglutination of known group A red cells by the unknown serum. Clarification in such cases is obtained by establishing the subgroup of A of the specimen (see p. 369) and by testing the unknown serum with suspensions of A_1 and A_2 cells. The latter test should be done at room temperature as well as at 4° C., since these antibodies as a rule act best at low temperatures. Group O cells must be included as control for presence of nonspecific cold agglutinins.

E. As mentioned previously, serums of newborn and young infants may not contain the isoagglutinins expected from the reactivity of their red cells (cf. p. 351); hence in infants use of the unknown serums is not a reliable procedure (cf. crossmatch tests, p. 393). Much less frequently isoagglutinins may be absent in older children and adults because of hypogammaglobulinemia or agammaglobulinemia or for unknown reasons.

COMMENTS

1. It is recommended that the serum be placed into the test tube first and that this be followed by the addition of the red cell suspension. In this way the error of omitting addition of the serum can be avoided.

2. The red cell suspensions of groups A, B, and O must be prepared freshly on the day of use. It is recommended that each suspension

be prepared from a pool of three different red cell specimens in order to reduce variations in individual reactivity and to guarantee that A_1 cells are present among the A cells. Some workers prefer to use only red cells known to be A_1 for this purpose.

Slide Grouping Tests

1. Prepare a 10 per cent suspension in saline of the red cells to be tested.
2. Mark the left side of a clean glass slide "anti-A" and the right side "anti-B."
3. Add to the left side a drop of anti-A grouping serum and to the right side a drop of anti-B grouping serum.
4. Next to the drops of anti-A serum and anti-B serum add 1 drop of the 10 per cent suspension of the unknown red cells. Be careful not to cause confluence of the drops on the left and right sides of the slide.
5. With one-half of an applicator stick, mix the red cell suspension with the anti-A serum, and with the other half mix the red cell suspension with the anti-B serum.
6. Gently rock the slide back and forth and observe the mixture for 1 minute unless agglutination occurs earlier.
7. Enter the results as "plus" for agglutination and as "minus" for absence of agglutination.
8. It is necessary to confirm the slide grouping by testing the unknown serum with the known red cell suspensions of groups A, B, and O as indicated in the previous section.

COMMENTS

1. Instead of a 10 per cent red cell suspension, small drops of blood obtained directly from skin punctures or whole oxalated or citrated blood not older than 24 hours may be used. In such cases one must avoid adding an excessive amount of blood to the antiserum, since this may interfere with adequate reading of the test and may also produce falsely negative results because of antigen excess.
2. Slow and weak agglutinations may occur with blood specimens of subgroups A_2, A_2B, A_3, A_3B, and so forth. This may result in falsely negative readings, since drying of the mixture may take place before the agglutination becomes clearly visible.
3. In some blood banks it is customary to do a preliminary ABO grouping for the donor record by adding to a drop of anti-A and anti-B serum 1 drop of blood from a skin puncture of the prospective donor. Results of such tests must be considered preliminary, since a certain percentage of weak subgroups of A and AB may erroneously be classified as O and B, respectively.

Determination of Subgroups of A and AB.

1. To a properly identified test tube add 1 drop of anti-A_1 reagent (absorbed anti-A serum or anti-A_1 lectin).
2. Add 1 drop of a 2 per cent red cell suspension in saline of the unknown specimen.
3. Let stand at room temperature for 15 minutes.
4. Centrifuge for one-half to 1 minute and check for presence of agglutination.
5. Controls with known red cells of group A_1 and group A_2 must be included with each test. Results are valid only if the expected positive and negative results are obtained with these controls.

Note: Some anti-A_1 reagents can be used for tube tests only, others for slide tests only. Instructions of the manufacturer for use of the reagent must be followed.

INTERPRETATION. Anti-A_1 serum or anti-A_1 lectin agglutinates only cells of group A_1 or A_1B. Specimens that are not agglutinated are most commonly group A_2 or A_2B. The rare subgroup A_3 or A_3B can be recognized by the fact that on microscopic examination only a few small agglutinates are found surrounded by large numbers of nonagglutinated red cells even when potent anti-A serums are tested with the unknown red cells. Red cells of the rare subgroup A_x have the property of being agglutinated by most anti-A,B serums (serums of group O persons), while anti-A serums are not capable of doing so.

Rh Typing

Determination of Rh_0 (D) Factor with Antiserums Containing IgG Rh Antibodies (Modified Slide Test Serums)

1. Prepare a 5 per cent red cell suspension of the unknown specimen in its own serum or in group AB serum found to be free of any agglutinins.
2. Into a properly labeled test tube place 1 drop of the antiserum.
3. Add 1 drop of the 5 per cent red cell suspension and mix well.
4. Incubate in a water bath for 30 minutes at 37° C.
5. Roll the tube gently in order to redisperse the red cells.
6. Check for agglutination with the scanning lens of the microscope. If agglutination is present, record the result after checking it microscopically.
7. If agglutination is absent, centrifuge for 1 to 2 minutes at 1500 r.p.m.
8. Resuspend the red cells as before and check for agglutination with the naked eye and the scanning lens. If agglutination is absent or doubtful, check by placing a drop of the mixture on a slide and examine with the 16 mm. objective of the microscope.
9. Enter the results in the workbook.

COMMENTS

1. Instead of centrifugation after a one-half hour incubation, the test may be incubated for 2 hours at 37° C. and read without centrifugation.

2. A modification of this test can be used by the experienced worker: Instead of preparing a 5 per cent suspension in their own serum of the unknown red cells, one may transfer with an applicator stick ("stick method") a sufficient number of red cells into the test tube containing the anti-Rh typing serum to make an approximately 5 per cent suspension.

3. Agglutinations with anti-Rh serums are less solid and more easily dispersed than those produced by anti-A and anti-B serums; hence, the serum red cell mixtures should never be shaken but should be gently twisted or rolled until the red cells are resuspended.

4. With each run of Rh typings, controls must be included in which the same antiserum is tested with specimens of known Rh-positive and Rh-negative red cells.

Rh Typing with Antiserums Containing IgM Antibodies (Saline Test Serums). The procedure is identical with the preceding one, except that a 2 per cent red cell suspension of the unknown specimen is prepared in saline. One drop of this suspension is added to 1 drop of the antiserum. Incubation of the serum-red cells mixture for 2 hours at 37° C. or incubation for 30 minutes followed by centrifugation may be used.

COMMENTS

1. In view of the limited availability of saline anti-Rh serums, their use should be restricted to special cases, such as checking doubtful results obtained with antiserums containing incomplete antibodies.

2. Saline Rh antiserums should not be used for Rh typing of newborn infants with hemolytic disease of the newborn; because of coating of red cells with Rh antibodies, falsely negative results may be obtained in such specimens.

3. Specimens of patients with autoimmune hemolytic disease (see p. 404) may be difficult to type with IgG Rh antibodies, since suspension of red cells in any serum may bring about agglutination. In this situation repeated washing of the red cells and use of the saline test is recommended.

Slide Test for Rh Typing

1. On a properly labeled glass slide place 1 drop of anti-Rh serum containing IgG Rh antibody.

2. To the drop of antiserum add 2 drops of either whole blood (either directly obtained from skin puncture or oxalated or citrated blood not older than 24 hours, or a 50 per cent cell suspension prepared from clotted blood in its own serum).

3. Mix serum and red cells and distribute over a large area of the slide.

4. Place the slide on a heated viewing box, bring the temperature of the mixture to 40 to 45° C.

5. Gently rock the slide back and forth and observe for agglutination.

6. Observe the test for 2 minutes unless agglutination occurs earlier.

7. At the end of the 2-minute period record presence of agglutination with a "plus" and absence of agglutination with a "minus" sign.

COMMENTS

1. Only Rh antiserums with IgG antibodies (blocking, albumin agglutinin, slide test serums) can be used.

2. Use of a too dilute red cell suspension or addition of a too small amount of red cell suspension to too much antiserum is a common source of falsely negative results.

3. Another important cause of falsely negative tests is inadequate warming of the mixture. The reaction may be speeded up by preheating glass slides on the viewing box.

4. Falsely positive results may result from autoagglutination or rouleaux formation.

5. Partial or complete drying of the mixture must be avoided, since this makes reading of the test difficult or impossible.

Tests for Weak Rh_0 Variants (D^u)

1. Prepare in saline a 2 per cent suspension of the red cells to be tested.

2. Add 2 drops of Rh antiserum with IgG antibodies to a properly labeled test tube.

3. Add to the test tube 2 drops of the 2 per cent red cell suspension.

4. Incubate the red cell serum mixture for 30 minutes in a water bath at 37° C.

5. Fill the test tube with physiologic saline and resuspend the red cell-serum mixture in the entire volume.

6. Centrifuge for 30 to 60 seconds.

7. Decant the supernatant as completely as possible and replace with physiologic saline.

8. Repeat such washing of red cells three times.

9. Remove the supernatant of the last washing as completely as possible.

10. Resuspend the packed red cells in 2 drops of physiologic saline.

11. Add 1 drop of antihuman globulin serum to the red cell suspension and mix.

12. Centrifuge for 1 minute.

13. Check for presence of agglutination.

Caution: Each test must be accompanied by a control consisting of 2 drops of a red cell suspension used in the main test *without* addition of IgG Rh antibodies; otherwise this control is treated in the same way as the test itself.

INTERPRETATION AND COMMENTS

1. Agglutination observed in the main test and absence of agglutination in the control indicate the presence of the weakly reacting $Rh_0(D^u)$ factor.

2. If the control also shows positive results, the test may be repeated in order to rule out a technical error. If the control continues to give positive results, this suggests coating of the red cells with autoantibody (positive direct antiglobulin test). Determination of the D^u

factor in a patient with a positive direct antiglobulin test is not possible.

3. Since there are many variants of the D^u factor differing from each other in reactivity, it is not uncommon that the red cells of the same persons may be found at one time to react as D^u, whereas subsequently when different anti-Rh serums are used they may be found as "regularly" Rh_0-(D)-positive in tests using the method described on p. 369. However, as a rule, negative results are obtained with such specimens when tested with the saline test tube method (p. 370).

4. In rare instances D^u specimens possess such weak reactivity that even the test just described fails to give a positive result. In some of these instances presence of D^u can be demonstrated if the cells are first treated with papain (cf. p. 374) and then subjected to incubation with anti-Rh serum, followed by the antiglobulin test as just described.

Rh Subtyping. In instances to be discussed in connection with pretransfusion (cf. p. 392) and prenatal testing (cf. p. 400), it is necessary to test for other Rh factors. Tests for rh′(C) and rh″(E) are usually done in persons negative for Rh_0(D), whereas Hr factors are of interest in connection with tests for Rh genotypes (cf. p. 407) or in cases of suspected isoimmunization.

The techniques are identical with tests for Rh_0(D). Test tube techniques are preferred and, depending on the availability of antiserums with IgM or IgG antibodies, tests are carried out with corresponding techniques.

Antiserums are also available that contain antibodies for the three Rh factors, Rh_0(D), rh′(C), and rh″(E). Such antiserums may be used parallel with anti-Rh_0(D) serum. If positive results are obtained with anti-Rh_0′″ (anti-CDE) serum and negative results with anti-Rh_0(D) serum, this indicates the presence of rh′(C) and/or rh″(E). Individual tests with anti-rh′(C) and anti-rh″(E) must be done in order to determine the exact type.

In subtyping for Rh and Hr factors, it is essential to include known positive and negative controls in order to assure validity of the tests.

The Antiglobulin Test

Direct Antiglobulin Test

1. Place 5 to 10 drops of blood in a test tube (100 mm. long, 13 mm. wide) and fill with physiologic saline.
2. Mix contents and centrifuge for 1 minute at 1500 r.p.m. in order to pack the red cells.
3. Decant the supernatant as completely as possible. Repeat the washing three times, each time removing as much of the supernatant as possible. Washing should be done immediately and without interruption.
4. Prepare a 2 per cent suspension of the red cells in saline.
5. In a test tube (75 mm. long, 10 mm. wide) place 2 drops of the antihuman globulin serum.
6. Add 2 drops of the red cell suspension and mix. Let stand for 5 minutes.
7. Centrifuge for 1 minute at 500 r.p.m. and check for agglutination with the naked eye and with the microscope.
8. Include controls, without which the test is valueless.

POSITIVE CONTROL

1. Prepare 2 per cent suspension in saline of known Rh-positive red cells of a healthy person.
2. Place into a small test tube 1 drop of an anti-Rh_0 (anti-D) slide test serum that meets the minimum requirements of the National Institutes of Health and dilute with saline two to four times.
3. Add 2 drops of the cell suspension.
4. Incubate for 30 minutes at 37° C.
5. Centrifuge the mixture of cells and serum and decant serum as completely as possible.
6. Wash cell sediment three times with tubefuls of saline, followed each time by centrifugation and by as complete removal of supernatant as possible.
7. After the third washing, add saline to the packed cells to the original volume.
8. Add 2 drops of anti-human serum to the cell suspension and let stand at room temperature for 5 minutes. If agglutination is observed, this is recorded.
9. If no agglutination is visible, centrifuge at low speed for 1 minute (500 r.p.m.). Check again for agglutination.

NEGATIVE CONTROL

Proceed in the same manner as with the positive control, but use known Rh-negative red cells of a healthy individual.

INTERPRETATION

1. A positive direct antiglobulin test is indicated by agglutination of the test and the positive control and absence of agglutination in the negative control. Although microscopic checking of doubtful results is recommended, the presence of a few small agglutinates visible only microscopically should be regarded as a doubtful result. In such cases the test should be repeated, preferably with a different antiglobulin reagent.
2. Coating of red cells of groups A and B with the corresponding isoagglutinins anti-A and anti-B in newborn infants is often difficult to detect by means of the direct antiglobulin test. For best results the test should be centrifuged immediately after addition of the antiglobulin serum. Specifically standardized antiglobulin reagents may prove most suitable.
3. Positive direct antiglobulin tests are most commonly found in infants with hemolytic disease of the newborn, in patients with auto-

immune hemolytic anemia, and in recipients of incompatible blood transfusions.

4. Drug-induced coating of red cells with positive direct antiglobulin tests is not uncommon in patients receiving some types of medication (e.g., penicillin, cephalothin, methyldopa).

Indirect Antiglobulin Test

1. Prepare a 2 per cent red cell suspension of the specimen to be used. (*Note*: This may be either a specimen of known antigenic composition if the test is to be used for demonstration of an unknown antibody, e.g., anti-Duffy or anti-Kell, or it may be a specimen of unknown antigenic composition if demonstration of an unknown antigen with a known antibody, such as anti-Duffy or anti-Kell, is intended.)

2. Into a properly labeled test tube place 2 drops of the serum to be used.

3. Add 2 drops of the red cell suspension.

4. Incubate the red cell-serum mixture for 30 minutes to 2 hours, depending on the reactivity and sensitivity of the serum.

5. If no agglutination has occurred after incubation, fill the test tube with physiologic saline and centrifuge.

6. Follow the same steps (Nos. 2, 3, and 5 to 7) as outlined for the direct antiglobulin test (p. 371).

7. In order to assure validity of the test, controls must be included in which either red cells of known antigenic composition or antibodies of known specificity are used in parallel with the main test.

COMMENTS

1. The indirect antiglobulin technique cannot be used with red cells known to give a positive direct antiglobulin test.

2. The indirect antiglobulin technique is frequently used for determination of certain blood factors, such as Duffy, Kell, and Kidd.

3. The indirect antiglobulin test may also be used for demonstration of antibodies for those blood factors.

4. The indirect antiglobulin test is one of the most reliable methods for crossmatching (cf. p. 382).

5. A modification of the indirect antiglobulin test, with increased sensitivity in some instances, is based on use of enzyme-treated red cells. However, this method cannot be used for demonstration of anti-Duffy, anti-S, and some other antibodies reacting with blood factors that are destroyed or weakened by proteolytic enzymes. Caution also must be exerted concerning falsely positive results owing to the great sensitivity of the technique.

Detection of coating of red cells by complement fixing antibodies requires use of "broad spectrum" antiglobulin serum. Such reagents contain antibody, specifically reacting with complement, in addition to antigamma globulin.

SOURCES OF ERROR IN ANTIGLOBULIN TESTS. False negative reactions may result from (1) neutralization of the antiglobulin reagent by human serum globulin because of failure of adequate washing of the red cell suspension or inadvertent addition of serum; (2) use of excessively high or excessively low concentration of red cells; and (3) inadequate periods of incubation in indirect antiglobulin tests. False positive reactions most commonly result from (1) bacterial contamination of specimens; (2) chemical contamination, particularly silica released from some glassware; (3) presence of a high percentage of reticulocytes. A true negative reaction may be recognized by addition of red cells intentionally coated with gamma globulin which should be agglutinated in tests properly performed.

Tests for Other Blood Factors

MN Typing

REAGENTS

The anti-M and anti-N typing serums commonly used are prepared by injecting rabbits with human red cells of type OM or ON and absorbing these immune serums with reciprocal red cells (N after injection of M cells; M after injection of N cells) until agglutination specific for one of the two types is obtained. A lectin with specificity of anti-N is also available. In using anti-M and anti-N typing serums, it is important to follow closely the instructions of the manufacturer, since specificity and sensitivity of the tests have been standardized for these conditions.

TECHNIQUE

1. Prepare a 2 per cent suspension in saline of the red cells of the unknown specimen. Controls of known blood groups and types must include M, N, and MN cells in combination with A, B, and O so that all groups, subgroups, and types are presented (for example: A_2M or A_2BM; A_1BMN or A_1MN; BM; ON).

EXAMPLE

TYPING SERUM	SUSPENSION OF UNKNOWN RED CELLS		
	(a)	(b)	(c)
1st row anti-M	+	−	+
2nd row anti-N	−	+	+
Results:	M	N	MN

TYPING SERUM	RED CELL SUSPENSIONS OF CONTROLS
1st row anti-M	A_2M (+) A_1BMN (+) BM (+) ON (−)
2nd row anti-N	A_2M (−) A_1BMN (+) BM (−) ON (+)

2. Set up two rows of five tubes each.
3. To each tube of the first row add 1 drop of anti-M serum.
4. To each tube of the second row add 1 drop of anti-N serum.
5. To the first tubes of each row add 1 drop of a 2 per cent suspension of the unknown cells.
6. To the second tubes of each row add 1 drop of the first control suspension. To the third tubes of each row add 1 drop of the second control suspension. To the fourth tubes of each row add 1 drop of the third control suspension. To the fifth tubes of each row add 1 drop of the fourth control suspension.
7. Shake. Incubate for 2 hours at room temperature (about 20° C.), shaking tubes at 15-minute intervals.
8. Shake tubes gently and check for agglutination with naked eye. If no clumping is visible, place the tube horizontally on the stage of the microscope and read with the scanning lens. Clumping of the unknown cells with the anti-M serum indicates the presence of factor M. Clumping of the unknown cells with the anti-N serum indicates the presence of factor N. If the unknown cells are clumped by both serums, both factors are present. The test is invalid unless the controls show the following results: Cells of type M must be clumped with anti-M serum, cells of type N with anti-N serum, and cells of type MN with both serums.

Kell and Duffy Typing

REAGENTS

Anti-Kell and anti-Duffy typing serums, as a rule, contain IgG antibodies, which react best in the antiglobulin technique.

TECHNIQUE

1. Prepare a 2 per cent suspension in saline of the red cells of the unknown specimen.
2. Into a properly labeled test tube, place 1 drop of anti-Kell (anti-Duffy) serum.
3. Add to the serum 2 drops of the 2 per cent red cell suspension.
4. Incubate for 1 hour in a water bath at 37° C.
5. Wash with physiologic saline three times and proceed as outlined in the direct antiglobulin test (p. 371, steps 5 to 7).

INTERPRETATION

1. Agglutination obtained in the test indicates that specimen is Kell-positive (K) or Duffy-positive (Fy^a), depending on the type of serum used.
2. Positive and negative controls, with red cells of known antigenic composition, must be included with each test, and the results are valid only if these controls give the expected results.

Miscellaneous Blood Factors. In certain conditions a variety of other blood factors may have to be determined, such as P_1, Lewis, and Lutheran factors. In all such instances availability of potent and reliable antiserums is critical. The reactivity of such antiserums must be known, specifically whether they contain IgM or IgG antibodies, and optimal conditions of time and temperature of incubation must be observed. Positive and negative controls must always be included in order to assure validity of the results.

Screening for and Identification of Isoantibodies. The following procedures are designed to detect and identify isoantibodies other than anti-A and anti-B in serum of persons of any of the ABO groups. Such tests, as a rule, are required in connection with either blood transfusion therapy or isoimmunization associated with pregnancy. Most commonly, these tests concern the presence of Rh antibodies in Rh_0(D)-negative persons. More rarely, antibodies for Rh factors other than Rh_0(D) may be detected in Rh-positive persons or antibodies for factors of other blood group systems in serum of Rh-negative and Rh-positive persons.

The following techniques deal mainly with tests for Rh antibodies. Modifications necessary for detection and identification of antibodies other than anti-Rh are discussed subsequently. One of two general approaches may be utilized for screening for Rh antibodies: (1) individual red cells of known Rh phenotypes may be used in order to detect presence and determine specificity of Rh antibodies, or (2) a pool of red cells prepared from two or three specimens possessing the commonly involved Rh factors may be employed for screening only. If positive results are obtained with pooled red cells, the test is repeated with individual red cells in order to provide information concerning specificity of the Rh antibodies. Whenever pooled red cells are used, it is important that at least 30 per cent of the red cells forming the pool contain each blood factor for which antibodies are sought.

Several methods may be employed in order to have available red cells of known antigenic composition whenever needed. Members of the blood bank staff, laboratory, or hospital may be typed for such blood factors and blood obtained at appropriate times. All such blood specimens should be of group O in order to eliminate any confusing results resulting from isoagglutination by anti-A and anti-B. Blood donors readily available when needed may be used in a similar fashion, or blood specimens recently drawn may be tested for presence of the blood factors needed in order to select specimens with the desired antigenic composition. Finally, panels of reagent red cells of known antigenic composition are available commercially with periods of usefulness ranging from two to four weeks (cf. p. 366 for preservative solutions suitable for such purposes).

Papain-treated Red Cell Technique (Kuhns and Bailey, 1950). This is one of the most sensitive techniques for demonstration of Rh-Hr antibodies.

REAGENTS

1. Stock solution of papain (1 per cent). Suspend 1 gm. of papain in 100 ml. of 0.9 per cent physiologic saline and, after vigorous shaking, filter. This suspension when stored at 4° C. is stable for one month.

2. Sörenson phosphate buffer. Mix 76.8 ml. of $^1/_{15}$M Na_2HPO_4 with 23.2 ml. of $^1/_{15}$M KH_2PO_4; expected pH: 7.3.

3. Buffered saline. Mix 9 volumes of physiologic saline with 1 volume of the buffer (2).

4. Working solution of papain (0.1 per cent). On the day of use mix 9 volumes of buffered saline (3) with 1 volume of the stock solution of papain (1). Keep refrigerated when not in use. This solution must be prepared fresh daily.

RED CELL SUSPENSIONS

1. Minimum requirement: O Rh_1Rh_2(CDE); O rh(cde).

2. If O Rh_1Rh_2 cells are not available, cells of types O Rh_1(CDe) and O Rh_2(cDE) may be either used individually or equal parts of their suspensions may be mixed.

3. For identification of specificity of Rh antibodies the following additional red cells are needed: rh′(Cde), Rh_0(cDe), and rh″(cdE).

TECHNIQUE

1. In a large test tube prepare red cell suspension in amount sufficient to yield 0.5 ml. of packed red cells.

2. Wash red cells three times with large volumes of physiologic saline and pack the cells after last washing.

3. Add 1.0 ml. of the buffered working solution of papain to 0.5 ml. of packed red cells and mix.

4. Incubate the red cell-papain mixture for 30 minutes in water bath of 37° C. Agitate mixture at frequent intervals.

5. Centrifuge mixture at moderate speed and remove supernatant.

6. Wash the red cell sediment three times with saline.

7. After the last washing remove the supernatant as completely as possible and add physiologic saline to make a 2 per cent suspension of the red cells.

Note: Papain-treated red cells react reliably only for 24 hours and, hence, must be prepared fresh on the day of use.

SCREENING TEST

1. Label with proper identification as many test tubes for each serum to be tested as different types of red cells are to be used.

Note: The minimum consists of two test cells: Rh-positive red cells for the main test and Rh-negative red cells as control (cf. Red cell suspensions).

2. Into each test tube place 2 drops of the unknown serum.

3. To each tube add 1 drop of the appropriate suspension of papain-treated red cells and mix.

4. Incubate all test tubes in a water bath of 37° C. for 30 minutes.

5. Check for agglutination with the naked eye and with the scanning lens. If results are doubtful, place 1 drop of suspension on a slide and check microscopically (16 mm. objective).

INTERPRETATION

1. Absence of agglutination in all tubes indicates absence of Rh antibodies.

2. Agglutination of Rh-positive cells in the absence of agglutination of Rh-negative cells indicates presence of Rh antibodies. Specificity of the antibodies can be determined by using test cells of different Rh phenotypes as shown in Table 5–11. Results of such tests also indicate whether antibodies react specifically with only one of the Rh factors or whether a combination of antibodies with different specificities is present.

3. The test is valid only if simultaneously run positive and negative controls—serums known to contain Rh antibodies or to be free of Rh antibodies, respectively—give the expected results.

4. In prenatal testing a red cell suspension of the husband should be included whenever available, provided his wife does not possess isoagglutinins reacting with AB blood factors present in the husband's red cells.

5. If agglutination occurs with Rh-positive and Rh-negative red cells, the following possibilities must be considered:

A. *Autoagglutinins* can be confirmed by finding a positive direct antiglobulin test on the red cells of the blood specimen tested; furthermore, the serum of the specimen tested with its own papain-treated red cells will produce agglutination.

B. *Unsuitability of test cells* may be due to bacterial contamination, coating with globulin, or improper preservation.

C. *Bacterial contamination* of the serum tested (cf. bacteriogenic agglutination, p. 388).

D. *Presence of antibody* owing to a factor (which is present in all test cells) other than Rh_0(D). One such antibody is anti-hr′(c). As indicated in Table 5–11, identification of anti-hr′(c) is possible if the panel includes red cells of type Rh_1Rh_1(CCDe), which are not agglutinated by this antibody. Analogously, anti-hr″ (anti-e) agglutinates all red cells except Rh_2Rh_2(cDEE).

CAUTIONS AND COMMENTS

1. The papain-treated red cells must not be incubated for periods exceeding 30 minutes, since falsely positive results may be obtained after prolonged incubation.

2. Other enzymes, such as trypsin, ficin, and

Table 5–11. INTERPRETATION OF SCREENING TESTS FOR Rh ANTIBODIES

	PANEL CELLS*						
Serum No.	rh cde	rh'rh Ccde	Rh_0 cDe	rh''rh cdEe	Rh_1Rh_1 CCDe	Rh_2Rh_2 cDEE	Antibodies Present for Factor(s)
I	–	–	–	–	–	–	none
II	–	–	+	–	+	+	Rh_0(D)
III	–	+	–	–	+	–	rh'(C)
IV	–	–	–	+	–	+	rh''(E)
V	+	+	+	+	–	+	hr'(c)
VI	+	+	+	+	+	–	hr''(e)
VII	–	+	+	–	+	+	Rh_0(D), rh'(C)
VIII	–	–	+	+	+	+	Rh_0(D), rh''(E)
IX	–	+	+	+	+	+	Rh_0(D), rh'(C), rh''(E)

*All cells group O.
+Agglutination.
–Absence of agglutination.

bromelin, may be used with similar results as papain. The techniques recommended for their use must be observed closely, whether or not centrifugation is indicated.

Indirect Antiglobulin Technique (Including Test for IgM Agglutinins). Test cells of similar composition as those mentioned for the papain technique are used.

TECHNIQUE

1. Prepare 2 per cent suspensions of the test cells in saline.
2. For each serum specimen to be tested, identify properly as many test tubes as test cells are to be used.
3. Into each test tube place 2 drops of the serum to be tested.
4. To each tube add 2 drops of the 2 per cent suspension of the appropriate test cell suspension.
5. Incubate the red cell serum mixtures in a water bath at 37° C. for 2 hours.
6. Check for agglutination with the naked eye and with the scanning lens, and microscopically if in doubt.
7. If no agglutination is observed, proceed with washing of red cell suspensions and addition of antiglobulin serum as outlined in section on antiglobulin test (p. 371).

INTERPRETATION

1. If agglutination is observed in step 6, this indicates presence of IgM Rh antibodies.
2. If agglutination is absent in step 6 and occurs after completion of step 7, this indicates presence of IgG Rh antibodies.
3. Presence and absence of agglutination observed with different test cells is interpreted as outlined for papain technique (Table 5–11).

Albumin Technique (Hattersley)

REAGENTS

1. Bovine or human albumin (22 or 30 per cent).
2. Test cells, as outlined in papain technique.

TECHNIQUE

1. Prepare a 2 per cent suspension of the test cells in bovine albumin.
2. For each serum specimen to be tested identify properly as many test tubes as test cells are used.
3. Into each test tube place 2 drops of the serum to be tested.
4. To each test tube add 1 drop of the appropriate suspension of the test cells in bovine albumin and mix.
5. Without waiting, centrifuge the red cell serum mixture for 3 minutes at 1200 r.p.m.
6. Check for agglutination macroscopically and with the scanning lens.
7. If no agglutination is noted, incubate test tubes for 1 hour in a water bath of 37° C.
8. Centrifuge for 1 minute at 500 r.p.m.
9. Gently resuspend the red cells and check for agglutination with the naked eye and microscopically.

INTERPRETATION AND COMMENTS

1. The centrifugation in step 5 is intended to eliminate false negative results caused by antibody excess, which may be responsible for a prozone phenomenon.

2. The following additional sets may also be included in the test: (A) red cells of the unknown specimen suspended in their own serum (2 per cent) and treated in the same way as the other tubes; (B) addition to 2 drops of the unknown serum of 1 drop of 2 per cent suspensions in saline of the test cells, run parallel with the test tubes containing albumin-suspended red cells. Positive results with red cells of set (A) indicate presence of auto-agglutinins. Positive results obtained with saline-suspended red cells suggest the presence of IgM (saline) Rh antibodies.

Slide Test (Diamond-Abelson)

REAGENTS

50 per cent suspension of O Rh-positive and O Rh-negative test cells.

TECHNIQUE

1. Place 1 drop each of the unknown serum on two glass slides, one of which is identified as "Rh+," and the other as "Rh–."

2. To the first slide add 2 drops of the 50 per cent suspension of O Rh-positive blood; to the second slide add 2 drops of the 50 per cent suspension of the O Rh-negative blood.

3. On each slide mix the serum with the cell suspension and spread over large area.

4. Place the slides on a heated viewing box.

5. Gently rock the slides back and forth, and observe up to 3 minutes unless agglutination occurs earlier.

INTERPRETATION. Agglutination of the Rh-positive red cells and absence of agglutination of Rh-negative red cells indicates the presence of Rh antibodies.

Note: The sensitivity of the techniques for detection of Rh antibodies decreases in this order of enumeration: papain technique, indirect antiglobulin technique, albumin technique, and Diamond-Abelson test.

Detection and Identification of Other Antibodies

TEST CELLS. Suspension of red cells possessing known blood factor and of red cells free of blood factors for which antibodies may be present in the serum tested.

TECHNIQUES. Whenever the presence of an irregular antibody is suspected in a serum, it should be tested with appropriate red cell suspensions by the following three techniques: saline-suspended red cells; indirect antiglobulin technique; and papain-treated red cells. Although the first part of the indirect antiglobulin test also permits evaluation of the presence of IgM antibodies reacting with saline-suspended red cells at 37° C., it is also advisable to test for the presence of IgM antibodies reactive at lower temperatures, specifically at 20 to 25° C. (room temperature) and at 4 to 6° C. A single set in which saline-suspended red cells are used may be first incubated and read at room temperature and then transferred to the refrigerator, preferably overnight. The general procedures for antibody screening are those outlined before. In some instances it also may be advisable to use bovine albumin-suspended test cells (see p. 375).

INTERPRETATION

1. Exclusion of antibody specificity: Presence of antibodies is conclusively ruled out for those blood factors that are represented by test cells not agglutinated by the unknown serum under the various testing conditions. For example, if test cells containing the Kell factor (K) are not agglutinated, this is evidence for absence of anti-K antibody in the serum under study.

2. Tentative identification of antibody specificity: This is facilitated by finding a "common denominator" in test cells that were agglutinated by the serum tested; e.g., if all test cells agglutinated contain the Duffy factor (Fy^a), this is presumptive evidence for presence of anti-Fy^a in the serum tested.

Figure 5–4 illustrates this approach schematically by the arbitrary assignment to red cells of six different blood group antigens, different combinations of which are present in each of five specimens of panel red cells. Since the serum with the unknown antibody failed to react with panel cells 1, 3, and 5, one can conclude that the antibody cannot be specific for five of the six antigens that are

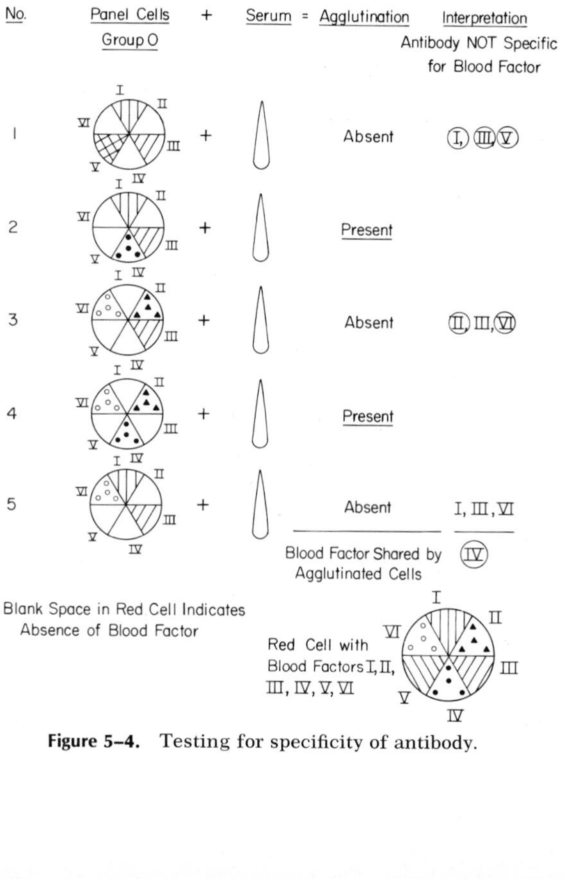

Figure 5–4. Testing for specificity of antibody.

Table 5–12. IDENTIFICATION OF ANTIBODIES: SERUM I

	PANEL CELL ANTIGENS*												REACTIONS TO TESTS**	
Panel Cell No.	Rh_0 D	rh′ C	rh″ E	hr′ c	M	N	S	s	P_1	K	Fy^a	Jk^a	*A*	*B*
1	+	+	−	+	+	+	+	+	−	−	−	+	−	−
2	+	−	−	+	+	−	−	+	+	−	+	−	+	−
3	+	−	+	+	−	+	−	+	+	+	−	+	−	−
4	−	−	−	+	+	+	+	+	+	+	−	−	−	−
5	+	+	−	−	−	+	+	+	−	+	+	+	+	−
6	−	−	−	+	+	−	+	−	−	+	+	−	+	−
7	−	+	−	+	−	+	−	+	+	−	+	+	+	−
8	+	+	−	−	+	+	+	+	+	−	+	−	+	−
9	−	−	+	+	+	−	+	−	+	−	−	+	−	−

*+ Present
− Absent
**++ Strong agglutination
+ Moderate agglutination
− No agglutination

Interpretations: Cross out antigens present in panel cells not agglutinated by the serum being tested; circle remaining antigen(s).

1. Antigens in panel: ~~Rh_0~~ ~~rh′~~ ~~rh″~~ ~~hr′~~ ~~M~~ ~~N~~ ~~S~~ ~~s~~ ~~P_1~~ ~~K~~ (Fy^a) ~~Jk^a~~
2. Antibody or antibodies not excluded for: Fy^a.
3. Is at least one of the blood group antigens not excluded in 2 present in all panel cells agglutinated by the serum? Yes.

Presumptive identification of antibody or antibodies: anti-Fy^a.

present in these red cells. On the other hand, antigen "IV," the only one not excluded, is present in panel cells 2 and 4, which reacted with the antibody. Thus, the presumptive identification of the specificity of the antibody is "anti-IV."

In Tables 5–12 and 5–13 these principles are applied to identification of antibodies by testing the serums with a panel of nine red cell specimens, each of which possesses a different combination of blood group antigens. The results shown in column *A* were obtained with the indirect antiglobulin technique, those in column *B* with enzyme-treated red cells. Additional techniques may have to be utilized as indicated. By elimination of antigens present in panel cells not agglutinated by either technique, it is possible to identify the antibody in the serum in Table 5–12 presumptively as anti-Fy^a. Results shown in Table 5–13 give presumptive evidence for presence of two antibodies – anti-Rh_0(D) and anti-K.

3. Definitive identification of antibody specificity: After a tentative identification of the antibody specificity has been made, a definitive identification should be attempted by the following methods:

A. The serum is tested with a minimum of six separate red cell specimens, three of which contain the antigen in question and three of which do not contain it (e.g., if tentative identification of anti-Kell antibody is made, test the serum with three Kell-positive and three Kell-negative red cell specimens). If agglutination is obtained with all red cell specimens containing the incriminated antigen and no agglutination is obtained with red cell specimens free of this antigen, the tentative antibody identification has been confirmed.

B. The serum is absorbed with red cell suspension containing the incriminated antigen (red cell suspension 1) and with red cell suspension free of this antigen (red cell suspension 2).

With the same red cell suspension as used for absorption (1), parallel titrations are set up with (a) the unabsorbed serum, (b) the serum after absorption with red cell suspension 1, and (c) the serum after absorption with red cell suspension 2.

If titrations 1 and 3 yield results differing only slightly from each other and if titration 2 yields significantly lower values or even disclosed disappearance of the antibody, this corroborates the tentative identification of the antibody.

The absorbed antibody may be eluted (cf. p. 385) from the red cells and the eluate may be tested for the expected specificity. This is particularly valuable when a serum contains two or more antibodies.

C. If at all possible, the complete blood formula of the red cells of the person with the antibody should be determined. With rare

Table 5–13. IDENTIFICATION OF ANTIBODIES: SERUM II

	PANEL CELL ANTIGENS*												REACTIONS TO TESTS**	
Panel Cell No.	Rh_0 D	rh′ C	rh″ E	hr′ c	M	N	S	s	P_1	K	Fy^a	Jk^a	*A*	*B*
1	+	+	−	+	+	+	+	+	−	−	−	+	+	+
2	+	−	−	+	+	−	−	+	+	−	+	−	+	+
3	+	−	+	+	−	+	−	+	+	+	−	+	++	+
4	−	−	−	+	+	+	+	+	+	+	−	−	+	−
5	+	+	−	−	−	+	+	+	−	+	+	+	++	++
6	−	−	−	+	+	−	+	−	−	+	+	−	+	−
7	−	+	−	+	−	+	−	+	+	−	+	+	−	−
8	+	+	−	−	+	+	+	+	+	−	+	−	+	++
9	−	−	+	+	+	−	+	−	+	−	−	+	−	−

*+ Present
− Absent
**++ Strong agglutination
+ Moderate agglutination
− No agglutination

Interpretations: Cross out antigens present in panel cells not agglutinated by the serum being tested; circle remaining antigen(s).

1. Antigens in panel: (Rh_0) ~~rh′~~ ~~rh″~~ ~~hr′~~ ~~M~~ ~~N~~ ~~S~~ ~~s~~ ~~P_1~~ (K) ~~Fy^a~~ ~~Jk^a~~
2. Antibody or antibodies not excluded for: Rh_0(D); K.
3. Is at least one of the blood group antigens not excluded in 2 present in all panel cells agglutinated by the serum? Yes.

Presumptive identification of antibody or antibodies: anti-Rh_0(D); anti-K.

exceptions the antigen for which the antibody is specific should be absent in the red cells of the sensitized person; e.g., a person with anti-rh″(E) antibody in the serum has red cells that are negative for rh″(E).

Controls, Sources of Error, and Supplementary Suggestions

1. One of the most common pitfalls in attempts to identify irregular hemoantibodies is caused by the presence of nonspecific agglutinins, which clump red cell specimens indiscriminately. The best method of detecting such antibodies is to include in each test the red cells of the same person whose serum is tested. Agglutination found in this suspension suggests the presence of nonspecific agglutinins (IgM or IgG cold agglutinins or warm autoagglutinins). In some of these cases the presence of autoantibodies may be confirmed by finding a positive direct antiglobulin test with the red cells of the specimen tested.

2. Cell controls: In order to be sure that test cells have not undergone some changes making them agglutinable in a nonspecific fashion, always include controls consisting of 2 drops of saline and 2 drops of the corresponding red cell suspension. Agglutination found in any of these "cell controls" invalidates results obtained in the main test.

3. Helpful information on probable identity of the antibody may be derived from its behavior at different temperatures and in different techniques:

A. Anti-P_1, anti-M, and anti-N most commonly react better, or only, at low temperatures and with saline-suspended red cells.

B. Anti-Fy^a antibodies, as a rule, react only with the indirect antiglobulin technique and give negative results with papain-treated red cells.

C. MN factors are destroyed by proteolytic enzymes and cannot be detected with this technique.

D. Rh-Hr antibodies react best with papain-treated red cells, and when present in low titer may give positive results only with this technique.

E. Antibodies resulting from isoimmunization by blood transfusions or pregnancy are, as a rule, IgG antibodies and give best results with papain and antiglobulin techniques; "natural" antibodies for which the cause of immunization is not known react best with saline-suspended red cells.

F. Some antibodies give much stronger reactions with red cells homozygous for the respective factor, while red cells heterozygous for the factor are agglutinated either weakly or not at all ("double dose effects"); e.g., anti-M may agglutinate MM cells much more strongly than MN cells.

4. More than one antibody may be present.

This possibility is suggested when in the course of the tentative antibody identification two or more test cell specimens agglutinated by the serum tested are found not to contain a common antigen (cf. Table 5–13). Definitive identification of multiple antibodies requires absorption tests.

5. Red cell suspensions should not be used for longer than 12 hours after preparation even if stored at 4° C.

Titration of Antibodies. Serial dilutions of the serum to be tested are prepared. To each serial dilution add the test cells containing the blood factor(s) reacting with the antibodies tested. After completion of the test, agglutinations are observed and recorded. The highest dilution of the serum showing agglutination is the reciprocal of the antibody titer; e.g., if agglutination is observed in the serum dilution of 1:32 but agglutination is absent in the serum dilution of 1:64, the titer is recorded as 32.

Results may be also expressed as "scores" based on the strength of agglutination observed in each dilution and converted into a numerical value. The following scheme for recording agglutinations may be used or modified: 5 (++++)–massive clumps of red cells releasing few free cells on shaking; 4 (+++)–massive clumps of red cells breaking up into large clumps on shaking; 3 (++)–numerous large clumps of red cells; 2 (+)–small clumps of red cells readily visible with naked eye; 1 (+w)–clumps of red cells barely visible with naked eye with numerous clumps visible microscopically; 0.5 (+vw)–clumps mixed with numerous unagglutinated cells and demonstrable only microscopically.

As demonstrated in Table 5–14, scoring of titrations permits more exact assessment of the potency of antibodies than do titers, since the score takes into account not only concentration, but also avidity of antibody. For most purposes, titers are sufficient. Scores are useful when precise comparison of different antiserums tested with the same red cell reagent is desired or when reactivities of different red cell reagents tested with the same antiserum are compared, especially when one investigates the "double dose effect" in red cells homozygous for a particular antigen.

The following techniques refer to titration of Rh antibodies. With suitable modification of the nature of test cells these techniques can be applied to titration of other isoantibodies.

Titration of IgM Rh Antibodies

TECHNIQUE

1. Prepare 2 per cent suspensions in saline of O Rh-positive test cells. Test cells of type O Rh_1Rh_2(CDE) or pooled test cells of types O Rh_1(CDe) and O Rh_2(cDE) may be used. If so desired, parallel titrations may also be done with separate suspensions of test cells; e.g., in order to compare titers obtained with Rh_1 (CDe) and with Rh_2(cDE) cells.

2. For each serum to be titrated set up as many rows of 10 test tubes as test cells are to be used.

3. Into the first tube of each row place 2 drops of the undiluted serum.

4. In a separate dilution tube prepare a 1:2 dilution of the serum by mixing an equal number of drops of serum and physiologic saline.

5. In separate dilution tubes an equal number of drops of the 1:2 serum dilution and physiologic saline are mixed, resulting in a dilution of 1:4. Such dilutions are continued until the dilution of 1:512 is reached.

6. Into the second tube of each row place 2 drops of serum dilution 1:2; into the third tube place 2 drops of serum dilution 1:4, and so on.

7. To each tube add 1 drop of the 2 per cent suspension of the appropriate test cells.

8. Mix the contents of the tubes and incubate in a water bath of 37° C. for 2 hours.

9. Check for agglutination with the naked eye, with the scanning lens of the microscope, and with the low-power objective (16 mm.) if result is doubtful.

Alternative Procedure to Steps 4 to 6. If only one test cell suspension is used, one may proceed as follows: (1) Into all but the first of the 10 tubes place 2 drops of saline. (2) To the second tube add 2 drops of the serum tested, and after mixing the contents transfer 2 drops to the third test tube. Continue with this procedure until the tenth test tube, from which, after mixing of contents, 2 drops are removed and discarded. Thus again a twofold serial dilution up to 1:512 has been prepared. If a high antibody titer is expected, one may

Table 5–14. COMPARISON OF TITERS AND SCORES

TITRATION NO.	RECIPROCAL OF DILUTION 1	2	4	8	16	32	64	TITER	SCORE
I	++	+	+	+	+w	+vw	–	32	10.5
II	++++	+++	+++	++	+	+w	–	32	19

prepare a primary serum dilution of 1:5 or 1:10 and then proceed with twofold serial dilutions; i.e., 1:5, 1:10, 1:20, and so on.

Indirect Antiglobulin Technique. The test is set up in the same way as outlined for IgM (saline) agglutinins. Serum-test cell mixtures remaining free of agglutination after the period of incubation are converted into the antiglobulin test by following the procedures outlined on page 375.

Albumin Technique. The procedure is identical with that described for IgM agglutinins, except that the suspending medium for the red cells is 20 to 30 per cent bovine albumin and the serum is diluted with serum of a person of group AB instead of with physiologic saline. The diluent serum must have been shown previously to be free of irregular agglutinins. The test is read after incubation for 2 hours in a water bath of 37° C.

Papain Technique. Papain-treated red cells are prepared as outlined in the technique on page 383 and added to serum dilutions prepared as outlined for the titration of saline agglutinins. The test is read for agglutination after incubation for 30 minutes in a water bath at 37° C.

Volumetric Titration. In most laboratory procedures use of capillary pipettes for titration is satisfactory; that is, the required number of drops of serum, serum dilutions, or red cell suspensions is delivered from pipettes with tips 1 to 2 mm. in diameter. For each red cell suspension and for each serum, a clean pipette must be used. Transfer of serial dilutions of the same serum may be carried out with the same capillary pipette provided the contents are expressed as completely as possible between each dilution and the pipette is rinsed each time by drawing up clean physiologic saline solution a few times and discarding the contents as completely as possible. This can be facilitated by setting up three containers with saline in which the pipettes are rinsed twice, transferred to the next, and kept in the third container. By having several pipettes available simultaneously, the transfer of serum is probably reduced to an insignificant minimum. Nevertheless, even with this technique traces of higher serum concentrations are transferred to the next dilution. In general, one must keep in mind that results of titrations are only quantitative approximations and by no means approach the accuracy of chemical quantitative tests.

Volumetric titrations provide for an increased accuracy. In this technique serums and red cell suspensions are measured in quantities of 0.1 ml.; a separate calibrated pipette is used each time; otherwise, the procedures are those outlined before. Volumetric techniques are mandatory for determination of the titer of antiserums used for blood grouping procedures, e.g., anti-A, anti-B, anti-Rh_0(D). Their use is also desirable when one wishes to obtain information on the comparative antibody titer of two different specimens, such as may be needed in prenatal tests. Such comparison of antibody titers is valid only when the two or more serum specimens are tested simultaneously by volumetric methods and the same test cell suspension. This is necessitated by the observation that, even in the same laboratory, titers run at different times may vary, depending on test cells and diluents used.

Titration of Isoagglutinins Anti-A and Anti-B. Because of special considerations given to anti-A and anti-B isoagglutinins in connection with selection of blood for transfusions and diagnosis of hemolytic disease of the newborn, the following methods of quantitative estimations are presented separately.

Screening Procedure for Elimination of "High-titered" Isoagglutinins. In order to avoid use of potentially "dangerous universal donors" (cf. p. 393), a screening procedure capable of detecting "high-titered" group O blood is carried out in most blood banks. There is no unanimity as to what represents a "high titer." The following procedure is based on the assumption that any agglutinating activity of anti-A and anti-B persisting in a 1:50 dilution is to be considered high titered.

TECHNIQUE

1. Into a large test tube place 4.9 ml. of physiologic saline.
2. To the test tube add 0.1 ml. of the serum to be tested with an accurately calibrated serologic pipette.
3. Mix carefully by expelling the contents of the pipette into the saline, drawing up fluid, and expelling it several times. Stopper and mix by inverting the tube. This produces a dilution of 1:50.
4. Identify one of two tubes as "A" and the other as "B."
5. Add 0.1 ml. of the diluted serum to each of the two tubes.
6. To the tube marked "A" add 0.1 ml. of a 2 per cent suspension of red cells of group A, and to the tube marked "B" add 0.1 ml. of a 2 per cent suspension of red cells of group B.
7. Let stand at room temperature for 15 minutes and centrifuge for 1 minute.
8. Check for presence of agglutination with the naked eye and, if in doubt or if result is negative to the naked eye, microscopically after placing a drop of the serum-cell mixture on a slide.

INTERPRETATION. If the diluted serum agglutinated A or B cells, the titer of anti-A or anti-B exceeds 50; such blood is designated as "high titered" and is eliminated from use as "universal donor." If the diluted serum did not agglutinate A or B red cells, it is designated as "low titered," and the blood may be selected for potential use as "universal donor."

Note: Specific tests are required before low-titered blood of group O can be safely given as universal donor (cf. Minor crossmatch for universal donor and recipient, p. 383).

If the presence of hemolysin for A or B cells has been noted in the ABO grouping (cf. Six-tube technique, p. 367), such blood should be designated as "high titered" (even if the saline dilution of 1:50 failed to agglutinate A or B cells) and be excluded from use as universal donor.

If the titer exceeded 50 for one blood group but not for the other, such blood may be considered for use as universal donor for a recipient of the blood group for which the titer did not exceed 50.

Detection and Titration of Isoagglutinins. Characteristics shown in Table 5–15 permit in many instances, distinguishing between "natural" and "immune" anti-A and anti-B isoagglutinins; as a rule, the latter result from specific antigenic stimulations, such as administration of incompatible blood, pregnancy of a woman with a fetus of an incompatible ABO group, or administration of antigens widely distributed in nature and chemically related to A and B group-specific substance. Since the properties differentiating IgM and IgG anti-A and anti-B cannot be demonstrated regularly, it is advisable to use more than one method in each instance. Techniques for titration of antibodies, using different media and temperatures, and enzyme-treated red cells have been described. The following outline presents a method for testing the neutralization of anti-A and anti-B by blood group subtances.

NEUTRALIZATION TECHNIQUE

1. Mix equal parts of the serum and of group-specific substances A and B.
2. For each test cell suspension (A_1, B, husband's red cells) to be used, prepare two sets of twofold serial dilutions of the mixture of the serum with group-specific substance, using physiologic saline as diluent for one set and serum of group AB for the other.
3. To each tube of the saline dilution series add 1 drop of the corresponding 2 per cent red cell suspension in saline (group A_1, group B, husband's red cells).
4. To each of the test tubes of the serum dilutions prepared with group AB serum, add 1 drop of the corresponding albumin-suspended red cells.
5. Incubate all titrations for 2 hours at room temperature.
6. Read and record the results.

Interpretation. As a rule, neutralization with group-specific substance reduces or completely inhibits the isoagglutination of saline-suspended red cells. On the other hand, in the presence of IgG anti-A and anti-B, testing of the neutralized mixture with albumin-suspended red cells shows unchanged strength of agglutination. Thus, absence of agglutination with saline-suspended red cells and presence of agglutination with albumin-suspended red cells exposed to serum mixed with group-specific substance speaks in favor of the presence of IgG isoagglutinin.

Note: If, after mixing equal parts of serum and group-specific substance, neutralization is incomplete, the proportion of group-specific substance should be increased, e.g., by adding 4 volumes of group-specific substance to 1 volume of serum. The subsequent procedures are analogous to those described.

The presence of IgG isoagglutinins in "neutralized" serum may also be demonstrated by means of the indirect antiglobulin test: serial dilutions of the neutralized serum are incubated with saline-suspended red cells in a water bath of 37° C. for 2 hours and checked for agglutination. Dilution tubes not

Table 5–15. CHARACTERISTICS OF "NATURAL" AND "IMMUNE" ANTI-A AND ANTI-B*

		NATURAL	IMMUNE
Immunization		Unknown	Transfusion or Pregnancy
Immunoglobulin class		IgM	IgG
Ability to pass placenta		No	Yes
Hemolysis *in vitro*		Rare	Often
Optimal conditions	a. Medium	Saline	Macromolecular
	b. Temperature	25° C. or below	37° C.
	c. Red cells	Untreated	Enzyme-treated
Neutralized by blood group substances		Completely	Incompletely
Avidity		Low	High
Sensitive to	a. Heating	Yes	No
	b. SH-compounds	Yes	No

*"Natural" anti-A,B in group O persons is usually IgG.

showing agglutination are converted into the indirect antiglobulin test. If the indirect antiglobulin test produces a significant increase of titer as compared with the first reading, this speaks in favor of presence of IgG isoagglutinins.

Detection of Incompatible Isoagglutinin in Serum of Newborn Infants. The direct antiglobulin test frequently fails to detect coating of red cells of newborn infants with anti-A or anti-B isoagglutinin. Nevertheless, the serum of such infants may contain incompatible isoagglutinin, e.g., anti-A in an infant A or anti-B in an infant B. For their detection the following methods are suitable.

REAGENTS

Test cell suspensions; see page 366, Reagents 3.

PROCEDURE

1. Into each of six properly identified test tubes place 2 drops of the serum to be tested.
2. To the first tube add 2 drops of saline-suspended red cells of group A_1; to the second, 2 drops of saline-suspended red cells of group B; and to the third, 2 drops of saline-suspended red cells of group O.
3. To the fourth, fifth, and sixth test tubes add 2 drops each of papain-treated red cells of groups A_1, B, and O, respectively.
4. Incubate the mixtures of serum and saline-suspended red cells in a water bath of 37° C. for 2 hours and check for presence of agglutination.
5. Test tubes not showing agglutination are converted into the indirect antiglobulin test and checked again for agglutination.
6. Test tubes with the serum and papain-treated red cells are incubated for 30 minutes in a water bath of 37° C.
7. The tubes are centrifuged for one-half minute and checked for agglutination.

INTERPRETATION

1. Presence of agglutination with saline-suspended red cells (step 4) before the indirect antiglobulin test indicates presence of IgM agglutinins.
2. Absence of agglutination before, and presence of agglutination after, the antiglobulin test as well as agglutination of papain-treated red cells, indicates presence of IgG agglutinins.
3. Presence of incompatible agglutinin is associated with subclinical or clinical hemolytic disease of the newborn caused by maternal isosensitization to A or B factors.

Note: Use of both antiglobulin and papain techniques is recommended, since in some instances only one of them may yield positive results. If so desired, titration of the isoagglutinins may be performed. Cells of group O serve as control for presence of isoantibodies other than anti-A and anti-B.

Crossmatching Tests. After blood has been selected for transfusion according to the principles detailed in a subsequent section (cf. p. 392), suitable tests *in vitro*—crossmatching tests—must be performed in each instance in order to insure absence of incompatibility between the blood to be transfused and the blood of the prospective recipient. Most importantly, one must make sure in the *"major crossmatch"* that the serum of the recipient does not contain isoantibodies capable of reacting with the transfused red cells. Of secondary, though sometimes considerable, importance in the *"minor crossmatch"* is absence in the transfused plasma of isoagglutinins capable of reacting with the recipient's red cells. It is essential that the tests be capable of detecting both IgM and IgG antibodies.

Note: The minor crossmatch test is not mandatory, provided adequate screening for presence of irregular antibodies has been done in blood of the donor. Nevertheless, routine inclusion of the minor crossmatch in compatibility testing is recommended in addition to screening for antibodies because it serves as an additional control capable of detecting some errors in ABO grouping of donor and recipient.

Major Crossmatch Tests

INDIRECT ANTIGLOBULIN TECHNIQUE

1. Prepare a 2 per cent suspension in saline of the red cells of the prospective donor.
2. Separate the serum of the recipient from a specimen of clotted blood obtained within 24 hours.
3. Into a properly identified test tube place 2 drops of the recipient's serum.
4. Add to the tube 2 drops of the 2 per cent suspension of the donor's red cells.
5. Centrifuge immediately for 1 minute.
6. Check for presence of agglutination.
7. If no agglutination is present, place in a water bath of 37° C. and incubate for 15 minutes.
8. Wash the red cells three times with tubefuls of saline, following the procedures outlined for the antiglobulin technique (cf. p. 371).
9. After the last washing, discard the supernatant and resuspend the red cells in the 1 drop of saline remaining in the tube.
10. Add 2 drops of the antiglobulin serum, centrifuge for 1 minute, and check for agglutination macroscopically and microscopically.

Interpretation

1. Agglutination observed in step 6 indicates incompatibility caused by IgM antibodies.
2. Agglutination that does not occur in step 6 but is found after performance of the antiglobulin test indicates incompatibility caused by IgG antibodies.

PROTEIN-ANTIGLOBULIN TECHNIQUE

1. Prepare a 5 per cent suspension in their own serum of the red cells of the prospective donor.

2. Into a properly identified test tube place 2 drops of the recipient's serum, 2 drops of the suspension of donor's red cells, and 2 drops of 22 per cent albumin.

3. Mix and centrifuge immediately.

4. Check for presence of agglutination.

5. If no agglutination is present, continue with steps 5 through 9 in the direct antiglobulin technique (p. 371).

Interpretation. Some IgG antibodies may produce agglutination in step 4, while others may be detectable only after application of the antiglobulin technique. Incubation of red cells with addition of albumin has been said to increase the sensitivity of the subsequent antiglobulin procedure (Griffitts *et al*, 1964; Stroup and MacIlroy, 1965).

ACTIVATED PAPAIN TECHNIQUE

Activated Papain Reagent. One gm. of papain is ground in a mortar with 100 ml of buffer (equal parts of $^{1}/_{15}$M Na_2HPO_4 and $^{1}/_{15}$M KH_2PO_4). After filtration of the solution, 0.3 gm. of 1-cysteine hydrochloride is added, and the mixture is incubated for 1 hour in a water bath of 37° C. The pH of the solution should be 6.4 to 6.7. The reagent is frozen in 2 ml. quantities, which are thawed as needed.

Technique

1. Into a properly identified test tube place 2 drops of the recipient's serum, 2 drops of the 2 per cent suspension in saline of the donor's red cells, and 2 drops of the activated papain reagent.

2. Incubate the test for 15 minutes in a water bath of 37° C.

3. Centrifuge for 30 seconds and check for agglutination macroscopically and microscopically.

Interpretation. Presence of agglutination indicates incompatibility caused by either IgM or IgG antibodies. This test is more sensitive than the indirect antiglobulin technique for detection of trace amounts of Rh-Hr antibodies. It may be converted into the indirect antiglobulin technique after the incubation period, thus detecting anti-Kell and some but not all anti-Duffy antibodies.

BROMELIN TECHNIQUE

Bromelin Reagent

Prepare buffer solution of pH 5.5 by mixing 96 ml. of $^{1}/_{15}$M KH_2PO_4 with 4 ml. of $^{1}/_{15}$M Na_2HPO_4. Suspend 0.5 gm. of bromelin in a mixture of 10 ml. of buffer and 90 ml. of saline. Add 0.1 gm. of sodium azide for prevention of bacterial and fungal growth. Dispense reagent into small tubes. These may be kept at 4° C. (stable for one month) or be stored at −20° C. (stable for four months or more).

Technique

1. Into a properly identified test tube place 2 drops of the recipient's serum, 1 drop of a 4 per cent suspension in saline of the donor's red cells, and 1 drop of the bromelin reagent. Mix.

2. Incubate at room temperature for 15 minutes.

3. Centrifuge and check for agglutination.

4. If no agglutination is present, incubate at 37° C. for 15 minutes.

5. Centrifuge and check for agglutination.

6. If no agglutination is present, the indirect antiglobulin test may be performed.

Interpretation. The bromelin technique gives results comparable to those obtained with the activated papain technique.

Minor Crossmatch Test. Proceed in the same way as outlined for the major crossmatch but use serum of the donor and red cell suspension of the recipient.

Note: In many laboratories the minor crossmatch is performed only through step 6 of the indirect antiglobulin technique. In this way only IgM agglutinins may be detected, and it is therefore important to prescreen serums of donors for presence of IgG antibodies, especially Rh antibodies in Rh-negative donors.

Crossmatch for Selection of Universal Donors and Transfusion of Universal Recipients. The blood to be selected should not have anti-A or anti-B hemolysin (cf. Six-tube technique, p. 367) and should have an anti-A or anti-B titer of less than 50 (cf. Screening procedure, p. 380). Nevertheless the minor crossmatch in such instances may always be expected to produce agglutination, since the serum of the donor contains an isoagglutinin reactive with the red cells of the recipient. The following technique (Grove-Rasmussen et al., 1953) is recommended for the minor crossmatch in order to avoid transfusion of potentially dangerous isoagglutinins.

1. To 0.1 ml. of the donor's serum add 0.3 ml. of solution of group-specific substances A and B.

2. Incubate the mixture at room temperature for 5 minutes.

3. To 0.1 ml. of this mixture add 0.1 ml. of a 2 per cent suspension in saline of the recipient's red cells.

4. Shake the tube and incubate for 15 minutes in a water bath of 37° C.

5. Convert into an indirect antiglobulin test.

INTERPRETATION. If agglutination is observed at the end of the test, it is not safe to transfuse the recipient with the blood selected.

Note: The modified minor crossmatch test and these considerations are not required if packed or resuspended red cells are to be transfused, that is, without the supernatant plasma. The test cannot be applied when the red cells of the recipient show a positive direct antiglobulin test.

Automated Procedures. Several models of a continuous-flow system are commercially available in the U.S.A. Basically, they consist of a sampler to pick up blood samples at given intervals, a proportional pump to advance selected amounts of samples and reagents through a continuous tubing system, a manifold made of glass coils and tubings to mix and incubate the reactants, and a recording device to record the results. Air bubbles are introduced into the system at a constant rate to mix reactants and to separate samples. Aggregates are decanted by gravity through a T-tube and thus separated from the free cells remaining in the main stream. Although the separation is incomplete, it does differentiate the reactive from the nonreactive sample. Three types of recording devices are available: (1) a continuously advancing strip of filter paper to receive the aggregates from the decanter, the most economical but least sensitive method; (2) a colorimeter-recorder and/or printer that indicates the level of hemoglobin liberated by a hemolyzing agent from red cells remaining in the main stream; and (3) an electronic counter-recorder and/or printer unit to compare the number of particles (aggregates and/or free cells) in the test samples with those in the control samples.

Two Immunochemical Approaches

ENZYME PROCEDURE. An enzyme, usually bromelin, is used to treat erythrocytes to enhance their reactivity. A rouleaux-forming reagent, usually PVP, is used to produce nonspecific aggregates of red blood cells; in the absence of specific antibody for the test cells, the aggregates are dispersed by isotonic sodium chloride solution, whereas presence of specific antibodies prevents dispersion of the aggregates.

LOW-ION MEDIUM PROCEDURE. Acidified low-ion medium is used to speed up attachment of antibodies to erythrocytes. A strongly positively charged agent, such as protamine or polybrene, is used to induce nonspecific aggregation of erythrocytes. Phosphate buffer or sodium citrate is used to disperse the aggregates without true antigen-antibody binding and, thus, to differentiate this reaction from a positive reaction induced by specific antibody.

Typing of Antigens

ROUTINE ABO AND RH TYPING. The enzyme procedure and filter paper recording system are being used. Reversed ABO typing and the automated reagin test (ART) for syphilis can be incorporated into the system. The 15-channel model with a capacity for handling 120 samples per hour has been found helpful in a large blood processing laboratory. Reagents to be used in the AutoAnalyzer have been licensed recently by the Bureau of Biological Standards.

SCREENING FOR RARE RED CELL ANTIGENS. Either the enzyme or low-ionic medium procedure can be used. A colorimeter-recorder or counter-recorder system is required to provide the necessary sensitivity. This technique has been found useful also for selection of "least incompatible blood" for patients with autoantibodies.

Detection and Identification of Antibodies

PRENATAL SCREENING TESTS. An automated system, either enzyme or low-ion medium technique, is more efficient for detection of Rh antibodies than are manual methods, espeially when a sensitive recording device is used. Titration of antibody in serum or in amniotic fluid can be carried out easily.

SCREENING OF BLOOD DONORS. Many laboratories screen the serum of every donor for irregular antibodies. Although automated procedures may not detect all antibodies, they have been found to be more sensitive than manual methods. They save a great deal of technologists' time, and the possibility of objective evaluation of recorded results of tests in parallel controls is a most desirable feature.

ANTIBODY IDENTIFICATION. A panel of red cells of known antigenic composition is placed in a sampler; as in manual methods, the specificity of the antibody in the test serum is demonstrated by the positive or negative reaction with each panel cell. When low-ion medium is used, the temperature of the bath surrounding the decanting section of coils and tubings may be increased slowly to initiate dissociation of antibodies from the cells. Under controlled conditions, antibodies of different specificity dissociate at different temperatures. Thus, an additional criterion for characterization of an antibody becomes available and may eliminate the need for the time-consuming absorption of cold agglutinins (Lee *et al.*, 1971; Berkman *et al.*, 1971).

Other Automated Procedures

THE DISCRETE SYSTEM. The French system is fully automated from sampling to print-out and is capable of handling 360 samples per hour. Reagents and properly identified samples are delivered into individual cuvettes, incubated, and centrifuged. Results are read optically, computed and printed out. This system is designed primarily for blood grouping.

AUTOMATED WASHERS FOR TRANSFUSION OF RED CELLS. At least three automated machines are available for washing red blood cells in a closed system. Usefulness of these devices has been established.

AUTOMATED WASHERS FOR TEST CELLS. Several table model centrifuges are capable of washing small numbers of cells automatically for antiglobulin and for other tests. One of these centrifuges can add antiglobulin serum automatically. These centrifuges have been found time-saving.

SPECIAL TECHNIQUES. The following techniques, initially developed for specialized research, may be of considerable help in the blood transfusion laboratory and do not demand excessive technical skill or facilities.

Absorption and Elution of Hemoantibodies. *Absorption* of hemoantibodies occurs in all hemagglutination reactions. When a particular antibody is to be removed from the serum as completely as possible, the following conditions must be met: red cells used for absorption should be as fresh as possible; they should contain the antigen reactive with the antibody, preferably in homozygous form ("double dose"); they must be free of antigens reacting with other antibodies present in the serum to be absorbed. Absorptions should be done at the temperature optimal for the particular antigen-antibody reaction. Absorption of hemoantibodies is required in order to (1) remove unwanted antibodies, e.g., cold agglutinins or anti-A and/or anti-B, from serums containing other hemoantibodies; (2) isolate an antibody, which after absorption can be eluted from the red cells; (3) separate mixtures of antibodies prior to identification of two or more antibodies present in the same serum.

TECHNIQUE

1. Wash red cells at least three times with large volumes of saline. After the last washing the supernatant should be colorless and transparent and should be removed as completely as possible.
2. Mix equal volumes of the packed red cells and the serum to be absorbed. Since absorption is more complete with large areas of contact, a container of sufficient size is to be used. Serums containing large amounts of antibody may have to be diluted prior to absorption.
3. Mix thoroughly and incubate at the desired temperature for a period of from 1 to 12 hours. The mixture should be frequently agitated.
4. After incubation, centrifuge and remove serum from the red cell sediment. If absorptions were carried out at 4° C., a refrigerated centrifuge or prechilled centrifuge cups should be used.
5. Test for presence of antibody in absorbed serum and, if present, compare its titer with that of the unabsorbed serum.
6. If *necessary*, repeat absorption.

Elution is the removal of antibodies absorbed by red cells *in vitro* or *in vivo.* Elutions are most commonly done in order to (1) isolate and identify antibodies after they were absorbed *in vitro;* (2) demonstrate antigen-antibody reactions which are too weak to yield unequivocal hemagglutination, e.g., agglutination of weak subgroups of A by anti-A antibody; (3) isolate and identify antibodies absorbed by red cells *in vivo,* e.g., maternal antibodies absorbed by fetal red cells of cord blood, antibodies responsible for hemolytic transfusion reactions, or autoantibodies coating red cells in autoimmune hemolytic anemia.

TECHNIQUE (LANDSTEINER'S HEAT ELUTION)

1. Wash the red cell suspension at least three times with large volumes of saline. If the supernatant of the third washing is found to contain antibody, washing must be continued until supernatant is free of antibody.
2. Mix equal volumes of the red cells to be eluted and saline. Serum of a person of group AB, free of hemoantibodies, may be substituted for saline, especially if one intends to store the eluted antibody for future use.
3. Place the mixture in a water bath of 56° C. for 10 minutes with frequent agitation.
4. Centrifuge the mixture at high speed in cups containing water of 56° C.
5. Remove supernatant and subject to proper tests.

Note: The eluate commonly shows evidence of hemolysis, which, as a rule, does not interfere with the subsequent tests. More complex techniques of elution have been described (see Technical Methods and Procedures of the American Association of Blood Banks, 1970, pp. 141–144).

Tests for Secretion of Blood-group Substances (A, B, H). Presence of substances with specificity of groups A, B, and H in saliva and other secretions is determined by a dominant Mendelian gene, called "secretor" (*Se*) (see page 351). The secretor property is tested in connection with unusual reactions of the ABO group antigens, in studies of the Lewis blood groups, and in genetic investigations. The principle of the test is the inhibition (neutralization) of anti-A, anti-B, or anti-H agglutinins by soluble blood group substance of the corresponding specificity.

TECHNIQUE

1. Preparation of saliva: Collect approximately 5 ml. of saliva. Place saliva into a clean test tube (10 by 15 mm.) and keep in a boiling water bath for 15 minutes. This procedure inactivates enzymes which are capable of hydrolyzing blood group specific substances. Centrifuge the boiled saliva and remove the clear supernatant. Unless test is done immediately, the specimen is to be kept frozen until use.
2. Antiserums: For persons of groups A and AB, anti-A serum; for persons of groups B and AB, anti-B serum; and for persons of any blood group, including group O, anti-H lectin can be used. Before use in the test, the highest dilution should be prepared which still yields readily visible agglutination consisting of many small clumps (++).
3. Place into each of four tubes 1 drop of the diluted antiserum. Add to tube 1, 1 drop of saline (positive serum control); to tube 2, 1

drop of saliva (test); to tube 3, 1 drop of saliva of known secretor (positive saliva control); to tube 4, 1 drop of saliva of known nonsecretor (negative saliva control). Mix and let stand for 10 minutes at room temperature.

4. To each of the four tubes add 1 drop of a 2 per cent suspension in saline of red cells of the proper group (A for anti-A serum, B for anti-B serum, O for anti-H lectin). Mix and centrifuge.

5. Read and record agglutination for each tube.

INTERPRETATION. Absence of agglutination in tube 2 indicates that the saliva donor is a secretor; presence of agglutination in tube 2 indicates that he is a nonsecretor. In order for the test to be valid, the control tubes must show the expected results: agglutination in tubes 1 and 4, no agglutination in tube 3.

Note: When the antiserum used is too strong and/or the soluble blood group substance is present in low concentration, inhibition may not be recognized and the person may be erroneously classified as a nonsecretor. In such instances more reliable results are obtained from quantitative tests in which the same amount of saliva is mixed with serial dilutions of the antiserum or the same amount of antiserum is mixed with different volumes or dilutions of saliva.

Long-term Preservation of Reagent Red Cells. Red cells possessing rare antigens or free of "universal" antigens (see page 364) may be preserved for prolonged periods in the frozen state by means of addition of glycerol. Small quantities of red cells can be preserved in liquid nitrogen without cryoprotective reagent.

REAGENTS FOR PRESERVATION WITH GLYCEROL

1. Citrate buffer. Dissolve 19.4 gm. of tribasic potassium citrate ($K_3C_6H_5O_7 \cdot H_2O$), 3.2 gm. of monobasic sodium phosphate ($NaH_2PO_4 \cdot 2H_2O$), and 2.9 gm. of dibasic anhydrous sodium phosphate (Na_2HPO_4) in 600 ml. of distilled water.
2. Glycerol (C.P. grade).
3. Buffered glycerol for freezing:
   - A. 60 per cent glycerol: Mix 40 ml. of citrate buffer with 60 ml. of glycerol.
   - B. 20 per cent glycerol: Mix 80 ml. of citrate buffer with 20 ml. of glycerol.
4. Buffered glycerol for deglycerolization:
   - A. 16 per cent glycerol citrate: 4 ml. of citrate buffer + 16 ml. of 20 per cent buffered glycerol.
   - B. 8 per cent glycerol citrate: 12 ml. of citrate buffer + 8 ml. of 20 per cent buffered glycerol.
   - C. 4 per cent glycerol citrate: 16 ml. of citrate buffer + 4 ml. of 20 per cent buffered glycerol.
   - D. 2 per cent glycerol citrate: 18 ml. of citrate buffer + 2 ml. of 20 per cent buffered glycerol.

Note: The glycerol reagents should be refrigerated when not in use.

TECHNIQUE

Freezing

1. Wash red cells three times with saline and remove supernatant after third centrifugation.
2. For each 10 ml. volume of packed red cells, add slowly and with constant mixing 5 ml. of 20 per cent buffered glycerol, followed by addition of 5 ml. of 60 per cent buffered glycerol.
3. Distribute mixture in small quantities (0.2 to 0.5 ml.) into small test tubes and store in deep freeze at –20° C. or lower temperatures.

Note: Tubes should be labeled with indelible ink and labels covered with cellophane.

Reconstitution

1. One or more tubes are removed from frozen storage and permitted to thaw at room temperature.
2. Centrifuge and remove supernatant.
3. Add a volume of 16 per cent buffered glycerol equal to the original volume, and mix well. Centrifuge and remove supernatant.
4. Repeat the procedure successively with 8 per cent, 4 per cent, and 2 per cent buffered glycerol, each time removing the supernatant before adding next solution.
5. After removing the last supernatant, wash three times with saline. Remove supernatant and suspend red cells in medium and concentration of choice.

Miscellaneous Tests. Several laboratory tests utilize hemagglutination, though they are not related to any of the specific blood factors described in the preceding sections: they may employ human red cells or red cells of a different species (heteroagglutinins). One important category is represented by autoagglutinins, i.e., antibodies capable of agglutinating the red cells of the same person from whom the serum is derived. They may be active either as "cold" or "warm" antibodies and be detectable by methods described for either IgM or IgG antibodies. These autoagglutinins are of particular importance in connection with the diagnosis of autoimmune hemolytic anemia. "Cold" autoagglutinins, usually referred to as cold agglutinins, form the basis of ancillary tests in diagnosis of atypical pneumonia (cf. p. 1229).

Heteroagglutinins for sheep red cells have been found to be increased in certain conditions, such as infectious mononucleosis, serum disease, and miscellaneous infections. Demonstration of increased titer and changes in absorption properties of sheep agglutinins is a part of the diagnostic test for infectious mononucleosis, as outlined in detail in another context (cf. p. 257).

Increased titers of agglutinin for sheep red cells previously sensitized with subthreshold amounts of antisheep hemolysin have been observed in serums of patients with rheumatoid arthritis (RA factor). As shown in subsequent work, other techniques can be used to detect this serum factor (cf. p. 1233).

Sources of Error in Hemagglutination Tests

False Negative Results

LACK OF SENSITIVITY OF AGGLUTINOGEN (BLOOD FACTOR) IN RED CELLS. Some agglutinogens, specifically A and B, are poorly developed in newborns and infants, reaching their full development with the age of approximately one year. Recent evidence has also been presented that such diseases as leukemia and cancer may in exceedingly rare cases change the reactivity of A and B factors. Reference to weakly reacting Rh factors has been made previously. An important extraneous factor lowering the reactivity of blood factors is the age of the blood specimen, especially if kept in a saline suspension and if not preserved at 4° C. Blood collected with an anticoagulant, as a rule, does not retain its full reactivity for more than one to two days. Clotted blood specimens properly preserved are fully reactive for at least five days, and the minimum reactivity needed for crossmatch tests is preserved for three weeks. Collection of blood in ACD solution has been found to provide better preservation of agglutinability of blood factors than is the case in clotted blood.

FAULTY CONCENTRATION OF RED CELL SUSPENSIONS. Too high a concentration may lead to an antigen excess, preventing union of the isoantibody with blood factors. On the other hand, a too dilute red cell suspension may interfere with observation of weak agglutinations.

FAULTY PROPORTION BETWEEN ANTIBODY AND RED CELL SUSPENSION. False negative reactions, representing prozone phenomena, may result from an excess of antibody in proportion to the amount of antigen present (i.e., quantity of red cells). Such "zoning" is especially common in undiluted serum with high titer of IgG Rh antibodies.

INADEQUATE ANTIBODY TITER IN SERUM. This is especially important in connection with blood grouping serums, such as anti-A, anti-B, and anti-Rh_0(D), for which minimum titers have been established by the Division of Biologics Standards of the National Institutes of Health (cf. p. 408). This assures the reliability of tests done with commercially distributed grouping serums. On the other hand, search for antibodies in unknown serums may give falsely negative results if the titer is below a certain threshold, especially if combined with a poorly reacting blood factor in the red cells used. Contrary to testing serums, the titers of antibodies in unknown serums are not subject to control. This makes it mandatory to use in such tests the most reactive form of red cell antigen available.

PRESENCE OF HEMOLYSIN. Since no agglutination for the specific blood factor tested may occur as a result of hemolysis, this may be interpreted erroneously as a negative result. Suspicion, however, should be raised by the absence or paucity of detectable red cells. Inactivation of such serum (30 minutes in water bath of 56° C.) destroys hemolytic reactivity so that agglutination can be observed in a test repeated with the inactivated specimen.

DEVIATION FROM OPTIMAL TEMPERATURE. Since some hemoantibodies react best at 4° C. and others at body temperature, it is important to observe such optimal temperatures in testing of low-titered antibodies in order not to miss weakly positive results.

INADEQUATE PERIODS OF INCUBATION. The lower the titer of the antibody and the poorer the reactivity of the blood factor (agglutinogen), the longer must be the periods of incubation in order to produce visible agglutination. Centrifugation and other forms of mechanical agitation may be used in order to shorten periods of incubation.

False Positive Results

PRESENCE IN THE SERUM OF UNSUSPECTED AGGLUTININS. This may occur with typing serums as well as with unknown specimens to be screened for presence of certain antibodies. Interfering antibodies most commonly encountered are cold agglutinins, warm autoagglutinins, and irregular agglutinins of specific nature, such as anti-P_1 and anti-Rh. Careful prescreening of grouping serums is a critical procedure. In the case of unknown serums, suitable red cell controls must be included in order to detect presence of unexpected agglutinins.

ROULEAUX FORMATION OR PSEUDOAGGLUTINATION. This is a reflection of the same phenomenon that is responsible for sedimentation of red cells in which the red cells adhere to each other, presenting a "stack of coins" appearance. Rouleaux formation is favored by the presence in serum of increased amounts of asymmetric protein molecules, such as fibrinogen and globulin, and by large surfaces, such as occurs in slide tests. Extreme rouleaux is commonly associated with certain diseases producing hyperproteinemia and hyperglobulinemia, such as multiple myeloma, kala-azar, Boeck's sarcoid, and cryoglobulinemia. The gross appearance of rouleaux may sometimes be difficult to differentiate from true agglutination, but as a rule the true nature of the phenomenon can be readily distinguished microscopically (cf. Fig. 5–5). In rouleaux formation individual red cells can be seen to separate readily from each other after mechanical agitation, such as tapping on the

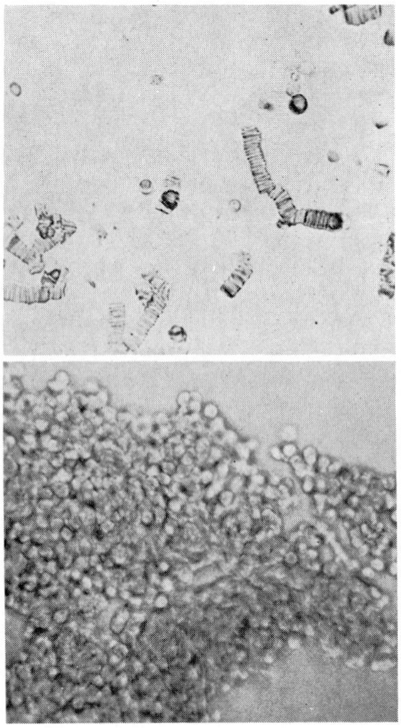

Figure 5-5. Microscopic appearance (×415) of rouleaux (*upper part*) and true agglutination (*lower part*).

slide, whereas this does not occur in true agglutinates. Actually, mechanical agitation favors true agglutination. Furthermore, red cell agglutinates exhibit deformation and discoloration of the red cells, while red cells in rouleaux retain the normal appearance. Dilution of serum with saline inhibits rouleaux formation, whereas true agglutination is not affected unless the titer is at a critically low level.

Large surface favors false agglutination such as rouleaux formation and may lead to errors; therefore, rouleaux formation is less pronounced in test tubes than on slides.

BACTERIAL CONTAMINATION. Certain microorganisms, such as *Vibrio cholerae,* "activate" receptors present in all red cells, designated as *"T agglutinogen,"* which react with the *T agglutinin* present in all serums except that of newborn infants. Such agglutination is independent of the presence or absence of any other blood factors (Hübener-Thomsen phenomenon). Bacterial contamination of the serum may impart to it the capacity to clump all red cells independent of presence or absense of any blood factors, a phenomenon called bacteriogenic hemagglutination (Davidsohn and Toharsky, 1942). It is obvious, therefore, that all precautions of asepsis must be taken in handling specimens and reagents used for hemagglutination.

PRACTICAL APPLICATIONS OF HEMAGGLUTINATION TESTS

Blood Transfusion. The numerous clinical considerations pertaining to hemotherapy cannot be discussed within the framework of this chapter. For information on this subject the reader is referred to monographs by Mollison (1972); "Standards for a Blood Transfusion Service," 1971–1972, and "Technical Methods and Procedures," 1970, published by the American Association of Blood Banks. The main purpose of the following outline is to discuss laboratory tests needed for the proper collection, processing, and selection of blood for transfusions.

Prescreening of Potential Blood Donors. The two main considerations in accepting potential blood donors are protection of the donor against any possible ill effects from the loss of blood and protection of the prospective recipient against any untoward effects from the transfusion. The first consideration necessitates that donors can be accepted only if they fulfill certain minimum requirements as to age, weight, and hemoglobin. In the most commonly employed screening test for hemoglobin, a drop of blood is permitted to fall into a solution of copper sulfate of known specific gravity. If the drop of blood descends to the bottom of the solution rather than floating or rising to the surface, the specific gravity of the blood is greater than that of the copper sulfate solution (see p. 110). Male donors should have a minimal hemoglobin concentration of 13.5 gm. per 100 ml.; that is, the drop of blood should have a specific gravity greater than a copper sulfate solution with specific gravity 1.055, while for female donors a minimal hemoglobin concentration of 12.5 gm. per 100 ml. is required, corresponding to a specific gravity exceeding that of a copper sulfate solution with specific gravity 1.053. Alternatively, determinations of the microhematocrit (p. 115) may be used for estimation of red cell mass in prospective donors. In order to be acceptable, male donors should have hematocrit of at least 41 per cent, female donors of at least 38 per cent. For his own protection a donor should not give blood more frequently than at intervals of eight to 10 weeks and not more often than five times a year. The second consideration—protection of the recipient—requires that the donor be free of any infectious or contagious disease, such as tuberculosis, rheumatic fever, or syphilis; and temperature, pulse, and blood pressure should be within the normal range. Donors who have had malaria or viral (infectious) hepatitis should never be accepted.

An adequate record of prescreening tests and answers to pertinent questions obtained from the prospective donor should be prepared and retained. Proper methods of identification of the donor and his record are of utmost importance prior to the collection of blood.

Collection of Blood. Although a variety of containers (glass, plastic) and methods (gravity, vacuum) can be employed for collection of blood and technical skill is important, the following precautions are essential: (1) elimination of any mistake in identity of donor and container assured by proper identification of the blood container and pilot tubes collected simultaneously; (2) aseptic handling of the collection and the container in order to avoid bacterial contamination; (3) use of proper anticoagulant and preservative solutions; (4) immediate refrigeration of the blood after collection; (5) storage of the blood in refrigeration equipment maintaining a temperature range of 2 to 4° C.; (6) addition of cryoprotective agents (glycerol), permitting storage of blood at −85° C. or below, or at −190° C. liquid nitrogen. Such blood can be used for transfusion for three years. This procedure is particularly useful for blood from "rare" donors and for autotransfusion.

Processing of Blood. The following tests are mandatory before blood can be released for transfusional use: (1) ABO grouping (p. 367); (2) Rh_0 typing (p. 370); (3) tests for presence of D^u (p. 370), when blood has been found to be Rh_0(D)-negative; (4) serologic test for syphilis; (5) test for hepatitis. Additional desirable tests are screening for high isoagglutinin titer in serum of group O blood (p. 380); screening for irregular antibodies of all serums, particularly for Rh antibodies in serums of Rh_0(D)-negative donors (p. 373); and identification of irregular antibodies when present (p. 376).

Note: There is no consensus on the need for testing Rh_0(D)-negative blood for presence of rh′(C) and rh″(E). In our opinion, only units of blood that contain neither Rh_0(D), including the weakly reactive variant D^u, nor rh′(C) and rh″(E), should be designated as "Rh-negative" and used for Rh_0(D)-negative recipients. The reason for this recommendation is not the remote hazard of isoimmunization to rh′(C) and/or rh″(E), but rather is based on the possibility that some prospective Rh_0(D)-negative recipients of transfusions, such as pregnant women or infants with hemolytic disease of the newborn, may have antibodies reactive with rh′(C) and/or rh″(E).

Only in special circumstances, such as unexplained difficulties in crossmatching or investigation of transfusion reactions (p. 395), is it necessary to carry out Rh subtyping (p. 371) of Rh_0(D)-positive blood or tests for subgroups of A in A and AB blood (p. 369).

At least once a day, and again before issuance, all units of blood should be inspected in order to detect any abnormal appearance, such as discoloration, hemolysis, and cloudiness, that may be an indication of faulty preservation or bacterial contamination. It is good practice to run bacterial cultures periodically on units of blood that have not been issued before the three-week period of useful shelf-life has ended or that have to be discarded for other reasons, such as positive serologic tests for syphilis. Results of such cultures provide information on the sterility of the collecting equipment and proper asepsis in handling and storage of blood.

Screening for Hepatitis B Antigen. Hepatitis associated antigen (HAA) is a term proposed in 1969 for an antigen that had been given three different names in the past: Australia (AU) antigen, serum hepatitis (SH) antigen, and hepatitis (H) antigen. Since the association of this antigen with Type B viral hepatitis became generally accepted, the term "Hepatitis B Antigen, HBAg" is being widely used.

HAA has been shown to be a large protein molecule with a trace of lipids but no carbohydrate and only a trace, if any, nucleic acids. Purified HAA has the electrophoretic mobility of an alpha globulin. HAA is found in all serum fractions except immunoglobulins. Presence of HAA in liver cells and glomeruli has been demonstrated by immunofluorescence and immunoelectron microscopy.

With electron microscopy, three important types of particles are demonstrable: (1) large spherical or hexagonal form (diameter about 42 nm.), with an inner core of about 27 nm. and an outer protein coat; it is known as the "Dane particle;" (2) spherical form (diameter from 18 to 25 nm.); and (3) spherical form (diameter about 27 nm.) found intranuclearly in hepatocytes ("Huang particle") and after treatment of Dane particles with Tween 80. Type 1 particle is considered to be the virus. Its protein coat resembles Type 2 particles. Two subtypes of HAA, Ad and Ay, have been demonstrated. With rare exceptions, only one of these subtypes has been found in an individual. In acute hepatitis, the incidence of each type is about equal; in chronic hepatitis or among blood donors, type Ad is prevalent, whereas type Ay is more frequent among drug users and in persons involved in renal dialysis. Positive cases in each outbreak show essentially only one of the two subtypes of HAA (see p. 1230).

Anti-HAA has been shown to be IgG; it is found in patients injected repeatedly with blood or blood components and rarely in apparently healthy persons. It was successfully produced by immunization in various animals.

BLOOD DONORS. General incidence of HAA is less than 0.5 per cent in North America and Europe. Incidence of HAA has been found consistently higher in paid donors as compared to voluntary donors.

HAA AND POST-TRANSFUSION HEPATITIS. About 7 million units of blood are used yearly in the USA. It is estimated that 150,000 recipients developed clinical or subclinical hepatitis, an incidence of over 2 per cent. When recipients of HAA-positive and HAA-negative blood were followed, the incidence of post-transfusion hepatitis was 50 per cent vs. 10 per cent in one report, and 16 per cent vs. 3 per cent in another. Thus, there is no doubt that use of HAA positive blood is associated with a much greater incidence of post-transfusion hepatitis. Therefore, the Bureau of Biological Standards requires, since October 1, 1971, that every unit of blood intended for transfusion and prepared in a licensed laboratory be tested for HAA.

The following recommendations may reduce the incidence of post-transfusion hepatitis: (1) prescribe blood transfusion only when it is definitely indicated; (2) consider autotransfusion; (3) use HAA-negative blood; (4) use blood of volunteer donors; and (5) use packed or washed red blood cells whenever feasible. (See page 393, Blood Component Therapy.)

Tests for HAA. Currently available tests for HAA are based on three types of immunologic reactions: precipitin formation, radioimmunoassay and complement fixation; only the first two types of tests are widely used.

Immunodiffusion Test for HAA. A precipitin line is formed when soluble antigen and its specific antibody diffuse toward each other and meet at a location where both reach optimal proportions. Thus, if their concentration is near their equivalent, a line is formed at an equal distance from their origins; if the concentration of one reagent is greater than that of the other, a line is formed closer to that with the lower concentration; if either concentration greatly exceeds the other, no lines form at all. A reagent composed of smaller molecules migrates quicker and forms a line curved toward the reagent consisting of larger molecules. The longer the distance between the two origins, the more time is needed to form a line. Normally one to seven days at room temperature are required to form the precipitin line. The size of wells accommodating the reagents and the total amount of reagent added will also affect the results.

Since neither monospecific anti-HAA antibody nor purified HAA are readily available, identification of the precipitin line requires simultaneous use of known antigen and antibody reacting side by side with the test serum. Fusion of precipitin lines of test serum and that of control serum indicates that test and control serums contain identical antigens; the formation of a spur, or spurs, indicates partial identity; two lines crossing each other indicate nonidentity. Detection and identification of HAA and anti-HAA can be accomplished in one operation if a known control serum is placed next to each test serum (Fig. 5–6). Fivefold concentration of the test serum increases the sensitivity of the test.

Electroimmunodiffusion Test for HAA. Electroimmunodiffusion is also known as

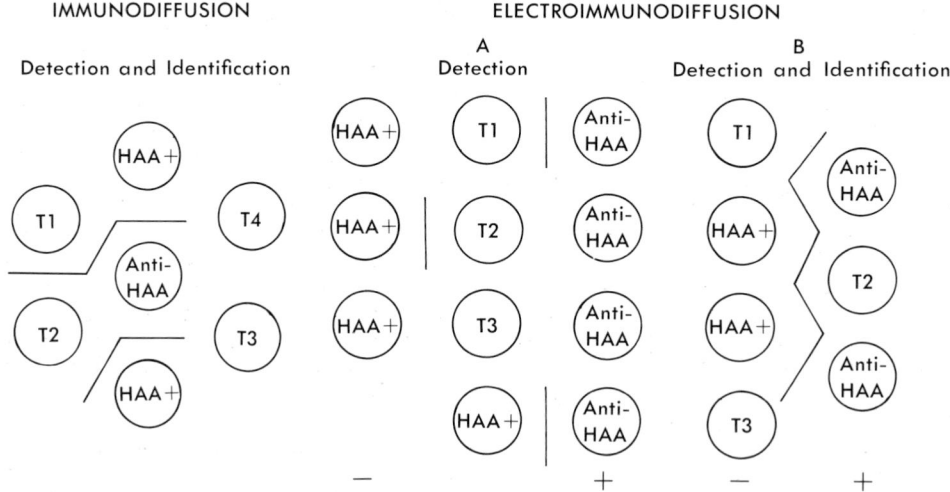

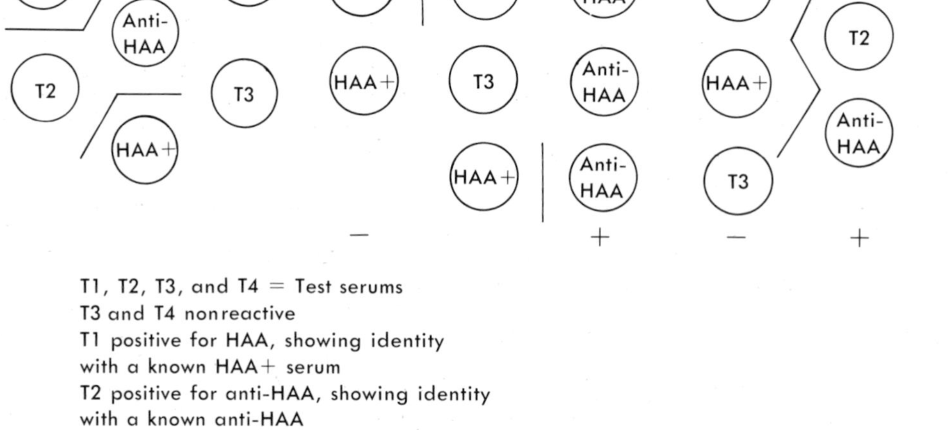

Figure 5–6. Tests for HAA and anti-HAA.

immunoelectroosmophoresis (IEOP), counter electrophoresis (CEP), or electroprecipitin (EP) test. Basically it is the application of electric current to speed up the process of immunodiffusion. There are a number of factors affecting this process. The power supply provides the driving force. Many laboratories obtain satisfactory results with a power supply providing 50 to 75 volts and 25 to 40 mA, measured at the ends of the agarose plate. Barbital or Tris buffer should have an ionic strength from 0.025 to 0.10 μ and a pH value from 8.2 to 9.0. Wicks made of a bath towel or sponges provide good conductivity; when sponges are used, the agarose plate should be placed face down. Household aluminum foil can be used as disposable electrodes. A properly designed disposable plastic box may be the most desirable type of electrophoretic chamber.

Serum proteins in an alkaline medium are negatively charged and migrate toward the positive pole in an electric field. Gamma globulins, which have a lesser negative charge, migrate toward the negative pole through the action of osmosis. Osmosis is created by the countermovement of the fluid in a supporting medium which is also negatively charged but unable to move toward the positive pole. The negative charges of agarose, a commonly used supporting medium, are derived from its impurity content; hence, a highly purified agarose may not be suitable for electroimmunodiffusion. Each brand and each lot of agarose should be tested before routine use.

Since anti-HAA is a gamma globulin and HAA is an alpha globulin, they migrate in different directions in an electric field. When they are properly placed, they migrate toward each other and form a precipitin line. Under influence of an electric current, both antigen and antibody move in narrow bands instead of diffusing into 360 degrees as in immunodiffusion; consequently, electroimmunodiffusion is not only faster but also more sensitive than immunodiffusion.

Agarose plates are prepared by spreading about 0.75 ml. of 1 per cent agarose per square inch on a glass or plastic plate. The size of the wells is usually from 2 to 3 mm. in diameter to accommodate about 5 to 10 μl. of reagents. The distance between two adjacent wells is from 3 to 5 mm.

For detection of HAA alone two wells are required per test serum; the addition of a third well near the negative pole to accommodate known HAA makes it possible to detect also anti-HAA in the test serum in the same operation (Fig. 5–6*A*).

The wells for concurrent detection and identification of HAA and anti-HAA by electroimmunodiffusion are arranged in the pattern shown in the diagram (Fig. 5–6*B*). Serum T-1 reacts with a known anti-HAA in forming a precipitin line showing identity with known HAA; thus, HAA in the T-1 serum is detected and identified. Anti-HAA in the T-2 serum is detected and identified in a similar fashion. Two additional advantages of this setup are sensitivity and economy: it is capable of showing identity of HAA not detectable by immunodiffusion technique; for two test serums only one well of anti-HAA is required instead of two wells in the normal pattern.

The time needed for electrophoresis varies with the particular setup. Using optimal conditions, it is unnecessary to run the test for more than 30 minutes, the minimum time required for crossmatching the same unit of blood.

Only anti-HAA approved by the Bureau of Biological Standards or of equivalent quality should be used. Excessive amounts of lipoprotein in the antiserum often interfere with the reading of results. Control HAA is equally important; preferably it should be weakly reactive and be included in each test plate.

The reading of faint precipitin lines requires some experience. The use of an oblique illumination against a dark background is definitely helpful; magnifying lenses or a dissection microscope of up to 10× magnification is a valuable aid. Staining is recommended for beginners to confirm preliminary readings. Any positive results should be repeated with an identity test if not done concurrently with detection.

Radioimmunoassay for HAA. The current radioimmunoassay procedure for HAA is based on a sandwich principle instead of competitive binding as in many other radioimmunoassay methods. Test samples are added to plastic tubes precoated with unlabeled anti-HAA antibodies. Tubes are incubated and washed. If HAA is present in the sample, it will become attached to the antibodies in the tube and will not be washed off. Anti-HAA serum labeled with ^{125}I is then added. After another period of incubation, tubes are washed and counted with a gamma counter. The presence of HAA is indicated by the higher counts derived from the radioactive antibodies retained by the HAA which are bound to the unlabeled antibodies in the tube, as compared with the negative controls. This procedure has been found highly sensitive and reproducible. However, it requires overnight incubation and may give false positive reactions when guinea pig anti-HAA is used as the source of antibodies.

None of the currently available tests for HAA can identify all donors capable of transmitting hepatitis; hence, a negative test for HAA does not exclude the possibility of transmitting hepatitis.

Since HAA is infectious material, it should be handled with great care. Tests are preferably done in a room restricted to this purpose. Drinking, eating, smoking, and pipetting by mouth are prohibited. If HAA-positive controls are kept in glass tubes, they should be placed into plastic bags or other forms of unbreakable containers. Whenever possible, disposable pipettes should be used for serum or whole blood. Gloves should be used to handle known HAA or HAA-contaminated utensils or instruments. Waste material should be disposed in a well-insulated container and preferably autoclaved before disposal (Symposium on Virus Hepatitis, 1970; Maugh, 1972; Lee *et al.*, 1971).

Selection of Blood. Adequate selection of blood requires close and intelligent cooperation between clinicians and blood bank staff. With rare exceptions, as explained later on, adequate pretransfusion tests are required for proper selection of blood. Clotted blood (quantities of 5 to 10 ml. are desirable) should be obtained from the prospective recipient, preferably within 24 hours before anticipated administration of blood. When the pretransfusion specimen is to be obtained from a patient receiving an intravenous infusion, care must be taken to collect the blood from another site. The blood is used for ABO grouping (p. 367) and Rh_0(D) typing (p. 370). In the case of infants or debilitated patients presenting difficulties for venipuncture, blood may be obtained by skin punctures in capillary tubes, which are centrifuged in order to yield red cell suspensions and serum for the crossmatch tests.

The primary consideration in selection of blood is to provide a unit of the same ABO group as that of the recipient. Furthermore, Rh_0(D)-positive recipients should receive Rh_0 (D)-positive blood, whereas for Rh_0(D)-negative recipients blood of type rh(cde) should be used. The pilot tube of a unit satisfying these criteria is then utilized for crossmatching tests as outlined previously (p. 382). Evidence of compatibility in major and minor crossmatch tests must be established before release of blood for transfusion.

It is important to screen the serum of the recipient for the presence of irregular antibodies concomitantly with or prior to crossmatching, since this may disclose irregular antibodies, including autoantibodies and cold agglutinins. If unexpected incompatibility is encountered in crossmatching tests, all possible sources of error should be investigated, preferably by repeating the test with a new specimen of the recipient and using other donor pilot tubes of suitable ABO and Rh type. Cold agglutinins are a common source of unexpected incompatibility, and their presence can be confirmed as outlined on p. 404. Selection of blood for patients with autoimmune hemolytic anemia often poses difficult problems, since complete compatibility can rarely be obtained. Testing with numerous units, usually by using serial dilutions of the patient's serum, may disclose some blood specimens that are less incompatible and, hence, presumably more suitable for transfusion. Crossmatching with serial dilutions of the recipient's serum is recommended in order to avoid the pitfall of prozone phenomena. The clinician should be advised of the findings before blood is released for transfusion. All specimens of pilot tubes of the units and of recipients used for crossmatching should be preserved under refrigeration for at least seven days after administration of the transfusion, since these specimens are indispensable for proper investigation of transfusion reactions if such occur (p. 395).

New specimens for crossmatching tests must be obtained from the recipient and used for selection of blood whenever more than 24 hours have elapsed since a previous transfusion. In other words, it would be a serious error to use a blood specimen obtained prior to a transfusion given two or three days before and to use it to select blood for a new transfusion, because subthreshold levels of irregular antibodies may have been present in the earlier specimen and may have escaped detection. The intervening transfusion then could have stimulated a rapid rise of such antibodies that could produce gross incompatibility with subsequently given blood, thus leading to serious hemolytic reactions.

In addition to serologic factors, there are other important considerations in selection of blood, such as the quantity of blood to be transfused. Basically this depends on medical judgment. Units commonly available contain 450 ml. of blood. In specific conditions it is advisable to give smaller amounts in order not to overload the circulation; on the other hand, much larger amounts may be needed for replacement of blood volume. Transfusion of a single unit of blood is only rarely indicated, except when it becomes apparent that a patient transfused with one unit does not require any additional blood. Nobody who is aware of the hazards of transmission of disease, isoimmunization, and similar potential untoward effects of blood transfusions can ever justify hemotherapy merely as a "tonic" or symptomatic treatment. Furthermore, blood is always in short supply and must be reserved for those in need of massive blood replacement during surgery, current demands being especially high in connection with open-heart surgery.

Close cooperation between clinician and hemotherapist is also required in connection with qualitative aspects of blood for transfusion, such as the age of stored blood. When replacement of blood volume is the indication for transfusion, blood of the appropriate type with the longest shelf-life is to be used so as to avoid excessive loss from overaging. On the other hand, for patients with certain diseases, blood within specified age limits is necessary or preferred. Patients needing blood because of inadequate erythropoiesis (aplastic or hypoplastic anemia) or excessive red cell destruction (hemolytic anemia) should be given blood not older than five days, since this will provide red cells with maximum survival. Likewise, transfusions to patients with hemorrhagic diseases should utilize blood not older than five to seven days, because some of the coagulation factors may deteriorate during more prolonged storage. Patients with advanced renal or cardiovascular disease should not receive blood older than seven days, since plasma potassium concentrations of blood increase with storage and may be injurious to such recipients. Analogous considerations hold true for patients with advanced liver disease in relation to rising ammonia levels in stored blood.

Finally, certain donors should be specifically excluded from use for certain patients: namely, the husband should never be a donor for his wife or a child for his mother. It is also not advisable to transfuse a patient with the blood of the same donor more than once. All these restrictions are based on the greater liability to isoimmunization that has been proved to be associated with these circumstances of transfusions.

Selection of Blood for Newborn and Young Infants. Because isoagglutinins are not formed until a few months after birth (cf. p. 351), reliable crossmatching tests cannot be performed with the serum of newborn or young infants. Any isoagglutinins present in such infants are derived from the maternal serum as a result of transplacental transmission. Hence, it is mandatory that the major crossmatching test in selection of blood for infants be carried out with the serum of the mother. If the child is between one to three months of age, the major crossmatch test should be done with both the serum of mother and the serum of infant, since passively transferred as well as actively formed isoagglutinins may be present at this age. Additional considerations apply to transfusion of infants with hemolytic disease of the newborn, as discussed in the subsequent section (p. 398).

"Universal" Donor and "Universal" Recipient. In some circumstances it may be necessary to deviate from the rule of administering blood of the same ABO group as the recipient (e.g., when Rh-negative blood of type B or AB is not available). Use of O Rh-negative blood is then necessary for recipients who are A or B, or AB Rh-negative recipients may be transfused with A or B Rh-negative blood. However, whenever a transfusion involves "universal donors" or "universal recipients," precautions must be taken in order to eliminate the risk of damaging the recipient's red cells by the transfused isoagglutinins. The safety of such transfusions should be established by the following criteria: The serum of the blood to be used should not possess hemolysin for the red cells of the prospective recipient; e.g., group O blood with anti-A hemolysin should not be used for a recipient of group A or AB. The titer of the reactive isoagglutinin should be less than 50 (cf. p. 380). The minor crossmatch test should be performed with the neutralized serum of the donor as outlined on p. 383. Only if this test fails to show agglutination is it safe to use the "universal" donor for a recipient of another blood group or to transfuse the "universal" recipient with the blood tentatively selected. Hazards associated with transfusions of "universal donor" blood can be minimized by partial or complete removal of the plasma whenever circumstances permit.

Another situation in which "universal" donor blood may have to be used is the "emergency" transfusion, when the urgency of replacement of blood volume precludes spending any time for pretransfusion tests. In this event it is best to use O Rh-negative (cde) blood with low titers of anti-A and anti-B that is free of any irregular antibodies. The decision to administer blood without pretransfusion tests must be made by the physician in charge, since it involves definite calculated risks: in rare instances the patient may already possess an antibody for one of the factors in the transfused blood. In addition, there is the delayed risk of isoimmunization. Obviously this procedure is therefore justifiable only in a true emergency but not in pseudoemergencies, such as failure to request on time or to prepare blood for surgery or similar circumstances.

"Blood Component Therapy." 1969; "A Prac-
of plastic containers with multiple tubings and the availability of large capacity refrigerated centrifuges make it possible to separate whole blood into different components and derivatives. In this way, each recipient receives the required component without unwanted and often undesirable components; each unit can be used effectively to fullfill the needs of several patients. Detailed information on this subject can be found in publications of the American Association of Blood Banks: "Manual of Blood Component Preparation," 1969; "Blood Component Therapy," 1969; "A Practical Workshop," Houston, Texas, 1969. A summary of blood component therapy is listed in Table 5–16.

Technique of Blood Transfusions. Although technical aspects cannot be dealt with in detail, it is important to be aware of the need for strict observance of the following precautions:

Table 5–16. BLOOD COMPONENT THERAPY

BLOOD OR BLOOD COMPONENTS	UNIT APPROX.	SHELF LIFE	INDICATIONS
1. Whole blood Hematocrit 40±%	510 ml.	21 days	Acute blood loss from injury, surgery, or disease
2. Red blood cells Hematocrit 70±% Packed	300 ml.	21 days 1 day (if open)	Anemias, especially in cardiovascular diseases (lower volume and lower potassium) and in liver and kidney diseases (less anticoagulant and less unwanted metabolites from storage)
3. Red blood cells, fresh or frozen Washed	200 ml.	1 day	Same as 2
4. Leukocyte concentrate	15 ml.	1 day	Agranulocytosis, granulocytopenia
5. Leukocyte-poor blood	200 ml.	1 day	Leukocyte antibodies; febrile transfusion reactions Potential recipient of tissue transplant
6. Platelet concentrate	15 ml.	3 days	Thrombocytopenia, qualitative platelet disorders
7. Single donor plasma, fresh frozen (−30° C.)	240 ml.	1 year	To maintain the blood volume To supply coagulation factors To supplement plasma for exchange transfusion
8. Cryoprecipitate	15 ml.	1 year	Hemophilia A, afibrinogenemia
9. Lyophilized anti-hemophilic factor	2–10 ml.	2 years	Hemophilia A
10. Fibrinogen	1 or 2 gm.	5 years	Hypofibrinogenemia, afibrinogenemia
11. Gamma globulin (Ig) Anti-Rh_0 (D) Ig	10 ml. 300 μg.	3 years 1½ years	Prophylaxis or treatment of some infections Prevention of Rh immunization
12. Albumin (60° C. 10 hr.)	5–25%	4 years	To maintain blood volume To bind unwanted metabolites, such as bilirubin, Hgb

REMARKS: Centrifugation: None for #1 and some #2; 5000 G 5 min. for #2, #3, #4, #5, #7 at 44° C. and for #6 at room temperature; 4100 G 10 min. at 4° C. for #8.
Implicated in hepatitis: Not reported for #11 and #12; very low for #3; yes for others.
Derivatives: #9, #10, #11, and #12 require special preparation not done in blood banks.

All safeguards must be taken to insure proper identity of the blood selected and of the patient to be transfused. Some of the most serious transfusion accidents have resulted from human errors in identification of recipient and donor blood. An error in blood grouping is fraught with greater danger than in any other laboratory procedure. Here are some of the reasons justifying such a statement. In most other tests the clinician has an opportunity to check the laboratory report with the clinical findings in the patient. When the white blood count or a blood sugar determination is high or when the serologic test for syphilis is positive, the clinician must not accept it if it does not agree with the findings in the patient; he does not have to base his treatment, be it medical or surgical, on the laboratory result without questioning. He may repeat the test or he may repeat the examination of the patient and find an explanation for the discrepancy without jeopardizing the patient's health. Not so in blood grouping. Here the test is done as a preliminary to transfusion. There is no relation between the blood group and the physical condition of a person; hence, the clinician has no means of checking the results. He is entirely dependent on the laboratory. If the result of the blood grouping or crossmatching test is incorrect, the error may become apparent too late to be corrected. There is no simple way of taking out the incompatible blood once it has been introduced into the patient's circulation. That is why accuracy, so important in all laboratory tests, is even more important in blood grouping and crossmatching tests. All possible checks should be included that may prevent errors and that may call attention to an error if it has crept in. This is the reason for emphasis on accuracy, on prevention of errors, and on detection of errors. The importance of speed in blood grouping and crossmatching tests is obvious. They are carried out in life-saving emergencies more often than any other laboratory test. However, the need for speed can be met in any well-organized laboratory by having a tray with all necessary reagents ready at all times and by having a blood grouping team so that one or more technicians can drop whatever task they are doing at the moment and work together to turn out the result in the shortest possible time without sacrificing accuracy. The trouble with some of the short-cut methods is that while they have something to recommend them in emergencies, when time is at a premium, they are used all too often when there is not the slightest indication for excessive speed. It must always be remembered that excessive speed invites errors. Strictest asepsis must be observed in administration of the blood. Excessive speed or excessively slow administration of blood must be avoided. No solution other than physiologic saline or glucose in physiologic saline should be administered through the same set as blood. Specifically, so-called isotonic glucose solution in water should be avoided, since it has been found capable of hemolyzing blood mixed with it. Finally, close observation of the patient during the transfusion is essential to detect as soon as possible any untoward reactions that may occur.

Investigation of Transfusion Reactions. The main purpose of such investigations is to rule out or to prove that a specific reaction reflects hemolysis of transfused red cells brought about by antibodies present in the recipient or, more rarely, destruction of recipient's red cells by transfused antibodies. Table 5–17 lists the common clinical symptoms as well as the classic laboratory findings that characterize the main categories of transfusion reactions. It must be stressed that absence of clinical symptoms does not conclusively eliminate a specific cause of a reaction. On the other hand, certain clinical findings, such as urticarial eruptions, may occur in more than one type of reaction and therefore by themselves do not permit definitive diagnosis. Finally, some reactions, including hemolytic ones, may be asymptomatic and escape detection unless there is careful follow-up of the recipient immediately or soon after the transfusion, preferably including a check of his hematologic status in order to obtain valid indications for survival of the transfused red cells.

The most common potential causes of hemolytic transfusion reactions are listed in Table 5–18 with reference to the ABO, Rh, and other blood group systems that may be involved.

As shown in Figure 5–7, a fairly constant chain of events takes place. Changes in serum bilirubin, bilirubinuria, azotemia, and urinary output follow a predictable course and are of great prognostic value for the ultimate fate of the patient. Hemoglobinemia and hemoglobinuria may be demonstrable within a few hours after administration of incompatible blood; peak values of this most direct evidence of intravascular hemolysis are found most frequently about 24 hours later, while 48 hours after the transfusion they can be detected only exceptionally. Jaundice and its corollary, bilirubinemia, become manifest approximately 24 to 48 hours later. Renal insufficiency, which may culminate in anuria, with resulting accumulation of nitrogenous wastes in the blood, may become noticeable any time after the first

Table 5–17. TRANSFUSION REACTIONS

TYPE OF REACTION	MOST CHARACTERISTIC CLINICAL SYMPTOMS	MOST CHARACTERISTIC LABORATORY FINDINGS
Hemolytic	Precordial pain Lumbar pain Chills Drop in blood pressure Oliguria → anuria Jaundice	Hemoglobinemia Hemoglobinuria Hypohaptoglobinemia Azotemia → uremia Elevation of indirect serum bilirubin
Pyrogenic (febrile)	Chills or fever	Isoleukoagglutinins
Allergic	Urticarial eruptions	———
Bacterial contamination	Severe hypotension Shock Anuria	Gram negative rods in direct smear of unit of transfused blood
Circulatory overload	Acute heart failure Pulmonary edema	———

Table 5–18. COMMON CAUSES OF HEMOLYTIC TRANSFUSION REACTIONS BASED ON BLOOD GROUP INCOMPATIBILITY

A. ANTIBODY PRESENT IN RECIPIENT

RECIPIENT WITH BLOOD GROUP	RECIPIENT WITH ANTIBODY	TRANSFUSED WITH BLOOD OF GROUP
O	anti-A and anti-B	A, B, or AB
A	anti-B	B or AB
B	anti-A	A or AB
rh(cde) rh′(Cde) rh″(cdE)	*anti-Rh_0(D)	Rh_1(CDe), Rh_0(cDe), Rh_2(cDE), or Rh_1Rh_2(CDE)
rh(cde)	*anti-rh′(C)	Rh_1(CDe), Rh_1Rh_2(CDE), or rh′(Cde)
rh(cde)	*anti-rh″(E)	Rh_2(cDE), Rh_1Rh_2(CDE), or rh″(cdE)
Rh_1(CDe)	*+anti-rh″(E)	Rh_2(cDE), Rh_1Rh_2(CDE), or rh″(cdE)
Rh_2(cDE)	*+anti-rh′(C)	Rh_1(CDe), Rh_1Rh_2(CDE), or rh′(Cde)
Rh_1Rh_1(CCDe)	*+anti-hr′(c)	rh(cde), Rh_0(cDe), Rh_1rh(CcDe), Rh_2(cDE), or Rh_1Rh_2hr′-positive (CcDE)
X-negative++	anti-X++	X-positive++

*Always result of isoimmunization.
+Occurs only exceptionally.
++Refers to blood factors such as Kell (K), Duffy (Fy^a), and so forth.

B. ANTIBODY PRESENT IN DONOR

DONOR WITH BLOOD GROUP	DONOR WITH ANTIBODY	TRANSFUSED INTO RECIPIENT HAVING BLOOD OF GROUP
O	"immune" or IgG anti-A or anti-B	A, B, or AB
A	"immune" or IgG anti-B	B or AB
B	"immune" or IgG anti-A	A or AB
rh(cde) rh′(Cde) rh″(cdE)	*anti-Rh_0(D)	Rh_1(CDe), Rh_2(cDE), Rh_0(cDe), or Rh_1Rh_2(CDE)
X-negative+	anti-X+	X-positive+

*Always result of isoimmunization.
+Refers to blood factors Kell (K), Duffy (Fy^a), and so forth.

24-hour interval following the transfusion. It is the complication which actually decides the ultimate fate of the patient; either subsiding with recovery of the patient, or proceeding toward a fatal outcome. Changes in the titer of the isoagglutinins responsible for the transfusion reaction are of considerable interest: immediately after administration of the blood a significant drop in antibody titer takes place because of removal by antigen-antibody union. Subsequently, that is within the next four to five days, the antibody rises, reaching a high titer within one to two weeks following administration of incompatible blood.

Whenever a patient exhibits untoward reactions during or following blood transfusion, such as chills and fever, skin eruptions, drop or rise in blood pressure, hemoglobinuria, jaundice within hours or a few days, and symptoms of renal failure such as oliguria and progressive azotemia, a complete and thorough investigation must be carried out. In order to make this possible, the pretransfusion specimen of the recipient and the pilot tube of the unit used must be preserved for at least seven days as mentioned previously. It is also desirable to return the container after conclusion of the transfusion to the blood bank so that blood remaining in it will be available for testing of identity and for detecting possible bacterial contamination.

As soon as a reaction is noted, a blood specimen of the recipient must be obtained and a urine specimen collected. Urinary output should be subsequently measured as long as indicated.

Table 5–19 lists the tests to be carried out on blood and urine specimens. Of particular importance are repeat tests for the ABO group and Rh type of the recipient's pre- and posttransfusion specimens, the donor pilot tube, and the blood remaining in the container if available. Crossmatching tests must be repeated with both pretransfusion and posttransfusion specimens, using sensitive methods for detection of incomplete antibodies. A finding lending strong support to diagnosis of a hemolytic transfusion reaction is a drop in concentration, or disappearance of serum haptoglobin observed in a posttransfusion specimen (Fink *et al.*, 1967).

It has recently been shown that some pyrogenic (febrile) reactions are caused by presence of leukoagglutinins in the recipient. Persons most likely to develop leukoagglutinins are recipients of multiple previous transfusions and multiparous women, the latter apparently being immunized by fetal leukocytic antigens (Dausset, 1954; Payne, 1957; and Brittingham and Chaplin, 1957). The presence of leukoagglutinins may be detected by tests described on page 411. Demonstration of this etiology of pyrogenic febrile transfusion reactions is im-

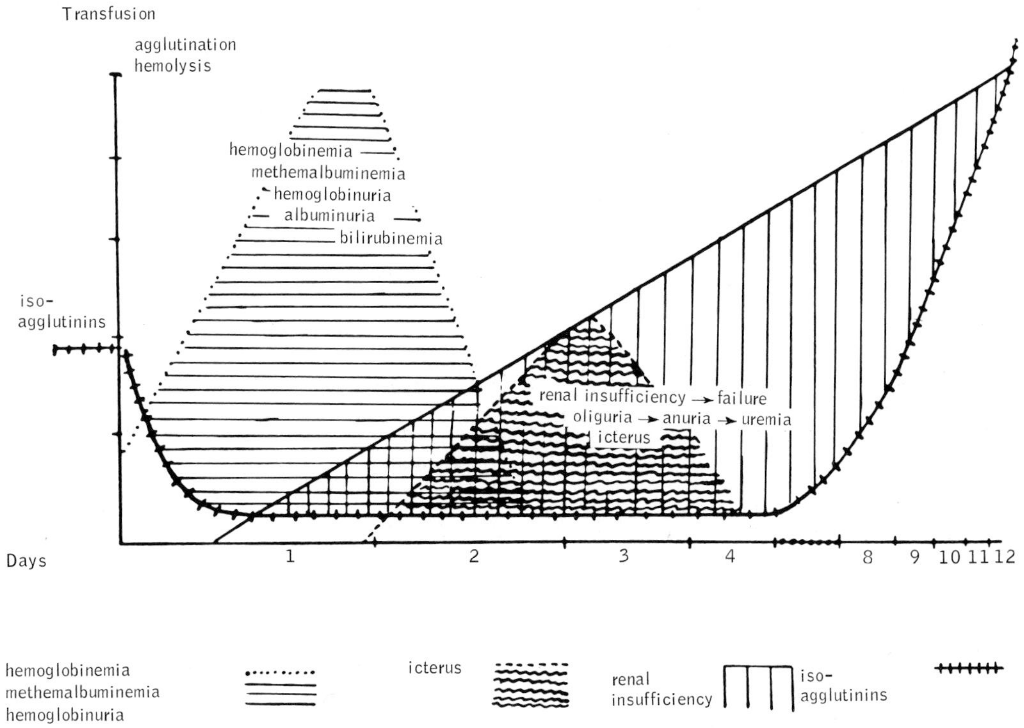

Figure 5–7. Course of laboratory and clinical findings in hemolytic transfusion reactions. (From Davidsohn, I. and Stern, K.: Diagnosis of hemolytic transfusion reactions. Am. J. Clin. Path., 25:381, 1955.)

Table 5–19. LABORATORY TESTS CAPABLE OF DETERMINING NATURE OF TRANSFUSION REACTION

A. ESSENTIAL TESTS

MATERIAL NEEDED			OPTIMUM TIME OF EXAMINATION AFTER REACTION		
RECIPIENT	DONOR	TEST(S)	FROM	TO	CAPABLE OF DETECTING
Pretransfusion blood specimen	Pilot tube; blood remaining in container	ABO and Rh typing	Immediate		Technical or clerical errors
Pretransfusion specimen	Pilot tube	Crossmatch	Immediate		Incompatibility
	Blood remaining in container	Bacteriologic study (smear, culture)	Immediate		Bacterial contamination
Posttransfusion blood specimen					
a. citrated or oxalated		Microscopic examination	Immediate	6-12 hours	Presence of clumps
b. red cell suspension		Direct anti-globulin test	Immediate	12-48 hours	Coating of red cells by antibody
c. plasma or serum		Hemoglobin	Immediate	48 hours	Hemoglobinemia (intravascular hemolysis)
d. serum		Indirect bilirubin	24 hours	72 hours	Hyperbilirubinemia*
e. serum		Urea N or NPN	36 hours		Azotemia
Urine		a. Hemoglobin	Immediate	48 hours	Hemoglobinuria (intravascular hemolysis)
		b. Volume	Immediate	Recovery	Oliguria (renal failure)

B. CORROBORATIVE TESTS

RECIPIENT	DONOR	TEST(S)	FROM	TO	CAPABLE OF DETECTING
Red cells		Complete typing	Immediate	6-12 hours	Blood factor incompatible with serum of donor
Serum		a. Antibody screening	Immediate	6-12 hours	Antibody specific for blood factor in red cells of donor
		b. Antibody titer	Immediate	4-5 days	Low titer (e.g., anti-A in B recipient after transfusion of A blood)
		c. Antibody titer	6 days	Several months	Rising titer (e.g., anti-A in B recipient after transfusion of A blood)
Urine		Protein	Immediate	Variable	Proteinuria
Kidney biopsy or autopsy		Histopathologic study	36 hours	10 days	Hemoglobinuric nephrosis

*To compare with pretransfusion specimen if possible.

portant practically, since considerable difficulties are encountered in hemotherapy of such patients, especially if they require repeated transfusions because of conditions such as aplastic anemia or myelofibrosis. If pyrogenic reactions are found to be associated with the presence of leukoagglutinins or if this mechanism is suspected even though it is not established, they can in most instances be readily eliminated by using for transfusion a red cell mass prepared in such a manner as to be practically free of leukocytes.

When it is suspected that a reaction may be due to bacterial contamination of the transfused blood, thorough bacteriologic examination must be carried out by means of direct smears as well as by culture of the blood. (For methods suitable for this purpose, see Chap. 18.) It must be specifically emphasized that such cultures must be incubated not only at 37° C. but also at 30 to 32° C. and preferably even at lower temperatures, since the contaminating organisms may be psychrophilic (that is, they may grow best, or exclusively, at low temperatures).

Hemolytic Disease of the Newborn (Fetal Erythroblastosis)

Etiology. Levine and associates (1941) advanced the hypothesis that hemolytic disease of the newborn may be the result of formation of Rh antibodies in an Rh-negative woman carrying an Rh-positive fetus. This has since been amply confirmed by numerous clinical and laboratory studies. One of the most direct pieces of evidence has been the demonstration of Rh-positive red cells, obviously derived from the fetus, in the peripheral blood of Rh-negative pregnant women by means of the acid elution technique (Kleihauer and Brandt, 1964).

Statistically, infants with clinical evidence of erythroblastosis are most frequently Rh-positive infants of Rh-negative mothers possessing Rh antibodies. It is now well known that, in addition to $Rh_0(D)$, fetomaternal differences in many other blood factors may induce maternal isoimmunization and hemolytic disease, although this occurs much more rarely. Of specific interest is ABO incompatibility as a cause of maternal isoimmunization: expectant mothers may form "immune" (IgG) antibodies in addition to "natural" isoagglutinins already present, and transplacental transmission of the antibodies may produce clinical symptoms similar to those resulting from other incompatible antibodies. As a rule, however, severe clinical disease owing to A and B immunization is much rarer than that caused by Rh immunization. Subclinical forms or mild disease expressed as slight jaundice appearing before the third day of life, spherocytosis, and moderate reticulocytosis are observed more frequently.

Pathogenesis. Entry into the maternal circulation of fetal red cells is especially common during and right after delivery. This may explain why Rh antibodies often are first detected a few weeks after delivery. As a rule, Rh antibodies do not develop during the first pregnancy of an Rh-negative woman bearing an Rh-positive fetus unless they were stimulated by preceding transfusion of Rh-positive blood. Most commonly two or three pregnancies are needed for development of Rh antibodies. Frequently even a much larger number of pregnancies with Rh-positive fetuses does not lead to formation of Rh antibodies in Rh-negative women. On the basis of statistical analyses of large series, only approximately one out of 10 Rh-negative women potentially exposed to Rh immunization by pregnancy actually develops antibodies.

Once antibodies are present they may pass to the fetus transplacentally provided they are IgG.

The most severe form of hemolytic disease (hydrops fetalis) is the result of damage to fetal red cells of sufficient extent to cause intrauterine death. If, on the other hand, the child is born alive, it may present one of two forms of disease. The first, more serious form is characterized by rapid development of jaundice resulting from the postnatal breakdown of red cells and entails the risk of damage of certain portions of the central nervous system by bilirubin (indirect, nonesterified) and other heme metabolites (nuclear jaundice, hyperbilirubinemic encephalopathy, generally known as kernicterus). This form is designated icterus gravis. The second, milder form of the disease is associated with a gradual destruction of the red cells coated with Rh antibody and leads to a hemolytic anemia similar to that found in patients with other causes of accelerated red cell breakdown. Figure 5–8 correlates the most important clinical, pathologic, and clinicopathologic findings in these three forms of hemolytic disease (Davidsohn, 1965). The pathogenesis of hemo-

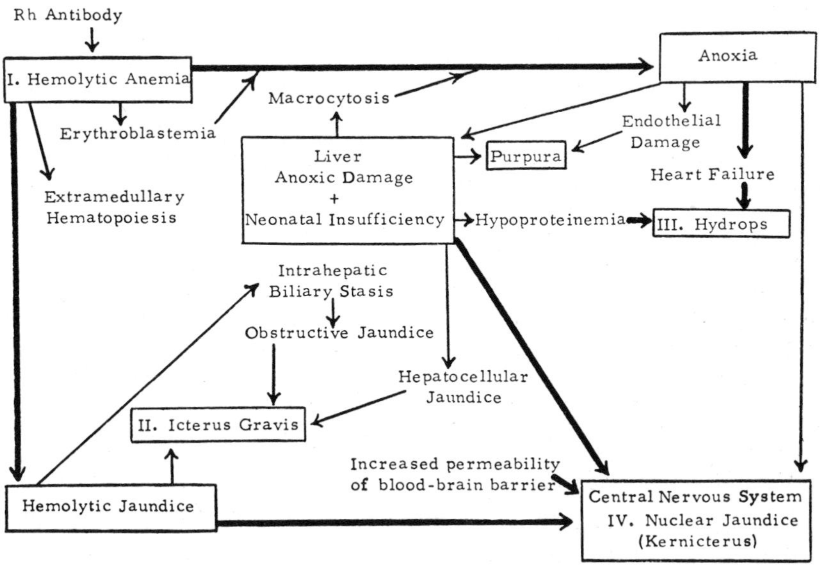

Figure 5–8. Pathogenesis of fetal erythroblastosis. (From Davidsohn, I.: Fetal erythroblastosis and the Rh and other blood factors. *In* Greenhill, J. P.: Obstetrics. 13th ed.)

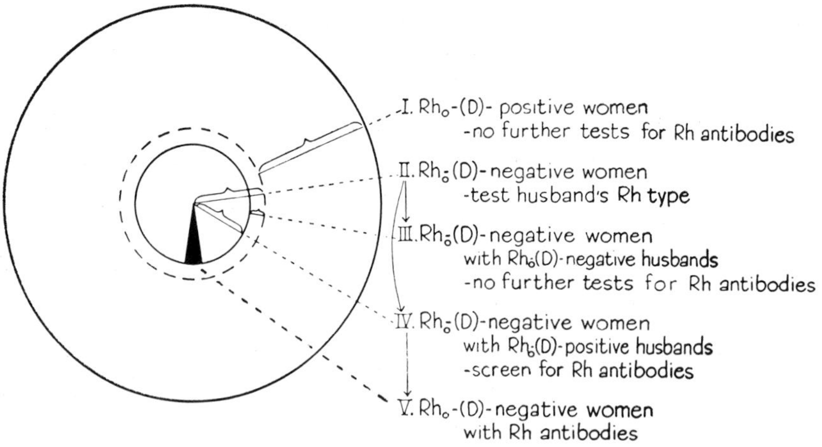
I. Rh₀-(D)- positive women
-no further tests for Rh antibodies
II. Rh₀(D)-negative women
-test husband's Rh type
III. Rh₀(D)-negative women
with Rh₀(D)-negative husbands
-no further tests for Rh antibodies
IV. Rh₀(D)-negative women
with Rh₀(D)-positive husbands
-screen for Rh antibodies
V. Rh₀-(D)-negative women
with Rh antibodies

Figure 5–9. Prenatal screening tests.

lytic disease caused by other forms of maternal isoimmunization is in all essential points analogous to that described for the disease associated with Rh immunization. At the same time it must be emphasized that none of the clinical, pathologic, and clinicopathologic findings is strictly specific for the disease, since they can also be found in a number of other conditions.

Prenatal Diagnosis. Because of the nonspecificity of clinical, pathologic, and hematologic findings in hemolytic disease of the newborn, the results of serologic tests are of paramount importance. Furthermore, if at all possible, the potential occurrence of the disease should be evaluated prenatally in order to be prepared for proper neonatal treatment without delay. For this reason certain prenatal tests should be carried out on all expectant mothers. According to the general scheme of such tests indicated in Figure 5–9, the first and crucial test is that for the Rh_0(D) factor. If the patient is found to be Rh_0(D)-positive, as a rule no further tests are necessary. On the other hand, all Rh_0(D)-negative women are potential candidates for Rh immunization provided their husbands are Rh_0(D)-positive. For that reason the serums of such patients should be screened for presence of Rh antibodies. The solid black segment in the innermost circle of Figure 5–9 represents the approximate percentage of Rh immunized women one may expect to detect upon prenatal testing. It is the infants of these women in whom hemolytic disease may become manifest provided they are Rh-positive.

Repeated screening for Rh antibodies is desirable, since a negative test early in pregnancy may induce a false sense of security responsible for failure to search for and detect subsequent development of Rh antibodies. On the other hand, if Rh antibody testing was done only close to term and showed a positive result, the length of exposure of the fetus to Rh antibodies cannot be established. Furthermore, repetition of antibody examinations during various stages of pregnancy may detect a rise in antibody titer. Such a rise can be accepted as significant only if the two specimens to be compared are tested simultaneously with the same technique, reagents, and test cells. Such titrations should preferably be done volumetrically (cf. p. 380). If in this manner a rise in antibodies is established, this can be taken as proving almost conclusively that the fetus carried in the respective pregnancy is Rh-positive, since presumably its red cells have provided the additional antigenic stimulus.

There is no unanimity of opinion whether or not valid prognostic information can be derived from the relative amounts – titers – of Rh antibodies in individual patients. Statistically they seem to be useful, inasmuch as "high" titers of Rh antibodies are more likely to be followed by manifest or severe disease in the newborn than "low" titers. What is to be considered as "high" or "low" titer depends on the techniques employed and therefore must be established empirically in each laboratory. Definite prognostic significance can be assigned only to the finding of IgM antibodies; they are unlikely to produce disease since they do not reach the fetus. Finally, the length of exposure to antibodies influences both the likelihood and degree of clinical disease; short periods of exposure are less likely to produce serious disease than longer periods. At the same time one must remember that these criteria have only general validity and that exceptions to the rule do occur. A change of opinion has taken place concerning the prognostic evaluation of the past obstetrical history. Undoubtedly a previous neonatal death attributable to maternal isoimmunization is an unfavorable factor. Nevertheless, in roughly one out of three or four pregnancies with an Rh-positive fetus following a previous stillbirth caused by Rh immunization, a live Rh-positive child may be delivered who, though diseased, may be treated successfully with replacement transfusion.

Once Rh immunization of an Rh-negative woman has taken place, the prognosis for subsequent pregnancies is significantly affected by the zygosity of her husband for the Rh factor. In this situation Rh genotyping (cf. tests outlined on p. 371) is of considerable importance because the results permit estimation of the odds for the likelihood of an Rh-negative child from a subsequent pregnancy (cf. Table 5–9).

Amniocentesis. Transabdominal insertion of a needle into the amniotic cavity has long been used for injection of radiopaque material for amniography and for injection of hypertonic saline solution in order to terminate pregnancy. Recently it has been widely used in prenatal diagnosis and prognosis of hemolytic disease of the newborn caused by Rh antibodies (Chap. 27).

Indications

1. Serum titer of anti-Rh_0(D) of 16 or higher by antiglobulin test in a pregnant woman with a history of previous stillbirth due to Rh immunization.
2. Serum titer of anti-Rh_0(D) of 32 or higher in a pregnant woman with history of a previous child who received exchange transfusions.
3. Progressive rise of anti-Rh_0(D) serum titer to 64 or higher in pregnant women without history of affected fetus or child.

The initial amniocentesis is usually done between 24 to 28 weeks of gestation, or 6 to 8 weeks before gestational age of previous fetal loss caused by Rh immunization. It is rarely done before 20 weeks of gestation, when the amniotic cavity is too small. Meaningful information usually requires at least two amniocenteses, at one to two weeks' interval, in order to confirm and compare the results of each tap.

The amniotic fluid should be protected against light which affects the level of pigments. The fluid portion should be separated as soon as possible from cellular and other sediment. Turbid fluid should be clarified by high speed centrifugation or by filtration before being tested.

Testing

1. Bilirubin Pigment. The level of bilirubinoid is by far the most important determination. The exact nature of this pigment and its pathway into the amniotic cavity are not yet known. Results of bilirubinoid determinations provide a high degree of accuracy in predicting outcome of the pregnancy in Rh immunization. Presence of bilirubin pigment leads to an abnormal elevation of optical density at 450 mμ in a spectrophotometric scan. The difference in optical density between baseline and peak of elevation is known as delta (Δ) O.D. The normal value of the Δ O.D. varies with gestational age; consequently, any value expressed must state the age of the fetus. Based upon analysis of 426 samples of amniotic fluid from 140 patients immunized to Rh_0(D), Queenan and Goetschel grouped all Δ O.D. values into three zones: (1) zone of "surviving infants" is below the line drawn from Δ O.D. of 0.15 at 20th week to a value of 0.05 at the 40th week; (2) zone of "dead fetuses" is above the line drawn from Δ O.D. of 0.3 at 20th week to 0.18 at 40th week; and (3) the zone between these two zones is less predictable, except that in a woman with a previously affected fetus or infant, the chance of having a dead fetus is greatly increased; an increase in O.D. value in a second or a third tap also implies an unfavorable outcome.

Increased optical density in a spectrophotometric scan of amniotic fluid may be due to material other than bilirubin. Blood, which is present in various amounts in about 50 per cent of the taps, produces a peak at 415 mμ; meconium gives high Δ O.D. below 425 mμ; urine gives a very high Δ O.D. below 400 mμ. A mixture of blood and bilirubin pigment can be differentiated by repetition of the scan after extraction of bilirubin with chloroform.

2. Anti-Rh_0 Titer. Comparison with the anti-Rh_0(D) titer of the maternal serum has been reported to be useful as prognostic index for viability of the fetus.

3. ABO Grouping can be done in three ways: (a) mixed agglutination of fetal epithelial cells using red blood cells of known group; (b) detection of soluble A, B, and H substances; or (c) direct grouping may be done provided the red cells have been shown to be of fetal origin by means of the Kleihauer test. Rh typing and direct antiglobulin test can also be done with fetal red blood cells.

4. Sex Determination. Presence of sex chromatin (Barr body) in desquamated fetal cells indicates a female fetus.

Complications

1. Fetal or maternal bleeding and fetal death following amniocentesis have been reported.
2. Fetal-maternal transfusion, inducing additional immunization of the mother.
3. Infection, essentially preventable.

Neonatal Tests. Certain tests should be done routinely on all infants born to Rh-negative women with Rh antibodies and on infants whose Rh-negative mothers have not been adequately tested prenatally. Special consideration must be given to infants whose mothers have a history of isoimmunization to blood factors other than Rh, including A and B. Finally, extensive testing is required when infants unexpectedly develop clinical symptoms suggestive of hemolytic disease. With exceedingly rare exceptions the presence of clinical hemolytic disease of the newborn owing to Rh incompatibility can be ruled out if the direct antiglobulin test is negative. On the other hand, a positive direct antiglobulin test may be associated not only with manifest disease but also with latent disease in which no other abnormal clinical or laboratory findings are obtained. Proper interpretation of laboratory tests is essential for establishing indication for treatment of hemolytic disease with replacement transfusion. (Detailed discussion of this problem may be found in monographs (Mollison, 1972; Queenan, 1967). The four critical laboratory tests are the direct antiglobulin test, hemoglobin or hematocrit of cord blood, reticulocyte count, and indirect serum bilirubin repeated every 6 hours through the first two to three days of life. Abnormalities in these tests together with abnormal clinical findings or history of a previously diseased child, as a rule, furnish the main indications for replacement transfusion, which is the treatment of choice, since it offers the greatest assurance of recovery and especially of prevention of bilirubin encephalopathy.

Controversial opinions have been expressed about the frequency with which a positive direct antiglobulin test is obtained in infants with AB hemolytic disease. Recent work has indicated that this variability reflects mainly the differences in selection of antiglobulin serums for the test; reagents particularly suitable for detection of coating of red cells with anti-A and anti-B can be prepared and give positive results. Another important confirmatory test for diagnosis of hemolytic disease of the newborn caused by AB sensitization is demonstration of the incompatible agglutinin in the serum of the infant, i.e., anti-A in infants of group A, anti-B in infants of group B, and so forth. These antibodies are, as a rule, demonstrable only by techniques suitable to detect incomplete antibodies, such as papain-treated red cells or the indirect antiglobulin technique (cf. p. 374).

Transfusion Therapy in Hemolytic Disease of the Newborn. The basic rule for selecting compatible blood for infants with hemolytic disease of the newborn is to use blood compatible with the mother. In other words, the major crossmatch is done with the serum of the mother and the red cells of the donor. Blood for replacement transfusions should preferably be not older than three days. If it differs in the ABO group from that of the infant, one must make sure that the isoagglutinin reactive with the infant's red cells is not of the "immune" type (cf. p. 381). For simple transfusions given merely to correct anemia, similar criteria for selection of blood apply. As to quantitative factors, successful replacement transfusions require at least 70 ml. of blood per pound of weight; in simple transfusions not more than 10 ml. of blood per pound should be given. For the latter purpose it may be preferable to use packed red cells rather than whole blood, since in this way more red cell mass can be administered.

After replacement transfusions or in untreated cases with latent disease the following laboratory tests are essential for follow-up purposes: direct antiglobulin test, indirect serum bilirubin, hemoglobin or hematocrit, and reticulocyte count. It is also recommended to test a postpartum specimen from an immunized mother about three to four weeks after delivery, since a rise in titer may occur at that time. Therefore, the antibody level ascertained at that time furnishes the most reliable baseline of comparison in future pregnancies.

SUPPLEMENTAL THERAPY. Infusion of albumin, administration of barbital, and phototherapy have been recommended to reduce the level of free serum bilirubin.

Intrauterine Transfusion. Intrauterine transfusion was made possible on the basis of (1) absorption of functional red blood cells from the peritoneal cavity into the general circulation; and (2) ability of the fetus to swallow radiopaque material, permitting visualization of the fetal peritoneal cavity by x-ray amniography. It offers a means of correcting severe fetal anemia in utero, thus preventing development of hydrops fetalis. However, it should be applied only in critically selected cases following timely and accurate diagnosis.

INDICATIONS. The following factors must be considered in making the decision for intrauterine transfusion: (1) previous history of stillbirth or exchange transfusion due to Rh immunization; (2) comparison of gestational age of previous fetal loss (stillbirth) with weeks of gestation of the current pregnancy; intrauterine transfusion, as a rule, is given between 20 to 33 weeks of gestation; (3) anti-$Rh_0(D)$ titer of maternal serum and bilirubin level in the amniotic fluid; and (4) when amniography discloses definite signs of hydrops, this is considered a contraindication. In these considerations it is not enough simply to decide which fetuses need transfusion, but more importantly, which do not.

SELECTION OF BLOOD. Group O Rh-negative packed red blood cells are generally used for intrauterine transfusion. Recently, frozen red blood cells have been recommended due to the fact that the washing process used for removal of the cryoprotective agent also reduces the chance of (1) transmitting hepatitis, (2) potassium intoxication, and (3) graft-versus-host reaction because of removal of most immunocompetent leukocytes. Very recently an automated machine for obtaining washed fresh red blood cells without buffy coat layer has become available; such fresh washed cells may be the choice for intrauterine transfusion.

The recommended volume to be injected is shown at the bottom of this page.

During the initial transfusion, a self-retaining Teflon catheter is inserted to facilitate subsequent transfusions which are usually repeated every two weeks until the infant can survive after delivery (more than 32 weeks of gestation).

RESULTS. The general survival rate of infants receiving intrauterine transfusion is about 30 per cent. In fetuses with some signs of hydrops, survival is less than 14 per cent, while it is 45 per cent in those without signs of hydrops.

COMPLICATIONS

1. *Fetal.* The mortality related to the procedure is about 14 per cent. Since premature labor is a common complication, many instances of fetal loss result from prematurity and associated respiratory distress syndrome. Injury to various parts of the fetus is not uncommon. Potassium intoxication, serum hepatitis, and graft-versus-host reaction have been reported. Exposure to x-ray should be reduced to minimal amounts.

2. *Maternal.* Infections developed in about 2 per cent of the patients and bleeding occurred in about 1 per cent (Queenan, 1967).

Prevention of Hemolytic Disease of the Newborn. As early as 1943 Levine noted a striking difference in incidence of ABO heterospecific and homospecific pregnancies in Rh-immunized as compared with nonimmunized Rh-negative women. Homospecific pregnancies are those in which the mother does not possess isoagglutinins (anti-A, anti-B) capable of reacting with the red cells of the fetus, whereas such isoagglutinins are present in heterospecific pregnancies. According to the distribution of ABO groups in the U.S. white population, approximately one-third of all pregnancies are expected to be heterospecific and the remaining two-thirds, homospecific. A much higher incidence – 80 to 85 per cent – of homospecific pregnancies was noted by Levine and many subsequent investigators in immunized Rh-negative women. Also, experimentally, it was confirmed that injection of ABO-incompatible, Rh-positive red cells is much less likely to induce Rh immunization than injection of ABO-compatible red cells (Stern, Davidsohn, and Masaitis, 1956). Thus, determination of the ABO group of husband and wife may also furnish information of prognostic significance. If the red cells of the husband are incompatible in the ABO system with the serum of his wife (heterospecific mating), this entails a lesser chance for Rh immunization than does a homospecific mating in which the serum of the wife is compatible with the red cells of her husband in the ABO system. For this reason Rh immunization is almost never found in O Rh-negative women married to AB Rh-positive husbands, since in this mating all children must be heterospecific, that is, incompatible in the ABO group with the mother.

Rh-negative men injected with Rh-positive red cells that have been coated *in vitro* with Rh antibodies do not develop Rh immunization (Stern, Goodman and Berger, 1961). When large doses of Rh antibodies are administered to Rh-negative men shortly after injection of Rh-positive red cells, the latter are rapidly removed from the circulation and Rh immunization does not occur (Finn *et al.*, 1961; Freda, Gorman, and Pollack, 1964). On the basis of these observations, it is now established practice to inject intramuscularly, within 72 hours after delivery, a suitable preparation of IgG anti-Rh_0(D) to all Rh-negative mothers of Rh-positive infants. This procedure presupposes absence of demonstrable Rh antibodies in the mother's serum and a negative direct antiglobulin test with the infant's red cells.

Hemotherapy of Autoimmune Hemolytic Anemia. Immunohematologic tests applied to this condition are significant for three reasons. First, the unequivocal diagnosis of the disease requires demonstration of autoantibodies. Second, autoantibodies may represent a source of error in the proper interpretation of results of ABO and Rh typing tests. Finally, hemotherapy of patients with this disease may meet with considerable difficulties and therefore necessitate modifications of laboratory tests used for selection of blood – specifically of crossmatching tests.

Diagnosis of autoimmune hemolytic anemia proceeds in three steps, as indicated in Figure 5–10: (1) establishment of accelerated destruc-

Weeks of gestation	20–22	23–24	25–26	27–29	30–31	32	33
Red blood cells (ml.) (hematocrit 70%)	20	30	35	40	50	60	70

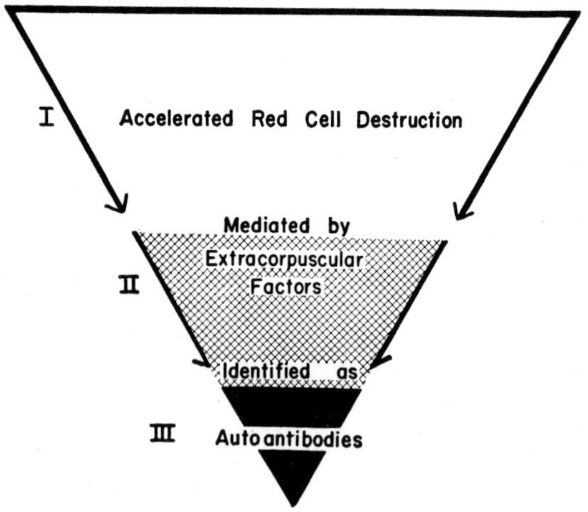

Figure 5–10. Steps in diagnosis of autoimmune hemolytic anemia.

tion or shortened survival of red cells; (2) demonstration of extracorpuscular factors as the cause of this red cell destruction; and (3) identification of the extracorpuscular factors as autoantibodies. Since most autoantibodies are IgG, the techniques most suitable for their detection are the indirect antiglobulin test and the use of enzyme-treated red cells. As a first step the direct antiglobulin test should always be done on the red cells of the patient. If this test is positive and does not reflect passive transfer of isoantibodies (e.g., hemolytic disease of the newborn) or transfusion of incompatible blood within the recent past, it is *prima facie* evidence for the presence of autoantibodies. On the other hand, negative direct antiglobulin tests are occasionally found in some cases of autoimmune hemolytic anemia, probably more frequently in patients during or after intensive steroid therapy. In such instances it is essential to test the serum of the patient for autoantibodies by having it act on random samples of cells of group O. Since most autoantibodies are of the "warm" type, these tests should be incubated at 37° C. In other instances "cold" autoantibodies are encountered, requiring incubation at 4° C. In either event, after incubation of saline-suspended red cells, the test is converted into the indirect antiglobulin technique (cf. p. 372); as an alternative the patient's serum may be tested with papain-treated red cells (cf. p. 374).

By merely suspending red cells that are heavily sensitized with autoantibodies in their own serum or in macromolecular medium, such as bovine albumin, agglutination may take place. Although this technique may be used for demonstrating the presence of autoantibodies, the phenomenon is more important as a source of error in ABO grouping and Rh typing. In such tests agglutinations may occur that are not the results of specific antigen-antibody reactions but merely reflect agglutination of antibody-coated cells in macromolecular medium. This is particularly prone to occur in slide techniques for ABO grouping, the nonspecific clumping leading to erroneous classification of a blood sample as AB. The error can be readily detected by suspending the red cells in their own serum or in the serum of a person of group AB. By the same token, nonspecific and frequently erroneous results may occur in Rh typing of "coated" red cells when these tests use IgG antibodies, necessitating suspension of red cells in macromolecular medium. For this reason it is preferable to use saline agglutinating antiserums for Rh typing of such samples in order to eliminate this source of error. In extreme cases it may be impossible to obtain reliable Rh types of such red cell specimens. Likewise, in the presence of a positive direct antiglobulin test, it is not possible to determine the blood factors that require, as a rule, the indirect antiglobulin technique, such as factors D^u, Kell, and Duffy.

Hemotherapy of patients with autoimmune hemolytic anemia depends primarily on medical decisions as to whether to transfuse at all and, if so, what quantities and what forms of blood to use. Since, as a rule, in severe cases of autoimmune hemolytic anemia it is not possible to find any blood that is completely compatible, one must attempt to select the least incompatible blood. For this purpose sensitive techniques, such as the indirect antiglobulin test or the use of enzyme-treated red cells, including the cysteine-papain technique (p. 374), are used with serial dilutions of the patient's serum. As a control one may use the red cells of the patient exposed to his own serum. In this way one is able to select among numerous units the one with the lowest titer or the weakest degree of agglutination. According to studies of several authors, some autoantibodies possess specificity for certain blood factors. Commonly, "warm" autoantibodies may be specific for Rh factors, including hr″(e) and hr′(c). "Cold" autoantibodies may have anti-I specificity (see p. 364). If such specificity is suspected or established, it is a helpful guide in selection of blood. The minor crossmatch in such cases cannot be carried out by means of the indirect antiglobulin test if the direct antiglobulin test on the patient's red cells is positive. For discussion of hematologic findings and their significance in the diagnosis and treatment of autoimmune hemolytic anemia, see chapter on hematology (p. 229).

Medicolegal Applications

Exclusion of Parentage. This application is based on the Mendelian inheritance of blood factors referred to previously. The following general principles must be understood in order to interpret properly blood grouping for possible exclusion of parentage:

1. Each person inherits one paternal and one maternal allele for each blood factor.

2. In logical consequence of this mode of inheritance a person can be either homozygous or heterozygous for each blood factor.

3. In the case of some blood factors it is possible to distinguish between homozygotes and heterozygotes, whereas for other blood factors this is not possible.

4. A person cannot possess a blood factor that is absent from the blood of both father and mother.

5. A blood factor cannot be absent in a person if one of his parents is homozygous for this factor.

6. If a parent is heterozygous for a factor of which both alleles can be demonstrated by suitable tests, his child must possess a blood factor corresponding to one of these two alleles.

By applying these principles to the ABO system, persons with certain ABO groups can be excluded from parentage as indicated in Figure 5–11. While such tests most commonly are utilized for exclusion of paternity, the same rules apply to exclusion of maternity. Therefore, the matings shown in Figure 5–11 are not specified as to sex of the person. Principle 4 mentioned in the preceding section permits formulation of the *first law of inheritance:*

> *Factors A or B cannot appear in a child unless present in one or both parents.*

Principle 6 applied to the ABO system permits formulation of the *second law of inheritance:*

> *A parent of group AB cannot have a child of group O.*

Finally, principle 5 adapted to the ABO system results in the *third law of inheritance:*

> *A parent of group O cannot have a child of group AB.*

In many thousands of tests done for medicolegal purposes or genetic studies no exception whatsoever was found to the first law of inheritance. On the other hand, two cases are on record of children of group O born to mothers of group A_2B without any possible doubt of maternity. Hence, exclusions based on the second and third laws of inheritance may have to be considered somewhat less stringent than those based on the first law of inheritance. Nevertheless, it must be realized that apparent violations of the second and third laws of inheritance are exceedingly rare; they possibly result from mutations or may result from chromosomal abnormalities, such as trisomy or translocation. This interpretation is supported by the finding that at least one of the infants of group O with an AB mother showed multiple congenital abnormalities.

Figure 5–12 summarizes possible exclusions from parentage of children of certain MN types. The laws of inheritance of MN factors may also be derived from general principles of Mendelian inheritance. Principle 4 applied to the MN system results in the *fourth law of inheritance:*

> *A child cannot possess M or N unless these factors are present in the blood of one or both parents.*

Principle 5 gives rise to the *fifth and sixth laws of inheritance:*

> *A parent of type M cannot have a child of type N.*
>
> *A parent of type N cannot have a child of type M.*

Because of the complexity of factors and phenotypes of the Rh system (cf. Table 5–8) Rh testing for exclusion of parentage requires additional considerations. If properly carried out it can contribute a great deal. As a rule,

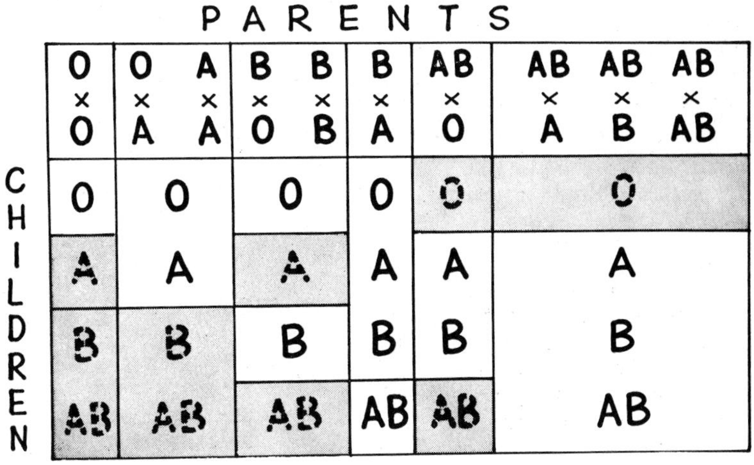

PARENTS
O × O
O × A
A × A
B × O
B × B
B × A
AB × O
AB × A
AB × B
AB × AB
CHILDREN
O
A
B
AB

Figure 5–11. Use of the ABO system for exclusion of parentage. Children of groups in shaded area are excluded.

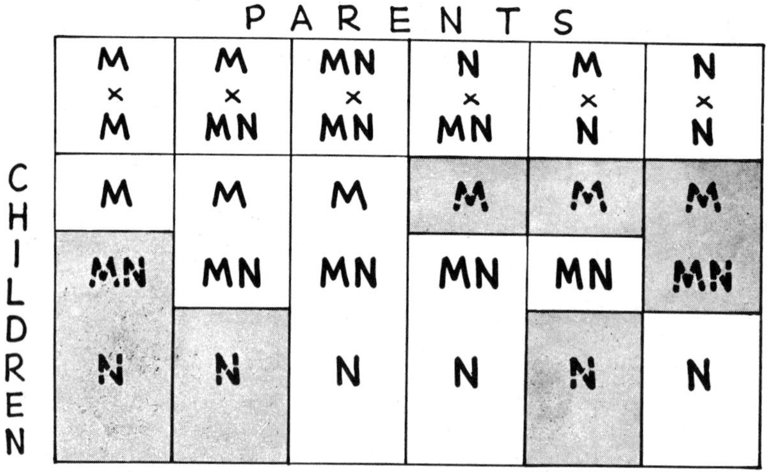

Figure 5–12. Use of the MN system for exclusion of parentage. Children of groups in shaded areas are excluded.

factors Rh_0(D), rh′(C), rh″(E), and hr′(c) are determined. Factor hr″(e) may also be determined provided reliable and potent antiserums are available. Results of such Rh tests, as interpreted by general principles of inheritance, permit the following conclusions:

1. None of the Rh factors [Rh_0(D), rh′(C), rh″(E), hr′(c), hr″(e)] can be present in a person unless one or both parents possess the corresponding factor.

2. A parent lacking the rh′(C) factor cannot have a child without the hr′(c) factor; vice versa, a parent lacking the hr′(c) factor cannot have a child without the rh′(C) factor.

3. A parent lacking the rh″(E) factor cannot have a child without the hr″(e) factor; vice versa, a parent lacking the hr″(e) factor cannot have a child without the rh″(E) factor.

The chances for excluding a person from parentage of a specific child are approximately 25 per cent by use of the ABO groups alone; the chances rise to 31 per cent when ABO and MN factors are determined and to approximately 50 per cent by testing for ABO, MN, and Rh factors. These figures are derived from tests on the U.S. white population and depend critically on the distribution of the factors in the population. The number of exclusions of parentage can be increased by tests for other blood group antigens. The feasibility and reliability of this approach depend critically on availability of adequate reagents. Such prerequisites are, as a rule, limited to specialized laboratories. This topic has been adequately presented (Wiener and Wexler, 1958; Sussman, 1968). Finally, it must be emphasized that blood grouping tests as described can be used only for exclusion of parentage but never for establishing parentage. Exceptions to this rule are exceedingly rare: if the child and one parent possess one of the unusual "private" or "family factors" (cf. p. 364), this may be considered as strong presumptive evidence for parentage.

Technical Considerations in Tests for Exclusion of Parentage. Although the techniques employed for this purpose are essentially the same as those described in the previous sections, it cannot be emphasized enough that proper performance of parentage tests requires a good deal of experience and expertise. Care must be taken in order to assure proper identification of the persons from whom the blood specimens are obtained. This may be supported by obtaining fingerprints of adults and older children or footprints of newborn and young children. It is also important that the parties identify each other, and photographs taken at the time of the interview have been recommended. Blood specimens must be reliably labeled and tested while in a good state of preservation. The validity of the test results must be secured in the following manner:

1. Each antiserum must be simultaneously tested with two control specimens of red cells, one of which contains the corresponding blood group antigen, while the other lacks it; the results obtained with these controls must conform to expectation.

2. Each blood factor [e.g., B, M, rh′(C)] must be tested with at least two different lots of antiserums, and concordant results must be obtained.

3. Tests should be set up in duplicate and read independently by two different persons.

The ABO grouping may be supplemented by use of anti-A_1 serum (cf. p. 369) in order to subgroup A and AB into A_1 and A_1B or into A_2 and A_2B. In this way it is possible to utilize consideration of inheritance of A_1 as an additional means for exclusion of parentage. As shown in Table 5–4, while persons of A_1 may be either homozygous or heterozygous for this factor, in either event their red cells react as A_1. Hence, one may derive an additional law of ABO inheritance:

A person of A_1B cannot have a child of group A_2; vice versa, a person of group A_2 cannot have a child of group A_1B.

CAUTIONS FOR INTERPRETATIONS OF EXCLUSIONS OF PARENTAGE. Apart from the exceedingly remote possibility that mutations or chromosomal abnormalities may be responsible for exceptions to laws of inheritance, some specific qualifications must be kept in mind when interpreting exclusion of parentage.

1. *ABO System.* Possible presence of weak subgroups of A must not be overlooked. Furthermore, exclusion based on differences in subgroups cannot be considered valid if it concerns a child under the age of one year, since tests for subgroups of A are unreliable at this age. Finally, exceedingly rare cases have been reported of "suppressor genes," which when present in one of the parents in homozygous form make it impossible to detect A or B factors in the red cells, although the factor may be present in the offspring, who is heterozygous for the suppressor gene (see p. 353).

2. *MN System.* A third allele, M^g, of exceedingly rare occurrence may lead to an apparent violation of the laws of inheritance of MN types, as described previously; e.g., a person who seemingly is type N but actually is type M^gN may have a child M from a mother M, the true type of the child being MM^g. Furthermore, there are weak subgroups of $N(N_2)$ that may be missed and thus lead to erroneous typing and interpretation.

3. *Rh System.* The apparent absence of $Rh_0(D)$ can be used only for exclusion of parentage provided suitable tests have also shown absence of Rh_0 variants (D^u factor). Otherwise, for example, a person could be erroneously excluded as the parent of an Rh-positive child because he and the other parent were found to be Rh-negative. This is especially important in connection with the Rh_0 variant (D^u) when it represents a suppression of reactivity of $Rh_0(D)$ because of presence of rh′(C). Particular caution must be used in arriving at exclusion of parentage on the basis of tests for rh′(C) and hr″(e), since variants of these blood factors may be encountered and cause atypical results with some antiserums (see p. 356).

Properly executed and interpreted blood grouping tests are now accepted as evidence for exclusion of parentage in the courts of some states.

Identification of Blood Stains and Secretions. Blood grouping tests can provide valuable evidence in connection with possible identity of blood stains found on clothing, utensils, and instruments presumably involved in assault or with the blood of persons involved in crime or accidents. However, such tests are by no means so simple as those routinely used, because only rarely is material available that is fresh enough to permit preparation of red cell suspensions capable of being reliably agglutinated by the corresponding antiserums. Most commonly it is necessary to prepare extracts of the blood stains or spots in which specific blood factors are demonstrated by mixing the extract with known antiserum (e.g., anti-A) and determining that in this mixture agglutinating activity has been inhibited or neutralized. Thus, material eluted from a blood stain and found capable of significantly inhibiting anti-A serum presumably has contained blood factor A. In order to control sources of error, such as nonspecific absorption of antibody, suitable controls must be included, and adequate performance and interpretation of these tests requires considerable experience. Similar considerations apply to the demonstration of A and B substances in the saliva of secretors. Presence of A and B in such saliva permits testing traces of saliva derived from sealing of envelopes. The sensitivity and specificity of such tests must be assured by proper controls. Because of the special expertness required, they should not be done in the average blood grouping laboratory. This may also apply to identification of blood by species; that is, in cases in which a blood stain might be of human or animal origin. Specific precipitin tests must be carried out in order to prove such identity. Presence of factors other than A, B, Le^a, and Le^b in secretions or in tissues other than blood has not been conclusively established and, hence, at present such tests are outside the area of practical application.

Anthropologic and Genetic Applications. Blood factors represent the most readily accessible and demonstrable genetic markers. This fact together with the significant differences in distribution of blood factors found in populations of different racial origin makes their study one of the most valuable and reliable means of anthropologic classification. Details of this fascinating discipline are outside the scope of this text; those interested in such information are specifically referred to the classic monograph on the subject (Mourant, 1954).

In general, the study of genetics of blood groups appears to offer outstanding opportunities for acquiring significant insights into mechanisms of inheritance in man. Some recent approaches to and observations in this area have been discussed previously (see pp. 351 and 352).

QUALITY CONTROL

Quality control in blood bank procedures is designed to reduce the technical and human errors to a minimum and thus to assure the accuracy of each procedure in producing reliable test results and providing the most suitable blood or blood components. For two obvious reasons quality control is even more important in blood banking than other branches of laboratory medicine because: (1) one deals mainly with immunologic reactions which exhibit wider variations than chemical or physical analyses, and (2) preparations are issued to patients on the basis of test results that cannot be evaluated by the physician, as is the case concerning other laboratory reports, and any error in the test may endanger the life of the recipient. While factors relating to specific procedures, including preparation of blood components, are described under each subject, general principles affecting more than one procedure are outlined below (Huestis, 1969; AABB, 1969).

Reagents

Antiserums. Antiserums such as anti-A, anti-B, anti-A,B, anti-Rh_0(D), anti-human globulin, and anti-HBAg serums must satisfy the minimum requirements regarding specificity, potency, and avidity, as established by the Division of Biological Standards of the Food and Drug Administration. Each reagent should be checked daily for reactivity with known antigens and the results should be recorded in the log book.

Antigens. Red blood cells of known antigenic composition, such as groups A, B, O, Rh_0(D)-positive, Rh_0(D)-negative, etc., should be prepared in the proper medium and proper concentration and be checked against known antiserums. Use of cells presensitized with anti-Rh_0 to confirm negative antiglobulin tests is highly recommended.

Reagin for testing syphilis and hepatitis B antigen of known specificity should be used and checked against known antiserums.

Solutions. Solutions, such as physiologic saline, buffers, enzyme preparations, and albumin solutions, should have the proper concentration and pH and be free of particles. They are to be stored at optimal temperatures.

Blood Specimens

Identification. Identification must be established for (1) person donating blood or specimen; (2) container for specimen; and (3) test tubes, plates, or plastic cups used in test.

Handling

1. Separate serum from clot as soon as possible to avoid hemolysis or release of enzymes or potassium from red cells.
2. Use the serum as fresh as possible, especially when complement is involved in the reaction.
3. Cover the specimen against light if bilirubin or bilirubin-like pigment is to be determined.
4. Keep the specimen warm, if cold agglutinins are to be tested.
5. Washed red blood cells are preferred for crossmatching.

Instruments and Supplies

Control temperature by

1. Selecting the right type of thermometer or sensor, placed in proper medium and at proper location.
2. Monitoring the temperature with a recorder.
3. Installing an alarm system with dual power supplies on a separate fuse (A.C.).
4. Auxiliary power supply for key refrigerators and freezers.
5. Adequate supply of liquid nitrogen for N_2 freezers.

The following equipment requires temperature regulation, including items referred to by numbers in parentheses:

a. Incubators, dry or wet, at 37° C., 56° C. or 60° C. (1).
b. Laboratory rooms, between 20 to 25° C. (1).
c. Refrigerators for storing blood preferably between 2 to 4° C., definitely within 1 to 6° C. (1, 2, 3 & 4).
d. Container for shipping blood, below 10° C. (1, 2, 3 & 4).
e. Electric freezers, –20° C., –30° C. or –85° C. (1, 2, 3 & 4).
f. Liquid nitrogen freezer, –190° C. (5).

Control centrifugation by

1. Selecting a specific relative centrifugal force (RCF or G) by using rotor of a known radius (r in cm) at a given speed (n as revolution per minute) where $G = 0.00001188\ rn^2$.
2. Selecting an optimal time, especially when a fixed speed centrifuge is being used; calibration should be done with each rotor. Heavier load and viscous medium may affect results.
3. Selecting an optimal temperature.

Balancing opposing loads is a must for all centrifugation. The following operations require regulation of centrifugation, including items referred to by number in parentheses:

a. Preparation of blood components (1, 2, & 3).

b. Preparation of reagents and samples for testing (2).
c. Enhancement of agglutination; especially for antiglobulin test, time should be calibrated in seconds (2).
d. Hematocrit determination (2).

Check each time:
1. pH meter with reference buffers.
2. Balance for level and zero.
3. Colorimeter or spectrophotometer for 0 to 100 per cent transmission.
4. Nonelectric timer for winding the spring.
5. Particle counters for noise level and patency of the aperture.
6. AutoAnalyzers for smooth flow and even air bubbling patterns.

Check periodically at specified intervals:
1. Vacuum pumps for water and oil traps.
2. Alarm systems for functional batteries.
3. Power supply for voltage and amperage.
4. AutoAnalyzer for worn-out tubings.
5. Speed of rotors and of proportional pumps.

Supplies:
1. Cleanliness: Disposable test tubes, pipettes and plastic cups are preferred.
2. Accuracy: Must be checked, especially for small volumes, for which disposable lambda pipettes are preferred.

Procedures

Written Procedure. A detailed description of each procedure should be available in each laboratory.

Controls. Controls for each series of tests, or for each plate in testing HBAg:
1. Positive (preferably weakly reactive).
2. Negative.
3. Autocontrol (in some tests).
4. Blank or albumin control (in certain tests).

Standards. Standards for quantitative analysis:

1. Individual dilutions are preferable to serial dilutions.

2. A reference sample or a previous sample of the same patient should be included for comparative titration.

3. In absence of a reference sample, a reference curve or table should be available.

4. Evaluation taking into consideration known frequency of specific antigens.

5. Satisfy the statistical evaluation, i.e., 95 per cent level of confidence in identification of a particular antibody with a panel of red cells requires a minimum of four negatives and three positives.

Reproducibility

1. Testing the specimen with the same or different reagents by more than one technologist.

2. Testing duplicate specimens by the same technologist.

3. Testing coded specimens of known specificity.

Reading and Recording of Results

1. Proper light for reading agglutination or precipitins.

2. A magnifier or a microscope for weak reactions.

3. Grading or scoring agglutination reactions.

4. Recording directly on the logbook or record sheet with initials.

IMMUNOHEMATOLOGY OF LEUKOCYTES

Immunohematology of leukocytes has been studied intensively in recent years. Important contributions have been made by J. Dausset, J. van Rood, R. Ceppellini, F. Kissmeyer-Nielsen, A. Amos, P. Lalezari, R. Payne, P. Terasaki, R. Walford and others.

The significance of leukocyte immunology has been related to:

1. Febrile reaction following blood transfusion.

2. Leukopenia following blood transfusion.

3. Leukopenia of newborns.

4. Rejection of transplants such as skin, kidney, heart, liver, lung, and bone marrow.

5. Evaluation of parentage and human genetics.

6. Different disease states such as acute leukemias, Hodgkin's disease, systemic lupus erythematosus and others.

Antigens. Among the many leukocyte antigens reported by various investigators, those of major importance belong to the HL-A system. The term "HL-A" was agreed upon by a committee of the World Health Organization and stands for human leukocyte locus-A, i.e., the first in the series. Results of intensive studies on members of many families are in agreement with the concept of two closely linked subloci, called first series (LA locus) and second series (Four locus). Each locus is occupied by one of many allelic genes, and each gene governs one HL-A antigen. At the Fifth Histocompatibility Workshop held in May, 1972, the following antigens were considered to be identifiable with currently used techniques:

1st series (LA):	HL-A1, HL-A2, HL-A3, HL-A9(W-23, W24), HL-A10(W25, W26), HL-A11, W19(W29, W30, W31, W32), (HL-A)28.
2nd series (Four):	HL-A5, HL-A7, HL-A8, HL-12, HL-A13 (HL-A)14, (HL-A)17, (HL-A)27, W16, W20, W21.

Since the accumulative gene frequency of each series is less than 100 per cent, at least one unidentifiable antigen has to be added to each series; hence, there should be a minimum of 14 allelic genes for the 1st and 12 for the 2nd locus.

Based on this minimum number of allelic genes, there would be $12 \times 14 = 168$ possible HL-A haplotypes on one chromosome and $168 \times (168 + 1) / 2 = 14,196$ possible genotypes on a pair of chromosomes. There would be $14 \times (14 + 1)/2 = 105$ phenotypes of the 1st series and $12 \times (12 + 1)/2 = 78$ of the 2nd series; a combination of both series would have $105 \times 78 = 8190$ phenotypes. This is far more complicated than the Rh-system of erythrocytes.

Each person may have a maximum of two HL-A antigens determined by one chromosome of a pair, and a total of four determined by both chromosomes of a pair. Individuals with only two or three HL-A detectable antigens may have the same allelic gene (homozygous) or may have an undetectable antigen(s). Since one chromosome of the pair is from the father and the other from the mother, their children have to belong to one of four possible genotypes (Fig. 5–13). Follow-up of recipients of transplants, such as bone marrow and kidney, disclosed that best results were achieved when the organ was obtained from siblings with identical HL-A types. The outcome was less favorable when there was partial identity of HL-A antigens between recipients and sibling donors, and the results were least favorable when unrelated donors with nonidentical HL-A types were used. Grading of donors by HL-A testing is listed in Table 5–20. It should be mentioned that two individuals may have the same HL-A phenotype (1, 3, 7, 8) but different genotype, e.g., 1, 7/3, 8 and 1, 8/3, 7.

Based upon the results obtained by mixed lymphocyte culture technique, a third locus close to the second locus has been proposed, and there is evidence for an additional fourth locus.

HL-A antigens have been demonstrated on the membranes of nucleated cells: different types of leukocytes, platelets, and cells in spleen, liver, kidney, skin, and placenta. Lipoproteins with HL-A2 and HL-A7 specificity have been demonstrated in plasma. Erythrocytes with DBG antigen have been shown to have also HL-A7 antigen.

Anti-HL-A antibodies have been found in polytransfused patients, in multiparous women, in recipients of allotransplants and in volunteers immunized with cells containing HL-A antigens.

Most of the antiserums contain multispecific antibodies. Monospecific antiserums are very rare and are difficult to prepare. Consequently, it is not easy to establish the antigenic composition on lymphocytes and microtechniques

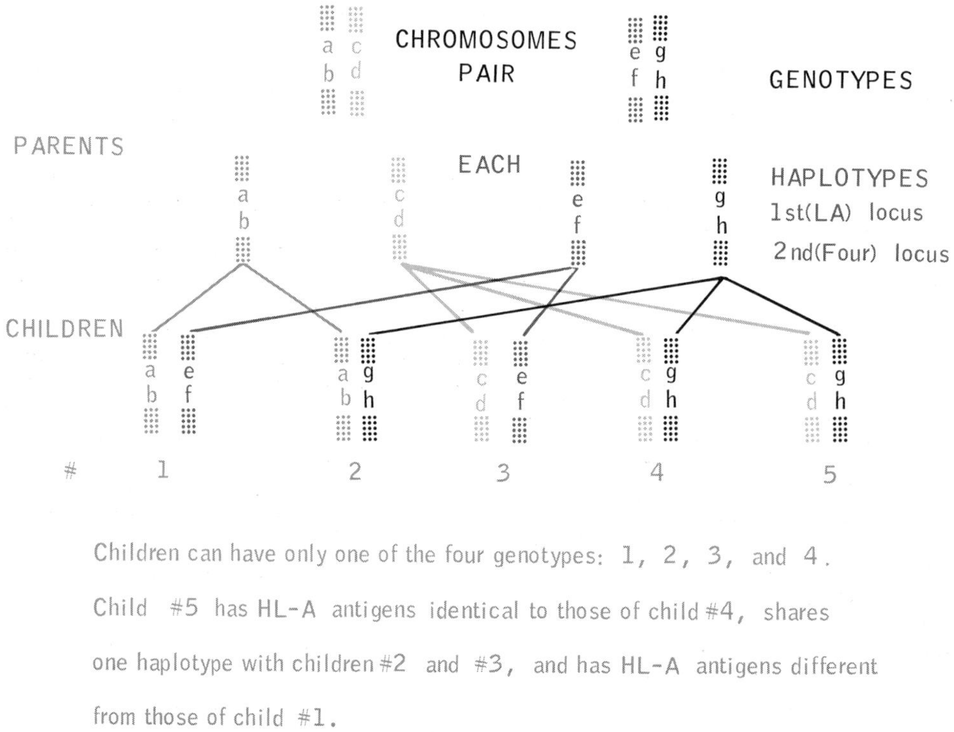

Figure 5–13. Inheritance of HL-A.

Table 5–20. GRADING IN HISTOCOMPATIBILITY TESTING

RESULTS OF TESTS ON HL-A ANTIGENS	MATCH GRADES U.S.A.	MATCH GRADES Europe	OUTCOME OF TRANSPLANT
Identical between donor and recipient	A	0	Favorable
1 antigen in recipient, not in donor	B	0	Favorable
1 antigen in donor, not in recipient	C	1	Less favorable
2–4 antigens in donor, not in recipient	D	2	Less favorable
Antibodies in recipient for antigens of donor (incompatible crossmatch)	E	3	Rejection

have to be used to conserve the limited amount of available satisfactory antiserum.

Histocompatibility Testing. Histocompatibility testing includes two basic steps:

1. Typing of HL-A antigens, which has been loosely referred to as tissue typing. Leukoagglutination, lymphocytotoxicity, and complement fixation are the procedures commonly used.

2. Crossmatching between the donor and the recipient is usually done with the lymphocytotoxicity test and occasionally with the mixed lymphocyte culture technique.

All these procedures have been carried out in selected laboratories with adequate staff and facilities, and are not recommended for every hospital. "Manual of Tissue Typing Techniques," April, 1972, is available on request from the Transplantation and Immunology Branch, Collaborative Research, National Institute of Allergy and Infectious Diseases, National Institutes of Health, Bethesda, Maryland 20014.

The leukoagglutinin test has long been used for studying febrile reaction following blood transfusion. Microtechniques have been developed for testing HL-A antigens. Although the leukoagglutinin test is not always reproducible, it is still used in some laboratories for detecting some HL-A antigens less readily demonstrable with other techniques.

Lymphocytotoxicity is by far the most widely used procedure for HL-A typing. It is based upon the principle that lymphocytes die quickly in the presence of specific antiserum and complement. Differentiation between live and dead lymphocytes can be established with:

1. ***A Phase Contrast Microscope.*** Dead cells appear dull and lack glowing luminescence.

2. ***Trypan Blue Dye.*** Live cells do not absorb the dye, whereas dead cells do.

3. ***Fluorochromasia.*** Esterase in live cells transforms nonfluorescent fluorescein-diacetate into a fluorescent compound visible under ultraviolet light.

4. ***^{51}Cr Exclusion.*** Dead cells release ^{51}Cr into the supernatant fluid.

Complement fixation using platelets as antigens offers several advantages: platelets are easily collected in large numbers and in reasonably pure suspension; viable platelets are not essential for the test; results are read macroscopically and are identical with those obtained with the lymphocytotoxicity test when suitable antiserums are available. However, scarce supply of reliable complement-fixing anti-HL-A antibodies prevents this technique from being widely adapted. Platelets have been found most useful in absorption of unwanted antibodies for preparation of monospecific antiserum for HL-A typing.

The mixed lymphocyte culture test is an *in vitro* measure of the immune response of living lymphocytes, stimulated by another group of lymphocytes which have been treated with mitomycin-C to block their mitosis. The degree of stimulation is assayed by measuring the amount of radioactive thymidine incorporated into the dividing cells during their DNA synthesis. Lymphocytes of siblings with identical HL-A types usually do not cause stimulation, whereas lymphocytes of unrelated donors not sharing common HL-A antigens always do. Thus, the mixed lymphocyte culture offers a means of direct compatibility testing between donor and recipient. Since the results become available only after several days, it cannot be used in situations where the time factor is of primary importance.

The presence of ABH antigens in addition to HL-A in tissues demands that only ABO compatible donors be used for organ transplantation. The significance of P antigen in organ transplantation has not yet been established.

IMMUNOHEMATOLOGY OF PLATELETS

Interest in platelet immunology has been growing in three areas:

1. HL-A antigens on platelets as described previously.
2. Antigens and antibodies specific for platelets.
3. Platelet transfusion.

Platelet Antigens. There are six antigens. Three pairs of nonlinked alleles have been shown with reasonable certainty to be unique to the platelets: Pl-Al, Pl-A2, Pl-El, Pl-E2 demonstrated by the complement fixation test; Ko^a, Ko^b demonstrated by the agglutination test. Although experimental production of specific antibodies against platelet antigens has been unsuccessful, isoimmunization to platelet antigens following pregnancy, transfusion, or transplantation is not uncommon. Specific anti-Pl-A or anti-Pl-E antibodies have been demonstrated in many cases of neonatal thrombocytopenic purpura due to maternal immunization; anti-HL-A2 antibodies have also been incriminated. Immunologic mechanisms may be involved in some drug-induced thrombocytopenias. Plasma or gamma globulin fractions from patients with chronic autoimmune thrombocytopenia often cause thrombocytopenia when injected into normal individuals. Procedures for study of platelet antigen and antibody reactions remain a research tool, at least at the present time.

Platelet Transfusion. Two factors may account for the increasing demand for platelet transfusion: the awareness of the usefulness of platelets in treating hemorrhages due to thrombocytopenias, and increasing numbers of thrombocytopenias caused by the frequent use of chemotherapy, radiation, and immunosuppression in modern medicine. Advances have been made in the preparation of platelets to meet the demand. Platelet donors should be advised not to take aspirin within three days before donation, since aspirin may affect the quality of the platelets and increase the bleeding time. Platelets collected in ACD (not acidified) or CPD are satisfactory, provided the platelet buttons are allowed to stay at room temperature for 60 minutes before resuspension. Platelets should be separated from other blood components, then shaken for 90 minutes, both at room temperature. Platelets prepared in this manner and stored at 4° C. without further agitation have been found satisfactory for up to three days. Preliminary reports indicated a normal yield of platelets even after storage of whole blood for 24 hours at 4° C., if a minute amount of prostaglandin E_1 is added during the collection. Survival rate of the platelets may be as high as 55 per cent in recipients transfused with platelets that have been stored in the frozen state.

While the presence of M, N, P_1, Rh, Fy^a, and K antigen on platelets has not yet been established, A and B antigens are undoubtedly present in platelets; therefore, platelets from ABO compatible donors are recommended for transfusion.

The best response was found in a recipient transfused with platelets from a sibling with identical HL-A types, whereas unsatisfactory responses were obtained with platelets from either siblings with nonidentical HL-A types or from a random donor.

REFERENCES

Allen, F. H., Jr.: "Minus minus" phenotypes. Transfusion *1*:209, 1961.

Allen, F. H., Jr., Corcoran, P. A., Kenton, H. B., and Breare, N.: M^g, a new blood group antigen in the MNS system. Vox Sang. *3*:81, 1958.

American Association of Blood Banks: A Practical Workshop. Presented by Committee on Workshops, Houston, Texas, November, 1969.

American Association of Blood Banks: Blood Component Therapy. Chicago, American Association of Blood Banks, 1969.

American Association of Blood Banks: Manual of Blood Component Preparation. Chicago, American Association of Blood Banks, 1969.

American Association of Blood Banks: Standards for a Blood Transfusion Service. 5th ed. Chicago, American Association of Blood Banks, 1971/72.

American Association of Blood Banks: Technical Methods and Procedures of the American Association of Blood Banks. 5th ed. Chicago, American Association of Blood Banks, 1970.

Aster, R. H.: Platelet antibodies, isoimmune thrombocytopenias, and platelet typing for HL-A factors. *In* Seminar on Histocompatibility Testing, 23rd Annual Meeting of American Association of Blood Banks, San Francisco, October, 1970, pp. 81–88.

Beattie, K. M., Seymour, D. S., and Scott, A.: Two further examples of acriflavin antibody causing ABO cell typing error. Transfusion *11*:107, 1971.

Berkman, E. M., Nusbacher, J., Kochwa, S., and Rosenfield, R. E.: Quantitative blood typing profiles of human erythrocytes. Transfusion *11*:317, 1971.

Brittingham, T. E., and Chaplin, H., Jr.: Febrile transfusion reactions caused by sensitivity to donor leukocytes and platelets. J.A.M.A. *165*:819, 1957.

Catino, M. L., Busch, S., Huestis, D. W., and Stern, K.: Transmission of the blood group genotype *pp* (Tj^a-negative) in a kinship with multiple consanguineous marriages. Amer. J. Human Genet. *17*:36, 1965.

Coombs, R. R. A., Mourant, A. E., and Race, R. R.: A new test for the detection of weak and incomplete Rh agglutinins. Brit. J. Exp. Path. *26*:255, 1945.

Dausset, J., Colombain, L., Legrand, N., Feingold, N., and Rapaport, F. T.: Genetic and biological aspects of HL-A system of human histocompatibility. Blood *35*:591, 1970.

Davidsohn, I: Fetal erythroblastosis and the Rh and other blood factors. *In* Greenhill, J. P.: Obstetrics. 13th ed. Philadelphia, W. B. Saunders Company, 1965.

Davidsohn, I.: Early immunologic diagnosis and prognosis of carcinoma. (Philip Levine Award Address.) Amer. J. Clin. Path. 57:715, 1972.

Davidsohn, I., Kovarik, S., and Lee, C. L.: A, B, and O substances in gastrointestinal carcinoma. Arch. Path. (Chicago) *81*:381, 1966.

Davidsohn, I., Kovarik, S., and Stejskal, R.: Ovarian cancer: Immunological aspects, influence on prognosis and treatment. UICC Monograph Series. Vol. *11*: Ovarian Cancer. Berlin, Springer-Verlag, 1968, pp. 105–121. (Presented at the International Union Against Cancer Symposium on Ovarian Tumors, Houston, Texas, October 12–15, 1966.)

Davidsohn, I., Norris, H. J., Stejskal, R., and Lill, P.: Metastatic squamous cell carcinoma of the cervix: The role of immunology in its pathogenesis. Arch. Path. *95*:132, 1973.

Davidsohn, I., and Stern, K.: Manual on Selected Topics in Immunohematology. Chicago, American Society of Clinical Pathologists, 1966.

Davidsohn, I., Stern, K., Strauser, E. R., and Spurrier, W.: Be, a new "private" blood factor. Blood *8*:747, 1953.

Davidsohn, I., and Toharsky, B.: Bacteriogenic hemagglutination. II. J. Immunol. *43*:213, 1942.

Fink, D. J., Petz, L. D., and Black, M. B.: Serum haptoglobin. A valuable diagnostic aid in suspected hemolytic transfusion reactions. J.A.M.A. *199*:615, 1967.

Finn, R., Clarke, C. A., Donohoe, W. T. A., McConnell, R. B., Sheppard, P. M., Lehane, D., and Kulke, W.: Experimental studies on the prevention of Rh haemolytic disease. Brit. Med. J. *i*:1486, 1961.

Freda, V. J., Gorman, J. G., and Pollack, W.: Successful prevention of experimental Rh sensitization in man by an anti-Rh $gamma_2$-globulin antibody preparation: a preliminary report. Transfusion *4*:26, 1964.

German, J. L., Walker, M. E., Stiefel, F. H., and Allen, F. H.: Autoradiographic studies of human chromosomes. II. Data concerning the position of the MN locus. Vox Sang *16*:130, 1969.

Giblett, E. R.: Js, a "new" blood group antigen found in Negroes. Nature *181*:1221, 1958.

Giblett, E. R.: Genetic Markers in Human Blood. Oxford, Blackwell Scientific Publications, 1969.

Griffitts, J. J., Frank, S., and Schmidt, R. P.: The influence of albumin in the antiglobulin crossmatch. Transfusion *4*:461, 1964.

Grove-Rasmussen, M., Shaw, R. S., and Marceau, E.: Hemolytic transfusion reaction in group A patient receiving group O blood. Am. J. Clin. Path. 23:828, 1953.

Huestis, D. W.: Quality Control in Blood Banking. Chicago, American Society of Clinical Pathologists, 1969.

Huestis, D. W., Bove, J. R., and Busch, S.: Practical Blood Transfusion. Boston, Little, Brown and Company, 1970.

Kabat, E. A.: Blood Group Substances. Their Chemistry and Immunochemistry. New York, Academic Press, Inc., 1956.

Kleihauer, E., and Brandt, G.: Zur Lebensdauer fetaler Erythrozyten im mütterlichen Kreislauf nach fetomaternaler Transfusion. Klin. Wschr. 42:458, 1964.

Kuhns, W. J., and Bailey, A.: Use of red cells modified by papain for detection of Rh antibodies. Am. J. Clin. Path. *20*:1067, 1950.

Landsteiner, K., and Wiener, A. S.: Studies on an agglutinogen (Rh) in human blood reacting with anti-rhesus sera and with human antibodies. J. Exper. Med. *74*:309, 1941.

Lee, C. L., Behzad, O., Froker, A., and Mandin, B.: Identification of erythrocyte antibodies with an AutoAnalyzer. *In* Technicon International Congress, 1970: Advances in Automated Analysis, Vol. *1*: Thurman Association, Miami, Florida, 1971, pp. 317–320.

Lee, C. L., Stejskal, F., and Behzad, O.: A rapid test for detecting and identifying hepatitis-associated antigen and its antibody. Lab. Med. 2(No. 2):39, 1971.

Levine, P., Celano, M. J., Falkowski, F., Chambers, J. W., Hunter, O. B., Jr., and English, C. T.: A second example of ---/--- or Rh_{null} blood. Transfusion 5:492, 1965.

Levine, P., Katzin, E. M., and Burnham, L.: Isoimmunization in pregnancy: Its possible bearing on the etiology of erythroblastosis fetalis. J.A.M.A. *116*:825, 1941.

Levine, P., and Stetson, R. E.: An unusual case of intragroup agglutination. J.A.M.A. *113*:126, 1939.

Maugh, T. H.: Hepatitis: A new understanding emerges. Science *176*:1225, 1972.

Miller, W. V., Holland, P., Sugarbaker, E., Strober, W., and Waldmann, A. W.: Anaphylactic reactions to IgA: A difficult transfusion problem. Amer. J. Clin. Path. 54:618, 1970.

Mollison, P. L.: Blood Transfusion in Clinical Medicine. 5th ed. Oxford, Blackwell Scientific Publications, 1972.

Morgan, W. T. J.: Molecular aspects of human blood-group specificity. Ann. N. Y. Acad. Sci. *169*:118, 1970.

Mourant, A. E.: The Distribution of Human Blood Groups. Springfield, Illinois, Charles C Thomas, 1954.

Owen, R. D., Stormont, C., Wexler, I. B., and Wiener, A. S.: Medicolegal applications of blood grouping tests. J.A.M.A. *164*:2036, 1957.

Payne, R.: Leukocyte agglutinins in human sera: Correlation between blood transfusions and their development. A.M.A. Arch. Intern. Med. *99*:587, 1957.

Public Health Service Regulations: Part 73: Section 73.300 to 73.306. Bethesda, Maryland, U.S. Department of Health, Education, and Welfare, 1958.

Queenan, J. T.: Modern Management of the Rh Problem. New York, Harper and Row, 1967.

Race, R. R., and Sanger, R.: Blood Groups in Man. 5th ed. Springfield, Illinois, Charles C Thomas, 1968 (also 4th edition, 1962).

Springer, G. F.: Relationship of Blood Groups to Disease: Certain Experimental Approaches to the Question of Blood Group-like Activity in Certain Bacteria and Plants. Procedures of John A. Hartford Foundation Conference on Blood Groups and Blood Transfusion. Bellevue, New York, New York, Better Bellevue Association, 1967.

Stern, K.: Clinical value of serologic examinations related to blood groups in pregnant patients. Amer. J. Obst. Gynec. *75*:369, 1958.

Stern, K.: Unusual blood types as a cause of disease. Med. Clin. N. Amer. *46*:277, 1962.

Stern, K., and Busch, S.: Report on a family with six Tj^a-negative siblings. Transfusion *3*:105, 1963.

Stern, K., Busch, S., and Buznitsky, A.: A cross-matching test using activated papain. Amer. J. Clin. Path. *27*:707, 1957.

Stern, K., Davidsohn, I., Jensen, F. G., and Muratore, R.: Immunologic studies on the Be^a factor. Vox Sang. *3*:425, 1958.

Stern, K., Davidsohn, I., and Masaitis, L.: Experimental studies on Rh immunization. Amer. J. Clin. Path. *26*:833, 1956.

Stern, K., Goodman, H. S., and Berger, M.: Experimental isoimmunization to hemoantigens in man. J. Immunol. *87*:189, 1961.

Stroup, M., and MacIlroy, M.: Evaluation of the albumin antiglobulin technic in antibody detection. Transfusion *5*:184, 1965.

Strumia, M. M., Crosby, W. H., Greenwalt, T. J., Gibson, J. G., and Krevans, J. R.: General principles of blood transfusion. Transfusion *3*:303, 1963.

Sturgeon, P.: Hematological observations on the anemia associated with blood type Rh_{null}. Blood *36*:310, 1970.

Sussman, L. N.: Blood Grouping Tests. Medico-legal Uses. Springfield, Ill., Charles C Thomas, 1968.

Symposium on Virus Hepatitis Antigens and Antibodies, Munich, August 1970: The Australia antigen, hepatitis associated antigen (HAA) and corresponding antibodies. Vox Sang. *19*:193, 1970.

Terasaki, P. I.: Histocompatibility Testing 1970. Baltimore, The Williams and Wilkins Co., 1970.

Vos, G. H., Vos, D., Kirk, R. L., and Sanger, R.: A sample of blood with no detectable Rh antigens. Lancet *1*:14, 1961.

Walford, R. L.: The Isoantigenic Systems of Human Leukocytes. Baltimore, The Williams and Wilkins Co., 1969.

Watkins, W. M.: Blood-group substances. Science *152*:172, 1966.

Wiener, A. S.: Rh-Hr Blood Types. New York, Grune & Stratton, 1954.

Wiener, A. S., Moor-Jankowski, J., and Gordon, E. B.: The relationship of the H substance to the A-B-O blood groups. Intern. Arch. Allerg. *29*:82, 1966.

Wiener, A. S., and Peters, H. R.: Hemolytic reactions following transfusion of blood of the homologous group. Ann. Intern. Med. *13*:2306, 1940.

Wiener, A. S., and Wexler, I. B.: Heredity of the Blood Groups. New York, Grune & Stratton, 1958.

Woodrow, J. C.: Rh immunization and its prevention. Ser. Haematol. 3:3, 1970.

Chapter 6

COAGULATION AND HEMOSTASIS

by ROBERT D. LANGDELL, M.D.

The vascular system is almost continually undergoing trauma. This results in defects in the wall of the vessel through which fluid can escape. Hemostasis is the process which retains fluid blood within the vascular system in spite of these injuries to the vessel wall. If the vascular discontinuity is sufficiently large, the relative effectiveness of the hemostatic mechanism will have little or no influence on the outcome. If the size of the defect is not too large, the defect in the wall is occluded almost immediately, and over a period of time, the defect is repaired. The immediate reaction to injury is vasoconstriction, which decreases the blood flow through the injured vessel. There is a simultaneous change which causes platelets in the area to clump together and to adhere to the inner surface of the injured vessel. The platelets thus serve as an emergency plug by occluding the defect. The plasma also undergoes a series of changes resulting in the formation of a fibrin clot which strengthens the platelet plug and serves as a framework for the process of fibroblastic repair. A bleeding tendency results from a defect in any of the phases of repair: (1) the vascular system itself may be unusually prone to injury; (2) platelets may be inadequate to form the emergency plug; (3) the fibrin clotting mechanism may be inadequate; or (4) fibroblastic repair may be inadequate. It has been emphasized by Jaques (1964) that excessive bleeding is usually the result of a combination of defects. When the vascular system is intact, blood does not usually escape, even though it is not able to coagulate. However, with an injury, the lack of coagulability results in excessive bleeding. This concept is of importance in understanding why all patients with congenital defects of the clotting mechanism do not exsanguinate at birth.

The formation of a clot is the result of fibrinogen, a soluble plasma protein, being transformed into an insoluble polymer, fibrin. In biologic systems, this polymerization results from the action of thrombin, a proteolytic enzyme, on the fibrinogen molecule. Parts of fibrinogen, called fibrinopeptides, are split from the molecule, and the resulting fibrin monomers then polymerize to form fibrin. In the presence of factor XIII, a fibrin-stabilizing factor, the polymerized fibrin forms a stable configuration.

The active enzyme, thrombin, is derived from a precursor substance, prothrombin. The complex mechanism of coagulation is involved in the transformation of prothrombin to thrombin in amounts adequate to act on fibrinogen molecules. The conversion of prothrombin to thrombin is accelerated by a number of factors which are collectively called procoagulants. Much of the knowledge of these procoagulants has been obtained from the study of patients with hereditary defects which result in a deficiency of one of the factors. Although much has been learned about each of the procoagulants, their mechanism of action is still speculative, and their chemical characterization is incomplete. In an attempt to improve communication, an international committee was formed in 1954 to standardize the nomenclature of the coagulation factors (Wright, 1962). Whenever possible this nomenclature will be used in this chapter.

In circulating blood there appears to be a balance between the forces which act to stimulate the formation of thrombin and the forces which tend to delay its formation or inhibit its action. This balance maintains blood in its fluid state. When injuries to the vascular system occur or when blood is removed from the vascular system, the balance is upset in favor of thrombin evolution and coagulation occurs. The balance is shifted toward delayed thrombin formation in patients with a defect in the coagulation mechanism. Injury to the vascular system of these individuals results in excessive bleeding because sufficient thrombin is not formed rapidly. Some individuals have a tendency to thromboembolic disorders; in these individuals the balance appears to be shifted toward excessive clot formation. Injury to the vascular integrity results in an overstimulation to the clotting mechanism, and excessive clotting results.

Many hypotheses have been proposed in an attempt to explain the sequence of events that leads to the development of a fibrin clot. Each hypothesis has been helpful by serving as a stimulus to investigators to test the concept. In order for a hypothesis to remain popular it must be consistent with new data. A hypothesis may remain popular because it is a true explanation of a natural phenomenon or because there is no way to design experiments to test its validity. As discussed by Popper (1963), only a hypothesis which asserts or implies that certain conceivable events will not happen is testable. With the procedures that are presently available only the final reaction, the formation of a visible fibrin clot, is directly measurable. It is therefore difficult to design experiments to disprove hypotheses concerning the reactions that occur early in the coagulation reaction. However, as an aid in remembering the data, many find it useful to have ideas expressed in the form of a diagram. The sequence of events resulting in the conversion of prothrombin to thrombin has been visualized as a waterfall by Davie and Ratnoff (1964) or cascade by Macfarlane (1964). It is believed that the procoagulants are substrates that are activated to become enzymes. This reaction series is unique in that at each step the substrate, when activated, catalyzes the next reaction. Such a series of reactions is visualized as shown above.

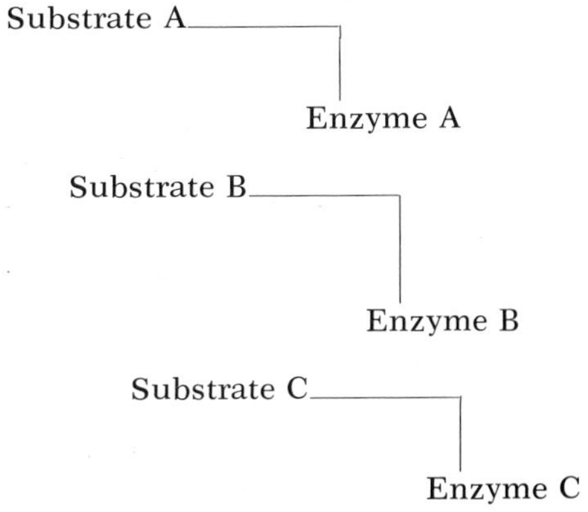

In the concept proposed by Davie and Ratnoff (1964), it is postulated that the procoagulants react in the following order: XII, XI, IX, VIII, X and V. Factor VII is believed to act independently on prothrombin. Although ionic calcium

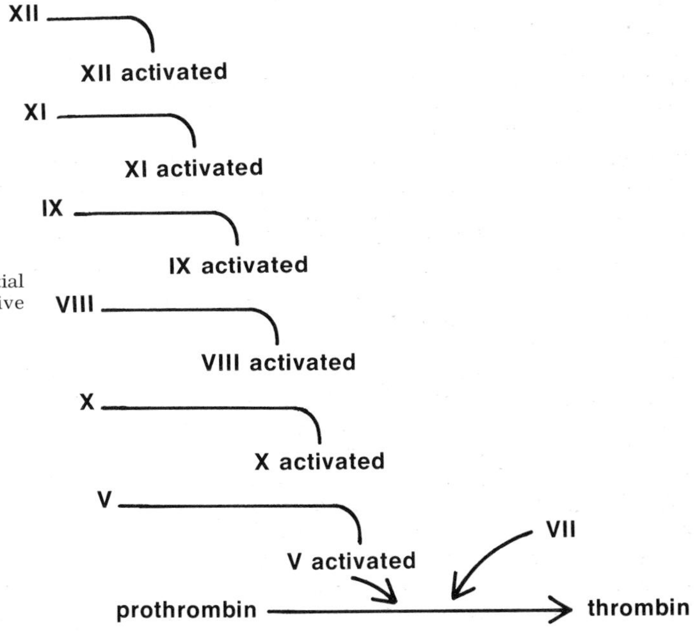

Figure 6–1. Intrinsic coagulation system (partial thromboplastin and calcium required). In the native blood, platelets furnish thromboplastin.

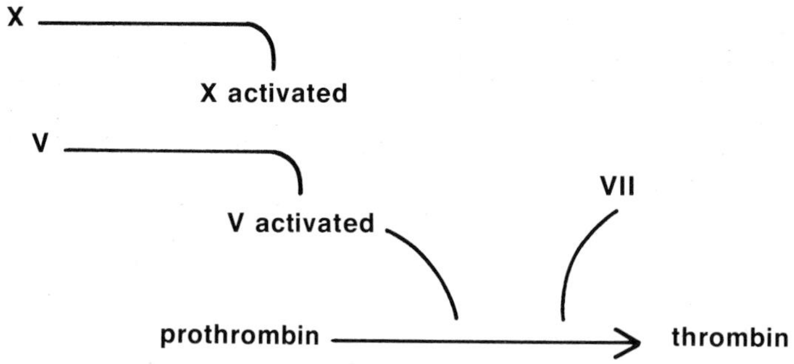

Figure 6–2. Extrinsic system (complete thromboplastin and calcium needed). The thromboplastin can be tissue thromboplastin as in the prothrombin time test or can be generated in native blood by the reactions of factors XII, XI, IX, VIII, partial thromboplastin and calcium.

and a source of partial thromboplastin are required, it is not clear which procoagulants can be activated in the absence of one or both of these substances. Exposure of blood to a wettable surface is thought to trigger the reaction sequence.

An earlier theory that was made popular by the introduction of the Thromboplastin Generation Test is not inconsistent with the data or the cascade theory. This hypothesis is based on the differences of reactivity of complete and partial thromboplastins. It is postulated that in the native system blood clots by the intrinsic system whereas in test procedures using tissue thromboplastin an alternate pathway, the extrinsic system, is utilized. Thus, factors XII, XI, IX and VIII are essential for the intrinsic pathway but do not influence the extrinsic pathway. The interaction of these procoagulants, calcium and partial thromboplastin from platelets is believed to result in the formation of blood thromboplastin which has the same activity as tissue thromboplastin. Thus, the final reactions of the intrinsic system and the extrinsic system are identical. The postulated sequence of events is illustrated in Figures 6–1 and 6–2.

The concepts described above are currently the most popular, but there are other ideas that are equally consistent with the accumulated data. Seegers (1962) has proposed that prothrombin is transformed into thrombin in a series of reactions and that some of the procoagulants are derived from the prothrombin molecule. The relationship of this theory and the cascade theory is discussed by Mammen (1971). Fortunately it is not essential to resolve the differences between the various concepts in order to establish a clinical diagnosis by laboratory methods. Although some theoretical aspects will be included, this chapter will deal mainly with information derived from clinical and laboratory observations of patients who have been found to have a deficiency in the hemostatic mechanism.

BLOOD PLATELETS

Blood platelets, or thrombocytes, are small (2 to 3 μ) discrete cell fragments present in circulating blood. They are bits of cytoplasm of megakaryocytes. In adults, megakaryocytes are found predominantly in the bone marrow, but they occur occasionally in other tissues, including the lungs. As megakaryocytes mature, their cytoplasm becomes granular and bits of cytoplasm break off and enter the blood in the form of blood platelets. These cell fragments circulate for four to six days before being removed by reticuloendothelial cells.

Normal blood contains 150,000 to 300,000 platelets per cubic millimeter. Following acute blood loss or surgical procedures, platelets are characteristically increased for several days.

Platelets have three major functions in hemostasis: aggregation and formation of a hemostatic plug, thromboplastic activity, and clot retraction.

Aggregation. Platelets circulate in the bloodstream as discrete bodies, but during the clotting process platelets clump together to form large masses. Platelets, like fibrinogen, have a built-in property of self-assembly. In the environment of circulating blood, platelets are separated by repulsive forces. When blood escapes from the vessel or when there is injury to the vessel wall, the environment is altered, and platelets aggregate together or adhere to the injured vessel wall. The exact circumstances under which platelets lose their repulsive forces is being studied by a number of investigators. Thrombin, collagen, and adenosine diphosphate (ADP) are currently being used to alter the platelet environment to stimulate platelet aggregation. An excellent study of the physical forces involved in erythrocyte agglutination by Pollack *et al.* (1965) suggests that similar forces could be of importance in platelet agglutination.

It is generally believed that this aggregation

of platelets to form a hemostatic plug at the site of injury to vessel walls is an important part of hemostasis. Unfortunately there are no procedures available at the present time that are adaptable for use in evaluation of this important function in patients, except as a research project.

Procoagulant Activity. Platelets have a procoagulant activity, as is demonstrated by the abnormal utilization of prothrombin in the clotting of platelet poor blood (Brinkhous, 1939). One of the procoagulant activities of platelets is to serve as a source of thromboplastin in native clotting systems. In this respect, platelets function as a partial thromboplastin. Other procoagulant activities have been found in platelets. These are described in detail by Seegers (1962). It is not clear which activities that can be demonstrated in platelets are integral parts of the thrombocyte and which are derived from the plasma environment. It has been suggested that platelets act as a sponge and acquire a certain amount of all constituents of plasma. The role of the nonthromboplastic procoagulant activity of the platelet in hemostasis is speculative.

Clot Retraction. When whole blood is allowed to clot and is observed over a period of time, the clot will be seen to decrease in size and clear serum will be expressed from the clot. This phenomenon is called clot retraction and is a function of platelets. The process is believed to be due to a rearrangement of the fibrin clot and is dependent upon intact functional platelets being present during formation of the clot. This phenomenon is essential to the formation of a firm hemostatic plug.

Thrombocytopenia. Whenever the number of circulating platelets decreases to 70,000 per cu. mm. or below, a clinically evident bleeding tendency exists. The syndrome is called thrombocytopenia. Although thrombocytopenia may be the result of diverse causes, the clinical and laboratory findings are a result of the severity of the thrombocytopenia.

The clinical manifestations of thrombocytopenia consist of easy bruising and excessive bleeding from minor lacerations. The bruising is frequently referred to as being spontaneous, but careful study of the history of the case usually reveals that trauma occurred but was so minor that the patient did not associate it with the appearance of the bruise.

The characteristic laboratory findings are (1) platelet count below 70,000 per cu. mm., (2) prolonged bleeding time, (3) poor clot retraction, (4) delayed utilization of prothrombin during clotting, and (5) increased capillary fragility.

Thrombocytopenia is the result of either decreased production or increased destruction of platelets. Since megakaryocytes are present principally in the bone marrow, any disorder involving the marrow can result in thrombocytopenia. Thus, thrombocytopenia is common in acute leukemia, total body irradiation, metastatic neoplasms involving bone, lipid storage diseases, lymphoma, and many other disorders in which the function of the marrow is impaired by a disease process. The thrombocytopenia frequently associated with untreated pernicious anemia may be an indication of the need of a maturation factor for platelets as well as erythrocytes.

Certain drugs and chemicals will cause sufficient marrow impairment to cause thrombocytopenia on a dose-related basis. The chemotherapeutic agents in use for control of malignant neoplasms are an example of these dose-related compounds. Other chemicals produce thrombocytopenia on a drug idiosyncrasy basis. Many isolated cases of thrombocytopenia due to drug idiosyncrasy have been reported, and the list of implicated compounds is long. To say that all drugs have been implicated would be only a slight overstatement. Some of the compounds have been shown to have a direct effect on the platelets rather than on the bone marrow. This was well documented for the drug Sedormid by Ackroyd (1955). Unfortunately such a clear-cut cause-and-effect relationship is demonstrated only infrequently. The drug sensitivity type of thrombocytopenia requires a considerable amount of detective work to determine the causative agent.

A syndrome of thrombocytopenia for which no exogenous toxic agent can be demonstrated is called *idiopathic thrombocytopenic purpura*. This syndrome occurs predominantly in young adults, although children and elderly individuals are also affected. The bone marrow contains abundant megakaryocytes, which has led some investigators to suggest that the defect is due to "maturation arrest." It was found that platelets from normal individuals had a decreased survival when transfused into patients with the disorder (Sprague *et al.*, 1952).

Since the thrombocytopenia was at least temporarily alleviated by splenectomy, it was felt that this was a disorder of the spleen. The work of Harrington *et al.* (1951) did much to indicate the pathogenesis of this syndrome.

Harrington *et al.* (1951) transfused plasma from patients with idiopathic thrombocytopenia into healthy volunteers, including the investigators, and produced a prompt and dramatic fall in the platelets in the blood of the recipients. In other studies (Harrington *et al.*, 1953) it was found that plasma from patients in remission following splenectomy would still cause thrombocytopenia when transfused into normal volunteers. Plasma from patients in spontaneous remission or steroid-induced remission did not cause thrombocytopenia when infused into normal subjects. It is clear from these excellent studies that patients with this form of thrombocytopenia have an antiplatelet factor in their plasma. It is felt that this factor is most likely an antiplatelet antibody. Work to demonstrate this by *in vitro* methods has been disappointing, although the data are consistent with the antibody concept. At the present time this form of thrombocytopenia is considered to be one of the autoimmune diseases. Isoantibodies have been demonstrated in the blood of patients receiving multiple transfusions, but it is felt that such isoantibodies have no relationship to idiopathic thrombocytopenia.

The role of the spleen in thrombocytopenia remains a provocative subject. In most disorders in which there is splenomegaly of any magnitude, there is also thrombocytopenia. Following splenectomy there is an increase in the number of circulating platelets. The duration of the thrombocytosis varies among individuals. This has led to the speculation that the spleen has a thrombocyte-regulating function and that some forms of thrombocytopenia are due to excessive splenic function—hypersplenism. A more attractive presumption is that the spleen and other reticuloendothelial tissues function by removing abnormal cells from circulation. The basic defect in thrombocytopenia characterized by decreased platelet life span could thus be thought of as being defective platelets. The defect could be due to abnormal formation or to damage produced by antibodies or other agents. It is likely that thrombocytopenia is a symptom caused by a wide variety of mechanisms.

Qualitative Platelet Defects. Information on the function of platelets in hemostasis has been derived from the study of patients with thrombocytopenia or from normal plasma that has been made platelet deficient by centrifugation. In these studies platelet function is directly related to the number of platelets in the test system. A few patients have been reported as having clinical and laboratory findings characteristic of decreased platelet function while having adequate numbers of platelets in circulation. These patients have qualitative platelet defects. Various eponyms have been used for isolated cases of this type. At the present time the various case reports are not clearly defined, so it is not clear which platelet function is lacking in each. For this reason it is preferable to consider qualitative platelet disorders as a syndrome and to subclassify on the basis of the specific platelet function that is deficient.

Qualitative platelet disorders will have abnormalities detectable by bleeding time, tourniquet test, clot retraction, or tests for thromboplastic function. The syndrome may appear as an isolated single disorder, or it may be a combined defect. The relationship of the platelet function and hemostasis has been discussed by Rodman and Mason (1967) and more recently by Roberts and Kroncke (1971).

Seegers (1962) considers the thromboplastic function as platelet factor 3. Patients with an isolated deficiency of this function have been reported (Ulutin, 1960). This activity is detected by substituting a suspension of platelets from the patient for the partial thromboplastin in one of the standard methods. Interpretation of results may be difficult because of technical problems in standardization of the technique of isolation of the platelets.

VASCULAR FACTORS

It is generally recognized that the integrity of the vessel wall is an important factor in hemostasis, but the procedures to evaluate vascular integrity are not adaptable to clinical use. As a result, this important aspect of hemostasis has remained for the most part a matter of speculation. Some information can be gained by estimating vascular fragility by the tourniquet test, but there remain a large group of disorders that cannot be evaluated by laboratory procedures. In these there is clinical evidence of a bleeding tendency, but all laboratory parameters are found to be in the normal range.

The importance of vascular integrity is obvious in traumatic wounds resulting in lacerations of major arteries. Blood coagulation is effective in these circumstances only after the defect of the artery has been repaired by surgical intervention. With injury to smaller size vessels, the action of platelets and plasma coagulation factors will promptly stop the flow of blood. On the basis of clinical observations, it is apparent that in some individuals bleeding from vascular injury continues in spite of normal platelet function and plasma coagulation activity. The nature of the vascular defect involved in these patients is not clear.

Unfortunately many patients are diagnosed as having a vascular defect because there is no other obvious cause of the symptoms presented. However, a few syndromes are sufficiently distinct that they are described briefly.

Vitamin C Deficiency. It has been known for many years that there is a bleeding tendency associated with scurvy. This takes the form of a tendency to bruise easily, with possible ecchymosis and frank hemorrhage into muscular tissues. In adults, tender bleeding gums is a frequent manifestation. Except for a positive reaction to a tourniquet test, the usual laboratory procedures for evaluating a bleeding tendency are of diagnostic importance only in that they exclude other possible causes of the bleeding tendency. Although frank scurvy is rare in this country at this time, a carefully obtained history will indicate a few individuals with dietary habits that result in an inadequate intake of vitamin C. These individuals have low plasma vitamin C levels, and their bleeding symptoms respond to administration of vitamin C. There are several specific procedures for the determination of blood ascorbic acid levels. These should be used in cases where the purpura suggests such a deficiency. The basic defect is believed to be due to increased capillary permeability and the inability to form a fibroblastic scar.

Vascular Purpura. In this group of disorders, the symptoms are those of a bleeding disorder characterized by a tendency to bruise easily, ecchymoses, and petechial hemorrhages. The laboratory findings are of importance mainly in that they exclude other disorders. The platelets are normal in number and function and the coagulation factors are characteristically present in normal amounts.

In most cases it appears that this syndrome is a result of an allergic response. Many different causative agents have been reported.

The purpura may be associated with abdominal complaints. Henoch (1874) noted the relationship between the abdominal pain and some types of purpura. Schönlein (1832) had previously noted joint pain and tenderness in association with purpura. The eponym Henoch-Schönlein purpura has been used for this syndrome.

The bleeding is not serious, and symptoms usually disappear spontaneously in about a week. Recurrent episodes are common unless the causative agent can be discovered and exposure avoided.

Hereditary Telangiectasis. This is a familial disorder characterized by a tendency to bleed from mucous surfaces at the site of vascular abnormalities. Although bleeding may be massive, platelets and plasma coagulation factors are normal. This defect appears to be transmitted as a somatic dominant trait. The vascular anomalies are characteristically small and appear clinically as telangiectases on the face, tongue, or oral mucosa. Bleeding from gastrointestinal vascular anomalies is frequently the presenting symptom. Diagnosis depends on family history, multiple telangiectases, and history of hemorrhage. Laboratory tests are usually of diagnostic value only in that other causes of a bleeding tendency are excluded.

PLASMA COAGULATION FACTORS

Blood coagulation is that phase of hemostasis involved in the formation of the fibrin clot. The various factors involved in the activation of prothrombin to form thrombin have been the basis of extensive research reviewed by Brinkhous, Langdell, and Wagner (1958). Certain characteristics of the plasma clotting factors appear to be well established, although their mechanism of action is still debated.

A major consideration in classification of the plasma clotting factors has been the discovery of patients with hereditary deficiencies of the procoagulants. In the following discussion the various factors will be considered on the basis of the disease states in which deficiencies of specific proteins appear to be the underlying abnormality. The role of the various factors in normal hemostasis will be inferred from the abnormalities resulting from their absence.

Fibrinogen

Nomenclature. Fibrinogen is the soluble precursor of the clot-forming protein, fibrin. This substance has been designated as factor I by the International Committee for the Nomenclature of Blood Clotting Factors (Wright, 1962). Since the term fibrinogen has been in general use for many years, the factor I designation is used only for completeness and is not frequently used for communication.

By the action of thrombin, peptides are split from the fibrinogen molecule. These peptides have been designated as fibrinopeptide A and fibrinopeptide B. The residual molecule has been designated as fibrin monomer. Under ordinary conditions the monomers polymerize to form a fibrin clot. Polymerized fibrin exists in at least two forms. In the presence of factor XIII (fibrin stabilizing factor), thrombin, and calcium, the fibrin polymer forms cross-links and the resulting clot is not soluble in urea. In the absence of factor XIII, cross-linking of fibrin filaments fails to occur and the resulting clot is soluble in urea and weak acids.

Pathophysiology of Defects Involving Fibrinogen Deficiency. Fibrinogen is essential for the formation of a blood clot, since it is the substance from which the clot is formed. It has been estimated that as long as fibrinogen is present in plasma at a level of 100 mg. per 100 ml. or higher, one-stage clotting tests will not be abnormally long. Hartman (1952) pointed out that in cases of polycythemia secondary to cyanotic heart disease it is important to consider the amount of fibrinogen in terms of whole blood.

Congenital deficiencies of fibrinogen have been found to be of three types: (1) afibrinogenemia, in which no fibrinogen can be measured by physicochemical methods; (2) hypofibrinogenemia, in which fibrinogen is present but in amounts of less than 100 mg. per 100 ml.; and (3) dysfibrinogenemia, in which fibrinogen is decreased as measured by its reaction to thrombin but is present in normal amounts when measured immunologically. It is of interest that although fibrinogen is obviously essential for clot formation, clinical symptoms of patients deficient in fibrinogen are less severe than are the symptoms of patients with a deficiency of one of the procoagulants.

Congenital Afibrinogenemia. Patients with reported congenital afibrinogenemia have been reviewed by Werder (1963). Blood from these patients does not form a visible clot either spontaneously or following the addition of thrombin. No fibrinogen can be demonstrated by physicochemical methods, but from immunologic studies it appears that a trace of fibrinogen is present.

Congenital Dysfibrinogenemia. A small group of patients reported with functionally abnormal fibrinogen were reviewed by Jackson, Beck, and Charache (1965). They used the term dysfibrinogenemia to designate the defect in this group of patients. A visible clot forms when blood is allowed to clot spontaneously. The amount of fibrinogen in the plasma is decreased, but exact amounts are dependent on the method used for determination. There appears to be deficient fibrinogen as measured by methods relying on the rate of clotting after addition of thrombin. It is estimated that congenital dysfibrinogenemia occurs more frequently than the small number of reported cases would indicate. If so, the knowledge that such a defect exists will stimulate other workers to investigate patients with a mild bleeding tendency who are not diagnosed by the usual methods.

Congenital Hypofibrinogenemia. Patients have been reported who have low but detectable fibrinogen. These tend to have a familial pattern. The relationship of such cases to afibrinogenemia and dysfibrinogenemia is not clear at this time. In most cases, bleeding symptoms do not occur unless the fibrinogen level decreases to a point below 100 mg. per 100 ml.

Acquired Deficiency of Fibrinogen. This occurs in a number of disorders affecting the liver—the site of fibrinogen synthesis. However, isolated fibrinogen deficiency is an uncommon complication of liver disease, since several procoagulants are also synthesized there. A group of disorders of fibrinogen have been described in patients with active fibrinolytic activity. These cases have been called fibrinogenolytic dysfibrinogenemias and were reviewed by Fletcher (1966).

Properties. Fibrinogen is a plasma protein with a molecular weight of about 340,000. It is present in plasma of normal persons in amounts of 300 to 400 mg. per 100 ml. It is less soluble than most of the other plasma proteins and can be precipitated from plasma by 25 per cent saturation with ammonium sulfate. When plasma is frozen and thawed, fibrinogen is present as particulate matter (Ware, Guest, and Seegers, 1947). A tyrosine residue has been present in all fibrinogens studied. Fibrinogen is denatured in plasma incubated at 56° C. for 3 minutes. The structure of fibrinogen has been studied by Hall and Slayter (1959). They estimate the molecule to be 475 Å in length and consist of three nodular structures connected by a thread. Two terminal nodules are about 65 Å in diameter, and the central nodule is slightly smaller.

Fibrinogen is not adsorbed from oxalate plasma by barium sulfate but is absent in serum. Estimates of plasma clearance of infused fibrinogen indicate half of the infused activity to be lost in three to four days (Werder, 1963).

Fibrinogen is changed to fibrin by the action of thrombin. According to Laki (1965), thrombin splits four peptide bonds of each fibrinogen molecule and four peptides are released. These are of two types—fibrinopeptide A and fibrinopeptide B. It appears that the presence of these peptides on the fibrinogen molecule inhibits polymerization because they act as repulsive forces. Following the release of the four peptides, aggregation of fibrin molecules takes place spontaneously. According to Laki (1965), the ionic conditions determine the type of aggregation. End-to-end aggregation is predominant at pH 8, and side-to-side aggregation is more common at pH 6.5. In the presence of factor XIII (fibrin stabilizing factor), the fibrin aggregates form cross-linkages by a transpeptidating mechanism (Lorand, 1965).

Genetic Aspects of Fibrinogen Deficiency. Fibrinogen appears to be controlled by an autosomal gene. Family studies of patients with congenital afibrinogenemia indicate that the disorder is transmitted by an autosomal recessive gene. Severely affected patients appear to be homozygous. There is an indication that low fibrinogen levels are present in persons heterozygous for the trait. Jackson *et al.* (1965) suggest that congenital hypofibrinogenemia may represent the heterozygous state of congenital afibrinogenemia. The pattern in family studies of congenital hypofibrinogenemia is also that of an autosomal recessive gene. Dysfibrinogenemia is apparently determined by an abnormal dominant gene (Jackson *et al.*, 1965). It remains to be demonstrated whether these disorders represent an abnormality at more than one locus.

Diagnosis of Fibrinogen Deficiency. A clinically evident bleeding tendency owing to fibrinogen deficiency can occur as a result of congenital deficiency, intravascular coagulation syndrome, liver disease, or active fibrinolysis. Although fibrinogen may be quite low, bleeding is usually not life threatening in the congenital form, so diagnosis is made on the basis of a quantitative assay of fibrinogen. Such studies should be done during a clinically quiet stage of the disease, since diagnosis of hypofibrinogenemia might not be made if the patient has recently received a transfusion of blood or plasma. The true fibrinogen level can be determined only when the patient is not actively bleeding and has had no transfusions for at least three to four weeks.

In emergency situations, such as the intravascular clotting syndrome occurring as an obstetrical complication, the bleeding may be life threatening. In such emergencies, it is important to make the correct diagnosis promptly, and quantitative fibrinogen determinations are too time consuming to be of immediate value. In such cases the thrombin clotting time is useful for the rapid estimation of fibrinogen. A sample of blood should be retained for a more quantitative measurement, but therapy should be instituted on the basis of the more rapid procedure.

Fibrinolysis may be a part of the intravascular clotting syndrome. It may not be possible to determine quickly whether the low fibrinogen is due to intravascular coagulation or fibrinolysis. One of the tests for fibrinolysis should be started, but the results will not be available for several hours. It should be assumed for the purpose of therapy that the primary defect is a deficiency of fibrinogen, and treatment should be started with a potent fibrinogen preparation. If it is later learned that fibrinolysis is the cause, specific therapy for this may be instituted.

At the present time the use of a number of procedures is required to distinguish dysfibrinogenemia from hypofibrinogenemia. Such a diagnosis should be suspected if there is a marked discrepancy between the thrombin clotting time and specific fibrinogen determinations. An immunologic method is necessary for the diagnosis (Jackson, Beck and Charache, 1965).

Prothrombin

Nomenclature. Prothrombin is the inactive precursor of the active proteolytic enzyme thrombin. This was designated factor II by the International Committee for the Nomenclature of Blood Clotting Factors (Wright, 1962). The term prothrombin has been in common use for many years and thus the term factor II is used only for completeness.

Pathophysiology of Defects Involving Prothrombin Deficiency. In normal plasma, there is an excess of prothrombin relative to the amount of thrombin needed to clot fibrinogen. It is known that in each milliliter of plasma there is the potential to form about 300 units of thrombin. This would be sufficient to clot the fibrinogen in 300 ml. of plasma in 15 seconds. Thus, the amount of prothrombin present would appear to be less critical to the clotting mechanism than the availability of factors necessary for its prompt conversion to thrombin. It is of interest that in studies done in which thrombin activity during clotting of blood was measured, not more than two units of thrombin could be detected at any time, although almost 300 units of prothrombin were utilized (Smith, 1943). At the time of visible clot formation in whole blood, the amount of prothrombin has decreased by less than five units (Langdell, Graham, and Brinkhous, 1950). These studies suggest that nature has provided a wide margin of safety for this important substance. A patient with an acquired isolated prothrombin deficiency reported by Karpatkin *et al.* (1962) had a severe bleeding tendency when no prothrombin was detectable by the two-stage method. Symptoms began to resolve when prothrombin became measurable. It is of interest that the prothrombin time and partial thromboplastin time were only slightly prolonged during the period when only a trace of prothrombin was measurable.

It is clear that prothrombin is synthesized by the liver and that vitamin K is essential for this process (Brinkhous, 1940). The relationship of prothrombin to the other vitamin K-dependent procoagulants is still a matter of speculation. When patients are treated with vitamin K-blocking drugs, such as Dicumarol, plasma prothrombin levels slowly decrease. With administration of vitamin K, plasma prothrombin levels slowly return toward normal. Although prothrombin deficiency occurs frequently in association with various disease states, there is almost always a concomitant decrease in other clotting factors as well.

Properties. Prothrombin is present in plasma in amounts of 10 to 15 mg. per 100 ml. It is utilized during the clotting process so that little remains in serum. Prothrombin is readily removed from oxalated plasma by various insoluble alkaline earths such as barium sulfate. The activity can be recovered from the precipitated material by elution with sodium citrate solution. The molecular weight of prothrombin has been calculated to be about 69,000 (Seegers, 1962). Prothrombin has an electrophoretic mobility between albumin and alpha globulins (Lewis *et al.*, 1958).

The prothrombin molecule is relatively unstable in that it tends to form the active enzyme thrombin. In plasma, this process depends upon the procoagulants for rapid evolution of thrombin. When isolated in purification procedures, thrombin evolution may be spontaneous. It is of interest that citrate acts in plasma to prevent the formation of thrombin, while purified prothrombin spontaneously converts to thrombin in high citrate concentration (Seegers, 1962).

The transformation of prothrombin molecules into thrombin molecules is under active investigation by a number of investigators. Seegers (1962) feels that this is a "step-wise" process in which clot accelerators that are not thrombin or precursors of thrombin are products of the reaction. He has called these substances autoprothrombins and has demonstrated types of activities similar to those of various procoagulants. Other investigators using different starting materials feel that prothrombin forms only one active enzyme—thrombin. There is no point in elaborating on these observations at this time, since the problem has still to be solved. It is clear, however, that one of the split products of prothrombin is thrombin.

Genetic Aspects of Prothrombin Deficiency. A number of patients have been reported who have congenital hypoprothrombinemia. Graham (1957), in reviewing these cases, felt that none met the criteria of isolated prothrombin deficiency.

Diagnosis of Prothrombin Deficiency. Prothrombin deficiency is almost always associated with a deficiency in other procoagulants. It is therefore difficult to determine whether the symptoms are due to the decreased prothrombin or a combination of deficiencies. The distinction is usually of only academic interest because therapy is the same. One-stage type clotting tests are affected by a number of factors in addition to prothrombin. The occasional case of true prothrombin deficiency can be diagnosed by the two-stage prothrombin method. This procedure will accurately measure prothrombin when other factors are also deficient.

Thromboplastin

The term thromboplastin was used by early workers to designate the clot accelerating action of extracts of tissue. Most of the tissue preparations had only weak clot promoting activity. Mills (1926) was able to prepare a potent tissue extract from lung tissue and believed that with such a preparation plasma prothrombin was not necessary for clotting. Some of the activity of his preparation was found to be due to contamination of the tissue extract with prothrombin and fibrinogen. Smith, Warner, and Brinkhous (1937) were able to prepare a potent thromboplastin from lung tissue that was free of prothrombin and fibrinogen. They demonstrated that calcium and tissue thromboplastin were necessary for conversion of plasma prothrombin to thrombin. Later, Quick found that a thromboplastin of similar potency could be prepared more easily from brain tissue.

It was noted by Quick (1947) that when active tissue thromboplastin was used, hemophilic plasma clotted as rapidly as normal plasma. This was in contrast to the earlier observation by Mills (1926) that crude cephalin preparations were relatively inactive when used with hemophilic plasma. In a study of the effect of antihemophilic factor on one-stage clotting tests, Langdell, Wagner, and Brinkhous (1953) found there were two types of thromboplastic activity. They confirmed the observation of Mills that crude cephalin preparations did not clot hemophilic plasma as rapidly as it did normal plasma. When active tissue thromboplastins were diluted or fractionated, these preparations had an activity similar to crude cephalin. On the basis of these findings, thromboplastin preparations could be described as complete or partial. Complete thromboplastins are able to produce clotting as rapidly with hemophilic plasma as with normal plasma. Partial thromboplastins clot hemophilic plasma less rapidly than they do normal plasma. This difference appears to be a matter of degree rather than chemical composition, since simple dilution changes a complete thromboplastin to a partial thromboplastin. Considerable insight into the complex coagulation mechanism can be gained if one understands the difference between complete and partial thromboplastins.

During clotting of whole blood, platelets appear to be the source of thromboplastin. Platelet suspensions behave as partial thromboplastins when used in one-stage clotting tests. An interesting theory is based on the assumption that platelets plus certain procoagulants interact to become complete thromboplastins during clotting (Biggs and Macfarlane, 1957). In spite of the popularity of this theory, the effects noted may be the result of impurities in the test system.

The clot accelerating activity of tissues has been assigned the term factor III by the International Committee for the Nomenclature of Blood Clotting Factors (Wright, 1962). This has not helped in communication, since each of the various tissue extracts has different activities in the clotting system. In this chapter the term tissue thromboplastin is used to designate the saline extract of tissues. The term partial thromboplastin is used to designate those reagents that are found to clot hemophilic plasma less rapidly than normal plasma.

Calcium

It has been known for many years that calcium is essential to the clotting process. The use of calcium binding anticoagulants makes it possible to store blood in blood banks and to study plasma. The exact mechanism by which calcium acts is not known. It may be necessary in more than one reaction. Although it is of great importance in *in vitro* studies of coagulation, it is very unlikely that hypocalcemia has been the cause of a clinical bleeding tendency except in a few cases in which massive transfusion of ACD blood was involved. This is because coagulation can take place with less calcium than that necessary for other physiologic functions. Clinical tetany occurs with higher levels than are necessary for adequate coagulation.

The influence of calcium is great in *in vitro* tests. In any type of procedure in which blood samples are of diverse origin, one must always consider whether the results obtained could be on the basis of variable calcium. In most tests of coagulation in which plasma is recalcified, the amount of calcium is a critical factor. The amount of calcium added to the various tests has been empirically determined to be in the optimal range when blood is mixed with standard quantities of anticoagulant solution. Nevertheless, calcium concentration must be considered whenever anticoagulants are used to obtain plasma for testing, since the ratio of plasma to cells may be a variable. If serum is used as a reagent, it must be taken into consideration that an anticoagulant is not usually used in obtaining serum. Thus, the amount of calcium to be added in order to recalcify a mixture of plasma and serum is different than the amount necessary to recalcify a mixture of plasmas.

It must be kept in mind that all anticoagulants do not act in the same manner. The soluble oxalate salts act as anticoagulants because, with calcium ions poorly soluble, calcium oxalate forms and precipitates. The amount of anticoagulant used in standard procedures results in an excess of soluble oxalate in solution. With recalcification, more calcium oxalate forms. Citrate salts are effective as anticoagulants because a soluble calcium-citrate complex is formed. Although calcium remains in solution, it appears to be unavailable for the clotting process. In standard tests, excess citrate is used. The chelates also bind calcium in a soluble complex. The neutralization of these multivalent ions is much more complex than is the neutralization of oxalate.

The term factor IV was assigned by the International Committee for the Nomenclature of Blood Clotting Factors (Wright, 1962) to calcium when it participates in the coagulation reaction. Since there is little confusion in respect to calcium, the term is seldom used.

Factor V

Nomenclature. A patient with a hereditary deficiency of this procoagulant was described by Owren (1947). He suggested the term parahemophilia for the deficiency state and the term factor V for the procoagulant. Stored plasma was found to become deficient in a nonprothrombin factor necessary for rapid clotting, which was called labile factor (Quick, 1947). Purified prothrombin preparations were found to require a plasma factor for effective thrombin formation (Fantl and Nance, 1946; Ware, Guest, and Seegers, 1947). The term accelerator globulin (Ac-globulin) was used for this plasma factor (Ware, Guest, and Seegers, 1947). It is now generally assumed that all of these observers were studying the same activity, and the term factor V has been assigned (Wright, 1962).

The terminology is still uncertain because some investigators have postulated that an inactive precursor becomes transformed to an active accelerator during coagulation. The terms factor VI, accelerin, and serum Ac-globulin have been used for a theoretically active substance, and factor V, proaccelerin, and plasma Ac-globulin for the inactive precursor.

Pathophysiology of Defects Involving Factor V Deficiency. Factor V is essential for the prompt conversion of prothrombin to thrombin in clotting of whole blood as well as in the presence of tissue thromboplastins. In the absence of factor V, abnormal results are obtained with each of the following test procedures: prothrombin time, partial thromboplastin time, whole blood clotting time, prothrombin utilization, and thromboplastin generation.

Patients with a congenital defect have a bleeding tendency of moderate severity. The reported cases were summarized by Fantl (1957). Symptoms consist of excessive bleeding from trauma, epistaxis, and gastrointestinal bleeding. Hemarthrosis is uncommon.

Factor V is believed to be formed by the liver, and acquired deficiencies have occurred in liver disease. When factor V levels decrease to 30 per cent of normal, bleeding manifestations occur. Purpura fulminans is a severe form of acquired factor V deficiency that occurs in association with an infectious disease such as scarlet fever. Factor V deficiency may result from the action of fibrinolysis in association with carcinoma of the prostate or other disorders involving increased fibrinolysis.

Factor V is retained in circulation longer than some of the procoagulants. In a study by Webster *et al.* (1964), it was found that half the activity achieved by transfusion of congenitally deficient patients was present 36 hours after infusion.

Properties. Factor V is a procoagulant present in human plasma but deficient in human serum. The activity decreases within a few hours when human blood or plasma is stored at room temperature or higher. It was for this reason that the term labile factor was used. However, as was pointed out by Fantl (1957), stability depends upon the conditions of storage. The relative lability of human factor V does not apply to other species. Although relatively little factor V activity is present in human blood after clotting, beef serum is a potent source of active material.

This is a trace protein, as indicated by the finding that electrophoretic patterns of normal and factor V deficient plasma appear identical. The activity can be salted out with the globulin fraction by 33 to 50 per cent ammonium sulfate saturation and is precipitated from dilute plasma at pH 5.0 to 5.5. It is thermolabile and is destroyed by trypsin.

Factor V activity in plasma can be separated from some of the procoagulants by treatment of the plasma with one of several insoluble alkaline earths such as barium sulfate. Factor V activity is not decreased by treatment of oxalated plasma with barium sulfate and similar prothrombin adsorbents. Plasma so treated is a useful reagent.

Genetic Aspects of Factor V Deficiency. The mode of inheritance of factor V deficiency has been reviewed by Fantl (1957) and Graham (1957). It appears to be an autosomal recessive trait. Seriously affected individuals are homozygous for the defective gene. There is some evidence that patients who are heterozygous for the trait have low levels of activity but do not have a bleeding tendency.

Diagnosis of Factor V Deficiency. Factor V deficiency should be suspected in any patient in whom the prothrombin time is found to be significantly prolonged. The results of the partial thromboplastin time will also be abnormal. The clotting defect is corrected by the addition of fresh normal plasma or fresh normal plasma treated with barium sulfate.

Some laboratories maintain a supply of plasma known to be deficient in this factor. Such plasma should not correct the patient's defect. Patients with liver disease may be deficient in factor V as well as in other procoagulants. In this case, simple mixing studies will not give unequivocal results. Also, a specific quantitative assay procedure is necessary for diagnosis.

Factor VII

Nomenclature. Alexander and associates (1951) used the term serum prothrombin conversion accelerator (SPCA) for the procoagulant that was deficient in a patient found to have a previously unrecognized bleeding tendency. It had been noted earlier by deVries, Alexander, and Goldstein (1949) that a factor, present in both plasma and serum, accelerated one-stage type clotting tests. This activity could be distinguished from prothrombin and factor V. Owren (1953) believed that the factor existed in two forms: an inactive precursor (proconvertin) and an active accelerator (convertin). There is some confusion in the literature about the characteristics of the disease state and the procoagulant, since factor X was not recognized as a distinct entity until 1957. Hougie, Barrow, and Graham (1957) pointed out that patients thought to have a deficiency of factor VII represented two separate and distinct deficiencies. The term factor VII was assigned by the International Committee for the Nomenclature of Blood Clotting Factors (Wright, 1962) to the procoagulant deficiency of the patient described by Alexander *et al.* (1951).

Pathophysiology of Defects Involving Factor VII Deficiency. Factor VII is essential for rapid clotting of plasma in procedures using tissue thromboplastin. Prothrombin utilization is normal in clotting of whole blood of patients deficient in the factor. Procedures using partial thromboplastin or native blood are unaffected by the absence of factor VII. With a deficiency of factor VII, characteristically only the prothrombin time is abnormal. Russell's viper venom (Stypven, Burroughs Wellcome & Co.), added to the prothrombin time procedure, will compensate for the deficiency.

The cases of congenital factor VII deficiency reported through 1964 have been reviewed by Marder and Shulman (1964). They noted a wide variation in hemorrhagic manifestations of patients with the same degree of deficiency. Bleeding in the reported cases has been in the form of epistaxis, easy bruising, and gingival bleeding. In women, severe menorrhagia is common.

Acquired deficiency of factor VII results from any disorder decreasing the synthesis of the factor in the liver, for which vitamin K is essential. Since other procoagulants are also affected, a pure acquired deficiency of factor VII is rare. It is estimated that manifestation of a hemorrhagic diathesis occurs with levels of factor VII below 15 per cent of normal. Hall *et al.* (1964) noted a paucity of bleeding episodes in factor VII deficient patients after surgical procedures other than tooth extractions.

Factor VII activity is cleared from the plasma rapidly. Following infusion of normal plasma into patients congenitally deficient in factor VII or during coumarin therapy, half the activity in the plasma disappears within 4 to 6 hours (Marder and Shulman, 1964). Synthesis also appears to be rapid, since factor VII activity returns to normal within 5 to 6 hours after adequate vitamin K has been administered to a patient with low plasma levels due to coumarin therapy.

Properties. Factor VII is a relatively stable procoagulant, although its activity in serum is destroyed at 56° C. within 3 minutes. It is present in high levels in stored blood as well as in serum. Unlike factors V and VIII, which decrease during clotting, there is evidence that suggests that factor VII activity may actually increase during the clotting process and during storage at 4° C. Factor VII is readily adsorbed from oxalated plasma by barium sulfate. The activity can be recovered by elution of the precipitated material with citrate solution.

Factor VII activity is not precipitated with the globulin fraction and is inactivated below pH 5 and above pH 9 (deVries *et al.*, 1949). It has been estimated that factor VII comprises less than 0.07 per cent of serum proteins (Alexander, 1961). In continuous flow electrophoresis, factor VII migrates with the alpha globulins (Lewis *et al.*, 1958).

Genetic Aspects of Factor VII Deficiency. The congenital deficiency of factor VII appears to result from a defective autosomal gene (Marder and Shulman, 1964). The severe bleeders are probably homozygous for the abnormal gene. In some family studies, a mild deficiency is present in persons heterozygous for the defect. These findings indicate that the defect is autosomal but only partially recessive (Marder and Shulman, 1964).

Diagnosis of Factor VII Deficiency. Factor VII deficiency should be suspected in any patient in whom prothrombin time is found to be significantly prolonged and other clotting parameters are in the normal range. The prothrombin time defect will be corrected by normal plasma and Russell's viper venom, but not by $BaSO_4$-adsorbed normal plasma.

Except for the rare congenital deficiency, most cases of factor VII deficiency will also be deficient in other vitamin K dependent procoagulants. In such cases, specific assay procedures are needed to evaluate the relative deficiencies.

Factor VIII

Nomenclature. Hemophilia refers to a sex-linked disorder described initially by Otto (Brinkhous, 1957). It has been demonstrated that the coagulation defect can be corrected by normal plasma (Patek and Taylor, 1937). The terms antihemophilic factor (AHF) and antihemophilic globulin (AHG) have been used to designate the procoagulant present in normal plasma but deficient in the plasma of patients with hemophilia. Because a number of other terms are used by various investigators to designate this activity, the term factor VIII was assigned by the International Committee for the Nomenclature of Blood Clotting Factors (Wright, 1962). The term hemophilia A is gradually being adopted to designate the hereditary disease.

Pathophysiology of Defects Involving Factor VIII Deficiency. Factor VIII is necessary for the prompt conversion of prothrombin to thrombin in native systems. Its activity can be compensated for by tissue thromboplastin. In the absence of factor VIII, abnormal results are obtained with the following test procedures: partial thromboplastin time, prothrombin utilization, whole blood clotting time, and thromboplastin generation.

Congenital deficiency of factor VIII occurs in three degrees of severity: (1) In the *severe form* of the disease, little or no factor VIII activity can be demonstrated in the plasma; (2) in the *moderate form* of the disease, factor VIII is present in the plasma in levels of about 5 per cent of normal; and (3) in the *mild form* of the disease, factor VIII is present in the plasma in levels of about 15 to 20 per cent of normal.

There is a close correlation between the severity of the bleeding symptoms and the level of factor VIII activity. The severe form of the disease is characterized by massive, life-threatening hemorrhage, hemarthrosis of weight-bearing joints, and excessive bleeding from minor injuries. The moderate form of the deficiency is associated with a definite bleeding tendency, but life-threatening hemorrhage and hemarthrosis are infrequently associated with this level of factor VIII. Excessive bleeding, requiring transfusion therapy, occurs following tooth extractions, minor surgical procedures, or moderate trauma. Patients with the mild form of the disorder are considered to be troublesome bleeders rather than serious bleeders. Although bleeding after tooth extractions, trauma, or surgical procedure is excessive, it tends to be in the form of a slow ooze rather than massive hemorrhage.

The site of origin of factor VIII is as yet not known, although the spleen appears to have a regulatory function (Weaver *et al.*, 1963). Only an occasional case of acquired factor VIII deficiency is reported. In these the lack of factor VIII activity appears to be the result of a specific inhibition rather than a true failure of synthesis. Active fibrinolysins have been found to destroy factor VIII, and an acquired deficiency may occur in association with fibrinolytic disorders. Factor VIII is unaffected by vitamin K deficiency and coumarin type drugs.

Factor VIII is lost rapidly from the blood stream; roughly one-half of the activity in plasma achieved by infusion disappears in 6 to 12 hours (Langdell *et al.*, 1955). This rapid clearance occurs in normal individuals as well as in patients with a congenital deficiency. It is of interest that factor VIII deficiency occurs in dogs as well as in humans (Graham *et al.*, 1949).

Properties. Factor VIII resembles fibrinogen in some of its properties in that both are present in various plasma fractions. Factor VIII activity precipitates from plasma, along with fibrinogen, at 25 per cent ammonium sulfate saturation. Factor VIII is not readily adsorbed from oxalated plasma by $BaSO_4$. However, $Al(OH)_3$ treatment of citrated plasma may remove appreciable factor VIII activity along with other procoagulants. Although factor VIII activity decreases in blood during the coagulation process, there may be sufficient factor VIII activity in fresh serum to influence most clotting tests. In addition, serum accelerator factors are present in serum; in some tests these appear to be factor VIII (Graham *et al.*, 1954). For these reasons, serum is not a satisfactory reagent in studies of factor VIII activity.

It is generally assumed that factor VIII is a labile procoagulant. However, when blood is properly drawn, factor VIII appears to be inactivated more rapidly by slow freezing than by storage at 4° C. or by rapid freezing and storage below –20° C. (Weaver and Langdell, 1966). About half of the factor VIII activity is lost from citrated plasma in 10 minutes at 56° C. (Wagner and Brinkhous, 1961). It has been estimated that factor VIII is present in normal plasma in an amount less than 5 mg. per 100 ml. (Brinkhous *et al.*, 1958). Factor VIII activity is decreased by thrombin, trypsin, and fibrinolytic agents.

Genetic Aspects of Factor VIII Deficiency. The heredity of classic hemophilia is that of a sex-linked recessive trait. Clinically affected individuals are males inheriting the hemophilic gene from mothers who are heterozygous for the disease. Clinically affected females are homozygous for the disorder. There is some indication that females who are heterozygous for the trait have low factor VIII activity (Parks *et al.*, 1965).

The mode of inheritance of moderate and mild hemophilia is unclear but appears not to be of the sex-linked recessive type (Graham *et al.*, 1953). Factor VIII deficiency in patients with vascular hemophilia is unique (see Vascular Hemophilia, p. 429).

It was demonstrated by Langdell *et al.* (1953) that there was a wide range of activity in normal individuals. This individual variation may be genetically determined (Brinkhous *et al.*, 1954).

Diagnosis of Factor VIII Deficiency. Factor VIII deficiency should be suspected in any patient with a bleeding tendency who is found to have a prolonged partial thromboplastin time and a normal prothrombin time. Fresh normal plasma and fresh $BaSO_4$-adsorbed normal plasma will correct the partial thromboplastin time defect.

The diagnosis of mild factor VIII deficiency will depend on failure of the patient's plasma to correct the partial thromboplastin time of plasma from a previously diagnosed factor VIII deficiency. The problem of distinguishing vascular hemophilia from mild hemophilia is covered in the discussion of vascular hemophilia (p. 429).

Results of some laboratory studies are apt to be in the normal range in moderate and mild deficiencies. It was demonstrated by Langdell (1957) that the whole blood clotting time and prothrombin utilization will be normal in blood containing at least 1 per cent of normal factor VIII activity. The partial thromboplastin time will be normal in blood containing above 15 to 20 per cent of the normal factor VIII.

Factor IX

Nomenclature. It was noted by Pavlovsky (1947) that patients thought to have hemophilia could be divided into two distinct types of coagulation defects. In 1952 three patients were reported, each with a sex-linked recessive bleeding tendency, with characteristics distinguishable from factor VIII deficiency. Aggeler and associates (1952) described a patient with the disorder and some of the biochemical characteristics of the procoagulant. They used the term plasma thromboplastin component (PTC) for the factor present in normal plasma but deficient in their patient. Schulman and Smith (1952) almost simultaneously described a patient with a similar defect. Several months later, Biggs *et al.* (1952) reported a patient with a similar deficiency and used the term Christmas disease for the hereditary bleeding disorder. The term factor IX was assigned by the International Committee for the Nomenclature of Blood Clotting Factors (Wright, 1962). The term hemophilia B is gradually being adopted for the hereditary disorder.

Pathophysiology of Defects Involving Factor IX Deficiency. Factor IX is essential for the prompt conversion of prothrombin to thrombin in native systems, but not in systems using tissue thromboplastin. In the absence of factor IX, abnormal results are obtained with the following: partial thromboplastin time, whole blood clotting time, prothrombin utilization, and thromboplastin generation.

The disease resembles factor VIII deficiency clinically, but mild deficiencies of factor IX appear to be more common. There appears to be a relationship of factor IX to vitamin K and coumarin type anticoagulants. Reduction of factor IX following the administration of coumarin has been reported (Loeliger *et al.*, 1964). However, the influence of decreased prothrombin, factor VII, and factor X on the test procedures used for measuring factor IX has not been established.

In metabolic studies, plasma and plasma fractions rich in factor IX have been infused into patients deficient in factor IX and into normal subjects. One-half of the plasma activity achieved is lost in 12 to 24 hours (Loeliger *et al.*, 1964). There is a wide range of activity in the plasma of healthy normal individuals. In a group of 61 women studied by Barrow *et al.* (1960) the range was found to be from 55 to 171 per cent of a standard control.

Properties. Factor IX is readily adsorbed from oxalated plasma by $BaSO_4$. Its activity is concentrated in the 45 to 50 per cent ammonium sulfate fraction of normal human plasma (White *et al.*, 1953). It is relatively stable over a wide pH range (4.2 to 10.1). It is generally considered to be a relatively stable procoagulant, since its activity remains high in blood stored under standard blood bank conditions (Geratz and Graham, 1960). However, it is completely inactivated in plasma heated at 56° C. for 10 minutes. In continuous flow electrophoresis, factor IX migrates with the alpha globulins (Lewis *et al.*, 1958).

Genetic Aspects of Factor IX Deficiency. Factor IX deficiency, like hemophilia, is inherited as a sex-linked recessive characteristic. There is evidence that persons who are heterozygous for the trait may have reduced factor IX levels (Barrow *et al.*, 1960).

Diagnosis of Factor IX Deficiency. Factor IX deficiency should be suspected in any patient with a bleeding tendency found to have an abnormal partial thromboplastin time and a normal prothrombin time. The partial thromboplastin time defect will be corrected by the addition of fresh normal plasma but not by $BaSO_4$-adsorbed normal plasma.

The differentiation between factor IX and factor XI deficiency will depend on the findings when plasma known to be deficient in factor IX is added to the partial thromboplastin time procedure.

The deficiency of factor IX in relation to vitamin K is quite complex. Specific assay methods are needed to evaluate this. The influence of mild deficiencies of other procoagulants on the assay procedure must be evaluated.

Factor X

Nomenclature. Lewis, Fresh, and Ferguson (1953) reported a patient with a bleeding tendency characterized by an abnormal prothrombin time not due to a deficiency of prothrombin, factor V, or fibrinogen. They felt this patient's coagulation defect was the same as that previously reported by Alexander *et al.* (1951). Hougie, Barrow, and Graham (1957) reviewed the previously reported cases of serum prothrombin accelerator deficiencies and pointed out that at least two types of coagulation anomaly were included. In direct mixing studies, they found that plasma from the patient reported by Lewis *et al.* (1953) corrected the deficiency of plasma from the patient reported by Alexander *et al.* (1951). Hougie *et al.* (1957) used the surname of the patient, Stuart, to identify the defect. The surname, Prower, of a patient described by Telfer, Denson, and Wright (1956) also has been used for the factor. The term factor X was adopted by the International Committee for the Nomenclature of Blood Clotting Factors (Wright, 1962).

Pathophysiology of Defects Involving Factor X Deficiency. Factor X is required for the prompt conversion of prothrombin to thrombin in both native systems and in procedures in which tissue thromboplastin is used. With a deficiency of factor X, abnormal results will occur with the following procedures: prothrombin time, partial thromboplastin time, whole blood clotting time, prothrombin utilization, and thromboplastin generation. Unlike factor VII deficiency, Russell's viper venom will not compensate for a deficiency of factor X. Only about 20 cases of congenital factor X deficiency have been reported. In these the symptoms have been those of a hemorrhagic diathesis including crippling hemarthrosis.

Acquired deficiency of factor X results from any disorder decreasing its synthesis in the liver for which vitamin K is essential. Since other procoagulants are also dependent on an intact liver and vitamin K, a pure acquired factor X deficiency is rare.

It has been estimated that following plasma transfusions to congenitally deficient patients, half the level reached in circulating plasma disappears in 20 to 42 hours (Roberts *et al.*, 1965).

Properties. Factor X is readily adsorbed from oxalated human plasma by $BaSO_4$ and can be recovered by citrate elution of the precipitate. It is relatively heat stable, although it is rapidly destroyed when serum is heated to 56° C. (Graham and Hougie, 1961). It is stable in blood stored under standard blood bank conditions. It is destroyed below pH 6.1 and above pH 9. It can be precipitated from plasma at between 55 and 65 per cent ammonium sulfate saturation. In electrophoresis it migrates as an alpha globulin ahead of prothrombin and factor VII. It has been separated from other procoagulants with continuous flow paper electrophoresis (Johnston *et al.*, 1959).

Genetic Aspects of Factor X Deficiency. Factor X deficiency is inherited as a highly penetrant but incompletely recessive autosomal characteristic (Graham, Barrow, and Hougie, 1957). There is evidence that persons heterozygous for the trait can be detected by specific assay methods (Graham, 1957).

Diagnosis of Factor X Deficiency. Factor X deficiency should be suspected in any patient with a bleeding tendency found to have an abnormal prothrombin time and partial thromboplastin. $BaSO_4$-adsorbed plasma will correct neither. The addition of Russell's viper venom will not correct coagulation defects due to factor X deficiency.

Except for the rare congenital deficiency, most patients with a deficiency of factor X will also be deficient in the vitamin K dependent procoagulants. Specific assay procedures are required to determine the quantitative defects in these cases.

Factor XI

Nomenclature. A patient with a previously unrecognized coagulation defect was reported by Rosenthal, Dreskin, and Rosenthal (1953). They used the term plasma thromboplastin antecedent (PTA) for the factor lacking in the plasma of the patient. The term factor XI was adopted by the International Committee for the Nomenclature of Blood Clotting Factors (Wright, 1962).

Pathophysiology of Defects Involving Factor XI Deficiency. Factor XI is essential to the prompt conversion of prothrombin to thrombin in native systems. The defect is compensated for by tissue thromboplastin. In the absence of factor XI, abnormal results are obtained with each of the following procedures: partial thromboplastin time, whole blood clotting time, prothrombin utilization, and thromboplastin generation.

Patients with a congenital deficiency have a mild bleeding tendency. The apparent mildness may indicate that partial deficiency is the common form. The symptoms and laboratory findings are not constant. On repeated observations of the same patient, the findings may not always be identical. This suggests that the levels of the plasma activity of this factor may be varying. Study of this disorder is especially difficult in view of the findings that plasma from a deficient patient will, after storage, correct the prothrombin utilization of a deficient patient (Rosenthal, 1957). It is probable that the apparently ubiquitous nature of the disorder can be attributed to the serum used in various studies. It is well known that serum is a relatively variable reagent because of incomplete loss of prothrombin, fibrinogen, and factor VIII in blood that is allowed to clot spontaneously. As more patients are discovered and studied by the many techniques available, the strange behavior of factor XI may come to be understood.

Properties. The properties of factor XI are not clear because of conflicting data reported by various investigators. (The various reports were summarized by de Nicola in 1962.) This appears to be due to the lack of standard assay procedures. Although factor XI activity can be recovered from the precipitate obtained following $BaSO_4$ treatment of normal plasma, it has been reported that $BaSO_4$ does not completely remove factor XI activity (Rosenthal, 1957). It is likely that the affinity of $BaSO_4$ for factor XI is intermediate between prothrombin and factor VIII. Factor XI is relatively stable at room temperature or below. Its activity has been reported to precipitate from plasma with levels of up to 50 per cent saturation by ammonium sulfate. In electrophoresis it migrates with the fast gamma globulins or between the beta and gamma globulins.

Genetic Aspects of Factor XI Deficiency. Factor XI deficiency is transmitted as a simple dominant trait with variable expression and penetrance (Rosenthal, 1957). The relative rarity of clinically severe deficiency of factor XI suggests that only the homozygous condition results in a bleeding tendency. Other data suggest that the gene for factor XI is incompletely recessive and the deficiency may occur as a major deficiency (homozygous) and minor deficiency (heterozygous) (Rapaport *et al.*, 1961).

Diagnosis of Factor XI Deficiency. Factor XI deficiency should be suspected in patients with a mild bleeding disorder in which the results of laboratory tests are intermittently abnormal. Poor consumption of prothrombin as measured by the one-stage method has been the most consistent finding. Mixing experiments in which plasma from a patient known to be deficient in factor XI fails to correct the clotting defect of the patient under study are the only means of diagnosis at present.

Factor XII

Nomenclature. A patient with a coagulation disorder but with no evidence of a bleeding tendency was described by Ratnoff and Colopy (1955). On the basis of the patient's surname, they used the terms Hageman trait for the disease state and Hageman factor for the deficiency in the plasma of the patient. The term factor XII was adopted by the International Committee for the Nomenclature of Blood Clotting Factors.

Pathophysiology of Defects Involving Factor XII Deficiency. Factor XII is essential for coagulation as measured by *in vitro* tests but is not needed for hemostasis. With a deficiency of factor XII, delayed clotting occurs as measured by the following: partial thromboplastin time, prothrombin utilization, whole blood clotting time, and thromboplastin generation.

It is generally believed that factor XII is activated by contact with glass or other surfaces. It is of interest that although the clotting time of factor XII deficient whole blood is abnormally long as measured in glass, it is not abnormally long when measured in silicone-treated glassware.

Properties. The properties reported for factor XII were summarized by deNicola (1962). Factor XII is not adsorbed from normal human plasma by $BaSO_4$ and is not reduced during the clotting process. It is relatively heat stable, with activity remaining in serum after 30 minutes at 60° C. It is stable in oxalated plasma stored at 4° C. for 12 weeks. The activity is precipitated at between 30 and 40 per cent ammonium sulfate saturation of plasma. By electrophoresis the activity migrates between the gamma and beta globulins. It has been estimated that factor XII activity accounts for no more than 0.2 mg. per 100 ml. of plasma protein.

Genetic Aspects of Factor XII Deficiency. The inheritance of factor XII deficiency was reviewed by McCain *et al.* (1959). They reported that factor XII deficiency is transmitted as an autosomal recessive trait. Some persons heterozygous for the trait have a mild deficiency.

Diagnosis of Factor XII Deficiency. Patients with factor XII deficiency have no history of a bleeding tendency. When coagulation tests are made as part of the preoperative routine, patients who have the deficiency will be discovered. Although the laboratory data suggest hemophilia, that is, a long partial thromboplastin time and a normal prothrombin time, a history of excessive bleeding is not found. In order to distinguish factor XII deficiency from true hemophilia, the effect of plasma known to be specifically deficient must be determined. This distinction is of considerable importance, since factor VIII deficiency is associated with a severe bleeding tendency and factor XII deficiency is associated with normal hemostasis.

Factor XIII

Nomenclature. It was noted by Robbins (1944) that fibrin derived from purified fibrinogen can be divided into two types: that which forms in the presence of a serum factor and is stable in weak acids and that which forms in the absence of the serum factor and is soluble in weak acids. It was pointed out by Laki and Lorand (1948) that solubility in urea is also a method of distinguishing the two types of fibrin. It was later found that the factor responsible for urea insolubility of fibrin is present in only trace amounts in serum and that high levels are present in the plasma (Lorand and Dickenman, 1955). The terms fibrinase and fibrin stabilizing factor (FSF) have been used for the factor. The term factor XIII was assigned by the International Committee for the Nomenclature of Blood Clotting Factors.

Pathophysiology of Defects Involving Factor XIII Deficiency. Factor XIII is essential for the formation of a stable fibrin clot. Although only a few patients with a deficiency of the factor have been reported, it appears that one of the manifestations of the deficiency is poor wound healing (Duckert *et al.*, 1960). Relative deficiencies of factor XIII have been observed in a number of disorders, including lead poisoning, pernicious anemia, and agammaglobulinemia (Lorand, 1962). The clinical importance of factor XIII is only beginning to be elucidated.

Properties. Factor XIII activity of plasma decreases during clotting, so that serum contains only a trace of activity. It precipitates with the globulins at 0° C. with 10 per cent ether at pH 5.4. Its molecular weight has been estimated to be about 130,000. A crude fraction can be obtained by precipitating plasma with 33 per cent saturation with ammonium sulfate.

Genetic Aspects of Factor XIII Deficiency. Only a few studies have been made on families of factor XIII deficient patients (Losowsky and Hall, 1966; Hampton and Bird, 1966). The method of genetic transmission is not completely clear at this time.

Diagnosis of Factor XIII Deficiency. Factor XIII deficiency should be suspected in patients with a mild bleeding tendency and poor wound healing capacity. A simple screening test of clot solubility has been suggested by Lorand (1962). Blood is allowed to clot. After 30 minutes, an equal volume of 2 per cent monochloracetic acid is added to the clot. The clot is inspected after 16 to 24 hours. Solubility of the clot indicates inadequate factor XIII activity.

VASCULAR HEMOPHILIA

Nomenclature. A hereditary bleeding disorder was found to occur with high frequency in the inhabitants of the Aland Islands by von Willebrand (1926). Unlike true hemophilia, this disease was characterized by an abnormal bleeding time and occurred in females. This disorder was called pseudohemophilia by von Willebrand (1926). Alexander and Goldstein (1953) found that patients with this disorder had reduced levels of factor VIII. There appear to be two defects in clinically affected individuals: a deficiency of a vascular factor and a low but measurable factor VIII. For this reason, the term vascular hemophilia has been used to distinguish this disorder from true hemophilia, the more severe but apparently pure deficiency of factor VIII.

Pathophysiology. Persons with this disorder appear to have two hemostatic defects; characteristically, affected persons have low but measurable factor VIII activity and a prolonged bleeding time. The prolonged bleeding time is thought to be due to a lack of a plasma factor necessary for normal vascular integrity. Transfusions of affected persons with normal plasma improves the abnormal bleeding time; however, quantitative relationships have not been established.

The symptoms of affected persons are those which would be expected from their plasma factor VIII levels. Although there is a definite bleeding tendency, massive life-threatening hemorrhage is uncommon.

The effect of plasma factor VIII levels following transfusion of normal plasma into patients with vascular hemophilia is of interest. It was shown by Langdell, Wagner, and Brinkhous (1955) that factor VIII activity rapidly disappears from the plasma of a classic hemophiliac following transfusion of whole blood plasma or plasma fractions. Nilsson *et al.* (1957) found that fraction 1-0 prepared from plasma of either normal or classic hemophiliac patients would produce an increase in factor VIII activity when transfused into patients with vascular hemophilia. The corrective effect of the fraction from a factor VIII deficient patient resulted in speculation that the plasma defect in vascular hemophilia was not factor VIII. It now appears that at least two factors are involved with plasma factor VIII activity hemophilia. In studies summarized by Caen (1964) it was shown that a two-phase response occurs in the plasma of a patient with vascular hemophilia following transfusion with normal plasma. In the first phase, occurring immediately after transfusion, plasma factor VIII activity is increased to levels that would be expected from the amount administered. During the next several hours, factor VIII in the plasma decreases as in classic hemophilia. However, in 12 to 24 hours after the transfusion, factor VIII activity in the plasma increases, so that the maximal activity is greater than the total amount initially infused. Plasma from a classic hemophiliac fails to produce the first phase of the response in vascular hemophilia but does produce the delayed response. Plasma from a patient with vascular hemophilia is ineffective in producing an increase in factor VIII when transfused into a patient with classic hemophilia. It has recently been shown by Barrow *et al.* (1965) that patients homozygous for the vascular hemophilia gene respond less to plasma of classic hemophilia than do patients heterozygous for the gene. It is believed that normal and hemophilic plasma contain some factor necessary for factor VIII synthesis in the patients with vascular hemophilia.

Genetics. The genetic aspects of vascular hemophilia have been reviewed by Barrow and Graham (1964). Males and females are equally affected, and transmission appears to be that of an autosomal dominant trait. The relationship of the hereditary transmission of plasma factor VIII activity and the factor(s) responsible for the long bleeding time is not clear. It is not clear what relationship the gene(s) controlling factor VIII in this disease has to the gene on the X chromosome controlling factor VIII in classic hemophilia. However, the information obtained from family studies of vascular hemophilia indicate that more than one gene is responsible for factor VIII activity.

Diagnosis. The deficiency of factor VIII in vascular hemophilia may be of a degree that is above the critical level of the usual test procedures. Although the partial thromboplastin time is sensitive for a wider range of factor VIII than are other methods (Langdell, 1957), it loses its sensitivity at levels above 20 per cent of normal. In patients suspected of having factor VIII deficiency above 20 per cent of normal, it is necessary to determine the effect of the patient's plasma on the coagulation defect of a known severe hemophiliac.

The differentiation between vascular hemophilia and mild factor VIII deficiency may be difficult. The bleeding time prolongation is helpful when present. However, the bleeding time results vary and at times may be normal in patients with vascular hemophilia. At the present time, the response of the patient to a transfusion of normal plasma appears to be the only method of differentiating mild classic hemophilia from vascular hemophilia if the bleeding time is not prolonged and family studies are inconclusive. Patients with mild classic hemophilia will not have the two-phase response to the administration of normal plasma.

VITAMIN K AND ANTIVITAMIN K DRUGS

Studies of the relationship between prothrombin and vitamin K were the subject of an excellent review by Brinkhous (1940). The elucidation of vitamin K and its relationship to blood coagulation emphasized the importance of hemostasis to all aspects of clinical medicine. This represented the beginning of a new era of research and clinical observation. Blood coagulation was no longer a laboratory curiosity but became a part of diagnosis and treatment in clinical medicine. All the important relationships between coagulation, liver disease, neonatal bleeding disorders, and vitamin K do not need to be reviewed at this time, but any serious student of hemostasis and blood coagulation will profit by studying these experiments.

Since 1940 it has been learned that prothrombin is not the only coagulation factor involved with vitamin K. Factors VII, IX, and X are dependent on the same synthesizing mechanism. Some of the apparent discrepancies in the earlier work were no doubt due to the varying influence of these factors on the test systems used by different investigators. It is still not clear which of the factors is of major importance in the pathogenesis of the hemorrhagic disease associated with vitamin K deficiency and which should be used as an index of hemostatic function.

It was ultimately demonstrated that the causative factor in spoiled sweet clover disease of cattle was a substance that blocked the action of vitamin K. This work, which was published in a number of articles between 1940 and 1946, was reviewed by Link (1948). It is now well known that Dicumarol and related prothrombinopenic drugs act by blocking the action of vitamin K. These drugs have been widely used in an attempt to decrease coagulation in patients prone to thromboembolic disorders. There continue to be differences of opinion as to which laboratory procedure should be used to evaluate the effects of therapy. Since several factors are influenced by the prothrombinopenic drugs, it should be obvious that no single test will be ideal under all circumstances. Most laboratories have utilized the one-stage prothrombin time as an index of therapy. This may not be the best on the basis of scientific evidence, but its almost universal use indicates its value in terms of convenience. It is not the aim of this chapter to resolve the various differences of opinion with regard to the drug of choice, the method of administration, the therapeutic level, or the method of testing in the use of anticoagulant drugs. It remains for the laboratory director and the physician responsible for the patient to determine what test or group of tests is best for their particular needs. This decision should be based on an understanding of all the problems involved.

Therapy with the prothrombinopenic drugs results in a deficiency of several procoagulants. Although the specific drug and method of administration contribute to the effect, in general, factor VII is most sensitive to the drug action. Factor VII decreases within a few hours after the drug is administered and is at low levels before prothrombin and factor X have decreased. The reverse is true when the drug action is stopped by therapy with vitamin K. Factor VII returns to normal levels within a few hours, while prothrombin and factor X require several days to recover from the effects of the drug. There is some evidence to suggest that during long-term therapy, factor VII may increase toward normal while prothrombin and factor X remain low. This may be the result of partial recovery of factor VII activity between doses of the drug. Although factor IX is reported to be influenced by the prothrombinopenic drugs, the extent of this has not been clearly established.

Hemorrhagic disease of the newborn, which was considered at length in the review by Brinkhous (1940), is now rarely seen because of the awareness of the cause and its treatment by obstetricians. However, such a possibility should be considered if symptoms of a bleeding tendency occur in the neonatal period. As demonstrated many years ago (Brinkhous, 1940), the newborn infant is unable to synthesize vitamin K and thus may have a temporary coagulation disorder.

An occasional diagnostic problem is presented to the laboratory by a patient who for some reason or another is taking Dicumarol or a similar drug and neglects to so inform the physician. The correct diagnosis can be established by administering vitamin K and noting the response.

The microorganisms responsible for vitamin K synthesis are normal inhabitants of the gastrointestinal tract. Symptoms and laboratory findings of a coagulation disorder are seen in patients receiving antibiotics orally.

DISSEMINATED INTRAVASCULAR COAGULATION

Nomenclature. An acquired bleeding disorder secondary to activation of the coagulation system *in vivo* has become a recognized syndrome. The concept has been popularized by McKay (1964). Although both activation of the coagulation system and fibrinolysis occur, it appears that fibrinolysis is a secondary response. A number of terms have been used for the syndrome, including consumption coagulopathy, defibrination syndrome, generalized Schwartzman reaction, and the thrombohemorrhagic syndrome.

Pathophysiology. As blood clots, some plasma procoagulants are activated while others decrease in activity. Fibrinogen, prothrombin, factor V, and factor VIII are characteristically present in low amounts in serum. Schneider

(1951) described a syndrome of excessive bleeding associated with fibrinogenopenia in patients with obstetric complications. A similar reaction can be produced experimentally in animals by injecting either tissue thromboplastin or dilute thrombin. Blood samples obtained from patients or experimental animals at the height of the disorder have characteristics of serum rather than of plasma. It is generally believed that the syndrome results from the activation of clotting within the blood vascular system. There appear to be a number of conditions that can initiate this reaction, such as the release of tissue thromboplastic materials into the blood stream, bacterial endotoxins, activation of certain proteolytic enzyme systems, the presence of particulate matter or certain colloids, antigen-antibody reactions and endothelial damage.

In addition to the changes in circulating blood, microthrombi occur primarily in capillaries. The renal glomeruli appear to be particularly prone to the formation of these thrombi.

With such a wide variety of conditions that appear to trigger intravascular coagulation it is not yet clear if one or more types of injury are the basic etiologic stimulus. Although the formation of thrombin appears to be a common factor in most, in some cases activation of other enzymes appears to produce the same result.

Diagnosis. As a number of disorders may be associated with the disseminated intravascular coagulation syndrome, diagnosis may be difficult. It should be suspected whenever excessive bleeding occurs in association with tissue necrosis, antigen-antibody reactions, or bacterial endotoxemia. Characteristically there is no previous history of a bleeding tendency. The blood platelet count is low, the prothrombin time is long, and the partial thromboplastin time is long. If specific assays are done there will be a low level of fibrinogen, factor V, and factor VIII. There may or may not be evidence of fibrinolysis. Since there is a decrease in fibrinogen, the thrombin clotting time will be long. The level of prothrombin is low in severe cases but may be normal. At the present time the laboratory diagnosis of this syndrome is circumstantial and the differentiation from primary fibrinolysis may be difficult and at times impossible, since the two may be occurring simultaneously. The presence of thrombocytopenia in addition to the decreased plasma clotting factors is considered to be strong circumstantial support for the diagnosis of intravascular coagulation. The therapeutic implications of the diagnosis of this disorder are discussed by McKay and Müller-Berghaus (1967).

ACQUIRED ANTICOAGULANTS

As indicated earlier, there are natural inhibitors present in the blood to keep the hemostatic mechanism in balance. The influence of these natural inhibitors appears to be neutralized rapidly in shed blood, so the clotting reaction proceeds rapidly as measured in the commonly used laboratory tests. Although these inhibitors may be found to be even more important than the procoagulants in the pathogenesis of thromboembolic disease, methods for evaluating the natural inhibitors are only beginning to evolve. The natural inhibitors have been reviewed by Soulier (1962).

An occasional patient will produce a circulating anticoagulant that either results in a hemostatic defect or is a complication of a preexisting coagulation disorder. The acquired inhibitors, reviewed by Deutsch (1962), occur in persons with previously normal hemostatic mechanism as a postpartum complication or in dysproteinemia associated with such disorders as lupus erythematosus or multiple myeloma. These may be specific anticoagulants in that the patient's plasma neutralizes a specific procoagulant, or they may be nonspecific in that several procoagulants are neutralized. The presence of a circulating anticoagulant of this type is distinguished from a procoagulant deficiency by the failure of normal plasma to correct the defect. Some anticoagulants require time to neutralize the normal clotting activity. To test for these time-dependent anticoagulants, the normal plasma should be incubated with plasma from the patient for 1 hour at 37° C. prior to proceeding to the next step of the test.

Circulating anticoagulants occur as a complication of a congenital deficiency of one of the procoagulants. In these cases, it appears that the anticoagulant is an isoantibody resulting from plasma therapy. It is believed that the procoagulant in the normal plasma used for transfusion acts as a foreign protein to the patient. The presence of such an anticoagulant makes further therapy poorly effective. The anticoagulant acts by neutralizing the procoagulant in the normal blood. Diagnosis of the basic congenital deficiency is made difficult by the presence of the anticoagulant. The failure of normal plasma to correct the patient's coagulation defect is evidence of an anticoagulant.

FIBRINOLYSIS

Nomenclature. The removal of fibrin once formed in the body is dependent upon a sequence of events that is as complex as that of the clotting mechanism. Whereas thrombin is the active enzyme for fibrin formation, plasmin is the active enzyme for fibrin removal. Plasmin is present in circulating blood in the form of an inactive precursor substance called plasminogen. The transformation of plasminogen to plasmin is produced by a proteolytic enzyme called plasminogen activator. The activator substance, in turn, is in part derived from proactivator. In addition to the plasmin activator system, normal plasma contains antiplasmins that will neutralize the activity produced. The fibrinolytic system has been the subject of two recent symposia (Ambrus *et al.*, 1966; Brinkhous *et al.*, 1970).

Pathophysiology. The active substance, plasmin, is a proteolytic enzyme capable of acting upon various proteins as well as on fibrin and fibrinogen. In contrast to the clotting reaction, which is rapid, the fibrinolytic process is slow. Most methods for measuring fibrinolysis require several hours to reach an endpoint. In the past, work has been difficult to interpret because of lack of pure preparations. For example, fibrinogen preparations frequently contain plasminogen; thus, materials thought to have plasmin activity were actually activators of the plasminogen in the fibrin substrate.

In addition to the obvious lytic effect on fibrin, the plasmin system may have a direct effect on the clotting mechanism (Fletcher, 1966). The split products resulting from plasmin action on fibrinogen are different than the fibrin monomer resulting from the action of thrombin. It appears that fibrin polymerization can be prevented when fibrin monomers combine with the atypical split products produced by the action of plasmin. This aspect of fibrinolysis has been discussed by Fletcher (1966).

Several clinical syndromes are associated with systemic fibrinolysis. These have been summarized by Sharp (1964). These include carcinoma of the prostate, obstetric complications, thoracic surgery, particularly in association with extracorporeal circulation, liver disease, and leukemias. Excessive fibrinolytic activity of a degree sufficient to cause spontaneous hemorrhage is not uncommon in patients with carcinoma of the prostate with metastasis. This appears to result from the production of plasminogen activator by the neoplastic tissues. Fibrinolysis in association with obstetrical complications is of complex etiology; it is probable that these result from tissue products entering the circulation. The tissue products have a thromboplastic action and produce intravascular coagulation. This results in fibrinogenemia and a bleeding tendency. The effects of intravascular coagulation may activate the lytic system. On the other hand, the tissue products contain activators that are capable of stimulating the formation of active plasmin. The fibrinolytic syndrome associated with thoracic operations is felt to be due in part to release of tissue activators into the systemic circulation, since the lung is a rich source of activator materials. There is some evidence that the heart-lung pump system may in itself cause activation of plasminogen. Patients with leukemia may have increased fibrinolytic activity. The mechanism of this is still unclear. The fibrinolysis associated with liver disease is complicated because the liver is the site of synthesis of fibrinogen as well as other clotting factors.

It is clear that excessive bleeding from the urinary tract is at times due to fibrinolysis. This is a manifestation of a local rather than a systemic process. The urine is rich in a plasminogen activator called urokinase. This substance activates plasminogen bound to fibrin which forms over an ulcerated mucosal surface. Thus, the effectiveness of the hemostatic clot is destroyed.

Streptokinase is an exogenous material that has a profound effect on fibrinolysis. It is a bacterial enzyme that activates proactivator in the human system. Streptokinase has been used for therapeutic purposes (McNicol and Douglas, 1964). Human plasma contains an antistreptokinase. The amount is variable and this may explain the variation in individual sensitivity to the material.

Epsilon-aminocaproic acid (EACA) is a synthetic amino acid that has been found to be a potent fibrinolytic inhibitor, the action of which has been reviewed by McNicol and Douglas (1964). The main action of EACA on the fibrinolytic system is competitive inhibition of plasminogen activation (Alkjaersig *et al.*, 1959). Although EACA has been used in the therapy of various bleeding disorders, its value has been confirmed only when used as an antidote for thrombolytic therapy and urinary tract bleeding. As the diagnosis of fibrinolytic disorders becomes more clearly established, the use of EACA as a therapeutic agent will also become established.

Diagnosis. The process of fibrinolysis is a part of the normal hemostatic mechanism. Although it is felt that excessive fibrinolytic activity can produce a hemorrhagic episode, it is difficult at the present time to evaluate what degree of activity is part of a normal physiologic process and when fibrinolysis becomes part of a pathologic syndrome. The laboratory procedures available require a relatively long incubation time, so rapid diagnosis is not possible. Ultimate diagnosis rests on the laboratory results and the clinical evaluation of the patient. Guest (1966) tends to minimize the clinical significance of fibrinolysis, while Fletcher (1966) suggests that pathological fibrinolysis is of major clinical significance.

The differentiation of primary fibrinolysis from disseminated intravascular clotting may be difficult. The action of fibrinolytic enzymes on fibrinogen results in split products that are different from fibrin monomer and fibrinpeptides A and B. In recent years immunologic procedures have been developed to demonstrate the presence of these split products in serum. These methods are not sufficiently standardized to be used for laboratory diagnosis. Although a few fibrinogen split products may be present in association with disseminated intravascular coagulation, these are more common in fibrinogenolysis.

PROCEDURES

The procedures used by investigators to study the various elements involved in the clotting reaction have been compiled in an excellent book by Tocantins and Kazal (1964) and in a more recent book by Bang *et al.* (1971). Each of the procedures has contributed much to the understanding of hemostasis. However, many of the procedures are technically difficult and highly specialized. Reliable results are obtained only when these specialized tests are performed frequently and a source of control reagents is available. Each laboratory must select a few procedures which will serve the needs of that laboratory. The limited number of procedures included in this chapter will serve the purpose of most laboratories that have diagnostic and therapeutic responsibilities. The procedures included are relatively simple, and most of the reagents are available from commercial sources. Although the information obtained by determining the whole blood clotting time is of limited value, the procedure is included since it is still used in a number of laboratories. On the other hand, only the principles and interpretation of results of the Thromboplastin Generation Test, the two-stage prothrombin assay, and the Prothrombin Utilization Test are included. These procedures are used in certain laboratories but are not essential for diagnosis and treatment. Even though it is not essential to know the details of these procedures, it is of value to be familiar with the principles on which they are based.

The procedures included are relatively simple to perform, but they require utmost attention to technique if results are to be of value. The procedure must be done in exactly the same way each time it is used if duplicate results are to be obtained. Short cuts and modifications should be avoided.

Automated Procedures

At the present time there are several equipment items commercially available that have been devised to mechanize the performance of clotting tests. Automated equipment for determining platelet counts has been available for several years. When properly adjusted and calibrated, these have been found to be satisfactory.

In addition there are several items of equipment designed for one-stage tests. Some of these are to detect the formation of a fibrin clot by electronic means. These are of some value in standardizing technique since the same endpoint is used each time. Such equipment is only semiautomatic, in that delivering the reagents to the container in which clotting is done is by manual techniques. The major advantage of such equipment is the relatively inexpensive cost and the standardization of the technique.

At least two completely automated methods for one-stage clotting tests are available. In both systems, after manual placement of the test sample in the proper container, the test is performed automatically. At the present time both systems appear promising, but it is still too early to evaluate them fully. As these become more widely used it will be possible to evaluate results obtained by both manual methods and the automated procedures. It is not within the scope of this chapter to make comparisons of the equipment currently available. However, it appears that in the near future, automated equipment will be available at reasonable cost for the performance of platelet counts, prothrombin time tests, and partial thromboplastin time tests. For a period of time it will be essential to do both manual and automated procedures to learn the sources of error in the systems. However, it appears that the results obtained by the automated procedures will be comparable to the currently used manual methods.

Collection of Blood. The results of most of the tests to evaluate the coagulation mechanism are dependent upon the technique used to obtain the blood sample. Blood must be obtained from a clean venipuncture, since probing of tissues contaminates the sample with tissue fluid which acts as a thromboplastin. For best results the two-syringe technique should be used. The first syringe, attached to the needle during the actual venipuncture, is used to obtain only enough blood to rinse the needle. A second syringe is then attached to the needle and used to collect the sample of blood to be used for testing. The blood should flow freely into the syringe; bubbles due to air leaks are to be avoided. Without delay the sample should be placed into an appropriate container and added to an appropriate anticoagulant solution. It is important that the sample and solution be mixed promptly and thoroughly. During the mixing, care should be taken to avoid air bubbles. If vacuum tubes are used for collection of blood, it is important that the exact volume of blood be collected for the amount of anticoagulant solution.

Once blood leaves the vascular system changes occur. Although actual clot formation can be prevented by the use of calcium binding anticoagulants, some reactions occur even in the presence of anticoagulants in excess. It is important to establish a routine for the collection and processing of blood so that comparative samples are tested. The one-stage prothrombin time is a widely used and relatively reliable test. It was found several years ago that varied results were obtained if the time blood stood in glass containers in the presence of anticoagulant prior to centrifugation was not standardized (Langdell, Graham, and Brinkhous, 1950).

Glassware. It has been known for many years that the surface to which blood is exposed has a significant effect on the speed of the clotting reaction. Early workers used paraffin lined containers to slow the clotting process. The finding that glassware could be made nonwettable by treatment with silicone (Jaques *et al.*, 1946) has had a major influence on experimental studies. The ability to prepare essentially incoagulable native plasma depends upon the availability of proper containers for the blood (Brinkhous, 1947).

In addition to the marked influence on the speed of the clotting reaction by silicone, there are subtle surface effects that must be standardized. Acid cleaning is generally considered the best method for cleaning laboratory glassware. Unless glassware so treated is rinsed many times with distilled water, the contents of the tube are influenced by the acid pH. Formalin is a general enzyme poison. Any glassware exposed to formalin is unsatisfactory for use in clotting tests. Thrombin is adsorbed to glass, and its influence persists through many rinses (Seegers, 1951; Quick, 1951).

Glassware used for coagulation studies must be chemically clean. It is best if this glassware is processed and stored separately from glassware used for other purposes in the laboratory. The availability of new, inexpensive glass and plastic containers may eliminate the problem of artifacts resulting from inadequately washed glassware. However, the surface quality of the "disposable" supplies may produce artifacts. The tubes should be inspected carefully to detect the oily film used by some manufacturers to coat the tubes. The soft glass used in disposable tubes is apt to have different surface properties than the hard glass used in standard laboratory glassware. The surface phenomena of plastics are quite variable. Results obtained with blood processed in plastic containers may not be comparable to results with the same blood processed in glass.

Anticoagulant Solutions. Plasma is a reagent in most tests used to evaluate clotting. This is obtained by adding calcium binding anticoagulant solutions to whole blood. Plasma thus obtained can be studied by the addition of sufficient calcium to neutralize the anticoagulant which was added. It must be understood that some reactions of the clotting system proceed in the presence of anticoagulant. Since the anticoagulant solutions act on the calcium in the plasma, the amount to be added depends on the plasma volume in the sample. The optimal amount of calcium necessary to cause the clotting reaction to proceed in anticoagulated plasma has a moderately wide range as determined empirically. However, under certain circumstances, erroneous results are obtained because of unusual hematocrit values, since the ratio of anticoagulant to plasma varies with packed cell volume.

Sodium Oxalate. One of the most widely used anticoagulant solutions is 0.1 M sodium oxalate. This is used in a ratio of 1 part oxalate solution to 9 parts whole blood. This solution is not isotonic. Oxalate combines with calcium of plasma to form insoluble calcium oxalate. Although this anticoagulant tends to increase the lability of the procoagulants, it is convenient to use, since with it $BaSO_4$ adsorption of plasma can be done if necessary. In one-stage clotting tests, the clotting mixture becomes cloudy with the addition of calcium because of the formation of calcium oxalate. When the fibrin forms, the cloudy mixture becomes clear because of incorporation of the calcium oxalate into the clot. This gives a sharp and easily detected endpoint.

Sodium Citrate. Another commonly used anticoagulant is sodium citrate. An isotonic solution of sodium citrate is 0.11 M. This is used in a ratio of 1 part citrate solution to 8 parts whole blood, Citrate acts by binding calcium in a soluble complex. When citrated plasma is recalcified, the clotting mixture remains clear. The endpoint is the formation of a filmy web of fibrin in a clear solution. Although this endpoint is sharp and distinct, it requires closer observation than does the endpoint with oxalate solution. Sodium citrate can be metabolized by the body and can be used to collect blood that is to be used for injection. Citrate has been found empirically to protect the labile procoagulants to a greater extent than oxalate. Plasma procoagulants are not easily adsorbed from citrated plasma.

EDTA Plasma. In recent years several chelating agents including ethylenediaminetetraacetic acid (EDTA) have been found to bind plasma calcium rapidly. The use of these agents has not offered any real advantage over oxalate or citrate. There appear to be several direct effects of EDTA on the clotting system that cannot be due to its calcium binding ability alone. This reagent is not a good substitute for oxalate or citrate, and EDTA should be reserved for specific procedures in which it has been shown to have an advantage.

Heparin. The use of heparin as an anticoagulant interferes with the clotting tests in which the speed of fibrin formation is measured. It should not be used except for a few specific procedures.

Adsorbed Plasma

PRINCIPLE. It has been known for many years that certain insoluble salts of alkaline earths will remove prothrombin from normal plasma. It is now known that other procoagulants are removed along with prothrombin. Plasma so treated makes a useful reagent for a number of procedures.

REAGENTS AND EQUIPMENT

1. 0.1 M sodium oxalate.
2. Equipment for collection of blood.
3. Glass test tubes which can be centrifuged.
4. Centrifuge.
5. Barium sulfate (C.P.).

PROCEDURE

1. Blood is collected in the usual manner and mixed with 0.1 M sodium oxalate solution in a ratio of 1 part oxalate solution to 9 parts whole blood.
2. After being mixed, the plasma is removed from the cellular elements by centrifugation.
3. A measured volume of plasma is placed in a glass tube that can be centrifuged.
4. 100 mg. of $BaSO_4$ is weighed out for each ml. of plasma to be treated and is added to the plasma.
5. The contents are mixed thoroughly. During the next 30 minutes, the contents of the tube should be mixed at least every 5 minutes.
6. At the end of 30 minutes, the tube is centrifuged at about 3000 r.p.m. for 20 minutes. The supernatant plasma should be clear.
7. The clear supernatant fluid is removed by aspiration. Care must be taken not to aspirate any of the $BaSO_4$. If the aspirated plasma is cloudy, it should be centrifuged again.
8. The supernatant plasma is tested by the prothrombin time procedure. No clot should form in 2 minutes. If clotting occurs in less time, the adsorption procedure should be repeated.

RESULTS. When properly done, most of the prothrombin, factor VII, factor IX, and factor X will be removed. It must be remembered that this results in a relative depletion of these factors, but a trace of activity remains. Factor V, factor VIII, and fibrinogen will not be decreased by this procedure.

MODIFICATIONS AND SOURCES OF ERROR

1. A number of compounds can be used in place of $BaSO_4$ and similar results obtained. $Ca(PO_4)_3$ has been used extensively by Quick, but this material has the disadvantage of necessitating the preparation and maintenance of a suspension.
2. The adsorption phenomenon is reversed by citrate; therefore, oxalate must be used as the anticoagulant.
3. Aluminum hydroxide gel will adsorb the same group of factors from citrated plasma. The amount of aluminum hydroxide gel is critical, since fibrinogen, factor V, and factor VIII can be removed with slightly greater amounts than are required to deplete the other factors.
4. The adsorption phenomenon is influenced by temperature: it is more rapid at higher temperatures. However, because of the thermolability of the procoagulants, it is best to carry out the adsorption procedure at 4° C.
5. If residual $BaSO_4$ is present in the plasma, it can adsorb the procoagulants of plasma with which it is mixed. This can cause erroneous results.
6. The results obtained by adsorption of plasma are not the same if serum is treated. If necessary to use serum, it should contain the usual ratio of oxalate.

Thromboplastin Preparations. There are several excellent thromboplastin suspensions available commercially for both the prothrombin time and the partial thromboplastin time procedures. If these reagents are used, the methods described by the manufacturer must be followed. Many of the tissue thromboplastins are packaged with $CaCl_2$ solution in the reagent. Many of the partial thromboplastins are packaged with an "activator" in the suspension. Although these packaged thromboplastins are convenient, their use is limited to procedures as described in the manufacturer's directions. Those wishing to use more sophisticated procedures may find it necessary to prepare their own reagents if the presence of $CaCl_2$ or artificial activators is undesirable.

Brain tissue is the most convenient source of both tissue and partial thromboplastin. Brain tissue from a number of mammalian species, including rabbit, cow, and man, is a good source of thromboplastin.

1. The meninges are removed and the brain is rinsed under tap water to wash off accumulated blood.
2. About 100 gm. of brain tissue is a convenient amount to process. This is placed in a large mortar and covered with acetone.
3. With the acetone present, the brain tissue is mashed with a pestle.
4. When the acetone becomes cloudy, it is decanted. More acetone is added and mashing is continued. The procedure is repeated until the tissue becomes dry and flaky and the acetone remains clear.
5. The acetone-dehydrated tissue is placed on filter paper in a large evaporating dish and air dried. It may be stored in the dry state at −20° C. as a stock material for tissue thromboplastin. This same material, when extracted with ether, is a partial thromboplastin reagent.

Saline Extraction (Tissue Thromboplastin)

1. Place approximately 100 mg. of the acetone-dehydrated brain reagent in a glass test tube.
2. Add 10 ml. of isotonic saline and mix contents thoroughly.
3. Place tube and contents in water bath (56° C.) for 10 minutes. During this time the contents of the tube must be mixed at frequent intervals.
4. The cloudy supernatant suspension is then aspirated. Centrifugation should be avoided, since some of the active material is easily sedimented.
5. An easy method by which to obtain active supernatant suspension is to place a ball of glass wool in the tube. This is gently submerged with the tip of a 5 ml. pipette. The suspension is drawn into the pipette with the ball of glass wool serving as a filter.
6. The saline suspension thus obtained is used as the thromboplastin reagent in the prothrombin time.
7. The saline suspension loses activity rapidly under most storage conditions. A fresh suspension should be prepared each day from the acetone-dehydrated tissue.

Ether Extraction (Partial Thromboplastin)

1. This material is relatively stable on storage at –20° C.; thus, a relatively large amount can be processed at one time.
2. The extraction procedure is not dependent on quantitative volumes, so any amount of acetone-dehydrated tissue can be processed. It is usually convenient to work with the dehydrated tissue obtained from 100 gm. of starting material.
3. Grind the acetone-dehydrated tissue with clean sand in a mortar.
4. Place the sand and tissue in an Erlenmeyer flask and add sufficient ether to cover the material.
5. Stopper the flask and, after thorough mixing, allow it to stand overnight. It is important to add sufficient ether so that the tissue remains covered by fluid at all times during this period.
6. Filter the material and discard the solid material.
7. Evaporate the ether-soluble material to dryness under vacuum in a rotary evaporator.
8. Wash the residue twice with acetone and then air dry.
9. The yield from about 100 gm. of brain tissue is usually 2 to 3 gm. of white, waxy material.
10. A 3 per cent stock suspension in saline is prepared by diluting 3 gm. of the waxy material to 100 ml. with normal saline (0.154 N NaCl). This is done by slowly adding saline and emulsifying with a glass stirring rod.
11. The 3 per cent stock suspension is stored in 1 ml. amounts at –20° C.
12. For use in the partial thromboplastin test, 1 ml. of this material is diluted with 10 ml. of normal saline. This 0.3 per cent suspension can be stored at –20° C. until used in the test.

Bleeding Time. The duration of bleeding from a standard puncture wound of the skin is a measure of the function of platelets as well as the integrity of the vessel wall.

Duke Method

EQUIPMENT

1. Stop watch.
2. Disposable lancet.*
3. Filter paper.
4. Glass slide.
5. Alcohol sponges.

PROCEDURE

1. The lobe of the ear should be cleaned with alcohol and allowed to dry.
2. The glass slide is placed behind the ear lobe and held firmly in place. This will furnish a firm site on which to make the puncture wound.
3. The lobe of the ear is pierced by a firm stroke against the glass slide. As soon as the puncture wound is made, the glass slide should be discarded and the stop watch should be started.
4. Bleeding of the wound is allowed to proceed without pressure, and the blood is allowed to drop onto the filter paper. The paper should be moved so that each drop will fall on a fresh area. When bleeding slows, the wound is touched gently with a fresh area of the filter paper at 30-second intervals. When blood no longer stains the filter paper, the watch is stopped and the time recorded.

RESULTS. The normal range is up to 6 minutes. Between 6 and 10 minutes, the results are borderline. Over 10 minutes is definitely abnormal.

MODIFICATIONS AND SOURCES OF ERROR

1. Some feel it is dangerous to puncture the ear lobe in patients suspected of having a bleeding tendency and that excessive bleeding can best be controlled from puncture wounds of the forearm. In small children, the heel may be used as the site.
2. Some feel that bleeding is artificially prolonged by touching the wound and that blood should be allowed to fall freely onto the paper or dry gauze sponge.
3. The size and depth of the wound may vary if one does not have a standardized technique.
4. If bleeding lasts for more than 15 minutes, it should be stopped by placing a dry gauze sponge over the site and applying finger pressure. The time is recorded as "greater than 15 minutes."
5. The filter paper used to collect the drops

*There are many individually wrapped sterile disposable lancets available commercially.

of blood can be dried and saved as a record of the procedure.

Ivy Method (Ivy *et al.*, 1935)

EQUIPMENT

1. Stop watch.
2. Disposable lancet.
3. Filter paper.
4. Blood pressure cuff.

PROCEDURE

1. The blood pressure cuff is put on the arm above the elbow and inflated to 40 mm. Hg.
2. An area of the forearm is cleaned with alcohol. The area selected should be free of visible veins.
3. After the area has dried, a puncture wound is made with the lancet and the timer started.
4. The puncture site is blotted gently with filter paper at 30-second intervals. When blood fails to stain the paper, the endpoint has been reached.

RESULTS. With this method the normal bleeding time is 2 to 3 minutes.

Clot Retraction

PRINCIPLE. When whole blood is allowed to clot spontaneously, the initial coagulum is composed of all elements of the blood. With time the coagulum reduces in mass, and fluid serum is expressed from the clot. This is due to an action of platelets on the fibrin network.

EQUIPMENT

1. Equipment for collection of blood.
2. Clean, dry, plain glass test tubes (10 by 75 mm.).
3. Timer.
4. Water bath (37° C.).

PROCEDURE

1. Blood is obtained with a standard two-syringe technique.
2. Approximately 1 ml. of blood is placed in each of two test tubes. The test tubes are then placed in the water bath.
3. One hour after clotting (as determined by the whole blood clotting time) the samples are inspected.
4. On the basis of a 0 to 4+ scale, the degree of reduction in the mass of the clot is estimated in both tubes. The average of the two estimations is the clot retraction.

RESULTS. The clot from a normal individual will be decreased to one-half the original mass within an hour after clotting (3 to 4+).

MODIFICATIONS AND SOURCES OF ERROR

1. There are an infinite number of variations. These include, among others, observations at time intervals and estimating the time when retraction is "complete," and measuring the volume of serum expressed.
2. When fibrinogen is reduced in amount, the clot may be very small and retraction may be interpreted as 4+ even though it is inadequate.
3. In the presence of active fibrinolytic activity the clot may dissolve.
4. In normal blood the exuded serum will be clear and free of erythrocytes. The presence of significant erythrocytes in the serum suggests fibrinolytic activity.
5. With a low hematocrit value, the mass of clot will be proportionately small and may give enormously high values.

Whole Blood Clotting Time

PRINCIPLE. Whole blood, when removed from the vascular system and exposed to a foreign surface, will form a solid clot. Within limits the time required for the formation of the solid clot is a measure of the coagulation system. The procedure was described initially by Lee and White (1913).

EQUIPMENT

1. Stop watch.
2. Equipment for collection of blood.
3. Clean, dry glass test tubes (10 by 75 mm.).
4. Water bath (37° C.).

PROCEDURE

1. Blood is collected with a standard two-syringe technique.
2. Approximately 1 ml. of blood is placed in each of two glass test tubes.
3. The stop watch is started as soon as the blood is placed in the tubes, and all tubes are placed in the water bath.
4. One of the glass tubes is inspected by gentle tilting every 30 seconds until it can be inverted and no blood flows down the side of the tube.
5. One should begin inspection by gentle tilting of the second tube at 15-second intervals until a solid clot is formed. Record the time, which is the clotting time.

RESULTS

1. In normal individuals a solid clot will be formed in the second glass tube in 5 to 8 minutes. Clotting in 8 to 10 minutes is suggestive of a coagulation defect. If more than 10 minutes is required for the formation of a solid clot, there is a definite abnormality.

MODIFICATIONS AND SOURCES OF ERROR

1. Most of the technical errors will tend to decrease the time required for clotting.
2. Air bubbles in the sample from excessively vigorous agitation of the sample during inspection will decrease the time required for clotting.
3. Two tubes are used to decrease agitation of the sample in the second tube. Any number of tubes can be used. The time required for clotting will vary directly with the number of tubes used.
4. Only small amounts of procoagulants are required for clotting to occur in the normal range. Langdell (1957) has shown that in volumetric mixing experiments only 1 to 2 per cent factor VIII is needed for normal

clotting in mixtures of normal and hemophilic blood.

5. The test can also be performed with silicone-coated tubes (Tocantins and Kazal, 1964). If silicone-treated glassware is used, special precautions must be taken to prevent confusion with plain glass.

Fibrinogen Determination

Quantitative Method

PRINCIPLE. It has been found that the tyrosine content of fibrinogen is relatively constant. Fibrinogen is converted to fibrin, and the clot is separated from the plasma. The clot is hydrolyzed by boiling with NaOH, and tyrosine is measured. The method is a slight modification of the method of Ratnoff and Menzie (1951).

EQUIPMENT AND REAGENTS

1. Equipment for collection of blood.
2. 0.1 M sodium oxalate solution.
3. Glass tubes which can be centrifuged.
4. 0.1 M $CaCl_2$ solution.
5. 10 per cent sodium hydroxide.
6. 20 per cent sodium carbonate.
7. Phenol reagent (Folin and Ciocalteu, 1927).
8. Tyrosine standard.
9. Spectrophotometer.
10. Glass funnels (2 inches in diameter).
11. Boiling water bath.
12. Graduated cylinder.
13. Centrifuge.
14. Topical Thrombin (Parke, Davis & Company) diluted to 100 units per ml.

PROCEDURE

1. A tyrosine standard calibration curve should be established prior to testing plasma samples. Dissolve 200 mg. tyrosine in 1000 ml. 0.1 N HCl. This gives a standard solution containing 20 mg. tyrosine per 100 ml. This reagent is added to a series of tubes in amounts of 0.1, 0.2, 0.3, 0.4, and 0.5 M. Distilled water is added to each tube to give a final volume of 9.5 ml. Then 0.5 ml. phenol reagent and 3 ml. sodium carbonate are added. After thorough mixing, let stand for 30 minutes to allow full development of color. Read at a wavelength of 650 mμ. Prepare a graph by plotting the tyrosine concentration against the spectrophotometric readings.

2. To a 50 ml. (25 × 150 mm.) test tube add 1 ml. plasma, 25 ml. saline, 2 ml. 0.1 M $CaCl_2$, and 0.2 ml. Topical Thrombin.

3. Mix thoroughly and then let stand 30 minutes.

4. Place a small ball (about 1 cm. in diameter) of glass wool in the funnel neck.

5. Pour the contents of the tube into the funnel. The glass wool will trap the fibrin.

6. Rinse the glass wool in the funnel with several applications of saline.

7. Place the glass wool with its trapped fibrin in a glass tube and add 1 ml. sodium hydroxide (10 per cent). Place the tube in a boiling water bath. Be certain the glass wool is completely submerged in the solution. Maintain in boiling water bath for 10 minutes.

8. Transfer the glass wool and the NaOH solution to a 25 ml. graduated cylinder. Rinse the tube with water and add washes to the cylinder. Enough water is used to reach the 25 ml. mark. Then mix the contents of the tube thoroughly.

9. Transfer 10 ml. of the fluid to a test tube and centrifuge for 5 minutes to precipitate any solid material.

10. Place 5 ml. of the clear supernatant fluid in a test tube and add 4.5 ml. water, 0.5 ml. phenol reagent, and 3 ml. sodium carbonate.

11. Mix contents thoroughly and then let stand for 30 minutes for full development of the blue color.

12. Place in spectrophotometer and read at a wavelength of 650 mμ.

CALCULATIONS

1. Fibrin from the original plasma sample was diluted to 25 ml. in step 8. Of this, 5 ml. is used to develop the color; thus, the results must be multiplied by a factor of 5.

2. The conversion factor of tyrosine to fibrin is 11.7. Thus, the tyrosine-like activity extrapolated from the standard calibration curve must be multiplied by a factor of 11.7.

3. The results are expressed in terms of mg. fibrinogen per 100 ml. Thus, the results must be multiplied by a factor of 100. Tyrosine equivalents × 11.7 × 5 × 100 = mg. fibrinogen per 100 ml. plasma.

MODIFICATIONS

1. There are many variations in obtaining the fibrin clot. Although it is possible to roll it onto a glass rod or applicator stick, it is difficult to be certain the entire clot is collected.

2. Ratnoff and Menzie (1951) suggest using different volumes and agitating the contents of the clotting mixture with powdered glass. The fibrin thus adheres to the glass particles.

3. There are many other methods available for determining the protein content of the clot. Any of these methods is satisfactory.

Rapid Method

PRINCIPLE. In some clinical syndromes it is of importance to determine the approximate fibrinogen level quickly. In these emergency situations the amount of fibrinogen in a blood sample can be estimated by the speed of clotting after the addition of standard amounts of thrombin. The method is a slight modification of that described by Bowman (1964).

REAGENTS AND EQUIPMENT

1. Equipment for collection of blood.
2. 0.1 M sodium oxalate solution or 0.11 M sodium citrate.
3. Topical Thrombin (Parke, Davis & Com-

pany) diluted with saline to 100 units per ml. (this should be stored at −20° C. in 1-ml. quantities) or Fibrindex (Ortho) made up to 100 units per ml.

4. Test tubes, 13 by 100 mm.
5. Serologic pipettes, 5 ml. and 1 ml.
6. 0.154 M sodium chloride (saline).

PROCEDURE

1. Obtain blood by standard technique.
2. Add immediately to sodium oxalate (or citrate) in a ratio of 1 part oxalate solution to 9 parts whole blood.
3. Centrifuge and collect plasma.
4. Make twofold serial dilutions of plasma with saline. Usually dilutions greater than 256 are not necessary.
5. To 1 ml. of each plasma dilution, 0.1 ml. thrombin solution is added. Mix each tube and allow to stand for 90 seconds.
6. Examine for the presence of a fibrin clot. The highest dilution in which a clot is present is the thrombin titer.

RESULTS

1. Normal healthy adults will form a clot at a dilution of 256. If a clot fails to form at a dilution of less than 128, the plasma fibrinogen is low. A titer below 1/64 is definitely abnormal.
2. The method should be standardized with plasma from several individuals prior to the emergency situation. In this standardization the actual amount of fibrinogen in each dilution can be calculated by testing the plasma samples by the quantitative fibrinogen method.

Fibrinolytic Activity. The fibrinolytic activity of blood depends on the action of plasmin. The amount of plasmin present at any one time is dependent upon the complex and constantly changing equilibrium between activator factors and inhibitory factors. Minor differences in technique and variable attention to the action of the accelerators and inhibitors have led to wide variation in the estimates of fibrinolytic activity. There are a number of quantitative procedures for the detection of each of the factors involved, but these are highly specialized and not readily adaptable to the usual diagnostic laboratory. The two tests described are measures of fibrinolytic activity in general and are influenced by many factors. These serve as screening procedures, but the specific contribution of the various factors must be determined by other means. The lack of suitable standards makes quantitative measurements unavailable for most diagnostic laboratories.

Euglobulin Lysis Time

PRINCIPLE. Euglobulin fraction of plasma contains fibrinogen and all the plasminogen activator and plasminogen of plasma but only traces of the antiplasmins (Kowalski *et al.*, 1959). The lysis of a fibrin clot formed by the addition of thrombin is a measure of the fibrinolytic activity.

REAGENTS AND EQUIPMENT

1. Equipment for the collection of blood.
2. Centrifuge.
3. 0.11 M sodium citrate.
4. Topical Thrombin (Parke, Davis & Company).
5. Serologic pipettes.
6. Carbon dioxide. A tank of CO_2 fitted with a valve to allow control of the rate of flow.

PROCEDURE

1. Blood is collected in the usual manner and mixed immediately with 0.11 M sodium citrate in a ratio of 1 part citrate solution to 8 parts blood.
2. Plasma is obtained by centrifugation.
3. 0.4 ml. plasma is placed in a test tube and 7.6 ml. distilled water is added.
4. Carbon dioxide is bubbled into the solution through a capillary tube for 30 seconds.
5. The precipitate which forms is collected by centrifugation at about 3000 r.p.m. for 15 minutes.
6. The precipitate is dissolved in 1 ml. M/15 phosphate buffer, pH 7.2.
7. To the euglobulin in phosphate buffer, 0.1 ml. thrombin (Topical Thrombin diluted to 100 units per ml. with saline) is added. The solution is mixed.
8. Clotting should be rapid. After clotting has occurred, the tube is placed in water bath (37° C.) and observed for lysis of clot, which is the endpoint.

RESULTS. In normal plasma a period of 2 to 4 hours is required for euglobulin clot lysis to occur.

MODIFICATIONS

1. Euglobulins can be precipitated from the plasma by other methods, such as dilute acetic acid.
2. The volume of plasma can be varied.
3. Since variability in handling the specimen is inevitable between laboratories, it is essential that the technique be standardized for each laboratory.

Dilute Blood Clot Lysis Time (Fearnley, 1960)

PRINCIPLE. Plasmin inhibitors lose activity on dilution to a greater extent than fibrinolytic activity. Whole blood is diluted with a buffer solution and clotted by the addition of thrombin. The clot is observed for lysis of the clot.

REAGENTS AND EQUIPMENT

1. Equipment for collection of blood sample.
2. Test tubes.
3. Timer.
4. Phosphate buffer, pH 7.4. To 1000 ml. distilled water, 9.47 gm. Na_2HPO_4 is added and dissolved. This is mixed with 250 ml. distilled water containing 3.02 gm. KH_2PO_4.
5. Topical Thrombin (Parke, Davis & Company) diluted to 100 units per ml. with normal saline.

PROCEDURE

1. Tubes containing 1.70 ml. buffer and 0.1 ml. thrombin solution are placed in an ice bath.

2. Collect blood in standard manner using a syringe that can deliver accurately 0.2 ml. aliquots of blood.

3. Add 0.2 ml. blood to each of two tubes containing buffer and thrombin and mix.

4. Clotting should occur promptly.

5. Tubes are placed in refrigerator (4° C.) for 30 minutes and then transferred to a water bath at 37° C.

6. The clots are observed for lysis. The end-point is fragmentation rather than complete dissolution of the clot.

RESULTS. Blood from a normal subject should not lyse in less than 6 to 10 hours. The test is qualitative. If results indicate rapid lysis of the clot, more quantitative methods are necessary. The fibrin plate method of Astrup and Mullertz (1952) should be incorporated as a procedure in laboratories requiring more than a qualitative screening test.

Platelet Count

PRINCIPLE. The number of platelets in a representative sample of blood can be determined with a calibrated chamber and phase microscopy (Brecher, Schneiderman, and Chronkite, 1953).

REAGENTS AND EQUIPMENT

1. Microscope and attachments for phase microscopy.

2. Hemocytometer. This must be of a special type with a flat undersurface.

3. Blood diluting pipettes (red cell type for 1:100 dilution and white cell type for 1:20 dilution).

4. Ammonium oxalate solution (1 per cent). This must be kept at 4° C. to prevent growth of microorganisms and filtered before use.

5. Equipment for collection of blood sample. Best results are obtained from venous blood, but capillary puncture can be used. For venous blood, disodium ethylenediaminetetraacetic acid (disodium EDTA) is used in dry form.

PROCEDURE

1. Blood is collected by a standard method. Venous blood mixed immediately with disodium EDTA will be satisfactory for 2 to 3 hours. Capillary blood must be drawn directly into the blood diluting pipette.

2. Blood is drawn to the 1 mark in an RBC diluting pipette. Ammonium oxalate (1 per cent) is immediately drawn into the pipette to the 100 mark. The contents are mixed in the standard manner.

3. Both wells of the hemocytometric chamber are filled in the standard manner. A No. 1 or 1½ coverslip is more satisfactory than the usual hemocytometer coverglass.

4. The filled chamber is placed in a Petri dish containing wet cotton or filter paper. The dish is covered, and the fluid in the chamber is left undisturbed for 10 to 15 minutes.

5. The chamber is placed on a microscope equipped for phase microscopy, and cells are counted as for the red blood cell count.

RESULTS. The mean normal platelet level is 250,000 per cu. mm. The range is between 150,000 and 450,000 per cu. mm.

SOURCES OF ERROR AND MODIFICATION

1. If mixing of the blood and oxalate is not adequate, platelet clumps occur. It is quite difficult to determine the exact number of platelets in a clump.

2. If the number of platelets is low, a dilution of less than 1:100 may be necessary. This can be done with the WBC diluting pipette.

3. The appearance of platelets in the phase field must be recognized. Extraneous material may be mistaken for platelets.

Prothrombin Determination (Two-stage Method)

PRINCIPLE. The procedure is based on the method of Warner, Brinkhous, and Smith (1934, 1936). Prothrombin in the presence of optimal procoagulants and calcium will form thrombin. The amount of thrombin formed can be calculated by determining the dilution of plasma that will clot a standard fibrinogen reagent in a specific period of time. The amount of thrombin formed is a measure of the amount of prothrombin present in the starting sample.

The test consists of two stages. In the first stage, prothrombin is incubated with a standard mixture containing thromboplastin, calcium, a buffer, and a source of procoagulants. In the second stage, samples of the incubating mixture are added to a standard fibrinogen solution and the clotting time is determined.

RESULTS

1. The object of the procedure is to determine the dilution of plasma from which will evolve one unit of thrombin under optimal conditions. A unit of thrombin is defined as that amount which will form a clot of 1 ml. of fibrinogen in 15 seconds under standard conditions.

2. If varying amounts of thrombin are added to standard amounts of fibrinogen, the clotting time of the mixture is an index of the thrombin concentration within a specific range. When thrombin concentrations are plotted against clotting times, the results describe a hyperbolic curve. With thrombin concentrations between 0.80 and 1.34 units, there is a good correlation between thrombin concentration and clotting time. With greater amounts of thrombin, there is little change in the speed of clotting, with relatively large changes in thrombin concentration. With lesser amounts of thrombin, small changes in thrombin concentration result in large changes in the speed of clotting.

Partial Thromboplastin Time

PRINCIPLE. Hemophilic plasma clots as rapidly as does normal plasma when recalcified in the presence of a potent tissue thromboplastin. It was demonstrated by Langdell, Wagner, and Brinkhous (1953) that certain thromboplastins lack the ability to compensate for the plasma defect of hemophilia. Such thromboplastins are called partial thromboplastins, and when such material is used in one-stage clotting tests, the procedure is called the partial thromboplastin time.

EQUIPMENT AND REAGENTS

1. Equipment for the collection of blood.
2. 0.1 M sodium oxalate solution.
3. Glass test tube which can be centrifuged.
4. Stop watch.
5. Water bath (37° C.).
6. Partial thromboplastin.
7. 0.02 M $CaCl_2$ solution.
8. Centrifuge.
9. Pipettes (blow-out type calibrated to deliver 0.1 ml.).
10. Clean dry glass test tubes (10 by 75 mm.).
11. Clean dry glass test tubes (13 by 100 mm.).
12. A good light source.
13. Plasma from a normal subject.

PROCEDURE

1. The plasma sample obtained for the prothrombin time can be used for the partial thromboplastin time (see Prothrombin Time for details of collection, p. 443).

2. For each sample to be tested, place approximately 0.4 ml. $CaCl_2$ solution in a clean glass test tube. In a separate tube place the same amount of partial thromboplastin suspension. Place both tubes in a water bath (37° C.).

3. Exactly 0.1 ml. plasma to be tested is measured into a clean, dry glass test tube (10 by 75 mm.), and the tube is placed in a water bath (37° C.).

4. After the plasma has incubated for 60 seconds, exactly 0.1 ml. of partial thromboplastin suspension and 0.1 ml. $CaCl_2$ solution are added to the tube in rapid sequence. The stop watch is started immediately after the addition of $CaCl_2$ solution.

5. The tube is tilted back and forth in front of a good light source and the contents observed for the appearance of a fibrin clot. The watch is stopped when the clot forms, and the time is recorded.

6. The procedure is repeated so that at least two recordings are obtained for each test and control sample. The average of the two determinations is the partial thromboplastin time of the sample.

RESULTS

1. The potency of partial thromboplastins is variable, so plasma known to be normal must be used as a control for interpretation of the results.

2. With most commercially available partial thromboplastins and with those prepared by the method described earlier, normal human plasma will clot in 60 to 70 seconds.

3. When the partial thromboplastin time is within 5 seconds of the control time, it should be considered normal. Results are to be considered as probably abnormal if 10 to 20 seconds longer than the control. Any results 20 or more seconds longer than the control indicate a definite deficiency of one of the plasma procoagulants.

4. The partial thromboplastin time will be long, with a significant plasma deficiency of any of the procoagulants other than factor VII.

MODIFICATIONS AND SOURCES OF ERROR

1. Consistent results will be obtained only by consistent technique. The simplicity of the test is apt to be delusive. Reproducible results can be obtained only by adhering to the principles of good technique.

2. Several minor modifications of the test have been suggested. These have been primarily for convenience and have not improved the quality of the results. Suggested modifications include (a) incubation of the plasma and thromboplastin solution at 37° C. for a standard time prior to the addition of calcium solution, (b) combining the thromboplastin and calcium solution (with some thromboplastins an insoluble precipitate forms if this is done), and (c) allowing the clotting mixture (plasma, thromboplastin, and calcium) to remain in the water bath for a standard time prior to an observation for the endpoint.

3. Major modifications have been suggested which are aimed at decreasing the time required for clotting. These are apt to change the specificity of the test.

A. *Activator Materials.* Clays and other silica compounds such as kaolin have been added to the procedure (Nye *et al.*, 1962). These have the general effect of decreasing the length of time between the addition of calcium and visible clotting. Although this increases the speed with which the test can be made, it decreases the differential in clotting between normal and procoagulant deficient plasma. In the nonactivated system, normal plasma will clot in about 70 seconds and hemophilic plasma will clot in about 130 seconds. In the activated system, normal plasma will clot in about 40 seconds and hemophilic plasma will clot in about 50 seconds. Thus, small differences in clotting time are of considerable importance in the activated systems.

B. *Active Accelerators.* A wide variety of materials derived from blood have the ability to shorten the partial thromboplastin time of both normal and deficient plasmas. In the original description of the method, it was shown that thrombin and serum accelerator in small amounts had this effect (Langdell, Wagner, and Brinkhous, 1953). Such materials should not be added to the partial thromboplastin time procedure except under carefully controlled conditions.

4. As in the prothrombin time, the collection and preparation of the plasma sample is of importance.

Prothrombin Time

PRINCIPLE. Plasma obtained from blood to which a calcium binding anticoagulant has been added will coagulate in a few seconds when recalcified in the presence of tissue thromboplastin. The elapsed time between the addition of calcium and the presence of a visible clot is the prothrombin time (Quick, Stanley-Brown, and Bancroft, 1935).

EQUIPMENT AND REAGENTS

1. Equipment for the collection of blood.
2. 0.1 M sodium oxalate solution.
3. Glass test tube which can be centrifuged.
4. Stop watch.
5. Water bath (37° C.).
6. Tissue thromboplastin.
7. 0.02 M calcium chloride solution.
8. Centrifuge.
9. Pipettes (blow-out type calibrated to deliver 0.1 ml.).
10. Clean, dry glass test tubes (10 by 75 mm.).
11. Clean, dry glass test tubes (13 by 100 mm.).
12. A good light source.
13. Plasma from a normal subject.

PROCEDURE

1. Prior to collection of blood, a clean, dry glass tube which can be centrifuged is calibrated so that a 5-ml. volume can be placed in the tube with accuracy.

2. 0.5 ml. of the 0.1 M sodium oxalate solution is placed in the tube.

3. Blood is obtained by standard venipuncture technique and immediately placed in the calibrated tube to the 5.0-ml. mark.

4. The blood and the oxalate solution are mixed thoroughly by gentle inversion of the tube.

5. The sample is allowed to stand for about 45 minutes at room temperature or in a refrigerator.

6. The tube and its contents are centrifuged at about 3000 r.p.m. for 15 to 20 minutes. The supernatant plasma is aspirated and transferred to a clean, dry glass test tube.

7. Plasma from a normal individual should be obtained and processed in exactly the same manner as the sample from the patient under study.

8. For each sample to be tested, place about 0.4 ml. of $CaCl_2$ solution in a clean test tube. In a separate tube, place the same amount of tissue thromboplastin suspension. Place both tubes in a water bath (37° C.).

9. Exactly 0.1 ml. plasma to be tested is measured into a clean, dry glass test tube (10 by 75 mm.), and the tube is placed in the water bath.

10. After the plasma has incubated for 60 seconds, exactly 0.1 ml. of tissue thromboplastin and 0.1 ml. of $CaCl_2$ solution are added to the tube in rapid sequence. The stop watch is started immediately after the addition of the $CaCl_2$ solution.

11. The tube is tilted back and forth in front of a good light source, and the contents observed for the appearance of a fibrin clot. The watch is stopped when the clot forms, and the time is recorded.

12. The procedure is repeated so that at least two recordings can be obtained for each test and control sample. The average of the two times is the prothrombin time of the sample.

RESULTS

1. Normal plasma should clot in 12 seconds following the addition of calcium with a potent tissue thromboplastin. The duplicate samples should clot within 0.3 second of each other.

2. The prothrombin time will be long with a deficiency of prothrombin, factor V, factor VII, or factor X, or a combination of deficiencies.

MODIFICATIONS AND SOURCES OF ERROR

1. Since the original description of the test there have been an infinite number of modifications. These have been for the convenience of the person doing the procedure and have not improved the quality of the results. The modifications include the following:

A. The thromboplastin and calcium solutions may be combined. These two reagents are then added simultaneously.
B. The plasma sample can be added to a tube containing a measured volume of 0.1 ml. of both the thromboplastin and the calcium.
C. The thromboplastin and plasma can be incubated for a standard time prior to the addition of calcium. Trace amounts of calcium in the thromboplastin suspension can cause artificially rapid clotting.

The choice of technique is probably of less importance than consistency of technique. If modifications are used, they should be used every time the test is performed.

2. Blood in contact with a glass surface produces a clot accelerating activity, even in the presence of adequate calcium binding anticoagulants. It requires about 45 minutes for this activity to reach its optimum level (Langdell, Graham, and Brinkhous, 1950). It is for this reason that blood is allowed to stand for 45 minutes prior to centrifugation. If testing is done sooner, abnormally long values are obtained.

3. Plasma standing at 37° C. rapidly loses

factor V activity. The samples must be tested promptly or stored in the frozen state to preserve factor V activity.

4. The results may be expressed as per cent activity rather than as the elapsed time in seconds. Prothrombin activity is calculated from a standard dilution curve obtained by a series of prothrombin times on volumetric mixtures of whole plasma and a solution known to be free of prothrombin activity. This is more difficult to do than it is generally believed to be. Some have suggested diluting plasma with isotonic saline. It is obvious that when this is done all clotting factors in the plasma are being diluted. The graph obtained when clotting time is plotted against plasma concentration has little or no relationship to the amount of prothrombin present in the mixture.

Prothrombin, factor VII, factor IX, and factor X can be quantitatively removed from plasma with certain insoluble alkaline earths, such as $BaSO_4$, $Ca(PO_4)_3$, and $Al(OH)_3$. Fibrinogen, factor V, and factor VIII remain in normal amounts following such treatment of plasma. Clotting times of volumetric dilutions of whole plasma with adsorbed plasma give a somewhat more meaningful standard curve for determining prothrombin activity. At least fibrinogen and factor V levels are constant in each dilution. Even so, the clotting time does not change significantly until the whole plasma has been reduced to a concentration of about 40 per cent of normal.

5. The results are a measure of several procoagulants other than prothrombin. Abnormally long prothrombin time results from deficiency of factor V, factor VII, and factor X, as well as prothrombin deficiency. As long as fibrinogen remains above about 100 mg. per 100 ml., the fibrinogen level does not influence the results. However, below this level, fibrinogen concentration becomes an important factor.

6. The procedure is standardized on the basis of standard amounts of $CaCl_2$ to neutralize the amount of anticoagulant added to the whole blood sample. When the ratio of anticoagulant to plasma is abnormal, as in severe anemia, the amount of calcium may not be optimal. Whenever the hematocrit value is significantly increased or decreased, the test should be modified to determine optimal calcium.

Prothrombin Utilization

Principle. During coagulation of blood, prothrombin is converted to thrombin. Although thrombin is formed during this process, it is inactivated rapidly so that at any one time only a few units of thrombin can be detected. An indirect measurement of the amount of thrombin formed is to determine the amount of prothrombin that is lost. Whole blood is allowed to clot, and at time intervals the reaction is stopped by the addition of an anticoagulant. The amount of prothrombin present is determined by either the prothrombin time or two-stage prothrombin method.

Results

1. In normal individuals little or no prothrombin will be present in the 60-minute sample as determined by the two-stage method.

2. In blood deficient in one of the procoagulants, 50 per cent or more prothrombin will be present in the 60-minute sample as measured by the two-stage method.

3. Blood with low platelet levels (below 70,000 per cu. mm.) will also have high prothrombin activity in the 30- and 60-minute sample.

4. The lack of prothrombin utilization is manifest in the one-stage procedure by clotting times as short as the control or shorter.

5. In normal individuals the modified prothrombin time of the 60-minute sample will be 20 seconds or longer.

6. In blood deficient in one of the procoagulants, the modified prothrombin time of the 60-minute sample will be 14 seconds or shorter.

Thromboplastin Generation Test

Principle. In native blood, clotting is relatively slow when compared to the rapid clot formation that occurs with the addition of tissue thromboplastin. It was noted by Biggs and Douglas (1953) that a mixture of dilute plasma, serum, partial thromboplastin, and calcium that was allowed to incubate caused rapid clotting when added to plasma. It was believed that during incubation, thromboplastin was generated. The test procedure consists of an incubation step and a clotting time determination.

Dilute adsorbed plasma, dilute serum, a partial thromboplastin and calcium are incubated together. At time intervals a sample of the incubating mixture and calcium solution are added simultaneously to plasma and the clotting time determined.

Results

1. The shortest clotting time that is obtained is the Thromboplastin Generation Time. In a complete system the clotting time is about the same as in the prothrombin time.

2. The adsorbed plasma is the source of factors V, VIII, and XII in the incubating mixture.

3. The serum is the source of factors VII, IX, X, and XI in the incubating mixture.

4. By using both control and test samples it is possible to determine if inadequate clot acceleration is due to a deficiency in the test plasma or test serum.

5. Platelets may be used as the partial throm-

boplastin in the incubating mixture. This can then be used to evaluate platelet function.

Tourniquet Test

PRINCIPLE. Capillary fragility is measured by maintaining pressure halfway between systolic and diastolic for a standard time interval. The lack of appearance of petechiae is an indication of normal vascular integrity.

EQUIPMENT

1. Blood pressure cuff.
2. Timer.
3. Skin marking pencil.

PROCEDURE

1. Examine the arm and note any skin blemishes that might be mistaken for petechiae.
2. Draw a circle 1½ inches in diameter on the volar surface of the arm, 3 to 4 inches below the antecubital fossa.
3. Apply the blood pressure cuff to the upper arm and inflate to the point midway between systolic and diastolic pressure.
4. Maintain pressure for 5 minutes and then deflate the cuff.
5. Examine the area enclosed in the circle for evidence of petechiae and record.

RESULTS. Normal subjects may form up to five petechiae. Any more than five is considered to be abnormal.

MODIFICATIONS. An infinite number of modifications are possible, all of which have some merit. The pressure can be maintained for a longer or shorter time interval. The area examined for petechiae can be increased in size.

One major deficiency of the method is that a series of tests cannot be done, since pressure is maintained in the entire forearm and petechiae occur at numerous sites. For this reason, a vacuum device has been suggested.

Screening Tests for Diagnosis of Procoagulant Deficiency

PRINCIPLE. Most of the coagulation disorders can be classified on the basis of the prothrombin time used in conjunction with the partial thromboplastin time (Langdell, 1961). The effect of $BaSO_4$-adsorbed normal plasma on the results of the abnormal test is of diagnostic significance.

REAGENTS AND EQUIPMENT

1. All reagents and equipment necessary for the prothrombin time and partial thromboplastin time.
2. $BaSO_4$-treated normal plasma.

PROCEDURE

1. The plasma under study is tested in the usual manner by both the prothrombin time and the partial thromboplastin time.
2. Mix equal volumes of the test plasma and normal control plasma. About 0.5 ml. of the mixture is needed.
3. Mix equal volumes of the test plasma and $BaSO_4$-treated normal plasma. About 0.5 ml. of the mixture is needed.
4. Determine the prothrombin time and the partial thromboplastin time of each of the mixtures.

RESULTS

1. If both the prothrombin time and the partial thromboplastin time are normal, it is doubtful that a clinically significant coagulation disorder is present.
2. If the normal plasma fails to correct an abnormal prothrombin time or partial thromboplastin time, it is likely that the patient has a circulating anticoagulant.
3. If normal plasma corrects either the prothrombin time or the partial thromboplastin time, the presumptive diagnosis is as indicated in the table at the bottom of this page.
4. Factor XII deficiency will have a pattern similar to that of factor VIII deficiency. The correct diagnosis can be further elucidated by the lack of a real bleeding tendency in the factor XII deficiency. Definite diagnosis can be established only by having available samples of plasma known to be specifically deficient in factor VIII and factor XII. Failure of correction of the patient's partial thromboplastin time by plasma known to be deficient in factor VIII establishes the diagnosis of hemophilia. Likewise, failure of correction of the patient's partial thromboplastin time by plasma known

PROTHROMBIN TIME		PARTIAL THROMBOPLASTIN TIME		PRESUMPTIVE DIAGNOSIS
Test Plasma Alone	Test Plasma Plus $BaSO_4$ Plasma	Test Plasma Alone	Test Plasma Plus $BaSO_4$ Plasma	Deficiency of Factor
Long	Normal	Long	Normal	V
Long	Long	Normal	Normal	VII
Normal	Normal	Long	Normal	VIII
Normal	Normal	Long	Long	IX
Long	Long	Long	Long	X

to be deficient in factor XII establishes the diagnosis of Hageman trait.

5. Factor XI deficiency may have a pattern similar to that of factor VIII or factor IX deficiency. The correct diagnosis can be further elucidated by the sex-linked recessive transmission of factor VIII or factor IX deficiency. Definitive diagnosis can be established only by having available samples of plasma known to be specifically deficient in factors VIII, IX, and XI. Failure of correction of the patient's partial thromboplastin time by plasma known to be deficient in factor XI establishes the diagnosis of factor XI deficiency.

The two-stage prothrombin method is required to distinguish a true deficiency of prothrombin from the pattern indicated for factor X deficiency.

A severe deficiency of fibrinogen will have a pattern similar to that of factor V deficiency. A quantitative method for fibrinogen is required to determine the fibrinogen level.

REFERENCES

Ackroyd, J. F.: Platelet agglutinins and lysins in the pathogenesis of thrombocytopenic purpura with a note on platelet group. Brit. Med. Bull. *11*:28, 1955.

Aggeler, P. M., White, S. G., Glendening, M. B., Page, E. W., Leake, T. B., and Bates, G.: Plasma thromboplastin component (PTC) deficiency: A new disease resembling hemophilia. Proc. Soc. Exp. Biol. Med. *79*:692, 1952.

Alexander, B.: Factor VII (proconvertin). Thromb. Diath. Haemorrh. 7:392, 1961.

Alexander, B., and Goldstein, R.: Dual hemostatic defect in pseudohemophilia. J. Clin. Invest. *32*:551, 1953.

Alexander, B., Goldstein, R., Landwehr, G., and Cook, C. D.: Congenital SPCA deficiency. J. Clin. Invest. *30*:596, 1951.

Alkjaersig, N., Fletcher, A. P., and Sherry, S.: ϵ-Aminocaproic acid: An inhibitor of plasminogen activation. J. Biol. Chem. *234*:832, 1959.

Ambrus, J. L.: Pharmacology society symposium. The fibrinolysin system. Fed. Proc. 25:28, 1966.

Astrup, T., and Mullertz, S.: Fibrin plate method for estimating fibrinolytic activity. Arch. Biochem. Biophys. *40*:346, 1952.

Bang, N. U., Beller, F. K., Deutsch, E., and Mammen, E. F.: Thrombosis and Bleeding Disorders. New York, Academic Press, Inc., 1971.

Barrow, E. M., Bullock, W. R., and Graham, J. B.: A study of the carrier state for plasma thromboplastin component (PTC Christmas factor) deficiency utilizing a new assay procedure. J. Lab. Clin. Med. 55:936, 1960.

Barrow, E. M., and Graham, J. B.: Von Willebrand's disease. *In* Moore, C. V., and Brown, E. B. (eds.): Progress in Hematology. New York, Grune & Stratton, Inc., 1964.

Barrow, E. M., Heindel, C. C., Roberts, H. R., and Graham, J. B.: Heterozygosity in von Willebrand's disease. Proc. Soc. Exp. Biol. Med. *118*:684, 1965.

Biggs, R., and Douglas, A. S.: The thromboplastin generation test. J. Clin. Path. 6:23, 1953.

Biggs, R., Douglas, A. S., Dacie, J. V., Pitney, W. R., Merskey, C., and O'Brien, J. R.: Christmas disease, a condition previously mistaken for hemophilia. Brit. Med. J. 2:1378, 1952.

Biggs, R., and Macfarlane, R. G.: Human Blood Coagulation and Its Disorders. Springfield, Illinois, Charles C Thomas, 1957.

Bowman, H. S.: Plasma fibrinogen titer ("thrombin titer"). *In* Tocantins, L. M., and Kazal, L. A. (eds.): Blood Coagulation, Hemorrhage and Thrombosis. New York, Grune & Stratton, Inc., 1964.

Brecher, G., Schneiderman, M., and Chronkite, E. P.: The reproducibility and constancy of the platelet count. Amer. J. Clin. Path. *23*:15, 1953.

Brinkhous, K. M.: A study of the clotting defect in hemophilia: The delayed formation of thrombin. Amer. J. Med. Sci. *198*:509, 1939.

Brinkhous, K. M.: Plasma prothrombin; vitamin K. Medicine *19*:329, 1940.

Brinkhous, K. M.: Clotting defect in hemophilia: Deficiency in a plasma factor required for platelet utilization. Proc. Soc. Exp. Biol. Med. *66*:117, 1947.

Brinkhous, K. M.: Chairman's opening remarks. *In* Brinkhous, K. M. (ed.): Hemophilia and Hemophilioid Diseases. Chapel Hill, North Carolina, University of North Carolina Press, 1957.

Brinkhous, K. M., Langdell, R. D., Penick, G. D., Graham, J. B., and Wagner, R. H.: Newer approaches to the study of hemophilia and hemophilioid states. J.A.M.A. *154*:481, 1954.

Brinkhous, K. M., Langdell, R. D., and Wagner, R. H.: Hemostatic disorders: Hemophilia and the hemophilioid diseases. Ann. Rev. Med. *9*:159, 1958.

Brinkhous, K. M., Roberts, H. R., Hinnoms, S., and Kiesselbach, T. H.: Fibrinogen: Structural, Metabolic and Pathophysiologic Aspects. Stuttgart, F. K. Schattauer-Verlag, 1970.

Caen, J.: Effect of normal and hemophilic plasma on AHG activity and long bleeding time in von Willebrand's disease. *In* Brinkhous, K. M. (ed.): The Hemophilias. Chapel Hill, North Carolina, University of North Carolina Press, 1964.

Davie, E. W., and Ratnoff, O. D.: Waterfall sequence for intrinsic blood clotting. Science *145*:1310, 1964.

de Nicola, P.: Report of the subcommittee on new clotting factors. Thromb. Diath. Haemorrh. 7:347, 1962.

Deutsch, E.: Acquired inhibitors. Thromb. Diath. Haemorrh. 7:112, 1962.

de Vries, A., Alexander, B., and Goldstein, R.: Factor in serum which accelerated conversion of prothrombin to thrombin. I. Its determination and some physiologic and biochemical properties. Blood *4*:247, 1949.

Duckert, F., Jung, E., and Shmerling, D. H.: A hitherto undescribed congenital haemorrhagic diathesis probably due to fibrin stabilizing factor deficiency. Thromb. Diath. Haemorrh. 5:179, 1960.

Fantl, P.: Parahemophilia (proaccelerin deficiency) occurrence and biochemistry. *In* Brinkhous, K. M. (ed.): Hemophilia and Hemophilioid Diseases. Chapel Hill, North Carolina, University of North Carolina Press, 1957.

Fantl, P., and Nance, M. H.: Acceleration of thrombin formation by a plasma component. Nature (London) *158*:708, 1946.

Fearnley, G. R.: Spontaneous fibrinolysis. Amer. J. Cardiol. 6:371, 1960.

Fletcher, A. P.: Pathological fibrinolysis. Fed. Proc. 25:84, 1966.

Folin, O., and Ciocalteu, V.: On tyrosine and tryptophane determinations in proteins. J. Biol. Chem. *73*:627, 1927.

Geratz, J. D., and Graham, J. B.: Plasma thromboplastin component (Christmas factor, factor IX) levels in stored human blood and plasma. Thromb. Diath. Haemorrh. *4*:376, 1960.

Graham, J. B.: Genetic problems. Hemophilia and allied diseases. *In* Brinkhous, K. M. (ed.): Hemophilia and Hemophilioid Diseases. Chapel Hill, North Carolina, University of North Carolina Press, 1957.

Graham, J. B., Barrow, E. M., and Hougie, C.: Stuart clotting defect. II. Genetic aspects of a 'new' hemorrhagic state. J. Clin. Invest. *36*:497, 1957.

Graham, J. B., Buckwalter, J. A., Hartley, L. J., and Brinkhous, K. M.: Canine hemophilia, observations on the course, the clotting anomaly, and the effect of blood transfusions. J. Exp. Med. *90*:97, 1949.

Graham, J. B., and Hougie, C.: Factor X (Stuart-Prower factor). Thromb. Diath. Haemorrh. 7:416, 1961.

Graham, J. B., Langdell, R. D., Morrison, F. C., and Brinkhous, K. M.: Serum accelerator factors and antihemo-

philic factor (AHF) in early phases of clotting. Proc. Soc. Exp. Biol. Med. *87*:45, 1954.
Graham, J. B., McLendon, W. W., and Brinkhous, K. M.: Mild hemophilia: An allelic form of the disease. Am. J. Med. Sci. *225*:46, 1953.
Guest, M. M.: Functional significance of the fibrinolytic enzyme system. Fed. Proc. *25*:73, 1966.
Hall, C. A., Rapaport, S. I., Ames, S. B., and DeGroot, J. A.: A clinical and family study of hereditary proconvertin (factor VII) deficiency. Amer. J. Med. *37*:172, 1964.
Hall, C. E., and Slayter, H. S.: The fibrinogen molecule, its size, shape and mode of polymerization. J. Biophys. Cytol. *5*:11, 1959.
Hampton, J. W., and Bird, R. M.: The pattern of inheritance of defective fibrinase. J. Lab. Clin. Med. *67*:914, 1966.
Harrington, W. J., Minnich, V., Hollingsworth, J. W., and Moore, C. V.: Demonstration of a thrombocytopenic factor in the blood of patients with thrombocytopenic purpura. J. Lab. Clin. Med. *38*:1, 1951.
Harrington, W. J., Sprague, C. C., Minnich, V., Moore, C. V., Ahlvin, R. C., and Dabach, R.: Immunologic mechanisms in idiopathic and neonatal thrombocytopenic purpura. Ann. Intern. Med. *38*:433, 1953.
Hartman, R. C.: A hemorrhagic disorder occurring in patients with cyanotic congenital heart disease. Bull. Hopkins Hosp. *91*:49, 1952.
Henoch, E.: Über eine eigenthümliche Form von Purpura. Berl. Klin. Wschr. *11*:641, 1874.
Hougie, C., Barrow, E. M., and Graham, J. B.: Stuart clotting defect. I. Segregation of an hereditary hemorrhagic state from the heterogeneous group heretofore called 'stable factor' (SPCA, proconvertin, factor VII) deficiency. J. Clin. Invest. *36*:485, 1957.
Ivy, A. C., Shapiro, P. F., and Melnick, P.: The bleeding tendency in jaundice. Surg. Gynec. Obstet. *60*:781, 1935.
Jackson, D. P., Beck, E. A., and Charache, P.: Congenital disorders of fibrinogen. Fed. Proc. *24*:816, 1965.
Jaques, L. B.: Stress and multiple factor etiology of bleeding. Ann. N.Y. Acad. Sci. *115*:78, 1964.
Jaques, L. B., Fidlar, E., Feldsted, E. T., and Macdonald, A. G.: Silicones and blood coagulation. Can. Med. Ass. J. *55*:26, 1946.
Johnston, C. C., Jr., Ferguson, J. H., O'Hanlan, F. A., and Payne, R. B.: Isolation of coagulation factors by continuous flow electrophoresis. Proc. Soc. Exp. Biol. Med. *101*: 747, 1959.
Karpatkin, S., Ingram, G. I. C., and Graham, J. B.: Severe isolated prothrombin deficiency: An acquired state with complete recovery. Thromb. Diath. Haemorrh. *8*:221, 1962.
Kowalski, E., Kopec, M., and Niewiarowski, S.: An evaluation of the euglobulin method for the determination of fibrinolysis. J. Clin. Path. *21*:215, 1959.
Laki, K.: Enzymatic effects of thrombin. Fed. Proc. *24*:794, 1965.
Laki, K., and Lorand, L.: On the solubility of fibrin clots. Science *108*:280, 1948.
Langdell, R. D.: Transfusion therapy in hemophilia. *In* Brinkhous, K. M. (ed.): Hemophilia and Hemophilioid Diseases. Chapel Hill, North Carolina, University of North Carolina Press, 1957.
Langdell, R. D.: Laboratory diagnosis of hemorrhagic disorders. South. Med. J. *54*:560, 1961.
Langdell, R. D., Graham, J. B., and Brinkhous, K. M.: Prothrombin utilization during clotting: Comparison of results with the two-stage and one-stage methods. Proc. Soc. Exp. Biol. Med. *74*:424, 1950.
Langdell, R. D., Wagner, R. H., and Brinkhous, K. M.: Effect of antihemophilic factor on one-stage clotting tests. J. Lab. Clin. Med. *41*:637, 1953.
Langdell, R. D., Wagner, R. H., and Brinkhous, K. M.: AHF levels following transfusion of blood, plasma and plasma fractions. Proc. Soc. Exp. Biol. Med. *88*:212, 1955.
Lee, R. I., and White, P. D.: A clinical study of the coagulation time of blood. Amer. J. Med. Sci. *145*:495, 1913.
Lewis, J. H., Fresh, J. W., and Ferguson, J. H.: Congenital hypoproconvertinemia. Proc. Soc. Exp. Biol. Med. *84*:651, 1953.
Lewis, J. H., Walters, D., Didisheim, P., and Merchant, W. R.: Application of continuous flow electrophoresis to the study of blood coagulation proteins and the fibrinolytic enzyme system. I. Normal human materials. J. Clin. Invest. *37*: 1323, 1958.
Link, K. P.: Dicumarol and the estimation of prothrombin. *In* Flynn, J. E. (ed.): Blood Clotting and Allied Problems. New York, Josiah Macy Jr. Foundation, 1948.
Loeliger, E. A., Hensen, A., Veltkamp, J. J., Van der Meer, J., and Hemker, H. C.: On the metabolism of factor IX. *In* Brinkhous, K. M. (ed.): The Hemophilias. Chapel Hill, North Carolina, University of North Carolina Press, 1964.
Lorand, L.: Properties and significance of the fibrin-stabilizing factor (FSF). Thromb. Diath. Haemorrh. *7*:238, 1962.
Lorand, L.: Physiological roles of fibrinogen and fibrin. Fed. Proc. *24*:784, 1965.
Lorand, L., and Dickenman, R. C.: Assay method for the "fibrin-stabilizing factor." Proc. Soc. Exp. Biol. Med. *89*: 45, 1955.
Losowsky, M. S., and Hall, R.: Estimation of plasma fibrin-stabilizing factor in families showing congenital deficiencies. Clin. Sci. *30*:171, 1966.
Macfarlane, R. G.: An enzyme cascade in blood clotting mechanism, and its function as a biochemical amplifier. Nature (London) *202*:498, 1964.
Mammen, E. F.: Physiology and biochemistry of blood coagulation. *In* Bang, N. U., Beller, F. K., Deutsch, E., and Mammen, E. F. (eds.): Thrombosis and Bleeding Disorders. New York, Academic Press, Inc., 1971.
Marder, V., and Shulman, N.: Clinical aspects of congenital factor VII deficiency. Amer. J. Med. *37*:182, 1964.
McCain, K. F., Chernoff, A. I., and Graham, J. B.: Establishment of the inheritance of Hageman defect as an autosomal recessive trait. *In* Brinkhous, K. M. (ed.): Hemophilia and Other Hemorrhagic States. Chapel Hill, North Carolina, University of North Carolina Press, 1959.
McKay, D. G.: Disseminated Intravascular Coagulation. New York, Hoeber Division, Harper and Row, 1964.
McKay, D. G., and Müller-Berghaus, G.: Therapeutic implications of disseminated intravascular coagulation. Amer. J. Cardiol. *20*:392, 1967.
McNicol, G. P., and Douglas, A. S.: ϵ-Aminocaproic acid and other inhibitors of fibrinolysis. Brit. Med. Bull. *20*:233, 1964.
Mertz, E. T., and Owen, C. A.: Imidazole buffer: Its use in blood clotting studies. Proc. Soc. Exp. Biol. Med. *43*:204, 1940.
Mills, C. A.: Blood clotting studies in hemophilia. Amer. J. Physiol. *76*:632, 1926.
Nilsson, I. M., Blombäck, M., Jorpes, E., Blombäck, B., and Johansson, S. A.: von Willebrand's disease and its correction with human plasma fraction 1-0. Acta Med. Scand. *159*:179, 1957.
Nye, S. W., Graham, J. B., and Brinkhous, K. M.: The partial thromboplastin time as a screening test for the detection of latent bleeders. Amer. J. Med. Sci. *243*:279, 1962.
Owren, P. A.: Parahemophilia: Hemorrhagic diathesis due to absence of previously unknown clotting factor. Lancet *1*:446, 1947.
Owren, P. A.: Prothrombin and accessory factors. Amer. J. Med. *14*:201, 1953.
Parks, B. J., Brinkhous, K. M., Harris, P. F., and Penick, G. D.: Laboratory detection of female carriers of canine hemophilia. Thromb. Diath. Haemorrh. *12*:368, 1965.
Patek, A. J., Jr., and Taylor, F. H. L.: Hemophilia: Some properties of substance obtained from normal human plasma effective in accelerating coagulation of hemophilic blood. J. Clin. Invest. *16*:113, 1937.
Pavlovsky, A.: Contribution to the pathogenesis of hemophilia. Blood 2:185, 1947.
Pollack, W., Hager, H. J., Reckel, R., Toren, D. A., and Singher, H. D.: A study of the forces involved in the second stage of hemagglutination. Transfusion 5:158, 1965.
Popper, K. R.: Science: Problems, aims, responsibilities. Fed. Proc. 22:961, 1963.
Quick, A. J.: Studies on the enigma of the hemostatic dysfunction of hemophilia. Amer. J. Med. Sci. *214*:272, 1947.
Quick, A. J.: *In* Flynn, J. E. (ed.): Blood Clotting and Allied Problems. New York, Josiah Macy Jr. Foundation, 1951.
Quick, A. J., Stanley-Brown, M., and Bancroft, F. W.: A study

of the coagulation defect in hemophilia and in jaundice. Amer. J. Med. Sci. *190*:501, 1935.

Rapaport, S. I., Proctor, R. R., Patch, M. J., and Yettra, M.: The mode of inheritance of PTA deficiency: Evidence for the existence of major PTA deficiency and minor PTA deficiency. Blood *18*:149, 1961.

Ratnoff, O. D., and Colopy, J. E.: A familial hemorrhagic trait associated with a deficiency of a clot promoting fraction of plasma. J. Clin. Invest. *34*:602, 1955.

Ratnoff, O. D., and Menzie, C.: A new method for the determination of fibrinogen in small samples of plasma. J. Lab. Clin. Med. *37*:316, 1951.

Robbins, K. C.: A study on the conversion of fibrinogen to fibrin. Amer. J. Physiol. *142*:581, 1944.

Roberts, H. R., and Kroncke, F. G., Jr.: Tests of platelet activity: Application to clinical diagnosis. *In* Brinkhous, K. M., and Shermer, R. W. (eds.): The Platelet. Baltimore, The Williams & Wilkins Company, 1971.

Roberts, H. R., Lechler, E., Webster, W. P., and Penick, G. D.: Survival of transfused factor X in patients with Stuart disease. Thromb. Diath. Haemorrh. *13*:305, 1965.

Rodman, N. F., and Mason, R. G.: Platelet-platelet interaction. Relationship to hemostasis and thrombosis. Fed. Proc. *26*:95, 1967.

Rosenthal, R. L.: The present status of plasma thromboplastin antecedent (PTA) deficiency. *In* Brinkhous, K. M. (ed.): Hemophilia and Hemophilioid Diseases. Chapel Hill, North Carolina, University of North Carolina Press, 1957.

Rosenthal, R. L., Dreskin, O. H., and Rosenthal, N.: New hemophilia-like disease caused by a deficiency of a third plasma thromboplastin factor. Proc. Soc. Exp. Biol. Med. *82*:171, 1953.

Schneider, C. L.: Fibrin embolism with defibrination as one of the end results during placenta abruptio. Surg. Gynec. Obstet. *92*:27, 1951.

Schönlein, J. L.: Allgemeine und spezielle Pathologie und Therapie. Vorlesungen niedergeschrieben und herausgegeben von einem seiner Zuhörer. 2. Bd. Würzburg, 1832.

Schulman, I., and Smith, C. H.: Hemorrhagic disease in an infant due to deficiency of a previously undescribed clotting factor. Blood *7*:794, 1952.

Seegers, W. H.: Antithrombin – alpha tocopherol. *In* Flynn, J. E. (ed.): Blood Clotting and Allied Problems. New York, Josiah Macy Jr. Foundation, 1951.

Seegers, W. H.: Prothrombin. Cambridge, Mass., Harvard University Press, 1962.

Sharp, A. A.: Pathological fibrinolysis. Brit. Med. Bull. *20*:240, 1964.

Smith, H. P.: The coagulation of blood: Quantitative viewpoints. *In* Essays in Biology. Berkeley, University of California Press, 1943.

Smith, H. P., Warner, E. D., and Brinkhous, K. M.: Prothrombin deficiency and the bleeding tendency in liver injury. J. Exper. Med. *66*:801, 1937.

Soulier, J. P.: Natural inhibitors. Thromb. Diath. Haemorrh. *7*:38, 1962.

Sprague, C. C., Harrington, W. J., Lange, R. D., and Shapleigh, J. B.: Platelet transfusions and pathogenesis of idiopathic thrombocytopenic purpura. J.A.M.A. *150*:1103, 1952.

Telfer, T. P., Denson, K. W., and Wright, D. R.: A "new" coagulation defect. Brit. J. Haemat. *2*:308, 1956.

Tocantins, L. M., and Kazal, L. A.: Blood Coagulation, Hemorrhage and Thrombosis, Methods of Study. New York, Grune & Stratton, Inc., 1964.

Ulutin, O. N.: The qualitative platelet diseases. *In* Johnson, S. A., *et al.* (eds.): Blood Platelets. Henry Ford Hospital International Symposium. Boston, Little, Brown, and Company, 1960.

von Willebrand, E. A. Hereditär Pseudohämofili. Finsk. Lakaresallsk. Handl. *68*:87, 1926.

Wagner, R. H., and Brinkhous, K. M.: Factor VIII (AHF). Thromb. Diath. Haemorrh. *7*:403, 1961.

Ware, A. G., Guest, M. M., and Seegers, W. H.: Fibrinogen: With special reference to its preparation and certain properties of the product. Arch. Biochem. *13*:231, 1947.

Ware, A. G., Guest, M. M., and Seegers, W. H.: Plasma accelerator factor and purified prothrombin activator. Science *106*:41, 1947.

Ware, A. G., and Seegers, W. H.: Two-stage procedure for the quantitative determination of prothrombin concentration. Amer. J. Clin. Path. *19*:471, 1949.

Warner, E. D., Brinkhous, K. M., and Smith, H. P.: The titration of prothrombin in certain plasmas. Arch. Path. *18*: 587, 1934.

Warner, E. D., Brinkhous, K. M., and Smith, H. P.: Quantitative determination of prothrombin in plasma. Amer. J. Physiol. *114*:667, 1936.

Weaver, R. A., and Langdell, R. D.: Antihemophilic factor (AHF) stability in fresh frozen blood bank plasma. Transfusion *6*:224, 1966.

Weaver, R. A., Price, R. E., and Langdell, R. D.: Antihemophilic factor in cross-circulated normal and hemophilic dogs. Amer. J. Physiol. *206*:335, 1963.

Webster, W. P., Roberts, H. R., and Penick, G. D.: Hemostasis in factor V deficiency. Amer. J. Med. Sci. *248*:194, 1964.

Werder, E.: Kongenitale Afibrinogenamie. Helv. Paediat. Acta *18*:208, 1963.

White, S. G., Aggeler, P. M., and Glendening, M. B.: Plasma thromboplastin component (PTC), a hitherto unrecognized blood coagulation factor. Blood *8*:101, 1953.

Wright, I. S.: The nomenclature of blood clotting factors. J.A.M.A. *180*:733, 1962.

Chapter 7

NUCLEAR MEDICINE PROCEDURES IN THE CLINICAL LABORATORY

by W. NEWLON TAUXE, M.D., and ALAN L. ORVIS, Ph.D.

After the x-ray was discovered by Röntgen in 1895, it was quickly applied by the medical profession to visualization of internal organs. Similarly, when radioactivity was discovered in 1896 by Becquerel and by Pierre and Marie Curie, followed in two years by the isolation of radium, a powerful tool for the irradiation of cancer became available to medicine.

Although some of the radioactive elements were early used to trace biologic pathways, those first available were the naturally occurring radioactive elements, most of which are isotopes of the very heavy elements. Thus, almost none of the common constituents of the body—hydrogen, oxygen, nitrogen, sulfur, phosphorus, iron, iodine, calcium, sodium, and magnesium—were available in a radioactive form.

The real beginning of diagnostic applications of the radionuclides was in 1934, when the daughter of Pierre and Marie Curie, Irène, and her husband, F. Joliot, were able to transmute aluminum into radioactive phosphorus. Quickly, and by a variety of techniques, radioactive isotopes of most of the elements in the periodic table were produced artificially. Many of these have already been used for medical research, but so far only a few have found a place in routine diagnostic procedures.

The diagnostic application of radionuclides began in 1938 with radioiodine, radiosodium, and radiopotassium. Later applications were based on radiophosphorus (1940), radioiron (1942), radioiodinated albumin (1944), and radiocobalt and radiochromium (1950).

Unfortunately no gamma-emitting isotopes of carbon, hydrogen, nitrogen, oxygen, phosphorus, or sulfur are readily available. Although tests involving the use of pure beta emitters is rapidly gaining ground, it is still the gamma emitter that plays the most important role in the average nuclear medicine laboratory today.

RADIONUCLIDE PHYSICS

Some knowledge of the characteristics of radioactive decay and of the interaction of radiation with matter is necessary for the proper selection and use of detection equipment. Furthermore, the choice of radionuclide for a given laboratory procedure depends on the half-life and the kind and energy of the emitted radiation as well as on the availability, chemical form, and cost.

Radioactive Decay. Each radioactive nuclide has unique decay characteristics which are unaffected by chemical form, temperature, pressure, or other environmental factors. Half-life is defined as the time required for disintegration of half of the radioactive nuclei initially present. Therefore, the amount of radioactivity present decreases by a factor of two for every half-life period that elapses. For example, technetium-99m has a half-life of 6 hours; therefore, with 16 mCi. (millicuries) initially, there will be 8 mCi. remaining at 6 hours, 4 mCi. at 12 hours, 2 mCi. at 18 hours, and 1 mCi. at 24 hours after the original time. The basic unit of radioactivity is the Curie (Ci), originally defined as the disintegration rate of 1 gm. radium (3.7×10^{10} disintegrations per second). It was later defined simply as 3.7×10^{10} disintegrations per second, without regard to radium. The millicurie (mCi) (10^{-3}Ci.) produces 3.7×10^{7} dps, and the microcurie (μCi. or 10^{-6} Ci.) 3.7×10^{4} dps.

Radioactive nuclei decay by emitting alpha particles (heavy particles with two units of positive charge), beta particles (single electrons, positively or negatively charged), or gamma rays (high-energy electromagnetic radiation) or by electron capture (capture of an orbital electron by the nucleus), or combinations of these modes. The energy of the emitted particles (or rays) and the combinations of emissions (e.g., negative beta followed by single gamma) are diagramed as plots against the atomic number of the atom to give the "decay scheme" of a given radionuclide, and each radionuclide has a unique decay scheme.

For example, carbon-14 decays by emission of a single beta particle, the daughter product being stable nitrogen:

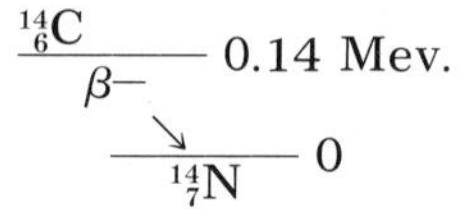

The maximal beta energy is 0.14 million electron volts (Mev.). Every disintegration of a carbon nucleus produces a beta particle. The decay of cobalt-60 is more complex:

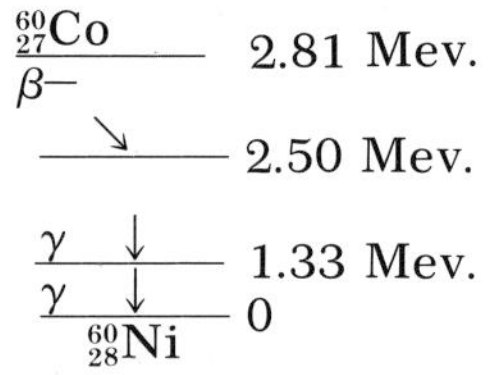

Each disintegration produces one beta particle followed in rapid succession by two emissions of gamma rays.

Chromium-51 decays by electron capture, with alternate possibilities: 91 per cent of the time, simple electron capture occurs with no measurable particle emission (other than a vanadium x-ray), but 9 per cent of the time a 0.32-Mev. gamma radiation results.

Sometimes the gamma ray in a decay sequence is not emitted immediately after the disintegration of the parent nuclide but is delayed a measurable amount of time. This is called an isomeric state of the daughter and is denoted by adding the letter *m* to the mass number of the nuclide. Thus, technetium-99m decays by delayed gamma emission, and the decay scheme includes the parent, molybdenum-99:

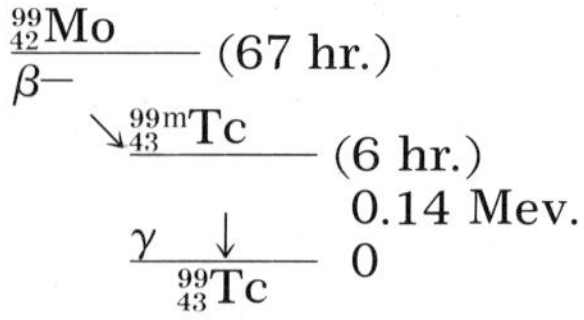

The relatively short half-life of ^{99m}Tc, the gamma ray of optimal energy for counting, the absence of a ^{99m}Tc beta particle, and the ease of chemical separation of technetium from the parent molybdenum combine to make ^{99m}Tc an ideal nuclide for many clinical applications.

Radionuclides with short half-lives are especially advantageous in the diagnostic laboratory for short-term studies because the reduced radiation exposure to the patient permits use of more millicuries, and studies may be repeated with less interference from previous procedures. Half-lives of less than 12 hours have formerly been impractical because of the decay during transportation from supplier to consumer. However, development of so-called generators has made available a number of radionuclides of fairly short half-life (Table 7–1). The short-lived materials are generated by longer lived radioactive parents, one example being ^{99}Mo (67 hr.)→^{99m}Tc (6 hr.). The daughter nuclide produced by the decay of the parent is chemically separated as needed. The shelf life corresponds to the life of the parent, but once the daughter nuclide is separated and put into use, the decay is characterized by the half-life of the daughter. Figure 7–1 shows an example of the build-up of ^{99m}Tc in

Table 7–1. RADIOISOTOPE GENERATORS

^{68}Ge (270 days)	⟶	^{68}Ga (68 min.)
^{87}Y (80 hr.)	⟶	^{87m}Sr (2.8 hr.)
^{90}Sr (28 yr.)	⟶	^{90}Y (64.2 hr.)
^{99}Mo (67 hr.)	⟶	^{99m}Tc (6 hr.)
^{132}Te (77 hr.)	⟶	^{132}I (2.3 hr.)
^{137}Cs (30 yr.)	⟶	^{137m}Ba (2.6 min.)

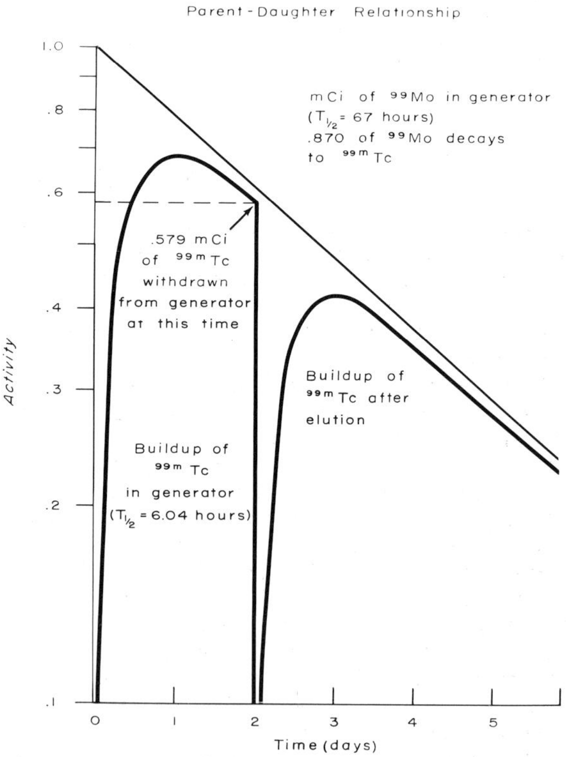

Figure 7–1. Parent-daughter relationship. Buildup of ^{99m}Tc (daughter) in solution with ^{99}Mo generator (parent) after separations at t = 0 and t = 2 days.

Table 7–2. DECAY CHARACTERISTICS OF RADIONUCLIDES

ISOTOPE	HALF-LIFE	DECAY MODE*	ENERGY (MEV.)†
Calcium-47	4.54 days	$\beta-$, γ	$\beta-$: 1.98 (18%), 0.67 (82%) γ : 1.31 (74%), others, daughter radiations from Scandium-47
Chromium-51	27.8 days	EC, γ	γ : V x-rays, 0.32 (9%), c.e.
Iron-59	45.6 days	$\beta-$, γ	$\beta-$: 0.46 (54%), 0.27 (46%) γ : 1.29 (43%), 1.10 (57%), others
Cobalt-57	271.3 days	EC, γ	γ : Fe x-rays, 0.122 (87%), 0.136 (11%), others, c.e.
Cobalt-60	5.26 years	$\beta-$, γ	$\beta-$: 0.31 γ : 1.33 (100%), 1.17 (100%)
Copper-64	12.8 hours	$\beta-$, $\beta+$, EC, γ	$\beta-$: 0.57 (39%), c.e. $\beta+$: 0.65 (19%) γ : Ni x-rays, 0.511 (38%, $\gamma\pm$), others
Copper-67	58.5 hours	$\beta-$, γ	$\beta-$: 0.39 (45%), others, c.e. γ : Zn x-rays, 0.092 (23% , 0.184 (40%)
Gallium-67	77.9 hours	EC, γ	γ : Zn x-rays, 0.093 (40%), 0.184 (24%), 0.296 (22%), 0.388 (7%), c.e.
Strontium-85	64 days	EC, γ	γ : Rb x-rays, 0.514 (100%), c.e.
Strontium-87m	2.83 hours	IT	γ : Sr x-rays, 0.388 (80%), c.e.
Technetium-99m	6.0 hours	IT	γ : Tc x-rays, 0.140 (90%), c.e.
Iodine-123	13.3 hours	EC, γ	γ : Te x-rays, 0.159 (83%), c.e.
Iodine-125	60 days	EC, γ	γ : Te x-rays, 0.035 (7%), c.e.
Iodine-131	8.05 days	$\beta-$, γ	$\beta-$: 0.61 (87%), 0.34 (9%), others γ : 0.64 (7%), 0.36 (82%), others
Xenon-133	5.27 days	$\beta-$, γ	$\beta-$: 0.35 (99%), c.e. γ : Cs x-rays, 0.081 (37%)

*EC = electron capture; IT = internal transition
†c.e. = conversion electrons

solution with ^{99}Mo after separations at t=0 and two days.

Table 7-2 lists decay characteristics of some of the more commonly used radionuclides.

Absorption of Radiation. Alpha and beta particles are electrically charged, and therefore they interact directly with the orbital electrons in all matter, continually losing their energy a little bit at a time in a series of many collisions. Particles with higher energy will travel farther than those with lower energy, and the maximal possible penetration at a given energy is called the range. Alpha particles are relatively massive and are readily stopped in tissue—for example, 5-Mev. alpha particles are completely stopped by less than 0.01 mm. of tissue.

Beta particles are considerably lighter than alpha particles and have half the electric charge, so the beta particles are not so readily absorbed. Table 7-3 lists the ranges in water of the radiations of some of the widely used beta emitters.

Gamma rays have no mass or electric charge and are able to lose energy only by chance collisions with single electrons in the material which they traverse. These energized electrons, in turn, cause the ionization which allows the gamma radiation to be detected and which can lead to radiation effects if living tissue is being irradiated. The probability of gamma absorption increases very rapidly with the atomic number of the absorber; hence, lead, with a high atomic number, stops gamma rays much more readily than does water. However, for any absorbing material, the likelihood of absorption decreases for higher energies, up to several million electron volts.

Table 7–3. RANGE OF BETA RADIATION FROM VARIOUS SOURCES

ISOTOPE	$E_{MAX.}$ (MEV.)	RANGE (MM. H_2O)
^{3}H	0.018	0.05
^{14}C	0.14	0.22
^{36}Cl	0.71	2.60
^{131}I	0.81	3.20
^{32}P	1.70	7.80
^{90}Sr-^{90}Y	2.18	10.50

Radioactive decay and gamma ray attenuation are both random processes and, mathematically, obey the so-called exponential law. Just as half-life was defined as the time required for half of the nuclei to decay, "half-value layer" (HVL) is defined as being that thickness of absorbing material necessary to reduce a beam of gamma rays to one-half its incident intensity. Table 7-4 gives half-value layer values for different energies of gamma radiation. For example, with ^{51}Cr shielded by aluminum, 2.5 cm. of aluminum will absorb 50 per cent of the 0.32 Mev. gamma radiation; therefore, 5 cm. will absorb 75 per cent, 7.5 cm. will absorb 87.5 per cent, 10 cm. will absorb 94.4 per cent, and so forth. A few gamma rays will penetrate very great thicknesses of material.

Counting Systems. The counting system consists of three components: (1) a radiation detector which converts the kinetic energy of the radiation into electrical impulses, (2) various electrical components which amplify the pulses and sort them according to their amplitudes, and (3) data-processing devices. Proper matching and selection of the elements of the counting system is important. The detectors must be selected for optimal response characteristics to count the given kind of radiation in the given circumstance. Detector design has become very specialized. Likewise, the electrical components must be matched to the detector output and to themselves with respect to pulse shape, pulse polarity, and repetition rate. Components of one manufacturer frequently are not interchangeable with those of another. The user must ascertain compatibility in each instance.

Detectors. The most important element of the counting system is the detector. There are three main types of detectors, categorized according to the principle involved in the conversion of radiation energy to electrical pulse. These are the Geiger counters, scintillation detectors, and solid-state detectors.

Table 7–4. HALF-VALUE LAYERS FOR GAMMA RADIATION

NUCLIDE	ENERGY (MEV.)	HALF-VALUE LAYER (CM.) WATER	ALUMINUM	LEAD
^{125}I	0.035	2.31	0.39	0.0087
^{99m}Tc	0.140	4.6	1.7	0.027
^{51}Cr	0.32	5.9	2.5	0.16
^{131}I	0.364 (82%) 0.723 (Max.)	6.2 8.4	2.7 3.6	0.22 0.61
^{87m}Sr	0.388	6.4	2.7	0.25
^{60}Co	1.17, 1.33	10.5	4.5	0.90

Historically, Geiger-Müller counters were the first to be used in the clinical nuclear medicine laboratory and were widely used for many years. Their use is now restricted to laboratory monitors, survey meters, and a few special beta counters. Most Geiger counters consist of a cylindric conducting shell (the cathode) and an axial wire at high electric potential (the anode), both in an atmosphere of a noble gas (helium or argon) and a small amount of a halogen impurity. The ionization produced in the gas by each incident particle of radiation initiates a gas discharge, and the resultant electrical pulse may be counted by a scaler, or the rate at which these pulses are occurring may be electrically calculated by a rate meter. Geiger counters are inexpensive, do not require elaborate electric circuitry, and are very efficient for routine beta counting. They are no longer widely used for gamma counting, however, because of their intrinsically low efficiency for detection of gamma radiation. Geiger counters may be constructed with a thin window of Mylar or mica at one end to allow entrance into the counting gas of beta particles with energies greater than 0.05 Mev. Such a device is called an "end-window Geiger counter" or a "thin-window β counter." Geiger probes may also be very small (and fragile), with the cathode very thin, in order to allow the entrance of beta particles from the side. Wall thickness requirements restrict the use of these needle probes (or tissue probes) to the counting of moderate or high-energy beta particles. The presence of material of high atomic number in the wall (bismuth wall counter) allows for enhanced gamma counting efficiency.

Scintillation counters are now the most universally used detectors in the clinical nuclear medicine laboratory. Figure 7–2 is a sketch of a scintillation detector and shows the two principal components, the scintillator (crystal) and the photomultiplier tube. Some of the gamma photons which strike the scintillator collide with electrons in the crystal, transferring some or all of their energy to the electron. This energy is, in turn, transformed into a scintillation, a very weak and fast flash of light. The intensity of the flash is proportional to the amount of energy lost by the gamma photon. The light travels through the scintillator to the photomultiplier tube, where it is converted into photoelectrons in the photosensitive layer (photocathode).

An external high-voltage supply is connected to the dynodes of the photomultiplier and causes the electrons to be accelerated and multiplied when they strike successive dynodes. The overall multiplication factor can be as large as a million, and the amplitude of the electric pulse coming from the phototube

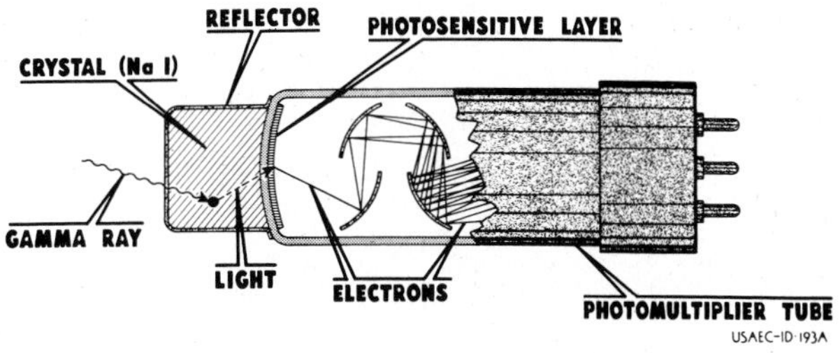

Figure 7-2. Scintillation detector. (Courtesy of U.S. Atomic Energy Commission.)

is proportional to the energy lost by the gamma photon in the scintillator. Therefore, a scintillation counter can be used to identify radionuclides by measuring the energy of their gamma emissions, as well as to count the number of gamma photons present.

Two classes of scintillators are available for gamma detection. Sodium iodide crystals activated with a trace of thallium [NaI (Tl)] are the most commonly used of the inorganic class. Organic scintillators may be of anthracene, an activated polyvinyltoluene plastic material, or any of a group of scintillating liquids.

NaI (Tl) crystals are the best general-purpose gamma detectors, principally because the atomic number of iodine is high enough to provide efficient photoelectric absorption and also because absorption of a given amount of energy results in the emission of a brighter flash of light than in other detectors.

Organic scintillators are much less expensive than NaI (Tl) and may be constructed in a greater variety of forms and shapes. Therefore, large-volume detectors, such as 2π and 4π whole-body counters, are made of organic detectors, despite the lesser gamma efficiency per unit volume than the highly expensive NaI (Tl) crystals would provide. However, low atomic number is a real disadvantage for general clinical gamma ray detection.

Liquid scintillators are often used to count low-energy beta emissions because the radioactive material to be assayed may be mixed directly with the scintillator for maximal counting efficiency.

The response of a scintillation counter to a given flux of gamma radiation may be characterized by the spectrum of the energies of the rays. Figure 7-3 shows the spectra of two different nuclides measured with an NaI (Tl) crystal. These are called differential spectra because the counting rate in a small increment of the energy range is plotted against the energy (which is proportional to the intensity of the light flash in the crystal). Spectra from nuclides emitting gamma rays of different energies are shown for comparison. The lower energy gamma rays from ^{137}Cs have a greater relative probability of being photoelectrically absorbed, so the total absorption region is larger with respect to the Compton region for ^{137}Cs gamma rays than it is for the ^{60}Co gamma rays. Differences in the spectra of different nuclides are exploited when mixtures of radionuclides are to be measured, as will be described later in this chapter.

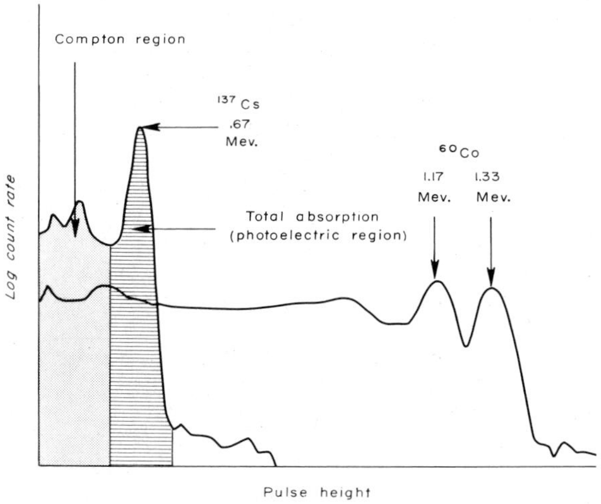

Figure 7-3. Differential spectra of gamma ray energies of ^{137}Cs and ^{60}Co, measured with a NaI (Tl) crystal.

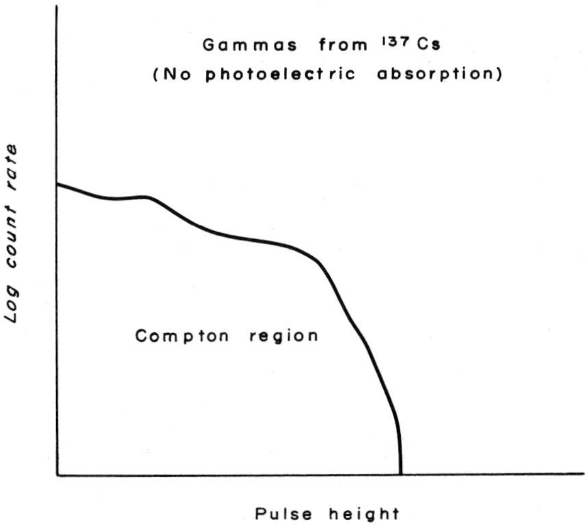

Figure 7-4. Differential spectrum of gamma ray energies of ^{137}Cs, measured with an organic scintillator (plastic, 4 by 4 inches).

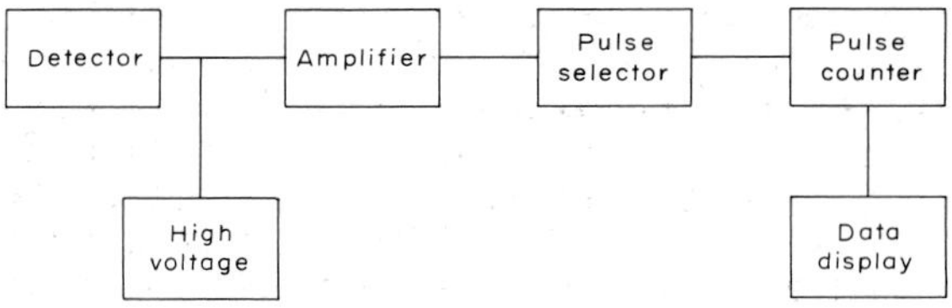

Figure 7–5. Electrical components of a counting system.

Figure 7–4 illustrates the spectrum obtained when 0.66-Mev. gamma rays from ^{137}Cs are counted with an organic scintillator. The Compton region is similar to that obtained with NaI (Tl), but there is virtually no photoelectric region because of the low atomic numbers in the organic material.

Another type of radiation detector that has recently been found to be useful is the solid-state detector. These transistor-like devices may be made small enough to form the tip of a catheter. They are beta sensitive and require only two lead wires to carry the signal and the applied voltage (5 to 100 volts).

Electrical Components. The principal elements of a counting system are shown in Figure 7-5. Each element is a special-function electronic device. The high-voltage supply provides a direct-current potential to the detector and must be particularly stable and ripple-free for scintillation counters. The amplifier must also provide a stable and drift-free gain because fluctuations in either the voltage applied to the detectors or the amplifier gain will cause changes in the pulse spectrum which enters the pulse selector, and the calibration (linearity) of the system will be affected. Figure 7-6 illustrates these effects. Increasing either the high-voltage supply to the detector or the gain of the amplifier causes the height of the output pulses to be increased, so that the spectrum will be stretched further along the abscissa but will retain the same general shape.

The pulse selector rejects unwanted pulses and passes the others to the counting device. Pulse selectors may be either integral or differential. Integral selectors (discrimination) reject pulses the amplitudes of which are less than the selected threshold value and allow all larger pulses to be counted. Figure 7-7 shows the portion of a spectrum that would be counted with the discriminator level as shown.

A differential selector (pulse-height analyzer) accepts only those pulses the amplitudes of which fall within a range of values, a "window." Those with amplitudes greater than the upper level in Figure 7-7 as well as those with amplitudes less than the lower level will be rejected. Pulse-height analyzers have two control knobs. One controls the lower level (base line). The other knob may select the upper level independently of the base line or may instead control the window width directly.

The pulse counter can be either a scaler or a rate meter. Scalers are generally fast, electronic decade registers and count the number of pulses arriving from the pulse selector in a measured interval of time. Rate meters, as the name implies, measure the rate at which pulses are received. There are two types of rate meters, digital and analog. In essence, digital rate meters are automatic recycling scalers: they count for a fixed period, report the information in units of rate, reset themselves, and repeat the process. Some digital rate meters concurrently accumulate counts in the scaler section while reporting out the information from the previous count which had been stored in a memory module.

Analog rate meters convert each input pulse into a fixed amount of electric charge which is stored in a capacitor. At equilibrium the leakage of current from the capacitor equals

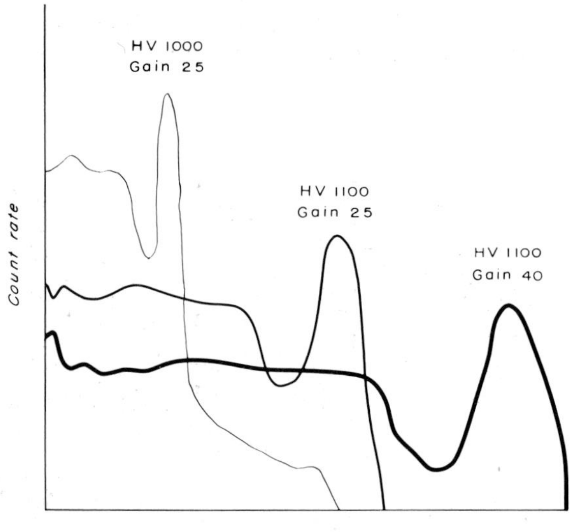

Figure 7–6. Effect of changes in high voltage or amplifier gain on response of counting system [NaI(Tl) detector].

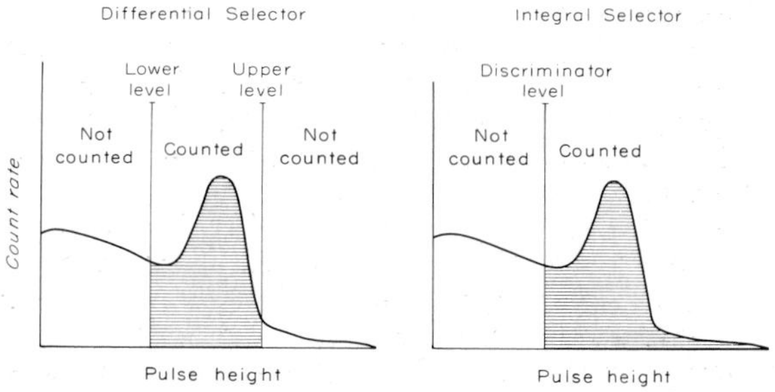

Figure 7–7. Effect of differential and integral selectors on count rate.

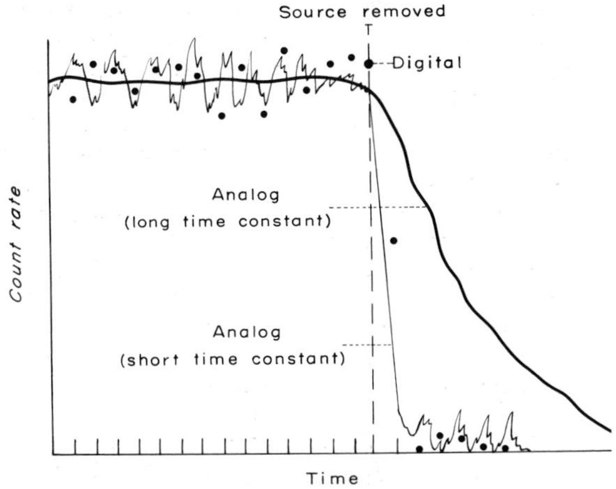

Figure 7–8. Response of rate meters to rapid withdrawal of a radioactive source. Digital rate meter (solid circles) reached base line almost instantly. When analog rate meter was set for rapid response (short time constant – thin line), large fluctuations in count rate occurred. When fluctuations were damped (longer time constant – heavy line), response was tardy.

the rate of storage of charge, and the voltage across the capacitor is proportional to the count rate, so that the device may be calibrated in units of count rate. The amount of time required to reach equilibrium, however, depends on the count rate and on the electric components in the circuit (the "R-C time constant"), so that if the count rates are changing the meter readings will lag and in some cases will give a distorted picture of the dynamic process being measured. This is the principal disadvantage of the analog rate meter, although time-constant corrections can be made. In any case, equilibrium should be established before the readings are taken. Most analog rate meters offer a choice of time constants, and the meter reading is linearly related to the input pulse rate. However, the circuits may be modified to provide an output that may be calibrated as the logarithm of the count rate. The statistical accuracy is the same at all rates, and therefore the time constant is a function of rate. One commercially available logarithmic rate meter has an effective time constant that goes from 15 seconds at 10^3 counts per minute (c.p.m.) to 0.15 second at 10^6 c.p.m.

Figure 7-8 compares the response of rate meters when a fixed source of radioactivity is being measured and is then rapidly removed. The digital rate meter requires only one time interval to reach the base line. The analog unit with the fast time constants also shows a rapid response, but data in the steady state show the large statistical fluctuations that result from the relatively few counts received, on the average, in 0.2 second. The longer time constant averages out the statistical fluctuations but distorts the dynamic characteristic of the curve.

Data display for a scaler or for a digital rate meter may consist simply of a visual indication of the total counts or may take the form of an automatic digital print-out. Paper tape punching may also be used if subsequent digital computer processing of the data is desired. Analog rate meters provide visual display of the rate and also supply a signal for conventional strip-chart recorders.

Collimators. A device that shields the detector from extraneous radiation (background) and restricts the detector's field to the organ being measured is called a "collimator." Although there are many designs, collimators can be categorized in one of four ways, flatfield or focusing, diverging or pinhole. The latter are used principally on scintillation cameras (Fig. 7–9). Flatfield collimators are used when the gross activity in a whole organ or region of the body is to be measured – for example, thyroid uptake. The collimator consists of an annulus, usually of lead or steel, surrounding the detector and part of the photomultiplier. The objective of its design is to make the detector as nearly as possible equally sensitive to radiation emanating throughout the volume of the organ and, at the same time, to prevent radiation that originates in other parts of the body from reaching the detector.

Focusing collimators are designed for sensitivity in a very limited region (Fig. 7-9) and are used with scanning devices to map the distribution of radioactivity in a region of the body. An insert of dense material containing a number of holes is placed before the detector in the annulus. The line of sight of the holes converges at some point along the axis of the collimator, perhaps 4 or 5 inches from the front of the device. The insert must be designed for the energy of radiation as well as for the depth of focus because high-energy radiations require greater thickness and maximal atomic number of absorber if good resolution is to be

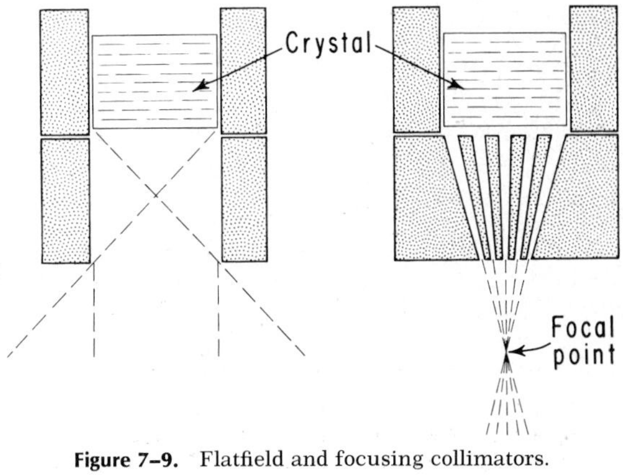

Figure 7–9. Flatfield and focusing collimators.

obtained. Inserts made of gold or tungsten have been built, but most are of lead because of the cost factor.

Imaging Detectors. The classic scanner provides a mechanism for moving the detector and focusing collimator back and forth over the region being mapped while recording the information from the pulse counter in a two-dimensional display of radioactivity contours. The resultant map provides a means of visualizing the shape of an organ or the variations of distribution of radioactivity within the organ. This information is not available by conventional roentgenographic techniques and thereby constitutes a major contribution of radionuclides to diagnostic medicine.

The scanner carriage transports the detector once across the organ laterally, advances it a short distance longitudinally, brings it back across the organ, advances it again, and so forth, producing a rectangular grid coverage of the region being scanned. The speed of the lateral motion of the detector (the scan speed) is one of the variables that must be adjusted for optimal visualization. Scan speed is usually set to be directly proportional to the amount of radioactivity in the organ.

The display of scintigraphic scan data may make use of one or more of a number of techniques. The classic and still widely used format is the so-called dot scan. A stylus, coupled to the motion of the detector, tracks over a piece of pressure-sensitive or current-sensitive paper. Pulses from the scaler activate the stylus, producing dots. The dot density on the paper is then proportional to the count rate at any given locus. The ratio of the number of pulses at the input of the scaler to the number of dots which are produced is called the scaling factor or dot factor. This factor may be adjusted to compensate for radionuclide concentration levels. With larger dot factors, more counts from the detector are necessary to produce a dot; thus, the statistical uncertainty associated with the spacing of the dots is less and contours are easier to discern.

In photorecording systems, a source of light is coupled to the motion of the detector and moves over a film. The light intensity is modulated by the output of the rate meter on the scaler, so that regions of maximal exposure correspond to maximal radionuclide concentration. Contrast with this system is superior to that of non-color-coded dot scans because of the nonlinear response characteristics of photographic film. By adjusting the light intensity to conform to film characteristics, the background exposure can be eliminated.

In some cases, type ribbons of various colors have been utilized in which a specific color is used to depict a certain counting rate interval.

Color scintigrams essentially combine the features of dot scans and photographic scans. Dots of different colors are produced, the color being controlled by a rate meter and the frequency of dots, by a scaler.

The pulse selector is an important part of any scintigraphic apparatus because radiation scattered into the detector after being emitted from activity outside the field of view of the detector will cause blurring of the image. The energy loss due to the scattering process allows this radiation to be rejected by proper adjustment of the pulse selector.

Different techniques are available for background subtraction. Except in special circumstances (such as the evaluation of "cold" nodules), this level should not be set so high that the peripheral parts of the active regions are eliminated. In fact, unless there is some specific reason for utilizing it, background subtraction in routine clinical use is to be avoided.

Radionuclide imaging is, in a sense, a procedure in which the interrelationships of scan speed, dot factor, contrast, background subtraction, total activity in the organ, organ depth, collimator characteristics, half-life, and redistribution within the body must always be considered, and compromises must be accepted.

At this writing, scintigraphic techniques are in a rapidly expanding phase. Particularly great strides are being made in several areas: (1) Special radiopharmaceuticals are being developed. (2) Larger crystals with special collimators are being used to increase efficiency and reduce imaging time. (3) Data display systems in which television or computer techniques or both are used are making more efficient use of the fundamental information content of the scan. (4) Stationary scintigraphic equipment (scintillation cameras) is available. These devices, using a large, flat crystal or a mosaic of crystals, function somewhat like a camera and view all the region being imaged at once; there is no mechanical motion of the detector and, thus, a cinema-like visualization of the changing distribution of radioactivity within an organ is possible.

The most widely used stationary scintigraphic apparatus, the scintillation (or Anger) camera, uses a sodium iodide crystal of large diameter (typically $11\frac{1}{2}''$ OD $\times$ $\frac{1}{2}''$ thick) which is viewed by an array of photomultiplier tubes (Fig. 7–10). Output from the phototubes goes to an electrical circuit which senses the location of the scintillation in the crystal, since each tube will receive a different fraction of the light produced, depending upon its distance from the original scintillation. The signal then goes to an image-readout device such as a storage oscilloscope, where the scintillation is recorded as a spot on the oscilloscope screen, with the location of the spot corresponding to the position of the generating scintillation in

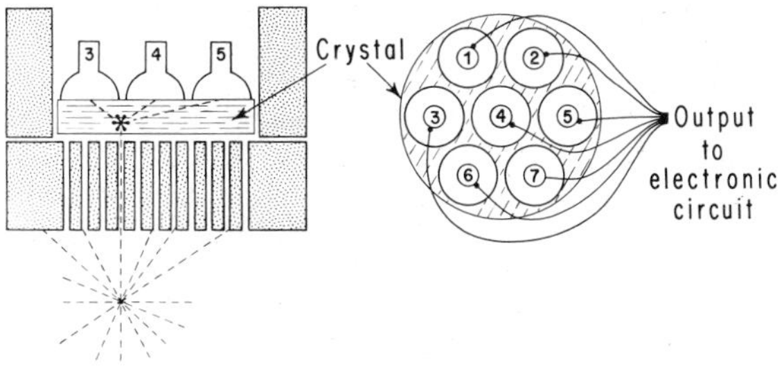

Figure 7–10. Diagram of mechanism of scintillation camera. A parallel hole collimator is attached.

the crystal. Various computer and other techniques may be employed to enhance the image, and rapid sequencing of images is possible for studies of dynamic function.

A special collimator, usually consisting of a large number of parallel holes (Fig. 7–10) but sometimes of a pinhole or of a divergent type (Fig. 7–11), preserves the spatial relationship between the distribution of radioactivity in the object and the area density of scintillations in the crystal.

(5) Positron imaging exploits the directional relationship between the 0.51-Mev. annihilation quanta resulting from positron-producing radionuclides, and the increasing availability of suitable radiopharmaceuticals is contributing to increased interest in this technique.

Measurement. The data provided by the counting system require correction for background and radioactive decay. Interpretation of these corrected data involves a consideration of counting statistics. Count rates can be converted into units of radioactivity, or per cent of dose, in an organ only if the counter is accurately calibrated.

Background Activity. Counts may be registered by a radiation detecting system even if no known source of radioactivity is present. Background activity is produced by cosmic rays, by natural radioactivity in the air, and by radioactivity in the soil and common building materials. Radioactivity from regions of the body other than the organ being measured may penetrate the collimator and produce background counts. Indeed, if the patient has received tracers previously, the residual activity in the organ should be considered as background relative to measurement of the most recent tracer dose. Extraneous background count rates may be measured when no patient is present and then subtracted from the count rate over the patient. Background due to collimator penetration may be evaluated by taking a count with the organ shielded. Residual background activity in that organ must be measured before administration of the study dose.

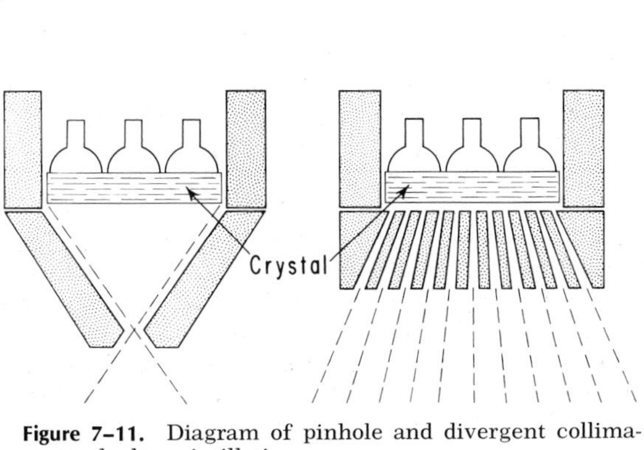

Figure 7–11. Diagram of pinhole and divergent collimators attached to scintillation cameras.

Statistics. Replicate measurements of the same radioactive source will yield a group of different numbers. The spread of the values obtained will depend only on the number of counts obtained in each counting time interval and on the number of times the measurement is repeated. If n_i equals the number of counts recorded in a single measurement and $\bar{n}$ is the mean of all the measurements, then the standard deviation of a single measurement is equal to $\sqrt{\bar{n}}$. That is to say, approximately two-thirds of the values of n_i will fall within the range defined by $\bar{n} \pm \sqrt{\bar{n}}$. For example, if a series of observations has 1600 counts as its mean value, then the standard deviation is $\sqrt{1600} = 40$ and two-thirds of the individual measurements would be expected to fall within the range defined by 1600 ± 40, or 1560 to 1640. The per cent standard deviation would be $\frac{100\sqrt{\bar{n}}}{\bar{n}}$ or, in the example given, $\frac{4000}{1600} = 2.5$ per cent. The error is numerically larger if $\bar{n}$ is a larger number, but the percentage deviation is smaller. For instance, if $\bar{n} = 160{,}000$, $\sqrt{\bar{n}} = 400$ but the deviation $= 0.25$ per cent.

If n_i counts are obtained in a measured time (t), then the count rate $r_i = \frac{n_i}{t}$. It can be shown that the standard deviation of the rate is $\sqrt{\frac{r}{t}}$. If, in our example, the counting time were 16 seconds, then $r = \frac{1600}{16} = 100$ c.p.s. (counts per second) and the standard deviation of the rate would be $\sqrt{\frac{100}{16}} = 2.5$ c.p.s., which is also 2.5 per cent of the rate (100 c.p.s.). We can see from this that counting for a longer period of time will reduce the error of measurement. A rate of 100 c.p.s. measured over a period of 1600 seconds will have a standard deviation of only 0.25 c.p.s. or 0.25 per cent.

However, the organ count rate must be calculated and the background count rate must be subtracted if conversion to microcuries or percentage of dose is desired. The cumulative errors should then be calculated by using statistically developed techniques for the propagation of errors. Suppose that the organ is counted for a time t_o, and the count rate is r_o. Background for time t_b is r_b. Then, the net count rate r_n is $r_o - r_b$. The standard deviation of r_n is then given by the expression $\sqrt{\frac{r_o}{t_o} + \frac{r_b}{t_b}}$. For example, an organ is counted for $t_o = 300$ seconds and the rate $r_o = 60$ c.p.s. Background, measured for 1000 seconds, is 20 c.p.s. The net rate will be $60 - 20 = 40$ c.p.s., and the standard deviation of this measurement will be $\sqrt{\frac{60}{300} + \frac{20}{1000}} = \sqrt{.22} = 0.47$ c.p.s. The result could then be expressed as 40 ± 0.47 c.p.s. or 40 c.p.s. $\pm$ 1.2 per cent.

Decay Correction. Radioactive decay may be expressed mathematically as an exponential function of time. If A is the activity remaining at time t and A_0 is the initial activity, then $A = A_0e^{-\lambda t}$, where λ is the decay constant for the particular radionuclide, an expression for the rate of decay. λ is related to the half-life, $\lambda = \frac{0.693}{t_{1/2}}$. The fraction remaining at time t may be written $A/A_0 = e^{-\lambda t}$. Values for A/A_0 as a function of t are given in decay tables for most of the clinical radionuclides. The quantity A is obtained from measurement over an area of the body or *in vitro* and must be corrected to A_0 by dividing it by the tabulated value of $e^{-\lambda t}$. For example, let us take a nuclide with a half-life of eight days, ^{131}I. A decay table would show that 16 days after $t = 0$, the decay fraction (A/A_0) is 0.25. Therefore, if 5 μCi. of ^{131}I is measured in a thyroid 16 days after administration of a dose of 50 μCi., the thyroid content corrected to the time of administration of the dose will be $\frac{5}{0.25} = 20$ μCi., and the uptake is $\frac{20}{50} \times 100 = 40$ per cent of the dose.

Calibration. Radiation emanating from a point source is dispersed according to the inverse square law. Therefore, the count rate measured by a detection system will decrease according to the square of the distance between source and detector, even though the source radioactivity remains constant. This is another way of saying that the calibration of the counter depends on the distance between source and detector. The calibration factor is the number by which count rate is multiplied to determine the actual radioactivity. Thus, if a small source containing 1 μCi. produces 50 c.p.s. at 20 cm. from a detector, $50 \times \left(\frac{20}{40}\right)^2 =$ 12.5 c.p.s., which will be measured at a distance of 40 cm. The calibration factor at 20 cm. would be 1/50 μCi./c.p.s. and at 40 cm. would be 1/12.5 μCi./c.p.s. However, organs measured *in vivo* are not point sources, so the effect of distance on counter calibration is not a simple function. Therefore, calibration of a counter for *in vivo* determinations usually requires that a model or phantom of the organ containing a known amount of radioactivity be constructed. This phantom should be measured under conditions which closely simulate the *in vivo* circumstances, since factors other than geometry also affect the calibration.

Two of these factors are scatter and self-absorption and are sketched in Figure 7–12. Radiation not originally directed toward the counter may be Compton-scattered in that direction by the tissues surrounding the organ. Therefore, count rate from an organ surrounded by tissue may be higher than if the organ were in air. The Compton effect decreases the energy of the scattered radiation, so that the influence of scattering on the calibration may be minimized by setting the pulse selector to exclude rays of lower energies. Another method sometimes used to eliminate scatter is placement of a thin filter of lead in front of the detector (the low-energy rays are much more efficiently absorbed by the lead than are the rays of higher energies).

Some of the radiation which is initially directed toward the detector never reaches it because some is absorbed by intervening tissues and some is scattered away from the detector. Correction for these artefacts may only be approximated by proper choice of an

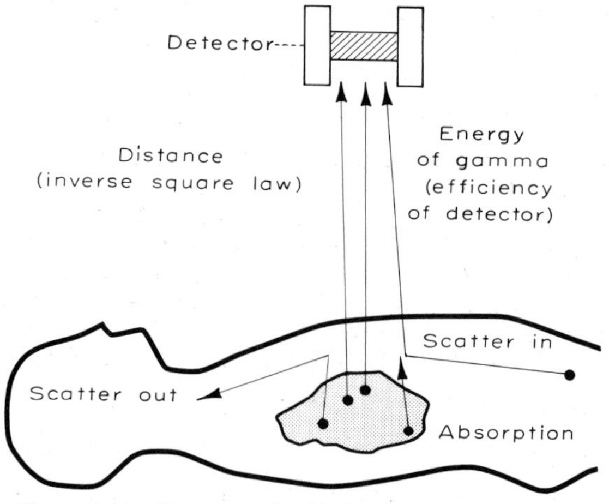

Figure 7–12. Scatter and self-absorption of gamma rays by passage through tissue and other factors affecting *in vivo* calibration.

organ-simulating phantom. This amounts to only a few per cent for counting ^{131}I in the thyroid, but it can be a factor that limits the usefulness of a nuclide whose gamma ray energy is low. ^{125}I has very restricted *in vivo* applications because self-absorption of its 0.035-Mev. gamma ray is critically dependent on the size of the patient and the location of the organ in the body, making calibration very uncertain.

The calibration of a counter with one nuclide is not necessarily applicable to measurement of a different radionuclide, because detector efficiency, scatter, and self-absorption all are critically dependent on gamma ray energy. For example, the c.p.s./μCi. for ^{51}Cr will be radically different from that of ^{24}Na in almost any counting system.

In vitro measurements of radionuclides also require consideration of the calibration factors discussed above, but the duplication of experimental conditions may usually be accomplished quite simply. Caution should be exercised, however. As an example, the volume (height) of material in the test tube to be counted will affect the sensitivity of the well-type scintillation counter and should be considered in the calibration.

Mathematical Concepts. Interpretation of the data may usually be accomplished after the application of standard mathematical procedures. Fractional uptake may be calculated by simply taking the ratio of net count (corrected for physical decay) to the dose administered (the dose should also be expressed in the appropriate units of count rate). Multiplication by 100 converts to percentage uptake.

Studies which assay the dilution of a radioactive tracer, such as measurements of blood volume and erythrocyte volume, and dynamic clinical studies, such as the renogram, require special consideration of the assumptions on which the mathematical analysis is based.

Radionuclide Dilution. Let the specific activity of the administered tracer be given as $S_0 = \frac{A_0}{M_0}$, in which A_0 is the amount of radioactivity and M_0 is the mass of labeled substance. The mass of the corresponding unlabeled material (mother substance) in the body is M, and this is the quantity to be measured. After administration of the tracer, the total mass will be $M_0 + M$, but the activity remains A_0 because the mother substance has no radioactivity. Therefore, the specific activity (S) after complete mixing will be given by $S = \frac{A_0}{M_0 + M}$; therefore, $M = M_0\left(\frac{S_0}{S} - 1\right)$. Thus, the mass of mother substance (M) can be measured if the specific activity (S) can be determined. M_0 is frequently quite small compared with M, and the previous expression is then simply $M = \frac{A_0}{S}$.

Several conditions must obtain if the results of radionuclide dilution studies are to be valid. First, the tracer must be in equilibrium with the mother substance at the time of sampling. Second, excretion of tracer (A_e) during the period of equilibration must be taken into account (that amount is subtracted from A_0, so that $M = \frac{A_0 - A_e}{S}$. Third, the purity of the administered material must be known. Many radioactively labeled organic substances suffer radiation damage and breakdown during storage.

Dynamic Systems. Clinical interpretation of the data from some dynamic studies frequently need be only qualitative; for instance, an experienced observer can determine abnormal aspects of a renogram by inspection. On the other hand, the use of complex mathematical transforms is sometimes necessary in order to calculate such things as mean transit time in circulation studies (this is beyond the scope of this chapter).

Some kinetic data yield readily to analysis if the assumption is made that the tracer is moving between discrete compartments in the body. These compartments may be anatomically defined, e.g., in the case of renal substances, the bladder. In many situations, however, anatomic or physiologic identification of a compartment may not be possible, even though the data are amenable to compartmental analysis.

This system is said to be in the steady state if mother substance is entering and leaving at the same rate. The steady state is assumed in most situations. Furthermore, rapid mixing of tracer is also required, so that specific activities in all regions of a compartment are the same at any given time.

The number of compartments chosen to define a system depends on the data available and on the information sought. For instance, a one-compartment "open" system (a system permitting efflux of tracer) is adequate to describe turnover of body water when tracers such as D_2O (heavy water) or tritiated water are administered. A plot of per cent initial tracer remaining in the body as a function of time will be a single-component exponential whose slope will be the fractional loss of body water per unit time. The half-time of this curve will be the biologic half-life of water in the body. However, if transfer rates of water between compartments within the body are desired, such as between extracellular and intracellular phases, then serial measurements of tracer specific activity must be obtained and analyzed by a multicompartment system.

We shall consider a two-compartment open system to illustrate in a general way the tech-

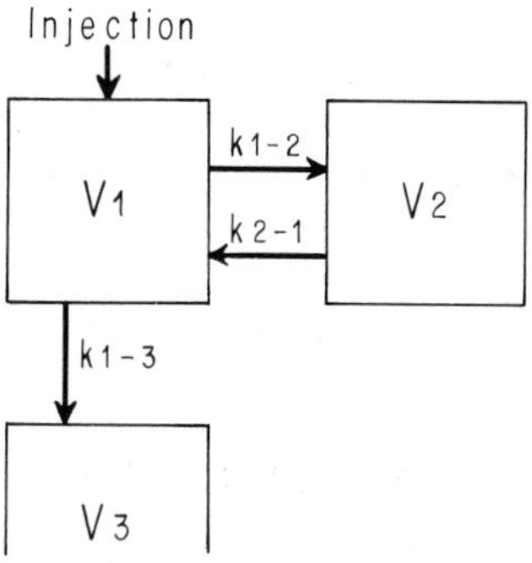

Figure 7–13. Model of open two-compartment system.

niques of compartmental analysis. Many substances used in measuring various body functions are handled in a way that is often well approximated by this model. Figure 7–13 shows such a system. In the steady state, mother substance enters and leaves through compartment V_1. Exchange between V_1 and V_2 is described by the rate constants $k_{1\text{-}2}$ and $k_{2\text{-}1}$, the fractional amounts leaving the respective compartments per unit time. k_{1-3} is the fraction of substance in V_1 that leaves the system per unit time. Total theoretical volume of distribution of the substance in the system is $V_1 + V_2$.

The measured curve of Figure 7–14 characterizes the disappearance of a tracer from V_1 after its introduction into the system by way of V_1, the central compartment. The ordinate is given as fraction of injected dose in V_1 but could just as well be in units of fraction of initial specific activity if the volume of the compartment remains constant, as would normally be the case. The measured curve is the sum of two exponentials, one with slope λ_a and intercept A and the other with slope λ_b and intercept B. The presence of more exponential components in the measured curve would indicate that more compartments would be required for the model. A two-compartment open system is always characterized by two exponentials. The time course of the tracer activity in V_2 would be represented by the difference between two exponentials, one with slope λ_a and the other with slope λ_b, but both with intercepts different from A and B.

The constants A, B, λ_a and λ_b may be obtained by simple extrapolation from the measured curve if the observations extend long enough to allow the contribution of the more rapidly decreasing exponential to become negligible relative to the other. The straight-line portion of the tail of the measured curve (when plotted on semilogarithmic paper) is extrapolated back to the origin to give intercept A. The slope, λ_a, of this straight line is then subtracted point by point from the measured curve, and these values are plotted to give the line with slope λ_b and intercept B.

Various parts of this model may be of use in several applications. For example, the flow ($F_{1\text{-}3}$) from V_1 into V_3 ($k_{1\text{-}3} \times V_1$) is of interest if one is studying the disappearance of ^{131}I-orthoiodohippurate from the body, for this closely approximates effective renal plasma flow (ERPF). The rest of the model is of little interest in this application.

On the other hand, in studies employing ^{131}I-human serum albumin, the intercompartmental clearances $k_{1\text{-}2} \times V_1$ or $k_{1\text{-}2} \times V_2$ may be of interest since these relate to the general capillary permeability of albumin and to extravascular albumin pools.

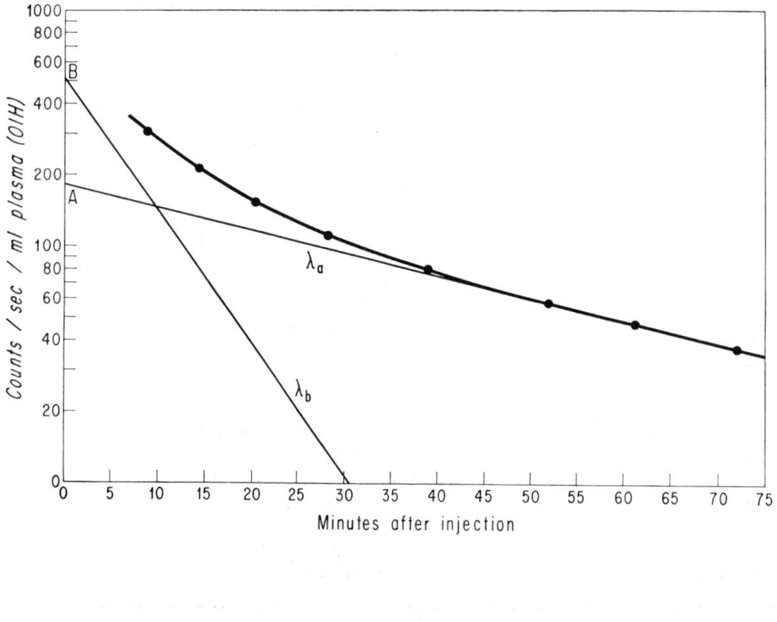

Figure 7–14. Disappearance of a radioactive tracer from the central compartment (V1, Fig. 7–13) of an open two-compartment system.

Formulas for all aspects of this model are as follows: (I = dose of tracer injected.)

$$F_{1\text{-}3} = \frac{I}{\int_0^\infty Ct'dt'} = \frac{I\lambda_a\lambda_b}{A\lambda_b + B\lambda_a}$$

$$V_1 = \frac{I}{A+B}$$

$$F_{1\text{-}2} = \frac{V_1\,[A\lambda_a + B\lambda_b]}{A+B} - F_{1\text{-}3}$$

$$V_2 = \frac{F_{1\text{-}3}F_{1\text{-}2}}{V_1\lambda_a\lambda_b}$$

$$k_{1\text{-}2} = \frac{F_{1\text{-}2}}{V_1} \quad \text{or} \quad \frac{AB(\lambda_b - \lambda_a)^2}{A \times \lambda_b + B \times \lambda_a}$$

$$k_{2\text{-}1} = \frac{F_{2\text{-}1}}{V_2} \quad \text{or} \quad A \times \lambda_b + B \times \lambda_a$$

$$k_{1\text{-}3} = \frac{F_{1\text{-}3}}{V_1} \quad \text{or} \quad A/\lambda_a + B/\lambda_b$$

If one wishes to know the precise fraction of the injected dose (X) in any compartment at any time, these formulas may be used.

$$X_1 = \frac{k_{2\text{-}1} - \lambda_a}{\lambda_b - \lambda_a}\,e^{-\lambda_a t} + \frac{k_{2\text{-}1} - \lambda_b}{\lambda_a - \lambda_b}\,e^{-\lambda_b t}$$

$$X_2 = \frac{k_{1\text{-}2}}{\lambda_b - \lambda_a}\,e^{-\lambda_a t} + \frac{k_{1\text{-}2}}{\lambda_a - \lambda_b}\,e^{-\lambda_b t}$$

$$X_3 = 1 - \left[\frac{k_{1\text{-}3}\,(k_{2\text{-}1} - \lambda_a)}{\lambda_a\,(\lambda_b - \lambda_a)}\,e^{-\lambda_a t} - \frac{k_{1\text{-}3}\,(k_{2\text{-}1} - \lambda_b)}{\lambda_b\,(\lambda_a - \lambda_b)}\,e^{-\lambda_b t}\right]$$

DIAGNOSTIC TESTS

In this section the widely accepted diagnostic radioisotope tests are described in detail, including the principles on which the tests are based and interpretation of results. Newer tests and others which are infrequently performed are described more briefly.

This section groups tests generally as *in vitro* or *in vivo* functions. The *in vivo* applications are grouped into kinetic, imaging, and body composition tests. The procedures will be grouped by organ and by technique.

Table 7–5 lists a few commonly employed radiopharmaceuticals used in scintigraphic tests.

Table 7–5. COMMON SCINTIGRAPHIC RADIOPHARMACEUTICALS

ORGAN	RADIOPHARMACEUTICAL	MECHANISM OF ACCUMULATION
Bone	^{99m}Tc-polyphosphate, ^{99m}Tc-phosphonate, ^{47}Ca, ^{18}F, ^{85}Sr, ^{87}Sr	Bone-seeking elements
Brain	^{99m}Tc-pertechnetate	Breakdown of blood-brain barrier
Heart	^{99m}Tc or ^{131}I human serum albumin	Remains in blood pool
Kidney	^{131}I-ortho-iodohippurate (OIH)	Measures effective renal plasma flow
	^{131}I-diatrizoate (DTZ)	Measures glomerular filtration rate
Liver	^{99m}Tc sulfur colloid	Trapped by reticuloendothelial system
	^{131}I rose bengal	Cleared like BSP
Lung	^{99m}Tc-microspheres	Trapped in pulmonary capillaries
	^{133}Xe	Traces pathway of inert gas
Marrow	^{59}Fe	Physiologic uptake
Pancreas	^{75}Se-selenomethionine	Uptake of methionine is physiologic
Placenta	$^{99m}TcO_4$ (for scintillation camera), ^{131}I human serum albumin, ^{99m}Tc-pertechnetate of human serum albumin	Remains in blood pool
Spleen	^{99m}Tc-sulfur colloid	Trapped by reticuloendothelial system
	^{51}Cr-labeled heat-damaged erythrocytes	Normal splenic trapping of effete erythrocytes
Thyroid	^{131}I	Physiologic uptake
	^{99m}Tc-pertechnetate	Behaves like halide

Tests of Thyroid Function

The metabolic state of the body is partially controlled by the activity of the thyroid gland, which in turn is closely linked to the metabolism of iodine. The availability of a suitable radioisotope of iodine (^{131}I) makes it possible to assess directly certain phases of thyroid function. Recently other radiopharmaceuticals that function as halides such as pertechnetate ($^{99m}TcO_4$) have become available. This substance accumulates in the thyroid trap but is not organified. It has proved useful for estimating the trapping mechanism and for imaging the thyroid gland (Table 11–21, p. 743).

Ingested iodine is rapidly absorbed from the intestine as iodide, whereupon it diffuses throughout the blood stream and the extravascular fluid compartments. As the iodide passes through the kidney, a portion is removed and excreted in the urine; a small amount is excreted into the stomach as hydroiodic acid along with hydrochloric acid, and some finds its way into the saliva. The iodide which reaches the thyroid gland is concentrated by that organ and coupled to amino acids yielding thyroxine, which is embedded in a large protein molecule (thyroglobulin). As the body needs thyroxine to maintain its metabolic activity, thyroxine is split from the thyroglobulin within the gland. The free thyroxine enters the blood stream and is promptly captured by the thyroxine-binding proteins. Presumably the thyroxine is carried to tissues which require its presence in order to increase the basal metabolic rate of the body. These target tissues are still unidentified and the biochemistry of thyroxine's metabolic effect is uncertain (p. 744).

A series of measurable activities can be detected based on this iodine pathway: the rate of uptake of iodine by the thyroid gland may be increased or decreased; the level of protein-bound iodine (PBI), essentially thyroxine iodine, can be measured chemically in the blood but now is usually measured by a radionuclide technique by competitive binding assay; the affinity of the thyroxine-binding proteins for thyroxine can be determined; and the overall activity can be estimated by the basal metabolic rate.

The availability of serum levels of both bound and free thyroxine and the thyroid-stimulating hormone (TSH) has in recent years effected a radical change in the handling of diagnostic problems involving the thyroid. In fact, they have all but eliminated the indications for the more conventional kinetic *in vivo* tests using radioiodine. Primary hyperthyroidism can best be diagnosed by the finding of elevated serum thyroxine levels coupled with depressed TSH levels. Primary hypothyroidism can in a reciprocal fashion best be diagnosed by the reverse. The presence of tumor, the suspicion of ectopic thyroid tissue, or the diagnosis of various forms of congenital hypothyroidism indicate the use of scintigraphic procedures. Although primary hypo- or hyperthyroidism can be diagnosed by *in vitro* procedures, the assessment of hyperthyroidism due to exogenous thyroxine really requires a thyroid uptake procedure. (This may be of importance in the diagnosis of factitial hyperthyroidism.) For this, a simple 6- to 24-hour uptake suffices. Use of all the array of variants of this procedure, the Berson clearance, the TSH stimulation test, the T3 uptake tests, the T3 and KI inhibition tests, and the conversion ratio, has become indicated only in unusual circumstances.

An occasional euthyroid patient will present with exceptionally low or high serum thyroxine levels. These are usually picked up incidentally. Since they may represent disorders of thyroid-binding proteins (TBP), it is sometimes necessary to perform tests to evaluate these proteins.

It is useful to group thyroid tests in the following way as described by Wahner:

- I. Tests that evaluate thyroid function
  - A. Tests that evaluate the feedback mechanism
    1. TSH stimulation tests
    2. T3 suppression test
    3. TSH immunoassay
  - B. Tests that measure iodide accumulation and turnover
    1. ^{131}I uptake ($^{99m}TcO_4$ uptake)
    2. Berson clearance
    3. PB ^{131}I conversion ratio
  - C. Tests that evaluate circulating thyronines
    1. Total thyronine
    2. Free thyronine
    3. T3 uptake
    4. Various TBP binding capacities
  - D. Tests that measure the interaction of thyronine and organism
    1. BMR
    2. Reflex relaxation time
  - E. Tests that measure functional anatomy
    1. ^{131}I or $^{99m}TcO_4$ images (scintigrams or scans)

Only the following radioiodine tests will be presented in detail (the serum thyroxine and TSH levels will be discussed under Radiobioassay techniques): (1) standard uptake of ^{131}I by the thyroid; (2) rate of clearance of ^{131}I from the blood (Berson test); (3) influence of thyroid-stimulating hormone on thyroidal uptake of ^{131}I (TSH test); (4) indirect test of the thyroxine-binding capacity of the binding proteins of the plasma (erythrocyte and resin T_3 tests); and (5) use of scintigraphic techniques in evaluation of the thyroid gland.

Standard 24-Hour Uptake of ^{131}I by Thyroid Gland. Probably the most common radionuclide test of thyroid function is the 24-hour uptake test. A dose of sodium ^{131}I-iodide is given orally, and 24 hours later the amount present in the thyroid gland is measured and compared with normal values. Since it is possible for a very thyrotoxic patient to achieve a peak concentration of ^{131}I in his thyroid within a few hours and to release significant amounts of labeled thyroxine before the 24-hour reading, some laboratories evaluate the uptake of ^{131}I during the first few hours as well as at 24 hours. Various intervals, up to 8 hours after the dose, have been recommended. We use 6 hours in our laboratory. Tests made earlier than 5 hours after administration of the dose need to take into consideration the relatively high neck background.

TECHNIQUE. ^{131}I is commercially available in capsules and in liquid form; the patient merely swallows a capsule with water as needed or a measured amount of ^{131}I in liquid form. At the time selected for measuring thyroidal uptake, the radioactivity in the neck, measured by a collimated NaI (Tl) crystal placed 20 to 30 cm. from the neck, is compared with the radioactivity in an identical capsule suitably housed to simulate the anatomy of the neck; plastic holders are available for this purpose. This technique obviates the need for calculating the decay of ^{131}I because it is the same in the capsule and in the body. The percentage uptake is simply $\frac{^{131}\text{I in the thyroid gland}}{^{131}\text{I in the dose}} \times 100$.

If ^{131}I is already in the thyroid gland before the test starts, the amount must be measured precisely and subtracted (after appropriate decay correction) from subsequent counts, just as in the case of other background.

We prefer to use solutions of ^{131}I because we can maintain a constant dose by increasing the volume administered. Our standard dose is 5 μCi. for adults and less, according to size, for children. For infants, the solution of ^{131}I, which is sterile, is given by intramuscular injection to insure precise dosage.

There has been a recent significant decrease of thyroid uptake values in the United States and Canada, probably owing to the generalized use of iodide as an additive in foods, salt, and vitamin preparations (see Table 11–25, p. 763).

The normal gland now accumulates approximately 5 to 15 per cent of an oral dose of ^{131}I at 6 hours and 12 to 35 per cent at 24 hours. In areas where iodide is not added to the diet, these values are much higher. It is therefore imperative to know where the patient lives and whether he uses preparations with iodide additives before evaluating the uptake value.

INTERPRETATION. We also collect all urine excreted during the 24-hour period, not only for diagnostic purposes but also as an internal check on the test. In normal or hyperthyroid patients, about 80 per cent of the dose should be accounted for in the urine and the thyroid gland. In hypothyroid patients the total may be somewhat less. If only about half the dose can be accounted for after 24 hours, the two most likely causes are technical error and congestive cardiac failure. On the other hand, if significantly more than 100 per cent of the dose is recovered, the two most likely causes are technical error and urinary excretion of a radioiodine which was administered to the patient previously. To minimize the chance of the latter occurring, we check for ^{131}I in the thyroid gland before our diagnostic tests are performed.

Berson Test of Thyroidal Clearance of Plasma Iodide. The Berson test estimates the rate of clearance of ^{131}I from the plasma by the thyroid gland. The results are usually expressed as milliliters of plasma cleared of iodide by the thyroid gland per minute. The main assumption in the calculation is that the ^{131}I in the plasma diminishes for three reasons during the half hour of the test: it is excreted by the kidney, it diffuses into the extracellular and intracellular spaces throughout the body, and it is trapped by the thyroid gland.

TECHNIQUE. Use of the Berson test requires a device which records change of radioactivity. Conventional renographic equipment is readily adaptable to this purpose. A dose of about 25 μCi. of ^{131}I is given intravenously and the ^{131}I in the neck is recorded continuously for 30 minutes. The urine is collected at the end of the half-hour recording period. The following data are needed to calculate the clearance: the patient's weight (to estimate the iodide space of the body); the dose given to the patient and the fraction of the dose excreted in the urine (both in microcuries); and two values calculated from the recording (identified by arrows in Figure 7–15). The initial, sharply increasing portion of the curve before the first arrow is initial extrathyroidal ^{131}I. The 30-minute uptake is the difference between the values at the two arrows. Each of these values must be converted from count rate to microcuries.

Calculation of clearance is actually simpler than the cumbersome equation suggests: Uptake of ^{131}I (μCi.) $= \text{Th} = \frac{(\text{D} \times \text{O})\ (\text{E} \times \text{U})}{(\text{D} - \text{E})}$, in which D is the dose (μCi.), O is the observed net uptake of ^{131}I during the half hour (μCi.), E is the extrathyroidal ^{131}I initially (μCi.), and U is the urinary ^{131}I (μCi.). D_{30} = residual ^{131}I in the body (except in the thyroid) after the half hour $= \text{D} - (\text{Th} + \text{U})$.

$\overline{\text{D}}$ = average dose in the body (except in the

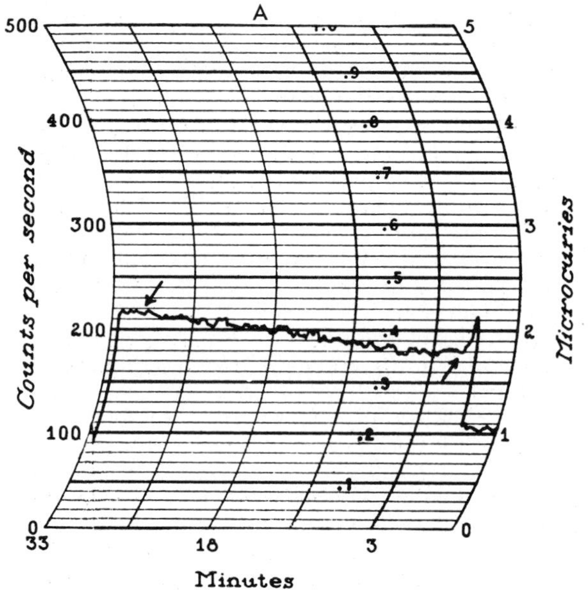

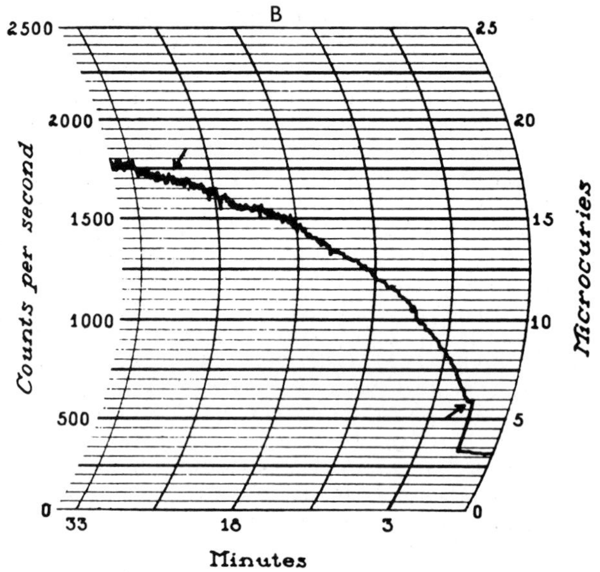

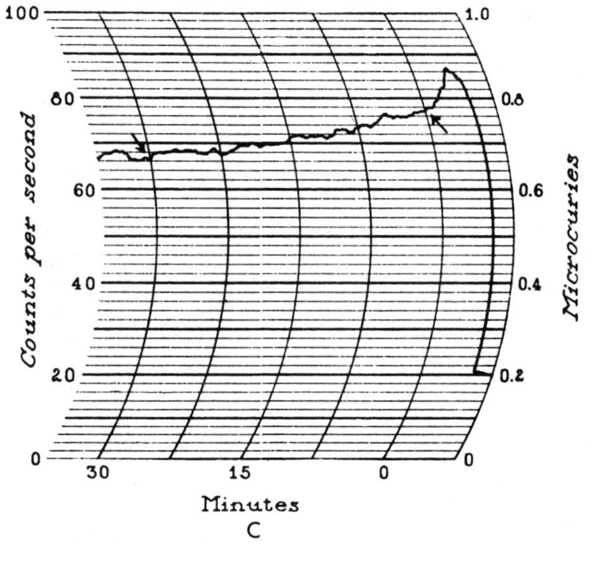

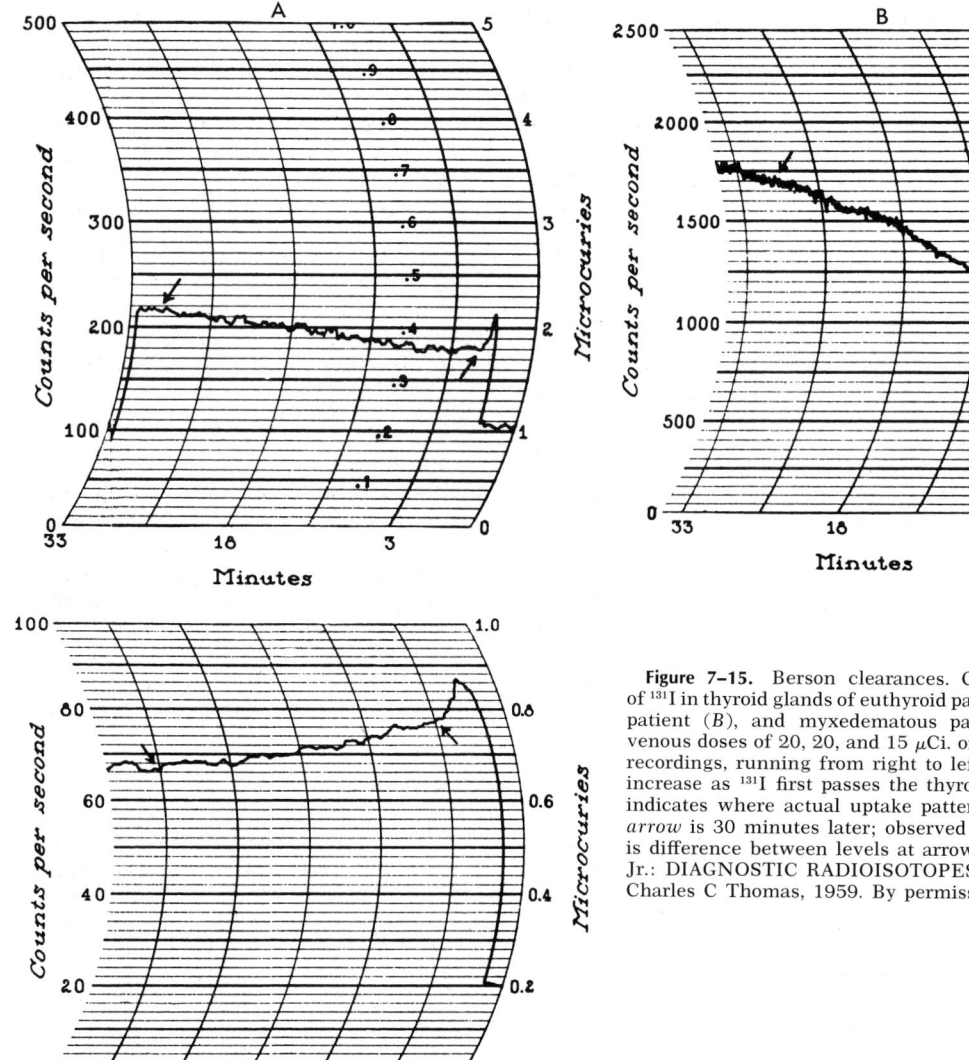

Figure 7–15. Berson clearances. Continuous recordings of ^{131}I in thyroid glands of euthyroid patient (*A*), hyperthyroid patient (*B*), and myxedematous patient (*C*) after intravenous doses of 20, 20, and 15 μCi. of ^{131}I, respectively. The recordings, running from right to left, show a rapid initial increase as ^{131}I first passes the thyroid gland. *First arrow* indicates where actual uptake pattern begins, and *second arrow* is 30 minutes later; observed uptake in 30 minutes is difference between levels at arrows. (From C. A. Owen, Jr.: DIAGNOSTIC RADIOISOTOPES. Springfield, Illinois, Charles C Thomas, 1959. By permission of the publisher.)

thyroid) during the half hour $= \frac{D + D^{30}}{2}$.

Cl_T = thyroidal clearance of ^{131}I from the plasma (ml./min.) $= \frac{Th \cdot W \cdot 200}{D \cdot 30}$, in which W = patient's weight (kg.), 200 = constant for estimating extrathyroidal iodide space of the body, and 30 = duration of the test (min.). The standardized thyroidal clearance (St. Cl_T) is the calculated clearance corrected for the surface area (SA) of the body (1.73 m.^{2} is considered standard).

$$\text{St. } Cl_T = Cl_T \times \frac{1.73}{SA} \text{ ml. per min.}$$

The surface area may be calculated from the patient's height and weight by using standard nomograms.

Interpretation. The normal thyroidal clearance of ^{131}I is about 8 to 10 ml. of plasma per minute (normal renal clearance of iodide is 30 to 40 ml. per min.). It is possible to calculate the Berson clearance at times less than 30 minutes by changing two numbers in the equation for Cl_T: the length of time in minutes and the extrathyroidal iodide compartment constant. At 5 minutes the constant is 137, at 10 minutes 157, at 15 minutes 169, at 20 minutes 180, and at 25 minutes 190.

TSH Test. Normally the thyroid gland is

under the control of thyrotropin or thyroid-stimulating hormone (TSH) produced by the pituitary gland. If the pituitary is diseased, the thyroid gland suffers from lack of TSH stimulation, and a myxedema develops which is difficult to distinguish from primary thyroidal myxedema. One way to distinguish the two types of myxedema is to administer TSH parenterally and determine if the thyroid gland regains its ability to take up radioiodine.

In actual practice the TSH test has been found to be more useful in a completely difrent way. If a patient is taking sufficient desiccated thyroid or thyroid hormones to satisfy the body's requirements, TSH production by the pituitary gland ceases and, in turn, synthesis of thyroxine by the thyroid stops. Since probably considerably more patients are receiving thyroid therapy than actually need it, distinguishing the euthyroid patient taking desiccated thyroid unnecessarily from the hypothyroid patient who requires the therapy may become important. The patient with primary myxedema cannot respond to exogenous TSH, while the euthyroid one can. Before TSH became commercially available the only sure way to distinguish these two groups of patients was to discontinue the desiccated thyroid and wait several weeks to see if the patient became myxedematous or remained euthyroid. With the TSH test, an evaluation of thyroidal function is possible within two or three days even though the desiccated thyroid treatment is continued.

Technique. An oral dose of 5 μCi. of ^{131}I is given, and 3 hours later the uptake by the thyroid gland is measured. Then an intramuscular injection of 10 units of commercial TSH is given, and 3 hours after this the thyroidal uptake is again measured. The next morning, the ^{131}I in the thyroid gland is measured again, a second dose of ^{131}I is given orally, and 3-, 6-, and 24-hour uptakes are determined and compared with the first set of uptake values. One may also collect blood before and after the administration of TSH to determine if changes (or lack of them) in the serum PBI level parallel changes in the ^{131}I uptake. We have not found this to be a necessary part of the test, however.

Interpretation. The various possible responses are shown in Figure 7–16. The normal gland responds to the injection of TSH. The gland which has a limited number of cells (post-thyroidectomy or post-^{131}I-irradiation) may have a normal ^{131}I uptake before injection of TSH but show no increase in uptake after the TSH. Primary myxedema is characterized by little thyroidal uptake of ^{131}I before or after the TSH. However, patients with adequate thyroid function which has been suppressed by exogenous thyroid drugs or who have pituitary failure show a markedly increased uptake of ^{131}I after the TSH test compared with their values before injection of TSH.

T_3 Uptake Test. ***TBP Estimations.*** Perhaps the simplest assessment of the state of the thyronine-binding proteins is the simple T-3 test. While the other radioiodine tests of thyroid function require administration of the nuclide to the patient, one test has been devised which merely requires taking a sample of the patient's blood and adding the radioiodine to the serum *in vitro*. This is the T_3 uptake test (T_3 stands for triiodothyronine).

The T_3 test measures the relative affinities of serum proteins and of an added competitive substance (erythrocytes or a resin) for radioactive T_3. Because the serum proteins have only a finite number of binding sites for thyroid hormone, the more sites occupied by endogenous thyroid hormones, the fewer there are to bind with any added radioactive hormone. The unbound or lightly bound ^{131}I-labeled T_3 then freely binds to the erythrocytes or resin added subsequently. In other words, the higher the endogenous thyroid hormone level, the greater the radioactivity which binds to added erythrocytes or resin, and the lower the serum thyroxine, the less the radioactivity which binds to the erythrocytes or resin.

The theoretic aspects of the test are complicated by several factors. There are at least four electrophoretically different proteins which have affinity for thyroxine: one moves even faster than albumin (TBPA or thyroxine-binding protein in the prealbumin zone), one is in the albumin zone (TBA), and two are in the α-globulin zone (thyroxine-binding globulins TBG I and TBG II). T_3 does not bind to TBPA at all and to TBG I only during preg-

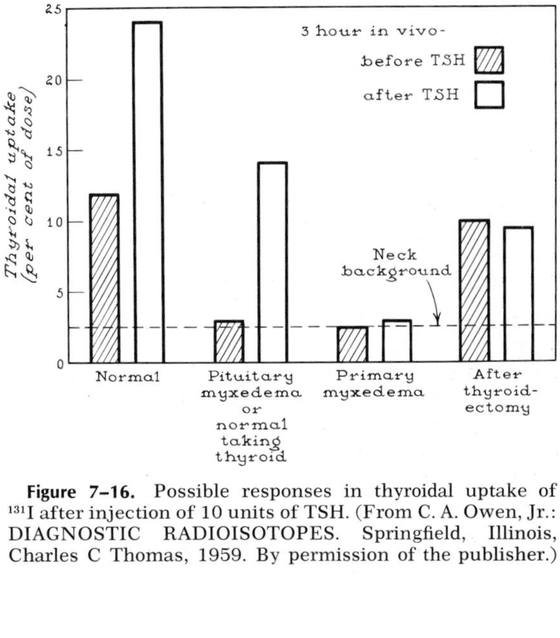

Figure 7–16. Possible responses in thyroidal uptake of ^{131}I after injection of 10 units of TSH. (From C. A. Owen, Jr.: DIAGNOSTIC RADIOISOTOPES. Springfield, Illinois, Charles C Thomas, 1959. By permission of the publisher.)

nancy or myxedema, so the addition of T_3 to serum does not truly reflect thyroxine binding. However, when radioactive thyroxine is added to serum, it tends to exchange with thyroxine already bound to protein, whereas added radioactive T_3 does not, so that T_3 does reflect more accurately the available thyronine-binding sites in those sites where it is known to bind.

Furthermore, differences exist between erythrocytes and resins as competitors in T_3 binding. For example, salicylate or diphenylhydantoin therapy produces marked depression in the serum thyroxine. This is reflected in increased T_3 uptake by erythrocytes but less by resins. Similarly, in diabetes mellitus some serum factor causes an increase in erythrocyte binding of T_3 without producing similar effects on resins. Another difference between erythrocytes and resins is the fact that l-thyroxine binds to resins but not to erythrocytes.

Which test is better? A clear answer cannot be given. In favor of resins is the fact that they are not subject to the effects of salicylates, diphenylhydantoin, or diabetes mellitus to the same degree as erythrocytes. However, the erythrocyte may represent more closely the actual physiologic state of the patient. If a low serum thyroxine value is accompanied by a low T_3 uptake by erythrocytes, myxedema is suggested; if the T_3 uptake by erythrocytes is increased, one should suspect TBP deficiency or medication with salicylate or diphenylhydantoin types of drugs. We prefer the erythrocyte uptake of T_3 also because we have found it to be much more reproducible than the test on resins. This reproducibility has been achieved by controlling several variables inherent in the test described by Hamolsky *et al.* (1959) and by expressing the result as a modification of the binding coefficient proposed by Adams and associates (1960). The erythrocyte uptake of triiodothyronine is more cumbersome to perform than are resin uptakes.

Because the probability is high that patients on whom T_3 uptake tests have been ordered may have had prior *in vivo* radioactive iodine tests, each sample of blood should be checked for radioactivity before the test is begun. The actual test should be done in suitable test tubes, for storage of blood in certain plastic test tubes causes spuriously high results (Tauxe and associates, 1966).

TECHNIQUE

1. Pipette 3 ml. of well-mixed heparinized blood into a 10-ml. stoppered Erlenmeyer flask.

2. Add 0.1 ml. of ^{131}I-l-triiodothyronine, made up with saline to a concentration of 0.12 μg. per ml.

3. Incubate in a shaking water bath at 37° C. for 2 hours.

4. Remove 2 ml. and place in a counting tube. Determine the net count per milliliter. Determine hematocrit value on the remaining incubation mixture.

5. After measurement of the radioactivity, centrifuge the counting tube for 5 minutes at 4° C. and 3000 r.p.m. (International Centrifuge, No. 2). Aspirate the supernatant fluid. Resuspend packed cells by ejecting from a filled 10-ml. syringe into the tube approximately 5 ml. of saline at 4° C., swirling mixture energetically for several seconds and then ejecting the saline remaining in the syringe and swirling the tube again. The time required for this step should be standardized and maintained constant for each test (it can be conveniently accomplished within 1 minute). Centrifuge again at 4° C. at 3000 r.p.m. for 5 minutes. Aspirate as before. Repeat these steps until the cells have been washed three times. Determine the net radioactivity of the cells per milliliter of incubation mixture by dividing by 2.

6. Calculate uptake by the following formula:

$$T_3 \text{ uptake coefficient} = \frac{F \times (1 - H)}{H \times (1 - F)} \times 100,$$

in which

$$F = \frac{\text{c.p.s./ml. after third wash}}{\text{c.p.s./ml. before washing}} \text{ and } H = \text{hematocrit value as a fraction of 1.}$$

INTERPRETATION. Normal coefficients in our laboratory are 8.7 to 13.5. If commercial resin kits are used instead of erythrocytes, normal values are higher—about 25 to 35. Lower T_3 uptakes occur with hypothyroidism, pregnancy, or therapy with estrogens or propylthiouracil. Higher T_3 uptakes are associated with hyperthyroidism, nephrosis, decreased plasma protein level, hepatitis, thyroid or T_3 medication, treatment with coumarin drugs, diphenylhydantoin or androgens, or TBG deficiency. The administration of iodides does not seem to affect the test (p. 759).

Thyroid Imaging. The distribution of radioiodide within thyroid gland tissue can easily be evaluated by scanning the organ after administering ^{131}I or $^{99m}TcO_4$ to the patient. Under most circumstances, with a 3-inch NaI (Tl) crystal there should be approximately 10 μCi. of ^{131}I in the gland, so the dose must be tailored to the thyroid uptake. Normally, approximately 50 μCi. of ^{131}I is administered, the thyroid being scanned 24 hours after administration.

With use of $^{99m}TcO_4$, which is preferable, considerably higher doses can be utilized with much less radiation to the patient. The energy level of the ^{99m}Tc permits imaging on a scintillation camera with a pinhole collimator, although a highly focused collimator (31 hole) used with the 3-inch scanner as described previously is generally preferable. One or 2 mCi. of $^{99m}TcO_4$ may be used and the thyroid

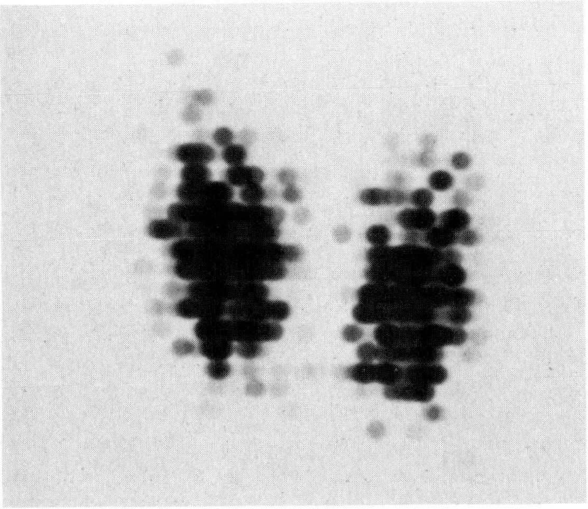

Figure 7–17. Photoscan of normal thyroid gland (^{131}I).

scanned approximately a half hour after injection.

There are at present few indications for thyroid imaging:

1. To assess the function of a palpable nodule.
2. To determine whether mediastinal or other ectopic tissues function as thyroid.
3. To determine the diagnosis and prognosis of infants and children with thyroid problems. Examples of various applications are illustrated in Figures 7–17 to 7–25.
4. To determine the effects of therapy.

A normal thyroid image is shown in Figure 7–17. The distribution is even, in the usual butterfly pattern. In the case of the palpable nodule, the clinical question is usually rather simple. Is the nodule functioning excessively as evidenced by depression of the rest of the gland (Fig. 7–18 *A*)? In this case the probability of malignancy is extremely low.

At times it may be helpful to prove depression of the rest of the gland by the administration of TSH followed by another scan. Figure 7–18 *B* illustrates this ability of the rest of the gland to be stimulated by TSH. This is not only usually unnecessary but unwise if radioiodine therapy is contemplated, since the normal erstwhile dormant portions of the thyroid may become irradiated unnecessarily.

If the nodule shows no or diminished function the probability of malignancy is on the order of 20 per cent (Fig. 7–19).

The locations of ectopic foci of thyroid uptake are often of clinical interest.

Figure 7–20 illustrates a case of pertechnetate uptake in the region of hilar shadows seen on a chest x-ray. In this case a positive identification of functioning thyroid tissue was achieved.

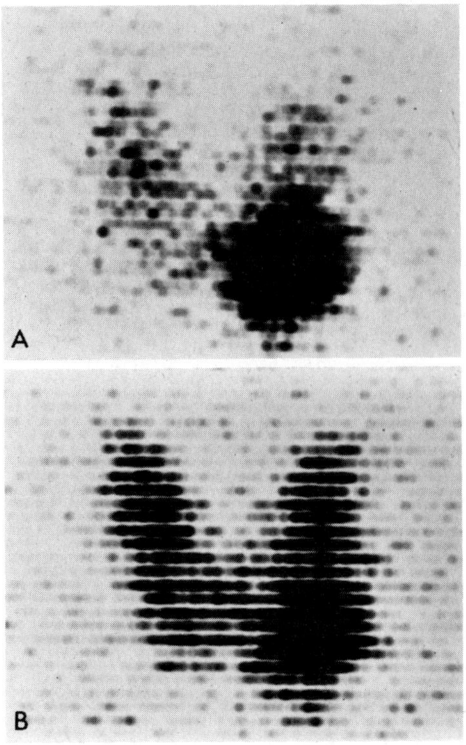

Figure 7–18. Scintigraphic image of thyroid containing autonomous ("hot") nodule. *A*, Before TSH stimulation. The rest of the gland appears depressed. *B*, After TSH stimulation. The rest of the gland is normally active.

It is sometimes necessary to evaluate lingual masses as shown in Figure 7–21 *A* and *B*, where a small focus of iodide uptake gave a positive identification of a mass as thyroid and indicated further that it was the only thyroid that the patient had.

In Figure 7–22 it may be seen that the ectopic thyroid follows the thyroglossal duct.

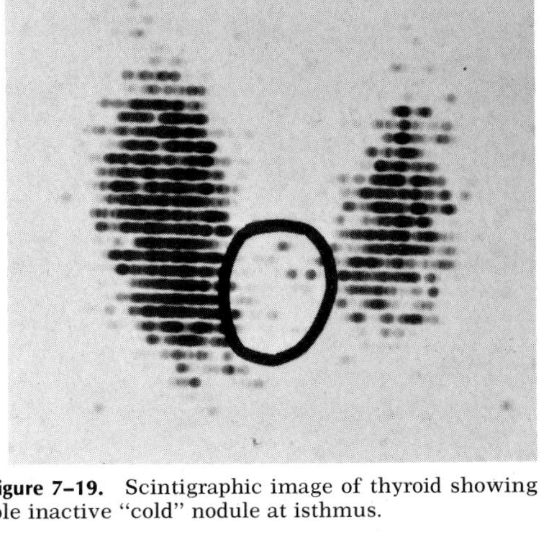

Figure 7–19. Scintigraphic image of thyroid showing palpable inactive "cold" nodule at isthmus.

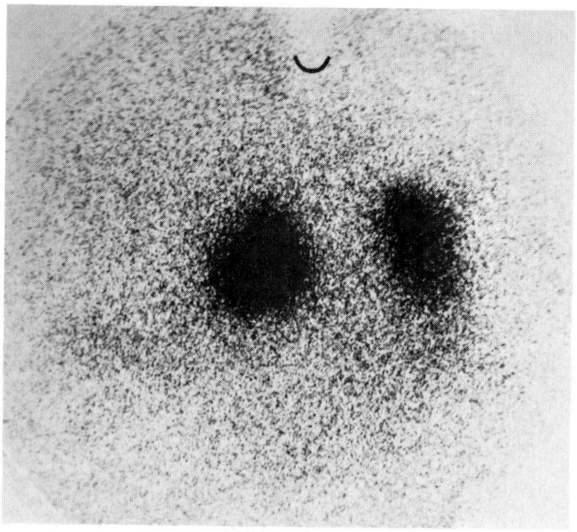

Figure 7–20. Scintigraphic image of chest seen anteriorly. Manubrial notch is indicated by marker. Bilateral hilar uptake of pertechnetate is depicted.

In the above two cases, the patients, both children, were euthyroid and were otherwise normal in their development.

The next two patients were retarded at birth. In the first (Fig. 7–23 *A* and *B*) a relatively good prognosis may be suspected with replacement treatment since a small bit of functioning gland was found in the tongue, as revealed by the pertechnetate image. A poor prognosis may be expected in the second (Fig. 7–24) because no thyroid tissue was detected. In both these patients, however, the parents need not fear that the disease is likely to appear in their other children. However, in the goitrous cretin in whom thyroid gland tissue may be observed in the normal place in the neck, the prognosis is not only poor for normal development, but the disease is likely to appear in other siblings. Therefore, scintigraphic studies of infants suspected of being hypothyroid is mandatory.

At times it is useful to determine the effects

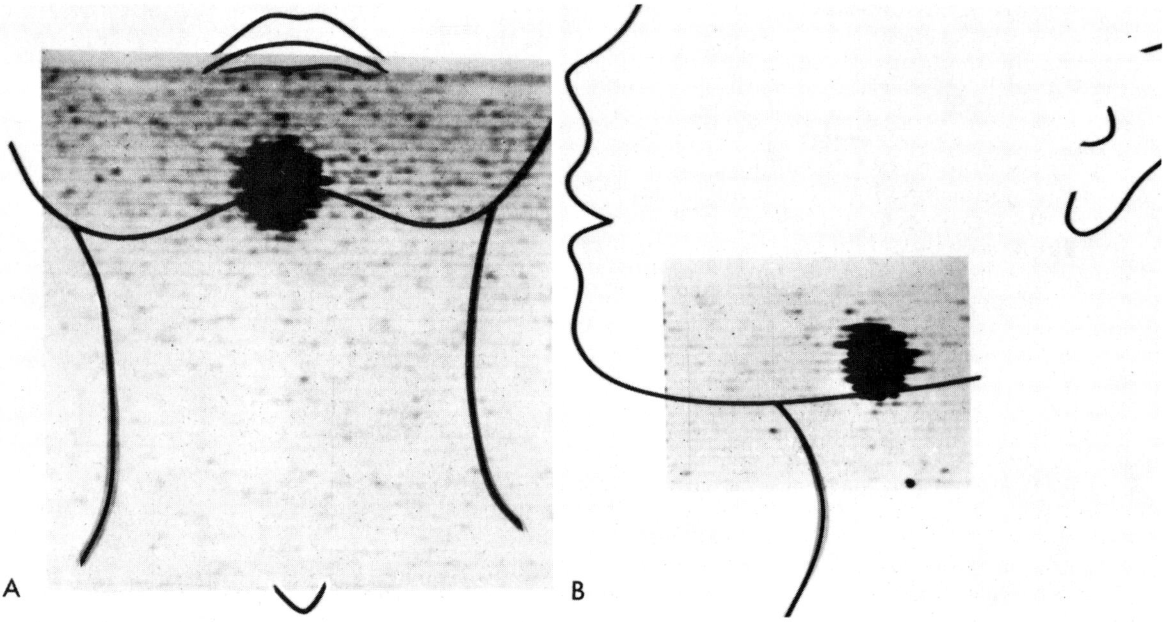

Figure 7–21. Anterior (*A*) and lateral (*B*) views of neck of child showing lingual thyroid. No other thyroid tissue is seen.

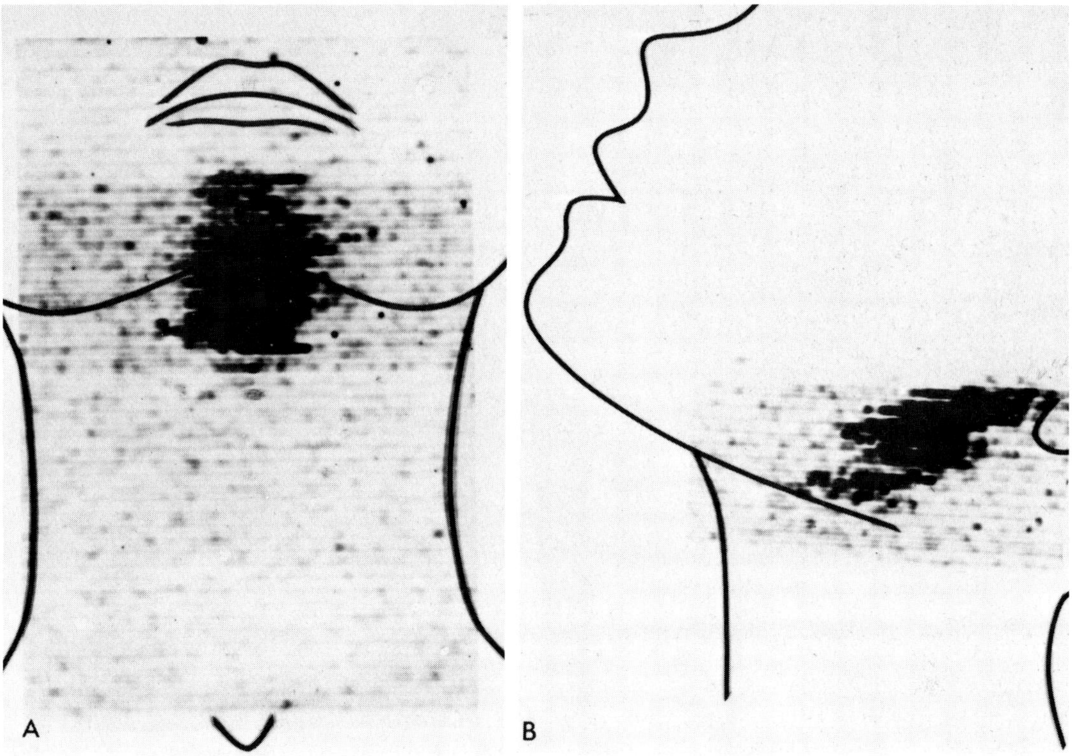

Figure 7–22. Anterior (*A*) and lateral (*B*) scintigrams of thyroid tissue in a child showing uptake only along thyroglossal canal. No thyroid is seen below hyoid bone.

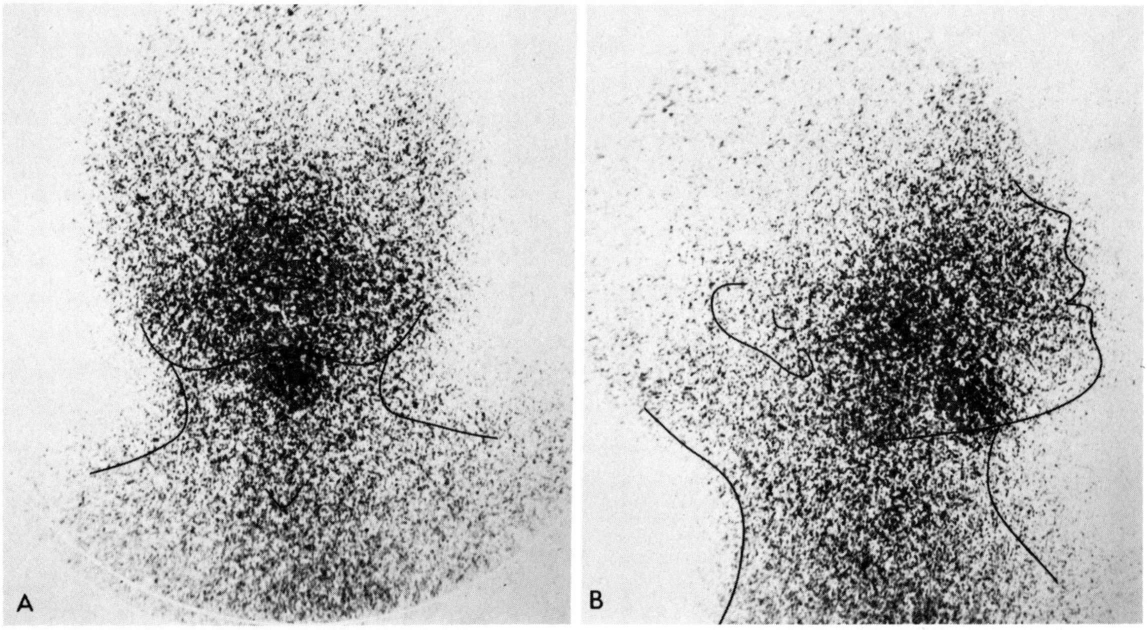

Figure 7–23. Anterior (*A*) and lateral (*B*) scintigraphic images of thyroid tissue in a child. There is only a small focus of uptake at the base of the tongue.

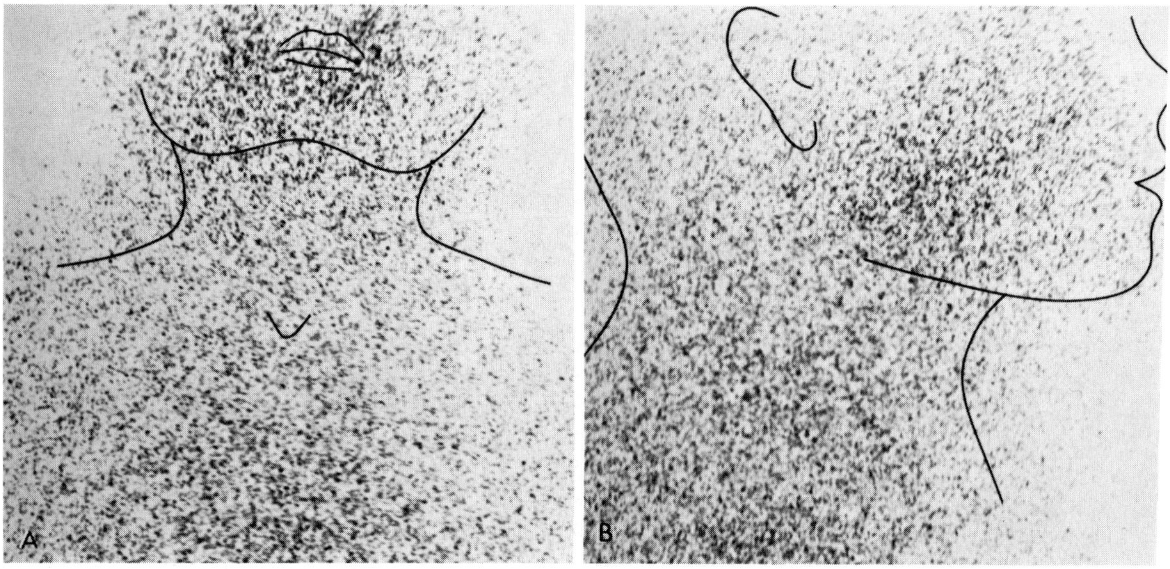

Figure 7–24. Anterior (*A*) and lateral (*B*) scintigraphic images of a completely athyreotic child.

of therapy. Figure 7–25 illustrates a patient in whom it was desired to ablate the functioning thyroid tissue in the neck. *A* and *B* show images before and after treatment.

It is mandatory to palpate the gland at the time of imaging and to mark on the dot-scan paper any tumors or scars. Landmarks, such as thyroid cartilage and the suprasternal notch, should also be identified.

Renal Tests

Three radioactive techniques have found wide application in evaluation of renal function: renal clearances, the renogram, and the renal scintigram.

Renal Clearances. Classically, para-aminohippurate (PAH) has been used to measure effective renal plasma flow (ERPF) because, at low concentrations, PAH is quantitatively

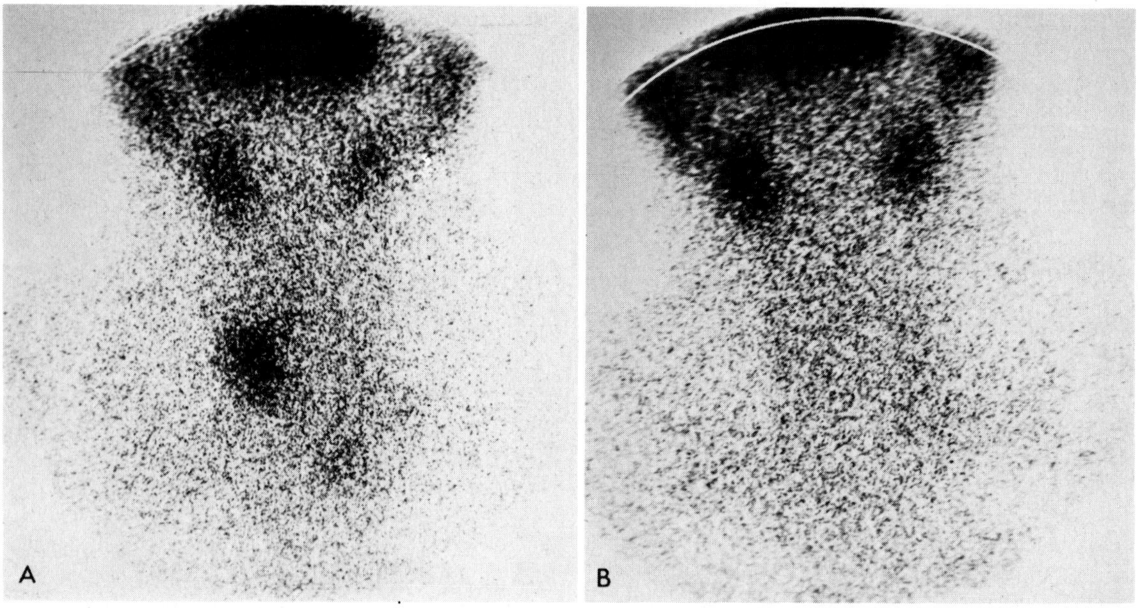

Figure 7–25. Anterior scintigraphic images of the neck in a patient before (*A*) and after (*B*) ablative treatment of the thyroid. At both times uptake is seen in salivary gland tissue.

removed from the blood passing through the kidney. Similarly, inulin has been used to evaluate glomerular filtration rate (GFR) because this substance has the same concentration in the glomerular filtrate as it has in the plasma and it is neither reabsorbed nor secreted by the renal tubule.

Radioiodinated counterparts of both PAH and inulin are available: ^{131}I-ortho-iodohippurate (OIH, Hippuran), like PAH, measures ERPF; and ^{131}I-diatrizoate (DTZ), like inulin, measures GFR. If the radioactive compounds are employed as their nonradioactive counterparts are—continuous intravenous infusion and catheterized collection of urine—the same values for ERPF and GFR are derived. Some simplification for calculating the ERPF has been suggested by Sapirstein and associates (1955). Their method eliminates continuous infusion of OIH and bladder catheterization and is now gaining wide acceptance as a diagnostic tool. By labeling OIH and DTZ with different isotopes of iodine (^{131}I and ^{125}I), both GFR and ERPF could be determined concurrently. At present, OIH is used primarily to determine the clearance of this compound from the blood, its concentration in the kidney, and its excretion in the urine.

A single injection of the radiopharmaceutical is made, and the plasma is sampled at approximately 10-minute intervals for an hour in the case of OIH, or for 90 minutes for GFR measurements. Counting rates from the plasma are obtained and expressed as percentage of the injected dose. They are then plotted on semilogarithmic paper and treated mathematically as shown in Figures 7–13 and 7–14. Flow is indicated by the passage from V_1 and V_3.

Recently we have published regression equations which relate the concentration at 40 minutes to the ERPF, thus further simplifying the test to the ease of a BSP.

TECHNIQUE. One injects a measured amount (I) of radioactive OIH and samples the concentration at 40 minutes (C_{40}). One then derives the theoretical volume of distribution X at this time (I/C_{40}) then substitutes into the following polynomial equation:

$$ERPF = -117 + 12.6x - 0.0589x^2$$

$$(Sy.x = 23.8 \text{ ml.})$$

In common with PAH clearances this technique may give invalid results when clearances are lower than 100 ml. per minute, levels at which the blood urea is clearly elevated and the estimation of ERPF is not really needed anyway (Tauxe *et al.*, 1971).

Radiohippurate Renography. Radiation detectors are focused at the kidneys while ^{131}I-OIH is injected intravenously. Continuous tracings from each kidney are recorded for one-half hour and the various upward and downward deflections are compared with the normal pattern. Although more precise interpretation of renograms is being sought, the present descriptive analysis has already found a firm place in the diagnostic laboratory.

Several technical problems must be considered in order to obtain consistently reproducible renograms. If the scintillation crystals are too small, they must be brought up close to the patient to increase the sensitivity. Results are erratic because slight changes in position cause significant changes in counting rate, by the inverse square law. Since renograms may have distinctly different contours when the patient is hydrated as compared to the dehydrated state, the choice of conditions becomes empirical. In our experience the likelihood of a renographic demonstration of renal artery stenosis is enhanced by maintaining the urinary flow rate at about 0.5 ml. per minute with the patient in a sitting position. Since certain renographic abnormalities may be accentuated by hydrating the patient and having him lie down, occasionally renograms may have to be repeated with changes in hydration and position.

The dose of ^{131}I-OIH depends on the efficiency of the radiation detection system used. Because the background is minimized by differential (pulse-height window) selectors, we prefer them to integral (discriminator) selectors. The same dose may be given to all patients, or the dose may be varied with the patient's surface area. We use the former system because of its technical simplicity.

It is generally agreed that the scintillation probes should be centered over the points of maximal radioactivity along the patient's back. Of the various methods for achieving this, we prefer an audiocontrol system in which the change in pitch of a whistling device indicates the intensity of radioactivity; the technician can center each probe within a few seconds after the injection of the radionuclide. Delay of up to a minute is not usually significant. Other localizing methods depend on prior roentgenography or administration of a preliminary dose of ^{125}I-OIH. The former will be inaccurate if the patient's position during renography is not the same as during roentgenography. The latter method delays the renogram until the sites of the kidneys are accurately defined.

TECHNIQUE. If the renogram is being made to assess renovascular hypertension, no food or drink is to be taken by the patient after the preceding midnight. Just before the test the patient empties his bladder. The patient assumes a comfortable sitting position, with his arms resting on a desk, and the collimators of the renal probes are placed next to the back at approximately the sites of the kidneys. With our equipment, the distance between the faces of the crystals and the back is 22 cm. ^{131}I-OIH (30 μCi.) is given intravenously, and the probes are positioned immediately. The patient is encouraged to sit quietly for one-half hour with the probes in place. At the conclusion of the test, the bladder is again emptied; the urine is assayed for ^{131}I, and its specific gravity and volume are checked to evaluate renal concentrating ability.

INTERPRETATION. Figure 7–26 depicts a normal renogram with key points indicated. Six indices based on these four points have been analyzed in normal subjects (Table 7–6). The two kidneys of a subject can be compared with each other or with those of another subject.

From a series of normal subjects we have calculated the indices with regard to the average value of B (the peak). In our laboratory, the average counting rate of B is 24,300 c.p.m. after a dose of 30 μCi. With other equipment and doses, once B is determined, the other indices can readily be calculated.

As a first approximation, the height of A is related to the size of the vascular bed (largely but not exclusively renal) beneath the probe; the slope from A to B is related to the ERPF and the slope from C to D, to the urinary flow rate as well as to ERPF.

Figure 7–27 illustrates a series of renograms from patients with progressively severe unilateral renal vascular stenosis. The upper left panel is normal. The upper center panel shows a modest functional impairment, but with clearance phases equal and normal; excretion in the right kidney is delayed. The upper right panel shows further derangement of function; uptake is diminished and excretion is delayed. The remaining panels show progressively more severe diminution of uptake.

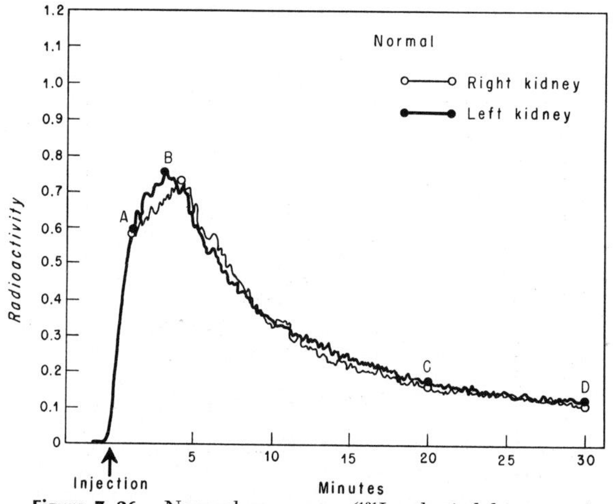

Figure 7–26. Normal renogram (^{131}I-ortho-iodohippurate). *A* represents end of sudden increase in radioactivity as vessels beneath probe fill with tracer; *B* is peak uptake; *C*, at 20 minutes, and *D*, at 30 minutes, arbitrarily define the slope of the decreasing curve. (From J. E. Wenzl, W. N. Tauxe, E. C. Burke, J. C. Hunt, and G. B. Stickler: Radioisotope renography in children. I. The renogram in children without renal disease. Pediatrics, *36*:120, 1965. By permission of the Charles C Thomas Publishing Company.)

Table 7–6. CHARACTERISTICS OF NORMAL RENOGRAM*

	MEAN HEIGHT (RANGE) AS PER CENT OF PEAK	NORMAL VARIATION BETWEEN SIDES AS PER CENT OF PEAK
A	62 (45-94)	25
B_{peak}†	100	26
B - A	35 (20-54)	18
C_{20}	27 (12-49)	15
D_{30}	17 (11-31)	7
t_o to B_{peak}	3.6 min. (2.5-6.0)	2.0 min.

*Patient dehydrated and in sitting position during measurement.

†Normal mean value for B is 24,300 by our technique; this has been assigned the value 100 per cent.

Renal Scintigraphy. Several labeled compounds have been used for imaging the kidneys. Two isotopes of mercury—^{203}Hg and ^{197}Hg—can be used to label chlormerodrin. The 46.6-day half-life of ^{203}Hg and the tendency of chlormerodrin to persist in the kidney for long periods render its use unwarranted. The half-life of ^{197}Hg is only 65 hours and its gamma ray energy is more suitable for imaging on scanner or scintillation camera. Figure 7–28 is a chlormerodrin scan showing normal renal tubular architecture.

When labeled with ^{131}I, the ortho-iodohippurate and diatrizoate can also be used for imaging. OIH, which generally yields the most informative scintigram, passes through the normal kidney so rapidly that a scintillation camera is used for this procedure. It is often interesting to sum the counts emitted over each kidney during the imaging process, i.e., to plot a renogram and to correlate the images with the renographic curves. Indeed, it is advantageous to sample the plasma at 40 minutes for the mathematical analysis described previously.

In this way one may derive from a single injection, renal images, renography, and an estimate of ERPF.

Figure 7–29 illustrates data from a case of ureteropelvic junction obstruction by such a technique.

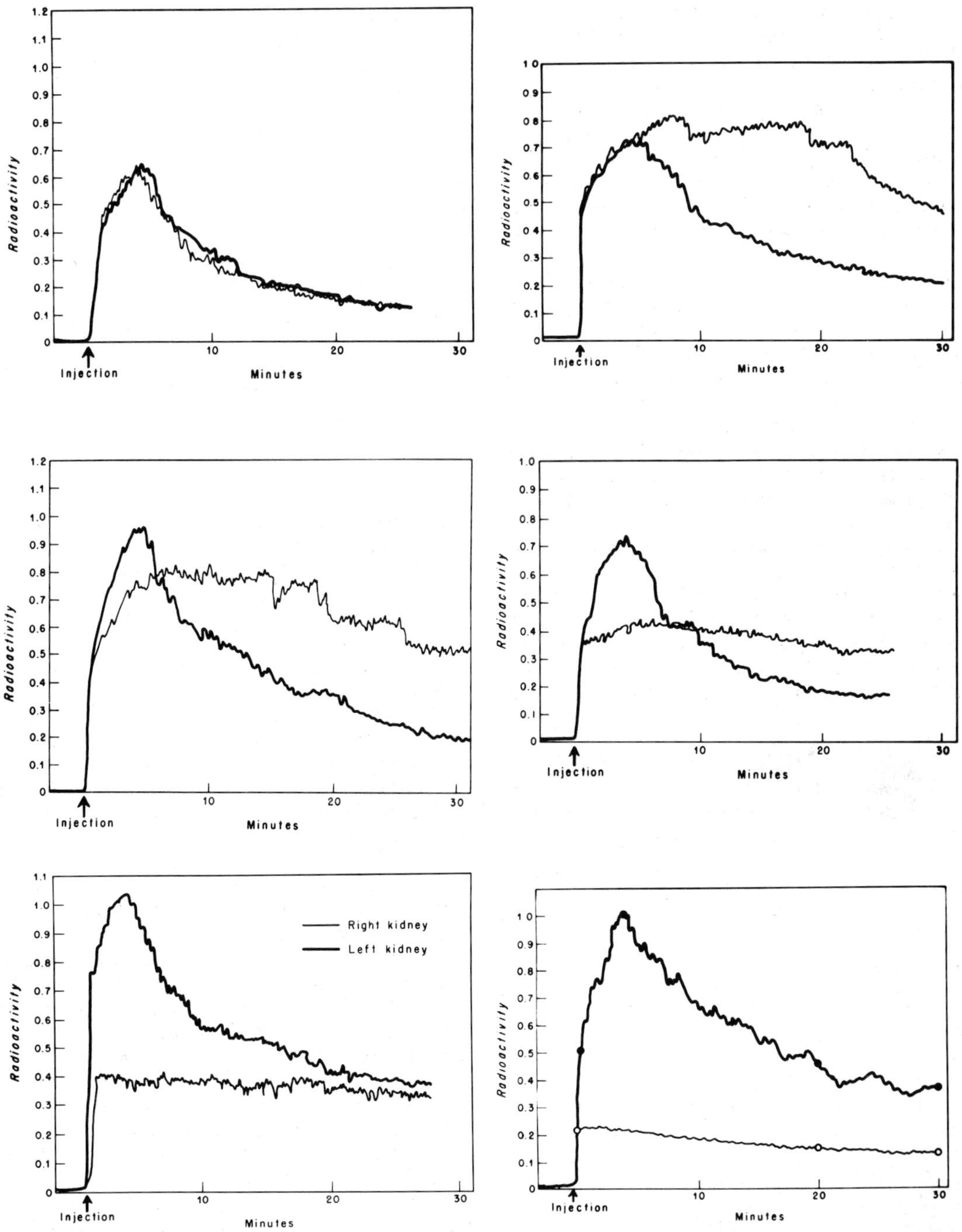

Figure 7–27. Series of ^{131}I-OIH renograms, progressively more abnormal from left to right in upper and then lower rows.

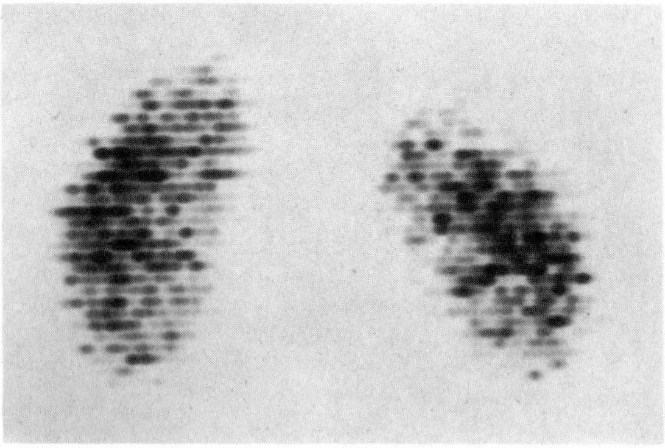

Figure 7–28. Scan of normal kidneys (^{197}Hg-chlormerodrin). (From W. N. Tauxe and J. C. Hunt: Evaluation of renal function by isotope techniques. Med. Clin. N. Amer., 50:937, 1966.)

Hematologic Tests

Plasma Volume. If a radioactive substance mixes readily with the plasma compartment of the body after intravenous injection, it affords a method for measuring the plasma volume by the principle of radionuclide dilution. The more rapidly the injected substance leaves the blood stream, the more difficult the estimation of the plasma volume. Thus, human albumin labeled with ^{131}I is currently the most popular indicator because it leaves the blood stream relatively slowly and can be measured accurately in small samples of blood. The patient need not be fasting, as is required for dye methods of estimating plasma volume.

TECHNIQUE. A reasonable approximation of the plasma volume may be made by collecting a single sample of blood about 15 minutes after injection of 25 μCi. of ^{131}I-albumin (^{131}IHSA, iodinated human serum albumin). If the interval is too short, mixing throughout the less accessible components of the vascular tree (such as the spleen) is incomplete. If the interval is too long, a significant amount of the label will have diffused into extravascular spaces and the apparent plasma volume will be too large.

For a degree of precision not usually required in clinical practice, two or preferably three samples of blood are collected at intervals (5, 10, and 20 minutes) after injection of the ^{131}IHSA. A line connecting the plotted values on semilogarithmic paper and extending back to the time of injection gives a very accurate estimation of the plasma volume because extrapolation to the concentration of ^{131}IHSA at zero time eliminates the effect of diffusion of the albumin out of the blood, yet the samples have been collected over a sufficient period to

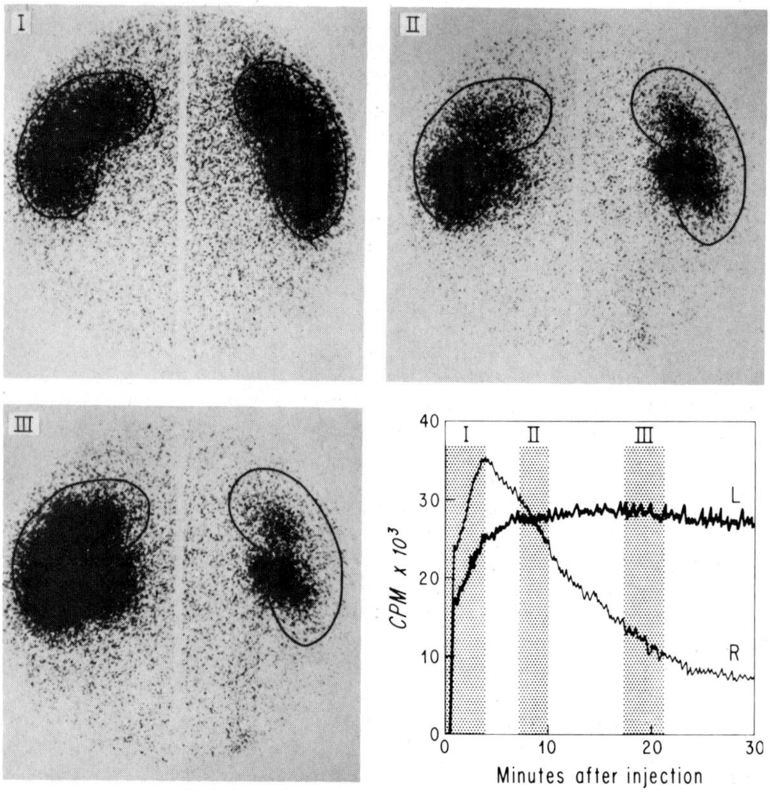

Figure 7–29. Simultaneous sequential scintigraphic images and renographic presentations after injection of ^{131}I-ortho-iodohippurate (OIH) in a patient with left ureteropelvic junction stricture. Shaded areas indicate imaging times and durations.

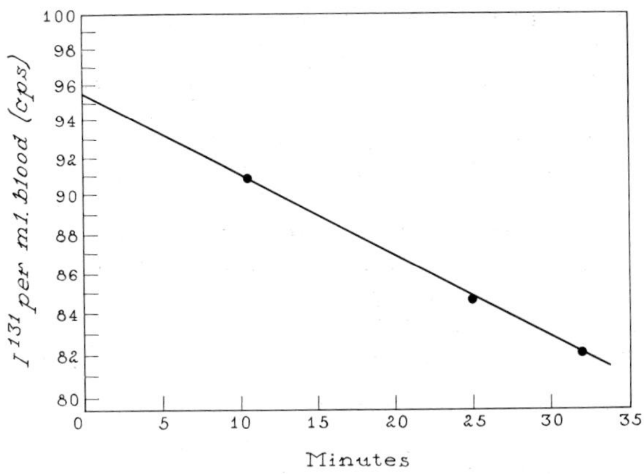

Figure 7–30. Disappearance of ^{131}I-labeled human serum albumin during estimation of plasma volume. (From C. A. Owen, Jr.: DIAGNOSTIC RADIOISOTOPES. Springfield, Illinois, Charles C Thomas, 1959. By permission of the publisher.)

permit reasonably thorough mixing (Fig. 7–30).

With either method the plasma volume (ml.)

$$= \frac{\text{net c.p.s. in dose}}{\text{net c.p.s. in 1 ml. of plasma}}.$$

Erythrocyte Volume. The principle for measuring the volume of circulating erythrocytes is the same as that for measuring the plasma volume: labeled erythrocytes are injected intravenously and the extent of dilution of the label, after thorough mixing, is a measure of the erythrocyte volume. However, the method is technically more difficult because the erythrocytes must be labeled *in vitro* with sterile precautions. On the other hand, erythrocytes do not diffuse out of the vascular tree, as do plasma proteins, so that a single withdrawal of blood is sufficient.

TECHNIQUE. The commonly used method consists of collecting blood into a citrate anticoagulant, labeling the erythrocytes with ^{51}Cr, returning the labeled cells to the circulation, sampling the blood after about 15 minutes, and calculating the extent of dilution of the injected label.

1. Under sterile conditions, withdraw 10 ml. of venous blood and inject into a sterile vial containing 2 ml. of Strumia ACD anticoagulant (2.55 gm. Na_2-citrate · H_2O, 0.80 gm. citric acid, and 1.20 gm. glucose made up to 100 ml. with water).

2. Add about 100 μCi. of sodium ^{51}Cr-chromate solution. Mix occasionally for 15 minutes, then convert all free chromate to chromic ion by adding 50 mg. of sterile ascorbic acid in solution. Mix thoroughly, but do not shake or permit foaming.

3. Inject 10 ml. of the labeled blood intravenously.

4. After 12 to 15 minutes, withdraw 6 to 7 ml. of blood with EDTA as anticoagulant. Determine hematocrit value.

5. Count the ^{51}Cr in 5 ml. of the second sample of blood and compare it with a standard of 1 ml. of a hundredfold dilution of the blood used for the dose (add 4 ml. of saline to the standard so that its volume is the same as that of the sample). The dose is 10 ml. × 100 × c.p.s. in the standard. The erythrocyte volume (ml.) is

$$\frac{\text{net c.p.s. in entire dose}}{\text{1/5 of net c.p.s. in 5-ml. sample of blood} \div \text{hematocrit}}$$

Normal values for plasma volume and red cell volume in liters may be expressed by the simple formulas shown in the table that follows. Surface area is expressed in square meters, derived from the standard DuBois equation.

Surface area (71.84) × (Ht. in cm.)$^{0.725}$ × (Wt. in kg.)$^{0.425}$

	MALES	FEMALES
Plasma volume	1.63 × SA (±.357)	1.41 × SA (±.241)
Red cell mass	1.1 × SA (±.208)	0.84 × SA (±.135)

Owing to the ease of measuring both plasma and erythrocyte volumes separately, it is no longer necessary to be encumbered with the quite large error of estimating the one from the other. In fact, modern clinical evaluation of patients with plasma or erythrocyte volume problems requires the greater precision afforded by the separately measured volumes.

TECHNIQUE

1. Withdraw 10 ml. of venous blood sterilely and leave the needle in the vein. Inject the blood into a sterile vial containing 2 ml. of Strumia ACD solution through one needle while air escapes through a second needle in the rubber stopper. Mix gently.

2. Inject an exactly known volume of ^{131}IHSA (about 25 μCi.) (prepared before step 1) through the needle left in the antecubital vein and withdraw the needle. Note the time.

3. Add about 100 μCi. of sodium ^{51}Cr-chromate solution to the vial containing the 10 ml. of blood and 2 ml. of anticoagulant. Swirl the vial gently and intermittently for 12 minutes. Stop the erythrocyte labeling process by adding a sterile solution containing 50 mg. of ascorbic acid.

4. Remove exactly 10 ml. of the well-mixed ^{51}Cr-labeled blood from the vial into a syringe and set the syringe aside.

5. Withdraw about 10 ml. of blood from the patient, but not from the vein used for the injection of the ^{131}IHSA. This sample, anticoagulated with EDTA, is to be used to determine the plasma volume and should be drawn 15 minutes after the injection of the ^{131}IHSA. Leave the needle in the vein.

6. Through the second needle left in the vein inject the 10 ml. of ^{51}Cr-labeled blood (from step 4).

7. After 12 to 15 minutes, withdraw 6 to 7 ml. of blood and anticoagulate it with EDTA. This sample is used to measure the erythrocyte volume. Determine the hematocrit value (Wintrobe or microhematocrit) on this sample.

8. *Preparation of standards.* Inject an amount of ^{131}IHSA identical to the dose given the patient (preferably from the same syringe; this can be done conveniently just before the syringe is refilled with the dose to be given to the patient) into a 200-ml. volumetric flask. Make up to volume with saline. Use a 1-ml. aliquot for the plasma volume standard (1/200th of the dose) and make up in the counting tube to 2 ml. by addition of 1 ml. of saline.

For the erythrocyte volume standard, thoroughly swirl the ^{51}Cr-labeled blood remaining in the labeling vial and then pipette 1 ml. into a 100-ml. volumetric flask. Make up to volume with saline. After thorough mixing, remove 5 ml. for the standard (1/200th of the dose). Centrifuge the aliquot and discard the supernatant fluid. Fill this tube with distilled water to the same height as the patient's packed red cells; hemolysis insures uniform distribution.

9. *Preparation of patient's plasma and erythrocytes.* Centrifuge the blood collected in step 5, pipette 2 ml. of the plasma into a counting tube, and count radioactivity. Centrifuge exactly 5 ml. of the blood collected in step 7. Remove the plasma. Wash the packed cells three times with saline to remove all ^{131}IHSA from the cells. The final packed cell mass is counted.

10. *Calculation.* Plasma volume (ml.) =

$$\frac{\text{net c.p.s. in plasma standard}}{\frac{1}{2}\text{ of net c.p.s. in 2 ml. of plasma}} \times 200.$$

Erythrocyte volume (ml.) =

$$\frac{\text{net c.p.s. in erythrocyte standard}}{\frac{1}{5}\text{ of net c.p.s. in erythrocytes from 5 ml.}}$$

× 200 × hematocrit value of patient's blood. (Multiplying the observed hematocrit value by 0.96 increases the accuracy because about 4 per cent of the packed erythrocyte mass is trapped plasma.)

Measurement of Blood Loss. In men, "invisible" loss of blood is restricted to the gastrointestinal tract because hematuria, hemoptysis, and epistaxis are readily apparent. In women, menstrual blood loss is often overlooked because most women have no standard against which to compare the volume of their menstrual flow. In patients with obscure hypochromic anemia, unwarranted loss of blood must also be considered in addition to the malabsorption problems. Although a careful history of menstrual blood loss and accurate chemical tests of fecal blood may solve a number of the clinical problems, occasionally quantitation of fecal and menstrual blood loss is clinically useful.

TECHNIQUE. Quantitation of blood loss involves labeling the circulating erythrocytes with ^{51}Cr, as for a blood volume estimation, except that 150 to 200 μCi. of ^{51}Cr is used. The radioactivity in fecal or menstrual material is then compared with that due to ^{51}Cr in the circulating blood so that the blood loss can be expressed in milliliters of blood.

Fecal radioactivity can be measured in an entire stool specimen. The reference standard is prepared by diluting 10 ml. of anticoagulated blood from the patient to about the same volume (height) and counting both the standard and the specimen in identical stool cartons. Menstrual blood is counted by placing the blood-soaked pads or tampons, wrapped in plastic film (Saran Wrap), in a stool carton; the reference standard (10 ml. of the patient's blood) may be placed on a pad or tampon to approximate the geometry of the sample. Increasing the distance between the tampon and the crystal increases the accuracy of the assay by minimizing the difference in counting efficiency between the edge and the center of the crystal. For precise analyses, a dome constructed to the curvature of the isointensity line passing through the edge of the crystal should be mounted over the crystal. This equalizes counting efficiency at all points over the surface of the crystal.

INTERPRETATION. The amount of ^{51}Cr in a 24-hour collection of feces usually approximates the ^{51}Cr in 1 to 2 ml. of blood; we do not consider the blood loss to be abnormal until it exceeds 3 ml. in 24 hours. A normal menstrual flow contains a total of only 30 to 60 ml. of blood; hypochromic anemia is not likely to occur unless more than 100 ml. is lost each month.

Iron-binding Capacity of Serum. A number of the plasma proteins function in a transport capacity. Of importance is the iron-carrying protein (iron-binding protein, transferrin, siderophilin). Iron entering the plasma pool binds to transferrin and is normally carried to the marrow (and iron-containing enzyme synthesizing sites). Nontransferrin bound iron is preferentially deposited in the liver.

The total iron-binding capacity (TIBC) is the sum of the serum iron level and the amount of iron which can be added to serum before the iron-binding capacity is saturated. Peters and co-workers (1956) have described a chemical method for measuring this capacity, based on supersaturating the iron-binding sites of serum with iron. The excess unbound iron is removed with a resin and the iron level in the serum (TIBC) is measured. The difference between the iron concentration in the serum before and after saturation is the latent iron-binding capacity (LIBC) or unbound iron-binding capacity (UIBC).

The ease with which ^{59}Fe can be measured suggests its use to indicate the amount of iron which must be added to serum to saturate the LIBC. This may be carried out as a modification of Peters' method.

TECHNIQUE

1. Pipette 1.0 ml. of serum into a test tube and add 1.0 ml. of ^{59}Fe-iron saturating solution.* Mix and let stand for 10 minutes at room temperature.
2. Add 5 ml. of barbiturate buffer† and not less than 120 mg. of treated IRA-410 resin.‡ Mix thoroughly for 15 minutes.
3. Centrifuge until the supernatant fluid is clear and pipette 4 ml. into a counting tube.
4. Prepare a standard by mixing 1 ml. of the ^{59}Fe-iron saturating solution with 6 ml. of water. Pipette 4 ml. into a counting tube.
5. Count the ^{59}Fe in the standard and serum samples.
6. Calculation:

$$\frac{\text{net c.p.s. of standard}}{\text{net c.p.s. of serum sample}} = \frac{\mu\text{g. Fe standard}}{\mu\text{g. added Fe bound to transferrin (LIBC)}}$$

or LIBC

$$= \frac{\text{c.p.s. of serum sample} \times \mu\text{g. Fe standard}}{\text{c.p.s. of standard}}$$

and TIBC = LIBC plus endogenous serum iron concentration.

INTERPRETATION. The TIBC of normal serum is about 300 to 350 μg. per 100 ml., of which about two-thirds is LIBC. Although the serum iron level fluctuates widely during the day, that expressing the serum iron concentration as a percentage of the TIBC provides some useful information.

*^{59}Fe-iron saturating solution. Pipette an amount of $^{59}FeCl_3$ equivalent to 250 to 300 μCi. into a 1000-ml. iron-free volumetric flask. Add 20 mg. of anhydrous $FeCl_3$ (or 33.3 mg. of $FeCl_3 \cdot 6H_2O$) (equivalent to 6.9 mg. of iron). Add 4 drops of concentrated ammonium hydroxide and wash down the sides with about 10 ml. of iron-free water. Warm the flask to about 56° C. and add enough citric acid to dissolve all the rust-colored precipitate, leaving a clear yellow solution. Add about 500 ml. of iron-free water and 4 drops of bromothymol blue indicator; the color should be deep yellow. Add dilute ammonium hydroxide (concentrated ammonium hydroxide diluted tenfold) until the solution is pale lime green. Fill the flask to the 1000-ml. mark and mix. The iron concentration is about 7 μg./ml. (6.9 plus 0.1 from the radioiron solution). The solution should be refrigerated.

†Barbiturate buffer. Put 6.4 gm. of NaCl and 2.3 gm. of sodium barbiturate (Veronal) into a 1000-ml. volumetric flask and dissolve them in 400 to 500 ml. of iron-free water. Add and dissolve 6 gm. of diethylbarbituric acid. Fill to the mark with iron-free water and mix. The pH is 7.5 and must not be permitted to fall below 7.

‡Resin. Only the larger particles (20 to 40 mesh) of IRA-410 anion resin are used. Suspend the resin in water and discard the slowly sedimenting particles. Wash the resin successively in 3 N HCl, iron-free water, and barbiturate buffer. Dry at 95° C. For the test, 120 mg. (half of a No. 1 Coor's scoop) is minimally adequate; two scoopfuls are used to insure complete removal of nonprotein-bound iron.

In iron deficiency anemias, the TIBC often increases to about 450 μg. per 100 ml. of serum. If the TIBC is lower than normal, liver damage and protein deprivation are likely possibilities. Saturation of the TIBC is often approached in hemolytic anemia, pernicious anemia, and aplastic anemia. It may also be saturated in hemochromatosis, cirrhosis, and certain refractory anemias, in which states iron is often deposited in the liver. The LIBC is characteristically increased during pregnancy and during therapy with estrogens (Table 9–66 and p. 654).

Erythrocyte Survival. The average life-span of normal human erythrocytes is approximately 120 days. When it is significantly shortened by hemolytic disease, there is usually direct evidence of hemolysis (increased serum bilirubin and fecal urobilinogen values). Milder hemolytic states may be obscure, so the ability to measure erythrocyte survival is occasionally useful.

^{51}Cr as chromate is currently the radionuclide of choice for labeling erythrocytes. This is because it has a gamma ray of convenient energy, it can attach itself to the hemoglobin of erythrocytes *in vitro*, and when erythrocytes are destroyed *in vivo*, the ^{51}Cr is no longer in the chromate form and cannot label other erythrocytes. However, it has one drawback: once the labeled cells are returned to the patient's circulation, some of the ^{51}Cr leaks out of intact erythrocytes. The ideal label should remain firmly bound to the cells until they disintegrate. ^{59}Fe is an example of such a nuclide, but it can label human erythrocytes only *in vivo;* furthermore, iron is reutilized when hemoglobin is released from effete erythrocytes. The simplicity of *in vitro* labeling of erythrocytes with ^{51}Cr is undoubtedly responsible for the wide use of this nuclide.

TECHNIQUE. An aliquot of the patient's blood is labeled with 150 to 250 μCi. of sodium ^{51}Cr-chromate, just as for a blood volume determination, and reinjected. Small samples of blood are drawn every 1 or 2 days for 10 to 14 days. These and an aliquot of the dose are counted at the same sitting. The ^{51}Cr of each sample can be compared with a single standard and no decay corrections are required.

The ^{51}Cr in each sample, expressed as per cent of dose per milliliter (or usually per liter in order to have whole numbers), is plotted on arithmetic paper, and a line is drawn through the dots, by visual fit.

If C_0 is the concentration of ^{51}Cr on day zero (by extrapolation) and C_{10} is the concentration on the tenth day, the percentage decrease per day is $\frac{C_0 - C_{10}}{10 \times C_0} \times 100$ or $\frac{C_0 - C_{20}}{20 \times C_0} \times 100$, etc.

INTERPRETATION. The laboratory technique

for evaluating erythrocyte survival with ^{51}Cr is simple. The interpretation is somewhat more complicated. Once the circulating erythrocytes are labeled, values for residual ^{51}Cr are determined frequently enough to establish a straight line, and the survival of erythrocytes is expressed as the slope of the line. The graphic presentation may be on arithmetic or on semilogarithmic paper. Neither method is actually correct because the disappearance of ^{51}Cr from the blood is the sum of two processes, an exponential one (^{51}Cr leaches from the cells at a rate of about 1 per cent per day) and an arithmetic one (erythrocyte death is normally about 0.8 per cent per day). The sum of an arithmetic curve and a logarithmic curve is not represented by either, so either form of presentation is simply a convenient compromise.

The logarithmic graphic presentation probably is the usual compromise. Normally the ^{51}Cr disappears from the blood with a half-time of about 30 to 40 days. This can be converted to per cent per day by the standard formula:

$\frac{\ln 2}{t_{1/2}}$ or $\frac{0.693}{t_{1/2}} \times 100$, or about 2 per cent per day normally.

We prefer arithmetic plotting of the data because of the ease of calculating the disappearance rate of the ^{51}Cr. It is simply the reduction of radioactivity between any two specific times divided by the number of days in the period, but this concept is valid for only the first 20 to 30 days. Thus, if the initial radioactivity decreases by 40 per cent in the first 20 days, the calculation is $\frac{40 \text{ per cent}}{20 \text{ days}} = 2$ per cent per day.

By either method of calculation a normal value of about 2 per cent per day is obtained. Since ^{51}Cr is leaching out at the rate of 1 per cent per day, erythrocytic senescence is assumed to account for the other 1 per cent per day, which is in reasonably good agreement with the accepted death rate of 0.8 per cent per day.

Three factors significantly complicate estimation of erythrocyte survival by the ^{51}Cr technique: blood loss, change in hematocrit value, and recent transfusions.

It is apparent that loss of blood (hemoptysis, melena, hematuria, epistaxis, menstruation) or extravasation of the labeled blood into tissues will reduce ^{51}Cr in the blood to the extent that labeled cells leave the circulation (Fig. 7–31). If the bleeding is unrecognized or unsuspected, apparently severe hemolytic disease will be interpreted incorrectly, as in continuous bleeding from esophageal varices. Because ^{51}Cr from labeled cells in the gut is essentially unabsorbable, measurement of fecal ^{51}Cr is an accurate method for estimating loss of blood by this route. It is wise to measure

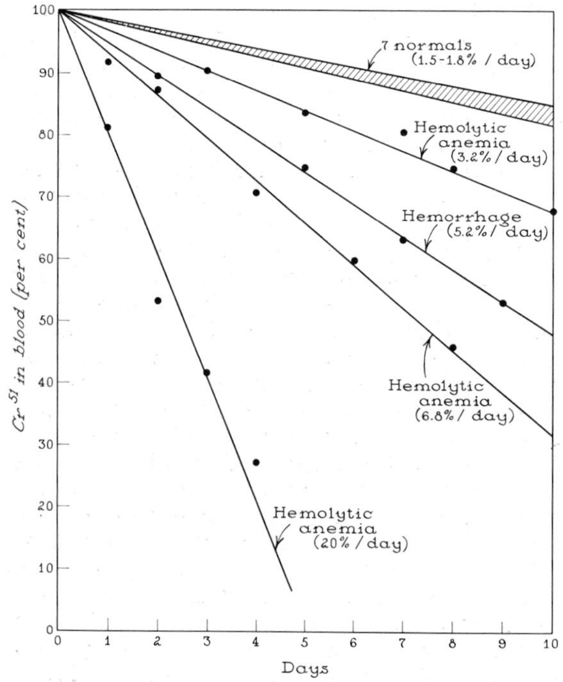

Figure 7–31. Accelerated rates of disappearance of ^{51}Cr-labeled erythrocytes from the blood of three patients with hemolytic anemia and one patient with gastrointestinal hemorrhage. (From C. A. Owen, Jr.: DIAGNOSTIC RADIOISOTOPES. Springfield, Illinois, Charles C Thomas, 1959. By permission of the publisher.)

fecal ^{51}Cr in any patient in whom erythrocyte survival seems to be shortened.

If the hematocrit value remains approximately constant, synthesis of new erythrocytes and loss of old ones is in equilibrium. In such circumstances, calculation of the rate of disappearance of ^{51}Cr from the blood is simple. In a patient with depressed synthesis of erythrocytes and normal erythrocyte survival, the hematocrit value decreases steadily and the ^{51}Cr disappearance curve is distorted as the plasma volume increases. The reverse situation occurs in an anemic patient when the hematocrit value is suddenly increased by transfusions. Survival times corrected for changing hematocrit values are not nearly so accurate as those obtained when no transfusions are given during the study. If the patient has received several units of blood shortly before erythrocyte survival is to be measured, it may be more appropriate to label normal erythrocytes for the test rather than the senescent, transfused cells circulating in the patient.

Recently Shih has described a simplified, faster, more accurate and more discriminating method of estimating red cell survival, based on urine counting. Furthermore, it permits a lower dosage of radioactivity to the patient. One labels the erythrocytes in the usual way, then collects complete urines for 5 days in 24-hour lots and expresses the radioactivity in each specimen in terms of percentage dosage injected. These values are subtracted successively from 100 per cent on day zero. A line is drawn through the points plotted on semilogarithmic paper; the half-life is derived. Half-life values in normal subjects were reported as 42 to 62 days. Values less than 42 days were seen in patients with accelerated hemolysis and values above 62 days were observed in patients with excessive loss (e.g., gastrointestinal or menstrual). We have found this test particularly helpful and have made it our basic routine procedure.

Disappearance of Plasma Iron. Whereas chromium studies are concerned with blood quantification and its destruction, the use of radioiron affords the capability of studying erythrocyte production.

Because of the differences of the gamma ray energies of ^{51}Cr and ^{59}Fe, one may be quantitated in the presence of the other.

When a soluble salt of ^{59}Fe mixed with plasma is injected intravenously, it disappears at the rate that unlabeled iron is being extracted from the plasma. The two controlling factors are the avidity of the tissues (normally, the marrow) for iron and the concentration of iron in the plasma. Because both factors are equally important in evaluating the turnover of plasma iron, both must be measured. The plasma iron concentration is measured chemically; the radioiron is measured by sampling the blood at 10- and 15-minute intervals for 2 to 3 hours after injection of the ^{59}Fe. The ^{59}Fe values in the plasma should decrease along a straight line when plotted on semilogarithmic paper. From the line the half-time is calculated and, in turn, the rate from the equation: rate $= \frac{\ln 2}{t_{1/2}} = \frac{0.693}{t_{1/2}}$, or $\frac{69.3}{t_{1/2}}$ if the rate is expressed as per cent. Thus, if the $t_{1/2}$ is 80 minutes, the rate of clearance of the ^{59}Fe from the plasma is 0.87 per cent per minute. This value multiplied by the concentration of iron in the serum yields the amount of iron cleared per minute. The usual expression converts the iron turnover to the amount removed from the entire plasma volume per 24 hours and is normally about 40 mg. of iron.

It is apparent that exactly the same amount of stable iron is being removed from the plasma if the plasma iron level is 100 μg per 100 ml. and the rate 2 per cent per minute or if the plasma iron level is 200 μg. per 100 ml. and the clearance rate is 1 per cent per minute or if the plasma iron level is 10 μg. per 100 ml. and the clearance rate is 20 per cent per minute. Thus, expressing iron turnover simply in terms of the radioiron disappearance rate alone is not very meaningful.

One important precaution in assessing the clearance of plasma iron is that the latent iron-binding capacity (LIBC) should not be exceeded by the amount of iron in the radioactive solution. The only sure method is to measure the LIBC beforehand. If it is small or nil, the radioactive iron may be mixed with normal plasma before injection. If the patient's LIBC is adequate, his plasma may be used to bind the labeled iron. In either case the iron should be incubated with plasma for about 15 minutes before injection to insure complete binding of the iron to the transferrin.

In Vivo Localization of Radioiron. After intravenous administration of ^{59}Fe, the destination of the radioiron leaving the plasma may be determined by external scintillation crystals directed toward marrow (manubrium, lower vertebrae, iliac crest), spleen (if this organ has regained erythropoietic function), or liver. If erythropoiesis is satisfactory, the tissue ^{59}Fe should begin decreasing by the second day and be matched by the appearance of labeled erythrocytes in the circulation.

^{59}Fe-labeled Erythrocytes. Regardless of the site of erythrocytic synthesis, the effectiveness of the mechanism can be evaluated by the rate and amount of ^{59}Fe returned to the blood in erythrocytes. Normally about 70 per cent of an intravenously injected dose of ^{59}Fe will have been returned to the circulation in labeled erythrocytes within 7 to 10 days. Higher values reflect iron-deficiency states; lower values are associated with abnormalities of erythropoiesis (vitamin B_{12} or folic acid deficiency or damaged or destroyed bone marrow). Accurate estimation of the amount of ^{59}Fe in erythrocytes depends on precise knowledge of erythrocyte volume; this should be estimated with ^{51}Cr before the radioiron study is begun.

Tests of Gastrointestinal Tract and Spleen

Absorption of orally administered substances may be demonstrated by detecting the substance in the blood, urine, or target organ (^{131}I in the thyroid gland or ^{57}Co-labeled vitamin B_{12} in the liver); it may be quantitated by measuring the amount excreted in the feces. Although the last method is the traditional one, it involves the assumption that all the test substance in the feces represents unabsorbed material, and this is not always true. For example, copper is absorbed from the gut but is also excreted, to a small extent, into the lumen, and a major excretory pathway is via the bile and thence the feces.

Tests of absorption of labeled vitamin B_{12} and labeled iron will be described in detail. These are the only tests of gastrointestinal absorption that have clinical application today.

Absorption of Vitamin B_{12} (Schilling Test). Because each molecule of vitamin B_{12} contains an atom of cobalt, vitamin B_{12} can be labeled with radiocobalt (^{60}Co initially, ^{57}Co now). Patients with pernicious anemia (deficient in intrinsic factor) are unable to absorb the vitamin. Although various tests to measure malabsorption of labeled vitamin B_{12} have been devised, only one is commonly used in the clinical laboratory. Measurement of fecal excretion of unabsorbed vitamin is accurate but requires 5 to 7 days. Hepatic concentration of labeled vitamin B_{12} can be assessed after all unabsorbed vitamin has disappeared from the intestinal tract, but the amount in the liver is hard to calculate quantitatively.

The Schilling test for evaluating absorption of vitamin B_{12} is an indirect one and does not actually measure the amount absorbed. The test consists of injecting a relatively massive dose of nonradioactive vitamin B_{12} (1000 μg.) 2 hours after an oral dose of the labeled vitamin. About one-third of the absorbed vitamin is "flushed" out of the blood into the urine. The presence of little or no radioactivity in the urine indicates negligible gastrointestinal absorption.

TECHNIQUE

First Day

1. Be sure patient has been fasting for at least 12 hours. No laxatives are to be used during the test.
2. Give 1 capsule of radioactive vitamin B_{12} (about 0.5 μg. of vitamin B_{12} and 0.5 μCi. of ^{57}Co) orally.
3. Two hours later, while the patient is still fasting, inject 1 mg. of nonradioactive vitamin B_{12} intramuscularly.
4. Start collection of urine after the injection and continue for 22 to 24 hours. Emphasize to the patient the importance of complete urine collection.

Second Day

1. Count standard solution* of ^{57}Co-labeled vitamin B_{12}.
2. Bring the patient's urine to a volume of 1800 ml. (or other designated volume) by addition of water. Count the ^{57}Co with a scaler equipped with a pulse-height selector (differential mode).
3. Divide the net c.p.s. in urine by the net c.p.s. of the standard and multiply by 100 to get percentage of the dose in the urine.
4. If the excretion is more than 8 per cent of the dose (normal), the test is completed. If it is less than 8 per cent (abnormal), the patient is given another capsule of the radioactive vitamin B_{12} plus a capsule of intrinsic factor. The injection of nonradioactive vitamin B_{12} is given 2 hours later and the 24-hour collection of urine is begun as before.

INTERPRETATION. Normal subjects excrete more than 8 per cent of a 0.5-μg. dose during a 24-hour period (range, 8 to 38 per cent) (Fig. 7–32).

Less than 8 per cent excretion may be interpreted as malabsorption (pernicious anemia, sprue or other malabsorptive syndromes, di-

*A standard solution should be made with each new shipment of capsules. One capsule is dissolved in 1800 ml. of water, or in some other convenient volume, in a bottle similar to the one given the patient. A wetting agent (Tergitol) is added to keep the standard in solution. Care should be taken to insure that any settled radioactive material is evenly distributed before counting.

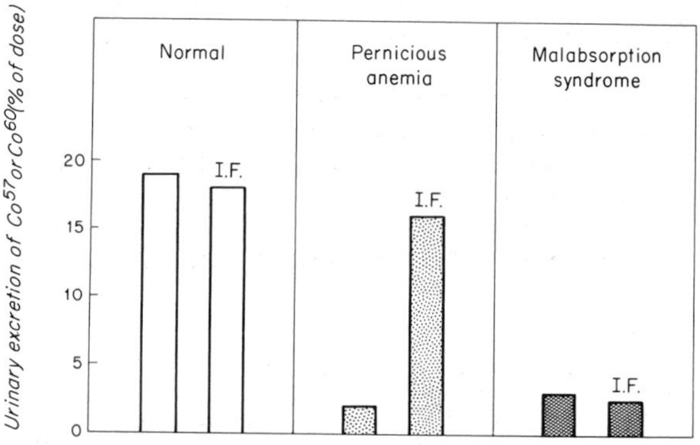

Figure 7–32. Responses to oral administration of intrinsic factor in the Schilling test of vitamin B_{12} absorption.

verticulosis, or infestation with *Diphyllobothrium latum*) or as inadequate excretion (which may occur in advanced uremia). In our experience the actual urinary excretion is less than 4 per cent of the dose in patients with pernicious anemia. Greater than 8 per cent excretion occurs after the administration of intrinsic factor in patients with pernicious anemia; this also occurs in patients with uremia when delayed excretion from the first day is carried over into the second day.

At times a patient with classic pernicious anemia may fail to show an adequate response to the dose of intrinsic factor if he has been taking it therapeutically. This presumably results from formation of antibodies to the intrinsic factor (which is usually of porcine origin). Such patients may absorb vitamin B_{12} if the oral dose is accompanied by human intrinsic factor. Generally this response is only about half that found in patients who have never been treated with intrinsic factor. Other conditions in which gray zone values are obtained include diabetes mellitus and Hashimoto's thyroiditis.

Iron Absorption. Bonnet and associates (1960) attempted to find an oral dose of iron which would lead to about 50 per cent absorption in normal persons and allow measurement of both hyperabsorption and hypoabsorption. The selected dose, 50 μg. of iron as a soluble salt, was absorbed by normal males to the extent of about 40 per cent and by normal menstruating females to about 60 per cent. Since there was no relationship between individual values and the hemoglobin level of the blood, it appears to be a true sex difference, perhaps related to the continued needs of the female for iron.

TECHNIQUE

1. Into a 50-ml. volumetric flask, place 100 μg. of iron from the stock solution,* about 2 μCi. of ^{59}Fe-ferrous citrate of high specific activity, and 600 mg. of ascorbic acid. Dilute to volume with distilled water.

2. Pipette 25 ml. into a plastic drinking cup. Have the patient drink the solution plus a rinse of the cup.

3. Collect all stools until any one specimen contains less than 1 per cent of the dose. Calculate fecal ^{59}Fe as per cent of dose (count an aliquot of the unused portion of the solution to determine the dose). The ^{59}Fe may be measured in whole stool specimens or in aliquots which have been homogenized with added water.

4. Absorption (per cent)

$$= \frac{\text{dose minus total fecal excretion}}{\text{dose}} \times 100.$$

INTERPRETATION. The average absorption is 40 per cent in men and 60 per cent in women. In iron deficiency, absorption may exceed 90 per cent of the dose; in steatorrhea, less than 10 per cent may be absorbed.

Scintigraphy of the Liver. A number of compounds which can be made radioactive tend to accumulate in the liver and are potentially useful for making hepatic scintigraphic images. Two general types are employed, radioactive dyes and radioactive particles. These obviously measure different hepatic functions. Advantages and disadvantages can be cited for both types. ^{131}I-labeled rose bengal has been most suitable in our experience for the former and technetium-labeled sulfur colloid most advantageous for the latter. The chief goal of both approaches is usually to determine whether tumors are present and to locate them.

The sulfur colloid images show the distribution of the reticuloendothelial system in both liver and spleen; this is usually an advantage, but at times images of the two organs are difficult to separate. In addition to its tumor-locating capability, the dye image provides information on the liver's capacity to clear dye from the blood stream (as a BSP clearance) and also provides information on the transit time through the liver and the location of post-hepatic bile pathways. Its chief disadvantage is the fact that it is labeled with ^{131}I, whose beta energy limits the dose that can be given to the patient (because of its high irradiation) and whose gamma ray energy is less efficiently detected and resolved on a scintillation camera than is that of ^{99m}Tc.

By far the most commonly used radiopharmaceutical at this time is technetium sulfur colloid (TSC); however, this may change if ^{123}I becomes available as a label for rose bengal.

TSC is most conveniently prepared from commercially available kits. Owing to the short half-life of ^{99m}Tc, labeling and preparation are usually carried out in the institution where the scintigraphy is made. Injection of 1 or 2 mCi. of the preparation will produce detectable images in 100 seconds.

Six images are usually carried out: liver–anterior, posterior, and right lateral; spleen–anterior, posterior, and right lateral. If rose bengal is used, imaging time is usually so long and the transit time through the liver so short that the use of six views is not feasible. Rather it is a good idea to use a scanner and to obtain multiple anterior views–one during the first

*Stock solution of iron. Make up 7.0213 gm. of $Fe(NH_4)_2(SO_4)_2 \cdot 6\,H_2O$ plus 3 ml. of concentrated sulfuric acid to 1000 ml. with distilled water (1 mg. iron/ml.). Dilute 1 ml. to 100 ml. with water (plus 2 to 3 drops of concentrated H_2SO_4) to yield a 10 μg./ml. stock solution.

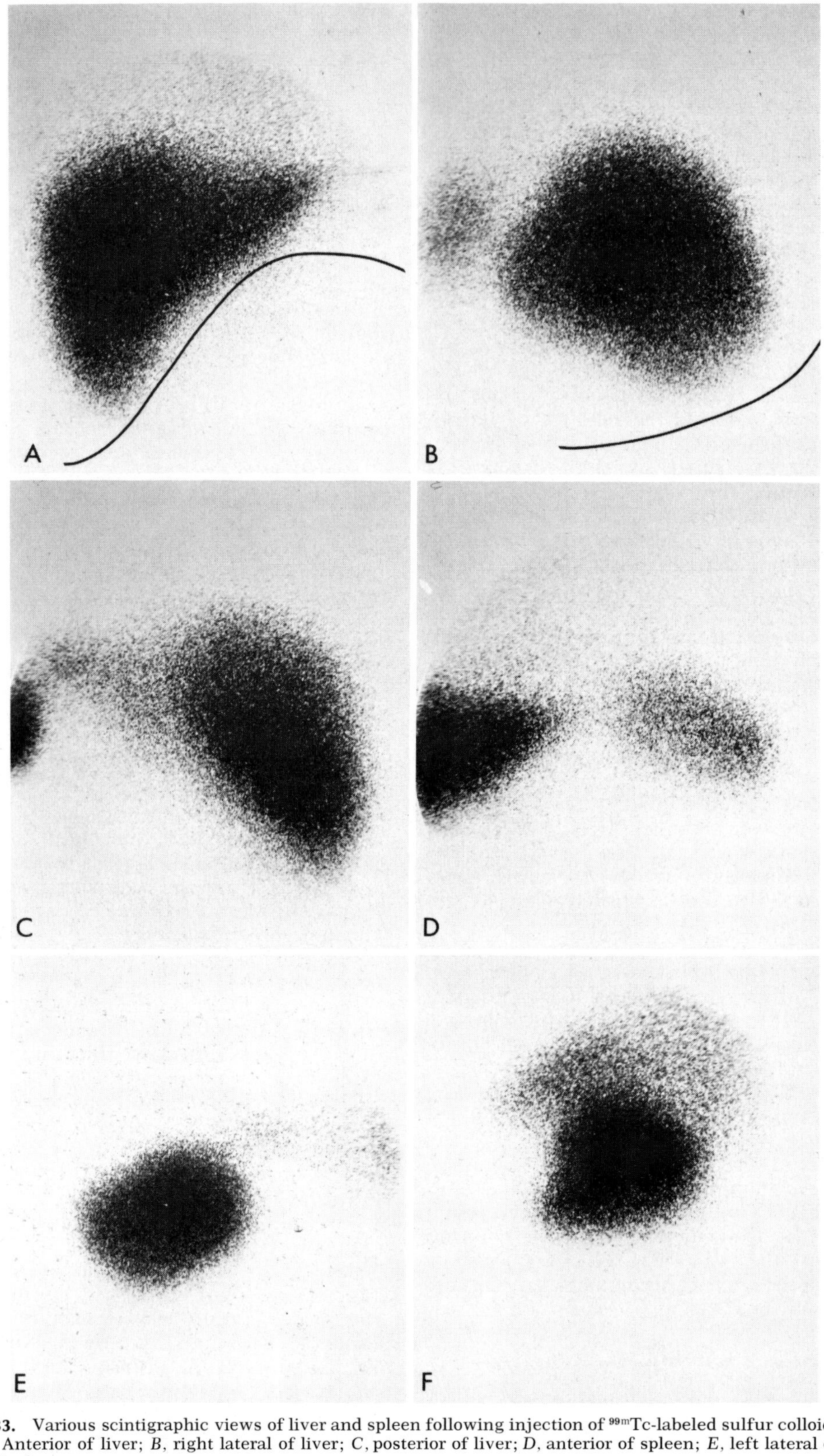

Figure 7–33. Various scintigraphic views of liver and spleen following injection of ^{99m}Tc-labeled sulfur colloid in a normal subject. *A*, Anterior of liver; *B*, right lateral of liver; *C*, posterior of liver; *D*, anterior of spleen; *E*, left lateral of spleen; *F*, posterior of spleen.

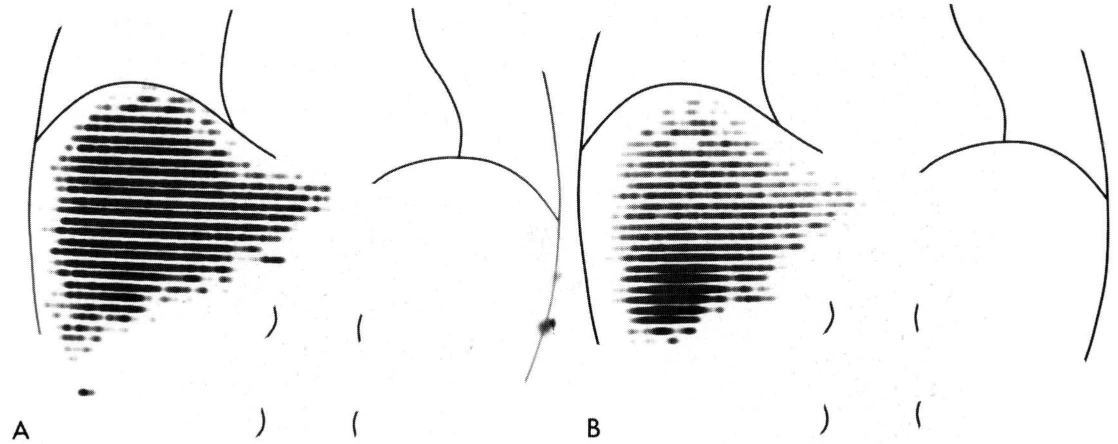

Figure 7–34. Anterior scintigraphic views of the liver made after the injection of ^{131}I-labeled rose bengal in a normal subject. *A*, First half hour only the liver is seen. *B*, Second half hour both liver and gallbladder are seen. The liver is paler.

half hour when maximal concentration occurs over the liver, and one during the second half hour after injection to permit the visualization of the bile pathways. Typical normal liver images following the injection of TSC and rose bengal are depicted in Figures 7–33 and 7–34.

When neoplastic disease of the liver is suspected, it is often convenient to apply a life-size representation of the liver against the patient's abdomen in order to guide a biopsy needle to the most likely spot for diagnosis. In such a case body landmarks must be utilized carefully. Figure 7–35 depicts an image of a typical liver containing metastatic cancer.

In cirrhosis, uptake is likely to be low over the liver and high over an enlarged spleen, as shown in Figure 7–36. When rose bengal is used, uptake over the liver is low and the transit time is delayed. Cysts, abscesses, and so forth, are likely to appear as voids in the liver image.

It is sometimes useful to assess the size of the spleen. Fischer has presented a regression equation for estimating splenic weight by the surface area of the left lateral view. We rou-

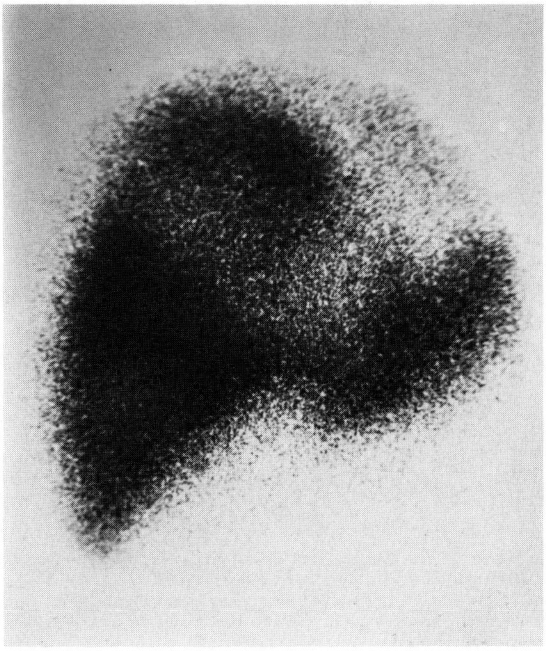

Figure 7–35. Anterior scintigram of the liver in a patient with hepatic metastatic disease. ^{99m}Tc-sulfur colloid was the radiopharmaceutical used.

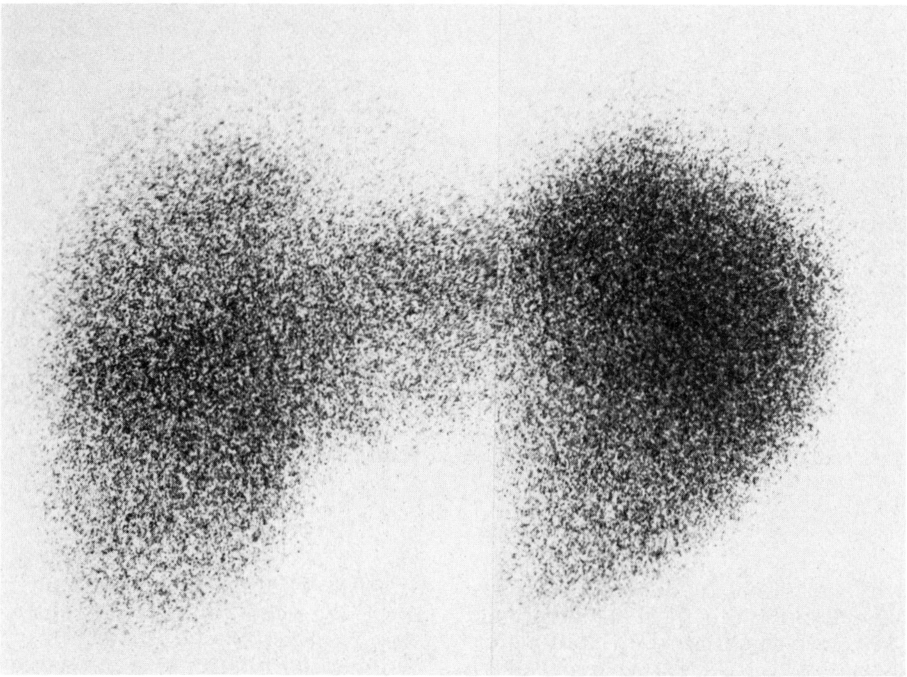

Figure 7-36. Anterior scintigram of the liver and spleen in cirrhotic patient after the injection of ^{99m}Tc-sulfur colloid. There is generally low uptake over the enlarged liver that is somewhat irregular. Uptake is elevated over the spleen and it is enlarged (estimated weight: 470 gm.).

tinely report these results and have found useful the graph shown in Figure 7-37.

Pancreas. Imaging of the pancreas using the methionine analog methoselenamine has proved occasionally useful, occasionally not. We have found that when the pancreas is clearly seen and appears to be normal, the chances are high that a normal gland will be found at surgery. If the pancreas is not clearly seen, the finding has little meaning (Fig. 7-38).

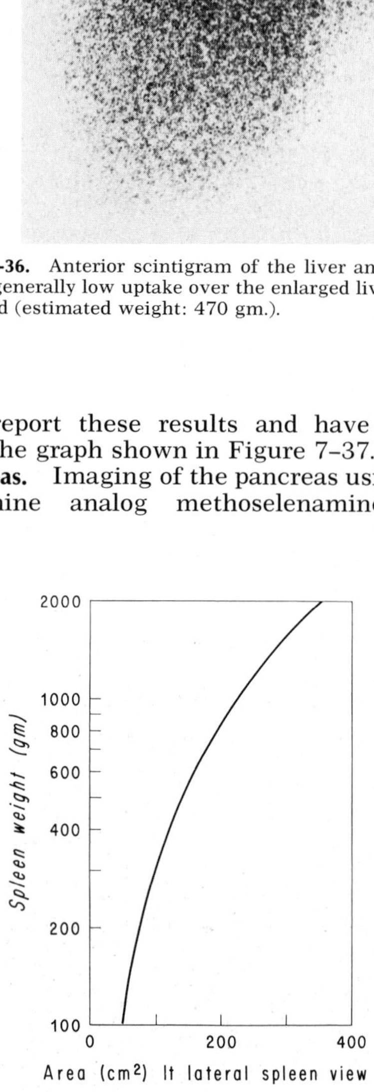

Figure 7-37. Estimation of spleen weight by Fischer's technique (Ref. Verh. Dtsch. Ges. Med. *69*:798, 1963.) The surface area of the spleen in the left lateral projection, obtained by planimetry, is related to weight by a power function from data derived empirically.

Neurological Applications

Brain Imaging. Over the years the brain has been imaged with numerous radiopharmaceuticals under a wide variety of circumstances. From this experience has developed a rather generally accepted technique.

We routinely use ^{99m}Tc as the pertechnetate and image both laterals, anterior and posterior, and the vertex 2 hours after injection. If vascular lesions are suspected we also image immediately after injection.

Indeed, one achieves two types of images. The one taken immediately after injection produces a picture principally of the blood pools of the head; the later one reflects the permeability of the blood vessels of the head, the point of interest being the fact that there is little uptake over the normal brain owing to the blood-brain barrier.

The vascularity of a given lesion may be assessed by early views, the permeability of

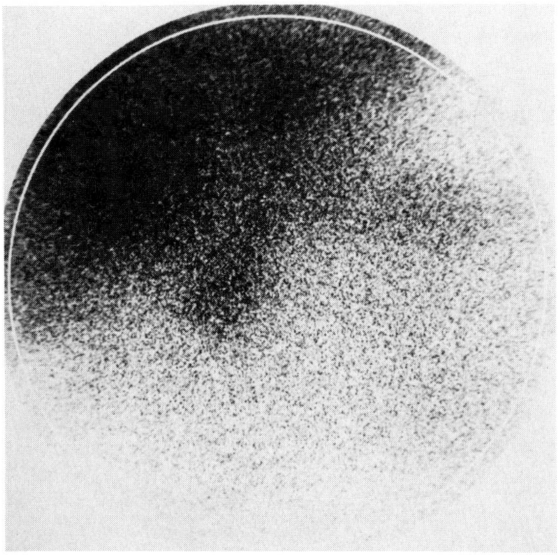

Figure 7–38. Scintigraphic image of the right upper quadrant in a normal subject after the injection of ^{75}Se-methselenamine ("selenomethionine"). Uptake is seen over protein-synthesizing structures, liver and pancreas. The detector is tipped 25 degrees from the horizontal and the two lower major gamma peaks of the ^{75}Se are summed. The image required 10 minutes.

the blood vessels by the later ones. Since even by using the scintillation camera, where individual views may take only from 100 to 300 seconds, scheduling problems may exist and one may have to choose an imaging time that will maximize the probability of detecting both vascular and cellular processes. We have found this to be from 2 to 3 hours after injection. One regularly finds early views that are negative in the face of positive 2-hour views, but the reverse is quite rare indeed. If one finds a positive 2-hour view and wishes to assess vascularity, it is a simple matter to repeat the process the next day.

Figure 7–39 depicts the normal brain (2-hour views). Note that the pertechnetate, being effectively a halide, accumulates in the salivary glands and, as has been noted, in the thyroid. It also has a tendency to accumulate in the choroid plexus, where false positive interpretations may occur. To block uptake by the plexus we routinely administer orally 30 minutes before pertechnetate dosing 30 ml. of a 1 per cent solution of potassium perchlorate syrup. Since this also interferes with the thyroid trapping mechanism, thyroid function studies using radioactive materials should precede brain

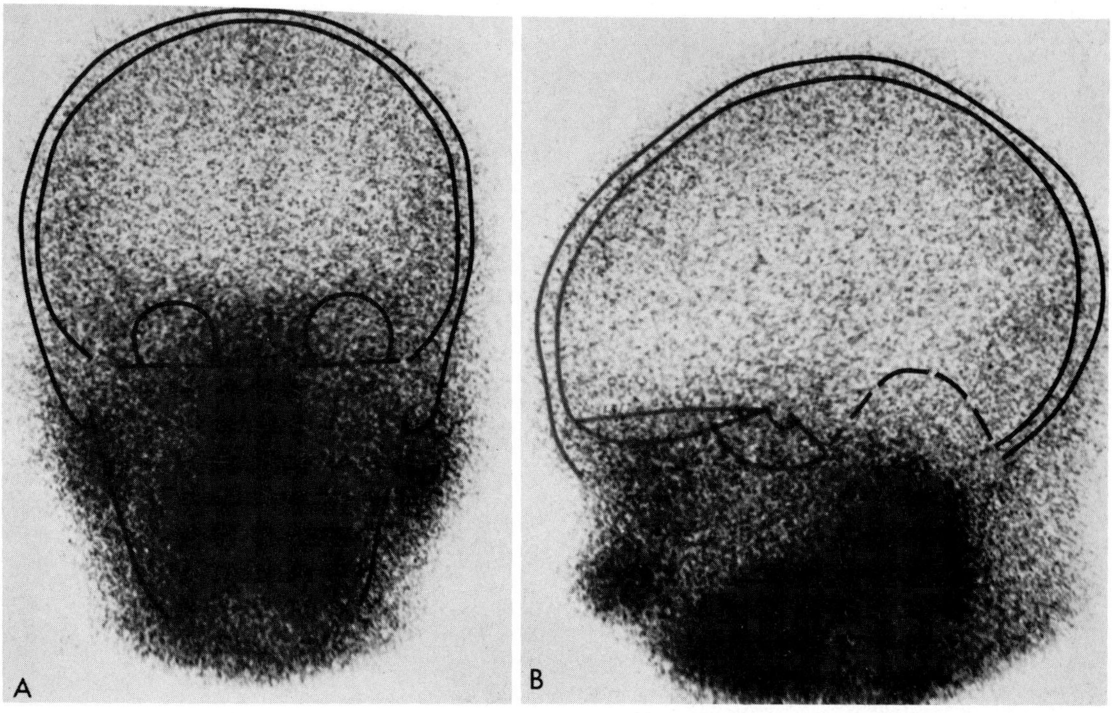

Figure 7–39. Scintigraphic images of the normal brain; anterior (*A*) and left lateral (*B*) made two hours after injection of pertechnetate.

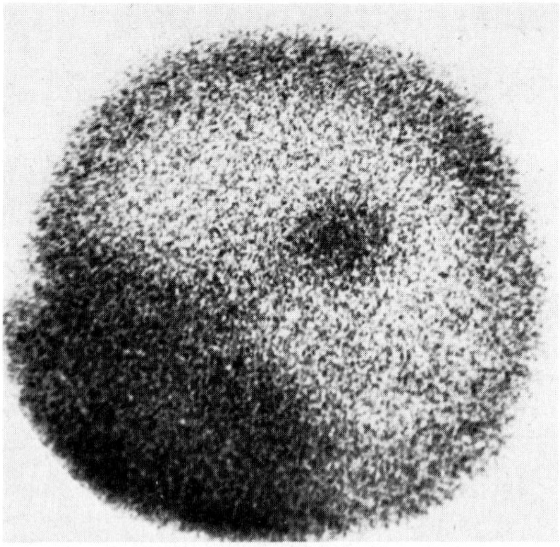

Figure 7–40. Left lateral scintigram of patient with meningioma after injection of pertechnetate.

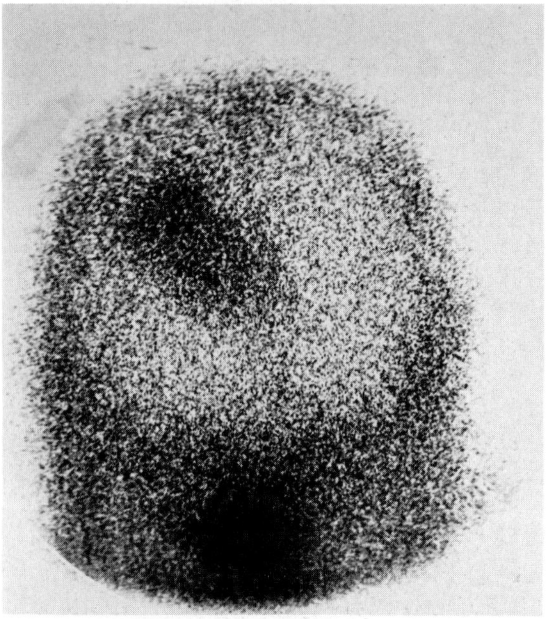

A

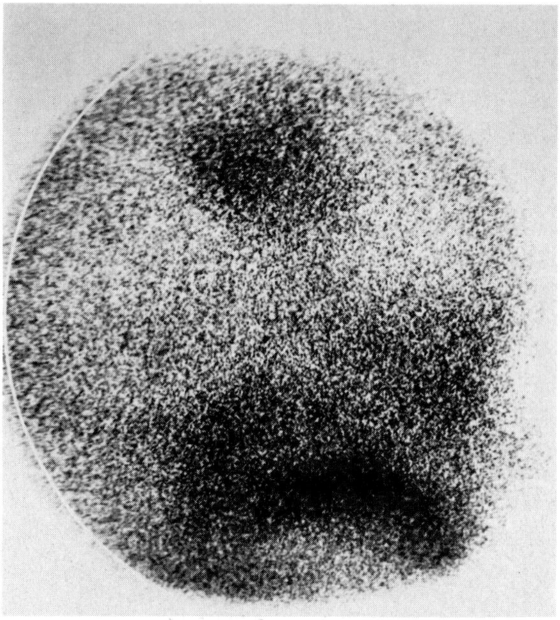

B

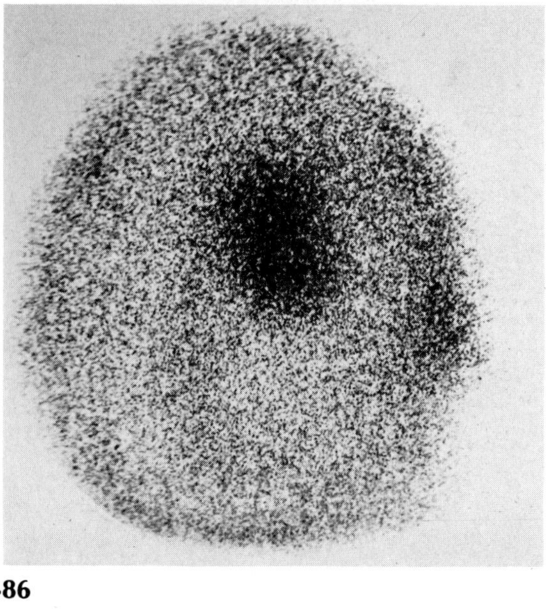

C

Figure 7–41. Anterior (*A*), right lateral (*B*), and vertex (*C*) views of a patient with an astrocytoma.

imaging. This dose does not completely block uptake of pertechnetate by the thyroid. When not in use, perchlorate should be kept in a sealed cabinet. It can explode!

Figure 7–40 illustrates the typical meningioma – spherical, near meninges, with intense uptake.

Figure 7–41 depicts the typical astrocytoma–irregular, generally slower to accumulate the radioactive material, and within the substance of the brain.

Subdural hematomas are usually more evident on later images. Early views (Figure 7–42) were completely negative. Later views (Figure 7–43) are strongly positive.

Metastatic lesions are often multiple (Fig. 7–44).

Brain abscesses, metastatic foci, strokes, and other tumors are usually positive. Simple cystic lesions are usually negative.

Cisternography. Recently the determination of the distribution of kinetics of cerebral spinal flow has become a test of clinical importance. Normally the CSF is assumed to be formed in the choroid plexus, to pass through the foramina of Luschka and Magendie, to bathe the spinal cord, and to exit via the pacchionian granulations.

If for any reason, the outflow pathways around the base of the skull become blocked prior to the passage of the CSF over the cerebral hemispheres, the CSF is diverted back into the ventricular system with a resultant communicating hydrocephalus whose clinical consequences (dementia and motor disturbances) can often be reversed by a shunting procedure. The use of scintigraphy in the diagnosis is therefore very important.

Since the CSF moves rather slowly, it is not possible to use the usual short-lived nuclides for imaging. Moreover, since the smaller molecules are thought to diffuse freely out of the subarachnoid space, it is recommended that macromolecules be used. Therefore, ^{131}I-labeled human serum albumin is the reagent of choice for this test.

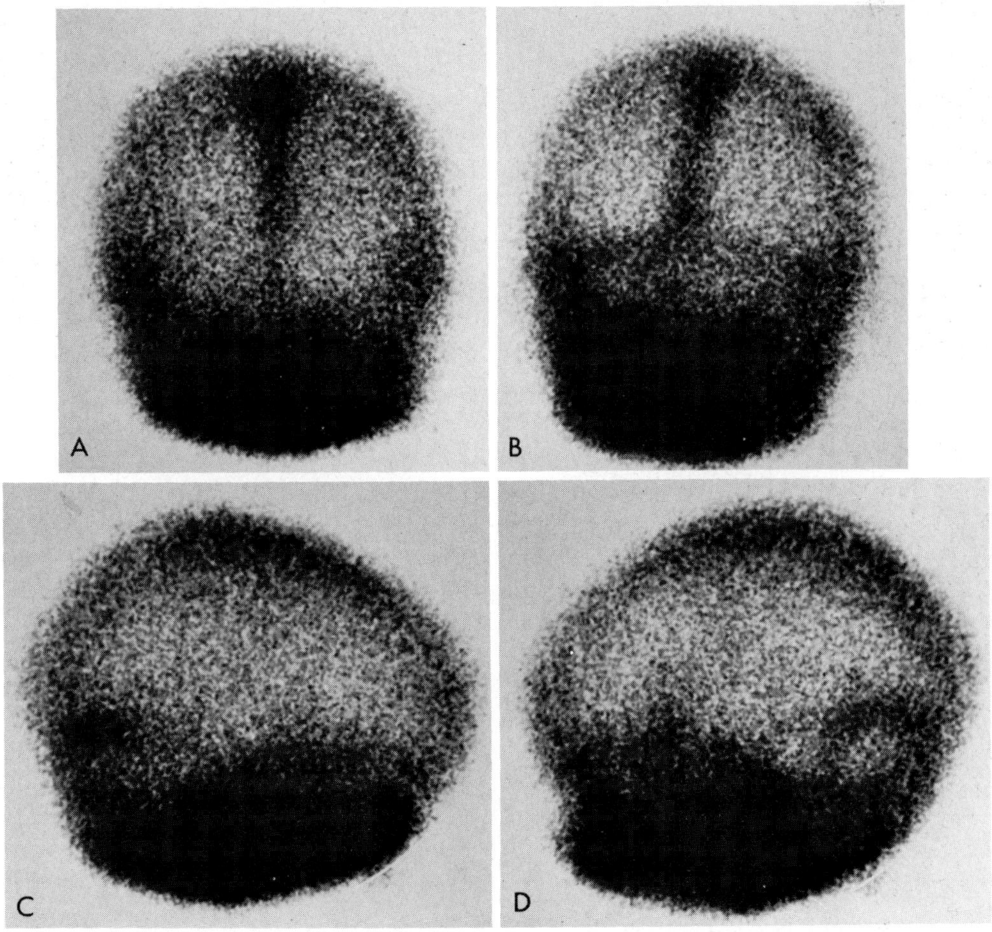

Figure 7–42. Images made in a patient with bilateral subdural hematoma. Anterior (*A*), posterior (*B*), right and left lateral (*C* and *D*) views made immediately after injection are negative.

To perform the test it is convenient to inject up to 200 μCi ^{131}I-HSA into the subarachnoid space by lumbar puncture. To avoid leakage around the site of injection, the patient should be placed in the Trendelenburg position for 3 hours and in a comfortable recumbent position for the next 3. Images made at 6 hours (Fig. 7–45*A*) normally show the radioactivity around the base of the brain. By 24 hours it is seen over the convexity and concentrated at the level of the pacchionian granulations (Figure 7–45*B*).

In Figure 7–46 may be seen the abnormal pathway into the lateral ventricles. It has been observed that the most favorable surgical results obtain when the activity remains in the lateral ventricles up to 48 hours. (At times it may be found there earlier, then over the convexity.) Surgery in such patients has, in general, not had striking results.

Lung. Scintigraphy of the lungs was first effected by the use of ^{131}I-macroaggregated human serum albumin. More recently ^{99m}Tc-

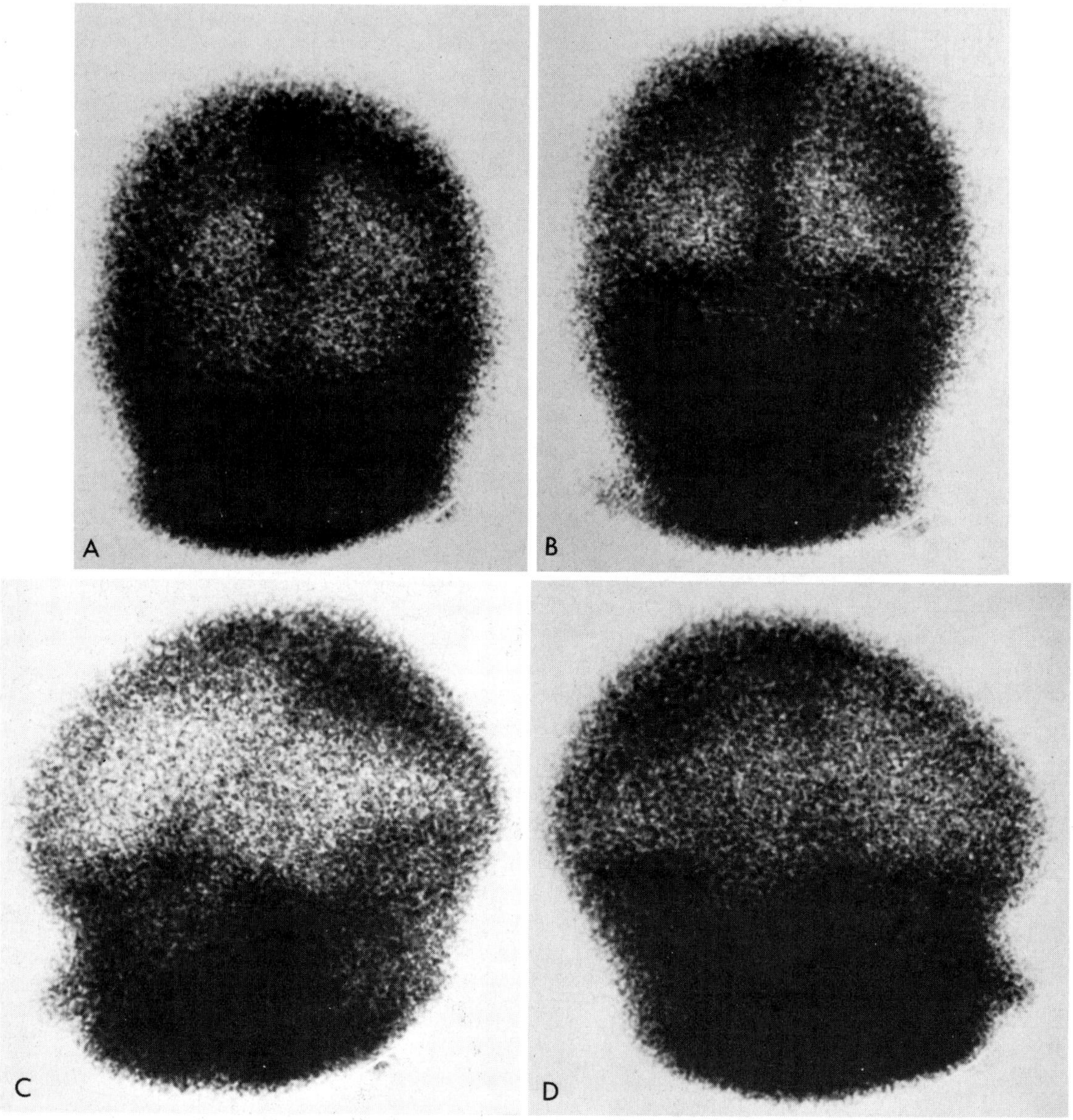

Figure 7–43. Images made in the patient with bilateral subdural hematoma shown in Figure 7–42. These views were made two hours after injection and clearly illustrate the crescent shaped peripheral lesions on all four views [anterior (*A*), posterior (*B*), right lateral (*C*), left lateral (*D*)].

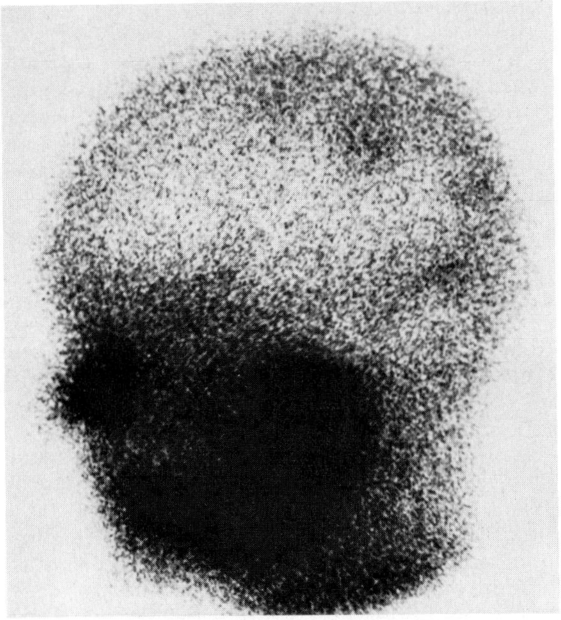

Figure 7-44. Left lateral image of a patient with metastatic disease of the brain made two hours after injection of pertechnetate. Multiple foci of uptake are evident.

labeled aggregates or microspheres have been found to be more efficacious; both may be conveniently prepared from commercially available kits.

Images made following the injection of these radiopharmaceuticals into the antecubital vein are possible because of temporary blockade of a minute fraction of the capillary bed in the lungs; therefore, they reflect the distribution patterns of pulmonary perfusion. Because of this, they are most useful in the diagnosis of pulmonary embolus, elevated pulmonary artery pressure, alpha-1 antitrypsin deficiency, and right-to-left shunts.

Perfusion images of the lungs can also be effected by the injection of xenon gas (^{133}Xe) dissolved in saline.

Ventilation patterns may be imaged after inhalation of the radioactive xenon gas. This technique allows for rapid sequence imaging and thus also permits kinetic studies of pulmonary function. These have proved useful in the diagnosis of pulmonary embolism, early emphysema, and early bronchial disease, as well as other diseases which have been difficult to diagnose in the past.

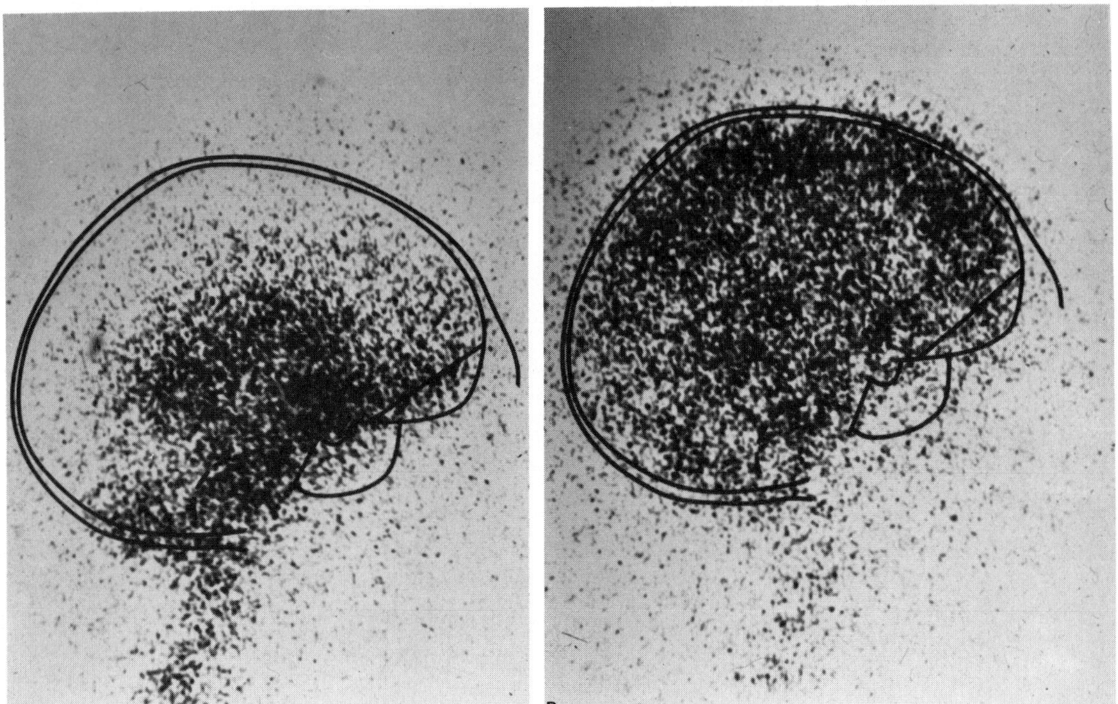

Figure 7-45. Cisternogram (right lateral view). Normal distribution of ^{131}I human serum albumin six (*A*) and 24 hours (*B*) after injection into the subarachnoid space in the lumbar region. Activity is seen over the basal cisterns in *A* and over the convexity of the brain, accumulating in the region of the pacchionian granulation in *B*.

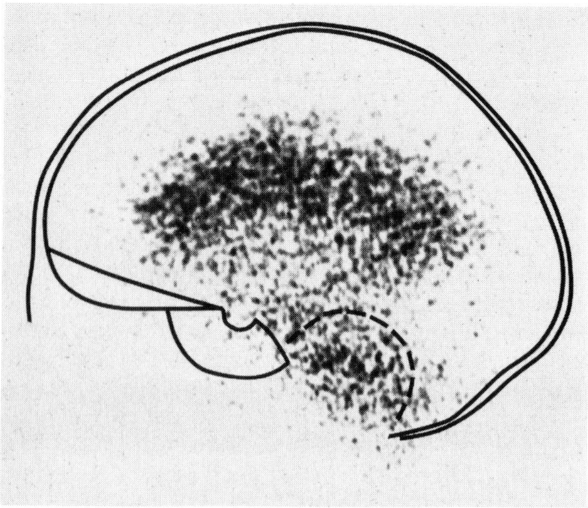

Figure 7–46. Abnormal cisternogram (left lateral view). Accumulation of ^{131}I albumin is seen in the lateral ventricles after injection into the lumbar subarachnoid space.

Figure 7–47 depicts perfusion (microspheres) and ventilation (inhaled xenon) studies in the normal lung. Figure 7–48 (*A* and *B*) depicts the distribution seen in a case of pulmonary embolization. This patient had, as is often the case, a normal chest roentgenogram.

Figure 7–48*A* reveals the normal xenon ventilation distribution characteristic of this process, whereas *B* reveals a highly abnormal perfusion pattern. In bronchial disease, both ventilation and distribution patterns are abnormal and usually identical.

Figure 7–49 illustrates a case of alpha-1 antitrypsin deficiency. In cases of right-to-left shunting, extrapulmonary activity may be seen to be high.

In order to know exactly the precise lung outlines at the time of a study it is often desirable to use a large plane source of a low energy emitter placed behind the patient. This is known as a *transmission* image. Figure 7–50 illustrates an example effected by use of technetium-99m.

Bone. Conventional x-rays have been shown to be diagnostic of something less than half of cases of neoplastic disease of bone. Scintigraphic procedures have been found to be positive in approximately 95 per cent; therefore, bone scintigraphy has obviously become of great importance in the nuclear medicine laboratory.

Numerous radiopharmaceuticals have been used, but for convenience, economy, low degree of radiation hazard, and availability we have found the reagent of choice to be ^{99m}Tc polyphosphate. Figure 7–51 shows a whole body camera image of a patient with multiple metastases. Roentgenographic findings in this case were negative.

^{99m}Technetium diphosphate yields similar scintigraphic images.

Healing fractures, Paget's disease, and lymphomas may also yield positive images.

Blood Pool Images. Frequently it is useful to make images of various blood pools: suspected aneurysms, the heart, or the placenta.

It is often difficult to diagnose abnormal accumulation of fluid in the pericardial sac by roentgenography alone because the heart and the fluid around it appear as a solid, even-textured shadow.

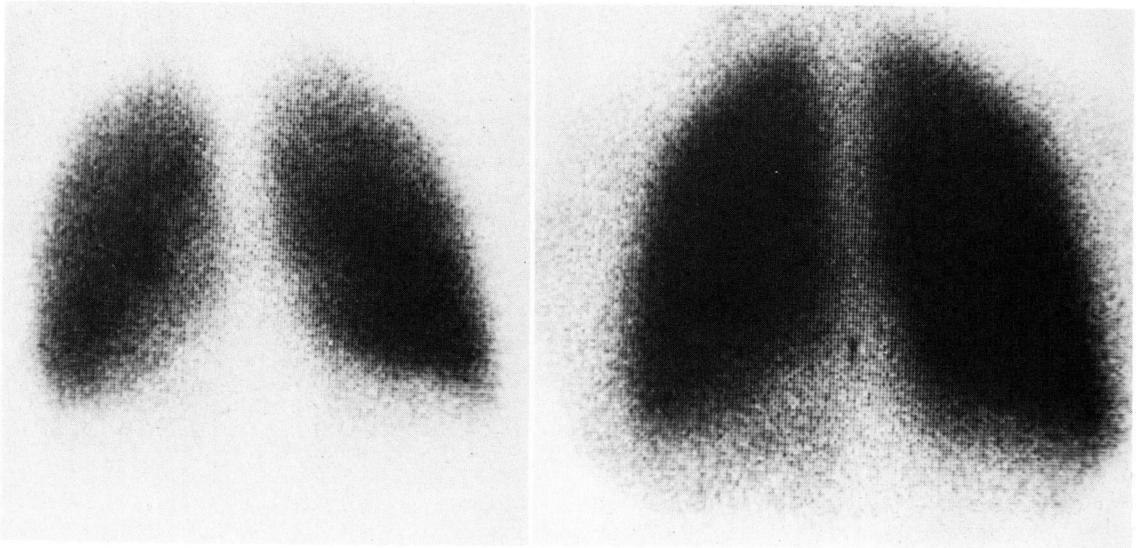

A B

Figure 7–47. Normal lung images made after the injection of technetium-labeled microspheres (*A*) and the inhalation of radioactive xenon (*B*) at equilibrium. These were viewed by the scintillation camera from the posterior aspect of the chest. No perfusion defects are noted.

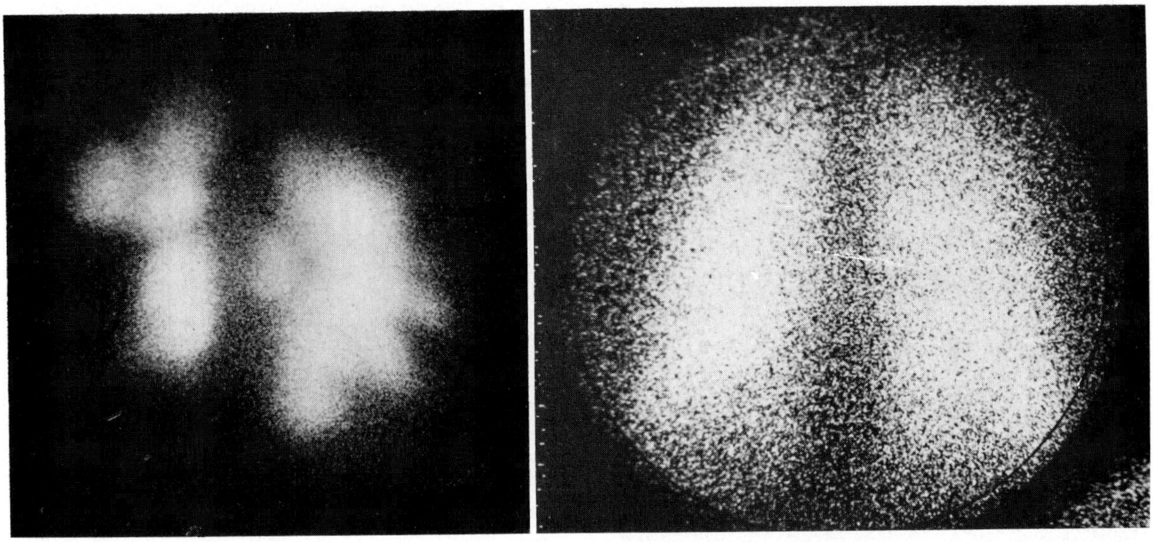

A B

Figure 7–48. Posterior perfusion (*A*) and ventilation (*B*) studies made in a patient with multiple pulmonary emboli. The perfusion image is highly irregular; the ventilation pattern, normal. This patient's chest x-ray was negative.

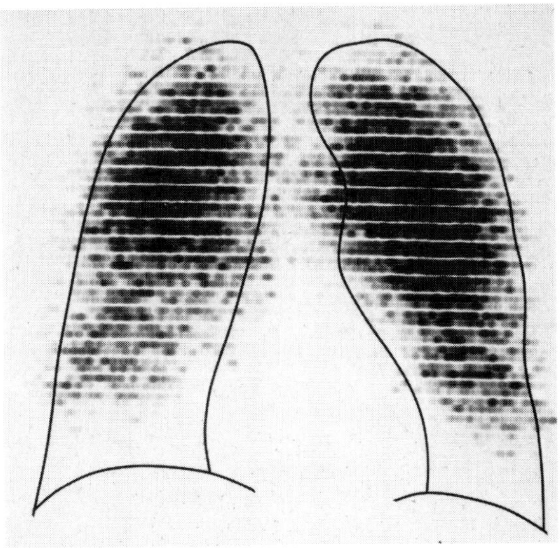

Figure 7–49. Anterior lung scan in a patient with alpha-1 antitrypsin deficiency. When injected in the upright position, the apices are seen to be preferentially perfused.

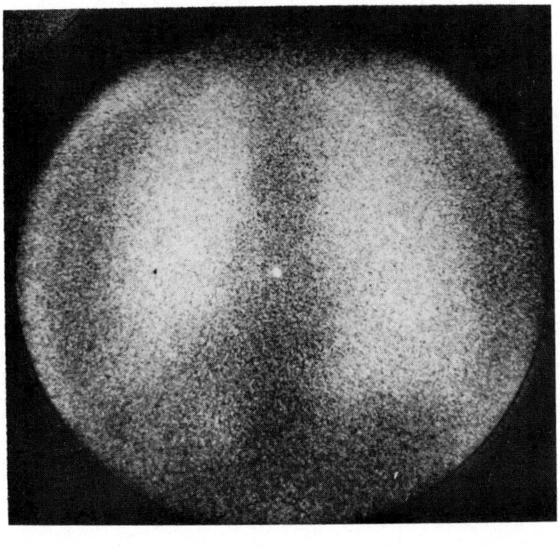

Figure 7–50. "Transmission" image to give general lung outlines in the position and at the magnification of the ventilation perfusion study. These were made from patient illustrated in Figure 7–48.

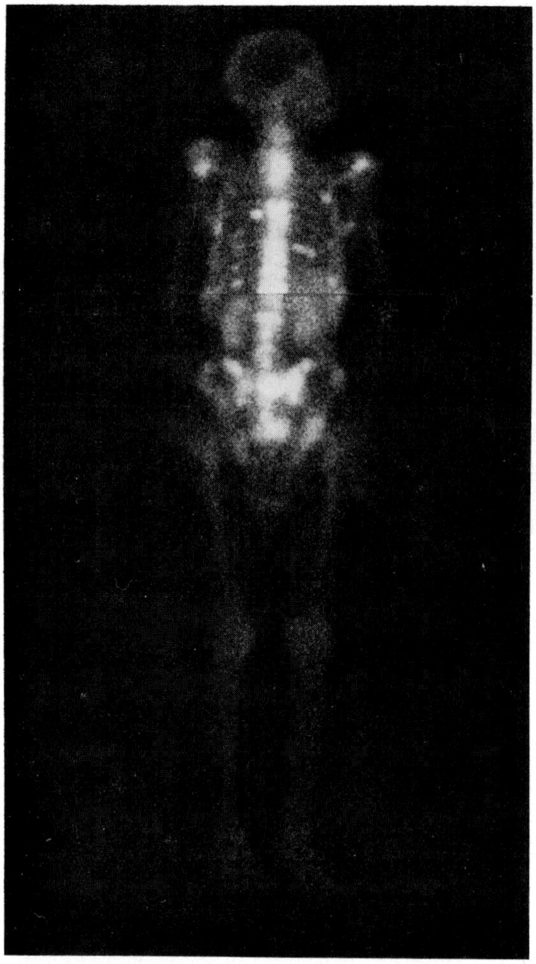

Figure 7–51. Whole body scintillation camera image of patient with widespread metastases. This was carried out three hours after injection of ^{99m}Tc-polyphosphate. It required seven minutes imaging time. This patient had a negative bone survey.

It is important to know the site of the placenta in a patient with third trimester vaginal bleeding. It is also essential to locate the placenta when fetal transfusion is contemplated.

Originally it was convenient to make use of labeled albumin owing to the long imaging time on scintillation scanners.

Figure 7–52 illustrates a normal heart image; Figure 7–53 a patient with pericardial effusion, for which the test is indicated; and Figure 7–54 a patient with an atrial myxoma.

With the availability of the scintillation camera, with which rapid sequencing is possible, useful images of only a few seconds' exposure time are possible with simple pertechnetate. Figure 7–55 depicts a placental image made in this way.

Positive Tumor Imaging. Edwards has recently described the use of radioactive gallium in the localization of tumors. Although still under investigation in many centers, it is clear that the substance has great promise in the detection of certain types of lesions. We have found variable results in several neoplasms of epithelial origin, but generally favorable results in patients with large cell lymphomas and connective tissue sarcomas.

Figure 7–56 illustrates an example of a reticulum cell sarcoma of the tonsil with

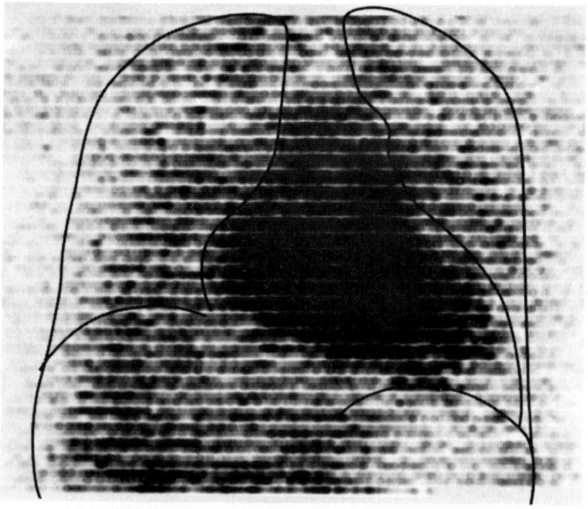

Figure 7–52. Scan of normal heart (^{99m}Tc-labeled albumin).

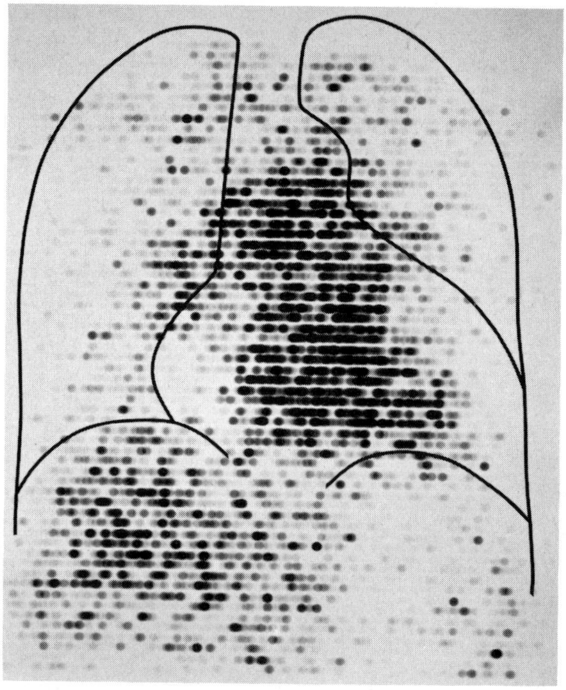

Figure 7–53. Scan of heart (^{131}I-IHSA) with pericardial effusion. Note the discrepancy between the left edge of the cardiac shadow and the outline of radioactivity.

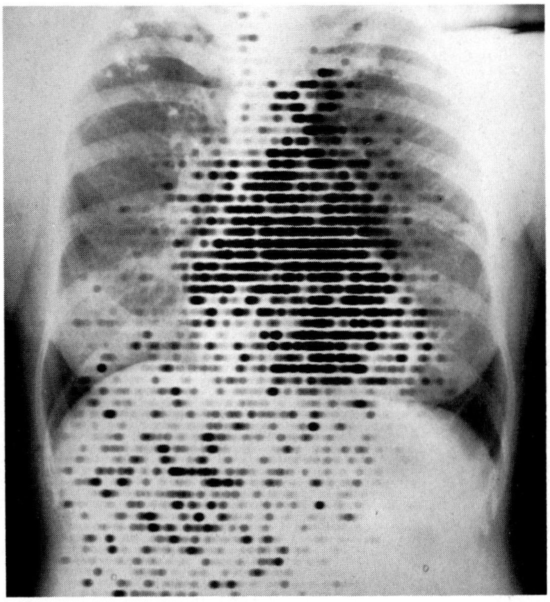

Figure 7–54. Scan of heart (^{131}I-IHSA) with filling defect due to a myoma.

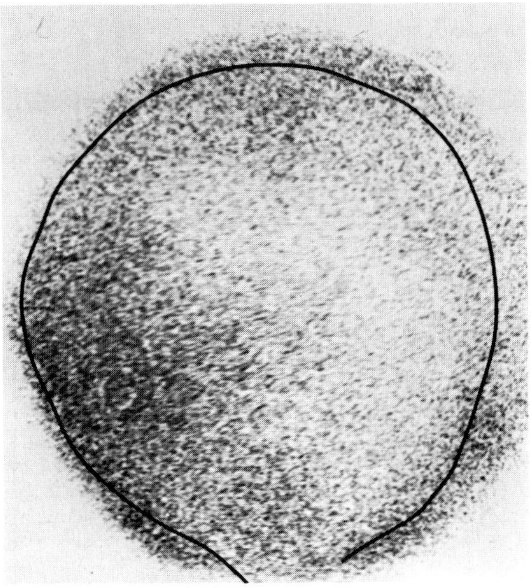

Figure 7–55. Scintillation camera image of the placenta made after antecubital vein injection of pertechnetate ($^{99m}TcO_4$). (From Emmett, J. L., and Witten, D. M.: Clinical Urography. 1971.)

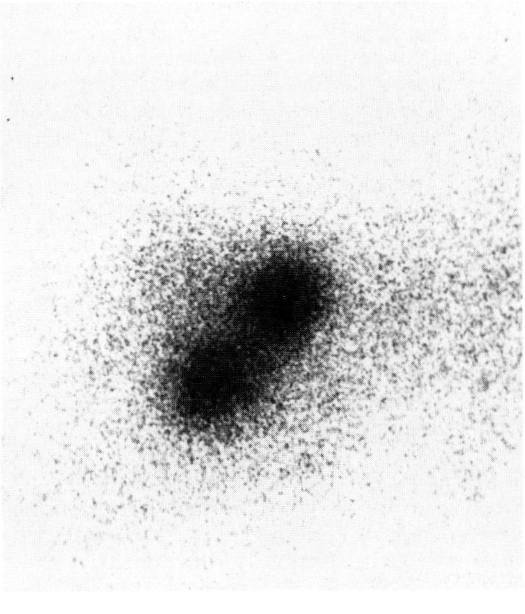

Figure 7–56. Scintillation camera image of the head (anterior aspect). Two foci of increased uptake of ^{67}Ga are seen. The medial one arises from a focus of reticulum cell sarcoma in the tonsil; the lateral one from a focus in a lymph node.

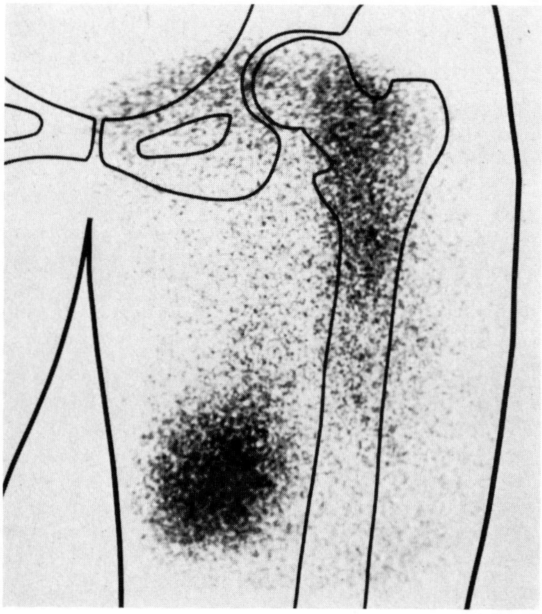

Figure 7–57. Scintigraphic image of the thigh of a patient with rhabdomyosarcoma. Uptake is clearly seen in the lesion and also in the marrow of the upper femur. This image was made 48 hours after the injection of ^{67}gallium as the citrate.

metastasis, and Figure 7–57, a picture of a rhabdomyosarcoma of the thigh.

The mechanism of such accumulation has not been elucidated. Other substances, particularly ^{57}Co-bleomycin, are under investigation.

Results of scintigraphy can be reported as simple narrative description. However, we reproduce the scintigrams by Polaroid camera and send the print with our interpretation; we include all the technical information (date and time of injection, radiopharmaceutical, lot number, dose, scan speed, settings, scan direction), so that a complete record is in the patient's file.

A note on reporting scintigraphy results to the patient's history: For many scintigraphic procedures it is imperative to relate the image to the anatomy of the patient. For the thyroid, this must be done with great care, since the usual question involves whether a given tumor is active or inactive. For heart, lungs, and bones, and often for the liver and the brain, it is imperative to know the outlines of the organ since lesions occurring around the edges may not be evident. In these problems it may be wise to make use of the transmission image mentioned above, i.e., a scintigraphic image performed by a plane source using a low energy emitter such as ^{99m}Tc or ^{241}Americium or, alternatively, to make use of magnification-free roentgenograms of the organ in question. Outlines from these films can be traced by wax crayon onto clear film for superimposition onto the scintigraphic film, using Lewall's technique.

Body Composition Studies

Whole body levels of various substances can be obtained by the use of a whole body counter or by the use of the dilution principle. (See Plasma Volume and Erythrocyte Volume.) Tests of this sort have been particularly interesting in assessing metal metabolism, electrolytes, and water.

Radioactive Copper and Wilson's Disease. Although the mechanisms underlying Wilson's disease are far from understood, they seem to be intimately related to the metabolism of copper. Accumulation of copper in Descemet's membrane is responsible for the Kayser-Fleischer ring, and accumulations in the lenticular portion of the brain and throughout the liver are closely related to the neurologic and cirrhotic symptoms that characterize hepatolenticular degeneration. The congenital absence of serum ceruloplasmin, a blue copper-protein oxidase, is suspected of being etiologically important in this disease, but the function of the enzyme is not known. Nonetheless, the metabolic pathways of copper can be traced accurately with ^{64}Cu or ^{67}Cu, and abnormalities are evident not only in the homozygous patient with Wilson's disease but also in the heterozygous carrier. Body retention studies have been particularly helpful in this area.

Body Sodium and Potassium. The availability of ^{24}Na and ^{42}K, both short-lived nuclides, makes it possible to estimate the total body sodium and potassium spaces of the body. The standard nuclide dilution technique is used; a known dose of each element is injected and the concentration of radioactive sodium in the plasma 6 hours later and the concentration of radioactive potassium 24 to 48 hours later reflects the extent of dilution. By measuring the sodium and potassium levels in the serum, the size of the electrolyte pools can be derived. The methods are valid only if the radiosodium and radiopotassium actually equilibrate with all sodium and potassium compartments of the body. Since this may not actually have happened within the period of study, the conservative term "total exchangeable electrolyte" is usually used instead of "total body electrolyte."

Normal values for total exchangeable sodium are about 41 mEq. per kg. for men and 39 mEq. per kg. for women. The corresponding potassium values are 47 and 41 mEq. per kg. The expression "per kilogram" is convenient but, like blood volumes, is not very accurate. It is preferable to express such values as a function of lean body mass. When expressed as ratios of sodium/potassium, normal values are about 0.87 in men and 0.95 in women. Much narrower ranges can be determined by the use of more complex anthropometric analysis, as reported by François. Another isotope of potassium, ^{43}K, is available. Its gamma-ray energy is more efficiently counted and its half-life is a little longer.

Whole Body Counters. Whole body counters are much too complicated and expensive for general use. Where one is available, measurements of very low levels of radioactivity are possible. One direct application of such a device is the measurement of body potassium, since all natural potassium contains a small amount of ^{40}K, a gamma-emitting isotope with a half-life of about 10^9 years. Precise measurement of absorption of gamma-emitting compounds from the intestinal tract should be considerably more accurate than conventional fecal collection and counting methods.

Competitive Binding Assay Procedures

Probably the most extensive nuclear medicine procedure in the future will be that of competitive binding assays. (See Table 11–11, p. 721.) This procedure is concerned with the *in vitro* quantification of a large number of substances that are present in trace quantities in the blood or other body fluids.

The basic procedure requires the following elements:

1. Labeled and unlabeled form of the substance to be tested.
2. A binding substance for the substance to be tested.
3. A means of separating bound and free forms.
4. A means of quantitating the label.
5. Preparation of a reference graph of bound to free ratios against known quantities of the material to be tested.

Frequently it may be necessary to extract the substance to be tested from natural binders in the body fluids.

Labeling of the substance is usually accomplished by employing a radioisotope of one of the elements in the substance, e.g., ^{131}I or ^{125}I for the thyronines, ^{57}Co for vitamin B_{12}, ^{3}H or ^{14}C for steroid, and so forth. Occasionally the test works if the test material is labeled in one other way, usually iodination, e.g., angiotensin, insulin.

The binders may be natural or artificially produced. Since some of these are antibodies, the test is referred to as radioimmunoassay.

Separation of free and bound forms can be accomplished in various ways: resins, Sephadex, paper chromatography, precipitation, use of a second antibody, and so forth.

In all cases the radioactive form of the test substances and varying known quantities of the unlabeled form are incubated with a fixed quantity of the binding substances. The fraction of the labeled material bound obviously decreases with the amount of unlabeled material added in proportion to the number of binding sites preempted. A curve is plotted of the percentage bound against the amount of unlabeled material added. Unknowns are measured by adding them also to the mixture of the labeled material and binder. The degree of displacement, i.e., the bound to free ratio, is compared with that seen on the graph and the amount present is read off.

While a comprehensive review of details of tests is beyond the scope of this text, several determinations are presented elsewhere (Chapter 11).

It should be noted that the availability of these tests has markedly changed the frequency with which other tests are ordered. The serum T4 and TSH have markedly reduced the indications for the PBI and the thyroid uptake; the serum vitamin B_{12} has replaced many demands for the Schilling test.

In the future, competitive binding assay procedures may provide convenient means of assaying blood levels of various drugs as well as hormones. Such procedures are already used to test digoxin levels. They may be serviceable for viruses, for example, a commercially available kit (Abbott) is quite useful in the detection of the virus of serum hepatitis.

SAFETY AND REGULATIONS

Absorption of energy from ionizing radiation can cause damage to tissue; therefore, principles of radiation safety must be strictly adhered to. Furthermore, the physician administering radioactive drugs must be able to estimate the radiation exposure to the patient and to evaluate the resultant biologic effects.

Protection of Personnel. The National Commission on Radiation Protection has published recommendations regarding maximal permissible exposure to radiation. For planning purposes, an upper limit of 5 rem per year for radiation workers, averaged over the adult years, is recommended. Although this amount of exposure is not expected to result in deleterious somatic effects, unnecessary exposure to radiation should always be avoided, and radiation levels in a laboratory should be kept as low as possible.

Two sources of exposure to personnel exist: One source consists of gamma-emitting radionuclides stored or being used in the laboratory. Persons working in the vicinity will be exposed to the radiations from these external sources. Also, the external sources will contribute to the background of the radiation detectors in the area. The other source consists of radionuclides which enter the body and irradiate the individual from within – internal sources. Amounts of radionuclides which are innocuous as external sources might constitute a serious hazard when taken into the body. Therefore, laboratory procedures must be established and observed faithfully to prevent ingestion of, inhalation of, or skin contact with the radioactive materials.

Protection against radiation from external sources involves consideration of three factors: time, shielding, and distance. Laboratory procedures should be carried out as rapidly as possible, lead shielding should be used where possible, and nuclides should be stored as far from working areas as is convenient.

Protection against internal sources may be achieved in the same way that laboratory workers protect themselves when handling dangerous chemicals such as acid.

Radiation survey meters should be available to measure radiation levels from external sources and to detect contamination of laboratory equipment. Personnel monitoring devices such as film badges are also helpful for evaluating external exposures.

Exposure of Patients. Estimation of the absorbed dose produced by internal sources of radioactivity is a complex matter beyond the scope of this chapter. The advice of an expert should be sought when specific calculations are desired. Generally, it is necessary to determine which organ of the body will be most affected by a given radioactive tracer; this is called the "critical organ." The radiation dose to a critical organ depends on its size, the distribution of radioactivity in the body (which depends on the initial chemical form of the administered material as well as subsequent physiologically altered forms), the decay scheme of the nuclide, the physical and biologic half-lives, and the radiosensitivity of the organ.

For example, a tracer dose of 20 μCi. of ^{132}I (half-life 2.3 hours) will deliver a dose of approximately 1 rem to a hyperfunctioning thyroid gland. The dose to the same thyroid from 20 μCi. of ^{131}I (half-life 8 days) will be nearly 40 rem, the difference being due to the longer half-life and different decay energies. Twenty microcuries of ^{42}K would result in a radiation dose to the whole body (the critical organ for K) of only 0.025 rem (or 25 mrem). This is slightly less than the radiation exposure produced by making a single standard thoracic roentgenogram.

Licensing. One by one the individual states are assuming the licensing and regulatory authority for the procurement and use of radioactive materials. This was formerly completely under the control of the Atomic Energy Commission. However, all state codes must, in general, conform to those of the AEC; Title 10, Chapter I, Code of Federal Regulations, contains all the basic information in this regard. Part 35 of the foregoing applies to human uses of by-product material. Some well-established procedures, such as thyroid uptake studies with ^{131}I, blood and blood plasma determinations with iodinated serum albumin (with ^{125}I or ^{131}I), measurement of intestinal absorption of ^{57}Co- and ^{60}Co-cyanocobalamin, and determination of erythrocyte volumes with ^{51}Cr, come under a so-called general license. Physicians may obtain licenses by simply completing Form AEC-482 for registration purposes and observing the restrictions listed in part 35. Other human uses require specific licenses, which are issued only to physicians submitting evidence of extensive personal experience with the proposed use.

DESIGN OF THE NUCLEAR MEDICINE LABORATORY

The physical layout of the nuclear medicine laboratory must be planned about the functions to be performed. There are three general categories of tests: (1) strictly *in vitro* tests, such as T_3-uptakes by erythrocytes or resins, competitive binding assay, iron-binding capacities of protein, thyroxine, and insulin; (2) *in vitro-in vivo* tests, which require the patient's presence for injections and withdrawals of blood but not for the test procedure itself nor for data processing, such as blood volume determination; and (3) *in vivo* tests, which require the patient's presence in the laboratory and in which the basic data gathering is performed on the patient after administration of some gamma-emitting substance (all scintigraphic procedures fall into this category), such as cardiac output or thyroid uptake studies. If measurement of endogenous radioactivity is planned, space must be reserved for a whole body counter.

The widespread use of radioactive gases, short-lived radionuclides with their pharmaceutical manipulation, necessitates a readily available radiopharmaceutical preparation area equipped with a good hood, well-shielded working area, sterilization area, and also dose quantitation equipment.

The design of the laboratory must allow for easy access to all parts by the technologists and for waiting rooms and a certain penetration of the laboratory by the patient, yet it must always consider the problem of confining radiation to protect both personnel and counting equipment from unwanted stray radiation. If the laboratory is near the site where radiotherapy is given, special precautions are needed to protect the diagnostic instruments from x-ray and cobalt devices and from patients who have received therapeutic doses of gamma-emitting nuclides.

Expansion of the laboratory is almost inevitable. Facilities are now needed for processing scintigraphic images; larger ones may be required if autoradiographic techniques become more popular. Since tests involving beta-emitting radionuclides seem certain to become popular as liquid scintillation counting improves, additional space for such equipment should be considered. The advantages of computer presentation of scintigrams as well as prompt calculation of function tests may well mean that access to a central computer is needed. When tests for viruses or bacteria are undertaken, care should be exercised for their confinement and for the elimination of contaminated material.

When tests for viruses or bacteria are undertaken, care should be exercised for their confinement and for the elimination of contaminated material.

Finally, attention should be paid to continually updating the laboratory's library.

REFERENCES

Achaval, A., Tauxe, W. N., and Gambill, E. E.: Scintillation scanning of the liver. Mayo Clin. Proc. *40*:206, 1965.

Adams, R., Specht, N., and Woodward, I.: Labeling of erythrocytes *in vitro* with radioiodine-tagged l-triiodothyronine as an index of thyroid function: An improved hematocrit correction. J. Clin. Endocr. *20*:1366, 1960.

Allen, H. C., Jr., Kelly, F. J., and Greene, J. A.: Observations on the nodular thyroid gland with the gammagraph. J. Clin. Endocr. *12*:1356. 1952.

Andrews, G. A., Kniseley, R. M., and Wagner, H. N.: Radioactive Pharmaceuticals: Proceedings of a Symposium at the Oak Ridge Institute of Nuclear Studies, Nov. 1-4, 1965. Oak Ridge, Tennessee, U.S. Atomic Energy Commission, Division of Technical Information, 1966.

Atwood, R. M., Burchell, H. B., and Tauxe, W. N.: Pulmonary scans achieved with macroaggregated radioiodinated albumin: Use in diagnosis of pulmonary artery agenesis. Amer. J. Med. Sci. *252*:84, 1966.

Bauer, F. K., Goodwin, W. E., Libby, R. L., and Cassen, B.: Visual delineation of thyroid glands in vivo. J. Lab. Clin. Med. *39*:153, 1952.

Beierwaltes, W. H., Johnson, P. C., and Solari, A. J.: Clinical Use of Radioisotopes. Philadelphia, W. B. Saunders Company, 1957.

Berson, S. A., Yalow, R. S., Sorrentino, J., and Roswit, B.: The determination of thyroidal and renal plasma ^{131}I clearance rates as a routine diagnostic test of thyroid dysfunction. J. Clin. Invest. *31*:141, 1952.

Bishopric, G. A., Garrett, N. H., and Nicholson, W. M.: Clinical value of the TSH test in the diagnosis of thyroid diseases. Amer. J. Med. *18*:15, 1955.

Blahd, W. H.: Nuclear Medicine. New York, McGraw-Hill Book Company, 1971.

Bonnet, J. D., Hagedorn, A. B., and Owen, C. A., Jr.: A quantitative method for measuring the gastrointestinal absorption of iron. Blood *15*:36, 1960.

Bull, F. E., Campbell, D. C., and Owen, C. A., Jr.: The diagnosis and treatment of pernicious anemia. Med. Clin. N. Amer. *40*:1005, 1956.

Burrows, B. A., and Ross, J. F.: The use of radiosodium and radiopotassium tracer studies in man. *In* Proceedings of the International Conference on the Peaceful Uses of Atomic Energy: Radioactive Isotopes and Nuclear Radiations in Medicine. New York, United Nations, 1956.

Bush, J. A., Mahoney, J. P., Markowitz, H., Gubler, C. J., Cartwright, G. E., and Wintrobe, M. M.: Studies on copper metabolism. XVI. Radioactive copper studies in normal subjects and in patients with hepatolenticular degeneration. J. Clin. Invest. *34*:1766, 1955.

Chase, G. D., and Rabinowitz, J. L.: Principles of Radioisotope Methodology. 3rd ed. Minneapolis, Burgess Publishing Company, 1967.

Chou, S. N., Aust, J. B., Moore, G. E., and Peyton, W. T.: Radioactive iodinated human serum albumin as tracer agent for diagnosing and localizing intracranial lesions. Proc. Soc. Exp. Biol. Med. 77:193, 1951.

Crispell, K. R., Porter, B., and Nieset, R. T.: Studies of plasma volume using human serum albumin tagged with radioactive iodine. J. Clin. Invest. *29*:513, 1950.

Ebaugh, F. G., Jr., Emerson, C. P., and Ross, J. F.: The use of radioactive chromium 51 as an erythrocyte tagging agent for the determination of red cell survival in vivo. J. Clin. Invest. *32*:1260, 1953.

Edwards, C. L., and Hayes, R. L.: Scanning malignant neoplasms with gallium 67. J.A.M.A. *212* (No. 7):1182, 1970.

Fabi, M. N., Stroebel, C. F., and Owen, C. A., Jr.: Some clinical uses of radioactive iron. Med. Clin. N. Amer. *40*:993, 1956.

Fields, T., and Seed, L.: Clinical Use of Radioisotopes: A Manual of Technique. Chicago, Year Book Medical Publishers, Inc., 1957.

Gray, S. J., and Sterling, K.: The tagging of red cells and plasma proteins with radioactive chromium. J. Clin. Invest. *29*:1604, 1950.

Hamolsky, M. W.: The plasma protein-thyroid hormone complex in thyrotoxicosis vs. euthyroidism in man. J. Clin. Invest. *34*:914, 1955.

Hamolsky, M. W., Golodetz, A., and Freedberg, A. S.: The plasma protein–thyroid hormone complex in man. III. Further studies on the use of the *in vitro* red blood cell uptake of ^{131}I-I-triiodothyronine as a diagnostic test of thyroid function. J. Clin. Endocr. *19*:103, 1959.

Harper, P. V., Beck, R., Charleston, D., and Lathrop, K. A.: Optimization of a scanning method using ^{99m}Tc. Nucleonics 22:50, 1964.

Hine, G. J.: Instrumentation in Nuclear Medicine. New York, Academic Press Inc., 1967.

Hine, G. J., and Brownell, G. L.: Radiation Dosimetry. New York, Academic Press, Inc., 1956.

Jefferies, W. M., Levy, R. P., Palmer, W. G., Storaasli, J. P., and Kelly, L. W., Jr.: The value of single injection of thyrotropin in the diagnosis of obscure hypothyroidism. New Eng. J. Med. *249*:876, 1953.

Kniseley, R. M., Andrews, G. A., and Harris, C. C.: Progress in Medical Radioisotope Scanning: Proceedings of a Symposium at the Medical Division of the Oak Ridge Institute of Nuclear Studies, Oct. 22–26, 1962. Oak Ridge, Tennessee, U.S. Atomic Energy Commission, Division of Technical Information, 1963.

Kniseley, R. M., Tauxe, W. N., and Anderson, E. B.: Dynamic Clinical Studies With Radioisotopes. Washington, D.C., U.S. Atomic Energy Commission, Division of Technical Information, 1964.

Lewall, D. B., and Tauxe, W. N.: A method for the elimination of magnification in roentgenograms. Amer. J. Clin. Path. *48*:568, 1967.

Matthews, C. M. E.: The theory of tracer experiments with ^{131}I-labelled plasma proteins. Phys. Med. Biol. 2:36, 1957.

Maytum, W. J., Goldstein, N. P., McGuckin, W. F., and Owen, C. A., Jr.: Copper metabolism in Wilson's disease, Laennec's cirrhosis and hemachromatosis: Studies with radiocopper (^{64}Cu). Proc. Staff Meet. Mayo Clin. *36*:641, 1961.

McAfee, J. G., Stern, H. S., Fueger, G. F., Baggish, M. S., Holzman, G. B., and Zolle, I.: ^{99m}Tc labeled serum albumin for scintillation scanning of the placenta. J. Nucl. Med. *5*:936, 1964.

Medical Radioisotope Scanning: Proceedings of the Symposium on Medical Radioisotope Scanning Held by the International Atomic Energy Agency in Athens, April 20–24, 1964. Vienna, International Atomic Energy Agency, 1964.

Moertel, C. G., Scudamore, H. H., Wollaeger, E. E., and Owen, C. A., Jr.: Limitations of the ^{131}I-labeled triolein tests in the diagnosis of steatorrhea. Gastroenterology *42*:16, 1962.

Moore, F. D., Olesen, K. H., McMurrey, J. D., Parker, H. V., Ball, M. R., and Boyden, C. M.: The Body Cell Mass and Its Supporting Environment: Body Composition in Health and Disease. Philadelphia, W. B. Saunders Company, 1963.

Moore, G. E.: Use of radioactive diiodofluorescein in the diagnosis and localization of brain tumors. Science *107*: 569, 1948.

Murphy, B. P., and Jachan, C.: The determination of thyroxine by competitive protein-binding analysis employing an anion-exchange resin and radiothyroxine. J. Lab. Clin. Med. *66*:161, 1965.

Murphy, B. P., and Pattee, C. J.: Determination of thyroxine utilizing the property of protein–binding. Medical Research Council Fellow, Medical Research Council, Canada.

Nagler, W., Bender, M. A., and Blau, M.: Radioisotope photoscanning of the liver. Gastroenterology *44*:36, 1963.

Necheles, T. F., Weinstein, I. M., and LeRoy, G. V.: Radioactive sodium chromate for the study of survival of red blood cells. I. The effect of radioactive sodium chromate on red cells. J. Lab. Clin. Med. *42*:358, 1953.

Orvis, A. L., and Albert, A.: Gamma counting of radiosodium and radiopotassium in the bioassay of aldosterone and related steroids. Endocrinology *56*:218, 1955.

Overman, R. T., and Clark, H. M.: Radioisotope Techniques. New York, McGraw-Hill Book Company, 1960.

Owen, C. A., Jr.: Measuring radioactivity in the diagnostic laboratory. *In* Diagnostic Radioisotopes. Springfield, Illinois, Charles C Thomas, 1959.

Owen, C. A., Jr.: Radioactive iron. *In* Diagnostic Radioisotopes. Springfield, Illinois, Charles C Thomas, 1959.

Owen, C. A., Jr., Bollman, J. L., and Grindlay, J. H.: Radiochromium-labeled erythrocytes for the detection of gastrointestinal hemorrhage. J. Lab. Clin. Med. *44*:238, 1954.

Owen, C. A., Jr., McCants, R. S., and McConahey, W. M.: Abbreviation of Berson technic for estimation of thyroidal clearance of plasma radioiodide: Use of Berson test to recognize thyroidal protein-binding defects. J. Clin. Invest. *39*:790, 1960.

Owen, C. A., Jr., McConahey, W. M., Keating, F. R., Jr., and Orvis, A. L.: Investigation of diseases of the thyroid gland by means of radioactive iodine. Fed. Proc. *14*:723, 1955.

Quimby, E. H.: Radioactive Isotopes in Medicine and Biology: Basic Physics and Instrumentation. Philadelphia, Lea & Febiger, 1963.

Quinn, J. L., III (ed.): The Yearbook of Nuclear Medicine. Chicago, Year Book Medical Publishers, Inc., 1973.

Radiological Health Handbook. Washington, D. C., U.S. Department of Health, Education, and Welfare, 1960.

Sapirstein, L. A., Vidt, D. G., Mandel, M. J., and Hanusek, G.: Volumes of distribution and clearances of intravenously injected creatinine in the dog. Amer. J. Physiol. *181*:330, 1955.

Schalch, D. S., and Parker, M. L.: A sensitive double antibody immunoassay for human growth hormone in plasma. Nature (London) *203*:1141, 1964.

Schilling, R. F.: Intrinsic factor studies. II. The effect of gastric juice on the urinary excretion of radioactivity after the oral administration of radioactive vitamin B_{12}. J. Lab. Clin. Med *42*:860, 1953.

Schilling, R. F., Clatanoff, D. V., and Korst, D. R.: Intrinsic factor studies. III. Further observations utilizing the urinary radioactivity test in subjects with achlorhydria, pernicious anemia, or a total gastrectomy. J. Lab. Clin. Med. *45*:926, 1955.

Sheppard, C. W.: Basic Principles of the Tracer Method: Introduction to Mathematical Tracer Kinetics. New York, John Wiley & Sons, Inc., 1962.

Shih, S. C., Fairbanks, V. F., and Tauxe, W. N.: The kinetics of urinary excretion of Chromium 51 from labeled erythrocytes in hemolytic anemia and the anemia of blood loss. Amer. J. Clin. Path. 55:431, 1971.

Shih, S. C., Tauxe, W. N., Fairbanks, V. F., and Taswell, H. F.: Urinary excretion of CR-51 from labeled erythrocytes. J.A.M.A. *220*:814, 1972.

Sklaroff, D. M., and Charkes, N. D.: Heart Pool Scanning. *In* Quinn, J. L., III: Scintillation Scanning in Clinical Medicine. Philadelphia, W. B. Saunders Company, 1964.

Sterling, K., and Gray, S. J.: Determination of the circulating red cell volume in man by radioactive chromium. J. Clin. Invest. *29*:1614, 1950.

Taplin, G. V., Johnson, D. E., Dore, E. K., and Kaplan, H. S.: Lung photoscans with macroaggregates of human serum radioalbumin: Experimental basis and initial clinical trials. Health Phys. *10*:1219, 1964.

Taplin, G. V., Meredith, O. M., Jr., Kade, H., and Winter, C. C.: The Radioisotope Renogram: An External Test for Individual Kidney Function and Upper Urinary Tract Patency. University of California (Los Angeles) School of Medicine, Atomic Energy Project No. 366, 1956.

Tauxe, W. N.: A rapid radioactive method for the determination of the serum iron-binding capacity. Amer. J. Clin. Path. *35*:403, 1961.

Tauxe, W. N.: Quantitation of menstrual blood loss: A radioactive method utilizing a counting dome. J. Nucl. Med. *3*:282, 1962.

Tauxe, W. N.: Urologic applications of radioactive material. *In* Emmett, J. L. and Witten, D. N.: Clinical Urography: An Atlas and Textbook of Roentgenologic Diagnosis. 3rd ed. Philadelphia, W. B. Saunders Company, 1971.

Tauxe, W. N., Becton, J. L., and Yamaguchi, M. Y.: Selection of formula for the expression of results of the uptake of l-triiodothyronine-I^{131} by red blood cells. Amer. J. Clin. Path. *39*:562, 1963.

Tauxe, W. N., Burbank, M. K., Maher, F. T., and Hunt, J. C.: Renal clearances of radioactive ortho-iodohippurate and diatrizoate. Mayo Clin. Proc. *39*:761, 1964.

Tauxe, W. N., Burchell, H. B., Chaapel, D. W., and Sprau, A.: Quantitating the effect of gravity on lung scans of macroaggregates of albumin-^{131}I. J. Appl. Physiol. *21*:1381, 1966.

Tauxe, W. N., Goldstein, N. P., Randall, R. V., and Gross, J. B.: Radiocopper studies in patients with Wilson's disease and their relatives. Amer. J. Med. *41*:375, 1966.

Tauxe, W. N., Hunt, J. C., and Burbank, M. K.: The radioisotope renogram (ortho-iodohippurate-^{131}I): Standardization of technic and expression of data. Amer. J. Clin. Path. *37*:567, 1962.

Tauxe, W. N., Jenkins, D., Stellmacher, V., and Cuklanz, E.: Increased red cell and resin uptake of l-triiodothyronine caused by use of acetate plastic test tubes. Amer. J. Clin. Path. *45*:139, 1966.

Tauxe, W. N., Maher, F. T., and Taylor, W. F.: Effective renal plasma flow: Estimation from theoretical volumes of distribution of intravenously injected ^{131}I orthoiodohippurate. Mayo Clin. Proc. *46*:524, 1971.

Tauxe, W. N., and Orvis, A. L.: The Mayo Clinic whole-body counter. Mayo Clin. Proc. *41*:18, 1966.

Tauxe, W. N., and Yamaguchi, M. Y.: Variants affecting results of red cell triiodothyronine uptake test. Amer. J. Clin. Path. *36*:1, 1961.

Van Vliet, P. D., Tauxe, W. N., Svien, H. J., and Jenkins, D. A.: The effect of craniotomy on the brain scan. J. Neurosurg. *23*:425, 1965.

Veall, N., and Vetter, H.: Radioisotope Techniques in Clinical Research and Diagnosis. London, Butterworth & Co., Ltd., 1958.

Wagner, H. N.: Radioisotope scanning of the spleen. *In* Kniseley, R. M., Andrews, G. A., and Harris, C. C.: Progress in Medical Radioisotope Scanning: Proceedings of a Symposium at the Medical Division of the Oak Ridge Institute of Nuclear Studies, Oct. 22–26, 1962. Oak Ridge, Tennessee, U.S. Atomic Energy Commission, Division of Technical Information, 1963.

Wahner, H. W.: Iodine metabolism in thyroid function. Minnesota Med. *55*:623, 1972.

Wahner, H. W., and Walser, A. H.: Measurements of thyroxine-plasma protein interactions. Med. Clin. N. Amer. *56* (No. 4): 849, 1972.

Wenzl, J. E., Tauxe, W. N., Burke, E. C., Hunt, J. C., and Stickler, G. B.: Radioisotope renography in children. I. The renogram in children without renal disease. Pediatrics *36*:120, 1965.

Werner, S. C., Quimby, E. H., and Schmidt, C.: The use of tracer doses of radioactive iodine, ^{131}I in the study of normal and disordered thyroid function in man. J. Clin. Endocr. *9*:342, 1949.

Yalow, R. S., and Berson, S. A.: Immunoassay of plasma insulin in man. Diabetes *10*:339, 1961.

Zipf, R. E., Webber, J. M., and Grove, G. R.: The application of the gravimetric technic to the simultaneous determination of plasma volume using radioiodinated human serum albumin and red cell mass using sodium radiochromate. Amer. J. Clin. Path. *26*:487, 1956.

Chapter 8

SPECTROPHOTOMETRIC INSTRUMENTATION

by ROBERT G. LANCASTER, M.D.

A great many measurements in clinical laboratories are facilitated by the use of instruments, some relatively simple and others quite complex. As the quest for more rapid diagnosis and for early delineation of clinical abnormalities continues, more and more instruments are being developed, and automation in one form or another is increasing by leaps and bounds. This is a double-edged sword, however. If one just introduces these devices into his laboratory and uses them with no basic understanding and by cookbook rote, one is never sure who is the master. More often than not, it turns out that the machine is consistently "one-up," and the human turns out to be an unhappy and frustrated slave who longs for the good old days when life wasn't so complicated.

It is the goal of this chapter to present an overall picture of the basics of operation of the commonly used spectrophotometric instruments found in a clinical laboratory. I feel quite strongly that such an understanding is essential on the part of laboratory directors, residents, and senior laboratory personnel. Once this is accomplished, the junior personnel become interested and quite capable in this regard. No one denies that knowing what knobs to turn in what order is important. However, understanding what the knobs are doing inside the black box and when and if a well-placed blow with the heel of the hand will stir a recalcitrant instrument to better efforts is more important. With basic understanding, common sense, a modicum of mechanical ability, and the will to be master most of the time, fully 90 per cent of the problems arising from the use of instruments can be solved. This chapter will attempt to supply the first of these. The remainder will have to be supplied by the reader.

SPECTROPHOTOMETRY

Classic spectrophotometry is by far the most useful instrumental method of measurement in the clinical laboratory, and it will doubtless remain so for a long time to come. Basically we are making use of the properties of atoms and molecules to absorb or emit electromagnetic energy in one of the many areas of the total electromagnetic spectrum. Table 8–1 illustrates this overall concept. In spectrophotometry, we are used to thinking in terms of light. In reality, the visible portion of the electromagnetic spectrum is by far the smallest arbitrary division. It is that portion which excites the retina and causes the phenomenon known as sight. In our understanding of the electromagnetic spectrum, this is often a disadvantage, since most people think about the entire electromagnetic spectrum in terms of light and color. It would be better if we could think about it in terms of energy because really that is what it is. The energy can be thought of as being propagated in the form of a wave, such as the wave produced by dropping a pebble into a pool of still water. Several crests form, with valleys between, and move out from the point of impact. Waves of electromagnetic energy are so constituted that the closer together the crests are, the greater the energy. One of the measurements of electromagnetic energy is the wavelength (λ), or the distance from one crest to another. This ranges from less than 1 angstrom unit (Å), or 0.1 nm., for gamma rays to over 25 cm. for radio waves (see Table 8–1). One nanometer (nm.) is equal to 1×10^{-9} meters. This preferred term should be no problem, since 1 nm. = 1mμ.

If we then think of these various instruments as composed of components which can be arranged and modified to fit a particular need, one can see more easily their similarities and differences. If a closer look is taken at a simple "colorimeter" (Fig. 8–1), which is really an abridged spectrophotometer, the components can be generally classified as follows:

1. A power supply to furnish appropriately regulated electrical energy for the operation of the instrument.
2. A source of radiant energy, usually containing a large group of wavelengths, e.g., a tungsten lamp.
3. A monochromator, which is a device for removing unwanted portions of radiant energy from the system, e.g., a filter, prism, or diffraction grating.
4. A sample container to hold the material being measured, e.g., a cuvette.
5. A detector system to detect the transmitted radiant energy and convert it into electrical energy so that it may be measured, e.g., a photocell.
6. A readout device to present the electrical current in a manner that allows it to be measured in useful units, e.g., a meter reading per cent T or absorbance.

Figure 8–1 is a diagrammatic illustration of a simple instrument. Any of the techniques listed in Table 8–1 can be accomplished by utilizing an instrument composed of several or all of these six components suitably modified. All these instruments measure either radiant energy emitted by atoms (e.g., flame emission photometry) or radiant energy absorbed by atoms or molecules (e.g., conventional filter photometry).

Now we can proceed to a much more detailed inspection of the components.

Components of a Spectrophotometer

Power Supplies. In order to make spectrophotometric measurements, the instrument itself must be in a stable state. The usual fluctuations of voltage and current from the electrical supply at the wall plug (mains) do not significantly upset the equilibrium of lamps, heaters, or motors. However, they are disastrous to the stable operation of measuring instruments. Therefore, a power supply capable of furnishing adequately regulated electrical energy for the particular needs of the instrument must be utilized. These power supplies fall into three general categories: batteries, magnetic voltage regulators, and electronic power supplies.

Batteries. Batteries, either wet or dry, produce stable voltages and are relatively inexpensive, but they do present some grave problems. Replacement of dry batteries is a nuisance, and they are not of sufficient capacity to operate most instruments completely. Over a long period the replacement expense becomes rather large. Dry cell batteries are used for the operation of some small photometers and radiation detectors, primarily to make them portable. Some other equipment now is available that utilizes nickel-cadmium or alkaline batteries. Here again portability is the chief concern, and these batteries are suitable only for instruments that require very little current. The nickel-cadmium type is rechargeable, and instruments containing them usually have also a small built in trickle charger.

Electronic Power Supplies. Fortunately the need for battery operated instruments now is quite small. This is due in large part to two factors: The first is the rather recent development of good, relatively inexpensive electric power supplies, most of them solid-state. The second is the close control of the frequency of commercially available electrical power.

This latter situation allows more widespread use of magnetic voltage regulators. These are essentially trouble free and have no vacuum tubes, transistors, moving parts, and so forth. They do a good job of regulating voltage, but are inherently and exquisitely sensitive to very small changes in frequency. As previously mentioned, close control of frequency by the power companies allows more widespread use of magnetic voltage stabilizers in many instruments. However, in outlying areas it may be well to check with the local power company before purchasing instruments to make certain that the frequency is held to within ± 0.5 per cent.

Some of the newer, more sophisticated instruments require a greater variety of stable voltages or more precise regulation than can be easily obtained from a magnetic voltage regulator. Situations may be encountered in which the frequency variations must be taken into account. This necessitates the use of an

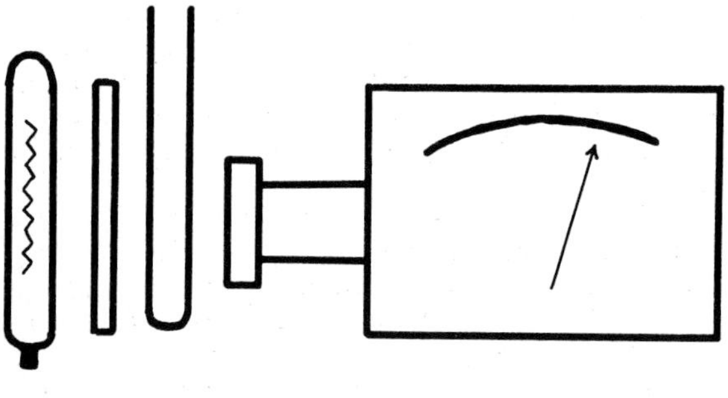

Figure 8–1. Simplified diagram of a simple colorimetric instrument. A, lamp; B, filter; C, cuvette; D, photocell; E, meter.

Table 8–1. CHARACTERISTICS OF DIFFERENT SPECTROPHOTOMETRIC INSTRUMENTS

REGION	RANGE nm.	OCCURRENCE	INSTRUMENT	COMMON CLINICAL MEASUREMENT USE
γ-rays	0.1	Nuclear energy transformations (radioactive isotopes)	Scintillation detector	γ-emitting isotopes
X-rays	0.1-10	Inner shell electron transitions	X-ray spectrometer	Limited at present
Vacuum U.V.	10-200	Ionization of atoms and molecules	Vacuum U.V. spectrophotometer	None
U.V.	200-400	Valence electron energy transitions	Spectrophotometer U.V. Flame photometer Atomic absorption	U.V. abs. substances e.g., DPNH, barbiturates
Visible	400-700	Valence electron energy transitions	Visible spectrophotometer Flame photometer Atomic absorption spectrophotometer	Most wet chemistry Na and K Most other metal elements
Infrared (I.R.)	700-25,000	Molecular vibrations stretching and bending	I.R. spectrophotometers	Toxicology Renal stones

electronic device to regulate and supply the desired voltages. These utilize either vacuum tube regulators or solid-state (transistorized) regulators. The latter are becoming much more common as a result of our rapidly advancing electronic technology. These devices are rather complex, and the average individual is usually not able to do more than replace a tube. Fortunately they are generally trouble free, but one should not put himself in the position of complete dependence on any one instrument or component. Also, power failures do occur occasionally, and every laboratory should have at least one instrument that is capable of being operated from a battery. One should also be sure that the proper connectors are at hand. A battery can always be found, but the proper plugs cannot. Remember that each cell of a lead acid battery delivers 2 volts, so if you need 6 volts, you can use three cells of a 12-volt auto battery. Parenthetically, hospitals having emergency generators should have provision for allowing operation of enough laboratory equipment to get through the emergency. Here again, frequency regulation may not be the best, and magnetic voltage regulators probably should not be used with emergency generators.

Some instruments use a magnetic regulator in front of an electronic regulator in order to provide precise regulation. At the other extreme, some instruments use no regulator but rely on matched twin detectors (e.g., Klett-Summerson) to compensate for voltage fluctuation. Although this is usually a satisfactory arrangement, we have observed occasional severe fluctuations in the Klett galvanometer. In this instance one photocell had begun to lose sensitivity in an instrument that was plugged into a heavily loaded electric circuit, and the voltage fluctuations apparently magnified the imbalance. One must always be on the alert.

Source of Radiant Energy. Before discussing sources of radiant energy, consideration should be given to the terms *continuous spectrum* and *discontinuous spectrum.* A continuous spectrum contains approximately equal representation of each wavelength present in a given region. The classic example of a source of continuous radiation is the tungsten lamp. In this case, wavelengths from about 350 to about 1000 nm. are represented, with more of the energy in the longer wavelengths than in the shorter wavelengths.

In order to increase energy output, at the shorter wavelengths particularly, some instruments are designed so that the lamp filament operates at a higher temperature than was intended by the designer. Although this does increase energy output, it greatly decreases lamp life. A continuous source allows selection of any desired wavelength for the purpose at hand.

The low-pressure mercury vapor lamp emits a discontinuous or line spectrum. This is very useful for calibration purposes but is not too practical for measurement purposes. Gamma-emitting radioisotopes can also be classed as sources of a discontinuous spectrum. Hydrogen and deuterium lamps are sources of both continuous and discontinuous spectra in the ultraviolet region, as are high-pressure mercury lamps. These sources are useful in ultraviolet absorption measurements and in producing fluorescence.

The main problems in this group are found in tungsten filament lamps. At the heat of the tungsten filament, some of the metal vaporizes and condenses on the inside of the relatively cool glass envelope. This coating acts as a neutral density filter and cuts down the intensity of the radiant energy. More important, it may change the spectrum sufficiently to alter instrument response. Since this coating is often uneven, instruments such as the AutoAnalyzer colorimeter, which has two photocells at right angles to the lamp, are susceptible to this type of interference. More widespread use of quartz-halogen lamps should eliminate this particular problem. Occasionally a bulb will leak air, and a white coating of tungsten oxide will form on the glass envelope. This is an interesting sight, but seldom presents a problem, since the lamp burns out instantly.

Many instruments are designed so that the lamps cannot be installed improperly. However, some are not so designed, and it does make a difference if the lamp filament is not centered and normal to the optical axis of the instrument both vertically and horizontally. In some instruments (e.g., the Klett), the filament support must be opposite the lens, or differences in readings can be observed. In the Coleman Junior, aging of the lamp can produce stray light effects with resultant measurement errors.

Occasionally it has been observed that chemical fumes will coat the outside of the bulb with a whitish coating. It has been shown that in the Coleman Junior this will effectively increase the band pass and may introduce errors in methods that have fairly critical band pass requirements. Periodic lamp inspection would appear a prudent precaution against most of these ills.

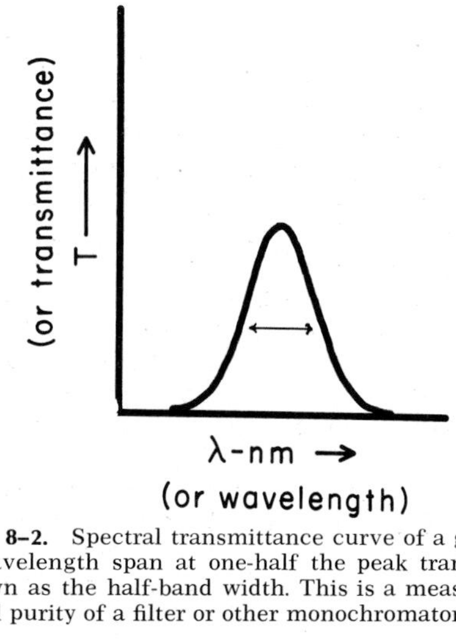

Figure 8–2. Spectral transmittance curve of a glass filter. The wavelength span at one-half the peak transmittance is known as the half-band width. This is a measure of the spectral purity of a filter or other monochromator.

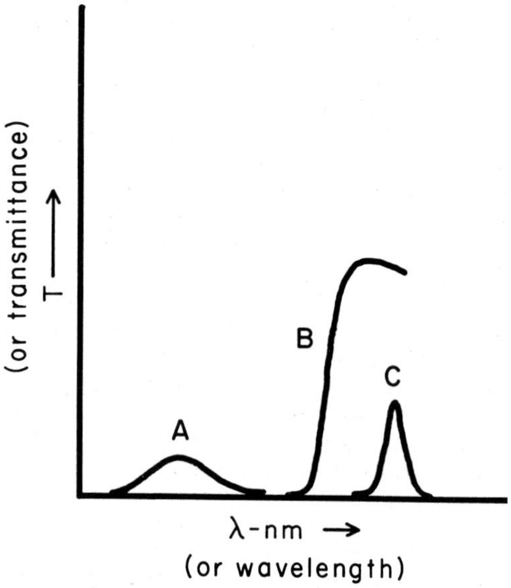

Figure 8–3. Types of filters. A is typical of a regular glass filter; B is typical of a sharp-cutoff glass filter; and C is typical of a narrow-band pass filter. An interference filter would have a curve similar to C, but the slopes would be steeper, and the half-band width would be narrower.

Monochromators. In measuring the absorption or emission of energy, it is necessary to be able to isolate the desired wavelengths of radiant energy and exclude the rest from the source. There are numerous ways of accomplishing this end, and the means chosen will depend on the use.

Filters. The simplest device is a filter which generally is composed of a metal complex dissolved or suspended in glass. For example, chromium salts in glass give it a red color, and cobalt salts produce blue. Photographic filters use dyed gelatin, and some of the early spectrophotometers contained flat-sided flasks filled with solutions of various colored salts. These last two types are no longer used in spectrophotometric instruments. Gelatin filters fade and are sensitive to heat, and if anything gets spilled on the filter edge, the gelatin either deteriorates or dissolves. Glass flasks filled with liquid have obvious disadvantages—they break. A glass filter is not really a monochromator, since it transmits a relatively wide range of wavelengths. The degree of monochromaticity of a filter or more sophisticated monochromator is designated by the half-band width. This is defined as the wavelength range transmitted at one-half of the peak transmittance of the filter (Fig. 8–2). Most commonly used glass filters have half-band widths in the neighborhood of 50 nm. This is perfectly adequate for many uses, and these filters are widely used. There are three main types of glass filters, the narrow-band pass, sharp-cutoff, and wide-band pass (Fig. 8-3). The designation of a glass filter by the instrument manufacturer often is not informative enough. No spectral transmittance curves or half-band widths are furnished with the filters, nor is the stated peak transmittance above suspicion. An example of this is the Klett No. 54 filter. This is supposed to have its peak transmission at 540 nm. Actually this filter has its peak at 525 nm., a fact that was noted many years ago, and which still is true. The type of filter is often important from a practical standpoint, as will be seen later. The narrow-band pass filters are usually composed of two or more sharp-cutoff or regular filters in an attempt to remove more of the unwanted radiation. For example, one can use an infrared absorbing filter and a sharp-cutoff filter to produce a narrow-band pass filter (Fig. 8-4).

Interference Filters. Another type of narrow-band pass filter is the interference filter. It is composed of a sandwich of two half-silvered pieces of glass with a dielectric material of carefully controlled thickness between the silvered layers (Fig. 8-5). The thickness of the dielectric layer determines the wavelength of energy that will pass through. Only energy of wavelengths that are multiples of this thickness will stay in phase as they reflect back and forth through the dielectric and finally emerge. Other wavelengths will cancel due to phase differences during the reflection process and will not be transmitted. These filters have very narrow half-band widths, commonly on the order of 5 to 10 nm.

They do require accessory glass filters, because they transmit harmonics, or multiples,

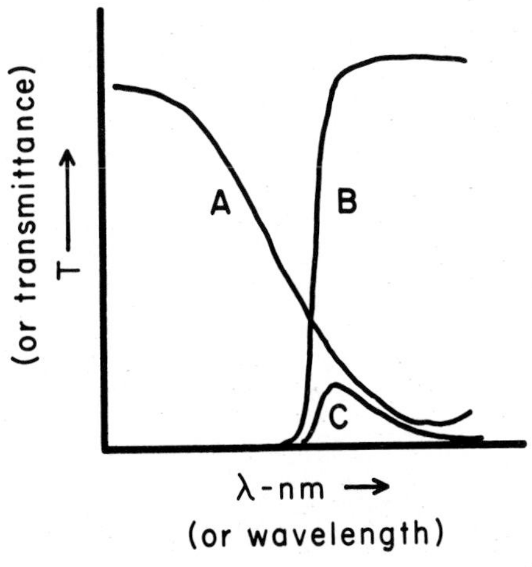

Figure 8-4. Combination filters. A is the spectral transmittance curve of an infrared absorbing filter, and B is the curve of a sharp-cutoff filter. C is the resultant curve of the combination.

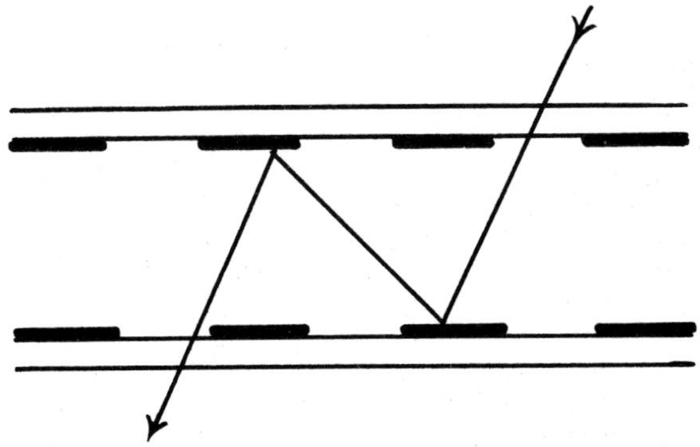

Figure 8-5. Diagrammatic representation of an interference filter. The glass outside supports are partially silvered (heavy black dashes) and are separated by the dielectric.

of the design wavelength. For example, an interference filter designed for 700 nm. will also transmit some radiation at 350 and 1400 nm. This necessitates the accessory filters to eliminate this transmission. They are used chiefly in flame emission photometry and are also used in the AutoAnalyzer colorimeter. A variation of an interference filter is one in which the dielectric is in the shape of a wedge. This allows wavelengths to be chosen at will by moving this wedge interference filter past a slit. This device is not in common use, however. One must be careful that interference filters are exactly normal (perpendicular) to the optical path, since any deviation or tilting of the filter will change the effective thickness of the dielectric and consequently change the wavelengths that are transmitted.

Prisms and Diffraction Gratings. Many instruments use prisms or diffraction gratings as monochromators. These devices separate the mixture of wavelengths emitted by sources such as a tungsten lamp by refraction or diffraction and present them as a spectrum from which the desired wavelengths may be selected.

Prisms use refraction, or the bending of radiant energy, according to wavelength to separate the wavelengths of a continuous spectrum source into a regular progression of wavelengths. Shorter wavelengths are bent, or refracted, to a greater degree than the longer wavelengths. This produces a nonlinear spectrum, with relative crowding of the longer wavelengths. In addition, a prism produces a curved spectrum. Both these inherent characteristics of a prism require relatively complex optical and mechanical devices to select a given spectral portion with a small half-band width.

On the other hand, diffraction gratings produce a linear, noncurved spectrum. Diffraction gratings are produced by evaporating a thin layer of speculum metal (an aluminum-copper alloy) onto the surface of an optically flat glass plate; then by means of an extremely accurate machine called a ruling engine, many grooves are ruled in the metal coating. These may vary from a few hundred to several hundred per inch. The more lines, or grooves, the greater the dispersion of the grating. Original gratings of high quality are much too expensive to be in common use. However, by applying a parting compound to the surface of an original grating, aluminizing it, and flowing on a layer of epoxy resin, an exact replica of the original may be formed. These replica gratings are utilized in all but the most exacting applications.

A diffraction grating is based on the principle that rays of radiant energy will bend (or refract) around a sharp corner, the degree of bending depending on the wavelength. Thus, with a beam of energy containing many wavelengths and a grating containing several hundred lines (and corners) per inch, a veritable plethora of tiny spectra is produced, one for each line of the grating that is illuminated. Here again the phase effect enters the picture. As the wavelengths move past the corners, wave fronts are formed (like dropping two pebbles in the pool). Where these cross, the wavelengths in phase reinforce one another, and those that are not in phase cancel out and disappear. What is left is a uniform display of wavelengths all neatly sorted out.

Some common grating monochromators have a half-band width of 35 nm., some 20 nm., and some (higher priced instruments) 0.5 nm. or less. However, gratings are plagued with more stray light difficulties than prisms. Stray light may be defined as radiant energy of unwanted wavelengths reaching the detector.

Minute imperfections in the optical surfaces of the monochromator cause stray light. A prism has only a few faces, and these can be polished to very close tolerances. A grating, on the other hand, has thousands of surfaces, the perfection of which is difficult to control. Also any imperfections in the master grating are transferred to the replica grating, plus a few new ones. In addition, most stray energy is at the longer wavelengths, which is generally a given detector's most sensitive region. This tends to magnify stray energy effects rather than minimize them.

In the less expensive instruments with wider half-band widths, a moderate amount of stray energy can be tolerated. However, in precision instruments, this becomes an intolerable situation. One solution to this, other than careful design and selection of high-quality replica gratings, is the use of a double monochromator. By passing the energy beam through two monochromators in series, most of the stray energy can be eliminated. This is an adequate, though expensive, solution.

Thus, it can be seen that a prism has a low stray energy output, but produces a curved nonlinear spectrum with its attendant complicated mechanical slit mechanism and varying half-band width. A grating has a linear straight spectrum and a constant half-band width, but sometimes it has excessive stray energy output unless a double monochromator is utilized. There are valid arguments and counterarguments for both systems.

Sample Container (Cuvette). This portion of a photometric system is probably one of the most neglected. A great many practical problems may arise here.

The most common cuvettes are of glass or silica and are round or square. Many infrared applications rely on the inclusion of solid material in a potassium bromide salt of high purity. This is then compressed into a tablet under high pressure, producing an I.R. transparent medium containing the material of interest which can be placed in the instrument. We need not concern ourselves further with this technique.

Square Cuvette. Let us first consider the square (or sometimes rectangular) cuvettes. These have plane-parallel optical faces and a constant light path. They are generally free of such optical aberrations as lens effect and variable refraction errors. This allows matching sets of cuvettes to very close tolerances. This type of cuvette is rather expensive, however, and is usually utilized in the more precise instruments. For precision work, this type of cell must be matched and always oriented in the instrument in the same way.

One must remember that the optically polished faces of a square cuvette can be scratched or etched and should not be roughly handled. Cleaning can be accomplished by a mild detergent or, if necessary, by a solution of one volume 3 N HCl and one volume ethanol. The gentle application of a cotton swab is often of value. Optical-grade cuvettes should not be allowed to soak for prolonged periods, and strong solutions such as dichromate cleaning solution should be avoided.

Round Cuvette. By far the most commonly used cuvette is the round test tube type. This type is fairly inexpensive and, if care is used, is adequate for most purposes. However it does have several drawbacks. In addition to reflection, refraction, and absorbance losses found in plane-parallel surface cuvettes that are fairly uniform, round cuvettes are prone to variable reflection and refraction errors as well as a lens effect.

Glass tubing is rarely round, being actually somewhat oval. In addition, the surfaces are not polished, so there is considerably more surface irregularity. These combine to make calibration and segregation of cuvettes into matched groups almost a must. Tube-type cuvettes are also very sensitive to position in the light path, and even if they are marked so they can be oriented in the light path the same way each time, small errors can be magnified considerably.

Calibration of Cuvettes. Reliance on commercial sources of cuvettes, without checking the degree of matching, can be hazardous. A fairly simple method of calibrating cuvettes (or even Pyrex culture tubes to be used as cuvettes) is as follows:

A solution of hemoglobin is made up roughly to a concentration of 50 mg. per 100 ml. Use a green filter or 540 nm. wavelength. (Obviously other stable solutions and wavelengths may be substituted.) One cuvette is filled with a hemoglobin solution and set in place, and the instrument is set to read 50 per cent T or, in the case of the Klett, at 150 Klett units. The same solution is then read in a series of cuvettes, rotating the cuvette. Those that match within 0.3 per cent T (or any other tolerance elected) are selected for use. A diamond pencil mark is made on the cuvette to indicate the proper alignment. One solution to the tube-type cuvette problem is the flow-through cuvette. At least two varieties are available commercially, the Celvac and the Thomas-Seligson units. Since the same cuvette is in the light path all the time, errors are compensated for by the blank, and highly reproducible results can be obtained. However, a source of vacuum is necessary to empty the cuvettes (once the sample has been poured in it cannot be reclaimed), and the rather small funnel tops of these units lead to spillage into and onto the instrument and resultant corrosion.

Several manufacturers have now produced flow-through systems with integral vacuum sources. Most of these systems have a cell volume in the neighborhood of 0.25 ml. and require a sample of 1.0 to 1.5 ml. for filling and washing.

Detectors. Electromagnetic energy can be detected and subsequently measured by first converting it to a different type of energy, namely, electrical energy. The conversion of one type of energy to another is accomplished by means of a transducer. Photocells, scintillation crystals, and so forth, are examples of transducers. Scintillation detectors are discussed in Chapter 7. Transducers used in the U.V.-visible-near-I.R. range are all photoconductive or photoemissive devices.

Photoconductive Devices. The photoconductive types are the simplest and generally can be considered to change their conductive properties under the influence of electromagnetic radiation.

PHOTOVOLTAIC CELL. The most common of the photoconductive types is the photovoltaic, or barrier layer, cell. This type requires no external voltage source but relies on internal electron transfers to produce a current in an external circuit. It is composed of an iron back plate and a layer of crystalline selenium or silicon on one surface.

Electrical contacts are made with the iron plate and an electrically conductive transparent coating on the front active layer. These cells are then sealed in a glass and plastic case to prevent chemical and physical damage to the very thin front coatings.

A photon striking one of the selenium or silicon atoms transfers its energy to an electron and raises it into a conduction band. This electron now can travel from the front to the back of the "barrier" and thus through the external circuit and back to the selenium or silicon layer. Thus, no electrons are ever really lost.

Theoretically a photovoltaic cell should last indefinitely. However, a wide gulf separates theory and practice, and these devices have a variable useful life: some will last for a long time in hard use, and others will go bad on the shelf. They are sensitive in the range of approximately 400 to 800 nm. They are more sensitive to the longer wavelengths, and failure is often first noticed at the less sensitive or shorter wavelengths.

The silicon types are more expensive but put out more current than the selenium types. The selenium types are more temperature sensitive than the silicon types. These cells tend to lose a certain degree of sensitivity in the first 5 to 10 minutes of operation and then become quite stable as thermal equilibrium is attained. It should also be realized that with instruments using fairly high energy levels, such as most filter photometers, a change of filter should be followed by a short equilibration period until the cell becomes "used to" the new wavelength. Similarly, if the instrument is inadvertently turned on with no filter in place, the cell will be blinded much as the human eye is and will require up to 30 minutes of rest before it will function properly.

PHOTORESISTORS. Another photoconductive type is the photoresistor. This is a small unit that consists of a band of a resistance material that decreases its resistance under the influence of electromagnetic energy. Photoresistors require an external source of current in order to operate, so instruments using them are electronically much more complex—less so, however, than those using photoemissive devices. With careful circuit design, the current flowing through a photoresistor can be made proportional to the intensity of electromagnetic energy striking the element. These cells have about the same sensitivity range as the photovoltaic cells.

Photoemissive Devices. Photoemissive cells, or phototubes, operate on a different principle than photoconductive elements.

In the simplest form, there are two electrodes in the tube, a curved negatively charged cathode, and a wire-like positively charged anode. The cathode is coated with a photoemissive compound such as cesium oxide. When a photon strikes this layer, it transfers its energy to an electron. In this excited state the electron can escape from the surface. Since the electron is negatively charged, it is repelled by the cathode and attracted by the anode. It then travels through the external circuit, with its fellows, as an electrical current. As previously mentioned, an external source of voltage is required. The main advantages of the phototube are high sensitivity to low energy levels and a certain latitude in altering the photosensitive surface to make the device more sensitive to radiant energy in a given wavelength region. However, the sensitivity to radiant energy is only slightly wider than that of the photoconductive types.

In the infrared regions the radiation produces a heating effect, so that thermocouples or similar devices may be used as transducers to convert the electromagnetic radiation into useful electrical energy.

Readout Devices. After the radiant energy passing through the sample has been detected, the resultant electrical current must be converted into some usable numerical form. Preferably this is one that relates to concentration, since that is what we are ultimately after. One of the most commonly used devices is a meter that is so calibrated that the current is presented as per cent transmittance and/or absorbance. Another commonly used indicator is a special kind of meter called a galvanometer. This device is designed not to measure the amount of current in the detector circuit, but actually the absence of it; i.e., it is a null indicator. More will be said about these types of circuits later.

Meters. Meters have some interesting characteristics, and it is also desirable to understand them a little better. A meter movement basically consists of a permanent horseshoe-shaped magnet with a movable frame and coil of wire suspended between its poles. This movable coil carries the current to be measured, and the axis of this coil is at right angles to the magnetic field between the poles of the permanent horseshoe magnet. An electrical current passing through a wire produces a magnetic field around the wire. The polarity of this field depends upon the direction of current flow. Therefore, a current passing through this suspended coil in the meter will produce a magnetic field of its own, and the field of the permanent magnet will attract the field of the coil, north pole attracting south pole, and vice versa. Since the coil is suspended and movable, this attraction results in rotation of the coil. If no counter force were applied, the field produced by any current, no matter how small, would result in the same amount of rotation, i.e., complete attraction of the coil's south pole with the permanent magnet's north pole and vice versa. This would not tell us very much, since the movement of the coil would be the same no matter what the current was. However, if counterforce is applied, either in the form of a taut-band suspension or coil-spring arrangement, the attraction of the two magnetic fields will at some point be balanced by the twisting of the taut-band suspension or tension on the coil-spring arrangement. Now, the more current flowing through the coil, the more powerful the magnetic field. This then produces rotation of the coil that is proportional to the magnetic field and therefore the current flow. If a pointer is attached to the coil, the amount of rotation of the coil is made known, and a suitable scale can be placed under the pointer.

At this point some of the problems become apparent. If the pointer is not in the same plane as the scale, parallax errors in reading can be made if the observer's eye is viewing the pointer from one side or the other. Some meters have a mirror next to the scale, so that if the pointer is superimposed on its mirror image, the eye of the beholder is properly positioned and fewer reading errors are made. The most important problems arise in the angle of rotation of the coil. The greater this angle, the greater the rotational error. This is primarily due to difficulties in manufacturing taut-bands and springs so that their tension is uniform throughout the angle of rotation necessary to move the pointer from one end of the scale to the other. Thus it can be seen that, after increasing the width of a meter to make it easier to read, any advantage may be obviated by increasing the angle of rotation, thus increasing the resultant angular errors.

One solution to this problem is to increase the length of the pointer. Thus, a small angle of rotation will produce a greater length of the arc at the tip of the pointer. Here again there is a limit to the length of the pointer, since it has weight, and soon a point is reached where more error is introduced from this source. The next step to a longer pointer is a weightless one, i.e., a beam of light. This system can be conveniently applied to the taut-band type suspensions. A small mirror is fixed to the suspension, and a beam of light is focused onto the mirror. The reflected beam is then projected onto a suitable scale on a translucent window. A hairline in the lens system is used to project a line shadow or indicator on this scale. This allows the pointer to be lengthened considerably, which then allows very small angles of rotation to be used. This decreases angular errors considerably. In addition, since the hairline is projected right onto the reading scale, parallax errors are also eliminated. Common examples of this type of arrangement are the Coleman Junior, with an effective pointer length of 13 inches, and the meters used with some of the Baird flame photometers and the Evelyn Colorimeter, which by reflecting the light beam back and forth inside the case attain a pointer length of about 3 feet. These problems of angular rotational error are also avoided by using the null type circuitry, in which the meter needle is always returned to the same position by other controlling devices. Since the meter is always returned to the same position, angular errors are eliminated. The most common example of this is in the Klett.

Servomechanisms. Considerable use is now being made of servomechanisms for readout devices. These are all null type devices in which the output of a separate current source is made to match the output of the detector. Here a special motor functions as a galvanometer and, by means of gears, the position of balance is either presented as a trace on a recorder or in digital form. A common example of the former is the AutoAnalyzer and of the latter is the flame photometer of Instrumentation Laboratories. More will be said about these types in the discussion of the null-type of circuit.

Digital Systems. More and more instruments are appearing with digital readouts. Although these are more complex and therefore both more expensive and prone to problems, they practically eliminate the various errors that may occur with meter movements. Most digital systems take the output voltage from the detector (analog signal) and convert it to an incremental (digital) signal which can be counted. The number of counts is then proportional to the original voltage. This process is called analog to digital (A-D) conversion.

In addition, accurate solid-state logarithmic amplifiers are now available allowing presentation in absorbance units, and slope controls allow presentation in concentration units. The addition of multiplication by a constant allows the presentation of kinetic enzyme measurements in appropriate units. Well-designed systems with some or all of the above features not only save time, but eliminate many sources of error, particularly those associated with calculations.

DIRECT READING AND NULL POINT SYSTEMS

Direct reading and null point systems are the two basic arrangements for presenting absorption or emission measurement data.

Direct Reading Systems. The simplest type is the direct reading system utilizing photovoltaic detectors and a meter readout. The output of this type of photocell is sufficient to drive a sensitive meter directly with no further amplification. Examples of this system are the Coleman Junior and the Leitz. Other direct reading instruments use detectors whose output is not sufficient to drive a meter directly. These utilize an amplifier to increase the output of the detector sufficiently to operate the readout. An example of this type is the Spectronic 20. Direct reading types of instruments all utilize a meter as the readout device, thus making the final result subject to any meter errors present, as has already been discussed. Generally the more expensive instruments do not use a direct reading system; but recently there appears to have been a resurgence of interest, and some fairly expensive instruments that use this type of readout have appeared on the market. Some newer meters are more accurate than those heretofore obtainable, but meters can present some real problems. Again it is well to keep in mind that a large, easy-to-read meter is not necessarily an accurate one. As was mentioned before, using a long light beam pointer to keep the rotational angle of the meter movement small is a great help.

Null Point System. The null point system is perhaps the one most commonly used. In this type of system the output of the detector is balanced against the "output" of another circuit. The meter is replaced by a galvanometer or a servomotor, which serves to indicate the state of balance. If the Klett is used as an example of this type of circuit, the basic concept can be more easily explained and understood.

The Klett utilizes two photovoltaic cells. One cell is known as the reference cell and has the shutter operating in front of it. The other cell, or sample cell, has the cuvette well in front of it. The outputs of these cells are connected to two resistors of equal resistance. One is fixed and the other is variable. The variable resistor, or potentiometer, is accurately made and has a logarithmic scale on the dial face. Thus far we have four components, forming the basis of the Wheatstone bridge type circuit, which is a classic null point system. The galvanometer is so connected that it will respond to any current flow in either direction, and only when both sides of the circuit are balanced electrically is the galvanometer pointer centered. Thus, when the blank is inserted in the cuvette well and the potentiometer is on zero absorbance (A) or Klett units (Klett units = A × 500), the circuit is balanced by increasing or decreasing the radiant energy that falls on the reference cells and thus electrical output. This is accomplished by adjusting the shutter. When the sample is placed in the cuvette well, the circuit is again unbalanced because of absorbance of the unknown.

The circuit now is brought into electrical balance by rotating the potentiometer dial until the null point is reached. The absorbance of the sample can now be read from the dial as Klett units. This system is inherently more accurate than direct reading systems because potentiometers can be made much more accurate than meters and angular errors of rotation are eliminated. When the circuit is balanced, the galvanometer needle is always in the same position. As a dividend in the Klett, the use of matched photocells to a large extent compensates for lamp intensity variations due to voltage fluctuations, making voltage regulation unnecessary. However, as the cells age, one cell may become less sensitive faster than the other, and severe voltage changes (e.g., a water bath on the same heavily loaded circuit turning off and on) can cause fluctuations in the outputs of the photocells. If this happens when one is using the instrument, errors can be introduced in the measurements.

Direct reading instruments such as the IL-143 Flame Photometer utilize this same basic bridge principle, except that the electronics are considerably more complex. Simply stated, for one channel only, the lithium phototube and sodium phototube take the place of the two photocells. A servomotor takes the place of the galvanometer. This motor will turn in either direction, depending on the direction of current flow, and will stop when the circuit is balanced (the null point). The motor is mechanically connected by a gear system to a potentiometer and to a digital counter. The components are arranged so that each digit is made equivalent to 1 mEq. per liter. This type of servo system seeks circuit balance automatically, and provision is made to set the blank and to adjust to the single standard value electrically.

One must remember, however, that in any single point standardization system one is assuming linearity. The linearity should be checked frequently with high- and low-value standards or controls. This principle is valid no matter how simple or complex the instrument happens to be. Other instruments with digital readout are becoming more and more common.

The AutoAnalyzer also depends on this basic bridge system of measurement. The AutoAnalyzer colorimeter has two photocells, one reference and one sample. The net output of these photocells is fed to the recorder, which contains a servomotor-potentiometer system, but instead of a digital readout, a pen is used to indicate the position of balance. This produces a series of curves, the peaks of which are proportional to the concentration of the unknowns that are passing through the colorimeter flowcell.

BEER'S LAW

The Lambert-Bouguer-Bunsen-Roscoe-Beer laws are essential to the understanding and intelligent use of absorption spectrophotometric methodology. The combination of laws for convenience is referred to as Beer's law. However, it should be realized that it is the combination of several laws, and that the above-named five persons all contributed to it. Bouguer stated that "equal thicknesses of an absorbing material will absorb a constant fraction of the energy incident upon it." This statement is the cornerstone of the whole law, and a real understanding of the meaning and scope of this statement is the key to correcting the confusion that Beer's law has created. With this in mind, let us examine this statement in greater detail.

"Equal thicknesses of an absorbing material . . ." It is easy to see a tangible example of this, e.g., several 1-mm. thick red glass plates stacked together. However, the real meaning is the concept of innumerable parallel monomolecular layers of the absorbing material situated normal (perpendicular) to the path of the beam of radiant energy. If we bring this to the molecular level, the whole concept becomes easier to understand.

". . . will absorb a constant fraction . . ." Again, at the molecular level, this is easier to understand. Each molecule that absorbs energy does so in a characteristic fashion. This added, or absorbed, energy is used generally to increase motion in the molecule. This type of motion change, e.g., valence electron changes or twisting of end groups on large molecules, determines what energy (wavelengths) will be absorbed. For a given molecule this absorption is related to the amount of energy presented. A specific fraction will be absorbed and the rest will be transmitted. This fraction is characteristic for a given molecule and is the basis of the concept of absorptivity.

". . . of the energy incident upon it." Again, let us use our molecular plate model. The energy incident on the first plate has a certain fraction absorbed. The remainder that is transmitted becomes the incident energy to the second plate, where the same fraction is absorbed. This sequence of events is repeated until that which is transmitted by the last plate is allowed to fall on the detector and be measured. Now we can use some terms and symbols to proceed further with our analysis of this part of the law. It can be seen from what has been said before that we are really measuring the energy that is transmitted by an absorbing material.

If we let P equal the transmitted energy and P_0 equal the incident energy, then the ratio $\frac{P}{P_0}$ represents the transmittance (T) of the absorbing material. If the material does not absorb at all, then P and P_0 are the same, and $\frac{P}{P_0} = T = 1$. This means that anything that absorbs must have a transmittance of less than 1. To avoid working consistently with decimals, the simple expedient of per cent, or multiplying by 100, was resorted to. Thus in our nonabsorbing example, when P and P_0 are the same, T = 1 and per cent T = 100.

Now we can examine the law thus far in greater detail. With some serious contemplation of this law, one may ascertain that the absorption of energy is logarithmic. This can be illustrated by the following example, with $\frac{1}{5}$ or 0.20 as the constant fraction absorbed and 0.80 as the fraction transmitted.

If P_0 starts out as 100 per cent of the original incident energy, then $0.80 \times 100 = 80$ per cent = P. This P then becomes P_0 for the next layer, and we repeat the calculation: $0.80 \times 80 = 64$ per cent = P. If we continue this process, the progression is 100, 80, 64, 52, 42, 36, 29, 23, etc. If one plots these values on coordinate graph paper, a logarithmic curve is produced. On semilog paper, a straight line is produced.

Once this part of the law is understood, the next two additions to it are easily seen. The first states that the thicker the absorbing material, the greater the absorption; the second states that the greater the concentration of absorbing molecules, the greater the absorption. If this is considered on the molecular scale, in both of these situations there are more absorbing molecules in the light path.

The Duboscq colorimeter varies the length of the light path, and matching with the standard occurs when the number of absorbing molecules is the same in standard and unknown cells. By visual matching the transmittance of both cells is brought to equality, and therefore concentration varies with the length of the light path. In spectrophotometers, the light path is held constant, and concentration varies with the transmittance.

The use of Beer's law could stop here, but all transmittance measurements would have to be read from semilog graphs, or logarithms would have to be used in calculating results. This presents difficulties. Logarithms are not easy for the average person to use, and mistakes in reading from semilog graphs are stated to be about three times as common as those made in reading from coordinate graphs. In addition, what we are measuring is energy transmitted, but what we are really interested in is energy absorbed. This is admittedly minor, since both T and $\frac{1}{T}$ vary with the concentration, as can be demonstrated by plotting the reciprocals of the earlier example on semilog paper.

However, to avoid all of these difficulties, some mathematic manipulation produces absorbance (A). This formerly was referred to as density (D) or optical density (OD). Further, by using the negative logarithm of T, measurements are transformed to the energy absorbed, $\frac{1}{T}$, which is less confusing and more esthetic. The equation now becomes $A = -\log T$, and since 2 is the log of 100 the per cent formula becomes $A = 2 - \log$ per cent T. Absorbance now is linearly related to concentration, allowing coordinate paper to be used, as well as relatively simple calculations. Both lead to fewer mistakes. Tables are available for conversion of per cent T to A, so constant reference to log tables is unnecessary.

Many instruments have both per cent transmittance and absorbance scales. The absorbance scale is of necessity logarithmic, and reading errors are more easily made, especially because it reads from right to left. For this reason it may be preferable to read per cent T and convert to A by means of a table. The Klett solves part of this problem by having only one scale and by being so constructed that it reads from left to right. As was stated, Klett units = $A \times 500$.

Now we are in a position to summarize the entire law as it is used in absorption spectrophotometry. The molecular constant of absorption or fraction absorbed at a given wavelength is called absorptivity (a). The thickness of the absorbing material, or length of the light path, is represented by the letter b. The concentration is represented by the letter c. Since the total absorbance is related to all of these, the formula becomes

$$A = a\,b\,c$$

Further, extinction coefficient (e) is defined as the absorbance of a molar or millimolar solution of the absorbing molecule, with the length of the light path being 1 cm. and the wavelength specified. Note that absorptivity is a general term, while extinction coefficient specifies a particular set of conditions. They both refer to the same molecular characteristic.

In routine use, the standard and unknown are the same material, so a is the same for both. The length of the light path (b) is held constant by measuring the standard and unknown in the same cuvette or in matched cuvettes. Therefore, in routine usage A is proportional to concentration (c).

This allows a further working simplification to be used to advantage. If the concentration of the standard is divided by the absorbance of the standard, a factor (F) can be derived.

$$\frac{c}{A} = F$$

The factor really contains units of concentration, as well as absorbance, such as

$$\frac{\text{mg./dl.}}{1\text{A}} \text{ or } \frac{\text{mg./dl.}}{1 \text{ Klett unit}}$$

Therefore, A of unknown × F = c of unknown. The factor also represents the slope of the calibration curve and assumes that this slope is constant, i.e., linear. This method can be used only with linear systems. In the common parlance of the laboratory, such a system is said to "follow Beer's law." Systems that are nonlinear must be used with a calibration curve and not with a factor.

In addition to use of a factor, the units of concentration used for the standard must represent those of the unknown sample. Factors such as differences in dilution, aliquoting during the chemical manipulations of the unknown but not the standard, and differences in final volume of the standard and sample must be taken into account. If these are not taken into account in the final representative concentration of the standard, they must be inserted in the A × F = c formula. The former procedure obviously is much more satisfactory in the long run.

Thorough understanding of the basic tenets of Beer's law will go a long way toward the intelligent use of absorption spectrophotometry.

FLAME PHOTOMETRY

The average clinical laboratory places great reliance on flame photometry, at least for measurement of sodium and potassium. We shall discuss the conventional flame photometers, which may also be referred to as flame emission photometers, as well as the newer atomic absorption spectrophotometers. These are complementary techniques, since flame emission photometry is the most practical method for sodium and potassium and atomic absorption can measure certain elements that cannot be measured easily by flame emission.

Flame Emission Photometry. Flame emission photometry is based on the principle that atoms of many metallic elements given sufficient energy in one form or another will emit this energy at particular wavelengths that are characteristic for the element. Note the similarity to fluorescence. Energy in flame emission photometry is supplied as heat or thermal energy, and energy in fluorescence is supplied as radiant energy that is generally in the ultraviolet region of the spectrum.

A particular amount or quantum of thermal energy is absorbed by an orbital electron, thus allowing it to occupy a higher, more energetic but less stable orbit. Being unstable, the electron returns almost instantaneously to its previous base or ground state and emits this quantum of absorbed energy in the form of a photon of a particular wavelength. For example, sodium emits energy primarily at 589 nm., with subsidiary emissions that are much less intense. In the average flame, only about 1 per cent of the atoms present undergo this transformation and emission of energy.

This very small proportion of atoms that emit, coupled with the relatively low intensity of emission of most elements, rather severely limits the biologic applications of this technique. Sodium and potassium are the only elements that have sufficiently high intensities to be measured with reasonable ease. Calcium has a fairly low intensity emission, but if very sensitive instruments are used, it can be measured reasonably well.

Components. What components make up a flame emission photometer? The main difference between a conventional photometer and a flame photometer is that the sample "container" and the source are the same, i.e., the flame. Also there must be an atomizer of some type to change the liquid sample into a fine mist that can be uniformly dispersed in the flame. The flame and atomizer are integrated partners, and although many design combinations are possible, the flame and atomizer must be considered as a single functioning unit. Flames can be generally classified as "hard" or "soft." A hard flame is small and hot, a common example being the flame of an oxyacetylene welding torch. The soft flame is larger and has a lower temperature. The best example of a soft flame is the flame of the Bunsen burner.

HARD FLAMES. Hard flames utilize oxygen with hydrogen, acetylene, or propane. The diluted fluid is aspirated directly into the flame. Hard flames are very susceptible to gas flow irregularities caused by dirt and dried salts.

They require frequent and careful maintenance and, probably for this reason, are no longer used to any extent.

SOFT FLAMES. The soft flames generally use compressed air and propane or natural gas. A modified Meker-type burner is commonly utilized, and several modifications have been attempted to stabilize the flame. Atomization of the diluted material is generally accomplished in an atomization chamber that is in the air supply line to the burner. This allows the larger droplets to settle out, and only the fine mist is carried into the flame, mixed with the air. If natural gas is used as fuel, further precautions are necessary. One should be sure that the pressure fluctuations in the gas line are not extreme (± 20 per cent probably is a reasonable range). A simple water manometer can be constructed and the pressure fluctuations can then be observed. In addition, many gas companies mix propane and/or manufactured gas with natural gas in cold weather. These gases all have different fuel-air ratios for optimum combustion, and mixtures will produce even further variations. These mixtures are barely tolerated by gas stoves and furnaces and present even more serious problems in precise burners that have been carefully designed for one gas only. If either of these situations is present, the best alternative is to use bottled propane. If gas composition is maintained fairly constant, but if the pressure fluctuation is intolerable or the pressure is too low, a pump and small reservoir can be set up in the gas line. This sometimes has to be resorted to when local fire codes do not allow propane.

Energy emitted by the atoms of interest, e.g., sodium, is passed through a filter (almost always an interference filter) to remove unwanted radiation from other emitting elements present and from the background emission of the flame itself. Interference filters lend themselves admirably to this application because of their narrow band pass, their ability to produce filters of any desired wavelength, and their relatively high transmission at that wavelength. The flame photometric attachments for the more sophisticated spectrophotometers use the grating or prism monochromator of the basic instrument to isolate the desired emission lines. The selected radiation is then presented to a detector, which can be one or another type of photoconductor, or a phototube, and the resultant electrical current is measured.

Direct and Internal Standards. Flame photometry may be performed either by the direct or internal standard methods. In the direct method, emission of only one element is measured, and by use of a standard curve the unknown values are obtained. The direct method is most commonly used with instruments having a so-called "hard" flame.

The internal standard method uses another element that is in all solutions at a constant concentration and the instrument makes a comparison of the emission of the desired element with the emission of the "reference" element. This reference element must be absent in biologic materials, must have a fairly high emission intensity, and must emit at a wavelength at which it can be separated adequately from the unknown elements. Lithium satisfies all of these conditions admirably and is used universally as the reference element. However, recently lithium salts have been used in the treatment of some psychotic disorders. Although the levels are low, approximately 3 mEq. per liter, this may be cause for concern.

The internal standard method is utilized with some intermediate flame instruments and should be used with all soft flame instruments. By using the internal standard, which is present in constant concentration, and measuring the emission of sodium against this reference, flame instability should be cancelled out. Theoretically whatever affects the sodium emission will also affect the lithium emission. Differences in atomization rates due to pressure fluctuation or solution viscosity may alter the results, however. Changes in atomization rates change the flame temperature, since more or less heat is required for more or less evaporation. Unfortunately the emission of lithium does not parallel that of sodium or potassium. Therefore, the internal standard method will compensate for small variations in flame stability and atomization rates but not large ones.

A wetting agent is often recommended for use in making dilutions. This tends to minimize the changes in atomizer flow rates due to differences in viscosity of the samples and helps to make flow rates more uniform. Obviously the same batch of lithium diluent must be used for blank, standards, controls, and unknowns or serious errors will be introduced. The atomizers must be kept clean and free of debris because of the above-mentioned flow rate effects. It is imperative that a good quality control program be utilized so that most problems can be recognized at as early a stage as possible.

Flame emission photometry presents a few unique problems also. Some ions have the property of enhancing or quenching radiation from other ions. Much work has been done on the effects of this type of interference, but no agreement has been reached. Fortunately the concentration of the various ions in serum does not vary too much, so the general practice is to ignore any interference effects. In urine, the concentrations vary rather widely, but here again no correction is made. Interference from this source can be checked for a particular instrument by constructing a calibration curve using pure solutions of the ion to be measured, and then measuring an unknown sample as well as a 1:2 or 1:4 dilution of the unknown sample. If the respective dilutions fall on the calibration curve where they are supposed to, significant interference is not present.

Atomic Absorption Spectrophotometry. In the past few years a different type of flame photometric technique, called atomic absorption spectrophotometry, has become rather widespread. As was previously mentioned, flame emission photometry utilizes only about 1 per cent of the atoms present, which is inadequate for most of the metals present in biologic material. This is due either to very low concentration or low emission intensities or both. What about the other 99 per cent?

Atoms in a flame are rendered active enough so that a large percentage of them will respond to radiant energy of their characteristic emission wavelengths and absorb it by a poorly understood process called resonance. Energy at these particular wavelengths can be supplied by a special type of lamp called a hollow cathode lamp.

The cathode is composed of or contains the desired metal. If we use our sodium example again, a hollow cathode lamp containing sodium can be made to emit energy at the 589 nm. wavelength of sodium emission. If this beam of energy is directed through a flame containing sodium atoms, this energy will be absorbed in proportion to the number of sodium atoms present. It is also necessary to have the temperature of the lamp higher than that of the flame, otherwise absorption of energy will not occur. Special burners are used for this technique, and the fuel, oxygen, and atomized sample are mixed together prior to burning. Considerable effort has been expended in the design of these burners, since the relatively low flow rates, large flame size, and the desire for low-temperature flames are all conducive to flashback and explosions in the burner. The sodium in the flame is also emitting some energy at 589 nm., and this now becomes unwanted radiation. This cannot be removed by a monochromator, since it is at the same wavelength as the energy from the lamp. The energy from the lamp is therefore made to act differently from the energy emitted by the flame. A rotating sector disc that produces pulses of lamp energy the frequency of which can be controlled by the shape and speed of the sector is placed between the lamp and the flame. The flame emission is steady at a given level and does not pulsate, at least at the same frequency as the lamp energy. The detector is allowed to look at both the pulsating and steady energy at 589 nm. through a monochromator set for this wavelength. The detector produces an electric current that corresponds to the pulsating energy from the lamp that is transmitted by the sample (flame). These two forms, really a D.C. signal with a superimposed A.C. signal, can be electronically separated so that the D.C. signal is rejected and only the A.C. signal is allowed to be measured. Thus, only absorption of 589 nm. lamp energy by the flame is measured, and all flame emission at 589 nm. is rejected.

Atomic absorption spectrophotometry is an extremely sensitive technique, so much so that it is not worthwhile for strong emitters like sodium or potassium, at least in the concentrations found in the average biologic sample. However, it makes possible for the first time the accurate measurement of such metals as calcium, iron, zinc, lead, copper, and magnesium that are present in essentially trace amounts in biologic samples and for which few if any other satisfactory methods are available. The detection limits of atomic absorption techniques depend more on the concentration of metal present and on the availability of satisfactory hollow cathode lamps than on any other factors.

FLUOROMETRY

A potentially very useful method for many applications in the clinical laboratory is the measurement of fluorescence. Fluorescence is a characteristic of a relatively small group of compounds, compared to the very large number of compounds that absorb energy. When certain compounds are presented with relatively intense radiant energy of a particular wavelength, a transformation occurs that is very similar to that occurring in flame emission and absorption. Absorption of a photon by a valence electron raises it to a higher unstable energy level. The electron returns to its ground state almost instantaneously (approximately 2×10^{-11} seconds) and emits a photon of energy.

Since there always is a slight amount of energy lost, the emitted wavelength is always longer than the exciting wavelength. This generally means that the exciting wavelengths are in the U.V. region and the emitted wavelengths are in the visible region. This is an extremely sensitive technique, measurement of quantities in the microgram to nanogram per milliliter ranges being easily attained. The only questions are: Does the material of interest fluoresce or can it be made to fluoresce, and is there any interference by other reagents in the system?

Basic Components. The basic instrument itself is composed of the basic components, which are suitably modified. The light source must be rich in ultraviolet and of fairly high intensity. Various types of mercury or xenon arc discharge lamps are most commonly used. This is termed the primary source, and the desired U.V. wavelength for excitation is selected, usually by a suitable U.V. transmitting filter termed the primary filter. More expensive instruments use a grating monochromator for selecting the primary or excitation wavelength. The energy is then directed through the sample cuvette or against a solid matrix, such as agar gel, and fluorescence of the unknown is produced. This fluorescent energy is emitted in all directions, so the detector is placed at right angles to the primary energy beam. Thus it does not see the transmitted U.V. energy. Since stray light is also present (reflection, refraction, etc.), a secondary filter that transmits only the fluorescent wavelength is interposed between the sample and the detector. Some instruments use a primary filter, but use a grating or prism monochromator for isolating the secondary emission. This system or a variant of it is commonly used in instruments that are basically spectrophotometers but have fluorescence accessory attachments. Both of these maneuvers eliminate all energy except the fluorescent wavelength. The fluorescent energy is detected and read out by the conventional mechanisms.

Because emission rather than absorption is measured, increasing the concentration will proportionately increase the emission, resulting in a linear relationship, just as in flame emission photometry.

THE ART AND SCIENCE OF SPECTROPHOTOMETRY

One of the major problems with spectrophotometric instruments is their tendency to have one component or another change or deteriorate slowly, so that instrumental inaccuracies creep up on one slowly. Occasionally this is so insidious that errors can be gradually introduced over a period of many days or weeks before it becomes apparent that something is wrong. If a component fails suddenly (e.g., the lamp burns out 2 minutes before you are going to read a critically timed procedure), there is considerable consternation, but repairs are made relatively easily, and the instrument is returned to its original operating condition. On the other hand, gradual component deterioration is not so easily recognized and occasionally is not so easily repaired.

Quality Control. One of the best all-round safeguards is a well-organized quality control program. The actual material used (homemade or commercial) is not as important as the design of the program. A drift of the control values may indicate subtle instrument changes. Remember that the use of a commercial serum preparation as the standard does not fulfill the criteria for a quality control program.

A daily reading of a known solution may be of value as long as the stability of the solution is known, orientation of the cuvette in the instrument is reproducible, and tender loving care is given to the outside surface of the cuvette. The Coleman Instrument Company has produced such a solution, and a good protocol for its use in the Coleman Junior. Other manufacturers have recently produced systems that are designed to test stray light, linearity of the instrument, and in some instruments a rough check of wavelength calibration. It is strongly recommended that one of these systems be used weekly or biweekly to check instrument function. As more information is obtained, better systems for checking instrument performance will evolve. Most instrument manuals contain a trouble-shooting guide, but this generally is not practical for a daily or weekly check—it is only practical for localizing the source of a problem after it has become apparent.

Calibration Curves. One must never take anything for granted. Calibration curves rarely stay constant year after year, and reliance on precalibration is indeed a poor procedure. It leads to a state of suspended animation of the common sense of the operator, as well as to forcing slavish conformation to the manufacturer's methodology. It must be realized that different batches of reagents, subtle changes in methodology (changes of a few hundredths of a degree in incubation temperatures will affect enzyme determinations, for example), and instrument changes all combine to make precalibration not only useless but dangerous. The best thing to do with the precalibration section of the instrument manual is to throw it out as soon as it is unpacked.

Methodology is being improved or replaced at a rapid rate, and the understanding of what can and what cannot be done with a given instrument is of paramount importance.

In particular, the requirements of the absorbing molecule in regard to the degree of monochromaticity necessary for adherence to Beer's law stands out. Sensitivity can be changed, and nonlinearity can sometimes be corrected, especially in filter instruments. A spectral transmittance curve can often allow proper selection of a filter or indicate the necessity for a narrow-band device, such as an interference filter, prism instrument, etc. These statements

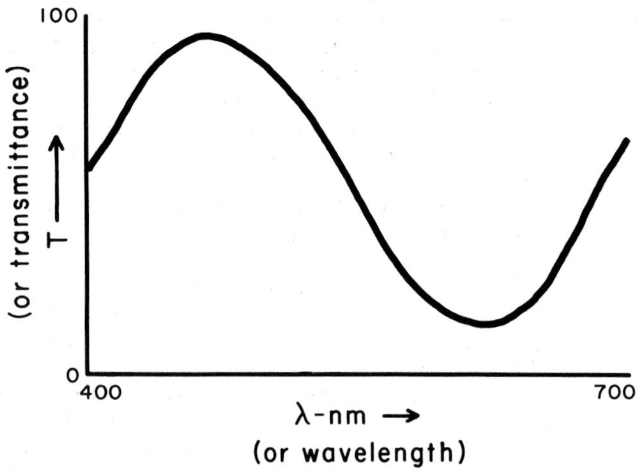

Figure 8–6. Spectral transmittance curve for the phenate-hypochlorite reaction for ammonia (Berthelot reaction).

can be amplified by some relatively simple examples.

The spectral transmittance curve of the Berthelot reaction for ammonia is shown in Figure 8–6. Inspection of this curve shows no real plateau but a smooth curve. If wavelengths in the 450 nm. region are selected, changes in concentration produce relatively small changes in absorbance. This situation leads to low sensitivity. If wavelengths at the other plateau (above 650 nm.) are used, the same changes in concentration will produce large changes in absorbance. Although this gives great sensitivity, its use for serum urea nitrogen would force an inordinate number of dilutions and redilutions. In this case great sensitivity is not necessary; in fact, it is undesirable because of the short range of measurable concentration. Therefore, a compromise of range and sensitivity is needed, and the only place that this is available is the long slope from about 480 nm. to about 600 nm.

This presents some more problems, however. When a wide area of a slope is measured, absorbance changes (related to concentration) at the two ends of the slope do not vary uniformly. The wider the half-band width of the filter, the greater the apparent deviation from Beer's law. This is an instance of instrumental deviation rather than chemical deviation from Beer's law. Figure 8–7 shows the 10 per cent departure from linearity with the Klett 54 filter, and the linear plot with a narrow-band pass instrument (0.5 nm. half-band width). One must therefore select an instrument that will produce a linear plot for the range desired or pick the point of deviation and use this as the highest absorbance to be used without dilution.

A somewhat different situation exists in the case of the O-toluidine glucose method. Inspection of this spectral transmittance curve shows a reasonable plateau at about 640 nm. that is of intermediate sensitivity. We should be able to get a reasonable range as well as adequate sensitivity. The absorption peak is symmetrical, so we should not have the nonlinearity problems encountered in the previous example. However, one must always check the linearity of the combined chemical system and instrument to be used to determine the point of nonlinearity.

These are examples of why the laboratorian should be able to refer to spectral absorbance curves of the method under consideration and why instrument manufacturers should supply a set of spectral absorbance curves with the glass filters supplied or available.

These problems are common with filter instruments, yet many of these instruments are quite adequate for most of the absorption

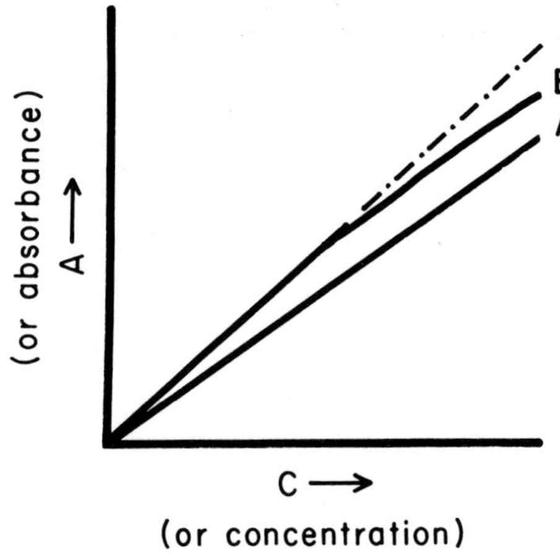

Figure 8–7. Concentration absorbance curve of ammonia (BUN) with the Berthelot reaction. B is the curve produced by a Klett 54 filter, and A is the curve produced by a grating monochromator.

spectrophotometry done in clinical laboratories. If one realizes that the entire instrument is not the cause of the problem, but only poor selection of a filter, then life becomes much simpler. It must also be remembered that the narrower the band pass, the more sensitive the instrument is to minor degrees of turbidity. This is becoming more and more important as more direct methods using serum or plasma are developed, and as the tendency to market narrow-band pass instruments increases. A rule of thumb is to use the widest band pass consistent with the range of instrumental linearity desired.

Photometric Errors. In general, photometric errors are excessive in the regions below 10 per cent T and above 80 per cent T (A of 1 and 0.11). This includes many small sources of error, and whenever possible, methods should be adjusted so that the more important readings are in a desirable range. If the value for a given procedure falls below 10 per cent T, two courses of action are possible. The course taken depends totally on the chemistry of the system. If sufficient amounts of reactants are present and complete reaction is assured, then the solution and blank may be diluted with an appropriate solvent and read. The answer is then multiplied by the dilution factor. However, if sufficient amounts of reactant are not present, a dilution of the starting material (e.g., serum) must be made and the procedure run again. The Gilford Instrument Company states that their instruments can measure an absorbance of 3 (0.1 per cent T) without significantly increasing the photometric error. Other instruments that have sufficient accuracy in the absorbance range of 1.0 to 2.0 are also becoming available. In some instruments, smaller diameter cuvettes can be used, but one should also read the standard and blank in the same size cuvette.

What is happening when we use a blank solution to set the readout to an arbitrary point? Really we are using a simple analog computer to subtract reagent absorbance and losses due to reflection, refraction, and absorbance of the cuvette and to compensate for the lens effect of round cuvettes. The arbitrary point selected is one that eliminates calculations, i.e., 100 per cent T (and 0.0 A) on the scale.

It must again be emphasized that cuvette mismatch will introduce gross errors in spectrophotometry.

Another thing that properly belongs to the art of spectrophotometry is the ability to read a given procedure on more than one instrument. When standards are used with each run, as they should be whenever possible, it is generally easy to shift instruments. However, for some procedures, calibration curves are necessary or may be adequate if the methodology is stable. This flexibility is invaluable in case of instrument failure.

There are many other specialized applications of the art of spectrophotometry. With a basic understanding, the interested person can progress as far as desired or necessary. The selected references contain additional information as well as more detailed discussion of many other aspects of this field.

REFERENCES

A Procedure for Monitoring the Performance Parameters of Coleman Junior Spectrophotometers. Coleman Technical Report No. T-198. Maywood, Illinois, Coleman Instruments Corp.

Glass Color Filters. Catalog No. CF3. Corning, New York, Corning Glass Works.

Henry, R. J.: Clinical Chemistry. New York, Hoeber Medical Division, Harper & Row, 1964.

Teloh, H. A.: Clinical Flame Photometry. Springfield, Illinois, Charles C Thomas, 1959.

Udenfriend, S.: Fluorescence Assay in Biology and Medicine. New York, Academic Press, Inc., 1962.

Willard, H. H., Merritt, L. L., Jr., and Dean, J. A.: Instrumental Methods of Analysis. 4th ed. Princeton, New Jersey, D. Van Nostrand Co., Inc., 1965.

Chapter 9

CLINICAL CHEMISTRY

by JOHN BERNARD HENRY, M.D.

Although other chapters review specific subjects within the realm of chemistry, general principles and techniques with clinicopathologic correlations will be presented with specific topics related to carbohydrates, proteins, and lipids. Selected inorganic ions and vitamins will also be reviewed briefly.

SPECIMEN COLLECTION AND PROCESSING

Chemical analysis of blood and other body fluids requires special attention to specimen collection and processing (Winston, 1965). Since blood is the most frequent specimen analyzed in clinical chemistry and other body fluids are reviewed in appropriate chapters, this specimen merits special consideration. With the exception of glucose, triglycerides, and inorganic phosphorus, most blood chemical constituents reveal no significant change after a standard breakfast, so it is not essential for the patient to be in an absolute fasting state prior to blood specimen collection (Annino and Relman, 1959).

However, lipemia (lactescence), caused by a transient rise in triglycerides as chylomicrons following a meal containing fat, may cause interference with a large number of chemical determinations because of turbidity. Hence, blood is most often collected from a patient in the postabsorptive state. This is usually accomplished with an overnight fast (12 to 14 hours, especially for lipids), although a four- to six-hour fast will usually suffice. Diurnal variation unrelated to eating is associated with a change in concentration of certain blood constituents such as iron and corticosteroids. Furthermore, dietary habits may influence blood concentration of uric acid, urea, and lipids. A glucose tolerance test procedure requires that the patient have an adequate carbohydrate intake (250 gm. per day) for three days prior to the glucose tolerance test.

Venipuncture with a Vacutainer system (Becton Dickinson, Rutherford, New Jersey 07070) is ideal in terms of direct sampling, economy, and efficiency (Figs. 9–1 and 9–2). This system provides flexibility in terms of specimen volume (2, 3, 5, 7, or 10 ml. per tube) and anticoagulant (heparin, oxalate, citrate, or ethylenediaminetetraacetic acid salts), as well as chemically clean or sterile glassware. Disposable needles eliminate the hazard of serum hepatitis transmission, and an adapter with holder may be used for selection of appropriate gauge needle when necessary. While rubber stoppers are color coded to distinguish whether the test tube contains a specific anticoagulant, is a plain tube, or is a special tube made chemically clean (e.g., for lead, iron, and iodine determinations), a color coded label may also be applied to insure appropriate tube selection and proper identification of specimen in terms of patient's name, hospital number, date, and time of collection. Serum is used for many analyses because of potential interference by the various anticoagulants. Whole blood with anticoagulant yields the frequently analyzed blood component or derivative known as plasma. Heparin in the form of a lithium salt is an effective anticoagulant in small quantities without significant effect on many determinations and is the ideal universal anticoagulant for blood from which plasma may be harvested (Table 9–1). For glucose measurements fluoride may be added to heparin. Fluoride impairs glycolysis of the blood cells that may otherwise destroy glucose at the rate of about 5 per cent per hour. In the presence of bacterial contamination of blood specimens, fluoride inhibition of glycolysis is neither adequate nor effective in preserving glucose concentration. Furthermore, prompt separation of plasma or serum from cells is important

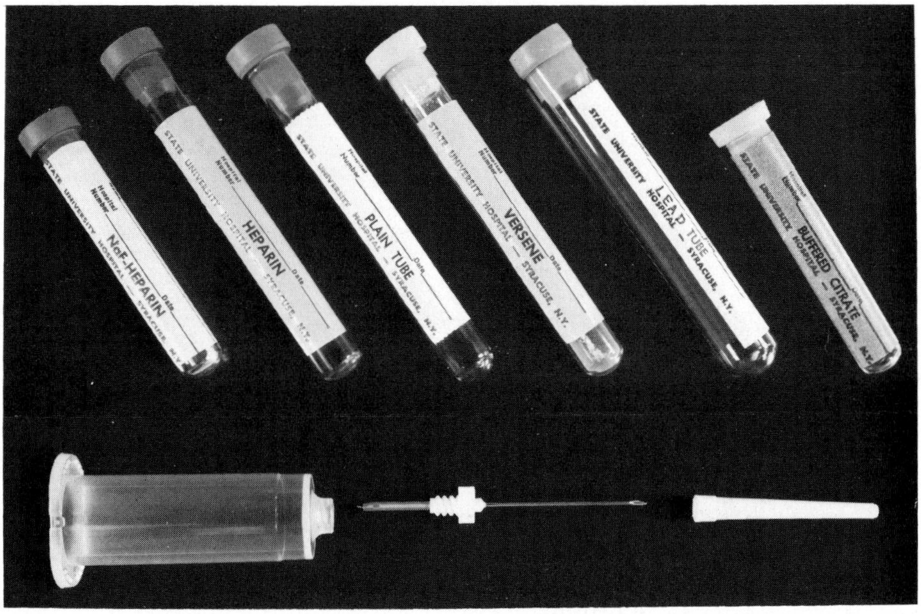

Figure 9–1. Vacutainer tubes with labels; Vacutainer holder, needle and needle cover are separate.

to yield a proper specimen for most chemical determinations.

While the pediatric Vacutainer system is practical for single or occasional blood specimen collections from infants after three months of age with small (2 or 3.5 ml.) volume tubes, a microsampling technique is required for newborn infants and children as well as for adults who require frequent blood specimen collections to evaluate repetitive sequential measurements and examinations (Figs. 9–2, 9–3). With aseptic technique, a deliberate skin puncture sufficient in depth to assure free blood flow from finger, big toe, or heel is made with either a long point microlance or regular microlance (Becton Dickinson, Rutherford,

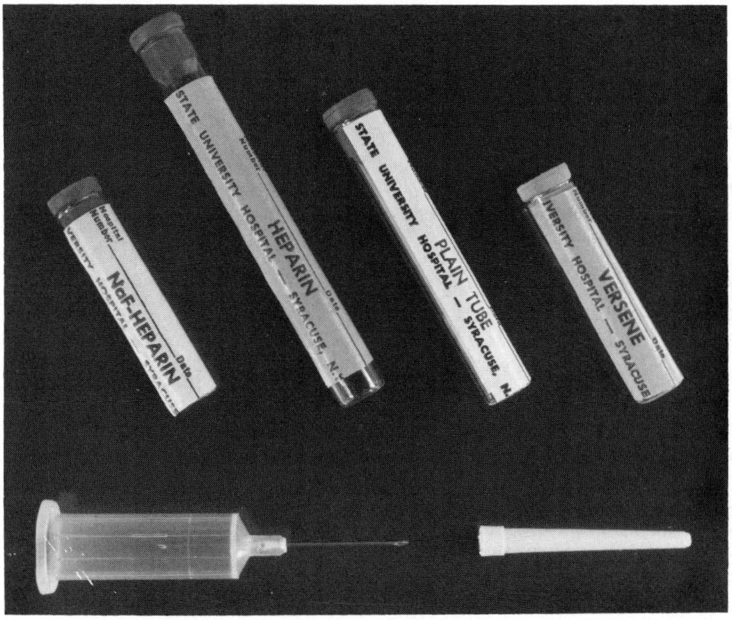

Figure 9–2. Vacutainer tubes for reduced specimen volumes (2 ml. and 3.5 ml.) and a holder-needle combination. This is also referred to as a pediatric Vacutainer system.

Table 9–1. GUIDE FOR PROPER SPECIMEN TUBE SELECTION*

CHEMISTRY—Plain Tube (red top)
Aldolase
Amylase
Blood Alcohol (drawn without alcohol swab)
Bilirubin
Barbiturate Screen (1 tube)
Barbiturate Level (2 tubes)
Bromide
B.S.P.
Calcium (Total & Ionized)
Carotenoid
Cholesterol
Copper (1 full)
Creatine (1 full)
CPK
Creatinine
Doriden (1 full)
Electrophoresis
Free Thyroxine (free T_4) (2 full tubes)
Iron & Iron Binding Capacity (2 full)
LAP (Leucine Aminopeptidase)
LDH & Isoenzymes
Lipase (1 full)
Lithium
Magnesium
Osmolality
Acid & Alkaline Phosphatase
Phosphorus
Total Protein
T_3 Uptake (1 full)
Total Thyroxine (Murphy-Pattee, T_4) (1 full)
Folate (2 full)
Dilantin (2 full)
TBG (2 full)
LATS & TSH (2 full)
Triglyceride
Salicylate
Sulfa Level
Electrolytes
BUN
Uric Acid
Vitamin B_{12} (2 full)
Vitamin B_{12} (combining power) (2 full)
SGOT
SGPT
Digoxin (1 full)
FSH
Pseudocholinesterase (1 full)

HEMATOLOGY—Plain Tube (red top)
Haptoglobin
LE Prep
Serum Viscosity (2 full tubes)

BLOOD BANK—Plain Tube (red top)
Crossmatch (1 full tube/4 units)
Prenatal Studies (2 full tubes)
Type & Hold (1 tube)
Coombs (2 tubes)
Antibody Identification (2 full tubes)
For Open Heart Surgery (3 full tubes)
Open Heart Work-up (2 full tubes)

SEROLOGY—Plain Tube (red top)
Alpha 1 Antitrypsin
Antihyaluronidase Titer
Antinuclear Antibody
Antistreptolysin O
Antithyroid Antibodies
Coccidioides Agglutinins
Ceruloplasmin
C-Reactive Protein
Cold Agglutinins
Cryoglobulin (keep at 37° C at all times)
Febrile Agglutinins (1 full)
FTA-ABS
Heterophile Test
Histoplasmosis Agglutinins (1 full)
Immunoglobulins
Leptospira Agglutinin Test
Rheumatoid Factor
Serum Complement Levels
Streptococcus MG Agglutinins
Toxoplasmosis Agglutinins (1 full)
Trichinella Latex Tube Test
VDRL
Australian Antigen (Au antigen)
Muramidase
Fetoglobulin

CHEMISTRY—NaF-Heparin (small—green top)
Glucose
Glucose Tolerance
Lactic Acid (on ice)
Pyruvic Acid
Lactose Tolerance

HEMATOLOGY—Versene (purple top)
CBC (WBC, RBC, Hgb, Hct, MCV, MCH, MCHC)
Differential Count
Total Eosinophil Count
Hgb Electrophoresis (1 full or 2 pediatric tubes)
G6PD Screen (1 pediatric tube)
Reticulocyte Count
Sed Rate (2 pediatric tubes or 1 full)
Sickle Cell
Platelets

HEMATOLOGY—Na citrate (gray top) TUBE MUST BE FULL FOR ALL TESTS
PTT
Prothrombin Time
Thrombin Time
Fibrinogen Titer
Fibrinogen Level
G6PD Assay (also 1 versene)

CHEMISTRY—Heparin (6 ml.—green top)
pH
Ammonia (on ice) (2 tubes)
RBC Potassium
Renin (2 full)
Plasma Testosterone (2 full)
Cholinesterase (1 full on ice)
Plasma Cortisol (2 full)
Methemoglobin
Plasma Hemoglobin

*Labels are color coded and identical to those affixed to Vacutainer tubes.

New Jersey 07070), depending on the amount of blood to be collected (Fig. 9–4). When 70 per cent alcohol-soaked sponges are used to prepare puncture site, a sterile 2 by 2-inch gauze pad should be applied to the site subsequently for final removal of all alcohol (when area is not dry) in order to prevent hemolysis of specimen and ensure that reasonable spherical bubbles of blood exude from the puncture site. Anhydrous ether or Wescodyne (West Chemical Products, Inc., Long Island City, New York) may be substituted for alcohol in preparation of skin; the latter is preferred when oxygen is being used in the area. From the puncture site, free-flowing blood may be collected in capillary tubes or Caraway microtubes, by capillary attraction, and gravity. For larger amounts of blood, Rasmussen disposable blood collectors may be used (Oakdale Company, P. O. Box 1111, South Bend, Indiana 46624).

We have found the Caraway micro blood-collecting tube No. A-2934 satisfactory (Clay Adams, Inc., 141 E. 25th Street, New York 10010)—length, 75 mm.; inside diameter, 2 mm.; outside diameter, 4 mm. (Fig. 9–4). However, microsampling techniques are best evolved to meet specific or predominant pa-

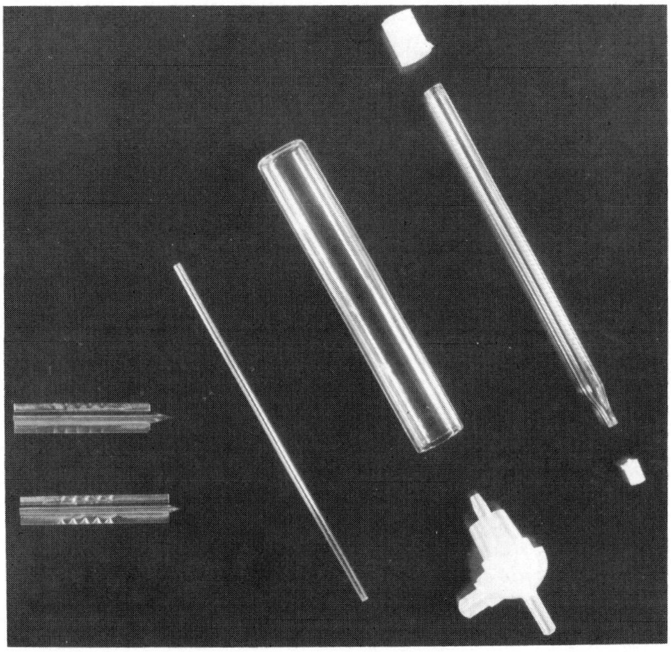

Figure 9–3. Equipment for finger stick blood drawing. Observing from left to right: long-point lancet over regular lancet; micro-hematocrit capillary tube; special cap and tube for micro-blood bank; Caraway tube and caps for microchemistry.

tient care requirements. This is especially true in regard to the selection of capillary tubes or other microcontainers. For the infant who requires a single total bilirubin measurement, a single capillary collection tube may suffice, but if several measurements are to be performed with a microsimultaneous automated system, a different type of microcontainer may be preferred. The skill or frequency of use by personnel is another factor that may prompt selection of other than capillary tubes, which are difficult to fill completely without

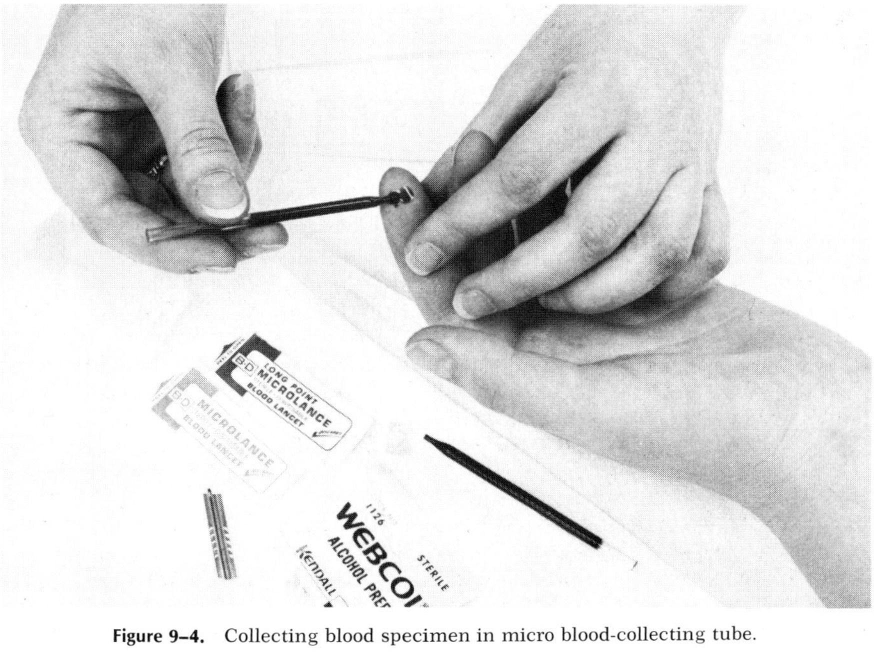

Figure 9–4. Collecting blood specimen in micro blood-collecting tube.

entrance of air bubbles and are fragile in processing. The specimen collection technique is a greater challenge than analysis or microliter measurements for many of the clinically useful determinations requiring 0.1 ml. (100 μl.) or less of specimen in the form of plasma, serum, or whole blood. Indeed, such a policy should prevail that all analyses be performed on minimal specimen volumes such as 20 to 100 μl. or less where possible and with maximal accuracy, precision, and efficiency, as well as compatibility with semiautomated or automated single or simultaneous measurements (Mabry *et al.*, 1966). This approach has obvious advantages to patients and personnel.

Arterial Punctures. Arterial punctures can be performed with the same ease and consideration given to venipuncture. While there is debate about the efficacy of local anesthesia with arterial punctures, it is apparent that, in addition to physicians, nurses and other paramedical personnel can perform such procedures with ease and safety (Sackner *et al.*, 1971). A tourniquet is not required and a patient will usually experience no more discomfort than with a venipuncture. In adults, the radial artery at the wrist is preferred, while the brachial artery, accessible at juncture of arm and forearm, may be used as a second choice. Application of a sterile 2 by 2-inch gauze pad to the puncture site with moderate pressure after removal of the needle is rarely required beyond 2 or 3 minutes. Although a syringe and needle combination displays pulsations of arterial blood upon penetration of the vessel, the Vacutainer system may also be used. A 1-ml. tuberculin syringe lubricated lightly with heparin (100,000 units per ml.) and a 20-gauge needle will suffice for most requirements; this will yield an adequate specimen volume for several measurements, including oxygen saturation, Po_2, Pco_2, and pH. The needle is closed by forcefully inserting it into a rubber stopper after removal from the artery to preclude entrance of air into the syringe.

Processing. Processing of blood specimens embraces that phase between collection of specimen and actual analysis. Ideally all measurements should be performed within 1 hour after collection. Whenever this is not practical, the specimen should be processed to a point at which it can be properly stored in order to preclude alterations of constituents to be measured. However, some whole blood specimens are initially processed by preparation of a protein-free filtrate with tungstic acid, trichloroacetic acid, or barium sulfate; such filtrates may be stored in a refrigerator at 4 to 6° C. if the interval prior to analysis exceeds 30 minutes. Plasma or serum is preferred to whole blood for most determinations because many constituents are distributed differently in erythrocytes and serum or plasma; also, the hematocrit or percentage of erythrocyte volume of whole blood varies significantly between individuals. Although the concentration of glucose and urea nitrogen is approximately the same in erythrocytes as in the plasma, analyses of whole blood give different results from those obtained in plasma because of a difference in water content between whole blood and plasma. Plasma or serum contains about 93 per cent water, whereas whole blood contains about 81 per cent water. The most efficient processing system generates a single or as few as possible blood fractions for analyses (Fig. 9–5). From this standpoint, plasma is virtually ideal when the anticoagulant is heparin. In medical chemistry, plasma can be used for virtually all measurements, although a few require serum (e.g., serum enzymes and protein electrophoresis), while whole blood can, for all practical purposes, be eliminated.

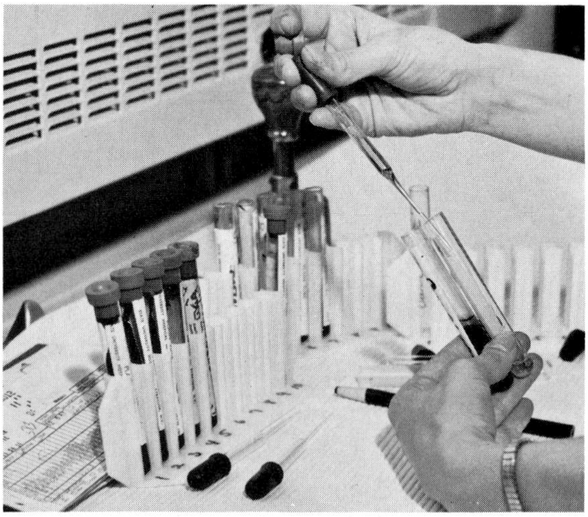

Figure 9–5. Processing blood specimens.

The actual steps in processing that must be followed for separation of whole blood into its fractions, components, or derivatives are as follows:

Whole Blood. Keep blood in the stoppered original container until ready for analysis, which should begin within 1 hour after drawing blood. If analysis is to be delayed, store the blood in a refrigerator at 4 to 6° C. (or if a protein-free filtrate is to be used, prepare it at once and refrigerate the filtrate). Mix blood gently by inversion or rotation immediately before analysis.

Plasma. Centrifuge blood within 1 hour after collection, preferably in the original container, for 10 minutes at a relative centrifugal force (RCF) of 850 to 1000,* keeping the container stoppered to prevent evaporation. Label plasma container and store in refrigerator at 4 to 5° C. until plasma is analyzed, or freeze at –20° C. if analysis is to be delayed more than 4 hours. The Caraway microcapillary tubes with a maximum volume of 350 μl. is occluded with microcaps or vinyl plaster putty at the tapered end prior to centrifugation for 1 minute at 5000 G.; this will yield about 150 μl. of plasma.†

*RCF of 1000 obtainable from IEC Nomograph (International Equipment Co., 300 Second Ave., Needham Heights, Massachusetts 02194) in (1) an International Clinical Centrifuge with 12-place angle head at 2700 r.p.m., (2) an International Model CM Centrifuge with 16-place angle head at 2500 r.p.m., (3) an International Size 1 Model SBV Centrifuge with 64-place multiple carrier swinging head at 2200 r.p.m., and (4) a Sorvall GLC-1 General Laboratory Centrifuge with an Omni-Carrier at 2340 r.p.m.

†International Micro-Hematocrit, Centrifuge Model MB with 16-place head. Sample slots are milled down to base. An embroidery hoop may be used as a gasket; tapered ends of Caraway tubes may cut standard rubber gasket (Mabry *et al.*, 1967).

Serum. Allow blood to clot in the original closed container at room temperature (usually 20 to 30 minutes). When clot has formed, gently loosen it at the top ("rim") with a fine glass rod or applicator stick, if necessary. Centrifuge blood 10 minutes at an RCF of 850 to 1000 in the stoppered container. Label and store the serum in a refrigerator at 4 to 6° C. until analyzed or freeze at –20° C. if analysis is to be delayed more than 4 hours.

Centrifugation. Centrifugation is of primary importance in blood processing to derive plasma or serum fractions. Conditions for centrifugation should specify both the time and centrifugal force. In selecting a centrifuge, one should look for the highest possible centrifugal force and not be misled by the high rotational speed. When the radius (r) is known, calculation of the relative centrifugal force (G) may be made from a nomogram (Fig. 9–6) or by the use of the following formula:

$$RCF = 1.118 \times 10^{-5} \times r \times (r.p.m.)^2$$

in which

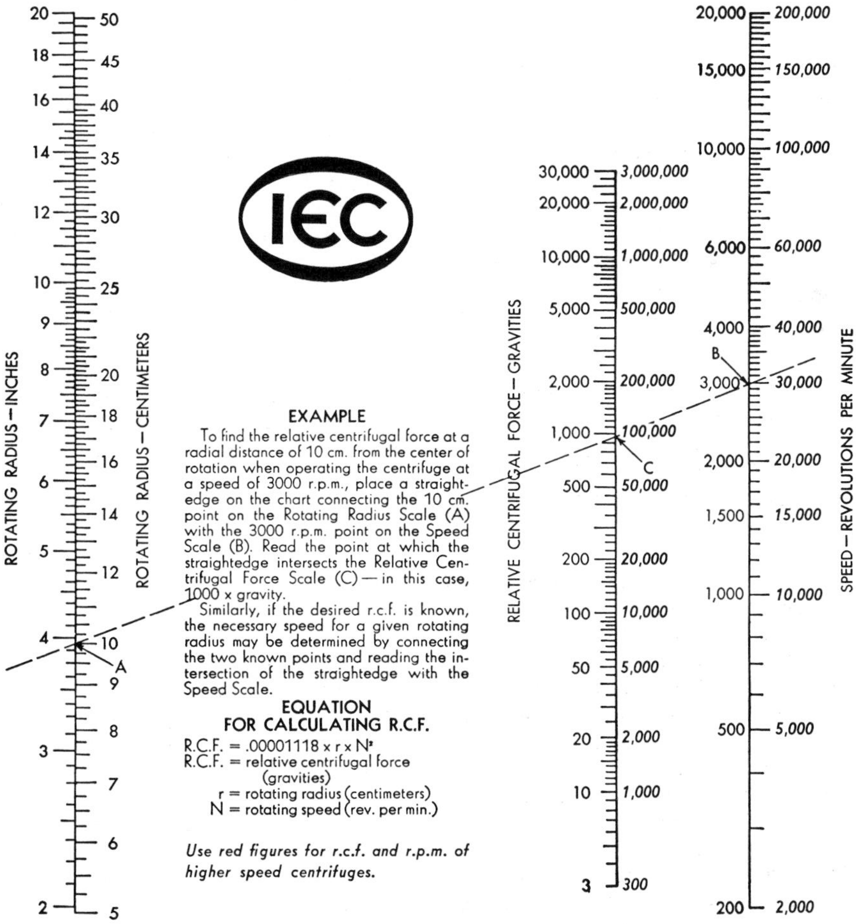

Figure 9–6. Nomogram for calculation of relative centrifugal force (G.). (Courtesy of International Equipment Corporation, Needham Heights, Massachusetts 02194.)

RCF	is the relative centrifugal force in units of G, i.e., multiples of the gravitational force,
1.118×10^{-5}	is a constant,
r	is the radius, expressed in centimeters, between the axis of rotation and the center of the centrifuge tube, and
r.p.m.	is the speed in revolutions per minute.

Several principles must be observed to avoid damage to the centrifuge or the specimen and danger to personnel.

Familiarity with the components of a centrifuge and a preventive maintenance schedule will insure maximum performance. Periodic lubrication of the shaft and inspection as well as replacement of brushes when necessary according to frequency and/or duration of use will prevent or reduce breakdown periods that may impair efficiency of patient care service. While certain manufacturers provide this service without charge, it is simple enough to assign to laboratory personnel, and this assures continued awareness of centrifuge care by all personnel. Unfortunately not all centrifuges lend themselves to regular external calibration with a tachometer to confirm revolutions per minute (r.p.m.).

The principle of "balance" must be observed. Tubes and carriers or shields of equal weight, shape, and size should be placed in opposing positions in the centrifuge head, with regard for a geometrically symmetrical arrangement, using water-filled tubes when necessary. With most biological liquid specimens, adequate overall balance can be obtained by placing visually matched approximately equal volumes of water into such matched equipment. Optimum care of a centrifuge dictates that opposing carriers be weighed for balance. In practice the demand of time is such that this is not feasible, with some sacrifice in life of the centrifuge. Mercury must never be placed in cups or shields for balancing.

Tubes should be supported by appropriately shaped rubber cushions in the carrier and shields. The latter should be selected from an adequate assortment to correspond closely in configuration and size to the tubes to be centrifuged, with adapters when necessary.

All glass tubes used should be inspected to eliminate those with cracks, chips, or other flaws. All tubes must be stoppered to prevent loss by evaporation due to heat and air flow.

When these precautions have been observed, the centrifuge is closed and slowly accelerated until the desired speed is attained. After 10 minutes the power is cut off either manually or by a timer. The centrifuge is allowed to come to rest without the use of the brake, which may cause resuspension of centrifugates. Braking is reserved for such emergencies as tube breakage.

Common Difficulties. In the collection and processing of blood, several common difficulties may be observed, and precautions must be taken. Although all tubes and syringes must be chemically clean, chemical analyses in general do not require sterile tubes. However, one should not assume that a sterile tube is chemically clean. Chemically cleans means free of actual or potential organic and/or inorganic constituents that may alter the result of a chemical analysis.

Hemolysis. Hemolysis must be avoided because it invalidates certain determinations through release of erythrocyte contents (e.g., lactate dehydrogenase, acid phosphatase, and potassium) or through color change, especially photometric measurements using shorter wavelengths of the visible spectrum (400 to 500 nm). Hemoglobin also interferes with specific chemical reactions (e.g., diazotization inhibition in bilirubin determination). Among the more common causes of hemolysis are the following (with some preventive measures).

COLLECTION OF BLOOD. Every effort should be made to avoid excessive venous stasis through prolonged application of the tourniquet. The combined effect of raised intravenous pressure and anoxia from sustained occlusion results in passage of water and small molecular size constituents from the lumen of a vein into the surrounding extracellular fluid, since erythrocytes and plasma proteins as well as other large molecules cannot pass through a vein wall; hence, their concentration rises. Some constituents such as hormones and calcium are bound to protein in the blood stream. Hence, prolonged stasis can falsely raise their concentration. With prolonged stasis, intracellular leakage of potassium, lactic acid, and other constituents may also cause false elevations. There may be moisture or contamination in needle, syringe, or blood container; avoid excessive traction on syringe plunger, particularly with small-lumen needles. The use of a 20-gauge needle is preferred when possible, and blood should be allowed to flow into the syringe gently, with minimal suction. Eliminate air leakage into the syringe during collection.

TRANSFER OF BLOOD. Expelling blood from a syringe through the needle and allowing blood to fall into container through the air are to be avoided. Do not shake blood in container to mix with anticoagulants. Mix by gentle repetitive inversion – approximately six or eight times. Agitation of whole blood not containing an anticoagulant is certain to produce hemolysis. Clotted specimens should be allowed to stand undisturbed for 15 to 20 minutes.

SEPARATION OF BLOOD. Avoid prolonged contact of serum or plasma with blood cells; prompt separation is essential to minimize, if not eliminate, glycolysis and/or a shift of constituents from cells (erythrocytes, leukocytes, and platelets) to serum or plasma.

Since many patients requiring blood specimen collection are receiving intravenous (I.V.) infusions, venipuncture in the same limb whether proximal or distal to infusion site (where the I.V. fluid drip may not have mixed with the entire blood volume) may cause local concentration of constituents to be unrepresentative of that circulating in the rest of the patient. However, blood taken from the opposite arm will yield a specimen that provides valid results.

Finally, blood specimens collected after hemodialysis may display profound alterations in the concentration of certain constituents, e.g., potassium and urea, when compared with blood specimens collected prior to hemodialysis. Relevant clinical information provided with such a specimen, e.g., "post-hemodialysis" rather than "renal failure" would account for such a discrepancy in sequential specimen analyses.

Refrigeration of freshly collected blood before clotting has occurred or freezing of whole blood before separation should be avoided. Separation of clot from container wall with stirring rod or applicator stick should be accomplished by a gentle "rimming" of clot only once, since excessive "rimming" may produce hemolysis. Refrain from overcentrifugation (RCF above 1500 for periods exceeding 15 minutes).

Lactescence. Milky or lipemic plasma and serum are frequently obtained with blood samples collected 1 to 2 hours after a fatty meal or from patients with certain metabolic diseases, most notably, primary and secondary hyperlipoproteinemias. It is associated with elevated blood neutral fat levels. This interferes with spectrophotometric measurements, e.g., uric acid and enzymes, and causes false elevations in fluorometric assays by nephelometry. It also produces false elevations when serum is used in the final test mixture but not in the reagent blanks (Caraway, 1962).

Concentration Changes. Changes in drawn blood samples from the original constituent concentrations occur through dilution or evaporation. Common sources of such errors are as follows:

Use of syringes and needles rinsed with saline solution, liquid anticoagulants, or otherwise not perfectly dry.

Use of anticoagulants in liquid form (prothrombin time determination is an exception, since the method is designed for the dilution present).

Allowing blood to stand in open containers for prolonged periods and centrifuging blood specimens in open containers. These should be avoided.

Composition Changes. The major sources of composition changes in blood specimens are bacterial and enzymatic effect, loss of volatile blood constituents by diffusion or evaporation, and interchange of substances between the liquid and cellular components of blood.

Protection from light is essential for certain constituents (e.g., bilirubin).

Bacterial Changes. These include ammonia formation from urea and are minimized by (1) sterile handling of blood when possible, (2) prompt separation of cells from plasma or serum, and (3) storage of the specimen at 4 to 6° C. until analyzed or freezing at –20° C. when possible.

Enzymatic Changes. Glycolysis is minimized by the same measures as bacterial changes, except that sterility has no effect unless an enzymatic method is employed. Use a fluoride-heparin anticoagulant if analysis of whole blood for glucose will be delayed for more than 1 hour.

Blood Gas Changes. A loss of CO_2 from specimens is minimized by filling the original container to capacity as nearly as possible with blood and keeping the container tightly closed; transfer plasma for total CO_2 content into small containers also filled to capacity. The CO_2 content loss is greatest during the first few minutes of exposure to air; it falls approximately 3 to 6 mM./L. during 1 to 2 hours (Gambino and Schreiber, 1966). Addition of alkali to plasma sample specimens that must stand for several hours has been shown to virtually preclude such CO_2 loss. To an empty Autoanalyzer cup, add one drop (0.035 ml.) of 1 N ammonium hydroxide with a disposable transfer pipette; then transfer 1 ml. of plasma to the cup; gentle swirling with tip of the transfer pipette permits mixing of alkali and plasma without bubble formation and foaming. Avoid rapid displacement or movement and mixing of separated fractions, e.g., plasma, to avoid loss of gases through air-specimen surface contacts.

Extravascular Interchange. The movements of substances between cells and plasma or serum is minimized by prompt separation of the liquid from the cells and avoidance of hemolysis. Potassium diffuses rapidly from the red blood cell to the plasma, as do cellular water, chloride, and phosphate; glucose is metabolized by erythrocytes and leukocytes.

Furthermore, the anticoagulant used must not affect the chemical analysis. This may happen in three ways: First, it may be additive, such as a sodium or potassium salt of anticoagulant to electrolyte analyses. Second, it may also remove the constituent to be measured, e.g., oxalate removes calcium from serum by forming an insoluble complex. Finally, the action of anticoagulants on enzymes is a function of enzymes as well as anticoagulant. In terms of inhibition of enzyme activity, oxalate has been reported for acid phosphatase, amylase, and lactate dehydrogenase, whereas fluoride inhibits urease but activates amylase.

In summary, the Vacutainer system lends itself to ideal, efficient blood collection and processing to yield plasma or serum.

Additional sources of error as well as specificity and the effect of various conditions and substances on clinical pathology determinations have been reported and should be familiar to all laboratory technical and professional personnel (see Caraway, 1962, 1965; Wirth and Thompson, 1965; Van Peenen and Files, 1969).

DRUG INTERFERENCE IN CLINICAL CHEMISTRY

The rapid growth in the last decade of pharmacotherapeutics in medicine has been paralleled only by the expansion and sophistication in the clinical laboratory. As the number of pharmacologic agents affecting a physiologic function has increased, so have the parameters of measuring this function.

Students of medicine for years have been aware that a drug cannot be applied intelligently or even safely without some understanding of mode of action, side effects, toxicity, and metabolism. Now it has become the responsibility of both the clinical and laboratory physician to be aware of drug interference with clinical laboratory tests. This applies not only to the inpatient or ambulatory patient, but to well people in multiphasic health testing or health evaluation, e.g., annual check-up.

Drug interference can be grouped into two general categories: First and foremost, pharmacologic interference, whereupon some action of the drug or its metabolite can cause an alteration (*in vivo*) in the concentration of the substance being measured by the test. Second, a so-called chemical interference, in which some physical or chemical property of the drug can alter the analyses directly (*in vitro*).

The listing of drugs affecting laboratory measurements and examinations is enormous and ever increasing. The tests most often altered by drugs appear to be those measuring hepatic function, perhaps because even subtle changes in hepatic function are measured easily and often are physically apparent.

Table 9–2 lists the common tests of hepatic function and the drugs implicated in pharmacologic interference.

Table 9–3 is an abridged compilation of common clinical chemistry tests, their direction of alteration, the offending drug, and the mode of interference in general terms.

A more complete listing of drug interaction with laboratory tests and their specific mechanism when known may be gleaned from reports of Christian (1970) and Young *et al.* (1972).

Table 9–2. SELECTED MEASUREMENTS OF HEPATIC FUNCTION AND A LIST OF DRUGS IMPLICATED IN PHARMACOLOGIC INTERFERENCE*

URINE:	Bilirubin: increased or false positive.
SERUM:	Alkaline phosphatase: increased or false positive
	Bilirubin: increased or false positive
	B.S.P.: increased or false positive
	Cephalin flocculation: increased or false positive
	Cholesterol: decreased or false negative
	Blood glucose: decreased or false negative
	SGOT and SGPT: increased or false positive
	Thymol turbidity: increased or false positive

Drugs That May Affect Liver Function Tests

Acetohexamide	Methyldopa
Acetophenetidin	Methylthiouracil
Allopurinol	Nicotinic acid
Aminosalicylic acid	Nitrofurantoin
Amodiaquin	Novobiocin
Amphotericin-B	Oleandomycin
Anabolic agents	Oxazepam
Androgens	Oxyphenbutazone
Chlorpropamide	Paraldehyde
Cyclophosphamide	Paramethadione
Desipramine	Phenacemide
Erythromycin	Phenothiazines
Glycopyrrolate	Phenylbutazone
Haloperidol	Progestrins
Halothane	Progestrins-estrogens (Oral B.S.P.'s)
Hydrazine	Propylthiouracil
Imipramine	Sulfonamides
Indomethacin	Tetracyclines
Isoniazid	Thiosemicarbazones
Lincomycin	Thiothizene
MAO inhibitors	Tolazamide
Mercaptopurine	Tolbutamide
Quinacrine (mepacrine)	Trimethadione
Metaxalone	Uracil mustard
Methoxalen	
Methoxyflurane	

*Modified from Martin, T. J.: The Pharmacologic Interactions with Laboratory Test Values, 1970. 596 Burnhamthorpe, Etobicoke, Ontario, Canada.

Table 9–3. AN ABRIDGED COMPILATION OF CHEMICAL MEASUREMENTS, THEIR DIRECTION OF ALTERATION, OFFENDING DRUG AND THE MODE OF INTERFERENCE IN GENERAL TERMS*

BLOOD VALUES	INCREASE	DECREASE
Amylase	Cholinergics (1) Ethanol (1) Narcotics (1)	Citrate (2) Oxalate (2)
Acid phosphatase	Androgens (in women) (1)	Fluorides (2) Oxalates (2)
Alkaline phosphatase	Refer to Table 9–2 Gold salts	Fluorides (2) Oxalates (2)
Bilirubin	Refer to Table 9–2 Chlordiazepoxide (1) Dextran (2) Gallbladder dyes (1)	Caffeine (2) Theophylline (2)
Bromsulphalein (BSP)	Refer to Table 9–2 Barbiturate (1) Clofibrate (1) Diphenylhydantoin (1) Heparin (2) Narcotics (1) (Opiates – meperidine and methadone) Phenazopyridine (2) Phenolphthalein (2) Probenecid (1) Phenolsulfonphthalein (PSP) (2)	
Calcium	Androgens (1) Calcified-activated (1) Calcium salts (1) Progestins-estrogens (1)	Citrate salts (2) Corticosteroids (1) EDTA (interferes with dye-binding methods) (2)
Chloride	Bromide (2) Chloride (1) Oxyphenbutazone (1) Phenylbutazone (1)	ACTH/corticosteroids (1) Diuretics (1)
Cholesterol	Refer to Table 9–2 ACTH (1) Bile salts (1) Bromide (2) Chlorpromazine (1)	Heparin (1) Thyroxine (1)
Creatinine	Amphotericin B (1) Ascorbic acid (2) Barbiturates (2) Glucose (2) Kanamycin (1) Levodopa (2) Methyldopa (2) PSP and BSP (2)	
Glucose	Drugs that alter the regulation of carbohydrate metabolism Ethacrynic acid (1) Furosemide (1) Thiazides (1)	

*Refer to key at bottom of page 528.

(Table 9–3 continues on following page.)

Table 9–3. AN ABRIDGED COMPILATION OF CHEMICAL MEASUREMENTS, THEIR DIRECTION OF ALTERATION, OFFENDING DRUG AND THE MODE OF INTERFERENCE IN GENERAL TERMS (*Continued*)

BLOOD VALUES	INCREASE	DECREASE
Lactate dehydrogenase (LDH)		Clofibrate Oxalate (2)
Lipase	Cholinergics (1) Ethanol (1) Narcotics (1)	
Potassium	Calcium (2) Heparin (1) Penicillin G Potassium (1) Spironolactone (1)	ACTH/corticosteroids (1) Amphotericin B (1) Oral diuretics (1) Salicylates (1) Tetracycline (1) (outdated)
Transaminases SGOT and SGPT	Refer to Table 9–2 Ampicillin (1) Colchicin (1) Cephalothin (1) Clofibrate (1) Gentamycin (1) Nafcillin (1) Opiates (1) Oxacillin (1)	
Sodium	Androgens (1) Rauwolfia alkaloids (1) Calcium (2) Corticosteroids (1) Methyldopa (1) Oxyphenbutazone (1) Phenylbutazone (1)	Ammonium chloride (1) Heparin (1) Mercurial diuretics Oral diuretics (1)
Urea nitrogen	Many drugs not listed are capable of renal toxicity in an individual whose renal function is already impaired or as an adverse reaction Alkaline antacids (1) Antimony salts (1) Arsenicals (1) Chloral hydrate (2) Chlorobutanol (2) Furosemide (1) Gentamycin (1) Kanamycin (1) Methyldopa (1)	
Uric acid	Adrenocortical steroids (1) Ascorbic acid (2) Busulfan (1) Ethacrynic acid (1) Glucose (2) Methyldopa (2) Nitrogen mustard (1) Purine analogue antimetabolites (1) Pyrazinamide (1) Quinethazone (1) Theophylline (2) Thiazides (1) Vincristine sulfate (1)	Acetylsalicylic acid Allopurinol (1) Oxyphenbutazone (1) Phenylbutazone (1) Probenecid (1)

(*Table 9–3 continues on opposite page.*)

Table 9–3. AN ABRIDGED COMPILATION OF CHEMICAL MEASUREMENTS, THEIR DIRECTION OF ALTERATION, OFFENDING DRUG AND THE MODE OF INTERFERENCE IN GENERAL TERMS *(Continued)*

URINE VALUES	INCREASE	DECREASE
Catecholamines	B-vitamin (high dose) (2)	MAO inhibitors
	Erythromycin (2)	
	Hydralazine (2)	
	Levodopa (2)	
	Methenamine hippurate (2)	
	Methenamine mandelate (2)	
	Methyldopa (2)	
	Nicotinic acid (2)	
	Nitroglycerin (1)	
	Phenothiazines (1)	
	Quinine-quinidine (2)	
	Salicylate (2)	
	Tetracyclines (2)	
Chloride	Bromide (2)	
Creatinine	Ascorbic acid (2)	
	Levodopa (2)	
	Methyldopa (2)	
	Nitrofuran derivatives (2)	
Glucose	Enzymatic method (Clinistix, Testape)	Ascorbic acid (2)
		Levodopa (2)
	Benedict's solution or Clinitest	
	Ascorbic acid (2)	
	Cephalosporins (2)	
Porphyrins	Not listed are several drugs that may precipitate acute porphyria	
	Acriflavine (2)	
	Ethoxazene (2)	
	Phenazopyridine (2)	
	Progestins-estrogens (1)	
	Procaine (2)	
	Sulfonamides (2)	
5-Hydroxyindolacetic acid (5-HIAA)	Mephenesin (2)	Phenothiazines (2)
	Methocarbamol (2)	
	Reserpine (1)	
		GROUP AFFECTED
17-Hydroxycorticosteroids (17-OH)	Meprobamate (2)	(17-OH, 17-KS, 17-KGS)
17-Ketogenic steroids (17-KGS)	Phenothiazines (2)	(17-OH, 17-KS, 17-KGS)
17-Ketosteroids (17-KS)	Spironolactone (2)	(17-OH, 17-KS, 17-KGS)
	Penicillin G (2)	(17-OH, 17-KS, 17-KGS)
	Anabolic steroids (1)	(17-KS)
	†Ascorbic acid (2)	(17-OH)
	†Chloral hydrate (2)	(17-OH)
	‡Chlordiazepoxide (2)	(17-OH)
	‡Hydroxyzine (2)	(17-OH)
	†Inorganic iodides (2)	(17-OH)
	§Methenamine (2)	(17-OH)
	Phenothiazines (2)	(17-KS)
	†Quinidine, quinine (2)	(17-OH)
	‡Reserpine (2)	(17-OH)

(Table 9–3 continues on following page.)

Table 9–3. AN ABRIDGED COMPILATION OF CHEMICAL MEASUREMENTS, THEIR DIRECTION OF ALTERATION, OFFENDING DRUG AND THE MODE OF INTERFERENCE IN GENERAL TERMS (*Continued*)

	DECREASE	GROUP AFFECTED
	Diphenylhydantoin (1)	(17-KS, 17-OH)
	Estrogens (1)	(17-KS, 17-OH)
	Ethacrynic acid (1)	(17-KS)
	Ethinamate (2)	(17-KS)
	Penicillin (1)	(17-KS, 17-KGS)
	Probenecid (1)	(17-KS)
	Thiazide diuretics (1)	(17-OH)

URINE VALUES	INCREASE	DECREASE
Pregnanediol	Mandelamine (2)	
Phenolsulfonphthalein (PSP)	Anthraquinone derivative (2) BSP (2) Ethoxazene (2) Phenozopyridine (2) Phenolphthalein (2)	Any drug capable of renal toxicity Penicillin (1) Probenecid (1) Salicylates (1) Sulfinpyrazone (1) Sulfonamides (1) Thiazide diuretics
Vanillylmandelic acid (VMA)	Anileridine (2) Caffeine (2) Epinephrine (1) Lithium carbonate (1) Mandelamine (2) ‖Methocarbamal (2) Nitroglycerin (1) Salicylates (2)	Chlorpromazine (1) Guanethidine (1) MAO inhibitors (1) Reserpine (1)

*Compiled from data in Martin, T. J.: The Pharmacologic Interactions with Laboratory Test Values, 1970.)
†With modification of Reddy, Jenkins, Thorn procedure.
‡With Glen-Nelson technique.
§With Reddy method.
‖Gitlow method.

KEY: (1) Alters blood or serum concentration of test substance.
(2) Chemical interference with test.
17OH = 17 hydroxycorticosteroids
17KS = 17 ketosteroids
17KGS = 17 ketogenic steroids

RECORDS AND REPORTING OF RESULTS

What is described for chemistry section of clinical pathology may also be applied to other sections, such as hematology, microscopy, and microbiology. Accurate and complete identification of specimen for processing and analysis is essential. A daily log and appropriate work sheets for individual or group (batch) analyses should be generated for transcription of patient's specimen(s) identification and determinations required (Figs. 9–7, 9–8). While the format of each may vary to meet local requirements, the principles underlying their use are universal. A daily log may serve as a source of statistical data in terms of workload and permit development of an accession number for use as specimen identification in analyses, a reference for retrieval of measurement results from a particular patient on a specific date (time), and a final focus for synthesis of analytical results with an individual patient. However, a third category of records that involves reporting of results for incorporation into patient's medical record may also serve as a focus for combining analytical data results with the individual patient if the accession number is transcribed onto this form. Because a single blood specimen or fraction such as plasma or serum may require use by different technologists for different methods, the need and use of work sheets for each different measurement or group of simultaneous analyses is apparent. This work sheet, as the name implies, also serves as a record of observations by personnel performing analyses. In addition to patient's identification by name and accession number, it should provide space for transcription of observed data, such as per cent transmission (T) or absorbance (O.D.) as well as calculations performed or results from direct readout or printout instrumental systems. Similar values for standards and reference control specimens for each measurement should be recorded on a work sheet for single measurements or batch analyses. An orderly sequential system of transcription of data and patient specimen identification proceeds from receipt of specimen with service request form to (1) log sheet, (2) work sheet(s) back to log sheet, and (3) report (cumulative report card) for photocopying and incorporation of copy into patient's medical record (Fig. 9–9).

For the attending physician, it is the final report that is important in terms of display for clarity and order of data presentation as well as contents of accurate and precise measurements. Cumulative report forms have several advantages for physician as well as clinical pathologist (Fig. 9–9). Chronology of data often reflects sequence of disease and serves as a form of quality control that can reduce or eliminate random error if previous measure-

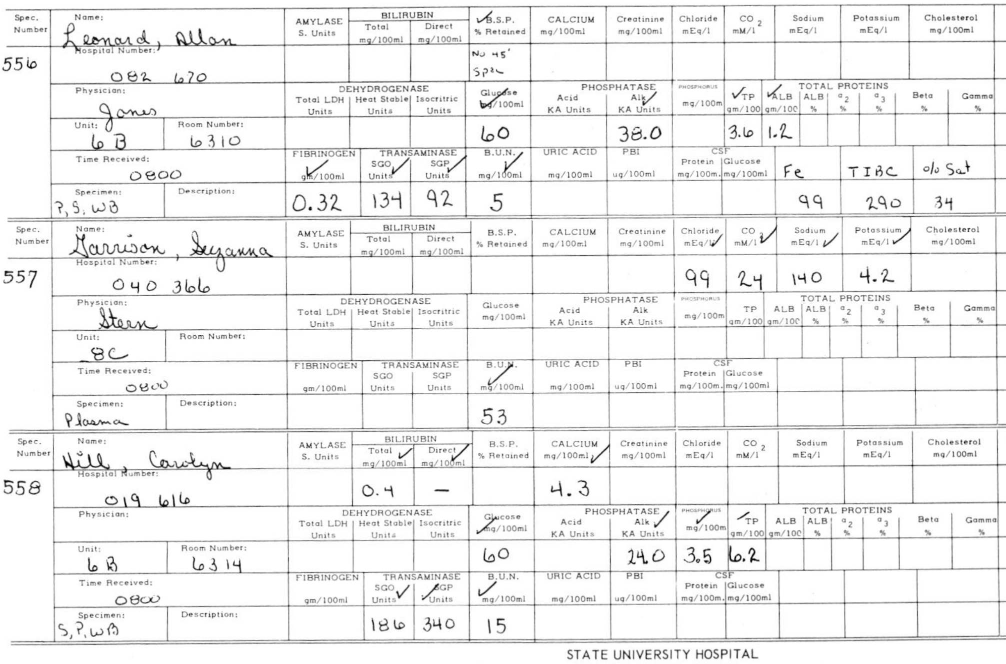
Spec. Number 556 — Name: Leonard, Allan — Hospital Number: 082 670 — Physician: Jones — Unit: 6 B — Room Number: 6310 — Time Received: 0800 — Specimen: P, S, WB — Description:
B.S.P. % Retained: No 45' Spec — Glucose mg/100ml: 60 — Phosphatase Alk KA Units: 38.0 — TP gm/100: 3.6 — ALB gm/100: 1.2 — Fibrinogen gm/100ml: 0.32 — Transaminase SGO Units: 134 — SGP Units: 92 — B.U.N. mg/100ml: 5 — Fe: 99 — TIBC: 290 — % Sat: 34

Spec. Number 557 — Name: Garrison, Suzanna — Hospital Number: 040 366 — Physician: Stern — Unit: 8C — Room Number: — Time Received: 0800 — Specimen: Plasma — Description:
Chloride mEq/l: 99 — CO2 mM/l: 24 — Sodium mEq/l: 140 — Potassium mEq/l: 4.2 — B.U.N. mg/100ml: 53

Spec. Number 558 — Name: Hill, Carolyn — Hospital Number: 019 616 — Physician: — Unit: 6 B — Room Number: 6314 — Time Received: 0800 — Specimen: S, P, WB — Description:
Bilirubin Total mg/100ml: 0.4 — Direct mg/100ml: — — Calcium mg/100ml: 4.3 — Glucose mg/100ml: 60 — Phosphatase Alk KA Units: 24.0 — Phosphorus mg/100m: 3.5 — TP gm/100: 6.2 — Transaminase SGO Units: 186 — SGP Units: 340 — B.U.N. mg/100ml: 15

Form columns: Amylase S. Units; Bilirubin Total mg/100ml, Direct mg/100ml; B.S.P. % Retained; Calcium mg/100ml; Creatinine mg/100ml; Chloride mEq/l; CO2 mM/l; Sodium mEq/l; Potassium mEq/l; Cholesterol mg/100ml; Dehydrogenase Total LDH Units, Heat Stable Units, Isocritric Units; Glucose mg/100ml; Phosphatase Acid KA Units, Alk KA Units; Phosphorus mg/100m; Total Proteins TP gm/100, ALB gm/100, ALB %, α_2 %, α_3 %, Beta %, Gamma %; Fibrinogen gm/100ml; Transaminase SGO Units, SGP Units; B.U.N. mg/100ml; Uric Acid mg/100ml; PBI ug/100ml; CSF Protein mg/100m., Glucose mg/100ml

STATE UNIVERSITY HOSPITAL
UPSTATE MEDICAL CENTER
CLINICAL PATHOLOGY – CHEMISTRY LOG BOOK

Figure 9–7. Daily log sheet for chemistry.

STATE UNIVERSITY HOSPITAL
UPSTATE MEDICAL CENTER

CLINICAL PATHOLOGY
CHEMISTRY

ELECTROLYTE WORK SHEET

DATE: January 5,1973 MEDICAL TECHNOLOGIST S. Klein MT(ASCP)

	QUALITY CONTROL	Cl mEq/l	CO_2 mM/l	Na mEq/l	K mEq/l	Glucose mg/100ml	Bun
	Reference Control Normal	105	14	142	4.2	105	17
	Reference Control Abnormal	117	2	153	5.7	207	48
SPECIMEN NUMBER	PATIENTS NAME					COMMENTS	
900	Blanden, K.	100	26	140	4.2	100	16
901	Martin, B.	103	23	135	3.5	99	18
902	Liss, C.	98	21	134	6.0 HEMO.	156	24
907	Putney, S.	86	33	125	4.8	104	15
908	Pickard, J.	103	27	140	4.4	95	13

STATE UNIVERSITY HOSPITAL
UPSTATE MEDICAL CENTER

CLINICAL PATHOLOGY
CHEMISTRY

WORK SHEET

DATE: January 5,1973 MEASUREMENT: Acid Phosphatase MEDICAL TECHNOLOGIST: S. Klein MT(ASCP)

SPECIMEN NUMBER	QUALITY CONTROL		% T	CALCULATIONS	RESULTS	COMMENTS
	Enzatrol	T	39	20.1	12.9	
		S	72	7.2		
	PATIENTS NAME					
899	Davis, B.	T	79	5.1	2.9	
		S	90	2.3		
957	Mosher, C.	T	66	9.0	6.2	
		S	88	2.8		
1001	Caputo, L.	T	81	4.6	2.3	
		S	90	2.3		

Figure 9–8. Work sheets for chemistry.

ments can be reviewed with current reports and work sheets. The grouping of measurements in terms of chemical pathology and the estimation of precision (± 3 S.D.) may be incorporated, as well as normal values. Color coding (e.g., red for hematology, green for chemistry, blue for microbiology, and yellow for microscopy) facilitates retrieval of specific information within the medical record. Furthermore, a photocopy system preserves original records in chemical pathology files from which copies may be made for incorporation

DOE, JOHN
99 00 27
M 3/31/01

6A______________

STATE UNIVERSITY HOSPITAL
UPSTATE MEDICAL CENTER

CLINICAL PATHOLOGY – CHEMISTRY

Last Reporting Date

1973 page 3

	Normal Values – Date	1-2	1-4	1-4	1-5
Specimen Description			H		
Glucose Fasting mg/100 ml	65-115				80
Glucose, 2 hr. P.C. mg/100 ml	70-120	75			
Urea Nitrogen mg/100 ml	8-18				10
Creatinine mg/100 ml	0.6-1.2				
Uric Acid mg/100 ml	Female 2.0-6.4 Male 2.1-7.8				
Chloride mEq/L	98-109		101		
CO_2 Content mM/L	24-30		27		
Sodium mEq/L	135-145		137		
Potassium mEq/L	4.0-4.8		6.0	4.5	
Blood pH units	Art. 7.38-7.44 Ven. 7.36-7.41				
Blood PCO_2 mmHg	Art. 35-40 Ven. 40-45				
Base Excess mEq/L	Female 3.3 to +1.2 Male 2.4 to +2.3				
Blood PO_2 mmHg	Art. 95-100				
Oxygen Saturation percent	Art. 94-100 Ven. 60-85				
Calcium mEq/L	4.5-5.4	4.6			
Inorganic Phosphorous mg/100 ml	Adult 2.0-5.2 Child 4.0-7.0	3.5			
Magnesium mEq/L	1.5-2.4				
Lithium mEq/L	0-1.5				
Bilirubin Total mg/100 ml	0.1-1.2	1.3			
Bilirubin Direct mg/100 ml	0.0-0.2	N			
B.S.P. % retained @ 45 min.	0.6				
Total Proteins gm/100 ml	6.7-8.3				
Albumin gm/100 ml	3.7-4.9				
Fibrinogen gm/100 ml	0.20-0.40				
Amylase Somogyi Units	60-160				100
Lactic Dehydrogenase IU/L @ 37° C	71-207				
Lactic Dehydrogenase Heat Stable %	20-40				
Acid Phosphatase K-A Units	0-4.0				
Alkaline Phosphatase K-A Units	Adult 4-13 Child 13-20				
SGO Transaminase IU/L @ 37° C	1-39				
SGP Transaminase IU/L @ 37° C	1-25				
C.P.K. IU/L @ 37° C	0-139				
Serum Iron mcgm/100 ml	50-150				
T.I.B.C. mcgm/100 ml	250-450				
Iron Saturation percent	20-55				
Cholesterol mg/100 ml	Age 20-30 120-240				
Triglyceride mg/100 ml	10-160				
Osmolality mOsm/kg	285-295				
T_3 Uptake percent	25-38				
Murphy Pattee mcgm/100 ml	3.4-6.4	6.7			
Free Thyroxine mcgm/100 ml	0.9-1.9				
Lipase Sigma-Tietz	0-1				0
Ionized Calcium mEq/L	2.0-2.6				
Acetone mg/100 ml	neg				
	Chem. Accession No	308	611	635	780
	Technologist	SK	SK	SK	SK

LEGEND

A. Laboratory Accident
B. Confirmed
C. Clotted
D. Moderate
E. Recollect specimen
F. Unit notified
G. Specimen not received
H. Hemolysis
J. Xanthochromic or icteric
K. Marked
L. Lactescence
M. Minimum
N. Not done-See schedule
P. Patient not available
Q. Quantity not sufficient
R. Patient uncooperative
S. Finger puncture
T. Improper labeled
U. Test cancelled by physician
W. Improper specimen
X. Report to follow
Y. Obscured by dye
< Less than
> Greater than

Date

Glucose Tolerance

TIME	mg/100ml	TIME	mg/100ml

Date

Glucose Tolerance

TIME	mg/100ml	TIME	mg/100ml

CEREBRO SPINAL FLUID

	Norm	Date
Protein mg/100 ml	15-45	
Glucose mg/100 ml	50-75	
Chloride mEq/L	122-132	
Globulin Total mg/100 ml	< 50%	

SPECIAL CHEMISTRY

40300

John B. Henry M.D.
Clinical Pathologist

12

Figure 9–9. Cumulative report card (CRC) for chemistry.

into the patient's medical record; previous reports are discarded so that only a single color-coded final copy is retained in the medical record. A duplicate photocopy may be made at time of discharge and sent to private physician for incorporation into his own file (Henry and Pruitt, 1964).

Data handling for laboratories with large workloads (in excess of one million measurements and examinations per year) requires electronic data processing equipment. (See Chapter 30.) From the service request form, all the forms and records reviewed can be made in such a manner as to reduce clerical workload and transcription errors, ensure accuracy and reliability of work, and bring about more prompt service with legible original compact reports. Some form of dedicated laboratory computer support with on-line capability is required, e.g., Berkeley Scientific Laboratory System (Clin-Data and Chem-Data), Digital Equipment Corporation (DEC Clini-Lab), B-D Spear Medical System (CLAS-300), and Diversified Numeric Application (DNA). Chapter 30, "Clinical Laboratory Computerization," should be consulted for a more detailed review of not only how computers work and handle massive amounts of data, but the current state of the art in terms of selecting an appropriate system. Several systems under development and operational in various centers should yield an economical and practical system that will enhance patient care and extend capability of clinical pathology (Johnson Associates, 1971; Krieg *et al.*, 1971; Westlake and Bennington, 1972).

MATHEMATICS AND CHEMICAL CALCULATIONS

Errors in patient or specimen identification as well as transcription errors may well constitute major problems, but errors in arithmetic warrant equal attention. A brief review of the mathematics most frequently utilized by laboratory personnel should clarify and identify principles so essential for accurate work (Rice, 1960).

Significant Figures. In addition, subtraction, multiplication, and division, calculation of data should retain as many significant figures as are contained in the quantity having the least number of significant figures.

Example: Sum of	65.12
	2.115
	1.2222
	68.4572
Answer:	68.46

Exponents. The use of exponential forms permits simple calculation involving large or small numbers.

$$5^2 = 5 \times 5 = 25$$

$$5^{-2} = \frac{1}{5^2}$$

$$5^0 = 1$$

$$5^2 \times 5^3 = 5^5$$

$$5^{1/2} = \sqrt{5^1} = \sqrt{5} = 2.23$$

$$5^{2/3} = \sqrt[3]{5^2} = \sqrt[3]{25} = 2.92$$

Logarithms. The common logarithm of a number is the exponent which must be applied to the base 10 in order to produce the number.

Example: $10^3 = 1000$. The exponent 3 is the common logarithm of 1000 since 3 applied as an exponent to $10 = 1000$.

In terms of logarithms, this is written as follows:

$\log_{10} 1000 = 3$ (logarithm of 1000 to the base 10 equals 3)

Exponents and Logarithms

$1 = 10^0$	$\log = 0$	$\log_{10} 1 = 0$
$10 = 10^1$	$\log = 1$	$\log_{10} 10 = 1$
$100 = 10^2$	$\log = 2$	$\log_{10} 100 = 2$
$1000 = 10^3$	$\log = 3$	$\log_{10} 1000 = 3$
$0.1 = 10^{-1}$	$\log = -1$	$\log_{10} 0.1 = -1$
$0.01 = 10^{-2}$	$\log = -2$	$\log_{10} 0.01 = -2$
$0.001 = 10^{-3}$	$\log = -3$	$\log_{10} 0.001 = -3$

A logarithm is composed of two parts: (1) the mantissa (found in logarithm tables), which is placed to the right of the decimal point, and (2) the characteristic, which is placed to the left of the decimal point. The mantissa gives the antilogarithm, or the number of which it is the logarithm. The characteristic identifies the decimal point in the antilogarithm. Logs simplify arithmetical calculations. For example:

1. To multiply two or more numbers, add their logs, then look up the antilog (antilog is the number which corresponds to a log).
2. To divide, subtract logs, then look up the antilog.
3. For roots and fractional exponents, multiply the log by the fractional exponent, then look up the antilog.

Examples:

$$\log (5 \times 2) = \log 5 + \log 2$$
$$\log 47/2 = \log 47 - \log 2$$
$$\log 76^{3/8} = {}^3/_8 \log 76$$

To find the characteristics:

Digits to the left of decimal point:	1	2	3	4	5	6
Characteristic is:	0	1	2	3	4	5

Zeros to right of decimal point and preceding first significant figure:	0 1 2 3 4
Characteristic is:	−1 −2 −3 −4 −5

Slide Rule. The C and D scales are used for multiplication and division. These scales are alike. In multiplication we add the lengths of these scales corresponding to the numbers we wish to multiply. In division, we subtract lengths of these scales.

Example: Multiply 2 by 2. Set the left index (1) of the C scale on 2 of the D scale. Find 2 on the C scale, and read the answer (4) on the D scale, beneath the 2 on the C scale.

The slide rule can be read to three significant figures and, with practice, can be used quickly and accurately. Position of the decimal point must be computed.

The L scale can be used as a log table to find the mantissa of the common logarithm for any number. Locate the number on the D scale and read the mantissa of its common log on the L scale.

A calculator may be used to shorten manual computation time and is more accurate than a slide rule (Fig. 9–10).

Metric System. The following prefixes are used:

nano-	10^{-9}, or 0.000000001
micro-	10^{-6}, or 0.000001
milli-	10^{-3}, or 0.001
centi-	10^{-2}, or 0.01
deci-	10^{-1}, or 1/10 or 0.1
deka-	10
hecto-	100
kilo-	1000

These prefixes, placed before any unit of measurement (length, weight, or volume), give smaller or larger units of the measurement.

Units of Length (Linear Measurement). The meter is defined by a standard platinum bar. An important relationship to English units is 2.54 centimeters = 1 inch. A meter is approximately 3.3 feet.

Common measurements are:

km.	1 kilometer = 1000 meters	= 0.62 miles
m.	1 meter	= 3.28 feet
cm.	1 centimeter	= 10^{-2} (0.01) meter
mm.	1 millimeter = 0.001 meter	= 10^{-3} meter
μm.	1 micrometer	= 10^{-6} meter
μ	1 micron*	= 10^{-6} meter
nm.	1 nanometer	= 10^{-9} meter
mμ	1 millimicron*	= 10^{-9} meter
Å	1 angstrom*	= 10^{-10} meter

*Obsolete according to the S.I. convention.

Units of Liquid Volume (Capacity or Volume Measurement). The liter is defined as the volume occupied by a mass of 1 kg. of pure water at its temperature of maximum density, 4° C., and under 1 atmosphere of pressure. One liter equals 1000.027 cubic centimeters. For most purposes, milliliters and cubic centimeters are used interchangeably, although there is a slight difference between them. The designation ml. is preferable to cc.

Although the mass of 1 cc. of water at 4° C. is equal to 1 gm. this varies slightly with temperature (Weast, 1965).

An important relationship to English units is 1 liter = 1.06 quarts. A gallon is slightly less than 4 liters.

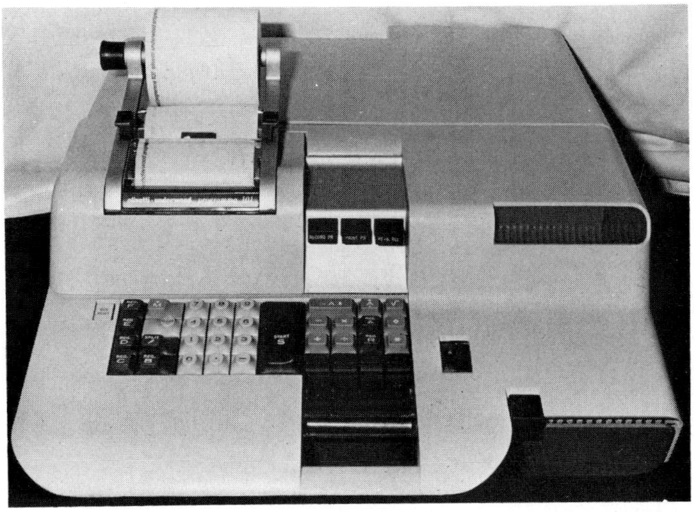

Figure 9–10. Calculator for rapid, accurate calculations. (Olivetti-Underwood, Programma 101)

	FAHRENHEIT (F.)	CENTIGRADE (C.)	ABSOLUTE or KELVIN (K.)
Boiling	212° F.	100° C.	373° K.
Freezing	32° F.	0° C.	273° K.
Absolute zero	–460° F.	–273° C.	0° K.

Common measurements are shown at the top of this page.

Units of Mass. The gram is 1/1000 of an arbitrary weight, the international kilogram. One ml. of water at 4° C. weighs approximately 1 gm. (or 1 g.). An important relationship to English units is 1 kilogram (kg.) = 2.2 pounds. The hypothetical average man is assumed to weigh 70 kg. Common measurements are shown at the bottom of this page.

Problems involving gases are solved by use of combined gas law formula:

$$\frac{P_1 V_1}{T_1} = \frac{P_2 V_2}{T_2}$$

Where P = pressure, V = volume, and T = absolute temperature.

Example: 500 ml. of air (or any other gas) at 27° C. and 720 mm. pressure is put under standard conditions of temperature and pressure (STP). The new volume (V_2) is:

$$\frac{720 \times 500}{300} = \frac{760 \times V_2}{273}$$

$$\text{or } V_2 = \frac{720 \times 500 \times 273}{300 \times 760} = 431 \text{ ml.}$$

Standard conditions are 760 mm. Hg and 0° C. (273° K.). Temperatures should be expressed in the absolute or Kelvin scale. If the gas is dry, its pressure may be read directly; if it has been exposed to or collected over water, it is necessary to subtract water vapor pressure from the gas pressure (tables are available to find water vapor pressure under different conditions).

Percentage Solutions. Weight in weight (w/w) solutions contain weight of an ingredient in 100 parts by weight of finished solution. This is rarely used.

Weight in volume (w/v) solutions contain weight of an ingredient in a given volume. If per cent and the volume are not specified, solute is made up to 100 parts by volume.

Example: (1) A 10 per cent (w/v) solution contains 10 gm. of solute in a final volume of 100 ml. of solution. (2) "Milligrams per cent" refers to milligrams of solute per 100 ml. of solution. This nomenclature is poor usage: "milligrams per 100 ml." is preferable. Milligrams per deciliter (dl.) has also been recommended.

Volume in volume (v/v) solutions contain a given volume of ingredient in 100 parts by volume of the finished solution. Per cent solutions of liquids in liquids are made up in this manner.

Example: Seventy per cent (v/v) solution of ethyl alcohol in water contains 70 ml. of absolute alcohol plus water sufficient to make up a final volume of 100 ml.

Atomic and Molecular Weights and Molar Solutions

Atomic Weight. Relative weight of atoms in terms of carbon-12, which has been arbitrarily chosen as a reference standard.

Example: Oxygen atom = 15.9994 ∴ O_2 = 31.9988 (molecular weight)
Hydrogen = 1.00797

Gram Atomic Weight. Gram atomic weight refers to atomic weight expressed in grams.

L.	1 liter	
dl.	1 deciliter	= 0.1 liter = 100 ml.
ml.	1 milliliter	= 0.001 liter
cc.	1 cubic centimeter	= 0.0009999 = 0.001 liter
μl. (λ)*	1 microliter (lambda)*	= 0.000001 liter = 1×10^{-6} liter
nl.	1 nanoliter	= 0.000000001 liter = 1×10^{-9} liter
pl.	1 picoliter	= 0.000000000001 liter = 1×10^{-12} liter

kg. or kilo	1 kilogram = 1,000 grams	
g.	1 gram	
mg.	1 milligram = 0.001 g.	= 1×10^{-3} g.
μg. (γ)	1 microgram (gamma)	= 1×10^{-6} g.
ng.	1 nanogram	= 1×10^{-9} g.
pg.	1 picogram	= 1×10^{-12} g.

*λ (lambda) obsolete according to S.I. convention.

Example: Atomic weight of carbon = 12.00. Gram atomic weight of carbon = 12.00 gm.

Gram Molecular Weight (GMW). GMW is the sum of the gram atomic weights of atomic constituents. An example is shown at the bottom of this page.

One gram molecular weight of a substance (GMW) is also called 1 mole of the substance. One mole of water (H_2O) = 18.015 gm.

$$\text{Moles} = \frac{\text{gm.}}{\text{GMW}}$$

A 1-molar (M) solution contains 1 mole of solute per liter of finished solution.

$$\text{Molarity} = \text{moles/liter} = \frac{\text{grams/liter}}{\text{GMW}}$$

A millimole (m mole) is 1/1000 of a mole.

$$\text{Millimoles per liter} = \frac{\text{milligrams/liter}}{\text{GMW}}$$

Although the use of m moles/L. instead of mM./L. has been recommended, the term mM./L. is still widely used.

Equivalent Weights and Normal Solutions. In ordinary usage, a gram equivalent weight is that weight of an element or compound which will combine with or replace 1 gm. of hydrogen (the special case of redox reactions will be discussed later). One gram equivalent weight of an element or compound equals the gram molecular weight divided by valence.

$$\text{Gram equivalent wt.} = \frac{\text{GMW}}{\text{valence}}$$

One gram equivalent weight of a substance is also called one *equivalent* of the substance.

$$\text{Number of equivalents} = \frac{\text{gm.}}{\text{gm. equiv. wt.}}$$

Example: $Ca(OH)_2$ (GMW 74)
Equivalent wt. = 74/2 = 37
1 mole = 2 equivalents

H_3PO_4 (GMW = 98)
Equivalent wt. = 98/3 = 32.7
1 mole = 3 equivalents

A one normal (N) solution contains 1 gm. equivalent weight of solute per liter of solution:

$$\text{Normality} = \text{equivalents/liter} = \frac{\text{gm./liter}}{\text{gm. equiv. wt.}}$$

A one normal solution of acid contains 1 gm. of hydrogen ion per liter; a one normal solution of alkali contains 17 gm. of hydroxyl ion per liter.

One gram of hydrogen ion will neutralize 17 gm. of hydroxyl ion; hence, a given number of milliliters of N acid is equivalent to the same number of milliliters of N alkali.

To determine the milliliters of acid required to neutralize a known amount of alkali, the following equation is used:

$$N_1 \times V_1 = N_2 \times V_2$$

N_1 and V_1 refer to the normality (concentration) and volume of the unknown, and N_2 and V_2 indicate corresponding known values.

One milliequivalent is 1/1000 of an equivalent.

$$\text{Number of milliequivalents} = \frac{\text{mg.}}{\text{gm. equiv. wt.}}$$

To convert mg./dl. to mEq. per liter:

$$\frac{\text{mg./liter}}{\text{eq. wt.}} = \text{mEq.}$$

$$\text{mg./dl.} \times 10 = \text{mg./liter}$$

$$\frac{\text{mg./dl.} \times 10}{\text{eq. wt.}} = \text{mEq./liter}$$

$$\text{Since eq. wt.} = \frac{\text{GMW}}{\text{valence}}$$

$$\text{mEq./liter} = \frac{\text{mg./dl.} \times 10}{\frac{\text{GMW}}{\text{valence}}}$$

Redox Reaction and Equivalent in Redox Reactions. Oxidation is defined as change of valence in an atom resulting from loss of electron(s). Reduction is the change in valence resulting from gain of electron(s). If a substance is oxidized in a reaction, another substance must be reduced in the same reaction; such reactions are termed redox reactions (reduction-oxidation). In such reactions, the oxidizing agent is reduced and the reducing agent is oxidized.

The equivalent weight of an oxidizing (reducing) agent equals its GMW divided by the electrons gained (lost) in the reaction:

$$\frac{\text{gram equivalent weight}}{\text{(as oxidant or reductant)}} = \frac{\text{formula weight (grams)}}{\text{oxidation state change}}$$

normality (in oxidation-reduction reaction) = molarity × oxidation state change

Example: In the Clark-Collip method, calcium is precipitated as the oxalate and titrated

---

Example: H_2O or water = 2 atoms of hydrogen 2 × 1.008 = 2.016
1 atom of oxygen 1 × 15.999 = 15.999
gram molecular weight = 18.015 gm.

with $KMnO_4$ as an oxidizing agent and indicator:

$$CaC_2O_4 + H_2SO_4 \rightleftarrows H_2C_2O_4 + CaSO_4$$

$$2\ KMnO_4 + 5\ H_2C_2O_4 + 3\ H_2SO_4 \rightarrow K_2SO_4 + 2\ MnSO_4 + 10\ CO_2\uparrow + 8\ H_2O$$

In the second reaction, Mn^{+7} (as MnO_4^- in which Mn has a valence of +7) goes to Mn^{++}, with a valence of +2. Hence, Mn has gained five electrons. The equivalent weight of $KMnO_4$ in this reaction is GMW/5.

Osmolal Solutions. Osmolality refers to osmotically active units expressed as moles per kilogram and is usually written as mOsm./kg.

An osmol is one osmotically active unit (molecule or ion), expressed as moles:

Osmols/liter = moles/liter × osmotically active units per molecule

A milliosmole is 1/1000 of an osmol. It is usually written as mOsm./liter.

milliosmoles/liter = millimoles/liter × osmotically active units per molecule

Example: NaCl dissociates completely in aqueous solution into two osmotically active units (ions). Hence:

osmoles/liter = moles/liter × 2

Glucose does not dissociate; osmolality of glucose solutions is the same as molarity until high concentrations are reached (interference effect).

Calculations Useful in Preparation of Solutions

To Reduce Solutions from Higher to Lower Concentrations

$$\text{Conc.}_1 \times \text{volume}_1 = \text{conc.}_2 \times \text{volume}_2$$

When the weight of salt to make 1 liter of solution is provided, to find weight required for more than or less than 1 liter use the following relationship:

$$w_1/v_1 = w_2/v_2$$

Dilutions are usually expressed as one unit of the original solution per total units of final solution. A 1:10 dilution requires that one unit of concentrated solution be diluted to a total volume of 10 units. To calculate the concentration of a solution, multiply by the dilution ratio. If several dilutions are made, multiply them together to arrive at final concentration.

Example: A 10 per cent solution is diluted 1:5, and is again diluted 1:5:

$$\text{Concentration} = 10\% \times 1/5 \times 1/5 = 0.4\%$$

Large dilutions which would be cumbersome to perform in one operation may be conveniently carried out by a series of dilutions.

Specific Gravity (sp. gr.). Specific gravity refers to weight per unit volume with respect to water, which has a sp. gr. of one.

$$\text{sp. gr.} = \frac{\text{weight in gm.}}{\text{volume in ml.}}$$

The specific gravity of a solution multiplied by its volume and again by the percentage of material in solution equals the weight of solute in solution.

To Prepare a Normal Solution of a Liquid. The amount of liquid in ml. to be diluted to 1 liter is given by the formula:

$$\frac{\text{GMW}}{\text{valence} \times \text{sp. gr.} \times \text{conc. (w./w.)}}$$

To make stronger than 1N, multiply by appropriate factor; to make weaker than 1 N dilute by appropriate factor.

Ionic Strength

$$\mu = \tfrac{1}{2}\ \Sigma\ (cZ^2)$$

where μ = ionic strength, c = molality, and Z = charge of the ion.

Example: For a 0.1 molal solution of Na_2SO_4:

$$\mu = \tfrac{1}{2}\ [(0.1 \times 1^2) + (0.1 \times 1^2) + (0.1 \times 2^2)] = \tfrac{1}{2}\ (0.1 + 0.1 + 0.4) = 0.3$$

Acids, Alkalis, and pH. An acid molecule yields hydrogen ions (protons) in aqueous solutions; an alkali accepts these. At room temperature in pure water:

$$[H^+] = [OH^-] = 1 \times 10^{-7}\ \text{molar}$$

In all aqueous solutions, both acid and alkaline:

$$K_W = [H^+] \times [OH^-] = 10^{-14}$$

In an acid solution $[H^+]$ is greater than 10^{-7} M. In an alkaline solution, $[H^+]$ is less than 10^{-7} M.

pH is the exponent which must be applied to 10 in order to give the value of $1/H^+$. That is,

$$pH = \log_{10} 1/H^+$$

When pH is	H^+ is	and OH^- is
1	10^{-1}	10^{-13}
2	10^{-2}	10^{-12}
4	10^{-4}	10^{-10}
6	10^{-6}	10^{-8}
10	10^{-10}	10^{-4}
13	10^{-13}	10^{-1}

A change of one pH unit indicates a tenfold change in H^+ concentration.

Buffer Solutions. A buffer is a solution of a weak acid and one of its salts. To prepare a buffer to a required pH, use the Henderson-Hasselbalch equation:

$$pH = pK + \log_{10} \frac{[\text{salt}]}{[\text{acid}]}$$

where pK = negative log of dissociation constant

When the concentration of salt and acid are equal (at pK), the buffer solution is most effective in resisting a change in pH. The pK can be found in tables published in Handbook of Chemistry and Physics (53rd Edition, 1972–73) and is a useful reference, since it defines pH where maximum buffering capacity is exerted.

LABORATORY SAFETY

The potential hazards in a medical chemistry laboratory warrant the attention of everyone who enters the environment. An attitude of safety and an awareness of hazards can help ensure the continued health and productivity of all personnel. While any development of this topic will focus on basic knowledge for prevention of accidents, it is recognized that most laboratory accidents are not due to ignorance but to carelessness or an attempt to take a shortcut by personnel under pressure to perform rapidly.

Safety devices should be available, and all personnel should be made familiar with their use. Fire drills and first aid instruction including cardiopulmonary resuscitation (CPR), should be conducted at regular intervals.

Knowledge about the properties of and proper handling procedures for chemicals in terms of use and storage should virtually eliminate danger of burns, explosions, fires, and toxic fumes. A manual on the handling of chemicals is available (*Safety in Handling Hazardous Chemicals,* Matheson, Coleman and Bell, Norwood, Ohio 45212). In addition, there are a large number of safety items that are reviewed in an excellent manual on laboratory safety (*Manual on Laboratory Safety,* Fisher Scientific Co., Pittsburgh, Pa. 15219).

Fire Extinguishers. Hand-size extinguishers should be located adjacent to each door and at various locations in the halls of the laboratory suite. These extinguishers should be of the dry powder type, so that they may be used for all types of fires (Fig. 9–11).

To operate these extinguishers, locate the small lever on the top that is sealed with a wire seal. The lever is simply raised to break the seal; the hose connection or nozzle is then aimed in the direction of the fire; and the large double handle is squeezed together to produce the extinguisher powder.

Notice on the front of each of these extinguishers a small dial with a safety zone indicated in green. If at any time these dials are not registering within these zones. they must be replenished. The physical plant department or other qualified personnel should maintain these extinguishers, and it should not be necessary to have them replenished at more frequent intervals than their inspection warrants (usually twice a year), unless they are used.

Fire Blanket. The fire blanket in the chemistry laboratory should be located just inside the hall door. Observe the rope handle jutting out from the case of this blanket; the blanket is rolled in such a way that by placing one's right arm through the rope loop and pulling

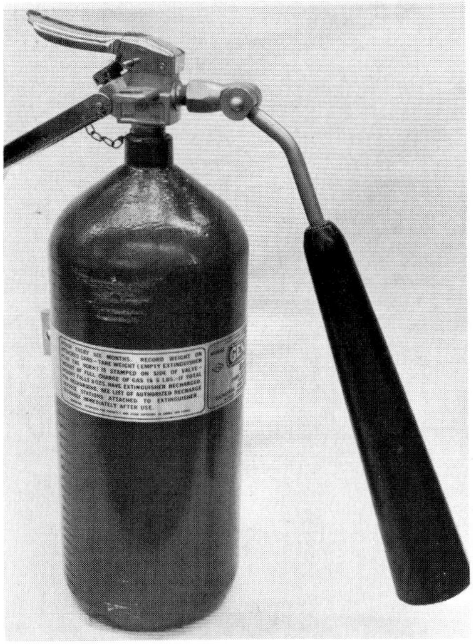

Figure 9–11.

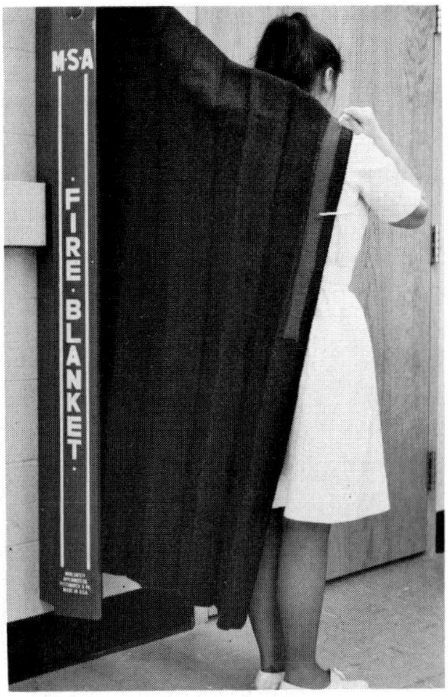

Figure 9–12.

Figure 9–11. Fire extinguisher (General Fire Extinguisher Corp., Detroit, Michigan).

Figure 9–12. Fire blanket (Mine Safety Appliances Co., Pittsburgh, Pennsylvania).

vigorously while turning to the left (counterclockwise) the blanket will unroll from the case and enwrap the subject. This blanket is intended for use when a flash fire has ignited clothing or parts of the body and a chemical extinguisher might be a hazard to the skin (Fig. 9-12). The blanket should be carefully rerolled on the rod within the case after use.

Safety Shower. A safety shower should be located immediately inside the hall door of the main chemistry laboratory and should be used to flush corrosives from the skin or clothing in case of accidental spillage or explosion. The shower is so designed that by pulling on the large handle hanging down from the shower head a large amount of water is released immediately and continues to flow only as long as the handle is held in the lowered position. As soon as the handle is released, the shower will stop running.

Gas Mask. A gas mask should be located on the right inside the door of the main chemistry laboratory. This is intended for use when large amounts of corrosive or poisonous gases have accidentally escaped into the working area and it becomes necessary to reenter the area to either turn off or neutralize the flow of gas.

It should be a canister-type mask that can be adapted to all faces and be supplied with a refillable cartridge. It should also be sealed with a small wire seal indicating that the canister is unused. The operation of this mask should be demonstrated to personnel at an early opportunity, and the cartridge should be replaced as soon as it is used.

Glassware. Any broken or chipped glassware should, if at all possible, be replaced. This is especially true of containers that are going to be used with stoppers or any kind of equipment that would exert pressure on the faulty glassware. Personnel should be especially careful of bottles, tubes, or any other glassware into which they are about to place corrosives of any sort, including acids, alkalis, or inflammable material. Indeed, safety glasses are not only desirable, but essential for many activities in the clinical laboratory (Fig. 9-13).

When inserting or extracting a glass rod or tubing from such items as stoppers and corks, it is important always to use some kind of protection—either hand towels or the rubber shields provided in the laboratory. Moistening the rod or tubing will in many instances facilitate insertion or extraction. If it becomes necessary to break a piece of glass rod or tubing, score it lightly with a metal file, moisten the area scored, and then, holding the tubing with both hands on either side of the scored area, break tubing with a firm tug while exerting a slight torque on the tubing.

When disposing of such items as needles, broken glassware, cans, and noncombustibles, always place in a specially marked container in order to avoid injury to janitorial staff personnel.

Inflammables. Inflammables may include such things as alcohols, ethers, and acetone. These should always be stored either in their original container or in special safety cans at room temperature in an unconfined area (Fig. 9-14). When pouring or otherwise measuring these inflammables, one should always check the area in which he is working to make certain there are no open flames. If spillage of these materials occurs either on individuals or parts of the laboratory, flush the area with water and wipe dry. When disposing of empty containers which have previously contained

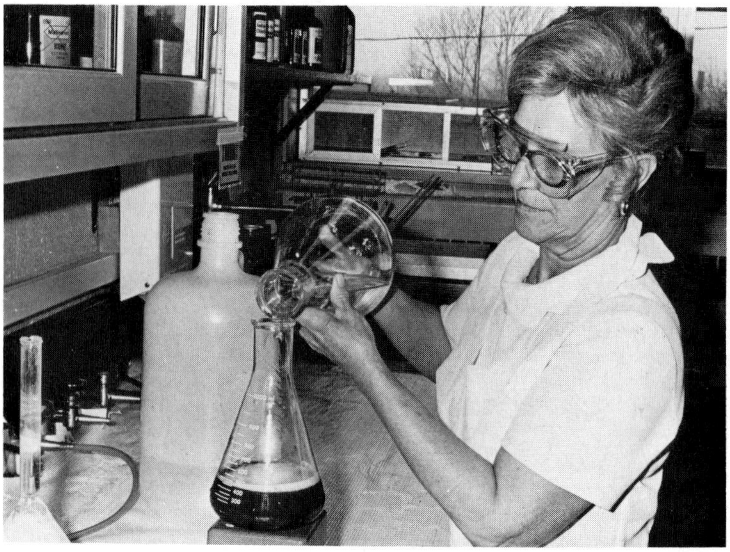

Figure 9-13. Safety glasses, required in many states for laboratory personnel, are especially important in handling corrosives that may splatter as well as glass and other materials that may fragment.

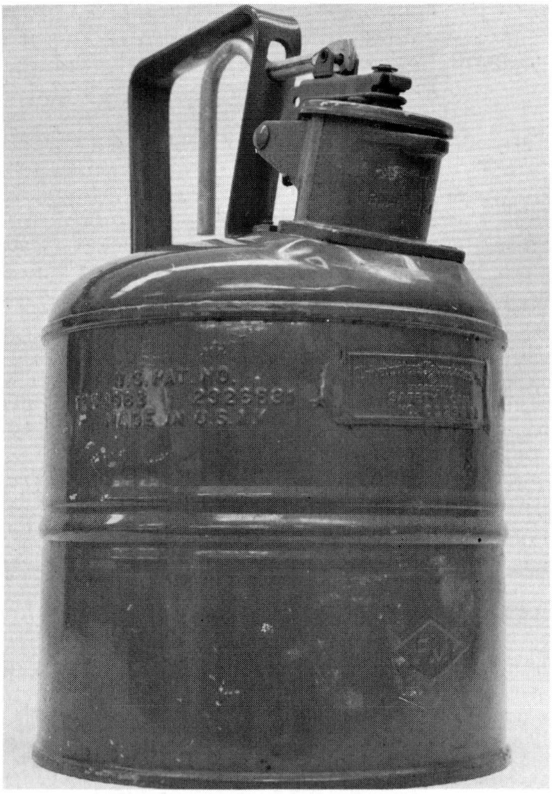

Figure 9–14. Special safety can for storage of inflammables (Justrite Mfg. Co., Chicago, Illinois).

inflammables, always fill the containers to overflowing several times with water to clear any trapped vapor. Drain the last of the rinse water completely out of the containers before placing them in specially provided disposal areas. Tanks of oxygen and propane gases should be located outside the laboratory working area, with special attention given to local fire regulations.

Contaminated Materials. When chemical determinations are performed on samples of blood or urine which are known to come from patients having infectious diseases, all materials used in the analysis, including glassware as well as the actual sample, must be autoclaved to prevent further spread of disease to unsuspecting persons, such as laboratory helpers processing the glassware. These items should be placed in a stainless steel receptacle, which can then be autoclaved completely before actual washing of containers occurs. The most common offender is the yellow (icteric) serum or urine which may come from a patient suffering from infectious hepatitis.

Accident Prevention

Location of Corrosive Chemicals. If at all possible, always place corrosives on lower shelves of storage area or on the back part of a counter where they cannot be easily knocked off by an elbow or hand reaching for some other material. Since many of these corrosives are procured in large bottles for reasons of economy, it is advisable to always store these on the lowest shelf available to avoid accidents in trying to lift a heavy bottle to or from an inconvenient height. Grasp bottles firmly around the body (never by the neck) with one or both hands, depending on size. In transporting a bottle of concentrated acid for distances of more than a few feet, use an acid bottle carrier. This is a polyethylene container into which the acid bottle fits, and prevents breaking of the acid container in transport.

Spillage. Always check caps or stoppers on all reagent bottles carefully to be sure they are tight. If reagents spill either on the outside of the bottle or on laboratory counters, wipe up immediately and wash carefully with water to avoid injury to other personnel using this same reagent later.

Pipetting Precautions. Inspect both ends of all pipettes used for chips or cracks to prevent either injury to the fingers or mouth when pipetting or inaccurate delivery from the tip when measuring reagents or samples. Always lay pipettes only on clean surfaces before using, and immediately after using place in jars provided for dirty pipettes. Do not place pipettes which have touched any other material back into a reagent bottle, thereby causing the whole bottle of reagent to be contaminated. Never pipette contaminated material or poisonous substances by mouth (Fig. 9–15); always use pipettes provided for this purpose. Examples of these would be blood from serum hepatitis patients or reagents such as sodium cyanide, which is lethal in small doses when ingested. When diluting acids, always add acid slowly to the water, with mixing; water should never be added to concentrated acid.

Electrical Equipment. Only grounded outlets and grounded plugs (three prong) should be used for electrical equipment in the laboratory. Special precautions for some high-voltage equipment (e.g., electrophoremeter cells or high-voltage electrophoretic tanks) are most important, but in general do not work with electrical equipment when hands are damp or counters, floors, or fuses and lamps are wet; always disconnect the equipment by removing the plug from the electrical outlet.

First Aid. If materials are accidentally pipetted into the mouth, rinse the mouth thoroughly with water immediately. If burning, itching, or other symptoms persist, report at once to the emergency room. If by accident, contaminated material such as spinal fluid is pipetted into the mouth, notify supervisor in order that prophylactic treatment may be begun if necessary.

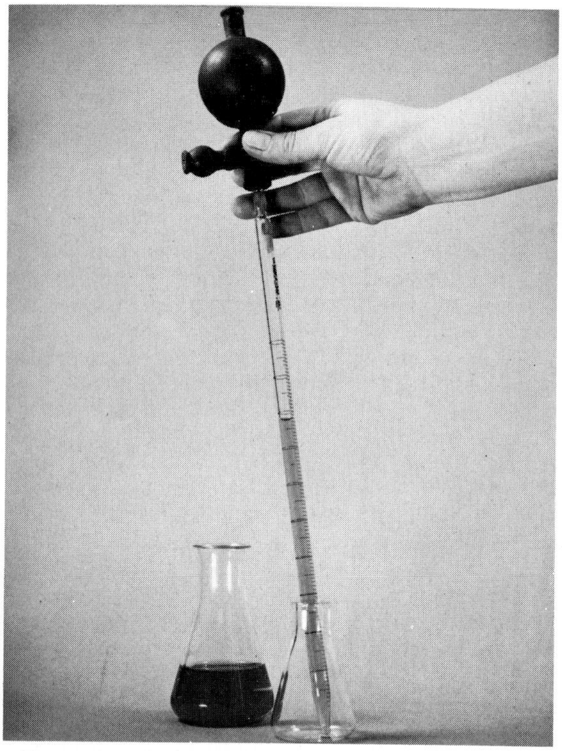

Figure 9–15. Propipette for transfer of contaminated or poisonous substances.

The best first aid for all types of alkaline or acid burns is to flush the area with water thoroughly as soon as possible. If actual burning does occur, report to the emergency room for medical attention.

Any type of cut or wound should be reported to the emergency room as soon as it occurs. Forms for this service as well as directions for follow-up work should be available in each laboratory, and procedures outlined there should be followed, even though the injury seems slight.

LABORATORY GLASSWARE

Types of Glassware. Most laboratory glassware should be made of borosilicate glass, which is a heat-resistant, hard glass manufactured by several companies.

Volumetric Glassware. This type of glassware is specially calibrated to either contain or deliver a given amount at a specified temperature following the standards set down by the National Bureau of Standards. There are many classifications of this type of glassware indicating accuracy of each piece. For example, you may find individually calibrated glassware certified by the National Bureau of Standards to be used for highly precise work with a very small tolerance allowed for error. Various gradations occur from there on down, including class A, student class, etc. Most glassware for medical chemistry use will be class A or better. Included in this category are such items as volumetric flasks ranging from 1 ml. to 5000 or 6000 ml., pipettes graduated to deliver or to contain a specified amount, and specially calibrated tubes for specific tests. Each manufacturer lists the specifications necessary to perform accurate work with their product. For example, most volumetric flasks will state the amount to contain at a specified temperature. Therefore, if the solution is made up to volume at a temperature either higher or lower than that specified, the concentration of the sample or reagent will be in error.

Pipettes manufactured in the United States have standard markings to indicate the proper way to use them. There are two main categories: (1) "to contain"—these will either be marked TC or "to contain," and this indicates that the solution being measured in the pipette must be rinsed thoroughly out of the pipette with the solution it is being added into; (2) "to deliver"—these will either be marked TD or "to deliver" and will also have the characteristic of either having a frosted ring (one or two) at the top of the pipette or no frosted ring (Figs. 9–16, 9–17). When the frosted ring appears on a pipette, this indicates that the last drop must be blown out of the pipette in order to have it measure correctly. When the ring is absent, the pipette is simply held against the side of the container into which the delivery is being made and most of the solution will be pulled out by capillary attraction. Allow 30 seconds for complete delivery. A small amount remains in the tip of the pipette to correct for this. Graduated pipettes are similarly marked. All volumetric glassware should be used by adjusting the lowest portion of the meniscus exactly on the calibration line when sighted at eye level, holding that portion of the glassware having the calibration line horizontal. Microliter pipettes are discussed subsequently (p. 554).

Special Glassware. Certain types of tubes, absorption cells, etc., will be found in the laboratory and may have special qualities such as spectrophotometrically matched sides or edges, or special size vials and tubes to be used in specific instruments.

Cleaning of Glassware. Immediately after use, glassware should be rinsed out and immersed completely in a hot detergent solution to facilitate cleansing. The glassware is then rinsed thoroughly in tap water, then distilled water, and in special cases demineralized water. When this is accomplished, the glass-

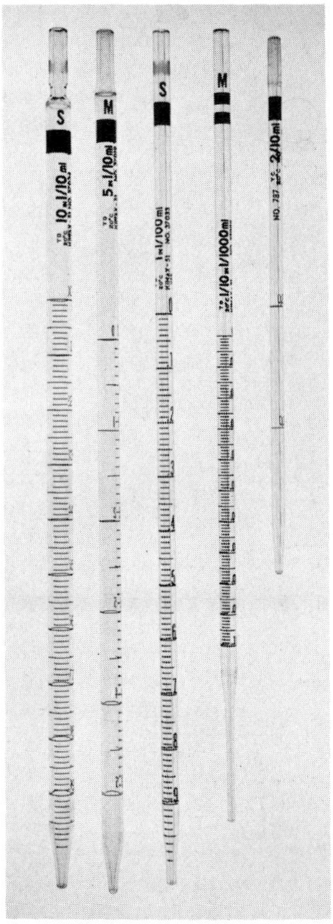

Figure 9–16.

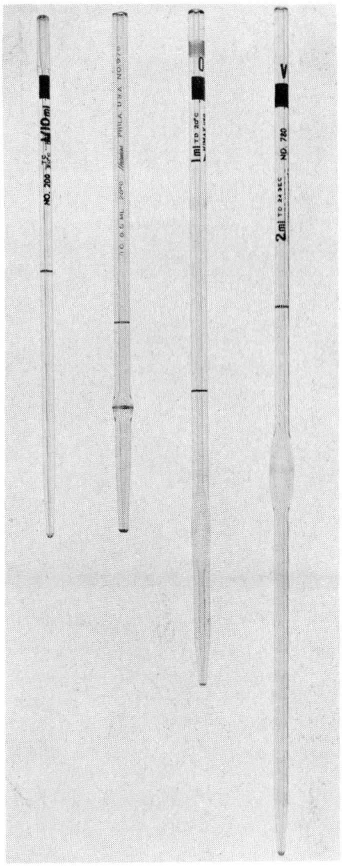

Figure 9–17.

Figure 9–16. To deliver (TD) and to contain (TC) pipettes.

Figure 9–17. Selection of volumetric pipettes.

ware should drain dry and be completely free of bubbles, water marks, etc., on the inside. If the water does not drain in this fashion, it may be necessary to clean this glassware with a chemical cleaning solution containing sodium dichromate and sulfuric acid. In most cases it is necessary that glassware be completely dry before being used. This is especially true of volumetric glassware, in which slight amounts of water will change the solution of the sample or reagent one is measuring.

LABORATORY EQUIPMENT AND MATERIALS

The principles of spectrophotometry and related instruments are the subject matter of Chapter 8. In addition to absorption and emission spectrophotometers, atomic absorption spectrophotometers, fluorometers, and several other instruments may be encountered in a medical chemistry laboratory. The centrifuge has been mentioned in regard to care and operation with preventive maintenance. Preventive maintenance of all instruments is of great importance. For selected instruments, more than one may be needed to ensure both manual emergency service and automated service of a continuing nature when transient breakdown or down-time may be anticipated.

Osmometers are referred to in Chapters 2 and 12. A modular arrangement in automated instrumental systems lends itself to trouble shooting and specific module replacement when warranted. Water baths and incubators, as well as automatic glassware washers and dryers, represent additional potential trouble areas if they are not given similar care and attention (Fig. 9–18). Familiarity with manufacturers' manuals for operation, maintenance, and trouble shooting pays dividends to laboratory personnel in terms of optimal sustained service and fewer crises. Such manuals should be kept with instrument logs nearby. A close working relationship with electronic and electrical personnel in the hospital or medical center can be rewarding for continuing operation and trouble-free instrument performance. Materials in the form of reagents, standards, glassware, and other disposable items require storage area and inventory to ensure availability at all times. Reagents and standards

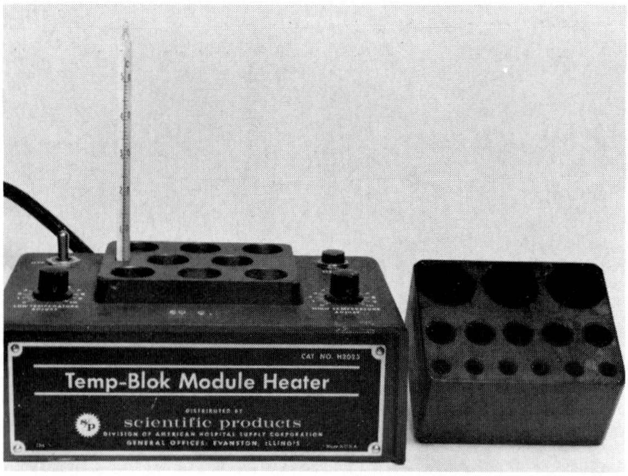

Figure 9–18. Dry heating unit to replace water bath.

are reviewed in specific chapters encompassing particular measurements and examinations.

Chemicals. Chemicals exist in varying degrees of purity. Even sodium chloride may contain a small amount of potassium sulfate or iodide. Meticulous attention to the label on a bottle as well as to the supplier's catalogue will frequently reveal the maximum limits of impurities in chemicals. Several companies show on the label the actual analysis so that one may identify the exact amount of an impurity present in a particular batch or bottle. For quantitative measurements and preparation of accurate standard solutions, it is important to use pure chemicals and to identify exact amounts of compound or elements desired, as well as amount of contaminants. The use of "reagent-grade" chemicals, although more expensive than less pure grades of chemicals, is essential to accuracy. Because several grades of chemicals are available, an awareness of the terms used widely is necessary. For the most highly purified chemicals, "reagent grade," "analytical grade," or "ACS" for having met the established standards of purity by the American Chemical Society are terms that should be identified on a label or in the catalogue. Less pure grades are referred to as "purified" and "technical."

U.S.P. and N.F. represent other grades of purity and mean that these chemicals meet the stipulations listed in the United States Pharmacopeia or the National Formulary; while they are adequate for human consumption, they may not be pure enough for specific chemical applications. Radin (1967) has reviewed the use and availability of standards with the limitations of so-called standards.

N.B.S., or National Bureau of Standards, and the College of American Pathologists (C.A.P.), along with several suppliers who list the exact composition or maximum limits of impurities in their chemicals, are preferred sources for preparation of many standards used in medical chemistry (Meinke, 1971). Proprietary reagents, such as drugs, of undisclosed composition should be avoided, even though they may give satisfactory results under the usual conditions. With abnormal specimens or under abnormal conditions, confusing results as well as invalid data may be caused by use of such proprietary reagents. It is important to know what compounds are being used in a specific determination to understand what reaction is taking place and to identify as well as anticipate and evaluate abnormal reactions or interferences.

Some reagent-grade chemicals contain less than 100 per cent of the desired compound. Where the assay is reported, one can identify the exact composition and note impurity, whether it be carbonate or even water in a bottle of sodium hydroxide. At other times it may be more important and necessary to select another reagent source, e.g., a bottle of a more pure acid or base without interfering compounds or elements to meet exact chemical assay requirements.

The degree of hydration or amount of water of crystallization in a compound should be evident. Although an anhydrous compound may be stable, it may have such an affinity for water that under usual atmospheric conditions it cannot be weighed accurately. The use of a stable hydrate form of the chemical compound is then essential. Although several degrees of hydration may exist for certain salts the most stable form should be selected for weighing, and appropriate calculations made to achieve desired final concentration as related to anhydrous salt form or specific degree of hydration (e.g., mono-, di-, pentahydrate) cited in the procedure. Disodium hydrogen phosphate ($Na_2HPO_4 \cdot 2\ H_2O$) as a dihydrate is the most stable form and thus is suitable for weighing, although heptahydrate ($Na_2HPO_4 \cdot 7\ H_2O$) and dodecahydrate ($Na_2HPO_4 \cdot 12\ H_2O$) as well as the anhydrous form are available. However, some compounds are available only in the hydrate form, such as sodium tungstate ($Na_2WO_4 \cdot 2\ H_2O$), and the concentration of final solution may be expressed in percentage of hydrate rather than anhydrous salt.

Desiccants. Drying agents have a variety of applications in the laboratory (Bermes and Forman, 1970). It is apparent in Table 9–4 that several are alkaline and one is strongly acidic. Selection of an appropriate desiccant or drying agent for absorption of moisture depends on the composition of materials or gases to be dried, convenience, efficiency, and cost. Some desiccants can be regenerated easily, e.g., silica gel by heating in a drying oven at 120° C.

Table 9–4. CHEMISTRY AND ACTIVITY OF DESICCANTS*

DRYING AGENT	ACTIVITY†	CAPACITY	DELIQUESCENCE	EASY REGENERATION	CHEMICAL REACTION
Phosphorus pentoxide	0.02	very low	yes	no	acidic
Barium oxide	0.6–0.8	moderate	no	no	alkaline
Alumina	0.8–1.2	low	no	yes	neutral
Magnesium perchlorate (anhydrous)	1.6–2.4	high	yes	no	neutral
Calcium sulfate (Drierite)	4–6	moderate	no	yes	neutral
Silica gel	2–10	low	no	yes	neutral
Potassium hydroxide (stick)	10–17	moderate	yes	no	alkaline
Calcium chloride (anhydrous)	330–380	high	yes	no	neutral

*From Bermes, E. W., Jr., and Forman, D. T.: Basic laboratory principles and procedures. *In* Tietz, N. W. (ed.): Fundamentals of Clinical Chemistry, 1970.
†Micrograms residual water per liter of air at 30° C.

BASIC TECHNIQUES

Potentiometry and gasometry are discussed in Chapter 12; absorption and emission spectrophotometry and fluorometry are presented in Chapter 8. Filtration may be used in place of centrifugation to separate solids from liquids. This is usually performed with paper folded properly. A funnel containing glass wool may be substituted for paper when acids or bases too strong for filter paper require filtering. Many types of filter paper with different degrees of porosity are available for selection according to requirements of separation by filtration (Table 9–5).

Mixing is readily accomplished with a Vortex mixer (Fig. 9–19). Mechanical devices employing air or electricity, including magnetic stirrers, with or without heat, aid in achieving solution when prolonged mixing is required (Fig. 9–20).

Table 9–5. TYPES AND CHARACTERISTICS OF FILTER PAPERS*

WHATMAN NO.	EQUIVALENT SCHLEICHER AND SCHUELL NO.	CHARACTERISTICS
		Unwashed
1	596	Medium; medium weight, speed, and retentiveness
2	597	Dense; more retentive, less rapid
3	598	Thick; heavy, strong, quite retentive
4	604	Soft; very rapid, less retentive
5	602	Very dense; very retentive, filters slowly
		Single acid washed (HCl)
30	497	Medium; fairly rapid and retentive
31	410	Soft; more rapid, less retentive
32	402	Retentive
		Double acid washed (HCl and HF)
40	589, white ribbon	Medium; medium speed and retentiveness
41	589, black ribbon	Soft; more rapid, less retentive
41H	589-IH	Hard, rapid, strong
42	589, blue ribbon	Dense; more retentive, less rapid
44	590	Thin; very retentive
		Hardened
50	507, 576	Retentive
52	589WH	Medium speed and retentiveness
54	589BH	More rapid, less retentive

*Courtesy of Dr. Ferrin B. Moreland.

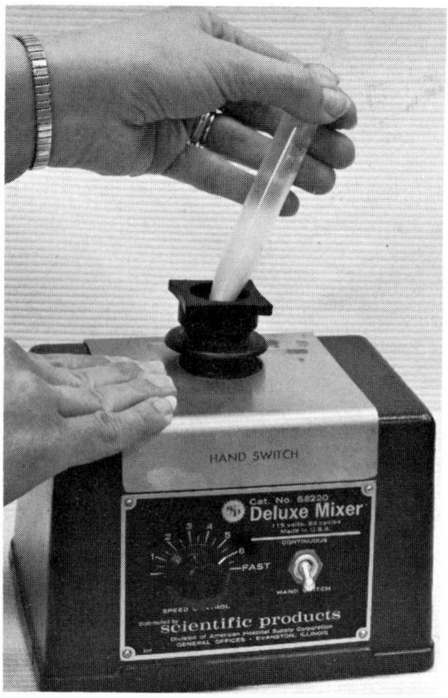

Figure 9-19.

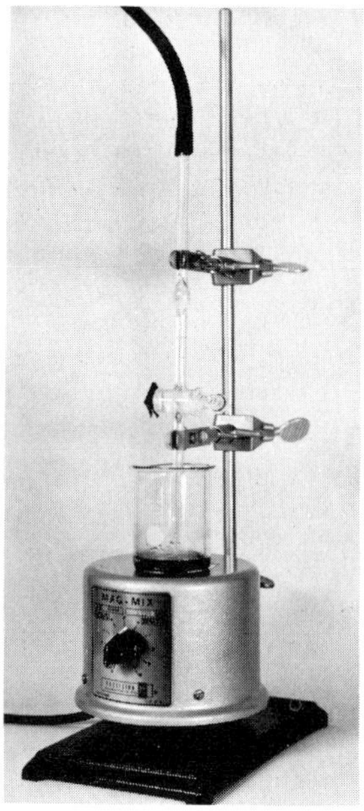

Figure 9-20.

Figure 9-19. Mixing contents of a test tube with a Vortex mixer.

Figure 9-20. Magnetic mixer with heat.

MASS OR WEIGHT

Measurement of mass or weight (gravimetric analysis) is most important for the preparation of reagents and standards for chemical determination. This underscores the need for a thorough background in quantitative analysis and understanding of the analytical balance. Care and maintenance of the analytical balance are of the utmost importance. With the exception of total serum lipids, virtually all medical chemical measurements are performed with other basic techniques; hence, methods of gravimetric analysis are not considered further, although they are important. The reader is encouraged to review a textbook of quantitative analysis for the details of operation and care of the analytical balance. For selection of a laboratory balance, the report of Hackler (1970) should be consulted.

VOLUME

Measurement of volume or volumetric analysis is familiar to every student who has had a course in quantitative analytical chemistry. While volumetric procedures may include neutralization, precipitation, and oxidation-reduction methods, as well as titrimetry, the amount of a substance in solution is determined by measuring the amount of a solution of known concentration that reacts with a premeasured amount of unknown solution. Meticulous selection and use of calibrated volumetric glassware, including pipettes, burettes, flasks, and cylinders, are most important. Several types of volumetric analysis are conducted in medical chemistry and will be discussed with the individual procedures. The analyst should be familiar with gravimetric (mass of mercury or water) and spectrophotometric methods for checking calibration of volumetric glassware as well as be attentive to tolerance limits specified by various manufacturers (Richterich, 1969).

TITRIMETRY

Acids and Bases. The preparation of commonly used acids and bases requires standard solutions of known accurate concentration or primary standards and an appropriate indicator or pH meter to identify the endpoint of titration. From constant boiling hydrochloric acid, a standard 0.100 N solution of hydrochloric acid (HCl) may be prepared (Annino, 1964); this primary standard can then be used to standardize bases and acids. A solid acid such as potassium acid phthalate ($KHC_8H_4O_4$) is suitable as a primary standard. With an equivalent weight of 204.23 either a 1 N or 0.100 N primary standard acid may be prepared as follows: weigh accurately 20.423 gm. of dry acid phthalate (National Bureau of Standards, or N.B.S.) and dissolve in water; dilute to the mark in a volumetric flask of 100-ml. volume (1 N) or 1000-ml. volume (0.100 N).

Tris (hydroxymethyl) aminomethane is suitable for a primary standard base. This organic compound is available as a highly purified, white crystalline solid (Sigma Chemical Co., 3500 DeKalb Street, St. Louis, Missouri 63118). As a monovalent base with an equivalent weight of 121.09, the empirical formula is $C_4H_{11}NO_3$, and the structural formula is as follows:

2-amino-2-hydroxymethyl-1,3-propanediol

```
              CH2—OH
               |
HO—CH2—C—CH2—OH
               |
              NH2
```

A standard solution of 0.100 N is prepared by dissolving 12.109 gm. of "tris" in water and diluting to the mark in a 1000-ml. volumetric flask. Rather than use an indicator, it is preferable to titrate to the equivalance point at pH 4.7, using a pH meter to standardize an acid with this solution.

With an appropriate primary standard acid or primary standard base, it is possible to prepare the commonly used acids and bases as secondary standards and to meet the requirements of a number of chemical measurements.

Solutions of sodium hydroxide (NaOH) in varying concentrations are frequently required and often used as a second standard. It is necessary to prepare a carbonate-free solution from the commercially available solid form that contains much sodium carbonate. Furthermore, special care is needed because of the avidity of sodium hydroxide for carbon dioxide present in the air. Sodium hydroxide solutions are prepared from a carbonate-free solution of concentrated sodium hydroxide (50 per cent w./w.) in a rubber- or plastic-stoppered borosilicate glass (Pyrex or Kimax) flask and protected from the air subsequently by a soda-lime tube. Solid reagent-grade sodium hydroxide is added to distilled water (1100 gm. to 1 liter) in a 2- or 3-liter flask. The flask is placed in a sink under running cold water and swirled intermittently until alkali is dissolved. Allow this stoppered, cool, saturated solution to stand for several days for the insoluble carbonate to settle out. Transfer by suction or decantation the supernatant alkali and store in a paraffin-lined glass or polyethylene tightly stoppered bottle, since alkali reacts with glass. This concentrated sodium hydroxide is approximately 17 N, but a measured volume (use a rubber bulb; do not pipette by mouth) should be diluted 1:200 with water (boiled and cooled promptly to free of CO_2) and the exact concentration determined by titration against a primary acid standard. The alkali should be in the burette during the acid-base titrations; etching of the burette and stopcock used with alkali can be avoided by rinsing with acetic acid and water after use.

Preparation of a Secondary Standard Solution of Sodium Hydroxide. Pipette 10 ml. of primary standard acid phthalate (0.100 N) into a 125-ml. Erlenmeyer flask; add 2 drops of 1 per cent (w./v.) phenolphthalein in 70 per cent (v./v.) ethyl alcohol. The concentrated sodium hydroxide is diluted as described to prepare an approximate 0.100 N solution: Solution 1 is concentrated sodium hydroxide, and solution 2 is dilute alkali.

$$N_1 V_1 = N_2 V_2$$

$$17 \times X = 0.1 \times 1000$$
$$17X = 100$$
$$X = 5.9$$

5.9 ml. of concentrated sodium hydroxide is diluted to 1000 ml. with distilled water to yield an approximate 0.100 N alkali solution.

Place this dilute sodium hydroxide in a 25-ml. burette; with continuous swirling of the flask containing 10 ml. of primary acid and indicator, add sodium hydroxide from the burette (Fig. 9–21). As the endpoint is ap-

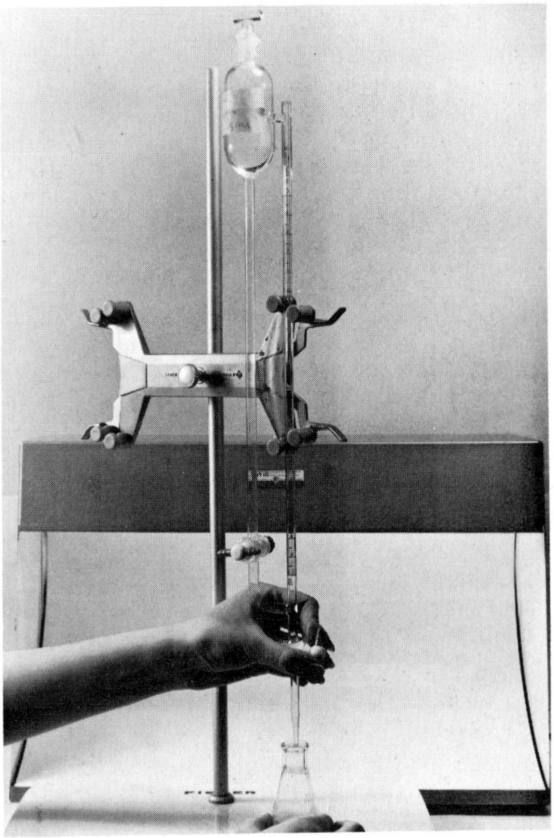

Figure 9–21. Proper technique for titration with a burette in acid-base standardization.

proached, the pink color that is observed where alkali stream enters the acid solution will disappear more slowly; at this point, decrease the flow rate of alkali until the endpoint is attained (pink remains for 15 seconds after mixing). The difference between the burette readings before and after the titration is the volume (ml.) of sodium hydroxide used. The concentration of NaOH is calculated as follows:

$$\text{Normality of NaOH} = \text{normality of acid } (0.100) \times \frac{10}{\text{ml. NaOH}}$$

If 9.5 ml. of NaOH solution was required to titrate to the endpoint 10 ml. of 0.1 N standard acid:

$$\text{Normality NaOH} = 0.1 \times \frac{10}{9.5}$$
$$\text{NaOH} = 0.1052 \text{ N}$$

To prepare an exact 0.100 N solution of NaOH, the concentrated alkali will have to be diluted appropriately and subsequently checked by a repeat titration. With volume of concentrated alkali solution as 1 and the dilution volume as 2, the exact normality may be calculated:

$$N_1 V_1 = N_2 V_2$$
$$N_1 \times 5.9 = 0.1052 \times 1000$$
$$N_1 = \frac{0.1052 \times 1000}{5.9}$$
$$N_1 = 17.831$$

Since concentrated NaOH is 17.831 N it will yield a 0.100 N solution by dilution as follows:

$$17.831 \times X = 0.100 \times 1000$$
$$X = 5.6$$

Therefore, 5.6 ml. of concentrated NaOH may be diluted to the mark in a 1000-ml. volumetric flask with distilled (boiled, cold water to render CO_2 free) to make a 0.100 N solution of sodium hydroxide that is subsequently transferred and stored in a tightly capped polyethylene bottle and appropriately labeled after repeat titration as described. An adequate standard or reagent label should indicate contents of bottle in terms of solution identification, concentration, date of preparation, and name or initials of person preparing solution.

Hydrochloric acid (HCl) solutions may be prepared from reagent grade concentrated hydrochloric acid; this is approximately 12 N. Inspection of the data on the label of analyzed brands of concentrated HCl will reveal the specific gravity, per cent (w./w.), grams (gm.) of reagent per ml., and molecular weight (m.w.).

With this information, the normality of the acid may be calculated:

$$\frac{\text{sp. gr.} \times \text{assay } (\% \text{ w./w.}) \times 10}{36.41 \text{ (equiv. wt. HCl)}}$$

Example:

$$\frac{1.19 \times 37 \times 10}{36.41} = 12.1 \text{ N}$$

To prepare 1 liter of 0.1 N HCl (N_2) from 12.1 N concentrated HCl (N_1), calculate the amount (ml.) of concentrated HCl (V_1) to dilute with water (V_2).

$$N_1 V_1 = N_2 V_2$$
$$12.1 \times V_1 = 0.1 \times 1000$$
$$V_1 = 8.26$$

Into a 1-liter volumetric flask filled to about half or two-thirds capacity with distilled water, add 8.26 ml. of concentrated HCl, and dilute to the mark with distilled water to make an approximate 0.1 N HCl solution.

If such a dilute HCl solution is to be standardized and adjusted to an exact 0.1 N, it is better to add a slight excess of concentrated HCl (about 2 per cent more than calculated) to avoid a weaker normality than desired.

Standardization of this approximate 0.1 N HCl is performed in a manner similar to that described for sodium hydroxide, using 10 ml. of HCl solution prepared rather than standard acid and titrating with standardized sodium hydroxide.

The preparation of other acid solutions, such as H_2SO_4 and HNO_3, may be carried out in manner similar to that described for HCl.

Oxidation-Reduction. Although these titrations are used infrequently in medical chemical determinations, their potential application should not be overlooked. While an indicator may be required, the color change of one of the compounds often reveals the endpoint. The Clark-Collip (1925) modification of the Kramer-Tisdall method for measurement of calcium represents a redox titration:

$$2\,MnO_4^- + 5\,C_2O_4^{--} + 16\,H^+ \longrightarrow 2\,Mn^{++} + 10\,CO_2 + 8\,H_2O$$

Calcium is precipitated as the oxalate salt, which is washed free of excess oxalate and then titrated in acid against $KMnO_4$. The dissolved oxalate precipitate is titrated in acid against permanganate. The manganese is reduced from a valence of +7 to +2, and carbon is oxidized from +3 to +4. When an excess of permanganate has been added, the purple color of permanganate shows as the endpoint.

Precipitation. Such titrations are used in the measurement of chloride with either mercuric nitrate or silver nitrate. In the mercurimetric procedure of Schales and Schales (1941), chloride combines with mercuric ions:

$$2\ Cl^- + Hg^{++} \longrightarrow HgCl_2$$

Although no precipitate is formed, the $HgCl_2$ is virtually un-ionized, so that the endpoint is identified by appearance of free Hg^{++} ions in solution when an indicator such as diphenylcarbazone is present. This indicator changes from colorless to light yellow to blue when combined with Hg^{++}, and the pH at the endpoint is between 4.5 and 6.0 (Asper, Schales, and Schales, 1947).

Coulometric Techniques. While coulometry involves the measurement of the quantity of electricity (in coulombs) at a fixed potential ($Q = I \times T$), potentiometric or electrometric techniques include the measurement of the potential (E) or electromotive force (EMF) between two electrodes in solution to quantitate the concentration of a particular substance. Potentiometric or electrometric titration of chloride was introduced and subsequently reviewed by Cotlove (1961); the instrumental system of analysis is referred to as chloridimeter or automatic chloride titrator. When the current is kept constant, the elapsed time is proportional to the total coulombs consumed. A coulomb is equal to a current flow of 1 amp sec. while a Faraday is defined as 96,500 coulombs and corresponds to the electrical charge carried by one gram equivalent of a substance; one equivalent is equal to 1 mole if only one electron is involved in the electrochemical reaction. Hence, the number of coulombs consumed can be related to the concentration of the unknown.

Solid silver, when placed into an acid solution, dissolves and generates silver ions until equilibrium is attained between silver in solid form and silver ion in solution (Ag^0/Ag^+). This generator, or coulometric system, will give rise to an electric current when connected with a second such system; the voltage produced when this half cell is part of an electrical system depends only on the silver ion concentration in solution. When chloride is also present in this solution, $Ag^+ + Cl^- \longrightarrow AgCl$, the equilibrium is forced to the right by insoluble silver chloride, and voltage is increased until all the chloride is combined (AgCl), with restoration of equilibrium and voltage drop. The time required for this to take place is monitored by an indicator (amperemetric) circuit which triggers a relay circuit to interrupt the titration and stop a timer with the appearance of free ions at the endpoint. This time is proportional to chloride concentration in an acidic solution. With reaction time values for reagent blank, chloride standard, and the unknown, appropriate calculations are made for the determination of chloride concentration in unknown biologic specimens. A direct readout device that eliminates calculations with such instruments has also been developed. This potentiometric chloride method has greater sensitivity than titration or spectrophotometric methods and is virtually automatic, with ease of operation.

Complexometric Techniques. A direct determination of calcium utilizes the formation of a chelate complex between calcium and ethylenediaminetetraacetic acid (EDTA). With certain indicators, a metal ion complexed or bound by a chelating agent no longer gives a color produced in the dissociated state (R. J. Henry, 1964). Titration of clear serum with a solution of EDTA under specified conditions and in the presence of an indicator such as ammonium purpurate (murexide) reveals a purple color until all free Ca^{++} is complexed or chelated with EDTA, at which point a pink color appears (absence of Ca^{++}). In an analogous manner, a fluorescent complexon (calcein) has an endpoint with fluorescence or a change of color. Like other visual titrimetric procedures, the endpoint may be obscured in the presence of bilirubin and hemoglobin; metals such as iron, zinc, magnesium, and copper may also interfere unless appropriate analytical conditions are attained.

CHROMATOGRAPHY

Chromatographic procedures based on one or more of the four physicochemical principles of adsorption, partition, ion exchange, and exclusion (molecular sieving) are observed in techniques such as column, paper, thin-layer, and gas chromatography (Cawley, 1965). Chromatography is used to separate or purify small amounts of closely related compounds from one another in a mixture. A mixture of two phases—mobile and stationary—comprise a chromatographic system. In the stationary phase a liquid or solid is fixed or motionless during the process of chromatography. In the mobile phase, a liquid or a gas moves through the system; ascending chromatography means the movement is upward, and descending chromatography refers to movement downward. The four possible chromatographic systems involving mobile and stationary phases are liquid-liquid, gas-liquid, liquid-solid, and gas-solid. Chromatography, then, represents a dynamic system of mobile and stationary phases that blend as an interphasing operation which is changing continuously (Cawley, 1965).

When the physicochemical principle of partitioning is involved, it is referred to as partition chromatography; this consists of liquid-liquid or gas-liquid phases. Partition liquid-liquid chromatography for the separation of most polar materials may be performed in column chromatography, paper chromatography, and thin-layer chromatography. A partition coefficient is the physical constant that characterizes the distribution of partitioning components (solute concentration relationship) between two immiscible phases. Usually the support medium (inert material) is impregnated or coated with a component of the stationary phase, while the mixture of solute materials or compounds to be separated is carried into the area by an appropriate liquid solvent in the mobile phase. Each compound is partitioned between the mobile phase and the stationary phase at a different site. Separation of a mixture of compounds according to the partition coefficient of each is based on their individual distribution between the mobile and stationary phases. The term *packing* refers to placing the inert support material in either liquid-column chromatography or gas chromatography. As the name implies, gas is the mobile phase in gas chromatography and liquid represents the stationary phase; hence, the term gas-liquid chromatography (GLC). The surface area in GLC is immense because small inert particles (packing) are coated with a liquid phase, and the efficiency of partitioning is enhanced. Paper chromatography is also an example of partitioning in most applications where water combines with cellulose fibers to form a stationary phase.

The physicochemical principle of adsorption in chromatography refers to the differential adsorption or adherence of materials at different locations, permitting separation on the solid stationary phase. This comes about because by gradually changing the environment (mobile phase) the compound under study is removed from the stationary solid phase; it then travels with the mobile phase to a specific point, at which it is redeposited according to its electrical charge and molecular size and shape. Adsorption chromatography (liquid-solid or gas-solid phases) is associated with techniques of column chromatography, gas chromatography, and thin-layer chromatography and may also play a role in paper chromatography.

Many separations are based on a combination of both adsorption and partition chromatography.

Column Chromatography. In column chromatography, the packing may be in the form of a finely divided solid. This may act as an adsorbent, or as an inert support material to be coated with a stationary liquid for partition chromatography. Columns are usually made of glass tubing drawn out at one end and usually fitted with stopcocks, glass plates, or other devices to make them more convenient to use (Fig. 9–22). The sample is introduced onto the column and an appropriate solvent system is allowed to wash through the column. The material that comes through the column is solvent or solvent containing separated compounds and is called eluent. Fractions of the eluent may be collected in separate tubes for analysis of a separated mixture of compounds. Automatic fraction collectors, employing volumetric or drop-counting devices or a timed flow method, will present a series of tubes to the effluent of the column to collect material for subsequent analysis. Under identical conditions, the same compounds will always take the same amount of time to elute from a particular column. This "elution time" can be used as a method of identification. Therefore, chromatography is not only ideal from an analytical standpoint in accomplishing *separation* of a mixture of compounds, but also provides tentative *identification* of individual compounds.

Paper Chromatography. Paper chromatography is a combination of both adsorption and

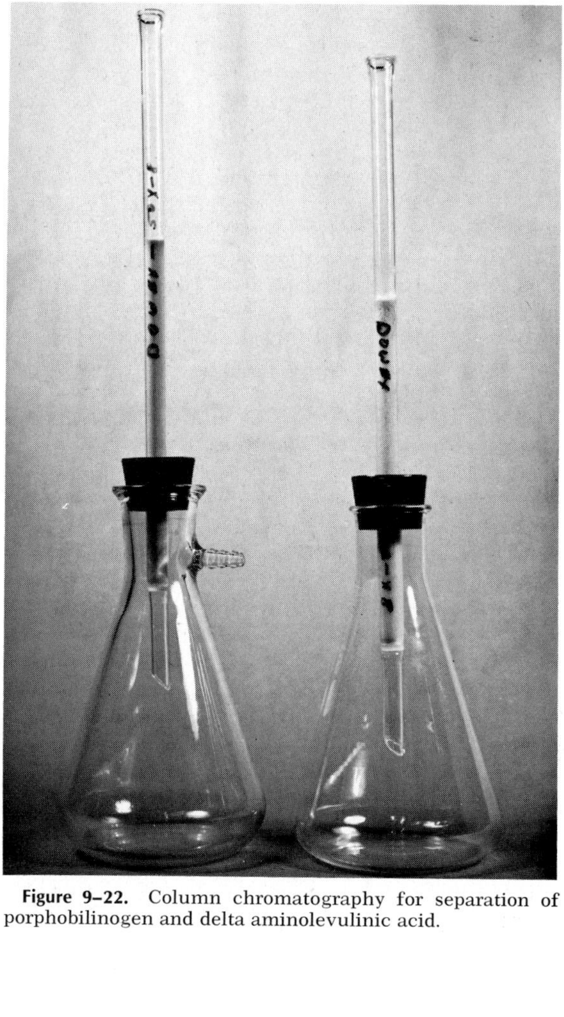

Figure 9–22. Column chromatography for separation of porphobilinogen and delta aminolevulinic acid.

partition chromatography, since the medium is a cellulose matrix containing entrapped water. The sample is applied in the form of a liquid spot or streak a few centimeters from one edge of the filter paper and allowed to dry. The solvent system is then allowed to flow over it from a solvent reservoir above the sample in descending chromatography or below the sample in ascending chromatography. The mobile liquid phase of solvent moves by capillary action over the sample (mixture of compounds), causing separation of the sample into individual spots (separated compounds) on the filter paper. The unit of measurement for this type of chromatography is Rf. Rf is a fraction which equals the distance a sample component travels in centimeters divided by the distance the solvent front has traveled. Under "identical conditions," the Rf of a particular compound is constant. Due to the number of variables, it is difficult to reproduce identical conditions or exact Rf values in paper chromatography, so an internal standard is incorporated as a reference point. Rg is then used as the unit of measurement and refers to the distance the component has traveled divided by the distance the standard (if the standard is glucose) has traveled. Two-dimensional chromatography is an example of more elaborate paper chromatography. After the initial regular run, with sample applied as a spot in the corner of the paper and separation made with suitable solvent or solvent system, the paper is dried and rotated 90 degrees, and another separation is made in a second perpendicular direction with the same or, usually, a different solvent. To visualize the separated compounds, it is often necessary to spray the paper with an appropriate stain. In addition to separation, tentative identification may be achieved, partly by specific chemical reaction between spray and spot. Quantification may be accomplished by densitometry or by elution followed by chemical methods.

Thin-layer Chromatography (TLC). This is similar in application to paper chromatography but usually employs the chromatographic principle of adsorption (liquid-solid) for separation of most nonpolar materials rather than partition (liquid-liquid chromatography) that separates most polar materials. It is more versatile, faster, and more sensitive for many substances than paper. TLC permits a choice of adsorbents from a maximum of adsorption to a minimum with increasing partition qualities. Alumina gel (aluminum oxide, Al_2O_3) reflects maximum adsorption, although silica gel (silica dioxide, SiO_2), when activated (dried by heat at 110° C.), approaches this state; it may reflect more partition qualities when dried in room air (variable humidity). Diatomaceous earth (Celite or kieselguhr) like cellulose favors partition (Stahl, 1969). Silica gel is acidic as well as active and useful to separate virtually all classes. Alumina is basic, with active properties, and is useful for separation of mainly bases and steroids (Stahl, 1969). Celite is neutral and inactive; it is used to separate sugars and pharmaceuticals (Stahl, 1969). Glass plates are thinly coated (wet film thickness of 0.25 mm. is common) with a slurry of one of the above materials, dried, and stored. With a capillary pipette, the prepared sample, usually in an organic solvent, is applied quantitatively to the dry or activated plate (Fig. 9–23). The actual run or development takes place in a closed environment (e.g., glass tank or chamber) to prevent evaporation. The bottom of the plate adjacent to but not on the application site is placed in the solvent system, which moves gradually up the thin layer (Fig. 9–24). Two-dimensional techniques (90-

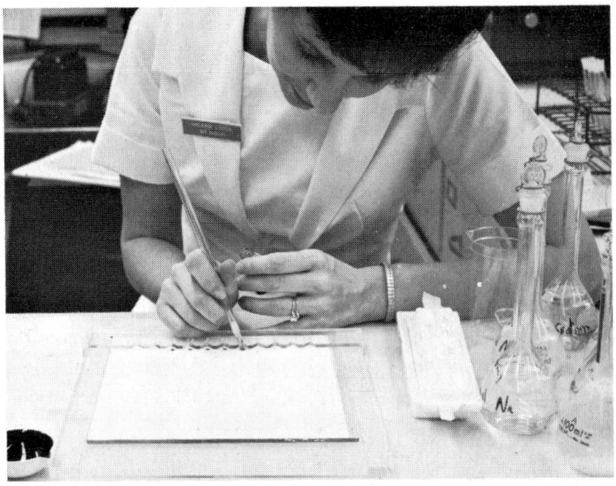

Figure 9–23. Thin-layer chromatography—application of sample.

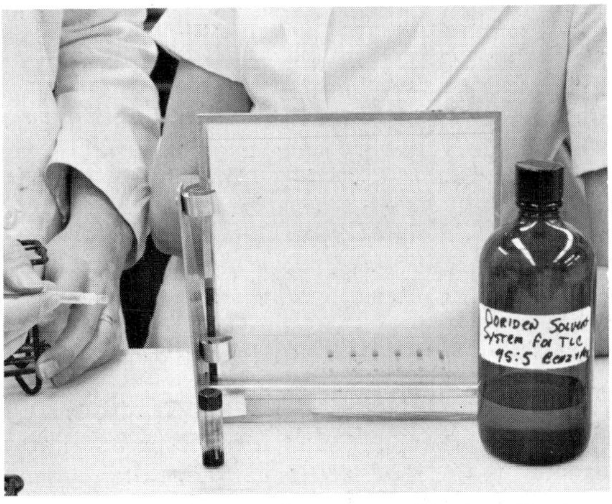

Figure 9–24. Thin-layer chromatographic plate after separation of specimen for glutethimide (Doriden) identification; note the solvent front that precedes the spots.

degree rotation of plate) with different solvents as well as thin-layer electrophoresis (TLE) have also been developed. Visualization of the resolved constituents is performed by spraying the plate with corrosives (e.g., H_2SO_4 when TLC adsorbent is inorganic) or suitable color-detecting systems. When the plate is exposed to short-wave (254 nm.) ultraviolet (U.V.) light, indicators in the adsorbent may be used to show chromatospots as nonfluorescing black spots; long-wave (350 to 366 nm.) ultraviolet light can be used to excite fluorescence in materials which absorb long ultraviolet and emit visible light, i.e., bright spots of fluorescence on a dark background (no fluorescent indicator in plate). $ZnSiO_4$ with $CdSO_4$ is a U.V. indicator that does not affect TLC when incorporated in the adsorbent. Identification by comparison with known standards is superior to Rf values that are less reproducible. When standards of different concentration are included, semiquantitative results are obtained. Scanning the plate directly or scanning the negative of a plate photograph has also been used; however, chemical analyses of the scraped off spot(s) are the most accurate means of quantitation. In regard to solvent systems, dilution is made according to the need for resolution of constituents by trial and error, by reference to elutropic solvent series, and by simple admixtures of two (polar *vs.* nonpolar) solvents (Janchen, 1967).

Instant Thin-layer Chromatography (ITLC). ITLC, although similar, differs from TLC. It is even more rapid, i.e., often less than 30 minutes instead of an hour or longer. Rather than a thin layer of chromatographic substances on a glass plate, a slurry of glass fiber microfilaments is combined with chromatographic substances to make a material which feels and handles like paper (Gelman Instruction Manual). Chromatographic materials entrapped in the glass microfibrils locked to each other include silica gel, potassium silicate, and alumina gel. Heat activation is required for some separations. Otherwise, sample application, development, and visualization are rather similar to TLC, although smaller tanks and even test tubes may be used when small strips of ITLC are used. ITLC capacity is about one-tenth of a TLC plate, since glass fibers affect adsorption. The sensitivity of ITLC is also about one-tenth that of TLC. ITLC uses different solvent systems than TLC because their partition coefficients differ; i.e., glass fibers serve as adsorbent (Hamilton, 1967). The clinical applications of ITLC and TLC are similar, i.e., steroids, including aldosterone, lipids, barbiturates, and alkaloids, as well as a variety of drugs, including phenothiazine derivatives, may be separated and identified. In toxicology, where the greatest potential use exists, TLC and ITLC are sensitive for screening purposes to achieve identification of drug(s) ingested and semiquantification of some compounds.

Gas Chromatography. Gas chromatography is similar to partition column chromatography but utilizes an inert carrier gas to replace a mobile liquid phase (Dal Nogare and Juvet, 1962). Nitrogen and helium are commonly used to carry a vaporized sample over a sorbent in and through a column. Gas chromatography (GC) reflects adsorbent and partition chromatographic principles in the two forms of gas-solid chromatography (GSC) and gas-liquid chromatography (GLC), respectively. In both categories the mobile phase or carrier gas is an inert gas which is made to flow at a constant rate through a packed column (a small diameter tube containing the sorbent). The sorbent is a solid of large surface area in GSC, but in GLC, the sorbent is a nonvolatile liquid coated on an inert solid support. Instrumental systems for GC, referred to as gas chromatographs, in general reveal similar features in regard to apparatus, gas sampling, detectors, etc., whether for GSC or GLC. Gas solid chromatography (GSC) is used primarily for gases (e.g., O_2, CO_2, N_2) or relatively nonpolar solutes of high volatility. Gas liquid chromatography (GLC) has broad applications not only to a wider range of solutes but also to both packed and capillary columns. A gas chromatograph, usually in modular form, reveals an injector device, column, and detector-recorder and has controls for temperature, gas flow rates, and electronic parts. In GLC a mixture in solution to be separated into its constituents is injected into one end of a long, heated column through which passes the carrier gas. At the inlet port (injector device) a small heater vaporizes the molecules, which are then carried by the gas down the length of the column for separation. The columns, often several feet in length and one-quarter inch or less in internal diameter, are packed with solid sorbent, a support such as microglass beads, or crushed firebrick. A variety of high boiling liquids are used to coat these inert particles. The particles coated with silicones or polyoxyethylene derivatives adsorb and then release passing molecules to a degree depending on the structural and charge characteristics of each particular compound. The net result is the separation of the molecules, which emerge individually from the far end of the column. In view of the tremendous surface area in GLC (small, inert particles coated with a liquid phase) the efficiency of partitioning (separation) is increased greatly. One of a number of detectors measures the presence and quantity of eluting substance(s). Electronic components maintain ideal conditions to detect the sample constituents as they elute from the column. The amplified detector signals drive a strip chart recorder which then shows a record of peaks of the signals; the location (elution time) of each peak characterizes a specified component (like Rf) and peak height and/or area is directly related to its relative concentration. In general, sample preparation prior to GLC analysis is extensive to attain purification and proper form. Sample aliquot for GLC rarely exceeds 5 to 10 μl. of specimen solution, of which solute components comprise only a small percentage; this emphasizes the tremendous sensitivity of GLC, as less than 1 μg. of substance on the column usually provides an adequate signal response.

Column temperatures range widely from ambient, but practical ranges usually do not exceed 300° C. Earlier systems employed a fixed temperature column for a specific analysis but these have been virtually replaced by temperature programming that provides predetermined and regulated degrees of gradual column heating; this permits analysis of complex solute mixtures wherein the slow, high boiling constituents can be eluted at high temperatures and at the same time allow separation of the low boiling, more rapidly eluting constituents. That detector most suitable for the type of compounds being separated is selected. Thermal conductivity detectors measure heat conduction of the effluxing gas and compare it with that of the pure carrier (greater the difference, greater the signal). These are used for the analysis of gases and low-boiling liquids. Ionization detectors are more sensitive. In these detectors the components leaving the column are ionized by either β-rays from a radioactive source or oxidation in a hydrogen flame. For materials of clinical significance, this detector is most often employed. Electron capture detectors depend on the electron affinity of specific atoms and molecular groups.

Virtually any substance that boils without decomposition or that can yield a volatile, stable derivative can be subjected to gas chromatographic analysis. Steroids, alcohols (methanol, ethanol, isopropanol), and drugs (barbiturates, anticonvulsants) can be separated readily and represent current practical applications of GLC in medical chemistry and toxicology (Creech, 1964). Clinical applications have yet to achieve the full potential of gas chromatography, the most sensitive of the chromatographic methods.

Ion Exchange Chromatography. Ion exchange chromatography utilizes resins to which are coupled either anions or cations which will exchange with other anions or cations in the material that is passed through their meshwork. These resins are highly insoluble synthetic polymers containing functional groups which are either basic ($-NH_2$, $-^{+}N(CH_3)_3$) or acidic ($-COOH$, $-SO_3H$). Deionization of water is a familiar application of ion exchange resins. Basically, two main types of resins are used: anionic, or diethylaminoethyl (DEAE), and cationic, or carboxymethyl (CM), cellulose resins. Dowex 50 and Amberlite IR 100 are cation exchange resins, since they have exchangeable basic groups. Separation may be facilitated by changing the pH or ionic strength or both of the buffer as well as temperature during the course of column chromatographic separation by gradient elution (changing slowly and continuously) or step-by-step elution (one elution system at a time). In essence, resins may be considered polyfunctional acids or bases that are insoluble. When a solution containing an amine salt is placed on a column pack with a cation exchange resin in acid form, the resin will take up the amine cation from the solution and generate a hydrogen cation. Subsequently the amine may be displaced by washing the column with a more acid solution. If a mixture of bases was applied initially, it would be possible to release them individually by the use of buffers of varying acidity and electrolyte content. A cation exchange resin in the sodium form will adsorb such ions as calcium and manganese in solution, with the release of sodium ions. Anion exchange resins saturated with chloride ions will replace weak organic acids in solution with chloride ion. Subsequently, the organic acids may be removed sequentially by appropriate application of selective solvents. A column of Amberlite MB-3 through which distilled water is passed yields a high standard of deionized water. Deionized water prepared in this manner and stored in polyethylene bottles with plastic aspirators is indispensable as "pure water" for the preparation of all aqueous solutions and as a diluent in virtually all methods (Nelson, 1961).

Exclusion Chromatography. Separation by the molecular sieve principle is based on molecular size. It is the size of the molecules that determines whether or not the molecular sieve principle will work and gel filtration can be applied. Sephadex (trademark of Pharmacia Laboratories Inc.) is the most frequently used component for this type of separation, which is quite commonly carried out on a column also. Sephadex, a modified dextran, is composed of dextran macromolecules cross-linked to give three-dimensional networks of polysaccharide chains that are formed into small microscopic beads. Sephadex is strongly hydrophilic, so the beads swell in water and electrolyte solutions. The types available differ in their swelling properties and one series (LH) is also lipophilic, and swells in organic solvents as well as in water. The degree of swelling characterizes the gel. Inside these small beads are openings that are adjusted so that a molecule is either excluded or permitted to enter the gel, depending upon the size of the molecule. Large molecules that are excluded pass readily through the column bed in the liquid phase outside the particle without restriction and are eluted first. Substances of small molecular weight penetrate the structure of the gel particles, depending on their size and shape. The term molecular sieve is somewhat misleading, since small particles are retained and large particles pass through. Molecules are eluted from a Sephadex bed in order of decreasing molecular size. The determination of molecular weight, e.g., of enzymes, and estimation of equilibrium constants can be achieved with relative ease by exclusion chromatography. Isolation and fractionation of serum, plasma, and cerebrospinal fluid proteins on the basis of molecular weight and size represent practical applications that have not been exploited fully in medical chemistry. Urine as well as other body fluids may be subjected to gel filtration to eliminate components which are adverse to a particular chemical reaction.

Affinity Chromatography. This involves procedures used to purify one of the components of a system consisting of two or more species whose reversible interactions reflect affinity with a high degree of biologic specificity (Cuatrecasas and Anfinsen, 1971). Originally it was used to describe simplest cases of such interacting substances, e.g., enzymes and competitive inhibitors. Purification of enzymes employing the principles of enzyme-substrate interactions has been used. The basic principle consists of immobilization of one of the components of the interacting system (e.g., the ligand) to an insoluble porous support which can then be used to selectively adsorb, in a chromatographic procedure, that component (e.g., enzyme) of the bathing medium with which it can selectively interact. Elution can then be achieved by any one of a number of procedures which result in dissociation of the complex. It appears that specific biologic properties of macromolecules may be exploited for purifications as much in the future as the physicochemical properties have been exploited in the past (Cuatrecasas and Anfinsen, 1971). It may be used to isolate specific substances, specific antibodies, enzymes, hormones, inhibitors, carrier proteins, and so forth, on the basis of their biospecific interactions with immobilized proteins.

ELECTROPHORESIS

The movement of colloidal particles in an electric field is called electrophoresis. In addition to the intensity of the electrical field, other factors that are very important include particle size and shape and electrical charge. Serum proteins are most commonly subjected to electrophoresis for identification and quantitation. In an electrical field, different proteins show different migration rates because they are different in electrical charge, size, and shape. The pH of the solution (usually a buffer) in which the protein comes in contact also plays a critical role in regard to the type (positive or negative) as well as number of charges on each colloidal protein particle.

When the electrical field is applied directly to a solution, it is called free electrophoresis. The moving boundary method of free electrophoresis is complex and requires expensive equipment for analyses; an optical system determining refractive indices monitors the proteins during the course of migration.

In zone electrophoresis, the charged particles are placed on a stabilizing medium which will contain the proteins after migration so they may be stained and examined sometime after the electrophoretic phase. Stabilizing media to trap the migrating proteins include filter paper, cellulose acetate, agar-gel, and agarose. Theoretically the support medium is inert and, like the liquid medium used in boundary electrophoresis, does not interact with protein. Hence, movement through the medium is related almost exclusively to electrophoretic mobility of the protein. However, with paper, some binding between cellulose fibers and protein occurs. Each of the different types of media has unique features which have led to their specific application. The time required for separation and the degree of resolution are the two major conditions for selection of one type of media or another. Hence, cellulose acetate has virtually replaced paper because it yields more rapid and distinct separation. Since it can be cleared, it has advantages in terms of optical superiority for visualization. Agar gel is also more rapid and complete than paper; it also produces an optically clear medium.

Two other media, starch gel and polyacrylamide gel, also exhibit a molecular sieve principle which in combination with electrophoretic mobility yields better separation of proteins. Instead of the usual five serum protein bands, as many as 25 bands can be identified using these more sensitive methods which separate protein molecules on the basis of molecular size and electrophoretic mobility (Cawley, 1969). In addition, the proteins may have a different position after electrophoresis with different media. In general, the procedure consists of immersing the media, such as cellulose acetate, with appropriate buffer solution (Kaplan and Savory, 1970). Although buffer pH 8.6 might be selected, buffers of other pH will yield a different electrophoretic migration of protein molecules. With a sample applicator very small aliquots (less than 10 μl.) are placed on the strip, and the ends of the strip are dipped

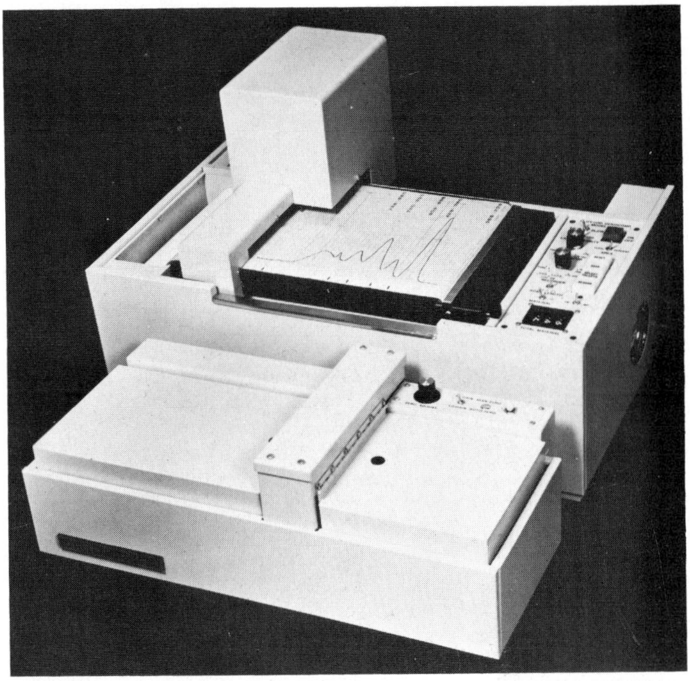

Figure 9–25. Electrophoresis Densitometer, Model 345. (Clifford Instruments, Inc.)

in buffer solution into which electrodes are placed. The chamber is sealed to prevent evaporation and appropriate voltage and current applied for a specific interval of time (approximately 30 minutes with cellulose acetate). Subsequently the strip is removed, fixed, stained, cleared, and dried. Quantification may be attained by measuring the intensity of the color of the several fractions. This can be accomplished by cutting out individual spots and eluting the protein into a solution for subsequent chemical measurement. More commonly the cellulose acetate paper strip is passed through a densitometer, and a record of the relative color intensities is recorded. This is usually performed by an electrical integrator which traces a curve that gives a quantitative measure of the individual component or protein fraction as well as a curve that is subject to clinical interpretation (Fig. 9–25).

A combination of electrophoresis and immunodiffusion is called immunoelectrophoresis (Cawley, 1969). In the first stage, antigen is subjected to electrophoresis in a medium of agar-gel or agarose (cellulose acetate may also be used). Subsequently, appropriate troughs are made in the agar along lines parallel to the axis of the original electrophoresis and antisera inserted. Over a period of time, diffusion of the antisera proceeds in a direction perpendicular to the trough into the zone of electrophoresis to react with the corresponding antigen. When an appropriate concentration of antibody and antigen is achieved, a precipitant arc appears as a wide band with clear transparent agar-gel or agarose in the background (Fig. 9–26). If polyvalent antisera and fresh serum for antigen are used, as many as 20 precipitin bands may be seen. Additional procedures may be performed to further characterize the bands.

Widespread application of electrophoresis has extended well beyond proteins of serum

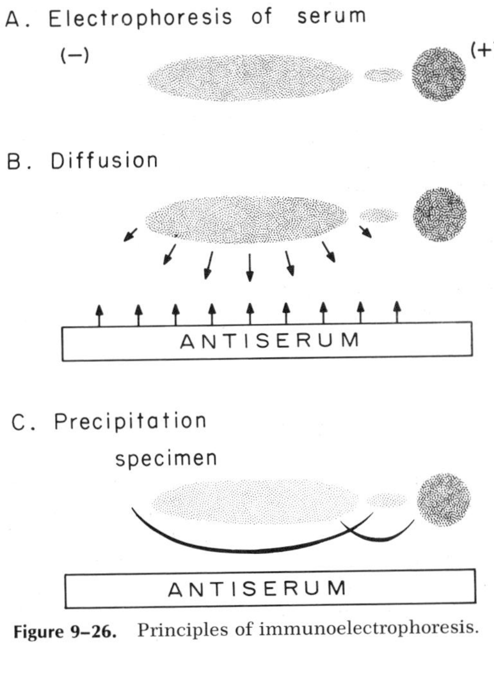

Figure 9–26. Principles of immunoelectrophoresis.

and hemoglobin to transferrins, haptoglobins, isoenzymes, and abnormal protein identification. The scope and application of these techniques will be discussed with individual procedures.

MICRO- AND ULTRAMICROANALYSIS

Ultramicromethods and techniques for the medical chemistry laboratory have been described by several authors (Sanz, 1957; O'Brien *et al.*, 1968). These procedures have not been widely adopted, despite the availability of complete analytical systems from commercial sources. Clayton and Jenkins (1966), among others, attribute this failure to inefficient ultramicro pipettes. Special training of technical personnel with emphasis on meticulous attention to detail as well as special equipment are required in addition to reliable, efficient microliter pipettes. In terms of specimen sample volume, methods may be classified as follows: macromethods, volumes of 1.0 ml. or more; micromethods, 0.1 to 0.9 ml.; ultramicro- or microliter methods, volumes of 0.09 to 0.01 ml. (90 to 10 μl.); and nanoliter methods, volumes of 0.009 to 0.001 ml. (9 to 1 μl.), or even less, i.e., 1 to 999 nl. pipettes and apparatus for nanoliter methods are under development and advocated by Sanz (1966). Ultramicro- or microliter methods, including pipettes and diluters, prevail.

Microliter pipettes may be divided into straight, constriction, and overflow types (Knights, MacDonald, and Ploompuu, 1962).

Today there are many types of microliter pipettes available commercially. It is important to appreciate the difference between "washout" and "blowout" pipettes. A "washout" type is also designated "t.c." (to contain). Since it is standardized on the volume contained, after delivery of the contents it must be washed out with the diluting solution. In contrast, a "blowout" or "t.d." (to deliver) pipette is calibrated to deliver the nominal volume into the diluting solution and is not washed out after delivery. For the most exact work, washout pipettes give better results. However, for work in which reproducibility is more important than absolute volume, and particularly in analyses wherein the sample of specimen and standard can be pipetted with the same pipette, the blowout type is easier to manipulate.

Slow aspiration automatically adjusts the volume at the point of narrowing of the capillary stem in a constriction pipette. Indeed, it is less difficult to draw up the desired volume to a constriction than to a calibration mark, since surface tension prevents drawing up the solution past the constriction.

Overflow pipettes are characterized by the fact that the volume is automatically adjusted, since any excess fluid overflows the top. They give extremely reproducible results but may be less exact for absolute measurements. Hence, it is preferable to use them only when the analytical sample of specimen and the standard can be measured with the same pipette. Since they are exclusively of the "blowout" type, they can be manipulated more quickly than the constriction type.

Although important in all absolute measurements, the error of the pipette is of no significance in methods in which the standard and the analytical sample of specimen are measured with the same pipette. Pipettes with a volume exceeding 20 microliters can be calibrated either gravimetrically or colorimetrically, but for volumes less than 20 microliters, the colorimetric calibration is more reliable. For details of pipette calibration, the reader is referred to the translation of Professor Richterich's Clinical Chemistry (1969), p. 105.

Caraway (1960) prefers the Lang-Levy self-adjusting constriction pipettes, with a curved tip calibrated to deliver (t.d.); they are also calibrated and available as to contain (t.c.) pipettes. Care and use of these pipettes and others are described by the authors mentioned as well as Natelson (1971), Mattenheimer (1970), and O'Brien *et al.* (1968). Indeed their textbooks should be consulted for additional information pertaining to techniques, methods, and apparatus used in micro- and ultramicroanalysis. Micro- or ultramicromethods are also presented with individual procedures described in this and other chapters. Methods in which 50 to 100 μl. are used, especially with automation, as proposed by the group at the University of Kentucky (Mabry *et al.*, 1968), are gaining popularity, since they are precise, practical, and efficient in meeting pediatric and adult clinical requirements.

AUTOMATION AND SEMIAUTOMATION

Reliability and precision of chemical measurements have been enhanced and accuracy sustained or improved by the utilization of instrumental systems or devices for manual methods that permit varying degrees of mechanical analyses or automation. Efficiency in terms of performance as well as capability to respond to peak demands and to increased workloads may be attained by incorporation of mechanized apparatus, or automation in the chemical laboratory (Westlake and Bennington, 1972).

Semiautomation of manual procedures can be achieved by the use of automatic diluent and/or reagent delivery or specimen sample measuring and delivery (with or without dilu-

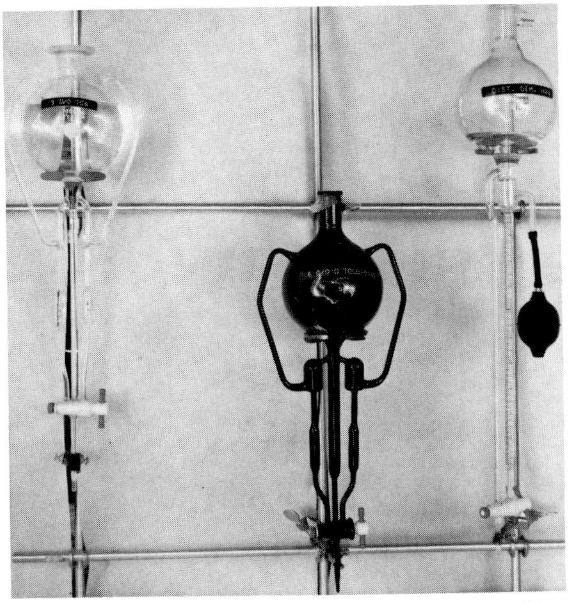

Figure 9–27. Delivery of diluent or reagent with Machlett automatic pipette (Scientific Products, 1210 Leon Place, Evanston, Illinois 60201).

ent) devices (Figs. 9–27, 9–28, and 9–29). Automatic pipettes, burettes, and titrators are examples. The Seligson pipette (A. H. Thomas, Philadelphia, Pennsylvania) can be applied to several methods with variable sample volumes ranging from microliters to milliliters (Fig. 9–29). A specimen sample may be washed with appropriate diluent or reagent into a volumetric flask or to the mark of a calibrated test tube. A variety of automatic specimen sample diluters are available that permit delivery of specimen volume followed by reagent or diluent (Fig. 9–30 and Table 9–6).

Automatic pipetting devices permit measuring out a whole series of equal volumes. Indeed, automatic pipetting and diluting apparatuses have evolved for ensuring the more efficient delivery of equal volumes of specimens followed by equivalent volumes of diluent. Such apparatus can be operated either manually or by a motor. Indeed, a manipulation that requires a certain volume, say of plasma, to be diluted with a known volume of reagent is a laborious manual procedure that requires two pipettings but can be greatly accelerated with the aid of dilution apparatus.

Commerical automatic pipettes are either of the sampling type (usually manually operated) or of the sampling-diluting type (usually electrically operated). Manually operated automatic pipettes are ordinarily of the air displacement variety. Since proper care and calibration are essential to precise, accurate sampling, it

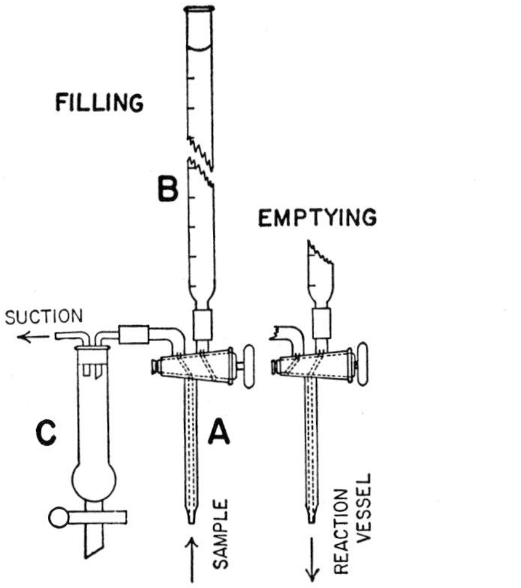

Figure 9–28. Significant features of the automatic pipette. A, pipette and three-way stopcock; B, calibrated tube; C, waste receiver. (From Seligson, D.: Amer. J. Clin. Path. 28:200, 1957.)

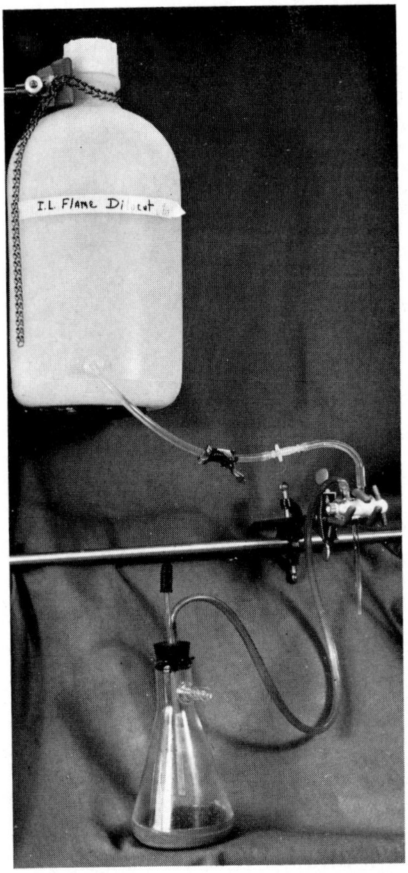

Figure 9–29. Sample measuring and diluent delivery with automatic pipette.

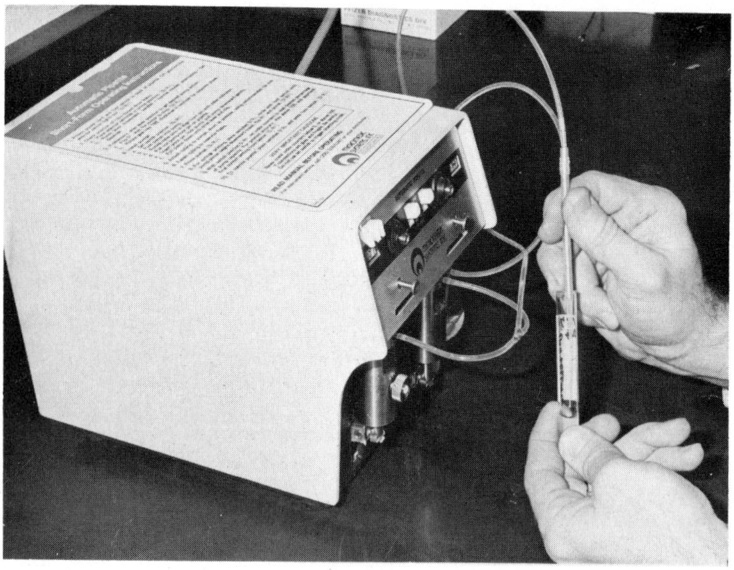

Figure 9–30. Micromedic Automatic Pipette. (See Table 9–6.)

Table 9–6. AUTOMATIC SAMPLER-DILUTERS

	PRINCIPLE OF SYSTEM	VOLUME RANGE*	
		SAMPLING	DILUTING
Brinkman Instruments, Inc. Cantiague Road Westbury, N.Y. 11590	Piston	0.1–5000 μl.	1–5000 μl.
Cordis Laboratories P.O. Box 684 Miami, Florida 33137	Piston	20–100 μl.	5–15 ml.
DADE Miami, Florida 33152	Piston	20–50 μl.	5–10 ml.
Fisher Scientific Co. 52 Fadem Road Springfield, N.J. 07081	Piston	10–1000 μl.	1–10 ml.
General Diagnostic Division Warner-Lambert Co. Morris Plains, N.J. 07950	Peristaltic	5 μl.–10 ml.	5 μl.–10 ml.
Hobbs Scientific, Inc. P.O. Box 600 S. Miami, Florida 33143	Piston	20–200 μl.	5–15 ml.
Micromedic Systems, Inc. Rohm and Haas Building 6th and Market Streets Philadelphia, Pa. 19105	Piston	2–1000 μl.	2–5000 μl.
Oxford Laboratories 1149 Chess Drive Foster City, Calif. 94404	Piston	10–100 μl.	0.5–20 ml.
Arthur H. Thomas Co. Vine Street at Third Philadelphia, Pa. 19105	Thomas-Seligson Pipette Vacuum Sampling-Gravity Dilution	0.02–1.0 ml.	Unspecified
York Instrument Corp. 150 Fifth Avenue New York, New York 10011	Piston	0–1 ml. (microliter ranges available)	0–25 ml.

*More than one model may be required to accomplish range indicated.

is important to read and follow the manufacturer's instructions. Two common errors are to allow a sample to aspirate into the barrel of the pipette, and to ignore lubrication of the piston. The sampling-dispensing automatic pipettes fall into three general classes: (1) the peristaltic type, (2) the piston type, and (3) the Seligson type, which uses a vacuum to aspirate, gravity to dispense, and a manually operated stopcock to separate the two phases of the cycle. Again, it is very important to follow the manufacturer's instructions in the operation and maintenance of these machines. Table 9–7 lists examples of automatic pipettes available commercially.

Automatic pipettes remove much of the tedium associated with repetitive sampling and dilution. Even for a limited number of samples, the speed of an automatic pipette is an advantage. Because operator fatigue is minimized, precision of multiple sampling and dilution is often improved with the automatic pipette. The micro-automatic pipettes, which can sample as little as 2 to 5 microliters, offer a unique advantage, especially for the expanding field of radioimmunoassays.

Manufacturers generally claim a pipetting and dilution accuracy in the range of 0.1 to 1.0 per cent. However, it is essential that automatic pipettes be calibrated when new and at regular intervals thereafter. Never assume that factory calibrations are accurate! One classic procedure for volume calibration is to weigh the volume of water that the pipette delivers, making an appropriate correction for the density of water at whatever its temperature. The same principle is applied to the calibration of an automatic pipette. For example, an automatic pipette of the sampling-diluting type was set to pick up 10 microliters and dispense

Table 9–7. AUTOMATIC MANUAL PIPETTES

	TRADEMARK	RANGE*
Brinkman Instruments, Inc. Cantiague Road Westbury, N.Y. 11590	Eppendorf	5–1000 μl.
Centaur Chemical Co. 4 West Kenosia Avenue Danbury, Conn. 06810	Centaur	5–1000 μl.
Clay-Adams 141 E. 25th Street New York, New York 10010	Aupette	10 μl–10 ml.
Dow Diagnostics 1200 Madison Avenue Indianapolis, Ind. 46225	MLA Precision Pipettes	10–1000 μl.
Labindustries 1802 Second Street Berkeley, Calif. 94710	Repipet	0.1 μl–50 ml.
Monostat 20 N. Moore Street New York, New York 10013	Vari-pet	10 μl.–30 ml.
Oxford Laboratories 1149 Chess Drive Foster City, Calif. 94404	Sampler	1–5000 μl.
Pfizer Diagnostics Division 300 W. 43rd Street New York, New York 10036	Micro Pipet	20–1000 μl.
Rainin Instrument Company 1030 Commonwealth Avenue Boston, Mass. 02215	Pipetman	0–1000 μl.
Schwarz/Mann Orangeburg, N.Y. 10962	Biopette	0.025–1.0 ml.

*More than one model may be required to accomplish range indicated.

a total of 1.00 ml. On the first cycle air was drawn into the tip without sample and water was dispensed into a glass-stoppered cuvette previously weighed on an analytical balance; 0.98582 gm. of water had been dispensed. On the second cycle water was sampled and dispensed with water; 0.99596 gm. of water had been dispensed. The difference of 0.01014 gm., divided by 0.9971 gm./ml. (density of water at 25° C.), equals 0.01017 ml. (10.17 μl.), which was the volume picked up by the automatic pipette. By the same logic, 0.9887 ml. of water was dispensed with the sample. Considering the accuracy of weighing to be ± 0.05 mg., the volume of sample picked up would be in the range of 10.04 to 10.24 μl. Precision of dilution can also be measured by spectrophotometric methods and by radioactive dilution.

In using an automatic pipette, the tip wiping technique is important in obtaining reproducibility. Aspirate the sample into the tip. Then wipe the tip with absorbent cloth or tissue with two downward strokes at 90 degrees with respect to one another. Each stroke should start above the level that the tip was immersed into the fluid sample and proceed downward past the tip. Do not actually touch the fluid in the tip as this will suck the fluid out of the tip.

With an automatic sampling-diluting pipette, the operator must always beware of possible carry-over. When a sample is introduced into the tip, diffusion of sample occurs. The washout by diluent may be insufficient to remove all the sample, and this then becomes mixed with the succeeding sample. The result is that any analyses performed on the first sample dilution are too low, and those done on the second are too high. In general, the ratio of diluent to sample must be at least 5:1 for quantitative washout. This must be increased if the sample is viscous or oily and the diluent is of an aqueous base. Also, certain components are adsorbed by the tip construction, and the washout must be increased. In general, a Teflon tip adsorbs less than a glass tip. Hormones, for example, have a higher affinity for glass.

Spectrophotometers with a direct readout displaying absorbance units or readings of concentration in any appropriate units and with a flow-through cuvette (100 μl. capacity) represent a second major application of automation to manual procedures (Fig. 9–31). The elimination of calculation errors and a net saving in time are realized, as is economy of glassware by elimination of cuvettes with use of such spectrophotometers. Each manual procedure should be scrutinized to identify potential application of one or both of these semiautomated improvements.

A variety of instruments have also been introduced that permit selective measurement of a single component with incorporation of automation from the time of sample introduction. These include the protein refractometer, for measurement of total protein concentration by refraction; the chloridimeter, for measuring serum chloride concentration; the hemoglobinometer, for measuring hemoglobin concentration of whole blood; apparatus for measuring directly pH, P_{CO_2}, and P_{O_2}; and flame photometers, for sodium and potassium. Microanalysis is also usually obtained with these selective instruments, since sample volumes require less than 0.1 ml. More sophisticated analytical systems achieving semiautomation have been developed by the combination of existing instruments. The Gilford Model 2000 unit (Gilford Instrument Laboratories, Inc., Oberlin, Ohio) incorporates a precision spectrophotometer with an automatic cuvette positioner and a recording unit. Rate reactions for many enzyme assays can be accomplished with this system, generating the

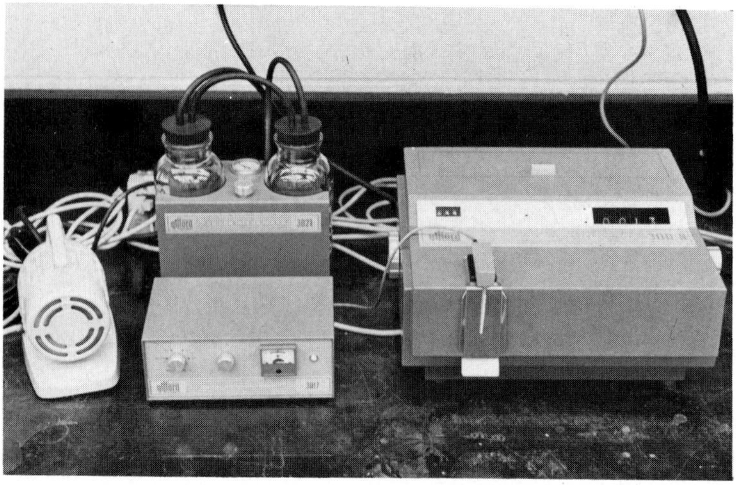

Figure 9–31. Gilford 300-N Spectrophotometer with Thermo-Cuvette.

most accurate measurements possible with greater efficiency and economy.

Full automation was introduced by Skeggs (1965) with the AutoAnalyzer (Technicon Instruments Corporation, Chauncey, New York) in 1957 (Vanderlinde, 1967). Over the past decade and a half it has been applied to a large number of different determinations singly and in combinations (multiple-channel techniques) to generate automatically and simultaneously as many as 12 different chemical measurements and in the near future 18 on one machine. The AutoAnalyzer reflects a continuous flow-through system rather than the discrete analyses usually performed in manual "wet" chemistry procedures. Flowing streams of reagents and samples are segmented by bubbles of air which assist in the washing process and prevent mixing of successive specimen samples. Running from one modular processing unit to another, the flowing streams are carried by tubing and glass coils for mixing. Dialysis replaces the protein-free filtrate preparation in many procedures. Continuous plotting of ratios, that is, the concentration ratio of the unknown against the known standard on a moving graph, displays measurement data. For this reason, it is not necessary to bring a reaction to completion.

The basic AutoAnalyzer consists of six modular units: (1) an automatic sampler for picking up specimens to be analyzed; (2) a proportioning pump, which maintains the flow of liquid in the system; (3) a dialyzer, which produces a dialysate for analysis; (4) a heating bath for color reaction development; (5) a spectrophotometer (colorimeter) with a flow-through cuvette; and (6) a recorder. A revolving tray displays different specimens or standards for sampling by aspiration at rates varying from 20 to 60 per hour to correspond with actual analytical values which appear after a suitable lag time interval for successive passage of specimen and reagents through the modules. Air bubbles maintain specimen sample integrity and provide good wash or cleansing of tubing. The internal diameter of tubing determines the flow volume of specimen sample and reagent.

Dialysis with temperature control permits diffusion of constituents across the membrane into a recipient stream where actual reagents may be combined with components for analyses. It is not essential that complete dialysis of individual components occur but rather that the rate of dialysis remain constant. Mixing is accomplished after the addition of reagents by movement of the stream through a tightly wound glass coil lying horizontally. The heating (temperature controlled) bath also contains a glass coil for circulating the flowing stream: it may be set at the temperature required or near boiling point at 95° C. When the color reaction has been completed, the air bubbles are removed from the stream so that a solid stream enters the spectrophotometer as a liquid segment into a continuous flow-through cell cuvette. The absorbance of the stream is continuously measured and the results recorded. Periodic replacement of dialyzer membrane and tubing is essential and represents a technical limitation of the AutoAnalyzer. An improved second generation AutoAnalyzer, the AAII (Technicon Instruments Corporation), is more compact and has corrected many of the technical limitations of the earlier system.

An endpoint device, such as a fluorometer, may be used in place of a colorimeter for measurement of calcium or magnesium. Furthermore, a flame photometer may be substituted for the determination of sodium and potassium; this in turn eliminates need for a heating bath and colorimeter. Other complex analytical processes have been adapted to continuous-flow operation and therefore are fully automated. Digestion as utilized in the protein-bound iodine is one example. Although Auto-Analyzers were originally a single-measurement system, dual-channel, quadruple channel, six-channel, and most recently 12- and 18-channel systems have been developed to produce more simultaneous automated analyses at a rate of 60 per hour. The admission chemical profile has gained wide application (Thiers *et al.*, 1966). Skeggs (1965) has reviewed the principles of automatic chemical analysis, and the interested reader should consult his comprehensive review for further details of operation and application. Thiers and Oglesby (1964), in an evaluation of an automatic continuous-flow system for six constituents, emphasized need for recognition of interaction between samples and instrumental drift with application of corrective techniques to improve accuracy and precision. In summary, the Auto-Analyzer is a reliable and rugged instrumental system for automated analyses that requires meticulous attention to kinetic parameters of continuous-flow analysis to enhance performance (Thiers *et al.*, 1967, 1971).

There are many other automated systems presently available (Couch, 1970); these are discrete sample analyzers. The relative merits of these two approaches, that is, discrete sample vs. flow-through analysis, have been debated, but unanimous agreement has not been reached. Since a comparison of the various systems is limited by both space and personal experience, these will only be listed: Autochemist (A.G.A. Corporation), DSA-560/564 Discrete Sample Analyzer (Beckman Instruments, Inc.), Robot Chemist (Diagnostic Sciences, Inc.), Du Pont Automatic Clinical Analyzer, ACA (E. I. du Pont de Nemours & Company, Inc.), Hycel Mark X/XVII (Hycel,

Inc.), Vickers Multi-Channel 300 (Medi-Computer Corp.), and Programachem 1040 (American Monitor Corp.). Coulter and Damon have also introduced new automated chemistry analyzers (Alpert, 1972).

A new concept in rapid analyses has recently been introduced into the clinical chemistry laboratory (Anderson, 1970; Gambino, 1971). This system allows the simultaneous analysis of microliter quantities of multiple sera for the same component and is based on the use of centrifugal force to move and mix samples and reagents concurrently (Gambino, 1971). Systems of this type include CentrifiChem (Union Carbide Corp.), Gemsaec (Electro-Nucleonics, Inc.), and Rotochem (American Instrument Company).

Our own experience with the Du Pont ACA has not only been most favorable as reported elsewhere, but it reflects many of the emerging characteristics of automation in clinical chemistry (Speicher *et al.*, 1972; Westgard and Lahmeyer, 1972). The Du Pont ACA performs discrete chemical analyses on blood serum and cerebrospinal fluid (Fig. 9–32). It has a basic capacity of 30 different measurements, with 26 currently available. Test results appear within seven minutes after insertion of test pack and aliquot of specimen. We have found the ACA especially useful for enzyme assays and emergency work as well as weekend and night workloads. However, we have also incorporated it into our regular day service for virtually all the measurements available.

As predicted in the previous edition, ion-selective electrodes have been marketed as continuous and automated systems for chemical analysis by Technicon Corporation for sodium, potassium, and chloride (Rechnitz, 1967).

Alpert (1972) in his excellent review projects more evolutionary developments, emphasizing the emerging characteristics of built-in computers, high test output, integrated sample identification, kinetic and 340 nm. measuring capability, microsampling and lower reagent consumption, and decreased demands on operator skill.

NITROGENOUS COMPOUNDS

The body constituents which have in common the element nitrogen are referred to as nitrogenous compounds. Proteins and nucleic acids are the chief macromolecules, while the small molecular constituents are crystalloids rather than colloids and are identified as a group by the term "nonprotein nitrogen" (NPN). In medical chemistry NPN has an analytical connotation, since it refers to that fraction of whole blood, plasma, or serum which is not precipitated by the usual protein-precipitating reagents (trichloroacetic acid, tungstic acid, or barium sulfate). With a normal NPN concentration of 10 to 40 mg./dl. of plasma, the more abundant NPN compounds expressed in percentage of NPN are approximately as follows:

Urea	55 per cent
Amino acids	20 per cent
Others, including creatinine, and NH_4	5 per cent

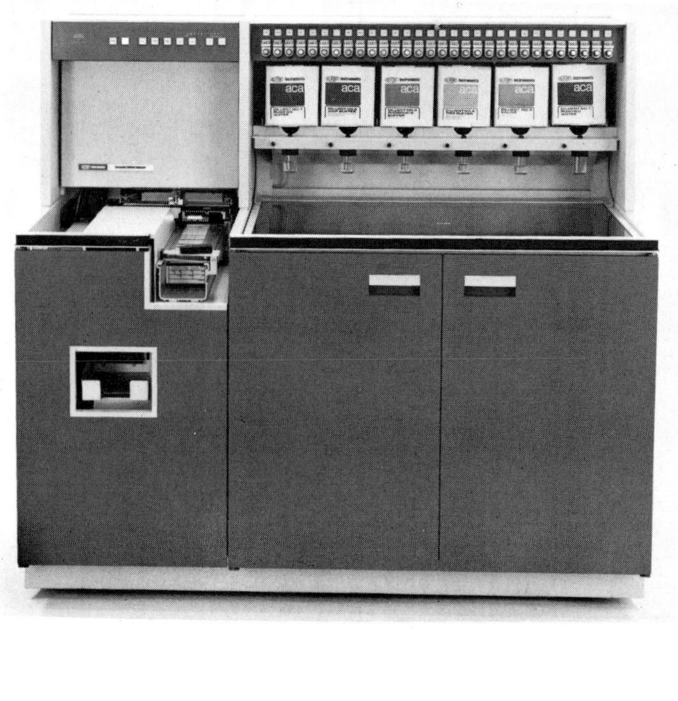

Figure 9–32. DuPont Automatic Clinical Analyzer (ACA).

As a determination, the NPN has generally been abandoned in view of the availability of specific measurements for individual components which have greater clinical pathologic significance.

Biochemistry

Proteins and nucleic acids are not only structural components of the cell, but also serve as biocatalysts (enzymes), regulators of metabolism (hormones), and preservers of genetic make up (chromosomes) of an individual. Amino acids are the building blocks of protein, while nucleotides are the distinct monomeric units for nucleic acid. Except in a few rare instances, natural amino acids are alpha and are of the L-configuration. Alpha amino refers to the position of the amino group on the alpha carbon of amino acids while L refers to steric configuration. An example of an L-α-amino acid is serine, or alpha-amino-beta-hydroxypropionic acid:

$$\begin{array}{c} \text{COOH} \\ | \\ \text{NH}_2-{}^*\text{CH} \\ | \\ {}^\dagger\text{CH}_2\text{OH} \\ \text{L-serine} \end{array}$$

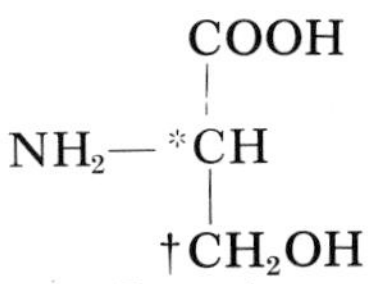

A carboxylic acid group is also attached to the same (α) carbon. With the structure of the side chain (R) in the general formula

$$\begin{array}{c} \text{H} \\ | \\ \text{R}-\text{C}-\text{COO}^- \\ | \\ \text{NH}_3{}^+ \end{array}$$

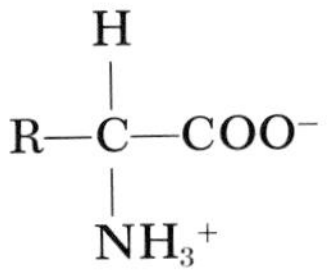

amino acids may be classified into seven groups of three categories (Fig. 9–33).

About 20 different α-amino acids are produced from protein hydrolysis, so that a large number of different proteins exist with varying amino acid composition (number and variety); cells, tissues, and organs reflect a spectrum of proteins as well as amino acids

---

*Alpha position.
†Beta position.

which serve to characterize them. By virtue of their acidic carboxyl (proton-donating) and basic amino (proton-accepting) groups, amino acids may act as acids and/or bases and thus are amphoteric. Amino acids display a variety of chemical reactions that are utilized in their identification, separation, and quantification.

Proteins are high molecular weight organic compounds composed of amino acids that are combined together to form polypeptide chains. The peptide linkage is formed by the condensation of the α-amino group of one with the carboxyl of another amino acid. An organic chemical reaction that splits out a molecule of water between a carboxyl group and an amino group yields an amide bond or peptide linkage and a dipeptide, as shown at the bottom of this page.

A continuation of this reaction produces further chain lengthening to form tripeptides (two peptide bonds), and higher peptides, eventually yielding long chain polymers known as polypeptides, or proteins. Polypeptides refer to short chains of amino acids (6 to 30) linked by peptide bonds while longer chains consisting of 40 or more amino acids linked together display the physical properties associated with proteins. In animal cells, these peptides are present in the free state, in which they may represent products of protein metabolism or hormones, such as insulin.

The application of enzymes which hydrolyze proteins (proteases) and peptide bonds of proteins has yielded valuable information regarding amino acid composition and sequence, as well as the biologically active component of hormones, including ACTH (adrenocorticotropic hormone), oxytocin, and vasopressin. The peptide bond comprises the backbone or basic structural bond as repeating links in proteins. Glutathione is one example of a polypeptide that is present intracellularly and in extracellular fluids, including blood:

$$\text{HOOC}-\underset{\text{H}}{\overset{\text{NH}_2}{\text{C}}}-\text{CH}_2-\text{CH}_2-\overset{\text{O}}{\overset{\|}{\text{C}}}-\text{NH}-\underset{\text{CH}_2\text{SH}}{\text{C}}-\overset{\text{H}}{\underset{}{\,}}\overset{\text{O}}{\overset{\|}{\text{C}}}-\text{NH}-\text{CH}_2-\text{COOH}$$

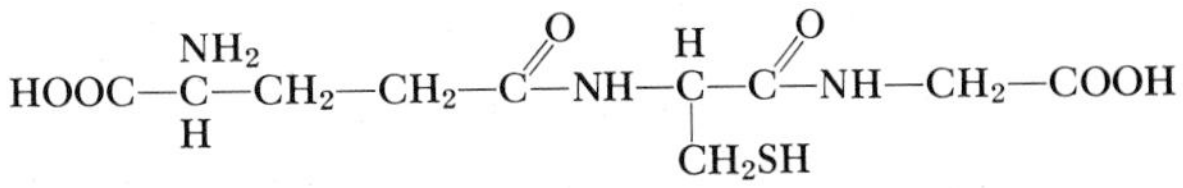

Glutathione

As a reduced sulfhydryl compound, it acts as an important reducing agent that may restore to full activity enzymes (proteins) with sulfhydryl (SH) groups that have been oxidized to disulfide linkages (S—S). The redox system of

---

$$\text{H}_2\text{N}-\underset{\text{R}_1}{\text{CH}}-\overset{\text{O}}{\overset{\|}{\text{C}}}-\boxed{\text{OH}+\text{H}}-\underset{\text{R}_2}{\overset{\text{H}}{\text{N}}}-\text{CH}-\text{COOH} \xrightarrow{\text{H}_2\text{O}} \text{H}_2\text{N}-\underset{\text{R}_1}{\text{CH}}-\boxed{\overset{\text{O}}{\overset{\|}{\text{C}}}-\text{NH}}-\underset{\text{R}_2}{\text{CH}}-\text{COOH}$$

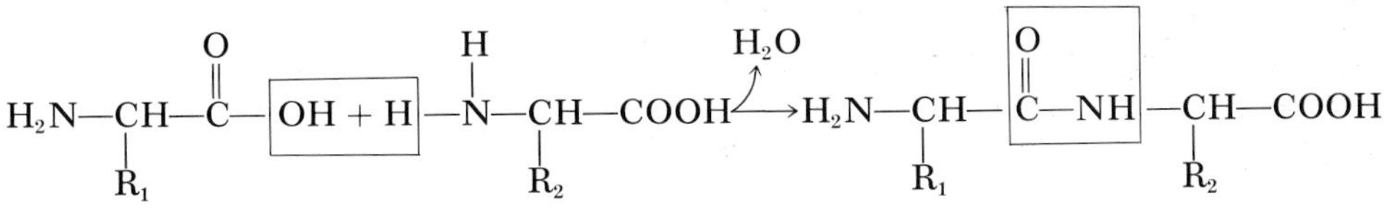

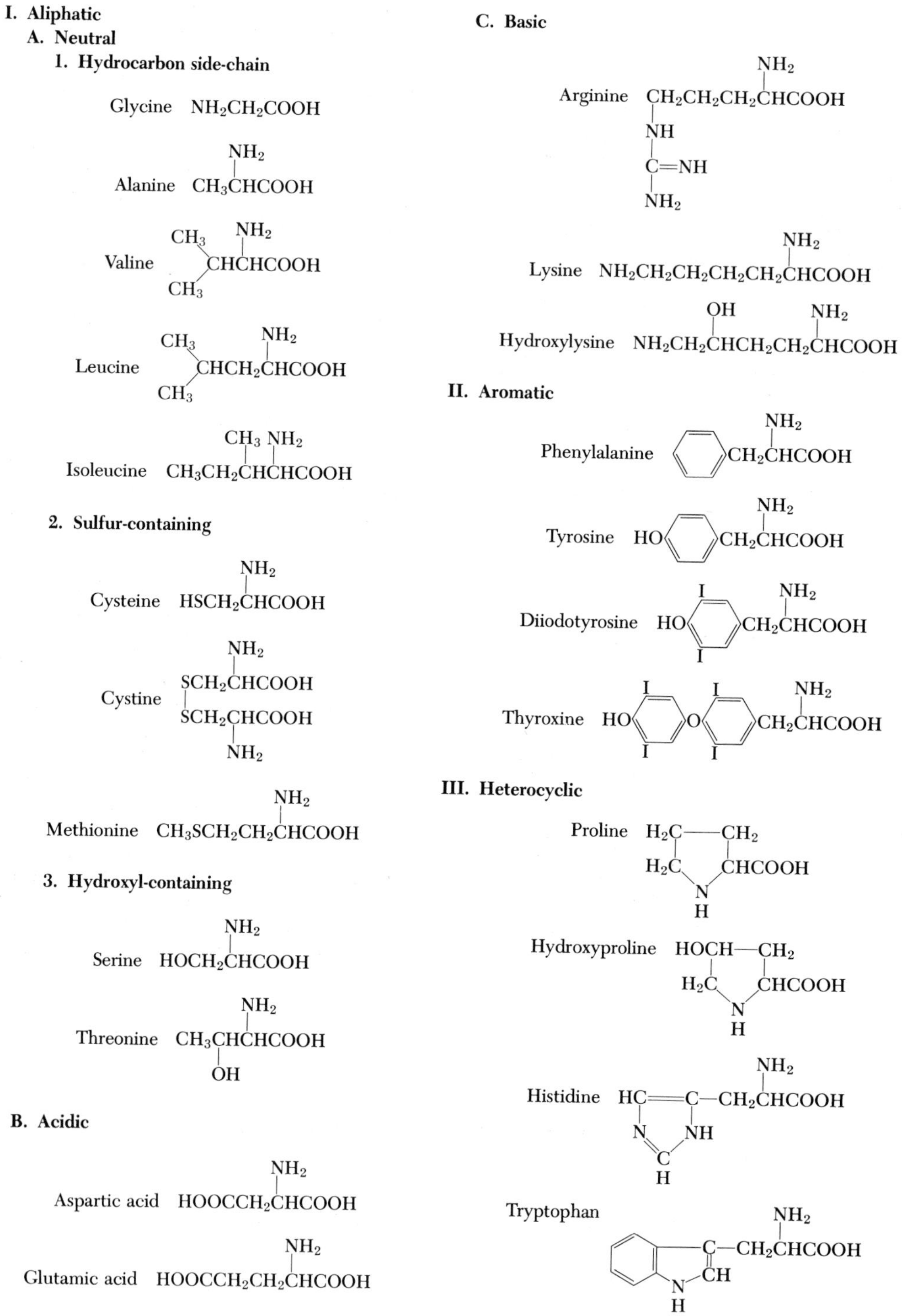

Figure 9–33. Classification and structure of amino acids. (From Cantarow and Schepartz: Biochemistry. 4th ed., 1967.)

erythrocytes (glutathione reductase) is one example: it is considered further in Chapters 4 and 14.

STRUCTURE

With an understanding of amino acids and their arrangement in long chains linked by peptide bonds forming polypeptides, the structure of proteins can be appreciated. The biologic activity of proteins lies in the unique structural arrangements of the polypeptide molecules. *Primary structure* refers to the number and order of the amino acids in the polypeptide chain (Harper, 1971). A relatively stable disulfide bond (S—S) may interconnect two parallel polypeptide chains. Another major force in preserving the structure of a protein molecule is the hydrogen bond. It is produced by the sharing of hydrogen atoms between the nitrogen and the carbonyl oxygen of the same or of different peptide chains. While the individual hydrogen bonds are weak, a large number of such bonds in a protein molecule produces a stable structure by virtue of reinforcement. The coiled structure (helix) of folded peptide chains in protein depends on the hydrogen bonds of a single peptide chain. In protein denaturation, these bonds are ruptured and result in unfolding of the peptide chains. *Secondary structure* of the protein refers to the folding of the peptide chains into a specific coiled structure held together by disulfide bonds and by hydrogen bonds (Harper, 1971). The arrangement and interrelationship of the twisted peptide chains of protein into specific layers, crystals, or fibers is called the *tertiary structure* of the protein (Harper, 1971). Some proteins display a fourth level of organization. Several units (each with appropriate primary, secondary, and tertiary organized structures, as described) may combine to form a quaternary structure; such a higher level of organization may be essential to the activity of enzyme protein.

A molecule of serum albumin (m.w., 69,000) consists of one long polypeptide chain (610 amino acids in primary structure) internally cross linked by many disulfide bonds (Murayama, 1965). The secondary structure appears to be one in which the single peptide chain is folded back upon itself to form layers that can be unfolded by lowering of the pH and refolded by raising the pH (Harper, 1971).

The major gamma globulin moiety (gamma-2 (γ_2), IgG) of the immunoglobulins in serum or plasma consists of two pairs of peptide chains, an identical "light" pair (m.w., about 20,000) and an identical "heavy" pair (m.w., about 53,000) joined by disulfide linkages as shown in the figure at the bottom of this page.

CLASSIFICATION

A useful although incomplete classification of proteins is given in Table 9–8. Composition and solubility features are imperfect but suffice for discussion. Albumin and globulin contain only amino acids. The solubility characteristics of albumins and globulins overlap but, in general, albumins are proteins that are soluble in water, while globulins require some salt to dissolve. While a half-saturated solution of ammonium sulfate will precipitate globulins, albumins require full saturation for precipitation. Precipitation of globulins is observed with addition of water and dialysis of serum that reduces salt concentration. Saline is preferable to water as a diluent for serum to avoid turbidity that is associated with precipitation of globulins. Both albumins and globulins are coagulated by heat. Their solubility is decreased by heat and they precipitate out of solution if the pH is adjusted to or near that at which there is no net ionic charge on

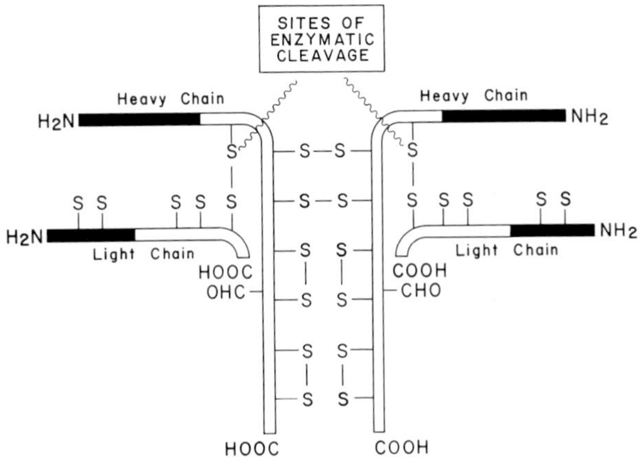

Table 9–8. CLASSIFICATION OF PROTEINS

Simple proteins
Albumin
Globulins
Conjugated proteins
Nucleoproteins
Porphyrinoproteins
Hemoglobin
Lipoproteins
Mucoproteins
Glycoproteins
Flavoproteins
Metalloproteins

the molecule (IEP, or isoelectric point). Cryoglobulins or cold precipitable globulins are reviewed subsequently.

On the basis of the length-width (axial) ratio, two general types of protein are identified—globular (axial ratio less than 10) and fibrous. The albumins and globulins of blood serum are globular proteins. Thus, the peptide chains are folded or coiled in a compact manner.

Denaturation of protein results in an alteration of the chemical, physical, and biologic characteristics of the protein. Physical and chemical agents denature proteins by disruption of the secondary, tertiary, and, if present, quaternary organization or structure of proteins. Heat, ultraviolet light, and surface action are physical denaturing agents. Chemical agents that denature proteins include acids, alkalis, organic solvents, urea, and detergents. Although deproteinization of a solution (e.g., serum or plasma) may be achieved by denaturation for subsequent inorganic analysis, in general, denaturation should be avoided prior to analysis of proteins such as serum proteins, enzymes, and hormones. Chromatography employing ion exchange and/or gel filtration principles has largely replaced the common precipitation and denaturation technique to separate proteins from small molecules and interfering substances. Dialysis is also a useful technique for purifying proteins. Albumins and especially globulins are heterogeneous. They are not single-protein species but families. At an acid pH, the usual single albumin fraction observed in serum protein electrophoresis with a buffer pH of 8.6 is occasionally resolved into more than one fraction (species). When different supporting media are used in serum protein electrophoresis, the globulins may be resolved into many fractions or species other than usual alpha (α_1, α_2), beta (β), and gamma (γ) components. Electrophoresis has virtually replaced salt fractionation (precipitation of globulins by Na_2SO_3, 26 per cent [w./v.]) of serum proteins in determinations of albumin and globulin content.

Conjugated proteins consist of protein combined with another moiety such as a lipid (lipoprotein), carbohydrate (muco- and glycoproteins), porphyrin (hemoglobin), and nucleic acids (DNA or RNA). Nucleic acids consist of the following:

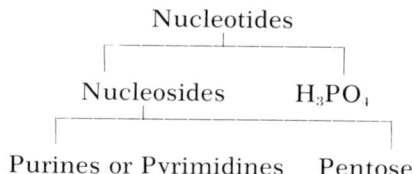

Nucleotides

Nucleosides H_3PO_4

Purines or Pyrimidines Pentose

Adenine and guanine are purines that give rise to uric acid in metabolism of nucleic acids.

METABOLISM AND NITROGEN BALANCE

Since nitrogen is one element that is characteristic of protein, much information concerning protein metabolism has been gained from the study of nitrogen metabolism. The term "nitrogen balance" is often used to reflect the anabolic and catabolic phases of the dynamic state of protein metabolism. Dietary protein represents most of the nitrogen intake, and most of the nitrogenous excretory products are derived from protein catabolism. Protein metabolism is reflected in the balance between nitrogen intake and output (urine, feces, menses). For normal serum proteins, 6.54 gm. of protein yield 1 gm. of nitrogen. Since normal proteins contain 15.3 per cent nitrogen, this is equivalent to a nitrogen factor of 6.54 (Sunderman, F. W., *et al.*, 1958, and Chiaraviglio *et al.*, 1963). Under genetic control, proteins are synthesized from dietary amino acids, amino acids from protein breakdown, or amino acids formed by amination of carbon fragments from lipid and carbohydrate metabolism. The intimate relationship of carbohydrate, lipid, and protein metabolism is also reflected by protein catabolism, wherein carbon fragments generated by deamination of amino acids form fatty acids and carbohydrates. In starvation and diabetes mellitus, the defect in carbohydrate metabolism precludes the usual major source of energy so that protein catabolism is increased, with a negative nitrogen balance. The proteins of the body are continuously undergoing breakdown to and resynthesis from their constituent free amino acids. Virtually all the dietary protein after digestion is absorbed from the small intestine in the form of amino acids that contribute to the general amino acid pool (Fig. 9–34). Synthesis (anabolism) and degradation (catabolism) of protein proceed from and to this pool. The specialized excretory products of protein metabolism are urea and ammonia. The

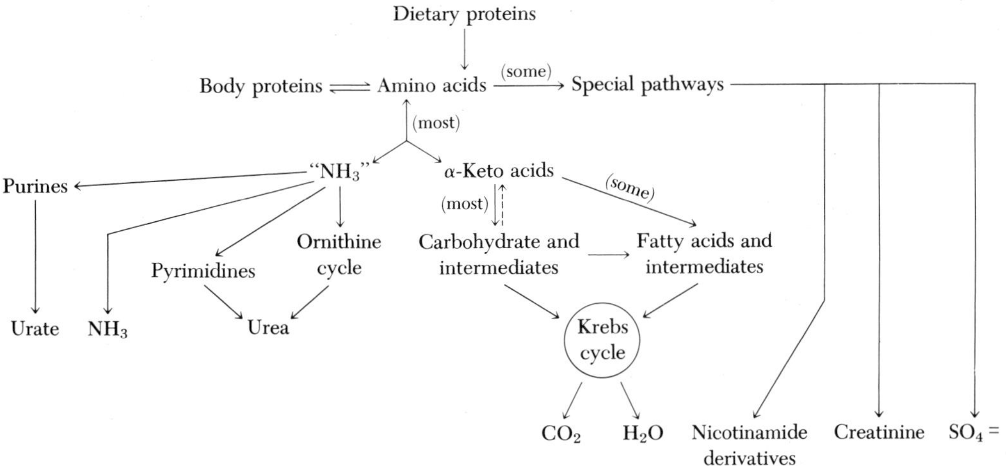

Figure 9–34. General pathways of protein and amino acid metabolism. Amino acids = amino acid pool. (From Cantarow and Schepartz: Biochemistry. 4th ed., 1967.)

ornithine cycle, which is primarily concentrated in the liver, removes the toxic substance NH_3 from the body to form urea; a simplified diagram of this complex cycle is outlined as follows (Cantarow and Schepartz, 1967):

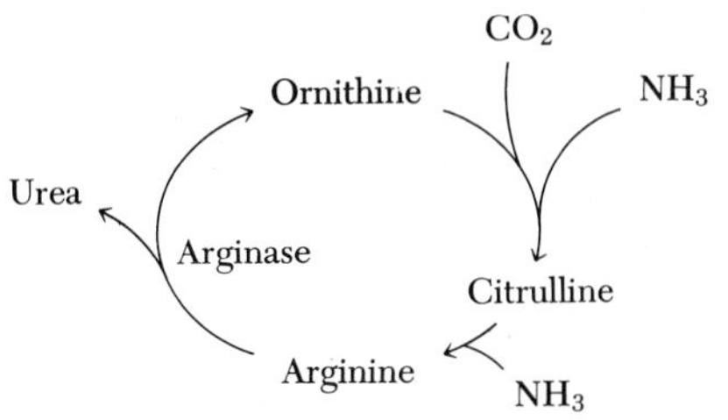

Urea is the major waste product of protein catabolism and, like other NPN constituents, is present in the blood and excreted in the urine. Synthesis of muscle phosphocreatine proceeds from blood creatine that has been formed by the liver or released from muscle. Creatinine, the anhydride of creatine, is formed from phosphocreatine and creatine largely in muscle and is also present in blood and urine. It represents a preliminary modification required for excretion of most of the creatine. Urinary creatinine reflects primarily muscle mass. Uric acid in the blood is an end product of purine catabolism (nucleic acids) and is excreted in the urine in the form of urate. Blood plasma amino acids may be considered in transit from one organ or tissue to another for synthesis or degradation. Only traces of amino acids are normally found in the urine.

From the standpoint of body economy, the three major categories of protein are tissue (organ) proteins, plasma proteins, and hemoglobin (Whipple, 1956). Liver, intestinal mucosa, and kidney have a high turnover rate of protein, while muscle protein is less labile. However, because of its great size, muscle mass provides the greatest amount of protein in conditions of deprivation. In terms of dynamic protein metabolism, a priority system appears to prevail in protein synthesis and breakdown. The plasma proteins do not reflect a significant decrease until tissue protein has been depleted, with clinical evidence of wasting in starvation or protein deprivation. When protein is ingested by individuals in the deprived state, hemoglobin has the highest priority for protein synthesis. Protein depletion with a negative nitrogen balance (output exceeds input) occurs on inadequate protein intake (fasting, undernutrition, malabsorption syndrome), on excessive protein loss (protein-losing gastroenteropathy, proteinuria of nephrotic syndrome, burns, plasmapheresis, sustained massive exudative lesions), and in states of accelerated catabolism of tissue protein (infections, wasting diseases, including some types of malignant disease, fever, hyperthyroidism, hyperadrenocorticism). The 11-oxysteroids and excess thyroid hormone provoke a protein catabolic effect, while androgens (testosterone) and growth hormone exert a protein anabolic effect.

Analytical Techniques for Protein Determination

Although recent developments in biochemistry have permitted the identification of a large number of discrete plasma proteins, a review of nomenclature and principles of more commonly used measurements will permit subsequent discussion of clinicopathologic correlations and methodology. For a more detailed presentation, the reader should consult comprehensive reviews present in several textbooks (R. J. Henry, 1964; Sunderman and Sunderman, 1964; Sandor and Kawerau, 1966; and Tietz, 1970).

Nitrogen Analysis. Since all protein molecules contain nitrogen, modifications of original Kjeldahl nitrogen analysis of protein materials represent classic methods for development of appropriate standards used in protein estimations as well as determination of serum protein nitrogen, NPN, total serum proteins (using nitrogen factor 6.54 mentioned previously), and plasma fibrinogen. Serum is devoid of fibrinogen. Hence, the total protein content of serum subtracted from the total protein content of plasma should approximate the fibrinogen concentration (0.2 to 0.4 gm./dl.). Plasma and urinary amino acid determinations are usually expressed as α-amino nitrogen (Goodwin, 1970). Kjeldahl nitrogen analysis involves digestion of specimen with concentrated sulfuric acid in the presence of a catalyst to yield oxidized carbonaceous material and nitrogen in the form of ammonium sulfate. Alkalinization and distillation of the ammonia into a known excess of standard acid is followed by titration of the residual acid. Alternatively, the ammonia liberated in digestion may be reacted directly with Nessler's reagent (a potassium mercuric iodide) to form a colored compound that is measured spectrophotometrically with appropriate standards.

Biuret Reaction. Although it is not very sensitive and, hence, is not suitable for analysis of specimens containing small amounts of protein (urine, cerebrospinal fluid), the biuret reaction for the determination of serum proteins is probably the most widely used procedure. It is 1/100th as sensitive as the Kjeldahl analysis. Because interfering substances in serum are present in minimal amounts with large amounts of protein, the reaction is virtually specific for protein. When an alkaline copper reagent reacts with substances containing two or more peptide bonds to produce a blue-violet color, it is called the biuret reaction. The complex between the cupric ion and two adjacent peptide chains produce the color (Cantarow and Schepartz, 1967):

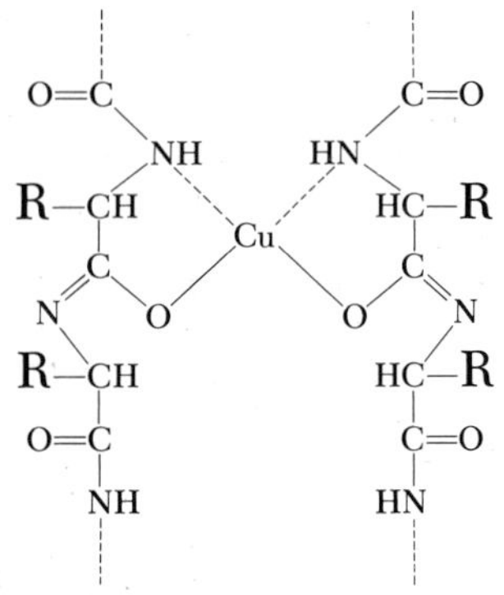

This color intensity is directly proportional to the number of peptide bonds over a wide range of measurements; i.e., it adheres to the Beer-Lambert law. The absorption maximum for proteins at 546 nm. is displaced slightly toward shorter wavelengths in peptides. Furthermore, different proteins yield very little difference in either wavelength maximum or absorptivity. Hence, biuret reaction gives reliable results with pathologic serum specimens also. Among others, Bennett (1967) has emphasized the limited specificity of this reaction for proteins; even ammonium salts give a positive biuret reaction, although NH_4^+ level in serum is too low to interfere. Bennett's (1967) procedure involves the analysis of protein separated from interfering substances so that greater specificity and sensitivity are achieved. Because of its simplicity, coupled with adequate precision and accuracy, the biuret method has become the method of choice for measuring total serum proteins.

Phenol Method. Another more sensitive colorimetric determination of protein employs the Folin and Ciocalteau reagent (lithium salts of phosphomolybdotungstic acid or phosphotungstic-phosphomolybdic acid). In an alkaline solution these compounds are reduced to a blue form in the presence of tyrosine and tryptophan. It is also referred to as a phenol method since phenol is the oxidizing group. Not only does the intensity of color development vary with different proteins in proportion to their amino acid composition of tyrosine and tryptophan, but many easily oxidizable substances can interfere. Lowry and associates' (1951) modification has extraordinary sensitivity (about 100 times more than biuret) but is a demanding technique.

Ninhydrin Reaction. Ninhydrin reacts with free amino groups of proteins to provide another colorimetric method for proteins as well as for amino acids.

Physicochemical Methods. Several physicochemical methods for estimation of serum proteins may be considered (Dubowski, 1964). The physical properties include refractive index, total solids, specific gravity or density, and ultraviolet light absorption of proteins.

In terms of rapidity and ease, refractometry has many advantages for total protein measurements (Naumann, 1964). It is reported to be as accurate and precise as biuret and Kjeldahl methods, with only slight interference from lipemic and icteric serums (Linese and Raine, 1970). Booij (1972) recommends that the A.O. Goldberg refractometer (American Optical Company, Buffalo, N.Y.) be standardized with measurements of fresh, clear serums of known protein concentration in view of an error in the calibration of the protein scale.

In view of a continual and increasing need for precision ultraviolet spectrophotometers for a wide variety of measurements, protein measurements based on ultraviolet (U.V.) light absorption should become more widely used. While ultraviolet light absorption of proteins in the 260 to 280 nm. range is attributed primarily to the content of aromatic amino acids, that between 200 and 250 nm. results principally from the peptide bonds with a greater absolute absorption or sensitivity (Dubowski, 1964). The excellent review by Dubowski should be consulted for further discussion and application of this principle.

Ionic Precipitation. Since proteins contain available amino acids, the ionic form plays an important role. Each amino acid or protein, depending on availability (end groups and side chains) and type of amino acid, displays amphoteric properties. This property to act as an acid or a base accounts for buffering capacity of proteins. At pH values that are acid to its isoelectric point (IEP), an amino acid carries a net positive charge, while at pH values that are basic to its IEP it carries a net negative charge. At a pH equal to its IEP (called pI), it exists as a doubly charged molecule with one positive and one negative charge, so it is electrically neutral. This is called a zwitterion, which when compared to other forms may be observed as follows:

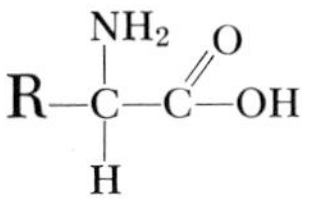

Classic structure

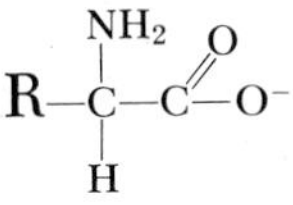

Anionic form

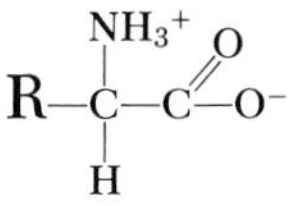

Zwitterion

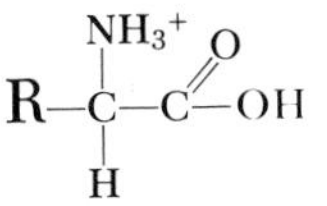

Cationic form

The numerical value of the pI is characteristic for individual amino acids and proteins. The form assumed by a protein or amino acid is dependent on the buffer solution (type and concentration of salt). In biologic specimens, such as plasma or serum, the fluid (salt solution) is slightly alkaline, so that most of these proteins are found in their negatively (anionic) charged forms. In protein analysis, this property underlies electrophoretic separation as well as anionic precipitation, cationic precipitation, and dye binding.

Anionic and Cationic Precipitation. When a protein is cationic in form (on the acid side of its isoelectric point), it will combine readily with an anion and precipitate. Turbidimetric methods for protein determination frequently employ anionic precipitants, such as trichloroacetic acid (trichloroacetate) and sulfosalicylic acid. Picric acid, tungstic acid, and anionic detergents yield a similar reaction. Barium (Ba^{++}) and zinc (Zn^{++}) are representative of cationic precipitants. The preparation of protein-free filtrates from whole blood, plasma, or serum involves a cationic or anionic precipitant.

Dye Binding. When pH indicators are added to protein solutions, a dye-binding effect on proteins is observed. This effect has generated several methods of protein estimation (de la Huerga, Smetters, and Sherrick, 1964). The familiar dip-stick tests for urinary protein take advantage of this principle, referred to as the "protein error" of indicators. Congo red, phenol red (phenolsulfonephthalein, or PSP), and tetrabromophenolphthalein are examples of dyes used. The Congo red test for amyloidosis as well as PSP renal function test are more familiar applications of these dyes, as is the Evans blue (T1824) dye plasma volume determination. Several of the methods have been adapted to the measurement of albumin rather than total serum proteins. Methyl orange, bromcresol green, and 2-(4′-hydroxyazobenzene) benzoic acid (HABA) are dyes used for albumin determinations. Bromcresol green appears to be free of pigment interference. Bilirubin concentrations over 5 mg./dl. of serum interfere with HABA procedures and, to a lesser degree, with methyl orange methods. Measurement of the reserve albumin-binding capacity in serum from newborn infants with hyperbilirubinemia (Porter and Waters, 1966) represents a modification of HABA determination of serum albumin. It has significant clinical correlation and serves as a model for the study of binding sites (affinity) of albumin for many drugs and antibiotics (Waters, 1967).

In the staining of proteins after electrophoretic separation and fixation, amido-schwartz (amido black), bromphenol blue, nigrosine, and Ponceau dyes are used. Fluorescent methods for albumin measurement depend upon certain dyes, e.g., vasoflavine, that become fluorescent when bound to protein (Betheil, 1960).

The measurement of methemalbumin subsequent to the reaction of ferriprotoporphyrin with albumin underscores the hematin-binding reaction for estimation of serum albumin proposed by Rosenfeld and Surgenor (1952). Shinowara and Walters (1963) reported an improved quantitative method.

Protein-free Filtrates. For many analyses, it is necessary to process the specimen in such a manner as to render it virtually free of protein. The term protein-free filtrate is applied to a solution resulting from treatment of a specimen to remove proteins. It is a relative term, since all the protein is usually not removed. Such precipitants remove not only most of the protein, which in itself may interfere with final reaction of the measurement, but other interfering substances as well, including many bound to protein. Turbidity, foaming, and precipitation are virtually eliminated in subsequent steps of analysis of protein-free filtrates. Anionic precipitants, discussed previously, and salting-out techniques, to be described subsequently, are most frequently used in the preparation of protein-free filtrates.

Chemical precipitation of serum, plasma, urine, or cerebrospinal fluid proteins is followed by either filtration or centrifugation and decantation of supernatant fluid to yield a crystal-clear protein-free filtrate. Precipitation generally results from protein dehydration or insoluble salt formation. Chloroform shaking and specific protein antigen-antibody reaction represent two other mechanisms for protein precipitation (R. J. Henry, 1964).

Dialysis of a specimen may also accomplish the same objective when conducted under controlled conditions of temperature, type of membrane, agitation, and removal of diffused components. Free-thyroxine assays and automated continuous-flow systems frequently employ dialysis. Chromatography has great potential for application to clinical specimens to achieve either protein-free filtrates or pure protein preparations. Small columns with or without gentle pressure devices should permit full exploitation of this approach. Patrick and Thiers' method (1963) for cerebrospinal fluid protein analysis represents an example, while Bennett's procedure (1967) makes use of membrane filtration on "Millipore" filters. Farese and Mager (1970) have applied membrane ultrafiltration to generate protein-free filtrates, which has eliminated precipitating methods and resulted in undiluted samples free of foreign ions.

Salting-out Techniques. Prior to the introduction of improved, rapid electrophoretic techniques, chemical analyses of serum or plasma proteins were performed most frequently by salting-out procedures according to the method of Howe (1921) or various modifications (Reinhold, 1953). Sodium sulfate in varying concentrations or a mixture of sulfate and sulfite has been the most commonly used salt. In essence, the hydration of salt added progressively removes water molecules so that protein becomes dehydrated, with a resultant decreased solubility. This precipitation of protein is called salting out (R. J. Henry, 1964). Since the protein is not denatured in either salting out or electrophoresis, it may be redissolved by lowering salt concentration or adding an appropriate aqueous diluent.

Total Protein and Albumin. In general, the serum total protein is measured as well as the serum albumin after precipitation of globulins with a colorimetric reaction (biuret). The difference between the total protein and albumin is reported as the globulin. The A/G ratio, representing albumin divided by globulin concentration, no longer has clinicopathologic significance, since it was originally based on Howe fractions that have been shown not to correlate with electrophoretic separation, because of incomplete separation (precipitation) of the globulin fractions from albumin. The term A/G ratio should be abandoned. Standardization of serum protein analyses should be based upon a reference preparation of bovine serum albumin such as crystalline bovine albumin available from the Armour Pharmaceutical Company (Chicago, Illinois). Commercial control serums should not be used in place of such a primary standard (Logan and Allen, 1968). Keyser and Cawson (1970) have reported a method for preparation of a stable pool of concentrated serum that is suitable as a reference standard in automated total protein and albumin procedures. A rapid, precise method for measurement of serum albumin employing bromcresol green that has also been adopted to continuous flow analysis appears to be replacing HABA as described by Doumas and Biggs, 1972.

Fibrinogen. Fibrinogen, a very large protein, constitutes normally about 5 per cent of the plasma proteins; it is virtually all removed in the clotting process, as plasma generates serum and a fibrin clot. The fibrin clot may be analyzed in terms of its nitrogen content or after resuspension by a colorimetric reaction, such as biuret. The incorporation of proteins other than fibrinogen in fibrin clots as well as fibrinolysis in an enzyme conversion method may occur to variable degrees. Fibrinogen can also be precipitated from plasma by chloride or sodium sulfate (salt fractionation) prior to quantification. However, proteins other than fibrinogen may also be precipitated in variable amounts. Immunologic techniques employing specific antisera have become available commercially, as have thrombin assays, wherein plasma fibrinogen serves as a substrate for enzyme analysis. Davey and colleagues (1972) have reported a comparison of rapid clottable fibrinogen assays.

The Plasma Proteins

Mammalian proteins may be simply classified as (1) tissue proteins, and (2) blood proteins. The blood proteins, in turn, can be separated into hemoglobin, the red cell protein, and plasma proteins.

While the tissue proteins are obviously of vital importance to the organism, the blood proteins, because of their accessibility, are most important in terms of clinical laboratory information. Not only can plasma proteins be sampled conveniently, but they occupy a central position in protein metabolism; they interact with virtually all body tissues or cells;

and they are intimately related to protein metabolism in the liver. Indeed, the liver is such a key organ in protein metabolism that hepatic disease is frequently associated with alterations in plasma proteins and disturbances of protein metabolism. In undernutrition and liver disease, the serum albumin level may be decreased by inadequate synthesis. Furthermore, plasma proteins have several important functions. Among these are transport functions (e.g., oxygen transport by hemoglobin); maintenance of osmotic balance (albumin); defense against infection (immunoglobulins, complement); hemostasis (the coagulation factors); contribution to nitrogen needs, and regulation of cellular activity and function (Putnam, 1960). Many of these are discussed in other chapters (3, 5, 6, 12). Others, including conjugated proteins, lipoproteins, glycoproteins, and metal binding proteins, will be reviewed subsequently in this chapter. Since albumin and γ-globulins are synthesized at slower rates than the α- and β-globulins, these fractions do not turn over at the same rate. Albumin probably has a half-life of about four weeks and the gamma globulins about one or two weeks. Approximately 15 to 20 gm. of plasma protein per day has been estimated to be formed and broken down by the hypothetic 70-kg. man (Cantarow and Schepartz, 1967). While the fate of the plasma proteins has not been clarified, the scant amount of albumin that penetrates capillary barrier into the extracellular space is returned to the vascular compartment by the lymphatic system. Destruction or elimination of gamma globulins probably takes place in the liver, intestinal tract, and kidneys. In this section we shall consider initially the major groups of serum proteins as they are determined by electrophoresis; subsequently we shall review the serum proteins defined by immunoelectrophoresis and radial immunodiffusion.

The technique of electrophoresis has already been described on page 552. At pH 8.6, electrophoresis on cellulose acetate separates the serum proteins into five fractions (Fig. 9–35). With agarose-gel electrophoresis, six distinct fractions appear. Albumin, because it is the smallest and has the largest number of negatively charged anionic groups, migrates most rapidly, followed by the globulins—alpha-1, alpha-2, beta and gamma, in that order. With agarose-gel, beta separates into beta-1 and

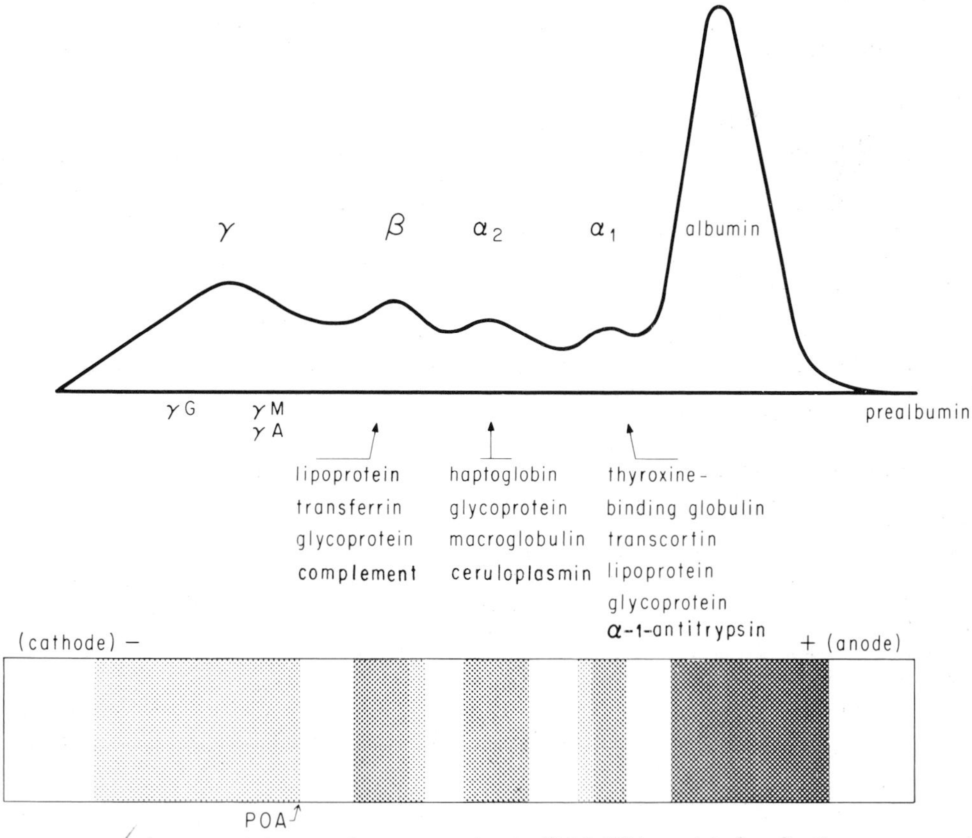

Figure 9–35. Electrophoresis of serum proteins at pH 8.6. POA = point of application.

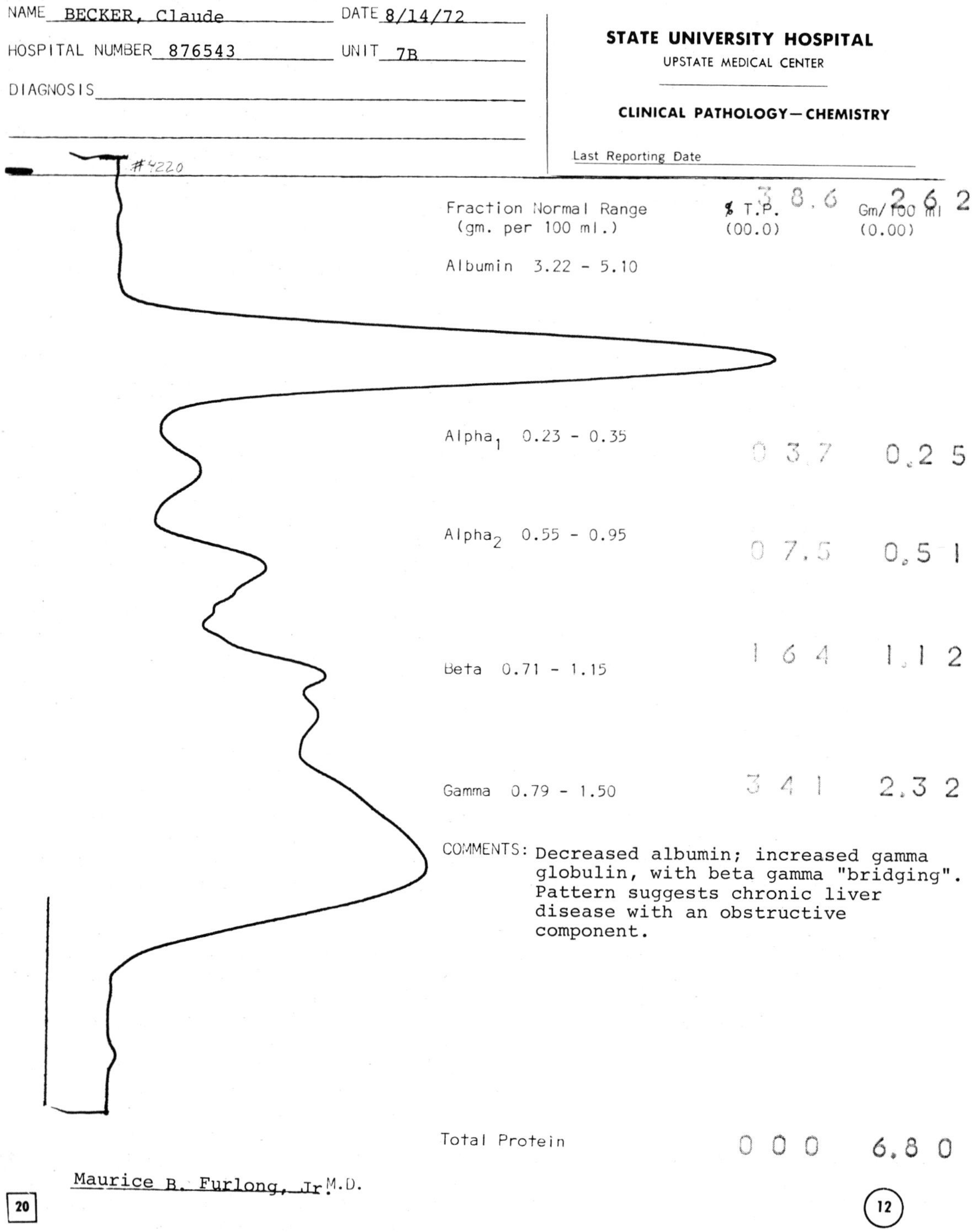

NAME BECKER, Claude DATE 8/14/72

HOSPITAL NUMBER 876543 UNIT 7B

DIAGNOSIS

STATE UNIVERSITY HOSPITAL

UPSTATE MEDICAL CENTER

CLINICAL PATHOLOGY—CHEMISTRY

Last Reporting Date

#4220

Fraction Normal Range (gm. per 100 ml.)	% T.P. (00.0)	Gm/100 ml (0.00)
Albumin 3.22 - 5.10	3 8.6	2.6 2
Alpha$_1$ 0.23 - 0.35	0 3.7	0.2 5
Alpha$_2$ 0.55 - 0.95	0 7.5	0.5 1
Beta 0.71 - 1.15	1 6 4	1.1 2
Gamma 0.79 - 1.50	3 4 1	2.3 2
Total Protein	0 0 0	6.8 0

COMMENTS: Decreased albumin; increased gamma globulin, with beta gamma "bridging". Pattern suggests chronic liver disease with an obstructive component.

Maurice B. Furlong, Jr. M.D.

20

12

Figure 9–36. Report form displaying electrophoresis scan and interpretation.

beta-2 fractions. In the clinical laboratory, these can be most easily quantitated by clearing and drying the membrane and scanning it with a densitometer, which is simply a scanning colorimeter. The Clifford densitometer traces the electrophoretic pattern (Fig. 9–36), automatically integrates each fraction, and prints out the amount of each fraction as a percentage of the total. When the total serum protein is known, the instrument will automatically calculate each protein fraction in gm./dl. Normal adult values of fractions separated by serum protein electrophoresis are shown in Table 9–9 and fractionated proteins are discussed subsequently.

Albumin. Albumin is the smallest and most abundant of the plasma proteins, normally constituting slightly over half of the total protein. The molecule (M.W. 69,000) has an asymmetry corresponding to that of an ellipsoid, with a diameter 38 Å and a length of 150 Å. It is synthesized in the liver and has a half-life of about four weeks; its exact metabolic fate has not been clarified, but presumably it is broken down in the liver to its constituent amino acids, which are then returned to the nitrogen pool. (See page 565.)

Because of its small size, albumin is the most osmotically active of the plasma proteins, accounting for 75 or 80 per cent of their total osmotic effect. It thus plays an important role in osmotic regulation, and indeed defines the intravascular compartment osmotically. Its second major role is as a transport molecule. Many substances only sparingly soluble in water are readily dissolved in serum or plasma, and it can be shown that these dissolved substances are actually bound to albumin. Among these are bilirubin, fatty acids, cortisol, thyroxine, and a number of drugs, including sulfonamides and barbiturates.

Alpha-1 Globulins. While albumin is a homogeneous molecule, all the globulin fractions consist of a number of different proteins, of similar electrophoretic mobility but otherwise unrelated chemically. The alpha-1 fraction, for example, includes a number of glycoproteins, orosomucoid, and several other components. Of clinical significance are the alpha-1 lipoproteins, important in lipid transport, which will be discussed in a later section of this chapter. Alpha-1 antitrypsin is an enzyme which has been found to be decreased in certain hereditary forms of chronic lung disease (e.g., emphysema). Transcortin, the cortisol-binding globulin, and thyroid-binding globulin (TBG) also migrate with the alpha-1 fraction.

Table 9–9. ADULT NORMAL VALUES OF SERUM PROTEINS (CELLULOSE ACETATE ELECTROPHORESIS)

Total protein	6.0-8.3 gm./100 ml.
Albumin	3.2-5.6 gm./100 ml.
α_1-globulin	0.1-0.4 gm./100 ml.
α_2-globulin	0.4-1.2 gm./100 ml.
β-globulin	0.5-1.1 gm./100 ml.
γ-globulin	0.5-1.6 gm./100 ml.

Alpha-2 Globulins. Like the alpha-1 globulins, this fraction consists largely of glycoproteins, including one of molecular weight 825,000 called alpha-2 macroglobulin. The clinically important components include haptoglobin, which binds free hemoglobin in the plasma, and ceruloplasmin, important in copper transport. In addition to erythropoietin, the enzymes, cholinesterase, lactate dehydrogenase, and alkaline phosphatase also migrate with this fraction.

Beta Globulins. These include the beta-lipoproteins, which are of lower density (LDL) than the alpha-lipoproteins (HDL) and will also be discussed in a later section. Hemopexin, which binds heme (but not hemoglobin), and plasminogen, the inactive form of plasmin (which lysis fibrin clots), also migrate in the beta-1 region. Furthermore, transferrin (siderophilin) which binds and transports iron in plasma, also migrates in the beta-1 region, as do many of the components of complement. C′3, the most abundant, is referred to as beta-1-C globulin. So-called beta-1-A globulin, as we will see, actually belongs to the group of globulins called the immunoglobulins. In the beta-2 region (seen clearly with agarose-gel electrophoresis) some of the other components of complement (C′2, C′6, C′7) travel, as do some glycoproteins of uncertain function.

Fibrinogen. This important component of the coagulation system, manufactured in the liver, is discussed in Chapter 6. It is not seen on routine serum protein electrophoresis, since it is consumed during clotting. However, if electrophoresis is performed on plasma (or incompletely clotted blood), fibrinogen will appear as a "spike" on the proximal side of the beta peak, i.e., between beta and gamma globulin region.

Gamma Globulins—The Immunoglobulins. Of all the plasma proteins, none have attracted such intensive investigation in recent years as the gamma globulins. Whereas the other globulin fractions consist of unrelated proteins which merely happen to share a common electrophoretic mobility, the gamma globulins have one vital property in common—that of antibody activity. This fact was demonstrated quite early with the observation of Tiselius and Kabat (1938) that immune serum had a higher level of gamma globulins than normal serum. It was also clear, even to these early investigators, that this "gamma globulin" was not one homogeneous protein but several. Heidelberger and Pedersen (1937), for example, found that rabbit antibody to pneumococcal polysaccharide had a sedimentation constant of approximately 7S and a molecular weight of 150,000 while horse antibody to the same antigen had a sedimentation constant of approximately 19S and a correspondingly greater molecular weight. Tiselius and Kabat (1938) showed that the 7S rabbit antibody migrated in the gamma fraction on electrophoresis while the 19S horse antibody migrated with a different fraction, in between beta and gamma fractions. It soon became clear that this antibody heterogeneity did not merely represent a species difference, but also existed within the same species. In fact, the same individual was found to respond to a single injection of antigen with two different antibodies, first 19S and then 7S. Still a third type of antibody, with 7S sedimentation coefficient but an electrophoretic mobility intermediate between beta and gamma was later demonstrated. Finally, in 1956 Gitlin and others showed by immunoelectrophoresis that not one but three proteins are absent from the serum of children with "agammaglobulinemia."

Numerous studies on these antibody globulins over the next 17 years resulted in a wealth of information about their physicochemical and functional characteristics, and also generated a profusion of conflicting nomenclatures and classifications (Edelman, 1973). Terms derived from molecular weights, electrophoretic mobility, and sedimentation coefficients were used interchangeably. To clarify matters, Heremans (1959) recommended the use of the term "immunoglobulins" to refer to the "system of closely related, though not identical proteins which are capable of acting as antibodies." Later, a uniform terminology was recommended by the World Health Organization in which each antibody fraction was indicated with a capital letter preceded by the letters "Ig" for immunoglobulin; IgG for immunoglobulin G; IgA for immunoglobulin A; IgM for immunoglobulin M; IgD for immunoglobulin D; and IgE for immunoglobulin E. Some of the properties of these five classes of immunoglobulins are indicated in Table 9–10. Their distribution in normal serum protein electrophoresis is shown in Figures 9–37 and 9–38.

Structure of Immunoglobulins. Only in the last dozen years has all of this information on the properties and classification of immunoglobulins been integrated into a unified model of antibody structure (Edelman, 1973). Three observations ushered in this new era.

1. Porter (1959) immunized rabbits against egg albumin and treated their gamma globulin with papain. This yielded three polypeptide fragments, two of which were almost identical in size, amino acid content, and behavior. Although they failed to precipitate when added to antigen (albumin), they did inhibit precipitation of antigen with *intact* antibody. Hence, these components apparently did bind antigen (though they did not precipitate it); the abbreviation Fab, or antigen-binding fragment, was subsequently applied to them. The other fragment was called Fc, because it crystallized out of solution (Fig. 9–39). Later, it became clear that while this piece did not bind antigen, it had several important properties, including complement fixation, cell binding, and placental transfer.

2. In 1960 Nisonoff and others attempted to repeat Porter's experiment using another proteolytic enzyme, pepsin. To their surprise, they obtained a fragment which *did* precipitate with antigen. It was then shown that this piece, referred to as $(Fab')_2$, could be split into two identical subunits, each of which was essentially identical to Porter's Fab. Now it was clear that Fab, while it binds antigen, cannot precipitate because it is *monovalent,* while the $(Fab')_2$, being bivalent, can form a lattice with antigen (Fig. 9–39).

3. Meanwhile, Edelman (1959) treated gamma globulin with mild reducing agents (which break disulfide bonds) in the presence of urea (which dissociates or cleaves immunoglobulin). By this technique, it was possible to separate polypeptide chains of two kinds by gel chromatography: a heavy (H) and light (L) chain. When treated similarly, the Fab was found to consist of an L chain and a portion of H chain; the Fc consisted of the remainder of the H chain. From these data, a model of the IgG molecule emerged (Fig. 9–40).

Four polypeptide chains, two H and two L, held together by covalent disulfide bonds, make up the symmetrical molecule. Both H and L chains participate in each of the two antigen-combining sites, as shown by experiments with radioactive-labeled antigen. The central portion of the H chain, called the "hinge region," allows the two "arms" of the molecule to bend to accommodate antigens of different sizes and conformations (Feinstein and Rowe, 1965).

Once the four-chain structure of the immunoglobulins had been established, protein chemists were eager to study the amino acid sequence, but a problem arose. Since antibodies, even those of a single specificity, consist of a heterogeneous group of molecules, as shown by their broad arc on electrophoresis, how then could one obtain a single molecular species for analysis? An experiment or accident of nature in the form of the disease multiple myeloma provided the answer (Edelman, 1973). Multiple myeloma is characterized by the presence in serum of a large amount of homogeneous gamma globulin. Polypeptide chains *can* be isolated in pure form from these proteins. When amino acid sequences were worked out for a number of these, an intriguing fact emerged. Approximately one-half of the L chain sequence and three-fourths of the H chain sequence were almost identical, or constant (invariant), from one myeloma protein to the next; the remainder of each chain was highly variable. *A priori,* one would expect

Table 9–10. PHYSICOCHEMICAL PROPERTIES AND BIOLOGIC FUNCTIONS OF IMMUNOGLOBULINS*

PROPERTIES	IgG	IgA	IgM	IgD	IgE
Light chain	κ, λ	κ, λ	κ, λ	κ, λ	κ, λ
Heavy chain	γ	α	μ	δ	ϵ
Heavy chain, class type	4 (G_1, G_2, G_3, G_4)	2	2	1	1
Molecular weight	160,000	170,000†	900,000‡	180,000	200,000
Sedimentation coefficient	7S	7S (9, 11, 13, 15, 17S)	19S	7S	8S
Electrophoretic mobility	Slow γ_2	Fast γ_1	Fast γ_1- Slow β_2	Fast γ_1– Slow β_2	Slow γ_2
Carbohydrate content (per cent)	2.9	7.5	11.8	–	10.7
Antibody activity	Major antibacterial and antiviral activity in serum	Major antibody of external secretions	Initial antibody formed to new antigens; antipolysaccharide	Unknown	Reaginic antibody
Complement fixation	+§	–	+	–	–
Placental transfer	+	–	–	–	–
Skin fixation	–	–	–	–	+
Seromucous secretions	–	+	–	–	–
Passive cutaneous anaphylaxis	+	–	–	–	–
Half-life (days)	23	6	5	2.8	2.4
Distribution (per cent of total in intravascular space)	45.0	42.0	76.0	75.0	51.0
Concentration mg./dl.	800–1600	50–250	40–120	0.5–3	0.01–0.04
Per cent of serum immunoglobulins	75%	15%	7%	0.2%	

*Modified from Harkness, D. R.: Postgrad. Med. *48*:68, 1970.
†Nonaggregated.
‡Consists of 5 monometric IgM units or an aggregate of 5 tetramers.
§Type specific: G_1 and G_3 fix complement well, G_2 fixes it poorly, and G_4 does not fix it at all.

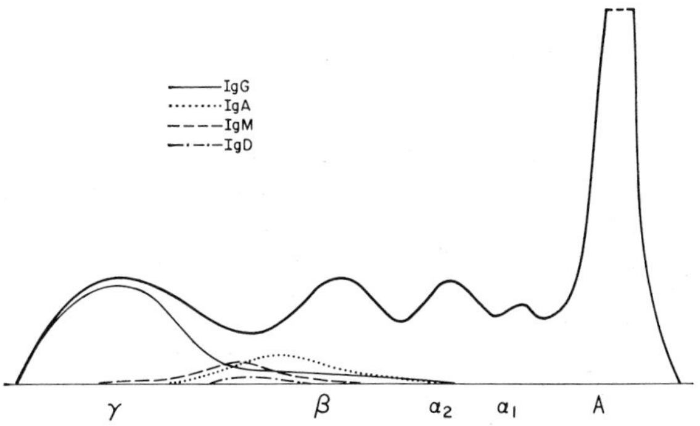

Figure 9–37. Distribution of immunoglobulins in normal human serum after electrophoresis. Areas under respective lines indicate relative amounts and electrophoretic distribution of IgG (7S γ_2-globulin), IgA (γ_1A; β_2A-globulin), IgM (18S γ_1-macroglobulin), and IgD (γD). (From Fahey, J. L.: J.A.M.A. *194*:183, 1965.)

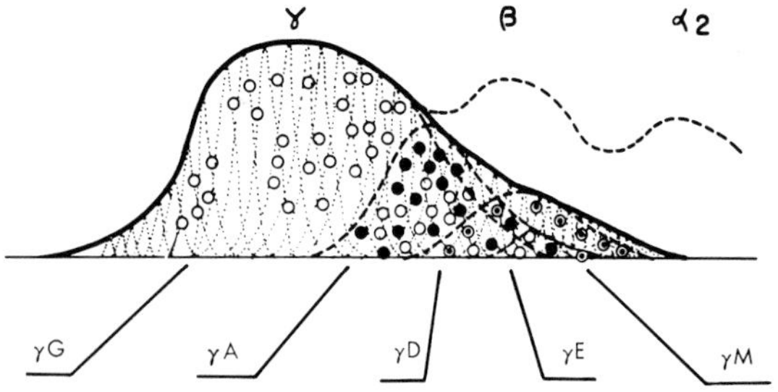

Figure 9–38.

Figure 9–38. Schematic representation of the cathodal end of a normal serum electrophoretic pattern showing the distribution of the four major classes of immunoglobulins (γG, γA, γD, γM, and γE). (From Osserman, E. F.: Plasma cell dyscrasia. In Beeson, P. B., and McDermott, W. (eds.): *Cecil-Loeb Textbook of Medicine.* 13th ed., 1971.)

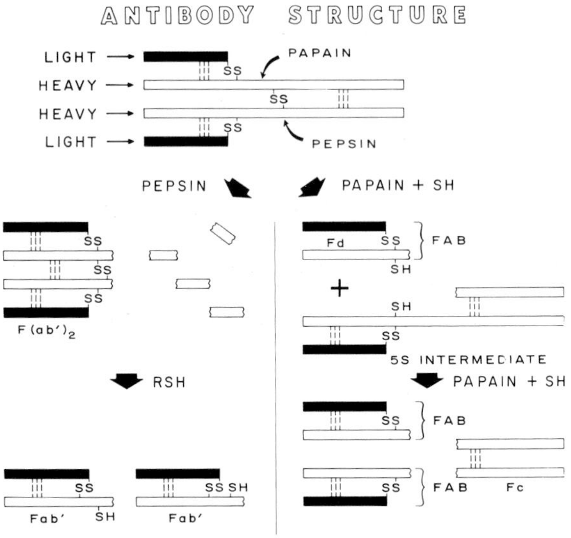

Figure 9–39.

Figure 9–39. Schematic diagram of the four-chained structure of γG immunoglobulins showing major interchain S-S bonds and regions susceptible to attack by papain and pepsin (arrows). That portion of the heavy chain within the Fab fragment is the Fd piece; hence, an Fab fragment consists of one light chain plus one Fd piece. (Modified from Davis, B. D., Dulbecco, R., Eisen, H. N., Ginsberg, H. S., and Wood, W. B., Jr. (eds.): *Microbiology*. New York, Harper & Row, 1967, Chapter 14, p. 422.)

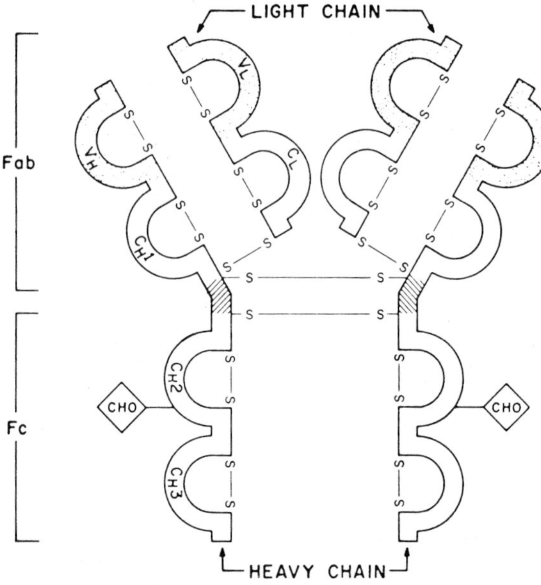

Figure 9–40.

Figure 9–40. Schematic diagram of the basic monomeric unit of all immunoglobulins. A notable feature of both the light chain and the heavy chain is the presence of a variant region, designated V_L and V_H in the light chain and heavy chain, respectively, and a constant region designated C_L and C_H. The V_L and C_L consist of approximately 107 amino acid residues each. The V_H contains approximately 121 residues, and the C_H (325 residues) consists of three homologous regions almost equal in length and designated C_H1, C_H2, and C_H3. Intrachain and interchain disulfide bonds are indicated by S-S. The hinge region between C_H1 and C_H2 is indicated by the hatched area; this region is particularly susceptible to proteolytic cleavage, which results in the production of fragments Fc and Fab, as indicated. The prosthetic carbohydrate group is designated by CHO. (Solomon, A., and McLaughlin, C. L.: Semin. Hematol. *10*:7, 1973.)

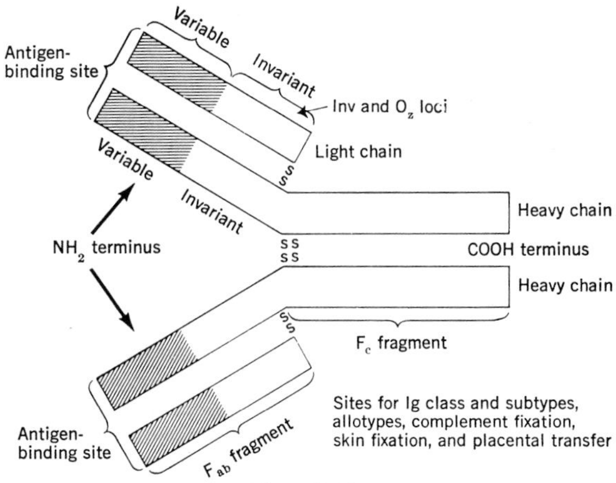

Figure 9–41.

Figure 9–41. Schematic diagram of an immunoglobulin molecule. (Harkness, D. R.: Postgrad. Med. *48*:66, 1970.)

the variable (V) region to be the site of the antigen-combining region and, indeed, this was shown experimentally (Fig. 9–41).

Myeloma provided other useful information. Many patients excrete in their urine a protein (Bence Jones or B-J protein) which is virtually a pure preparation of light chains. By injecting this protein into animals, anti-light chain antisera could be prepared. Many such antisera were prepared and tested for cross-reactivity against other Bence Jones proteins. It soon became clear that all light chains could be classified into two antigenic groups, called κ (kappa) and λ (lambda) (Fig. 9–42). These antigenic specificities reside in the invariant or constant (C) portion of the L chain (Fig. 9–41). Later, when pure preparations of H chain became available, it was found that H chains could also be classified into several antigenic groups, with their antigenic specificities determined by small but significant differences in the invariant or constant (C) portion of the polypeptide (Fig. 9–41). The H chain of IgG is called γ (gamma) chain and includes several subtypes (γ1, γ2, γ3, etc.). The H chain of IgM is called μ (mu) chain; that of IgA, α (alpha) chain; that of IgD, δ (delta) chain, and that of IgE, ϵ (epsilon) chain (Fig. 9–42).

Thus, the various classes of immunoglobulins are characterized on the molecular level by specific types of H chain (γ, α, μ, δ, or ϵ). Each class in addition has two subclasses, based on the type of L chain (κ or λ). For example, IgA-K is made up of two α (alpha) chains and two κ (kappa) chains; IgG-L, two gamma chains and two λ (lambda) chains (Fig. 9–42 and Tables 9–10 and 9–11).

In recent years further information about the function and quarternary structure of immunoglobulins has accumulated. IgM, for example, was shown to consist of five subunits (Fig. 9–43), each of these containing two H chains and two L chains (Miller and Metzger, 1965). IgM macroglobulin units (specifically a pentamer of the four chain model) can be dis-

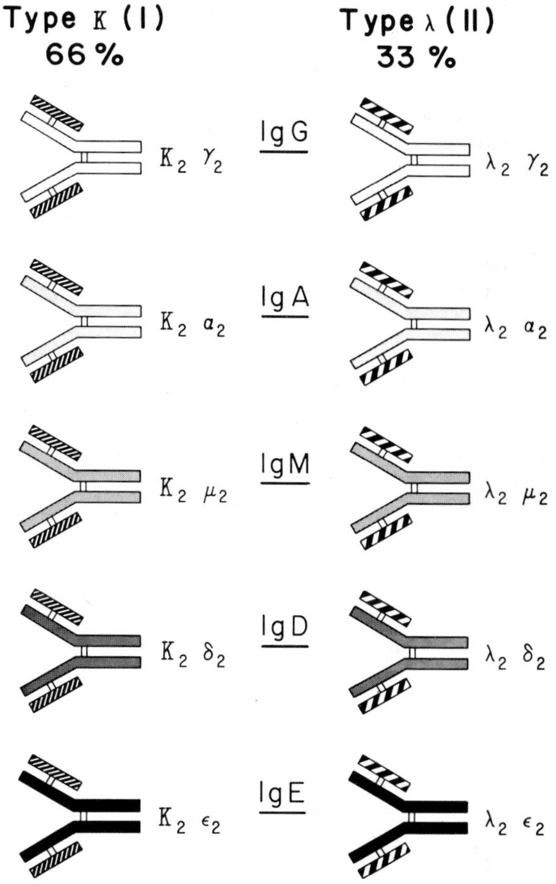

Figure 9–42. Ten classes of human immunoglobulins. (Modified from Harkness, D. R.: Postgrad. Med. *48*:65, 1970.)

Table 9–11. CLASSIFICATION OF HUMAN IMMUNOGLOBULINS*

IMMUNOGLOBULIN	IgG	IgA	IgM	IgD	IgE
Heavy chain					
Classes	gamma, γ	alpha, α	mu, μ	delta, δ	epsilon, ϵ
Subclasses	γ1, γ2, γ3, γ4	α1, α2	μ1, μ2	—	—
Light chain					
Type	kappa, κ	κ	κ	κ	κ
	lambda, λ	λ	λ	λ	λ
Molecular formula	$\gamma_2\ \kappa_2$	$(\alpha_2\ \kappa_2)_n$	$(\mu_2\ \kappa_2)5$	$\delta_2\ \kappa_2$	$\epsilon_2\ \kappa_2$
	$\gamma_2\ \lambda_2$	$(\alpha_2\ \lambda_2)_n$	$(\mu_2\ \lambda_2)5$	$\delta_2\ \lambda_2$	$\epsilon_2\ \lambda_2$
		n = 1,2,3 . . .			
Designation	IgG (κ)	IgA (κ)	IgM (κ)	IgD (κ)	IgE (κ)
	IgG (λ)	IgA (λ)	IgM (λ)	IgD (λ)	IgE (λ)

*Solomon, A., and McLaughlin, C. L.: Semin. Hematol. *10*:4, 1973.

sociated by sulfhydryl reagents into subunits by adding beta-mercaptoethanol (BME) to the serum prior to electrophoresis (10 λ of a 1:10 dilution of BME to 100 λ of serum); this breaks the disulfide bonds which link the five subunits together so that IgM after reduction has the same molecular weight as IgG and IgA. Recent electron microscopic observations suggest that this large molecule (pentamer) may be quite flexible, bending its five "arms" this way and that in crab-like fashion, to bind several antigenic units at once (Feinstein *et al.,* 1971). IgA shows a great tendency to aggregate in dimers and trimers, on electron microscopy (Fig. 9–43). They also tend to form complexes (protein:protein interactions) with other serum proteins including coagulation factors. Tomasi and others (1968) have shown that this immunoglobulin is found in high concentration in external secretions such as tears, saliva, nasal mucus, bronchial secretions, and stool or succus entericus. In these locations, the immunoglobulin is of 11S rather than 7S sedimentation and carries an additional glycoprotein fragment, called "secretory or transport piece," or "T component," which serves to facilitate transport of this IgA molecule across mucosal surfaces into the secretions. This transport piece, however, is found only in mucosal cells and not in cells which synthesize IgA globulins. Meanwhile, IgE has been identified as reaginic antibody, responsible for skin sensitization in atopic allergy. Elevated

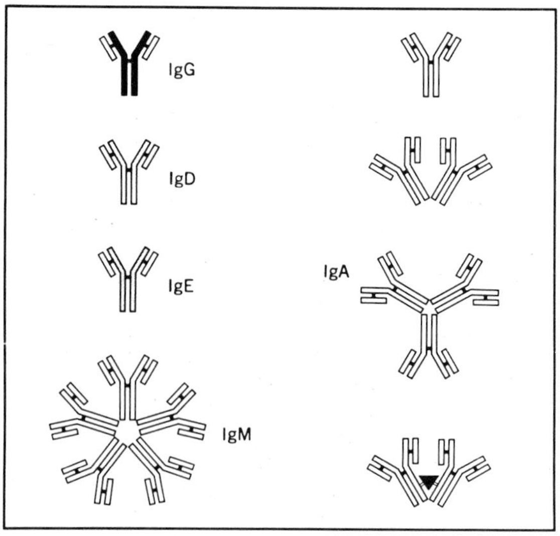

Figure 9–43. Primary forms of circulating immunoglobulins. IgG, IgD and IgE exist as single tetramers, IgM as aggregates of five tetramers, and IgA is variable. The IgA molecule (lower right) is the secretory form; the black triangle represents the transport piece. (Modified from Harkness, D. R.: Postgrad. Med. *48*:65, 1970.)

levels of serum IgE have been found in patients with various allergies, extrinsic asthma, and worm infestation. The physiologic significance of IgD remains unknown.

Analytical Techniques. Several techniques are suitable for measuring and identifying immunoglobulins (Cawley *et al.,* 1972; Iammarino, 1972). Immunoelectrophoresis, described on page 553, will identify the presence or absence of the major immunoglobulins as well as a myriad of other proteins; it also shows qualitative abnormalities in the precipitin arcs (Figs. 9–44 and 9–45), but provides virtually no quantitative information. With the use of a single-component or monospecific antiserum (e.g., IgG) in the trough opposite the trough containing multiple serum components or polyspecific antiserum (antihuman serum or a mixture of IgG, IgM, IgA) and patient's serum in the center well, specificity and further characterization of a deficiency or an excess of a specific protein component may be achieved. Clinical immunoelectrophoresis is described by Iammarino (1972) and Penn and Davis (1972), who are excellent resources and should be consulted for details of methodology, including use of commercial antisera.

As a quantitative technique, radial immunodiffusion has recently gained popularity. In addition to immunoglobulins (IgG, IgA, IgM, IgD, IgE), complement C′3, transferrin, alpha-1 antitrypsin and alpha-2 macroglobulin can be quantitated with this technique. In this method, antibody or specific antisera to human immunoglobulins is incorporated into agarose-gel, and wells for serum and known standards are cut into the gel (Cawley *et al.,* 1972). When the wells are filled with a known volume of serum (specimen) and plates incubated for 16 hours in a moist environment at room temperature, proteins diffuse out into the medium, and eventually the protein being measured forms a circular precipitin line with the antibody. The diameters of the precipitant rings produced are proportional to the concentration of the individual immunoglobulin in the serum (Cawley, 1969, 1972). Manual nephelometric methods for immunochemical determination of IgG, IgA, and IgM correlate well with radial immunodiffusion or automated immunochemical procedures, according to Killingsworth and Savory (1972).

Normal values of serum immunoglobulins vary in infancy, in childhood, and in adults (Stiehm and Fudenberg, 1966; Cawley, 1969). Two important normal deviations from the adult pattern may be observed in children: First, gamma globulin is normal (by adult standards) at birth owing to its passage across the placental barrier from the maternal to the fetal circulation. However, it decreases rapidly during the first three months of life; then, it

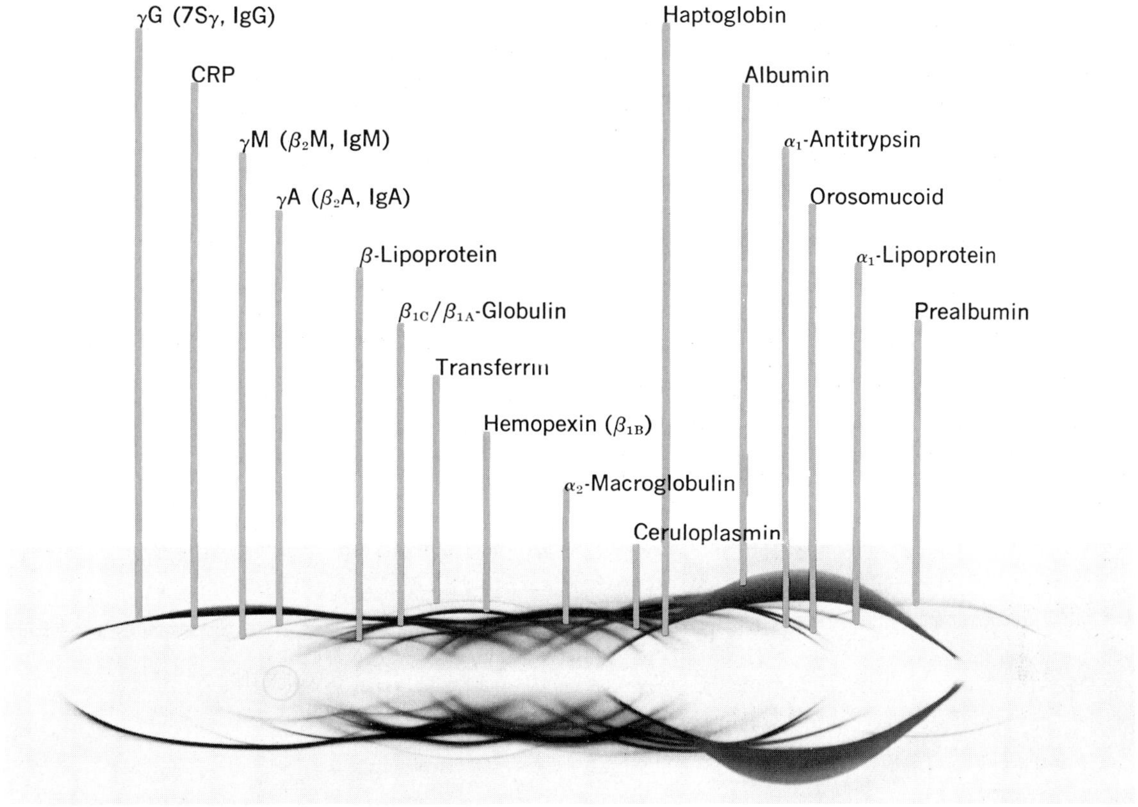

Figure 9–44. Typical immunoelectrophoresis pattern of parallel troughs of antiserum (horse) against pooled human serum in center well. (Courtesy of Hyland, Division Travenol Laboratories, Inc., 4501 Colorado Blvd., Los Angeles, California 90039.)

gradually increases as the child's own mechanism of gamma globulin production (by plasma cells and lymphocytes) matures, so that about 60 per cent of the adult level is reached by the age of two years. By the fifth to 10th year normal adult levels are attained. The second normal deviation is that alpha-2 globulin is high, frequently exceeding the beta globulin on serum protein electrophoresis; however, it falls off gradually to adult levels at about the 12th year. Claman and Merrill (1965) have reviewed some of the difficulties encountered in attempts to establish precise and accurate "normal" serum immunoglobulin concentrations; among others, these include population sample (age, race, sex), constant potency of monospecific antiserum, "standard" antigen preparations, and criteria used to delineate hyper- and hypo- conditions.

Clinicopathologic Correlations

In disease, the plasma proteins may fluctuate as components of a metabolically dynamic system. Hence, much clinical information is expressed in terms of examination and measurement of plasma proteins, the most conveniently obtained sample of available body protein.

Total Proteins. The determination of total proteins is most useful when done in conjunction with fractionation of serum proteins by electrophoresis. Since the serum total proteins represents the sum total of many different proteins resolved by electrophoretic separation, it is not a sensitive indicator of abnormal elevations or depressions of individual fractions. With advanced undernutrition or prolonged protein deprivation, the serum total protein concentration may be decreased. It tends to decrease also with hemorrhage, massive proteinuria, and protein-losing gastroenteropathy. A rare condition, idiopathic hypoproteinemia, is characterized by a profound depression of total serum proteins (both albumin and globulins), edema, and often hypocalcemia; it is relatively more frequent in infancy, although it affects all ages (Sandor, 1966). In general, the α-globulin level is raised in all conditions of hypoproteinemia.

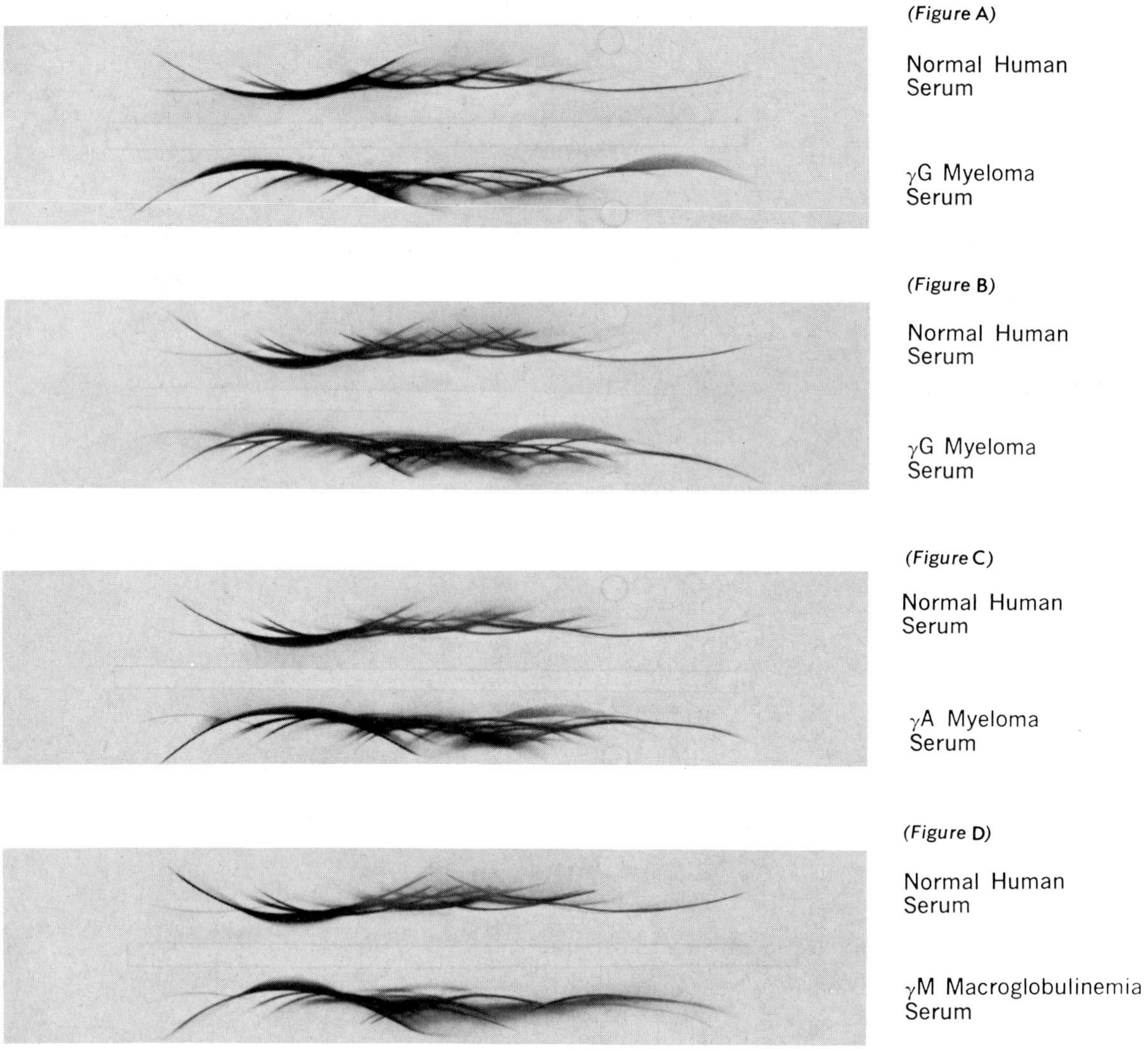

Figure 9–45. Diagnostic applications of immunoelectrophoresis. Normal serum control at top of each specimen: *A*, γG-myeloma; *B*, γG-myeloma; *C*, γA-myeloma; *D*, γM-macroglobulinemia. (Courtesy of Hyland, Division Travenol Laboratories, Inc., 4501 Colorado Blvd., Los Angeles, California 90039.)

Electrophoretic Patterns. When total protein is known, electrophoresis enables one to calculate the concentration of each individual serum protein fraction. In many cases, however, the overall electrophoretic pattern is more informative than the numerical concentrations of the individual fractions. In a study by Breckenridge and Csillay (1962) of 900 patients with a variety of diseases, several patterns emerged. Patients with acute infections, or acute tissue injury of any type, revealed a slight decrease in albumin and a prominent rise in alpha-1 and alpha-2 globulins. This has become known as the "immediate response pattern" (Fig. 9–46) and may be observed also with tissue inflammation or necrosis, such as burns, trauma, and malignant neoplasm in addition to infections. Chronic infection tends to lower the albumin still more and also produces a rise in the gamma fraction, "delayed response pattern" (Fig. 9–46). A so-called stress pattern, consisting of decreased albumin, increased alpha-1 and alpha-2 globulins with or without a slight relative polyclonal gamma increase, is a nonspecific pattern observed in hospitalized patients, especially postsurgically; it disappears when the patient recovers. More specific patterns are associated with multiple myeloma or macroglobulinemia, nephrosis, protein-losing enteropathy, and hepatic cirrhosis (Fig. 9–46). With cirrhosis of the liver, the characteristic polyclonal gamma elevation with "beta-gamma bridging" or smearing of the gamma into the beta region is usually associated with a decreased albumin and an increased alpha-2 globulin. A pattern that occurs in nephrotic syndrome and protein-losing enteropathy consists of a decreased albumin and gamma globulin but increased alpha-2 globulin; beta-1 globulin may also be increased. Although a discussion of individual serum protein fractions with regard to alterations in disease follows, it must be kept in mind that the serum protein patterns are usually more informative than isolated absolute values of individual fractions (Werner *et al.*, 1972).

Albumin. Because it comprises the major component of total serum proteins, albumin concentration alterations parallel many clinicopathologic correlations cited for total serum proteins. Hydration changes probably contribute to decrease of serum albumin concentration (and total protein) during the early phase of pregnancy. However, other factors may contribute to this change in the last trimester when normal total serum protein concentrations are observed; this is most likely the result of corresponding elevations of alpha and beta globulins with sustained decrease in serum albumin and fall in gamma globulins. Apparently the normal rate of catabolism cannot be met by synthesis in protein deprivation, starvation, or malnutrition with resultant low serum albumin levels. A similar decrease in

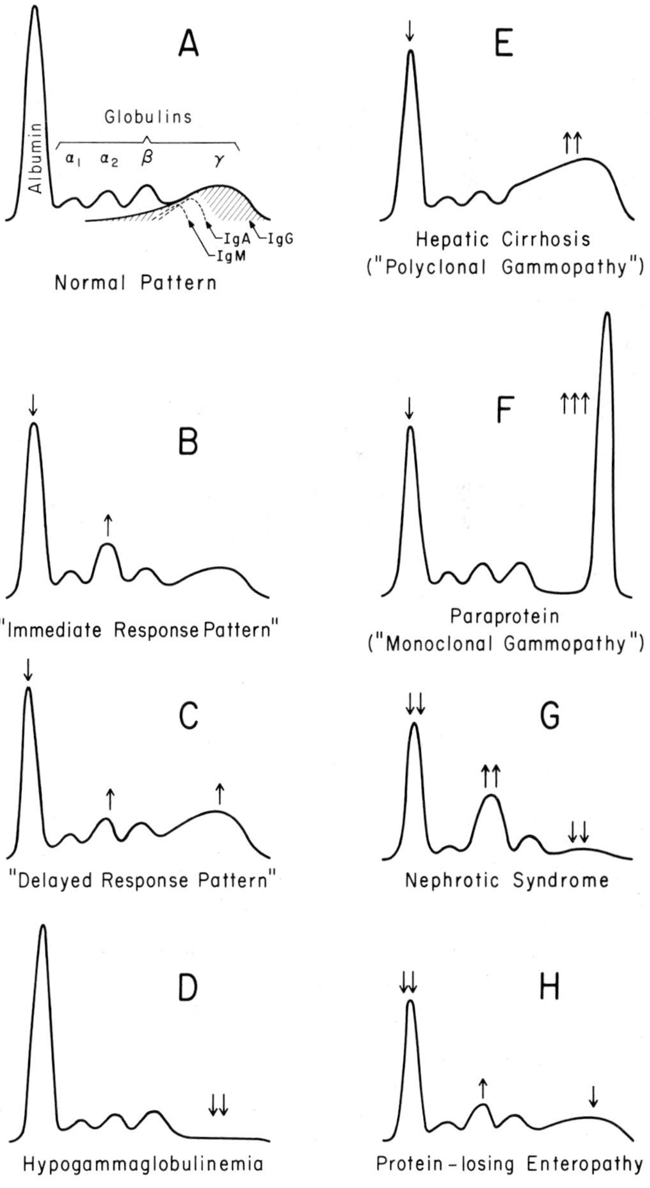

Figure 9–46. Serum protein electrophoresis: clinicopathologic correlations. (Courtesy of Dr. A. F. Krieg.)

serum albumin concentration is observed in the nephrotic syndrome; despite accelerated synthesis, the massive urinary loss of albumin (proteinuria) accounts for reduced serum albumin concentration. A negative nitrogen balance may also be incriminated in other examples of reduced serum albumin concentration, e.g., major infections, surgical and accidental trauma, eclampsia, uremia, gastrointestinal diseases (sprue, protein-losing enteropathy), and myocardial infarction (Sandor and Kawerau, 1966). An appreciable but variable fall in albumin is observed with chronic liver disease (cirrhosis). Since the plasma cell dyscrasias (myeloma and macroglobulinemia) are associated with larger falls in albumin than acute hepatitis, Sandor and Kawerau (1966) have questioned the evidence that supports the hepatic origin of albumin. At any rate, the serum albumin level represents the net result of distribution, degradation and synthesis; hence, it is not a good index of hepatic albumin synthesizing ability nor of the overall functional capabilities of the liver. A generalized decrease in serum albumin is a rather common finding in hospitalized patients.

Analbuminemia, characterized by the virtual absence of serum albumin and mild edema, has been reported in five subjects, including a pair of siblings (Earle, 1967). It appears to reflect a failure in production rather than in increased rate of removal. An interesting anomaly but rare condition is bisalbuminemia (double albumin); this condition is characterized by a double albumin peak on serum electrophoresis. Such genetic variants of albumin occur in two forms that are disclosed by electrophoresis: (1) presence of a variant albumin with a difference in electron charge, and (2) a form characterized by the occurrence of albumin dimers (Bearn and Cleve, 1972). The double albumin is made up of approximately half normal and half abnormal albumin in the first form, with varying mobility or migration of abnormal albumin. The additional albumin component in the dimer form represents only 10 to 15 per cent of the total albumin and is immunologically indistinguishable from normal albumin. Baisden and colleagues (1969) reported two families in which bisalbuminemia and diabetes mellitus were coexistent, although no disease entity has been linked definitely with bisalbuminemia.

Alpha (α) Globulins. The serum alpha globulins are elevated in hypoproteinemia (hypoalbuminemia) as a general rule. Since the glycoproteins migrate with α-globulins, hyperalphaglobulinemia may also reflect elevated glycoprotein concentration. Many of these glycoproteins, such as C-reactive protein, are "acute phase reactants," and this accounts for the rise in alpha globulins in the "immediate" or "acute response pattern." This may be especially true for alterations observed in disseminated carcinoma; although no diagnostic pattern has evolved, hyperalphaglobulinemia is often observed in patients with metastatic disease. Acute cellular necrosis (e.g., myocardial infarction) is often associated with elevated alpha globulins, especially α_2. Acute hepatocellular necrosis is frequently associated with a decrease in serum alpha globulins; this may be seen in acute, subacute, and chronic liver diseases. Haptoglobin binding to released hemoglobin and removal by the reticuloendothelial system may account for low levels of α-globulins in intravascular hemolytic anemia, since haptoglobin may comprise as much as 25 per cent of α_2-globulin. Finally, a low level of alpha-1-globulin suggests α_1-antitrypsin deficiency and should be followed up by specific assay for this protein, particularly in patients with pulmonary disease, especially emphysema or chronic obstructive pulmonary disease (Lieberman *et al.*, 1969; Sharp, 1971). Hepatic cirrhosis has also been associated with α_1-antitrypsin deficiency in childhood liver disease (Johnson and Alper, 1970).

Beta (β) Globulins. Of all the protein fractions, beta globulins are least frequently associated with specific pathologic disorders (Table 9–12). The increase associated with pregnancy may be attributed to lipoprotein changes, since lipid as well as protein changes occur in pregnancy; β-lipoprotein migrates with beta globulins. Since transferrin is associated with this fraction also, it is not surprising that conditions of iron deficiency provoke elevations of this fraction. In a similar manner, low transferrin levels or shortened life span of transferrin are associated with severe forms of infection, some neoplastic diseases, viral hepatitis, and cirrhosis, which reflect a depression of beta globulins. The beta globulin elevation often observed in patients with obstructive jaundice, uncontrolled diabetes mellitus, and nephrotic syndrome may also reflect beta lipoprotein alterations and disturbances in lipoprotein metabolism.

Fibrinogen. Bleeding disorders associated with decreased plasma fibrinogen concentration or activity are discussed in Chapter 6. The intravascular defibrination syndrome observed in several complications of pregnancy, in massive thrombosis, and after transfusion of several hundred milliliters of incompatible blood represent uncommon but nevertheless important recently recognized clinical entities associated with hypofibrinogenemia. Hypofibrinogenemia may also occur in sepsis, neoplastic disease, and surgery with extracorporeal circulation.

Gamma (γ) Globulins. Although defined electrophoretically as a single entity, the clinicopathologic correlations of the immunoglob-

Table 9–12. CLINICOPATHOLOGIC CORRELATIONS OF THE PLASMA PROTEINS*

PROTEIN	ADULT NORMAL CONCENTRATION RANGE	CLINICOPATHOLOGIC CORRELATIONS
Albumin	3.2-5.7 gm./100 ml.	↓ Nephrotic syndrome ↓ Malnutrition (starvation) ↓ Plasma cell dyscrasias (myeloma) ↓ Cirrhosis of the liver ↓ Major infections ↓ Surgical and accidental trauma ↓ Exudative enteropathy ↓ Eclampsia, uremia ↓ Acute infectious hepatitis ↓ Severe congestive heart failure ↓ Mesenteric lymphatic diseases ↓ Idiopathic hypoalbuminemia (hypoproteinemia)
α_1-globulin	0.1-0.4 gm./100 ml.	↑ Hypoproteinemia (hypoalbuminemia) ↑ Acute and chronic infections ↑ Lupus erythematosus
α_2-globulin	0.4-1.2 gm./100 ml.	↑ Rheumatoid arthritis ↑ Myocardial infarction ↓ Acute hepatocellular necrosis
Fibrinogen	0.20-0.40 gm./100 ml.	↓ Congenital afibrinogenemia ↓ Acquired hypofibrinogenemia
IgG (γG-globulin)	0.80-1.50 gm./100 ml.	↑ γG-myeloma ↑ Cirrhosis of the liver ↓ Agammaglobulinemia, congenital and acquired ↓ Hypogammaglobulinemia, transient ↓ Dysgammaglobulinemia ↓ Protein-losing enteropathies ↓ Nephrotic syndrome
IgA (γA-globulin)	0.05-0.20 gm./100 ml.	↑ γA-myeloma ↓ Ataxia telangiectasia ↓ Agammaglobulinemia ↓ Hypogammaglobulinemia, transient ↓ Dysgammaglobulinemia ↓ Protein-losing enteropathies
IgM (γM-globulin)	0.04-0.12 gm./100 ml.	↑ Waldenstrom's macroglobulinemia ↑ Parasitic diseases ↓ Agammaglobulinemia ↓ Hypogammaglobulinemia ↓ Dysgammaglobulinemia ↓ Protein-losing enteropathies
IgD (γD-globulin)	0.5-3 mg./100 ml.	↑ γD-myeloma
Ceruloplasmin	27-63 mg./100 ml.	↓ Wilson's disease (hepatolenticular degeneration)
C3 (third component of complement)	100-190 mg./100 ml.	↓ Acute glomerulonephritis ↓ Systemic lupus erythematosus ↓ Lupus nephritis
C4 (fourth component of complement)	3-5 mg./100 ml.	↓ Angioneurotic edema
α_2-macroglobulin	230-260 mg./100 ml.	↑ Nephrotic syndrome
α_1-antitrypsin	210-500 mg./100 ml.	↓ Familial alpha$_1$-antitrypsin deficiency (cause of pulmonary emphysema)
Transferrin	275-350 mg./100 ml.	↑ Iron lack conditions ↓ Atransferrinemia

*↑ = elevated concentration; ↓ = decreased concentration.

ulins (IgG, IgM, IgA, IgD, IgE) that comprise this group are outlined in Table 9–12. However, a diffuse or broad-based hypergammaglobulinemia may be observed in many infectious diseases, sarcoidosis, amyloidosis, subacute and chronic liver disease (especially cirrhosis), struma lymphomatosa (or Hashimoto's disease, an autoimmune disease), rheumatoid arthritis, lupus erythematosus, myelocytic and monocytic leukemias, and Hodgkin's disease. In some cases of chronic lymphatic leukemia and lymphoma, as well as nephrotic syndrome and scleroderma, hypogammaglobulinemia prevails. While a diagnosis of hypogammaglobulinemia or agammaglobulinemia may be confirmed by electrophoresis, immunoelectrophoresis and radial immunodiffusion are more sensitive, specific, and precise in regard to identification of immunoglobulin deficiency states.

Hypogammaglobulinemia and Agammaglobulinemia. Rosen and Janeway (1966) have classified the antibody deficiency syndromes in a comprehensive and lucid manner (Table 9–13). Although the human fetus is capable of forming antibodies (IgM and at times IgA), the transplacental passage of IgG accounts for the major component of the newborn infant's immunoglobulins; the infant usually forms and has attained about 60 per cent of adult normal concentrations of immunoglobulins by the end of the second year, with normal adult levels attained by the fifth to 10th year. Transient hypogammaglobulinemia is attributed to an abnormal delay in synthesis of normal γ-globulins by newborn infants. Increased susceptibility to infection characterizes this disorder, from which infants usually recover by nine to 15 months. The physiologic failure to produce γ-globulins in infancy (first two to three months) is called congenital agammaglobulinemia. Exaggerated susceptibility to infection does not usually appear in such infants during the first nine months of life, since maternal IgG probably protects infants during this period. During the second year of life, frequent and severe bacterial infections are the most common presenting complaints. Hypersensitivity and allergic manifestations

Table 9–13. THE ANTIBODY DEFICIENCY SYNDROMES*

DESCRIPTION
Transient hypogammaglobulinemia
Congenital agammaglobulinemia
Sex-linked, recessive
Sporadic (?) autosomal recessive
Acquired agammaglobulinemia
Primary
Secondary
Congenital and acquired dysgammaglobulinemia
Absent γG and γA, elevated γM (type I)
Absent γA and γM, normal γG (type II)
Absent γA, normal γG and γM (type III, ataxia telangiectasia)
Specific immunologic unresponsiveness
Hereditary thymic aplasia
(Alymphocytosis) ("Swiss-type" agammaglobulinemia)

*From F. S. Rosen and C. A. Janeway: New Eng. J. Med., *275*:709, 769, 1967.

as well as a condition similar to rheumatoid arthritis may be observed in congenital agammaglobulinemia. Quantitative measurement of immunoglobulins by radial immunodiffusion is required to establish the diagnosis; less than 100 mg./dl. of IgG with concentrations less than 1 per cent of adult normal serum values for IgA and IgM are observed (Rosen and Janeway, 1966). The absence of plasma cells from usual sites (lymph nodes, spleen, and bone marrow) is the most noteworthy anatomic pathologic feature in agammaglobulinemia.

An acquired form of agammaglobulinemia in adults without apparent cause separates this category from secondary acquired agammaglobulinemia. Susceptibility to infections, especially in adults with chronic progressive bronchiectasis and others with malabsorption syndrome, should prompt serum immunoelectrophoresis; IgG is less than 500 mg./dl. serum for confirmation of acquired agammaglobulinemia (Rosen and Janeway, 1966); plasma cells are also absent. In secondary agammaglobulinemia, defective synthesis of globulins may be associated with lymphosarcoma, reticulum cell sarcoma, chronic lymphocytic leukemia, and Hodgkin's disease. Depressed serum globulins are found regularly in patients with nephrotic syndrome, protein-losing enteropathy, and exfoliative dermatitides; severe malnutrition as well as hypercatabolic states may occasionally reflect similar changes.

As shown in Table 9–13, the congenital and acquired dysgammaglobulinemias comprise three distinct types in which immunochemical techniques are needed to confirm a diagnosis. Type 1 is the most common. An exaggerated susceptibility to infection as well as manifestations of autoimmune disorders (thrombocytopenia, neutropenia, anemia, and renal lesions) characterize this type which is inherited as an X-gene linkage appearing in boys and also appearing as a primary acquired form in adult females. Type II dysgammaglobulinemia is probably very rare; it is associated with normal IgG but decreased or absent IgM and IgA. A failure in antibody production to an antigenic stimulus in the congenital form and malabsorption syndrome in acquired form reflect major clinical features of type II. Type III dysgammaglobulinemia may occur in a small proportion of otherwise normal human subjects. Hence, an increased susceptibility to infection may not be seen. It is found in most patients with hereditary ataxia telangiectasia.

The most severe immunologic defect known is thymic dysplasia with agammaglobulinemia of Swiss type; it is characterized by defects in both cell-mediated and humoral immunity (Bellanti, 1971). The early onset of severe infections (pyogenic and enteric pathogenic as well as viral and fungal agents) in infants characterizes this disorder, with deficiencies in serum immunoglobulins, no antibody response after antitrypsin stimulation, severe lymphopenia, absent delayed hypersensitivity, delayed homograft rejection, and impaired *in vitro* lymphocyte responses to various stimuli including specific antigens. While the concept of thymic dependent (T cell) and bursa equivalent (B cell) lymphocytes is presented elsewhere (p. 150), the absence of both lymphocytes (T and B cells) and plasma cells in peripheral lymphatic tissue and a rudimentary thymus represent salient autopsy findings.

An isolated deficiency of IgA requires an analysis of secretory IgA in external secretions; immunohistologic studies of IgA-type plasma cells in mucosal biopsies may be more sensitive than serologic detections. With complete absence of IgA, an individual is exposed to a potentially severe transfusion reaction since he has the capacity to develop anti-IgA antibodies.

Hypergammaglobulinemia. By electrophoresis, hypergammaglobulinemia may take one of three forms: (1) a diffuse, serrated, or broad-base area; (2) a round hump or broad band with a round peak; and (3) a narrow band with a sharp peak or spike (Fig. 9–46). The gamma region (cathode area) or beta-gamma regions are the most frequent positions of the three configurations or patterns of hyperglobulinemia.

The gamma globulins were shown by Coons to be synthesized by cells of the plasma cell-lymphocyte series. A clone of such cells is a group or population derived by repeated mitosis from a single cell. Cells from a single clone synthesize only one type of antibody in response to an antigenic stimulus; this antibody, therefore, consists of a homogeneous protein identical in both C (constant or invariant) and V (variable) regions (Figs. 9–40 and 9–41). The variety of antibody molecules present in normal serum is the product of many such clones of antibody-producing cells. However, this is more complex as reviewed by Edelman (1973) with regard to the relationship of antibody structure and molecular immunology to clonal selection theory.

The clonal concept permits consideration of hyperglobulinemia (or "gammopathy") as monoclonal or polyclonal varieties indicating single or multiple clones and homogeneous or heterogeneous globulins formed. Monoclonal refers to one cell type from a single clone and one specific protein of gamma globulin with a high degree of intraclass specificity, i.e., a single type of IgG or even a IgG-K (or IgG-L) rather than heterogeneous assortment of IgG or an exaggeration of normal IgG. On electrophoresis, this appears as a narrow "M peak" (M-component) or "spike" (Figs. 9–46 and 9–47). "M" is derived from myeloma, macroglobulinemia, or malignancy. Polyclonal gammopathy, or hypergammaglobulinemia, refers to a diffuse increase in antibody protein, produced by many clones of cells and, therefore, of varying molecular structure. This is manifest on electrophoresis as a broad, diffuse elevation in the gamma and beta-gamma regions (Fig. 9–36). Intermediate varieties between monoclonal and polyclonal include so-called biclonal, triclonal, and oligoclonal types. This terminology emphasizes the relationship between cells and the proteins they synthesize, in the context of clonal theory.

Other terms that are used to describe these abnormalities include paraproteinemia and plasma cell dyscrasia. The variety of terms illustrates the basic debate about whether the underlying abnormality is protein or cellular in origin. In terms of a primary cellular lesion, abnormalities in cell types (histopathologic changes) from a variety of insults may cause abnormal protein elaboration. On the other hand, a protein lesion, whether at a genetic, molecular, or metabolic level, from a physical, chemical, or biologic insult may involve cells as a vehicle or secondary phenomenon. A third possibility that has also not been eliminated is a combined cellular and protein lesion, in view of the intimate association of protein synthesis within cells.

TERMINOLOGY. In summary several terms are used to describe serum protein alterations in hyper-γ-globulinemia: (1) diffuse hyper-γ-globulinemia, or polyclonal gammopathy, and (2) spike or narrow-peaked band of hyper-γ-globulinemia, or monoclonal gammopathy, M-components or monoclonal proteins associated with (a) malignant disorders (neoplastic, lymphoid, or plasma cell disease), (b) other diseases (cancer, collagen diseases, diabetes mellitus, etc.), or (c) no associated disease. Plasma cell dyscrasia describes a pathologic condition associated with spike, M-component, or monoclonal gammopathy. Dysproteinemia refers to analbuminemia and dysgammaglobulinemia or agammaglobulinemia.

POLYCLONAL GAMMOPATHY. A diffuse type of hyper-γ-globulinemia is frequently encountered on serum electrophoresis. It is most often observed in patients with chronic infections, granulomatous disorders, hepatic diseases (including cirrhosis or lupoid hepatitis), collagen diseases, and autoimmune diseases. On immunoelectrophoresis, the increment is observed in several species of immunoglobulins, most frequently a variety of IgG elevations (Fig. 9–45). With serum electrophoresis, a broad-based, rounded, or serrated configuration is most striking in the gamma region (Fig. 9–46). However, it often overlaps or is associated with an increase in β-globulin fraction because of an elevation of immunoglobulins normally located in small quantities in this

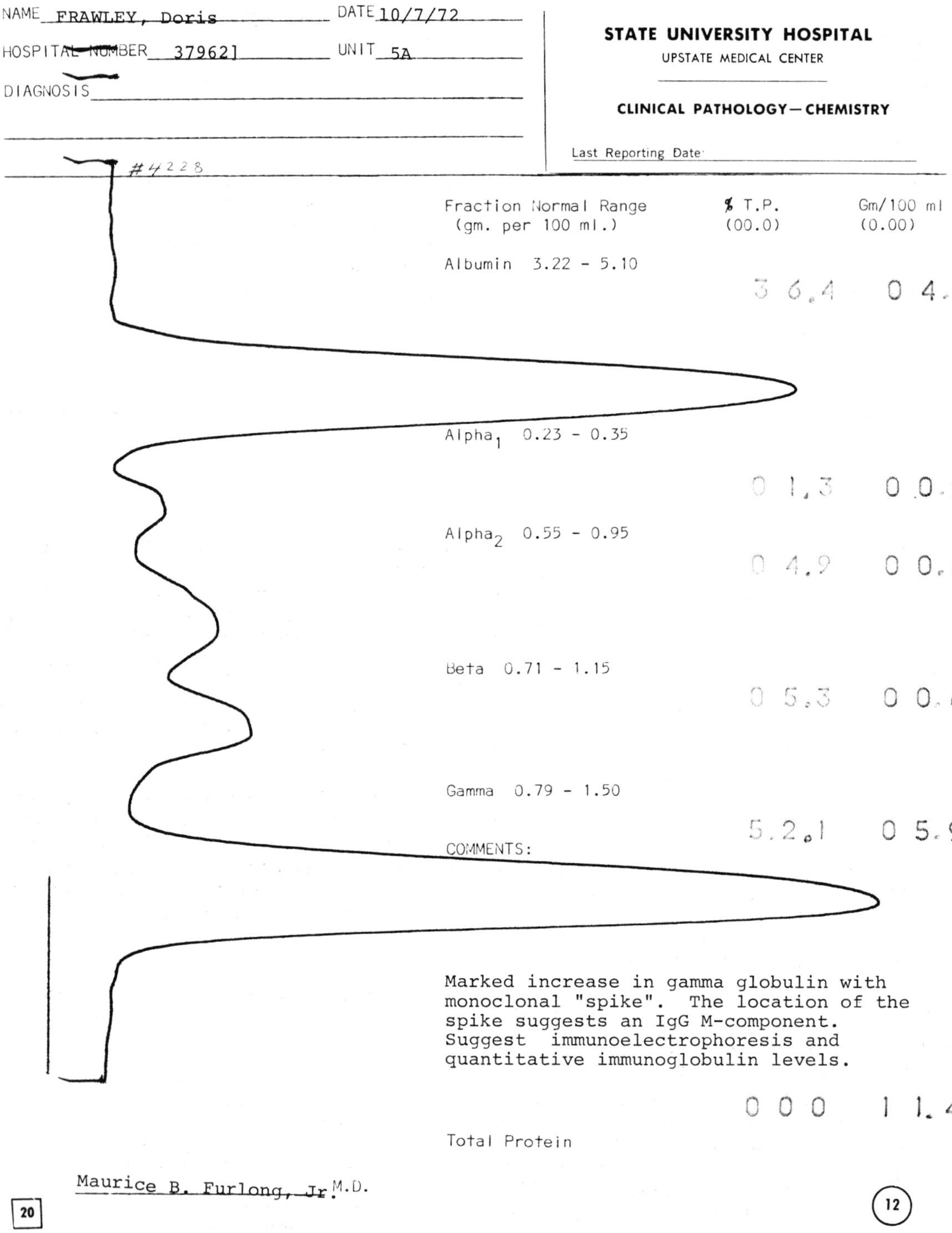

NAME FRAWLEY, Doris DATE 10/7/72

HOSPITAL NUMBER 379621 UNIT 5A

DIAGNOSIS

#4228

STATE UNIVERSITY HOSPITAL

UPSTATE MEDICAL CENTER

CLINICAL PATHOLOGY—CHEMISTRY

Last Reporting Date

Fraction Normal Range (gm. per 100 ml.)	% T.P. (00.0)	Gm/100 ml (0.00)
Albumin 3.22 - 5.10	36.4	04.1
$Alpha_1$ 0.23 - 0.35	01.3	00.2
$Alpha_2$ 0.55 - 0.95	04.9	00.6
Beta 0.71 - 1.15	05.3	00.6
Gamma 0.79 - 1.50	52.1	05.9
Total Protein	000	11.4

COMMENTS:

Marked increase in gamma globulin with monoclonal "spike". The location of the spike suggests an IgG M-component. Suggest immunoelectrophoresis and quantitative immunoglobulin levels.

Maurice B. Furlong, Jr. M.D.

20

12

Figure 9–47. Electrophoresis scan and interpretation of an "M peak" (M-component) or "spike."

Table 9–14. POLYCLONAL GAMMOPATHIES

- Hepatic parenchymal disease
  - Subacute or chronic hepatitis
  - Lupoid hepatitis
  - Laennec's cirrhosis
  - Postnecrotic cirrhosis
- Collagen disorders
  - Rheumatoid arthritis
  - Lupus erythematosus
  - Sjögren's syndrome
  - Polyarteritis nodosa*
  - Scleroderma*
  - Dermatomyositis*
- Infections
  - Acute and chronic infections*
  - Suppurative and subacute infections†
  - Bronchiectasis, chronic osteomyelitis†
  - Chronic pyelonephritis†
  - Tuberculosis and leprosy†
  - Syphilis, lymphogranuloma venereum†
  - Sarcoidosis*
  - Malaria, toxoplasmosis, and kala-azar†
- Malignant diseases*
  - Acute monocytic and myelocytic leukemia†
  - Hodgkin's disease and malignant lymphoma (lymphocytic)*
  - Carcinoma*
- Idiopathic polyclonal gammopathy
- Miscellaneous
  - Starvation, extreme*
  - Kwashiorkor*
  - Allergies*
  - Purpura, hyperglobulinemia (Waldenström)
  - Purpura, thrombocytopenic*
  - Purpura, nonthrombocytopenic*
  - Allergic or hyperimmune reactions*
  - Hypothyroidism*
  - Acquired hemolytic anemia*

*Variable.
†Frequent.

position. This beta-gamma overlap, fusion, linking, or bridging is commonly seen in hepatic cirrhosis (Fig. 9–36). A variant of polyclonal gammopathy called oligoclonal gammopathy refers to an increase in fewer species of individual immunoglobulins. Characteristically it shows a narrow, tall band with variable degrees of serration at its peak. Such a configuration or electrophoretic pattern is observed frequently in lupoid hepatitis and conditions with increased rheumatoid factor activity, e.g., Sjögren's syndrome, rheumatoid arthritis, and lupus erythematosus (elevated IgM). It may also be called a pseudo-M-component, since it mimics and may be mistaken for an M-component or monoclonal proteins.

In general, polyclonal gammopathy is observed with many diseases as a nonspecific serum protein abnormality; it does not permit a specific disease identification or diagnosis. The configurations observed in electrophoretograms are merely representative patterns and not diagnostic or typical of a specific disease. With this in mind, a summary of diseases and protein alterations are presented schematically in Figure 9–46 and outlined in Table 9–14.

Monoclonal Gammopathy. Monoclonal gammopathy is present in the plasmocytic dyscrasias characterized by Osserman (1971) as follows: (1) a proliferation of plasma cells (or immunologically competent cells) in the absence of an identifiable antigenic stimulus; (2) elaboration of electrophoretically and structurally (antigenic) homogeneous M-type or M-component (myeloma, macroglobulinemia) gamma globulins and/or excessive quantities of comparably homogeneous polypeptide subunits of these proteins, i.e., Bence Jones proteins, H-chains (Fc fragment), etc.; and (3) commonly an associated deficiency in the synthesis of normal immunoglobulins. The variants of monoclonal gammopathy, i.e., diclonal or biclonal and perhaps triclonal gammopathies, probably also reflect the criteria of Osserman. The major clinical patterns associated with plasma cell dyscrasias are listed in Tables 9–15 and 9–16. Osserman recommends use of the inclusive term "plasma cell dyscrasia" modified by the clinical pattern, e.g., myeloma, Waldenström's macroglobulinemia, amyloidosis, etc., when these are evident. However, when an M-type protein is observed in the absence of a recognizable

Table 9–15. PLASMA CELL DYSCRASIAS*

Clinically overt
- Multiple myeloma
- Waldenström's macroglobulinemia
- "Primary" amyloidosis
- Lichen myxedematosus
- γG (Fc fragment) heavy chain disease
- γA (α chain) heavy chain disease

Clinically occult
- Plasma cell dyscrasia
  - Of unknown significance
  - Associated with chronic RES stimulation
  - Associated with nonreticular neoplasms

*Osserman, E. F.: Plasma cell dyscrasias. *In* Beeson, P. B., and McDermott, W. (eds.): Cecil-Loeb Textbook of Medicine. 13th ed., 1971.

Table 9–16. ETIOLOGIC CLASSIFICATION OF MONOCLONAL GAMMOPATHIES*

A. Monoclonal gammopathies associated with neoplastic lymphoid or plasma cell disease:
1. Multiple myeloma
2. Macroglobulinemia (Waldenström's)
3. Lymphoma and lymphatic leukemia
4. Heavy chain disease (Franklin)

B. Monoclonal gammopathies associated with other diseases (cancer, hepatic cirrhosis, collagen diseases, diabetes mellitus, etc.). Also referred to as secondary monoclonal gammopathies.

C. Monoclonal gammopathies with no associated disease (idiopathic).

*Modified from Cannon, D. C.: Postgrad. Med. *46*:3, 1969.

clinical pattern, it should be classified as a plasma cell dyscrasia of unknown significance. Because an overlap may be seen in these categories and transition from asymptomatic to symptomatic forms may occur, these groupings or categories, though tentative, have considerable merit (Table 9–16). Amyloidosis may be a prominent feature of plasma cell dyscrasia. Hence, the magnitude of amyloid infiltration of tissues permits classification as primary amyloidosis or myeloma with amyloid. An individual with hyperproteinemia (9 gm./dl. or higher) may be asymptomatic initially but subsequently develop myeloma, macroglobulinemia, or amyloidosis. Furthermore, an M-type protein (M-component) may be associated with another disease, such as chronic infection (especially tuberculosis), recurrent cholecystitis, and cholelithiasis, or a nonreticular neoplasm such as adenocarcinoma of the rectum. Finally, M-components have been documented for 20 or more years with progression to a symptomatic plasma cell dyscrasia (multiple myeloma, macroglobulinemia, amyloidosis, etc.).

Serum electrophoresis is adequate for the detection of monoclonal gammopathies in most cases (Fig. 9–47). The spike pattern or configuration is most often present in the γ-globulin fraction but may appear in and between α_2, β, and γ regions; it is present rarely in the α_1 globulin position. Spikes in the β-γ regions usually indicate M-components but do not identify class of immunoglobulin present (Tables 9–17 and 9–18).

Immunoelectrophoresis and radial immunodiffusion are necessary to classify or characterize further M-components observed with serum electrophoresis. The abnormal or M-components in almost all cases may then be established as IgG, IgM, IgA, IgD, IgE, light chain (κ or λ), or heavy chain (α, γ, μ, δ, and ϵ) gammopathies (Table 9–11). Typical immunoelectrophoretic patterns are shown in Figure 9–45. For screening purposes polyvalent antisera to normal human serum are often sufficient in immunoelectrophoresis of patient's serum. In addition to characterization of M-components (e.g., IgG in myeloma or IgM in macroglobulinemia), it may also reveal deficiencies of the other normal immunoglobulins (Table 9–17). Monospecific antisera, specific for each of the classes of immunoglobulins, i.e., IgG, IgM, IgA, and IgD plus light chains (κ and λ) and perhaps heavy chains (γ, α, μ), are often necessary for confirmation of suspected abnormalities and characterization of M-components (Figs. 9–45 and 9–46). Greater sensitivity is achieved with use of such monospecific antiserum rather than polyvalent serum; this may be required in the presence of low concentrations of abnormal proteins as well as by inherent nature of abnormal protein to exclude a specific class (IgG, IgM, IgA) and suggest Bence Jones, or disorders such as IgD or heavy chain (Fc fragment) disease of Franklin *et al.* (1964). Although specificity and stability leave something to be desired, specific antisera to light polypeptide chains of immunoglobulins or Bence Jones proteins, type K (kappa) or L (lambda), although not readily available, are used for characterization of serum and urinary Bence Jones proteins,

Table 9–17. EVALUATION OF SERUM M-COMPONENTS OR MONOCLONAL PROTEINS IN BENIGN AND MALIGNANT DISORDERS

FACTOR	BENIGN	MALIGNANT
IgG M-component	< 2.0 gm./dl.	> 2.0 gm./dl.
IgA M-component	< 1.0 gm/dl.	> 1.0 gm./dl.
IgM M-component	Variable*	> 1.0 gm./dl.
Concentration of normal immunoglobulins of same type as M-component, and the other immunoglobulins	Not decreased	Decreased†
Variation in concentration of serum M-component with time	Tends to be stable	Tends to rise during course of disease
Bence Jones (BJ) protein in urine B-J concentration	Present < 6.0 mg./dl.	Present > 6.0 mg./dl.

*Although a majority of patients with Waldenström's macroglobulinemia have 1 gm./dl. or more of IgM M-component, some have only a few hundred milligrams. Virtually all M-components above 4 gm./dl. are associated with myeloma or Waldenström's macroglobulins.

†Normal levels of nonmonoclonal immunoglobulins may occur in patients with multiple myeloma.

< = less tham
> = greater than

Table 9–18. MONOCLONAL GAMMOPATHIES IN 126 PATIENTS*

	NO. CASES	%
Myeloma		
IgG	43	34.2
IgA	27	21.4
Bence Jones	24	19.0
IgD	2	1.6
Nonsecretory	2	1.6
TOTAL	98	77.8
Macroglobulinemia	18	14.2
Heavy chain disease	1	0.8
Monoclonal gammopathy without myeloma		
IgG	8	6.4
IgA	1	0.8
TOTAL	9	7.2

*Murphy, W. M., and Deodhar, S. D.: Studies in multiple myeloma. I. Characteristics by immunoglobulin class. Cleveland Clin. Quart. *40*:2, 1973.

light chain typing of M-components, and quantification of light chains. Since the normal concentration of immunoglobulins reveals a 2:1 ratio of K-L types of chains, when a serum with an abnormal protein is studied with L-chain specific antiserum, it is possible to estimate K-L type chains ratio and hence normal and presumably active antibodies (Fig. 9–42). This ratio is increased severalfold in many monoclonal gammopathies, indicating possible nonactive antibodies as globulins. Murphy and Deodhar (1973) have reported the occurrence and distribution of light chains (both free and in association with intact immunoglobulin molecules) and their prognostic significance in 98 patients with multiple myeloma (Table 9–19). Murphy and Deodhar's study of 126 cases of monoclonal gammopathies were classified as shown in Table 9–18. IgE as an M-component has also been described in multiple myeloma, so all five classes have been identified with this disease, although for all practical purposes, IgG and IgA comprise M-components in almost all cases of myeloma.

M-COMPONENTS. "Monoclonal component" or "M-component" is not peculiar to multiple myeloma or Waldenström's macroglobulinemia. It also occurs in two other groups of patients: (1) "secondary" patients with a specific disease other than multiple myeloma or macroglobulinemia (e.g., liver disease, lymphoma, chronic lymphocytic leukemia, carcinoma, subacute bacterial endocarditis, systemic lupus erythematosus, cold agglutinins, pulmonary tuberculosis, penicillin hypersensitivity, and cold urticaria); and (2) idiopathic—no underlying disease detectable. Abramson and Shattil (1973) found among 59 hospitalized patients: 18 (30 per cent) with a diagnosis of multiple myeloma or macroglobulinemia; "secondary," 24 patients (41 per cent); and idiopathic (essential), 17 (29 per cent). The majority of patients in the idiopathic group and 15 in the secondary group had M-components under 2.5 gm. per dl.; however, three patients in the myeloma-macroglobulinemia group were also in that range. All M-components above 4 gm. were associated with the myeloma-macroglobulinemia group. Table 9–20 shows the initial M-component size and heavy chain class. It should be noted that of the myeloma group, nine had an IgG component, one had IgA, and four had light chains only in serum or urine. However, four patients had an M-component in serum and concomitant Bence Jones proteinuria. In the secondary group, 11 of 21 patients had IgM M-components. This was the highest in the liver disease subgroup, in which five of seven patients had a IgM M-component. In the idiopathic or essential group (benign monoclonal), the gammopathy frequency of distribution of immunoglobulin class (IgG, IgA,

Table 9–19. CHARACTERISTICS OF MULTIPLE MYELOMA*

Ig CLASS	NO. CASES	MEAN AGE	LIGHT CHAINS κ	LIGHT CHAINS λ	BONE LESIONS	SERUM M-PROTEIN MOBILITY γ	SERUM M-PROTEIN MOBILITY β	ANEMIA	CHARACTERISTIC BONE MARROW
IgG	43	64	31	12	31	39	4	37	36
IgA	27	60	13	14	19	13	12	23	27
Bence Jones	24	55	10	12	21	1	—	24	20

*From Murphy, W. M., and Deodhar, S. D.: Cleveland Clin. Quart. *40*:3, 1973.

Table 9–20. INITIAL M-COMPONENT SIZE AND HEAVY CHAIN CLASS*

	INITIAL M-COMPONENT 2.5 gm./100 ml. (NO. OF CASES/ TOTAL CASES)	HEAVY CHAIN CLASS (NO. OF CASES†)		
		IgG	IgA	IgM
Multiple myeloma	3/15	9	1	–
Waldenström's macroglobulinemia	0/3	–	–	3
Idiopathic	12/17	9	4	2
Secondary	15/24	9	1	11
Liver Disease		2	0	5
Lymphoma		2	1	2
Chronic lymphocytic leukemia		0	0	2
Carcinoma		2	0	0
Subacute bacterial endocarditis		1	0	1
Cold agglutinins		0	0	1
Systemic lupus erythematosus		1	0	0
Penicillin hypersensitivity		1	0	0
Total		27	6	16

*Abramson, N., and Shattil, S. J.: J.A.M.A. *223*:156, 1973.
†Four patients with myeloma had light chains only in the serum or urine.

IgM) was 9:4:2; i.e., rather similar to related quantities of these classes in normal serum. Just as M-components can progress or evolve over a course of a year to malignant monoclonal gammopathy, other patients may survive for years with M-components and display no underlying disease. This is especially true in elderly patients.

Asymptomatic M-components or M-type protein abnormalities are more commonly observed in elderly subjects, many of whom have a background of tuberculosis, syphilis, or chronic biliary tract disease or a nonreticular neoplasm, especially of the large bowel, breast, oral, pharyngeal, and biliary tract carcinomas. Osserman (1971) has indicated that there is increasing evidence that certain plasma cell dyscrasias may be induced by diverse forms of protracted reticuloendothelial stimuli and, hence, a careful search for an occult infection or neoplasm should be periodically carried out in all patients with asymptomatic M-components with particular attention to the bowel and biliary tracts. Osserman prefers the terminology "plasma cell dyscrasia of unknown significance" to "premyeloma" or essential or benign monoclonal gammopathy or even idiopathic, because one can tell, if the patient lives long enough, whether the condition is truly benign or essential or develops a plasma cell dyscrasia. Finally, M-components or diffuse hyperglobulinemia or both have been observed in several cases of monocytic leukemia not associated with myeloma. They are often seen in patients who have had protracted chronic illnesses, especially chronic pulmonary infections, tuberculosis, and osteomyelitis similar to that found in plasma cell dyscrasias. Furthermore, monocytic leukemia develops late in the course of a small but significant number of cases of long-standing plasma cell myelomas, usually several years after effective control of the myeloma.

The hypogammaglobulinemia that prevails in the presence of an M-component for the myeloma-macroglobulinemia group is much less likely to be present in the "secondary" or idiopathic categories with M-components. Finally, in view of the fact that myeloma may occur without a large M-component and the M-component may be found in the absence of manifest disease, the use of laboratory test results as pathognomonic criteria is hazardous. Hence, clinical evidence is essential for a valid diagnosis, which should not be based solely upon the presence of the protein abnormality and plasma cell infiltration of bone marrow. Furthermore, a correct diagnosis is important since the idiopathic or essential variety of M-component is associated infrequently with disease, while the secondary M-component does not require chemotherapy but may disappear. Furthermore, when more sensitive techniques than paper or cellulose acetate electrophoresis (e.g., agarose-gel) are used for screening, more small M-components will be detected; then one is likely to encounter specimens of serum which display M-components from the idiopathic and/or secondary categories more frequently than the myeloma-macroglobulin groups, as reported by Abramson and Shattil (1973).

Bence Jones Proteins in Urine and Serum. Bence Jones protein and light chain (kappa and lambda) are synonymous terms. In regard to Bence Jones protein in urine (L-chains – kappa or lambda), concentration of the urine may be essential to characterize the urine protein on electrophoresis. The same relative homogeneity and electrophoretic mobility ranging from slow gamma through beta into the alpha-2 mobility range is observed on urine electrophoresis for Bence Jones proteins. Indeed, urine electrophoresis is a more reliable method for detection than the usual heat precipitation procedures. Bence Jones proteinuria occurs in a lesser percentage (10 to 20 per cent) of macroglobulinemia cases than of multiple myeloma (50 to 60 per cent). It should also be noted that Bence Jones proteinemia is usually not detectable by conventional electrophoresis, although it is always demonstrable by the more sensitive immunoelectrophoresis when Bence Jones proteinuria is present. In regard to multiple myeloma, about half the patients will have demonstrable Bence Jones proteinuria in addition to an M-component. The myeloma variant displaying Bence Jones proteinuria exclusively will occur in less than 20 per cent of the cases of myeloma and, in general, the Bence Jones protein will also be detectable in the serum.

With regard to heavy (H) chain (Fc fragment) disease, because these proteins are relatively larger than Bence Jones protein, their renal clearance is much less and they are retained in the serum in relatively high concentrations to be detected by conventional electrophoretic analyses. However, the abnormal serum and urinary protein peaks are of identical mobility and electrophoretically somewhat more polydisbursed than the abnormal peaks in other plasma cell dyscrasias. Since the urinary protein pattern is indistinguishable from the patterns observed with Bence Jones proteinuria, identification of the abnormal protein as related to the H-chain (Fc fragment) and unrelated Bence Jones proteins or light chains must be accomplished with appropriate radial immunodiffusion techniques utilizing monospecific sera accordingly; i.e., light chain sera (kappa and lambda) as well as γM, γG, or γA. The use of γD or γE antisera may be necessary when characterization has not been defined with aforementioned sera.

It should be stressed that in "benign" monoclonal gammopathy, the amount of Bence Jones proteinuria does not exceed 60 mg. per liter in most instances, which is lower than in multiple myeloma or macroglobulinemia. It should be stressed that abnormal proteins identical to those found in malignant plasmacytic, lymphocytic disorders also appear in the urine in other than malignant conditions.

Multiple myeloma is characterized by the development of painful bone tumors, soft tissue tumor masses disseminated widely, pathologic fractures, and anemia. The M-component is most often IgG or, less frequently, IgA or Bence Jones and rarely IgD (Table 9–18). In some patients without a myeloma-type globulin, their normal serum gammaglobulin is decreased markedly, but urine contains large amounts of Bence Jones protein (L chain). L chains in urine (or when present in serum) are either kappa (κ) or lambda (λ); presumably, they result from excessive synthesis in malignant cell (rather than breakdown of molecules in the serum) and appear in addition to serum M-component or as the sole protein abnormality. Light chain disease then refers to a variant of multiple myeloma in which κ or λ is the sole protein abnormality. Murphy and Deodhar (1973) emphasize that at least some malignant IgG- and IgA-producing plasma cells synthesizing lambda chains are more likely to make excessive amounts than those producing kappa chains. Furthermore, renal complications of multiple myeloma have been related to the amount and duration of free light chains excreted. Although macroglobulinemia (greater than 5 to 10 per cent macroglobulins) has been observed in several diseases (neoplastic, collagen, amyloidosis, cirrhosis, and chronic infections), *Waldenström's primary macroglobulinemia* is characterized by lymphadenopathy, anemia, hepatosplenomegaly and large amounts of monoclonal macroglobulin (IgM) in the serum, apparently produced by abnormally proliferating lymphocytes (Bhoopalam *et al.*, 1971). Since there are a pair of light chains (either κ type of the λ type), the macroglubulin in the serum reflects either $(\mu_2\ \kappa_2)_5$ or $(\mu_2\ \lambda_2)_5$. Bence Jones protein is present in 20 to 30 per cent of such patients (κ or λ). Macroglobulinemia has variable morphologic manifestations, i.e., peripheral lymphocytosis or normal numbers of lymphocytes and bone marrow with characteristic lymphocytic infiltrations.

Viscosity-related manifestations of disease include circulatory impairment of central nervous system with transient variable neurologic deficits, cardiac decompensation, and pulmonary symptoms. Protein-protein interaction with formation of complexes between paraprotein or M-component and coagulation factors undoubtedly contributes to bleeding diathesis.

Of the M-proteins, IgM is the most likely to give rise to thrombosis, bleeding diathesis, and hyperviscosity syndrome. IgA and IgG type M-proteins can also give rise to these conditions, but a much higher level of protein is usually required to produce similar symptoms. Occasionally an IgA or IgG paraprotein will have physicochemical properties similar to an IgM-paraprotein, and even here the severity of symptoms will be less than in cases of IgM-paraprotein of comparable levels (MacKenzie *et al.*, 1970).

Chronic recurrent infections are common

in both myeloma and primary macroglobulinemia. This susceptibility may be attributed to a decreased concentration of IgG or a lesser amount of immunologically competent IgG found on electrophoresis in both these diseases despite hyper-γ-globulinemia with M-component.

In addition to appropriate hematologic studies, including a bone marrow examination after serum protein electrophoresis, immunoelectrophoresis and radial immunodiffusion are necessary for an accurate diagnosis (Fig. 9–45). Serum uric acid and erythrocyte sedimentation rate are often elevated; additional laboratory abnormalities may include false positive serologic reactions and positive rheumatoid factors as well as increased serum viscosity and presence of cryoglobulins.

The rare *heavy chain disease* reflects an aberration of IgG synthesis in which an excess of heavy chains or portions thereof are produced and secreted into the circulation (Murphy *et al.*, 1972). Clinically, it simulates a lymphoma in middle-aged men with lymphadenopathy, hepatosplenomegaly, and mild anemia, invariably associated with moderate to severe proteinuria and hyperglobulinemia. Although picturesque, the name "heavy chain disease" is probably inaccurate, as the abnormal protein resembles more the Fc fragment of IgG. Its characterization requires sensitive and specific immunochemical techniques to differentiate it from Bence Jones protein and other L chain (κ, λ) polypeptides, as well as define it as γ-chain disease, α-chain disease or μ-chain disease. Lee and his colleagues (1971), in reporting a case of "heavy chain disease" of the μ-chain (μ) variety, characterize a syndrome of slowly progressive chronic lymphocytic leukemia with hepatosplenomegaly, pathologic fractures, apparent hypogammaglobulinemia, Bence Jones proteinuria, and an abnormal negatively charged IgM fragment on serum immunoelectrophoresis. They ascribe the biochemical defect to a lack of proper coupling in the cells rather than an overproduction of heavy chains, as in the case of alpha- and gamma-type heavy chain diseases.

Amyloidosis clinically manifests itself by multiple system involvement in association with a variety of chronic diseases (e.g., tuberculosis and osteomyelitis). In this secondary type, amyloid infiltration of liver, kidneys, and, rarely, adrenal cortices can produce hepatosplenomegaly, nephrosis, or hypoadrenocorticism. In the primary type unassociated with chronic diseases, heart, gastrointestinal tract, and skin, infiltrations may cause cardiac failure or a malabsorptive syndrome. In addition to the hematologic studies mentioned above, a biopsy of tongue or rectum may reveal a typical infiltrate that stains with Congo red or thioflavine T. Immunochemical as well as other appropriate chemical determinations may show an immunoglobulin deficiency, Bence Jones proteinuria, or specific hepatic and renal functional alterations. Osserman (1971) has emphasized that evidence of a plasma cell dyscrasia can be found in the majority of cases of apparently "primary" amyloidosis and, furthermore, secondary amyloidosis in certain cases is associated with a plasmacytic dyscrasia.

Lichen Myxedematosus. This is a rare skin disease, chronic in nature, in which an unusual paraprotein has been found rather consistently. It appears to be always IgG-L without Bence Jones proteinuria, but with a serum paraprotein level that would qualify as a benign paraprotein. With immunofluorescent studies, IgG has been localized in the skin lesions which also conform to type L; hence, it is suggested that IgG-L is a monoclonal antibody related to the skin disease in a manner similar to the way IgM-K appears to relate to primary cold agglutinin disease.

Cryoglobulins. This term refers to serum globulins that precipitate on cooling (4° C.) and redissolve on warming; these serum globulins may occur in a variety of clinical disorders. The immunoglobulin constituents identified in cryoglobulins have been either IgG or, occasionally, IgM alone, but more frequently they have consisted of mixtures of immunoglobulins and complement components (Barnett, 1970). Serologic factors that have been demonstrated to be either present or concentrated selectively in cryoglobulins include the following: anti-IgG "rheumatoid" factors, antinuclear antibodies, anticytomegalovirus antibodies, anti-erythrocyte antibodies ("cold agglutinins"), and anticomplementary activity. Several mechanisms have been proposed for mixtures of immunoglobulins precipitating at reduced temperature, which suggest that IgG components may represent autoantigens and IgM, IgG or IgA components may represent the antibodies; these mixtures of autoantigens and autoantibodies plus certain cofactors including complement may then precipitate at reduced temperatures (Barnett, 1970). In some cases it has been speculated that their presence may be a manifestation of immune complex disease.

Idiopathic cryoglobulinemia is characterized by cryoglobulins in the blood of patients who frequently present with purpura, urticaria, Raynaud's phenomenon, or gangrene. However, cryoglobulinemia has been demonstrated in a large number of clinical conditions, including leukemia, multiple myeloma, macroglobulinemia, systemic lupus erythematosus, polyarteritis nodosa, rheumatoid arthritis, Sjögren's syndrome, hemolytic anemia, polycythemia vera, subacute bacterial endocarditis, infectious mononucleosis, syphilis, cytomegalovirus mononucleosis, acute glomerulonephritis, hepatitis, cirrhosis, and coronary artery disease. Secondary cryoglobulinemia is the term used to describe cryoglobulinemia present in these conditions. There are several techniques for study of serum in these conditions to further characterize the cryoglobulins beyond their precipitation at 4° C. (Gokcen, 1966; Cawley, 1969).

Nonprotein Nitrogenous (NPN) Compounds

The more abundant NPN constituents referred to previously include urea, creatinine, creatine, uric acid, ammonium, and amino acids. The NPN as a determination has been virtually replaced by measurements for the individual compounds because of simplicity and precision of methodology, as well as clinicopathologic significance. Amino acids are reviewed in Chapter 2, while ammonia is considered in Chapter 13.

Biochemistry. Urea, the major end product of protein metabolism in man, is derived principally from the amino groups of amino acids. The liver is probably the major organ capable of urea synthesis via the ornithine cycle described previously (p. 565).

The molecular weight of urea ($NH_2 \cdot CO \cdot NH_2$) is 60. The urea molecule contains two nitrogen atoms with a total weight of 28. The concentration of urea in biologic fluids is usually expressed as urea nitrogen in the United States but as urea in European nations. This fact should be kept in mind in reviewing the literature. The urea nitrogen of blood is often referred to as BUN. Conversion of a urea nitrogen value to urea is performed by multiplying BUN by $\frac{60}{28}$ (2.14); thus, a BUN of 20 mg./dl. is equal to a urea of 20×2.14 or 42.80 mg./dl. Therefore, the concentration of BUN is approximately one-half that of urea.

After urea is formed in the liver, it passes into the blood and is excreted in the urine. Urea diffuses freely through capillary walls and cell membranes. It is present in virtually identical concentrations per unit of water in extracellular and intracellular fluids, i.e., plasma, serum, cerebrospinal fluid, saliva, perspiration, and intestinal secretions. However, the concentration of urea nitrogen in whole blood varies with the proportion (per cent) of erythrocytes in blood owing to the difference in per cent water concentration of plasma (serum) and erythrocytes. Because of this variability in water concentration between cells and plasma, serum or plasma is preferred for the BUN analysis.

BUN depends upon the relationship between urea production (protein ingestion and catabolism) and urea excretion; the minor amount of urea destroyed by microorganisms in the intestinal tract may be disregarded. The normal BUN ranges from 6 to 22 mg./dl. of plasma and varies directly with the nitrogen intake. Variation in protein intake contributes to the spread of normal range that is not eliminated by specimen collection under the usual fasting conditions. A second important factor contributing to the wide normal range of BUN arises from variations in urine volume, which in turn is dependent upon the fluid intake of the individual.

Urea is excreted by glomerular filtration. About 40 per cent of the urea in the glomerular filtrate is reabsorbed by the tubules. The extent of urea reabsorption by passive diffusion depends on the amount of water reabsorbed and on the urea concentration gradient between the glomerular filtrate and renal tubular intracellular as well as interstitial fluid. Because the gradient is larger and time for back-diffusion or passive reabsorption is longer when the urine volume is minimal, the rate of urea removal or clearance from the blood increases with the urine volume excreted or rate of urine formation (urine flow). A minimal water intake by individuals with a normal protein ingestion contributes to the spread at the extreme normal upper limits of BUN.

Urea constitutes about one-half (25 gm.) of the total urinary solids. Its excretion is related to protein intake and catabolism. Normally urea comprises 80 to 90 per cent of the total urinary nitrogen. The ability to concentrate NPN constituents ($50 \times$ urea, $20 \times$ uric acid, and $50 \times$ creatinine as high as in the blood) and other solutes constitutes one of the most important renal functions. Compensation for a diminution in this renal concentration function is attained by the elimination of increased quantities of water (osmotic diuresis) with a large urine volume of low specific gravity. When this compensatory mechanism fails or with concomitant dehydration, blood urea nitrogen (BUN) rises to pathologic levels referred to as azotemia.

The hormones that influence protein metabolism may also contribute to variations in BUN. Androgens and growth hormone by virtue of their anabolic effect may lower BUN, while the corticosteroids and an excess of thyroxine as well as a deficiency of insulin may contribute to an elevated BUN by enhancement of catabolism.

Clinicopathologic Correlations. Elevations of BUN referred to as azotemia may be produced by dehydration, with a decreased plasma volume. In gastrointestinal diseases, especially with intestinal obstruction, azotemia may be striking. When there is massive hemorrhage into the gastrointestinal tract, the azotemia caused by a low blood plasma volume is a more important factor than that produced by high protein (hemoglobin) "meal" (Young *et al.*, 1957). In such clinical conditions, a decrease in plasma volume secondary to dehydration, blood loss, hypotension, or shock is often referred to as prerenal azotemia. A decrease in renal blood flow is a consequence of a diminished plasma volume. Prerenal deviation of water has a profound effect on BUN retention that is most striking in the presence of renal disease. Two groups of conditions that invariably contribute to prerenal deviation of water include those producing edema and those resulting in dehydration. Edema may accompany myocardial insufficiency with congestive heart failure, while hypoproteinemia may occur with nephrosis or malnutrition. Dehydration can result from protracted vomiting, profuse diarrhea, excessive perspiration (febrile disorders), and water deprivation.

Excessive protein catabolism may also increase NPN constituents, especially urea nitrogen. This occurs most often with impairment of renal function or reduced renal excretion of the NPN constituents. Conditions that may be associated with excessive protein catabolism include the following: uncontrolled diabetes mellitus, thyrotoxicosis, adrenocortical hyperfunction, infections, and some neoplastic diseases.

In summary, BUN retention in the presence of renal disease depends essentially upon three factors: (1) prerenal deviation of water, (2) excessive protein catabolism, and (3) degree of renal functional impairment.

Pathologic lesions that may cause a decrease in renal function involve the following mechanisms: (1) decreased renal blood flow, (2) glomerular injury or destruction, (3) tubular injury or destruction, and (4) increased pressure in glomerular capsular space often associated with obstruction to the egress of urine such as a stricture, calculus or neoplasm.

One or more of these mechanisms is usually operative in virtually all clinically important forms of diffuse kidney diseases (see Chaps. 2 and 3, pp. 47, 89). Such mechanisms are also operative in congestive heart failure, arteriosclerosis or thrombosis, bilateral urinary tract obstruction, and hypotension (shock). Excessive tubular reabsorption of urea and several other NPN constituents may play a role in diseases producing acute tubular necrosis.

The only method by which the kidney can compensate for diminution in its concentrating ability is by the elimination of increased quantities of water with the urine, these being of large volume and low specific gravity. In the absence of extrarenal factors, BUN rises when the renal lesion fails to eliminate sufficient water to compensate for diminution in its power of concentration. Hence, with renal decompensation, the urine is consistently low in specific gravity, regardless of the volume of water eliminated. The nature and extent of the renal lesion (pathologic process) determines the degree of functional impairment and BUN retention. At normal rates of protein catabolism, an increase of the BUN above the normal range occurs when the glomerular filtration rate (GFR) is reduced to 30 to 40 per cent of normal, that is, a 60 to 70 per cent decrease in renal function.

Creatinine and urea are eliminated principally by glomerular filtration, but urea is partially reabsorbed by the tubules. The estimation of the serum BUN/creatinine ratio is useful in evaluating an increased BUN as to whether it is prerenal, renal, or postrenal. Elevated ratios result primarily from slow urine flow through the tubules, allowing for greater reabsorption of urea. For example, in obstructive uropathy, the increase in hydrostatic back pressure will slow urine flow in the tubules, allowing for greater urea absorption, but would not affect serum creatinine. Hence, an elevated ratio, greater than (>) 20, would be present. Table 9–21 characterizes further BUN/creatinine ratios (Sullivan *et al.*, 1972). Serum BUN/creatinine ratios may indicate the relative role of obstruction in cases of impaired renal function and be of practical value as a part of the differential renal function evaluation for hypertension (Marshall, 1964).

Uremia is a clinical syndrome resulting from severe reduction in renal excretory function; it reflects the end stage toward which all progressive renal diseases move. Uremia is characterized by variable degrees of severe azotemia, acidosis, water and electrolyte imbalance, lassitude, and mental depression that progresses to coma (Merrill and Hampers, 1970). The elevated BUN varies in magnitude but usually is in excess of 100 mg./dl. or approaching 200 mg./dl. with deep coma or stupor. The progressively rising but at times fluctuating

Table 9–21. SERUM BUN/CREATININE RATIOS IN VARIOUS CONDITIONS

BUN/CREATININE > 20×*	BUN/CREATININE < 10×*
Blood in GI tract	Chronic glomerulonephritis with protein deficiency
Dehydration	Overhydration
Early acute glomerulonephritis	Rapid rehydration
Intraperitoneal extravasation of urine	Repeated hemodialysis
Malignant nephrosclerosis	Severe hepatic insufficiency
Muscle wasting diseases	
Obstructive uropathy	
Prerenal underperfusion	
Severe tissue trauma	
Urinary-enteric fistula	

*× = times

BUN is in contrast to slower rising creatinine that rarely exceeds 20 mg./dl. and uric acid that in the absence of gout does not usually rise above 12 mg./dl. in chronic renal failure.

Although abnormally low levels of BUN have been attributed to liver failure, Gallagher and Seligson (1962) observed values of 5 mg./dl. or less in 1 per cent of 16,000 determinations; this is not a rare finding today, and its significance should not be overlooked. Low BUN values occurred in patients who were either rapidly rehydrated with solutions free of nitrogenous compounds after initial presentation with dehydration and in those who were overhydrated and were experiencing a diuresis. Low BUN levels were observed at the time of increasing urinary outflow and etiologically were attributed to low protein catabolism and increasing urine output with its concomitant increased elimination (clearance) of urea. Indeed these authors have suggested that a low BUN may be a good prognostic sign in that it indicates an adequate diuresis with good renal function. BUN is consistently low in pregnancy, and in eclampsia uric acid is a more sensitive NPN component reflection of disease than the BUN.

Methods. Urease, a very stable enzyme, is frequently employed for urea nitrogen measurements because of its absolute specificity. Indeed, it is a prototype for the use of enzymes as analytical reagents. The enzyme urease converts urea by hydrolysis ultimately to carbonic acid and NH_3.

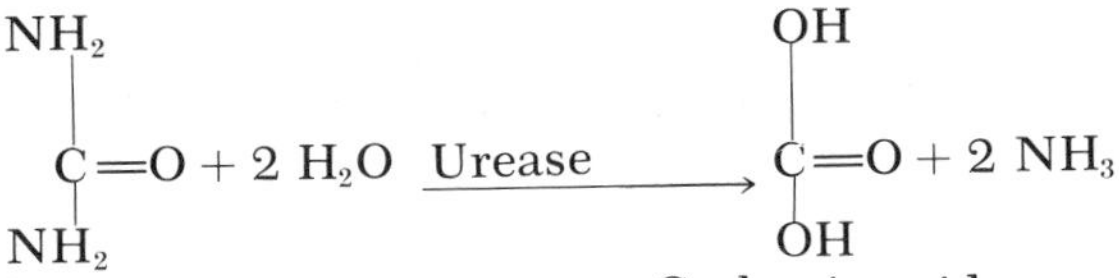

Urea Carbonic acid

Rigorous attention to requirements for an enzyme assay including temperature, pH, and time as well as contaminants must be followed.

The ammonia liberated is measured photometrically after reaction with phenol in the presence of hypochlorite (Berthelot reaction) or after nesslerization as shown at the bottom of this page.

While nesslerization techniques are widely used, methods employing Berthelot's reaction are becoming increasingly popular because of their greater sensitivity (Kaplan, 1965). Inaccurate results may be generated with Nessler's reagent unless meticulous attention is given to eliminating nitrogen contamination. Turbidity may also be a problem when the final reaction measurement is delayed or with some specimens. Although we have found a modification of Karr's method (1924) satisfactory for a manual procedure, the method of Chaney and Marbach (1962) is also recommended as a microanalytical method. In this procedure, urease liberates ammonia directly from an aliquot of specimen; the ammonia is measured after reaction with phenolhypochlorite (Berthelot's reaction) in the presence of sodium nitroprusside (catalyst); the stable blue color reaction product is determined photometrically. Creno *et al.* (1970) have described an automated micromeasurement of urea using urease and the Berthelot reaction.

Diacetyl monoxime reacts directly with urea as well as dibasic amino acids and perhaps other peptides that are present in insignificant quantities in normal blood. Manual and automated procedures have been developed. An acid solution and heat promote the reaction that usually incorporates an oxidant such as ferric ammonium sulfate to destroy hydroxylamine which may be formed. The alpha diketone reaction consists of the following:

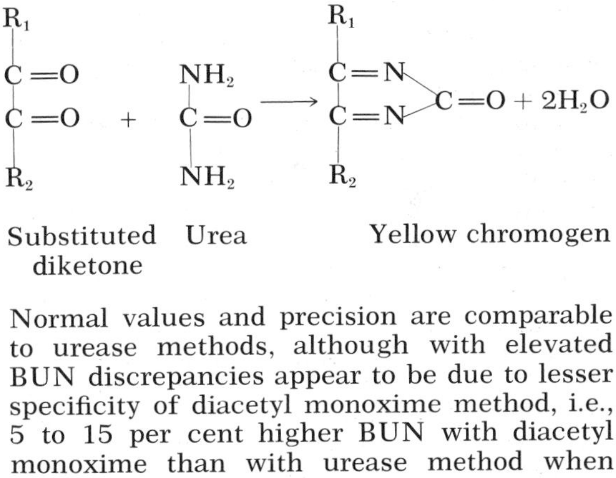

Substituted diketone Urea Yellow chromogen

Normal values and precision are comparable to urease methods, although with elevated BUN discrepancies appear to be due to lesser specificity of diacetyl monoxime method, i.e., 5 to 15 per cent higher BUN with diacetyl monoxime than with urease method when BUN exceeds 100 mg./dl.

In the method of Talke and Schubert (1965), ammonia liberated from urea following urease hydrolysis is combined with α-ketoglutaric acid in the presence of NADH and the enzyme glutamic acid dehydrogenase. The products of this reaction are glutamic

---

$$NH_4OH + 2\,(KI)_2HgI_2 + KOH \longrightarrow NH_2Hg_2I_3 + 5KI + 2H_2O$$

Nessler's salt — Ammonium dimercuric iodide, yellow orange

acid, water and NAD. The amount of NADH converted to NAD (read at 340 nm.) is proportional to the urea concentration as shown in the formula below.

This method has been automated and is available on several of the newer high speed batch instruments, such as the Du Pont Automatic Clinical Analyzer (ACA). Further information regarding selection of methodology with pitfalls and advantages may be found in several textbooks listed in references but especially Clinical Chemistry (R. J. Henry, 1964), Standard Methods of Clinical Chemistry (Kaplan, 1965), and October, 1966, Proficiency Test Service (Sunderman and Sunderman, 1972).

CREATINE AND CREATININE

Biochemistry. The synthesis of creatine from glycine and parts of two other amino acids (arginine and methionine) is a two-step enzymatic controlled process, as shown in Figure 9–48. Guanidoacetate (glycocyamine) is formed by transamidination primarily in the kidneys; this is a reversible reaction mediated by transamidinase which is subject to feedback inhibition of dietary creatine (Cantarow and Schepartz, 1967). Glycocyamine (guanidoacetate) is then methylated with a second reaction requiring transmethylase and activated methionine in the liver to form creatine (Fig. 9–48). Creatine in the free state and as phosphocreatine is distributed from liver via blood to muscle and brain with trace amounts in the urine. Phosphocreatine exists in high concentrations, especially in muscle, where it is an important form of high-energy phosphate storage. Creatinine is an anhydride of creatine formed by the two reactions shown in Figure 9–48. The spontaneous loss of phosphoric acid from phosphocreatine in muscle under physiologic conditions with ring closure is the major reaction that produces creatinine; the nonenzymatic slower reaction consisting of a loss of water from creatine also forms creatinine in muscle. Free creatinine appearing in the blood and urine is not reutilized. Creatinine is ultimately excreted in the urine at a remarkably constant rate. The formation of creatinine may represent a required preliminary step for excretion of creatine, since creatine is normally reabsorbed from the glomerular filtrate by renal tubules. Urinary creatinine, which under normal physiologic conditions represents glomerular filtration and active tubular excretion, is formed from creatine in rather constant amounts (women, 0.6 to 1.5 gm. and men, 1.0 to 2.0 gm. per 24-hour urine collection). Unlike urea it does not reflect dietary protein intake or urine volume; it is more related to creatine content of body or muscle mass. Creatinine output, however, is not constant in the same individual. In a study by Scott and Hurley (1968), the coefficient of variation averaged 10 per cent in the same individual and 29 per cent between individuals. Several other workers have also studied daily urinary creatinine excretion and have concluded that it is an unreliable measurement of the completeness or accuracy of a 24-hour urine specimen collection (Tocci *et al.*, 1972). Hence, the practice of using urinary creatinine excretion as a reference value for expressing rates of excretion of other urinary constituents leaves much to be desired; however, it is as reliable as anything we have available currently.

The blood levels of creatinine in normal subjects appear to be more constant than urinary excretion. It is also preferable to BUN, since it is virtually independent of protein metabolism and rate of urine formation under normal conditions. However, with substantial protein ingestion that includes a considerable quantity of meat and intensive exercise over extended periods, we have observed in healthy young men urinary creatinine excretion in the range of 2.5 to 2.7 gm. per 24-hour specimen but normal blood levels (0.6 to 1.2 mg./dl. of serum).

Clinicopathologic Correlations. The pathophysiologic changes described for BUN may also be applied to blood serum or plasma creatinine. Its variation in renal disease is also discussed in Chapter 3, where clearance is reviewed in detail. Because of its virtual independence from protein metabolism and hydration with resultant variation in urine volumes, the serum creatinine is preferable to BUN as a screening test for renal function evaluation. It appears to rise more slowly in the presence of renal disease than the BUN. It is less useful than the BUN to assess effectiveness of hemodialysis in the treatment of renal failure, since it does not decrease as rapidly as BUN.

Creatine is increased in the blood above normal range of 0.6 or less mg./dl. serum in the

$$\text{UREA} + 2\,H_2O \xrightarrow{\text{urease}} \text{CARBONIC ACID} + 2\,NH_3$$

$$NH_3 + \text{NADH} + \alpha\text{-ketoglutarate} \xrightarrow[\text{dehydrogenase}]{\text{glutamic acid}} \text{NAD} + H_2O + \text{L-glutamic acid}$$

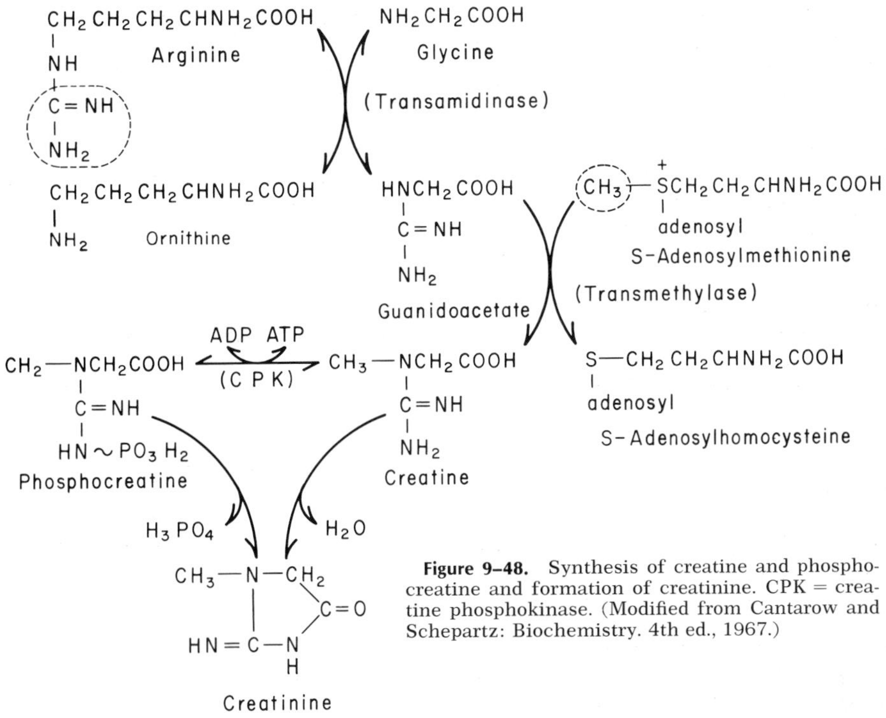

Figure 9–48. Synthesis of creatine and phosphocreatine and formation of creatinine. CPK = creatine phosphokinase. (Modified from Cantarow and Schepartz: Biochemistry. 4th ed., 1967.)

presence of severe muscle disease, including muscular dystrophy, atrophy, and myositis. In hyperthyroidism, serum creatine is also elevated; this may also be attributed to muscular atrophy with wasting observed in this disease.

Creatinuria occurs in children and in pregnancy, including puerperium, as well as in conditions described for hypercreatinemia; apparently the tubular reabsorption capacity is then exceeded. Urinary creatine elevations are more sensitive than serum creatine-creatinine ratios to identify muscle disease that reflects essentially a decrease in normal muscle mass. In view of the feedback mechanism described, in which the creatine level may repress the enzyme transamidinase (Fig. 9–48), it is not surprising that creatine measurements do not correlate well with degree or duration of muscle disease. The serum creatine phosphokinase (CPK) assay is the most sensitive reflection of certain types of muscular dystrophy and is described in Chapter 14.

Methods. Although a variety of methods have been described for the estimation of creatinine, the most popular method is based on the reaction described originally by Jaffé, in which creatinine treated with an alkaline picrate solution yields a bright orange-red solution (Sunderman and Sunderman, 1973a). Several modifications of the Jaffé reaction have been introduced to reduce sources of error associated with a lack of specificity and sensitivity to such variables as temperature, pH, and duration of reaction. Lloyd's reagent, an aluminum silicate, is frequently used to adsorb creatinine from a specimen in order to separate it from nonspecific chromogenic substances prior to Jaffé reaction. Preliminary treatment of urine by ether extraction eliminates the interference of glucose, protein, and acetone to increase specificity of Jaffé reaction.

A specific method for assay of urinary creatinine involves separation of creatinine from other urinary components by Sephadex gel filtration and measurement at 235 nm. More precise methods of creatinine measurement include the dinitrobenzoic acid and ortho-nitrobenzaldehyde methods. In our laboratory we prefer the latter method of Van Pilsum (1956) in which creatinine is converted to methylguanidine by ortho-nitrobenzaldehyde and the concentration of methylguanidine is determined colorimetrically by a modification of the Sakaguchi reaction. The method of Polar and Metcoff (1965), which depends on a strong cation exchange resin followed by a Jaffé reaction on the eluate, can be automated. This is recommended if precise creatinine clearance measurements are needed in diabetics or patients with high noncreatinine chromogens. An enzymatic (creatinine-amido-hydrolipase) method generates creatine which, in turn, is measured by creatine kinase coupled with pyruvate kinase and lactate dehydrogenase through NADH consumption. Creatininase, which converts creatinine to urea and methylhydantoin, also allows measurement of Jaffé chromogens before and after enzymatic destruction of creatinine (Sunderman and Sunderman, 1973a). With a specific enzyme method that destroys creatinine, Miller and Dubos (1937) found that all the Jaffé-reacting chromogenic material in normal urine was creatinine, as was 80 to 90 per cent in normal plasma.

Creatine is usually measured as creatinine subsequent to specimen treatment with heat for conversion of creatine to creatinine; in essence this requires two creatinine measurements per specimen and calculation of the difference between total creatinine (creatine + creatinine) and creatinine. Brinkerink (1961) has shown that the assumption of all creatine being converted to creatinine is incorrect; in the presence of high physiological concentrations of creatinine, a portion of creatine escapes conversion to creatinine. A specific method employing creatinine kinase is also available.

Terms such as "total chromogen," "alkaline picrate reactive material," and "apparent creatinine" have been employed to distinguish creatinine and "true creatinine." Extraction procedures as well as removal of interfering substances by adsorption with Lloyd's reagent in conjunction with the Jaffé reaction approach the estimation of true creatinine as determined by specific enzymatic methods. In our laboratories, the Jaffé reaction is applied according to a modification devised by Folin (1904) to reduce the variations produced in the development and stability of the chromogen by external and internal influences. A trichloroacetic acid (TCA) filtrate of serum or plasma is used without preliminary treatment. Appreciable amounts of noncreatinine chromogens are normally present in the erythrocytes, while only relatively small amounts are found in the serum or plasma. For this reason, serum or heparinized plasma is preferred to whole blood for creatinine analysis. According to Doolan *et al.* (1962), the noncreatinine chromogen does not introduce any greater variability in the measurement of serum creatinine within a single person or a group of persons than is encountered with the measurement of true creatinine, nor does it increase the range of normal values for clearance of creatinine as opposed to true creatinine.

It should be emphasized, however, that in the process of specimen collection attention should be given to the following substances, which may interfere with the Jaffé reaction: acetone, acetoacetic acid, ascorbic acid, pyruvic acid, barbiturates, phenolsulfonphthalein, Bromsulphalein, and protein. Since proteinuria is common in patients with renal disease, the urine should be tested. If positive, a 1 to 10 dilution should be made as in preparation for a protein-free filtrate. The specimen is then treated like a serum filtrate and the final result multiplied by 10, the dilution factor.

Furthermore, creatinine, especially in urine, is a relatively unstable compound; destruction can be reduced most effectively by short periods of urine collection and freezing of separated serum or urine.

The introduction of automated methods based on the Jaffé reaction for serum and urine creatinine determinations has resulted in greater clinical use of this measurement for blood, clearance studies, and a check (although not completely reliable, see p. 594) to monitor accuracy of 24-hour urine collections submitted for hormone assays.

URIC ACID

Gutman (1967) has pointed out that uric acid (urate) as a nitrogenous waste should be considered a product of amino acid metabolism by way of purines. The molecular structure of urate supports his view, since the carbons and nitrogens arise from several amino acids directly or indirectly.

Biochemistry. The catabolism of purine nucleosides to urate is illustrated in Figure 9–49. Hydrolysis of nucleic acids derived from cellular nucleoproteins yields mononucleotides, which are in turn broken down by phosphomonoesterases to the nucleosides, adenosine and guanosine. From the subsequent steps illustrated in Figure 9–49, it is apparent that xanthine is an important merger compound of the two nucleosides. The presence of xanthine oxidase in the liver and to a lesser extent in the intestinal mucosa underscores the hepatic site and role of urate synthesis in man. Uricase or urate oxidase is virtually absent in primates, so urate is indeed the major end product of nucleic acid or purine metabolism in man.

The concentration of urate in serum is approximately twice the concentration in erythrocytes. In serum or plasma, urate is present in two forms – free and bound to albumin; the affinity of urate for albumin differs in normal and pathologic serum (Morris, 1958). The normal adult urate pool (total uric acid) is about 1.0 gm., with normal serum values ranging from 2 to 7.8 mg./dl. Hence, a major portion of the body's urate exists in body fluids outside the vascular system. The daily urinary excretion of uric acid (0.4 to 0.8 gm.) reflects nucleoside (purine) catabolism. It is influenced by the dietary intake of purine-rich foods (e.g., meat, especially liver, and legumes, mushrooms, and spinach) as well as the rate of endogenous purine catabolism or intensity of nuclear metabolism. However, the urinary urate excretion does not account for the total

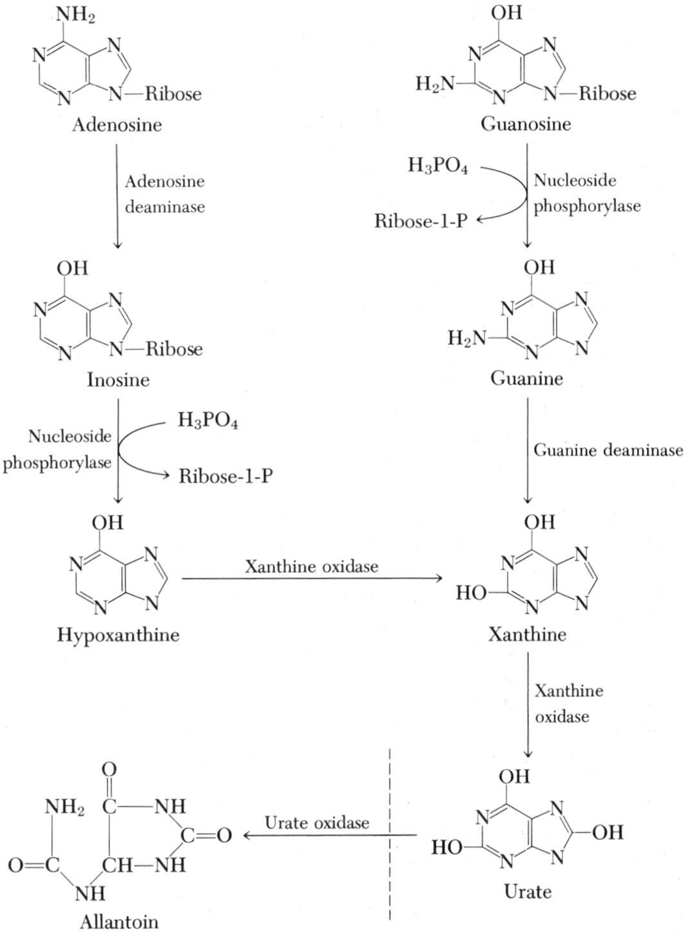

Figure 9–49. Catabolism of purine nucleosides. (From Cantarow and Schepartz: Biochemistry. 4th ed., 1967.)

quantity of urate formed or that converted from dietary purines, so there are probably other catabolic routes, one of which may be bacterial decomposition in the intestinal tract.

The renal excretion of uric acid has been investigated intensively, but remains controversial as to which mechanism is more important, i.e., filtration, reabsorption, or excretion. Uric acid clearance in the normal man is 10 per cent less than that of inulin. Data available suggest uric acid is freely filtered at the glomerulus; hence, in the tubule it must be reabsorbed and/or secreted. Berliner *et al.* (1950) have defined an approximate renal reabsorptive maximum of 15 mg. per minute. No sharp threshold was found above which uric acid was excreted and below which it was completely reabsorbed. At very low levels of filtered uric acid, uric acid excretion continued. Approximately 2 per cent of the filtered uric acid not reabsorbed accounts for 20 per cent of the urinary uric acid.

Various approaches are used to augment the excretion of uric acid by the kidney. One avenue has been to increase flow in the renal tubule and increase uric acid excretion by osmotic diuresis. Organic acids interfere with the tubular transport of uric acid. Drugs with a uricosuric action are probenecid, phenylbutazone, glucocorticoids, sulfinpyrazone and high doses of salicylates.

Yu and Gutman (1959) have shown that in most patients, salicylate causes urate retention at doses of up to 2 gm. per day and uricosuria at doses above 3 gm. per day. They investigated these effects of salicylates on discrete renal functions and concluded that a low concentration of unconjugated salicylate in the renal tubules may act by blocking a postulated tubular secretion of urate. Varying degrees of urate retention are produced in most gouty patients by moderate doses of salicylate. Indeed, a salicylate-induced urate retention may contribute to an erroneous diagnosis of gout in patients with rheumatoid arthritis.

An alkaline urine with a pH greater than 6.0 is desirable for patients prone to form uric acid calculi; urates are insoluble in more acid solutions. Also, alkalinization of the urine does not alter uric acid excretion, but accelerates the excretion of uricosuric agents such as probenecid. Of the alkali salts of the urate ion, ammonium salts are the least soluble; increasing solubility occurs with sodium, potassium, and lithium salts. While the urate ion form prevails in serum owing to the high pH, in urine, uric acid is the more common form.

Uric acid metabolism has been the subject of excellent reviews by Gutman and Yu (1965) and Rastegar and Thier (1972).

Clinicopathologic Correlations. In order to evaluate the clinical significance of a uric acid determination in a patient, an appreciation of its variability in different populations is necessary. For a detailed account of this subject, the reader is referred to the comprehensive report of Mikkelsen and his colleagues (1965), whose data were based upon the analysis of urate levels in a large population unselected as to gout or hyperuricemia. A trend for mean uric acid values was observed, with a rise as age increased and a difference in values between the sexes from the period of adolescence to the fifth decade. Many references list the upper limit of normal for serum uric acid as 6 mg./dl. for males and 5 mg./dl. for females. If these normal values are accepted, 21 per cent of all male subjects aged four years and over in the study quoted above had hyperuricemia (uric acid greater than 6 mg./dl.), while 22 per cent of all females aged four years and over had uric acids of 5 mg./dl. or greater. The data reported indicate clearly that age and sex have a definite bearing on serum uric acid concentration, but they also suggest that the arbitrary cut-off point for the diagnosis of hyperuricemia (which implies that an abnormal state exists in relation to uric acid) of 6 mg./dl. in males and 5 mg./dl. in females is too low. For these reasons, we have revised upward our normal values for serum uric acid, as suggested by the report of Brøchner-Mortensen, Cobb, and Rose (1963) on criteria for diagnosis of gout in surveys. Our revised normal values are as follows: males, 2.1 to 7.8 mg./dl.; females, 2.0 to 6.4 mg./dl.

In patients with renal failure, the uric acid level rises slowly as the GFR decreases. When the GFR is less than 10 ml./min., the filtered load of urate drops markedly. Also, the reabsorbing mechanism is defective along with the secretory mechanism. The defect in the secretory mechanism appears to be of greater significance in leading to hyperuricemia.

Serum uric acid may be considerably increased (two times normal) in starvation; this is due to accelerated tissue cell turnover and to decreased uric acid renal excretion, probably resulting from the acidosis that usually accompanies starvation. However, depletion of hepatic glycogen and the resulting gluconeogenesis (with formation of purine breakdown products) may explain the hyperuricemia of high fat diets, starvation, and nondiabetic ketosis. Diminished excretion with increased blood levels has also been observed in uremia as well as in nephritis and other conditions associated with obstruction or suppression of urinary flow. Violent muscular exercise may also raise the serum uric acid slightly. A transient serum uric acid elevation has been observed in pregnant women with the onset of labor. In eclampsia, the uric acid level is considerably elevated; the cause is not understood. In polycythemia, lobar pneumonia, and remissions in pernicious anemia, augmented nuclear catabolism (rapid cell turnover with nucleoprotein breakdown) probably contributes to serum uric acid elevations. Hyperuricemia may also be seen in coronary artery disease and hypertension due to physiological mechanisms not yet well defined.

On a purine-free diet, some uric acid is constantly excreted in the urine (0.2 to 0.5 gm. per day for an adult). The intensity of nuclear metabolism is frequently reflected in the urinary uric acid output. Thus, in polycythemia vera or in leukemia and therapy of leukemia and lymphoma with cytotoxic agents, there is considerable nuclear catabolism, and uric acid excretion is markedly increased. Uric acid calculi may ensue unless appropriate pH regulation of the urine is maintained together with adequate hydration.

Primary gout, as an undefined inborn error of metabolism, is characterized by hyperuricemia, recurrent attacks of acute arthritis, and eventually by tophaceous deposits of urate (tophi) in many instances (Gutman, 1967). Middle-aged men are most frequently the victims of primary gout. Two distinct groups of gouty patients have been described. One consists of patients with a moderately increased total pool size of uric acid and a normal turnover rate, and a second with a markedly increased pool size (>2400 mg.) and turnover rate (>1200 mg./day). Allopurinol reduces urate production by inhibiting xanthine oxidase and is used for treatment in both groups. Uricosuric agents should not be used in the increased pool group, as stones are easily precipitated in the early course of treatment.

In secondary gout, similar symptoms may be acquired. This may be observed in conditions in which there is an expansion and increased turnover of the nucleic acid pool. Polycythemia vera and other myeloproliferative disorders, including leukemia, have been reported as examples infrequently as well as the treatment of malignant tumors, renal failure, and psoriasis. A variety of drugs (e.g., thiazide diuretics) and conditions mentioned above must also be considered in the presence of hyperuricemia, which may be asymptomatic as well as familial. In addition to elevated blood urate levels, uric acid may also be demonstrated in the tophi, joint fluid, and synovial tissue of patients with gout (Chap. 25).

Hypouricemia, usually unimportant and rare, is a major finding in Fanconi's syndrome and may occur as a result of treatment of hyperuricemia. With xanthinuria, a very rare inborn error (deficiency of xanthine oxidase), the block results in elevated urinary excretion of xanthine, which may lead to xanthine stones.

Methods. The reference method for measurement of uric acid in biologic fluids employs the enzyme uricase and ultraviolet light absorption at 293 nm. (Liddle, Seegmiller, and Laster, 1959). Buffered enzyme at an alkaline pH and serum are the reactants. The initial uric acid absorption is followed over a 20-minute period, during which time urate is converted to its principal product allantoin, which does not absorb light in the ultraviolet range. The decrease in absorption is proportional to the urate present originally. If the assay is performed with appropriate controls, inhibitors in the specimen and other possible sources of error, such as an inactive enzyme preparation or an excess of substrate, will be identified. The precision and accuracy of this method as well as specificity are excellent, but it is a time-consuming procedure. Uricase methods yield values about 0.1 to 0.4 mg./dl. less than those obtained by phosphotungstic acid assays.

A vast array of analytical procedures are based upon the reducing properties of urate. Practically all the photometric methods depend on phosphotungstic acid reduction; tungstic acid protein-free filtrate of serum or plasma eliminates interference due to reducing agents (glutathione and ergothioneine) of erythrocytes. The ascorbic acid interference of fresh serum is eliminated by more sensitive cyanide methods, as well as by sufficient incubation with adequate carbonate. In view of the potential hazards of cyanide, instability of cyanide solution, and high blank values, it has been virtually abandoned in uric acid methods despite greater sensitivity. However, with the addition of sufficient carbonate to bring the final pH of reaction mixture between 10.0 and 10.4, full color development has been achieved (Caraway, 1963b, 1966). Jung and Parekh's (1970) modification employs phosphotungstic acid as the protein precipitant, trisodium phosphate to destroy serum nonurate chromogens and a triethanolamine-carbonate-urea reagent to increase stability of the final colored solution; the authors report 99 per cent recovery of uric acid in serum by their method. A combination of enzyme and photometric techniques has been incorporated into an automated procedure (Morgenstern, Flor, Kaufman, and Klein, 1966). Additional approaches into uric acid methodology include chromatography, ion exchange resins, and polyacrylamide gels.

CARBOHYDRATES

Carbohydrates, organic compounds containing the elements carbon, hydrogen, and oxygen, serve as an important source of energy. Chemically they are aldehyde or ketone derivatives of the polyhydric alcohols or compounds that yield these derivatives on hydrolysis. Glucose is the most important sugar or carbohydrate in medical chemistry. However, it cannot be appreciated fully without a review of carbohydrates that are intimately related although less frequently clinically significant.

Classification. Monosaccharides have the empirical formula $C_nH_{2n}O_n$, or $C_n(H_2O)_n$. These simple sugars are the basic units of more complex carbohydrates, including disaccharides, trisaccharides, and polysaccharides. The monosaccharides are the ultimate hydrolytic products of these higher molecular weight carbohydrates. The number of carbon atoms and presence of an aldehyde or ketone functional group in the molecule permit subdivision of this carbohydrate class as shown at the bottom of this page.

	FORMULA	EXAMPLES OF ALDO SUGAR	EXAMPLES OF KETO SUGAR
Triose (3 carbons)	$C_3H_6O_3$	glyceraldehyde (glycerose)	dihydroxyacetone
Tetrose (4 carbons)	$C_4H_8O_4$	erythrose	erythrulose
Pentose (5 carbons)	$C_5H_{10}O_5$	ribose	ribulose
Hexose	$C_6H_{12}O_6$	glucose	fructose

Organic compounds with carbon atoms having no plane of symmetry have isomers which differ only in their spatial relationship. These nonsuperimposable mirror image forms are called stereoisomers. The number of isomers given by a compound with N asymmetric carbon atoms is 2^n. Thus, a compound like glucose, with four asymmetric carbon atoms, has 16 stereoisomeric forms. The penultimate carbon atom of monosaccharides is the one adjacent to the carbon atom having a primary alcohol function. In ketoses this refers to the primary alcohol farthest from the keto function. The configuration of the penultimate carbon atom determines whether the molecule belongs to the D-series or the L-series. Most naturally occurring monosaccharides possess the D-configuration, as the following hexoses:

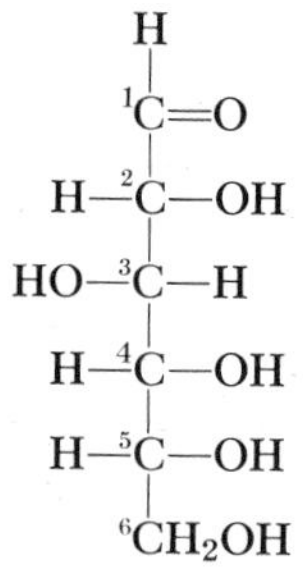

D-Glucose
(aldose)

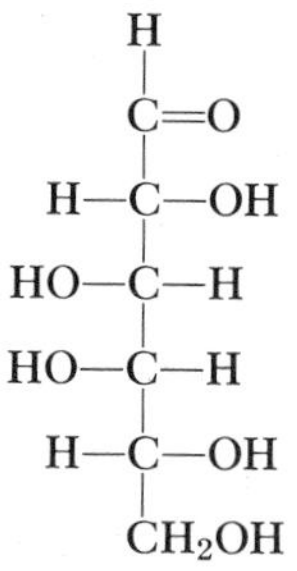

D-Galactose
(aldose)

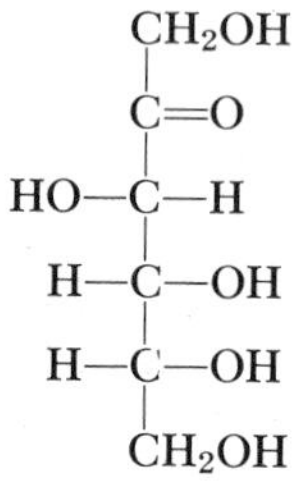

D-Fructose
(ketose)

Carbon number 5 is adjacent to the primary alcohol of each hexose; the hydroxyl (OH) group is on the right side of this carbon in the above D-series. Because glucose and galactose differ from one another only in configuration around a single carbon atom, i.e., number 4 in regard to position of hydroxyl group, they are called epimers. While glucose and galactose are aldohexoses, fructose is a ketohexose that lacks an aldehyde group and is therefore not a reducing compound, in contrast to the other two monosaccharides. In addition to the open chain formulas shown above, cyclic formulas are used to further characterize carbohydrates.

Carbohydrates which yield more than two molecules of monosaccharides are further classified as follows:

Disaccharides with the general formula $C_n(H_2O)_{n-1}$ may be hydrolyzed to two molecules of the same or of different monosaccharides. Three commonly occurring disaccharides are sucrose, lactose, and maltose.

Oligosaccharides yield two to 10 monosaccharides on hydrolysis. Polysaccharides contain more than 10 monosaccharide units, e.g., glycogen, starch, and dextrins.

Maltose is a disaccharide composed of two glucose molecules united by an α-1,4′ glycosidic linkage that may be visualized in a cyclic formula as follows:

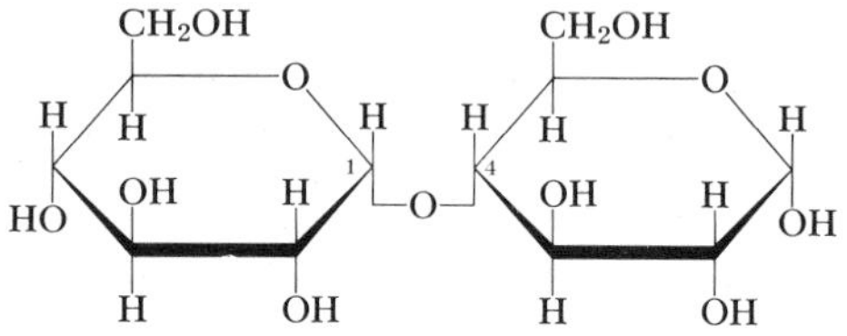

Maltose

The alpha (α) or beta (β) linkage refers to the spacial configuration of the glucosidic hydroxyl group on the carbon 1 atom when glucose is in the ring structure. Thus, in a cyclic formula for glucose, the hydroxyl group on carbon 1 is below the plane in the α-configuration and is above the plane of the ring in the β-configuration.

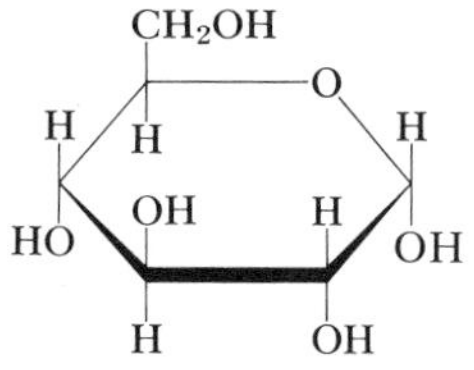

α-D-Glucopyranose

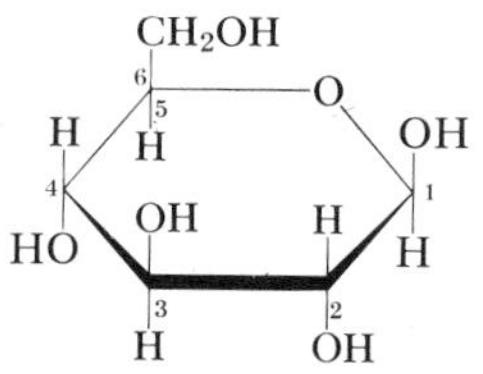

β-D-Glucopyranose

This type ring structure is the result of an intramolecular condensation of an aldehyde group and a hydroxyl group, yielding a structure known as a hemiacetal. When the hydrogen of the hemiacetal hydroxyl is replaced by a noncarbohydrate group, the compound formed is a glycoside. The substituting group is called the aglycone, and the sugar radical is the glycosyl group. Enzymes that cleave glycosidic linkages are known as glycosidases and may be alpha or beta in specificity.

Starch, composed of many molecules of glucose in chains, is the most common food source of carbohydrate, e.g., potatoes and cereals. It yields only glucose on complete hydrolysis and is formed of an α-glucosidic chain. Starch contains mostly amylose as straight-chain α-1,4 glucosidic linkages, while amylopectin has highly branched chains with many α-1,6 and α-1,4 glucosidic linkages. Branching occurs at α-1,6 linkages:

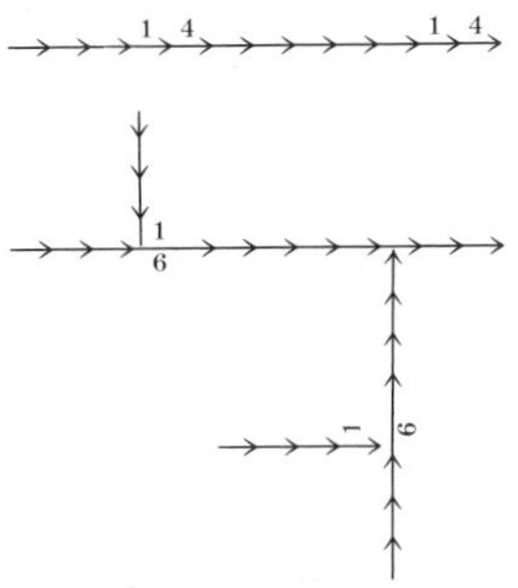

Glycogen is a polysaccharide similar to the amylopectin fraction of starch, except that it has an even higher degree of branching. It is often referred to as animal starch and in humans is concentrated in the liver and muscle as a storage form of carbohydrate for energy.

GLUCOSE

Metabolism. A review of glucose metabolism is essential in order to appreciate blood glucose concentration variations that may reflect primary abnormalities of carbohydrate metabolism as well as secondary abnormalities accompanying other diseases.

Digestion and Absorption. Enzymes (amylase, disaccharidases) liberated by salivary glands, the small intestine, and pancreas break down starch, the major polysaccharide ingested, and disaccharides (maltose, lactose, and sucrose) to hexoses (glucose, fructose, and galactose) or pentoses. By active transport (sodium dependent) and, to a lesser extent, simple diffusion (concentration gradient) monosaccharides are absorbed in the small intestine with the major portion passing into the portal blood for transport to the liver.

Gastrointestinal diseases that reduce absorptive surface or enzymes referred to above may decrease absorption of hexoses. Thyroxine accelerates absorption of hexoses so that alterations in thyroid function with disease, as well as adrenocortical function, may affect rate and quantity of hexoses absorbed.

Peripheral carbohydrate metabolism can be considered virtually entirely in terms of glucose, since the utilization of fructose and galactose by extrahepatic tissues is negligible.

Liver. Hepatic cells are freely permeable to glucose. The other hexoses, fructose and galactose, are also withdrawn from the portal blood by the liver, at which point they are converted to glucose by the hepatic cells. In addition to direct uptake of hexoses, other hepatic mechanisms are intimately related to carbohydrate withdrawal from the blood as follows: (1) Glycogenesis (conversion of glucose to glycogen), or formation of glycogen for storage, is promoted by insulin or elevated blood glucose concentration, and (2) glucose utilization for energy production by oxidation to CO_2 and water or for synthesis of fatty acids and specific amino acids is also promoted by insulin.

The liver can also manufacture glucose from certain amino acids (proteins) and glycerol, mostly of fat origin. Decreased blood glucose concentration (hypoglycemia) and diminished carbohydrates in the cells (glycogen storage) are the basic stimuli of this process, called gluconeogenesis, which is promoted by glucocorticoid hormones (cortisol). Systemic blood leaving the liver in the hepatic veins contains hexoses not picked up by the hepatic cells from portal blood as well as glucose released by the liver from glycogenolysis. Glycogenolysis refers to the breakdown of glycogen that yields blood glucose. Pyruvic and lactic acids are formed in muscle and liver by a sequence of reactions referred to as glycolysis, and they may also be the terminal products of glycogenolysis. While hepatic glycogenolysis is the major source of blood glucose, the hepatic cells also dispense glucose derived from gluconeogenesis and conversion of other hexoses (e.g., fructose and galactose) to glucose.

Blood Glucose: Hepatic and Extrahepatic Contributions. In the systemic circulation, blood glucose is available for utilization by the extrahepatic tissues. Glucose is transported to virtually all the cells in the body through the interstitial and extracellular fluids. Glucose oxidation is the major source of cellular energy so important for growth, development, division, and maintenance of body cells in tissues and organs of the body. Since only a limited amount of carbohydrates ingested can be stored as glycogen, when the essential physiological demands for energy or transformation to specialized carbohydrate products is exceeded, excess glucose is converted to fatty acids for storage as triglycerides in body fat (adipose tissue). A major portion of the glucose derived from dietary carbohydrate after absorption is converted to fat by adipose tissue and to a lesser extent by the liver. Obesity as a health hazard is apparent when one considers that in the average diet carbohydrate comprises more than half of the total caloric intake. Insulin is essential for maximal lipogenesis in the liver and adipose tissue. Furthermore, dietary carbohydrate stimulates lipogenesis and glucose utilization. Both lipogenesis and glucose oxidation are, however, diminished in adipose tissue by a high fat diet and by fasting (mechanism of starvation diabetes).

Although muscle stores glycogen, it does not contribute glucose to blood, because of the absence of glucose-6-phosphatase. This enzyme, required to split glucose-6-phosphate, is present in liver and kidney. Several hormones influence the activity of the liver in maintaining normoglycemia. Insulin reduces the concentration of glucose by enhancing lipogenesis, glycogenesis, and glucose oxidation. The primary effect of insulin is to convert extracellular glucose into metabolizable glucose-6-phosphate. Whether this is accomplished through an enhancement of the hexokinase (glucokinase) reaction in cellular uptake of glucose or through an increase in permeability of the cell membrane to glucose, or both, remains uncertain. Insulin also inhibits the hepatic release of glucose. Certain hormones of the anterior pituitary gland (growth hormone, ACTH) tend to produce hyperglycemia. A number of steroid hormones from the adrenal cortex stimulate gluconeogenesis. Epinephrine and glucagon increase the concentration of blood glucose by activating hepatic phosphorylase with resulting glycogenolysis. Both hormones are important in the normal homeostatic control of blood glucose. Thyroid hormone (thyroxine) may also influence the concentration of blood glucose through its effect on the rate of absorption from the gastrointestinal tract. However, glucose utilization is usually normal in patients with hyperthyroidism and decreased in those with hypothyroidism.

Glucose, for all practical purposes, is the only sugar that is present in the blood. After a meal, however, rarely more than 10 to 20 per cent of the total monosaccharides absorbed into the blood are hexoses (e.g., fructose and galactose) other than glucose. These other hexoses are usually taken up by the hepatic cells within 90 minutes of carbohydrate ingestion and converted to glucose or at least phosphorylated to a stage in which they cannot normally return from the cells to the blood. A typical blood glucose tolerance curve displays alterations in the blood concentration of "true glucose" after carbohydrate ingestion (100 gm. glucose) as a function of time. Peak levels (hyperglycemia) observed during the latter part of the first hour progress with time through relative hypoglycemic and finally normoglycemic phases (Fig. 9–50).

After absorption of glucose into the blood, the normal fasting level, ranging from 60 to 90 mg./dl. of blood, rises to 120 to 150 mg./dl. or even higher. In normal subjects these glucose levels soon decline from the peak values, so that after 1 hour and 30 minutes to two hours the fasting levels are once again attained. However, the diabetic is unable to efficiently utilize the administered glucose, and blood levels after ingestion of glucose return to a base level only after an extended period of time. The constancy of blood glucose concentration between meals is achieved through a balance between glucose utilization by tissues and glycogenolysis. A portion of blood glucose is converted by the liver to glycogen (glycogenesis). Some glucose is utilized directly for energy, but most of the glucose derived from digestion of dietary carbohydrate is converted to fat as described previously.

In summary, the sugar of blood is glucose derived from three sources: (1) the digestion of starches and sugars produces glucose, which is absorbed from the intestine; (2) the conversion of noncarbohydrate precursors into glucose, i.e., amino acids, intermediates in the breakdown of glucose (lactic, pyruvic, and succinic acids), and glycerol derived from hydrolysis of neutral fat; and (3) glycogenolysis (hydrolysis of glycogen stored in the liver).

Blood glucose concentration also reflects extrahepatic utilization of glucose as follows: (1) source of energy (glucose oxidation); (2) conversion to fat and glycogen; and (3) transformation to specific essential carbohydrate forms, e.g., glycolipids, lactose (milk), glycoproteins, mucopolysaccharides, glucuronic acid, and pentose sugars of nucleic acids.

Glucose, continually filtered by the glomeruli, is returned completely to the blood by the reabsorptive system of the renal tubules. The capacity of the tubular system to reabsorb glucose (phosphorylation) is limited by the concentration of the enzymatic components of the tubular cell to a rate of about 250 mg. per minute. Hence, with hyperglycemia, glycosuria may appear. In individuals with normal renal function, glycosuria occurs when the blood glucose concentration exceeds about

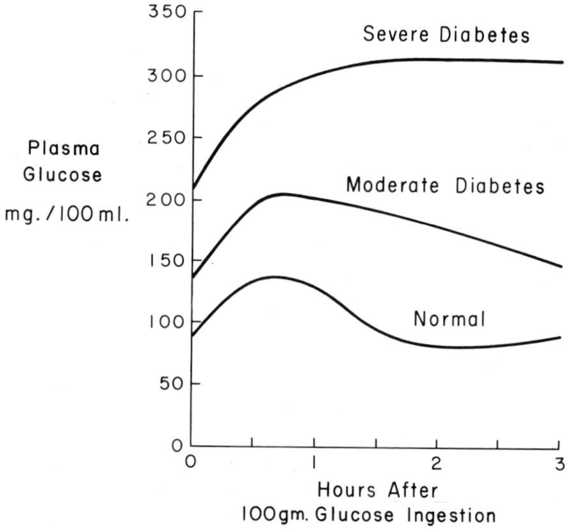

Figure 9–50. Oral glucose tolerance tests.

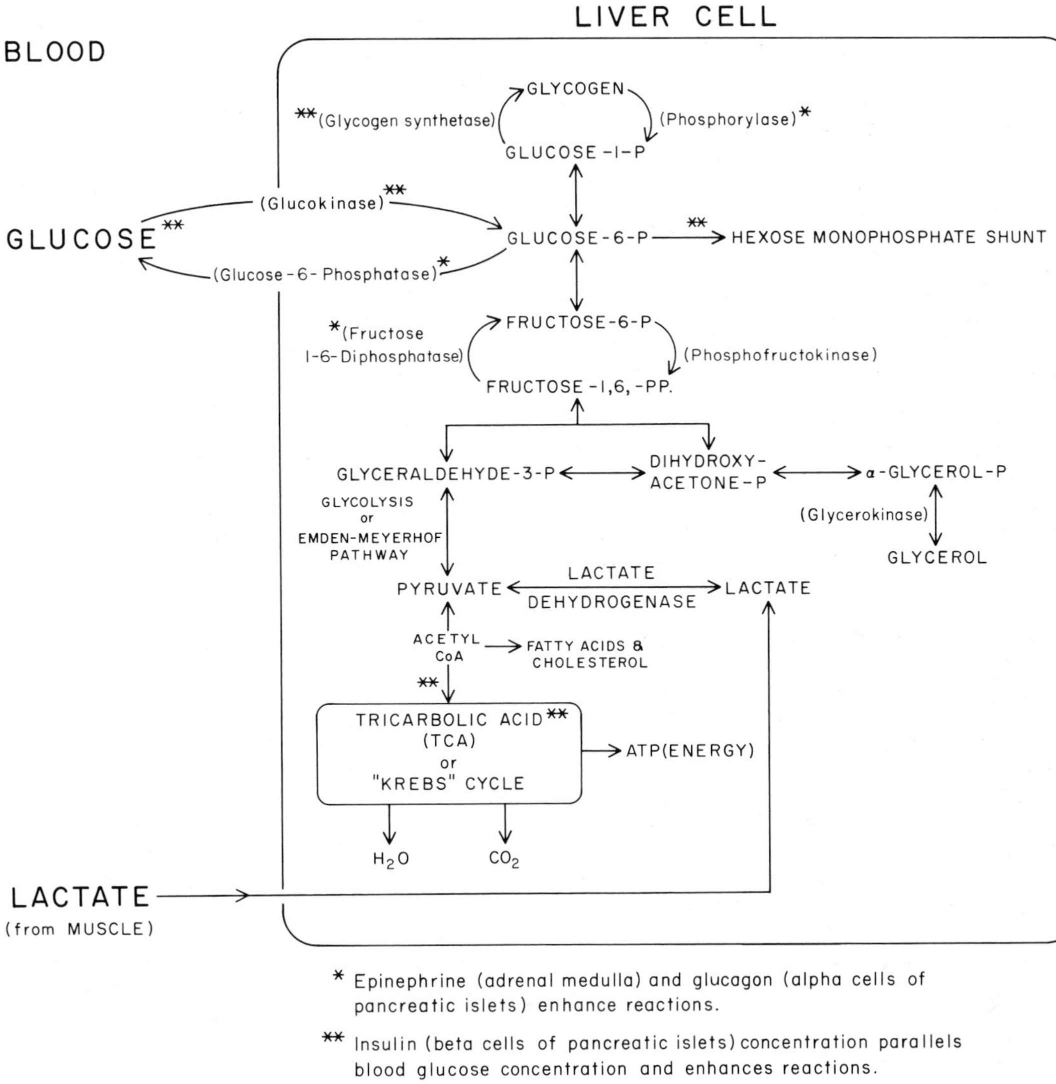

Figure 9–51. Intracellular metabolism of glucose (liver cell).

160 mg./dl. This is referred to as the renal threshold of glucose. However, defects in the renal tubule may produce glycosuria in the presence of normoglycemia. Glycosuria of renal origin may result from inherited defects or may be acquired as a result of disease processes described in Chapter 2. Diabetics with associated renal disease may have a "high threshold," with glycosuria appearing only with a blood glucose concentration well over 250 mg./dl.

Intracellular Metabolism of Glucose. Cells of the liver and kidney metabolize glucose in a similar manner, as outlined schematically in an abbreviated, simplified form shown in Figure 9–51. Glucose enters cells under the influence of insulin and the enzyme glucokinase to form glucose-6-phosphate intracellularly, a key pivot compound that may proceed in one of three directions. Glycogenesis and glycolysis through the tricarboxylic acid (TCA) cycle are the two major pathways, while a variable portion of glucose-6-phosphate may enter the alternative oxidative pathway called the hexose monophosphate shunt (HMP shunt). Energy requirements for generation of high energy phosphate compounds (ATP or adenosine triphosphate) probably have first call with demands from glycogen (glycogenolysis) when needed. Glycogen may also generate blood glucose, as noted in Figure 9–51, and glycogenesis may proceed when energy requirements are met.

About 90 per cent of the erythrocyte's energy is provided from glycolysis, so the alternative oxidation pathway (HMP shunt) plays a key role in the erythrocyte, which lacks a tricarboxylic acid cycle (Fig. 9–51). It is also an important metabolic pathway in the liver, adipose tissue, lactating mammary gland, thyroid, adrenal cortex, and testis. The sequence of reactions in the HMP shunt leads to the production of reduced nicotinamide adenine dinucleotide phosphate (NADPH), thereby generating reducing power in the extramitochondrial cytoplasm. (See Chapter 4 and Fig. 4–51.) This NADPH is utilized in the synthesis of fatty acids, steroids, and certain amino acids. The pathway also provides pentoses for the synthesis of nucleotides and nucleic acids.

Erythrocyte metabolism of glucose via glycolysis produces 2,3-diphosphoglycerate (2,3-DPG), which is essential for the normal functioning of hemoglobin. (See Chapters 4, 5, and 12.) 2,3-DPG, produced from 1,3-diphosphoglycerate by diphosphoglycerate (DPG) mutase, is returned to the Emden-Meyerhof pathway as 3-phosphoglycerate after cleavage of a phosphate group by a phosphatase. (See Fig. 4–51.) DPG mutase is strongly product inhibited and is further inhibited by a low intracellular pH. Since 2,3-DPG binds unsaturated hemoglobin (deoxyhemoglobin) within normal erythrocytes, in any condition in which the amount of deoxyhemoglobin increases, the amount of free 2,3-DPG decreases. By its binding to deoxyhemoglobin, 2,3-DPG produces a decreased affinity of hemoglobin for oxygen and a right shift of the oxyhemoglobin dissociation curve. An increased level of deoxyhemoglobin results in a decreased free level of 2,3-DPG, which lessens the product inhibition of DPG mutase. Such conditions occur in anoxic anemias, in patients moving to high altitudes, and in cyanotic heart disease. 2,3-DPG also acts as a nondiffusible anion, so that its binding to deoxyhemoglobin must be compensated for by a decrease in hydrogen ion concentration in red cells. This raises the intracellular pH and further increases the role of synthesis of 2,3-DPG as well as the activity of the entire Emden-Meyerhof pathway. Old erythrocytes have a tendency to lose 2,3-DPG as a function of age as a result of a loss of synthetic ability of senescent red cells. Banked blood also can be low in 2,3-DPG, particularly when stored in acid-citrate-dextrose solution, while citrate-phosphate-dextrose solution significantly improves 2,3-DPG retention in banked blood. Hence, a left shifted oxyhemoglobin dissociation curve is observed with massive transfusions of stored blood. This phenomenon is also seen in acidemia, septic shock, and respiratory distress syndrome of newborn for reasons that are not yet known.

Gluconeogenesis or formation of glucose from noncarbohydrate precursors may also be seen in Figure 9–51. The glycerol moiety of triglycerides (fat) can be seen to enter the glycolytic pathway. Certain amino acids (protein) enter the tricarboxylic acid cycle, while alanine may be converted to pyruvate. Glucocorticoids (adrenocortical hormones) promote gluconeogenesis, usually at the expense of protein.

In contrast to liver and kidney, muscle does not contain the essential enzyme for liberation of glucose into the blood, i.e., glucose-6-phosphatase. However, it can take up glucose from the blood for glycogenesis or glycolysis and further oxidation as described in Figure 9–51. Under relative anaerobic conditions, lactate formation is favored. Lactate of muscle may then contribute to blood lactate levels and enter liver cells for further metabolism as outlined (Fig. 9–51). Only through this mechanism can muscle glycogen contribute to blood glucose.

The neurons of the brain and cardiac muscle cells are especially dependent on glucose for energy and therefore are most sensitive to hypoglycemia in terms of duration and depth.

Clinicopathologic Correlations. Hyperglycemia encountered in patients with diabetes mellitus is more common than hypoglycemic (<50 mg./dl. blood) states. Glycogen storage disorders and lactic acidosis are other examples of disorders of carbohydrate metabolism. Lactic acidosis is considered in Chapter 12 (p. 780).

Diabetes mellitus is a chronic metabolic disorder with vascular components that is characterized by disturbances in carbohydrate, lipid, and protein metabolism. It usually develops in subjects with a hereditary predisposition and manifests itself by varying degrees of weakness, weight loss or failure to grow, lassitude, polyuria, and polydipsia. A relative or absolute deficiency of insulin for the requirements of tissues is central in the two theories that are currently held regarding pathogeneses: a decrease in transmembranal glucose transport *vs.* a shift intracellularly in glucose enzymatic equilibrium reactions. While most cases of diabetes mellitus are of an unknown cause, an abnormality of insulin secretion or some imbalance between the production of insulin and the demand for the hormone may be responsible. At any rate, hyperglycemia and glycosuria reflect the major metabolic lesion in carbohydrate metabolism, with secondary metabolic disturbances in proteins (gluconeogenesis) and lipids (ketosis and hypercholesterolemia).

The chemical pathologic reflections of carbohydrate metabolism in diabetes mellitus are shown in Figure 9–52. With hyperglycemia, renal glycosuria occurs with an osmotic diuresis. Sustained osmotic diuresis (polyuria) ultimately leads to dehydration and associated polydipsia (increased thirst). Glycogenolysis

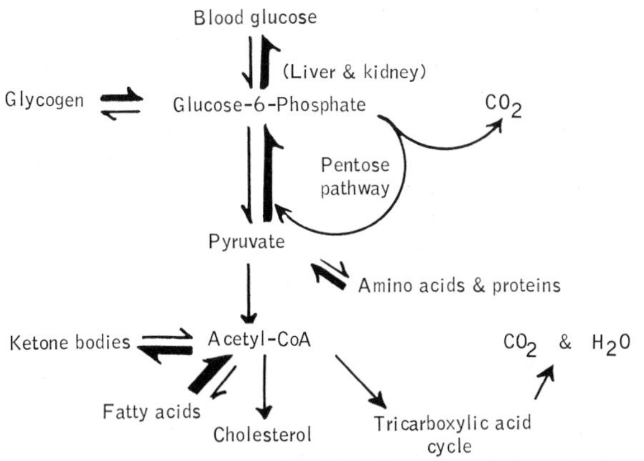

Figure 9–52. Diagram of carbohydrate metabolism in diabetes mellitus. (From Bondy, P. K.: Disorders of carbohydrate metabolism. *In* Beeson, P. B., and McDermott, W. (eds.): *Cecil-Loeb Textbook of Medicine.* 13th ed., 1971.)

and gluconeogenesis (protein depletion) are augmented to generate glucose that contributes to or sustains hyperglycemia. As mentioned previously, muscle glycogen cannot contribute glucose directly to the blood because of the absence of glucose-6-phosphatase. A failure of glucose to penetrate adipose tissue cells mobilizes fat and produces a rise in the free fatty acids and triglycerides of the plasma and of the triglycerides in the liver (Bondy, 1971). A diabetic fatty liver may result from the absence of lipoprotein synthesis when protein synthesis is compromised by accelerated gluconeogenesis (negative nitrogen balance). When glucose oxidation is impaired, fatty acids form the major source of energy and generate an excess of acetyl coenzyme A that cannot be oxidized to water and carbon dioxide or be disposed of in other metabolic routes. The condensation of two carbon fragments of acetyl coenzyme A results in formation of ketone bodies, ketonemia and ketonuria as shown at the bottom of this page.

All three substances are referred to as ketone bodies. Ketonuria is detectable when hepatic ketogenesis exceeds tissue utilization of ketones; when ketogenesis exceeds both tissue utilization and renal clearance, ketonemia appears. β-Hydroxybutyric acid is generally present in a concentration forty times that of acetone and acetoacetic acid is usually ten times as concentrated as acetone. With continual urinary excretion, buffer cations (especially sodium and potassium) are eventually depleted and acidosis ensues. Ketoacidosis is the hallmark of a potentially fatal complication of diabetes mellitus. The major complications of diabetes mellitus include ketoacidosis, retinopathy, neuropathy, nephropathy, arteriosclerosis, and an increased susceptibility to bacterial and fungal infections.

A classification of diabetes is outlined in Table 9–22. Primary diabetes mellitus of the maturity-onset (adult) type is by far the most common variety and mild in form compared to the juvenile type, which shows wide fluctuations in blood glucose and an increased predisposition to ketoacidosis. Indeed, the course of the disease can be divided into four stages, as recommended by the American Diabetes Association: (1) prediabetes, (2) suspected diabetes, (3) chemical or latent diabetes, and (4) overt diabetes. The period from birth until the first evidence of the disease characterizes prediabetes. In suspected diabetes, the patient displays an abnormal glucose tolerance test or even diabetic symptoms after stressful influences (e.g., obesity, pregnancy, trauma, infections), but usually is normal in all respects. In chemical or latent diabetes, there are no signs or symptoms of disease, but an abnormal glucose tolerance test or fasting hyperglycemia are evident when the patient is not under stress. With overt diabetes, symptoms of polyuria, polydipsia, and weight loss (and possibly ketoacidosis) are often associated with fasting hyperglycemia and glycosuria.

Although the mode of inheritance is not established, it is probably homozygous (genetic recessive) when the disease is manifest and heterozygous as a diabetic trait. As much as 2 or 3 per cent (2 million or 3 million) of the population may have diabetes mellitus with

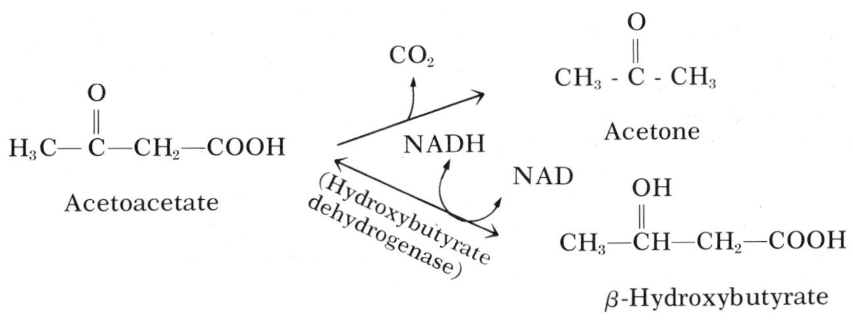

Table 9–22. CLASSIFICATION OF DIABETES

Primary
Maturity-onset (adult) type
Growth-onset (juvenile) type
Endocrine origin
Hyperpituitarism
Pituitary basophilism
Acromegaly
Hyperadrenalism
Cortical – Cushing's syndrome; aldosteronism
Medullary – Pheochromocytoma
Hyperthyroidism
Therapy induced
Corticosteroids and ACTH
Growth hormone
Thyroid extract and triiodothyronine
Destruction of pancreatic islets
Surgical removal of pancreas
Hemochromatosis
Fibrocystic disease of pancreas (mucoviscidosis)
Neoplasm
Miscellaneous
Diuretics and derivatives (thiazide therapy)
Stress reactions, surgery, and pregnancy
Starvation and low carbohydrate intake

diagnosis established in less than half. As a cause of death or contributor to other fatal diseases (coronary artery disease and hypertension), diabetes ranks in the top 10. In view of the frequency of associated morbidity and mortality, routine screening procedures for detection of diabetes have been accepted. The currently accepted empirical diagnostic tests are based primarily on the demonstration of impaired glucose tolerance. In those individuals with marked glucose intolerance, the demonstration of glycosuria and fasting hyperglycemia (confirmed) establishes the diagnosis, and provocative tests are not necessary; these are the usual findings in the "juvenile-onset" (insulin-requiring) diabetic. In most diabetics (approximately 90 per cent), the disease is detected in the adult years at a time when they have neither glycosuria nor fasting hyperglycemia. In this group, provocative tests may be required to demonstrate impaired glucose tolerance. Glycosuria associated with ketonuria is almost always pathognomonic of diabetes mellitus.

Screening Tests. Screening tests for detection of diabetes mellitus include blood and urine glucose measurements.

URINE GLUCOSE. Glucose in the urine may be estimated by use of Clinitest tablets (quantitative estimation of urinary reducing substances via alkali reduction of Cu^{++} to Cu_2O – not specific for glucose) or by use of Combistix, a glucose-oxidase-impregnated paper strip (Ames Company, Division Miles Laboratories, Inc., Elkhart, Indiana 46504) which specifically detects glucose in the urine (see Chapter 2, p. 55). In evaluating glycosuria, it should be remembered that venous "true glucose" must exceed 160 mg./dl. of blood before any glucose will spill over into the urine ("renal threshold"). In diabetic nephropathy, the renal threshold may be elevated considerably without glycosuria in the presence of hyperglycemia. Also, the renal threshold increases with age, and in some elderly patients no glycosuria will be present with serum levels of 200 mg./dl. of glucose.

FASTING BLOOD GLUCOSE. Glucose can be measured by one of several methods that will be discussed subsequently. Plasma is the blood fraction of choice. Fasting plasma glucose values in excess of 120 mg./dl. ("true glucose") are considered indicative of diabetes mellitus; values between 110 and 120 mg./dl. are equivocal and should be confirmed with a standard glucose tolerance test. Most patients with mild diabetes or adult onset diabetes will have a fasting blood glucose which falls in the normal range. Fasting blood sugar (glucose) as a screening test is less sensitive than the 2-hour postprandial glucose determinations. Indeed, the fasting blood glucose should be replaced by 2-hour postprandial (pp) glucose measurement as a screening test. Emotional hyperglycemia from secretion of epinephrine as well as cerebral lesions (skull fractures, tumors, vascular accident, and encephalitis) and carbon monoxide poisoning, which often provoke hyperglycemia and glycosuria, must be considered in the evaluation of blood glucose measurements.

TWO-HOUR POSTPRANDIAL BLOOD GLUCOSE. After an overnight fast (12 hours) the patient is given a breakfast of 100 gm. of carbohydrate or a 100-gm. glucose load. Previous to the test, the patient should have been on an adequate carbohydrate diet (300 gm. daily) and all medications that influence glucose tolerance should have been discontinued three days prior to the test. Two hours later (2 hours pp or pc, post cibum) a single sample of blood is withdrawn for analysis. A value within normal limits makes the diagnosis of diabetes mellitus unlikely; plasma glucose values ranging from 110 to 120 are suspicious, and in excess of 120 mg./dl. ("true glucose"), diagnosis is most likely and should be confirmed by a standard glucose tolerance test, especially if there is any doubt or suspicion. The limitations of a single 2-hour pc glucose value includes the following: (1) slow absorption, which may delay the peak level; (2) rapid absorption with early hyperglycemia, rapid fall in the concentration of blood glucose (due to insulin release), and then a second hyperglycemic peak due to the effects of counterregulatory responses (epinephrine, glucagon, growth hormone); and (3) errors in timing specimen collection. While a 1-hour postprandial glucose measurement is more sensitive for detection of diabetes, it also yields a higher percentage of false positive diagnoses, i.e., less specific than the 2-hour pc test.

Diagnostic Tests. Oral glucose tolerance tests (OGTT) are performed to establish a diagnosis (1) in patients with transient or sustained glucosuria who have no clinical symptoms of diabetes (polyuria) and with normal fasting and postprandial blood glucose levels, (2) in patients with symptoms of diabetes but with no glycosuria and normal fasting level, (3) in persons with a strong family history of diabetes but with no overt symptoms, (4) in patients whose glycosuria is associated with pregnancy, thyrotoxicosis, liver disease, and/or infections, (5) in women who have characteristically large (>9 lbs.) babies or individuals who were large babies, and (6) in patients with neuropathies and retinopathies of undetermined origin.

PROCEDURE. The American Diabetes Association Committee on Statistics has issued a report on the Standardization of the Oral Glucose Tolerance Test (OGTT) which is excellent, and the reader should refer to it as reference material for the OGTT (Klimt *et al.*, 1969). It is essential that patients ingest at least 300 gm. of carbohydrate daily for three days or more prior to OGTT. Hence, a glucose tolerance should not be determined routinely during hospitalization of an acutely ill patient whose dietary intake has been low. Criteria for interpretation of carbohydrate (glucose) tolerance tests are based on values obtained in the ambulatory patient. When possible, the test should be performed after the patient has resumed normal activity. If a slightly abnormal test is observed with an illness requiring bed rest, the glucose tolerance test should be repeated after the patient recovers. A diurnal variation in glucose tolerance with tolerance in the afternoon significantly decreased from that in the morning has prompted suggestions that OGTT be performed in the morning (Bowen and Reeves, 1967; Ravel, 1967). Various malignancies, fever, cachexia, liver dysfunction, and renal failure may be associated with mild to moderate degrees of abnormal glucose tolerance. There appears to be an age-linked decrease in glucose tolerance that makes interpretation of OGTT in elderly subjects a challenge (Searcy *et al.*, 1966). Timing of glucose administration and blood sampling must be accurate. The same source of blood (venous or capillary) must be used throughout the test and same analytical method applied to each specimen sample. Samples of urine and whole blood are taken at fasting, 30 minutes, 1, 1½, 2, 3, and 4 hours after ingestion of the carbohydrate meal. The American Diabetes Association recommends the following test dose of glucose in 25 per cent (w./v.) solution:

Age	*Dose*
0–18 mos.	2.5 gm./kg.
1½–3 yrs.	2.0 gm./kg.
8–12 yrs.	1.75 gm./kg.
>12 yrs.	1.25 gm./kg.

Some individuals tolerate a glucose load poorly; any associated nausea or vomiting influences the interpretation of results.

There are three popular methods of evaluation of the glucose tolerance test for diabetes mellitus:

1. Wilkerson point system

Time	*mg./dl. plasma*	*Points*
Fasting	130 or more	1
1 hr.	195 or more	½
2 hr.	140 or more	½
3 hr.	130 or more	1

Two or more points are judged diagnostic of diabetes mellitus (D.M.).

2. The Fajans-Conn Criteria (numeric values adjusted per Niejadlik *et al.*, 1973)

Time	*mg./dl. plasma*
Fasting	
1 hr.	185 or more
1½ hr.	165 or more
2 hr.	140 or more

A diagnosis of D.M. in otherwise healthy and ambulatory individuals under age 50 is made if the above criteria are met.

3. The University Group Diabetes Mellitus Program. The fasting, 1-hr., 2-hr., and 3-hr. blood glucose levels are adjusted for plasma glucose as above, and the subject is judged diabetic if the sum of values obtained equals 500 or more (Klimt *et al.*, 1967).

Abnormally high values in the first hour with a rapid fall to normal values or a flat curve with no appreciable rise usually reflect primary alterations in intestinal absorption of glucose; the former is characteristic of hyperthyroidism and the latter of hypothyroidism or malabsorptive states. A very flat rise in blood glucose followed by a prolonged and pronounced hypoglycemic phase may be observed in primary (islet cell adenoma or hyperplasia) and secondary hyperinsulinism (hypoadrenocorticism). Since there is an age-linked decrease in glucose tolerance with the hyperglycemic tendency becoming more conspicuous with increasing age in both sexes, but especially in females, interpretation of OGTT must be made in light of what is an apparent age-dependent carbohydrate intolerance (Searcy *et al.*, 1966).

An intravenous glucose tolerance test may supplement or replace the oral tolerance study in patients with gastrointestinal diseases, including sprue or malabsorption syndrome and in postgastrectomy patients or those suspected of having a disturbance in intestinal absorption. A sterile glucose solution is administered intravenously (20 per cent w./v.) over a 30-minute period in an amount of 0.5 gm. per kg. of ideal body weight. Similar blood collection intervals, including fasting specimen, are followed, and a curve is plotted for evaluation (½, 1, 1½, 2, 2½, and 3 hours). In normal subjects, the control specimen of blood contains a normal amount of glucose; the concentration of any single specimen does not exceed 250 mg./dl.; and by 1 hour 30 minutes to 2 hours, the blood glucose level approximates fasting values. Fajans (1960), among others, has reported that this test is a less sensitive indicator of mild abnormalities of carbohydrate tolerance than the standard oral glucose tolerance test (OGTT).

A rapid intravenous (50 per cent w./v.) glucose tolerance test (0.5 gm. glucose per kg. ideal body weight) to a maximum dose of 25 gm. may also be administered over a 3- to 4-minute period. Blood samples are obtained at intervals of 10 minutes for at least 1 hour. Under these conditions, disappearance of glucose from blood follows an exponential curve and a glucose disappearance constant can be calculated. In normal subjects glucose disappearance usually exceeds 1.5 per cent of the administered dose per minute; values below 1 per cent are compatible with diabetes mellitus.

The cortisone glucose tolerance test may reveal "prediabetic" patients, especially in relatives of known diabetics. Cortisone promotes gluconeogenesis that may accentuate carbohydrate intolerance in a latent or mild diabetic. After performance of an initial glucose tolerance study a standard dose of cortisone for adults (50 mg.) is administered parenterally 8 hours and 30 minutes and again 2 hours before a regular glucose tolerance procedure. A positive test shows a blood glucose concentration of 140 mg./dl. or higher with 2-hour specimen. Follow-up studies are necessary for such individuals.

Parenteral administration of glucagon or epinephrine will cause a slight elevation of blood glucose concentration from glycogenolysis in normal subjects: this is much greater and more sustained in diabetics. It is also a measure of glycogen storage and release, so it may be used to study patients suspected of having a glycogen storage disease.

The administration of an oral hypoglycemic agent in the intravenous tolbutamide test normally results in the elaboration of insulin from the pancreas. This principle is taken advantage of to indicate available (active) insulin reserve in patients. Sodium tolbutamide (1 gm.) is given intravenously in 20 ml. of saline over two minutes to a fasting (12 hour) subject. A control preinjection blood specimen and postinjection samples at 2, 5, 10, 20, 30, 60, 120 and 180 minutes are collected for glucose analyses (Fig. 9–53). Serum insulin assays may also be helpful. Juvenile (prematurity-onset) diabetics (insulinopenic) reveal virtually no response, while adult (maturity-onset) diabetics show a delayed decrease in blood glucose concentrations. Patients with an insulin-secreting tumor (islet cell adenoma or hyperplasia) reveal a profound depression of blood glucose values which persists below 50 mg./dl. at 2 hours; this is associated with maximum insulin values (33–2,267 μU./ml.) as early as 15 minutes. Appropriate medical precautionary measures must

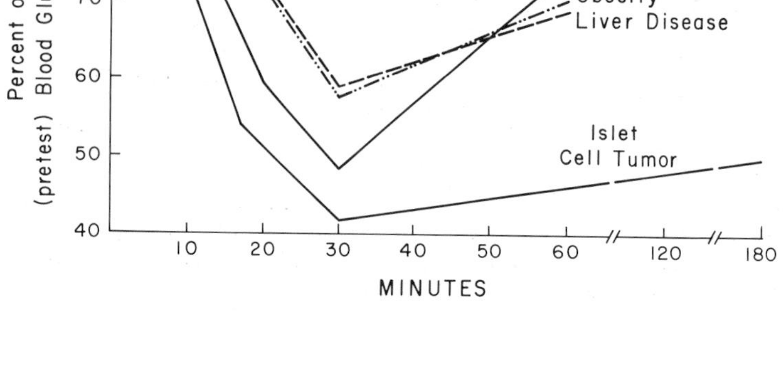

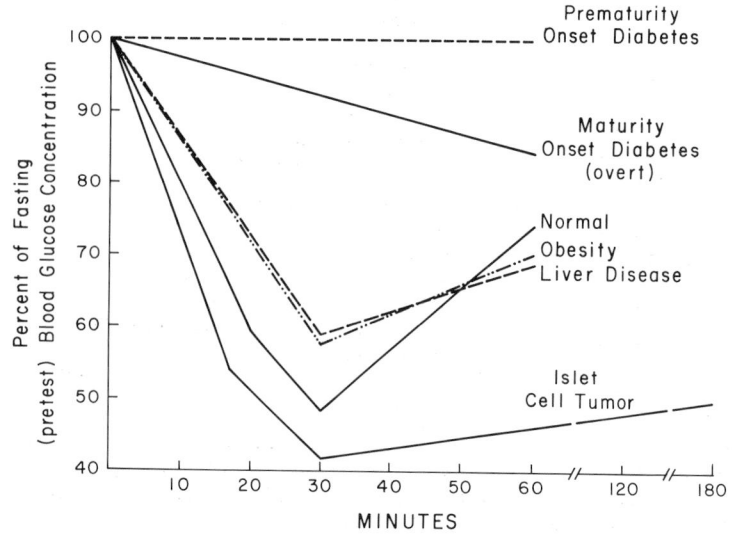

Figure 9–53. Intravenous tolbutamide tolerance test that may indicate available (active) insulin reserve as reflected by blood concentration changes.

be readily available (sterile glucose solution) and used promptly with any stress tolerance test whenever a patient's condition warrants intervention and cessation of test.

In the intravenous insulin (0.1 unit per kg. of ideal body weight) tolerance test administered in the fasting state, blood specimens are collected at appropriate intervals over a 2-hour period for glucose analyses. Within 30 minutes the blood glucose concentration falls to about 50 or 60 per cent of the fasting level and returns to normal fasting levels between 1 hour 30 minutes and 2 hours. A failure to observe such a depression in blood glucose concentration may indicate insulin resistance. This may be seen occasionally in adult-type diabetes, as well as in acromegaly and Cushing's syndrome. In panhypopituitarism and adrenocortical insufficiency (Addison's disease) a more profound and sustained decrease in blood glucose may be observed, so caution should be exercised in testing patients suspected of having these disorders. Although insulin radioassays have become available, measuring plasma insulin along with glucose has not yet proved of practical value (Bondy, 1971). However, Cerasi and his colleagues (1973) stress the inadequate insulin response to orally administered glucose by prediabetic and diabetic subjects. If not in diabetes mellitus, insulin assays may be helpful for diagnosis of islet cell tumor (free fasting levels) in which they are relatively high in relation to the hypoglycemia.

Management of Diabetic Patients: Laboratory Aspects. A 24-hour as well as fractional (freshly voided) urine collection may be analyzed for ketone bodies and glucose to indicate glucose loss (total grams) and serve as a guide to therapy and dietary regulation. The labile diabetic can be managed most effectively with the aid of such quantitative urinary glucose measurements.

When therapy requires additional guide line information, especially in the absence of glucosuria, blood specimens for glucose analyses collected at intervals throughout the day 2 or 3 hours after each meal (7 A.M., 11 A.M., 3 P.M., and 8 P.M.) are of great value (Somogyi, 1959). Again the labile diabetic receives maximum benefit, which is also helpful with rapidly changing insulin dosage and delineation of a suspected fluctuation from hypoglycemia to hyperglycemia.

In view of the disturbance in lipid metabolism of diabetics, serum cholesterol and triglyceride, measurements should be documented at intervals during treatment. Periodic serum lipoprotein electrophoresis determinations are important when a demonstrated elevation of cholesterol and/or triglycerides exists. Hypercholesterolemia may be a presenting manifestation, and approximately half of the "treated" diabetics show hypercholesterolemia. The concentration of serum cholesterol changes more slowly than does glucose and, hence, is an important indicator of inadequate treatment for prolonged periods.

Ketone estimation in serum is helpful in assessing severity of ketoacidosis and estimating insulin requirements during therapy. Ketonemia is not observed until ketonuria is marked (3+ to 4+). Furthermore, plasma or serum ketone levels decrease prior to a diminution in ketonuria with successful diabetic management. Estimation of ketone bodies in serum or plasma is similar to that described for urine in Chapter 2.

Hypoglycemia. With increased or excessive insulin levels, hypoglycemia (by definition less than 50 mg./dl.) is likely to occur. Increased peripheral uptake of glucose and reduced gluconeogenesis are factors that may contribute to the induced form of hypoglycemia (Table 9–23). With spontaneous hypoglycemia, in addition to excessive insulin of endogenous

Table 9–23. CLASSIFICATION OF HYPOGLYCEMIA*

I. Spontaneous (Fasting) Hypoglycemia
  A. Excessive insulin
    1. Insulinoma or insulin-secreting carcinoma
    2. Erythroblastosis fetalis
  B. Nonendocrine tumor (usually large retroperitoneal sarcoma)
  C. Glycogen storage disease of the liver
  D. Malnutrition or malabsorption
  E. Adrenocortical or pituitary failure
  F. Liver necrosis
  G. Hereditary galactosemia
  H. Reye's syndrome and other forms of ketotic hypoglycemia in children
II. Induced Hypoglycemia
  A. Excessive insulin
    1. Overtreated diabetic
    2. Leucine (includes some islet cell tumors)
    3. Sulfonylureas
    4. Functional
      a. Prediabetic
      b. Postgastrectomy
      c. Hemodialysis with hypertonic glucose
      d. Idiopathic
  B. Reduced gluconeogenesis
    1. Ethanol
    2. Hypoglycin
    3. Hereditary fructose intolerance
    4. Failure of glucagon secretion
  C. Persistent increase of peripheral glucose uptake
    1. Failure of catecholamine secretion
    2. Propranolol blockade of catecholamine effect
  D. Cause uncertain
    Pentamidine

*Bondy, P. K.: Hypoglycemic states. *In* Beeson, P. B., and McDermott, W. (eds.): Cecil-Loeb Textbook of Medicine. 13th ed., 1971.

origin, other contributing factors include a depression of glycogenesis with a decreased rate of hepatic formation and release of glucose, massive hepatic necrosis, and glycogen storage disease. Either a loss of glycogen stores or inability to release glucose (absence of glucose-6-phosphatase in liver) can account for hypoglycemia in these conditions. A comprehensive classification of hypoglycemia proposed by Doctor P. K. Bondy (1971) is shown in Table 9–23.

COLLECTION AND PRESERVATION OF BLOOD FOR GLUCOSE ANALYSIS. At room temperature, glucose in blood undergoes glycolysis at a rate of approximately 5 per cent each hour and may disappear completely from blood in as short a period as six hours. Leukocytosis and bacterial contamination tend to increase glycolysis greatly. Whole blood should be analyzed ½ hour after collection, or a preservative such as fluoride must be added. If the blood is refrigerated, 2 mg. of fluoride per ml. of blood will prevent glycolysis for 48 hours. Preservation for longer periods requires the addition of 10 mg. of sodium fluoride (NaF) per ml. of blood, along with the addition of thymol in the amount of 5 per cent of fluoride.

In contrast, the glucose concentration in a protein-free filtrate is relatively stable for a period of 48 hours in a refrigerated environment. Prompt separation of plasma or serum from the cells is essential. In our laboratory we use the Vacutainer system, which contains 20 mg. NaF and 143 USP units heparin (see p. 518).

Plasma or serum is used almost exclusively in glucose analysis instead of whole blood for many reasons: Glucose concentration is uniform in the water phase of plasma and red blood cells. Hematocrit will not interfere with plasma glucose, as whole blood glucose increases 3–4 mg./dl. with each 10 unit decrease. Finally, plasma or serum is more suitable for automated methods.

The concentration of glucose in arterial blood is generally higher than in venous blood from the same individual. Since capillary blood usually approximates arterial blood, the differences must be taken into consideration in clinical interpretations.

A cerebrospinal fluid (CSF) glucose value requires a measurement of blood glucose collected simultaneously for optimal interpretation and identification of low CSF glucose, since the brain-blood barrier reflects exchange of glucose between two compartments; i.e., CSF is about two-thirds plasma glucose normally, and normal blood plasma glucose has a wide range (Greenawald *et al.*, 1973).

Methods for Estimation of Glucose. The diagnosis of diabetes mellitus is based primarily on the proper interpretation of one or a group of blood glucose measurements, either as fasting 2-hr. postprandial (pp) or as glucose tolerance test specimens. With so much emphasis on glucose values reported by the clinical laboratory, the diagnostician involved should be well aware of the method or methods of glucose analyses being utilized. Niejadlik *et al.* (1973) derived linear regression equations for three methods: Nelson-Somogyi on whole blood glucose, copper reduction (neocuproine) on plasma glucose, and hexokinase on plasma glucose. Plasma glucose by the copper reduction method is approximately 17 per cent higher than whole blood glucose and consistently 5 mg./dl. higher than plasma glucose measured by the hexokinase method (Table 9–24). The Cu reduction methods may give even higher values than hexokinase; in azotemic patients, the discrepancy may be greater than 25 mg./dl.

Although several methods for glucose determination have evolved, most are nonspecific and depend on the reduction of selected heavy metals (especially Cu^{++}) or nitroaromatic acids by the aldehyde group of glucose.

The Folin-Wu method employs a tungstic acid filtrate of whole blood that is heated with an alkaline copper solution with reduction of cupric ions to cuprous ions. The cuprous ions are then measured photometrically (colorimetrically) by the addition of an excess of phosphomolybdic acid to form molybdenum blue. The wide range and high normal values (80 to 120 mg./dl.) reflect the nonspecificity of the reaction, which measures nonglucose-reducing substances (the "saccharoids"–

Table 9–24. CONVERSION OF WHOLE BLOOD GLUCOSE TO PLASMA GLUCOSE*

NELSON-SOMOGYI WHOLE BLOOD GLUCOSE	COPPER-REDUCING METHOD (NEOCUPROINE)	HEXOKINASE METHOD
mg./dl. whole blood	*mg./dl. plasma*	*mg./dl. plasma*
80	95	90
90	107	102
100	118	113
110	129	124
120	141	136
130	152	147
140	164	159
150	175	170
160	186	181

*Niejadlik, D., Dube, A., and Adamko, S.: J.A.M.A. *225*:1734, 1973.

glutathione, glucuronic acid, ergothioneine, ascorbic acid, etc.) as well as other hexoses in blood; as such, this method does not estimate "true glucose" values.

Nelson-Somogyi procedure utilizes a barium hydroxide–zinc sulfate filtrate, which is virtually free of nonglucose-reducing substances. The cuprous ion formed by heating this filtrate with an alkaline copper solution is measured photometrically by the addition of arsenomolybdic acid that forms a colored complex. Normal values range from 60 to 100 mg./dl.; this method is a measure of "true glucose" values.

Ferricyanide methods are based upon the reduction of yellow ferricyanide ions to colorless ferrocyanide ions by glucose at an alkaline pH. With the AutoAnalyzer, dialysis separates glucose from red blood cells and protein. The dialyzed glucose decolorizes potassium ferricyanide to the ferro form, and the disappearance of color, which is proportional to the glucose concentration, is measured photometrically. The values obtained are equivalent to "true glucose." However, ferricyanide values are 5–10 mg./dl. greater than hexokinase or glucose-oxidase values, to be described subsequently. Klein and his associates (1966) have described a modified automated procedure.

When neocuproine is substituted for phosphomolybdic or arsenomolybdic acid, an improved colorimetric copper reduction procedure is achieved. A cupric-neocuproine copper reduction procedure is used widely with the SMA-12 AutoAnalyzer. Plasma glucose measurements of normal subjects average 6 mg./dl. higher than by glucose oxidase measurements. Furthermore, such automated cupric-neocuproine measurements of azotemic serums yield values which average 40 mg./dl. higher than by glucose oxidase procedure (Sunderman and Sunderman, 1972). Part of this large discrepancy is also due to a lowering of the glucose value measured by glucose oxidase in azotemic sera caused by hyperuricemia. This is emphasized in a recent report by Miskiewicz and colleagues (1973). It appears that uric acid competes for the chromogen with the oxygen released during the peroxidase step of the reaction.

The ortho-toluidine method devised by Hultman in 1959 is based upon color reaction obtained by the condensation of aldosaccharides with ortho-toluidine in glacial acetic acid. A number of modifications of Hultman's method have been introduced recently (Cooper and McDaniel, 1970). The rapidity, sensitivity, accuracy, and relative simplicity, coupled with hexose specificity of Dubowski's method (1962), make it an ideal manual procedure; it can be used for emergency as well as regular determinations. To a trichloroacetic acid filtrate of blood, ortho-toluidine dissolved in glacial acetic acid is added, and the mixture is heated at 100° C. for 10 minutes; the stable green color that develops is measured spectrophotometrically. Wenk and colleagues (1969) have reported an automated micromethod. The values obtained with this method are 9 per cent less than with ferricyanide automated procedure (Ceriotti, 1971). An O-toluidine method is frequently performed on plasma or serum without the use of protein precipitation. AutoAnalyzer methods are also available without using dialysis.

Enzymatic methods for glucose determination provide the ultimate degree of specificity in estimating true blood glucose. Glucose oxidase catalyzes the oxidation of glucose to gluconic acid and hydrogen peroxide. A coupled glucose-oxidase-peroxidase-enzyme system for glucose determination in biologic fluids introduced by Keston in 1956 has undergone several modifications in recent years. The hydrogen peroxide produced by glucose oxidase is estimated in the presence of peroxidase that catalyzes transfer of oxygen from peroxide (H_2O_2) to a chromogenic oxygen acceptor such as ortho-tolidine or ortho-dianisidine as shown at the bottom of this page.

The second step, involving peroxidase, is less specific. Various reducing substances inhibit the reactions by competing with the chromagen for oxygen from H_2O_2. Most of these interfering substances are eliminated by use of a Somogyi-Nelson filtrate. Recent advances in technology circumvent the peroxi-

---

$$\text{1. Glucose} \xrightarrow[\text{oxidase}]{\text{glucose}} \text{gluconolactone} \xrightarrow[O_2]{H_2O} \text{gluconic acid} + H_2O_2$$

$$\text{2. } H_2O_2 + \text{Ortho-tolidine or Ortho-dianisidine (chromogenic } O_2 \text{ receptors)} \xrightarrow{\text{peroxidase}} \text{blue color (chromogen)} + H_2O$$

dase step by directly measuring the amount of O_2 generated by the glucose oxidase.

A hexokinase method provides the ultimate degree of specificity in estimating true blood glucose. Hexokinase acts in the following way (Neeley, 1972):

1. $\text{Glucose} + \text{ATP} \xrightarrow{\text{hexokinase}} \text{glucose-6-phosphate (G-6-P)} + \text{ADP}$

2. $\text{G-6-P} + \text{NADP} \xrightarrow{\text{G-6-P dehydrogenase}} \text{6 phosphogluconolactone} + \text{NADPH} + H^+$

For every mole of glucose reduction, there is a reduction of one mole of NADP to NADPH, which is measured spectrophotometrically. In view of occasional impurities in commercial hexokinase preparations, the substitution of acyl phosphate for substrate and acyl-phosphate-glucose-6-phosphotransferase as the first stage enzyme in lieu of hexokinase has been recommended by Bergmeyer and Moellering (1966) as shown in the formula below.

The second stage reaction as shown above is used to generate reduced NAD that is measured spectrophotometrically.

The current state of the art for glucose methodology, in view of the limitations cited, prompts our selection of an enzymatic method (e.g., hexokinase) or ortho-toluidine method for plasma glucose measurements (Mitchell and Rydalch, 1968; Cooper and McDaniel, 1970). Peterson (1968) has described a hexokinase method for urinary glucose measurements as specific, accurate, and reliable.

LIPIDS

Biochemistry. Lipids are organic substances that contain mostly carbon and hydrogen and some oxygen; several of the compound lipids also contain nitrogen and phosphorus. They are, in general, insoluble in water and soluble in such organic solvents as hydrocarbons (petroleum ether and benzene), halogenated hydrocarbons (chloroform, carbon tetrachloride, and dichloroethane), and ether. As fatty or greasy compounds, they are chemically related to fatty acids as esters, either actually or potentially (Harper, 1971).

Classification. In Table 9–25, a general but simplified classification of lipids is presented. Naturally occurring fats, such as triglycerides (neutral fats), are formed by esterification (alcohol plus an acid) as follows:

Table 9–25. CLASSIFICATION OF LIPIDS

- Simple lipids—esters of fatty acids and an alcohol
  - Fats (true or neutral fats)—alcohol is glycerol
    - Triglycerides
  - Waxes—alcohol other than glycerol
    - Sterol esters (cholesterol)
- Compound or conjugated lipids—esters of fatty acids that contain groups in addition to an alcohol and fatty acid such as phosphoric acid, nitrogenous moiety, or carbohydrate
  - Phospholipids
    - Lecithins—one fatty acid esterified to glycerol is replaced by phosphoric acid and choline (nitrogenous moiety)
    - Cephalins—nitrogenous moiety is serine or ethanolamine in place of choline
    - Sphingomyelins—no glycerol present
  - Glycolipids (cerebrosides)—fatty acids and carbohydrates (galactose or glucose) with nitrogen but no glycerol
  - Others (aminolipids and sulfolipids)
    - Lipoproteins
- Derived lipids—hydrolytic derivatives of the above substances
  - Fatty acids
    - Saturated
    - Unsaturated
  - Glycerol alcohol
  - Other alcohols
    - Sterols
    - Steroids

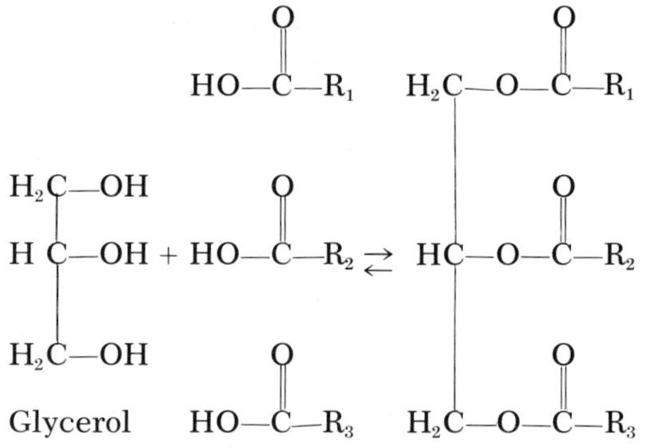

Glycerol — Three fatty acids, R_1, R_2, and R_3 — Triglyceride

Step-by-step hydrolysis of a triglyceride, in turn, yields a diglyceride, monoglyceride, and

---

$$\text{Glucose} + \text{acyl phosphate} \xrightarrow{\text{acyl-phosphate-G-6-P-transferase}} \text{G-6-P} + \text{acyl}$$

finally all constituent fatty acids and glycerol by a reverse of the above reaction. Since there may be three different fatty acids rather than one fatty acid esterified to glycerol, this compound is often referred to as a mixed glyceride. When the alcohol is of a higher molecular weight than glycerol, the compound is called a wax. Naturally occurring fatty acids usually have an even number of carbon atoms and are straight chains. Unsaturation refers to the presence of one or more double bonds, in contrast to saturated fatty acids that contain no double bonds. Palmitic acid ($CH_3(CH_2)_{14}$-$COOH$), with 16 carbon atoms, and stearic acid ($CH_3(CH_2)_{16}COOH$), with 18 carbon atoms, are saturated fatty acids, while oleic acid (CH_3-$(CH_2)_7CH = CH\ (CH_2)_7\ COOH$), with 18 carbon atoms, is an unsaturated fatty acid (one double bond). These three fatty acids are the most common types present in human adipose tissue or depot fat (Cantarow and Schepartz, 1967). Fat not only yields the highest caloric value compared to protein and carbohydrate but lends itself to a stored form of energy in organs and tissues. The composition of dietary fat is important, since it influences greatly the composition of depot fat and provides several essential unsaturated fatty acids not synthesized by humans. The essential fatty acids are shown at the bottom of this page.

The degree of unsaturation of dietary fat may also play an important role in the development of atherosclerosis, which will be discussed subsequently.

Steroids have a structure similar to cholesterol but lack an alcohol group. They include bile acids and a number of hormones, reviewed with their structure in Chapter 11.

The phospholipids like lecithin and cephalin are distributed in a variety of tissues; they are particularly important in the structure of cells and metabolism of fat by the liver. An example of a lecithin (phosphatidyl choline) is as follows:

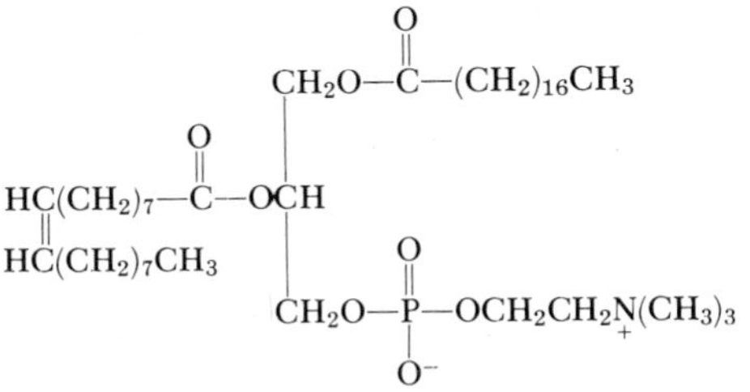

A lecithin
(phosphatidyl choline)

Choline is the nitrogenous moiety in lecithin. In cephalins, the nitrogenous moiety is either serine or ethanolamine in place of choline (Cantarow and Schepartz, 1967).

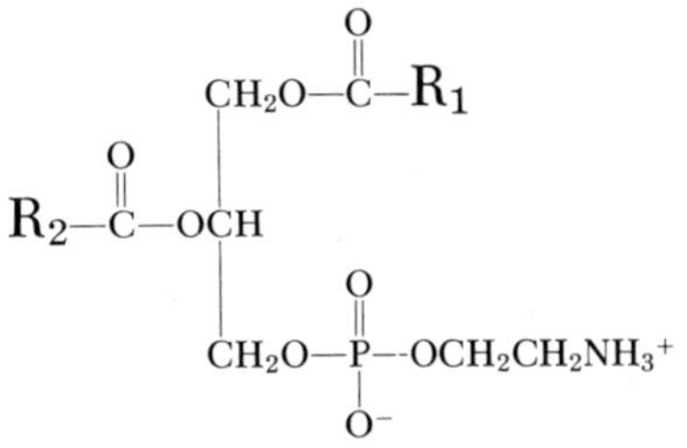

An ethanolamine-cephalin
(phosphatidyl ethanolamine)

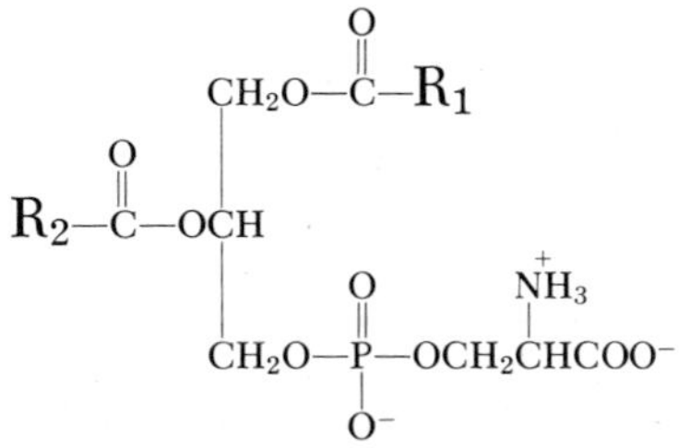

A serine-cephalin
(phosphatidyl serine)

Sphingomyelins contain a complex base (amino alcohol), sphingosine, in addition to a fatty acid, choline, and phosphoric acid. They are most abundant in the brain and nervous tissue. Niemann-Pick disease is associated with a widespread increase in sphingomyelin and cholesterol in many tissues of the body, especially in the reticuloendothelial system. Glycolipids have been considered as cerebrosides and gangliosides to emphasize their neural tissue distribution, but they are more complex and closely related as a family of glycolipids (Cantarow and Schepartz, 1967). In Gaucher's disease, high concentrations of cerebrosides are present in the spleen, liver, and bone marrow (Brady, 1972).

Other techniques, including electrophoresis and immunoelectrophoresis, have also yielded separation and identification of lipoproteins. According to Fredrickson and others (1967), four lipoprotein groups have been identified as follows:

High density (HDL) 1.063–1.21 or α (alpha) lipoprotein

Low density (LDL) 1.006–1.063 (S_f 0–12 and 12–20), or β (beta) lipoprotein

---

Linoleic (C-18)	$CH_3\ (CH_2)_4\ CH = CHCH_2CH = CH(CH_2)_7COOH$
Linolenic (C-18)	$CH_3CH_2CH = CHCH_2CH = CHCH_2CH = CH(CH_2)_7COOH$
Arachidonic (C-20)	$CH_3(CH_2)_4\ (CH{=}CHCH_2)_4\ (CH_2)_2COOH$

Very low density (VLDL) < 1.006 (S_f 20–400, 400–40,000), or pre-beta lipoprotein

Chylomicrons (extremely low density) < 1.00

For the sake of completeness, albumin-bound free fatty acids (FFA) may be considered a fifth group of lipoproteins. In alpha and beta lipoproteins, there is a characteristic HDL-apoprotein (A protein of alpha lipoprotein) and an LDL-apoprotein (B protein of beta lipoprotein), respectively. Both apoproteins are found in VLDL (pre-β) and chylomicrons. However, other proteins have been found in the VLDL fraction. The apoproteins lend immunologic specificity to lipoproteins. Chylomicrons and VLDL consist of a core of triglyceride and cholesterol ester surrounded by a more polar layer of protein, phospholipid, and cholesterol; since carbohydrate has been detected in most lipoproteins, they probably also contain glycoprotein components (Mayes, 1971). Alterations in the concentration of one or more of these classes have been identified in various clinical conditions, so it is important to appreciate this characterization of serum lipoproteins, which will be developed further.

To separate the lipoproteins, advantage is taken of their low density. Because of their differing sedimentation or flotation behavior in the ultracentrifuge, the serum lipoproteins have been prepared, purified, and classified. The rate of flotation of a lipoprotein in an ultracentrifuge is related to the density of lipoprotein; these are expressed as negative Svedberg units ($S = 1 \times 10^{-13}$ cm./second dyne/G. at 26° C.) or flotation S units, i.e., S_f value. As the proportion of lipid to protein increases, the density of lipoprotein decreases ($S_f \uparrow$) or the density of lipoproteins increases as the proportion of protein to lipid increases ($S_f \downarrow$). Much of the carbohydrate we ingest is converted to fat before it is utilized as a source of energy. Not only is fat a major source of energy for many tissues but, in certain organs, fat may be used preferentially to carbohydrate (Mayes, 1971).

Chemical Reactions of Lipids. Lipases (esterases) are enzymes that hydrolyze a neutral fat (triglyceride) to glycerol and fatty acids. The corresponding enzymes (esterases) that split other lipids are lecithinases and cerebrosidases. Alkali (KOH) hydrolysis of a fat or saponification liberates glycerol and alkali salts of fatty acids used in cleansing agents, called soaps, which have an emulsifying action. On the other hand, acid hydrolysis of a fat yields glycerol and free fatty acids. Unsaturated fats react with iodine in proportion to number and degree of unsaturation in fatty acid constituents. In a similar manner, hydrogenation converts vegetable fats from liquids at room temperature (attributed to number and extent of unsaturation in fatty acids) to solid fats (like animal fats) that are virtually completely saturated.

Metabolism. As a large concentrated form of stored energy (9.3 cal./gm.) and a major source of energy consumed in humans, body fat is in a dynamic state with continuing utilization and synthesis from carbohydrates or lipids.

Lipoproteins exercise an important role in determining the structure of several animal membranes and also regulate important enzyme reactions, such as electron transport in mitochondria. Certain hydrophobic proteins in the presence of phospholipid associate to form morphologic membranes. Lipoproteins are found in such subcellular structures as microsomes, mitochondria as well as the nucleus and in plasma are responsible for transport of most of the blood lipids.

The association of more insoluble (hydrophobic) lipids (triglycerides) with more soluble (hydrophilic) or polar lipids (phospholipids) in combination with hydrophilic lipoprotein complex permits transport of lipids in the blood (Table 9–26). Chylomicrons represent triglycerides derived predominantly from intestinal absorption (dietary source or exogenous), while very low density lipoproteins (VLDL) reflect transport of triglycerides derived from synthesis within the body, i.e., primarily the liver (endogenous origin). Lipoproteins synthesized primarily in the liver and intestine as a group have a turnover in the blood of about four days, faster than the turnover of any other plasma protein except fibrinogen (Mayes, 1971).

Adipose tissue yields fat in the form of free fatty acids (FFA) that are transported (unesterified) in the serum or plasma as an albumin-FFA complex. Hence, FFA in blood are classified as lipoproteins and consist primarily of long-chain fatty acids derived from lipolysis of stored triglycerides in adipose tissue (palmitic, stearic, oleic, palmitoleic, linoleic, etc.). The second source of plasma FFA, derived from the breakdown of triglyceride-laden lipoproteins (by lipoprotein lipase) during the uptake of plasma triglycerides into the tissues, represents a rather minor contribution to the total circulating pool of FFA. Despite a tremendous amount of FFA mobilization each day, the rate of removal of FFA from the blood is so very rapid that FFA contribute relatively little to the total circulating plasma lipid content at a given time (Fig. 9–54 and Table 9–26).

The FFA are taken up by cells of many tissues and virtually all major organs for oxidation to acetyl coenzyme A that is broken down to CO_2 and water with further generation of ATP in the tricarboxylic acid (TCA) or Krebs cycle. Oxidation of FFA is a complex system of reactions prior to formation of acetyl coenzyme A (acetyl-CoA) that also generates ATP

Table 9–26. TRANSPORT OF BLOOD LIPIDS AND A CLASSIFICATION OF LIPOPROTEINS*

CLASSIFICATION OF BLOOD LIPIDS	SUBDIVISIONS OF LIPOPROTEINS	DENSITY (gm./ml.)†	S_f	SIZE Å (diameters)	LIPID CONTENT PER CENT (w./w.) TC	TG	PL	PROTEIN CONTENT PER CENT (w./w.)
Albumin-bound free fatty acids (FFA)								99
Phospholipid-protein complexes		> 1.21 (very high)						
Alpha-(α) lipoproteins	High density lipoprotein (HDL)							
	HDL1‡	1.063 (high)						
	HDL2	1.063 to 1.112 (high)	0–2	95	18	2	30	45–55
	HDL3	1.112 to 1.21 (high)		65				
Beta-(β) lipoproteins (from liver and intestines)	Low density lipoproteins (LDL)							
	LDL1	1.019 to 1.063 (low)	0–12	215–220	43	10	22	25
	LDL2	1.006 to 1.019 (low)	12–20					
Pre-beta-(β) lipoproteins (very low density particles predominantly from liver or endogenous origin)	Very low density lipoproteins (VLDL)	0.94 to 1.006 (very low)	20–400	280–750	15	45	25	15
			> 400		15	55	20	10
Chylomicrons (particles 0.5 μ in diameter predominantly from intestine or exogenous origin)	Chylomicra	< 0.94 (extremely low)	> 400	750–12,000	2	93	3	1–2

*Compiled from data in Fredrickson, D. S., Gotto, A. M., and Levy, R. I.: Familial lipoprotein deficiency. *In* Stanbury, J. B., Wyngaarden, J. B., and Fredrickson, D. S. (eds.): The Metabolic Basis of Inherited Disease. New York, McGraw-Hill Book Company, 1972, Chapter 26.

†Density is proportional to protein concentration and inversely related to lipid concentration. > = greater than; < = less than; TC = total cholesterol; PL = phospholipids; TG = triglycerides.

‡Quantitatively an insignificant fraction.

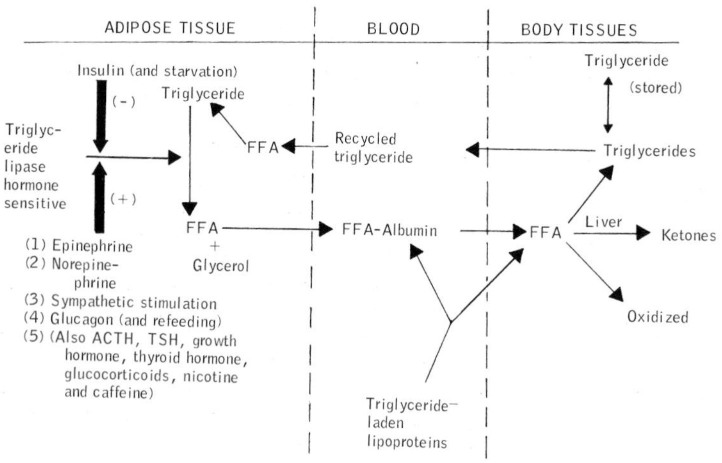

Figure 9–54. Schematic summary of FFA (free fatty acid) mobilization and transport. Those factors that stimulate the hormone-sensitive triglyceride lipase are indicated by the symbol (+); those that inhibit, by the symbol (−). (Courtesy of Frank Provato, M.D.)

for energy and takes place in the mitochondria, as does the TCA cycle. Through this mechanism, it is estimated that 25 to 90 per cent of the body's energy requirements in the fasting state may be met by FFA, i.e., uptake by tissues and subsequent beta oxidation to acetyl-CoA for use in the citric acid cycle. Synthesis of fatty acids from acetyl coenzyme A is also complex and takes place in extramitochondrial systems of reactions with further lengthening of fatty acid chain within mitochondria (Mayes, 1971). Lipogenesis reflects synthesis of fatty acids and ultimately lipids (triglycerides and phospholipids) from glucose and intermediates (pyruvate and acetyl-CoA). Lipolysis (hydrolysis) of triglycerides in adipose tissue by lipase yields FFA and glycerol, which are metabolized further in other tissues as described; re-esterification (fatty acids plus glycerol) replenishes triglycerides of adipose tissue, which reflects a dynamic state. FFA concentration and turnover in plasma is critical in terms of dynamics of lipid metabolism, which is intimately related to carbohydrate metabolism. Insulin promotes lipogenesis and inhibits release of FFA from adipose tissue. In other words, insulin (and starvation) inhibit hormone-sensitive lipoprotein lipase. Lipolysis with a release of FFA from adipose tissue and an elevation of plasma FFA may be enhanced, possibly through stimulation of hormone-sensitive lipoprotein lipase, by several pituitary hormones (ACTH, or adrenocorticotropic hormone; TSH, or thyroid-stimulating hormone; GH, or growth hormone; and vasopressin) in the presence of glucocorticoids (cortisol), thyroid hormones plus glucagon, epinephrine, and norepinephrine, as well as nicotine and caffeine.

Triglycerides transported predominantly in chylomicrons from intestinal absorption or as extremely low density lipoproteins (VLDL) undergo hydrolysis prior to uptake by adipose tissue. A lipoprotein lipase (clearing factor) is a critical enzyme for hydrolysis of triglycerides and cellular uptake as FFA and glycerol, which are disposed of in a manner described previously.

Lipolysis of triglycerides in adipose tissue may be associated with a different lipoprotein (triglyceride) lipase (i.e., more hormone sensitive) which is responsible for fat mobilization (Fig. 9–54). Its action and that of the other lipoprotein lipase enzyme concerned with tissue uptake of triglycerides account for free fatty acids (FFA) in plasma as NEFA (nonesterified fatty acids). This latter source of FFA (breakdown of triglyceride-laden lipoproteins during uptake into the tissues), as noted previously, represents a rather minor contribution to the total circulating pool of FFA. Furthermore, FFA that comprise dietary fat do not enter the blood as FFA, but instead, following breakdown of triglycerides in the intestine, the constituent fatty acids are resynthesized into new triglycerides and then released into the blood. There is a very rapid turnover (removal and uptake by tissues) of FFA related to FFA concentration (bound to plasma albumin), which in turn depends on production of FFA by adipose tissue. As we have noted, because the rate of removal of FFA from the blood is so very rapid, FFA contribute relatively little to the total circulating plasma lipids at any particular time (Fig. 9–54).

Hepatic Role in Lipid Metabolism. Although the paramount role of adipose tissue in lipid metabolism has been referred to previously and adipose tissue is very active metabolically as are other tissues, the liver is of major importance. It is the source of plasma endogenous (VLDL) lipoproteins and synthesizes triglycerides, phospholipids, and cholesterol. Furthermore, the liver oxidizes and synthesizes fatty acids with conversion of fatty acids to ketone bodies (ketogenesis), already described. By the production of bile containing cholesterol and bile salts (emulsifying agents) from hepatic synthesis, it enhances digestion and absorption of lipids and fat soluble vitamins within the small intestine. The chylomicrons (exogenous triglycerides) absorbed from the intestine are transported in the lymphatics as chyle to enter, via the thoracic duct, the vena cava and ultimately portal blood, where they are acted upon by the hepatocytes and processed as described previously.

Fatty Liver (Fatty Degeneration). Fatty infiltration (metamorphosis) of liver has been the subject of extensive and intensive investigation. It is of special interest to the pathologist because of its frequent appearance at autopsy in a variety of diseases and its relation to cirrhosis. The pale, greasy, enlarged liver shows mainly triglyceride accumulation in the hepatocytes. A fatty liver may occur when the production of lipoprotein does not keep pace with triglyceride synthesis in hepatocytes presented with an excess of free fatty acids (elevated concentration of plasma fatty acids). This is caused by a mobilization of fat from adipose tissue or extrahepatic tissue lipoprotein lipase action (hydrolysis) on lipoproteins or chylomicron triglycerides (Mayes, 1971). Diabetes mellitus (uncontrolled) and starvation as well as high-fat diets may induce this type of fatty liver. In another type of fatty liver, associated with a failure to produce or release plasma lipoproteins, the metabolic lesion may be at one or more sites within the cell concerned with lipoprotein apoprotein (A, B, ?C, etc.) synthesis, combination of protein with lipid, or hepatocyte transport and secretion of lipoprotein (Mayes, 1971). A deficiency of one or more lipotropic factors (choline, betaine, and methionine) that donate methyl groups is often associated with the production of this second type of fatty liver wherein triglycerides accumulate intracellularly with a normal uptake of FFA and synthesis of fatty acids. Malnutrition, protein deprivation, or a diet poor in methionine and choline (lecithins) may thus cause a fatty liver. An impairment of protein synthesis and fatty liver development occur with several substances, including ethionine (methionine analogue), chloroform, carbon tetrachloride, and phosphorus. A deficiency of vitamins (especially B group and E) and essential fatty acids (for phospholipid synthesis) are also associated with fatty infiltration of the liver. How alcoholism contributes to fatty liver development is not clear.

The ketone bodies mentioned with carbohydrate metabolism and diabetes mellitus are produced by the liver and released into the blood when there is a high rate of fatty acid oxidation. Several organs and many extrahepatic tissues utilize ketone bodies in the tricarboxylic acid cycle. With excess production or diminished utilization (less likely) ketoacidosis occurs, e.g., starvation and uncontrolled diabetes mellitus.

Triglyceride Metabolism. About 1 to 2 gm. per kg. of body weight of glycerides are ingested daily. In the intestinal lumen these are hydrolyzed, absorbed, and in the intestinal mucosa are reformed into triglycerides (long-chain fatty acid esters). These triglycerides are then incorporated into the extremely low density chylomicrons (presumably small amounts of pre-beta lipoproteins [VLDL] are also formed). The triglyceride-rich (about 88 per cent) chylomicrons are released into the mesenteric lymphatics and carried via the thoracic duct to the blood stream for distribution to most tissues where they are either utilized for energy or are stored, e.g., in adipose tissue, heart, and muscle. A notable exception to this tissue storage is the liver which, owing to the absence of the lipoprotein-splitting enzyme (lipoprotein lipase), is unable to take up significant amounts of chylomicrons. Medium-chain triglycerides and short-chain fatty acids absorbed in the gut do not participate in the formation of chylomicrons but are transported directly to the liver via the portal venous system. Triglyceride levels, as chylomicrons, peak in the blood two to six hours after ingestion of a meal and are generally cleared from the plasma by 10 to 12 hours after eating. Persistence of chylomicrons in the fasting state constitutes an exogenous hyperlipoproteinemia. As stated previously, chylomicrons are cleaved by the enzyme lipoprotein lipase at the tissue sites, liberating glycerol and free fatty acids to the tissues. Lipoprotein lipase may be located within the capillary endothelial wall of extrahepatic tissues (Fig. 9–55). Since lipoprotein lipase is stimulated not only by insulin but also by heparin, a diagnostic test for assay of this enzyme is referred to as the postheparin lipolytic activity or PHLA measurement. It involves administering heparin to a patient and then assessing the ability of his plasma to split free fatty acids from a prepared emulsion of fats or an estimation of the clearing of plasma specimens collected at 0 minutes and again at 10 minutes. Any factor which decreases the PHLA will result in an increased plasma chylomicron level.

Endogenous triglycerides derived from the liver constitute the major source of plasma triglycerides. Triglycerides are synthesized from free fatty acids taken up by the liver or from acetyl coenzyme A derived from carbohydrate metabolism. Before these triglycerides are released into the blood stream, they are put together or packaged primarily as pre-beta lipoproteins (VLDL), presumably by combining triglyceride with both alpha and beta lipopro-

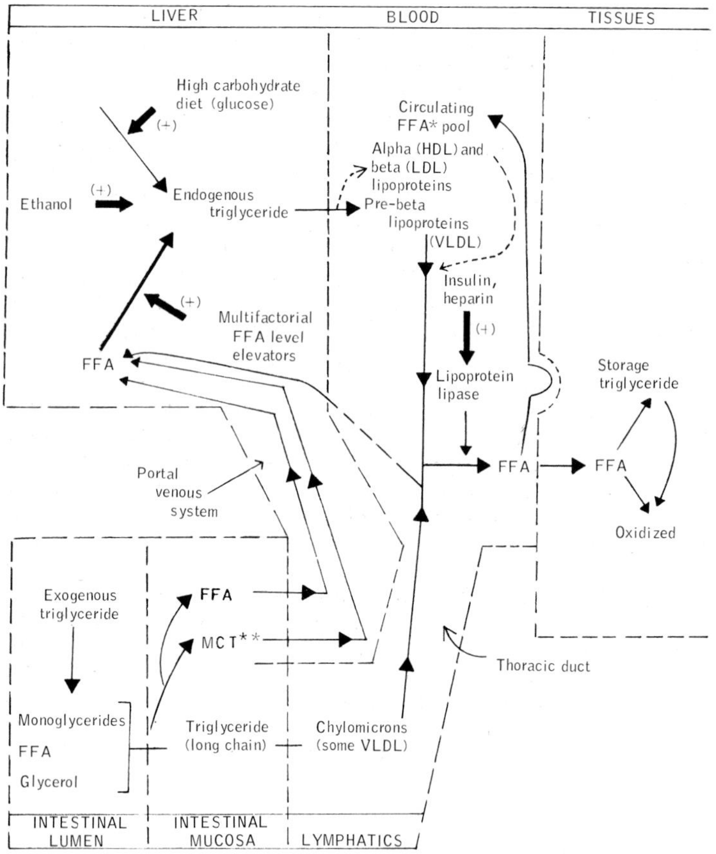

Figure 9–55. Exogenous and endogenous triglyceride transport and distribution. (Courtesy of Frank Provato, M.D.)
*FFA = Free Fatty Acid.
**MCT = Medium Chain Triglycerides.

teins (HDL and LDL). A very small amount of the endogenously synthesized triglycerides are transported as pure alpha lipoprotein (HDL) and beta lipoprotein (LDL). The contribution of the various lipoproteins to the transport of triglycerides may be noted in the following schematic outline (modified from Lees and Wilson, 1971):

Exogenous and endogenous triglyceride transport and distribution are shown in Figure 9–55.

Ethanol consumption and any of the factors that elevate plasma free fatty acids will enhance the synthesis and secretion of the triglyceride-rich pre-beta lipoproteins (VLDL), as shown in Figure 9–55. A carbohydrate-rich diet (especially sucrose and fructose) will also

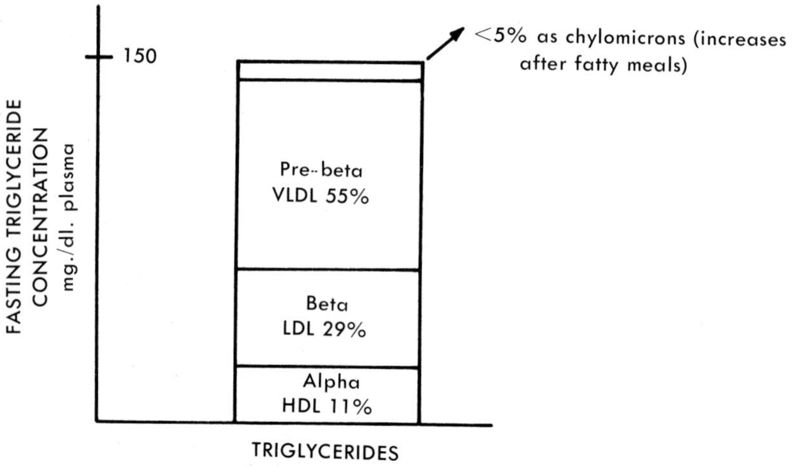

elevate plasma pre-beta lipoprotein (VLDL) and triglyceride levels. Such "carbohydrate induction" is a normal occurrence. In normal subjects, however, with the severalfold elevation of plasma triglyceride levels that ensues three to 10 days following initiation of a high carbohydrate diet, the lipid values usually fall thereafter even if the high carbohydrate diet is sustained. Individuals who show an increased sensitivity to high carbohydrate diets such that, following initiation of a high carbohydrate diet, the plasma triglyceride levels rise to sustained high levels, reflect "carbohydrate intolerance." The implications of this will be reviewed subsequently with discussion of hyperlipoproteinemias. Levy and Langor (1970) emphasize the normal half-life of the pre-beta lipoproteins (VLDL) in the plasma of about six to 12 hours. Although hypertriglyceridemia with elevation of pre-beta lipoproteinemia may be induced by alcohol (ethanol) and also by carbohydrates, it is interesting to note that if hypertriglyceridemia is induced in a patient by carbohydrate, it cannot be induced in the same patient by alcohol, and vice versa (Jones, 1973).

Cholesterol Metabolism. The average diet (meat and egg yolks especially) contributes a lesser portion (exogenous origin) to the total body cholesterol (endogenous plus exogenous origins). In contrast to endogenous synthesis of about 1 gm. per day, about 0.3 gm. per day arises from the average diet (exogenous). Cholesterol, in association with chylomicrons, after intestinal absorption eventually enters the portal blood. The liver extracts much of the exogenous cholesterol. However, chylomicrons are distributed to tissue sites where cholesterol is released to the cells; the uncertain role of lipoprotein lipase in cholesterol uptake is shown in Figure 9–56. Cholesterol synthesis takes place primarily in the liver but also may be found in many tissues, including the adrenal cortex, aorta, skin, intestines, and testes (Mayes, 1971). Actual synthesis involves a complex series of reactions with acetyl coenzyme A as a source of all the carbon atoms and several important intermediates, including squalene and lanosterol. Conversion to bile acids and excretion of neutral steroids that exit in bile and feces reflect the important role of the liver, which accounts for major pathways (90 per cent) of cholesterol excretion. An enterohepatic circulation of cholesterol and bile salts underscores the intestinal participation in cholesterol metabolism. Cholesterol is of great importance in synthesis of steroid hormones, the conjugated and degradative products of which are eliminated in the urine as a minor excretory pathway of

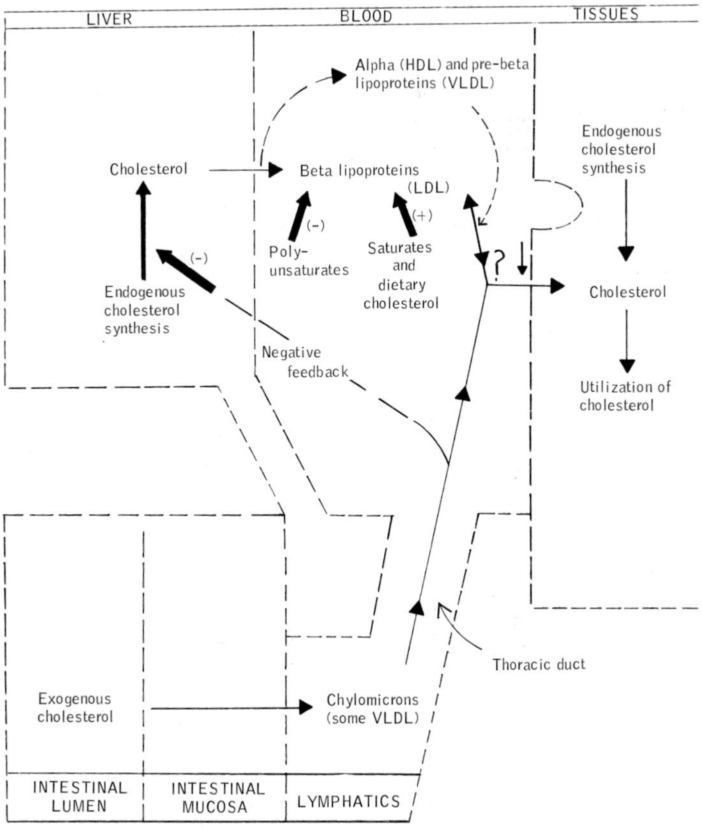

Figure 9–56. Exogenous and endogenous cholesterol transport and distribution. (Courtesy of Frank Provato, M.D.)

cholesterol. The few if any extrahepatic tissues not capable of synthesis may receive their cholesterol transported in the form of α- and β-lipoproteins (serum). Cholesterol synthesized within the body is transported in the plasma mainly as beta lipoprotein or LDL. The contribution of the various lipoproteins to the transport of cholesterol is shown schematically below (modified from Lees and Wilson, 1971).

Cholesterol in the blood has a wide normal concentration range that varies with age (approximately 150 to 300 mg./dl. serum). Although it may not be synthesized in all tissues, cholesterol is ubiquitous in its tissue or cellular distribution. Bile and pancreatic juice are necessary for digestion and absorption of cholesterol in the intestines. Nearly three-fourths of total serum cholesterol is esterified (by liver) and transported with low-density (LDL or beta) lipoproteins of blood for delivery to tissues (Fig. 9–56).

Lecithin cholesterol acyl transferase (LCAT), with highest activity in serum, has a key role in the metabolism of lipoproteins through formation of cholesterol esters, i.e., in conjunction with lipoprotein lipase, LCAT participates in the removal of triglycerides from plasma. In other words, as lipoprotein triglycerides are hydrolyzed by lipoprotein lipase, cholesterol esters formed through LCAT reaction may stabilize the lipoprotein structure. A second role postulated emphasizes that LCAT may promote a clearance of unesterified cholesterol from peripheral tissues. Unesterified cholesterol is diffusible in contrast to cholesterol esters, which are relatively "fixed" in lipoproteins (Jones, 1972). In the second role, unesterified cholesterol from peripheral tissue diffuses into the lymph and blood stream where, in contact with LCAT and HDL, it is esterified. Subsequently, cholesterol esters are transported to the liver where they are hydrolyzed and excreted. In combination these two key roles allow one to visualize the exchange of lipids between lipoproteins with cholesterol esterified in HDL diffusing to LDL. This dual role model combines the notions that LCAT reaction not only influences lipoprotein stability, but also participates in the transfer of cholesterol from peripheral tissue to the liver (Jones, 1972).

The substitution of a high content (absolute and relative) of polyunsaturated fatty acids for saturated fatty acids in the diet produces a reduction in total serum lipids (cholesterol, phospholipids, and triglycerides); the mechanism is not clear. Saturated fatty acids, especially lauric (C_{12}), myristic (C_{14}), and palmitic (C_{16}), are potent hypercholesterolemic agents, being twice as effective in increasing plasma cholesterol as polyunsaturates are in reducing plasma cholesterol. Sufficient polyunsaturates, with a limitation on saturates and cholesterol in the diet, will achieve a reduction in plasma cholesterol concentration. Saturated fatty acids with less than 12 carbons have no effect on plasma lipid levels. This may be related to the fact that medium-chain and short-chain triglycerides are absorbed directly into the portal venous system and transported to the liver where they are oxidized and reshuffled into new triglycerides. However, catabolism and excretion of cholesterol as bile salts and sterols are augmented by infusion of unsaturated fatty acids (Lewis, 1959). Drugs have been introduced to lower serum lipids; these interfere with synthesis, accelerate metabolism or decrease absorption with variable effectiveness (Table 9–27). The interest in lowering serum lipids is due to the attempt to reduce and reverse atherosclerosis, a disease that is characterized by lipid deposition (especially cholesterol) in the subintimal layer of arterial walls and tends to obliterate the vascular lumen (Taylor *et al.*, 1972).

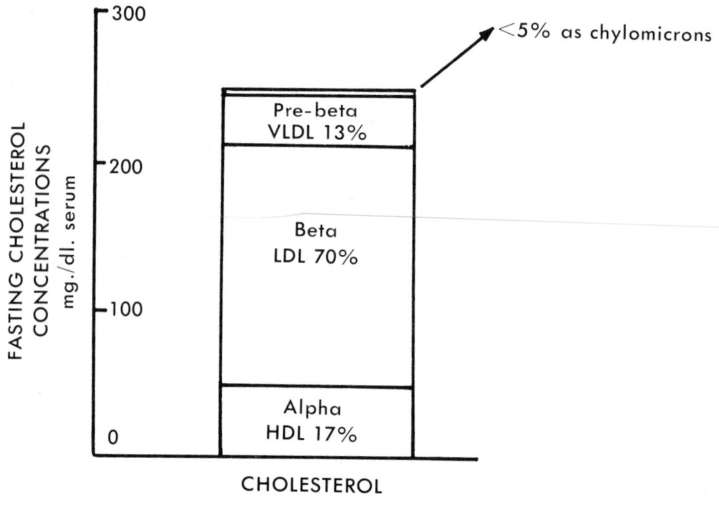

Table 9–27. PARTIAL LIST OF AGENTS SHOWN TO LOWER BLOOD CHOLESTEROL ACCORDING TO THEIR PROBABLE PRINCIPAL MODE OF ACTION*†

Inhibition of cholesterol absorption
- **Bile acid-binding resin (cholestyramine)**
- **β-Sitosterol (Cytellin)**
- Neomycin
- Brain extract (cerebrosides)
- Aluminum oxide (Gelusil)
- Androgenic steroids
- Competing sterols (dihydrocholesterol)
- Ferric sulfate

Inhibition of cholesterol synthesis
- **Phenylbutyrates (clofibrate)**
- **Nicotinic acid (Heparinoid)**
- Estrogenic substances
- Triparanol (MER-29)
- Aza sterols (7-aza-5 β-cholestan-3 β-ol)
- Ubiquinone
- Hydroxylamines (benzyloxy acetamide)
- Cholestane-triol analogues
- Benzmalacene

Enhancement of cholesterol excretion
- **Thyroactive substances (dextrothyroxin)**
- Salicylates
- Linoleamides
- Sulfaguanidine
- "Lipotropic" agents (choline)

Unknown mechanism
- Avocados
- Artichokes
- Mucopolysaccharides (mucin)
- Pancreatic extract
- Phenothiazines
- Vanadium

*Jones, R. J.: Med. Clin. N. Amer. 57:47, 1973.
†Agents in **boldface** type are those now considered to be clinically useful and commercially available. Individual examples are given in parentheses.

Blood Lipids. The total serum or plasma lipid measurements in healthy individuals of different age and sex reveal a distribution as shown at the bottom of this page.

Usual values and upper limits are more meaningful terms for consideration of lipid fraction concentrations than normal values because of wide ranges with different age groups. The absolute and relative concentrations of individual fractions (cholesterol, triglycerides, and phospholipids) is more significant than total serum lipids. Hyperlipidemia, by definition an elevation of one or more blood lipids, may be reflected by an opalescent to milky or turbid appearance of serum (called lactescence) and may indicate the usual postprandial rise or an abnormal elevation of triglycerides. It is possible, however, to have an elevation of this fraction as VLDL (endogenous origin) without lactescence. Phospholipids comprise the largest fraction of serum lipids (70 per cent phosphatidylcholine, 20 per cent sphingomyelin) and provide an adjunct to protein in the transport of other lipids.

Cholesterol, as the second largest serum lipid fraction, may also enhance the stabilization achieved by phospholipids. As mentioned previously, about three-fourths of serum cholesterol is esterified (liver) to long-chain fatty acids (mainly unsaturated). In chylomicrons, the ratio of free to ester forms of cholesterol is higher than in the remainder of lipoproteins.

Glycerides, virtually all as triglycerides (small amounts of mono- and diglycerides), comprise the third highest serum lipid fraction concentration. Fatty acid transport by glycerides is of primary importance. As described previously with triglyceride metabolism, exogenous and endogenous sources of triglycerides can be delineated. The former reflect dietary source absorbed from small intestine (1 gm. per kg. body weight or more per day), with initial appearance in chylomicrons. These are particles, 0.5 μ in diameter, composed of about 90 per cent triglycerides and associated with small amounts of cholesterol and phospholipids plus alpha and beta lipoproteins to stabilize them in aqueous solution. Endogenous triglycerides reflect synthesis and transport from the liver to adipose tissue and other organs in lipoproteins or 0.1-μ particles of protein, triglyceride,

		RANGE
Total lipids	600 mg./dl.	400–800 mg./dl.
Phospholipids	250 mg./dl.	150–380 mg./dl.
Cholesterol, total	250 mg./dl.	115–340 mg./dl.
Free	50 mg./dl.	
Esters	200 mg./dl.	
Triglycerides (neutral fat)	100 mg./dl.	25–190 mg./dl.
Free fatty acids (NEFA)	0.4 mEq./liter	0.3–0.8 mEq./liter

cholesterol, and phospholipids. Alpha (HDL) and beta (LDL) lipoproteins are frequently associated with endogenous triglycerides. As shown in Figure 9–55, these endogenous glycerides appear in the liver from at least three sources: (1) conversion of glucose, (2) conversion of free fatty acids issuing from adipose tissue in amounts exceeding need or capacity for oxidation, and (3) exogenous glyceride, which may be held temporarily by the liver and later retransported in the same manner as newly synthesized glyceride. The pre-beta lipoproteins (VLDL) are responsible for the normal levels of plasma triglycerides in the fasting state for normal subjects.

Although they represent only a few per cent of total serum lipids, free fatty acids contribute the greatest net transport of serum lipid. As described previously, adipose tissue liberates FFA when glucose and insulin levels are decreased; FFA are then transported (albumin carrier) to liver, muscle, and other tissues.

Lipoproteins. Serum proteins associated with lipid transport include albumin and alpha (α) and beta (β) polypeptides as well as other polypeptides. As mentioned, albumin is a carrier of FFA. The α- and β-polypeptides, named after electrophoretic mobility of lipoproteins, migrate with alpha globulins and beta globulins on serum protein electrophoresis. They differ in amino acid composition, antigenicity, genetic control, and presumably in their role in lipid transport (Fredrickson *et al.*, 1972). The lipoprotein peptides combine with variable concentrations of phospholipids, triglycerides, and cholesterol to form stable complexes; these combinations are identified by the terms alpha (HDL) and beta (LDL) lipoproteins and are a heterogeneous mixture. Ultracentrifugation (S_f) and electrophoresis as stated previously, are the techniques employed to characterize and measure lipoproteins, since fat solvent extraction techniques destroy them (Fig. 9–57).

In Table 9–26, the transport of lipids in blood and the characterization of lipoproteins are shown in a simplified tabular form. Four major subdivisions of lipoproteins which also manifest important biologic differences include high density (HDL) or alpha lipoproteins, the low density (LDL) or beta lipoproteins, the very low density (VLDL) or pre-beta lipoproteins, and the chylomicron fraction or $S_f > 400$ lipoproteins (Fig. 9–58). The LDL or β-lipoproteins transport most of the cholesterol and, to a lesser extent, phospholipids, which increase in concentration with age. In fasting subjects, the triglycerides are transported mainly by the VLDL or pre-β-lipoproteins; the pre-β-lipoproteins display their characteristic migration because they contain at least α-polypeptide as well as β-polypeptides (Fredrickson *et al.*, 1972).

Between the alpha and beta lipoproteins, there is a clear-cut, distinct separation by either centrifugation (on basis of size and density) or electrophoresis (on the basis of charge and size). The latter is shown in Figure 9–57. In the ultracentrifuge, high density lipoproteins display three distinct peaks, although usually subdivided into two fractions of HDL_2 and HDL_3, since HDL_1 is present in an insignificant quantity. In contrast to HDL_2, HDL_3 contains relatively more protein and less total cholesterol but a higher ratio of esterified to unesterified cholesterol. Between LDL and VLDL, the dividing line in the preparative centrifuge is arbitrary, with the more popular division made at 1.0×10^8 G min. at density 1.006 (Jones, 1973). However, there is a rather sharp separation between LDL and VLDL on paper, cellulose acetate, or agarose-gel electrophoresis, but on polyacrylamide-gel (PAG), multiple VLDL bands may be seen. As

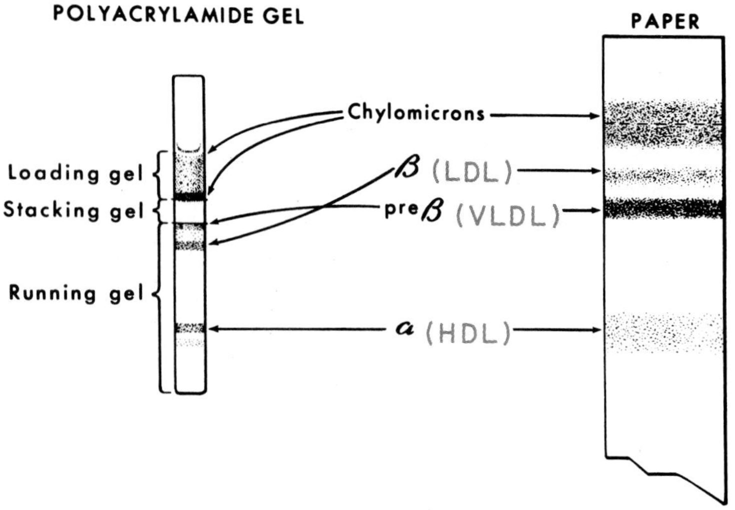

Figure 9–57. Migration of plasma lipoprotein families on polyacrylamide gel and paper electrophoresis. (Modified from Fredrickson, D. S., and Levy, R. I.: Familial hyperlipoproteinemia. *In* Stanbury, J. B., Wyngaarden, J. B., and Fredrickson, D. S.: The Metabolic Basis of Inherited Disease. New York, McGraw-Hill Book Company, Inc., 1972.)

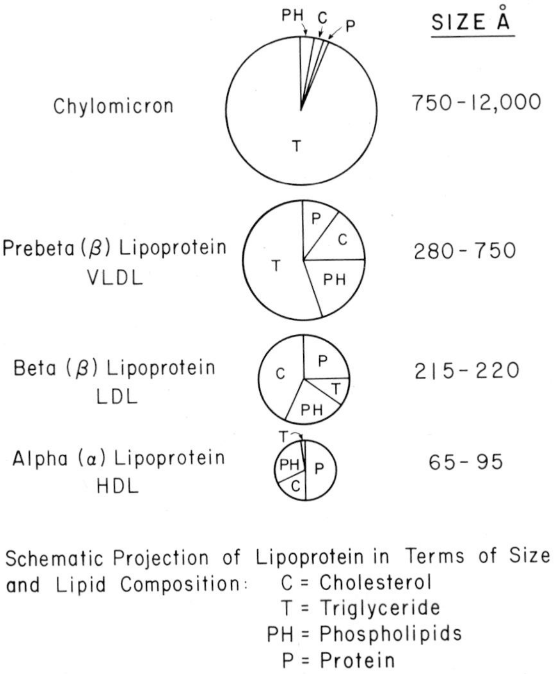

Figure 9–58. Schematic properties of lipoproteins in terms of size and relative lipid composition: C = cholesterol; T = triglyceride; PL = phospholipid; P = protein.

shown in Table 9–26, an LDL molecule contains about 75 per cent lipid and 25 per cent protein by dry weight. In regard to total cholesterol (TC) of 43 per cent in the LDL molecule, the cholesterol ester content is about five times that of unesterified cholesterol OR:

TC = 43% < 36% cholesterol ester; 7% unesterified

To four-fifths of cholesterol esterified in LDL, about one-third is esterified in VLDL, in which total cholesterol is much less but triglycerides predominate (Table 9–26). VLDL (in contrast to rather homogeneous LDL) is also heterogeneous with respect to size, density, and flotation rate (S_f), so it overlaps (at the lower end of its density range) with the chylomicron fraction and merges with LDL (at the higher end of its density range). It is not yet possible to get good separation of chylomicrons from VLDL because of this overlapping in size and density of primary (chylomicron or exogenous triglycerides) particles derived from lymph (but originating in the intestinal mucosa) and secondary (pre-beta, VLDL, or endogenous) particles made in the liver. Although the origin of LDL has not been elucidated, it is likely that LDL comes primarily from the liver also, although it is currently considered that considerable LDL may come from the metabolism of VLDL through removal of much of the glyceride and virtually all the apoproteins (Fredrickson *et al.*, 1972). With regard to HDL synthesis, which is primarily independent of LDL, it may occur in the same organs, the liver again being most likely the principal site. Alterations in lipoprotein concentration may be attributed to changes in production (increased turnover rate) or clearance (decreased turnover rate) as shown in Figure 9-59.

With electrophoresis of lipoproteins, Fredrickson *et al.* (1972) revealed several types of abnormal lipid and lipoprotein patterns in patients with familial hyperlipoproteinemia (Fig. 9–60).

Abnormal or Unusual Lipoproteins. Abnormal or unusual lipoproteins that may appear in plasma include: (1) "floating beta," (2) "sinking pre-beta," (3) lipoprotein X (Lp-X), and (4) complexes of normal lipoproteins with other globulins. Beta migrating VLDL, referred to as "floating beta" lipoproteins, have also been called broad-beta or beta-VLDL and are now

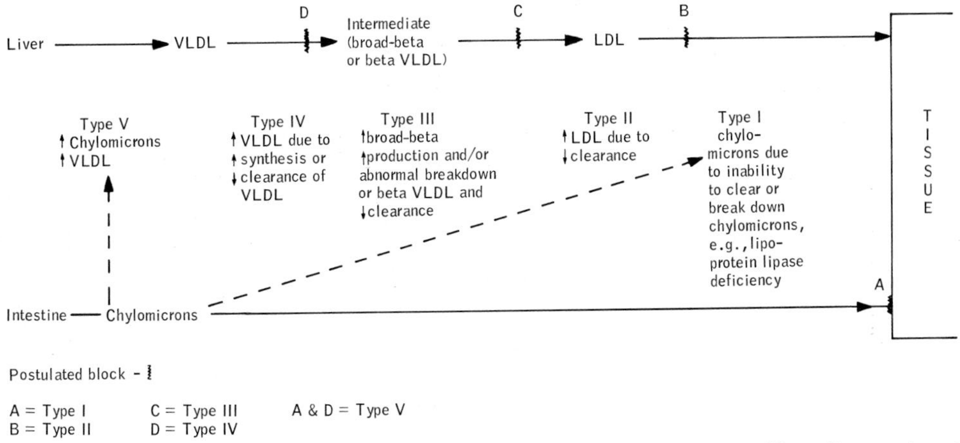

Figure 9–59. Schematic illustration of possible mechanisms for the development of hyperlipoproteinemia.

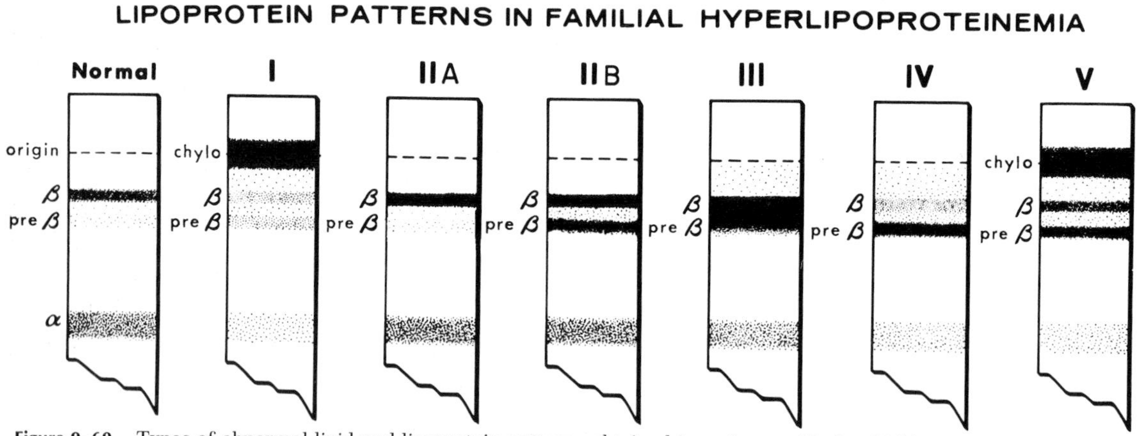

Figure 9–60. Types of abnormal lipid and lipoprotein patterns obtained in patients with familial hyperlipoproteinemia by paper electrophoresis. (Modified in part from Fredrickson, D. S., Lees, R. S., and Levy, R. I.: Genetically determined abnormalities in lipid transport. In *Progress in Biochemical Pharmacology*. Vol. 3. Basel, S. Karger, 1967.)

identified as either (1) lipoproteins of beta mobility floating at density 1.006 after 16 hours at 100,000 G, or (2) an inversion of the usual concentrations of S_f 0–20 and S_f 20–100 lipoprotein as measured in the analytical ultracentrifuge. While an absolute definition of this anomaly requires the ultracentrifuge, simpler methods that allow recognition include a combination of agarose-gel electrophoresis and polyacrylamide-gel (PAG) electrophoresis. In the latter form of electrophoresis (PAG), with a reversion of the distribution of the pre-beta (VLDL), there is clear separation and recognition of what appears to be a broad-beta on the agarose-gel. This abnormal lipoprotein is observed with the unusual form of hyperlipoproteinemia referred to as type 3, primary in etiology and often familial, to be discussed subsequently. In rare instances, a floating beta may be secondary to other diseases such as uncontrolled diabetes mellitus. However, a floating beta may prove to be a normal lipoprotein that is present in only trace concentrations, since with the use of electrophoresis after ultracentrifugation, it has been observed in patients homozygous for familial HDL deficiency (Tangier disease) as well as with type 3, hyperlipoproteinemia.

The sinking pre-beta lipoprotein (SBL) is an apparently normal variant pre-β-lipoprotein that has a higher density than conventional VLDL; SBL has a density of 1.050 to 1.080 (Fredrickson and Levy, 1972). This pre-beta band (SBL) on electrophoresis may sometimes arise from the HDL instead of VLDL (Jones, 1973).

Lipoprotein X (Lp-X) consists of complexes mainly of phospholipid, unesterified cholesterol and VLDL lipoproteins (including the delipidated proteins from VLDL) formed in patients with obstructive liver disease. It may be identified with an antibody which also reacts with apo-VLDL on paper and agarose. Lp-X migrates slower than beta because it contains free cholesterol and phospholipids. Since it contains free cholesterol and phospholipids, it stains poorly with lipid stains (oil red O or Sudan red dyes).

Between lipoproteins and immunoglobulins or macroglobulins, complexes, some representing antigen-antibody reactions, may occur. Certain IgA and IgG myeloma proteins react with lipoproteins; no consistent or definitive electrophoretic or ultracentrifugal test is available for their recognition. Finally, there are a few infrequently encountered, extremely rare abnormal lipoproteins that include HDL_+ or alpha T lipoproteins, while others which include HDL and VLDL have abnormal chemical compositions in familial lecithin cholesterol acyl transferase (LCAT) deficiency.

Clinical Pathologic Correlations

Hyperlipemia means a lactescent appearance of plasma caused by increased concentration of triglycerides in either VLDL or chylomicrons. Hyperlipidemia, on the other hand, means an increase in concentration of any plasma lipid constituent, which for practical purposes is usually confined to cholesterol or triglycerides or both. Hyperlipoproteinemia refers to an increase in plasma concentration of one or more lipoprotein families and is nearly always accompanied by hyperlipidemia. The patterns in which the four major lipoproteins appear in certain subjects resulted in the Fredrickson, Levy and Lees (1967) classification of hyperlipoproteinemias, which has been adopted in its latest modification by a committee of the World Health Organization (1972). This is shown in Table 9–28.

Table 9–28. FAMILIAL HYPERLIPOPROTEINEMIAS AND ABNORMAL LIPOPROTEIN PATTERNS

TYPE (WHO CLASSIFICATION)	SYNONYMS	CAUSE	LIPOPROTEIN ABNORMALITIES AND DIAGNOSTIC CRITERIA	APPEARANCE OF PLASMA†	USUAL CHANGES IN LIPID CONCENTRATION†	THERAPEUTIC PRINCIPLE
I (rare)	Essential hyperlipemia Familial hypertriglyceridemia Fat-induced hyperlipemia Exogenous dietary hypertriglyceridemia Familial hyperchylomicronemia Exogenous hyperlipemia	Dietary fat not cleared from plasma	1. Dense chylomicron band 2. VLDL, LDL, HDL normal or decreased 3. ↓ PHLA*** 4. Genetic basis – recessive	Cream layer on top, clear below	C ↑, TG ↑ (C/TG < 0.2)**	Restrict fat intake Medium chain triglycerides
IIa (common)	Essential hypercholesterolemia Familial hypercholesterolemia (with xanthoma tendinosum) Hyperbetalipoproteinemia Xanthoma tuberosum multiplex	Delay in removal of LDL ? Hereditary metabolic defect	1. ↑ LDL 2. VLDL normal 3. Dense beta band on electrophoresis 4. Tendon xanthomata or family history 5. Autosomal dominant	Usually clear, may be slightly turbid	C ↑, TG normal or ↑ (C/TG usually > 1.5)	Chemotherapy‡ Attain and maintain normal weight
IIb	Mixed hyperlipoproteinemia Overindulgence hyperlipemia	Long-term dietary excess ?+Hereditary element occasionally	1. Pre-beta band in addition to the above (IIa) 2. ↑ VLDL	Slightly turbid	C ↑, TG ↑	Diet alone probably adequate but may need reinforcement with chemotherapy
III (less common than Types II and IV)	Broad beta disease Floating beta lipoproteins Familial hyperlipemia	Hereditary metabolic defect	1. Wide beta-band on electrophoresis 2. β-VLDL ("floating beta", LDL of abnormal lipid composition) 3. Beta-mobility of VLDL, isolated by centrifugation 4. Absence of beta-band on polyacrylamide gel (not paper) 5. C/TG, VLDL > 0.4	Usually turbid, often with faint cream layer	C ↑, TG ↑ (C/TG variable, often = 1)	Diet and chemotherapy – reduction to ideal body weight
IV (probably most common type)	Hyperprebetalipoproteinemia Carbohydrate-induced hyperlipemia Endogenous hyperlipemia Endogenous hypertriglyceridemia	Disordered carbohydrate metabolism or excessive intake of carbohydrates or ↑ production of VLDL	1. ↑ Pre-beta band 2. ↑ VLDL 3. Normal or low LDL 4. Chylomicrons absent	Usually turbid, no cream layer	C ↑ or normal, TG ↑ (C/TG variable)	Weight reduction diet Reduced carbohydrate intake Limited alcohol
V (uncommon)	Mixed hyperlipidemia Mixed Types I and IV Exogenous/endogenous Hypertriglyceridemia	?Metabolic defect ↑ production VLDL	1. ↑ VLDL 2. ↑ Pre-beta band 3. Chylomicrons present 4. Exclude other types (PHLA normal) 5. Recessive	Cream layer on top, turbid below	C ↑, TG ↑ (C/TG usually > 0.15 and < 0.6)	Diet and chemotherapy

*C, cholesterol; TG, triglycerides
**G/TG = Cholesterol/triglyceride ratio
***PHLA = Post heparin lipolytic activity
† = After standing at 4°C for 18 hr or more
↑ = Increased
↓ = Decreased
> = Greater than
< = Less than
‡ = Chemotherapy may be in the form of clofibrate, D-thyroxine, nicotinic acid, cholestyramine, or iron-exchange resins as appropriate.

Table 9–29. TYPES OF HYPERLIPOPROTEINEMIA ASSOCIATED WITH SELECTED DISEASES*

DISORDER	TYPES OF HYPERLIPOPROTEINEMIA†
Acute intermittent porphyria	II
Alcoholism	I, IV, V
Autoimmune hyperlipidemia	I, III, IV, V, (II)
Biliary obstruction	Not associated predictably with any of the major types
Diabetes mellitus (insulin-dependent, uncontrolled)	I, III, IV, V, (II)
Dysglobulinemias	I, II, III, IV, (V)
Glycogen storage diseases	IV
Hepatic disease	II, III
Hypercalcemia (idiopathic)	II, IV
Hyperestrogenemia	I, IV
Hypothyroidism (myxedema)	I, II, III, IV (especially II and IV)
Nephrotic syndrome	II, IV, (V)
Pancreatitis	I, IV, V

*Taken in part from WHO Memorandum: Classification of Hyperlipidaemias and Hyperlipoproteinaemias. In Cooper, G. R. (ed.): Standard Methods of Clinical Chemistry. Vol. 7. New York, Academic Press, 1972.

†Secondary hyperlipoproteinemias are shown in parentheses.

Primary disorders of lipid metabolism reflecting familial or primary hyperlipoproteinemia or hyperlipoproteinemia secondary to known diseases or associated with selected common diseases are shown in Tables 9–28 and 9–29 and Figure 9–60. The secondary form is that caused by other known diseases, e.g., insulin-dependent diabetes mellitus (uncontrolled), dysglobulinemia, and autoimmune diseases as shown in Table 9–29. This table also denotes the types of hyperlipoproteinemia associated with several common diseases. Finally, the primary hyperlipoproteinemias must be differentiated into heritable and nonheritable forms. They may be evaluated through the following maneuvers: (1) simple inspection of serum or plasma that has been stored in the refrigerator, unfrozen, for 18 to 24 hours (most sensitive technique for the detection of chylomicrons); (2) specific measurements of serum cholesterol and plasma triglycerides; and (3) lipoprotein analysis including paper, agarose-gel, or polyacrylamide-gel electrophoresis (PGE), ultracentrifugation, and immunochemical techniques (e.g., LDL measurement).

Usually a combination of measurements is applied; namely, inspection of plasma specimen, serum cholesterol and plasma triglyceride determinations, and if either or both lipids are abnormal, lipoprotein electrophoresis most often employing agarose-gel and, if necessary, polyacrylamide-gel (PGE) for further resolution of possible type 3 patterns.

Plasma or serum specimens must be collected under minimum standard conditions that include the subject's having not eaten for 12 to 14 hours before blood is drawn, usually in the morning. His last meal (6:00 P.M.) should have been modest in fat. For two weeks prior to the blood specimen collection, he should not have gained or lost weight or have been on a diet unusual for his population group (i.e., a metabolically stable subject on an isocaloric United States diet). Finally, the patient must not be taking medications known to affect plasma lipid or lipoprotein concentrations. Preferably individuals should not have consumed any alcoholic beverages or taken any of several drugs in the previous 24 hours.

As stated previously, when the diagnosis of a primary disorder of lipid metabolism is suspected, serum cholesterol and plasma triglyceride measurements should be performed. If these are within normal limits, a primary disorder of lipid metabolism can be virtually ruled out for all practical purposes. However, if the fasting serum cholesterol or triglycerides or both are elevated, further study of the disorder and lipid metabolism must be pursued. A detailed history, physical examination, and carefully chosen laboratory studies will often distinguish primary from secondary hyperlipoproteinemias. To establish the familial nature of a hyperlipoproteinemia, the same abnormality must be shown in a first degree relative. Definitions and characterizations of hyperlipoproteinemias are noted in Table 9–28.

Not only is the abnormality in a lipoprotein pattern dependent upon quantitation of the serum cholesterol and triglyceride levels of the patient, but such determinations under appropriate circumstances may be sufficient in many cases for diagnosis. Indeed, a patient with a serum cholesterol above the normal limits who has a fasting triglyceride concentration within normal range most likely has a type II phenotype. With a family history of type II or the presence of tendon xanthomatosis (or xanthelasma), this is the genotype. Although electrophoresis may be helpful in confirming this pattern, it is not absolutely necessary. These observations emphasize the close correlation of serum lipid measurements with lipoprotein alterations; for example, cholesterol as a reflection of LDL concentration and triglycerides as a reflection of VLDL or chylomicron levels.

As shown in Table 9–30, a modest elevation of fasting plasma triglycerides associated with a normal serum cholesterol is seen in type IV or type V; pronounced hypertriglyceridemia in type I or type V and a combined but modest elevation of cholesterol and triglyceride in type IIB, type III, or type IV. While reference to the cholesterol-triglyceride

Table 9–30. PRIMARY HYPERLIPOPROTEINEMIAS*

TYPE AND APPEARANCE OF PLASMA	TRIGLYCERIDE CONCENTRATION (mg./dl.)	CHOLESTEROL CONCENTRATION (mg./dl.)	ADDITIONAL MEASUREMENTS AND EXAMINATIONS†	HYPERLIPOPROTEINEMIAS SECONDARY TO OR ASSOCIATED WITH SPECIFIC DISORDERS
I (milky, or cream layer over clear infranatant)	1000–30,000 (markedly elevated)	50–1000 (normal to moderately elevated)	Plasma post-heparin lipolytic activity, or PHLA (usually decreased) GTT‡ (normal)	Uncontrolled diabetes mellitus Pancreatitis Acute alcoholism Hypothyroidism Hyperestrogenemia
II (clear)	150–500 (normal to elevated)	300–1800 (markedly elevated)	GTT‡ (usually normal) PHLA (normal)	Diet (high saturated fats and/or cholesterol) Hypothyroidism Obstructive hepatic diseases Hypoproteinemia (nephrotic syndrome, etc.) Multiple myeloma Macroglobinemia Hypercalcemia Acute intermittent porphyria
III (turbid or milky)	175–1500 (variable to elevated)	200–1400 (moderately elevated)	GTT‡ (usually abnormal) Ultracentrifugation§	Hypothyroidism Dysglobulinemias Hepatic disease Diabetes mellitus
IV (turbid, clear or milky)	175–10,000 (usually elevated)	150–2000 (slightly elevated to elevated)	GTT‡ (usually abnormal)	Diabetes mellitus Pancreatitis Acute alcoholism Glycogen storage disease Hypothyroidism Nephrotic syndrome Hyperglobulinemia (monoclonal) Pregnancy Progesterone analogues along with estrogens Gout Gaucher's disease
V (turbid or milky; i.e., cream layer over turbid infranatant)	175–10,000 (usually moderately elevated)	300–1500 (elevated)	GTT‡ (usually abnormal) PHLA (plasma post-heparin lipolytic activity) normal to low	Diabetes mellitus Acute alcoholism Chronic pancreatitis

*Compiled in part from data in Fredrickson, D. S., Levy, R. I., and Lees, R. S.: New Eng. J. Med. *276*:148; 215; 273; 1967.
†Lipoprotein electrophoresis is an important aid in all of these disorders.
‡GTT = glucose tolerance test.
§Necessary for definitive diagnosis of type III hyperlipoproteinemia to identify very low density lipoproteins with a beta migration pattern on electrophoresis.

ratio (C/T) can often sort out these patterns, electrophoresis is a more appropriate maneuver.

The broad-beta or floating beta of the type III pattern on paper, cellulose acetate, or agarose-gel can be characterized in terms of this abnormal or unusual lipoprotein recognition through polyacrylamide-gel electrophoresis (PGE). In contrast to paper, cellulose acetate or agarose-gel, VLDL migrate behind instead of before LDL; HDL migrate to the most advanced position, as they do on other media, while chylomicrons remain at the origin in the loading gel of PGE (Fig. 9–57). On starch-gel electrophoresis, a migration similar to that of PGE is observed for lipoproteins. With type III, on paper, cellulose acetate, or agarose-gel there is usually a broad-beta band extending from the beta position into the pre-beta position. Indeed, this occurs in about two-thirds of plasma specimens containing a floating beta. A distinct pre-beta band is sometimes present and may be increased in intensity, whereas the alpha lipoproteins are usually decreased. A faint chylomicron band is often present even during periods of very low fat intake. However, on PGE electrophoresis, a broadened VLDL band is present, and no lipoproteins are seen in the usual position occupied by LDL on this medium. The presence of beta migrating lipoproteins on paper, cellulose acetate, or agarose-gel, but their absence on polyacrylamide-gel, is a presumptive test for the type III anomaly that is about 95 per cent accurate. Indeed, this combination of electrophoretic tests is often considered diagnostic. However, the definitive diagnostic test for the demonstration of beta migrating lipoprotein at a density less than 1.006 or floating beta requires ultracentrifugation at a density of 1.006 followed by paper, cellulose acetate, or agarose-gel electrophoresis of the supernatant fraction, demonstrating beta migrating lipoproteins. Normally only pre-beta lipoproteins and chylomicrons float at this density; thus, pre-beta migrating lipoproteins are present in the lipoprotein fraction with a density of less than 1.006. The type III anomaly may indicate the production of an abnormal LDL with an increased affinity for triglycerides; the increased triglyceride would account for reduction in the density of the beta lipoprotein (LDL) without altering the charge sufficiently to affect electrophoretic migration. An alternative explanation and mechanism suggests an abnormality in the normal breakdown of pre-beta lipoprotein such that an abnormal beta lipoprotein with very low density and heavily laden with triglycerides results. Finally, it has been suggested that there exists an intermediate of pre-beta lipoprotein metabolism, which normally is present in fleeting, small amounts but which persists in type III hyperlipoproteinemia (Levy and Langer, 1970). It should be suspected from a cholesterol/triglyceride ratio (C/T) of one (but ratio may vary from 0.3 to greater than two) and a broad-beta band appearing on conventional electrophoresis.

Type II appears to represent a dominant genetic trait, sometimes with reduced penetrance (Jones, 1973). Homozygous patients with serum cholesterol elevations three to four times normal die before adulthood of atherosclerotic complications. Heterozygous patients with type II pattern reveal a serum cholesterol value about two times normal and often have manifestations of coronary disease in their 20's and 30's (Jones, 1973). In addition, there may be a *forme fruste* that is dependent on a high fat diet for its appearance. Type II patients often show not only premature ischemic coronary artery heart disease, but also arcus senilis, xanthelasma and tendon xanthomatosis. Not only is there an increase in LDL, but the LDL cholesterol concentration is usually higher than the normal 170–210 mg./dl. (Friedewald *et al.*, 1972; Jones, 1973). As shown in Table 9–28, type IIB patients have an LDL cholesterol also greater than 170–210 mg./dl. in addition to an elevation of VLDL. With elevations of both cholesterol and triglyceride in their serum, the VLDL often responds to restriction of carbohydrates in the diet. Hence, type IIB patients should be treated as though they had abnormalities of both type II and type IV.

Table 9–30 demonstrates common changes in fasting plasma levels of triglycerides and cholesterol in primary disorders of lipid metabolism. Ancillary investigations are suggested that may help in the classification of the disease and other diseases that may give a similar lipid pattern in the plasma; these, of course, must be ruled out before a diagnosis of primary hyperlipoproteinemia can be established. Wilson and colleagues (1969) have reviewed postheparin lipolytic activity (PHLA) assays employing artificial substrates and human chylomicrons.

While the exact etiology and pathogenesis are not established, a schematic outline of possible mechanisms provides a point of departure for greater understanding of hyperlipoproteinemias (Fig. 9–59). Hence, hyperlipoproteinemia, type I, with an accumulation of chylomicrons as shown in Figure 9–59, may be attributed to a deficiency of lipoprotein lipase with a failure to take up the chylomicrons into the cell and, hence, a decreased clearance. On the other hand, an increased production of VLDL may well characterize type IV and type V. As one proceeds from VLDL to LDL, an intermediate variety may appear; it is associated with type III and may be related to an increased production or a failure in removal or clearance. Such an intermediate has been referred to as a broad-beta or floating beta. When it comes to LDL or low density lipoprotein (beta lipoprotein) observed in type II, familial hyperlipoproteinemia, there appears to be a defect in removal of LDL (i.e., rather than three to four days, seven to 11 days pass before disappearance), or decreased clearance.

Measurements of triglycerides and cholesterol are useful only insofar as they help to classify and assist in the management or treatment of diseases. Unfortunately, a disease may not always fit the classification proposed, and as more is learned about diseases, classifications may change. Synonyms for various disorders of lipid metabolism have proliferated rapidly over the past several years. Hence, a useful classification of disorders of lipid metabolism was greatly needed (Table 9–28).

In terms of secondary or associated disorders of lipid metabolism, elevations of serum cholesterol have been identified more frequently or more attention has been given to this lipid fraction than to phospholipids and triglycerides. In the third trimester of pregnancy, the serum cholesterol concentration rises, with sustained elevations until several weeks after delivery. In the nephrotic syndrome, an elevated serum cholesterol with lipiduria can be demonstrated; however, phospholipids and triglycerides are even more consistently and strikingly elevated. The mechanisms for these elevations of serum cholesterol are not clear. However, hyperestrogenemia (oral contraceptives and pregnancy) may result in an elevated alpha lipoprotein (HDL) with a rise in serum cholesterol. In the nephrotic syndrome there may be an overproduction and/or defects in interconversion of LDL and VLDL, so both are elevated. With intrahepatic (e.g., biliary cirrhosis) and posthepatic obstructive jaundice, moderate to marked elevations of serum cholesterol and phospholipids (greater) are observed; this is attributed to an interference with biliary excretion and enterohepatic circulation of cholesterol in the form of bile salts and neutral sterols. The unusual lipoproteins, Lp-X (rich in unesterified cholesterol and phospholipids), occur only in chronic biliary obstruction (Fredrickson and Levy, 1972). Estimation of cholesterol esters is an insensitive measurement of hepatic function. In hypothyroidism a moderate elevation of serum cholesterol that may reflect depression in overall metabolism is almost always demonstrable. Adrenocortical hormone therapy and Cushing's syndrome may be associated with slight elevations of serum cholesterol. As mentioned previously, diabetes mellitus (uncontrolled or inadequately managed) invariably reflects a moderate increase in serum cholesterol; this has been implicated as a contributing factor if not an etiologic factor in the development of vascular disease (atherosclerosis with coronary artery disease) and other complications in diabetics. Diabetic patients with atherosclerosis have higher triglyceride (including elevated VLDL) and cholesterol levels than diabetic patients without atherosclerosis or control subjects (Santen *et al.*, 1972). Table 9–29 summarizes the type of hyperlipoproteinemia that may be encountered in a variety of disorders.

In view of the histopathologic lesion in atherosclerosis (especially coronary artery disease and cerebrovascular disease) that shows a high cholesterol content in the lipid deposit (plaques), a disorder of lipid metabolism and particularly cholesterol or LDL has been incriminated as a causative factor. A high fat diet (saturated fats) and/or increased cholesterol ingestion may augment serum cholesterol and LDL levels to variable degrees. The ratio of phospholipids to cholesterol may be important, since phospholipids enhance the solubility and transport of serum lipids. In patients less than 40 years of age with suspected coronary artery disease investigated by coronary arteriography, those with cholesterols of 150 mg./dl. showed a lesser incidence of coronary atherosclerosis, while patients with cholesterol of 300 mg./dl. showed an extremely high incidence; however, triglycerides are elevated more frequently than cholesterol in such patients with coronary artery disease (Crowley, 1971). With moderate hypercholesteremia (i.e., plasma cholesterol level between 250 and 350 mg. per 100 ml.), Friedman (1966) has pointed out that it is statistically valid to consider such patients subject to three to five times greater risk of developing vascular accidents than normocholesteremic individuals. In addition, a patient exhibiting severe hypercholesteremia (above 350 mg. per 100 ml.) may not escape from prematurely occurring vascular accidents involving the heart and brain (Friedman, 1966). Undoubtedly, type IIa and type IIb patients can be associated with such elevated serum cholesterol values and early death or morbidity from atherosclerotic complications (especially coronary artery disease) and cardiovascular accidents. Early diagnosis of type II may be achieved with cord blood cholesterol measurements (Glueck *et al.*, 1971).

Kuo (1967) has stressed the value of serum lipid measurements (cholesterol, phospholipid, and triglyceride determinations) and serum lipoprotein analysis (paper electrophoresis) in obtaining an etiologic classification of hyperlipidemia in patients with atherosclerosis. More than 90 per cent of 286 patients studied by Kuo (1967) were found to have hyperglyceridemia derived from increased endogenous lipogenesis from carbohydrate; a carbohydrate-sensitive hyperglyceridemia was frequently found in association with hypercholesterolemia (type III). A variable lipogenic response to carbohydrate ingestion that may be profound in patients with atherosclerosis has therapeutic implications and underscores the interrelationship of carbohydrate and lipid metabolism in lipogenesis.

According to Jones (1973), type II and type IV patients are most often afflicted with serious atherosclerotic disease. In addition, types II and III primary disorders of lipid metabolism are frequently observed with atherosclerosis that may be premature, progressive, and severe, with vascular complications (Table 9-30). Taylor and colleagues (1972) have reviewed the risk factors in the pathogenesis of atherosclerotic heart disease and generalized atherosclerosis. They emphasize that regardless of age, one should never consider it too late to eliminate risk factors (e.g., hypercholesterolemia and beta hyperlipoproteinemia), not only to stop progression of disease, but to reverse it.

One or another serum lipid abnormality was seen in 80 per cent of patients studied under age 50 who showed abnormal coronary arteriography (Jones, 1973). When expressed in terms of myocardial infarction survivors, these appear to be almost equally divided between type II and type IV lipoprotein patterns (Table 9-31). Although the general incidence of type II and type IV patterns in the population as a whole is not yet established, in one study it was found that of a well population, 3.7 per cent had type II and 8.9 per cent had type IV patterns (Jones, 1973). The incidence of type I, type IIb, and type III patients may also be seen in Table 9-31 (referring to item D). In view of the reports that type II or type III patients will manifest arteriosclerotic cardiovascular complications in about 70 per cent, whereas type IV patients will show them in only about 21 per cent, type II appears to be much more "atherogenic" than the more common type IV abnormality (Jones, 1973). In Table 9-31, with particular attention to item C, the various phenotypes observed in an NIH referral clinic may be observed. Since these patients had secondary hyperlipidemias excluded, this selection may explain the difference in relative proportion of subjects with type II and type IV patterns from the other groups (Jones, 1973). The bulk of hyperlipidemias in a medical practice will be type II or type IV; the odd ones, types I, III and V are sufficiently rare to be numerically of little importance (Jones, 1973).

However, a type IV pattern is often associated with diabetes mellitus. Type IV is perhaps more common than types I and V in patients presenting with acute pancreatitis (Table 9-30).

Since dietary and drug therapy can modify lipoprotein patterns, brief consideration is in order. Type IV and V patterns frequently return to normal with a weight reduction or low carbohydrate diet. Type II patients will usually respond incompletely to even a strict low animal fat, low cholesterol diet. Since dietary fat from any source is responsible for the chylomicronemia in type I and type V patients, they may require particularly strict attention to dietary fat intake (Jones, 1973). Hence, diet therapy should be tailored to the lipoprotein pattern. The serum level of beta lipoprotein varies directly with the level of animal fat and

Table 9-31. FREQUENCY OF TYPES OF HYPERLIPOPROTEINEMIA*

<table>
<tr><th rowspan="2">TYPE, AGE, AND SEX</th><th rowspan="2">REFERENCE NO.</th><th colspan="6">TYPE (%)</th><th rowspan="2">NUMBER</th></tr>
<tr><th>I</th><th>IIa</th><th>IIb</th><th>III</th><th>IV</th><th>V</th></tr>
<tr><td colspan="9">A. Coronary artery disease</td></tr>
<tr><td>20–79, M and F</td><td>14</td><td>0</td><td colspan="2">28.1</td><td>0</td><td>25.2</td><td>0</td><td>126</td></tr>
<tr><td>20–49, M and F</td><td>14</td><td>0</td><td colspan="2">39.2</td><td>0</td><td>41.0</td><td>0</td><td>51</td></tr>
<tr><td colspan="9">B. Myocardial infarction survivors</td></tr>
<tr><td><55, M</td><td>31</td><td>0</td><td colspan="2">14.9</td><td>0</td><td>14.9</td><td>0</td><td>54</td></tr>
<tr><td><65, F</td><td>31</td><td>0</td><td colspan="2">19.1</td><td>0</td><td>17.0</td><td>0</td><td>47</td></tr>
<tr><td colspan="9">C. Familial hyperlipemics† (referred)</td></tr>
<tr><td>M and F</td><td>9</td><td>1.9</td><td colspan="2">64.2</td><td>8.9</td><td>17.7</td><td>7.3</td><td>966</td></tr>
<tr><td colspan="9">D. Normals</td></tr>
<tr><td>25–80, M</td><td>42</td><td>0</td><td>2.8</td><td>1.6</td><td>0.2</td><td>13.0</td><td>0.2</td><td>494</td></tr>
<tr><td>25–80, F</td><td>42</td><td>0</td><td>4.6</td><td>1.4</td><td>0.2</td><td>4.8</td><td>0.2</td><td>497</td></tr>
</table>

*Jones, R. J.: Med. Clin. N. Amer. 57:47, 1973.

†These numbers include only "primary" or familial Type IV patients.

cholesterol in the diet, while the pre-beta lipoprotein concentration depends directly upon the level of carbohydrate in the diet, especially fructose. Because ethanol may be responsible for some pre-beta lipoprotein elevation, it may be necessary to restrict it also.

Drug treatment may be used when dietary management is not completely successful (Table 9–27). The bile acid-binding resin, cholestyramine, inhibits the absorption of cholesterol; simultaneously it stimulates an increased conversion of cholesterol to bile acids. In Jones' experience this resin has lowered the serum cholesterol dramatically, even reducing serum cholesterol of some type II patients to normal levels. Because of a fairly selective effect on the LDL of the serum, serum VLDL cholesterol and triglyceride were sometimes increased enough to more than compensate for any reduction in LDL in patients with type IIb, III, or IV. This drug has been suggested as the treatment of choice for patients with hyper-beta lipoproteinemia. Clofibrate, which inhibits cholesterol synthesis, is another drug which is receiving much consideration in therapeutic trials. Clofibrate has little effect upon the serum beta lipoproteins but operates selectively to reduce the pre-beta lipoproteins; hence, it is more effective in lowering the triglycerides than the cholesterol, yet it can lower both cholesterol and triglycerides because the pre-beta lipoproteins contain both lipids (Jones, 1973). It appears to work most effectively to normalize patients with type IIb, III, or IV phenotypes who may not respond completely to dietary management, yet it has minimal effect in type IIa patients. Thyroactive substances such as dextrothyroxine enhance the cholesterol excretion, while nicotinic acid also inhibits cholesterol synthesis. In summary, cholestyramine will lower LDL (as in type IIa) and clofibrate will lower VLDL (as in types II and IV). Combined therapy, i.e., cholestyramine and clofibrate, may be indicated if both beta and pre-beta lipoproteins are elevated, i.e., type IIb. In view of the dietary and drug therapeutic benefits, it is essential that the physician screen all atherosclerotic patients for hyperlipoproteinemia before making dietary recommendations or inaugurating drug therapy. An awareness of these drug and dietary effects is useful in the interpretation of lipoprotein electrophoretograms in the course of patient management (Table 9–27).

While the phenotypes noted in Tables 9–28 and 9–29 may be seen in pure genetic expression as primary hyperlipoproteinemias, they are more often seen as secondary to some underlying disease or associated with some other disorders. Dietary influenced, i.e., carbohydrate or alcohol-sensitive, hypertriglyceridemia occurs rather frequently. With such dietary influences, patients may change from a type IV to a type V or from a type IIb to a type IIa or a type IV or even to a normolipidemic pattern (Jones, 1973).

Although all the phenotypes may have a genetic basis (particularly types I, II, and III), the environmental contribution in terms of diet, alcohol, drugs, physiological "stress," and disease remains significant in all; it is often predominant in types IV and V. With a weight reduction program or a low animal fat, low cholesterol diet, patients with elevated cholesterol levels will sometimes attain normal levels. A caloric excess or high carbohydrate diet will lead to an increase in serum triglycerides reflected in VLDL. While this carbohydrate-induced increase of VLDL is a universal phenomenon, it is exaggerated in patients with type IV patterns. On a weight reduction program, hyperpre-beta lipoproteinemia ($\uparrow$ VLDL) will often subside completely (normalize), so caloric balance is equally important. Jones (1973) has pointed out that the frequency with which minor elevations of fasting serum triglycerides and VLDL may be attributed to modest but regular consumption of alcoholic beverages remains unaltered.

Lipid Storage Diseases. The sphingolipidoses have been reviewed by Brady (1972). Enzymatic defects in cerebroside catabolism and their application to diagnosis are shown in Figure 9–61 and reviewed in detail by Brady (1972). Major signs and symptoms to correlate with the metabolic lesion of sphingolipidosis are shown in Table 9–32.

For the other diseases of the diffuse histiocytoses and lipidoses, defects may involve either synthetic or degradative pathways. A partial tentative classification of the lipidotic histiocytoses may be seen in Table 9–33. The lipoprotein deficiency states are reviewed succinctly in Table 9–34.

Familial Lecithin:Cholesterol Acyl Transferase Deficiency. Familial lecithin:cholesterol acyl transferase deficiency is a rare disease characterized by corneal infiltration, anemia, proteinuria, reduced plasma cholesterol esters and lysol lecithin, increased plasma unesterified cholesterol and lecithin, and absent or near absent levels of the enzyme in plasma (Norum, Glomset and Gjone, 1972). Peripheral blood smears reveal target cells, while erythrocytes contain increased amounts of cholesterol and lecithin. Erythropoiesis is decreased and erythrocyte destruction is increased (Norum, Glomset and Gjone, 1972). The very low density lipoproteins of the plasma appear to migrate in the beta position, while the high density lipoproteins are in the alpha-2 position. The elevated level of unesterified cholesterol and lecithin in the plasma may be attributed to the lack of the transferase. The erythrocyte abnormality may well be the result of changes

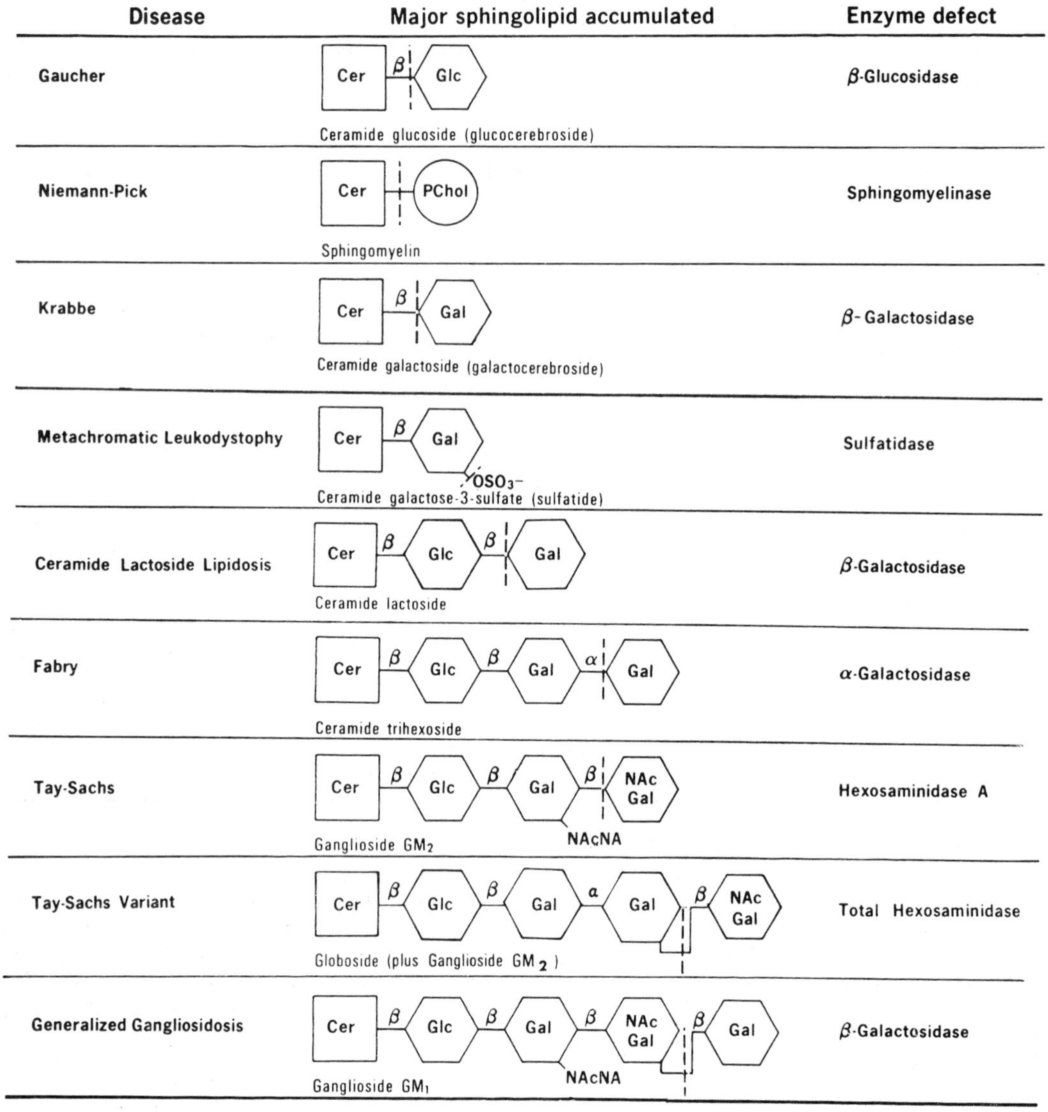

Cer = N-Acyl Sphingosine (Ceramide) Glc=Glucose PChol=Phosphorylcholine Gal=Galactose

NAcNA = N-Acetylneuraminic Acid NAcGal=N-Acetylgalactosamine

Figure 9–61. Metabolic lesions in the sphingolipidoses. (Brady, R. O.: Ann. Clin. Lab. Sci. 2:288, 1972.)

in the plasma environment resulting from the enzyme deficiency, while many of the clinical features can be attributed to abnormalities in plasma membranes resulting from the plasma deficiency of transferase activity. The feasibility of multiple successive plasma transfusions as a therapeutic maneuver remains to be explored further. Multiple transfusions may be of value in reversing some of the changes in this disease. While the genetic data are very sparse, it appears to be an expression of the homozygous state of an autosomal recessive trait.

Methods. The analysis of total serum lipids is less useful medically than the determination of individual lipid fractions. An appreciation of the principles employed in such analyses, however, provides much understanding in terms of individual lipid fraction measurements. While several techniques have been developed, we prefer a gravimetric method for serum total lipids and a titrimetric (acidimetric) estimation of fatty acids for fecal fat (described in Chap. 17). Bloor's mixture (three parts absolute ethanol plus one part ethyl ether) as a solvent, when added to serum with

Table 9–32. MAJOR SIGNS AND SYMPTOMS OF THE SPHINGOLIPIDOSES*

Gaucher's disease	Mental retardation (infantile form only), hepatosplenomegaly, hip and long bone involvement, Oil-red-O and PAS-positive lipid-laden cells in bone marrow, increased serum acid phosphatase, mild anemia, and thrombocytopenia
Niemann-Pick disease	Generally similar to Gaucher's disease; 30 per cent with cherry-red spot in macula; marrow cells (foam cells) stain for both lipid and phosphorus, cachexia
Globoid leukodystrophy (Krabbe's disease)	Mental retardation; almost total absence of myelin, severe gliosis, and multinucleated "globoid bodies" in white matter
Metachromatic leukodystrophy	Mental retardation; psychological disturbances (adult form); decreased nerve conduction time; nerve biopsy shows yellow-brown droplets when stained with cresyl violet (metachromasia)
Ceramide lactoside lipidosis	Slowly progressing CNS impairment; hepatosplenomegaly; macrocytic anemia, leukopenia and thrombocytopenia due to involvement of bone marrow and spleen
Fabry's disease	Reddish purple maculopapular rash in umbilical, inguinal and scrotal areas; renal impairment; corneal opacities; peripheral neuralgias and abnormalities of EKG
Tay-Sachs disease	Mental retardation, amaurosis, cherry-red spot in macula, macrocephaly, neuronal cells distended with "membranous cytoplasmic bodies"
Generalized gangliosidosis	Mental retardation, cherry-red spot in macula (50 per cent of patients), hepatosplenomegaly, foam cells in bone marrow, rarefaction of all bones and skeletal deformities

*Brady, R. O.: Ann. Clin. Lab. Sci. *2*:286, 1972.

the aid of heat, permits extraction of lipids and precipitation of proteins (separated by filtration). Virtually all serum lipids are bound to protein (lipoproteins); this solvent insures their complete dissociation as well as extraction. Since the filtered extract contains nonlipid substances (e.g., glucose, uric acid, urea, creatinine, glutathione, and inorganic salts), it must be dried and reextracted with petroleum ether; this extract is filtered again, with elimination of all the nonlipid constituents (R. J. Henry, 1964). A final drying with aid of infrared light of filtered petroleum ether extracts (pooled) in a preweighed beaker precedes gravimetric estimation in the final step. Several other extraction techniques yield a nonoxidized lipid residue that is reduced by dichromate for spectrophotometric analysis (Bragdon, 1960). In view of the heterogeneity of serum lipids with varying reducing capabilities, the selection of an appropriate standard (e.g., palmitate) for a spectrophotometric procedure is arbitrary. Nevertheless, satisfactory precision if not optimal accuracy can be achieved for total serum lipids by several methods (R. J. Henry, 1964; Sunderman and Sunderman, 1964).

The inherent difficulties and need for improved accurate, precise, and rapid methods for analysis of the individual lipid fractions has undoubtedly contributed to the vast amount of literature published in the past decade. Chromatographic techniques, includ-

Table 9–33. CLASSIFICATION OF LIPIDOTIC HISTIOCYTOSES*

Differentiated Lipidoses
- Strict neurolipidoses (cerebromacular degenerations)
  - Congenital amaurotic idiocy
  - Infantile Tay-Sachs disease
  - Childhood Jansky-Bielschowsky disease
  - Juvenile Spielmeyer-Vogt disease
  - Adult Kufs-Sjögren disease
- Neuroreticuloendothelial lipidoses (symptoms follow lipid storage)
  - Niemann-Pick disease; Wolman's disease
  - Gaucher's disease (acute infantile, chronic childhood, benign adult)
  - Metachromatic leukodystrophy
  - Lipidemic amentia
  - Generalized gangliosidosis
  - Fabry's disease
- Differentiated progressive histiocytoses (lipid storage follows symptoms)
- Histiocytosis "X" group: (1) Letterer-Siwe (acute), (2) Hand-Schüller-Christian (chronic), (3) solitary eosinophilic granuloma

*Courtesy of Robert E. Wenk, M.D.

Table 9–34. FAMILIAL LIPOPROTEIN DEFICIENCY STATES*

DISEASE(S)	CHOLESTEROL (mg./dl. plasma)	TRIGLYCERIDES (mg./dl. plasma)	PHOSPHOLIPID (mg./dl. plasma)	ADDITIONAL MEASUREMENTS AND EXAMINATIONS
Abetalipoproteinemia CLINICAL FEATURES: retarded growth and fat malabsorption in infancy; progressive neurologic (especially ataxia) deficits in late childhood, and retinitis pigmentosa	20–80 (very low)	0–20 (very low)	35–95 (very low)	Acanthocytosis on peripheral blood smear; liver biopsy and intestinal biopsy reveal foamy and vacuolated cells; lipoprotein electrophoresis shows absence of beta (LDL) lipoproteins, pre-beta (VLDL) and chylomicrons; only α lipoprotein (HDL) persist
Hypobetalipoproteinemia (familial low density lipoprotein (LDL) deficiency) CLINICAL FEATURES: progressive neuromuscular difficulties in adulthood	55–150 (low to very low)	15–75 (low to normal)	110–170 (low, normal, or borderline)	Erythrocyte fragility test, intestinal absorption studies; lipoprotein electrophoresis reveals a deficiency of LDL as reflected by a faint beta lipoprotein band; VLDL and HDL are normal
Familial high density lipoprotein (HDL) deficiency or alpha-lipoprotein deficiency (Tangier disease) CLINICAL FEATURES: enlarged orange-yellow coloration of tonsils; peripheral neuropathy; splenomegaly; occasionally hepatomegaly and lymphadenopathy	30–125 (low)	150–330 (normal or elevated)	70–140 (abnormally low)	Tonsillar biopsy (cholesterol lipid as foam cell accumulation); lipoprotein electrophoresis reveals virtual absence of high density lipoproteins (HDL) but a broad beta band due to abnormal β-migrating (LDL) lipoprotein in the VLDL fraction of plasma or anomaly of type III hyperlipoproteinemia

*Compiled from data in Fredrickson, D. S., Levy, R. I., and Lees, R. S.: New Eng. J. Med. *276*:37, 94, 1967; and Fredrickson, D. S., Gotto, A. M., and Levy, R. I.: Familial lipoprotein deficiencies. *In* Stanbury, J. B., Wyngaarden, J. B., and Fredrickson, D. S. (eds.): *The Metabolic Basis of Inherited Disease.* New York, McGraw-Hill Book Company, 1972, Chapter 26.

ing thin layer, gas liquid, paper, and column, represent powerful tools for estimation of lipids that have been proposed but not generally accepted for daily service application (Skipski, Peterson, and Barclay, 1964; Hamilton *et al.*, 1961).

Cholesterol Assays. Cholesterol, because of its medical importance, has probably prompted the development of more methods for its measurement than the other lipid fractions. Improved accuracy and precision as well as rapidity and practicality of analysis have been the goals of various methods that have evolved. Extraction of serum with an organic solvent (e.g., ethanol-ether, isopropanol, chloroform, or acetone) with particular attention to temperature and proportions (solvent and serum) separates the lipid from protein and denatures proteins (precipitation). A great deal of attention has been given to the selection of solvent systems that represent the initial step or preliminary procedure in many determinations; however, several methods have been developed to bypass this first step and substitute a direct reaction mixture. Digitonin is used to separate the extracted free cholesterol (digitonide precipitate) from esterified cholesterol when total cholesterol and cholesterol ester determinations are requested. The hydroxyl group on the third carbon atom of the A ring in the steroid nucleus reacts with digitonin to form an insoluble complex in most solvents. Since the specificity is not absolute and the medical importance of cholesterol esters has declined (insensitive test of hepatic function), this step is of historical interest only. In some procedures, however, an alkali hydrolysis (saponification) step has been incorporated to allow digitonide precipitation of all the cholesterol or to yield more complete extraction into certain organic solvents such as petroleum ether (R. J. Henry, 1964). The final step for spectrophotometric analysis most often requires a complete colorimetric reaction that is dependent on many variables, such as concentration of reactants (type and concentration of oxidizing agents), solvents, temperature, time, and light (R. J. Henry, 1964). The most popular if not the most common is the Lieberman-Burchard color reaction, in which a chloroform solution of cholesterol is admixed with concentrated sulfuric acid (H_2SO_4) in acetic anhydride to produce a green color with a maximum absorption peak at 620 nm. The names of Bloor, Schoenheimer, and Sperry and Abell and associates (1958), among others, reflect advances in lipid chemistry and cholesterol methodology. The method of Abell *et al.* (1958) has secured a firm position as a reference method and is practical as well as precise and accurate; it involves (1) ethanolic alkali (KOH) to liberate the cholesterol from protein complexes (lipoproteins) and saponify the cholesterol esters, (2) extraction of the cholesterol into petroleum ether after an aqueous dilution of alcoholic solution, and (3) measurement of the cholesterol in a portion of the petroleum ether layer after the Lieberman-Burchard reaction (Abell *et al.*, 1958). Honing and coworkers (1968), employing the Autoanalyzer, have automated the method of Abell. This appears to be a most accurate procedure with a standard error of analysis of 1.5 per cent.

The Lieberman-Burchard reaction may be applied directly to serum without an initial organic solvent extraction step. In the method of Pearson, Stern, and McGavach (1953), paratoluenesulfonic acid liberates cholesterol from lipoproteins for direct reaction with sulfuric acid in the presence of acetic anhydride and acetic acid.

A direct colorimetric method using a ferric chloride sulfuric acid reagent and glacial acetic acid solution of cholesterol has become increasingly popular in recent years, especially with automation (Zlatkis, Zak, and Boyle, 1953; Zak, Epstein, and Baginski, 1972). It is a more sensitive reaction that yields a more intense and stable color than the Lieberman-Burchard color reaction; however, it is also light sensitive. A modification of Zlatkis iron color reagent with isopropanol extraction of serum cholesterol (and precipitation of proteins) by Leffler and McDougald (1963) enhanced the specificity of this color reaction by elimination of several interfering substances (especially bilirubin and bromide); a second extraction with petroleum ether followed by the addition of sodium hydroxide, evaporation to dryness, and resuspension in isopropanol represents an alternate procedure for icteric serum that eliminates completely interference from bilirubin and bromide. Bilirubin is also removed by adsorbent aluminum hydroxide gel in a modification described by Babson *et al.* (1962). The improved iron color reaction procedures are comparable to the reference method of Abell *et al.* (1958) and with increasing automation are gaining widespread application (Block *et al.*, 1966). Jung and Parekh (1971) have described a direct method employing ferric acetate–uranium acetate and sulfuric acid–ferrous sulfate reagents. The ferric acetate–uranium acetate is a unique precipitating agent that removes bilirubin with proteins, clears the serum of lipids, and extracts cholesterol without need of solvents. When the acetate reagent extract is mixed with sulfuric acid–ferrous sulfate reagent, it produces a purple color with a maximum absorbance at 560 nm. and maximum color development within 15 minutes; it is stable for at least 1 hour. It also correlates well with analyses by the Abell technique and appears to be practically free from interference. According to Sunderman and Sunderman

(1972), it may well prove to be the method of choice for clinical laboratories.

The importance of pure cholesterol standards cannot be overemphasized; this has been reviewed critically by Radin and Gramza (1963), who recommend a dibromide method for cholesterol recrystallization, followed by estimation of molar absorptivity (Radin, 1965; Witter *et al.*, 1970). NBS (National Bureau of Standards) and CAP (College of American Pathologists) offer cholesterol standards for standardization of methods.

An immunochemical method for estimation of beta lipoprotein (LDL) is commercially available (BETA-L Test Kit, Hyland Laboratories, Los Angeles, California). It has been evaluated and recommended as an additional procedure for studies of serum lipid (Reveno and MacDonald, 1964). VLDL must be removed by ultracentrifugation before LDL can be measured immunochemically, since VLDL and LDL share antigenic determinants (Lees, 1970). However, Friedewald, Levy and Fredrickson (1972) described a method for estimation of LDL cholesterol in plasma without use of the preparative ultracentrifuge.

Serum should be used for cholesterol analysis, since anticoagulants may dilute plasma with cell water (by increasing osmotic pressure), causing falsely depressed values. Since hemolysis liberates cholesterol from erythrocytes, a hemolyzed serum specimen must be avoided to eliminate false positive elevations. Despite a general lack of agreement as to normal values for total serum cholesterol, Keys *et al.* (1950) have reported normal values for males as follows:

AGE (YEARS)	RANGE (mg./dl. SERUM)
20	101–189
30	108–218
40	128–237
50	145–270
60	165–258
70	129–246

Cord blood cholesterol values have been reported to range from 20 to 196 mg. per dl., with a mean of 63.8 and SD $\pm$ 18.7; this yields a normal cutoff at about 130 mg. per dl. (Glueck *et al.*, 1971). With direct serum cholesterol measurements as performed on the SMA 12–60, serum cholesterol values may be as high as 10 per cent greater when compared with a serum cholesterol extraction method. With an elevated level, e.g., 300 mg. per dl., there may be as high as a 30 mg. per cent difference in the methods.

Sperry and Schoenheimer (1935) have reported normal values for males to range from 150 to above 350 mg. per 100 ml. Adult females have somewhat lower normal ranges than adult males until they are postmenopausal, at which time they are approximately the same for matched age groups; this may reflect an estrogen effect on the relative concentration of alpha lipoproteins (HDL). The "normal limits" of Fredrickson and his colleagues (1972) are presented in Table 9–35. Cholesterol appears to vary not only with age and sex but also with race, geographic location, diet, seasonal factors, physical activity, and occupational stress.

Troxler and co-workers (1972) studied serum cholesterol in 1000 male flyers age 20 to 50 screened for coronary artery disease by treadmill EKGs at the USAF School of Aerospace Medicine. The mean serum cholesterol per age group was consistent with data reported in studies by Keys *et al.*, (1950) and by Fredrickson *et al.* (1967). The data were compiled in percentiles for 5 mg./dl. increments of cholesterol and five-year age groups (Table 9–36).

Triglyceride Assays. Witter and Whitner (1972) emphasize three basic methods for determination of triglycerides: enzymatic; colorimetric, in which the glycerol is oxidized to formaldehyde; and fluorometric, which measures formed formaldehyde. Specificity is gained by initial extraction of lipids from

Table 9–35. PLASMA CHOLESTEROL, TRIGLYCERIDE CONCENTRATIONS AND CHOLESTEROL CONCENTRATION OF MAJOR LIPOPROTEIN FRACTIONS AS SUGGESTED "NORMAL" LIMITS ACCORDING TO AGE*

AGE (yrs.)	TOTAL CHOLESTEROL (mg./dl.)	TRIGLYCERIDE (mg./dl.)	PRE-BETA CHOLESTEROL (VLDL) (mg./dl.)	BETA CHOLESTEROL (LDL) (mg./dl.)	ALPHA CHOLESTEROL (HDL) (mg./dl.) Males	ALPHA CHOLESTEROL (HDL) (mg./dl.) Females
0–19	230	140	25	170	65	70
20–29	240	140	25	170	70	75
30–39	270	150	35	190	65	80
40–49	310	160	35	190	65	85
50–59	330	190	40	210	65	85

*From Fredrickson, D. S., and Levy, R. I.: Familial hyperlipoproteinemia. *In* Stanbury, J. B., Wyngaarden, J. B., and Fredrickson, D. S. (eds.): *The Metabolic Basis of Inherited Disease.* 3rd ed., New York, McGraw-Hill Book Company, 1972, p. 531.

Table 9–36. SERUM CHOLESTEROL PERCENTILE DISTRIBUTION BY AGE GROUP*

SERUM CHOLESTEROL mg./dl.	AGE IN YEARS						
	20–24	25–29	30–34	35–39	40–44	45–49	50+
110	0.01	<0.01	0.01	<0.01	<0.01	<0.01	<0.01
125	0.03	<0.01	0.02	0.01	<0.01	<0.01	<0.01
130	0.03	0.02	0.03	0.01	0.01	<0.01	<0.01
135	0.05	0.02	0.04	0.01	0.01	0.01	<0.01
140	0.14	0.07	0.04	0.03	0.01	0.01	0.02
145	0.15	0.09	0.05	0.03	0.02	0.01	0.02
150	0.19	0.12	0.08	0.06	0.02	0.01	0.02
155	0.22	0.15	0.09	0.09	0.03	0.04	0.02
160	0.24	0.19	0.18	0.13	0.05	0.05	0.07
165	0.33	0.24	0.22	0.17	0.07	0.08	0.09
170	0.36	0.29	0.26	0.22	0.11	0.09	0.12
175	0.42	0.34	0.32	0.24	0.16	0.11	0.14
180	0.50	0.45	0.37	0.32	0.18	0.14	0.19
185	0.61	0.49	0.42	0.38	0.22	0.18	0.21
190	0.68	0.56	0.48	0.46	0.31	0.26	0.26
195	0.71	0.59	0.53	0.53	0.34	0.29	0.26
200	0.77	0.64	0.62	0.58	0.45	0.34	0.41
205	0.77	0.69	0.64	0.62	0.49	0.39	0.43
210	0.80	0.75	0.69	0.67	0.55	0.48	0.43
215	0.82	0.80	0.72	0.70	0.59	0.51	0.43
220	0.82	0.84	0.76	0.75	0.63	0.56	0.46
225	0.85	0.87	0.78	0.77	0.66	0.59	0.48
230	0.87	0.91	0.82	0.81	0.69	0.65	0.48
235	0.87	0.93	0.86	0.85	0.70	0.68	0.56
240	0.89	0.94	0.89	0.86	0.72	0.74	0.60
245	0.91	0.94	0.91	0.87	0.76	0.75	0.63
250	0.91	0.95	0.92	0.88	0.83	0.80	0.68
255	0.94	0.97	0.93	0.89	0.86	0.82	0.73
260	0.96	0.97	0.95	0.91	0.94	0.84	0.73
265	0.96	0.97	0.96	0.92	0.95	0.85	0.75
270	0.96	0.98	0.96	0.94	0.95	0.90	0.80
275	0.96	0.98	0.97	0.94	0.96	0.90	0.82
280	0.96	0.98	0.98	0.96	0.97	0.92	0.95
285	0.96	0.98	0.99	0.97	0.97	0.94	0.95
290	0.96	0.99	>0.99	0.97	0.98	0.95	0.97
295	0.96	>0.99	>0.99	0.97	0.99	0.96	0.99
300	0.98	>0.99	>0.99	0.98	>0.99	0.97	>0.99
305	0.98	>0.99	>0.99	0.98	>0.99	0.98	>0.99
310	0.98	>0.99	>0.99	0.99	>0.99	0.98	>0.99
315	0.98	>0.99	>0.99	>0.99	>0.99	0.99	>0.99
320	0.99	>0.99	>0.99	>0.99	>0.99	>0.99	>0.99

*Courtesy of Raymond G. Troxler, Major, USAF, MC. See text.

serum or plasma, separation of phospholipids and glucose and, finally, hydrolysis of the isolated triglycerides prior to determination of glycerol. Since all three procedures are based on determination of glycerol, and all include steps to control interfering substances, comparable results are obtained. Standards and reference materials are available (Witter *et al.*, 1970).

Triglycerides, then, are most often measured in terms of their glycerol content after preliminary separation from phospholipids by adsorption to a zeolite mixture or by chromatography on silicic acid. Saponification of triglycerides yields glycerol, which can be oxidized to formaldehyde by periodic acid; the formaldehyde liberated may be determined spectrophotometrically by the chromotropic acid reaction (R. J. Henry, 1964) or fluorometrically when condensed with diacetylacetone and ammonia to give a fluorescent product 3,5-diacetyl-1,4-dehydrolutidine in the Hantzsch condensation (Kessler and Lederer, 1966). The semiautomated fluorometric procedure described by Kessler and Lederer (1966) represents a significant improvement and is recommended (Edwards *et al.*, 1972). With a 1:20 manual dilution (0.5 ml. serum plus 9.5 ml. isopropanol) step, extraction yields complete recovery of triglycerides, phospholipids, and cholesterol. The incorporation of Lloyd's Reagent in the zeolite mixture removes bilirubin and other serum chromogens as well as the phospholipids; glucose which can be oxidized to formaldehyde by periodate is also eliminated in this procedure by a copper-lime treatment with the zeolite mixture. By omitting the saponification step, a serum blank determination is carried out for each specimen to delineate any interference from the many drugs, reagents, and detergents that have fluorescent properties. Nevertheless, a net rate of 20 determinations per hour can be achieved. Furthermore, the same isopropanol extract can be used for automated cholesterol determinations (Block *et al.*, 1966) and the estimation of phospholipids. Since all acetylacetone reagents formulated to date are unstable and rapidly develop a yellow color on standing, a new periodate and acetylacetone reagent formulation stable for at least six months should generate interest (Foster and Dunn, 1973). Alumina is used to adsorb interfering substances and the glycerol content of triglycerides is determined colorimetrically. Fredrickson and his colleagues have recommended the "normal limits" for plasma lipid and lipoprotein concentrations presented in Table 9–35. Physicians should be aware of the higher values (approximately 7 to 10 per cent) obtained with direct serum cholesterol measurements (e.g., SMA 12–60) in contrast to serum cholesterol extraction procedures, which are also automated.

Phospholipid Assays. Phospholipids are most frequently estimated in terms of lipid phosphorus. An organic solvent extraction of serum, such as isopropanol described for triglycerides, is performed initially to recover the phospholipid fraction, which is subsequently brought to dryness. A wet acid digestion step is then usually carried out to destroy all organic materials prior to final determination of phosphorus in the residue (Heinmiller, 1964). Since lipid phosphorus represents about one twenty-fifth of the weight of the phospholipid molecule, a factor of 25.0 is used to convert the concentration of lipid phosphorus to phospholipid (Sunderman and Sunderman, 1973b). Adult normal serum phospholipid values range from 200 to 300 mg. per 100 ml. and vary with age, as does cholesterol; the values for premenopausal women tend to be slightly higher than in men. The estrogen hormones may account for the higher alpha lipoprotein concentration with associated greater phospholipid values. Further information pertaining to lipid phosphorus methodology is available in several excellent reviews (Sunderman and Sunderman, 1960; Frings and Dunn, 1972).

Free Fatty Acid (FFA) Assays. Soloni and Sardina (1973) have reported recently a simplified, sensitive, accurate and specific colorimetric method for microdetermination of free fatty acids. Normal values are rather low, i.e., 10.5 ± 9.4 mg./dl. Gas chromatographic, titrimetric and thin layer chromatographic methods are also available.

Lipoprotein Electrophoresis. According to Fredrickson and his colleagues (1967), for a qualitative assessment of lipoprotein patterns, electrophoresis should be performed. Plasma separated from blood collected without venostasis with the patient at rest and anticoagulated with EDTA (ethylenediaminetetraacetate) is ideal for lipoprotein electrophoresis. EDTA delays deterioration of lipoproteins, possibly by inactivation of lipoprotein lipase.

At any rate, fresh plasma (same day collection) yields an ideal specimen for lipoprotein electrophoresis. Stability of human serum lipoproteins *in vitro* has been reported recently (Bermes and McDonald, 1972). Even with storage at 2 to 4° C., there is a disappearance of lipoproteins (especially VLDL) after 24 hours. Freezing plasma irreversibly alters lipoprotein patterns, especially LDL, but has no effect on triglyceride and cholesterol values. In view of the effect of stress on lipoproteins, patients who have had a myocardial infarction should not have a whole blood specimen analyzed for at least two to three months after infarction.

On the basis of electrophoretic migration, there are several useful methods for separating the four plasma lipoprotein families. Although usually a semiquantitative technique, quantification is feasible by staining of the lipoprotein bands and measurement of intensity of staining by densitometry before or after elution. Agar-agarose gel has virtually replaced paper electrophoresis of lipoproteins (Papadopoulos, 1971; Irwin and Campbell, 1972). It provides sharper bands and it more often resolves the pre-beta lipoprotein and alpha-lipoprotein into several bands; however, no pathologic significance has yet been given to these subbands. Cellulose acetate does not yield the clear pattern seen with agar-agarose gel (Fletcher, 1970). Furthermore, in some preparations, chylomicrons do not remain at the origin but migrate with pre-beta lipoproteins as they do on free electrophoresis. Starch-gel electrophoresis is impractical in view of the time and effort required; furthermore, similar merger of chylomicrons and pre-beta lipoproteins occurs. While these electrophoretic systems separate the lipoproteins mainly by differences in charge, they may not be valuable in identifying several unusual kinds of lipoproteins discussed previously, i.e., floating beta, sinking pre-beta, and Lp-X.

Polyacrylamide-gel electrophoresis (PGE) separates lipoproteins on the basis of both their size and charge (Frings *et al.*, 1971). It is a rapid, easily standardized, and sensitive method. As shown in Figure 9–57, the migration of two of the lipoprotein families differs from that on other electrophoretic media. On PGE, VLDL runs behind LDL; it sometimes stays in the loading gel. This phenomenon plus the prestaining technique used with PGE often suggests the presence of chylomicrons not observed by other methods. PGE is also useful, as previously described, in the diagnosis of type III hyperlipoproteinemia in view of the pre-beta VLDL migration. Brilliant electrophoresis on a slab of polyacrylamide gel provides information comparable to that obtained from more expensive and prolonged studies by preparative ultracentrifugation (Bautovich *et al.*, 1973).

Lipoprotein electrophoresis on paper, cellulose acetate, and agar-agarose gel employs fat stains such as oil red O or sudan dyes. It should be emphasized that these dyes dissolve into triglycerides and cholesterol esters only. Hence, such stains do not reflect lipids associated with increases of free cholesterol or phospholipids. Therefore, dissociation between individual blood lipid measurements and electrophoresis can be appreciated in selected cases. Hence, one cannot go directly to lipoprotein electrophoresis without available quantitative information for serum cholesterol and triglyceride measurements.

Werner and Jones (1972) have analyzed lipoproteins after electrophoresis, employing immunochemical and electron microscopic studies to detect individual differences not apparent immediately in the electrophoretic pattern; the authors anticipate that this approach may provide a new insight into the classification of hyperlipoproteinemias.

INORGANIC IONS

Sodium (Na^+), potassium (K^+), chloride (Cl^-), carbon dioxide (HCO_3^-), and magnesium (Mg^{++}) are reviewed in Chapter 12. Calcium (Ca^{++}) and phosphorus (HPO_4^{--}), as well as iron and copper, represent other inorganic ions that warrant special consideration.

Biochemistry of Calcium and Phosphorus

Bones and teeth contain over 99 per cent of the body calcium and 80 to 85 per cent of the phosphorus. Calcium ions (Ca^{++}) are essential for the preservation of skeletal structure, the activation of several enzymes, blood coagulation, muscle contraction, and transmission of nerve impulses. Furthermore, Ca^{++} (ions) decrease cell membrane and capillary permeability and depress neuromuscular excitability (Cantarow and Schepartz, 1967). The important functions of phosphorus have been mentioned in reference to their contribution to carbohydrate metabolism as major intermediates and high-energy phosphate bonds (ATP). Phosphorus is also an important constituent of nucleic acids, phospholipids, nucleotides (NAD, NADP), and other moieties, as well as bone.

Residing in the stored phosphate radicals in bone is a buffering capacity of considerable magnitude. Because the serum bicarbonate and phosphate buffer systems constitute the primary circulating buffer mechanism, and since protection against acidemia (acidosis) contributed by mobilized bone phosphate is theoretically considerable, and because a phosphate radical accompanies every calcium ion into the circulation when parathyroid hormone-mediated bone mobilization occurs, Barzel (1971) has renewed interest in the concept of bone phosphate as a buffer for acid.

Milk and milk products are the major sources of dietary calcium. Cow's milk contains more phosphorus than calcium; otherwise, the food distribution for both ions is similar. Many factors account for the variable absorption of calcium (Ca^{++}) and phosphate (HPO_4^{--}), from such foods in the small intestine. A high calcium concentration, low pH, vitamin D, which is essential, and parathyroid hormone (dependent on vitamin D) promote intestinal absorption of calcium. A dietary concentration ratio (Ca:P) in excess of 2:1 and phytic acid that occurs in cereal grains impair absorption; several substances (e.g., iron, lead, manganese) that form insoluble phosphates also interfere with the absorption of phosphate. In steatorrhea, fatty acids form insoluble soaps with calcium and are then lost in the feces; intestinal secretion of calcium also contributes to fecal loss in addition to unabsorbed dietary calcium. Vitamin D, which is fat soluble, is absorbed poorly in the presence of steatorrhea; since vitamin D is essential for normal intestinal absorption of calcium, calcium-fecal loss is enhanced, with a resulting low plasma calcium. With a calcium intake of 1 gm. per day, approximately 15 per cent is absorbed. During childhood, pregnancy, and lactation, the dietary requirement (0.8 gm. per day) should be augmented from 25 to 75 per cent to maintain calcium balance; this is essential for metabolic requirements, especially bone growth and development.

Blood. Since erythrocytes are virtually devoid of calcium, serum or plasma accounts for calcium concentration, which varies normally from 9.0 to 10.4 mg./dl. (4.5 to 5.2 mEq. per liter). Serum calcium is present, however, in three different forms: (1) about 45 per cent (2.2 mEq. per liter) is bound to the serum proteins, especially albumin, and is consequently nondiffusible through the capillary membrane; (2) about 5 per cent of the calcium (0.2 to 0.3 mEq. per liter) is complexed, with citrate, phosphate, etc., so that it is not ionized; and (3) the remaining 50 per cent of serum calcium (2.3 to 2.4 mEq. per liter) is in the ionic (free) form and diffuses through the capillary membrane as shown at the bottom of this page.

The ionic fraction of calcium is most important in terms of physiologic functions described and bone formation (osteogenesis) or resorption (osteolysis). It also accounts for nearly all the extravascular fluid concentration of calcium, e.g., cerebrospinal fluid (2.3 to 2.4 mEq. per liter). Blood pH and protein concentration are important factors that control calcium fraction concentration; acidosis promotes an increase in the ionic fraction concentration, while alkalosis causes a decrease in the ionic calcium fraction concentration. Hyperproteinemia is associated with an increase in the total serum calcium concentration, the greatest increment being in the protein-bound calcium form; the total serum calcium concentration is depressed with hypoproteinemia.

The interpretation of a serum calcium measurement, then, must take into consideration the concentration of serum proteins and acid-base status of the patient. For example, if alkalosis causes a reduction in the circulating ionic calcium fraction, tetany may occur in the presence of normal total serum calcium levels if alkalosis is present. Conversely, since an acid pH enhances ionization of calcium salts, a normal total calcium level in states of chronic acidosis may falsely obscure the cause of the nebulous symptoms of hypercalcemia (fatigue, weakness, confusion, polyuria, constipation, nausea, vomiting); here an elevated ionized calcium fraction must be suspected. An occult increase in the ionized calcium fraction is suggested by a normal total calcium level in the presence of significant hypoproteinemia. For practical purposes, an elevated protein-bound calcium level in the presence of normal ionized calcium concentration occurs in only one clinical condition, i.e., dehydration with hemoconcentration. The total calcium elevation is mild and proportional to the relative hyperproteinemia. Rehydration restores normocalcemia. Artefactual hemoconcentration produced by prolonged venous stasis during blood collection may increase slightly the protein bound fraction and, hence, the total calcium level. However, Li and Piechocki

---

Protein-bound calcium ⟷ Ca^{++} or Ionic
Nondialyzable
45 per cent
4.2–4.4 mg./dl.
2.1–2.2 mEq./liter

Ca^{++} or Ionic
Dialyzable
50 per cent
4.6–4.8 mg./dl.
2.3–2.4 mEq./liter

Complexed calcium
(phosphate, citrate, carbonate, sulfate)
5 per cent
0.4–0.6 mg./dl.
0.2–0.3 mEq./liter

(1971) demonstrated virtually no effect on the serum ionized calcium when compared with controls collected without a tourniquet. The secretion of hormones that influence calcium metabolism is also most sensitive to variations in concentration of the ionized calcium fraction, i.e., a decrease in the circulating ionic fraction normally causes release of parathyroid hormone, and increased ionized calcium levels stimulate release of calcitonin (Harris and DeMets, 1971).

Serum phosphorus consists of inorganic phosphate in the form of HPO_4^{--} and $H_2PO_4^-$ as the two predominant species (a third is $PO_4^{\equiv}$); the distribution of three phosphate species is pH dependent. At pH 7.4, the ratio of $[HPO_4^{=}]$ to $[H_2PO_4^{-}]$ is about 4:1. A more acid pH favors an increase in the latter and a decrease in the former, while the opposite takes place with alkalosis. Because of the variations in blood pH and analytical difficulties inherent in the determination of the two phosphate fractions, the determination is expressed as phosphorus in milligrams per dl. The conversion of serum inorganic phosphorus values from mg. per dl. to mEq./L. over a wide pH range by use of a factor permits the utilization of phosphorus in the interpretation of acid-base equilibria (Sunderman and Sunderman, 1973b) (see Table 9–37).

Serum phosphorus normally ranges in adults from 3.2 to 4.3 mg./dl. Higher serum phosphorus levels are observed in growing children (4 to 7 mg./dl.). Growth hormone causes serum inorganic phosphate levels to be elevated. In addition to serum phosphorus variation as a function of age, with a substantial increase in children as compared to adults, there is a demonstrated circadian rhythmicity; this is in contrast to serum calcium level which varies to a minimal degree during the day. Hence, serum phosphorus values should be interpreted only with reference to normal values at each time of day (Goldsmith, 1972). In addition, dietary carbohydrate and phosphorus intakes may influence serum phosphorus values for the first few hours after a meal. Therefore, normal values or clinical limits of serum phosphorus should be defined with reference to a specific time of day, usually early morning and with the patient fasting. With an increase in carbohydrate metabolism, e.g., glucose absorption or parenteral administration, there is a decrease in serum phosphorus (HPO_4^{--}) concentration.

Except when active bone formation is taking place (children and pregnancy), the average daily urinary excretion of calcium of about 125 mg. approximates the net intestinal absorption of calcium. With an increased concentration of serum ionized calcium, the renal loss of calcium increases proportionately. When the ionized calcium concentration of serum is decreased, there is a corresponding decrease in urinary calcium loss. This is attributed to renal tubular reabsorption of filtered ionized calcium; this is enhanced by parathyroid hormone, which in turn is liberated in response to low serum calcium ionized fraction concentrations. Growth hormone also causes an increased renal excretion of calcium.

Virtually all the dietary phosphorus (phosphate) not excreted in the feces in combination with calcium is absorbed from the small intestine into the blood and excreted subsequently in the urine (0.5 gm. per 24 hours). As a threshold substance, urinary phosphate loss is dependent on serum phosphate concentration; it disappears from the urine when the serum phosphorus is below 3.2 mg./dl., and above this critical level it is lost in the urine in direct proportion to the serum phosphorus concentration. Therefore, serum phosphorus (phosphate) concentration variations govern the renal loss of phosphate, which in turn regulates phosphorus concentration in the extracellular fluid, including serum. An increase in parathyroid hormone causes increased urinary excretion of phosphate by decreasing the renal tubular reabsorption of phosphate; a decreased parathyroid hormone level causes an elevation of serum phosphorus by a retention of phosphate in extracellular fluids. Although the action of vitamin D on the kidney is not fully understood, there is evidence that it may enhance tubular reabsorption of phosphate, both directly and indirectly, by decreasing parathormone secretion (Raisz *et al.*, 1972). In large doses, however, vitamin D causes increased renal excretion of phosphate; to this extent its renal effect resembles parathormone. Moreover, thyrocalcitonin (TCT)

Table 9–37. pH CONVERSION FACTORS FOR INORGANIC PHOSPHORUS*

pH	FACTOR
7.10	0.537
7.15	0.546
7.20	0.555
7.25	0.563
7.30	0.570
7.35	0.577
7.40	0.583
7.45	0.589
7.50	0.594
7.55	0.599
7.60	0.603
7.70	0.611

*Milligrans per deciliter × factor = mEq. per liter. (With permission of Sunderman, F. W.: Inorganic Phosphorus, Proficiency Test Service, April, 1973, p. 3.)

causes an increased renal excretion of phosphate.

Bone. With a major portion of body calcium stored in bone, it is important to review the composition and role of the skeletal system in calcium metabolism. The average compact skeletal bone contains by dry weight about 75 per cent inorganic mineral salts and approximately 25 per cent organic matrix. The crystalline salts are deposited in the organic matrix of bone, as shown at the bottom of this page.

The formula for the major crystalline salt may resemble the naturally occurring mineral hydroxyapatite: $[Ca_3(PO_4)_2]_3 \cdot Ca(OH)_2$. The small amounts of other elements present may be absorbed to the surface of the hydroxyapatite crystal lattice structure in bone (Guyton, 1966). Magnesium, sodium and potassium may, however, replace calcium; fluoride may replace hydroxide (Harper, 1971). Prior to the typical hydroxyapatite crystal formation, the initial calcium salt deposited with bone formation (ossification) in the organic matrix is most likely $CaHPO_4$. The solubility product (Ksp) of $Ca^{++} \times HPO_4^{--}$ is then critical. Since the ionic composition of the extracellular fluid can affect bone growth, a high $Ca^{++} \times HPO_4^{--}$ product is important to initiate mineralization. A pyrophosphatase enzyme, alkaline phosphatase, present in osteoblasts (bone-forming cells) liberates from organic phosphate esters the required inorganic phosphate to react with calcium to form insoluble calcium phosphate. Two critical factors thought to influence bone formation are phosphate and parathyroid hormone (Rasmussen and Tenenhouse, 1967). In addition to enhancing mineral accretion, phosphate may also favorably alter collagen formation through the proposed function of the osteoblastic curtain (Rasmussen and Tenenhouse, 1967). Inorganic pyrophosphate, detectable in normal plasma ultrafiltrates (1 to 4 nanograms per liter), may be the critical factor that both inhibits crystal growth and retards crystal dissolution by "coating" the crystal and, hence, altering the physical and chemical characteristics of hydroxyapatite (Harris and Heany, 1969). Parathyroid hormone inhibits both collagen formation and pyrophosphatase activity; it mobilizes mineral salts (Ca^{++}) by enhancing bone resorption (Pechet, 1967; Rasmussen and Tenenhouse, 1967). The dissolution of bone in bone resorption reflects a loss of inorganic mineral salts primarily in osteomalacia; however, with osteoporosis in which organic protein matrix loss is fundamental, there is also a loss of inorganic mineral salts. Osteoclasts are the multinucleated giant cells of bone associated with bone resorption. Bone resorption is intimately related to local ion concentrations in bone, which in turn are influenced by hormones and the extracellular fluid, including serum, concentrations of calcium and phosphate (HPO); this relationship is emphasized in the model proposed by Rasmussen and Tenenhouse (1967) and shown in Figure 9–62.

Raisz (1970) has reviewed the physiologic and pharmacologic factors that influence bone resorption as demonstrated by either *in vitro* techniques, i.e., tissue culture, or *in vivo* techniques, i.e., assessment of appropriate morphologic or kinetic responses (Table 9–38).

The excellent symposium edited by Pechet (1967) on thyrocalcitonin provides much information and understanding pertaining to calcium homeostasis. A decrease in serum calcium (ionized fraction) promotes an increase in parathyroid hormone secretion to sustain calcium homeostasis.

Parathormone (PTH). Secretion of parathormone (PTH) from the parathyroid glands is under negative feedback control and is inversely proportional to the total activity of divalent cations (especially calcium and magnesium) which bathe the glands (Raisz *et al.*, 1972). It undergoes rapid degradation, with a half-life of minutes, although it is not clear which organs are responsible or whether all the degraded fragments are biologically inactive (Raisz *et al.*, 1972). Parathyroid hormone

---

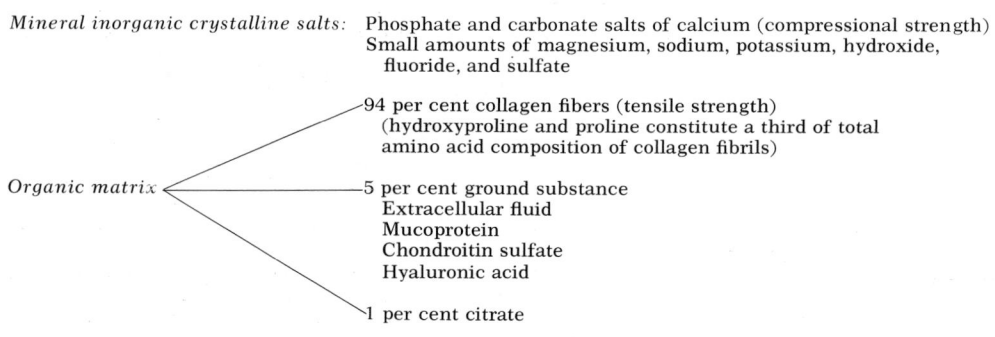

Mineral inorganic crystalline salts: Phosphate and carbonate salts of calcium (compressional strength)
Small amounts of magnesium, sodium, potassium, hydroxide, fluoride, and sulfate

Organic matrix
- 94 per cent collagen fibers (tensile strength) (hydroxyproline and proline constitute a third of total amino acid composition of collagen fibrils)
- 5 per cent ground substance
  - Extracellular fluid
  - Mucoprotein
  - Chondroitin sulfate
  - Hyaluronic acid
- 1 per cent citrate

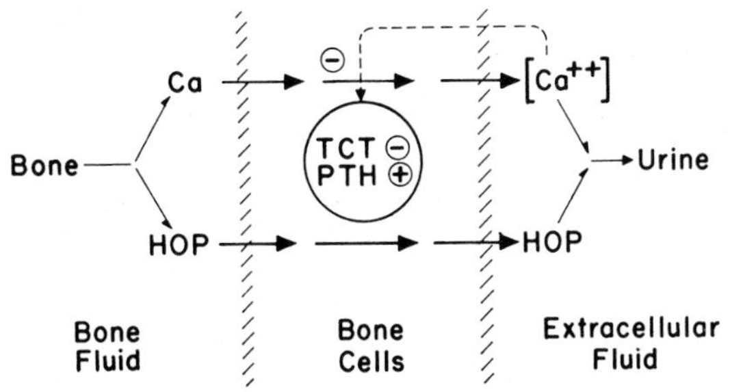

Figure 9–62. A model of the control of bone resorption emphasizing the importance of changes in extracellular fluid calcium and hormonal factors (TCT = thyrocalcitonin, and PTH = parathyroid hormones). Local control operates in a setting or concentration determined by hormones. (From Rasmussen, H., and Tenenhouse, A.: Amer. J. Med. *43*:711, 1967.)

has three target organs: bone, kidney, and intestinal mucosa. PTH causes an early increase of cyclic AMP content of bone and kidney cells.

Mobilization of calcium from bone is the major action that assists in restoring extracellular fluid (serum) calcium concentration to a normal range; while it may require hours to begin, the capacity is almost infinite. Parathyroid hormone (PTH)-induced resorption appears to occur in two phases: (1) osteocytic osteolysis – the initial phase of calcium release from bone mediated by osteocytes and characterized by its rapid onset after PTH administration and its limited capacity, i.e., PTH does not increase the number of osteocytes; this is the major system involved in mineral homeostasis (Rasmussen, 1971); and (2) osteoclastic osteolysis – the resorption phase mediated by osteoclasts characterized by delayed onset and infinite capacity, i.e., PTH-induced mesenchymal proliferation resulting in an increased number of osteoclasts and increased osteolytic function; this appears to be the principal effect of PTH and the phase primarily concerned with skeletal remodeling (Harris and Heany, 1969). Under normal circumstances this phase is of no consequence to mineral homeostasis; however, under abnormal conditions osteoclastic osteolysis assumes a major role in mineral homeostasis (Rasmussen, 1971).

The kidney, via the effect of PTH on renal tubular cells, assists in elevating extracellular calcium concentration by enhancing renal tubular reabsorption of calcium and increasing urinary loss of phosphate (decrease in tubular reabsorption). The latter tends to depress the serum phosphorus level to correspond with the altered serum calcium concentration, which might otherwise exceed the solubility product of two ions ($Ca^{++} \times HPO_4^{--}$) in extracellular fluids, leading to precipitation of insoluble salts ($CaHPO_4$). The least sensitive target organ of parathyroid hormone is the intestine, in which it may promote absorption of dietary calcium.

Vitamin D. The primary physiologic function of vitamin D or its metabolites is to elevate serum calcium and phosphate, which leads to normal mineralization of bone (DeLuca, 1969b; and Palmisano, 1973). This is primarily accomplished by two processes: intestinal transport of dietary calcium (facilitates absorption); and bone mineral mobilization (facilitates bone resorption). To achieve optimal intestinal absorption and bone resorption *in vivo,* both

Table 9–38. FACTORS INFLUENCING BONE RESORPTION*†

			POSSIBLE PATHOLOGIC & THERAPEUTIC FACTORS	
PHYSIOLOGIC STIMULATOR	PHYSIOLOGIC INHIBITOR	INTRACELLULAR MEDIATOR	Stimulator of Bone Resorption	Inhibitor of Bone Resorption
PTH Vitamin D (active form, HCC)	Thyrocalcitonin or calcitonin (TCT) Extracellular PO_4 concentration	cAMP Ca^{++} or specific Ca-BP calcium protein complexes	Acidosis Bacterial endotoxins Fatty acids Heparin and other polyanions Hyperoxia Serum proteins: Albumin Antiserums Globulins Sucrose Thyroxine Vitamin A	Alkalosis Antibiotics: Dactinomycin Mithramycin Estrogen & androgens Fluoride Glucagon Glucocorticoids Magnesium depletion Protamine Pyrophosphate and diphosphonates

*Raisz, L. G.: New Eng. J. Med. *282*:910, 1970.

†The agents listed have been shown either to affect bone resorption in tissue culture or to produce appropriate or kinetic responses in vivo. For many agents both types of data are available. Other agents, which can affect serum calcium concentration in vivo but for which there is not sufficient evidence to indicate whether the effect is mediated by changes in bone resorption, have not been listed.

vitamin D and parathyroid hormone are essential. This applies to physiologic conditions and treatment with physiologic doses in deficiency diseases. Whereas vitamin D is the major determinant in the intestine, parathyroid hormone assumes the primary role in stimulating bone resorption. In contrast, the primary function of vitamin D in bone is to promote formation of bone, i.e., it is necessary for the initial calcification of bone matrix, also known as osteoid calcification. Thus, these two hormones manifest complementary functions in achieving increased bone turnover, i.e., increased formation (vitamin D) and increased resorption (PTH), while their action on the intestine is supplementary. In contrast, vitamin D is not required for parathyroid hormone-directed, renal tubular reabsorption of phosphate.

Vitamin D is a generic designation for a family of sterols that possess similar functional and structural characteristics. The only members of human importance are vitamin D_2 (calciferol), vitamin D_3 (cholecalciferol), and dihydrotachysterol. Endogenous vitamin D is now considered to be a hormone (Alvioli, 1972; Talmage and Munson, 1972), while the exogenous D compounds in the diet retain the vitamin status. Ultraviolet radiation of the precursors ergosterol (derived from plant sources), or 7-dehydrocholesterol (from animals), whether in plant or in animal tissues (skin), results in formation of ergocalciferol (D_2) and cholecalciferol (D_3), respectively. Ultraviolet radiation of integumentary 7-dehydrocholecholesterol, producing cholecalciferol (D_3), appears to be the major human biosynthetic pathway. Most of D_2 and D_3 (94 per cent) circulates bound to an inter-alpha globulin (M.W. 60,000). Excess vitamin D may be stored in tissues or metabolized to inactive products that are excreted.

Ingested vitamin D is absorbed as a fat soluble vitamin in the jejunum and transported to liver bound to chylomicrons in the portal blood (Kimberg, 1969). Whether of exogenous or endogenous origin, vitamin D compounds are converted to biologically active metabolites that possess greater antirachitic properties and achieve more rapid action than their parent compound in effecting intestinal calcium absorption and bone mineral mobilization (DeLuca, 1969a; and Palmisano, 1973). The two important metabolites are 25-hydroxycholecalciferol (25-HCC) and 1,25-dihydrocholecalciferol (1,25-DHCC). A flow diagram of probable events in metabolism of vitamin D is shown in Figure 9–63. Specific hydroxylases in the liver convert vitamin D_3 to 25-HCC; while 1,25-DHCC appears to be generated exclusively in the kidney (DeLuca, 1971). The function of 1,25-DHCC and 25-HCC is currently debated, but a few generalizations apply. The most potent compound in terms of intestinal calcium transport is 1,25-DHCC. It stimulates synthesis of a calcium-binding protein and a calcium-dependent ATP'ase in the intestinal mucosal cell. The former is probably responsible for providing cation selectivity, while energy requirements for active transport may be linked to the ATP'ase. Although conflict exists on whether 25-HCC exerts a greater effect than 1,25-DHCC on bone mineral resorption and mineralization, it is generally agreed that either metabolite is more active than parent vitamin D compounds *in vivo* and *in vitro.* It tends to increase both serum calcium and phosphate concentrations, which increases the product of their ion activities, i.e., Ca × PO_4 with calcium phosphate product (Raisz *et al.,* 1972). The pathogenetic, diagnostic, and therapeutic implications of these active metabolites have been reported by Palmisano (1973). Primary application will be in the diseases characterized by resistance to vitamin D; namely, familial hypophosphatemia, vitamin D resistant rickets, and so forth. Circulating 25-HCC levels, as measured by competitive protein binding (Alvioli, 1972), have been noted to be increased with prolonged sun exposure, normal in osteoporosis and sarcoidosis, and decreased in chronic renal disease and biliary cirrhosis.

Calcitonin (Thyrocalcitonin). Since parathy-

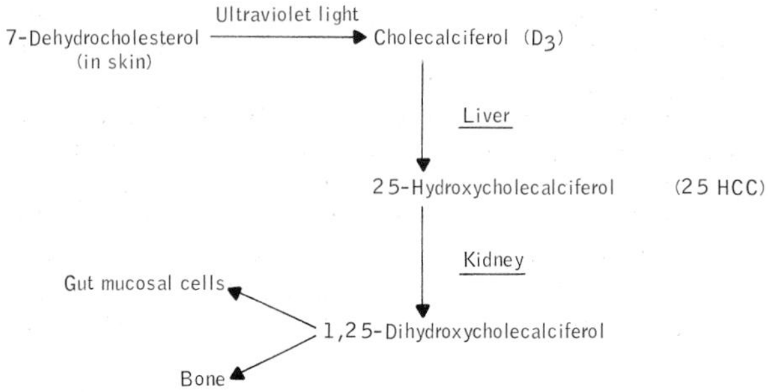

Figure 9–63. Flow diagram of probable events in metabolism of vitamin D. (Palmisano, P. A.: J.A.M.A. 224:1527, 1973.)

Table 9–39. SUMMARY OF ACTIONS AND STIMULI OF FACTORS THAT ARE IMPORTANT IN CALCIUM AND PHOSPHORUS HOMEOSTASIS*

		ACTIONS			BLOOD		URINE	
FACTOR	STIMULUS	BONE	KIDNEY	GI TRACT	Ca^{++}	HPO_4^{--}	Ca^{++}	HPO_4^{--}
Parathyroid hormone	↓ Serum calcium (hypocalcemia)	↑ Resorption;† inhibits pyrophosphatase activity, slow but infinite release of Ca^{++} to extracellular fluids	Hyperphosphaturia† Hypocalciuria (immediately); later with hypercalcemia there is hypercalciuria	↑ Ca^{++} absorption	↑	↓	↑	↑
Vitamin D		↑ Resorption	Hyperphosphaturia	↑ Ca^{++} absorption†	↑	↑	↑	↑
Calcitonin	↑ Serum calcium (hypercalcemia)	Blocks resorption†	Phosphaturia Hypocalciuria	↓ Ca absorption	↓	↓	↓	↑

* ↑ = increase; ↓ = decrease.
†Dominant.

roid hormone responds to hypocalcemia as described, calcitonin, which responds to hypercalcemia, may then be called a hypercalcemic factor (Copp *et al.*, 1962). Calcitonin secretion, then, can be stimulated directly by increased calcium concentrations. While calcium is more potent than magnesium, there can also be direct stimulation of calcitonin secretion by other hormones (e.g., gastrin, pancreozymin-cholecystokinin, and glucagon). A hypocalcemic response to calcitonin is augmented when serum phosphorus concentration is high or after injections of phosphate. This hormone is stored in and liberated by the parafollicular or "C" cells of the thyroid gland in response to an elevated serum calcium (ionized fraction) concentration (Pechet, 1967; and Raisz *et al.*, 1972). The major biologic action of calcitonin is the inhibition of bone resorption, but an action on bone formation cannot be excluded; it suppresses osteoclastic activity associated with bone resorption (Pechet, 1967). Calcitonin negates parathyroid hormone (PTH) and vitamin D action on bone resorption, including osteocytic and osteoclastic osteolysis (Pechet, 1967). A dynamic state with a continuum of bone remodeling is undoubtedly influenced by calcitonin. Calcitonin causes a decrease in urinary excretion of calcium, magnesium, and hydroxyproline. While Pechet (1967) notes the conflicting results regarding urinary phosphate excretion, it apparently does not suppress PTH action on intestines and kidneys, so calcitonin cannot be considered simply as an inhibitor of parathyroid hormone. However, several other actions of calcitonin may include: increased urinary excretion of sodium, phosphate, and chloride in the proximal tubule; increased calcium deposition in bone; and decreased intestinal absorption of calcium (Raisz *et al.*, 1972). An outline of the actions, stimuli, and effects of these three important factors in calcium homeostasis is presented in Table 9–39.

Glucocorticoids can inhibit calcium absorption in the gut and enhance calcium and phosphate excretion in the kidney, with a resultant PTH stimulation and increased bone resorption.

Gonadal hormones (androgens and estrogens) also depress bone resorption, while growth hormone (GH) increases both intestinal absorption and renal excretion of calcium; since GH stimulates metabolic activity of bone with growth of long bones at the epiphyses, there is an overall increase in calcium retention.

In summary, calcium homeostasis may be thought of as a dynamic interplay of forces at three levels of structural organization: (1) *ionic*–Ca^{++}, $PO_4^{\equiv}$, Mg^{++}, pH; (2) *molecular* (a) extracellular messenger system (hormones)–vitamin D, parathyroid hormone, calcitonin, gonadal hormones (estrogens, androgen), and growth hormone; (b) intracellular "second" messenger–cyclic AMP; (c) plasma proteins; and (3) *cellular*–(a) endocrine organs–parathyroid glands, parafollicular (C-cells) cells of the thyroid gland, and integument; (b) target organs–bone (osteocyte, osteoclast, osteoblast), kidneys (renal tubular cells), and intestine (mucosal cells of jejunum and ileum). This is more readily envisioned when organized into a schematic diagram (Fig. 9–64). Homeostasis is achieved by three physiologic processes: intestinal transport and absorption, renal tubular reabsorption, and bone resorption.

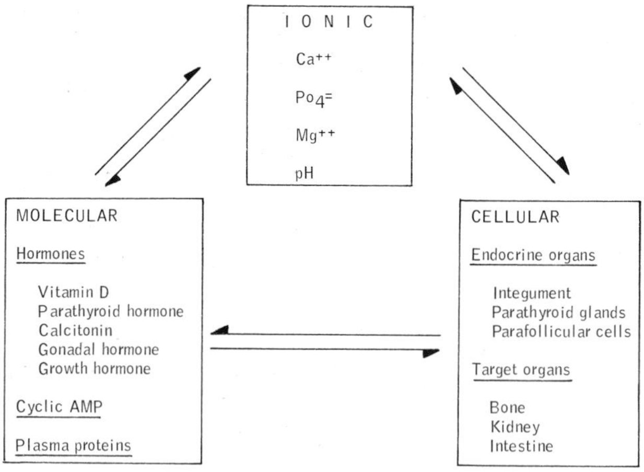

Figure 9–64. Calcium homeostasis—a dynamic interplay of forces at three levels of structural organization involving three major physiologic processes: intestinal absorption, renal tubular reabsorption, and bone resorption. (Courtesy of Donald McGovern, M.D.)

Clinicopathologic Correlations

From the foregoing discussion it is apparent that several measurements relating to serum and urine calcium, phosphorus (phosphate), serum alkaline phosphatase, and urinary hydroxyproline may show alterations that reflect (1) medical (generalized) bone disease, (2) endocrine dysfunction (parathyroid), and (3) dietary intake or absorption of calcium, as well as vitamin D. Interpretation of such data against a background of a complete history and physical examination of the patient is most likely to yield a definitive diagnosis when coupled with appropriate roentgenographic and histopathologic examinations. The limitations in terms of specificity, accuracy, and precision of various chemical measurements will be discussed subsequently with the methods. Critical attention to the patient's history, with the delineation of malabsorption syndrome and renal insufficiency, is important for proper assessment of significant chemical findings. In addition, urine calcium measurements require collection of a 24-hour urine specimen after a low calcium diet (at least free of dairy products) to render maximum information. With a regular diet, urinary calcium in normal subjects may be as high as 250 to 300 mg. per 24 hours, but with a low calcium intake urine calcium should not exceed 150 mg. per 24 hours. Urinary calcium, phosphate, phosphate clearance, and tubular reabsorption of phosphate examinations are discussed in Chapters 2 and 3. Serum phosphorus (phosphate) measurements must be performed on specimens collected after overnight fasting to preclude carbohydrate metabolic alterations. An iliac crest percutaneous needle biopsy for a specimen of bone is useful in the study of patients with generalized metabolic bone disease. A hematoxylin and eosin stained histologic preparation without prior decalcification and avoidance of formalin as a fixative is suitable for study of cellular detail and estimation of number and thickness of osteoid seams (Heaney, 1967). The value of such a bone biopsy can be enhanced greatly, according to Heaney (1967), when the patient is given a full therapeutic dose of a tetracycline prior to biopsy (one to three days at an interval of five days to two weeks earlier); fluorescent microscopic examination of such a histologic specimen can then yield a quantitative estimation of fractional bone turnover, as fluorescent bands are present between regular seams with bone formation during the interval before the biopsy was taken.

Three abnormalities in calcium metabolism emphasized by Howard and Thomas (1963) are presented in Table 9–40. Since blood calcium measurements are frequently reviewed as the initial source of data, this approach is useful despite overlaps that may exist due to duration or severity of single or multiple pathologic lesions. From this outline we can also proceed to review briefly the salient features with emphasis on chemical abnormalities, of specific diseases that may cause abnormalities in calcium metabolism.

BONE DISEASES

Osteoporosis refers to a deficiency of bone tissue per unit of mass (volume) of bone. It may reflect a dominance of resorption in the dynamic state of bone remodeling with continual formation and resorption. This absence of a normal quantity of bone is also described as bone atrophy and may reflect a deficient production of bone matrix. However, despite a decrease in bone mass, the mineral content is grossly normal and there is no excess of osteoid. Histopathologic features include a thin cortex with small fine bony trabeculae that are not only thin but decreased in number. A fragile structure of bone can be inferred from this picture; this can account for an increased susceptibility to fractures from compression forces. Vertebral bone compression fractures associated with back pain are common in patients with extensive osteoporosis. It is probably the most common variety of generalized metabolic bone disease. While the cause of postmenopausal or senile osteoporosis is unknown, a deficiency of gonadal hormones and a decrease in calcium absorption and/or dietary intake (calories and protein) may contribute to and accentuate a tendency to bone resorption in this group. Bone marrow examination and biopsy of bone provide necessary information to exclude other diseases (e.g., metastatic malignant tumors, multiple myeloma, hyperparathyroidism). Although urinary calcium may be increased, the serum and urine calcium and phosphorus measurements are usually within normal limits. Serum alkaline phosphatase activity is within normal limits or slightly depressed. Specific osteoporosis occurs in two endocrine disorders: hyperthyroidism and Cushing's syndrome (Heaney, 1971).

Table 9–40. ABNORMALITIES IN CALCIUM METABOLISM*

Calcium loss with normocalcemia
- Vitamin D deficiency
  - Rickets
  - Osteomalacia (other factors than vitamin D in adults)
- Malabsorption syndrome (steatorrhea)
- Osteoporosis
  - Senile and postmenopausal
  - Ovarian agenesis
  - Disuse
  - Nutritional deficiency (protein and calories)
  - Hyperthyroidism
  - Cushing's syndrome
  - Chronic metabolic acidosis

Calcium loss with hypercalcemia
- Hyperparathyroidism
  - Adenoma – 90 per cent – usually solitary but multiple in 10 per cent
  - Hyperplasia, clear cell and chief cell – 9 per cent
  - Carcinoma – 1 per cent
- Vitamin D intoxication
- Neoplasms
  - Metastatic or lytic tumors involving bone
    - Carcinoma of breast
    - Multiple myeloma
    - Lymphomas and leukemia
  - Various neoplasms without evidence of direct bone involvement
    - Parathyroid hormone-secreting tumors, e.g., carcinoma of lung (squamous cell), breast, kidney (hypernephroma), bladder, pancreas, esophagus and other organs
- Sarcoidosis (30 to 60 per cent of patients)
- Milk-alkali syndrome
- Miscellaneous
  - Idiopathic hypercalcemia of infancy
  - Disuse atrophy with a major portion of the body immobilized
  - Hyperthyroidism
  - Addison's disease

Hypocalcemia
- Hypoparathyroidism
  - Inadvertent surgical removal of parathyroids or damage during thyroidectomy
  - Idiopathic with or without systemic infections, e.g., candidiasis
  - ? autoimmune disease, when associated with Addison's disease, or Hashimoto's thyroiditis
- Pseudohypoparathyroidism (end-organ failure)
- Advanced and sustained vitamin D deficiency
  - Rickets
  - Osteomalacia
- Renal failure
  - Acute (anuria)
  - Chronic
- Renal tubular acidosis or Fanconi syndrome
- Acute pancreatitis
- Pituitary insufficiency
- ? Thyrocalcitonin excess

*Data from Howard, J. E., and Thomas, W. C., Jr.: Medicine *42*:25, 1963.

Osteomalacia may be associated with normal, increased, or decreased bone mass, but the proportion of uncalcified bone (osteoid) tissue with an increase in number and thickness of osteoid seams is larger. Usually, osteomalacia reflects a decrease in mineralized bone mass in which unmineralized matrix or osteoid is present in excess; this is usually because the $Ca^{++} \times PO_4^{\equiv}$ product is too low (Raisz *et al.*, 1972). Since a large proportion of the osteoid tissue is not calcified (mineralized), the bones are soft; skeletal deformities may then ensue, with severe bone pain as the prominent clinical feature. In childhood the term rickets associated with vitamin D deficiency denotes similar findings but also reveals a pronounced lack of calcification of the primary ossification line; this gives rise to retarded growth and more striking deformities due to a disturbance in the epiphyseal growth plates. Rickets, then, is osteomalacia that occurs before the epiphyses are closed; compensatory overgrowth or epiphyseal cartilage occurs, and wide bands of cartilage remain unmineralized and unresorbed.

In contrast to children with rickets due to a deficiency in vitamin D when bone growth demands are maximum, osteomalacia in adults is almost never associated with a vitamin D deficiency, and factors causing it are more obscure. Although vitamin D and phosphate deficiency generally produce osteomalacia, calcium deficiency alone is more likely to produce osteitis, but it may produce osteomalacia. Abnormalities in the matrix of bone that preclude normal mineralization as well as an insufficient concentration of calcium and phosphorus in the extracellular fluids have been incriminated to varying degrees; both defects may be responsible (Heaney, 1971). Renal tubular acidosis, hypophosphatasia, and dietary deficiency or a failure in absorption of calcium and vitamin D as well as other causes of increased loss of calcium must be considered in patients with osteomalacia. Normocalcemia or a depressed Ca × P product may be observed (Chalmers *et al.*, 1967). Hypocalcemia and hyperphosphatemia, however, may be present separately or in combination. If osteomalacia is associated with hypocalcemia, there is initially some osteitis because of secondary hyperparathyroidism (Raisz *et al.*, 1972). The striking tremendous increase in serum alkaline phosphatase activity observed in children with rickets is more variable, but this also appears in adults with osteomalacia; alkaline phosphatase represents the single most sensitive indicator of active disease. Urinary calcium and hydroxyproline may be increased in patients with osteomalacia (Kocher, 1966).

Vitamin D resistant rickets (familial hypophosphatemia, or phosphate diabetes) has virtually all the manifestations of rickets, except that it occurs in older infants or children. Low levels of serum phosphorus are observed with a normal or slightly depressed serum calcium and moderate elevations of serum alkaline phosphatase; hyperphosphaturia and a normal or decreased urinary calcium are present. The designation vitamin D resistant is not appropriate, since these patients are not completely refractory to vitamin D. Treatment with a combination of phosphate and vitamin D is commonly employed, but it is not known whether this is more effective than supplemental phosphate alone (Heaney, 1971).

Hypophosphatasia also expresses itself primarily as rickets and osteomalacia (Heaney, 1971). It is a rare inherited disorder transmitted as an autosomal recessive trait (Heaney, 1971). The most characteristic chemical pathologic finding is a profound depression of serum alkaline phosphatase. The leukocyte alkaline phosphatase is also depressed, and this enzyme deficiency is observed in virtually all other cells examined. Intermittent hypercalcemia may be observed in these patients, who also demonstrate an increase in phosphoethanolamine in their blood and urine.

Osteitis deformans, or Paget's disease of bone, is a rare chronic progressive acquired bone disorder of unknown cause that is characterized by bone destruction (osteolysis), with resorption and repair or replacement (osteogenesis) with poorly mineralized osteoid tissue and variable amounts of fibrous tissue. Localized or generalized bony enlargements of variable size that are soft, structurally weak, and deformed with stress are apparent most often in weight-bearing bones of men after the age of 30. Ultimately, it may spread to involve a major fraction of the skeleton. In addition to an increased susceptibility to fractures at bony deformities, patients with Paget's disease may develop osteogenic sarcomas in these lesions as a relatively infrequent but fatal complication. The highest elevations of serum alkaline phosphatase observed are noted in patients with osteitis deformans; serum and urine calcium and phosphorus values are usually within normal limits.

As mentioned previously and shown in Table 9–40, patients with osteolytic metastatic neoplasms (especially with active or extensive lesions) may display hypercalcemia and hypercalciuria which can be further complicated by nephrocalcinosis and renal failure. In general, osteolytic bone lesions are associated with an increased calcium loss in the urine and hypercalcemia; however, osteoblastic lesions do not reflect an excess calcium but show a striking elevation of serum alkaline phosphatase. Furthermore, several tumors without bone involvement may also cause hypercalcemia (Table 9–40).

Osteitis fibrosa cystica generalisata, or Recklinghausen's disease of bone, represents the pathologic skeletal changes observed with prolonged or severe primary or secondary hyperparathyroidism (to be discussed subsequently). In addition to features of severe bone resorption with increased osteoclastic activity yielding thinning of cortical and cancellous bone, there is fibrous tissue replacement with microscopic and gross cystic changes. Skeletal fractures and deformities with joint pain and dysfunction, especially of weight-bearing bones, ensue. These chemical and clinicopathologic features are often less conspicuous than the manifestation of the underlying disease, such as primary hyperparathyroidism or renal failure with secondary hyperparathyroidism.

Renal osteodystrophy is a term used to indicate that patients with progressive or chronic renal failure tend to develop bone lesions (Raisz *et al.*, 1972). The varied osseous manifestations of chronic renal failure which have become more common with the increasing use of maintenance hemodialysis and renal transplantation include osteomalacia and osteitis fibrosa; osteosclerosis (increased bone density) is common but usually asymptomatic, whereas osteoporosis, rare in the undialyzed patient, may be the principal lesion in some patients on maintenance hemodialysis (Parfitt and Chir, 1972).

PARATHYROID DISEASES

In hyperparathyroidism associated with the pathologic lesions shown in Table 9–40, hypercalcemia of greater than 5.3 mEq. per liter or 10.5 mg./dl. is probably the most important single diagnostic aid; an elevation of ionic calcium is virtually always present, and associated generally with a low serum phosphorus (although hypophosphatemia is not invariable), except in advanced renal failure (Nordin, 1964; Low *et al.*, 1973). The accuracy and precision of multiple serum calcium determinations are of the utmost importance in the detection of this disease in patients who might otherwise be asymptomatic or have nonspecific complaints, such as nausea, vomiting, anorexia, dyspepsia, constipation, weight loss, weakness, or sensorial changes that may progress from somnolence or psychosis to coma. Nephrolithiasis or, less frequently, nephrocalcinosis and acute pancreatitis may represent presenting manifestations, while osteitis fibrosa cystica generalisata reflects longstanding severe disease and an inadequate calcium intake or absorption. A pathophysiologic overproduction of parathyroid hormone (PTH) accentuates bone resorption, which in turn causes hypercalcemia and hypercalciuria as well as a decrease in renal tubular phosphorus reabsorption, with an ensuing low serum phosphorus concentration. With severe bone involvement, the serum alkaline phosphatase activity increases along with urinary calcium and hydroxyproline; eventually, renal failure may develop from nephrocalcinosis and/or nephrolithiasis complicated further by pyelonephritis. When the disease has progressed to the renal failure stage, the classic serum calcium elevation and phosphorus depression may be obscured, since renal disease causes a retention of phosphorus and a decrease in serum calcium; this in turn stimulates parathyroids to secrete hormone. Indeed, the differential diagnosis between primary hyperparathyroidism with renal failure and secondary hyperparathyroidism due to chronic renal disease (with failure) may be extremely difficult and at times virtually impossible.

The widespread and increased application of biochemical screening, i.e., chemical profiles or metabolic organ panels which include serum calcium measurements, has made primary hyperthyroidism a more frequently encountered and hence common endocrine disorder manifest by hypercalcemia (even though the most common cause of hypercalcemia is a nonparathyroid neoplasm). Boonstro and Jackson (1971) reported a ratio of one case of hyperparathyroidism per 1000 individuals surveyed (i.e., about 50 cases in 50,000 clinic patients over a 10-year period). When these workers performed serum calcium measurements for the relatives of all patients with hyperparathyroidism found in their survey, an additional 24 patients in seven families with hyperparathyroidism were encountered. In addition to familial hyperparathyroidism, genetic implications are also undoubtedly present in the hyperparathyroidism of multiple endocrine neoplasia type I – pituitary (chromophobe adenoma), pancreas (insulinoma or Zollinger-Ellison syndrome) and also type II – adrenal (pheochromocytoma), thyroid parafollicular cell (medullary) carcinoma (Raisz *et al.*, 1972).

Secondary hyperparathyroidism, associated most frequently with progressive chronic renal failure, is attributed to retention of phosphorus. An elevated serum phosphorus, in turn, stimulates parathyroids to secrete more hormone, which promotes bone resorption with an elevation of serum calcium as well as phosphaturia; however, the chemical hallmarks are an elevated serum phosphorus and a depressed serum calcium. In essence, both primary and secondary hyperparathyroidism have elevated PTH levels, but the presence of renal disease mitigates the renal phosphaturic effect of hormone in a manner analogous to end-organ (renal tubular) failure.

As noted in Table 9–40, hypercalcemia is also present in other diseases, including vitamin D intoxication and, with a prolonged or excessive intake of calcium and alkali, the milk-alkali syndrome. In Table 9–41, other conditions with associated chemicopathologic findings are presented.

While there is poor correlation between the severity of the clinical manifestations and the degree of hypercalcemia, clinical evidence is nearly always present, with serum calcium levels exceeding 15 mg./dl.; at levels above 18 mg./dl., patients are so very ill that death may occur from cardiac arrest. The most frequent cause of hypercalcemia is neoplasia (especially bony metastases with highest levels); like that associated with prolonged immobilization of patients, the hypercalcemia is accompanied by normal or elevated serum phosphorus levels.

With medullary carcinoma of the thyroid, patients have high serum calcitonin levels, usually without any abnormality of calcium metabolism.

In hypoparathyroidism there is a decrease in parathyroid hormone secretion that causes (1) an increase in renal tubular phosphorus reabsorption, (2) an elevation in serum phosphorus concentration, and (3) a depression in serum calcium concentration. Hypocalcemia, reflecting a decrease in the ionized fraction concentration, is associated clinically with tetany and other physical signs (Chvostek and Trousseau) on examination due to an increased excitability of peripheral nerves and ganglia

Table 9–41. SUMMARY OF CHEMICAL PATHOLOGIC FINDINGS IN PARATHYROID AND BONE DISEASES*

CONDITION	SERUM Ca^{++}	SERUM HPO_4^{--}	URINE Ca^{++}	URINE HPO_4^{--}	SERUM ALKALINE PHOSPHATASE
Primary hyperparathyroidism	↑	↓	↑	↑	N or ↑
Secondary hyperparathyroidism	↓	↑	↑ or N	↓ or N	N or ↑
Hypoparathyroidism	↓	↑	↓	↓	N
Pseudohypoparathyroidism	↓	↑	↓	↓	N
Rickets or adult osteomalacia (advanced)	↓	↓	↓	↓	↑
Vitamin D resistant rickets (familial hypophosphatemia)	N(↓)	↓	N	↑	↑
Renal tubular acidosis or Fanconi syndrome	N(↓)	↓	↑	↑	↑
Vitamin D intoxication	↑	↑, N, ↓	↑	↑	N
Paget's disease (osteitis deformans)	N(↑)	N	N(↑)	N	↑↑
Fibrous dysplasia of bone	N	N	N	N	↑

*N = normal; ↑ = elevation; ↓ = depression.

with hyperactivity of the autonomic nervous system. Thinning of the hair with a patchy scalp distribution and scant or absent eyebrows as well as papilledema (increased intracranial pressure) and dry coarse skin are other classic signs frequently observed in patients with hypoparathyroidism. The chemical pathologic changes are shown in Table 9–41, and differential diagnoses under hypocalcemia are shown in Table 9–40.

Although primary hypoparathyroidism is an uncommon cause of hypocalcemia, slight hypocalcemia (without a disorder in calcium regulation) is most frequently associated with a decreased serum protein concentration; however, ionic calcium concentration is normal and only protein-bound calcium is decreased (Raisz *et al.*, 1972). Hypocalcemia may be observed not only in patients on very low calcium intakes, but also in many with osteomalacia. An explanation for development of hypocalcemia in patients with magnesium deficiency revolves around a magnesium requirement for PTH synthesis, so that with a chronic deficiency, insufficient PTH is produced. Hence, it is important to treat magnesium deficiency initially prior to an expected response from calcium, PTH, or vitamin D therapy (Raisz *et al.*, 1972).

Pseudohypoparathyroidism, with all the features described for hypoparathyroidism plus somatic and skeletal abnormalities, such as short, thick-set body, round face, and irregular, shortened metatarsal and metacarpal bones with calcification of soft tissues and basal ganglia, represents an end-organ (renal tubular) defect. It is a rare cause of hypocalcemia. These patients are refractory to parathyroid hormone administration. A failure to respond to the administration of parathyroid hormone by such patients is used as a definitive diagnostic test.

Hypocalcemia is observed rather frequently in infants; such neonatal hypocalcemia appears to be associated with diabetes, prematurity, and other complications of pregnancy that may be ascribed to inadequate development of the parathyroid glands (Raisz *et al.*, 1972). It can also occur when the mother is hyperparathyroid, apparently because high calcium levels are also present in the fetus, so the infant's parathyroids do not develop normally (Raisz *et al.*, 1972). Infants on cow's milk with a high phosphate content may also develop hypocalcemia.

METHODS

Calcium. While several methods have been introduced for serum calcium determinations, the Clark and Collip (1925) procedure has been regarded until recent years as the classic reference method. This technique involves precipitation of calcium directly from serum with ammonium oxalate. The addition of sulfuric acid dissolves calcium oxalate precipitate and yields oxalic acid, which is measured in the final step by a redox titration with potassium permanganate (oxidant); a pink color, which appears with an excess of permanganate, represents the endpoint. Meticulous technique is essential to insure optimum precision, and the procedure is time consuming, so a number of other methods have been developed.

Complexometric techniques employing ethylenediaminetetraacetic acid (EDTA) as a chelating agent are less tedious. EDTA binds calcium as well as other alkaline earth metals. When calcium is complexed (bound) with EDTA, certain indicators (e.g., Cal-Red, eriochrome black T, and ammonium purpurate) change color in the absence of ionized calcium (Ca^{++}); pH is critical to minimize reaction with other divalent ions (especially magnesium), and the presence of bilirubin and hemolysis interferes with the endpoint in titrimetry; photometric adaptations have also been developed. Normal values with EDTA techniques may be slightly lower than with the Clark-Collip method.

Hill (1965) introduced an automated fluorometric method that gives results comparable to Clark-Collip permanganate titration. Fluorescein-complexone or calcein fluoresces in a strongly alkaline solution in the presence of calcium but not in the presence of magnesium. The fluorometric calcium procedure described by Meites (1970) requires only 20 μl. of serum and little analytical time; hence, this method is suitable for pediatric and emergency service requirements. However, as Meites points out, the main disadvantages are possible unsuspected interference in assay and potential variation in calcein from lot to lot.

Precipitation of serum calcium with chloranilic acid yields an insoluble precipitate (calcium chloranilate) that is dissolved in EDTA at a high pH to liberate chloranilate for spectrophotometric determination (Ferro and Ham, 1957). In the method described by Sherrick and de la Huerga (1963), hydroxynaphthalimide precipitates calcium from serum for subsequent measurement of yellow color spectrophotometrically after calcium hydroxynaphthalimide precipitate is dissolved with EDTA; in their micromethod (0.05 ml. serum), a ferric nitrate solution is added to the EDTA solution of dissolved precipitate to yield a ferric complex in a hydroxamin-iron reaction with a more intense amber color.

The application of flame photometry to calcium measurements has not been as successful as with sodium and potassium determinations. Teloh (1963) has reported a satisfactory procedure with careful attention to prerequisites for emission spectrophotometry. The normal values are slightly higher than in the Clark-Collip method.

Atomic absorption spectroscopy is recommended as the method of choice as well as a reference method for serum calcium determinations (Willis, 1960; Zettner and Seligson, 1964; Bowers and Pybus, 1972). An intense hot flame is required to excite a very small fraction of the total atomic population, with the remainder in the ground state. While atomic absorption is free of spectral interference, chemical interferences are eliminated or compensated for in calibration standards. The anions, phosphate and sulfate, tend to depress absorption in the flame; the addition of lanthanum chloride to samples and standards controls this because lanthanum competes with calcium for phosphate and sulfate. The excellent report of Zettner and Seligson (1964) as well as the presentation of a standard method by Bowers (1972) should be consulted for further details.

In the reports of Klein and Kaufman (1967) and Mabry and Wyles (1967), a procedure for the automated simultaneous determination of phosphorus and calcium is described; atomic absorption spectrophotometry is used in the calcium assay of Klein and Kaufman (1967). Gambino and Fonseco (1971) have reported comparable results for serum calcium measurements by SMA 12/60 and atomic absorption spectrophotometry.

Improved glass electrodes for accurate measurements of ionized or ionic calcium are available (Seamonds *et al.*, 1972; Low *et al.*, 1973). This system supplements and complements total serum calcium measurements, in view of the significance of the ionic calcium fraction, especially its greater sensitivity in defining hypercalcemia of hyperparathyroidism and also normal ionic fraction with depressed serum calcium observed with hypoproteinemia.

Fresh serum (less than 24 hours) is necessary for accurate and precise calcium measurements to preclude erratic results, which are observed when serum is stored.

Phosphorus (HPO_4^{--}) measurements require a serum specimen free of hemolysis. The separation of serum from whole blood should be performed as quickly as possible after collection to preclude any contribution to serum inorganic phosphate from the large organic phosphorus fraction in erythrocytes. Furthermore, a fasting state prior to morning blood collection will eliminate any circadian rhythmicity and effect of carbohydrate metabolism that may cause variation in serum phosphorus concentration.

Nearly all the serum inorganic phosphate is free or not bound to protein. Thus, dialysis as well as protein precipitation may be used to prepare a protein-free filtrate for phosphorus analysis. Traditionally phosphate is reacted with molybdate under appropriate conditions to form a phosphomolybdate complex; the addition of a suitable reducing agent that reacts with the phosphomolybdate complex causes the formation of a blue color of molybdenum; this is proportional to the amount of phosphate present and can then be determined spectrophotometrically. The most commonly used procedure is that of Fiske and Subbarow (1925). Ammonium molybdate in an acid medium of serum protein-free filtrate forms phosphomolybdic acid; reduction by para-aminonaphtholsulfonic acid reagent then yields phosphomolybdous acid with blue molybdenum for photometric determination. A variety of reducing agents with greater sensitivity and several modifications have been introduced; these are reviewed critically by Sunderman and Sunderman (1964, 1973b).

In the method of Parekh and Jung (1970b), molybdic acid is combined with trichloracetic acid as one reagent (to save technical steps) and a new reagent, p-phenylenediamine dihydrochloride is used for color development; this results in a stable molybdenum blue complex obeying Beer's Law and yielding such good reproducibility and accuracy that it is recommended by Sunderman and Sunderman (1973b).

Urinary hydroxyproline measurements reflecting collagen turnover (primarily bone resorption) have yielded considerable clinical information, as shown in Table 9–42 (Niejadlik, 1972). An elevation is most valuable in assessing bone disease, whether it be primary, metabolic, or metastatic. In terms of precision, accuracy, and rapidity of analyses, the method described by Parekh and Jung (1970a) has been well received. A methodology review by Klein and Kaufman (1967) should also be consulted for further details.

Urinary cyclic AMP measurements have proved most useful in differentiation of hypoparathyroidism from pseudohypoparathyroidism (Goldsmith, 1972). Since the latter disease does not show a renal response to PTH, cyclic AMP does not appear in the urine, as it would with PTH administration to a subject with primary hypoparathyroidism.

According to Goldsmith (1972), the development of radioimmunoassays for estimation of serum or plasma parathyroid hormone (PTH) concentrations distinguishes between normal and hyperparathyroid subjects. However, there are differences among assays, probably because of two circulating forms of biologically active PTH and perhaps also immunoreactive but biologically inactive fragments as well. Until recently either bovine or porcine hormone had to be relied on for serum human PTH assays (Brewer *et al.*, 1972). Since the biologically active segment of human parathyroid hormone (HPTH) has been delineated (Brewer *et al.*, 1972), more accurate diagnostic assay procedures should be forthcoming.

Calcitonin serum radioimmunoassays have been reported most recently with regard to their special value in detection of medullary thyroid cancer in families (Jackson *et al.*, 1973). Raisz *et al.*, (1972) have reported a tissue culture bioassay.

Goldsmith (1972) has reviewed other laboratory aids in the diagnosis of metabolic bone disease, including renal tubular reabsorption of phosphorus, phosphorus deprivation tests, calcium and PTH infusion tests, bone biopsy, and morphometry.

Table 9–42. ELEVATION OF URINARY HYDROXYPROLINE IN DISEASE*

Marked
Paget's disease
Fibrous dysplasia
Osteomalacia
Neoplastic bone disease
Rickets
Hyperthyroidism
Hyperparathyroidism (primary and secondary)
Severe burns
Acute osteomyelitis
Congenital hypophosphatasia
Moderate
Acromegaly
Marfan's syndrome
Active rheumatoid arthritis
Active scleroderma
Normal to slight
Inflammatory skin diseases
Osteoporosis
Pregnancy
Aseptic bone necrosis
Diabetes mellitus
Renal disease

*Niejadlik, D. C.: Postgrad. Med. *51* (No. 5):214, 1972.

Iron. Since iron metabolism is reviewed in Chapter 4, only the salient features will be presented (Fig. 9–65). For additional information, several excellent textbooks may be consulted (Bothwell and Finch, 1962; Fairbanks *et al.*, 1971; Gross, 1964; Harris and Kellermeyer, 1970).

The element iron is essential to most living organisms. Iron is present in many enzymes and oxygen-carrying pigments. It readily undergoes oxidation and reduction; therefore, iron is an important constituent of enzymes engaged in electron transport. The distribution of iron in the body is best explained in Table 9–43.

Only 11 to 14 per cent of dietary iron (12 to 18 mg. per day) is absorbed in the gastrointestinal tract (Moore, 1965, 1967). In iron deficiency states and during growth and pregnancy, however, the normal retention of 0.6 to 1.8 mg. daily is increased two- or threefold (1.2 to 4.8 mg. daily). The excellent review by Moore (1965) should be consulted for further information pertaining to iron nutrition and requirements.

Iron is lost through the skin by sweat and exfoliation of squamous cells, in feces and urine, and, in the female, through menstruation (2 to 79 mg. of iron per period). Pregnancy results in maternal losses of approximately 280 mg. to the fetus and approximately 100 mg. at the time of parturition (Bothwell and Finch, 1962). Lactation is also a drain on maternal iron stores. Generally iron losses are about 0.6 mg. per day in adult males and nonmenstruating females, with an additional 1.22 mg. per day loss in menstruating women (Moore, 1967).

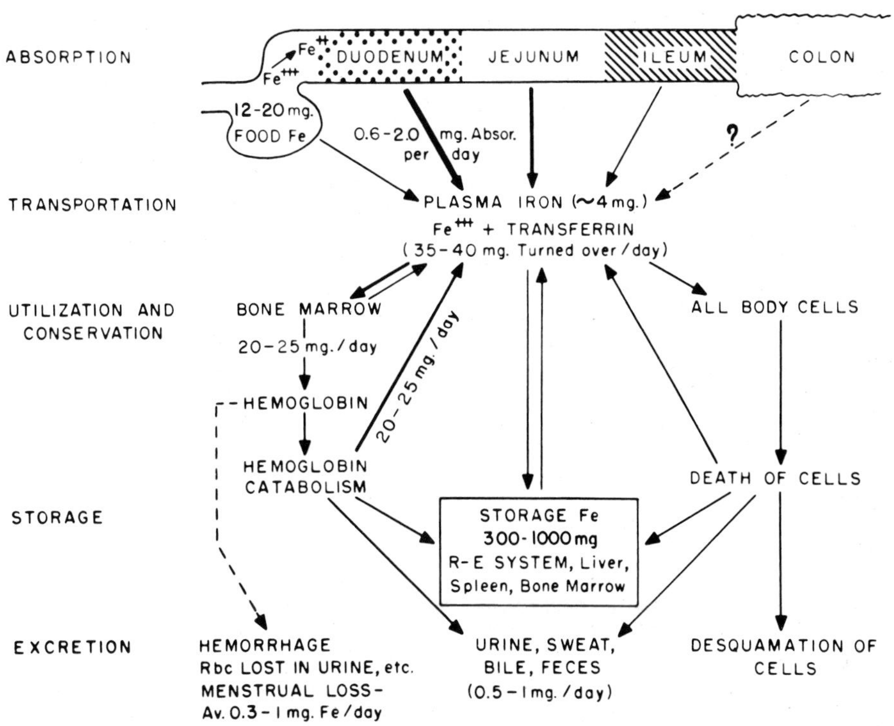

Figure 9–65. Schematic outline of iron metabolism in adult. (From C. V. Moore: Hypochromic anemias. *In* Beeson, P. B., and McDermott, W. (eds.): *Cecil-Loeb Textbook of Medicine*. 12th ed., 1967.)

The method for the regulation of iron absorption through the gut is largely unknown. Iron, however, is absorbed through the upper portion of the small bowel directly into the blood rather than through the lymphatics. While entry of iron at the brush border of mucosal cells appears to be by passive diffusion, exit from the cells to the plasma transferrin probably requires energy for active transport.

Table 9–43. DISTRIBUTION OF BODY IRON IN THE AVERAGE ADULT MALE*

COMPOUND	TOTAL IN BODY (MG.)	TOTAL IRON IN COMPOUND (MG.)	PER CENT OF TOTAL BODY IRON
Hemoglobin	900.0	3060.0	72.90
Myoglobin	40.0	140.0	3.30
Cytochrome	0.8	3.4	0.08
Catalase	5.0	4.5	0.11
Ferritin	3.0	690.0	16.40
Siderophilin (transferrin)	7.5	3.0	0.07
Total organic iron		3900.0	92.90
Remaining iron (by difference)		300.0	7.10

*From Beutler, Fairbanks, and Fahey: In *Clinical Disorders of Iron Metabolism.* New York, Grune & Stratton, Inc., 1963. Used by permission of the publisher.

When iron traverses the bowel mucosa, it enters the blood and is rapidly bound to transferrin (siderophilin). This protein has the electrophoretic mobility of a beta-1 globulin and is formed in the liver. Transferrin is a species of molecules which migrates at different electrophoretic mobilities. To date, there are 19 genetic variants of transferrin. The molecular weight of transferrin is approximately 90,000, and each molecule is able to bind two atoms of ferric iron (Bearn and Parker, 1964). The half-life of this protein is about 10 days. By contrast, the iron in the plasma pool has a half life of 60 to 120 minutes.

Iron, after absorption, finds its way largely to bone marrow, liver, and, in smaller amounts, other tissues. Transferrin is not itself assimilated by the receptor tissues. Indeed, transferrin may bind briefly to normoblast membrane and release its iron load (Fairbanks *et al.*, 1971). Iron is then taken up by normoblasts and incorporated into heme. Subsequently transferrin returns to plasma to take up unbound iron. From effete erythrocytes, iron is split from hemoglobin by reticuloendothelial system (RES) cells; most of it returns to plasma, where it is again bound by transferrin (Fairbanks *et al.*, 1971). Iron may be found in small quantities on the membranes of the young red blood cells (reticulocytes) and may be found in larger quantities in the reticuloendothelial cells. From the studies of Morgan (1966), however, no appreciable transferrin was bound to reticuloendothelial (RE) cells. However, transferrin that has given up its iron to immature erythrocytes acquires more iron from the storage sites, so that the cycle may repeat itself (Katz and Jandl, 1964).

Approximately 25 per cent of the iron in the body is in storage form as ferritin and hemosiderin (hepatic parenchymal cells and reticuloendothelial cells of the bone marrow, liver, and spleen). This represents a ready reserve of iron which can be called upon whenever the need arises. Transferrin is measured by the amount of iron which it can bind; this is referred to as the total iron-binding capacity (TIBC). Approximately one-third of the iron binding sites of transferrin contain iron; this is measured in serum iron determinations. The unsaturated iron-binding capacity (UIBC), or latent iron-binding capacity (LIBC), is that amount of iron which transferrin can bind above the iron with which it is already complexed. This relationship can be expressed as TIBC = UIBC + serum iron.

Another useful expression of this relationship is per cent saturation, which relates the amount of iron present in the serum to the amount of transferrin present. The formula for this relationship is:

$$\%\ \text{saturation} = \frac{\text{serum iron}}{\text{TIBC}} \times 100$$

The relationship between serum iron and transferrin (TIBC) is graphically illustrated as it occurs in various conditions and diseases in Figure 9–66. Additional clinical pathologic correlations are reviewed in Chapter 4.

The TIBC in normal adults averages between 300 and 340 μg. per dl. The normal per cent saturation is between 30 and 35 per cent. There is no diurnal fluctuation in the level of the TIBC as there is for the serum iron. Values, however, decrease with age (250 μg. per dl. of TIBC between 70 and 80 years of age). At birth the average newborn levels are about 225 μg. per dl. and reach a peak by the eighth month. Common causes for an increase in serum iron-binding capacity include iron deficiency anemia, pregnancy, infancy, ingestion of oral contraceptive drugs, and possibly hepatitis (Fig. 9–66). Low levels are found with diseases in which there has been a decrease in plasma protein through reduced protein synthesis or by direct loss as in nephrosis, or secondary to increased catabolism as seen in malignancy, starvation, and various chronic inflammatory states. Patients with blood transfusional iron overload show transferrin depression.

Serum iron, coupled to transferrin, is transport iron. Free hemoglobin is rarely present in sufficient quantity to affect the serum iron determination; if hemolysis is severe, the serum iron values will be falsely elevated. In acute iron poisoning, much nontransferrin-bound iron may be present also. Both of these conditions, however, are uncommon. The

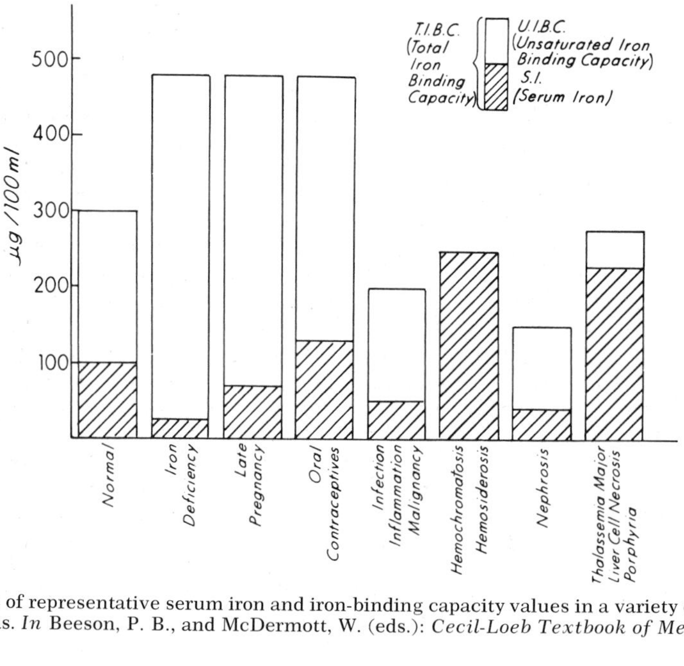

Figure 9–66. Examples of representative serum iron and iron-binding capacity values in a variety of conditions. (Brown, E. B.: Hypochromic anemias. *In* Beeson, P. B., and McDermott, W. (eds.): *Cecil-Loeb Textbook of Medicine*. 13th ed., 1971.)

average serum iron level has been established at about 125 μg. per dl. in adult males and 110 μg. per dl. in adult females. The range is wide and varies between 60 and 200 μg. per dl. Several authors have shown that the average day-to day variation in plasma iron may be as high as 30 per cent. There is no seasonal variation of iron levels, although a diurnal variation has been noted. In the evening there is often a fall in levels of nearly 32 per cent or, stated differently, serum iron may be one-third higher in the morning. As old age approaches, however, the serum iron level falls to 60 to 80 μg. per dl. The average plasma iron levels at birth are about 195 μg. per dl. There is a drop to about 45 μg. per dl. during the first few hours of life that is followed during the first two weeks by a rise to 125 μg. per dl. In pathologic states, serum iron is elevated during conditions of increased erythrocyte destruction, decreased blood formation, and increased release of iron from the body stores. If the incorporation of iron into heme is blocked, for example, in conditions such as lead poisoning or pyridoxine deficiency, the serum iron will be high. In acute hepatic cell necrosis, serum iron levels are high because of a sudden release of stored iron from the necrotic hepatic cells. Serum iron is high in both hemochromatosis and in transfusion siderosis.

There are two ways in which a depression of serum iron can be produced; there may be a decreased release of iron into the plasma or a deficiency in the total amount of iron present in the body. In cases of infection, the serum iron level is greatly reduced because of impaired release of iron from the reticuloendothelial system. Moderate serum iron depression is seen in cancer, chronic renal disease, and rheumatoid arthritis.

The ratio of serum iron level to plasma transferrin level (per cent saturation) varies in disease. An increase in the saturation of transferrin can occur in conditions of decreased circulating protein (chronic liver disease, nephrosis, kwashiorkor), in conditions associated with ineffective erythropoiesis or blocks in hemoglobin synthesis (thalassemia, lead poisoning, pyridoxine anemia), in diseases associated with iron overload (idiopathic hemochromatosis and hemosiderosis), and in acute blood loss. A decrease in the percentage of saturation (values less than 15 per cent) is present in iron deficiency anemia and in late pregnancy. In conditions such as infection and malignancies, both serum iron and total iron-binding capacity are decreased, but the serum iron depression is proportionately greater, so the percentage of saturation is reduced.

In the evaluation of patients for suspected disorders of iron lack or iron excess, the most useful clinical supporting data in addition to a complete hematologic workup, including an examination of peripheral blood smear, can be obtained from measurements of both serum iron and iron-binding capacity (TIBC), with calculation of per cent saturation. A single measurement of serum iron is usually inadequate for confirmation of iron excess or iron lack conditions. Pediatric patients with iron intoxication represent an exception: in these cases a serum iron value alone is sufficient.

Urinary iron measurements may evolve as important determinations in the assessment of total body iron. A simplified deferoxamine test has been reported by Rosen and Tullis (1966) that may prove valuable in the identification of patients with iron overload (for example, hemochromatosis). Deferoxamine (deferrioxamine) is a chelating agent with a high affinity for iron. It has been used therapeutically for iron intoxication and in a variety of diagnostic tests for excessive iron stores (Rosen and Tullis, 1966). Two 6-hour urinary specimens for iron analyses are collected; each urine collection represents a specimen before and after intramuscular injection of a 500-mg. dose of deferoxamine mesylate. With iron overload, patients display iron elevations in both specimens, but it is more striking in the postdeferoxamine urine collection.

In the various colorimetric methods for determination of serum iron, the initial step usually involves separating iron from its combination with transferrin (Giovanniello and Peters, 1963). The addition of hydrochloric acid with a reducing agent such as thioglycolic or ascorbic acid is used to release iron from transferrin and convert ferric ion to the ferrous ion for a colorimetric reaction with an iron reagent. Protein precipitation or extraction of reduced iron may be used prior to or with iron colorimetric reaction for photometric measurement. The more sensitive reagents available for the colorimetric determination of iron include bathophenanthroline, tripyridyltriazine (TPTZ), and ferrozine (Carter, 1971). In a critical comparison of the sensitivity and specificity of iron chromogens, Zak and colleagues (1971) concluded that terosite is the optimal ligand. In the micromethod proposed by Caraway (1963a), iron is simultaneously reduced and detached from serum protein with the aid of ascorbic acid and hydrochloric acid; proteins are precipitated with trichloroacetic acid in the presence of chloroform, and TPTZ is added to an aliquot of supernatant at an optimum pH for color development. The manual method of Fischer and Price (1964) also employs the chromogen tripyridyl-s-triazine (TPTZ), as does the automated procedure described by Young and Hicks (1965).

Although Zettner and co-workers (1965, 1966) have described atomic absorption methods for serum iron and iron-binding capacity as well as urinary iron determinations, the method of Olson and Hamlin (1969) has also been found to be rapid, accurate, and reliable (Sunderman and Sunderman, 1972).

The International Committee for Standardization in Hematology has recommended a method utilizing bathophenanthroline sulfonate as a chromagen to be used as a reference method for serum iron (Lewis, 1971). The risk of contamination in iron assays should always be kept in mind, with attention given to avoidance of hemolysis and substitution of glassware by disposable plastic tubes (most types are iron free) and the use of metal-free reagent dispensers (Cook, 1970).

While a serum iron determination reflects iron bound to transferrin, this transport protein is usually only 30 per cent saturated with iron, so the latent or unsaturated iron-binding capacity (LIBC or UIBC) is estimated also in measurements of total iron-binding capacity (TIBC). UIBC may be estimated directly by the measurement of absorbance increase produced by addition of iron to serum with formation of a red-colored iron-transferrin complex. Radioactive iron (^{59}Fe) can also be used to estimate UIBC directly (Koepke, 1965); an alternative approach involves actual measurement of iron in excess of that required to saturate transferrin.

More commonly the UIBC is determined indirectly by subtracting the serum iron from the TIBC. TIBC is determined by saturating transferrin with excess iron, removing the excess unbound iron with an iron absorbent, and performing a conventional iron determination on the supernate. Absorbents serve to remove any unbound iron excess and ideally should not remove iron which has become bound to the transferrin molecule (Cook, 1970). Although charcoal and $MgCO_3$ absorbents are comparable in reproducibility, resin appears to be less satisfactory (Cook, 1970). Koepke (1965) studied two commonly used iron absorbents: Amberlite resin sponge and light magnesium carbonate; the magnesium carbonate removed relatively large amounts of transferrin-bound iron, while the resin sponge was found to be an efficient and complete iron absorbent with minimal disturbance of iron bound to transferrin.

A commercially available immunologic method (Immunoplate, Hyland Laboratories, Los Angeles, California) employs an antiserum specific for human transferrin and immunodiffusion followed by measurement of precipitin ring diameter; the concentration of transferrin is expressed in micrograms of iron-binding capacity per dl. of serum.

Burrows (1967) has reported a comparison of three methods designed to measure transferrin and iron-binding capacity of serum. He found the immunodiffusion method to underestimate the IBC, while a radioisotopic method (Irosorb-59, Abbott Laboratories, North Chicago, Illinois) and the Fischer and Price colorimetric procedure (1964) were similar in accuracy and precision if allowance for the difference in iron absorbents was made.

Manual and automated techniques for measurement of serum iron and total iron-binding capacity have been reported recently by Giovanniello and Pecci (1972); for details of methods, this reference should be consulted. Zettner's unpublished colorimetric modification of his bathophenanthroline atomic absorption procedure (1966) is also recommended as reported in the October, 1972, Proficiency Test Service by Dr. F. W. Sunderman.

Copper. Copper, along with iron, is required for hemoglobin synthesis. It is a constituent of the enzymes cytochrome oxidase (so important in cellular respiration), monoamine oxidase, uricase, and tyrosinase (involved in melanin formation) (Harper, 1971).

Erythrocuprein is the copper-containing protein found in erythrocytes. While the erythrocyte copper content is rather constant at 93 to 114 μg. per dl., the serum copper level is more variable, averaging about 90 μg. per dl. (Harper, 1971). In serum, copper is distributed as follows: (1) about 96 per cent is firmly bound to α_2-globulin, which because of its blue color is called ceruloplasmin (20 to 35 mg. per dl.), (2) nearly 4 per cent is less firmly bound to albumin, and (3) a scant amount is free or dialyzable (Cantarow and Schepartz, 1967). The greatest oxidase activity of ceruloplasmin has been demonstrated with the substrate paraphenylenediamine. Ceruloplasmin is the main transport form of copper; however, amino acids may facilitate copper transport into erythrocytes (Neumann and Silverberg, 1967). Hypercupremia is usually observed during pregnancy, with a twofold increase in ceruloplasmin at term. Increases have also been seen in certain malignancies, acute and chronic infections, rheumatoid arthritis, biliary cirrhosis, and thyrotoxicosis.

Although copper deficiency is infrequent in severely malnourished infants and rarely may be a complication of severe chronic intestinal malabsorption, the clinicopathologic findings of hypocupremia, anemia, neutropenia, and bone changes similar to those observed in scurvy have been emphasized (Cordano and Graham, 1966). A low serum ceruloplasmin is present normally in the first six months of life and may be observed in patients with nephrotic syndrome, malabsorption syndrome, and severe malnutrition.

Wilson's disease or hepatolenticular degeneration is a more important abnormality of copper transport (Walshe, 1967). The accumulation of excess copper in the tissues of patients with Wilson's disease is the major chemical pathologic lesion. While the brain, particularly the basal ganglia, bears the brunt of the insult, the liver may be initially or even exclusively involved (Walshe, 1967). With an autosomal recessive mode of inheritance, this rare disease is characterized by degenerative changes of basal ganglia and cirrhosis of the liver, with onset sometimes during childhood but more often during the second and third decades of life and, rarely, in the fourth decade. Tremor, with purposeful ataxia, choreoathetosis, and incoordination reflect central nervous system dysfunction; jaundice may be an early complaint, but the other clinical features of hepatic disease are less likely to appear, despite underlying cirrhosis. In the hepatic form of Wilson's disease, neurologic signs are often minor or absent (Bearn, 1972). Sternlieb and Scheinberg (1972) have called attention to chronic hepatitis as a first manifestation of Wilson's disease; they recommend a serum ceruloplasmin measurement in every child and young adult with idiopathic chronic hepatitis. A brown ring at the corneal margin, referred to as the Kayser-Fleischer ring, is pathognomonic of Wilson's disease; it probably reflects excessive copper deposition in Descemet's membrane of the cornea. Renal tubular damage may result from excess copper accumulation; aminoaciduria may then appear.

A depression of serum ceruloplasmin to less than 20 mg. per dl. is almost always observed in Wilson's disease. This is associated with a low serum copper concentration and increased urinary copper excretion and tissue deposition, especially hepatic copper. Failure to synthesize this major copper transport protein is associated initially with an increase in copper-albumin serum fraction; since the copper is less firmly bound to albumin, it appears in the urine along with tissue accumulations. The possibility that the small amount of ceruloplasmin synthesized by most patients with Wilson's disease is structurally abnormal has not been excluded (Bearn, 1972). Some patients with Wilson's disease, however, excrete relatively small amounts of copper in their urine, and some have normal or near normal concentrations of ceruloplasmin in their serum (Scheinberg and Sternlieb, 1963).

While a serum ceruloplasmin estimation (Wallace, 1964) is more readily performed, measurements of urine and hepatic tissue copper can be performed with great accuracy (Sunderman and Roszel, 1967) and be valuable adjuncts in delineating this disorder (Arras, 1969). For the diagnosis of Wilson's disease, laboratory confirmation requires demonstration of a serum ceruloplasmin concentration of less than 20 mg. per dl., a urinary copper excretion of more than 100 μg. per 24 hours and a hepatic copper concentration greater than 100 μg. per gm. of dry liver (or 50 μg. per gm. wet weight). However, in both primary biliary cirrhosis and longstanding large bile duct obstruction, including biliary atresia, copper levels are well within those seen in Wilson's disease (Ozsoylu, 1971). With the use of penicillamine as a chelating agent for the removal of copper, urinary and serum copper measurements can be followed to ascertain the effectiveness of therapy. Indeed, if the disease can be diagnosed before the onset of irreversible damage, no patient receiving appropriate therapy should die subsequently of hepatolenticular disease (Walshe, 1967).

REFERENCES

Abell, L. L., Levy, B. B., Brodie, B. B., and Kendall, F. E.: Cholesterol in serum. In Seligson, D. (ed.): Standard Methods of Clinical Chemistry. Vol. 2. New York, Academic Press, Inc., 1958.

Abramson, N., and Shattil, S. J.: M-Components. J.A.M.A. 223:156, 1973.

Alpert, N. L.: Automated clinical chemistry analyzers: An overview of emerging patterns in laboratory automation. Lab World, February, 1972.

Alvioli, L.: Overview: Vitamin D. *In* International Symposium: Clinical Aspect of Metabolic Bone Disease, June, 1972, Detroit, Michigan. Amsterdam, Excerpta Medica. In Press.

Anderson, N. G.: Clinical analyzer moves into market place. Chem. Eng. News, August 3, 1970.

Annino, J. S.: Clinical Chemistry, Principles and Procedures. 3rd ed. Boston, Little, Brown and Company, 1964.

Annino, J. S., and Relman, A. S.: The effect of eating on some of the clinically important chemical constituents of blood. Amer. J. Clin. Path. *31*:155, 1959.

Arras, M. J.: Clinical pathologic correlations of copper. Postgrad. Med. *45*:55, 1969.

Asper, S. P., Jr., Schales, O., and Schales, S. S.: Importance of controlling pH in the Schales and Schales method of chloride determination. J. Biol. Chem. *168*:779, 1947.

Babson, A. L., Shapiro, P. O., and Phillips, G. E.: A new assay for cholesterol and cholesterol esters in serum which is not affected by bilirubin. Clin. Chim. Acta 7:800, 1962.

Baisden, R., Conn, R. B., Jr., and Anido, V.: Heterogeneity of human serum albumin: Report of two cases of bisalbuminemia. Amer. J. Clin. Path. *51*:760, 1969.

Barnett, E. V.: Cryoglobulinemia and disease. Ann. Intern. Med. 73:95, 1970.

Barzel, U. S.: Parathyroid hormone, blood phosphorus, and acid-base metabolism. Lancet *1*:1329, 1971.

Bautovich, G. J., Dash, M. J., Hensley, W. J., and Turtle, J. R.: Gradient gel electrophoresis of human plasma lipoproteins. Clin. Chem. *19*:415, 1973.

Bearn, A. G.: Wilson's disease. *In* Stanbury, J. B., Wyngaarden, J. B., and Fredrickson, D. S. (eds.): The Metabolic Basis of Inherited Disease. 3rd ed. New York, McGraw-Hill Book Company, 1972.

Bearn, A. G., and Cleve, H.: Genetic variations of plasma proteins. *In* Stanbury, J. B., Wyngaarden, J. B., and Fredrickson, D. S. (eds.): The Metabolic Basis of Inherited Disease. 3rd ed. New York, McGraw-Hill Book Company, 1972.

Bearn, A. G., and Parker, W. C.: Some observations on

transferrin. *In* Gross, F. (ed.): Iron Metabolism. Berlin, Springer-Verlag, 1964.

Bellanti, J. A.: Immunology. Philadelphia, W. B. Saunders Company, 1971.

Bennett, T. P.: Membrane filtration for determining protein in the presence of interfering substances. Nature (London) *213*:1131, 1967.

Bergmeyer, H. U., and Moellering, H.: Enzymatische Glucose-bestimmung mit Acylphosphat: D-glucose-6-phosphotransferase. Clin. Chim. Acta *14*:74, 1966.

Berliner, R. W., Hilton, J. G., Yu, T. F., and Kennedy, T. J., Jr.: The renal mechanism for urate excretion in man. J. Clin. Invest. *29*:396, 1950.

Bermes, E. W., Jr., and Forman, D. T.: Basic laboratory principles and procedures. *In* Tietz, N. W. (ed.): Fundamentals of Clinical Chemistry, Philadelphia, W. B. Saunders Company, 1970.

Bermes, E. W., Jr., and McDonald, H. J.: The stability of human serum lipoproteins, in vitro. Ann. Clin. Lab. Sci. *2*:226, 1972.

Betheil, J. J.: Fluorometric microdetermination of human serum albumin. Anal. Chem. *32*:560, 1960.

Bhoopalam, N., Lee, B. M., and Yakulis, V. J.: IgM heavy chain fragments in Waldenström's macroglobulinemia. Arch. Intern. Med. *128*:437, 1971.

Block, W. D., Jarrett, K. J., Jr., and Levine, J. B.: Use of a single color reagent to improve the automated determination of serum total cholesterol. *In* Skeggs, L. T., Jr. (ed.): Automation in Analytical Chemistry. Technicon Symposia, 1965. New York, Mediad, Inc., 1966.

Bondy, P. K.: Diabetes mellitus. *In* Beeson, P. B., and McDermott, W. (eds.): Cecil-Loeb Textbook of Medicine. 13th ed. Philadelphia, W. B. Saunders Company, 1971.

Booij, J.: Some divergent results of protein standardization. Clin. Chim. Acta *38*:355, 1972.

Boonstra, C. E., and Jackson, C. E.: Serum calcium survey for hyperparathyroidism: Results in 50,000 clinic patients. Amer. J. Clin. Path. *55*:523, 1971.

Bothwell, T. H., and Finch, C. A.: Iron Metabolism. Boston, Little, Brown and Company, 1962.

Bowen, A. J., and Reeves, R. L.: Diurnal variation in glucose tolerance. Arch. Intern. Med. *119*:261, 1967.

Bowers, G. N., and Pybus, J.: Total calcium in serum by atomic absorption spectrophotometry. *In* Cooper, G. R. (ed.): Standard Methods of Clinical Chemistry. Vol. 7. New York, Academic Press, Inc., 1972.

Brady, R. O.: Enzyme defects in the sphingolipidoses and their application to diagnosis. Ann. Clin. Lab. Sci. *2*:285, 1972.

Bragdon, J. H.: Determination of total lipids and of triglycerides by difference. *In* Sunderman, F. W., Jr., and Sunderman, F. W. (eds.): Lipids and the Steroid Hormones in Clinical Medicine. Philadelphia, J. B. Lippincott Co., 1960.

Breckenridge, D. J., and Csillay, E. R.: A quantitative electrophoretic survey of serum protein fractions in health and disease. Acta Med. Scand. Suppl. *172*:383, 1962.

Brewer, H. B., Fairwell, T., Ronan, R., Sizemore, G. W., and Arnaud, C. D.: Human parathyroid hormone: Amino-acid sequence of the amino-terminal. Proc. Nat. Acad. Sci. *69*:3585, 1972.

Brinkerink, P. C.: Determination of creatine in urine: Inadequacies of present methods based on the conversion of creatine to creatinine: Significance of the creatine-creatinine equilibrium. Clin. Chim. Acta *6*:531, 1961.

Brochner-Mortensen, K., Cobb, S., and Rose, B. S.: Report of subcommittee on criteria for the diagnosis of gout in surveys. *In* Kellgren, J. H., Jeffrey, M. R., and Ball, J. (eds.): The Epidemiology of Chronic Rheumatism. Vol. 1. Philadelphia, F. A. Davis Company, 1963.

Brown, E. B.: Iron deficiency anemia. *In* Beeson, P. B., and McDermott, W. (eds.): Cecil-Loeb Textbook of Medicine. 13th ed. Philadelphia, W. B. Saunders Company, 1971.

Burrows, S.: Comparison of methods designed to measure transferrin and iron-binding capacity of serum. Amer. J. Clin. Path. *47*:326, 1967.

Cantarow, A., and Schepartz, B.: Biochemistry. 4th ed. Philadelphia, W. B. Saunders Company, 1967.

Caraway, W. T.: Microchemical Methods for Blood Analysis. Springfield, Illinois, Charles C Thomas, 1960.

Caraway, W. T.: Chemical and diagnostic specificity of laboratory tests. Amer. J. Clin. Path. *37*:445, 1962.

Caraway, W. T.: Macro and micro methods for the determination of serum iron and iron-binding capacity. Clin. Chem. *9*:188, 1963a.

Caraway, W. T.: Uric acid. *In* Seligson, D. (ed.): Standard Methods of Clinical Chemistry. Vol. 4. New York, Academic Press, Inc., 1963b.

Caraway, W. T.: Sources of error in clinical chemistry. *In* Meites, S. (ed.): Standard Methods of Clinical Chemistry. Vol. 5. New York, Academic Press, Inc., 1965.

Caraway, W. T., and Marable, H.: Comparison of carbonate and uricase-carbonate methods for the determination of uric acid in serum. Clin. Chem. *12*:18, 1966.

Carter, P.: Spectrophotometric determination of serum iron at the submicrogram level with a new reagent (ferrozine). Anal. Biochem. *40*:450, 1971.

Cawley, L. P.: Principles of chromatography. *In* Manual for Workshop on Chromatography. Chicago, American Society of Clinical Pathologists, 1965.

Cawley, L. P.: Electrophoresis and Immunoelectrophoresis. Boston, Little, Brown and Company, 1969.

Cawley, L. P., Penn, G. M., Itano, M., Bell, H. E., and Minard, B.: Basic Electrophoresis, Immunoelectrophoresis and Immunochemistry. Chicago, American Society of Clinical Pathologists, Commission on Continuing Education, 1972.

Cerasi, E., Efendic, S., and Luft, R.: Dose-response relation between plasma-insulin and blood-glucose levels during oral glucose loads in prediabetic and diabetic subjects. Lancet *1*:794, 1973.

Ceriotti, G.: Blood glucose determination without deproteinization, of O-toluidine in dilute acetic acid. Clin. Chem. *17*:440, 1971.

Chalmers, J., Conacher, W. D. H., Gardner, D. L., and Scott, P. J.: Osteomalacia: A common disease in elderly women. J. Bone Joint Surg. *49*B:403, 1967.

Chaney, A. L., and Marbach, E. P.: Modified reagents for determination of urea and ammonia. Clin. Chem. *8*:130, 1962.

Chiaraviglio, E. C., Wolf, A. V., and Prentiss, P. G.: Total protein/protein nitrogen ratio of human serum: A factor consistent with total solids. Amer. J. Clin. Path. *39*:42, 1963.

Christian, D. G.: Drug interference with laboratory blood chemistry determinations. Amer. J. Clin. Path. *54*:118, 1970.

Claman, H. N., and Merrill, D.: Hypergammaglobulinemia: The role of the immunoglobulins (γG, γA, γM). J. Allerg. *36*:463, 1965.

Clark, E. P., and Collip, J. B.: A study of the Tisdall method for determination of blood serum calcium with a suggested modification. J. Biol. Chem. *63*:461, 1925.

Clayton, B. E., and Jenkins, P.: Micro methods and micro apparatus for chemical pathology with special reference to pediatrics. J. Clin. Path. *19*:293, 1966.

Cook, J. D.: Methods to determine plasma iron and total iron-binding capacity. *In* Hallberg, L., Harwerth, H.-G., and Vannotti, A. (eds.): Iron Deficiency: Pathogenesis—Clinical Aspects—Therapy. New York, Academic Press, Inc., 1970.

Cooper, G. R., and McDaniel, V.: The determination of glucose by the orthotoluidine method (filtrate and direct procedure). *In* MacDonald, R. P. (ed.): Standard Methods of Clinical Chemistry. Vol. 6. New York, Academic Press, Inc., 1970.

Copp, D. H., Cameron, E. C., Cheney, B. A., Davidson, A. G. F., and Henze, K. G.: Evidence for calcitonin: A new hormone from the parathyroid that lowers blood calcium. Endocrinology *70*:638, 1962.

Cordano, A., and Graham, G. G.: Copper deficiency complicating severe chronic intestinal malabsorption. Pediatrics *38*:596, 1966.

Cotlove, E.: Chloride. *In* Seligson, D. (ed.): Standard Methods of Clinical Chemistry. Vol. 3. New York, Academic Press, Inc., 1961.

Couch, R. D. (ed.): Summary Report. American Society of Clinical Pathologists. Vol. VII, Nos. 7 & 8, July & August, 1970.

Creech, B. G.: Separation and determination of ketosteroids, pregnanediol and pregnanetriol on one column. J. Gas Chromatog. 2:194, 1964.

Creno, R. J., Wenk, R. E., and Bohlig, P.: Automated micromeasurement of urea using urease and the Berthelot reaction. Amer. J. Clin. Path. *54*:828, 1970.

Crowley, L. V.: Serum lipid concentrations in patients with coronary arteriosclerosis demonstrated by coronary arteriography. Clin. Chem. *17*:206, 1971.

Cuatrecasas, P., and Anfinsen, C. B.: Affinity chromatography. Ann. Rev. Biochem. *40*:259, 1971.

Dal Nogare, S., and Juvet, R. S.: Gas Liquid Chromatography—Theory and Practice. New York, Interscience Publishers, Inc., 1962.

Davey, F. R., Carrington, C. E., and Nelson, D. A.: Comparison of rapid clottable fibrinogen assays. Clin. Chem. *18*: 1360, 1972.

de la Huerga, J., Smetters, G. W., and Sherrick, J. C.: Colorimetric determination of serum proteins: The biuret reaction. *In* Sunderman, F. W., and Sunderman, F. W., Jr. (eds.): Serum Proteins and the Dysproteinemias. Philadelphia, J. B. Lippincott Co., 1964.

DeLuca, H. F.: 25-Hydroxycholecalciferol. Arch. Intern. Med. *124*:442, 1969a.

DeLuca, H. F.: Vitamin D. New Eng. J. Med. *281*:1103, 1969b.

DeLuca, H. F.: Role of kidney tissue in metabolism of vitamin D. New Eng. J. Med. *284*:554, 1971.

Doolan, P. D., Alpen, E. L., and Theil, G. B.: A clinical appraisal of the plasma concentration and endogenous clearance of creatinine. Amer. J. Med. *32*:65, 1962.

Doumas, B. T., and Biggs, H. G.: Determination of serum albumin. *In* Cooper, G. R. (ed.): Standard Methods of Clinical Chemistry. Vol. 7. New York, Academic Press, Inc., 1972.

Dubowski, K. M.: An O-toluidine method for body fluid glucose determination. Clin. Chem. *8*:215, 1962.

Dubowski, K. M.: Measurements of hemoglobin derivatives. *In* Sunderman, F. W., and Sunderman, F. W., Jr. (eds.): Hemoglobin: Its Precursors and Metabolites. Philadelphia, J. B. Lippincott Co., 1964a.

Dubowski, K. M.: Physical-chemical measurements of serum proteins. A. General considerations, C. Determinations of proteins by ultraviolet absorbance measurements. *In* Sunderman, F. W., and Sunderman, F. W., Jr. (eds.): Serum Proteins and the Dysproteinemias. Philadelphia, J. B. Lippincott Co., 1964b.

Earle, D. P.: Abnormal albumins. *In* Beeson, P. B., and McDermott, W. (eds.): Cecil-Loeb Textbook of Medicine. 12th ed. Philadelphia, W. B. Saunders Company, 1967.

Edelman, G. M.: Dissociation of γ-globulin. J. Amer. Chem. Soc. *81*:3155, 1959.

Edelman, G. M.: Antibody structure and molecular immunology. Science *180*:830, 1973.

Edelman, G. M., and Poulik, M. D.: Studies on structural units of the γ-globulin. J. Exp. Med. *113*:861, 1961.

Edwards, L., Falkowski, C., and Chilcote, M. E.: Semiautomated fluorometric measurement of triglycerides. *In* Cooper, G. R. (ed.): Standard Methods of Clinical Chemistry. Vol. 7. New York, Academic Press, Inc., 1972.

Fairbanks, V. F., Fahey, J. L., and Beutler, E.: Clinical Disorders of Iron Metabolism. New York, Grune & Stratton, 1971.

Fajans, S. S.: Diagnostic tests for diabetes mellitus. *In* Williams, R. H. (ed.): Diabetes. New York, Paul B. Hoeber, Inc., 1960.

Farese, G., and Mager, M.: Protein-free filtrates obtained by membrane ultrafiltration: Application to the determination of serum constituents. Clin. Chem. *16*:280, 1970.

Farquhar, J. W., and Ways, P.: Abetalipoproteinemia. *In* Stanbury, J. B., Wyngaarden, J. B., and Fredrickson, D. S. (eds.): The Metabolic Basis of Inherited Disease. 3rd ed. New York, McGraw-Hill Book Company, 1972.

Feinstein, A., Munn, E. A., and Richardson, N. E.: The three-dimensional conformation of IgM or IgA globulin molecules. Ann. New York Acad. Sci. *190*:104, 1971.

Feinstein, A., and Rowe, A. J.: Molecular mechanism of formation of an antigen-antibody complex. Nature (London) *205*:147, 1965.

Ferro, P. V., and Ham. A. B.: A simple spectrophotometric method for the determination of calcium. Amer. J. Clin. Path. *28*:208, 1957.

Fischer, D. S., and Price, D. C.: A simple serum iron method using the new sensitive chromogen tripyridyl-s-triazine. Clin. Chem. *10*:21, 1964.

Fiske, C. H., and Subbarow, Y.: The colorimetric determination of phosphorus. J. Biol. Chem. *66*:375, 1925.

Fletcher, M. J., and Styliou, H. A.: A simple method for separating serum lipoproteins by electrophoresis on cellulose acetate. Clin. Chem. *16*:362, 1970.

Folin, O.: Beitrag zur Chemie des Kreatinins and Kreatins im Harne. Z. Physiol. Chemie *41*:223, 1904.

Foster, L. B., and Dunn, R. T.: Stable reagents for determination of serum triglycerides by a colorimetric Hantzach condensation method. Clin. Chem. *19*:338, 1973.

Franklin, E. C., Lowenstein, J., Bigelow, B., and Meltzer, M.: Heavy chain disease: A new disorder of serum γ-globulins. Amer. J. Med. *37*:332, 1964.

Fredrickson, D. S., Gotto, A. M., and Levy, R. I.: Familial lipoprotein deficiency (abetalipoproteinemia, hypobetalipoproteinemia, and Tangier disease). *In* Stanbury, J. B., Wyngaarden, J. B., and Fredrickson, D. S. (eds.): The Metabolic Basis of Inherited Disease. 3rd ed. New York, McGraw-Hill Book Company, 1972.

Fredrickson, D. S., and Levy, R. I.: Familial hyperlipoproteinemia. *In* Stanbury, J. B., Wyngaarden, J. B., and Fredrickson, D. S. (eds.): The Metabolic Basis of Inherited Disease. 3rd ed. New York, McGraw-Hill Book Company, 1972.

Fredrickson, D. S., Levy, R. I., and Lees, R. S.: Fat transport in lipoproteins: An integrated approach to mechanisms and disorders. New Eng. J. Med. *276*:34; 94; 148; 215; 273, 1967.

Friedewald, W. T., Levy, R. I., and Fredrickson, D. S.: Estimation of the concentration of low-density lipoprotein cholesterol in plasma, without use of the preparative ultracentrifuge. Clin. Chem. *18*:499, 1972.

Friedman, M.: Plasma cholesterol concentration. J.A.M.A. *198*:657, 1966.

Frings, C. S., and Dunn, R. T.: Measurement of phospholipids in serum. *In* Cooper, G. R. (ed.): Standard Methods of Clinical Chemistry. Vol. 7. New York, Academic Press, Inc., 1972.

Frings, C. S., Foster, L. B., and Cohen, P. S.: Electrophoretic separation of serum lipoproteins in polyacrylamide gel. Clin. Chem. *17*:111, 1971.

Gallagher, J. C., and Seligson, D.: Significance of abnormally low blood urea levels. New Eng. J. Med. *266*:492, 1962.

Gambino, S. R.: Met and unmet needs of the automated clinical laboratory. Anal. Chem. *43*:21, 1971.

Gambino, S. R., and Fonseca, I.: Comparison of serum calcium measurements obtained with the SMA 12/60 and by atomic absorption spectrophotometry. Clin. Chem. *17*:1047, 1971.

Gambino, S. R., and Schreiber, H.: The measurement of CO_2 content with the autoanalyzer: A comparison with three standard methods and a description of a new method (alkalinization) for preventing loss of CO_2 from open cups. Amer. J. Clin. Path. *45*:406, 1966.

Giovanniello, T. J., and Pecci, J.: Measurement of serum iron and total iron-binding capacity: Manual and automated techniques. *In* Cooper, G. R. (ed.): Standard Methods of Clinical Chemistry. Vol. 7. New York, Academic Press, Inc., 1972.

Giovanniello, T. J., and Peters, T., Jr.: Serum iron and serum iron-binding capacity. *In* Seligson, D. (ed.): Standard Methods of Clinical Chemistry. Vol. 4. New York, Academic Press, Inc., 1963.

Gitlin, D., Hitzig, W. H., and Janeway, C. A.: Multiple serum protein deficiencies in congenital and acquired agammaglobulinemia. J. Clin. Invest. *35*:1199, 1956.

Glueck, C. J., Heckman, F., Schoenfeld, M., Steiner, P., and Pearce, W.: Neonatal familial type II hyperlipoproteinemia: Cord blood cholesterol in 1800 births. Metabolism *20*:597, 1971.

Gokcen, M.: Cryoglobulins behaving as "cold autoantibodies." Postgrad. Med. *39*:A68, 1966.

Goldsmith, R. S.: Laboratory aids in the diagnosis of metabolic bone disease. Orthoped. Clin. N. Amer. *3*:545, 1972.

Goodwin, J. F.: Spectrophotometric quantitation of plasma and urinary amino nitrogen with fluorodinitrobenzene. *In* MacDonald, R. P. (ed.): Standard Methods of Clinical Chemistry. Vol. 6. New York, Academic Press, Inc., 1970.

Greenawald, K. A., Speicher, C. E., Evers, W., and Henry, J. B.: Glucose content in cerebrospinal fluid: A comparison with glucose levels in serum as determined by copper reduction and hexokinase methods. Amer. J. Clin. Path. *59*:518, 1973.

Gross, F. (ed.): Iron Metabolism. Berlin, Springer-Verlag, 1964.

Gutman, A. B.: Gout. *In* Beeson, P. B., and McDermott, W. (eds.): Cecil-Loeb Textbook of Medicine. 12th ed. Philadelphia, W. B. Saunders Company, 1967.

Gutman, A. B., and Yu, T. F.: Uric acid metabolism in normal man and in primary gout. New Eng. J. Med. *273*:252, 313, 1965.

Guyton, A. C.: Textbook of Medical Physiology. 4th ed. Philadelphia, W. B. Saunders Company, 1971.

Hackler, M.: How to choose a laboratory balance. American Laboratory, March, 1970.

Hamilton, J. B.: Personal communication at Gelman Eastern Regional TLC, ITLC Workshop in New York, April 11, 1967.

Hamilton, J. G., Swartwout, J. R., Miller, O. N., and Muldrey, J. E.: A silica gel impregnated glass fiber filter paper and its use for the separation of cholesterol, triglycerides and the cholesteryl and methyl esters of fatty acids. Biochem. Res. Commun. *5*:226, 1961.

Harkness, D. R.: Structure and function of immunoglobulins. Postgrad. Med. *48*:64, 1970.

Harper, H. A.: Review of Physiologic Chemistry. Los Altos, California, Lange Medical Publications, 1971.

Harris, E. K., and DeMets, D. L.: Biological and analytic components of variation in long-term studies of serum constituents in normal subjects. V. Estimated biological variations in ionized calcium. Clin. Chem. *17*:983, 1971.

Harris, J. W., and Kellermeyer, R. W.: The red cell production, metabolism, destruction: Normal and abnormal. Revised ed. Cambridge, Harvard University Press, 1970.

Harris, W. H., and Heaney, R. P.: Skeletal renewal and metabolic bone disease. New Eng. J. Med. *280*:253, 1969.

Heaney, R. P.: Bone physiology and calcium homeostasis. *In* Beeson, P. B., and McDermott, W. (eds.): Cecil-Loeb Textbook of Medicine. 12th ed. Philadelphia, W. B. Saunders Company, 1967.

Heaney, R. P.: Diseases of bone: Bone physiology and calcium homeostasis. *In* Beeson, P. B., and McDermott, W. (eds.): Cecil-Loeb Textbook of Medicine. 13th ed. Philadelphia, W. B. Saunders Company, 1971.

Heidelberger, M., and Pedersen, O. O.: The molecular weight of antibodies. J. Exp. Med. *65*:393, 1937.

Heinmiller, E. C.: Phospholipids in serum. *In* Sunderman, F. W., and Sunderman, F. W., Jr. (eds.): Lipids and the Steroid Hormones in Clinical Medicine. Philadelphia, J. B. Lippincott Co., 1964.

Henry, J. B., and Pruitt, C. T.: This report system reduces lab errors. Mod. Hosp. *104*:118, 1964.

Henry, R. J.: Clinical Chemistry: Principles and Techniques. New York, Hoeber Medical Division, Harper & Row, 1964.

Heremans, J. F.: Immunochemical studies on protein pathology: The immunoglobulin concept. Clin. Chim. Acta *4*:639, 1959.

Hill, J. B.: Automated fluorometric method for determination of serum calcium. Clin. Chem. *11*:122, 1965.

Honing, J. V. D., Saarloos, C. C., and Stip, J.: Method for fully automated determination of total cholesterol in blood serum, including saponification and extraction. Clin. Chem. *14*:960, 1968.

Howard, J. E., and Thomas, W. C., Jr.: Clinical disorders of calcium homeostasis. Medicine *42*:25, 1963.

Howe, P. E.: The use of sodium sulfate as the globulin precipitant in the determination of proteins in blood. J. Biol. Chem. *49*:93, 1921.

Hultman, E.: Rapid specific method for determination of aldosaccharides in body fluids. Nature (London) *183*:108, 1959.

Iammarino, R. M.: Proteins and amino acids: Technique of immunoelectrophoresis. *In* Cooper, G. R. (ed.): Standard Methods of Clinical Chemistry. Vol. 7. New York, Academic Press, Inc., 1972.

Irwin, W. C., and Campbell, D. J.: Agarose gel electrophoresis of lipoproteins. *In* Cooper, G. R. (ed.): Standard Methods of Clinical Chemistry. Vol. 7. New York, Academic Press, Inc., 1972.

Jackson, C. E., Tashjian, A. H., Jr., and Block, M. A.: Detection of medullary thyroid cancer by calcitonin assay in families. Ann. Intern. Med. *78*:845, 1973.

Janchen, D.: Personal communication at Gelman Eastern Regional TLC, ITLC Workshop in New York City, April 11, 1967.

Johnson, A. M., and Alper, C. A.: Deficiency of alpha-antitrypsin in childhood liver disease. Pediatrics *46*:921, 1970.

Johnson (J. Lloyd) Associates: Clinical Laboratory Computer Systems: A Comprehensive Evaluation. Prepared for the College of American Pathologists, 1971.

Jones, D. P.: Lecithin cholesterol acyl transferase (LCAT). Ann. Clin. Lab. Sci. *2*:93, 1972.

Jones, R. J.: The hyperlipoproteinemias: Detection, diagnosis and management. Med. Clin. N. Amer. *57*:47, 1973.

Jung, D. H., and Parekh, A. C.: An improved reagent system for the measurement of serum uric acid. Clin. Chem. *16*:247, 1970.

Kaplan, A.: Urea nitrogen and urinary ammonia. *In* Meites, S. (ed.): Standard Methods of Clinical Chemistry. Vol. 5. New York, Academic Press, Inc., 1965.

Kaplan, A., and Savory, J.: Cellulose acetate electrophoresis of proteins of serum, cerebrospinal fluid, and urine. *In* MacDonald, R. P. (ed.): Standard Methods of Clinical Chemistry. Vol. 6. New York, Academic Press, Inc., 1970.

Katz, J. H., and Jandl, J. H.: The role of transferrin in the transport of iron into the developing red cells. *In* Gross, F. (ed.): Iron Metabolism. Berlin, Springer-Verlag, 1964.

Kessler, G., and Lederer, H.: Fluorometric measurements of triglycerides. *In* Skeggs, L. T., Jr. (ed.): Technicon Symposia Automation in Analytical Chemistry, 1965. New York, Mediad, Inc., 1966.

Keston, A. S.: Specific colorimetric enzymatic analytical reagents for glucose. Abstracts of papers of the 129th Meeting of the American Chemical Society, Dallas, Texas, April, 1956.

Keys, A., Mickelsen, O., Miller, E., Hayes, E., and Todd, R.: Concentration of cholesterol in blood serum of normal man and its relation to age. J. Clin. Invest. *29*:1347, 1950.

Keyser, J. W., and Cawson, M.: A serum reference standard for automated total protein and albumin procedures. Clin. Chem. *16*:147, 1970.

Killingsworth, L. M., and Savory, J.: Manual nephelometric methods for immunochemical determination of immunoglobulins IgG, IgA, and IgM in human serum. Clin. Chem. *18*:335, 1972.

Kimberg, D. V.: Effects of vitamin D and steroid hormones on the active transport of calcium by the intestine. New Eng. J. Med. *280*:1396, 1969.

Klein, B., and Kaufman, J. H.: Automated atomic absorption

spectrophotometry. IV. Simultaneous determination of calcium and phosphate. Clin. Chem. *13*:1079, 1967.

Klein, B., Morgenstein, S., and Kaufman, J. H.: A modified automated ferricyanide-phosphomolybdic acid procedure for serum or plasma glucose. Clin. Chem. *12*:816, 1966.

Klimt, C. R., Prout, T. E., Bradley, R. F., Dolger, H., Fisher, G., Gastineau, C. F., Marks, H., Meinert, C. L., and Schumacher, O. P.: Standardization of the oral glucose tolerance test: Report of the Committee on Statistics of the American Diabetes Association, June 14, 1968. Diabetes *18*:299, 1969.

Knights, E. M., MacDonald, R. P., and Ploompuu, J.: Ultramicro Methods for Clinical Laboratories. 2nd ed. New York, Grune & Stratton, Inc., 1962.

Kocher, P.: Étude de l'hydroxyproline-urie dans les osteopathies. Path. Biol. *14*:1020, 1966.

Koepke, J. A.: Comparison of light magnesium carbonate and amberlite sponge adsorbants in the measurement of the latent iron-binding capacity of serum. Amer. J. Clin. Path. *44*:77, 1965.

Krieg, A. F., Johnson, T. J., Jr., McDonald, C., and Cotlove, E.: Clinical Laboratory Computerization. Baltimore, University Park Press, 1971.

Kuo, P. T.: Hyperglyceridemia in coronary artery disease and its management. J.A.M.A. *201*:101, 1967.

Lee, S. L., Rosner, F., Ruberman, W., and Glasberg, S.: Mu-Chain disease. Ann. Intern. Med. *75*:407, 1971.

Lees, R. S.: Protein component of LDL linked with atherosclerosis. J.A.M.A. *211*:581, 1970.

Lees, R. S., and Wilson, D. E.: The treatment of hyperlipidemia. New Eng. J. Med. *284*:186, 1971.

Leffler, H. H., and McDougald, C. H.: Estimation of cholesterol in serum. Amer. J. Clin. Path. *39*:311, 1963.

Levy, R. I., and Langer, T.: Mechanisms involved in hyperlipidemia. Mod. Treat. 6:1313, 1970.

Lewis, B.: The metabolism of cholesterol. Postgrad. Med. *35*:208, 1959.

Lewis, S. M.: Proposed recommendations for measurement of serum iron in human blood. J. Clin. Path. *24*:334, 1971.

Li, T. K., and Piechocki, J. T.: Determination of serum ionic calcium with an ion-selective electrode: Evaluation of methodology and normal values. Clin. Chem. *17*:411, 1971.

Liddle, L. L., Seegmiller, J. E., and Laster, L.: The enzymatic spectrophotometric method for determination of uric acid. J. Lab. Clin. Med. *54*:903, 1959.

Lieberman, J., Mittman, C., and Schneider, A. S.: Screening for homozygous and heterozygous l-antitrypsin deficiency. J.A.M.A. *210*:2055, 1969.

Linese, J. G., and Raine, D. M.: Ann. Clin. Biol. 7:6, 1970.

Logan, J. E., and Allen, R. H.: Control serum preparations. Clin. Chem. *14*:437, 1968.

Low, J. C., Schaaf, M., Earll, J. M., Piechocki, J. T., and Li, T. K.: Ionic calcium determination in primary hyperparathyroidism. J.A.M.A. *223*:152, 1973.

Lowry, O. H., Rosebrough, N. J., Farr, A. L., and Randall, R. J.: Protein measurements with the folin phenol reagent. J. Biol. Chem. *193*:265, 1951.

Mabry, C. C., Gevedon, R. E., Roeckel, I. E., and Gochman, N.: Automated submicrochemistries. A system of rapid submicrochemical analysis for the measurement of sodium, potassium chloride, carbon dioxide, sugar urea nitrogen, total and direct-reacting bilirubin and total protein. Amer. J. Clin. Path. *46*:265, 1966.

Mabry, C. C., Roeckel, I. E., Gevedon, R. E., and Koepke, J. A.: Recent Advances in Pediatric Clinical Pathology. Lexington, Kentucky, The University of Kentucky Medical Center, 1967.

Mabry, C. C., Roeckel, I. E., Gevedon, R. E., and Koepke, J. A.: Recent Advances in Pediatric Clinical Pathology. New York, Grune & Stratton, 1968.

Mabry, C. C., and Wyles, P.: Micro automated parallel measurement of serum calcium and phosphorus. Amer. J. Clin. Path. *47*:395, 1967.

MacKenzie, M. R., Fudenberg, H. H., and O'Reilly, R. A.: The hyperviscosity syndrome. I. In IgG myeloma. The role of protein concentration and molecular shape. J. Clin. Invest. *49*:15, 1970.

Marshall, S.: Urea-creatinine ratio in obstructive uropathy and renal hypertension. J.A.M.A. *190*:109, 1964.

Martin, T. J.: The Pharmacologic Interactions with Laboratory Test Values. August, 1970, 596 Burnhamthorpe, Etobicoke, Ontario, Canada.

Mattenheimer, H.: Micromethods for the Clinical and Biochemical Laboratory. Ann Arbor, Michigan, Ann Arbor Science Publishers, Inc., 1970.

Mayes, P.: Lipids. *In* Harper, H. A. (ed.): Review of Physiological Chemistry. 13th Edition. Los Altos, California, Lange Medical Publications, 1971.

Meinke, W. W.: Standard reference materials for clinical measurements. Anal. Chem. *43*:28A, 1971.

Meites, S.: Calcium (fluorometric). *In* MacDonald, R. P. (ed.): Standard Methods of Clinical Chemistry. Vol. 6. New York, Academic Press, Inc., 1970.

Merrill, J. P., and Hampers, C. L.: Uremia. New Eng. J. Med. *282*:953; 1014, 1970.

Mikkelsen, W. M., Dodge, H. J., and Valkenburg, H.: The distribution of serum uric acid values in a population unselected as to gout or hyperuricemia. Amer. J. Med. *35*:242, 1965.

Miller, B. F., and Dubos, R.: Studies on the presence of creatinine in human blood. J. Biol. Chem. *121*:447; 457, 1937.

Miller, F., and Metzger, H.: Characterization of a human macroglobulin. II. Distribution of the disulfide bonds. J. Biol. Chem. *240*:4740, 1965.

Miskiewicz, S. J., Arnett, B. B., and Simon, G. E.: Evaluation of a glucose oxidase-peroxidase method adapted to the single-channel autoanalyzer and SMA 12/60. Clin. Chem. *19*:253, 1973.

Mitchell, T., and Rydalch, V.: An evaluation of a true glucose procedure utilizing the enzyme hexokinase. Amer. J. Clin. Path. *50*:401, 1968.

Moore, C. V.: Iron nutrition and requirements. Scand. J. Haemat. (Suppl.), 6:1, 1965.

Moore, C. V.: Hypochromic anemias. *In* Beeson, P. B., and McDermott, W. (eds.): Cecil-Loeb Textbook of Medicine. 12th ed. Philadelphia, W. B. Saunders Company, 1967.

Morgan, E. H.: Transferrin and albumin distribution and turnover in the rat. Amer. J. Physiol. *211*:1486, 1966.

Morgenstern, S., Flor, R. V., Kaufman, J. H., and Klein, B.: The automated determination of serum uric acid. Clin. Chem. *12*:748, 1966.

Morris, J. E.: The transport of uric acid in serum. Amer. J. Med. Sci. 235:43, 1958.

Murayama, M.: The structure of serum albumin. *In* Sunderman, F. W., and Sunderman, F. W., Jr. (eds.): Serum Proteins and the Dysproteinemias. Philadelphia, J. B. Lippincott Co., 1964.

Murphy, W. M., and Deodhar, S. D.: Studies in multiple myeloma. I. Characteristics by immunoglobulin class. Cleveland Clin. Quart. *40*:1, 1973a.

Murphy, W. M., and Deodhar, S. D.: Studies in multiple myeloma. II. Light chains. Cleveland Clin. Quart. *40*:9, 1973b.

Murphy, W. M., Deodhar, S. D., and Battle, J. D., Jr.: Heavy chain disease. Cleveland Clin. Quart. *39*:73, 1972.

Natelson, S.: Techniques of Clinical Chemistry. 3rd ed. Springfield, Illinois, Charles C Thomas, 1971.

Naumann, H. N.: Determination of total serum proteins by refractometry. *In* Sunderman, F. W., and Sunderman, F. W., Jr. (eds.): Serum Proteins and the Dysproteinemias. Philadelphia, J. B. Lippincott Co., 1964.

Neeley, W. E.: Simple automated determination of serum or plasma glucose by a hexokinase/glucose-6-phosphate dehydrogenase method. Clin. Chem. *18*:509, 1972.

Nelson, D. A.: Pure water. Postgrad. Med. (Part I) *30*:A36; (Part II) *30*:A20, 1961.

Neumann, P. Z., and Silverberg, M.: Metabolic pathways of red blood cell copper in normal humans and in Wilson's disease. Nature (London) *213*:775, 1967.

Niejadlik, D. C.: Hydroxyproline. Postgrad. Med. *51*:213, 1972.

Niejadlik, D. C., Dube, A. H., and Adamko, S. M.: Glucose measurements and clinical correlations. J.A.M.A. *224*: 1734, 1973.

Nisonoff, A., Wissler, F. C., and Lipman, L. N.: Properties of the major components of a peptic digest of rabbit antibody. Science *132*:1770, 1960.

Nisonoff, A., Wissler, F. C., Lipman, L. N., and Woernley, D. L.: Separation of univalent fragments from the bivalent rabbit antibody molecule by reduction of disulfide bonds. Arch. Biochem. Biophys. *89*:230, 1960.

Nordin, B. E. C.: Tests for parathyroid function. Postgrad. Med. *35*:A42, 1964.

Norum, K. R., Glomset, J. A., and Gjone, E.: Familial lecithin: cholesterol acyl transferase deficiency. *In* Stanbury, J. B., Wyngaarden, J. B., and Fredrickson, D. S. (eds.): The Metabolic Basis of Inherited Disease. 3rd ed. New York, McGraw-Hill Book Company, 1972.

O'Brien, D., Ibbott, F. A., and Rodgerson, D. O.: Laboratory Manual of Pediatric Micro-biochemical Techniques. 4th ed. New York, Hoeber Medical Division, Harper & Row, 1968.

Olson, A. D., and Hamlin, W. B.: A new method for serum iron and total iron-binding capacity by atomic absorption spectrophotometry. Clin. Chem. *15*:438, 1969.

Osserman, E. F.: Plasma cell dyscrasias. *In* Beeson, P. B., and McDermott, W. (eds.): Cecil-Loeb Textbook of Medicine. 13th ed. Philadelphia, W. B. Saunders Company, 1971.

Ozsoylu, S.: Diagnosis of Wilson's disease. New Eng. J. Med. *284*:1159, 1971.

Palmisano, P. A.: Vitamin D: A reawakening. J.A.M.A. *224*:1526, 1973.

Papadopoulos, N. M., and Kintzios, J. A.: Varieties of human serum lipoprotein pattern: Evaluation by agarose gel electrophoresis. Clin. Chem. *17*:427, 1971.

Parekh, A. C., and Jung, D.: An improved method for determination of total hydroxyproline in urine. Biochem. Med. *4*:446, 1970a.

Parekh, A. C., and Jung, D. H.: Serum inorganic phosphorus determination using p-phenylenediamine as a reducing agent. Clin. Chim. Acta *27*:373, 1970b.

Parfitt, A. M., and Chir, B.: Renal osteodystrophy. Orthoped. Clin. N. Amer. *3*:681, 1972.

Patrick, R. L., and Thiers, R. E.: The direct spectrophotometric determination of protein in cerebrospinal fluid. Clin. Chem. *9*:283, 1963.

Pearson, S., Stern, S., and McGavack, T. M.: A rapid accurate method for the determination of total cholesterol in serum. Anal. Chem. *25*:813, 1953.

Pechet, M. M.: Symposium on thyrocalcitonin. Amer. J. Med. *43*:645, 1967.

Penn, G., and Davis, T.: Clinical immunoelectrophoresis. *In* Cawley, L. P., Penn, G. M., Itano, M., Bell, H. E., and Minard, B.: Basic Electrophoresis, Immunoelectrophoresis and Immunochemistry. Chicago, American Society of Clinical Pathologists, Commission on Continuing Education, 1972.

Peterson, J. I.: Urinary glucose measurement. Clin. Chem. *14*:513, 1968.

Polar, E., and Metcoff, J.: "True" creatinine chromogen determination in serum and urine by semi-automated analyses. Clin. Chem. *11*:763, 1965.

Porter, E. G., and Waters, W. J.: A rapid micromethod for measuring reserve albumin binding capacity in serum from newborn infants with hyperbilirubinemia. J. Lab. Clin. Med. *67*:660, 1966.

Porter, R. R.: The hydrolysis of rabbit γ-globulin and antibodies with crystalline papain. Biochem. J. *73*:119, 1959.

Putnam, F. W. (ed.): The Plasma Proteins. New York, Academic Press, Inc., 1960.

Radin, N.: Cholesterol (primary standard). *In* Meites, S. (ed.): Standard Methods of Clinical Chemistry. Vol. 5. New York, Academic Press, Inc., 1965.

Radin, N.: What is a standard? Clin. Chem. *13*:55, 1967.

Radin, N., and Gramza, A. L.: Standard of purity for cholesterol. Clin. Chem. *9*:121, 1963.

Raisz, L. G.: Physiologic and pharmacologic regulation of bone resorption. New Eng. J. Med. *282*:909, 1970.

Raisz, L. G., Au, W. Y. W., and Simmons, H.: Calcitonin in human serum: Detection by tissue culture bioassay in medullary carcinoma of the thyroid and other disorders. Arch. Intern. Med. *129*:889, 1972.

Rasmussen, H.: Ionic and hormonal control of calcium homeostasis. Amer. J. Med. *50*:567, 1971.

Rasmussen, H., and Tenenhouse, A.: Thyrocalcitonin, osteoporosis and osteolysis. Amer. J. Med. *43*:711, 1967.

Rastegar, A., and Thier, S. O.: The physiologic approach to hyperuricemia. New Eng. J. Med. *286*:470, 1972.

Ravel, R.: Current methods for diagnosing diabetes mellitus. Postgrad. Med. (Part I) *42*:A40; (Part II) *42*:A46, 1967.

Rechnitz, G. A.: Ion-selective electrodes. Chem. Eng. News *45*:146, 1967.

Reinhold, J. G.: Total protein, albumin and globulin. *In* Reiner, M. (ed.): Standard Methods of Clinical Chemistry. Vol. 1. New York, Academic Press, Inc., 1953.

Reveno, W. S., and MacDonald, R. P.: Values for serum α-lipoprotein and cholesterol. Amer. J. Clin. Path. *41*:366, 1964.

Rice, E. W.: Principles and Methods of Clinical Chemistry for Medical Technologists. Springfield, Illinois, Charles C Thomas, 1960.

Richterich, R.: Clinical Chemistry: Theory and Practice. New York, Academic Press, Inc., 1969.

Rosen, B. J., and Tullis, J. L.: Simplified deferoxamine test in normal, diabetic, and iron-overload patients. J.A.M.A. *195*:261, 1966.

Rosen, F. S., and Janeway, A. C.: The gamma globulins. III. The antibody deficiency syndrome (concluded). New Eng. J. Med. *275*:769, 1966.

Rosenfeld, M., and Surgenor, D. M.: The hematin-binding reaction as a basis for serum albumin determination. J. Biol. Chem. *199*:911, 1952.

Sackner, M. A., Avery, W. G., and Sokolowski, J.: Arterial Punctures by Nurses. Chest *59*:97, 1971.

Sandor, G., and Kawerau, E.: Serum Proteins in Health and Disease. London, Chapman and Hall, Ltd., 1966.

Santen, R. J., Willis, P. W., III, and Fajans, S. S.: Atherosclerosis in diabetes mellitus: Correlations with serum lipid levels, adiposity, and serum insulin level. Arch. Intern. Med. *130*:833, 1972.

Sanz, M. C.: Ultramicro methods and standardization of equipment. Clin. Chem. *3*:406, 1957.

Sanz, M. C.: Personal communication, 1966.

Schales, O., and Schales, S. S.: Simple and accurate method for the determination of chloride in biological fluids. J. Biol. Chem. *140*:879, 1941.

Scheinberg, I. H., and Sternlieb, I.: The dual role of the liver in Wilson's disease. Med. Clin. N. Amer. *47*:815, 1963.

Scott, P. J., and Hurley, P. J.: Demonstration of individual variation in constancy of 24-hour urinary creatinine excretion. Clin. Chim. Acta *21*:411, 1968.

Seamonds, B., Towfighi, J., and Arvan, D. A.: Determination of ionized calcium in serum by use of an ion-selective electrode. I. Determination of normal values under physiologic conditions with comments on the effects of food ingestion and hyperventilation. Clin. Chem. *18*:155, 1972.

Searcy, R. L., Low, E. M. Y., and Simms, N. M.: Age, glucose tolerance and insulin. Lancet *1*:1040, 1966.

Sharp, H. L.: Alpha-1-antitrypsin deficiency. Hosp. Pract. *5*:83, 1971.

Sherrick, J. C., and de la Huerga, J.: N-Hydroxynaphthalimide method for calcium in serum. *In* Sunderman, F. W., and Sunderman, F. W., Jr. (eds.): Evaluation of Thyroid and Parathyroid Function. Philadelphia, J. B. Lippincott Co., 1963.

Shinowara, G. Y., and Walters, M. I.: Hematin-studies on protein complexes and determination in human plasma. Amer. J. Clin. Path. *40*:113, 1963.

Skeggs, L. T.: Principles of automatic chemical analysis. *In* Meites, S. (ed.): Standard Methods of Clinical Chemistry. Vol. 5. New York, Academic Press, Inc., 1965.

Skipski, V. P., Peterson, R. F., and Barclay, M.: Quantitative analysis of phospholipids by thin-layer chromatography. Biochem. J. *90*:374, 1964.

Soloni, F. G., and Sardina, L. C.: Colorimetric microdetermination of free fatty acids. Clin. Chem. *19*:419, 1973.
Somogyi, M.: Quantitative relationship between insulin dosage and amount of carbohydrates utilized in diabetic persons. Amer. J. Med. *26*:165, 1959.
Speicher, C. E., Fetrat, M., Fiske, M. L., and Henry, J. B.: The Automatic Clinical Analyzer (ACA): Critical Evaluation. Amer. J. Clin. Path. *57*:643, 1972.
Sperry, W. M., and Schoenheimer, R.: A comparison of serum heparinized plasma and oxalated plasma in regard to cholesterol content. J. Biol. Chem. *110*:655, 1935.
Stahl, E. C. (ed.): Thin-Layer Chromatography: A Laboratory Handbook. 2nd ed. Ashworth, M. R. (tr.). New York, Springer-Verlag, 1969.
Sternlieb, I., and Scheinberg, I. H.: Chronic hepatitis as a first manifestation of Wilson's disease. Ann. Intern. Med. *76*:59, 1972.
Stiehm, E. R., and Fudenberg, H. H.: Clinical and immunologic features of dysgammaglobulinemia type I. Report of a case diagnosed in the first year of life. Amer. J. Med. *40*:805, 1966.
Sullivan, M. J., Lackner, L. H., and Banowsky, L. H. W.: Intraperitoneal extravasation of urine: BUN/serum creatinine disproportion. J.A.M.A. *221*:491, 1972.
Sunderman, F. W., and Sunderman, F. W., Jr.: Serum Proteins and the Dysproteinemias. Philadelphia. J. B. Lippincott Co., 1964.
Sunderman, F. W., and Sunderman, F. W., Jr.: Cholesterol. Proficiency Test Service, July. Philadelphia, Institute for Clinical Science, Inc., 1972a.
Sunderman, F. W., and Sunderman, F. W., Jr.: Total Serum Proteins and Serum Iron. Proficiency Test Service, October. Philadelphia, Institute for Clinical Science, Inc., 1972b.
Sunderman, F. W., and Sunderman, F. W., Jr.: Creatinine. Proficiency Test Service, February. Philadelphia, Institute for Clinical Science, Inc., 1973a.
Sunderman, F. W., and Sunderman, F. W., Jr.: Inorganic Phosphorus. Proficiency Test Service, April. Philadelphia, Institute for Clinical Science, Inc., 1973b.
Sunderman, F. W., and Sunderman, F. W., Jr.: Glucose. Proficiency Test Service, June. Philadelphia, Institute for Clinical Service, Inc., 1973c.
Sunderman, F. W., Sunderman, F. W., Jr., Falvo, E. A., and Kallick, C. J.: Studies of the serum proteins. II, The nitrogen content of purified serum proteins separated by continuous flow electrophoresis. Amer. J. Clin. Path. *30*:112, 1958.
Sunderman, F. W., Jr., and Roszel, N. O.: Measurements of copper in biologic materials by atomic absorption spectrometry. Amer. J. Clin. Path. *48*:286, 1967.
Talke, H., and Schubert, G. E.: Enzymatische Harnstoffbestimmung in Blut und Serum im optischen Test nach WARBURG. Klin. Woch. *43*:174, 1965.
Talmage, R. V., and Munson, P. L. (eds.): Calcium, Parathyroid Hormone and the Calcitonins. Proceedings of the Fourth Parathyroid Conference, 1971. Amsterdam, Excerpta Medica, 1972.
Taylor, C. B., Hass, G. M., Ho, K. J., and Liu, L. B.: Risk factors in the pathogenesis of atherosclerotic heart disease and generalized atherosclerosis. Ann. Clin. Lab. Sci. *2*:239, 1972.
Teloh, H. A.: Flame photometric method for serum calcium and magnesium. *In* Sunderman, F. W., and Sunderman, F. W., Jr. (eds.): Evaluation of Thyroid and Parathyroid Function. Philadelphia, J. B. Lippincott Co., 1963.
Thiers, R. E., Bryan, J., and Oglesby, K.: A multichannel continuous-flow analyzer. Clin. Chem. *12*:120, 1966.
Thiers, R. E., Cole, R. R., and Kirsch, W. J.: Kinetic parameter of continuous flow analysis. Clin. Chem. *13*:451, 1967.
Thiers, R. E., and Oglesby, K. M.: The precision, accuracy and inherent errors of automatic continuous flow methods. Clin. Chem. *10*:246, 1964.
Thiers, R. E., Reed, A. H., and Delander, K.: Origin of the lag phase of continuous flow analysis curves. Clin. Chem. *17*:42, 1971.
Tietz, N. W. (ed.): Fundamentals of Clinical Chemistry. Philadelphia, W. B. Saunders Company, 1970.
Tiselius, A., and Kabat, E. A.: Electrophoresis of immune serum. Science *87*:416, 1938.
Tocci, P. M., Phillips, J., and Sager, R.: The effect of diet upon the excretion of parahydroxyphenylacetic acid and creatinine in man. Clin. Chim. Acta *40*:449, 1972.
Tomasi, T. B., Tan, E. M., Solomon, A., and Prendergast, R. A.: Characteristics of an immune system common to certain external secretions. J. Exp. Med. *121*:101, 1965.
Troxler, R. G.: Personal communication, 1972.
Vanderlinde, R. E.: Why automation in clinical chemistry? Health News *44*:4, 1967.
Van Peenen, H. J., and Files, J. B.: The effect of medication on laboratory test results. Amer. J. Clin. Path. *52*:666, 1969.
VanPilsum, J. F., Martin, R. P., Kito, E., and Hess, J.: Determination of creatine, creatinine, arginine, guanido-acetic acid, guanidine, and methyl guanidine in biological fluids. J. Biol. Chem. *222*:225, 1956.
Wallace, J. M.: Ceruloplasmin. *In* Pre-Workshop Manual, Workshop on Clinical Enzymology. Chicago, American Society of Clinical Pathologists, 1964a.
Wallace, J. M.: Ceruloplasmin. *In* Technical Manual, Workshop on Clinical Enzymology. Chicago, American Society of Clinical Pathologists, 1964b.
Walshe, J. M.: The physiology of copper in man and its relation to Wilson's disease. Brain *90*:149, 1967.
Waters, W. J.: The reserve albumin binding capacity as a criterion for exchange transfusion. J. Pediat. *70*:185, 1967.
Weast, R. C. (ed.): Handbook of Chemistry and Physics. 48th ed. Cleveland, The Chemical Rubber Co., 1965.
Wenk, R. E., Creno, R. J., Loock, V., and Henry, J. B.: Automated micro measurement of glucose by means of O-toluidine. Clin. Chem. *15*:1162, 1969.
Werner, M., Brooks, S. H., and Cohnen, G.: Diagnostic effectiveness of electrophoresis and specific protein assays, evaluated by discriminate analysis. Clin. Chem. *18*:116, 1972.
Werner, M., and Jones, A. L.: Characterization of electrophoretic lipoprotein fractions: Immunochemical and electron microscopic studies. Clin. Chem. *18*:534, 1972.
Westgard, J. O., and Lahmeyer, B. L.: Comparison of results from the Du Pont "ACA" and Technicon "SMA 12/60." Clin. Chem. *18*:340, 1972.
Westlake, G. E., and Bennington, J. L.: Automation and Management in the Clinical Laboratory. Baltimore, University Park Press, 1972.
Whipple, G. H.: The Dynamic Equilibrium of Body Proteins; Hemoglobin, Plasma Proteins, Organs and Tissue Proteins. Springfield, Illinois, Charles C Thomas, 1956.
WHO Memorandum: Classification of hyperlipidemias and hyperlipoproteinemias. Circulation *45*:501, 1972.
Willis, J. B.: The determination of metals in blood serum by atomic absorption spectroscopy. I. Spectrochim. Acta *16*:259, 1960.
Wilson, D. E., Schreibman, P. H., and Arky, R. A.: Postheparin lipolytic activity in diabetic patients with a history of mixed hyperlipemia: Relative rates against artificial substrates and human chylomicrons. Diabetes *18*:562, 1969.
Winsten, S.: Collection and preservation of specimens. *In* Meites, S. (ed.): Standard Methods of Clinical Chemistry. Vol. 5. New York, Academic Press, Inc., 1965.
Wirth, W. A., and Thompson, R. L.: The effect of various conditions and substances on the results of laboratory procedures. Amer. J. Clin. Path. *43*:579, 1965.
Witter, R. F., Kuchmak, M., Williams, J. H., Whitner, V. S., and Winn, C. L.: Lipids of commerical serum products offered as controls or "standards" for cholesterol and triglyceride determinations. Clin. Chem. *16*:743, 1970.
Witter, R. F., and Whitner, V. S.: Determination of serum or plasma triglycerides. *In* Nelson, G. L., and Rouser, G. (eds.): Blood Lipids and Lipoproteins. New York, John Wiley & Sons, Inc., 1972.
Young, D. S., and Gochman, N.: Methods for assuring quality data from continuous flow analyzers. *In* Cooper, G. R. (ed.): Standard Methods of Clinical Chemistry. Vol. 7. New York, Academic Press, Inc., 1972.
Young, D. S., and Hicks, J. M.: Method for the automatic

determination of serum iron. J. Clin. Path. *18*:98, 1965.
Young, D. S., Thomas, D. W., Friedman, R. B., and Pestaner, L. C.: Effects of drugs on clinical laboratory tests. Clin. Chem. *18*:1041, 1972.
Young, P. C., Burnside, C. R., Knowles, H. C., Jr., and Schiff, L.: The effects of intragastric administration of whole blood on the concentration of blood ammonia in patients with liver disease. J. Lab. Clin. Med. *50*:11, 1957.
Yu, T. F., and Gutman, A. B.: Study of the paradoxical effects of salicylate in low, intermediate and high dosage on the renal mechanisms for excretion of urate in man. J. Clin. Invest. *38*:1298, 1959.
Zak, B., Baginski, E. S., Epstein, E., and Weiner, L. M.: Comparisons of sensitivity and specificity of iron chromogens: Measurement of serum iron with a new aqueous color reagent. Ann. Clin. Lab. Sci. *1*:14, 1971.
Zak, B., Epstein, E., and Baginski, E. S.: Review and critique of cholesterol methodology. Ann. Clin. Lab. Sci. *2*:101, 1972.
Zettner, A., and Mansbach, L.: Application of atomic absorption spectrophotometry in the determination of iron in urine. Amer. J. Clin. Path. *44*:517, 1965.
Zettner, A., and Mensch, A. H.: Molar absorptivity of cyanmethemoglobin based on iron analysis by atom in absorption spectroscopy. Presented at the Fifth National Meeting of Society for Applied Spectroscopy. June, 1966.
Zettner, A., and Seligson, D.: Application of atomic absorption spectrophotometry in the determination of calcium in serum. Clin. Chem. *10*:869, 1964.
Zettner, A., Sylvia, L. C., and Capacho-Delgado, L.: The determination of serum iron and iron-binding capacity by atomic absorption spectroscopy. Amer. J. Clin. Path. *45*:533, 1966.
Zlatkis, A., Zak, B., and Boyle, A. J.: A new method for the direct determination of cholesterol. J. Lab. Clin. Med. *41*:486, 1953.

Chapter 10

CLINICAL TOXICOLOGY AND DRUG ASSAYS

by DENNIS L. ALLEN, M.D., and JOHN BERNARD HENRY, M.D.

Until recent years the field of clinical toxicology was a discipline concerned with retrospective investigation into cause of death in cases suspected of having been related to poisoning. The methods available were generally lengthy and consequently offered little to patient care in the acute situation. The multitude of potentially toxic substances now available has complicated the problem of dealing with an unknown poisoning. Techniques are presently available which are rapid, sensitive, and specific enough to play a direct role in patient care.

The majority of poisonings today are a result of accidents or suicidal intent rather than homicide. It is estimated that in the United States and Britain, 5 to 19 per cent of acute medical admissions to city hospitals involve poisoning. The majority of fatal poisonings are due to one or a combination of four agents—barbiturates, carbon monoxide, ethyl alcohol, and salicylates (Loomis, 1968). In the United States accidental poisonings in children account for almost half the fatal accidents in that population.

Recent advances in therapeutic blood level monitoring for drugs have especially benefited patients receiving antiepileptic or cardiac glycoside therapy, thereby preventing toxic side effects.

Recognizing the high incidence of poisoning in the United States, it is incumbent on the clinician to hold a high index of suspicion, particularly when faced with a patient in coma or manifesting other sensorial derangement. The clinician may obtain most rapid confirmation of his impression by furnishing with his request for toxicologic analyses, pertinent information such as level of consciousness, medications for which the patient has been known to have prescriptions, and the suspected drug or drugs involved. This warrants a special toxicology report which may be rapidly submitted to those responsible for the patient's care. In acute poisoning the clinical pathology laboratory can play a meaningful role only when the necessary data can be generated in a few hours or less and when facilities and personnel are available every day around the clock.

For clinical applications whole blood, serum, plasma, and urine are the preferred specimens. The analysis of gastric aspirate may be worthwhile in some circumstances. Urine is used for many screening procedures. The harmfulness or safety of a chemical compound is related primarily to the amount of that compound in the body. For this reason blood, or its fractions, is preferred for quantitative analysis. Rapid qualitative screens serve to rule in or out the presence of potentially toxic substances in body fluids. (See Description of Methods, p. 690.) Quantitative analysis provides information on which a cause and effect relationship between the amount of substance present in body tissues or fluids and the clinical symptoms may be based. It may aid in evaluation of prognosis and perhaps influence the therapeutic approach. The pathologist and attending physician must ensure that appropriate specimen collection is instituted and that the chain of evidence be preserved through identification, seals, and handling. Consult Table 10–1 for recommended specimens for clinical and postmortem investigation.

The modern, well-equipped clinical toxicology laboratory should include thin-layer chromatographic materials, ultraviolet spectrophotometer, gas liquid chromatograph, atomic absorption spectrometer, and radiation counter

Table 10–1. RECOMMENDED SPECIMENS FOR TOXICOLOGIC ANALYSIS*

SPECIMEN	MINIMAL QUANTITY	IDENTIFICATION AND QUANTIFICATION	REMARKS
Blood	Living: 10 ml.	1. All gaseous poisons 2. All volatile poisons 3. Most drugs 4. Sedatives, hypnotics, ataractics 5. Fluoride 6. Lead 7. Hemoglobin derivatives 8. Alcohols 9. Cardiac glycosides 10. Antiepileptics	Particularly indicated for alcohol, barbiturates, carbon monoxide, salicylates, antiepileptics, cardiac glycosides 6. Use lead-free plastic container 7. Use heparinized whole blood
Urine	Drug screen: 50 ml. Heavy metals: 24-hr. urine Deceased: All available	1. Nearly all drugs and poisons 2. Lead 3. Heavy metals 4. Tranquilizers, ataractics, stimulants, narcotics	2. Use lead-free plastic container Particularly indicated for drug screening and quantitation of heavy metals
Gastric contents	Living: Entire aspirate and first 50 cc. lavage Deceased: All available	All ingested substances within 0 to 6 hours after ingestion	Useful only to prove ingestion or to identify poison; cannot establish toxic cause-effect relationship
Brain	1000 gm. (for ethyl alcohol only: 5 gm.)	1. Alcohols, other volatiles 2. Sedatives, hypnotics 3. Narcotics	
Liver	1000 gm.	1. Narcotics 2. Metals 3. Barbiturates 4. Phenothiazines	
Kidney	1 kidney	1. Metals 2. Sulfonamides	Particularly useful in mercury poisoning
Hair and nails	All available	Arsenic Lead	Useful only in chronic arsenic and lead poisoning
Lung	500 gm.	1. All inhaled poisons except carbon monoxide 2. Narcotics (heroin, cocaine)	For proof of entry site
Muscle	500 gm.	1. Heavy metals 2. Carbon monoxide 3. Most other poisons	Useful when internal organs are badly decomposed
Heart blood	5–10 ml. from each atrium	Electrolytes: sodium, potassium, magnesium, chloride	Useful in questionable drownings

*Courtesy of Kurt M. Dubowski, Ph.D., F.A.I.C.

as well as ancillary equipment items, materials, space, and personnel.

This chapter is intended to cover the commonest sources of poisoning for which the effects are dose related. Additional general and specific information may be found in the following references: Bensley and Joron, 1963; Curry, 1969; Deichmann and Gerarde, 1964; Driesbach, 1971; Gleason *et al.*, 1963; Goodman and Gilman, 1965; Kaye, 1970; Loomis, 1968; Meyers, Jawetz, and Goldfein, 1972; Polson and Tattersall, 1969; Stewart and Stolman, 1960; Sunderman and Sunderman, 1970; Sunshine, 1969; Swidler, 1971; Thienes and Haley, 1972, Williams, 1959.

An approach to the "general unknown toxin"

may be found in the American Society of Clinical Pathologists Clinical Toxicology Workshop, Denver, 1972.

ALCOHOLS AND OTHER VOLATILES

Ethanol

Clinical Indications and Correlations. The effect of ethyl alcohol on the central nervous system is similar to that of a general anesthetic, but because of its high solubility in water, the concentration required to produce narcosis is far greater than that usually consumed. In practice, ethanol has only slight effects on the brain. These slight effects, however, assume greater significance, since it is generally agreed that even small amounts of alcohol in blood are sufficient to impair the performance of tasks requiring skill and accuracy. When the performance of the task or tasks, e.g., driving a car, exposes others to risk, the impaired ability becomes a social problem. Because of this, many states have adopted a statutory limit on the amount of alcohol a driver may have in his blood. Thus, for medicolegal purposes, the quantitative determination of ethanol has great practical importance.

In addition to medicolegal purposes, it may be important to determine alcohol concentrations in body fluids in patients presenting with other medical problems, i.e., diabetic coma, central nervous system trauma, coma of unknown cause, or in any case of drug overdose in which symptoms are more profound than expected on the basis of type and quantity of drug present in the body. It should be realized that alcohol need not be ingested to produce toxicity. Fatalities have occurred from breathing alcoholic vapors in distilleries.

The dose of alcohol required to produce a given degree of intoxication or death varies considerably from one case to another. This variable response may be due to the type of alcoholic beverage consumed, the subject's previous experience with alcohol (chronic alcoholics, for example, are often able to tolerate doses which might be fatal in other persons), or the concomitant ingestion of potentiating drugs. In general, however, 75 to 80 gm. of alcohol (150 to 200 ml. of whiskey) will produce definite symptoms, and three times this amount causes stupor in a 70-kg. man (Thienes and Haley, 1972). DuPan, quoted by Moeschlin (1965), established the relationship between blood alcohol content and clinical changes for relatively mild cases, with young persons and persons not habituated to alcohol revealing more severe changes at equal concentrations than chronic alcoholics (shown at the bottom of this page). The fatal dose may vary from 250 to 500 gm. of alcohol (500 to 1000 ml. of whiskey) in an adult.

Metabolism. The action of any drug depends largely upon the concentration that it attains at its site of action. Therefore, the effects of alcohol upon the human body can best be explained if the metabolism of ingested alcohol is understood: absorption, distribution, and elimination (Committee on Medicolegal Problems, 1970).

There are many factors that may affect the rate of alcohol absorption. Among these are the quantity ingested, its concentration in the drink, the nature and quantity of the diluting material in the stomach, and the duration of its presence in the stomach. When ingested in one draught following a light breakfast, the absorption of 60 to 100 ml. of ethanol is usually rapid enough to produce a peak alcohol concentration in the blood in about 30 minutes (Payne *et al.*, 1966). When 150 to 360 ml. of 70-proof spirits were ingested by nine volunteers over a 30- to 60-minute period, the highest concentration of blood alcohol was noted between 8 and 35 minutes from the end of ingestion

CONCENTRATION	INFLUENCE
0.01 to 0.05 per cent (10 to 50 mg./100 ml.)	No influence
0.05 to 0.1 per cent (50 to 100 mg./100 ml.)	Merely influence on stereoscopic vision and dark adaptation
0.1 to 0.15 per cent (100 to 150 mg./100 ml.)	Euphoria, disappearance of inhibitions, prolonged reaction time
0.15 to 0.2 per cent (150 to 200 mg./100 ml.)	Moderately severe poisoning; reaction time greatly prolonged, loss of inhibition and slight disturbances in equilibrium and coordination
0.2 to 0.25 per cent (200 to 250 mg./100 ml.)	Severe degree of poisoning; disturbances in equilibrium and coordination; retardation of the thought processes and clouding of consciousness
0.35 to 0.4 per cent (350 to 400 mg./100 ml.)	Deep, possibly fatal coma

(Payne *et al.*, 1966). By the end of about 1 hour, about 90 per cent of the alcohol had been absorbed; approximately 20 per cent of this was absorbed through the gastric mucosa and the remainder was absorbed at a rapid rate from the small intestine (Thienes and Haley, 1972). Alcohol is one of the few substances absorbed through the stomach.

Because it is readily diffusible, ethanol is rapidly distributed to all the tissues in nearly equal concentration according to their water content. The organs of the body that have the highest water content will have the highest alcohol concentration, while those with the lowest water content will have the lowest alcohol concentration. An equilibrium is established between the alcohol concentration in blood and parenchymatous cells of brain, kidney, or liver after approximately 10 minutes (Moeschlin, 1965). At equilibrium the brain contains slightly more alcohol than the blood; the urine, 1.3 times as much as the blood (Thienes and Haley, 1972). Thus, if the alcohol content of one tissue can be determined, the ethanol content of any tissue can be approximated by direct ratio calculations; in this way, the alcohol content of the brain may be estimated by measuring the alcohol content of blood or urine.

Elimination by metabolism and urinary excretion occurs at about half the rate of absorption (Polson and Tattersall, 1969). Less than 10 per cent of ingested alcohol is eliminated unchanged, in part by the lungs (0.5 to 5.0 per cent) and partly by the kidneys (0.2 to 10.0 per cent) (Moeschlin, 1965). The remainder is burned (oxidized) in the body to CO_2 + H_2O at a rate of about 8 gm. per hour. This rate of elimination varies from person to person, but for any one individual it is reasonably constant. The average 150-pound (68-kg.) man can eliminate approximately one third of an ounce of alcohol per hour.

$$2\ C_2H_5OH + 7\ O_2 \longrightarrow 4\ CO_2 + 6\ H_2O$$

The exact mechanisms for the destruction of alcohol are not completely understood. However, it has been established that acetaldehyde and acetic acid are intermediates in this oxidation. The initial oxidative step occurs primarily in the liver and is dependent upon the enzyme, alcohol dehydrogenase, which converts ethanol quantitatively to acetaldehyde.

$$CH_3CH_2OH + NAD \rightleftarrows CH_3CHO + NADH$$

The conversion of acetaldehyde to acetic acid has also been shown to be catalyzed by the enzyme, acetaldehyde dehydrogenase. This reaction is virtually irreversible.

$$CH_3CHO + H_2O + NAD \longrightarrow CH_3COOH + NADH$$

Subsequently, the reaction presumably enters the metabolic pool of 2-carbon compounds, with CO_2 the final product. The step-by-step reaction may be summarized as shown at the bottom of this page.

Interaction with Other Drugs. Inhibition of drug-metabolizing liver enzymes by ethanol contributes to increased sensitivity to barbiturates. It is also synergistic with meprobamate, phenothiazines, and other central nervous system depressants. Alcohol increases the metabolism of diphenylhydantoin, possibly by stimulation of the hepatic microsomal enzyme system, rendering a standard dose less effective than expected (Swidler, 1971). Antabuse and a number of other substances presumably inhibit the oxidation of ethyl alcohol at the stage of acetaldehyde and promote the accumulation of this toxic substance; the patient thus becomes too ill to continue imbibing after one or two drinks.

Specimen. Studies by Payne and his colleagues (1966, 1968) should be consulted for detailed information regarding choice of specimen for analysis. In general, the systemic effects of alcohol have been best correlated with blood alcohol concentrations, and blood is the preferred specimen for analysis. From their experimental studies in dogs and human volunteers, these authors concluded that venous blood samples collected from a forearm vein give values for blood alcohol concentration not significantly different from arterial samples.

The relationship between the alcohol concentration of the urine and the alcohol content of blood is ordinarily quite constant and therefore affords, with certain precautions, a reliable index for the indirect measurement of blood alcohol concentration.

In practice, the urine alcohol content times the factor 1.32 reflects the alcohol concentration in blood only when the peak urine alcohol concentration has been passed and when the bladder has been emptied within the preceding 30 minutes. Since the urine peak may not be reached for up to three hours after drinking, the application is limited. In practice, at least

$$\underset{\text{Ethanol}}{CH_3CH_2OH} \xrightarrow{(O)} \underset{\text{Acetaldehyde}}{CH_3CHO} \xrightarrow{(O)} \underset{\text{Acetic acid}}{CH_3COOH} \xrightarrow{(O)} \underset{\text{Metabolic pool}}{\text{2-carbon} \rightarrow CO_2}$$

two urine samples are needed, about 30 minutes apart. The first is only a reference point, but, if the alcohol concentration in the second is below that in the first specimen, it may be used to provide substantial corroborative evidence in doubtful cases. If the second sample is higher than the first, it is of less value and may have to be discarded.

Breath analysis for alcohol content is based on the principle that the amount of alcohol in the expired air is representative of the amount in the blood at the time the sample is taken. Breath analysis is frequently employed for law enforcement purposes. Techniques for breath analysis generally tend to underestimate the true blood alcohol concentration (Payne *et al.*, 1966). Furthermore, falsely elevated values may be obtained in some circumstances, i.e., residual alcohol in mouth or if analysis is done following an episode of belching or vomiting.

Arterial, venous, or capillary blood properly collected in a closed system is preferred. Avoidance of contamination of skin, syringe, needle, or container with alcohol is mandatory. Cleansing of the site for vessel puncture should be done with a nonalcoholic solution (preferably green or surgical soap removed with sterile water or aqueous Zephiran). Whole blood with heparin, potassium oxalate, or citrate may be used. Serum or plasma may be used, but values average 1.18 times the whole blood values. Whole blood may be stored in a refrigerator for nine to ten months without significant change.

Methods. Detection and quantitation of ethanol in body fluids has been achieved by three different approaches – dichromate methods, enzymatic (alcohol dehydrogenase) methods, and gas chromatographic methods. Consult the following references for more detailed information: Curry, 1969; Sunderman and Sunderman, 1970; Savory *et al.*, 1968; Bonnichsen and Theorell, 1951; Stiles *et al.*, 1966.

The dichromate method is used in the analysis of last phase breath air, blood, or urine. Quantitation depends on the development of a green color by reduction of dichromate in acid solution by ethanol (see chemical equation). The amount of color development read as O.D. absorbance at 600 nm. is proportional to the concentration of alcohol. The test may be performed with inexpensive equipment. The method is relatively nonspecific in that other alcohols, ketones, and aldehydes also reduce dichromate and produce false positives and falsely elevated concentrations of ethanol. (See Description of Methods.)

Chemical equation for dichromate reaction:

$$\underset{\text{(yellow)}}{2\,K_2Cr_2O_7} + 8\,H_2SO_4 + 3\,C_2H_5OH \longrightarrow \underset{\text{(green)}}{2\,Cr_2(SO_4)_3} + 2\,K_2SO_4 + 3\,CH_3COOH + 11\,H_2O$$

The alcohol dehydrogenase method is simple, accurate, and specific. Other primary and secondary aliphatic alcohols yield false positives to a lesser degree, but methanol, ketones, and aldehydes do not. Ethanol is converted to acetaldehyde by alcohol dehydrogenase (ADH) and NAD, which is correspondingly reduced to NADH. The reaction is driven to the right by removal of acetaldehyde by semicarbazide. The NADH produced is proportional to the total ethanol originally present. The NADH is measured by an increase in O.D. at 340 mμ:

$$CH_3CH_2OH + NAD^+ \text{ (nonabsorbing at 340 m}\mu\text{)} \xrightarrow{ADH} CH_3CHO + NADH \text{ (absorbing at 340 nm.)} + H^+$$

Gas chromatography is the method of choice for rapid, direct, and specific qualitative and quantitative analysis. In comparison to the other methods this involves more expensive and sophisticated instrumentation and specially qualified personnel. The assay may be accomplished by head space analysis (Curry *et al.*, 1962), by simple extraction of blood according to Laessig, or by direct injection of blood onto the column (Baker *et al.*, 1969) (Fig. 10–1).

The presence of volatile substances other than ethanol may be identified and quantitated by gas chromatography.

Interpretation. Because the conversion of blood or urine alcohol levels into quantity consumed is not possible scientifically, legal authorities in many states have established blood concentrations as their most important criteria for determining fitness to drive a motor vehicle (Camps, 1965).

The committees of the National Safety Council and the American Medical Association and the legislatures of several states have in general recognized the following (Turner *et al.*, 1959):

1. Persons having a blood alcohol concentration of 0.05 per cent (50 mg./100 ml.) or less shall be considered not to be under the influence of alcohol.
2. Those having a blood alcohol concentration of 0.150 per cent (150 mg./100 ml.) or more shall be presumed to be under the influence of alcohol.
3. Persons having blood alcohol concentrations between 0.050 per cent (50 mg./100 ml.) and 0.150 per cent (150 mg./100 ml.) may or may not be under the influence, depending on other signs and symptoms of intoxication which may be observed at that time.

Most European countries have set their lower limit of being under the influence of ethanol as 0.100 per cent (100 mg./100 ml.). The Committee on Medical Legal Problems of

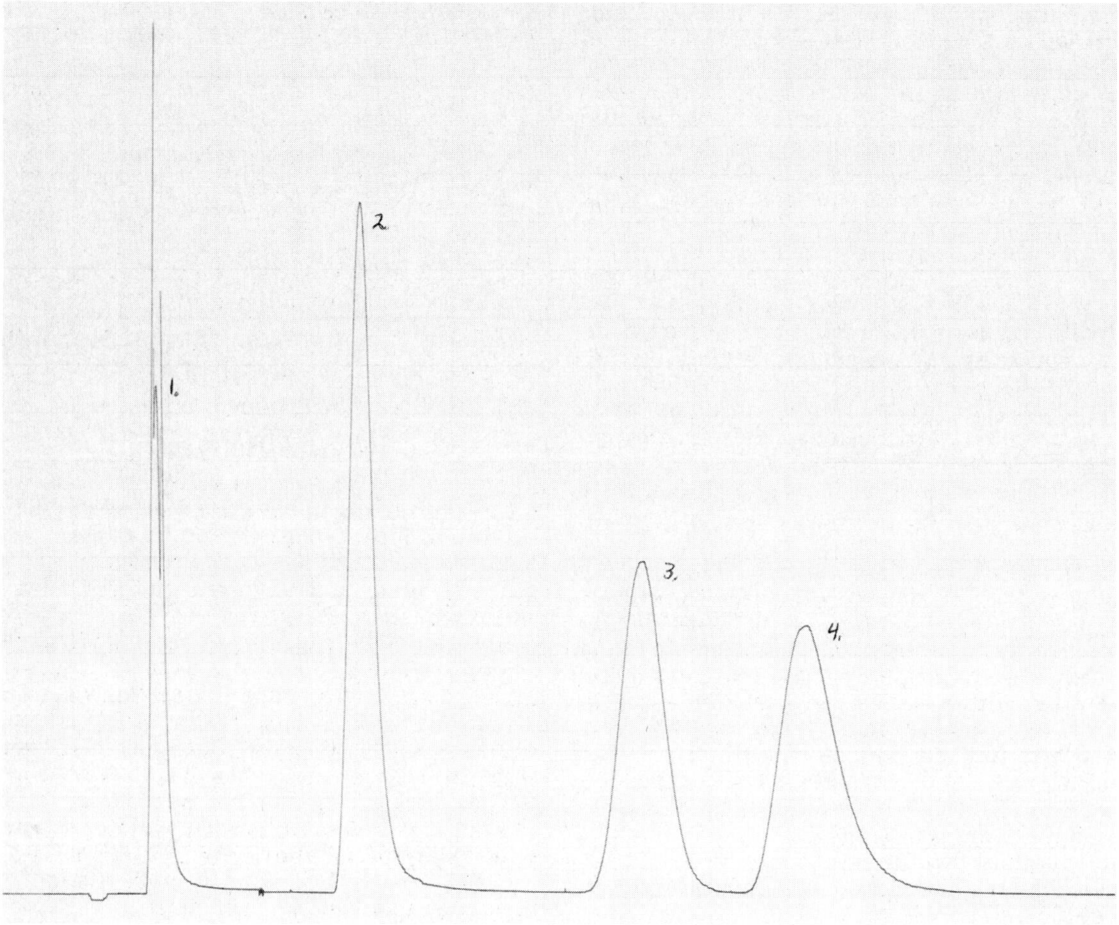

Figure 10–1. Gas chromatogram of 1, methanol; 2, ethanol; 3, acetone; and 4, isopropanol. Six-foot column Porapak Q at 118° C., N_2 flow 60 ml./min. Total time 30 minutes.

The American Medical Association (1960) has modified its original position with adoption of the following policy statement: "Blood alcohol of 0.10 per cent may be accepted as *prima facie* evidence of alcoholic intoxication recognizing that many individuals are under the influence in the 0.05 per cent to 0.10 per cent range" (Hall, 1960; Committee on Medicolegal Problems, 1970).

Methanol

Clinical Indications and Correlations. Methyl alcohol, also called methanol and wood alcohol, is the simplest of the alcohols. It is of interest because accidental poisoning results from its ingestion as a substitute for or as an adulterant of ethyl alcohol (Sunshine, 1961).

Blindness may occur after a single dose or after a series of small nontoxic doses. A fatal dose appears to be between 30 and 100 gm. (Copeman and Venter, 1956). Symptoms of toxicity include drowsiness, photophobia, headache, nausea, vomiting, and blurred vision. Pupils become dilated and poorly reactive. Convulsions and respiratory failure occur as a terminal event. This diagnostic possibility should be investigated in confirmed alcoholics manifesting these symptoms and in any case of severe acidosis unexplained by more common causes.

Metabolism. Following absorption, methanol is widely distributed in the body tissues, with its concentration in cerebrospinal fluid exceeding that in blood. Most is excreted unchanged by the lungs. The remainder is oxidized to formic acid and possibly formaldehyde as an intermediary. The rate of oxidation of methanol is only one-seventh that of ethanol; hence, complete oxidation and excretion of methanol requires several days. Because of its very slow elimination, repeated small doses may accumulate to produce toxic manifestations of insidious onset.

Specimen. Five milliliters of blood with heparin, oxalate, or citrate anticoagulant, serum, or urine may be used.

Methods. A technique employing microdistillation for isolation of methanol followed by oxidation of methanol to formaldehyde and photometric determination of chromotropic acid and formaldehyde reaction product has been reported (Hindberg and Wieth, 1963). Gas chromatography provides the most rapid and specific identification and quantitation (Roeckel and Talbert, 1970). (See Figure 10–1.)

Interpretation. A blood level of 80 mg./100 ml. is regarded as dangerous (Curry, 1969). Levels above 100 mg./100 ml. may warrant dialysis and levels above 400 mg./100 ml. result in anesthetic death (Erlanson *et al.*, 1965).

Other Volatiles

Other volatiles which may be identified and quantitated by gas chromatography include ether, acetaldehyde, acetone, isopropanol, paraldehyde, carbon tetrachloride, ethchlorvynol (Placidyl) (Curry *et al.*, 1962). A rapid colorimetric method for ethchlorvynol in urine and serum has been reported (Frings and Cohen, 1970).

AMPHETAMINES

Clinical Indications and Correlations. Amphetamines are powerful central nervous system stimulants which are chemically related to catecholamines. They have rather limited use in modern medicine but have been used to reduce appetite and produce cerebral stimulation. Known as "uppers" to the drug culture, they have become a commonly abused group of drugs. Symptoms of intoxication proceed from restlessness, agitation, elation, intense but purposeless activity, tachycardia, hyperthermia, and euphoria to hallucinations and panic states followed by exhaustion. The pupils become dilated but reactive. Symptoms may persist as long as five days after large doses (Polson and Tattersall, 1969). Tolerance may occur, and very high daily intakes without apparent ill effects have been reported. Patients in methadone maintenance programs are necessarily screened for abuse of these drugs, which include amphetamine, dextroamphetamine, and methamphetamine. Correlations between toxic blood level and clinical symptoms are not yet available.

Metabolism. About 20 per cent of an ingested dose is excreted unchanged in the urine (Schweitzer and Friedhoff, 1970). Methamphetamine is partially demethylated such that part of it is eliminated as amphetamine in the urine. The rate of excretion is dependent on blood levels and urine pH (Beckett *et al.*, 1969a). Additional details of amphetamine metabolism and elimination are not presently available.

Interaction with Other Drugs. Amphetamines interact with guanethidine and monoamine oxidase inhibitors such that large quantities of norepinephrine are released at nerve endings. This may precipitate a hypertensive crisis.

Specimen. Fifty milliliters of urine or 5 ml. of serum are adequate quantities for analysis.

Methods. Urine may be screened concurrently for the presence of amphetamines and other commonly abused drugs utilizing simple thin-layer chromatographic procedures (Davidow *et al.*, 1968; Dole *et al.*, 1972). (See also Table 10–5.) This is a necessary part of therapeutic monitoring for methadone maintenance programs. Although the method requires a matter of hours to perform, it is especially suited for the processing of multiple specimens efficiently in nonemergency situations.

For purposes of rapid qualitative analysis and the additional information of quantitative results in an emergency situation, gas chromatography is the method of choice (Lebish *et al.*, 1970; Schweitzer and Friedhoff, 1970). If nanogram quantities are present and chromatographic amplification is adequate, urine may be directly applied to the column, thus eliminating any additional specimen processing (Beckett *et al.*, 1967). If sample processing is required, one must avoid subjecting the specimen to heat because these compounds are volatile and significant losses can occur.

Interpretation. Thin-layer chromatographic methods reveal the presence of amphetamines and are sensitive to 0.5 μg./ml., depending on the quantity of urine extracted and the care taken in sample processing. Therapeutic blood levels as measured by gas chromatography are about 0.04 μg./ml. Blood levels in persons abusing amphetamines are at least twice that amount and their urine contains at least ten times the amount found in urine after administration of a single therapeutic dose (Lebish *et al.*, 1970; Schweitzer and Friedhoff, 1970).

ANTIEPILEPTICS

Clinical Indications and Correlations. A variety of drugs are used as antiepileptic agents. Diphenylhydantoin and phenobarbital are most commonly used. In the past, dosage of these drugs was regulated on the basis of giving the drug until signs of toxicity were reached and then decreasing the dose enough to avoid toxicity and hopefully obtain adequate seizure control. However, during the past decade, the value of blood level determinations has been demonstrated by many investigators (Rose, Smith, and Penry, 1971). The recent monograph, *Antiepileptic Drugs*, edited by D. M. Woodbury, J. K. Penry and R. P. Schmidt (1972), is an excellent source.

Common symptoms of diphenylhydantoin toxicity include nystagmus, ataxia, drowsiness, slurring of speech, diplopia, blurred vision, tremors and headache; nausea and vomiting sometimes occur. Deaths are rare. Assays are indicated in patients who show signs and symptoms of intoxication, show unexpected toxicity on multiple drugs, or fail to respond to therapeutic doses of a drug whether secondary to unreliable drug intake or abnormal absorption, metabolism, or excretion.

The presence of ethyl and phenyl groups at the C_5 position of the barbituric acid nucleus confers selective anticonvulsant activity on phenobarbital. Barbiturates depress the activity of nerve, skeletal muscle, smooth muscle, and cardiac muscle (Goodman and Gilman, 1965). They are frequently consumed with suicidal intent. Symptoms of toxicity, metabolism, and methods of assay are discussed in the section on barbiturates.

Metabolism of Diphenylhydantoin. The major metabolite of diphenylhydantoin is 5-(p-hydroxyphenyl)-5-phenylhydantoin (HPPH), which is produced in the liver by hydroxylation by a nonspecific oxidative enzyme system. It is then conjugated with glucuronic acid and excreted in the urine.

The rate of disappearance of diphenylhydantoin is dose dependent (Dayton *et al.*, 1967). Body fat serves as a reservoir for the drug, thus affecting the onset of therapeutic blood levels and the prolongation of therapeutic and toxic effects after discontinuance of the drug. Practically all the drug is eliminated in the urine within 48 hours.

Interaction with Other Drugs. Phenobarbital can significantly lower blood levels of diphenylhydantoin (Dilantin) by induction of liver microsomal enzyme activity; however, this is somewhat compensated for by its own antiepileptic activity. Isoniazid, para-aminosalicylic acid, and dicoumarol depress the metabolism and thus raise serum levels of diphenylhydantoin and may induce symptoms of overdose (Swidler, 1971).

Specimen. Five milliliters of whole blood or serum is adequate for most assay methods. Urine is not recommended for therapeutic monitoring.

Methods. Ultraviolet spectrophotometry has been used to quantify a variety of antiepileptic drugs, including barbiturates and diphenylhydantoin (Huisman, 1966; Bock and Sherwin, 1971). These methods are rapid and require relatively simple equipment; however, they are subject to interference in the patient on several drugs and do not lend themselves to simultaneous assay of more than one anticonvulsant. Thin-layer chromatography has also been used. Gas-liquid chromatography is the method of

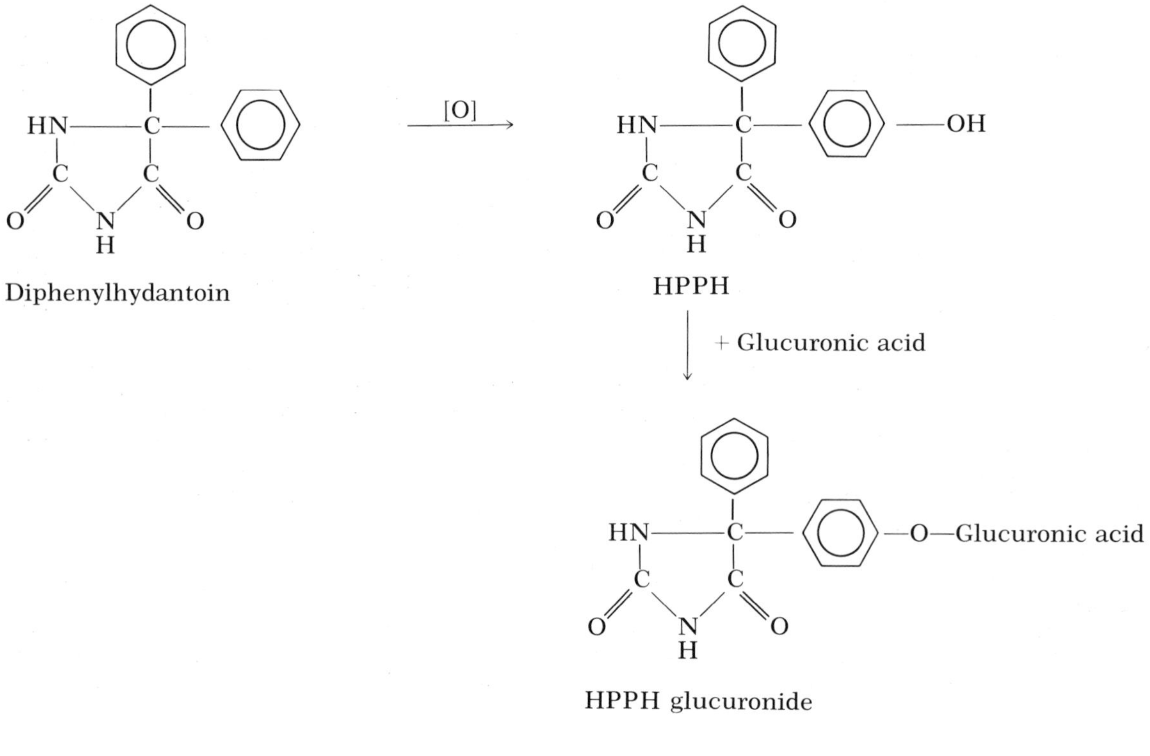

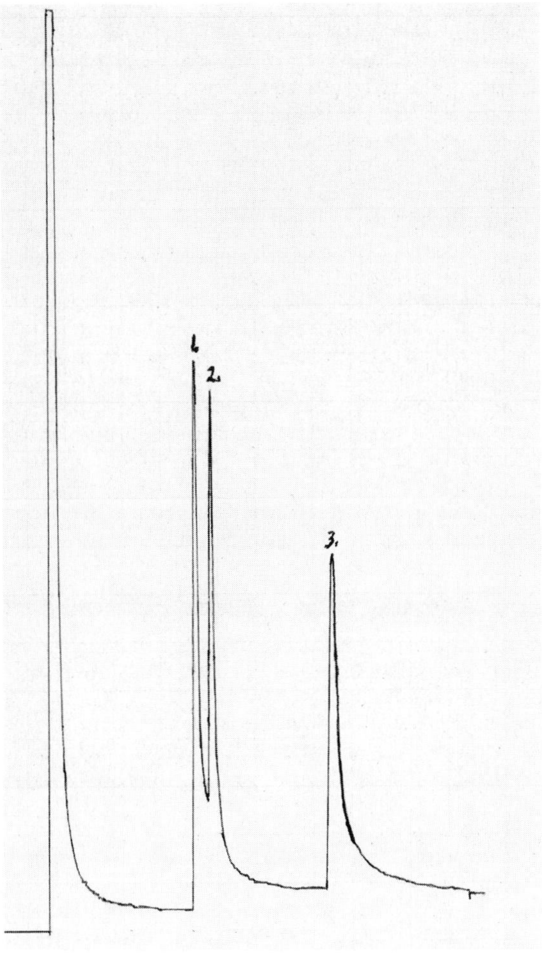

Figure 10–2. Gas chromatogram of 1, phenobarbital; 2, heptabarbital (internal standard); 3, diphenylhydantoin. Six-foot column 3 per cent OV-17 on Gas Chrom. Q at 200 to 277° C. at 15°/minute, N_2 flow 60 ml./min. Total time 8 minutes.

choice when available. Rapid, sensitive, specific, precise assays of single or multiple drugs may be accomplished (Barrett, 1971; Evenson *et al.*, 1970; Sampson *et al.*, 1971; Allen, unpublished) (Fig. 10–2).

Interpretation. Blood levels must be correlated with the clinical findings for each patient (Table 10–2). It is desirable to establish the effective level for the patient and to repeat the assay if seizure activity or symptoms of toxicity appear. Changes may occur on the basis of unreliable drug taking, interaction with other drugs, or a change in metabolism and elimination.

Adequate seizure control for most patients is obtained with diphenylhydantoin levels of 15–20 μg./ml. (Buchthal *et al.*, 1960). Children and patients with generalized major seizures may require higher levels (Melchior, 1965; Friedman *et al.*, 1960; Svensmark and Buchthal, 1964). Diphenylhydantoin has also been used in the treatment of cardiac arrhythmias (ventricular irritability) with levels of 10–18 μg./ml. (Bigger *et al.*, 1966).

Gas chromatographic techniques for the simultaneous analysis of the major anticonvulsant drugs diphenylhydantoin, phenobarbital, primidone, trimethadone, and ethosuximide are also available (Woodbury, Penry, and Schmidt, 1972).

BARBITURATES AND GLUTETHIMIDE

Barbiturates

Clinical Indications and Correlations. Barbiturates are general depressants that probably account for most clinical toxic reactions (both fatal and nonfatal), with the possible exception of carbon monoxide.

The formula of barbituric acid is as follows:

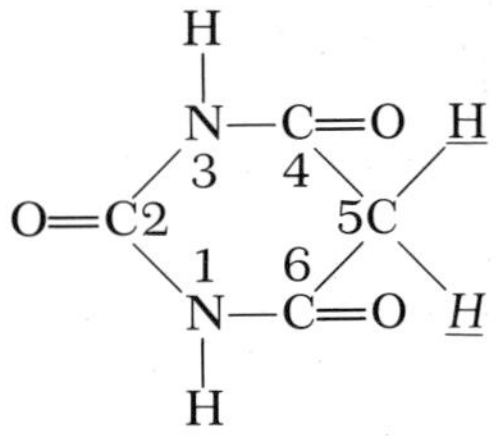

When the two underlined hydrogens are replaced by various radicals, the derivatives formed are referred to as barbiturates. Most barbiturates used clinically have alkyl groups substituted in the barbituric acid nucleus. Other radicals may be substituted, and in certain members, a cyclohexenyl radical replaces hydrogen. Substituents can also be added to one or both of the nitrogens (especially number 3, as a methyl group, in place of a hydrogen). When a sulfur atom replaces the carbonyl oxygen at C_2, an entirely new series of barbiturates results – this barbiturate is in contrast to the oxybarbiturate series. A reactive alkyl group, or a phenyl group at C_5, confers selective anticonvulsant activity on the barbiturate,

Table 10–2. DIPHENYLHYDANTOIN LEVELS CORRELATED WITH CLINICAL SIGNS*

14–20 μg./ml.	Nystagmus on far lateral gaze, usually adequate seizure control
30 μg./ml.	Ataxia
40 μg./ml.	Mental changes, lethargy, inability to concentrate

*Modified from Kutt, H., Winters, W., Kokenge, R., and McDowell, F.: Arch. Neurol. *11*:642–648, 1964.

as is the case with phenobarbital and mephobarbital (Sharpless, 1965).

Symptoms of acute poisoning include various degrees of respiratory depression, hypotension, coma, pupillary contraction, or dilation with poor reactivity, depressed deep tendon reflexes, extensor plantar responses, and may progress to hypothermia, cyanosis, pulmonary edema, apnea, and circulatory collapse. Rapid diagnostic confirmation or exclusion should be available for any suspected case of overdose. Most cases of barbiturate overdose are observed in suicidal patients. However, many cases of "drug automatism" have been reported wherein a confused patient may unwittingly continue to take frequent doses of the drug, resulting in toxic levels (Jansson, 1961). Patients who have high blood alcohol levels associated with barbiturate overdose are especially likely to have a fatal outcome, as are individuals who have also ingested other depressants such as glutethimide, meprobamate, phenothiazines, or methadone. Hence, blood ethanol determination as well as barbiturate analyses and selected tests for the presence of other drugs may be important in some patients.

Patients receiving phenobarbital or mephobarbital for purposes of seizure control may be monitored by following serum levels according to indications listed under antiepileptics.

The barbiturates may be classified on the basis of duration of hypnotic action, which has clinical and therapeutic significance (Table 10–3).

Metabolism. In general, the rate of absorption from the stomach and small intestine parallels the duration of action; the long-acting barbiturates are absorbed slowly, and the short-acting, rapidly. After their absorption from the alimentary tract or after intravenous administration, the barbiturates are found in the blood and throughout all the tissues of the body. The concentration of barbiturates in the tissues depends to a great extent on the concentration in the blood.

Table 10–3. CLASSIFICATION OF SELECTED BARBITURATES ON THE BASIS OF DURATION OF HYPNOTIC ACTION AFTER AVERAGE ORAL DOSE*

Long acting (6 or more hours)
Barbital (Veronal)
Diallylbarbituric acid (Dial)
Mephobarbital (Mebaral)
Phenobarbital (Luminal)
Intermediate acting (3 to 6 hours)
Amobarbital (Amytal)
Butabarbital (Butisol)
Hexethal (Ortal)
Probarbital (Ipral)
Vinbarbital (Delvinal)
Short acting (less than 3 hours)
Cyclobarbital (Phanodorn)
Pentobarbital (Nembutal)
Secobarbital (Seconal)
Ultrashort acting (intravenous anesthetic use)
Hexobarbital (Evipal)
Methohexital (Brevital)
Thiamylal (Surital)
Thiopental (Pentothal)

*Commercial name or synonym is given in parentheses.

Only small quantities of phenobarbital and minimal amounts of barbital are bound to plasma proteins, in contrast to other barbiturates, such as secobarbital, pentobarbital, and thiopental, which may fluctuate in the range of 50 per cent or higher protein-bound form. Binding by tissue proteins appears to parallel that of plasma proteins. The maximum concentration of drug in the tissues is reached a short time after its intravenous administration, and there are usually no great differences between the concentrations of the drug in the tissues and the concentration in the blood. Adipose tissue, however, is an exception to this rule. The maximum concentration of barbiturate is not found in fatty tissues until sometime after its administration, and this maximum may be several times higher than that of the blood. The immediate result of this fixation is the removal of a large proportion of the drug circulating in the blood and the formation of a fat deposit for the drug, from which it is later released.

In general, the short-acting barbiturates have much higher relative concentrations in blood than in body fat; with long-acting barbiturates, the concentrations in blood and adipose tissue are approximately equal.

In summary, the concentration of barbiturates in different tissues depends upon the dose administration, the blood supply to the tissue, the specific chemical and physical affinities of the tissue for the drug, the particular barbiturate administered, and the time of observation.

Complete information concerning the fate of each individual barbiturate in man is not yet known; however, two major pathways can be delineated in eliminating these drugs: (1) destruction in the tissues, and (2) excretion through the kidneys. A few barbiturates are excreted predominantly by the kidney (barbital and phenobarbital); others are destroyed in the body, particularly by the liver (secobarbital and pentobarbital); and still others are partly excreted and partly destroyed. There are several chemical reactions that may be involved in the metabolic fate of barbiturates. These mechanisms include: (1) oxidation of radicals in position 5 with the formation of keto, hydroxy, and carboxy barbituric acids; (2) loss of N-alkyl radicals; (3) desulfuration of thiobarbiturates; and (4) hydrolytic opening of the barbiturate ring.

Table 10–4. PATHWAYS OF ELIMINATION FOR SELECTED BARBITURATES*

Renal excretion primarily	Long acting ↑
Barbital	
Phenobarbital	
Hepatic degradation and renal excretion	
Cyclobarbital	
Diallylbarbituric acid	
Mephobarbital	
Vinbarbital	
Hepatic degradation primarily	
Amobarbital	
Hexethal	
Pentobarbital	
Secobarbital	
Adipose tissue deposition but ultimately hepatic degradation and renal excretion	
Hexobarbital	↓
Thiopental	Short acting

*Toxic levels may result in decreased metabolic degradation or renovascular collapse causing altered pathways of elimination.

In Table 10–4 several of the clinically important barbiturates are classified on the basis of the degree of their elimination, which depends on renal excretion, liver degradation, or both.

Primidone (Mysoline), a commonly used antiepileptic drug, is metabolized partly to phenobarbital, which is believed to be the source of its antiepileptic activity (Butler and Waddell, 1956).

Interactions with Other Drugs. The effects of barbiturate and alcohol are additive in proportion to blood levels. A blood alcohol of half the fatal level reduces the amount of lethal barbiturate by about half. They also react synergistically with other central nervous system depressants, including glutethimide, phenothiazines, meprobamate, methadone, and others (Swidler, 1971).

Specimen. Blood and its fractions, urine, or gastric contents in quantities of 5 ml. may be used for screening purposes. For meaningful quantitative results, 5 ml. of blood or serum is the preferred specimen.

Methods. A simple, sensitive, and rapid qualitative screening may be done on serum, whole blood, urine, or gastric contents (Curry, 1969). The test is sensitive to 1 mg. per cent and should be available at any hour for acute situations in which confirmation or exclusion of barbiturate overdose is needed. (See Description of Methods.) A positive reaction also occurs with glutethimide and meprobamate. If a positive reaction occurs, both specific identification of the barbiturate, glutethimide, meprobamate (or combinations) and quantitation should be done.

Thin-layer chromatographic methods are useful for screening of multiple specimens in nonemergency situations such as therapeutic monitoring in methadone maintenance programs (Schweda, 1967; Davidow *et al.*, 1968; Dole *et al.*, 1972). (See Table 10–5.) They may be used in conjunction with gas chromatographic methods for additional confirmatory evidence. Thin-layer chromatography provides differentiation of short-acting, intermediate-acting, long-acting barbiturates and Doriden and meprobamate.

Quantitative analysis for total barbiturate concentration may be done by Sunshine's method (1961), which is based on the method of Goldbaum (1952). The method is relatively time-consuming and does not indicate specific identification or individual concentrations if more than one drug is present.

Gas-liquid chromatography is the method of choice for rapid, specific, quantitative results. The test should be available at all times if any benefit is to be obtained in terms of patient management. A single analysis may be completed in 30 to 60 minutes. It requires sophisticated equipment and skilled personnel (Thompson and Decker, 1968; Brochmann-Hanssen and Svendsen, 1962; Reid *et al.*, 1970; Allen, unpublished) (Fig. 10–3). It is also the method of choice for therapeutic monitoring of antiepileptic therapy (Rose *et al.*, 1971).

Interpretation. Coma that may be associated with shock may be observed with blood levels ranging from 3 mg./100 ml. whole blood for short-acting barbiturates to 9 mg./100 ml. for long-acting barbiturates in fatal cases (Bernstein, 1966). There is wide individual variation in reaction to blood levels of barbiturates, so concentration alone is not definitive in evaluation of individual patients. Short-acting barbiturates are more potent and more toxic than long-acting barbiturates; however, the short-acting drugs are eliminated faster from the body and the direct effects of the drug may last a matter of hours, whereas the effects of long-acting drugs may persist for days.

Antiepileptic control with phenobarbital has been reported in the 10–40 μg./ml. range (Svensmark and Buchthal, 1964).

Glutethimide

Glutethimide (Doriden) use has increased markedly in the past decade as an alternative drug to barbiturates. Its action is similar to barbiturates, and coma often precedes death from shock in fatal cases of suicidal overdose. Glutethimide absorption is irregular and variable. Since the drug is poorly soluble in water, gastric lavage is valuable in cases of suspected poisoning. It is rapidly taken up by body adipose tissue after absorption and subsequently gradually released into the blood. Blood, body

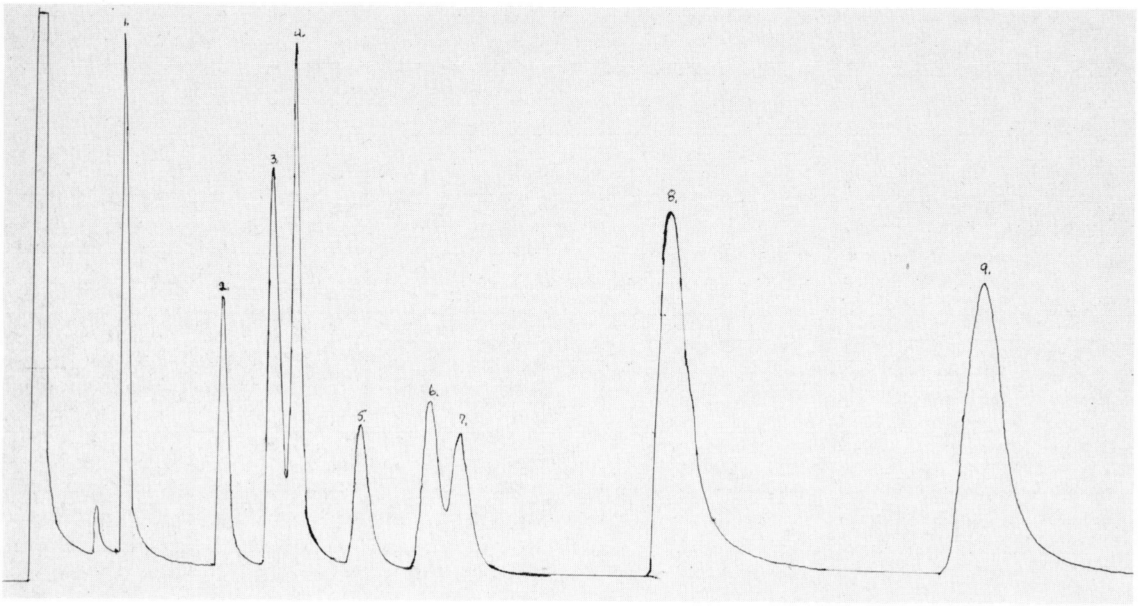

Figure 10–3. Gas chromatogram of 1, barbital; 2, butabarbital; 3, amobarbital; 4, pentabarbital; 5, secobarbital; 6, glutethimide; 7, hexabarbital; 8, phenobarbital; 9, heptabarbital (internal standard). Six-foot column 5 per cent SE-30 on Gas Chrom. Q at 175° C., N_2 flow 50 ml./min. Total time 18 minutes.

fat, and liver are ideal specimens for analysis of glutethimide concentration. Hepatic degradation yields inactive metabolites that are excreted in urine and bile.

With a history of ingestion of as much as 10 gm. or blood levels of 3 mg. per 100 ml., hemodialysis has been recommended by Maher and Schreiner (1965). Since the concentration of drug in body fat is several times that in the blood, there is often an influx of active drug into the blood, with progression of coma after transitory reduction in glutethimide blood levels by hemodialysis.

Because of the relative insolubility of the drug, hemodialysis may not improve prognosis. A lipid dialysate system utilizing soybean oil has been developed and is reported to be effective, nontoxic, inexpensive, and readily available. It has been employed for treatment of glutethimide, secobarbital, pentobarbital, trifluoperazine, and camphor intoxication. There is no unanimity among the experts in this area; indeed, others feel that while lipid dialysis may avoid the solubility limitations, many practical problems are incurred with its use (Ginn et al., 1968).

Özdemir and Tannenberg (1972) indicate that peritoneal dialysis may have a place in early treatment of glutethimide intoxication when used in tandem with hemodialysis.

In contrast to barbiturate intoxication with a small mortality rate, glutethimide intoxication has a high mortality rate. Individual variation in susceptibility and alcohol potentiation are also apparent with glutethimide as with barbiturates. It has thus received even greater clinical importance. Cardiovascular depression is greater than the respiratory depression that precedes death with toxic doses.

The rapid screening test of barbiturates by Curry (see Description of Methods) should be the first step in the confirmation or exclusion of a diagnosis of glutethimide intoxication. A thin-layer chromatographic method may be used for specific identification and semiquantitative analysis of glutethimide (Korzun *et al.*, 1966). A quantitative spectrophotometric method has been reported (Rieder and Zervas, 1965). Gas chromatographic methods are preferred for rapid specific identification and quantitation after a preliminary diagnosis of overdose has been made either by history and physical or by the above screen (Thompson and Decker, 1968; Allen, unpublished). (See Figure 10–3.)

BROMIDES

The alkaline salts of bromine, especially sodium, may exist in a variety of proprietary mixtures (for example, Bromo-Seltzer) but appear to be less frequently used with the increasing availability of other hypnotic agents and sedatives. Although fatalities may occur with accidental ingestion by children, they are rare, and chronic toxicity is more likely to be encountered. Bromides displace chlorides from body fluids and cells to produce central nervous system depression. Although bromide excretion is initially rapid, it subsequently proceeds at a slow rate, so that a cumulative effect may be noted. Complete excretion may even require as long as three weeks after cessation of bromide ingestion. Alcoholics appear to be especially susceptible to bromide intoxication. The response to bromide varies in individuals; however, in general, concentrations between 100 mg. and 200 mg. per 100 ml. of serum are associated with toxic manifestations.

In addition to suspected cases of bromide intoxication, serum bromide measurements are useful in patients with delirium and organic neurologic manifestations, since these patients often have bromide intoxication.

Bromide concentration of Bromo-Seltzer and Sleep-eze were recently redefined by Serpe (1972) in his interesting report of a case of bromism.

Method. A protein-free filtrate of serum or plasma is most commonly reacted with gold chloride to form a brown-red orange color that is proportional to bromide concentration. With the exception of iodides, the method is specific for bromides. Coprecipitation of bromide with protein precipitant varies with protein and bromide concentration of serum specimen. Chloride methods often reflect bromide as well as chloride present in a biologic fluid, so an appropriate correction in chloride measurement for bromide content should be made.

CARDIAC GLYCOSIDES

Clinical Indications and Correlations. The digitalis glycosides, of which there are several, have a powerful effect on increasing the force of myocardial contraction in the decompensating heart. They are most frequently used in the treatment of congestive heart failure. Although they are highly specific and effective in their activity, their toxic-therapeutic ratio is among the lowest of any drug. Consequently, toxicity secondary to digitalis glycosides occurs in about 7 to 20 per cent of hospitalized patients, and the mortality rate among toxic patients is very high at about 44 per cent (Sodeman, 1965; Rodensky and Wasserman, 1961; Beller *et al.*, 1970). Symptoms of toxicity include anorexia, nausea, vomiting, diarrhea, visual disturbances characterized by blurred vision and by objects appearing green or yellow, and cardiac effects which may be manifest in a variety of ways including ventricular extrasystoles, atrioventricular block, paroxysmal atrial tachycardia, ventricular tachycardia, ventricular fibrillation, and others. However, these symptoms may also occur as a result of the underlying disease process, unrelated to drug excess. Therefore, blood levels of these drugs could aid in confirming or excluding the diagnosis of glycoside intoxication. Patients with severe myocardial ischemia, hypoxia, hypokalemia, or poor renal function are especially susceptible to toxicity. The test is also indicated in situations of presumed underdosage, whether on the basis of unreliable drug taking, variable glycoside concentration in particular concentration, or unusually efficient metabolism and elimination.

Several clinical correlative studies with blood levels have been done on the most commonly used cardiac glycosides, digoxin and digitoxin (Jelliffe, 1968; Beller *et al.*, 1971; Smith and Haber, 1971; Chamberlain *et al.*, 1970). The discussion in this section is limited to these two drugs.

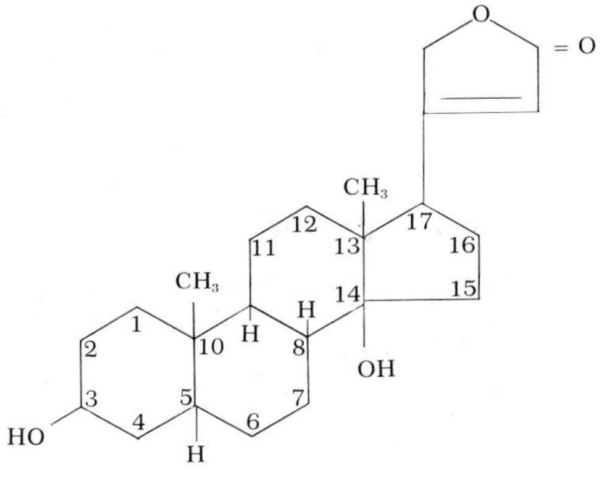

Digitoxin: $C_{18}H_{31}O_9$ at 3 position $(Digitoxose)_3$

Digoxin: $C_{12}H_{31}O_9$ at 3 position $(Digitoxose)_3$ OH at 12 position.

Basic nucleus of cardiac glycosides

Metabolism. Approximately 90 per cent of an oral dose of digoxin and all of digitoxin is absorbed in the intestinal tract within two hours. They are significantly bound to plasma albumin, heart muscle, skeletal muscle, and liver. Digitoxin is metabolized chiefly in the liver to several products—one of which is digoxin—which are excreted with a half-life of about five days. Digoxin is excreted by the kidneys unchanged with a half-life of about 1.6 days or longer if renal function is poor (Doherty, 1968).

Interaction with Other Drugs. Hypoxia and abnormalities in acid-base balance predispose to glycoside toxicity. Any drugs which produce potassium depletion such as diuretics and adrenocorticosteroids may precipitate signs of toxicity. Simultaneous administration of reserpine or parenteral calcium may result in arrhythmias (Swidler, 1971).

Specimen. One milliliter of serum or plasma from heparinized or oxalated blood is adequate for most methods. Plasma and serum give identical results (Smith and Haber, 1971).

Methods. Smith and Haber (1970) have critically reviewed several methods for assay of digoxin and digitoxin. To date, radioimmunoassay techniques appear to be the most sensitive, rapid, specific, and reliable and are currently available in kit form.

Separate assays are done for each glycoside. An antibody to the specific glycoside (digoxin or digitoxin) is produced in an animal (rabbit). The antibody is combined with the patient's serum which also contains a known amount of the radioactive-labeled glycoside. Either tritium or radioactive iodine labels are used. Competition between labeled and unlabeled glycoside for the antibody takes place over a finite period of time. The free labeled and unlabeled glycoside is separated from the bound glycoside by adsorption onto another substrate or binder (e.g., dextran-coated charcoal). The glycoside bound to the antibody is then counted in a suitable radiation detector or scintillation counter and the per cent labeled bound glycoside is determined. A calibration curve is prepared with unlabeled glycoside standards, using this procedure. Quantification of unknowns is then determined by the procedure according to the corresponding per cent labeled glycoside on the calibration curve (Oliver *et al.*, 1971; Smith *et al.*, 1969; Smith and Haber, 1971).

Assays may be run within one hour. The results should be generated within 24 hours to be clinically useful.

Interpretation. False positives do not occur. There is no cross reaction with physiologic steroids which have chemical structures similar to digitalis glycosides. When digitoxin antibody is used for serum containing digoxin, some cross reaction does occur and apparent digitoxin levels are extremely small (about one-tenth of the therapeutic range). The clinician, therefore, must be certain to request the specific assay according to the glycoside being administered to the patient.

Most patients on digoxin show evidence of toxicity with levels above 2 ng. per ml., while most patients with levels less than 2 ng. per ml. show no toxicity. Older people and patients with severe coronary artery disease tend to become toxic on lower levels. Infants can tolerate higher blood levels than adults. Patients receiving antiarrhythmic drugs such as quinidine and propranolol tend to tolerate levels over 2 ng. per ml. without toxicity (Smith and Haber, 1971).

No digitoxin level clearly differentiates toxic and nontoxic states. The average levels for nontoxic and toxic patients are 17 ng. per ml. and 34 ng. per ml., respectively, with significant overlap at 26 ng. per ml. (Smith and Haber, 1971).

HALLUCINOGENS

Clinical Indications, Correlations, and Metabolism. Hallucinogenic or psychotogenic drugs have very limited if any medical uses. They have been used primarily by cults of individuals for religious rites or "mind-expanding" experiences. They are commonly derived from plant sources and include psilocybin, peyote, mescaline, and lysergic acid diethylamide (LSD). They produce euphoria, dysphoria, disturbance of time and space sense, extroversion, visual and auditory hyperesthesia, visual hallucinations, mydriasis, facial congestion, asthenia, bradycardia, hyperactive reflexes, vertigo, and tremor. Their direct effects are not characteristically lethal. Fatalities are usually a result of accidents, which occur while the person is under the influence of the drug. The induced psychotic states are sometimes irreversible or may recur as late as three weeks following ingestion (Horowitz, 1969).

The usual oral dose of mescaline is 5 mg./kg. for induction of psychosis. LSD is about 400 times more potent than mescaline, and ingestion of as little as 25 μg. is sufficient to produce psychosis (Goodman and Gilman, 1965).

Little is known about the metabolism of hallucinogens. LSD is rapidly absorbed and concentrated in the liver, with relatively little found in the brain. It is excreted by the liver as 2-oxy-LSD (Axelrod *et al.*, 1957).

Interaction with Other Drugs. The effects of the hallucinogens may be counteracted with phenothiazines. Reserpine exacerbates the symptoms produced by LSD.

Specimen and Methods. Because of the high

potency of LSD, blood levels of the drug in intoxicated patients are generally beyond the sensitivity of readily available qualitative and quantitative techniques. Thin-layer chromatography and fluorimetry have been used for qualitative and quantitative analysis of LSD (Aghajanian and Bing, 1964; Dal Cortivo *et al.*, 1966). However, the toxicology laboratory may be called upon to analyze carrying media (e.g., sugar cubes, blotting paper) for the presence of hallucinogens. A variety of hallucinogens may be identified by the method of Clarke (1967) utilizing paper and thin-layer chromatography. Crystal examination of pure hallucinogenic drugs has also been used in identification (Clarke, 1957).

METALS

Arsenic

Clinical Indications and Correlations. Arsenical intoxication is caused mostly by accidental ingestion of household or garden insecticides containing arsenous oxide, copper acetoarsenite (Paris green), or calcium or lead arsenate. Toxic amounts of arsenic have also been ingested from the consumption of fruits and vegetables sprayed with arsenic-containing insecticides. Individual susceptibility to arsenical intoxication varies considerably and appears to depend largely upon the amount and duration of exposure. Organic arsenicals release arsenic slowly and therefore are less likely to cause toxicity. Toxicity is attributed to combination of arsenic with tissue sulfhydryl (–SH) groups, especially of enzymes, that ultimately results in cell death.

In acute poisoning, nausea, vomiting, and diarrhea occur suddenly; and in severe cases this may be followed shortly by circulatory collapse or death. Within a few days or weeks, hyperkeratotic lesions of the skin usually develop, along with evidence of peripheral neuropathy and transverse white striae in the fingernails (Mee's lines). Patients with chronic exposure to arsenic may not exhibit the acute gastrointestinal symptoms; the first signs are usually those of peripheral nervous system involvement or nonspecific manifestations, such as fatigue, prostration, muscular weakness, and personality changes (Heyman *et al.*, 1956).

Metabolism. Arsenic can be absorbed by ingestion, inhalation, or through the skin. It is deposited in the liver, spleen, and kidneys. There is also preferential binding to sulfhydryl groups in skin, hair, and nails. The concentration in hair is higher than in any other tissue. It can be detected in the hair in high levels many months after exposure. This depends upon the portion of hair tested, the rate of growth, the quantity of arsenic absorbed, the duration of exposure, and the interval after poisoning. Arsenic provokes vomiting when ingested in sufficient quantities and, via its irritant action on the intestine, is eliminated in vomitus and diarrhea. It is also eliminated unchanged in the urine.

Specimen and Methods. Urine and gastric contents are preferred for qualitative analysis by the Reinsch test. (See Description of Methods.) A 24-hour urine collection is used for quantitative analysis in acute clinical situations. For postmortem investigation, kidney, liver, and hair roots may be analyzed. The Reinsch test should be done first as a preliminary screening which detects arsenic, mercury, bismuth, and antimony. If a positive screen is obtained, the appropriate contact reagent may be applied according to the method of Stolman (1960) for specific identification of arsenic. These tests are sensitive to 0.050 mg. arsenic. Quantitative chemical and spectrophotometric methods may then be used to more clearly document a cause and effect relationship (Leifheit, 1961; Kauffman and Sunderman, 1970). Neutron activation analysis has also been used in quantifying arsenic in tissue (Smith, 1959).

Interpretation. Hair has been found to contain arsenic within 30 hours of ingestion. Normal subjects have shown an average of 0.05 mg. of arsenic per 100 gm. of hair. In chronic poisoning the concentration ranges from 0.1 mg. to 0.5 mg. per 100 gm. of hair, and levels as high as 1 to 3 mg. have been found in acute cases.

Confirmation of absorption of arsenic is usually based on the measurement of 24-hour urinary excretion. Normal persons without known exposure have been found to excrete an average of 0.015 mg. of arsenic per liter of urine, while those ingesting fruit sprayed with arsenic-containing insecticides may have values of 0.05 mg. of arsenic per liter of urine. Because the exact level of urinary arsenic indicative of poisoning cannot be established, a more realistic value of clinical arsenical intoxication is about 0.1 mg. or greater per 24-hour urinary excretion (Leifheit, 1961).

Iron

Acute iron toxicity in children who ingest their mother's iron tablets because the tablets look like candy can be a serious and dramatic medical emergency. It should be suspected in any child with symptoms of abdominal discomfort, vomiting, and diarrhea of black tarry or bloody stools. Iron damages the gastric and intestinal mucosa, causing pain, ulceration, and hemorrhage, which can sometimes be massive. Iron absorbed in a toxic amount causes acidosis and cardiovascular collapse with coma within a short period of time. Lethal doses of ferrous sulfate have varied from 3 to 18 gm., although survival has been reported after doses as high as 15 gm. In about 20 per cent of children who ingest large amounts, death occurs in four to six hours. Those who survive this early period enter a second phase in which improvement occurs, whether spontaneously or in response to treatment. Such improvement may progress to complete recovery, but often this lull in symptoms is disrupted after 18 to 24 hours by a third phase of progressive cardiovascular collapse, convulsions, coma, and often death. Finally, a fourth phase of gastrointestinal obstruction from scarring of the stomach or small intestine as a result of the direct damage of the iron to the mucosa may occur weeks or months after the initial episode of acute intoxication.

The metabolism and methods of analysis of iron are discussed in Chapter 9, Clinical Chemistry. (See also Description of Methods.)

Serum or plasma must be used for analysis because whole blood contains about 50 mg. per 100 ml., most of which is in the red cells. Toxic serum levels are above 600 μg. per 100 ml. (Fischer, 1967).

Lead

Clinical Indications, Correlations, and Metabolism. Lead is present in a number of alloys. Salts of lead (Pb^{++}), such as lead acetate and lead carbonate, are used in ointments; lead sulfate is present in some fabrics. Lead, or some form of lead, is used in many and varied industries, e.g., in paints, storage batteries, solder, ceramics, chinaware (especially in the unglazed), gasoline (as an additive), and insecticides.

Lead, like mercury, combines with the sulfhydryl groups of proteins, including enzymes, to cause cellular death. All forms of lead are dangerous, but they are dangerous in varying degrees, depending on their solubility. Consequently, lead compounds such as basic carbonate and lead subdioxide (PbO_2), being very soluble, are extremely toxic. Compounds such as lead acetate, lead chloride, and lead nitrate are soluble to a lesser extent but are, nevertheless, still toxic. Lead sulfate, chromate, and sulfide are insoluble and therefore theoretically harmless; but they are potentially dangerous, since they may be transformed into soluble forms by the action of gastric juice. (The salt may be converted by the gastric juice to the chloride, which is readily absorbed).

Lead poisoning may be observed in the acute or chronic form. (It is also reviewed in Chapter 4, The Blood.) Most cases of acute poisoning are accidental and seldom homicidal. Acute cases result from the ingestion of large amounts of a soluble salt (acetate or nitrate) or many small doses at intervals. Retention of lead is cumulative, so that a sudden acute attack may occur after a long period of administration. The continued intake of small doses, when released suddenly by the body stores, may give rise abruptly to a type of poisoning similar to that which follows the ingestion of a large amount. Removal of old paint by workers in a closed environment or with minimal ventilation may be responsible for on-the-job lead poisoning. Ingestion of lead-containing paint and plaster by children accounts for many cases.

Although the symptoms of acute poisoning are varied, the patient may complain of a metallic taste, a dry or burning sensation in the throat, cramps, retching, and persistent vomiting; hematemesis and melena may occur.

Most lead poisoning cases are chronic and invariably are incurred accidentally, most frequently from exposure to lead compounds in industry. Lead, after absorption, is carried by the blood to different organs, where it produces a multiform symptomatology. Hence, the signs and symptoms are sundry, e.g., anorexia, loss of weight, abdominal colic, weakness, constipation, icterus, anemia, backache, arthralgia, headache, hypertension, and others, including various neurologic signs. In addition to the above mentioned nonspecific signs and symptoms, there may appear a black lead line on the gums, produced by a deposit of black lead sulfide at the tips of the gum papillae; poor oral hygiene promotes development of this sign.

In most cases a greater proportion of lead is stored in the bones, where it is harmless as long as it remains in combination with the osseous tissue. In children the absorbed lead is deposited near the epiphyseal ends of the bones and may be demonstrated on roentgenograms as a dark zone adjacent to the cartilage. In the adult it is stored in the trabeculae of bone and later deposited in the cortex as the less soluble tertiary phosphate. High serum calcium tends to favor the storage of lead, whereas low calcium tends to release it in the blood. An acid-base shift may alter mobilization and storage relationships. Lead stored in bones is always potentially dangerous, since acidosis may release lead into the circulation in excess and produce symptoms.

Specimen and Methods. Coproporphyrins and delta-aminolevulinic acid elevations are observed with lead poisoning. Coproporphyrins are normal constituents of urine, types I and

III occurring naturally. In lead poisoning there is an increase of the urinary coproporphyrins—principally type III—with a concomitant increase of type I. Porphyrinuria is often the first sign of lead poisoning. (See Description of Methods.)

Other laboratory features are anemia and basophilic stippling of erythrocytes. During the absorption of lead, dark blue granules appear in some of the erythrocytes and produce a stippling. These stippled cells are considered diagnostic, for though they may appear rarely in other conditions, they occur in erythrocytes of those suffering from lead poisoning in large numbers (about 100 in every million red blood corpuscles).

Whole blood is the specimen of choice for quantitative analysis because lead is bound primarily to protein in the erythrocytes. Only heparin should be used, because other anticoagulants such as EDTA chelate the lead, which makes it unavailable for analysis by commonly used methods. Care must be used not to contaminate the specimen. Use lead-free glass containers and process the specimen in a dust-free environment. Urine should also be assayed for lead after EDTA stimulation of the patient to avoid false negative results.

Lead analysis can be performed by atomic absorption spectrophotometry, although dithizone methods are prevalent (Rice *et al.*, 1965). The sample, usually urine or blood, is digested; the alkalinized digest is then extracted with a toluene solution of dithizone. Dithizone reacts with lead, forming a red-colored lead diethizone complex; the intensity is directly proportional to the amount of lead present and is measured spectrophotometrically (Stolman and Stewart, 1960). A rapid urinary lead assay reported by Forman and Garvin (1965) should be valuable for screening individuals exposed to lead. An analysis of lead in hair has also been proposed for screening children exposed to possible lead intoxication (Kopito *et al.*, 1967; Rice *et al.*, 1965; Lubran, 1970).

Interpretation. Lead is regularly present in all the tissues and fluids of the human body. It is a natural constituent of the soil and consequently appears in plant and animal products, so that man ingests traces of lead with his food and drink. The amount of lead found in normal human tissues is small, ranging between 0 and 0.20 mg. of lead per 100 gm. of fresh tissue.

The normal content of lead in urine ranges between 0.01 and 0.15 mg. per day and in whole blood between 0.01 and 0.08 mg. per 100 ml. (Westerman *et al.*, 1965). Most of the blood lead, 50 per cent or more, is found in the erythrocytes.

Chronic lead poisoning coexists with normal blood and urine levels because of deposition in the bones which, during treatment with chelating agents, may be mobilized, resulting in increased levels during treatment.

Lithium

Lithium ion in the carbonate form (Li_2CO_3) is administered as an alternative or supplement to the major tranquilizers in the control of the manic stage of manic-depressive illness. Administered orally, it is well absorbed and distributed throughout the body water. At a therapeutic dosage it has a half-life of 24 hours and is excreted by the kidneys. About 80 per cent of the lithium in the glomerular filtrate is reabsorbed by the tubules and this fraction is not influenced by diuretics. Lithium ion displaces sodium and potassium ions, producing a hyperkalemic-like electrocardiogram, a diabetes insipidus-like diuresis, and a general loss of body sodium and potassium. Lithium has been reported to have teratogenic effects in animals. Consequently, lithium treatment is contraindicated in patients who have cardiac or renal disease and in women who may bear children.

Because of the delay in action, requiring several days after initiation of therapy (average six to ten days elapse before peak effect is reached), patients are given initial doses of 600 mg. of lithium carbonate three times daily for a week so that the same level does not exceed 1.5 mEq. per liter. Maintenance dose subsequently is 300 mg. three times a day to give serum levels of 0.5 to 1.0 mEq. per liter of serum (therapeutic levels).

Side effects are generally mild with a serum lithium level less than 1.5 mEq. per liter. However, when serum lithium exceeds 2 mEq. per liter, acute toxic manifestations such as the following may be noted: transient nausea and fine tremor (mild grade); anorexia, vomiting, diarrhea, thirst and polyuria, tremor, muscle weakness, twitching, sedation, ataxia (moderate grade); chorea, athetosis, confusion, stupor, and convulsions (severe grade); and coma terminally. Irreversible and fatal toxicity is associated with levels from 4 to 6 mEq. per liter. Chronic administration of lithium may lead to the development of a goiter; however, only isolated cases of hypothyroidism have been reported (Luby *et al.*, 1967). Lithium should not be administered to patients without access to a facility providing serum lithium level determinations. Close, regular monitoring of lithium levels in plasma or serum is necessary in any patient receiving lithium carbonate, especially in the elderly, in epileptics, or in those with poor general health, for example, diabetics. Toxicity or disappearance of toxic effects occurs within 24 hours of the effective dose in view of the half-life of 24 hours.

Lithium measurements are performed by either emission spectrophotometry (flame photometry) or atomic absorption spectrophotometry. The latter is preferred and is considered the reference method. If emission spectrophotometry is used, lithium standards should contain approximately normal serum concentrations for sodium, potassium, and calcium since lithium emission is reduced significantly without these other ions. Reduced emission standards tend to produce false elevations of patient lithium values. Indeed, flame photometry has been criticized as a less than ideal methodology for lithium that may undoubtedly be associated with this phenomenon. In addition, since lithium serves as an internal standard in widely used flame photometers, the electrical amplifiers and filters of potassium and lithium must be changed so that potassium is used as the internal standard. This prevents simultaneous measurement of potassium with lithium. Because of these difficulties and the precise, accurate estimations available by atomic absorption spectrophotometry, we recommend this analytical system.

Lithium therapy has notable effects upon other clinical pathology measurements. These vary from a pronounced increase in the leukocyte count, with increased neutrophils in the peripheral smear, to toxic lesions of the bone marrow with a shift to the left of myelopoiesis, erythropoiesis, and thrombopoiesis. Disturbances in mitosis with karyorrhexis of the erythroblasts, clumping of chromosomes, and megaloblastic changes have been reported. Fasting blood glucose increases, though not usually to diabetic proportions. Urinary sodium and potassium tend to increase while serum values are reduced. BUN may rise with acute toxicity and renal failure.

Mercury

Clinical Indications and Correlations. Acute mercurial poisoning may occur following: (1) ingestion of simple salts of mercury, particularly the more soluble salts such as mercuric chloride (corrosive sublimate); (2) the ingestion or injection of complex mercurials, such as the mercurial diuretics; or (3) exposure to simple organic mercurials, such as the methyl and ethyl mercury salts. Classically it is described following the ingestion of mercuric chloride; ingestion is followed by an astringent burning taste, a burning sensation retrosternally, and intense epigastric pain that spreads over the entire abdomen. Vomiting is usually marked and may become hemorrhagic. Edema of the larynx and fauces may occur rapidly, producing asphyxia. The local symptoms, severe at first, usually subside after 24 to 48 hours. Other symptoms that may occur during the first few hours after absorption include excitement, restlessness, disorientation, stupor, and coma. Mercuric chloride is the salt responsible for most of the acute deaths; a minimal lethal dose is about 180 mg.

Chronic mercury poisoning may occur following prolonged exposure to metallic mercury, either as vapor or fine dust, or after continued exposure to mercury salts in low concentration. Industrial contamination of waterways has led to high concentrations of methyl mercury in fish. Methyl mercury is several hundred times more toxic than inorganic alkyl mercury compounds. The biologic half-life in man is about 70 days; therefore, it accumulates and produces symptoms of chronic toxicity (Felton *et al.,* 1972). Fine tremors, initially local, progress to involve all the extremities, head, and trunk. These progress to a coarse tremor and ataxia associated with emotional disturbances. Mercury is found in the urine of all these patients, but the quantity excreted is not related to the severity of symptoms. Mercury excretion continues for months in the absence of further exposure. There is a variation in the content of mercury in the urine, with a rather indefinite association with the severity of the clinical syndrome. All excretion figures are reported as micrograms of mercury, no notice being taken as to the nature of the compound. Thus, after injections of a mercurial diuretic, the urine contains massive quantities of mercury estimated as the metallic mercury, though in fact the patient shows no evidence of mercury poisoning.

In general, mercurous compounds are less lethal than mercuric. Exposure to metallic mercury as a vapor or fine dust may produce chronic mercury poisoning, since metallic mercury vaporizes appreciably at ordinary room temperatures. Hence, the potential danger of insidious poisoning is present in every laboratory in which mercury is used, especially with gasometric analysis. Since ingested metallic mercury (for example, that in thermometers) is not absorbed, it is not toxic.

Metabolism. All dissociable mercurial compounds act by a single basic mechanism—the reaction of the mercury with sulfhydryl groups to form mercaptides with depression of tissue enzymes and cell death. Acute renal tubular necrosis is the most prominent pathologic finding.

Mercury is eliminated primarily by the kidneys at a rate of about 100–300 μg./L., and elimination begins immediately after absorption. It is also eliminated in significant amounts by the large bowel and salivary glands (ptyalism).

Specimen and Methods. The Reinsch test for heavy metal screening detects 0.020 mg. mercury in urine or gastric secretions. Specific qualitative analysis may be done by the method of Stolman (1960). Quantitative analysis may be done by the dithizone method of Gray (1952) or by atomic absorption spectrometry (Willis, 1962). A 24-hour urine must be collected for quantitation because of extremely variable excretion rates.

Interpretation. Normal tissue levels have been reported by Howie and Smith (1967). Urine and blood levels vary considerably in a single patient, and among patients with symptoms. A large study of nonexposed normal patients showed urine concentrations of mercury less than 20 μg. per liter and blood levels less than 3 μg. per liter (Jacobs *et al.*, 1964). Symptoms of mercury toxicity occur with urine excretion of 30 to 100 μg. per day (Rodger and Smith, 1967).

Other metals may give a positive Reinsch test and be specifically identified by the method of Stolman (1960). The substances and sensitivities are as follows: bismuth, 0.010 mg.; antimony, 0.010 mg.; tellurium, 0.050 mg.; sulfur, 0.050 mg. Quantitative methods and clinical correlations are not yet available for these substances.

HEMOGLOBIN DERIVATIVES

Carboxyhemoglobin

Clinical Indications, Correlations, and Metabolism. Carbon monoxide (CO), ordinarily a relatively inert gas, is clinically significant because of its ability to combine with hemoglobin to form carboxyhemoglobin (HbCO) and thereby prevent the normal transport of oxygen. The CO combines with the iron atom of hemoglobin by a bondage similar to that of oxygen (O_2) in oxyhemoglobin (See Chapter 4.) The affinity of hemoglobin for CO, however, is over 200 times as great as for O_2. Therefore, if the concentration of CO in the air is minimal (1/210) compared to that of O_2, the blood will contain, after equilibrium has been established, an equal mixture of oxyhemoglobin and carboxyhemoglobin. Air contains about 20 per cent oxygen. Hence this condition will be reached if the air contains 0.1 per cent CO. The toxic effect of CO is primarily due to oxygen deprivation. Not only is there a diminished amount of hemoglobin that can combine with oxygen, but there is a shift to the left of the oxygen dissociation curve because of the carboxyhemoglobin, so that, at low oxygen tensions, more than a normal amount of oxygen remains combined with the hemoglobin. The anoxia is first reflected in the brain, where it produces headache and throbbing of the temples, followed by syncope, deep coma, respiratory failure, and death. The clinical diagnosis can be made from a history of exposure and from the cherry red discoloration of the nailbeds and mucous membranes. Inadequate ventilation and incomplete combustion in home and automobile heating systems may be responsible. Administration of oxygen represents essential therapy and takes advantage of the law of mass action:

$$HbO_2 + CO \rightleftarrows HbCO + O_2$$

Despite the fact that the reaction is predominantly to the right, a considerable excess of O_2 will drive it to the left.

Specimen and Methods. Five milliliters of heparinized blood, preferably arterial, is used for qualitative and quantitative analysis. The specimen must be assayed within two days for reliable quantitative results. Katayama's test (1888) is simple and rapid and may be used for rapid screening when spectroscopy is unavailable. (See Description of Methods.) It is described in Chapter 4, The Blood. Spectroscopic identification (see absorption pattern, Fig. 10–4) involves less sophisticated instrumentation but is not so satisfactory as a spectral absorption curve of a diluted blood specimen (Stolman and Stewart, 1960). Carboxyhemoglobin and oxyhemoglobin give almost identical absorption spectra (maximum absorption near 535 and 575 nm.). There are two major points of differentiation. Oxyhemoglobin has a greater absorption at 570 nm. and lesser absorption at 535 nm., whereas carboxyhemoglobin is the reverse. With the addition of a reducing agent, oxyhemoglobin is also converted to reduced hemoglobin and the two bands are replaced by one broad band which shifts slightly to the left; however, with carboxyhemoglobin, no such change occurs. Quantitative analysis spectrophotometrically should be performed after identification (Amenta, 1963; Dubowski, 1964). Automated instruments which process specimens and compute results as per cent oxyhemoglobin, per cent carboxyhemoglobin, and total hemoglobin are available (Instrumentation Laboratory, Lexington, Massachusetts). Gas chromatographic methods for qualitative and quantitative analysis have been developed but are generally cumbersome (Rodkey, 1970).

Interpretation. Twenty-five per cent saturation of hemoglobin with carbon monoxide is associated with major symptoms of poisoning. If significant anemia is present, death may occur at lower per cent saturation.

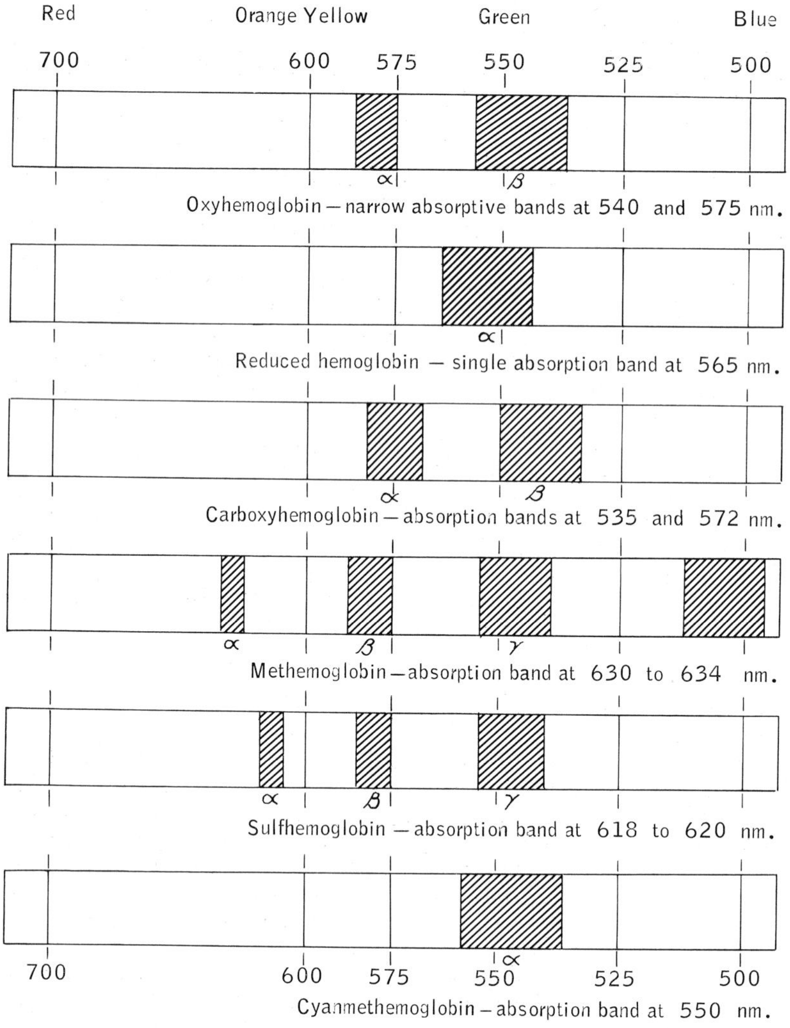

Figure 10–4. Characteristic spectrums of hemoglobin derivatives; absorption maxima in nanometers (nm.) are shown in darkened area.

Cyanmethemoglobin and Cyanide

Clinical Indications, Correlations, and Metabolism. Cyanide poisoning does not produce cyanmethemoglobinemia. Cyanide, even in very small doses, produces histotoxic anoxia by poisoning the cytochrome system and other respiratory enzymes. Cyanosis is absent in cyanide poisoning; cyanosis is produced by an excessive concentration (over 5 gm. per 100 ml.) of reduced hemoglobin. When anoxia is due to cellular intoxication, there is no anoxemia or excessive accumulation of reduced hemoglobin. Cyanide poisoning is produced by inhalation of hydrocyanic acid gas or by ingestion of inorganic cyanides. Laboratory personnel should be alert to potential chemical changes when using cyanide salts in order to prevent formation of hydrocyanic acid. The treatment of cyanide poisoning is to induce the production of cyanmethemoglobin; this diverts the cyanide from its toxic effect on the cellular enzymes. Suicide by ingestion of cyanide or inhalation of hydrocyanic acid is not uncommon in individuals with chemical knowledge.

Specimen and Methods. Five milliliters of heparinized blood is used for spectral analysis. The characteristic absorption pattern is a single band at 550 nm. (See absorption patterns, Fig. 10–4.) Cyanide may be screened for and quantified by the method of Gettler and Goldbaum (1947). Toxicity occurs with whole blood levels above 100 μg./100 ml.

Methemoglobin

Clinical Indications, Correlations, and Metabolism. When the ferrous atom of the hemoglobin molecule is converted to the ferric state, the hemoglobin is converted to methemoglobin. Normally the physiologic methemoglobinemia is continuously resisted by the reducing enzymes associated with the hexose-monophosphate shunt in the erythrocytes. In the rare disease of congenital methemoglobinemia, there is an inborn deficiency of one or more of the reducing enzymes in the erythrocytes, so that instead of having a normal methemoglobin concentration of less than 1.5 per cent of the total hemoglobin, erythrocytes contain from 10 to 40 per cent methemoglobin. The commoner condition of acquired acute methemoglobinemia is caused by ingestion, inhalation, or absorption through the skin of a variety of drugs and inorganic as well as organic nitrites and nitrates; the latter, particularly from drinking well water, is most frequent in infants. Less commonly involved are chlorates, ferricyanide, pyrogallol, sulfonal, and hydrogen peroxide. The oxyhemoglobin is first deoxygenated to form reduced hemoglobin, and this is then oxidized to methemoglobin. A number of compounds which produce methemoglobin are not oxidizing but reducing agents; they produce methemoglobin *in vivo* by unknown mechanism(s), although oxidation may occur initially. The symptoms of methemoglobinemia are due to the diminished oxygen uptake caused by the inactivation of a large proportion of the hemoglobin. Diagnosis is based on the history of exposure to well water or drug ingestion, and the brown cyanosis, which is caused by a combination of brown methemoglobin and bluish red reduced hemoglobin, and on the finding of excessive quantities of methemoglobin in the blood.

Specimen and Methods. Five milliliters of heparinized blood are used. The characteristic absorption maxima are at 535, 575, and 630 nm. (See absorption patterns, Fig. 10–4.) Addition of sodium cyanide abolishes the absorption band at 630 nm. The resulting change in optical density at 630 nm. is directly proportional to the concentration of methemoglobin. Quantitation may be carried out by the method of Dubowski (1964). Refer to Chapter 4, The Blood, for further discussion on interpretation of results.

Sulfhemoglobin

Clinical Indications, Correlations, and Metabolism. Many drugs which produce methemoglobin also produce sulfhemoglobin. Sulfhemoglobin has an unknown structure. Sulfhemoglobin is stable and cannot be reduced to methemoglobin, nor can it be converted *in vivo* to cyanmethemoglobin. Hence, erythrocyte destruction is the only means for removal of sulfhemoglobin. Sulfhemoglobin and methemoglobinemia are seen together in poisoning with sulfanilamide, acetanilide, and sulfonal. The symptoms and findings are similar, but there is no specific treatment for sulfhemoglobinemia. Ascorbic acid and methylene blue or other reducing drugs do not affect its concentration in the blood as they do with methemoglobinemia. Therapy is directed toward methemoglobinemia, while the sulfhemoglobinemia disappears spontaneously.

Specimen and Methods. Five milliliters of heparinized blood may be used for spectroscopic analysis. Sulfhemoglobin has absorption peaks in the 535, 575, and 620 nm. range. Addition of sodium cyanide has no effect on the 620 nm. band as opposed to abolishment of the 630 nm. band of methemoglobin. (See absorption patterns, Fig. 10–4.) The concentration of sulfhemoglobin is proportional to the residual optical density after the methemoglobin has been converted to cyanmethemoglobin by the addition of sodium cyanide. Refer to Chapter 4, The Blood, for interpretation of results.

NARCOTICS

The term narcotic is a legal one defined according to the Federal Narcotic–Internal Revenue Regulations (i.e., Harrison Narcotic Act) as any drug derived from opium or coca, or any of their natural or synthetic derivatives or drugs which have properties similar to those of morphine. The drugs are categorized and regulated according to their addiction liability.

The past decade has seen widespread abuse of these drugs to the extent that it has become a major medical and social problem. The problem manifests itself by an increasing incidence of death secondary to overdose, particularly involving youth, and by an increase in crime which appears to be related to the addict's resorting to any method in order to secure economic means to satisfy his need for the drug, which has become his central, if not only, concern.

Cocaine

Clinical Indications and Correlations. Cocaine is a derivative of coca and classified with the opiates as a narcotic with high addiction liability. It presently has very limited medical use. Its systemic effect is central nervous system stimulation, producing symptoms generally opposite those secondary to opiates. Cocaine is one of the commonly abused narcotics and is taken by intranasal inhalation or hypodermic.

Symptoms of toxicity include excitement, restlessness, garrulousness, anxiety, confusion, hyperreflexia, headache, tachycardia, hyperthermia, mydriasis, nausea, vomiting, abdominal pain, Cheyne-Stokes respiration, and convulsions. Lethal doses produce death rapidly, i.e., within one hour of appearance of symptoms.

Metabolism. Cocaine is absorbed well through the mucous membranes. It is hydrolyzed and deactivated in the gastrointestinal tract. It is rapidly metabolized in the liver, resulting in very little unchanged drug being excreted in the urine.

Opiates

Clinical Indications and Correlations. The most commonly abused opiate is heroin, which has no approved medical use. It is the diacetylated derivative of morphine. Other abused opiates include morphine, codeine, methadone, meperidine, and propoxyphene.

Symptoms of toxicity include various degrees of analgesia, drowsiness, mood changes (usually euphoria, occasionally dysphoria), mental clouding, nausea, vomiting, constipation, miosis (except meperidine which produces mydriasis), respiratory depression, decreased urine output, hypothermia, shock, and coma. Death occurs secondary to respiratory arrest.

Rehabilitation of the narcotic addict has been approached by several methods. One approach which does not solve the problem of physical addiction but does aid in rehabilitation of the addict is methadone maintenance (Dole and Nyswander, 1967). Methadone addiction is preferred under such circumstances for the following reasons: (1) a single dose gives the desired effect (euphoria) lasting 24 hours versus four to six hours for morphine or heroin; (2) absence of extremes of mood between withdrawal symptoms ("sick") and euphoria ("high"); (3) cross tolerance between methadone and heroin such that a patient on methadone receives no added effect from a superimposed dose of heroin; and (4) the desired effect is obtained from an oral dose of methadone, thus eliminating the complications attendant on use of needles. All these factors enable the individual to turn his attention to socially productive activity, which is an integral part of methadone maintenance programs, rather than being constantly concerned with the highs, the lows, and the acquisition of heroin.

Unfortunately the widespread utilization of methadone maintenance has presented secondary problems, including black marketing and increasing illicit use of methadone outside the context of a program of social rehabilitation and an increasing incidence of fatal overdose of children who accidentally ingest it.

Testing of urine specimens from patients is an important part of therapeutic monitoring for methadone maintenance programs. The tests give the following information: (1) confirmation that the patient has taken methadone; (2) the presence or absence of other narcotics; (3) the presence or absence of other abused drugs, including amphetamines and barbiturates, as drug abuse more often than not involves multiple drugs. Obviously quality control of the highest order is a necessity, as the results of such tests may affect an individual's participation in such programs or may be used as evidence in his prosecution.

Metabolism. The opiates are well absorbed parenterally and erratically absorbed from the gastrointestinal tract. Heroin is usually taken by intranasal inhalation ("snorting"), intravenously ("shooting"), or subcutaneously ("skin-popping"). Heroin is rapidly hydrolyzed to 6-monoacetyl-morphine and morphine which is excreted free and conjugated. The others are N-dealkylated and conjugated with glucuronic acid in the liver. Codeine is O-dealkylated to produce morphine to a small extent. The metabolic products and very little of the unchanged drugs are excreted in the urine almost completely within 24 hours (Way and Adler, 1962).

Interactions with Other Drugs. Any sedatives, particularly phenothiazines and barbiturates, enhance the effects of analgesia, respiratory depression, sedation, and hypotension of narcotics.

Quinine

Quinine sulfate, although not a narcotic, is a commonly used diluent for heroin. Its presence in urine may be detected as late as five days following use, whereas heroin and morphine are eliminated generally within two days.

Symptoms of quinine intoxication are nausea, vomiting, headache, deafness, tinnitus, blurred vision, confusion, delirium, convulsions, hypotension, respiratory failure, and cardiac arrest.

It is rapidly metabolized by the liver, yielding several metabolic products detectable in the urine. Its presence in addition to the presence of morphine in urine is strong evidence that the patient has taken heroin diluted with quinine.

Specimens, Methods, and Interpretation

Therapeutic monitoring of patients on methadone maintenance programs is best done by analysis of a randomly collected urine specimen. At least 50 ml. of urine collected under supervision is the preferred specimen. Rapid and specific identification of narcotics for therapeutic monitoring and in diagnosis of overdose is of more practical importance than quantitation. When available, 5 ml. of serum may be submitted for quantitative analysis.

Several spot tests have been developed for qualitative analysis of drugs in relatively pure and concentrated form. They may be used to identify substances in the patient's possession (Carlton and Quittner, 1970).

For therapeutic monitoring in methadone maintenance programs, thin-layer chromatography by the methods of Davidow (1968), Mulé (1969) or Dole *et al.* (1972) have been most widely used. By these methods an experienced technician may identify a variety of commonly abused drugs, including morphine (metabolic product of heroin), amphetamines, barbiturates, codeine, methadone, and phenothiazines.

Following separation in a thin-layer chromatographic developing system, the drugs are specifically identified by their migration on the plate (Rf) and characteristic color obtained with a series of sequential sprays (Table 10–5). A fluorescent indicator incorporated in the TLC plate enables detection of quinine and its metabolites.

Because many specimens may be chromatographed and sprayed on the same TLC plate, the procedure lends itself to efficient processing of multiple specimens, as is required in monitoring a large methadone maintenance program. It is apparent that strict quality control is a necessity.

Although far from ideal, the TLC method is sufficiently rapid (about two hours) that it may be used in the acute overdose situation. Care must be taken not to heat the specimen excessively with resultant loss of amphetamine. Although urine may be hydrolyzed to release greater amounts of conjugated morphine, this treatment also cleaves the O-methyl bond on codeine, resulting in a false positive morphine if codeine should be present.

The use of more than one TLC solvent developing system aids in confirmation of the presence of certain drugs. It is especially helpful in differentiating between methadone and cocaine, which have similar Rf and color reactions by the above methods (Bastos *et al.*, 1970; Jansen and Bickers, 1971).

Sensitive immunoassay techniques for detection of abused drugs are now available. These include the free radical assay technique (FRAT) and the Emit technique (Syva Co., Palo Alto, California) in which the active site of an enzyme is exposed after a drug-antibody interaction. The rate at which the enzyme cleaves a substrate is proportional to drug concentration. These techniques have the following advantages over thin-layer chromatography: (1) no extraction of the urine is required, (2) sensitivity is greater, and (3) sample volume is small. The major disadvantages are: (1) expense, (2) possible antibody cross reactivity, (3) only drugs for which antibodies are available can be detected, and (4) it is a less comprehensive "screen" than TLC.

A radioimmunoassay technique for detection of morphine is also available (Abuscreen™ Radioimmunoassay for Morphine (^{125}I), Roche Diagnostics, Division of Hoffman-LaRoche, Inc., Nutley, New Jersey). This technique

Table 10–5. THIN-LAYER CHROMATOGRAPHIC DATA FOR VARIOUS DRUGS EXTRACTABLE FROM URINE*

	Rf	NINHYDRIN	DIPHENYLCARBAZONE $HgSO_4$	OVEN	ULTRAVIOLET LIGHT	IODOPLATINATE DRAGONDORFF
Cocaine	0.96					OR
Propoxyphene	0.90					O
Glutethimide	0.99		P			
Phenobarbital	0.46		P			
Secobarbital	0.75		P			
Codeine	0.54					RV
Morphine	0.32					DB
Meperidine	0.90					RV
Methadone	0.99					OR
Amphetamine	0.78	P	P	P		
Chlorpromazine	0.96			P		BV
Quinine	0.65				LB	RV

B = blue; D = dark; L = light; P = pink; R = red; O = orange; V = violet.
*From Davidow, B., Petri, N. L., and Quarne, B.: Amer. J. Clin. Path. *50*:714, 1968.

provides the most sensitive detection limits—25 ng. per ml. (Catlin *et al.*, 1973).

Several quantitative methods for opiates have been developed and critically reviewed (Ehrlich-Rogazinsky and Cheronis, 1963; Way and Adler, 1962). A fluorometric assay for morphine has been developed (Kupferberg *et al.*, 1964). Gas-liquid chromatographic methods of analysis for narcotics and related drugs have been developed and are used primarily as confirmatory methods for TLC results. With further development, it may become the method of choice for quantitative analysis (Mulé, 1971).

Limits of detection using 10 ml. urine and the Davidow TLC procedure are as follows: methadone and morphine—5 μg.; barbiturates, glutethimide, amphetamines, phenothiazines—50 μg.; and quinine by fluorescence—1 μg. A positive test for quinine occurs if the patient has ingested tonic water or the cardiac antiarrhythmic quinidine within five days of specimen collection. Clinical correlations with serum levels of narcotics are not presently available.

PHENOTHIAZINES

Clinical Indications and Correlations. A multitude of phenothiazine derivatives are available and have become extremely popular as psychotherapeutic, antiemetic, and antipruritic agents, with variable induction of sedation, hypotension, and depression of motor activity. A classification of examples of these drugs is shown in Table 10–6.

Table 10–6. CLASSIFICATION OF PSYCHOTHERAPEUTIC AGENTS, PHENOTHIAZINE DERIVATIVES, OR NONBARBITURATE SEDATIVES

Chlorpromazine-like
Chlorpromazine (Thorazine)
Promazine (Sparine)
Triflupromazine (Vesprin)
Methoxypromazine (Tentone)
Promethazine (Phenergan)
Trimeprazine (Temaril)
Piperazine group
Prochlorperazine (Compazine)
Trifluoperazine (Stelazine)
Perphenazine (Trilafon)
Piperidine group
Mepazine (Pacatal)
Thioridazine (Mellaril)
Minor tranquilizers
Meprobamate (Equanil, Miltown)
Chlordiazepoxide (Librium)
Diazepam (Valium)
Antidepressant drugs
Imipramine (Tofranil)
Amitriptyline (Elavil)
Phenelzine (Nardil) (monoamine oxidase inhibitor)

The phenothiazines have a high toxic-therapeutic ratio. The most common side effects are hypersensitivity reactions. They have been incriminated as hepatotoxic agents producing characteristic jaundice, abnormal hepatic function tests, and histopathologic changes. Extremely large amounts are needed to produce toxicity in adults; however, toxicity is marked in infants and young adults, and in patients who are febrile and dehydrated. Hollister (1964) has reviewed the adverse effects of phenothiazines. Symptoms of toxicity include dystonia, oculogyrus, torticollis, trismus, facial grimace, athetoid spasms, opisthotonus, frequency of micturition, ptyalism, motor restlessness, difficulty in sitting still, and orthostatic hypotension (Duffy, 1971).

The dibenzasepine antidepressants, imipramine and amitriptyline, have atropine-like side effects, i.e., dry mouth, constipation, dizziness, blurred vision, urinary retention, postural hypotension, and tremors. Cardiac arrest has been related to large overdoses (Williams and Sherter, 1971).

Metabolism. Absorption from the gastrointestinal tract is rapid, with widespread tissue distribution. Hepatic degradation includes demethylation, hydroxylation, formation of sulfoxides, side chain alterations, and conjugation. About half the metabolites are excreted in the urine and the rest in the stool. Metabolites of phenothiazines have been detected in tissues up to 12 months after discontinuing the drug.

Interaction with Other Drugs. The action of alcohol and barbiturates is prolonged by phenothiazines. Other interesting interactions and sequelae are reviewed by Kline and Baer, 1972.

Specimen, Methods, and Interpretation. Rapid qualitative screening for phenothiazines and tricyclic antidepressants may be done on as little as 3 ml. urine. (See Description of Methods.) These tests should be available at all times (Forrest, Forrest and Mason, 1961; Forrest and Forrest, 1960). Phenothiazines may be detected in urine by the thin-layer chromatographic methods for drug screening. (See section on Narcotics.) Total phenothiazine concentration may be quantitated in urine, blood, or tissue by UV spectrophotometry (Wallace and Biggs, 1971). Gas-liquid chromatographic methods have been developed for specific identification and quantitation of a large number of sedatives and tranquilizers (Proelss and Lohmann, 1971) (Fig. 10–5).

Clinical correlations of the various tranquilizers with toxic serum drug levels have not been reported. Therapeutic levels depend on

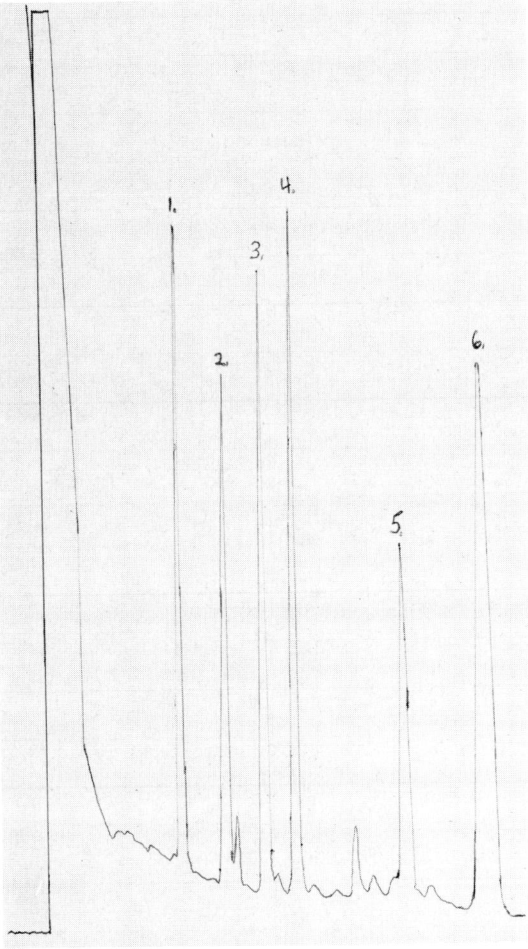

Figure 10–5. Gas chromatogram of 1, Vesprin; 2, Sparine; 3, Thorazine; 4, Stelazine; 5, Compazine; 6, Mellaril. Four-foot column 3 per cent OV-17 on Gas Chrom. Q at 200° to 300° C. at 15°/min., N_2 flow 60 ml./min. Total time 15 minutes.

the specific drug used. In the future, quantitative analysis may be used to monitor therapy with tranquilizers and antidepressants as is now done with antiepileptics.

SALICYLATES

Clinical Indications and Correlations. The availability of salicylates makes this group of drugs the most important cause of accidental poisoning in children. A significant number of attempted suicides in adults are also associated with salicylates.

Salicylate, primarily aspirin, is probably the most prevalent drug in homes. It is an effective analgesic and antipyretic. Salicylic acid is used externally as a keratolytic agent, and methyl salicylate (oil of wintergreen), as a counterirritant, is a common constituent of liniments.

Symptoms of toxicity ("salicylism") include headache, dizziness, tinnitus, deafness, decreased vision, confusion, lassitude, drowsiness, sweating, thirst, nausea, vomiting, and hyperventilation.

Salicylates stimulate the medullary respiratory center, causing increased tidal volume and tachypnea, which produce an initial decrease in carbon dioxide and a respiratory alkalosis (Winters *et al.*, 1959). These effects are potentiated by preexistent fever or dehydration. The respiratory alkalosis is roughly proportional to the dose of salicylate and lags two to four hours behind rising plasma levels.

With continued intoxication, an increased metabolic rate is noted (salicylates uncouple oxidative phosphorylation) and hyperthermia ensues. The PCO_2 tends to rise, but the respiratory loss of CO_2 is so great that the increased production of CO_2 may be unnoticed. Metabolic dysfunction can be recognized by other clinicopathologic reflections, including hyperglycemia, glycosuria, ketosis, and increased lactate and pyruvate levels; such measurements indicate a "salicylate diabetes." Ketosis rarely exceeds 20 mg. acetoacetic acid per 100 ml. serum, contrasted with diabetic ketosis of usually over 50 mg. per 100 ml. Carbohydrate derangement is also reflected in increased hepatic glycogenolysis. Rarely "exhaustion" hypoglycemia may be noted. The end result of the metabolic effects is a metabolic acidosis, which comes about mainly as a consequence of the severe bicarbonate (HCO_3^-) depletion resulting from renal compensation of the initial respiratory alkalosis. In other words, the metabolic effects of salicylate would not produce an acidosis if sufficient bicarbonate were available (Done, 1960). Nevertheless, many children are first seen when they are in metabolic acidosis (Tschetter, 1963).

Frank bleeding caused by salicylates is uncommon. It may be related to local gastrointestinal irritation, capillary damage, reduced platelet aggregation and stickiness, antifibrinogenic action, and decreased utilization of vitamin K by the liver. Bleeding is more apt to occur in chronic toxicity (therapy for rheumatoid arthritis, "aspirin eaters") when salicylism is superimposed on severe liver diseases or peptic ulcer, or in warfarin therapy.

Metabolism. Salicylates are rapidly absorbed from the gastrointestinal tract, with peak tissue and blood levels occurring about two hours after ingestion. Toxic amounts of salicylate and salicylic acid may be absorbed through the skin. Aspirin and methyl salicylate are rapidly hydrolyzed to salicylic acid, the majority of which is bound to plasma proteins. Metabolism occurs in many tissues but primarily in the liver. The unchanged salicylate and metabolic products are excreted by the kidneys with a serum half-life of about 20 hours.

Drug Interactions. Salicylates produce an additive effect with anticoagulants which may result in spontaneous bleeding, primarily from the gastrointestinal tract. Drugs such as acetazolamide, para-aminohippurate, and probenecid compete for tubular transport mechanisms with salicylate and result in sustained blood levels of both drugs.

Specimen, Methods, and Interpretation. Urine may be qualitatively screened for salicylates, which are excreted beginning about 30 minutes after absorption. (See Description of Methods.) This test is extremely sensitive and may be positive after the ingestion of one aspirin tablet (0.3 gm.). If Trinder's reagent (ferric chloride) is used in screening urine, rare false positives may occur after phenacetin ingestion or in ketonuria secondary to diabetes mellitus. Boiling an aliquot of urine eliminates false positives caused by acetoacetic acid in diabetes. Occasional false negatives are noted in markedly acid urine containing large amounts of phosphates. An excess of ferric reagent eliminates this source of error. Salicylates of any kind are excreted for as long as 24 to 48 hours after absorption, depending to some extent upon the dose.

Salicylates may be semiquantitatively determined on 1.0 ml. serum (or plasma) by the ferric chloride method of Trinder as modified by Furman and Finberg (1967). In serum (or plasma) false negative reactions do not occur. Rare false positives may occur in cases of poisoning by phenolic compounds.

More exact concentrations may be determined spectrophotometrically on 0.2 ml. of serum by a ferric nitrate method (Natelson, 1961, p. 372).

Toxicity is associated with plasma salicylate levels of about 30 mg. per 100 ml. (Tschetter, 1963), but severe toxic effects in terms of acid-base imbalance, gastrointestinal irritability, hyperthermia, and ketosis are noted when serum levels reach 50 mg. per 100 ml. Death occurs when 12 to 30 gm. of salicylate are absorbed or with serum levels of 45 to 75 mg. per 100 ml. (Brown *et al.*, 1967).

Older children and adults show good correlation between serum salicylate levels and severity of toxic state, but young children display variable sensitivity to salicylate levels. There may be severe effects that bear no relation to serum salicylate levels unless the interval between the time of ingestion and the determination of the blood level is taken into consideration, as in the nomogram of Done (1960) that is shown in Figure 10–6.

DESCRIPTION OF METHODS*

Barbiturates and Glutethimide (Curry, 1969)

REAGENTS

1. Dithizone in chloroform: 3.75 mg./100 ml. for stock solution and dilute 1:2 with chloroform to give an optical density at 605 nm. (1 cm. cell) of 1. This should be stored at 4° C. and made fresh every two weeks.
2. Mercury Reagents: 0.5 gm. mercuric chloride is dissolved in 50 ml. water with 3 drops concentrated nitric acid. One ml. of this solution is diluted to 50 ml. with water and 0.42 gm. $NaHCO_3$ is added.
3. Phosphate buffer: (M/15, pH 6.95) : 6.24 gm. $Na_2HPO_4 \cdot 2\,H_2O$ and 3.63 gm. KH_2PO_4 are made up to a volume of 1000 ml. with water.
4. Reagent grade chloroform.

PROCEDURE

1. Add 10 ml. chloroform to each of three 100-ml. beakers resting on magnetic stirrers—one labeled patient, one labeled positive, and one labeled negative control.
2. Add 2 ml. of patient sample (serum, blood, urine, gastric washings), positive, and negative controls to respective beakers. Stir vigorously for 2 minutes by magnetic stirring. Allow layers to separate and remove upper layer by suction.
3. Wash each chloroform extract three times with 50 ml. water.
4. Add 1 ml. mercury reagent to each beaker and stir for 2 minutes.
5. Perform two 40 ml. washes with distilled water. After each addition of water, stir vigorously for about 10 seconds. Allow layers to separate and remove aqueous layer by suction.
6. While stirring extract, add 1 ml. dithizone reagent by pipette under the chloroform remaining in the beaker.
7. Observe color immediately. Unchanged green is a negative test while a clear orange color is seen with barbiturates and glutethimide. Meprobamate produces a pink-colored complex.
8. Test is sensitive to 1 mg./100 ml. barbiturate.

Carbon Monoxide. Carbon monoxide imparts a bright cherry red color (carboxyhemoglobin) to blood.

MATERIALS AND REAGENTS

1. Blood containing carbon monoxide, control normal blood.
2. Thirty per cent sodium hydroxide.
3. Test tube and rack, medicine droppers, graduated cylinder.

---

*Several methods courtesy of Sidney Kaye from Kaye, S.: Rapid, simple, reliable tests for poisons. Lab. Med. (5) 3: 28–41, 1972.

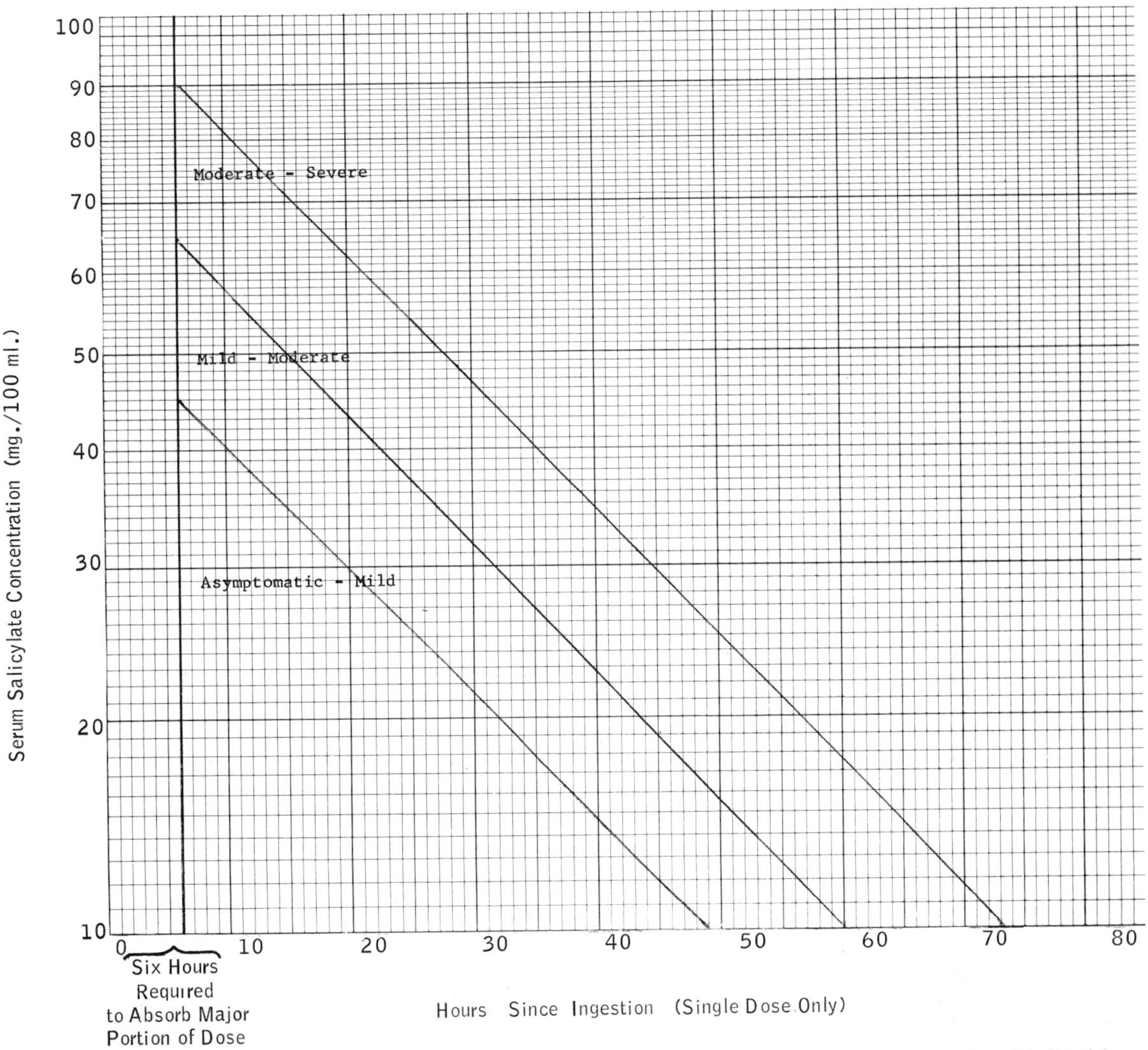

Figure 10–6. Toxicity in children (salicylism) *vs.* serum concentration as related to time since ingestion. (Modified from A. K. Done: Pediatrics 26:800, 1960.)

PROCEDURE

1. Dilute 1 or 2 drops of blood with about 15 ml. of water in a test tube so that the solution is now faint pink. If the pink color is more than faint, add a little more water. This variance depends upon the hemoglobin concentration in the blood.

2. Simultaneously have prepared a positive control, a normal blank, and the unknown specimen; to each one add about 5 drops of 30 per cent sodium hydroxide. Quickly cap with thumb and shake and observe if the original faint pink persists for a while or if it immediately changes to straw yellow.

3. If the blood is negative or contains less than 20 per cent carboxyhemoglobin, the pink color will immediately turn a straw yellow. If the pink color persists for several seconds or more, this indicates the presence of carbon monoxide in excess of 20 per cent. However, even with high (80 per cent) concentration of carbon monoxide, this also (within 60 seconds or so) will eventually turn a straw yellow color.

4. The intensity of the pink color and its persistence before turning yellow will give a rough approximation of the concentration.

5. This test is specific for carboxyhemoglobin; only fetal blood behaves similarly.

6. Evaluation: Below 10 per cent is normal; 10 to 20 per cent is subclinical; 20 per cent and above may be toxic; 40 per cent and above is lethal.

Ethanol. Modification of the microdiffusion technique (Conway-Feldstein-Klendshoj).

PROCEDURE

1. Sealer: 2 ml. of potassium carbonate (saturated) is placed in the small groove of rim of the microdiffusion cell.

2. Reactant: 2 ml. of Ansties reagent is placed in the center chamber. Ansties: Dissolve 3.70 gm. of potassium dichromate c.p. in 150 ml. of distilled water. Add slowly, with constant stirring, 280 ml. of sulfuric acid c.p. Finally dilute to 500 ml. with distilled water.

3. One ml. of blood or urine is spread in the outer chamber.

4. Spread 1 ml. of potassium carbonate (saturated) on top of the blood and quickly seal with the lid.

5. Put the lid in place and gently twist to obtain a liquid seal. Then gently swirl entire unit to mix specimen and liberating agent. Diffusion is started.

6. Allow to diffuse at least 1 hour at room temperature (30° C.).

7. Ethanol standards may be used: 1 ml. of 95 per cent ethanol in 250 ml. of water makes a stock solution.

STOCK SOLUTION		APPROX. GM. PER 100 ML. OF BLOOD	COLOR OF ANSTIES SOLUTION
0.00 ml	0	0.00	yellow-canary
0.25	+	0.08	yellow-yellow-green
0.50	++	0.15	yellow-green
0.75	+++	0.23	yellow-green-green
1.00	++++	0.30 (dangerous)	green
		(above 0.40 is dangerous to life)	blue

8. Terminal blood-alcohol levels may sometimes be low if survival time permitted metabolism and elimination or presence of other depressant drugs acting synergistically.

9. Methanol and isopropanol also give this reaction: 0.05 per cent methanol or 0.22 per cent isopropanol will give readings equivalent to 0.09 per cent using ethanol standards. Differentiation should therefore be made, because treatment is quite different.

Ferrous Sulfate

MATERIALS

1. Stomach contents containing ferrous sulfate; control stomach contents.

2. Ten per cent potassium ferricyanide.

3. Hydrochloric acid.

4. Test tube rack, test tubes, small funnel, filter paper.

PROCEDURE

1. Stomach content is diluted with distilled water to make it just barely fluid. Filter and transfer 5 ml. to a test tube; add 2 drops of hydrochloric acid.

2. To this filtrate add 1 ml. of potassium ferricyanide.

3. The presence of even traces of ferrous sulfate will produce an intense Prussian blue.

NOTE: Ferrous sulfate may change (in part) to ferric sulfate in the body.

Ferrous ion + potassium ferricyanide – intense blue.

Ferric ion + potassium ferrocyanide – intense blue.

Heavy Metals

MATERIALS AND REAGENTS

1. Macerated liver or urine containing heavy metal standards for positive control; and a negative macerated liver or urine for a blank control.

2. Hydrochloric acid (conc.).

3. Ten per cent potassium cyanide.

4. Five per cent sodium sulfite (Na_2SO_3).

5. Fifteen per cent nitric acid.

6. Bismuth test reagent: 1 gm. of quinine sulfate is dissolved in 100 ml. of 0.5 per cent nitric acid; then dissolve 2 gm. potassium iodide into solution.

7. Test tubes and rack, flasks, hot plate or water bath.

8. Copper sheet 5 × 10 mm. or copper wire (spiral).

PROCEDURE

1. Ten ml. of macerated liver or kidney (kidney is best for mercury) or urine, gastric contents, etc., is placed in a small Erlenmeyer flask. At the same time, set up a positive and negative urine for control comparison.

2. Two ml. of concentrated hydrochloric acid and a small copper sheet (5 × 10 mm.) are added. The copper must be shiny clean to show clearly a contrast of a deposition of a heavy metal, when positive. If sheet copper is not available, a small copper wire spiral may be used.

3. Cover the flask with a watch glass and heat gently for about 1 hour; boiling is to be avoided to prevent too rapid evaporation. If large amounts (over 0.100 mg.) are present, deposition will take place in less than 1 hour. In 1 hour deposition will then demonstrate the small traces.

HEAVY METAL	APPEARANCE OF COPPER	SENSITIVITY OF TEST (at least)
Mercury	shiny-silver deposit	0.050 mg./10 ml.
Arsenic	dull black deposit	0.010 mg./10 ml.
Bismuth	shiny black deposit	0.020 mg./10 ml.
Antimony	dark purple sheen	0.020 mg./10 ml.

Report amount present as: Negative, small, moderate, or large

To differentiate the dark deposits from each other:

Mercury: Silver – self-evident

Arsenic: Dull black – place copper in a small test tube and add about 15 drops of 10 per cent potassium cyanide. The dark deposit due to arsenic dissolves; large amounts of arsenic will require more cyanide to dissolve. Antimony or bismuth dark deposit does not dissolve. This test for arsenic is very sensitive; less than 0.010 mg. can be detected.

Bismuth: Shiny black – place the copper and deposit into a small test tube and add about 15 drops of 5 per cent sodium sulfite and 1 ml. of 15 per cent nitric acid. The deposit due to bismuth dissolves. Arsenic or antimony does not dissolve. To the dissolved bismuth solution add 1 ml. of water and 1 ml. of bismuth test reagent – orange turbidity. This test is specific and sensitive to 20 μg. of bismuth.

Bismuth originally takes a little longer to deposit on the copper than the others.

Antimony: Purple shiny deposit – unchanged by both of the above treatments.

Lead

Coproporphyrin III, acid ether – soluble fraction. Five ml. of fresh urine, 10 drops of acetic acid, and 5 drops of hydrogen peroxide (3 per cent) are gently shaken with 5 ml. of ether in a test tube. Allow to separate and discard the urine layer. To the ether add 1 ml. of 1 N hydrochloric acid and observe under ultraviolet light (Wood's filter). Blue (green) fluorescence is normal; pink (red) is positive. Iron-deficiency anemias may also give positive results.

Determination of lead in urine and blood should be made by the dithizone or atomic absorption technique as a follow-up.

Phenothiazine Compounds in Urine (Forrest *et al.*, 1960, 1961). Prochlorperazine (Compazine); perphenazine (Trilafon); thiopropazate (Dartal); trifluoromethylated derivatives (Stelazine and Prolixin); trifluoropromazine (Vesprin); chlorpromazine (Thorazine); promazine (Sparine); or mepazine (Pacatal).

MATERIALS AND REAGENTS

1. Urine containing Thorazine, etc.; control blank urine.
2. Sulfuric acid (conc.).
3. Ferric chloride 10 per cent.
4. Test tubes and rack, medicine dropper.
5. FPN (5 ml. of ferric chloride 5 per cent; 45 ml. of perchloric acid 20 per cent; 50 ml. of nitric acid 50 per cent; all w/v).

PROCEDURE

1. To 2 ml. of urine add 6 drops of sulfuric acid and 2 drops of 10 per cent ferric chloride. A light pink to purple color indicates a positive reaction for a phenothiazine compound. Salicylates do not interfere.
2. One ml. of urine plus 1 ml. of FPN reagent:
   a. Lilac color – chlorinated derivatives
   b. Flesh color – fluorinated derivatives
   c. Blue color – sulfurated derivatives
   d. Orange color – Sparine

NOTE: Color fades rapidly. Ignore color that does not appear in seconds.

3. Remarks:

Order of toxicity of the different derivatives is:

   a. Fluorinated
   b. Chlorinated
   c. Sulfurated

Salicylates

Salicylates: Urine

MATERIALS AND REAGENTS

1. Ten per cent ferric chloride.
2. Test tubes and rack, graduated cylinder.

PROCEDURE. To 3 ml. of urine add 1 ml. of 10 per cent ferric chloride. If salicylate is present, a purple color will appear and persist. This test is very sensitive and is positive in urine after the ingestion of only one 0.3 gm. (5 gr.) aspirin tablet. This test is positive for aspirin, sodium, phenyl, or methyl salicylates, or phenol derivatives.

Paper strip test (Phenistix) may also be used. Whereas a positive test is suggestive, a negative test is certain.

Salicylates: Serum (Natelson, 1961)

REAGENTS

1. Ferric nitrate: 1 per cent in 0.07 N nitric acid.
2. Nitric acid: 0.07 N (4.69 ml. of nitric acid sp. gr. 1.42 and 70.5 per cent; made up to 1 liter).
3. Salicylate standard: 25 mg./100 ml.: 29 mg. of sodium salicylate; or 25 mg. of salicylic acid/100 ml. H_2O.

PROCEDURE

Qualitative. Serum or urine, 0.01 ml., is placed in a small white evaporating dish; then add 1 drop 1 per cent nitrate (in 0.07 N nitric acid). A purple color is positive for salicylates.

Report amount present as: Negative, faint, moderate, or large.

Tricyclic Antidepressant Drugs. To 1 ml. of urine add 1 ml. of the following reagent: 10 ml. each of potassium dichromate (0.2 per cent w/v), sulfuric acid (30 per cent w/v), perchloric acid (20 per cent w/v), and nitric acid (50 per cent w/v).

Green color suggests the presence of imipramine, trimipramine, or desipramine.

REFERENCES

Aghajanian, G. K., and Bing, O. H. L.: Persistence of lysergic acid diethylamide in the plasma of human subjects. Clin. Pharmacol. Ther. 5:611, 1964.

Allen, D.: A rapid qualitative and quantitative analysis of commonly abused barbiturates and glutethimide by gas liquid chromatography. Unpublished, 1971.

Allen, D.: A rapid simultaneous assay of diphenylhydantoin and phenobarbital by gas liquid chromatography. Unpublished, 1972.

Amdisen, A.: Serum lithium determinations for clinical use. Scand. J. Clin. Lab. Invest. *20*:104, 1967.

Amenta, J. S.: The spectrophotometric determination of carbon monoxide in blood. *In* Seligson, D. (ed.): Standard Methods of Clinical Chemistry. Vol. 4. New York, Academic Press, Inc., 1963.

Axelrod, J., Brady, R. O., Witkop, B., and Evarts, E. V.: The distribution and metabolism of lysergic acid diethylamide. Ann. N.Y. Acad. Sci. *66*:435, 1957.

Baker, R. N., Alenty, A. L., and Zack, J. F., Jr.: Simultaneous determination of lower alcohols, acetone, and acetaldehyde in blood by gas chromatography. J. Chrom. Sci. 7:312–319, 1969.

Barrett, M. J.: Determination of serum levels of Dilantin by gas liquid chromatography. Clin. Chem. Newsletter *3*:16, 1971.

Bastos, M. L., Kananen, G. E., Young, R. M., Monforte, J. R., and Sunshine, I.: Detection of basic organic drugs and their metabolites in urine. Clin. Chem. *16*:931, 1970.

Beckett, A. H., Salmon, J. A., and Mitchard, M.: The relation between blood levels and urinary excretion of amphetamine under controlled acidic and under fluctuating urinary pH values, using [^{14}C] amphetamine. J. Pharm. Pharmacol. *21*:251, 1969a.

Beckett, A. H., Tucker, G. T., and Moffat, A. C.: Amphetamine and other stimulants (gas chromatography). *In* Curry, A. S.: Poison Detection in Human Organs. 2nd ed. Springfield, Ill., Charles C Thomas, 1969b, p. 156.

Beckett, A. H., Tucker, G. T., and Moffat, R. C.: Routine detection and identification in urine of stimulants and other drugs some of which may be used to modify performance in sport. J. Pharm. Pharmacol. *19*:273, 1967.

Beller, G. A., Hood, W. B., Jr., Abelmann, W. H., Haber, E., and Smith, T. W.: Digitalis intoxication: A prospective clinical study with serum level correlations. Circulation *42* (Suppl. 3):110, 1970. (Abstract.)

Beller, G. A., Smith, T. W., Abelmann, W. H., Haber, E., and Hood, W. B.: Digitalis intoxication: A prospective clinical study with serum level correlations. New Eng. J. Med. *284*:989, 1971.

Bensley, E. H., and Joron, G. E.: Handbook of Treatment of Acute Poisoning. Baltimore, The Williams & Wilkins Company, 1963.

Bernstein, Z. L.: Treatment of barbiturate coma. New York J. Med. *66*:2290, 1966.

Bigger, J. T., Jr., Schmidt, D. H., and Kutt, H.: The relationship between the antiarrhythmic effect and the plasma level of diphenylhydantoin sodium (Dilantin). Bull. N.Y. Acad. Med. *42*:1039, 1966.

Blijenberg, B. G., and Leijnse, B.: The determination of lithium in serum by atomic absorption spectroscopy and flame emission spectroscopy. Clin. Chim. Acta *19*:97, 1968.

Bock, G. W., and Sherwin, A. L.: The rapid quantitative determination of diphenylhydantoin in plasma, serum, and whole blood of patients with epilepsy. Clin. Chim. Acta *34*:97, 1971.

Bonnichsen, R., and Theorell, H.: An enzymatic method for the microdetermination of ethanol. Scand. J. Clin. Lab. Invest. *3*:58–62, 1951.

Brochmann-Hanssen, E., and Svendsen, A. B.: Separation and identification of barbiturates and some related compounds by means of gas-liquid chromatography. J. Pharm. Sci. *51*:318, 1962.

Brown, S. S., Cameron, J. C., and Matthew, H.: Plasma salicylate levels in acute poisoning in adults. Brit. Med. J. *2*:738, 1967.

Buchthal, F., Svensmark, O., and Schiller, P. J.: Clinical electroencephalographic correlations with serum levels of diphenylhydantoin. Arch. Neurol. *2*:624, 1960.

Butler, T. C., and Waddell, W. J.: Metabolic conversion of primidone (Mysoline) to phenobarbital. Proc. Soc. Exp. Biol. Med. *93*:544, 1956.

Camps, F. E.: Chemical tests for alcoholic intoxication. Practitioner *195*:342, 1965.

Carlton, R. F., and Quittner, H.: Narcotics, dangerous drugs and the clinical laboratory. *In* Sunderman, F. W., and Sunderman, F. W., Jr. (eds.): Laboratory Diagnosis of Diseases Caused by Toxic Agents. St. Louis, Warren H. Green, Inc., 1970, Chapter 23.

Catlin, D., Cleeland, R., and Grunberg, E.: A sensitive, rapid radioimmunoassay for morphine and immunologically related substances in urine and serum. Clin. Chem. *19*:216–220, 1973.

Chamberlain, D. A., White, R. J., Howard, M. R., and Smith, T. W.: Plasma digoxin concentrations in patients with atrial fibrillation. Brit. Med. J. *3*:429, 1970.

Clarke, E. G. C.: The identification of some prescribed psychedelic drugs. For. Sci. Soc. J. 7:46, 1967.

Clarke, E. G. C.: Microchemical identification of some less common alkaloids. J. Pharm. Pharmacol. *9*:187, 1957.

Clinical Toxicology Workshop, American Society of Clinical Pathologists, Denver, Colorado, 1972.

Coleman, A. B., and Alpert, J. J. (eds.): Poisoning in Children. Pediat. Clin. N. Amer. *17*:471–753, 1970.

Committee on Medicolegal Problems, A.M.A.: Alcohol and the Impaired Driver. Chicago, American Medical Association, 1970.

Copeman, P. R., and Venter, J. A.: Poisoning by "alcohol." Particularly methyl alcohol. J. Forensic Med. *31*:131, 1956.

Council on Drugs: Evaluation of lithium carbonate for treatment of manic-depressive psychosis. J.A.M.A. *215*:1486–1488, 1971.

Curry, A. S.: Poison Detection in Human Organs. 2nd ed. Springfield, Ill., Charles C Thomas, 1969.

Curry, A. S., Hurst, G., Kent, N. R., and Powell, H.: Rapid screening of blood samples for volatile poisons by gas chromatography. Nature (London) *195*:603, 1962.

Dal Cortivo, L. A., Broich, J. R., Dihrberg, A., and Newman, B.: Identification and estimation of lysergic acid diethylamide by thin layer chromatography and fluorimetry. Anal. Chem. *38*:1959, 1966.

Davidow, B., Petri, N. L., and Quame, B.: A thin-layer chromatographic screening procedure for detecting drug abuse. Amer. J. Clin. Path. *50*:714, 1968.

Dayton, T. C., Cucinell, S. A., Weiss, M., *et al.*: Dose dependence of drug plasma level decline in dogs. J. Pharmacol. Exp. Ther. *158*:305–316, 1967.

Deichmann, W. B., and Gerarde, H. W.: Symptomatology and Therapy of Toxicological Emergencies. New York, Academic Press, Inc., 1964.

Doherty, J. E.: The clinical pharmacology of digitalis glycosides: A review. Amer. J. Med. Sci. *255*:382, 1968.

Dole, V. P., Crowther, A., Johnson, J., Monsalvatge, M., Biller, B., and Nelson, S. S.: Detection of narcotic, sedative and amphetamine drugs in urine. New York J. Med. *72*: 471, 1972.

Dole, V. P., and Nyswander, M. E.: Rehabilitation of the street addict. Arch. Environ. Health (Chicago) *14*:477, 1967.

Done, A. K.: Salicylate intoxication, significance of measurements of salicylate in blood in cases of acute ingestion. Pediatrics *26*:800, 1960.

Dreisbach, R. H.: Handbook of Poisoning: Diagnosis and Treatment. 7th ed. Los Altos, Lange Medical Publications, 1971.

Dubowski, K. M.: Measurements of hemoglobin derivatives. *In* Sunderman, F. W., and Sunderman, F. W., Jr. (eds.): Hemoglobin: Its Precursors and Metabolites. Philadelphia, J. B. Lippincott Co., 1964.

Duffy, B.: Acute phenothiazine intoxication in children. Med. J. Aust. *1*:676, 1971.

Ehrlich-Rogazinsky, S., and Cheronis, N. D.: The identification and determination of morphine. Microchem. J. 7:336, 1963.

Erlanson, P., Fritz, H., Hagstam, K., Liljenberg, B., Tryding, N., and Voigt, G.: Severe methanol intoxication. Acta Med. Scand. *177*:393, 1965.

Evenson, M. A., Jones, P., and Darcey, B.: Simultaneous measurement of diphenylhydantoin and primidone in serum by gas-liquid chromatography. Clin. Chem. *16*: 107, 1970.

Feldstein, M., and Klendshoj, N. C.: The determination of volatile substances by micro diffusion analysis. J. Forensic Sci. Soc. 2:39, 1957.

Felton, J. S., Kahn, E., Salick, B., Van Natta, F. C., and Whitehouse, M. W.: Heavy metal poisoning: Mercury and lead. Ann. Intern. Med. *76*:779–792, 1972.

Fischer, D. S.: A method for the rapid detection of acute iron toxicity. Clin. Chem. *13*:11, 1967.

Forman, D. T., and Garvin, J. E.: Rapid determination of lead in urine by ion exchange. Clin. Chem. *11*:1, 1965.

Forrest, I. S., and Forrest, F. M.: A rapid urine color test for imipramine (Tofranil, Geigy). Amer. J. Psychiat. *116*:840, 1960.

Forrest, F. M., Forrest, I. S., and Mason, A. S.: Review of rapid urine tests for phenothiazines and related drugs. Amer. J. Psychiat. *118*:300, 1961.

Frings, C. S., and Cohen, P. S.: Rapid colorimetric method for the quantitative determination of ethchlorvynol (Placidyl) in serum and urine. Amer. J. Clin. Path. *54*: 833, 1970.

Furman, M., and Finberg, L.: A rapid method for estimation of salicylate in serum. J. Pediat. *70*:287, 1967.

Gettler, A. O., and Goldbaum, L. R.: Detection and estimation of microquantities of cyanide. Anal. Chem. *19*:270, 1947.

Ginn, H. E., Matter, B. J., and Shinaberger, J. A.: Clinical experience with lipid dialysis. J. Clin. Invest. *47*:40a, 1968.

Gleason, M. N., Gosselin, R. E., and Hodge, H. C.: Clinical Toxicology of Commercial Products: Acute Poisoning, Home and Farm. 2nd ed. Baltimore, The Williams & Wilkins Co., 1963.

Goldbaum, L. R.: Determination of barbiturates; ultraviolet spectrophotometric method with differentiation of several barbiturates. Anal. Chem. *24*:1604, 1952.

Goodman, L. S., and Gilman, A.: The Pharmacological Basis of Therapeutics. 3rd ed. New York, The Macmillan Co., 1965.

Gray, D. J. S.: The determination of traces of mercury in urine by the reversion technique. Analyst *77*:436, 1952.

Hall, G. E.: Medicolegal aspects of chemical tests. *In* Chemical Tests for Intoxication Manual. Chicago, American Medical Association, 1959, Addendum to Chapter 8, 1960.

Heyman, A., Pfeiffer, J. B., Jr., Willett, R. W., and Taylor, H. M.: Peripheral neuropathy caused by arsenical intoxication. New Eng. J. Med. *254*:401, 1956.

Hindberg, J., and Wieth, J. O.: Quantitative determination of methanol in biologic fluids. J. Lab. Clin. Med. *61*:355, 1963.

Hollister, L. E.: Adverse reactions to phenothiazines. J.A.M.A. *189*:311, 1964.

Horowitz, M. J.: Flashbacks: Recurrent intrusive images after the use of LSD. Amer. J. Psychiat. *126*:565, 1969.

Howie, R. A., and Smith, H.: Mercury in human tissue. J. For. Sci. Soc. *7*:90, 1967.

Huisman, J. W.: The estimation of some important anticonvulsant drugs in serum. Clin. Chim. Acta *13*:323, 1966.

Jacobs, M. B., Ladd, A. C., and Goldwater, L. I.: Absorption and excretion of mercury in man. Arch. Environ. Health *9*:454–463, 1964.

Jansen, G., and Bickers, I.: Rapid method for simultaneous qualitative assay of narcotics, cocaine, quinine, and propoxyphene in the urine. Southern Med. J. *64*:1072, 1971.

Jansson, B.: Drug automatism as a cause of pseudosuicide. Postgrad. Med. *30*:A–34, 1961.

Jelliffe, R. W.: An improved method of digoxin therapy. Ann. Intern. Med. *69*:703, 1968.

Katayama, K.: Übèr eine neue Blutprobe bei der Kohlenoxydvergiftung. Virchows Arch. Path. Anat. *114*:53, 1888.

Kauffman, J. M., and Sunderman, F. W.: Determination of arsenic in urine. *In* Sunderman, F. W., and Sunderman, F. W., Jr. (eds.): Laboratory Diagnosis of Diseases Caused by Toxic Agents. St. Louis, Warren H. Green, Inc., 1970.

Kaye, S.: Handbook of Emergency Toxicology. 3rd ed. Springfield, Ill., Charles C Thomas, 1970.

Kaye, S.: Rapid, simple, reliable tests for poisons. Lab. Med. *3*:28, 1972.

Kline, N. S., and Baer, L.: Psychotropic Drugs. New York J. Med. *72*(17):2170–2173, 1972.

Kopito, L., Byers, R. K., and Shwachman, H.: Lead in hair of children with chronic lead poisoning. New Eng. J. Med. *276*:949, 1967.

Korzun, B. P., Brody, S. M., Keegan, P. G., Luders, R. C., and Rehm, C. R.: Rapid chromatographic method for the identification and estimation of glutethimide (Doriden) in blood. J. Lab. Clin. Med. *68*:333, 1966.

Kupferberg, H., Burkhalter, A., and Wax, E. L.: A sensitive fluorometric assay for morphine in plasma and brain. J. Pharmacol. Exp. Ther. *145*:247, 1964.

Laessig, R. H.: Submicro sampling and solvent extraction system for rapid gas chromatographic determination of blood alcohol. Anal. Chem. *40*:2205–2207, 1968.

Lebish, P., Finkle, B. S., and Brackett, J. W., Jr.: Determination of amphetamines, metamphetamines and related amines in blood and urine by gas chromatography with hydrogen-flame ionization detector. Clin. Chem. *16*:195, 1970.

Leifheit, H. C.: Arsenic in biological materials. *In* Seligson, D. (ed.): Standard Methods of Clinical Chemistry. Vol. 3. New York, Academic Press, Inc., 1961.

Loomis, T. A.: Essentials of Toxicology. Philadelphia, Lea & Febiger, 1968.

Lubran, M.: Determination of lead by atomic absorption spectrophotometry. *In* Sunderman, F. W., and Sunderman, F. W., Jr. (eds.): Laboratory Diagnosis of Diseases Caused by Toxic Agents. St. Louis, Warren H. Green, Inc., 1970.

Luby, E. D., Schwartz, D., and Rosenbaum, H.: Lithium-carbonate-induced myxedema. J.A.M.A. *20*:104, 1967.

Lynn, E. J., Satloff, A., and Tinling, D. C.: Mania and the use of lithium: A three-year study. Amer. J. Psychiat. *127*: 1176–1180, 1971.

Maher, J. F., and Schreiner, G. E.: Hazards and complications of dialysis. New Eng. J. Med. *273*:370, 1965.

Melchior, J. C.: The clinical use of serum determinations of phenytoin and phenobarbital in children. Develop. Med. Child Neurol. *7*:387, 1965.

Meyers, F. H., Jawetz, E., and Goldfine, A.: Antipsychotic tranquilizers. *In* Review of Medical Pharmacology. Los Altos, California, Lange Medical Publications, 1972, Chapter 25, pp. 247–248.

Meyers, F. H., Jawetz, E., and Goldfine, A.: Toxicology. *In* Review of Medical Pharmacology. Los Altos, California, Lange Medical Publications, 1972, Part VIII, pp. 620–642.

Moeschlin, S.: Poisoning: Diagnosis and Treatment. New York, Grune & Stratton, 1965.

Mulé, S. J.: Identification of narcotics, barbiturates, amphetamines, tranquilizers, and psychomimetics in human urine. J. Chromatog. *39*:302, 1969.

Mulé, S. J.: Routine identification of drugs and abuse in urine. (I.) Application of fluorometry, thin-layer and gas-liquid chromatography. J. Chromatog. *55*:255, 1971.

Natelson, S.: Microtechniques of Clinical Chemistry for the Routine Laboratory. 2nd ed. Springfield, Ill., Charles C Thomas, 1961.

Nobel, S.: Toxicology in a general hospital. *In* MacDonald, R. P. (ed.): Standard Methods of Clinical Chemistry. Vol. 6. New York, Academic Press, New York, 1970.

Oliver, G. C., Parker, B. M., and Parker, C. W.: Radioimmunoassay for digoxin. Amer. J. Med. *51*:186, 1971.

Özdemir, A., and Tannenberg, A. M.: Peritoneal and hemodialysis for acute glutethimide overdosage. New York J. Med. *72*(16):2076–2079, 1972.

Payne, J. P., Hill, D. W., and King, N. W.: Observations on the distribution of alcohol in blood, breath, and urine. Brit. Med. J. *1*:196, 1966.

Payne, J. P., Hill, D. W., and Wood, D. G. L.: Distribution of ethanol between plasma and erythrocytes in whole blood. Nature (London) *217*:963–964, 1968.

Polson, C. J., and Tattersall, R. N.: Clinical Toxicology. 2nd ed. Philadelphia, J. B. Lippincott Co., 1969.

Proelss, H. F., and Lohmann, H. J.: Profile of sedatives and tranquilizers in serum as measured by gas-liquid chromatography. Clin. Chem. *17*:222, 1971.

Pybus, J., and Bowers, G. N., Jr.: Serum lithium determination by atomic absorption spectroscopy. *In* MacDonald, R. P. (ed.): Standard Methods of Clinical Chemistry. Vol. 6. New York, Academic Press, 1970, pp. 189–192.

Reid, R. W., Katzen, R., and Clinger, J. M.: Analysis of blood and other body fluids by gas chromatography. Amer. J. Clin. Path. *53*:462, 1970.

Rice, E. W., Fletcher, D. C., and Stumpff, A.: Lead in blood and urine. *In* Meites, S. (ed.): Standard Methods of Clinical Chemistry. Vol. 5. New York, Academic Press, Inc., 1965.

Rieder, S. V., and Zervas, M.: The assay of glutethimide. Amer. J. Clin. Path. *44*:520, 1965.

Rodensky, P. L., and Wasserman, F.: Observations on digitalis intoxication. Arch. Intern. Med. *108*:171, 1961.

Rodger, W. J., and Smith, H.: Mercury absorption by fingerprint officers using grey powder. J. Forsenic Sci. Soc. 7:86, 1967.

Rodkey, F. L.: The measurement of carbon monoxide in biological fluids. *In* Sunderman, F. W., and Sunderman, F. W., Jr. (eds.): Laboratory Diagnosis of Disease Caused by Toxic Agents. St. Louis, Warren H. Green, Inc., 1970.

Roeckel, I. E., and Talbert, W. M., Jr.: Measurement of methanol in biological fluids. *In* Sunderman, F. W., and Sunderman, F. W., Jr. (eds.): Laboratory Diagnosis of Diseases Caused by Toxic Agents. St. Louis, Warren H. Green, Inc., 1970.

Rose, S. W., Smith, L. D., and Penry, J. K.: Blood level determinations of antiepileptic drugs, clinical value and methods. Bethesda, Maryland, Section on Epilepsy, National Institute of Neurological Diseases and Stroke, National Institutes of Health, 1971.

Rossi, G. V.: LSD – A pharmacologic profile. Amer. J. Pharmacol. *143*:38, 1971.

Sampson, D., Harasymiv, I., and Hensley, W. J.: Gas chromatographic assay of underivatized 5,5-diphenylhydantoin (Dilantin) in plasma extracts. Clin. Chem. *17*:382, 1971.

Savory, J., Sunderman, F. W., Jr., Roszel, N. O., and Mushak, P.: An improved procedure for the determination of serum ethanol by gas chromatography. Clin. Chem. *14*:132–144, 1968.

Schweda, P.: Thin layer chromatography of toxicologically significant substances on silica gel coated glass plates and polyester sheets. Anal. Chem. *39*:1019, 1967.

Schweitzer, J. W., and Friedhoff, A. J.: Amphetamines in human urine: Rapid estimation by gas-liquid chromatography. Clin. Chem. *16*:786, 1970.

Serpe, S. J.: Bromide intoxication. New York J. Med. *72*(16): 2086–2088, 1972.

Sharpless, S. K.: Hypnotics and sedatives. I. Barbiturates. *In* Goodman, L. S., and Gilman, A. (eds.): The Pharmacological Basis of Therapeutics. 3rd ed. New York, The Macmillan Co., 1965.

Smith, H.: Estimation of arsenic in biological tissue by activation analysis. Anal. Chem. *31*:1361, 1959.

Smith, T. W., Butler, V. P., and Haber, E.: Determination of therapeutic and toxic serum digoxin concentrations by radioimmunoassay. New Eng. J. Med. *281*:1212, 1969.

Smith, T. W., and Haber, E.: Current techniques for serum or plasma digitalis assay and their potential clinical application. Amer. J. Med. Sci. *259*:301, 1970.

Smith, T. W., and Haber, E.: The clinical value of serum digitalis glycoside concentrations in the evaluation of drug toxicity. Ann. N.Y. Acad. Sci. *179*:322, 1971.

Sodeman, W. A.: Diagnosis and treatment of digitalis toxicity. New Eng. J. Med. *273*:35, 1965.

Stewart, C. P., and Stolman, A.: Toxicology: Mechanisms and Analytical Methods. Vol. I. New York, Academic Press, Inc., 1960.

Stiles, D., Batsakis, J. G., Kremers, B., and Briere, R. O.: The evaluation of ethanol measurements with alcohol dehydrogenase. Amer. J. Clin. Path. *46*:608–611, 1966.

Stolman, A., and Stewart, C. P.: Metallic poisons. *In* Stewart, C. P., and Stolman, A. (eds.): Toxicology, Mechanisms and Analytical Methods. Vol. 1. New York, Academic Press, Inc., 1960.

Sunderman, F. W., and Sunderman, F. W., Jr. (eds.): Laboratory Diagnosis of Diseases Caused by Toxic Agents. St. Louis, Warren H. Green, Inc., 1970.

Sunshine, I.: Alcohol in biological materials. *In* Seligson, D. (ed.): Standard Methods of Clinical Chemistry. Vol. 3. New York, Academic Press, Inc., 1961.

Sunshine, I.: Barbiturate. *In* Seligson, D. (ed.): Standard Methods of Clinical Chemistry. Vol. 3. New York, Academic Press, Inc., 1961.

Sunshine, I. (ed.): Handbook of Analytical Toxicology. Cleveland, Chemical Rubber Co., 1969.

Svensmark, O., and Buchthal, F.: Diphenylhydantoin and phenobarbital serum levels in children. Amer. J. Dis. Child. *108*:82, 1964.

Swidler, G. D.: Handbook of Drug Interactions. New York, John Wiley & Sons, Inc., 1971.

Thienes, C. H., and Haley, T. J.: Clinical Toxicology. 5th ed. Philadelphia, Lea & Febiger, 1972.

Thompson, H. L., and Decker, W. J.: Analysis of blood, a simplified gas chromatographic approach for toxicologic purposes. Amer. J. Clin. Path. *49*:103, 1968.

Triedman, H. M., Fishman, R. A., and Yahr, M. D.: Determination of plasma and cerebrospinal fluid levels of Dilantin in the human. Trans. Amer. Neurol. Ass. *85*:166, 1960.

Tschetter, P. N.: Salicylism. Amer. J. Dis. Child. *106*:334, 1963.

Turner, R. F., Heise, H. A., and Muehlberger, C. W.: Interpretation of tests for intoxication. *In* Chemical Tests for Intoxication Manual. Chicago, American Medical Association, 1959.

Wallace, J. E., and Biggs, J. D.: Determination of phenothiazine compounds in biologic specimens by UV spectrophotometry. J. Pharmacol. Sci. *60*:1346, 1971.

Way, E. L., and Adler, T. K.: The biological disposition of morphine and its surrogates. 4. Bull. WHO *27*:359, 1962.

Westerman, M. P., Pfitzer, E., Ellis, L. D., and Jensen, W. N.: Concentrations of lead in bone in plumbism. New Eng. J. Med. *273*:1246, 1965.

Williams, R. B., Jr., and Sherter, C.: Cardiac complications of tricyclic antidepressant therapy. Ann. Intern. Med. *74*:395, 1971.

Williams, R. T.: Detoxication Mechanisms: The Metabolism and Detoxication of Drugs, Toxic Substances and Other Organic Compounds. 2nd ed. New York, John Wiley & Sons, Inc., 1959.

Willis, J. B.: Determination of lead and other heavy metals in urine by atomic absorption spectroscopy. Anal. Chem. *34*:614, 1962.

Winters, R. W., White, J. S., Hughes, M. C., and Ordway, N. K.: Disturbances of acid-base equilibrium in salicylate intoxication. Pediatrics *23*:260, 1959.

Woodbury, D. M., Penry, J. K., and Schmidt, R. P. (eds.): Antiepileptic Drugs. New York, Raven Press, 1972.

Chapter 11

ENDOCRINE MEASUREMENTS

by JOHN BERNARD HENRY, M.D., and ARTHUR F. KRIEG, M.D.

Hormones are chemical substances that are formed in one organ and exert their influence on other organs or tissues, in effect acting as a chemical communications system (Cantarow and Schepartz, 1967). Endocrine measurements provide quantitation of hormones or their metabolites in blood or urine, thus aiding in identification of diseases associated with deficient or excess hormone secretion. The following organs comprise the established endocrine system: anterior and posterior pituitary, thyroid, parathyroids, adrenal cortex and medulla, pancreatic islets of Langerhans, ovaries, testes, and placenta.

The skin is now considered an endocrine organ by numerous investigators of vitamin D metabolism because it elaborates, by irradiation of 7-dehydrocholesterol, vitamin D_3 (cholecalciferol), a chemical that exerts its influence on distant organs, i.e., intestine and bone (De Luca, 1969). For details, refer to discussion of vitamin D in Chapter 9 on biochemistry of calcium and phosphorus and the reviews by Alvioli (1972) and Raisz (1972).

In addition to hypothalamus with its several releasing factors, the gastrointestinal tract is associated with the hormones listed below and reviewed in Chapter 16.

HORMONE	SITE OF ACTION	PRINCIPAL ACTIONS
Secretin and pancreozymin	Pancreas	Secretion of alkaline fluid and digestive enzymes
Cholecystokinin	Gallbladder	Contraction and emptying
Enterogastrone	Stomach	Inhibition of motility and secretion
Gastrin	Stomach	Secretion of acid

Production and secretion of thyroid, adrenocortical, and gonadal hormones are under control of pituitary trophic hormones: thyroid-stimulating hormone (TSH), adrenocorticotrophic hormone (ACTH), follicle-stimulating hormone (FSH), and interstitial cell-stimulating hormone (ICSH). Production and/or secretion of these pituitary trophic hormones is influenced by neurohumoral (releasing) factors from the hypothalamus, which in turn is influenced by stimuli from the cerebral cortex. Neural regulation appears to be superimposed upon a negative feedback mechanism: as concentration of the circulating target hormone rises, secretion of the corresponding pituitary hormone is depressed; as concentration of the target hormone falls, secretion of the trophic hormone increases. This negative feedback system appears to be of great importance in maintaining normal blood levels of thyroid, adrenocortical, and gonadal hormones. Simpler negative feedback systems provide regulation of blood glucose and calcium without the intervention of a mediating hormone; increased glucose causes increased secretion of insulin, and decreased calcium causes increased secretion of parathyroid hormone.

Several hormones are transported largely in combination with plasma proteins, including thyroxine bound to thyroxine-binding globulin (TBG), cortisol bound to transcortin, estrogen bound to albumin, and vitamin D bound to an inter-alpha globulin of approximately 60,000 M.W. The protein-bound hormone apparently exists in equilibrium with free, or unbound, hormone. Because of the relative nondiffusibility of the protein-bound hormone, it is not lost in the urine by passage across the glomerular membrane, but neither does it readily pass across cell membranes. Thus it is free, or unbound, hormone which is physiologically active with respect to the responsive organ or tissue.

The liver occupies a key role in terms of hormone metabolism. Vitamin D_3 is hydroxylated to the metabolite 25-hydroxycholecalciferol ($25OHD_3$). De Luca (1969) has shown that "hepatectomy" prevents this conversion. Thyroxine, androgens and estrogens, progesterone, corticosteroids, insulin, and epinephrine are either excreted by the liver or metabolized to physiologically less active or inactive compounds. In addition, TBG and transcortin are produced in the liver. Obviously liver disease can have important effects upon hormone metabolism and may cause difficulty in interpretation of endocrine measurements.

The kidney is also a key organ where transformation of vitamin D occurs. Here, $25OHD_3$ is hydroxylated further to 1,25-dihydroxycholecalciferol also called 1,25-dihydroxy vitamin D_3 ($1{,}25(OH)_2D_3$), the final active metabolite of vitamin D_3 (Raisz, 1972).

In the target organs or tissues, hormones exert their final action in control of metabolic events and transport processes; the mode of action at this level is not fully understood but through cyclic AMP probably is related to activation, inhibition, or altered production of intracellular enzymes and/or coenzymes. At this level hormones may undergo transformation into compounds of different biologic activity before returning to the blood as relatively inactive metabolites which may be excreted in urine directly or metabolized further by the liver.

CYCLIC AMP

Adenosine 3′, 5′ monophosphate, commonly referred to as "cyclic AMP," is a cyclic nucleotide (Fig. 11–1) found primarily within the soluble portion of the cytoplasm of vertebrates, invertebrates, and bacteria. It is generated from adenosine triphosphate (ATP) in the presence of adenyl cyclase, with liberation of a pyrophosphate byproduct. Hormone receptor sites

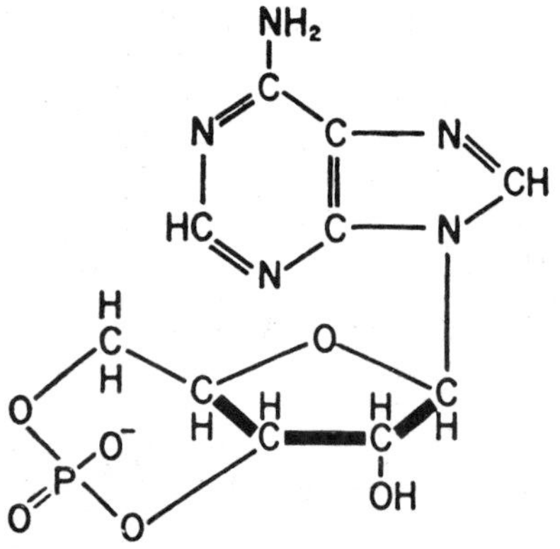

Figure 11-1. Cyclic AMP (adenosine 3′,5′ (cyclic) monophosphate).

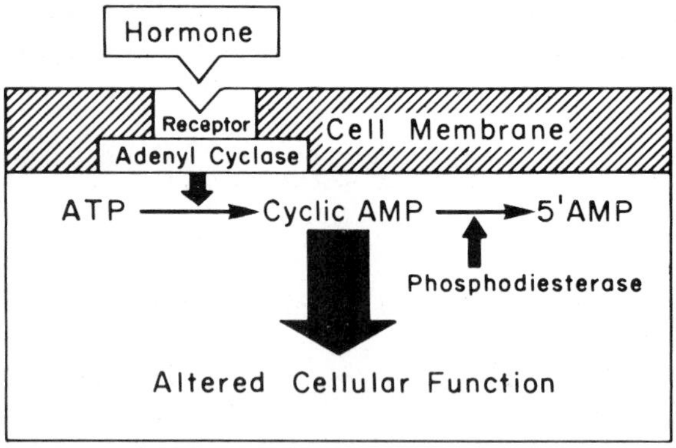

Figure 11-2. Diagrammatic representation of the role of cyclic AMP as a "second messenger" in the actions of many hormones. (With permission of Liddle, G. W., and Hardman, J. G.: New Eng. J. Med. *285*:560, 1971.)

in the cell membranes of endocrine target organs have been closely associated with this adenyl cyclase enzyme system which is also located in the cell membrane (Sutherland *et al.*, 1965). In order to explain the selective nature of hormone interaction with target organs, Liddle and Hardman (1971) have suggested that hormone specificity may be conferred by the chemical properties of the receptor-cyclase system. Also postulated is an adenyl cyclase model composed of a receptor subunit, programmed for specific hormone interaction, and a catalytic subunit that accelerates the conversion of ATP to cyclic AMP within the cell (Fig. 11–2). The authors concluded that although the functional and anatomic associations are strong, there is no current evidence to define how the hormone receptor spatially relates to the adenyl cyclase molecule in the cell membrane.

The major effect of cyclic AMP appears to be the modification of intracellular enzyme systems, particularly protein kinases. According to a general theory of cyclic AMP action (Walsh *et al.*, 1970), the transfer of phosphate from ATP to certain proteins is enhanced when a protein kinase (e.g., phosphorylase kinase) is activated by cyclic AMP.

$$\begin{array}{c}\text{Cyclic AMP}\\ +\end{array}$$
$$\text{Protein} + \text{ATP} \xrightarrow{\text{Protein kinase}} \text{Protein phosphate} + \text{ADP}$$

The phosphorylated proteins, manifesting varied biologic properties not present in the dephosphorylated state, subsequently evoke the metabolic events that have classically been used as parameters of hormone-target cell interaction. Because cyclic AMP is rapidly inactivated by cyclic nucleotide phosphodiesterase, these metabolic alterations are evanescent unless the receptor-cyclase system is continually exposed to hormone (Butcher and Sutherland, 1962). The phosphodiesterase-mediated degradation consists of an opening of the phosphate-ribose ring of cyclic AMP to yield a noncyclic nucleotide, 5′-AMP.

The "Second Messenger" Concept

In the early 1960's Sutherland and associates formulated the "second messenger" concept to explain the mechanism of action of hormones at the cellular level (Sutherland, 1970). According to this concept, the blood-borne hormones are the first transporters of messages emanating from endocrine organs (Fig. 11–3). Having reached the target tissues, the hormones pass on the message by modifying the intracellular concentration of a second messenger, cyclic AMP, which in turn evokes the characteristic metabolic changes. The following hormones have been established as exerting their effect by increasing intracellular cyclic AMP concentrations: glucagon, catecholamines (beta component), ACTH, luteinizing hormone (LH), melanocyte-stimulating hormone (MSH), vasopressin, parathyroid hormone, calcitonin, and others. In contrast, insulin and catecholamines (alpha component) act by decreasing cytoplasmic cyclic AMP concentration (Liddle and Hardman, 1971). Nonendocrine modifiers of intracellular cyclic AMP concentration include ionized calcium (Rasmussen *et al.*, 1972) and pharmacologic inhibitors of phosphodiesterase, e.g., caffeine and theophylline (Liddle and Hardman, 1971). A hypothetical model of interaction between cyclic AMP and ionized calcium in achieving cell activation has recently been published by Rasmussen and his associates (1971, 1972).

Clinicopathologic Correlations

Two basic methods have been employed in the determination of cyclic AMP levels:

1. Biochemical assay, which measures the augmentation of an enzymatic reaction that is sensitive to cyclic AMP, e.g., conversion of inactive to active phosphorylase.

2. Competitive protein binding (Gilman, 1970). Measurement before and after incubation with phosphodiesterase, the specific cyclic AMP inactivator, is suggested as a specificity check (Liddle and Hardman, 1971).

Cyclic AMP levels have been determined in tissue, plasma, and urine. Approximately 60 per cent of urinary cyclic AMP is derived from the plasma by glomerular filtration. The remaining 40 per cent is derived from the kidney by direct secretion ("nephrogenous" cyclic AMP). Under basal conditions, normal plasma cyclic AMP concentrations have ranged from 10 to 25 nanomoles per liter (Broadus *et al.*, 1972). Normal urinary cyclic AMP levels have ranged from 2 nanomoles to 9 nanomoles per day (Sutherland, 1970). A departure from basal levels has been demonstrated by Liddle and Hardman (1971) with the following:

1. *Glucagon* is capable of inducing a thirtyfold increase in both plasma and urinary cyclic AMP levels.

2. *Parathyroid hormone* elicits a maximal urinary response (up to fortyfold increase), and a minimal plasma response (approximately threefold increase).

3. *Calcitonin* evokes a minimal response in both plasma and urine (two- to threefold increase of cyclic AMP levels in urine and plasma).

In general, the measurement of cyclic AMP levels is currently limited to the fields of basic and clinical research. Recently it has been recommended as an auxiliary but potentially

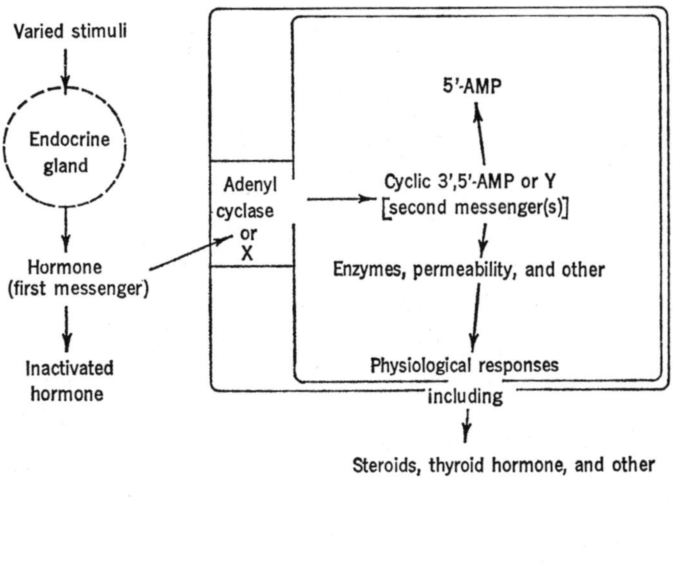

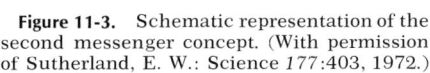

Figure 11-3. Schematic representation of the second messenger concept. (With permission of Sutherland, E. W.: Science *177*:403, 1972.)

useful procedure in differentiating hypercalcemia of various causes. The authors, Murad and Pak (1972), correlated urinary cyclic AMP levels in normal controls and in patients with: (1) hypercalcemic hyperparathyroidism, (2) normocalcemic hyperparathyroidism, (3) hypoparathyroidism (idiopathic, pseudo-, or postparathyroidectomy), (4) hypercalcemia secondary to osseous metastasis from carcinoma, and (5) sarcoid hypercalcemia. The measurement appeared useful in detecting cases of normocalcemic hyperparathyroidism with elevated urinary cyclic AMP levels, and in distinguishing hypercalcemia of hyperparathyroidism from hypercalcemia of carcinoma. Variability within and between groups was reduced by normalizing the amount of urinary cyclic AMP for the amount of creatinine in a 24-hour urine specimen. Low urinary cyclic AMP levels in hypoparathyroidism corroborated a previous study of Chase, Melson, and Aurbach (1969).

HORMONES OF THE HYPOTHALAMUS

The interrelationship between the pituitary gland, the hypothalamus, and the target organs is shown in Figure 11-4. The "releasing factors" originating in the brain regulate the anterior pituitary gland which, in turn, controls the peripheral endocrine glands (Guillemin and Burgus, 1972). Since the pituitary gland is attached by a stalk to the region in the base of the brain known as the hypothalamus, the fact that the hypothalamus and the pituitary act in concert can be more readily appreciated. Two of these hypothalamic hormones have now been isolated, chemically identified, and synthesized. Thyroid-stimulating hormone (TSH), a pituitary hormone, is associated with the hypothalamic hormone called TSH-releasing factor or TRF. Hence, the hypothalamic hormone, TRF, is the critical factor that triggers the release of the pituitary hormone, thyrotropin (TSH).

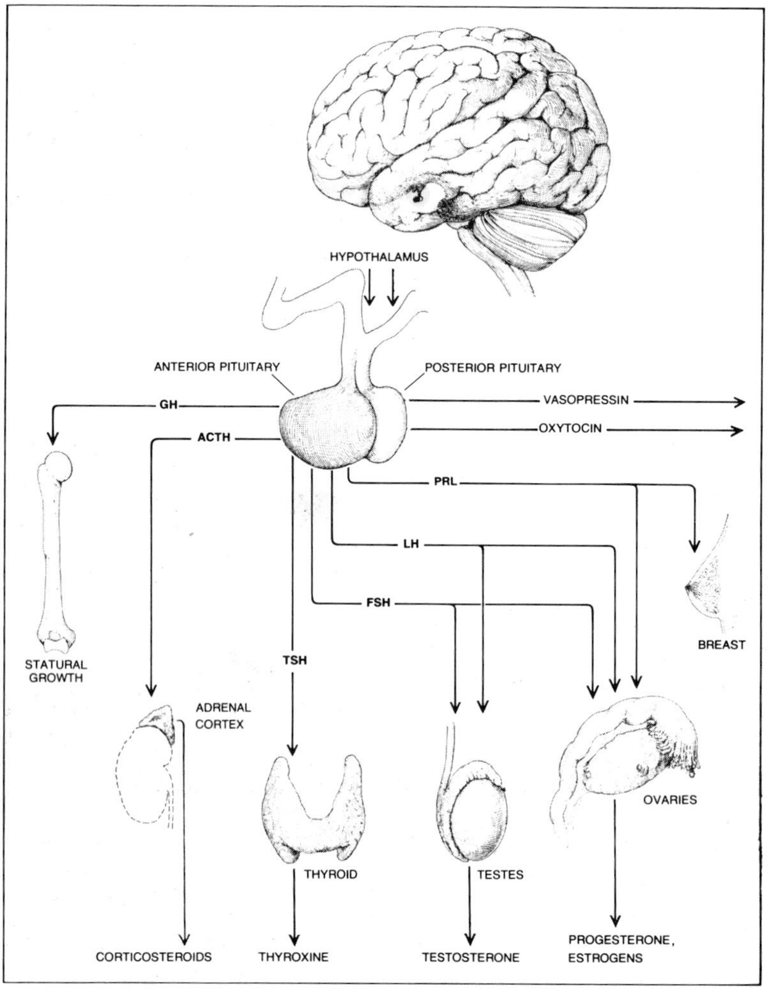

Figure 11-4. Interrelationship between the pituitary gland, hypothalamus, and target organs. (With permission of Guillemin, R., and Burgus, R.: Sci. Amer. 227:26, 1972.)

The other hypothalamic hormone that has been characterized so well is LRF. RF refers to "releasing factor" while L indicates the gonadotropic pituitary hormone, LH, or luteinizing hormone. Although a third gonadotropic hormone from the anterior pituitary FSH (follicle-stimulating hormone), may have its own hypothalamic releasing factor, or FRF, this has not yet been demonstrated. Indeed, the hypothalamic hormone LRF appears to stimulate the release of FSH as well as LH. Several other hypothalamic hormones are known to exist, although they have not yet been isolated. One of these regulates the secretion of adrenocorticotropin (ACTH), the pituitary hormone whose target is the adrenal cortex. Release of the pituitary hormone prolactin appears to be regulated by another hormone (possibly two hormones with opposing actions). Prolactin is involved in pregnancy and lactation. Another hormone, again possibly two hormones with opposing actions, regulates the release of the pituitary hormone involved in growth and structural development, called growth hormone (GH).

Indeed, the anterior pituitary is made up of at least six different secretory types of cells, each capable of functioning independently of one another. A singular specific pituitary deficiency (monotropic) in the secretion of growth hormone (GH), thyrotropic hormone (TSH), adrenocorticotropic hormone (ACTH), and prolactin has been recognized in addition to combined deficits in secretion of the gonadotropic hormones, i.e., luteinizing hormone, LH, and follicle-stimulating hormone, FSH (Reichlin, 1972). Rabin and his colleagues (1972) have reported a case of primary amenorrhea in which the gonadotropin deficit was shown to be of only one of the gonadotropins; that is, an absolute primary deficiency of FSH with the predictable observation of undeveloped ovarian follicles, estrogen secretion undetectable; in the absence of appreciable quantities of estrogen, the negative feedback control system of the pituitary was activated, leading to hypersecretion of LH. This FSH deficit appeared to be congenital in nature in view of the appearance of anti-FSH antibodies (but not anti-LH antibodies) after exposure to human gonadotropins. Three pituitary glycoprotein hormones (FSH, LH, and TSH) are secreted by basophil cells which, on the basis of immunohistochemical and ultrastructural work, suggests that each of these cells is morphologically distinct (Reichlin, 1972). However, there is some evidence that a minority of cells may secrete LH and FSH.

The hypothalamic hormones, TRF and LRF, available by synthesis in virtually unlimited quantities, are highly active in stimulating pituitary functions in humans (Guillemin and Burgus, 1972). TRF is used to delineate abnormalities of pituitary function insofar as TSH release is concerned. Furthermore, both hormones may be used for replacement therapy in situations in which there appear to be hypothalamic rather than pituitary deficiencies. Ovulation can be induced in women by the administration of synthetic LRF. Moreover, women who have no ovulatory menstrual cycle and who show no pituitary or ovarian defect often begin to secrete normal amounts of the gonadotropins LH and FSH after the administration of LRF. Hence, LRF has great potential for treatment of those cases of infertility in which the functional defect resides in the hypothalamus-pituitary system. Furthermore, analogues of LRF have been reported as antagonists of LRF; it is possible that LRF antagonists may be used as contraceptives in the future.

In summary, there is clear evidence for separate releasing factors that can excite and inhibit the release of the following pituitary hormones:

1. Growth hormone (GH)
2. Prolactin
3. Melanocyte-stimulating hormone (MSH)

and can stimulate the release of:

4. Thyroid-stimulating hormone (TSH)
5. Adrenocorticotropic hormone (ACTH)
6. One or both gonadotropins (FSH, LH)

Undoubtedly other factors will be identified. In the future it may be possible to delineate selective failure of each pituitary cell type and its relevant hypothalamic hypophysiotropic hormone (Reichlin, 1972).

Pituitary Hormones

As may be noted in Figure 11–4, two hormones are secreted by the posterior pituitary: (1) vasopressin (antidiuretic hormone – ADH), and (2) oxytocin. Both hormones are octapeptides and, as shown by Du Vigneaud's group (1953), six of the eight amino acids in the two molecules of hormones are identical. This explains their closely related physical-chemical properties and similar biologic activity. Hence, both hormones exhibit, although in different ratios, all the major biologic effects attributed to them separately, i.e., the reabsorption of water from the kidney into the blood stream, the stimulation of uterine contractions, and the release of milk.

The hormones secreted by the posterior lobe of the pituitary (vasopressin and oxytocin) are actually manufactured in some specialized nerve cells in the hypothalamus, from which they flow slowly down the pituitary stalk to the posterior pituitary through the long fibers of the hypothalamic nerve cells. In essence, the posterior pituitary is a storage organ rather than a manufacturing site from which vasopressin and oxytocin are secreted into the blood stream on the proper physiologic stimulus. The secretion of vasopressin is regulated by plasma osmolality (when osmolality is increased, vasopressin is secreted) and by changes in extracellular fluid volume (vasopressin is secreted when extracellular fluid volume is depleted).

Diabetes insipidus is characterized by lack of ADH, resulting in sudden onset of progressive polyuria, nocturia, and polydipsia that may be incapacitating within a few days (Utiger, 1969). A radioimmunoassay for ADH has permitted delineation of those pathophysiologic entities associated with ADH insufficiency due to pituitary disease such as vascular compromise, tumor, trauma, or microbiologic destruction. The use of ADH measurements may be helpful in differentiating polyuric states, including diabetes insipidus of end-organ (renal tubular) failure associated with pyelonephritis (nephrogenic diabetes insipidus) from pituitary failure (idiopathic or secondary to neurologic disease) (Moses and Miller, 1972.)

Usually, random simultaneous urinary and plasma osmolalities are employed for screening rather than dehydration with injection of aqueous Pitressin to differentiate diabetes insipidus, nephrogenic diabetes insipidus, and primary (psychogenic) polydipsia. ADH assay is only an adjunct and not widely available (Table 11–1). Excessive ADH excretion with inappropriate antidiuresis and dilutional hyponatremia (as a consequence of water retention characterized by a low plasma osmolality with a concentrated urine) has been associated with oat-cell carcinoma of the lung.

In terms of the anterior pituitary gland, growth hormone (GH), thyrotropin (TSH), and gonadotropin measurements by radioimmunoassay are presently used for detection and diagnosis of disease.

Although elevated plasma GH levels occur with liver and kidney disease as well as other conditions, an excess secretion of GH is observed in patients with eosinophilic adenomas of the pituitary resulting in gigantism or, later in life, acromegaly. Although baseline levels of human growth hormone are elevated in patients with acromegaly, it is imperative to demonstrate a lack of suppressibility of elevated GH levels with a standard dose of glucose administered, since growth hormone concentrations in normals vary greatly with state of wakefulness and virtually all kinds of activity (Katz, 1969). Measurements of GH during the course of a glucose tolerance test are satisfactory. After 100 gm. of glucose by mouth, normal persons will have serum growth hormone levels less than 1 ng./ml. an hour later. In contrast, acromegalic patients demonstrate little, if any, suppression of the fasting growth hormone and almost invariably never below 1 ng./ml. Unfortunately successful management of acromegaly is not necessarily accompanied by normalization of growth hormone measurements. GH levels may remain elevated despite good clinical response to therapy, although levels often are lower than before therapy (Katz, 1969).

The diagnosis of panhypopituitarism or pituitary dwarfism can be established by plasma growth hormone (GH) levels. Measurements of a depressed absolute GH level should be supplemented by the evaluation of the response to insulin or hypoglycemic stimulus which will

Table 11–1. RESPONSES TO DEHYDRATION TEST IN NORMAL SUBJECTS AND IN PATIENTS WITH POLYURIC SYNDROMES*

CLINICAL STATE	URINE OSMOLALITY AT PLATEAU (mOsm./kg.)†	INCREASE IN URINE OSMOLALITY AFTER ADH INJECTION (%)	PLASMA OSMOLALITY AT PLATEAU (mOsm./kg.)†
Normal	800 ± 200	< 5	290 ± 5
Diabetes insipidus (severe)	168 ± 59	> 50	306 ± 12
Diabetes insipidus (partial)	438 ± 116	> 9	294 ± 4
Nephrogenic diabetes insipidus	96–151 (range)	< 50	302–320 (range)
Primary polydipsia	696 ± 140	< 5	289 ± 5

*With permission of Moses, A. M., and Miller, M.: Postgrad. Med. *52*:190, 1972.
†Mean ± S.D.
< = less than
> = greater than

Table 11–2. CLINICAL INTERPRETATION OF HUMAN GROWTH HORMONE (HGH) RESULTS*

PROVOCATIVE TEST	DOSAGE	BLOOD SPECIMEN INTERVALS (minutes)‡	RESPONSE		
			Normal	Hypopituitarism	Acromegaly
Insulin	0.1 unit per kg. body wt. intravenously	0†, 30, 45, 60	> 10 ng./ml. at 30–45 min.	< 7 ng./ml. at 30–45 min.	Usually autonomous, occasionally hyper-responsive
Arginine	0.5 g per kg. body wt. in 0.85% NaCl and H_2O infused over 30 min. (Response enhanced by oral propanolol 2 hr. before)	0†, 30, 60, 90	> 10 ng./ml. at 60 min.	< 7 ng./ml. at 60 min.	Not applicable
Glucagon	1 mg. subcut.	0†, 45, 90, 120, 150	> 10 ng./ml. at 2 hr.	< 10 ng./ml. at 2 hr.	Not applicable
Glucose	1 gm. per kg. body wt. (orally)	0†, 60, 120, 180	< 5 ng./ml. (men), < 10 ng./ml. (women) at 2 hr.	None detectable at 2 hr.	< 50% fall, or HGH levels > 5 ng./ml. at 2 hr.

*With permission of Sherwood, L. M.: Clinical use of human pituitary growth hormone (HGH) assays. Clinchem Comments, prepared by Clin-Chem Laboratories, 1106 Commonwealth Avenue, Boston, Massachusetts 02215.

†These samples are obtained in the fasting state before administration of the test solution.

‡These intervals are measured from the beginning of the administration of the test solution.

normally increase the secretion of the GH (Table 11–2). Insulin hypoglycemia produced with administration of 0.1 unit insulin per kilogram intravenously to children (up to 0.15 units/kg. in adults) is utilized to elicit increase in growth hormone excretion (Katz, 1969). Within 30 to 60 minutes of the administration of insulin and adequate hypoglycemia, i.e., 40 to 45 mg. per cent plasma glucose, normal persons have a substantial increase in plasma growth hormone. However, other conditions in addition to hypopituitarism are associated with an inability to increase plasma growth hormone level in response to insulin hypoglycemia; for example, hypothyroidism (especially in children), hyperadrenocorticism, hypogonadism, and corticosteroid administration in adults. Obese patients may also display a blunted response (VanderLaan *et al.*, 1970). Patients with hypopituitarism are extremely sensitive to insulin, often resulting in a persistent hypoglycemia. Hence, smaller doses of insulin are frequently utilized and patients must be carefully observed for severe hypoglycemic reactions. The use of arginine as a stimulus for growth hormone secretion avoids the consequences of poor tolerance to hypoglycemia in the diagnosis of pituitary dwarfism (Table 11–2). Half a gram per kilogram of body weight of neutralized arginine hydrochloride given intravenously over 30 minutes stimulates normal persons to produce plasma GH levels greater than 10 ng./ml., whereas pituitary dwarfs do not respond (Katz, 1969). A screening test for the ability to secrete GH in children has also been proposed (Wolfsdorf *et al.*, 1967): this consists of a rise in growth hormone concentration at the end of a glucose tolerance test (3½ to 4 hours).

Thyrotropin (TSH) assays are also determined by radioimmunoassay. Elevations of peripheral plasma levels of TSH appear in most patients with myxedema. Indeed, this may be the most sensitive single test for primary hypothyroidism, i.e., elevated TSH levels with destruction of thyroid gland, e.g., thyroiditis (intrinsic thyroid disease).

The TSH stimulation test is used to differentiate hypothyroidism due to intrinsic thyroid disease from hypothyroidism secondary to a lack of pituitary secretion of TSH. A baseline serum thyroxine (T_4) and a 24-hour RAI or ^{131}I uptake are determined. Subsequently the patient receives 10 units of bovine TSH daily for three successive days. Then a serum thyroxine (T_4) and the ^{131}I uptake are repeated. A one-dose test procedure has also been suggested (Fore and Wynn, 1966). With primary disease of the thyroid gland, patients show no change in serum thyroxine (T_4) or the RAI uptake. In most patients with hypothyroidism secondary to pituitary insufficiency, the serum thyroxine (T_4) and RAI rise to normal or supernormal levels. With severe longstanding secondary atrophy of the thyroid gland, an occasional patient with pituitary insufficiency must receive TSH for a longer period to stimulate thyroid tissue to near normal activity. Caution should be exercised in administering TSH to some patients in whom the increase in thyroid hormone secretion may precipitate cardiac failure or angina pectoris with coexisting coronary artery disease (Katz, 1969). In addition, a prompt sudden increase in circulating thyroid hormone may precipitate more severe relative adrenal insufficiency in persons with Addison's disease or hypopituitarism. Treatment of such patients with corticosteroids as well as TSH may be indicated if clinical suggestion of adrenal insufficiency occurs with TSH administration. The administration of TSH is occasionally associated with such effects as a mild reaction at the injection site, nausea, vomiting, urticaria, and transitory hypotension or thyroid swelling; hence, only one or two doses of TSH may be desirable for an individual.

Gonadotropins

Pituitary gonadotropins may be measured collectively by classic bioassay procedures. However, more recently radioimmunoassays specific for follicle-stimulating hormone (FSH) and luteinizing or interstitial cell-stimulating hormone (LH or ICSH) have become available.

FSH stimulates the ovarian follicle to increase in size and to mature, while in the male it is associated with the stimulation and maintenance of spermatogenesis. LH in the female causes ovulation and steroid (estrogen and progesterone) production by the corpus luteum, while in the male LH stimulates the interstitial cells (Leydig cells) to produce androgens and estrogens. However, small quantities of LH are also necessary to promote estrogen production by the FSH-stimulated maturing follicle (Northcutt and Albert, 1969).

Pituitary gonadotropins are increased in primary hypogonadism. A female with primary ovarian failure (e.g., Turner's syndrome) shows increased gonadotropins, whereas hypopituitarism is characterized by diminished gonadotropin levels in the urine. Pituitary gonadotropin assay also permits delineation of male hypogonadotropic eunuchoidism due to testicular insufficiency (e.g., Klinefelter's syndrome) from hypogonadism due to pituitary failure or selected adults' seminiferous tubular "failures." Diminished gonadotropin excretion may also be observed in patients with anorexia nervosa (Katz, 1969).

Serum radioimmunoassay values of FSH and LH are shown in Table 11–3. The metabolic fate of secreted pituitary gonadotropins is largely unknown; however, only about 5 per cent of the total FSH and LH entering the circulation appears in the urine as biologically active material. In contrast to adult human males, in whom FSH and LH secretion rates are relatively fixed in a tonic control mechanism depending on the status of testicular function, in women during their productive life span more complex cycling of gonado-hypothalamic-pituitary interaction occurs. During the menstrual cycle, FSH secretion rises during the follicular or proliferative phase and then falls, but may rise again at mid-cycle, declining to low levels during the luteal phase. LH, on the other hand, is secreted at low levels throughout the menstrual cycle except for a surge of secretion occurring just prior to and initiating ovulation and corpus luteum formation. Very high levels of FSH and LH secretion which exceed five- to fifteenfold those of normal men and women occur with castration as well as with loss of gonadal function in the menopause. In men a singular loss of germinal epithelial function following testicular irradiation or in the "Sertoli cell only" syndrome is associated with elevated FSH but normal LH.

Disturbances of the hypothalamus may result in decreased secretion of both FSH and LH. This is also observed with central nervous system disorders and following administration of certain depressant drugs such as phenothiazine tranquilizers. Gonadotropin hypersecretion disproportionate to the patient's chronologic age may be observed in precocious puberty, a disturbance perhaps of the central

Table 11–3. RADIOIMMUNOASSAY VALUES OF SERUM FSH AND LH*

				WOMEN		
				Ovulatory Menses		Postmenopausal
HORMONE	UNITS	CHILDREN PREPUBERTAL BOTH SEXES	MEN	Luteal and Follicular Phases	Midcycle	
FSH	μg./100 ml. serum	4 (0–20)	25 (10–60)	25 (10–50)	40 (25–45)	250 (150–400)
LH	μg./100 ml. serum	4 (1–12)	12 (4–24)	15 (8–27)	50 (30–80)	60 (40–70)

*Modified from Northcutt, R. C., and Albert, A.: J.A.M.A. *210*:2387, 1969.

Table 11–4. TUMORS ASSOCIATED WITH SPECIFIC ECTOPIC HORMONE SYNDROMES*

SYNDROME	HORMONE	SITES
Cushing's syndrome	ACTH (adrenocorticotrophic hormone)	Lung (oat cell carcinoma; bronchial adenoma carcinoids); thymus; pancreas; thyroid (medullary)
Hyperparathyroidism	PTH (parathormone)	Kidney; lung (squamous); pancreas; ovary; many squamous sites
Inappropriate antidiuresis	Arginine-vasopressin (ADH)	Lung (oat cell)
Erythrocytosis	Erythropoietin	Cerebellum (hemangiomas); liver; uterus
Zollinger-Ellison syndrome	Gastrin	Pancreas (non-beta-islet-cell adenomas)
Gynecomastia (adults) precocious puberty	Gonadotropins	Lung (large cell) Liver
Hyperthyroidism	Thyrotropin	Trophoblast; lung
Hypoglycemia	Unknown	Retroperitoneal mesoderm; liver

*Modified from Omenn, G. S.: Ann. Intern. Med. *72*:137, 1970.

nervous system control of gonadotropin secretion. Here, normal adult levels of gonadotropins and gonadal function may be noted in the "fertile eunuch" syndrome, and the inability to elaborate the ovulatory surge of LH may be observed in a certain variety of anovulatory menses with specific LH deficiency (Northcutt and Albert, 1969). Specific measurements of FSH and LH are necessary for the diagnosis of these and other rare disorders.

Corticotropin (ACTH)

Although ACTH can be measured in plasma by radioimmunoassay, less complex clinical procedures can be utilized to demonstrate normal or abnormal ability to release ACTH (See p. 731.)

Polypeptide Hormone Production by Tumors

In Table 11–4 tumors associated with specific ectopic hormone syndromes are shown. Rapid clinical deterioration in a cancer patient may be attributed to hormonal causes that, in turn, reflect the production and release of excessive amounts of hormone by the underlying tumor, with additive effects of metabolic derangements to the neoplastic illness (Omenn, 1970). While the clinical manifestations of the ectopic hormone syndromes vary with the amount of hormone produced and with the course of the underlying neoplastic disease, profound minimal or insidious deleterious effects of hormones may be observed. For example, with oat-cell bronchogenic carcinoma producing ectopic ACTH, most patients have hypokalemia, weakness, impaired glucose tolerance, edema, and hypertension due to hypercortisolism (Omenn, 1970). With more slowly growing malignancies and over a longer period, signs of Cushing's syndrome such as centripetal obesity, cutaneous striae, and osteoporosis may appear. With ectopic parathyroid hormone production, weakness, nausea, vomiting, loss of appetite, and weight loss due to hypercalcemia may occur, while over longer periods, renal stones, duodenal ulcer, pancreatitis, and bone disease may appear. These neoplasms are usually unresponsive to the physiologic feedback; hence, extremely high hormone concentrations and profound symptoms have been associated with tumor-produced syndromes. In obscure diagnostic problems, excessive hormone production by tumors should be kept in mind.

A clue to an unrecognized resectable primary tumor may occasionally be noted through one of these syndromes (Table 11–4). Furthermore, surgical removal of a tumor or effective radiation therapy to the tumor may "cure the endocrinopathy" as well as the underlying neoplasm. This has been most successful with malignancies associated with parathyroid hormone production. Tumor recurrence may also be reflected by estimations, both clinically and chemically, of hormonal secretion.

Liddle (1968), in reviewing progress in the characterization of tumor extracts and their comparison with normal hormones in terms of immunologic, biologic, and physical-chemical assays, noted no distinguishing features between tumor extracts and the normal hormones of parathyroid hormone, ACTH, and antidiuretic hormone. Furthermore, gonadotropin, thyrotropin, gastrin, and erythropoietin activities also resemble their normal hormone counterparts.

Although massive retroperitoneal tumors may be associated with hypoglycemia, there is no supporting evidence that these tumors produce insulin hypoglycemic mechanisms in such cases may include impaired gluconeogenesis and glucose consumption. The possibility that some of these tumors produce proinsulin, the form in which insulin is normally synthesized in the pancreas and not detectable by assay methods, remains to be established.

ADRENAL CORTEX

To appreciate fully the laboratory evaluation of adrenocortical function, a review of steroid nomenclature is essential. A group of biologically active organic compounds, to which the term steroid is applied, have in common a cyclopentanophenanthrene nucleus consisting of a five-carbon cyclopentane ring (D) fused to a phenanthrene (rings A, B, and C):

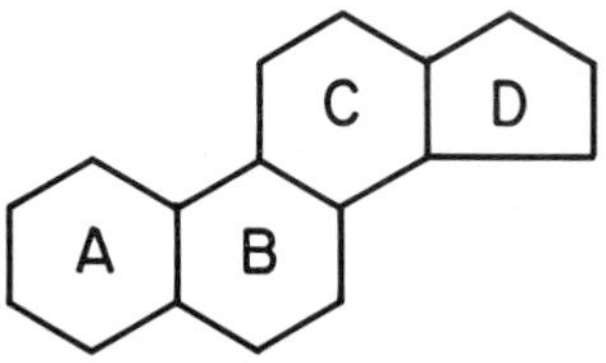

A standard numbering system is used to identify constituents in the nucleus and the frequently associated side chains.

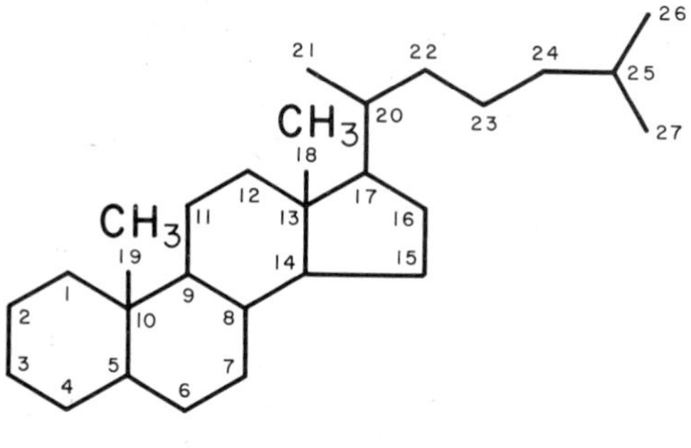

Unless otherwise indicated, it is assumed that the full complement of valence bonds for each carbon atom is satisfied by hydrogen and/or carbon atoms. Unsaturated carbons are indicated by double bonds. Angular methyl groups (18 and 19) are at the junctures of the A and B and C and D rings. Six asymmetric carbon atoms are common to two different rings:

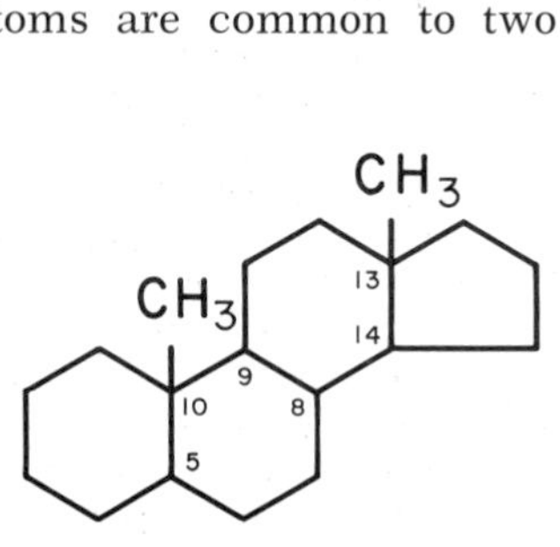

Although four of the six asymmetric carbon atoms are linked to three carbon atoms and carry only one hydrogen atom, carbons 10 and 13 (attached to angular methyl groups 18 and 19) are linked to four carbon atoms and carry no hydrogen atoms. Steroid molecules can be visualized as virtually flat structures with some substituents projecting below (away from the observer) and others projecting above (toward the observer). The angular methyl groups (18 and 19) are important reference points. The use of a solid line to attach them to carbons 10 and 13 indicates that carbons 18 and 19 are above the plane of the molecule; the use of a dotted line indicates that any constituent directly attached to the ring structure lies below this plane. Other groups connected to the nucleus by solid lines indicate a spatial configuration similar to the angular methyl groups; that is, they lie on the same side of the molecule. When a broken line is used to connect other groups to the phenanthrene nucleus, it means that they lie below the plane of the molecule and project downward. Groups that project in the same direction from the plane of the nucleus are stated to be *cis* to each other; those that project in different directions are *trans* to each other. Groups that are cis to the methyl reference group at position 19 are designated as β and are shown by solid valence lines; groups that are trans to the same points are designated as α and are dotted valence lines. The methyl groups at positions C-10 and C-13 are β in natural steroids, as is the chain attached at C-17 and the 11-hydroxyl group in certain adrenocorticosteroids. Many steroids have a hydroxyl group at C-3, which can exist in the two isomeric forms. The side chain attached at C-17 is written vertically to agree with the geometric configuration. Substituents attached to the side chain do not have geometric orientation, since the C-C bond attaching C-17 and C-20 is free to rotate. Groups attached to the side chain are given orientation in relation to those directly attached to the ring structure. By convention, the groups written to the right of the side chain are α oriented; those written to the left are β oriented.

The terminology can be better understood by a review of prefixes and suffixes used in steroid nomenclature (Table 11–5).

It is very desirable to employ chemical names of steroid compounds which have intrinsic meaning. Unfortunately the terminology is confused by use of other than chemical names for many compounds. Due to usage, these have become established and must also be recognized.

The parent structural compounds which are closely related to major physiological functions are shown in Figure 11–5.

Table 11–5. SUFFIXES AND PREFIXES FOR STEROIDS*

SUFFIX OR PREFIX	MEANING
Suffix	
-ane	Saturated hydrocarbon
-ene	Unsaturated hydrocarbon
-ol	Hydroxyl group, as in an alcohol or phenol
-one	Ketone group
Prefix	
hydroxy- (oxy-)	Hydroxyl group
keto- (oxo-)	Ketone group
deoxy-	Loss of an oxygen atom
dehydro-	Loss of two hydrogen atoms
dihydro-	Gain of two hydrogen atoms
cis-	Refers to spatial arrangement of two groups on the same side of the molecule
trans-	Refers to spatial arrangement of two groups on opposite sides of the molecule
α-	Refers to group which is *trans* to the methyl at C-10
β-	Refers to group which is *cis* to the methyl at C-10
epi-	Isomeric in configuration to a reference compound; specifically α at location C-3
iso-	Similar to epi-, but not restricted to C-3
allo-	Differing from reference compound in having 5α instead of 5β configuration; rings A and B in *trans* instead of *cis* relation to each other
etio-	Refers to final degradation product of a more complex molecule which still retains the essential chemical character of the original molecule
nor-	Refers to compound similar chemically to reference substance, but having one less carbon atom in side-chain
Δ	Indicates position of unsaturated linkage

*From A. Cantarow and B. Schepartz: Biochemistry. 4th edition. Philadelphia, W. B. Saunders Company, 1967.

The adrenal cortex, ovary, testis, and placenta form steroid compounds. The number of carbons permits characterization of three categories: (1) C-18 estrogens, (2) C-19 androgens, and (3) C-21 progestins and adrenal steroids or corticosteroids (Fig. 11–5). Further identification of compounds within these categories may be seen in Figures 11–6, 11–7, and 11–8. It is important to note that the A ring of estrogens is completely unsaturated (benzene ring). The C-19 steroids (C-19 compounds) in Figure 11–8 are of testicular and adrenocortical origin; they give rise to the urinary 17-ketosteroid assay substances. With this background, we can review the hormones of the adrenal cortex in reference to structure, biosynthesis, and metabolic action as related to laboratory measurements. In Figure 11–9 the adrenocortical hormones are separated into three groups vertically and two horizontally. The intermediate compound desoxycorticosterone with the addition of a hydroxyl group at C-11 becomes corticosterone, and with the loss of hydrogen it becomes dehydrocorticosterone. In a similar manner deoxycortisone (which is similar to desoxycorticosterone but has a hydroxyl group at C-17) with the addition of a hydroxyl becomes hydrocortisone (cortisol, compound F), and when the hydrogen is lost it becomes cortisone. In addition to the ketone at C-3, the C-4–C-5 bond is unsaturated in all these compounds. The difference between corticosterone series and hydrocortisone series (two horizontal groups) is at the 17 position, where a hydroxyl exists for hydrocortisone series. A great difference in function is apparent when the compounds are separated vertically into three groups. From a functional standpoint, these three vertical groups could be considered two pairs rather than three, although there is an overlap between the two. The column on

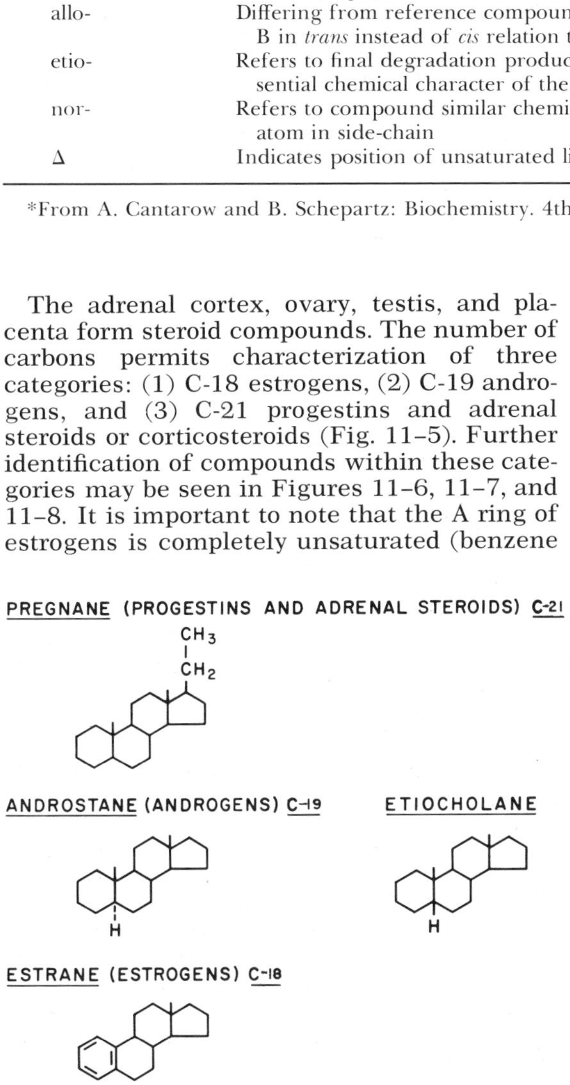

Figure 11-5. Parent structural compounds.

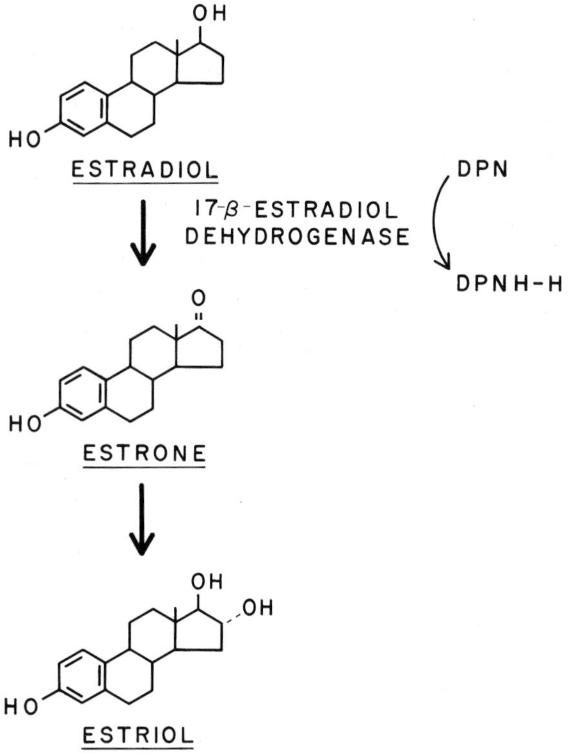

Figure 11-6. Estrogenic steroid hormones (C-18).

the left, which includes aldosterone, represents the mineralocorticoids, while the center column represents anti-inflammatory or glucocorticoid activity; those in the right column are degradative materials (Fig. 11–9).

Biosynthesis

The biosynthesis of adrenocorticosteroids may be seen in Figure 11–10. Cholesterol, the chief corticosteroid precursor, is synthesized in the adrenal cortex from acetate and also extracted from circulating blood. Biosynthesis proceeds so that the androgens and corticosteroid pathways are derived from Δ-5-pregnenolone. In man the major metabolic pathway involves the following steps successively: (1) 17-hydroxylation of progesterone to form 17-hydroxyprogesterone, (2) 21-hydroxylation of 17-hydroxyprogesterone to form 11-deoxycortisone (cortexolone, "S"), (3) 11-hydroxylation of deoxycortisone to form hydrocortisone (cortisol). Another pathway is (1) 17-hydroxylation of pregnenolone, (2) oxidation to form 17-hydroxyprogesterone, and then the subsequent steps to form cortisol. An alternate minor pathway involves successively: (1) 21-hydroxylation of progesterone to form desoxycorticosterone, (2) 11-hydroxylation of latter to corticosterone, (3) 18-hydroxylation of corticosterone that in turn is converted to aldosterone. The series of hydroxylation reactions (17, 21 and 11-hydroxylases) is preserved in both pathways, although the first step of hydroxylation (17) is omitted in the alternate minor pathway. These enzymes play a key role in the biosynthesis of the adrenocortical hormones. An appreciation of singular deficiencies in any one of these enzymes forms a basis for understanding the metabolic abnormalities and clinical manifestations of congenital adrenal hyperplasia (adrenogenital syndrome, or virilizing adrenal hyperplasia) which will be discussed later in this chapter.

In Figure 11–10 the formation of androgens and estrogens may also be identified. Pregnenolone undergoes 17-hydroxylation to form 17-hydroxypregnenolone; this compound enters into the formation of hydrocortisone (cortisol) as described previously (21- and 11-hydroxylation steps) and formation of androgens and estrogens by loss of the side chain to form dehydroepiandrosterone and oxidation to androstenedione.

Regulation of Adrenocorticosteroid Secretion. Zonal segregation of secretory activity is present in the adrenal cortex. Hydrocortisone (cortisol, or compound F), a glucocorticoid, is produced in zona fasciculata. In the zona

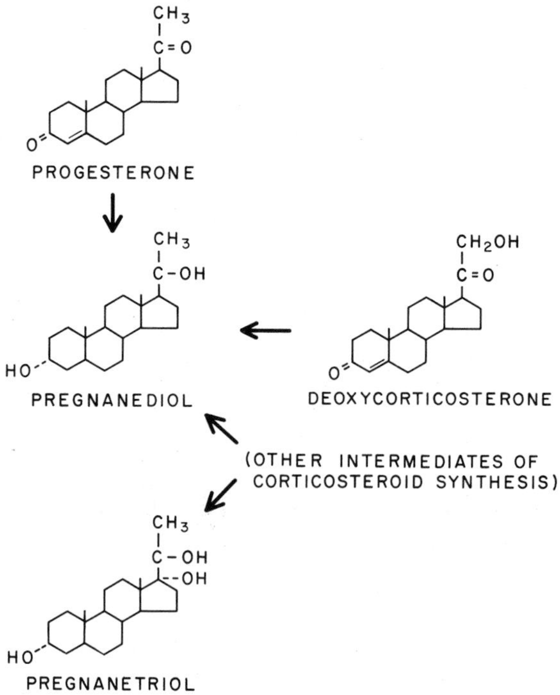

Figure 11-7. Pregnane progesterone steroid hormones (C-21).

TESTICULAR PRECURSORS
(17-KETOSTEROIDS)

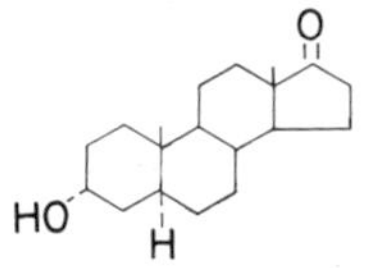

ANDROSTERONE

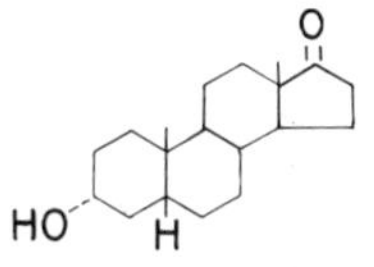

ETIOCHOLANOLONE

ADRENOCORTICAL PRECURSORS
(17-KETOSTEROIDS)

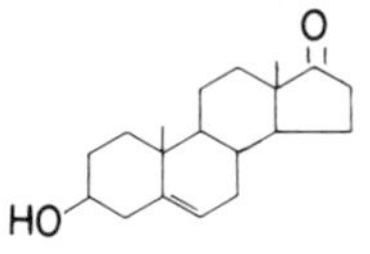

DEHYDROEPI-
ANDROSTERONE (DHA)

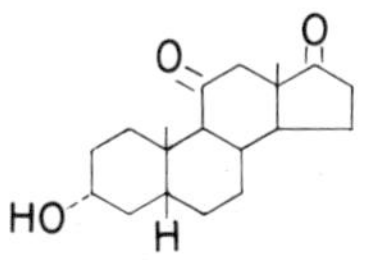

11-KETO-
ETIOCHOLANOLONE

TESTOSTERONE COMPOUNDS

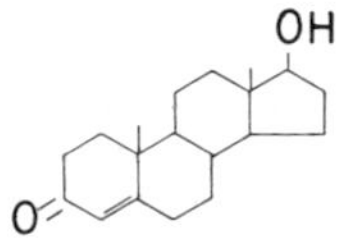

TESTOSTERONE

Figure 11-8. Androgenic steroid hormones (C-19).

reticularis, androgen production, especially dehydroepiandrosterone (DHA), is evident. Aldosterone, a mineralocorticoid, is produced in the zona glomerulosa. Corticosterone (compound B) is produced in all three zones. Apparently, 18-hydroxylase is present in significant quantities only in the zona glomerulosa and 17-hydroxylase only in the other two zones.

ACTH (adrenocorticotrophic hormone) stimulates the zona fasciculata most strikingly and results in a marked increase in the concentration of glucocorticoids in the blood and increased excretion of these hormones and their metabolites in the urine. The converse is observed after hypophysectomy. Adrenal cortisol secretion is regulated principally by ACTH. The rate-limiting step (conversion of cholesterol to pregnenolone) is influenced by ACTH, and cyclic AMP appears to be the intracellular mediator of the steroidogenic action of ACTH. An increase in the blood concentration of glucocorticoids causes a depression of ACTH secretion; if sufficiently high and for sufficient duration, it can result in adrenocortical atrophy comparable to that following hypophysectomy. A decrease in the concentration of blood glucocorticoids results in an increased secretion of ACTH.

The relative effectiveness of different adrenocortical hormones varies: hydrocortisone (cortisol, or compound F), the major physiological glucocorticoid in man, is most active. The negative *feedback mechanism* (ACTH versus compound F) appears to be the major and first controlling factor in normal subjects. Adrenalectomy results in elevated blood levels of ACTH. Hypothalamic CRF (corticotrophin releasing factor) provokes or controls the release of ACTH from the pituitary. The hypothalamic center is sensitive both to cortisol blood (tissue) levels and to stress (e.g., major surgical trauma, pyrogens, hypoglycemia, or electroshock). The latter, i.e., *stress*, appears to prevail, since minimal supraphysiologic quantities of cortisol suppress ACTH secretion in nonstressed subjects, but fail to control ACTH secretion during *major stress*. A third regulator of ACTH secretion is related to *sleep-wake habits* and results in an ACTH diurnal rhythm secretion. High levels of ACTH and, therefore, high levels of cortisol are observed usually at about the time of awakening, and low levels at about the time of sleep (Liddle, 1971). A fourth level of control, direct mediation by the adrenal cortex, may also exist.

Although ACTH is involved in the synthesis or production of aldosterone via corticosterone in biosynthesis, the secretion or release of aldosterone from the adrenal glands is also controlled by the renin-angiotensin system and by plasma potassium concentration. Possibly pituitary factors (other than ACTH) are necessary for a maximal adrenal aldosterone response.

The renin-angiotensin system is a major physiologic mechanism that controls body fluid volume by regulation of aldosterone secretion (Figs. 11–11 and 11–12). According to the excellent comprehensive review of the physiology of adrenal cortical function by Liddle (1971), cyclic AMP may be the intracellular mediator of the renin-stimulating action of catecholamines produced by reflex sympathetic nervous system activity from sodium loss (diuretic administration or salt restriction), blood loss or hemorrhage, and changes in posture through sequestration of venous blood (as occurs during the upright posture). In regard to the extrarenal mechanism for control of renin release, volume depletion appears to be a common denominator (Liddle, 1971). Aldosterone secretion is inversely related to extracellular fluid (especially plasma) volume and to the total body (especially serum) sodium. Sodium deprivation in man (low sodium diet) causes a fivefold increase in aldosterone secretion (e.g., 100 to 500 μg. per 24 hours), whereas a high sodium diet reduces secretion profoundly, e.g., 50 μg. or less per 24 hours. The renin-angiotensin sys-

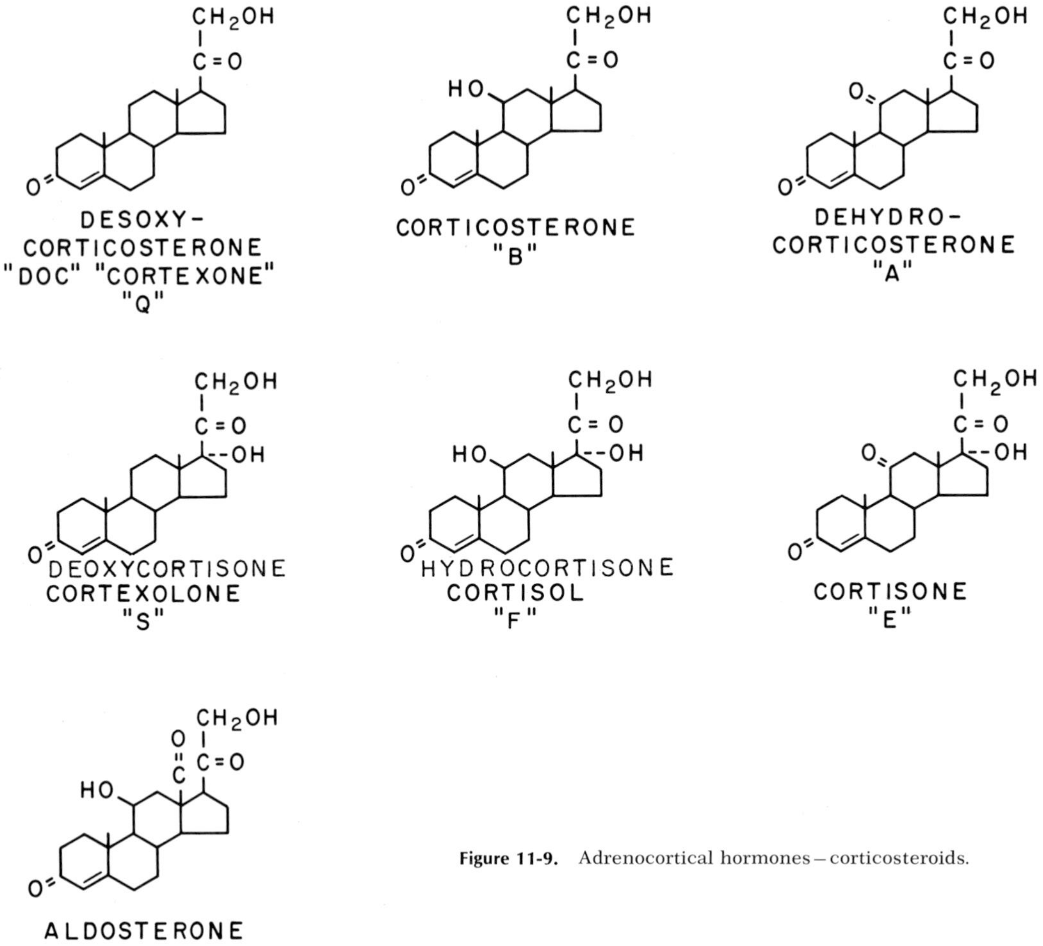

Figure 11-9. Adrenocortical hormones – corticosteroids.

tem (angiotensin II) stimulates aldosterone secretion as it does also glucocorticoid secretion. A low plasma volume or serum sodium will stimulate release of renin from the kidneys (juxtaglomerular apparatus) into the blood; renin (a proteolytic enzyme) in turn hydrolyzes angiotensinogen, an α-2-serum globulin produced in the liver, with formation of angiotensin I. A peptidase in normal blood plasma (pulmonary circulation) liberates angiotensin II from angiotensin I. Normally angiotensin II is rapidly destroyed by peptidases present in virtually all tissues (Figs. 11–11 and 11–12). Since it is the most powerful known vasopressor agent (direct action on peripheral arterioles), the persistence of angiotensin II may account for certain forms of hypertension. It is also the most potent stimulus for the production and release of aldosterone by the zona glomerulosa (Fig. 11–11). Indeed, a classic negative feedback control mechanism exists, with elevation of angiotensin inhibiting the production of renin with a consequent diminution in further generation of angiotensin (Liddle, 1971). A normal diurnal rhythm in renin secretion (exclusive of diurnal variations in posture and intake of fluid and food) is reflected in relatively high plasma renin activity levels during the night and morning with lower levels during the afternoon in normal subjects. This rhythm in renin levels also accounts for the lower aldosterone secretion during the afternoon than at other times of the day.

An increase in plasma potassium concentration causes an increase in aldosterone levels. This direct stimulation of adrenocortical production of aldosterone (presumably a transmembrane effect) reflects a potassium-mediated aldosterone control system in parallel with the renin-angiotensin system (Liddle, 1971). In renal failure, this potassium-mediated aldosterone control may be of even greater importance than the renin-angiotensin system. The fact that the renin-angiotensin

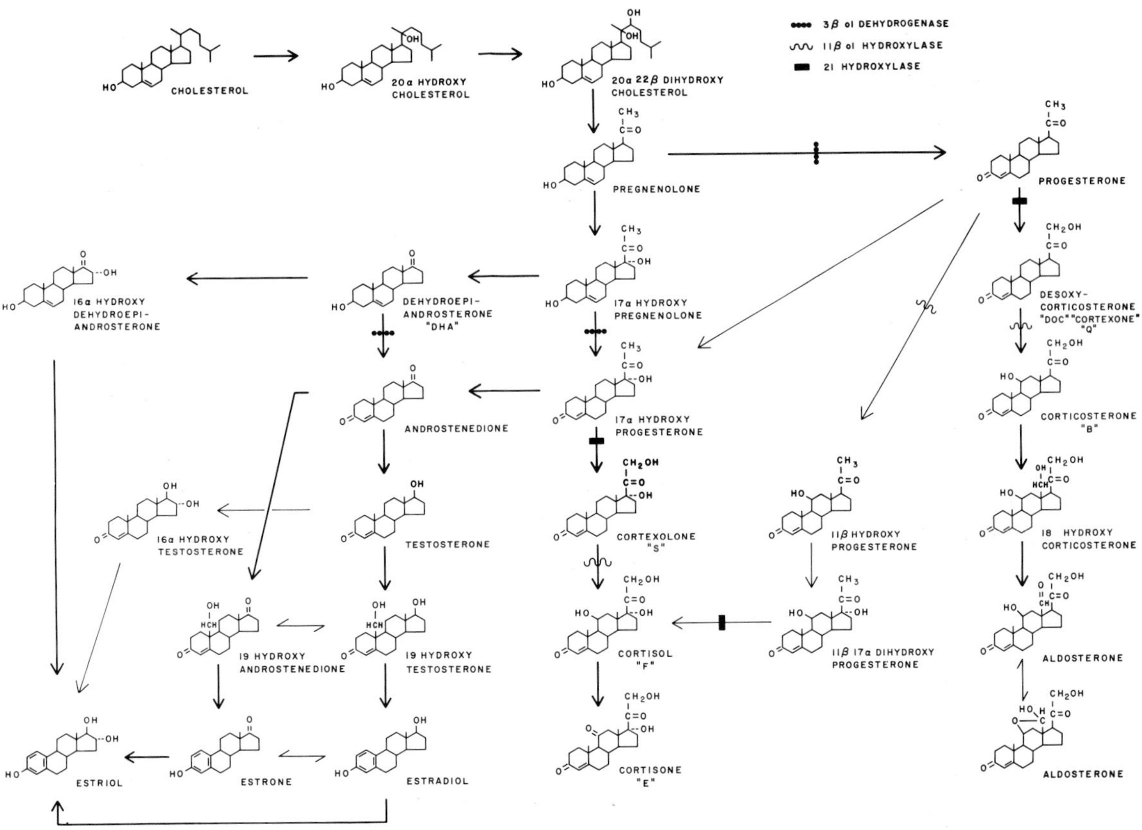

Figure 11–10. Synthesis and metabolism of adrenocortical hormones. (Courtesy of Dr. Ross Jacobs.)

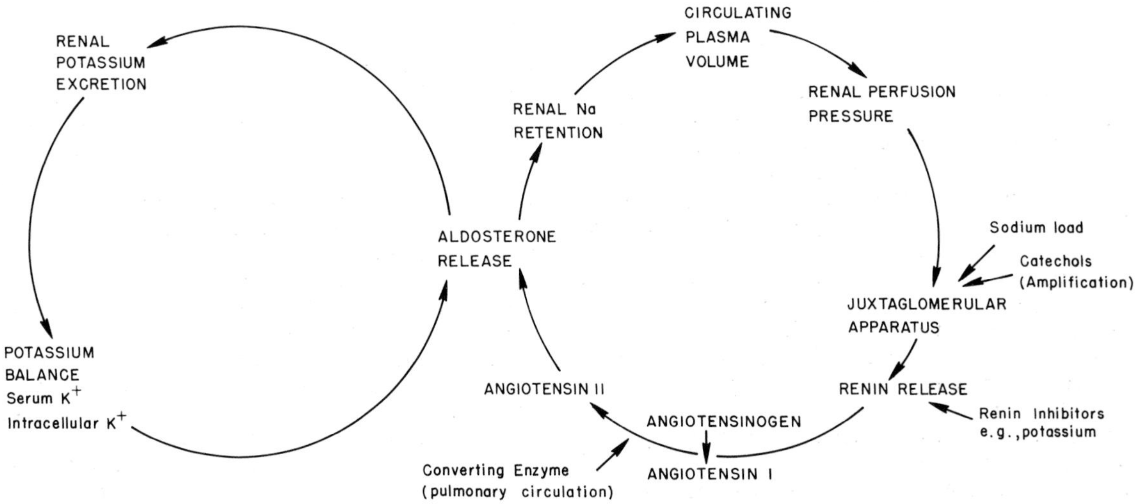

Figure 11-11. The interrelationship of the volume and potassium feedback loops on aldosterone secretion. Integration of signals from each loop determines the level of aldosterone secretion. Heparin and heparinoids inhibit aldosterone secretion through cytochemical alterations in the zona glomerulosa. (Modified from Williams, G. H., and Dluhy, R. G.: Amer. J. Med. 53:603, 1972.)

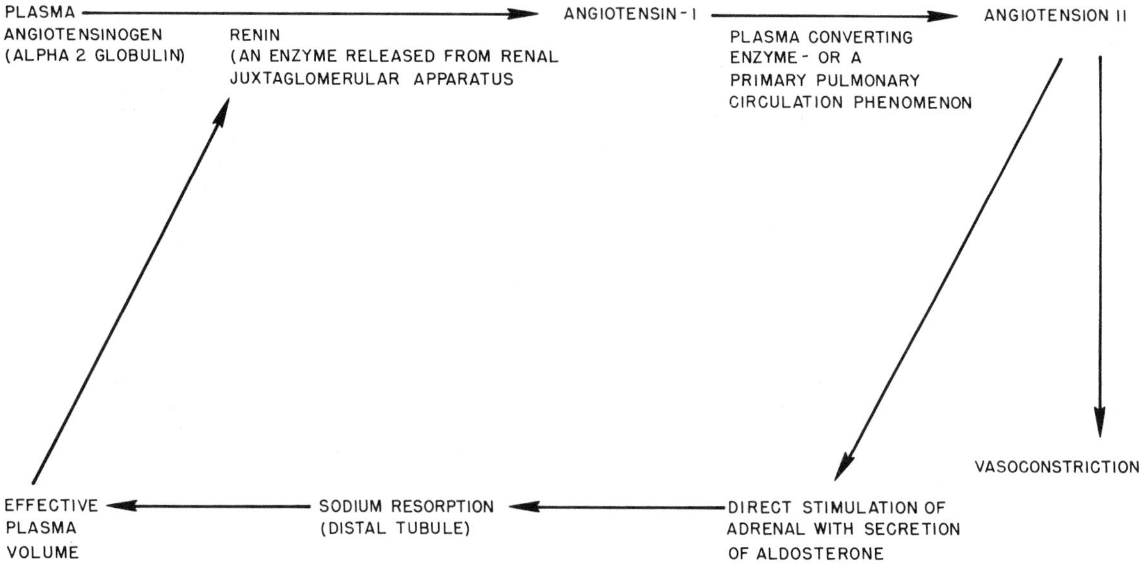

Figure 11-12. The renin-angiotensin system and aldosterone.

system is related to control of adrenal mineralocorticoid and glucocorticoid secretions permits one to understand clinical features of adrenal cortex disorders.

Transport, Metabolism, and Excretion. Salient features of transport, metabolism, and excretion are shown in Table 11-6. While the adrenal vein blood shows concentrations of about 300 μg. hydrocortisone and 80 μg. of corticosterone per 100 ml., the average blood plasma concentrations are as follows: hydrocortisone (cortisol, or compound F) 12 (5 to 25) μg. per 100 ml.; corticosterone (compound B) 1.0 (0.04 to 2.0) μg. per 100 ml.; aldosterone 0.05 (0.03 to 0.08) μg. per 100 ml.; DHA 0.5 (0.4 to 0.6) μg. per 100 ml. With normal plasma concentrations, about 10 per cent of the hydrocortisone is free, and 90 per cent is bound to protein (1/3 to albumin and 2/3 to α-2-globulin-transcortin); with elevated blood hydrocortisone levels, the binding capacity of transcortin (20 μg. per 100 ml.) is exceeded and the proportions bound to albumin and free increase. Protein binding not only facilitates plasma transport of corticoids; it may protect target organs from possible toxic effects of free hormone, and may prevent loss of hormones via glomerular filtration. Elevations of plasma cortisol following administration of estrogens (or contraceptive drugs with estrogenic activity) and during the third trimester of pregnancy are not associated with manifestations of hyperadrenocorticism since estrogen stimulates increased transcortin similar to the well known increase in thyroxine-binding globulin (TBG). Plasma cortisol concentration exhibits a diurnal rhythm in humans with maximum values at 8 A.M., falling subsequently to about 50 per cent or less between 4 P.M. and midnight. Because of this diurnal rhythm, plasma cortisol measurements sequentially should be performed on specimens collected at exactly the same hour each day.

The adrenocortical hormones are metabolized rapidly with loss of biologic activity (Table 11-6). Saturation of the A ring by hepatic reduction of the 4-5 double bond with formation of dihydro cortisol and further reduction of the 3-oxo group to form tetrahydro cortisol and finally conjugation of reduced steroid with glucuronic acid. The formation of a conjugate involves a 3-glucosiduronate or a 3-sulfate. Conjugates are water soluble and therefore are readily excreted by the kidneys. The major identifiable end-products of cortisol metabolism are tetrahydrocortisol (THF) glucuronide and tetrahydrocortisone (THE) glucuronide. However, urinary unconjugated cortisol parallels the level of unbound or free cortisol in the blood, and less than 1 per cent of daily cortisol secretion appears unaltered in the urine. Hence, urinary free corticoid assay (measuring urinary free cortisol, free cortisone, substance S, corticosterone, progesterone, and 17-hydroxyprogesterone) ranging between 16 and 71 μg./24 hours (average 33 μg./24 hours) in normal subjects may be the most important test for assessment of the physiologic status of adrenal glands in patients suspected of having either hypercortisolism or adrenal insufficiency (Hsu and Bledsoe, 1970).

In liver disease, e.g., cirrhosis and hypothyroidism, a relative hyperadrenocorticism is attributed to a prolonged "half-life" of corticoids; the major defect appears to be a decreased rate of reduction of the A ring and

Table 11–6. METABOLIC FATE OF CORTICOSTEROIDS

	GLUCOCORTICOIDS	MINERALOCORTICOIDS	ANDROGENS
Corticoids	Hydrocortisone (compound F, or cortisol) Corticosterone (compound B)	Aldosterone	Androstenedione Dehydroepiandrosterone (DHA) Adrenosterone (17-ketosteroids; weakly androgenic)
Blood	90 per cent protein bound (α globulin – 2/3 transcortin and 1/3 serum albumin) 10 per cent free (unbound)	Protein binding is minimal and primarily to albumin in a loose fashion	Two-thirds protein bound One-third unbound (free)
Liver	Reduced to biologically inactive dihydro and tetrahydro derivatives and conjugated with glucuronic acid Reduction of 3-ketone group and ring A Formation of dihydro and tetrahydro derivatives	Similar to glucocorticoids, but aldosterone is also conjugated at the 18 position with glucuronic acid	Similar to glucocorticoids plus conjugation with sulfate
Intestine	25 per cent excreted in bile as free and conjugated corticoids with enterohepatic circulation		
Kidneys	Excreted in urine mainly as inactive conjugates of tetrahydro derivatives Very little free corticoids in urine	Similar to glucocorticoids, but aldosterone is conjugated with glucuronic acid at the 18 position	Excreted in urine as glucuronide and sulfate conjugates DHA excreted partly unchanged
Conjugates			

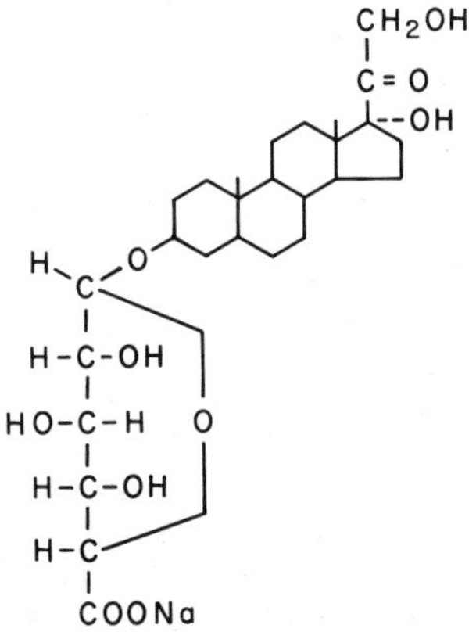

GLUCOSIDURONATE

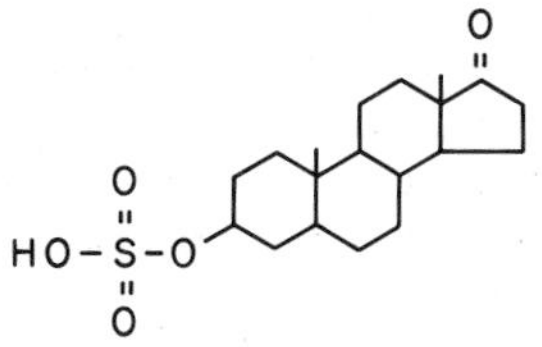

SULFATE

	HORMONES	PRINCIPAL METABOLITES
Male	Testosterone* (androgens)	Androsterone Etiocholanolone
Female	Follicular – estradiol Luteal – progesterone	Estrone and estriol† Pregnanediol‡

*Some biliary excretion.
†Excreted in urine as sulfates and glucuronides.
‡Excreted in urine as glucuronides.

conjugation with glucuronic acid. The turnover of plasma cortisol, however, is increased in hyperthyroidism and in simple obesity, i.e., decrease in half-life of disappearance of cortisol from plasma. Hence, through the action of the pituitary-adrenal negative feedback control system, there is a compensatory change in secretion, i.e., obese patients have high cortisol secretion rates and hypothyroid subjects have low secretion rates. Thus, "low" levels of plasma cortisol may be physiologic in patients with hepatic disease or hypothyroidism, while "high" levels may be physiologic in patients with simple obesity or hyperthyroidism. Furthermore, in severe renal disease, low urinary levels of corticosteroids do not signify hypoadrenalism, since renal excretion is impaired.

Hydrocortisone (cortisol, or compound F), cortisone (compound E), and deoxycortisone (compound S, or cortexolone) give rise to essentially similar metabolites. In part they are excreted in the urine unchanged except largely conjugated (glucuronide). Reduction at carbons 3, 4, and 5 and in part also at C-20 ketone (glycerol configuration) yields a saturated A ring as dihydro and tetrahydro derivatives, plus cortolone and cortol (Fig. 11–13); these are excreted in the urine as glucosiduronides. With removal of the side chain by virtue of the 17-hydroxy group, 17-ketosteroids of the C-19 type (11-hydroxy and 11-keto androsterones and etiocholanolone) are excreted in the urine mainly as sulfates and glucuronides. They account for about 10 per cent of the cortisol excreted. The androgenic effects of cortisol and cortisone when administered in large amounts are due to androsterone.

Corticosterone (compound B) also undergoes reduction to dihydro and tetrahydro derivatives that are biologically inactive due to loss of the α, β-unsaturated 3-ketone grouping in the A ring. Because it lacks a 17-hydroxy group, corticosterone cannot give rise to 17-ketosteroids.

Aldosterone also undergoes hepatic reduction to tetrahydro aldosterone and conjugation with a glucuronic acid which is excreted readily in the urine. In addition, both kidney and liver conjugate aldosterone at the 18 position with glucuronic acid, yielding a water soluble substance which is also readily excreted in the urine. This glucuronide is referred to as the "acid hydrolyzable" conjugate of aldosterone.

In summary, adrenocorticoids and their metabolites exist in urine mainly in the following forms: (1) biologically active compounds in their original forms (cortisol, corticosterone, aldosterone), (2) biologically inactive reduction products, free and mostly conjugated, (3) 17-ketosteroids, mainly conjugated (sulfates, glucosiduronides), with some biologically active (androgenic) and others inactive, (4) biologically inactive pregnanediol. In the adrenogenital syndrome, pregnanetriol may be excreted in the urine in significant amounts; this results from a congenital defect (absence) in hydroxylation reaction, i.e., absence of 11-hydroxylase or 21-hydroxylase.

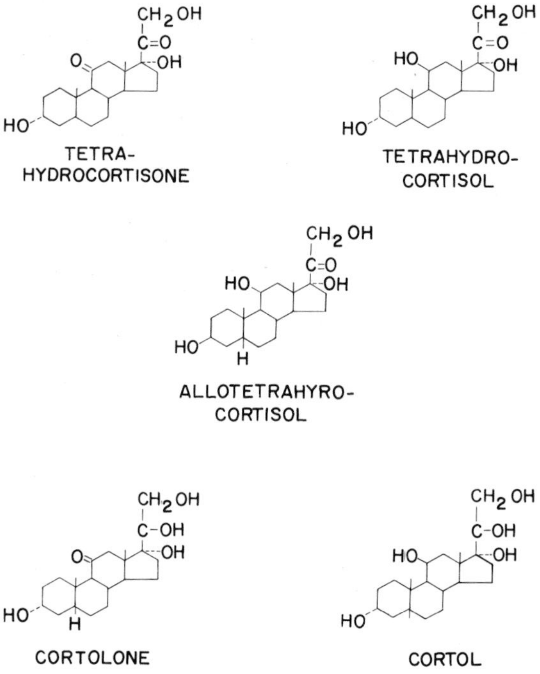

Figure 11-13. Urinary corticoids.

Evaluation of adrenocortical functional activity is usually carried out by measuring urinary excretion of these substances, so it is important to understand their origin and fate for a critical appraisal of data.

Biological Effects and Diagnostic Methods

A consideration of the biological effects or actions of corticosteroids permits a diagnostic approach to evaluation of adrenocortical function (Table 11–7).

Cortisol (compound F, or hydrocortisone) is quantitatively the major circulating C-21 adrenocorticosteroid and exemplifies glucocorticoid effects with characteristic metabolic changes in carbohydrate, protein, and fat metabolism.

Aldosterone is the principal mineralocorticoid that reflects electrolyte and water metabolic changes; it is 20 to 50 times more potent than desoxycorticosterone (DOC) in sodium-retaining influence at the distal tubular level of the kidneys.

A quantitative as well as qualitative overlap exists between these two broad categories in metabolic effects. Hence, glucocorticoids have an important effect upon sodium and water metabolism; it may be synergistic and thus critical but of a lesser magnitude. Furthermore, aldosterone causes glycogen deposition but its activity is about one-third that of cortisone and two-thirds that of corticosterone (Fig. 11–9).

A summary of major biologic effects of a representative hormone from each of the three functional categories with suggested diagnostic procedure is presented in Table 11–7.

At the cellular level, aldosterone promotes a shift of potassium (K^+) ions from intracellular to extracellular fluid compartments in exchange for Na^+ and H^+ ions which pass in the opposite direction. At the renal level, aldosterone enhances Na^+ reabsorption from ascending loop of Henle and promotes in the distal convoluted tubular cell reabsorption of Na with bicarbonate and water by exchange with K^+ and H^+ ions; it also enhances Na^+ exchange for NH_4^+ in collecting duct cells. Hence, the plasma sodium concentration elevation with hypervolemia (which may be modified by hydration) is associated with a hypokalemic

Table 11–7. ADRENOCORTICAL HORMONES: EFFECTS AND DIAGNOSTIC APPROACH

REPRESENTATIVE HORMONE	BIOLOGICAL EFFECTS	DIAGNOSTIC PROCEDURES
Cortisol (compound F or hydrocortisone)	Gluconeogenesis Protein nitrogen catabolism increase and anabolism decrease Increased blood glucose concentration Decreased glucose tolerance Increased liver glycogen Increased liver glycogenolysis Decreased peripheral uptake and utilization of glucose Decrease synthesis of acid sulfated mucopolysaccharides Fat synthesis and redistribution Cellular or tissue effects Anti-inflammatory (retardation of inflammatory reactions) Dissolution of lymphoid tissue Lymphopenia Eosinopenia Increased erythropoiesis Alteration of cellular permeability, especially decreased membrane permeability to water Increased gastric (HCl and pepsin) secretion	Carbohydrate (glucose tolerance) function test Eosinophil count Water load test Urine calcium with low calcium intake Plasma and urinary hydroxycorticoids plus ACTH stimulation or specific suppressive tests
Aldosterone	Electrolyte regulation Sodium (Na) retention Potassium (K) excretion Retention of water and expansion of extracellular fluid volume Hypertension	Na:K ratio in saliva and sweat Plasma electrolytes Urine electrolytes (Na, K) with low sodium intake EKG for K effect Urinary aldosterone
Androgens (C-19 compounds, adrenosterone)	Protein nitrogen anabolism Growth and maturation—osseous and muscular Body hair (pubic and axillary) Seborrhea	Urinary 17-ketosteroids Dehydroepiandrosterone (DHA)

alkalosis; urinary sodium excretion is decreased but urinary potassium excretion is increased. Similar effects are observed in regard to decreased Na but increased K concentrations in salivary, sweat, and intestinal secretions.

In regard to water, adrenocortical insufficiency (Addison's disease or hypoadrenocorticism) is characterized by hypernatruria (excessive sodium excretion) with inability to excrete a large water load at a normal rate; normal excretion is restored by glucocorticoids (cortisol) but not by aldosterone or desoxycorticosterone. At least in part, this action is dependent on a cortisol-facilitated control of permeability in the distal tubule, and also in part, is secondary to the maintenance of a normal distribution of body water between the extracellular (ECV) and intracellular (ICV) compartments. Indeed, there is extracellular dehydration, intracellular overhydration, and an increase in total body water in the absence of cortisol. A decrease in plasma volume (ECV or extracellular volume) associated with dehydration or loss of body water may lead to hypotension (shock) with hyperkalemia and metabolic acidosis in classic severe Addison's disease (Addisonian crisis).

Tests of water-loading measure the percentage excretion of a given water load over a specified period of time, e.g., over 50 per cent of 1500 ml. of water ingested is excreted within 4 hours in normal subjects. Patients with hypoadrenocorticism will retain the water for an abnormally long period of time.

Cortisol (compound F, or hydrocortisone) is the most potent glucocorticoid; cortisone (compound E) is about two-thirds as active; and corticosterone (compound A) is about one-third as active. In addition to gluconeogenesis by cortisol, insulin may be antagonized by glucocorticoids, since an increased sensitivity to insulin is noted with hypoadrenocorticism that ameliorates diabetes produced by pancreatectomy or alloxan. Administration of cortisol and hyperadrenocorticism (Cushing's syndrome) aggravates (may unmask) diabetes mellitus. Hence, there is diagnostic importance of blood glucose measurements with hypoglycemia in Addison's disease and diabetes in Cushing's syndrome.

Cortisol may also be antagonistic in terms of physiologic effects with two other hormones. Such consideration at least helps one to understand the clinical features of Addison's disease. The release of posterior pituitary antidiuretic hormone (ADH) appears to be opposed by cortisol, perhaps through plasma volume expansion. Secondly, a reciprocal relationship between plasma cortisol concentration upon release of melanocyte-stimulating hormone (MSH) from anterior pituitary is analogous to that between cortisol (hydrocortisone) and ACTH. Thus, increased skin pigmentation in Addison's disease may be due to high plasma concentrations of MSH in presence of decreased cortisol levels that fail to suppress MSH release. Administration of cortisol decreases MSH plasma levels in such conditions. There is also some evidence that ACTH *per se* may have a melanocyte-stimulating action, due to structural similarities between ACTH and MSH.

Osteoporosis observed with administration of glucocorticoids and in hyperadrenocorticism may be attributed to the following: (1) a possible decrease in synthesis of acid mucopolysaccharides (chondroitin sulfate), (2) protein catabolism and antianabolism, (3) hypercalciuria secondary to loss of bone matrix from above effects, and (4) decreased intestinal absorption of calcium secondary to interference with the effect of reactive metabolite of vitamin D on the mucosal transport mechanism (Kimberg, 1969).

Measurement of Adrenocorticosteroids (Corticoids, Corticosteroids)

Plasma and 24-hour urine specimens are most frequently used for such steroid measurements. From the standpoint of methodology, three determinations may be considered with a separate discussion of aldosterone with the renin-angiotensin system.

17-Ketosteroids (17-KS, Neutral 17-Ketosteroids). These are substances that are determined colorimetrically (Zimmermann reaction) and reflect metabolites of adrenal and testicular steroids excreted as 17-ketones in the urine. In normal adults the adrenal cortex is responsible for about two-thirds to three-fourths of the total 17-ketosteroids in men (one-fourth from testes) and for practically the total quantity in women; ovarian stroma may contribute a trace amount. While the 17-ketosteroids arise from secretion of C-19 type corticoids (androgens), they can also result from the catabolism of C-21 type corticoids (e.g., 17-hydroxyprogesterone and pregnenolone), as may be seen in Figure 11–10. The major 17-ketosteroids (17-KS) isolated from urine of normal humans are shown in Figure 11–8. They may be grouped into the alpha fraction (principally androsterone and etiocholanolone) and a beta fraction (principally dehydroepiandrosterone or DHA) as reflected by stereoisomers formed by a hydroxyl group (OH) on carbon-3 (i.e., lines dotted for alpha and solid for beta). Since these compounds possess very weak androgenic properties, urinary 17-ketosteroid measurements may not yield confirmatory data in appropriate clinical conditions.

Table 11–8. SULFATE AND GLUCURONIDE CONJUGATES OF ANDROGENS IN HUMAN PLASMA*

ANDROGENS	CONJUGATED ANDROGENS IN PLASMA (μg./100 ml.)				
	Adult Males	Adult Females	Females at Delivery	Umbilical Cord	Prepuberty Children <7 yr.
Sulfates					
Dehydroepiandrosterone	126 ± 34	113 ± 28	38 ± 20	91 ± 37	6.0 ± 4.5
Androsterone	43 ± 12	36 ± 9	28 ± 9	33 ± 10	1.5 ± 0.6
Etiocholanolone	1.5 ± 0.4	1.7 ± 0.6	—	—	—
Testosterone	0.11 ± 0.05	0.02 ± 0.01	—	—	—
Glucuronides					
Androsterone	2.2 ± 0.6	1.5 ± 0.3	—	—	—
Etiocholanolone	1.8 ± 0.7	1.5 ± 0.5	—	—	—

*Modified from Migeon, C. J.: Amer. J. Med. *53*:612, 1972.

However, the 17-ketosteroids serve as a rough guide to androgenic activity, since androsterone and dehydroepiandrosterone (DHA) cause some stimulation of secondary male characteristics. However, urinary 17-KS assay does not measure biologically active androgenic hormones but their metabolites, and only a fraction are excreted as urinary 17-KS. Testosterone (perhaps dihydrotestosterone), the most potent androgen, is not a 17-ketosteroid, so it is not reflected in 17-ketosteroid assays. Demetriou and Austin (1970) have reported a competitive protein-binding assay for plasma testosterone requiring small volumes of specimen and apparent ease in performance.

Table 11–8 shows the conjugated androgens found in normal subjects' peripheral blood plasma. Of all the androgens present in peripheral plasma, DHA (dehydroepiandrosterone or dehydroisoandrosterone) and androsterone are present in the largest concentrations as sulfate conjugates (Migeon, 1972). The glucuronide conjugates of androsterone and etiocholanolone are present in the next largest amount in the circulation. Gas-liquid chromatography using a flame ionization detector is employed to measure conjugates after hydrolysis and extraction. Among the plasma unconjugated androgens, testosterone arises mainly from testes in men and from the peripheral conversion of androstenedione in women (Table 11–9). Rather than testosterone, dihydrotestosterone, mainly a product of testosterone metabolism in men (i.e., testosterone, 60 per cent; androstenedione, 15 per cent; and balance, 25 per cent direct secretion from testes), but in women virtually all from androstenedione, might be the biologically active form of androgens in adults (Migeon, 1972). Hence, in women androstenedione of adrenal origin contributes significantly to the level of androgenic activity, while in men this contribution is nil (Migeon, 1972). Androstenedione and its 11-β-hydroxy derivative and dehydroepiandrosterone are derived mainly from the adrenal, while androsterone and etiocholanolone are metabolites primarily of androstenedione (Migeon, 1972).

Radioimmunoassay is the best technique to measure plasma or serum testosterone and dihydrotestosterone levels as well as dehydroepiandrosterone (DHA) and other androgens (Migeon, 1972). Urinary methods are not reliable indicators of androgen secretion because

Table 11–9. UNCONJUGATED ANDROGENS IN HUMAN PLASMA* †

ANDROGENS	UNCONJUGATED ANDROGENS IN PLASMA (ng./100 ml.)					
	Adult Males	Adult Females	Pregnant Females	Females at Delivery	Umbilical Cord	Prepuberty Children <7 yr.
Testosterone	559 ± 151	48 ± 14	114 ± 38	134 ± 72	46 ± 24	11.5 ± 4.5
Androstenedione	114 ± 21	180 ± 58	249 ± 82	387 ± 176	126 ± 58	21 ± 12
Dehydroepiandrosterone	553 ± 178	534 ± 157	363 ± 233	1016 ± 806	203 ± 139	39 ± 28
Dihydrotestosterone	50 ± 14	22 ± 4	—	—	—	—
11β-OH-Androstenedione	200 ± 80	180 ± 80	—	—	—	—

*Modified from Migeon, C. J.: Amer. J. Med. *53*:616, 1172.

†Androsterone (160 ± 80 ng./100 ml. in men; 70 ± 30 ng./100 ml. in women) and etiocholanolone (70 ± 60 ng./100 ml. in men; 180 ± 80 ng./100 ml. in women) also present in plasma.

of the interconversion of androgens and dynamics of metabolism. Free testosterone plus protein-bound testosterone comprise total plasma testosterone that, in turn, reflects changes in binding protein concentration, i.e., elevation with pregnancy and administration of contraceptives containing estrogen. Since terminal hair growth and acne have been found in patients without elevated plasma testosterone, it has been suggested that there may be an elevated free fraction of testosterone since this is the physiologically active component (Ettinger *et al.*, 1973); other mechanisms suggested include increased testosterone, turnover, another active androgen, e.g., dihydrotestosterone, and increased end-organ sensitivity characterized by elevated local production of follicular testosterone and dihydrotestosterone.

A flow chart for urinary 17-ketosteroid determination is shown in Figure 11-14. With gas chromatographic measurements, the individual 17-ketosteroid as well as pregnanediol and pregnanetriol compounds can be identified and quantitated so that ketonic fractionation, if not the entire procedure, may be abandoned in the future (Chattoraj, 1970). With the usual endpoint of most determinations at the neutral fraction level, the Zimmermann reaction is applied. It is shown as follows as a reaction between the metadinitrobenzene and an active methylene group (carbon 16) of 17-ketosteroids.

A blue-violet color reaction product is also given by compounds with a ketone at carbon 11.

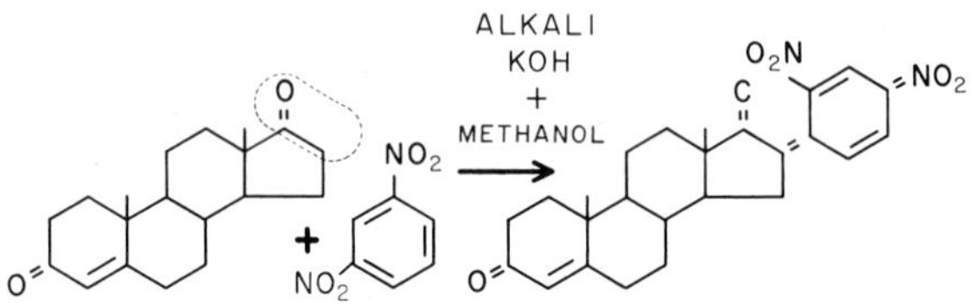

After age 60 the adult values shown in Figure 11-14 decline progressively. A signifi-

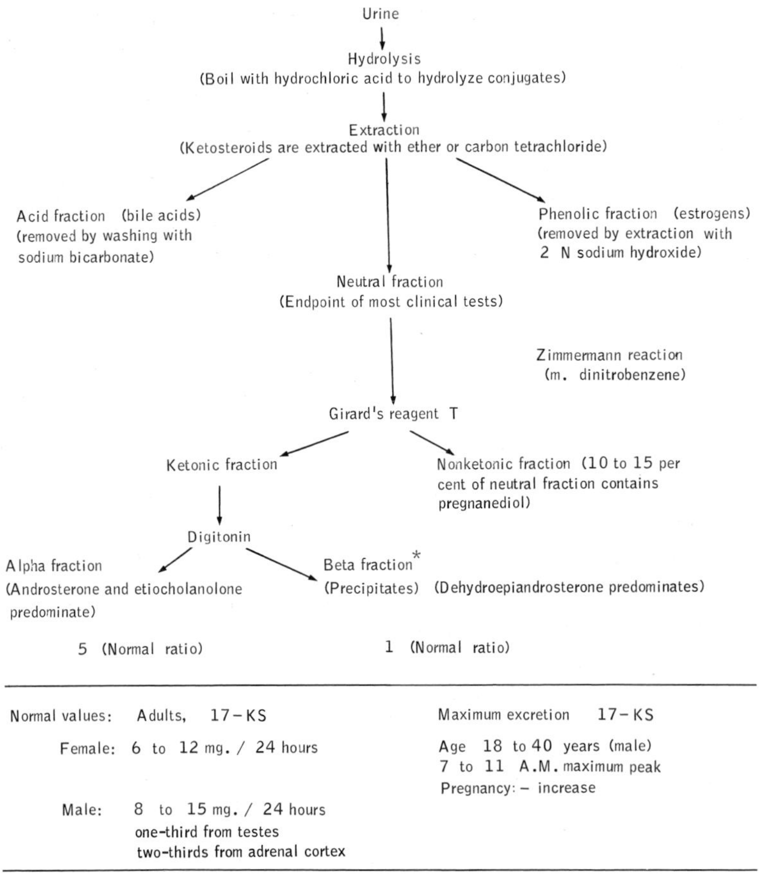

Figure 11-14. Flow chart for extraction of 17-ketosteroids (17-KS) from urine. *In carcinoma of adrenal cortex, beta fraction predominates.

cant daily variation in urinary 17-ketosteroids is observed in individual subjects. Furthermore, in children of both sexes a range of normal values are found as follows:

First year – less than 1 mg. per 24-hour urine
1 to 4 years – less than 2 mg. per 24-hour urine
5 to 8 years – less than 3 mg. per 24-hour urine
13 to 16 years – 3 to 10 mg. per 24-hour urine

Clinical correlations of urinary 17-ketosteroids measurements are shown in Table 11–10. Increased values are most striking with adrenocortical tumors, especially malignant forms (usually 30 to 100 mg., but as high as 1000 mg. per 24 hours). In adrenal carcinoma there is an increase in the beta fraction, usually due to an increase in DHA (dehydroepiandrosterone). Relatively low levels are often associated with benign tumors. If hyperplasia develops before puberty, the elevation of 17-ketosteroids is greater than if hyperplasia develops after puberty. The Cushing syndrome or adrenogenital syndrome may show adenoma, hyperplasia, or, rarely, carcinoma as the pathologic lesion responsible for functional derangement; hyperplasia is the most frequent cause of the adrenogenital syndrome. In Addison's disease the most profound depression of 17-ketosteroid levels (1 to 5 mg. per 24 hours) is observed, as they are also in panhypopituitarism. The decreased levels in other disorders listed show progressively lesser depressions of urinary 17-ketosteroid values.

17-Hydroxycorticosteroids (17-OH-Corticoids or Porter-Silber Chromogens). C-21 adrenocorticosteroids containing a dihydroxyacetone group at carbons 19, 20, and 21 react with phenylhydrazine in the Porter-Silber reaction:

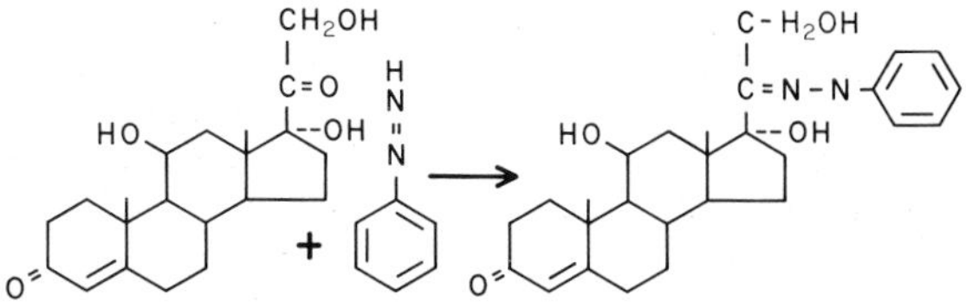

This determination is a sensitive index of adrenocortical function, since it measures a major portion of corticoid secretion in adrenal vein, i.e., hydrocortisone (cortisol, or compound F) and deoxycortisone (compound S), as well as their tetrahydroderivatives (THF, THE, and THS). In addition to urine 17-OH-corticoids, this method is also used for blood corticoids, since cortisol (compound F, or hydrocortisone) is the major component of blood corticoids.

Since the dihydroxyacetone side chain is labile to acid hydrolysis employed in urinary 17-ketosteroid assay, an aliquot of urine is subjected to β-glucuronidase in order to hydrolyze the conjugates of cortisol (hydrocortisone, compound F), cortisone (compound E), and deoxycortisone (compound S) and their tetrahydro derivatives (THF, THE and THS). Subsequent organic solvent extraction of urine and/or purification by column chromatography isolates free steroids that are subjected to Porter-Silber reagent (phenylhydrazine-sulfuric acid) and measured spectrophotometrically (Fig. 11–13).

This method does not measure all the 17-OH-corticosteroids excreted in certain pathologic states, i.e., pregnanetriol and other 20-OH compounds which may be strikingly increased and comprise a major fraction of the total urinary 17-hydroxycorticosteroids.

Urinary free (unconjugated) cortisol (30 to

Table 11–10. CLINICAL CORRELATIONS: URINARY 17-KETOSTEROIDS

INCREASED VALUES	DECREASED VALUES
Adrenocortical carcinoma Adrenocortical adenoma Adrenocortical hyperplasia	Addison's disease Panhypopituitarism Myxedema
Acromegaly (vary from low, normal to high)	Nephrotic syndrome
Virilizing ovarian syndrome (arrhenoblastoma, hilar cell tumor, adrenal rest tumor, Stein-Leventhal syndrome)	Chronic illness with debility
Testicular tumors (teratoma, interstitial cell) gonadotropin-producing tumors in male	Gout
Pregnancy – last trimester	Castration of male or eunuchoidism
Hirsutism, occasionally ACTH therapy Stress, severe	Thyrotoxicosis Female hypogonadism Diabetes mellitus

150 μg. per 24 hours) is the urinary reflection of the unbound plasma 17-hydroxycorticoids. Even though it is in the range of 1 per cent of the adrenal production of cortisol excreted, the amount not only correlates with the amount secreted, but also is a better reflection of the mean nonprotein-bound (free) plasma cortisol for the period during which the collection is made than are plasma cortisol or plasma 17-hydroxycorticosteroids. Because of the fluctuating plasma cortisol levels during much of the day, and since the diffusable or free cortisol is the component which is metabolically active, urinary cortisol level is a more valid estimate of adrenal cortical activity (Tyler and West, 1972). The measurement of urinary free corticoids by competitive protein-binding radioassay appears to represent the best single test to assess adrenal cortical function in patients suspected of having either hypercortisolism or adrenal insufficiency (Hsu and Bledsoe, 1970). In normal subjects urinary free corticoids excretion ranged between 16 and 71 μg. per 24 hours, with an average of 33 μg.

Plasma hydroxycorticosteroid measurements employing fluorescence (Mattingly, 1962) are more sensitive, requiring smaller specimen volumes, but are less specific than the Porter-Silber reaction. From heparinized whole blood, the plasma must be separated promptly because erythrocyte uptake of corticosteroids increases on standing; nor should plasma be frozen (store at 1 to 4° C.), since this may produce a precipitate which may trap or absorb steroids, causing low results. In one of the many procedures described free and protein-bound cortisol are extracted from plasma with dichloromethane; the organic extract shaken with a sulfuric acid-ethanol reagent with subsequent removal of supernatant dichloromethane yields a fluorescence of acid solution that is read fluorimetrically at a specific time with specific excitation and emission wavelengths and compared with that of a known concentration of cortisol treated in the same manner. Corticosteroids measured include cortisol, corticosterone, and 20-dihydrocortisol, but the last two steroids normally are not present in amounts comparable to cortisol. Estrogens (especially estradiol), which fortunately are present in negligible quantities even in the plasma of pregnant women, also produce fluorescence. Since the emission spectrum of spironolactone is identical to cortisol, misleading elevations of plasma cortisol levels have been observed in patients treated with spironolactone (Lurie, 1970). Therapy with triparanol may also lead to falsely high values. Patients taking contraceptive drugs (estrogenic compounds) which increase cortisol-binding globulin (CBG) also show spuriously high results, as with other plasma cortisol methods. Plasma cortisol is also determined by the method of Murphy (1967), employing competitive protein-binding or displacement technique described subsequently. Utilizing the steroid-binding properties of corticosteroid-binding globulin (CBG, transcortin) has permitted an increased sensitivity and specificity with little or no preliminary purification for plasma or urine. Other steroids, including corticosterone, cortisone, 11-desoxycortisol, corticoids (F, B, S), progesterone, and 17 α-OH-progesterone may be measured by this technique (Murphy, 1967).

In addition to great sensitivity, the particular advantage of competitive protein-binding (CPB) analyses is the virtual absence of effects due to nonsteroidal substances, making special preparation of reagents and special handling of glassware virtually unnecessary. CPB radioassays employ three basic steps, as shown in Table 11–11. First, the binding proteins in the plasma must be removed; otherwise, they would act in the same way as the assay protein. Second, the extracted hormone is then mixed with a known amount of CBG (cortisol-binding globulin) and radioactive tracer hormone. Assay conditions are chosen so that the CBG is just saturated with tracer steroid. Because the tracer steroid bound to the CBG is in dynamic equilibrium with unbound tracer steroid, the steroid of the sample displaces a portion of the tracer and the percentage of tracer bound to the CBG falls proportionally. Third, the protein-bound and unbound fractions are separated and the distribution of the tracer is determined. Quantification of the steroid in the sample is achieved by comparing its displacement of tracer with that caused by known amounts of the same steroid. A curve may be drawn by plotting the percentage of bound tracer against the amount of steroid added. If the reciprocal of the per cent bound steroid is used, essentially a straight line relationship is obtained over the most usable range. Because time required to count the protein-bound fraction to a preset number of counts is proportional to the reciprocal of the per cent bound steroid, it is much more convenient to plot the time required to reach a preset count vs. the amount of steroid added, since no calculations are necessary (Murphy, 1967).

Normal values are presented in Table 11–12. Low or low normal values are present in Addison's disease, myxedema, and hypopituitarism. The most striking elevations are observed in Cushing's syndrome (not all cases), in which diurnal plasma cortisol variation is absent, and in extreme stress, as well as in eclampsia and acute pancreatitis. Slight increases are seen in the first trimester of pregnancy, virilism, obesity, hyperthyroidism, and in severe hypertension. Moderate elevations

Table 11–11. COMPETITIVE PROTEIN-BINDING ANALYSIS*

STEP	PURPOSE	MEANS
A. Deproteinization	Destroys or removes binding protein from sample	Heat Alcohol Methylene chloride
B. Quantitation: 1. Equilibration with tracer and assay	Sample steroid displaces tracer from assay protein in proportion to the amount present	Mix at room temperature, cool to 10° C. or lower (binding varies with temperature)
2. Separation of protein-bound and unbound steroid	Permits one or both fractions to be counted	Dialysis Electrophoresis Gel filtration Ion exchange resins Protein precipitation Adsorption of unbound fraction to insoluble particles e.g., Fuller's earth } aluminum Lloyd;s reagent } silicates Florisil – magnesium silicate Coated charcoal

*With permission of Murphy, B. E. P.: J. Clin. Endocr. *27*:974, 1967.

may be associated with stress of infectious diseases, surgery, and burns.

17-Ketogenic Steroids (17-KGS, Ketogenic Corticoids, Ketogenics, and Total Ketogenic Corticoids). The Porter-Silber reaction does not measure all the 17-hydroxycorticoids, such as C-20 reduced derivatives of compounds F, E, and S and abnormal elevations of the following corticoids frequently seen in adrenogenital syndrome and occasionally in Cushing's syndrome: pregnanetriol, 17-hydroxyprogesterone, and 17-hydroxypregnenolone. Hence, a meas-

Table 11–12. NORMAL URINARY STEROID VALUES EXPRESSED AS MILLIGRAMS PER 24 HOURS IN RELATION TO AGE AND SEX

	AGE (YR.)	MEN	WOMEN
17 Ketosteroids (17-KS)	2–5	<2	<2
	5–10	3–6	3–6
	10–15	6–15	5–11
	15–60	8–20	5–15
	60–90	5–20	3–13
17 Hydroxycorticosteroids			
1. Ketogenic steroids (17-KGS)	2–5	1–5	1–5
	5–10	2–9	2–9
	20–50	11–22	7–18
	over 50	14–24	10–22
2. Porter-Silber chromogens (17-OH corticosteroids or 17-21 dihydroxy-20 ketosteroids)	0–2	2–4	2–4
	2–6	3–6	3–6
	6–10	4–8	4–8
	10–14	4–10	4–10
	Adult	5–15	5–13
Progesterone derivatives			
Pregnanetriol	0–6	<0.2	<0.2
	7–16	<1.1	<1.1
	16-Adult	<3.5	<3.5
	Late Pregnancy	Up to 7.2	Up to 7.2

urement that will include a more total assessment of adrenocorticoid secretion was evolved as urinary 17-ketogenic steroid assay. Two conversion steps consisting of reduction followed by oxidation are carried out as follows:

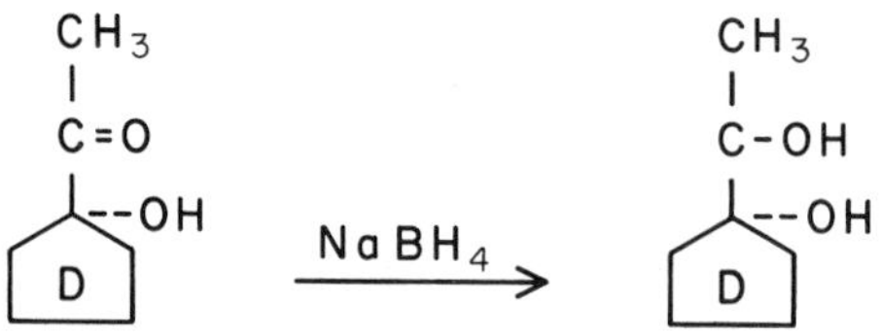

21-DEOXYKETOL
17-OH-PROGESTERONE

GLYCOL

Borohydride reduces 17-OH-corticosteroids with a hydroxyl at carbon 17, a ketone at C-20, and a C-21 methyl. This configuration is not oxidized by bismuthate or periodate (next step) to the 17-keto. After reduction to 17, 20, diol, these compounds are oxidized by bis-

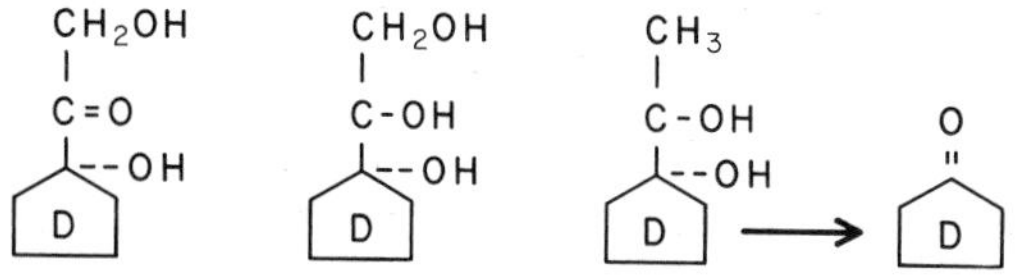

DIHYDROXY ACETONE	GLYCEROL	GLYCOL	17-KETO
Cortisone (Compound E) Cortisol or Hydroxycortisone (Compound F) tetrahydro derivatives of compounds E, F, and S	Cortol Cortolone	Pregnanetriol Pregnane 11-keto (17-hydroxyprogesterone and 17-hydroxypregnenolone after borohydride reduction)	

muthate or periodate. The borohydride also removes the chromogenic property of the original 17-ketosteroids present by reducing the 17-ketone to a 17-hydroxyl group. In essence, this initial reduction step eliminates existing urinary 17-ketosteroids before subsequent oxidation of C-21 compounds to C-19 17-ketosteroids.

The Zimmermann reaction (metadinitrobenzene) for 17-ketosteroids is applied to final extracted products. Since reduction with borohydride is followed by oxidation with bismuthate or periodate, the original 17-ketosteroids are no longer included in the final colored products or reaction; a more total estimation of 17-hydroxycorticoids and adrenocortical function is thus achieved with 17-ketogenic steroid assay. The normal values vary with the procedure followed but, in general, are about 30 per cent higher than the urinary Porter-Silber (17-hydroxycorticosteroids) reaction values (Table 11–12).

Although the urinary 17-hydroxycorticosteroids determination (Porter-Silber chromogens) is a sensitive index of adrenocortical function, the 17-ketogenic steroid assay is more sensitive and especially valuable in adrenogenital syndrome and rare examples of Cushing's syndrome in which 17-hydroxycorticosteroids (e.g., cortisol) may be within normal range. This is attributed to the absence of hydroxylase enzymes in the adrenogenital syndrome. Recalling the biosynthetic pathway of adrenocortical hormones (Fig. 11–10), the sequence of hydroxylation is 17, 21, and 11. Cases of adrenogenital syndrome have been most frequently associated with absence of one of the latter two enzymes (21-hydroxylase and 11-hydroxylase), as noted in Table 11–13. In either example there is a decreased production of hydrocortisone (compound F, or cortisol) with decreased plasma cortisol. This causes increased ACTH, with adrenal hyperplasia and increased production of compounds proximal to enzyme deficiency, including pregnanetriol. This is most prominent with a 21-hydroxylase deficiency, which results in 17-hydroxycorticosteroid values within normal or below normal range. Management of adrenogenital syndrome with administration of cortisone and cortisol inhibits ACTH secretion and restores normal adrenocortical function. Adrenogenital syndrome androgenic or virilizing features (precocious puberty in the male and pseudohermaphroditism in the female) are also attributed to hydroxylase deficiency (21 and 11) with exaggeration of pathway that in addition to pregnanetriol over-production leads to increased secretion of androstenedione with peripheral conversion of this steroid to testosterone; hence, the striking elevation of plasma testosterone levels (Fig. 11–10). With a deficiency of 11-hydroxylase, adrenogenital syndrome patients often show hypertension that is not seen with a 21-hydroxylase deficiency. Cortexolone or Cpd S and deoxycorticosterone (DOC), mineralocorticoids, with their tetrahydro derivatives accumulate in increased quantity with 11-hydroxylase deficiency but not in 21-hydroxylase deficiency. Indeed, some virilizing adrenogenital syndrome patients may exhibit a mineralocorticoid deficiency with salt losing due to a 21-hydroxylase deficiency and simulate Addison's disease. There is also a deficiency of aldosterone as well as cortisol in the salt losing form. The variety of adrenocortical disorders with elevated urinary 17-KS and alterations in DHA and androsterone are shown in Tables 11–14 and 11–10.

Aldosterone. In contrast to methods for 17-ketosteroids and 17-hydroxycorticosteroids, which are within the province of the clinical

Table 11-13. CATEGORIES OF ADRENOGENITAL SYNDROME*

I. Virilizing (elevated urinary 17-ketosteroids)
  A. 21-Hydroxylase deficiency (90% of all cases)—elevated urinary pregnanetriol and plasma 17-OH progesterone
    1. Compensated (incomplete)
    2. Salt losing (complete)
  B. 11-Hydroxylase deficiency
    1. Hypertensive—elevated plasma Cpd S and urinary tetrahydro S and DOC
    2. Nonhypertensive (?)

II. Mixed
    3 β-Hydroxysteroid dehydrogenase deficiency (rare and usually salt losing)

III. Nonvirilizing
  A. 17-Hydroxylase deficiency with hypertension (elevated corticosterone and DOC and low testosterone)
  B. Desmolase deficiency (salt losing)—lipoid adrenal hyperplasia

*Modified from A. Bongiovanni: *In* Stanbury, J. B., Wyngaarden, J. B., and Fredrickson, D. S. (eds.): The Metabolic Basis of Inherited Disease. 3rd ed. New York, McGraw-Hill Book Co., 1972.

pathology laboratory, assays for urinary aldosterone until recently have been most complex and demanding. Chromatography after a double isotope derivative procedure (Kliman and Peterson, 1960) depends on the acetylation of aldosterone with tritium-labeled acetic anhydride of known specific activity to permit recovery of an aldosterone derivative of specific activity. C^{14} isotope-labeled aldosterone diacetate added early in the method permits calculation of aldosterone concentration present initially. Normal ranges appear to be between 2 and 26 μg. per 24-hour urine. To insure stability of this hormone, an acidified urine (pH 3 to 4) collection is required, and patients should have adequate sodium intake. Radioimmunoassays for aldosterone offer much promise and may eventually replace the more difficult double isotope derivative procedure. In addition to 24-hour urinary aldosterone measurements, peripheral and adrenal venous blood specimens for aldosterone radioimmunoassay are useful for diagnosis and localization in primary aldosteronism (Horton and Finck, 1972). Normal supine aldosterone venous blood values range from 3 to 7 ng/100 ml. plasma with a coefficient of variation (C.V.) of less than 10 per cent. Primary aldosteronism (Conn's syndrome) and secondary aldosteronism show elevated urinary aldosterone levels.

Clinical features of primary aldosteronism include *hypertension*, polyuria, muscular pains, cramps, weakness, and tetany. Laboratory findings in this condition include *low plasma potassium* with slightly elevated sodium, alkalemia, suppressed plasma renin activity, and nonsuppressible aldosterone secretion. Sodium retention with excessive urinary potassium loss accounts for plasma electrolyte abnormalities. Consequences of urinary potassium loss include: (1) decreased carbohydrate tolerance in about one-half of all

Table 11-14. ADRENOCORTICAL DISORDERS WITH INCREASED EXCRETION OF URINARY 17-KS*

	ANDROSTERONE	DHA-S	11-OXYGENATED 17-KS	SUPPRESSION OF 17-KS IN SUPPRESSION TEST
Congenital adrenal hyperplasia				
Simple virilizing form	3+	In proportion to total 17-KS	2+	Yes
Salt-losing	3+	Same	2+	Yes
Hypertensive	3+†	Same	—	Yes
3β-ol-dehydrogenase deficiency	—	3+	—	Yes
Lipoid hyperplasia	—	—	—	Low control 17-KS
Virilizing adrenal tumor	1+	3+	N	No
Feminizing adrenal tumor	N to 2+	N to 2+	N	No
Cushing's syndrome				
Bilateral hyperplasia	1+	1+	1+	Partial
Adrenal adenoma	—	—	1+	Often low control 17-KS
Adrenal carcinoma	1+ to 3+	1+	1+ to 3+	No

NOTE: N = normal levels; — = lower than normal; 1+ to 3+ = higher than normal.
*With permission of Migeon, C. J.: Amer. J. Med. *53*:612, 1972.
†Etiocholanolone.

patients with primary aldosteronism (related to impairment of insulin release secondary to K depletion); (2) loss of renal concentrating ability (tubular vacuolation and pyelonephritis appear to be due to K depletion); and (3) blunting of circulatory reflex response (postural hypotension without tachycardia). Hence, an assay for aldosterone is often considered in evaluation of patients with hypertension in whom the incidence of primary aldosteronism has been variably assessed at from 0.5 to 10 per cent (Biglieri and Stockigt, 1971). While the majority of patients with Conn's syndrome have an aldosterone-producing adrenocortical adenoma (APA), about 20 per cent may have nodular hyperplasia; carcinoma of adrenal cortex has also been reported infrequently. Although patients with bilateral hyperplasia tend to have less severe hypokalemia, lower aldosterone secretion and plasma renin (PRA), differentiating such patients from those patients with APA is difficult; bilateral adrenal vein sampling for plasma aldosterone has been suggested (Carey *et al.*, 1972).

The clinical and physiological conditions associated with elevated urinary aldosterone levels without an intrinsic adrenal lesion are called secondary aldosteronism and include nephrosis and cardiac failure with sodium retention, cirrhosis of the liver with ascites, pregnancy increasing to term, potassium loading, and salt depletion affecting extracellular fluid compartments. According to Streeten's excellent review (1971), secondary aldosteronism manifests itself clinically three principal ways: edema, hypertension, and hypokalemia. Patients who are receiving diuretics, especially thiazides, and excrete large amounts of salt can have hypokalemia and, hence, if they are also hypertensive, may mimic aldosteronism.

Since angiotensin II stimulates aldosterone production as described previously (p. 710 and Figs. 11–11 and 11–12), secondary aldosteronism may be traced to the renin-angiotensin system. In severe renovascular disease and especially in patients with primary renovascular hypertension (hypertension of renal origin), increased urinary aldosterone excretion is associated with elevated plasma renin levels. Plasma renin levels are, however, depressed in primary aldosteronism (Gunnells *et al.*, 1967). It is therefore important to differentiate between hyperaldosteronism due to renal disease and hyperaldosteronism of adrenocortical origin. Plasma renin or angiotensin I measurements in conjunction with urinary aldosterone determination may be required in addition to previously described studies in selected patients to make this distinction.

Renin radioimmunoassay is available commercially as well as in kit form; it is within the scope of most medium- to large-sized hospital laboratories, provided the principles of radioimmunoassay are understood and appropriate technical assistance is available. Measurement of renin activity by immunoassay for angiotensin I eliminates need to depend on the converting enzyme which was required for procedures based on angiotensin II assays. In the presence of enzymatic inhibitors (EDTA, dimercaptol, and 8-OH-quinoline) angiotensin I remains stable, and this method has largely replaced techniques based on angiotensin II.

Evaluation of Hypertensive Patient. Ambulatory patients with hypertension subjected to screening for primary aldosteronism require a comprehensive workup that should initially include a careful determination of electrolytes. Serum sodium is usually normal or elevated, while potassium wasting is indicated by a urinary excretion of greater than 50 mEq. of K^+ per 24 hours when the serum K^+ is 3 mEq. per liter or less. In view of the fact that a major action of aldosterone is to facilitate K^+ exchange for Na^+ in the distal renal tubules, K^+ loss is retarded if Na^+ delivery to the distal tubular exchange site is diminished by salt restriction. Indeed, K^+ depletion can be corrected significantly in patients with primary aldosteronism by a combination of Na^+ restriction and ingestion of food with a high K^+ content. Hence, *salt loading* can be used to good advantage to produce the characteristic electrolyte patterns of primary aldosteronism, especially when initial serum K^+ is questionable or equivocal, i.e., low normal K^+ versus slight serum K^+ depression. To accomplish salt loading, patient should ingest 2 gm. of sodium chloride three times daily for three days with a regular diet. Salt intake is raised to about 200 mEq. per day. After the fourth day a serum sodium, potassium, chloride, and carbon dioxide are determined to observe development of hypokalemia. Evaluation of 24-hour urinary potassium excretion is also an integral part of electrolyte studies; with a low or borderline serum potassium and over 50 mEq. excretion of K^+ per 24 hours, the patient has renal potassium wasting and is a strong suspect for primary aldosteronism.

If these studies are abnormal, spironolactone screening test can be conducted as follows:

Short Test. Four hundred milligrams of spironolactone is administered orally each day for four days with serum and urinary K^+ determined at three intervals: before therapy, at the end of four days, and a week after cessation of the drug. If urinary K^+ falls to less than 20 mEq. per 24 hours and serum K^+ increases during therapy, but serum K^+ falls with an increase in urinary K^+ after spironolactone is stopped, a presumptive diagnosis of primary aldosteronism can be made with strong evidence that the aldosterone effect on the renal tubules was temporarily interrupted.

Long Test. Four hundred milligrams of spironolactone is administered orally daily for three to four weeks. If both serum K^+ and blood pressure return to normal, there is good evidence for diagnosis, but if no antihypertensive effect is observed, suspect secondary aldosteronism.

If the spironolactone test is abnormal, mineralocorticoid administration (400 μg. 9 α-fluorohydrocortisone in divided doses orally daily for four days) may be conducted while the ambulatory patient is receiving at least 100 mEq. dietary sodium daily. A normal response shows a 50 per cent decrease in 24-hour urinary aldosterone; a decrease of variable degree (suppression) is also seen in secondary hyperaldosteronism as well as hyperaldosteronism seen occasionally in hypertensive outpatients. However, patients with primary aldosteronism show no fall in aldosterone.

When an outpatient demonstrates high urinary aldosterone levels after sodium loading and after administration of mineralocorticoid, hospital evaluation is in order. While detailed studies are usually made, according to Biglieri and Stockigt (1971), the most important procedures in the diagnosis of an APA (aldosterone-producing adrenal cortical adenoma) are the administration of desoxycorticosterone acetate (DOCA) with measurement of urinary aldosterone and plasma renin. With a daily sodium intake of greater than 100 mEq. per day, 10 mg. desoxycorticosterone acetate is administered intramuscularly every 12 hours for three consecutive days. Urinary aldosterone measurement of 24-hour specimens are collected before DOCA administration (control specimen) and on the third day; at least 50 per cent suppression of aldosterone excretion is normal, but minimal or no suppression is presumptive evidence of primary aldosteronism. In patients with accelerated or renovascular hypertension or in those taking estrogen-containing oral contraceptives, the secondarily increased aldosterone levels are reduced to normal with this maneuver.

In normal subjects plasma renin activity (PRA) estimations change with aldosterone in a parallel fashion during the foregoing maneuvers, but when primary overproduction or excretion of aldosterone occurs, extracellular fluid expansion leads to suppression of PRA. This discrepancy between aldosterone level and PRA value (↓ PRA and ↑ aldosterone levels) is diagnostically important. In primary aldosteronism the autonomous secretion of aldosterone by an aldosterone-producing adrenal adenoma (APA) leads to sodium retention, expansion of extracellular fluid volume, and suppression of renin production by the kidneys (Fig. 11–11). In contrast to primary aldosteronism, with secondary aldosteronism the production of abnormally large quantities of aldosterone is secondary to increased renin production; hence, ↑ PRA and ↑ aldosterone levels are typical of secondary aldosteronism. Secondary aldosteronism may be observed with renovascular or malignant hypertension, oral contraceptives (may persist four weeks or more after cessation of intake), or in the "aldosterone rebound" phase following vigorous diuretic therapy.

Because of the parallel response of PRA and aldosterone in normal subjects to various stimuli (e.g., excess salt intake yields ↓ PRA, ↓ aldosterone and low salt intake yields ↑ PRA and ↑ aldosterone), the conditions for specimen collection must be appreciated and adhered to rigidly to determine PRA and aldosterone for critical evaluation (Figs. 11–11 and 11–12). With the beginning point of a urinary aldosterone assay, body position and salt intake can be considered. Urinary aldosterone measurements should be made after five days of a 300 mEq. sodium intake (salt excess), whereas plasma renin activity should be measured after four days of salt restriction (10 mEq. Na^+ daily for four days) or a mild diuretic to accentuate or achieve maximal stimulus of PRA and with patient recumbent (before arising, 7 to 8 A.M.) as well as upright (following four hours of quiet activity, upright about 12 noon). The plasma sample for PRA drawn after the patient is upright should achieve maximal stimulation, while the recumbent specimen is for comparison as a control without PRA stimulation. A normal response is a two- to threefold rise in PRA after four hours of ambulation. With APA, patients typically show PRA values of less than 20 per cent of normal (30 to 330 ng. per 100 ml. plasma) under comparable conditions. With increased aldosterone, a subnormal renin is strong evidence for diagnosis of primary aldosteronism. The mild elevations of PRA (335 to 870 ng. per 100 ml. plasma) in the recumbent specimen of the patient with renovascular hypertension are also usually elevated in the upright specimen, while marked elevations (450 to 4000 ng. per 100 ml. plasma) of PRA in malignant hypertension (recumbent) are also markedly elevated with the upright specimen. Very low, approaching zero, PRA is noted in both recumbent and upright specimens of patients with frank primary aldosteronism. In addition to secondary aldosteronism, an elevated PRA may be observed in the following: low salt diet, primary-salt-losing nephropathy, upright posture, Addison's disease, diuretic therapy, hemorrhage, pregnancy, antihypertensive drug therapy including reserpine and hydralazine and also diazoxide. In addition to primary aldosteronism, a depressed PRA can be seen with the following: increased salt intake, salt-retaining steroid therapy, antidiuretic hormone therapy, after a period of recumbency, blood transfusion, drug therapy with methyl-dopa, L-dopa, and guanethidine, and with diurnal variation lower from noon to 6 P.M. than 8 A.M. to noon, independent of postural changes.

The measurement of renal-vein renin appears to have predictive value in several types of renal hypertension (Stockigt *et al.*, 1972).

The schematic outline at the bottom of the page (slightly modified from Biglieri and Stockigt, 1971) emphasizes the importance of plasma renin activity (PRA) measurements in the diagnosis of primary aldosteronism.

With elevated aldosterone levels, renin measurements (A, B) will show whether the patient has primary or secondary aldosteronism. Some hypertensive patients with low aldosterone and low PRA (after four hours in an upright position), respond to high dose spironolactone therapy (400 mg per day for five weeks) with normalization of blood pressure and significant weight loss (Spark and Melby, 1971). It has been suggested that a yet unidentified mineralocorticoid could be responsible for suppressed PRA, low aldosterone, and hypertension in these patients. Carey *et al.*, (1972) also have suggested that hypertensive patients with suppressed PRA may have a mineralocorticoid excess; the hypertension in such patients may respond favorably to spironolactone.

Bartter's syndrome is characterized by hyperaldosteronism, increased PRA, normal blood pressure without edema, and hypokalemia. These patients are insensitive to the pressor effect of infused angiotensin (White, 1972). The normal blood pressure distinguishes Bartter's syndrome patients from those patients with renal artery stenosis or malignant hypertension who otherwise have a similar increase in PRA and angiotensin insensitivity. Except for the absence of edema and more severe hypokalemia, Bartter's syndrome patients resemble patients with secondary hyperaldosteronism. This syndrome may be the result of renal tubular defects in handling sodium and potassium.

Because aldosterone production is sensitive or responsive to potassium (K^+) balance (serum K^+ and total body K^+), normal subjects with a depressed serum K^+ and reduction of body K^+ show a decrease in aldosterone production. Hence, it is possible that in a patient with primary aldosteronism (e.g., APA), severe potassium depletion may yield a urinary aldosterone excretion within normal range even though production may still be abnormally high for the magnitude of potassium depletion. In patients who are strong suspects for primary aldosteronism, it is important to initiate vigorous potassium repletion and observe the effect on aldosterone excretion. In such patients, K^+ repletion may produce a severalfold (five to ten times) increase in aldosterone excretion and establish the diagnosis of primary aldosteronism.

Clinical Pathology Correlations. The diseases associated with increased and decreased corticoid production are shown in Table 11–15.

The basic steroid measurements to identify hyper- and hypoadrenocortical function include 17-ketosteroids, 17-hydroxycorticosteroids, total ketogenic corticosteroids and urinary free cortisol or preferably urinary free corticoids (Hsu and Bledsoe, 1970).

In hypoadrenocortical function (Addison's disease), the 17-hydroxycorticosteroid (urine

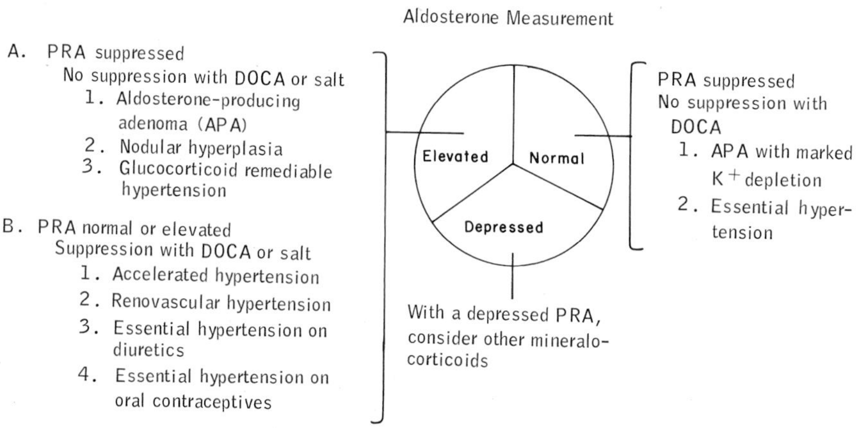

Table 11–15. CLINICAL PATHOLOGY CORRELATIONS*

HYPERSECRETORY STEROID ENDOCRINOPATHIES	HISTOLOGICAL ENTITIES
Cushing's syndrome	Adrenocortical hyperplasia (70%) Primary Secondary to hypothalamic lesions Secondary to ACTH-producing tumor Pituitary adenoma Nonpituitary tumor Carcinoma of lung (oat cell) Other carcinoma: breast, prostate, ovary, pancreas, parotid, liver, esophagus, thymus, thyroid Bronchial adenoma Adrenocortical adenoma (15%) Adrenocortical carcinoma (10%) Adrenal rest tumors
Aldosteronism (primary)	Adrenocortical adenoma (80%) Adrenocortical hyperplasia (15%) Adrenocortical carcinoma (5%)
Aldosteronism (secondary)	Pinealoma (animals only)
Virilism	*Adrenal Lesions* Congenital adrenal hyperplasia (common) Adrenocortical carcinoma Adrenocortical adenoma (rare) *Nonadrenal Lesions* Ovarian neoplasms (arrhenoblastoma, adrenal rest tumor, hilar cell tumor, granulosa cell tumor, Brenner tumor) Testicular neoplasms (interstitial cell tumor, adrenal rest tumor, others)
Feminization	Adrenocortical carcinoma Testicular tumors (various)
Mixed endocrinopathies	Adrenocortical carcinoma
HYPOSECRETORY STEROID ENDOCRINOPATHIES	**HISTOLOGICAL ENTITIES**
Adrenal insufficiency (primary)	*Destructive Adrenal Lesions* Idiopathic atrophy (most common cause) Infectious (tuberculosis, histoplasmosis, coccidioidomycosis, cryptococcosis) Bilateral metastases (lung carcinoma) Hemorrhage (sepsis, trauma, vascular disease) Surgical removal *Partial Adrenal Metabolic Failure* Cortical hyperplasia (virilizing) Hyperplasia secondary to enzyme inhibitors: metyrapone (specific), amphenone (nonspecific) Necrosis secondary to cytotoxic agents: ortho-para-DDD
Adrenal insufficiency (secondary)	*Destructive Pituitary Lesions* Necrosis secondary to shock (post partum) Hemorrhage Infections Neoplasms (metastases from breast, lungs) Hypoplasia (iatrogenic suppression)

*Modified from T. R. Harrison, R. D. Adams, I. L. Bennett, W. H. Resnik, G. W. Thorn, and M. M. Wintrobe: *Principles of Internal Medicine.* 5th edition. New York, McGraw-Hill Book Company, 1966.

and/or plasma cortisol and urinary free cortisol) assay should confirm the clinical picture (Table 11–16). A plasma cortisol assay followed by ACTH infusion tests reveals in patients with Addison's disease no significant response to exogenous ACTH because the gland, if any remains, is already stimulated maximally by elevated endogenous ACTH (Thorn, 1971). A metyrapone test should only be considered with an adequate adrenal cortical response to ACTH (Table 11–16). A low plasma sodium without features of dilutional syndromes but normal or elevated potassium may also be observed, depending on the patient's hydration. Acutely ill patients with Addison's disease may show hyperpotassemia, moderate urea retention, hypoglycemia, and evidence of hypovolemia (Tyler and West, 1972).

In hyperadrenocortical function, the steroid assay selected should fit the clinical picture. Four different pathologic mechanisms result in Cushing's syndrome: (1) adrenal hyperplasia associated with hypothalamic-pituitary dysfunction; (2) adrenal tumor; (3) ectopic ACTH-secreting tumor; and (4) exogenous steroid administration. Persistent excessive ACTH secretion presumably is the mechanism for the first type, although the exact mechanism is controversial: an analogy to a reset thermostat regulation for excessive ACTH has been used. Adrenal tumors suppress ACTH secretion in Cushing's syndrome. Thus, in hyperplasia an ACTH elevation is observed in contrast to virtual absence in adrenal tumors. Ectopic ACTH-secreting tumors also reveal elevated plasma ACTH levels. Indeed, Cushing's syndrome may be classified as follows:

ACTH dependent
- Pituitary ACTH excess
  - Tumor (10 per cent)
  - Nontumor (65 per cent)
- Ectopic ACTH-secreting tumor (1 per cent)
- Exogenous ACTH administration

Table 11-16. STEROID MEASUREMENTS IN ADRENOCORTICAL HYPOFUNCTION AND OTHER SELECTED DISORDERS

CLINICAL CONDITION	BASAL LEVEL			ACTH STIMULATION*			METYRAPONE†			SUPPRESSION‡			PLASMA CORTISOL LEVELS
	PS	KGS	17 KS	PS	KGS	17 KS	PS	KGS	17 KS	PS	KGS	17 KS	
Normal	See Table 11-12			3-5 fold increase		2-3 fold increase	D	2 fold increase		50% of basal level			10-20 μg./100 ml. at 8 A.M. 5-10 μg./100 ml. at 5 P.M.
Primary chronic cortical atrophy or inflammatory necrosis	Very low (5% may be normal)			D-SI	D-SI	D-SI	Test not performed			Test not performed			
Secondary atrophy due to prolonged cortisone administration	Very low			Pt. continued on cortisone, given ACTH gel 5 days Compare 1st & 5th day excretion (Addison's: No rise)			Test not performed			Test not performed			
Panhypopituitarism	Very low			2-3 fold increase			Test not performed			Test not performed			
Hyperthyroidism	May be 2-fold increase			3-5 fold increase		2-3 fold increase	D	2 fold increase		50% decrease			10-20 μg./100 ml.
Hypothyroidism	Low			3-5 fold increase		2-3 fold increase	D	2 fold increase		Test not performed			
Gout	Low						D						
Simple hirsutism	Normal	Normal	Upper limit normal	3-5 fold increase		2-3 fold increase	D	2 fold increase		50% of normal			
	Normal	Slight increase	Upper limit normal	5 fold increase			D	2 fold increase§		50% decrease			

*ACTH Stimulation: 20 units in 500 ml. dextrose in 8 hour I.V.; 80 units gel I.M. for two successive days
†Suppression: Dexamethasone or equivalent: Low level, 0.5 mg., q. 6 h. for two days; high level, 2.0 mg., q. 6 h. for two or three days 750 mg., q. 4 h. for 24 hours. or 30 mg./kg. as a single dose at midnight
‡Pregnanetriol increase suggests congenital adrenal hyperplasia
PS = 17-21 dihydroxy 20 ketosteroids (Porter Silber chromogens) or 17 hydroxycorticosteroids
KGS = Ketogenic steroids
17 KS = 17 ketosteroids
D = Decrease
SI = Slight increase

Table 11-17 CUSHING'S SYNDROME (PURE METABOLIC; MIXED PATTERN WITH VIRILIZATION OR DEMASCULINIZATION): DIAGNOSTIC APPROACH EMPHASIZING STEROID MEASUREMENTS AND APPROPRIATE MANEUVERS

ADRENAL LESION	BASAL LEVEL			ACTH STIMULATION*			METYRAPONE†			SUPPRESSION DEXAMETHASONE			X-RAY WITH OR WITHOUT GAS INSUFFLATION MAY REVEAL
	PS	KGS	17 KS	PS	KGS	17 KS	PS	KGS	17 KS	PS	KGS	17 KS	
None	I	I	N	I	I	I	D	I	N	D‡	D‡	D‡	No masses
Hyperplasia	I	I	N-SI	I	I	I	D-NC	I	I	NC‡ D§	NC‡ D§	NC‡ D§	Bilateral masses
				Greater than 5X									
Adenoma	I	I	D-N	I	I	I	NC	I-NC	I-NC	NC‡ NC§	NC‡ NC§	NC‡ NC§	Unilateral mass
Carcinoma	I	I	I	NC	NC	NC	NC	NC	NC	NC§	NC§	NC§	Unilateral mass
Extraadrenal tumors	I	I	I	I-NC	I-NC	I-NC	NC	NC	NC	NC	NC	NC	

*ACTH Stimulation: 20 units in 500 ml. dextrose in 8 hour I.V.; 80 units gel I.M. for two successive days.
†750 mg. q. 4 h. for 24 hr. or 30 mg./kg. p.o. at midnight.
‡2 mg./day for three days.
§8 mg./day for two days.
PS = 17-21 dihydroxy 20 ketosteroids (Porter Silber chromogens) or 17-hydroxycorticosteroids
KGS = Ketogenic steroids
17 KS = 17 ketosteroids
N = Normal
D = Decreased
I = Increased
NC = No change

ACTH independent
- Carcinoma (10 per cent)
- Adenoma (10 per cent)
- Adrenal cortical hyperplasia
- Adrenal cortical rest tumors
- Exogenous glucocorticoid administration

In Cushing's syndrome, with excess of glucocorticoids, the 17-hydroxycorticosteroid assay should confirm the diagnosis. If it does not, ketogenics should be performed. In most patients with Cushing's syndrome, blood cortisol (17-hydroxycorticosteroid) measurements do not show the normal diurnal variation, an afternoon (5 P.M.) specimen's concentration being about 50 per cent of the morning value.

Although urinary free cortisol or, preferably, urinary free corticoids with urinary creatinine determinations are probably the most valuable measurements for hyperadrenalcortical secretory states, suppression tests are the best technique for laboratory identification of Cushing's syndrome, especially in patients with borderline or slightly elevated urinary or plasma cortisol measurements. Table 11–17 shows typical results and principle as well as further details of the dexamethasone suppression test considered subsequently. The response to metyrapone is also useful in differentiating hyperplasia from other adrenal abnormalities (differentiating types of Cushing's syndrome) and is about equally successful as dexamethasone suppression. It is also described subsequently under suppression test and shown in Table 11–17. The exogenous ACTH stimulation test has also been used to differentiate the types of Cushing's syndrome, although Tyler and West (1972) emphasize that the responses may be variable at times (Table 11–17).

In the adrenogenital syndrome (virilizing and 21- or 11-hydroxylase deficiency), the ketogenic assay is the best single determination, although 17-ketosteroids will probably confirm the majority of cases. An increase in urinary 17-ketosteroids is observed with hyperadrenalcorticism in the conditions shown in Table 11–14. In addition, testicular tumors (teratoma, interstitial cell tumors) as well as gonadotropin-producing tumors in males are also accompanied by an increased excretion of urinary 17-KS, as is also often the case in virilizing ovarian syndromes – arrhenoblastoma hilar cell tumor, adrenal rest tumor, Stein-Leventhal syndrome (Migeon, 1972).

Several stimulation and suppression or inhibition procedures have also been introduced in conjunction with steroid assays. (Tables 11–17 and 11–18).

ACTH is used to stimulate the adrenal cortex for differentiation of primary and secondary hypoadrenocortical function. A number of techniques have been used (Tyler and West, 1972). These vary in amount, duration, and manner of ACTH administration, with 24-hour urine collections prior to and after such stimulation. Blood specimens have also been used alone or in conjunction with urine specimens for corticoid assays. In hypopituitarism, in contrast to primary destruction of adrenal cortex (Addison's disease), the urine and blood corticoids (e.g., 17-hydroxycorticosteroids) ap-

Table 11-18 ADRENOGENITAL SYNDROME: LABORATORY DIAGNOSTIC APPROACH (INCLUDING VIRILIZATION IN FEMALE, CONGENITAL OR ACQUIRED, WITH OR WITHOUT PSEUDOHERMAPHRODITISM; VIRILIZATION IN MALE, FEMINIZATION OF MALE; HIRSUTISM; STEIN-LEVENTHAL SYNDROME)

ADRENAL LESION	BASAL LEVEL				ACTH STIMULATION*				METYRAPONE†				DEXAMETHASONE SUPPRESSION at highest level 2 mg. p.o. q. 6 h. for 2-3 days			
	PS	KGS	17 KS	P_3	PS	KGS	17 KS	P_3	PS	KGS	17 KS	P_3	PS	KGS	17 KS	P_3
Hyperplasia	SD or N	I	I	Cg:I Ac:N	SI	SI	SI	SI	D	I	I	I	D	D	D	D
Adenoma	D-N	I	I	N-	NC-SI	NC-SI	NC-SI	NC-SI	D	NC	NC	NC	NC	NC	NC	NC
Carcinoma	D-N	I	I	I	NC	NC	NC	NC	NC	NC	NC	NC	NC	NC	NC	NC
Virilizing tumors, not adrenal‡	N	N-I	N-I	N	NC§	NC§	I§	NC§	NC§	NC§	NC§	NC§	NC§	NC§	NC§	NC§

*ACTH Stimulation: 20 units in 500 ml. dextrose in 8 hr. I.V.; 80 units gel I.M. for 2 successive days.
†750 mg. q. 4 h. for 24 hr. or 30 mg./kg. p.o. at midnight.
‡Severe virilization by testosterone from tumor not reflected in 17 KS or KGS assays.
§Response of normal adrenal may mask.

PS = 17-21 dihydroxy 20 ketosteroids (Porter-Silber chromogens)
KGS = Ketogenic steroids
17 KS = 17 ketosteroids
P_3 = Pregnanetriol
N = Normal
D = Decreased
I = Increased
S = Slightly
NC = No change
Cg. = Congenital
Ac. = Acquired

proach normal levels after ACTH stimulation. A baseline prestimulation urine and/or blood collection is essential for proper interpretation of the ACTH stimulation test.

Adrenal suppression or cortisol suppression, depending on substitution of a drug, may be used. Cortisol (compound F, or hydrocortisone) suppresses adrenocorticosteroid production and secretion via the negative feedback ACTH mechanism of plasma cortisol. Again, a baseline specimen collection for determination of urinary 17-hydroxycorticosteroids, 17-ketogenics, or urinary free corticoids (less frequently 17-ketosteroids), or plasma cortisol is a prerequisite. The most commonly employed suppressive agent is 9α-fluoro-16α-methylprednisolone (dexamethasone). Normal persons show a depression of plasma and urinary 17-hydroxycorticoids (cortisol) after the oral administration of dexamethasone (low level or dosage—0.5 mg. given every 6 hours for eight times, i.e., 2 mg. per day for two days). Hence, adrenal suppression with dexamethasone can be a valuable aid in the identification of patients with minimal or borderline hyperfunction of the adrenal cortex who fail to show a depression in urinary steroid excretion (17-OH, 17-KGS, free corticoids or, less frequently, 17-KS) or plasma cortisol. Equally satisfactory results on outpatients are obtained if 1.0 mg. of dexamethasone is given at 11:00 P.M. or midnight and plasma cortisol determined the ensuing morning (Tyler and West, 1972). It is also used in patients with hyperadrenocortical function (Cushing's syndrome) to delineate adrenocortical hyperplasia from autonomous adrenocortical adenoma or carcinoma and ectopic ACTH-secreting tumors. In most patients with adrenocortical hyperplasia, suppression by dexamethasone in higher dosage (2.0 mg. given every 6 hours eight times, i.e., 8 mg. per day for two days) causes a decrease of about 50 per cent in the elevated urinary 17-hydroxycorticosteroids (compared to baseline) while in patients with autonomous tumors (adrenal tumor or ectopic tumor ACTH production) baseline elevated values persist. Therefore, adenoma and carcinoma of the adrenal cortex causing hyperadrenocorticism (Cushing's syndrome, or virilizing adrenocortical tumor) do not usually reveal suppression, as demonstrated by a decrease in elevated urinary hydroxycorticoids, ketogenics, or free corticoids, or plasma cortisol. Some patients with adrenocortical hyperplasia secondary to an ACTH-secreting tumor (pituitary or nonpituitary—see Table 11–15) may not show such suppression when given large doses of dexamethasone. This has been attributed to intermittent function with a periodicity of days

(Tyler and West, 1972). In the adrenogenital syndrome, suppression should also occur but would more likely be reflected in the urinary 17-ketosteroids or ketogenics with a deficiency of one of the hydroxylase enzymes in steroidogenesis. The 11-hydroxylase deficiency type of adrenogenital syndrome is associated with increased amounts of compound S (cortexolone) that react in the urinary total ketogenic assay; with a 21-hydroxylase deficiency type, there is a decrease or absence of cortexolone, but pregnanetriol accumulates and also reacts in the urinary total ketogenic assay.

Adrenal inhibition employs the inhibitory agent metyrapone, which is used to assess anterior pituitary ACTH reserve or demonstrate a deficient function of the pituitary-adrenal axis and to differentiate between adrenocortical tumor and hyperplasia. Metyrapone is a selective inhibitor of the 11-hydroxylation step in biosynthesis (blocks 11-hydroxylase), the final hydroxylation reaction that forms cortisol (hydrocortisone, or compound F); hence, there is a secretion of Cpd S (11-deoxycortisol) instead of cortisol with an accumulation of cortexolone (compound S, or deoxycortisol) that does not so effectively block ACTH in the negative feedback mechanism usually attributed to cortisol (hydrocortisone, or compound F). In normal subjects, ACTH is secreted as the plasma and tissue cortisol fall below a critical level (Jubiz *et al.*, 1970). Therefore, administration of metyrapone causes more ACTH production (pituitary reserve) in the normal individual, and a total ketogenic assay will show an increased excretion. Cortisol is the major compound reflected in the 17-hydroxycorticosteroid assay, and its production is blocked with metyrapone. However, cortexolone (compound S) is produced, and it is measured nonspecifically as increased urinary 17-hydroxycorticosteroids or total ketogenic (17-KGS) or specifically as tetrahydro S or plasma S (deoxycortisol). With this block, cortexolone and other corticoids proximal to it in the biosynthetic pathway accumulate, and many more of these metabolites are measured with the total ketogenic corticosteroid assay than with the 17-hydroxycorticoid assay.

Metyrapone is usually given in doses of 750 mg. every 4 hours for 24 hours, but since the system is more critically responsive at night, a larger single dose (30 mg./kg.) is required in the evening and should be given with food to improve tolerance for larger dose and delay absorption so that adequate blockade is present during the early morning hours. Plasma compound S and plasma cortisol should be determined on 8:00 A.M. specimens when normals show plasma S elevated to 7–18 μg./dl. but depressed plasma cortisol levels (Tyler and West, 1972). With inadequate absorption of metyrapone or acceleration of its metabolism by other drugs (e.g., diphenylhydantoin) or by hyperthyroidism, insufficient blockade and continued cortisol secretion may result without stimulation of ACTH or an effective function test of pituitary-adrenal axis.

The metyrapone test employing a baseline and two postadministration 24-hour urinary collections for total ketogenic corticosteroids or 17-hydroxycorticosteroids (Porter-Silber reaction) may also be used to delineate the adrenocortical lesion. In the presence of hyperplasia of the adrenal cortex, the elevated urinary total ketogenics often increase as much as twofold, while carcinoma reveals no change and an adenoma may show a minimal depression or no change. The metyrapone test for hypothalamic-pituitary integrity and responsiveness with the release of ACTH may be impaired in patients with Cushing's syndrome due to adrenocortical carcinoma or adenoma but not in cases of adrenocortical hyperplasia; the sustained elevations of cortisol from such autonomous tumors may have impaired this responsiveness and reduced the pituitary reserve when challenged by metyrapone.

Pituitary ACTH deficiency, somewhat more common than Addison's disease, may be caused by a wide variety of pituitary and hypothalamic abnormalities, including the effects of pharmacologic doses of glucocorticoids administered to patients for many and sundry reasons. With the overnight metyrapone test, patients with pituitary insufficiency show rather consistently little response, although some response not reaching normal levels may occur. Furthermore, pituitary ACTH deficiency is frequently partial in contrast to primary adrenal insufficiency (Addison's disease). Ideally measurement of cortisol and ACTH simultaneously should permit differentiation of pituitary from adrenal disease. However, plasma ACTH determinations are not readily available, so an ACTH infusion test is required to demonstrate the adrenal's ability to produce cortisol. However, when the ACTH deficiency has been severe and prolonged, the resulting profound adrenal atrophy may preclude an adequate response to initial ACTH infusion of 25 units intravenously over a six-hour interval (and measurement of plasma cortisol at five and six hours) and require intramuscular injections. Because anaphylactic reactions to ACTH have been reported in several patients, including a few deaths, Tyler and West (1972) recommend administration of 1.0 mg. of dexamethasone at midnight and 0.5 mg. at the start of the infusion. Despite the fact that intramuscular (I.M.) ACTH (40 units of long-acting) injection is occasionally misleading because of irregular absorption or tissue destruction of ACTH, it may be used and may be preferable (i.e., 40 units long-acting ACTH I.M. for three days) to intravenous infusions (daily for three days) in selected situations, e.g., sustained and severe ACTH deficiency with marked adrenal atrophy.

Hirsutism (excessive facial and body hair) and virilism manifested by deepened voice, amenorrhea, acne, increased libido and rate of hair growth with variable degrees of greater muscular build, decreased feminine fat, male hair distribution and texture, as well as clitoral hypertrophy suggest a variety of etiologies that may be classified as follows (modified from Bledsoe and Longscope, 1972):

Constitutional (? end-organ sensitivity)
Adrenogenital
- Enzyme defects (congenital virilizing adrenal hyperplasia)
- Adrenal tumor (adenoma or carcinoma)
- Cushing's syndrome (tumor or hyperplasia)
- Obesity stress syndrome
- Psychic stress (emotional instability with repeated psychic stress)

Ovarian
- Stein-Leventhal (? ovarian and adrenal disorder or ? hypothalamic-pituitary etiology)
- Ovarian tumors (arrhenoblastoma, hilar cell tumor, luteoma of pregnancy, lipoid cell tumor, dermoid cyst with androgenic stroma)
- Hyperplasia (hilar cells)
- Gonadal dysgenesis (chromatin negative variant, ambiguous genitalia)
- Feminizing testes (incomplete form)
- True hermaphroditism (ambiguous genitalia)

Although masculinizing and feminizing syndromes induced by adrenal gland abnormalities have been considered in two groups, i.e., (1) those caused by adrenal cortex tumors with estrogen or androgen excess, and (2) those caused by an adrenal cortical enzymatic defect with androgen excess, it is necessary to rule out or consider other causes (Bondy, 1971). Gynecomastia, the major sign of *estrogen excess* in prepubertal children and men, prompts consideration of testicular tumors, Klinefelter's syndrome, liver disease, and other causes of hyperestrogenism before making a diagnosis of an adrenal lesion. Since most women with Cushing's syndrome due to an adrenal lesion have both amenorrhea and elevated urinary estrogens, at least one factor that contributes to amenorrhea may be the estrogen excess with a negative feedback inhibition of pituitary gonadotropins (e.g., FSH). With such a lesion in postmenopausal women, uterine bleeding resumes; this may be associated with endometrial hyperplasia (polypoid), suggesting estrogen excess.

With *androgen excess* in Cushing's syndrome due to adrenal tumor, the anabolic effects may mask some of the usual features (catabolic manifestations) of Cushing's syndrome, i.e., diminution of osteoporosis and abdominal striae but persistence of rounded face and dorsal fat pad.

Androgen-induced hirsutism and amenorrhea in women warrants consideration of ovaries and adrenal cortices as the sources of excessive androgen. Plasma testosterone determinations reflecting baseline values and results after ACTH stimulation and dexamethasone suppression should delineate the origin by virtue of the fact that adrenal testosterone secretion is often stimulated and suppressed by these maneuvers. With Stein-Leventhal ovaries reflecting thickened capsule and multiple abortive cysts, ovarian excessive testosterone secretion can usually be suppressed by administration of estrogens and stimulated with chorionic gonadotropin. Apparently adrenal and ovarian hormones can suppress testosterone in both glands; hence, the suppression tests cannot be relied upon to reveal the source of androgen (Ettinger *et al.*, 1973). Virilization with luteoma of pregnancy is a rare entity associated with elevated urinary 17-KS and markedly increased plasma testosterone levels (Wolff *et al.*, 1973).

With virilizing adrenal tumors, the androgenic manifestations are acquired in contrast to congenital adrenal hyperplasia. The 17-KS output is often markedly increased (e.g., 100 mg. or more per 24 hours) with dehydroandrosterone (DHA) also increased, representing 50 per cent or more of the total urinary 17-KS. Androsterone and testosterone are also secreted but in much lesser amounts than DHA. Furthermore, with virilizing adrenal tumors, dexamethasone suppression of total urinary 17-KS and DHA is virtually absent. This maneuver should differentiate patients with adrenal tumors from those with congenital adrenal hyperplasia.

Urinary 17-Ketosteroids*

PRINCIPLE. Urine is subjected to acid hydrolysis and the steroids are extracted with ethylene dichloride. A solvent aliquot is evaporated to dryness under a nitrogen stream, and the resultant residue is reacted with m-dinitrobenzene (Zimmermann reaction), which in the presence of alkali gives a red color with compounds containing an active methylene group. This color obtained with the 17-ketosteroids has an absorption maximum at 520 mμ, and the interfering chromogens, as well as the 3-, 11-, 20-ketosteroids, are corrected for by means of the Allen correction factor.

---

*I. J. Drekter, A. Heisler, C. R. Scism, S. Stern, S. Pearson, and T. H. McGavack: The determination of urinary steroids. J. Clin. Endocr., *12*:55, 1952. Modification by Dr. R. Jacobs, Upstate Medical Center, Syracuse, New York. Personal communication, 1965.

SPECIMEN. A 24-hour urine is collected with refrigeration during collection. No preservative is added. Total volume is noted, and an aliquot is removed and refrigerated upon receipt in laboratory.

METHOD. See Davidsohn, I., and Henry, J. B. (eds.): *Todd-Sanford Clinical Diagnosis by Laboratory Methods.* 14th ed. 1969, Chapter 11, p. 617.

17-Hydroxycorticoids*

PRINCIPLE (Porter-Silber reaction). The glucuronide conjugates of urinary corticosteroids are hydrolyzed with β-glucuronidase. The "freed" steroids and free steroids (i.e., tetra and dihydro derivatives) normally present in the urine are extracted in methylene chloride. This extract is washed with a dilute aqueous alkali to remove a considerable amount of "blank material" which consists of estrogens, bile acids, and other interfering chromogens. A portion of methylene chloride is shaken with a phenylhydrazine hydrochloride–sulfuric-acid–ethanol reagent. For correction of the residual blank material, another portion of the extract is shaken with just the sulfuric-acid–ethanol reagent. The upper layer of methylene chloride is removed, and the lower phase after color development is measured spectrophotometrically at 410 mμ. The reacting steroids which have a dihydroxyacetone group on the 17 carbon (i.e., 17, 21-dihydroxy, 20-ketosteroids) have nearly the same molar absorbancy index with this procedure.

SPECIMEN. Urine, 24-hour refrigerated collection. Specimens to be assayed for Porter-Silber chromogens should be collected without preservative but refrigerated during collection. Since the test of drugs interfering with the determination is incomplete, all medications should be interrupted 48 hours prior to urine collection.

METHOD. See Davidsohn, I., and Henry, J. B. (eds.): *Todd-Sanford Clinical Diagnosis by Laboratory Methods.* 14th ed. 1969, Chapter 11, pp. 618–619.

ESTROGEN AND PROGESTERONE

Secretion of ovarian estrogen and progesterone is coordinated with pituitary follicle-stimulating hormone (FSH) and luteinizing hormone (LH) (Mishell *et al.*, 1971). At the beginning of each cycle, low estrogen levels coincide with release of pituitary FSH, which acts upon thecal cells, causing follicular growth and increased estrogen secretion. As

*R. Peterson, A. Karrer, and S. L. Guerra: Evaluation of Silber-Porter procedure for determination of plasma hydrocortisone. Anal. Chem., 29:144, 1957. R. Peterson, National Institutes of Health, Personal communication, June, 1959.

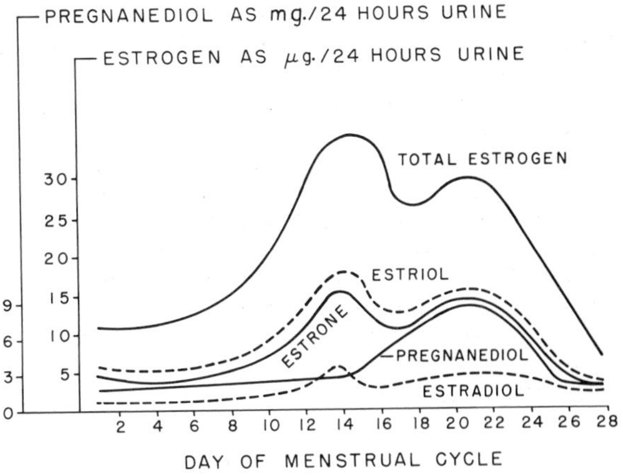

Figure 11-15. Urinary hormone excretion during the menstrual cycle.

estrogen increases, there is a slight decrease in circulating FSH. The increased estrogen, which peaks shortly before midcycle, causes a rapid release of LH which presumably is responsible for initiation of ovulation at midcycle. A sharp FSH peak is concomitant with the LH peak.

Immediately after ovulation, there is a transient fall in estrogen excretion. However, under the influence of slightly elevated LH, the granulosa cells undergo luteinization and produce progesterone and a secondary estrogen peak (Fig. 11–15).

Response of the corpus luteum to LH and FSH apparently depends upon its age: a corpus luteum only a few days old responds with secretory activity, while a corpus luteum which has started to regress will not respond to any great extent. Blood levels of progesterone seem largely independent of LH concentration. Causes for regression of the corpus luteum are not understood well. It has been postulated that unless pregnancy occurs, late progestational endometrium may secrete a "luteolysin." Regression of the corpus luteum produces regular menstrual bleeding.

Estrogen

Although over 20 estrogens have been identified, urinary estrogen is chiefly estriol (E3) with smaller amounts of estradiol (E2) and estrone (E1). E2 is believed to be the primary estrogenic hormone and is formed from androstenedione within ovarian stroma, follicles, and the corpus luteum. E1 is also formed from androstenedione; in addition, E1 and E2 apparently undergo interconversion (Fig. 11–16). E3, formed from E2 and E1 in the liver, is conjugated with glucuronide and excreted in urine and bile. If biologic activity of E2 is

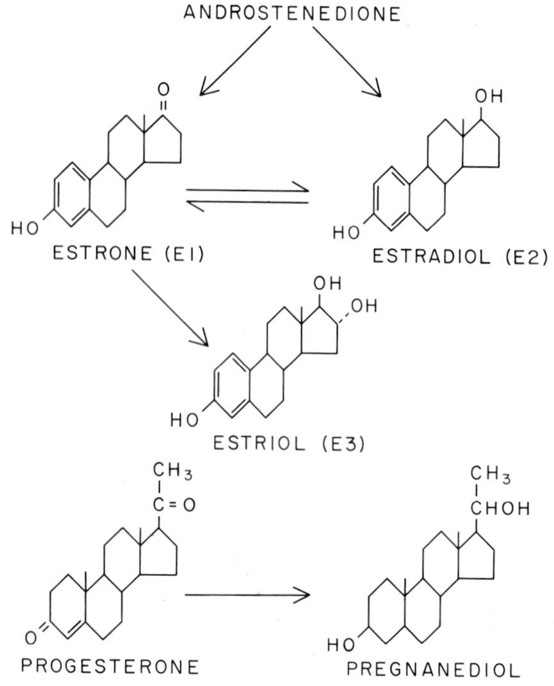

Figure 11-16. Relationships of estrone, estradiol, estriol, progesterone, and pregnanediol.

expressed as 100 per cent, E1 may be expressed as 20 per cent and E3 as less than 1 per cent. Failure of the liver to convert E1 and E2 to E3 accounts for signs of feminization which may accompany severe hepatic disease.

Because of marked variations in physiologic activity of different estrogens and a repressive effect of E3 on biologic activity of E2, results of bioassays on urinary extracts are not comparable to chemical measurements.

It is important to remember that patients on oral diethylstilbestrol or progestational agents have decreased urinary estrogen excretion, since these compounds cause decreased pituitary stimulation of the ovary.

Urinary estrogen determinations may be clinically useful in evaluating whether amenorrhea is due to pituitary, ovarian, or end-organ failure. With pituitary failure, FSH and estrogen levels are low, administration of gonadotrophin causes an increase in urinary estrogen, and secretory endometrium is found on biopsy following estrogen-progesterone therapy. With primary ovarian failure, FSH is increased and estrogen levels are low; gonadotrophins fail to increase the urinary estrogen, but estrogen-progesterone therapy results in secretory endometrium. With end-organ failure (e.g., uterine agenesis), FSH and estrogen are normal. A combination of endometrial biopsy with measurements of urinary estrogen, pregnanediol, and FSH provides a complete picture of end-organ response and endogenous hormonal stimulus in diagnostic problems (Nesbitt *et al.*, 1965).

Urinary estrogen measurements may also be helpful in evaluating hyperestrinism which may be due to gonadal or adrenal neoplasm (see p. 732). Simultaneous study of vaginal smears, urinary pregnanediol, and urinary FSH may provide a complete picture of pituitary, ovarian, and end-organ response.

The greatest clinical value of estrogen measurement may be in diagnosis of fetal distress during pregnancy. After the twelfth week of pregnancy, HCG levels gradually decline, while levels of urinary estrogen (and pregnanediol) gradually increase. About 90 per cent of the urinary estrogen during pregnancy is E3 (Fig. 11–17). Indeed, estriol (E3) is the principal estrogen found in the urine of pregnant women and in the placenta.

After the twenty-fifth week, urinary estrogen and pregnanediol continue to increase, but at a more rapid rate. E1, E2, and E3 are produced in the placenta from a number of intermediates, including dehydroepiandrostenedione (DHA), which is formed in the X-zone of the fetal adrenals. Perhaps because of decreased DHA, urinary estrogen levels tend to decrease with fetal distress and are very low with atrophy of fetal adrenals in most cases of anencephaly (cf. Chapter 27 on Amniotic Fluid).

Decreased E3 (and, hence, decreased total estrogen) is found with fetal distress due to many conditions, including pre-eclampsia, placental insufficiency, and poorly controlled diabetes mellitus. Low maternal urinary estrogens can occur with normal infants. Low urinary E3 may be observed with growth retarded fetuses. *Increased* E3 has been reported with erythroblastosis fetalis, but decreased levels do occur when this condition becomes severe.

Because of marked day-to-day and individual variations, there is a broad "low normal" range, and consecutive measurements of estrogens and/or E3 are needed unless initial measurements are markedly decreased (less than 30 per cent of normal). In general, a day-to-day decrease of 40 to 50 per cent or a week-to-week decrease of 20 to 30 per cent is considered significant. Furthermore, a steady consistent decrease in urinary estrogen values is significant irrespective of the per cent decrease.

Patients with a high fetal risk may be followed with successive E3 or total estrogen measurements after the thirty-second week; if persistently low or decreasing levels are found, premature delivery may offer increased probability of fetal survival (Magendantz *et al.*, 1968). The potential value of measuring maternal urinary 15-α hydroxy compounds

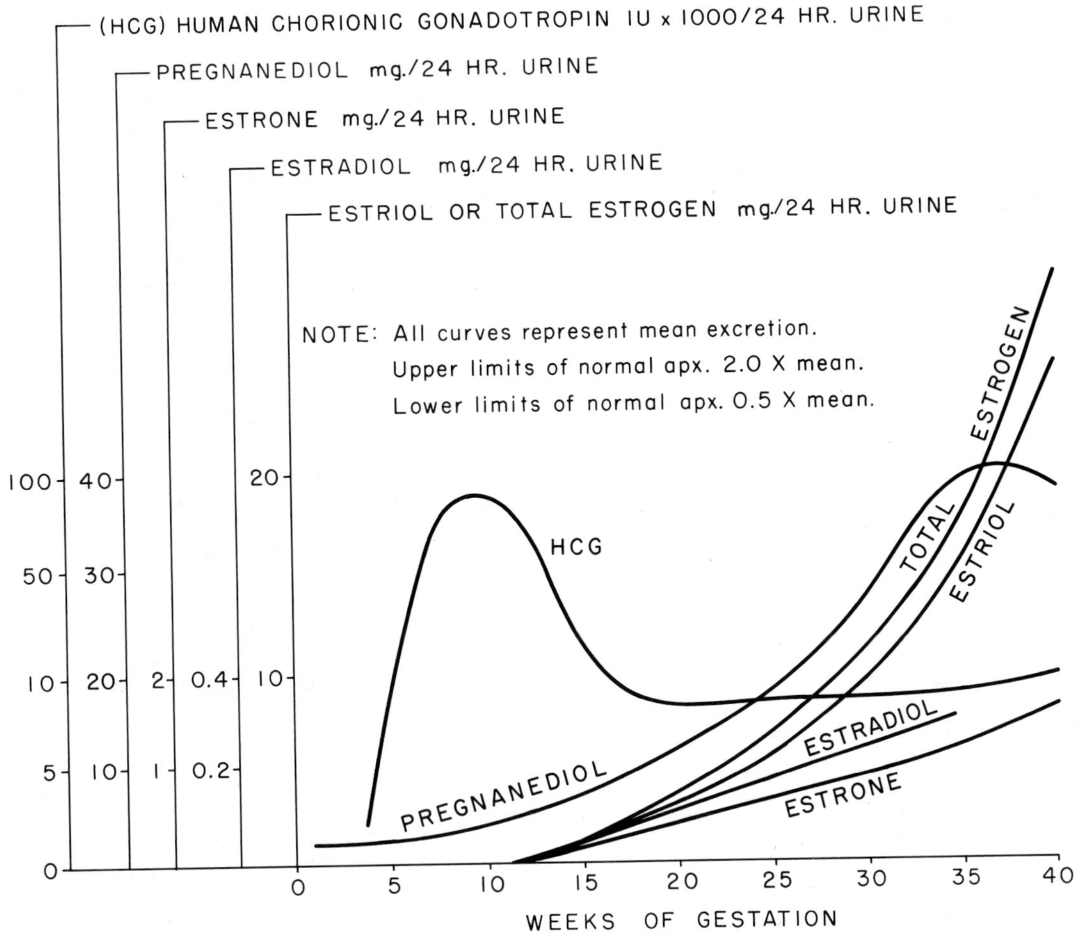

Figure 11-17. Urinary hormone excretion during pregnancy.

more specific to the fetus than E3 remains to be established.

During the past few years, gas chromatography has opened new dimensions in steroid analysis. Sensitive and specific measurement of urinary E3 is available. During the past two or three years, competitive protein binding has become a sensitive, specific assay method to determine plasma 17-β estradiol (Knox and France, 1972). The procedure is based on the ability of the patient's extracted estrogen to displace radiolabeled E2 from a carrier protein or adsorbent. Measurement of plasma E2 may be more clinically useful than urine E3, but this remains to be established.

Progesterone

Progesterone is produced by the ovary and placenta and is also formed in the adrenals as an intermediate in cortisone and aldosterone synthesis. Like estrogen, progesterone is metabolized in the liver; its biologically inert metabolite, pregnanediol, is conjugated with glucuronide and excreted in urine. If progesterone is given orally or parenterally, only about 10 per cent is recovered as pregnanediol; hence, urinary pregnanediol is not helpful in evaluating physiologic effects of exogenous progesterone (evaluation of vaginal cytology has been used for this purpose, cf. Chapter 25). However, urinary pregnanediol measurements serve as an index of endogenous progesterone production and correlate well with the majority of clinical conditions.

As with estrogen, there is considerable day-to-day variation and a broad "low normal" range. Bed rest helps to eliminate fluctuations due to activity and insures complete urine collections.

During the first half of the menstrual cycle, only a small amount of urinary pregnanediol is excreted; this may be derived from ovarian stroma and/or the adrenals. Following ovulation, there is a rapid increase in urine pregnanediol (Fig. 11–15). In the absence of pregnancy, this falls abruptly about three days prior to menstruation.

Measurements of urinary pregnanediol have been employed for detection of ovulation. A single measurement consistent with normal postovulatory levels may be misleading because increased pregnanediol may accompany luteinized granulosa or thecal cell tumors, diffuse thecal luteinization, metastatic carcinoma to ovary, adrenal hyperplasia, or ACTH administration. Maximal clinical information is obtained by multiple measurements and examinations, including basal body temperature, at least two pregnanediol measurements, several vaginal cell spreads, and endometrial biopsy.

Urinary pregnanediol is also useful in detection and diagnosis of placental dysfunction. Like estrogen, pregnanediol increases gradually between the twelfth and twenty-fifth weeks of pregnancy; after 25 weeks, the rate of increase becomes more rapid. Unlike estrogen, a maximum at about the thirty-seventh week is followed by a slight decrease prior to delivery (Fig. 11–17). Pregnanediol levels during pregnancy reflect placental function rather than fetal status. Indeed, even after fetal death, pregnanediol levels remain normal if maternal circulation to the placenta is intact. With hydatidiform mole, pregnanediol may be either normal or low, but total estrogen and E3 are invariably decreased.

Pregnanediol measurements may be clinically helpful in threatened abortion and premature delivery. A marked or progressive decrease in urinary pregnanediol is suggestive evidence of placental insufficiency. With normal pregnanediol, there is no benefit from progesterone therapy, while with decreased pregnanediol, progesterone therapy may be helpful. In patients with repeated abortions, pregnanediol measurements early in pregnancy may be helpful.

The measurement of human placental lactogen (HPL) has also been successfully utilized in the evaluation of placental function (Genazzani *et al.*, 1969) and may be the best test in early pregnancy. The placental fraction of alkaline phosphatase is more easily measured in maternal serum but is probably of limited value.

Testosterone

Testosterone, the principal androgen responsible for development and maintenance of male secondary sex characteristics, is produced chiefly by the Leydig cells of the testis. It is also produced in ovarian tissue and the adrenal cortex. Other androgens are formed by metabolism of testosterone and as intermediates in adrenal steroid synthesis: these include androsterone, epiandrosterone, and etiocholanolone (cf. p. 709). For clinical purposes, the determination of urinary 17-ketosteroids has been commonly employed to evaluate androgen production. However, the 17-ketosteroids represent a variety of end products, none of which is a specific metabolite of testosterone. Details of interrelationship were reviewed previously in this chapter under adrenal cortex and may be found on p. 717.

A number of chromatographic techniques are available for the separation of testosterone from urinary and plasma extracts; these include thin-layer and gas-liquid chromatography. Final quantitation of testosterone may be accomplished by several methods, including flame-ionization detection (gas-liquid chromatography), double-isotope derivative techniques, acid fluorescence, and competitive protein binding. The last procedure is probably the method of choice in the clinical laboratory.

In males testosterone excretion has been found decreased in hypogonadal subjects and Klinefelter's syndrome. In females testosterone excretion may be increased in the adrenogenital syndrome, in those cases of Stein-Leventhal syndrome that include associated virilization, and in some cases of hirsutism. However, measurements of testosterone excretion are not widely available, and for the present, this must be considered a research procedure.

FSH and LH

Measurements of LH and FSH are now possible by radioimmunoassay. Clinically, LH measurement is as useful as FSH in separating primary from secondary gonadal failure (see FSH p. 704) and, further, has been used to measure human chorionic gonadotropin (HCG) because of its frequent cross reactivity with HCG, and its greater sensitivity in following therapy or disease progress in patients with trophoblastic or gonadal tumors. These measurements in terms of clinical pathologic correlation are considered on p. 704, earlier in this chapter.

ADRENAL MEDULLA

The medullary portion of the adrenal gland rises from the neural crest and represents a modified postganglionic neuron. It can be viewed as a sympathetic ganglion lacking postsynaptic fibers with cells able to synthesize not only norepinephrine (NE) but also epinephrine (E). Epinephrine (80 to 90 per cent) and norepinephrine (10 to 20 per cent) make up its hormonal secretions. These hormones are designated catecholamines. Norepinephrine is also the mediator of the adrenergic fibers of the sympathetic nervous system. Because it stains brown with chromic acid or its salts, the adrenal medulla is referred to as chromaffin, or chromaphil tissue. While catecholamine production has been identified within these chromaffin cells, it is uncertain whether the two hormone secretions of the medulla represent a secretion of the granules from a single cell or from separate cell types. Chromaphil cells are also found in association with the sympathetic chain ganglia, in which case they are called paraganglia. Extra-adrenal chromaffin tissue, such as the Zuckerkandl's bodies (situated near the bifurcation of the aorta), chromaphil tissue located ventral to the abdominal aorta (slightly above the mesenteric artery), and the carotid body, function independently of the adrenal medulla. However, they may account for the large amount of catecholamines noted during fetal life. Normal values of urinary catecholamines and their metabolites during infancy and childhood warrant special consideration (Voorhess, 1967); daily urinary excretion increases from birth to adolescence, so that measurements of these compounds should be correlated with age during infancy and childhood.

A rare cause of hypertension (less than 1 per cent of patients with hypertension), important because of its curability in selected cases, is due to a secreting tumor of adrenal medulla or extra-adrenal chromaphil tissue called a pheochromocytoma (Fig. 11–18). Although such tumors are usually solitary benign adenomas, about 5 per cent are malignant, and at least 10 per cent are multiple. Over 80 per cent of all pheochromocytomas arise from the adrenal medulla; most of the others are found in sympathetic ganglia or embryologic rests found along the aorta in the abdomen and pelvis. Less than 1 per cent of pheochromocytomas arise outside the abdomen; they are most common in the intrathoracic sympathetic chain. While they may be encountered at any age from infancy to senility, they are observed most frequently between the ages of 20 and 50. The classic clinical picture with paroxysms of hypertension associated with the release into the blood of a variable mixture of epinephrine and norepinephrine is found in approximately one-third of patients with pheochromocytoma. In the remaining cases, persistent hypertension, often with postural variations, is observed. While the majority (80 to 90 per cent) of pheochromocytoma patients appear as sporadic cases, the remainder comprise familial groups with certain associated neuroectodermal tissue disease (Engelman and Sjoerdsma, 1971). Pheochromocytoma may be associated with neurofibromatosis (von Recklinghausen's disease), Lindau-von Hippel disease, or tuberous sclerosis, and also with multiple endocrine tumors of the pituitary, pancreas, and parathyroid, or with medullary carcinoma of the thyroid. Multiple adrenal pheochromocytomas and amyloid-containing medullary thyroid carcinoma with autosomal dominant inheritance have been described.

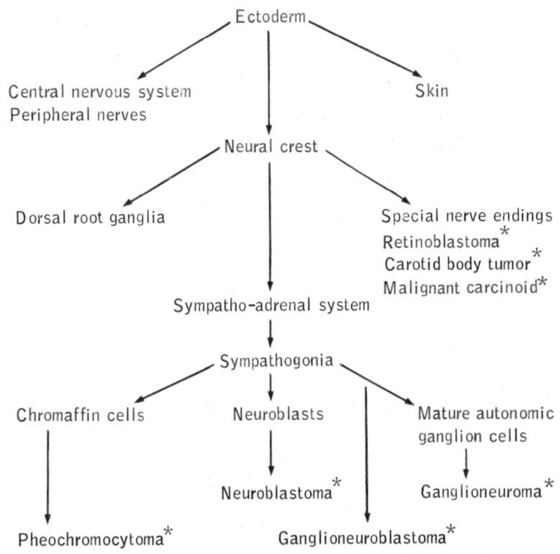

Figure 11-18. Origin of tumors that produce sympatho-adrenal hormones. *Hormone production that may yield elevated urinary catecholamines, vanilmandelic acid, metanephrines, and/or homovanillic acid.

In addition to pheochromocytoma, other disorders of the adrenal medulla associated with hormone release include the malignant neuroblastoma of children as well as ganglioneuroblastomas and ganglioneuromas (Fig. 11–18).

In summary, pheochromocytoma and neuroblastoma are the two major pathologic entities associated with chemical pathologic reflections of adrenomedullary disorders.

Biochemical and Physiologic Considerations

The biosynthesis and metabolism of adrenomedullary hormones are shown in Figures 11–19 and 11–20. Although dopamine is present in small amounts in the adrenal medulla, larger amounts are present in the sympathetic nerve fibers. Tyrosine is the major precursor of dopamine, epinephrine, and norepinephrine present in the gland (Axelrod and Weinshilboum, 1972). The naturally occurring hormones are levorotatory. Dopamine, epinephrine, and norepinephrine are classified chemically as catecholamines (catechol=dihydroxybenzene), although this term usually refers only to norepinephrine and epinephrine. Because the catecholamines are readily oxidized, it has been inferred that the large concentration of ascorbic acid in the adrenal medulla maintains these compounds in the reduced state. With sympathetic nerve stimulation, catecholamines are released from the secretory granules of adrenal medullary cells and from storage (synaptic) vesicles in sympathetic nerve fiber endings. After release into the adrenal vein circulation epinephrine and norepinephrine are metabolized preferentially in the liver by catechol-O-methyl transferase. Epinephrine and norepinephrine are converted to their physiologically inert 3-methoxy derivatives (metanephrine and normetanephrine, respectively) in the presence of the enzyme catechol-O-methyl transferase. Subsequently, these compounds, metanephrine and normetanephrine, are either excreted in the urine or metabolized in many body cells by a second major enzyme, monoamine oxidase, to 3-methoxy-4-hydroxymandelic acid (vanillylmandelic acid, vanilmandelic acid, or VMA). An alternative pathway with sequence of action of these two enzymes reversed exists in which 3,4-dihydroxymandelic acid is produced as an intermediate. About 75 per cent of the total urinary catecholamine metabolites is VMA. Metanephrines contribute about 10 per cent and free catecholamines about 1 per cent (Engelman and Sjoerdsma, 1971); hence, the determination of the catabolite VMA in urine serves as a sensitive measure of catecholamine production. The administration of monoamine oxidase inhibitors (iproniazid and some related hydrazine derivatives) produce a marked increase in metanephrines and normetanephrines at the

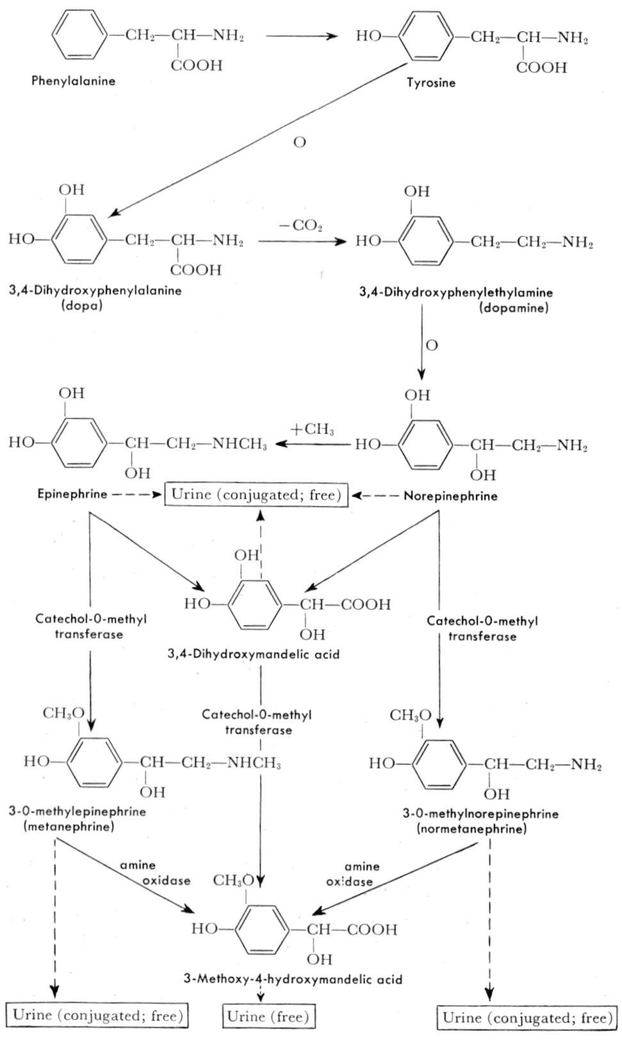

Figure 11-19. Biosynthesis and metabolism of adrenomedullary hormones.

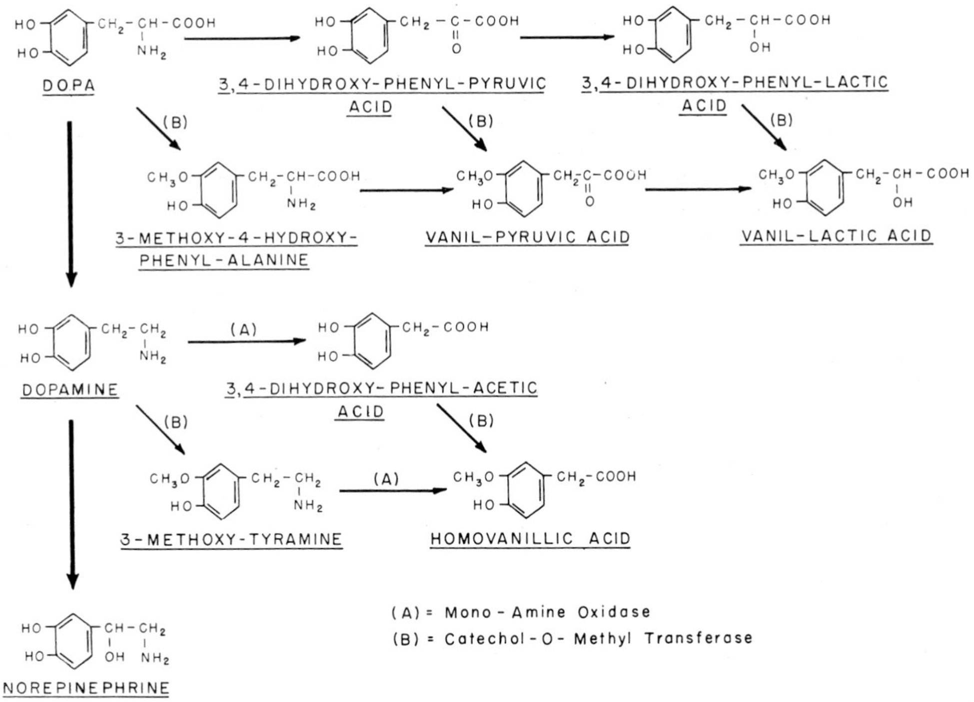

Figure 11-20. Pathways of dihydroxyphenylalanine (DOPA) metabolism. (From Sunderman, F. W., Jr.: Amer. J. Clin. Path. 42:481, 1964.)

expense of VMA. Dopamine, the other major catecholamine, may also be converted by a series of reactions analogous to those just described to compounds which ultimately yield homovanillic acid (HVA) (Fig. 11-20). VMA and HVA constitute the main urinary metabolites of the catecholamines. These as well as unchanged catecholamines are excreted partly in the free form and partly conjugated with sulphuric and glucuronic acids. Because of the minute concentration of catecholamines in blood (microgram quantity), the urine is assayed for these hormones or their metabolites in assessment of the state of adrenomedullary function.

Catecholamines of the adrenal medulla participate with the autonomic nervous system reactions to sudden emergencies and prepare the individual for "flight or fight." Pain, heat, cold, emotional stress, hypoglycemia, injury, hemorrhage and asphyxia, a variety of drugs, and undoubtedly other factors stimulate the release of catecholamines and produce many of the effects observed with stress. Epinephrine and norepinephrine stimulate the action of the sympathetic nervous system and exert numerous wide and varied effects on many functions of the body. However, the physiologic actions of epinephrine and norepinephrine differ in many respects; the stimuli for their release may also differ. Norepinephrine exerts its primary effect on the circulatory system, with elevation of both systolic and diastolic blood pressure but without the significant change in pulse rate produced by epinephrine. Norepinephrine produces an increase of total peripheral resistance, while epinephrine does not. Hyperglycemia and eosinopenia are attributed to epinephrine rather than norepinephrine.

Clinical Pathology Correlations

Unlike the adrenal cortex in which extirpation results in death of humans without replacement therapy, the medulla is expendable. Hence, there is no need to consider assessment of hypoadrenomedullary function. The usual indications for study of adrenomedullary function are evaluation of patients with hypertension to identify individuals with pheochromocytoma and evaluation of children to confirm the diagnosis of neuroblastoma or related tumors derived from sympathetic cells.

Bioassay techniques for the determination of epinephrine and norepinephrine have been replaced by simpler, less costly, more sensitive and more specific chemical methods. Four measurements are employed in the laboratory evaluation of adrenomedullary function: total catecholamines, vanilmandelic acid (VMA), metanephrines, and homovanillic acid. A differential catecholamine assay may also be used but is rarely indicated.

Total Catecholamines. Fluorometric determination of catecholamines in 24-hour urine specimens is frequently used (Sandhu and Freed, 1972). The diurnal variation in excretion with output decreasing during sleeping hours precludes less than a 24-hour specimen. The normal range for adults varies with the individual method but in general is up to 14 μg. per 100 ml. or 100 μg. per 24-hour urine. Elevations reveal a high degree of correlation with patients demonstrated to have a pheochromocytoma. However, an occasional patient with a pheochromocytoma may fail to have significantly increased urinary catecholamines. Patients with a neuroblastoma may also have a striking elevation of urinary catecholamines. Spurious elevations may be due to fluorescent urinary excretion products of medications including adrenaline or adrenaline-like drugs, antibiotics such as tetracyclines, quinidine, and selected antihypertensive agents (e.g., methyldopa); hence, specificity is not absolute, and false elevations may be encountered. Furthermore, patients with widespread burns, individuals undergoing vigorous exercise, and patients with progressive muscular dystrophy and myasthenia gravis may also show elevations of urinary catecholamines; a decreased excretion may be observed in familial dysautonomia, malnutrition, and transection of cervical spinal cord. Since catecholamines represent a very small fraction of total urinary excretion products from the adrenal medulla, increased sensitivity may be obtained by other measurements.

Vanillylmandelic Acid (3-Methoxy-4-hydroxymandelic Acid, Vanilmandelic Acid, VMA). Since the major urinary metabolite of norepinephrine and epinephrine is VMA, urinary VMA excretion is considerably higher than total catecholamines. The normal range of VMA in a 24-hour urine is up to 7 mg. or less than 7 μg. per mg. of creatinine, depending on the specific procedure. Several methods have been employed. Unfortunately many nonspecific VMA colorimetric or electrophoretic techniques of poor quality have been in vogue, yielding unreliable data and misinformation with high normal value ranges, e.g., 10 to 15 mg. per 24 hours. Urine is a frequent manifestation of such nonspecific tests, often markedly affected by diet. Organic extraction of VMA from the urine, oxidation to vanillin, and measurement of vanillin at 360 mμ are critical steps of the assay we recommend at the end of this section (Pisano *et al.*, 1962). Although this assay is not significantly affected by dietary constituents, the results may be altered by certain drug therapy. The antibiotic nalidixic acid (NegGram) increases the apparent VMA value by producing an interfering drug metabolite. Others have reported that clofibrate (Atromid-S) will decrease the apparent VMA excretion by reducing recovery of the assay (Engelman and Sjoerdsma, 1971). To preclude false elevations of urinary VMA, all medications and foods which may give rise to phenoxy acids in the urine should be excluded for several days before, as well as during, collection of the specimen. Coffee, fruits (especially bananas), and many drugs (including aspirin) may yield specimens with false positive elevations. From the standpoint of laboratory methodology. VMA is preferable to total catecholamine estimation, although it can hardly be called a simple procedure. VMA has been shown to be normal in some patients with pheochromocytoma and normal urinary catecholamines, while some patients with neuroblastoma may have a normal VMA but elevated urinary catecholamines. Since pheochromocytoma may be familial, VMA should be measured in relatives. Because of the frequency of multiple tumors and the occasional malignant recurrence of pheochromocytoma, as well as neuroblastoma, serial postoperative measurements are also indicated.

Metanephrines. Metanephrines represent 3-methoxy metabolites of the catecholamines; urinary levels are greater than total catecholamines but less than VMA, as reflected by the normal range up to 1 mg. in a 24-hour specimen. In tumors, however, variations in metabolic pathways may cause an increase in metanephrines alone. Hence, a few patients with pheochromocytoma may have elevated urinary metanephrines but normal catecholamines and VMA. Methods available for urinary metanephrines include chromatoelectrophoretic, fluorometric, and colorimetric assays, with the latter based on chemical conversion of the metanephrine to vanillin. Gitlow and colleagues (1970) have employed successfully a column chromatographic method for total metanephrines, reporting adult normal control values from 0.001 to 2.2 μg./mg. creatinine. However, a major limitation of this assay is due to the variability of catecholamine excretion during illnesses associated with severe stress, e.g., hemorrhagic shock, sepsis, widespread metastatic disease, and so forth. Hence, an elevated level of total metanephrines was not specific for pheochromocytoma, although a normal level ruled out the presence of this tumor. Patients receiving monoamine oxidase (MAO) inhibitors (drugs for depression and hypertension) display significantly increased excretions yielding false positive tests.

Homovanillic Acid (HVA). Since dopamine is present in sympathetic nervous tissue as a precursor of norepinephrine, and since it has a separate metabolic pathway that yields HVA, tumors such as neuroblastomas may cause elevations of urinary dopamine and its metabolite, HVA; in some cases these elevations have been observed with normal levels of VMA, total catecholamines, and metanephrines. Urinary HVA is usually normal in patients with pheochromocytoma. Neuroblastomas and ganglioneuromas probably should not be ruled out in individual patients without an estimation of HVA, although cases have been observed with normal levels of HVA and all other metabolites cited above. While colorimetric procedures have been employed for measurement of HVA, gas chromatography appears to have more promise as an ideal method. Indeed, gas chromatography permits simultaneous assay of VMA and HVA; these represent the best single combination of determinations available for the study of the majority of patients (Williams and Greer, 1965).

Differential Catecholamine Assay. Although extra-adrenal pheochromocytomas often are pure norepinephrine secretors, the more common adrenal tumors may secrete a mixture of catecholamines. In problem cases not resolved by other measurements (VMA, total metanephrines and/or catecholamines), a differential determination of epinephrine and norepinephrine may be helpful as a diagnostic acid (Hunter *et al.*, 1963; Sandhu and Freed, 1972).

Summary. While most patients undergoing laboratory investigation for suspected pheochromocytoma will reveal elevated urinary total metanephrines, the vast majority will also have an elevated VMA. Total metanephrines by column chromatography is the best single measurement for pheochromocytoma, with a sensitivity of 100 per cent and a specificity of 98 per cent (Gitlow *et al.*, 1970); however, urinary VMA is almost as sensitive and specific and is more widely available. If equivocal or negative VMA results are obtained and there exists strong clinical suspicion, three subsequent VMA and total metanephrine assays on 24-hour urines should be performed. In problem cases, as well as in patients with neuroblastoma, HVA and dopamine measurement may be helpful. If equivocal results persist, metanephrines may be determined; if this result is also negative or equivocal, the differential catecholamine assay may be helpful. For patients being evaluated for neuroblastoma and related tumors, HVA assay and VMA or total catecholamines are ordinarily measured.

METHOD.* Urinary 3-methoxy-4-hydroxymandelic acid (VMA).

PRINCIPLE. The procedure involves an extraction with ethyl acetate of 3-methoxy-4-hydroxymandelic acid along with other phenolic acids, oxidation of the potassium carbonate extract with 3-methoxy-4-hydroxymandelic acid by periodate to vanillin, extraction of the vanillin from the other phenolic acids into toluene, and finally the spectrophotometric determination of the vanillin with an absorption peak at 360 mμ.

REAGENTS

1. 2 per cent w/v sodium metaperiodate in distilled water. This solution is stable one week at room temperature.
2. 10 per cent w/v sodium metabisulfite in distilled water. This solution is stable one week if refrigerated.
3. 6 N hydrochloric acid.
4. 1 M potassium carbonate.
5. 5 N acetic acid.
6. 1 M phosphate buffer, pH 7.4, approximately 45 ml. of 1 M potassium hydroxide plus 50 ml. 1 M potassium dihydrogen phosphate. Adjust with 1 N potassium hydroxide until pH is 7.4.
7. Ethyl acetate, A. R.
8. Sodium chloride, A. R.
9. Toluene, A. R.
10. Stock standard 3-methoxy-4-hydroxymandelic acid 1 mg. per ml. in distilled water. This solution is stable three months if refrigerated.
11. Working standard VMA solution (10 μg. per ml.). Prepare immediately prior to use by diluting 1 ml. of the stock standard up to 100 ml. with distilled water in a 100 ml. volumetric flask.

SPECIMEN. No dietary restriction pertaining to coffee, chocolate, bananas, vanilla-containing foods, and citrus fruits is necessary. However, dietary restriction pertaining to drugs (especially antihypertensive agents and inhibitors of monoamine oxidase) three days prior to and during collection is necessary. Prior to collection, place 25 ml. of 6 N HCl into a 2-liter dark brown bottle. The total volume is measured and recorded with a 100-ml. aliquot stored at 4° C. for subsequent analysis. The specimen appears to be stable for several weeks at this temperature.

PROCEDURE

1. For each test specimen and reference control specimen, pipette 0.2 per cent of the 24-hour volume into four screw-cap 50-ml. centrifuge tubes, so that each urine blank and test is in duplicate. In addition, select two determinations and pipette in duplicate the same amount into two 50-ml. tubes each. These are used as internal standards.
2. To those tubes selected as internal standards, pipette 1 ml. of the working standard and proceed as with the rest of the test.
3. Dilute all these tubes to 5.5 ml. with distilled water, and further acidify with 0.5 ml. 6 N hydrochloric acid.
4. Saturate each tube with approximately

*From J. J. Pisano, R. J. Crout, and D. Abraham: Determination of 3-methoxy-4-hydroxymandelic acid in urine. Clin. Chim. Acta, 7:285, 1962 and Broadsheet Number 44. British Society of Clinical Pathologists.

3 gm. of sodium chloride. Mix well on Vortex* mixer.

5. To each tube add 30 ml. ethyl acetate. Cap tightly, shake mechanically for 5 minutes and centrifuge for 5 minutes.

6. Pipette 25 ml. of the ethyl acetate (upper) phase into a second screw-cap 50-ml. centrifuge tube which contains 1.5 ml. 1 M potassium carbonate.

7. Cap tightly, shake mechanically for 3 minutes and centrifuge for 5 minutes.

8. Transfer 1 ml. of the carbonate (lower) phase to a third screw-cap centrifuge tube.

9. To all the tests and standards add 0.1 ml. of the 2 per cent sodium metaperiodate. Mix contents of tubes and cap loosely; place all tubes into a 50° C. water bath for 30 minutes.

10. At the end of incubation interval, remove tubes and allow them to come to room temperature.

11. To all tubes add 0.1 ml. 10 per cent metabisulfite to reduce residual periodate.

12. To blank tubes add 0.1 ml. 2 per cent sodium metaperiodate and mix well.

13. To neutralize, add 0.3 ml. 5 N acetic acid and mix well to release CO_2, using a Vortex mixer.

14. To all tubes, add 0.6 ml. 1 M phosphate buffer pH 7.4.

15. Extract contents of each tube with 20 ml. toluene by shaking mechanically for 3 minutes and centrifuging for 5 minutes.

16. Pipette 15 ml. of the toluene (upper) layer into a fourth screw-cap centrifuge tube containing 3.5 ml. 1 M potassium carbonate.

17. Cap tightly, shake mechanically for 3 minutes and centrifuge for 5 minutes.

18. Use 10 mm. lightpath Beckman cuvettes and a Beckman DU or comparable spectrophotometer; read against a water blank. Determine the absorbance of the carbonate (lower) layer for contents of each tube at 360 mμ.

CALCULATIONS

A_b = absorbance of the urine blank.
A_t = absorbance of the test.
A_{st} = absorbance of the standard plus test.

$$\frac{A_t - A_b}{A_{st} - A_t} \times 5 = \text{mg. VMA excreted per 24 hours.}$$

To determine other tests without an internal standard:

A_u = absorbance of other test.
A_{ub} = absorbance of the other urine blank.

$$\frac{(A_u - A_{ub})}{(A_{st} - A_t)} \times 5 = \text{mg. VMA excreted per 24 hours.}$$

NORMAL VALUES. The normal adult excretion of VMA lies below 7 mg. per 24 hours. Values exceeding 10 mg. per 24 hours are diagnostic of catecholamine-secreting tumor.

*Scientific Products, Raritan, New Jersey.

THYROID

Normal Anatomy

The thyroid gland consists of two lobes connected by an isthmus. Normally the right lobe is slightly larger than the left. Absence of the isthmus is a normal variant (perhaps 2 per cent). About 50 per cent of normal persons have a third pyramidal lobe, arising from the isthmus. Weight of this gland is influenced by diet; in North Americans the "normal range" is 15 to 25 gm.* Blood supply is from two superior thyroid arteries (arising from the external carotids) and two inferior thyroid arteries (arising from the subclavians). Normal blood flow is about 100 ml. per minute, but with hyperplasia this may exceed 1000 ml. per minute, presenting serious problems during surgery.

During fetal development thyroid tissue arises near the foramen cecum at the base of the tongue and migrates along the thyroglossal duct to its final position below the larynx. Abnormal migration may cause location of thyroid tissue at the foramen cecum, along the thyroglossal duct, or in the mediastinum. Unfused thyroid nodules – small masses of thyroid tissue immediately adjacent to the main gland – can be found in about 10 per cent of autopsies. Normal-appearing thyroid tissue found within carotid lymph nodes usually represents metastasis from well-differentiated thyroid carcinoma; however, a few such cases may represent benign ectopic glandular rests.

Microscopically the thyroid consists of follicles with low cuboidal cells arranged about protein-rich colloid. Parafollicular cells (believed to secrete calcitonin), ganglion cells, and blood vessels are found in the surrounding stroma.

Thyroid Hormone Synthesis

The first step in synthesis is absorption of dietary iodide in the small intestine (Fig. 11–21). Average intake in the U.S.A. is about 200 μg./day, but this varies from about 50 to 2000 μg./day. Intake typically is low in central or mountainous areas and high near the seacoast – possibly on the basis of soil iodide content. Minimum daily requirement for iodide is usually given as 100 μg./day. Ingested iodide

*In the U.S. "goiter belt," normal range has been reported as 20 to 40 gm.

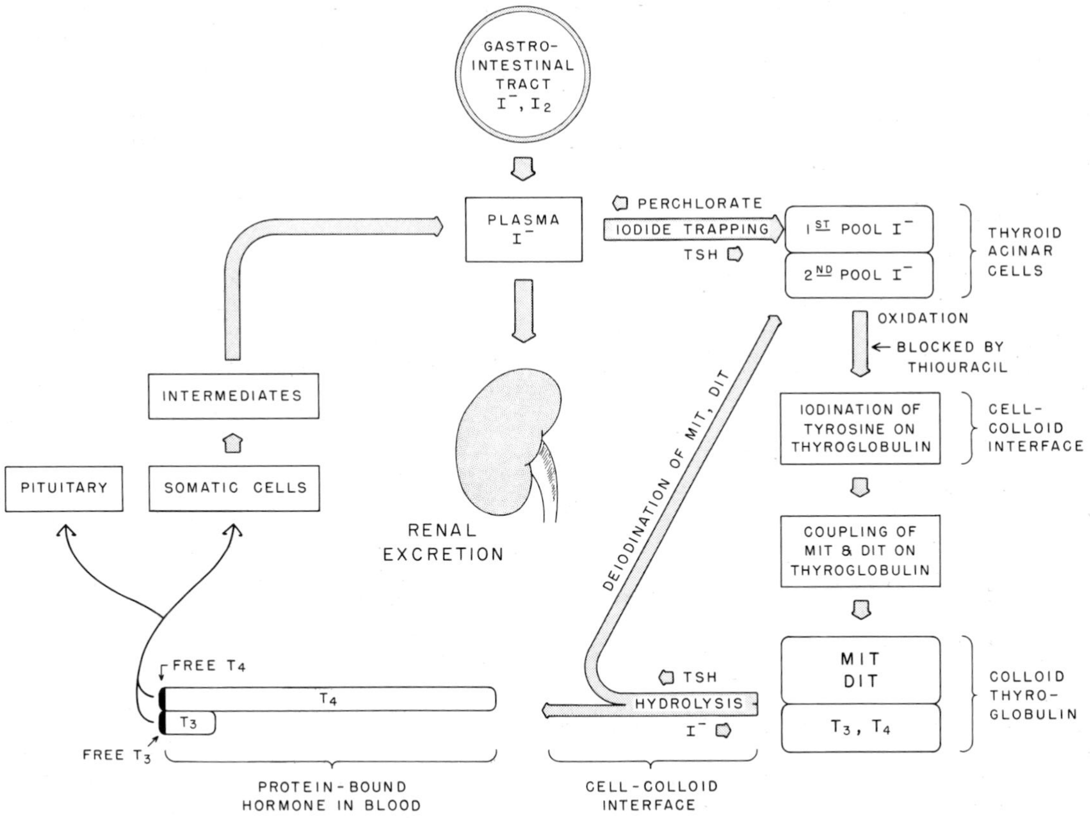

Figure 11-21. Outline of iodine metabolism in relation to thyroid function.

is almost completely absorbed, distributed in extracellular fluid and plasma, then cleared by the thyroid (about 20 ml./min.) and kidney (about 40 ml./min.). Renal clearance is via glomerular filtration; thyroid clearance is via active iodide transport or "trapping."

Iodide transport by the thyroid normally produces a thyroid: plasma iodide ratio of about 40:1; however, this may vary from 20:1 to 200:1, depending on: (1) stimulation of iodide transport by thyroid stimulating hormone (TSH); or (2) iodide stores in the thyroid (low intrathyroidal iodine increases iodide transport). Other tissues which also concentrate iodide include salivary gland, gastric mucosa, mammary gland, placenta, choroid plexus, and ciliary body (perhaps 1 per cent of total iodide clearance). After entering the thyroid, iodide must be oxidized and combined with tyrosine on thyroglobulin, after which the iodotyrosines are coupled and the thyroglobulin stored as colloid (Fig. 11-22).

Thyroglobulin, a glycoprotein of about 660,000 G.M.W., is formed on ribosomes of thyroid acinar cells and passes to the "cell-colloid interface" (Fig. 11-22), which includes vacuoles of thyroglobulin near the apices of acinar cells and portions of colloid between villi of acinar cells. There are about 125 tyrosyl residues per molecule: only about 20 of these are iodinated to monoiodotyrosine (MIT) or diiodotyrosine (DIT), and only about three undergo coupling to form T3 or T4. Oxidation of iodide and incorporation into tyrosine on thyroglobulin are believed to proceed simultaneously. Coupling of MIT and DIT occurs shortly thereafter.

It is suggested that thyroid peroxidase may mediate oxidation of iodide, iodination of tyrosine, and coupling of iodotyrosines to form thyroxine (T4) and triiodothyronine (T3); the H_2O_2 required for these reactions may be generated in the thyroid via oxidation of NADPH (DeGroot *et al.,* 1972). It is possible that coupling may be regulated by TSH; the ratio of iodotyrosine:iodothyronine increases with hypophysectomy and is restored to normal by TSH.

The thyroglobulin, with incorporated MIT, DIT, T3, and T4, is stored as colloid.

The thyroid is unique among endocrines owing to its large amount of stored hormone (as thyroglobulin) and its slow rate of hormone turnover. Both T3 and T4 reach peripheral circulation by hydrolysis of thyroglobulin. Colloid droplets near the apical plasma mem-

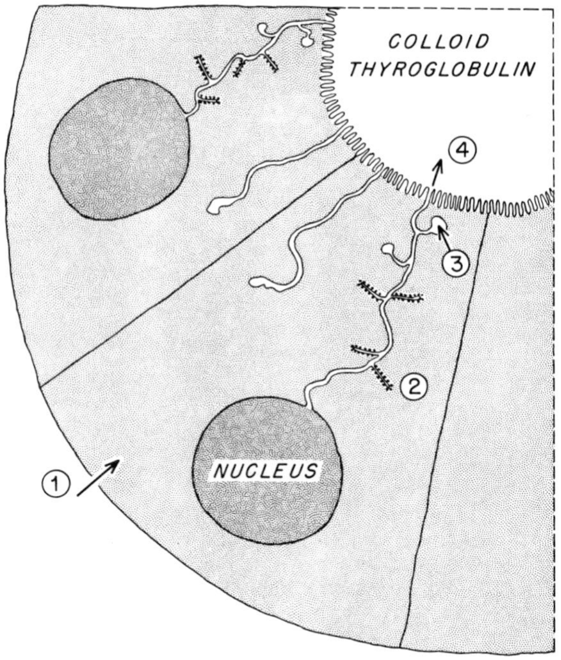

Figure 11-22. The thyroid acinar cell. 1, Iodide trapping mechanism, or "iodide pump"; 2, formation of thyroglobulin on ribosomes; 3, droplets of thyroglobulin within acinar cells; iodination of thyroglobulin here and in colloid adjacent to villi; 4, passage of iodinated thyroglobulin into colloid. (Modified from Means, De Groot, and Stanbury: *The Thyroid and Its Diseases.* New York, McGraw-Hill Book Co., Inc., 1963.)

brane are liquefied by phagolysosomes to release iodotyrosines, iodothyronines, and non-iodinated fragments of the thyroglobulin molecule. This hydrolysis appears to be under control of TSH, and proceeds in three stages: (1) phagocytosis of thyroglobulin droplets by lysosomes, (2) proteolysis of thyroglobulin, and (3) movement of lysosomes toward basal end of the cell, with discharge of T3 and T4 into blood stream.

The iodotyrosines are deiodinated by an enzyme system called iodotyrosine deiodinase. This microsomal system, specific for free iodotyrosine, is stimulated by TSH. Iodide released on deiodination of iodotyrosines enters a "second iodide pool" within the thyroid, (Fig. 11-21); unlike the "first iodide pool" (trapped iodide prior to oxidation or organification), this is not dischargeable by perchlorate or thiocyanate.

Serum Transport of Thyroid Hormones

Serum normally contains free iodide (about 0.1–0.6 μg./dl.), iodotyrosines (about 0.3 μg./dl.), thyroxine (about 6–12 μg./dl.), and triiodothyronine (about 0.2–0.3 μg./dl. or 200–300 ng./dl.).

Thyroxine (T4) is bound to three serum proteins: thyroxine-binding globulin (TBG), thyroxine-binding prealbumin (TBPA), and albumin. About 0.02 per cent of T4 is free, and about 99.98 per cent bound. About 60 per cent of T4 is bound to TBG, about 30 per cent to TBPA, and about 10 per cent to albumin. Of these binding proteins, TBG has the lowest T4 capacity (15–25 μg./dl.) and highest affinity; TBPA has intermediate T4 capacity (200–300 μg./dl.) and intermediate affinity; albumin has greatest T4 capacity and least affinity. The absolute free thyroxine (FT4) may be calculated as T4 multiplied by per cent free thyroxine (per cent FT4):

$$\begin{aligned} FT4 &= T4 \times \%\ FT4 \\ &= 9000\ \text{ng./dl.} \times 0.0002 \\ &= 1.8\ \text{ng./dl.} \end{aligned}$$

Triiodothyronine (T3) is bound to TBG and albumin, but not to TBPA. About 0.2 per cent of T3 is free and about 99.8 per cent bound. The absolute free triiodothyronine (FT3) may be calculated as T3 multiplied by per cent free triiodothyronine (per cent FT3):

$$\begin{aligned} FT3 &= T3 \times \%\ FT3 \\ &= 250\ \text{ng./dl.} \times 0.002 \\ &= 0.5\ \text{ng./dl.} \end{aligned}$$

Thus, concentration of free T4 in serum is about four times that of free T3 (Fig. 11-23). However, it appears that FT3 is several times more active than FT4, and that effects of these two hormones on target organs may be approximately equal. Perhaps 10 per cent of plasma T3 and T4 is excreted by the liver in bile, then reabsorbed from the intestinal tract; it has been suggested that this pathway occasionally may be of clinical importance in man.

Peripheral Actions of Thyroid Hormones

Like many other endocrine secretions, the two thyroid hormones, triiodothyronine (T3) and thyroxine (T4), have several effects (Table 11-19). Actions of the two hormones are similar, although T3 has a shorter latent period and a shorter duration of action and is more potent than T4. Primary hormone action may be at a mitochondrial level, but several pathways probably are involved, since after hormone administration increased heart rate has a short latent period (12 to 24 hours), increased basal metabolic rate (BMR) an intermediate latent period (2 to 3 days), and decreased body weight a long latent period (several weeks). The bound hormones are believed to be physiologically inactive. It is the free hormone which diffuses into cells, to cause the physiologic effects of T3 and T4 (Table 11-19). The exact site and mechanism of action for free T3 and T4 are not established, but effects on mitochondria and enzyme systems have been described.

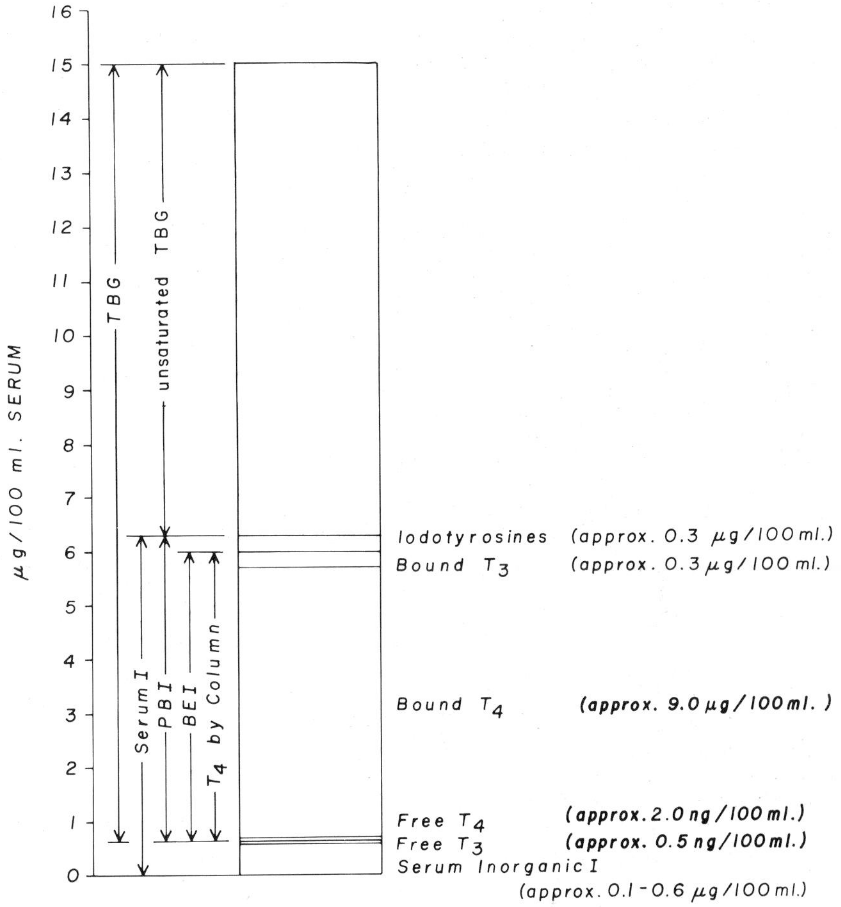

Figure 11-23. Relationships between total thyroxine-binding globulin (TBG), protein-bound iodine (PBI), butanol-extractable iodine (BEI), T4 by column, and iodotyrosines.

Table 11-19. SOME EFFECTS OF THYROXINE (T4) AND TRIIODOTHYRONINE (T3)

Required for normal growth and maturation, especially skeletal and central nervous system; cretinism occurs with lack of hormone in early life.
Generalized increase in oxygen consumption (BMR), causing increased heat production and symptoms of heat intolerance.
Increased anabolism (small amounts of hormone); larger amounts of hormone cause increased catabolism, with weight loss despite increased food intake.
Cardiac effects: increased pulse, increased pulse pressure, and increased cardiac output; may result in high output failure.
Increased sensitivity to epinephrine, causing tremors and emotional lability (reserpine and guanethidine may be helpful in treatment).
Impaired formation of phosphocreatine; causes muscle weakness and decreased creatine tolerance.
Increased glucose absorption from gastrointestinal tract; may cause diabetic-type glucose tolerance curve.
Increased lipid catabolism; may cause decreased serum cholesterol.
Increased bone resorption; may cause increased serum calcium.
Stimulation of various enzyme systems.

There is some evidence that T4 may be converted to T3 in peripheral tissues (Sterling *et al.*, 1970); additional data are needed to confirm these findings and establish their significance.

Within peripheral tissues, thyroid hormones are: (1) excreted by hepatocytes in bile, and reabsorbed in the small bowel (enterohepatic circulation), and (2) deiodinated, and inorganic iodide released into plasma.

Regulation of Thyroid Gland

The thyroid feedback system consists of three main components: hypothalamus (secretes TRF), anterior pituitary (secretes TSH), and thyroid gland (secretes T3 and T4).

Thyrotropin-releasing factor (TRF) is a tripeptide, L-pyroglutamyl-L-histidyl-L-proline amide, of molecular weight 362, secreted by nerve endings in the hypothalamus. On secretion, TRF diffuses into the capillary plexus of the median eminence and is carried by veins of the pituitary stalk to sinusoids of the anterior pituitary. In the pituitary, TRF appears to have two actions: it stimulates release of preformed TSH, and it causes synthesis of new TSH.

Thyroid hormone blocks these effects of TRF on the pituitary, possibly by stimulating formation of an inhibitor (Hershman and Pittman, 1971). Thyroid hormone may also act directly on the hypothalamus, with high levels inhibiting, and low levels stimulating, TRF formation or release.

Thyroid-stimulating hormone (TSH) is a glycoprotein of molecular weight 26,000 secreted by basophil cells in the pituitary. TSH apparently consists of two nonidentical polypeptide units, designated α and β: the α subunit has a structure similar to the α subunit of LH and HCG, while the β subunit confers TSH specificity (Hall, 1972).

Normal TSH level in serum is 0–10 μU./ml. (Nelson *et al.*, 1972). Effects of TSH on the thyroid gland may include: increased iodide trapping, coupling of iodotyrosines on thyroglobulin, hydrolysis of thyroglobulin, ratio of T3 to T4, and size and vascularity of thyroid gland.

In addition to TRF, circulating levels of free T3 and free T4 control TSH release at the pituitary: low levels of free hormone cause TSH release, while increased free hormone prevents TSH release, possibly by causing synthesis of an inhibitor. Although free T3 and free T4 may also influence TRF release from the hypothalamus, this is not yet proved. Thus, normal levels of free hormone are maintained by a negative feedback effect: increased free hormone causes decreased TSH secretion, hence decreases in iodide trapping, hydrolysis of thyroglobulin, and total hormone. The decrease in total hormone tends to reduce free hormone levels to normal. Decreased free hormone causes increased TSH secretion, hence increases in iodide trapping, hydrolysis of thyroglobulin, and total hormone. The increase in total hormone tends to raise free hormone levels to normal.

In addition to pituitary and hypothalamic effects, there is some degree of autoregulation within the thyroid gland itself. Large amounts of iodide cause decreased iodide trapping, oxidation-organification, and coupling, while depletion of iodide causes increased iodide trapping, increased T3:T4 ratio, and increased responsiveness to TSH.

The physiologic effect of a given blood level of "thyroid hormone" depends upon the concentration of TBG, the T3:T4 ratio, and the sensitivity of peripheral tissues to free hormone. Increased T3:T4 ratio may be due to decreased dietary iodide, exogenous T3, or (possibly) increased TSH (Greer, 1972). Variations in peripheral tissue response have been reported but are believed to be rare.

Pathophysiology

GENERAL CONSIDERATIONS

The response of an endocrine gland to disease is limited. Clinical effects of a pathologic lesion usually depend upon the answers to five fundamental questions:

1. Is there too much or too little hormone?
2. Is the disease "primary," "secondary," or related to failure of the target organ?
3. Is the diseased gland normally responsive, is its responsiveness altered, or is it entirely autonomous?
4. Does the disease have local mechanical consequences?
5. Does the altered hormonal function affect other endocrine organs?

An excess or deficiency of hormone might seem rather obvious; however this is not necessarily the case. Rates of hormone release vary widely; there is no single "normal" level, but rather a range of responses, each appropriate to a particular feedback signal. For example:

1. "Normal" TSH levels vary from 0 to 10 μU./ml. A level of TSH in this range is "normal" with a serum thyroxine of 10.0 μg./ml. but "abnormal" with a serum thyroxine of 2.0 μg./dl.
2. Levels of plasma cortisol which are "normal" at 0800 hours may be abnormal at 1800 hours.
3. Levels of serum thyroxine which are within normal limits for a normal TBG may be abnormal if TBG is either increased or decreased.
4. A damaged endocrine gland may produce normal levels of hormone under "routine" conditions, but may be unable to respond further when stressed; failure of serum thyroxine to rise following TSH indicates "limited reserve" and probable thyroid dysfunction.

The question of "primary," "secondary," or target organ failure applies to all endocrine glands. Dysfunction may represent: (1) failure of the endocrine gland; (2) failure of the feedback mechanism (pituitary and/or hypothalamus); (3) after prolonged secondary hyperfunction, an endocrine gland may enlarge and undergo transformation to autonomous hyperfunction; or (4) inability of the target organ to respond (i.e., peripheral tissues).

Endocrine disease frequently is associated with altered response to normal stimuli or autonomous function. For example, primary hyperthyroidism typically is associated with autonomous hyperfunction; hyperadrenalism is characterized by abnormal response to ACTH.

Local mechanical and hormonal consequences are most dramatic with the pituitary, where tumors or cysts may cause compression of the optic chiasma, and/or lack of tropic hormones, with generalized endocrine insufficiency. Tumors or inflammation of the thyroid may involve the recurrent laryngeal nerve and cause compression of the trachea, even if hormone output remains normal.

Effects of one endocrine gland upon others are most marked for the pituitary but also occur with the thyroid. Thyroxine accelerates hepatic conversion of cortisol to inactive tetrahydrocortisol, causing increased output of urinary 17-hydroxycorticosteroids, as well as 17-ketogenic steroids.

Classification of Thyroid Disease

Diseases Primarily Characterized by Euthyroidism

1. Diffuse goiter
   a. Sporadic – idiopathic
   b. Sporadic – known cause (congenital defect in hormone synthesis; chemical goitrogen; iodine deficiency or excess)
   c. Endemic – idiopathic
   d. Endemic – known cause (iodine deficiency; dietary goitrogens)
2. Uninodular goiter
   a. Functional (hot nodule)
   b. Nonfunctional (cold nodule)
3. Multinodular goiter
   a. Sporadic – idiopathic
   b. Sporadic – known cause (similar to diffuse goiter above)
   c. Endemic – idiopathic
   d. Endemic – known cause (similar to diffuse goiter above)
4. Tumors
   a. Benign – follicular adenoma, atypical adenoma, teratoma
   b. Malignant – follicular adenocarcinoma, papillary adenocarcinoma, medullary carcinoma, undifferentiated carcinoma
5. Thyroiditis
   a. Acute (bacterial or viral)
   b. Subacute (giant cell thyroiditis)
   c. Chronic (Hashimoto's disease)
6. Congenital anomaly
   a. Thyroglossal duct cyst
   b. Abnormal location of thyroid gland

Diseases Primarily Characterized by Hyperthyroidism

1. Diffuse toxic goiter (Graves' disease)
2. Toxic goiter
   a. Uninodular
   b. Multinodular
3. Exogenous thyroid hormone
4. Tumors
   a. Follicular adenoma
   b. Follicular carcinoma
   c. Secretion of TSH-like substance (choriocarcinoma, hydatidiform mole, embryonal carcinoma of testis)

Diseases Primarily Characterized by Hypothyroidism

1. Idiopathic
   a. Adult
   b. Childhood, including congenital aplasia
2. Loss of thyroid mass
   a. Hashimoto's thyroiditis
   b. Surgery
   c. Radioiodine
3. Biochemical lesions
   a. Iodide deficiency
   b. Goitrogens
   c. Inborn error of metabolism
4. TSH deficiency
   a. Isolated
   b. Panhypopituitarism
5. TRF deficiency due to hypothalamic injury or disease

Disease Characterized by Decreased Thyroid Reserve

1. Idiopathic
2. Loss of thyroid mass (see above)
3. Biochemical lesions (see above)
4. TSH deficiency
5. TRF deficiency

Goiter

Goiter refers to enlargement of the thyroid, which may be diffuse, uninodular, or multinodular. It is not a single disease, but a group of diseases with varying etiology. The patient may be euthyroid ("compensatory goiter"), hyperthyroid ("toxic goiter"), or hypothyroid. On the basis of gross and microscopic appearance, goiter may be classified as: diffuse, uninodular, multinodular, tumor, thyroiditis, or diffuse toxic goiter (Graves' disease).

Most patients with goiter are euthyroid; the thyroid enlargement represents a compensatory response. Diffuse, uninodular, or multinodular goiter may be caused by a variety of diseases with a final common pathologic pathway and two characteristics in common: (1) the thyroid gland is anatomically normal at the outset; and (2) one or more factors impair capacity of the thyroid to synthesize hormone. Causes for such compensatory goiter are listed in Table 11–20. The sequence of events is believed to be:

1. Impaired thyroid function causes decreased free thyroxine, resulting in
2. Increased TSH, which causes
3. Hypertrophy and papillary hyperplasia of thyroid, with
4. Restoration of normal free thyroxine, followed by

Table 11-20. CAUSES FOR COMPENSATORY GOITER

Extrinsic
- Diet: Iodide deficiency
  - Dietary goitrogens which block oxidation and organification: cabbage, turnips, kale, rutabaga, cauliflower, milk from cattle fed on certain grasses
- Drugs: Block iodide trapping: chlorate, perchlorate, hypochlorite, nitrate, thiocyanate
  - Block oxidation and organification: amphenone, carbimazole, cobalt, methimazole, methylthiouracil, para-aminosalicylate, phenylbutazone, phenylindanedione, propylthiouracil, resorcinol
  - Block gastrointestinal reabsorption of thyroxine: soybean milk formulas for infants
  - Block thyroglobulin hydrolysis: iodide (especially in Graves' disease; occasionally in other patients)

Intrinsic
- Increased physiologic demand for hormone: puberty, pregnancy
- Partial or complete metabolic block: if severe, may cause goitrous hypothyroidism during infancy; if mild, may cause nontoxic goiter developing during adolescence or later adult life
  1. Failure of iodide trapping: RAI is low and large doses of iodide cause regression of goiter in early stages before scarring has occurred
  2. Failure of oxidation and organification: RAI is normal but discharged by perchlorate; abnormal discharge test also seen with thiouracil treatment or Hashimoto's thyroiditis
  3. Impaired coupling of MIT and DIT: RAI is high; PBI may be high owing to escape of MIT and DIT into plasma; serum thyroxine normal or low
  4. Lack of iodotyrosine deiodinase: RAI initially high, but low at 24 hours; MIT and DIT may be present in plasma and urine
  5. Production and release of abnormal, metabolically hypoactive, iodinated proteins: RAI and PBI high; serum thyroxine low (may also occur with thyroiditis or thyroid carcinoma)

5. Involution of thyroid, with formation of colloid nodules, and later
6. Recurrence of impaired thyroid function with decreased free thyroxine,
7. Recurrence of increased TSH*, hypertrophy, hyperplasia, and formation of hyperplastic nodules,
8. Restoration of normal free thyroxine,
9. Focal involution of thyroid, with more colloid nodule formation, hemorrhage, scarring, and
10. Repetition of cycle.

If compensation is incomplete, the patient will be hypothyroid, or may have "decreased thyroid reserve." In some patients the hyperplastic nodules may develop autonomous function, resulting in hyperthyroidism ("toxic nodular goiter").

*This postulated increase in TSH has not been confirmed by recent studies; possibly some other mechanism may be involved.

Probably the most common cause of goiter is iodide deficiency, which was prevalent in the central U.S.A. as well as Switzerland prior to use of iodized salt. Today iodide deficiency remains endemic in portions of central Africa and South America (especially the Andes Mountains). Goitrogenous hypothyroidism may be associated with this condition, depending on severity of the iodide deficiency.

In the U.S.A., iodide excess is probably more frequent than iodide deficiency. For a small number of susceptible individuals, iodide excess inhibits oxidation-organification and thyroglobulin hydrolysis. The mechanism is not known; however, this response may occur in the fetuses of mothers given iodide during pregnancy. Goiter is four to eight times more common in women than men, except in endemic areas where the incidence is about equal. This possibly may reflect recurrent stimulation throughout the menstrual cycle, as well as during pregnancy.

Estimates on prevalence of compensatory goiter in the U.S.A. vary widely, from less than 1 per cent to over 4 per cent. The statistics are influenced by region, by age, and by sex. At autopsy, nodularity may be found in about 20 per cent of thyroid glands at age 20 (women), increasing to about 60 per cent at age 60 (women): incidence in men is about 10 per cent lower. There has been considerable controversy over the proper treatment of "thyroid nodules." The fact that over 50 per cent of clinical "solitary nodules" may prove to be multinodular goiters at operation contributes to this confusion. Thus, a "solitary nodule" may prove to be: a colloid nodule, a multinodular goiter, an adenoma, a benign cyst, or carcinoma. Reported incidence of carcinoma in solitary thyroid nodules ranges from 3 to 25 per cent, and in multinodular glands, from 2 to 18 per cent. The lower figures are probably closer to a true estimate, since there is a tendency for reports to originate from referral centers where there is a high degree of patient selectivity.

There is no simple approach to treatment of nodular goiter. Solitary nodules in children or males probably should be excised; solitary nodules in women should be excised if the lesion does not regress with suppressive doses of thyroid hormone given over a period of two to four months. Patients with stony hard nodules, symptomatic tracheal or esophageal compression, or cervical lymphadenopathy probably should have surgery.

Thyroid scans may be of some help in evaluating solitary nodules. Using this approach, thyroid nodules can be placed in four functional categories:

1. Hyperfunctional (hot) nodules which concentrate more radioactivity than normal portions of the gland.
2. Functional (warm) nodules which concen-

trate radioactivity to the same extent as normal thyroid.

3. Hypofunctional (cool) nodules which concentrate radioactivity to a lesser extent than normal thyroid.

4. Nonfunctional (cold) nodules which do not concentrate radioactivity.

Widely divergent results have been reported on the value of scans for differentiating benign from malignant lesions: incidence of carcinoma in solitary "cold" nodules ranges from 7 to 58 per cent (Zacharewicz, 1968). In older patients the incidence tends to be low (about 10 per cent), while in younger patients incidence of carcinoma in solitary cold nodules may be 40 to 50 per cent. "Hot" nodules are almost never malignant, and "warm" nodules, rarely so.

The treatment of diffuse or multinodular goiter is even less well standardized than for solitary nodules. If the enlarged gland presents a cosmetic problem, if there are pressure symptoms, or if the patient is hyperthyroid, surgery may be indicated. In other patients medical treatment with suppressive doses of thyroid is recommended. However, multinodular glands frequently contain autonomous functional nodules; in such patients "suppressive" thyroid therapy may produce clinical hyperthyroidism (Miller and Block, 1970).

Thyroid Tumors

Adenomas of the thyroid are benign, encapsulated lesions which usually present as an asymptomatic solitary nodule. Hemorrhage or degeneration in an adenoma can cause pain and/or rapid enlargement, which may lead the patient to seek medical advice. Of all clinical "single nodules," about 60 per cent represent single or multiple colloid nodules, about 30 per cent adenomas, and about 10 per cent carcinomas. Since the incidence of colloid nodules increases with age, a solitary nodule is more likely to represent tumor in patients under age 30 than in older individuals (over age 50). On the basis of histologic appearance, adenomas are classified as: (1) follicular, (2) fetal (small closed follicles), (3) embryonal (cells in cords without follicles), (4) atypical (rare; histologic pattern easily confused with carcinoma), or (5) papillary (? low grade malignant potential).

Follicular adenomas typically present as solitary "cool" or "cold" nodules; however, they also may be "warm" or even "hot," causing clinical hyperthyroidism. Such "hot nodules" may have autonomous function and may suppress RAI uptake of surrounding normal thyroid tissue. Distinction between follicular adenoma and well-differentiated carcinoma is difficult and requires study of many histologic secretions.

Fetal adenomas are seldom functional; as with follicular adenomas, histologic diagnosis may be difficult. Embryonal adenomas are infrequent and almost never functional. These are easily confused with thyroid carcinoma.

Atypical adenomas are very cellular and histologically may be confused with undifferentiated carcinoma. The benign behavior of these lesions was not recognized until the late 1960's.

Papillary adenomas, like follicular adenomas, can be distinguished from well-differentiated carcinoma only by absence of invasion (capsular and vascular) and clinical follow-up. There is some question whether all papillary adenomas may not represent low grade malignancies.

Carcinoma of the thyroid is classified as: papillary adenocarcinoma, follicular adenocarcinoma, undifferentiated carcinoma, or medullary carcinoma. Thyroid carcinoma may arise either de novo or from a preexisting nodule of many years' duration; thus adenomas, as well as single or multiple "compensatory nodules," may have a low grade "premalignant" potential.

Papillary adenocarcinoma comprises about 60 per cent of all thyroid cancers. Peak incidence is in young females (3:1 female:male ratio); however, the tumor may also occur in males and in children. The usual presenting symptom is an asymptomatic neck mass, diagnosed as "cold" nodule on scan. Extension is by local invasion and metastasis to regional lymph nodes. Distant metastases are rare. Treatment is local resection, followed by replacement therapy. Progress is good, with a 10 year survival of about 80 to 90 per cent. The primary tumor as well as lymph node metastases may regress with thyroid therapy.

Follicular adenocarcinoma comprises about 20 per cent of all thyroid cancers. Peak incidence is in older females, about age 40 to 60. There is a history of preexisting goiter in many cases, implying transition either from adenoma or "compensatory" adenomatous goiter. Scan typically reveals a "cool" or "cold" nodule. Extension is via blood stream invasion, and initial symptoms may be from metastases to bone or lungs. Histologic appearance may be well differentiated and indistinguishable from normal thyroid tissue, moderately differentiated, or poorly differentiated. In some cases histologic blood vascular invasion may be the only evidence of malignancy. Those follicular adenocarcinomas which present as "cool" nodules may be treated with radioiodine following thyroidectomy and TSH. Treatment with thyroid hormone may also be effective, since this suppresses TSH stimulation of the malignancy. Prognosis varies according to degree of differentiation and extent of the lesion when discovered: patients with well-differentiated lesions and only microscopic evidence of blood vascular invasion may have a five-year survival of 60 to 80 per cent, while patients with less well-differentiated lesions have five-year survivals in the 20 to 40 per cent range.

Undifferentiated carcinoma comprises about 15 per cent of all thyroid malignancies. Peak incidence is in elderly persons. Presenting symptoms may include a rapidly growing mass fixed to other tissues in the neck, with dyspnea and vocal cord paralysis. Surgery is not indicated, and radiation provides only temporary relief; the prognosis is poor, and most patients die within a year of diagnosis.

Medullary carcinoma with amyloid stroma has only recently been recognized as separate from undifferentiated carcinoma. This rare tumor (comprises about 5 per cent of thyroid cancers) is believed to arise from parafollicular cells rather than thyroid acini. Secretion of calcitonin, serotonin, and ACTH has been reported; the clinical picture may resemble carcinoid or Cushing's syndrome. Despite production of calcitonin, most of these patients are normocalcemic. A familial incidence has been reported, as well as an association with pheochromocytoma (coexists in 10 per cent of medullary carcinomas). Measurement of calcitonin as a "screening test" for medullary carcinoma has been suggested in patients with a familial history of this disease.

Thyroiditis

Thyroiditis typically presents with neck pain and/or enlarged thyroid gland. Differential diagnosis includes: (1) hemorrhagic degeneration of multiple colloid nodules in a "compensatory" goiter; (2) diffuse nontoxic goiter; and (3) neoplasm. Classification of thyroiditis as acute, subacute, or chronic is based on histopathology and laboratory findings, as well as clinical findings and duration.

"Acute thyroiditis" refers to suppurative disease, caused by bacteria, as well as nonspecific acute inflammation, presumably viral in etiology. Suppurative thyroiditis may be related to sepsis, or attempted injection into the jugular vein, while nonsuppurative acute thyroiditis may be related to a respiratory or systemic viral illness. Regardless of the etiology, the patient usually has fever, neck pain, tenderness, swelling, elevated sedimentation rate, and leukocytosis. Suppurative thyroiditis is best treated with antibiotics or surgical drainage if a fluctuant area develops, while treatment of nonsuppurative thyroiditis is nonspecific.

"Subacute thyroiditis" is also known as giant cell thyroiditis, granulomatous thyroiditis, or de Quervain's disease. Etiology is unknown, possibly being viral. Pathologic examination reveals irregular granulomatous inflammation with rupture of follicles and thyroglobulin release. Clinically, onset may be gradual or abrupt, accompanied by pain in the thyroid which may radiate to the ears, jaw, or head. Both serum thyroxine and PBI may be elevated (Christiansen *et al.*, 1969); in some cases PBI exceeds serum thyroxine, suggesting release of abnormal iodinated protein. The sedimentation rate typically is elevated and offers a useful index of progress. In some cases it may be helpful to confirm the diagnosis with needle biopsy. Treatment of most cases is nonspecific; if this is ineffective, corticosteroids or radiotherapy (300 to 400 R) may be used. This disease usually subsides spontaneously within a few months; about 10 per cent of patients may follow a prolonged course ending in hypothyroidism, and another 10 per cent may remain euthyroid after developing compensatory goiter.

"Hashimoto's thyroiditis" is also known as "autoimmune thyroiditis" or "chronic thyroiditis." During the last 40 years there has been a fiftyfold increase in incidence of this disease (McConahey, 1972). Although less common than thyrotoxicosis, Hashimoto's thyroiditis is over ten times more frequent than acute or subacute thyroiditis. Peak incidence is in middle-aged women, although children and males may be affected. The female:male ratio is over 10:1. Clinically the patient usually has painless diffuse enlargement of the thyroid; however, the presenting picture may be either (1) diffuse painful enlargement; (2) diffuse enlargement associated with thyrotoxicosis; or (3) diffuse enlargement associated with hypothyroidism. Anatomic pathology findings include: diffusely enlarged thyroid which appears pale and firm on section, and a diffuse lymphocytic infiltrate, with lymphoid follicles and large eosinophilic acinar cells (Hürthle or Askanazy cells); fibrosis may also be present.

Etiology is unknown, but an autoimmune process is postulated. The following antibodies have been described in sera of patients with this disease:

1. Antibodies to thyroglobulin:
   a. Precipitating antibodies
   b. Agglutinating antibodies
   c. Complement fixing antibodies
2. Complement fixing antibodies to thyroid acinar cell microsomes.
3. Antibodies reacting with nuclei of thyroid acinar cells (demonstrable by fluorescence microscopy).
4. Antibodies reacting with colloid antigens other than thyroglobulin (demonstrable by fluorescence microscopy).

5. Cytotoxic antibodies that destroy normal thyroid cells grown in tissue culture.

The thyroglobulin antibodies may be detected and measured by: (1) agglutination of tanned red cells; (2) agglutination of latex particles coated with thyroglobulin. Of these two procedures, tanned red cell agglutination is the more sensitive.

About 95 per cent of patients with Hashimoto's disease have detectable antibody, as determined by the tanned red cell agglutination test; however, this finding is NOT specific, since antibody is also present in myxedema (about 80 per cent), thyrotoxicosis (about 60 per cent), nontoxic nodular goiter (about 30 per cent), and thyroid carcinoma (about 25 per cent).

In the latex particle test, sensitivity is decreased but specificity increased: about 60 per cent of patients with Hashimoto's disease and about 20 per cent of patients with myxedema have a "positive" reaction.

Initial symptoms of Hashimoto's thyroiditis range from hyperthyroidism, to euthyroidism, to hypothyroidism. A few patients may have clinical and histologic findings intermediate between Graves' disease and Hashimoto's thyroiditis (Fatourechi *et al.*, 1971). Prognosis varies from: (1) complete recovery; (2) recovery with euthyroidism but decreased thyroid reserve; to (3) permanent damage, with hypothyroidism. Thus, a patient may initially present with hyperthyroidism, progressing gradually to euthyroidism and, finally, myxedema. The percentage of patients with Hashimoto's disease who finally become hypothyroid is not known but may be in the range of 20 to 30 per cent.

Graves' Disease

This is a multisystem disease, clinically characterized by one or more of the following: hyperthyroidism with diffuse hyperplasia of the thyroid gland, infiltrative ophthalmopathy (exophthalmos), and/or infiltrative dermopathy (pretibial myxedema).

Thyrotoxicosis is NOT identical to Graves' disease, but is a syndrome which may be caused by: Graves' disease, multiple colloid adenomatous goiter ("toxic goiter" or Plummer's disease), follicular adenoma, follicular adenocarcinoma, excessive production of TSH or similar substance (pituitary tumors, choriocarcinoma, hydatidiform mole, embryonal carcinoma of testis), Hashimoto's disease, or exogenous thyroid hormone (factitious thyrotoxicosis).

With the exception of Graves' disease, thyrotoxicosis is NOT associated with ophthalmopathy or dermopathy. Onset of Graves' disease varies from abrupt to insidious; the course varies from fulminant to chronic or recurrent; severity ranges from virulent to barely detectable. There is no constant temporal relationship between the three cardinal features: ophthalmopathy may occur before, during, after, or without hyperthyroidism—and so may dermopathy.

Graves' disease is more common in women than in men (ratio about 10:1), with a peak incidence at about 20 to 40 years; however, the condition may occur at any age. There appears to be a hereditary tendency, but this is not well defined.

Etiology of Graves' disease is unknown. An abnormal gamma globulin called long-acting thyroid stimulator (LATS) can be demonstrated in the serum of about 20 to 60 per cent of patients with Graves' disease (Solomon and Chopra, 1972); however, presence of LATS does not correlate reliably with the severity of hyperthyroidism, ophthalmopathy, or dermopathy (Silverstein and Burke, 1970). LATS has also been reported in asymptomatic relatives of patients with Graves' disease and in occasional patients with Hashimoto's thyroiditis.

There is suggestive evidence that Graves' disease may be an autoimmune disorder:

1. Immunoglobulins as well as complement are localized in connective tissue of the thyroid (Werner *et al.*, 1972).
2. Clinical improvement occurs on treatment with steroids and immunosuppressive agents.
3. Thyroid autoantibodies are found in patients and relatives.
4. "Autoimmune diseases" have increased incidence in patients and relatives (Hashimoto's thyroiditis, pernicious anemia, idiopathic adrenal insufficiency, systemic lupus erythematosus).
5. Splenomegaly, lymph node enlargement, thymic hyperplasia, and peripheral lymphocytosis are frequent.

However, these immunologic abnormalities do not establish autoimmune pathogenesis, and etiology remains unproved at this time.

Two disturbances in thyroid function are characteristic of Graves' disease: (1) administration of T3 does not suppress serum thyroxine or RAI uptake, and (2) administration of iodide causes decreased hydrolysis of colloid, with enlargement of the thyroid gland and decreased serum thyroxine.

Administration of T3 to a normal individual causes suppression of pituitary TSH, decreased RAI uptake, and decreased serum thyroxine. Normally RAI uptake and serum thyroxine fall to 60 per cent (or less) of the original value (Henneman and Bussemaker, 1969); (Williams *et al.*, 1969). Alternatively, a single oral dose of L-thyroxine may be used, with a second RAI uptake measurement one week later (Wallack *et al.*, 1970); the advantage of a "single dose" is offset by the fact that serum thyroxine measurements cannot be used for verification of thyroid suppressibility. Patients with active Graves' disease almost invariably fail to suppress RAI uptake and serum thyroxine following T3. In about 30 to 50 per cent of patients this abnormality persists for up to 20 years following reversion to euthyroidism. Until recently it was thought that nonsuppressibility was due to LATS; however, some patients without LATS may fail to suppress, and some patients with LATS may show normal suppressibility: at present, the cause for autonomous hyperfunction in Graves' disease remains unknown. Other causes for an abnormal T3 (or T4) suppression test include: Hashimoto's thyroiditis; relatives of patients with Graves' disease (? preclinical state); "toxic goiter" due to multiple colloid adenomatous goiter, follicular adenoma, or follicular adenocarcinoma; and ectopic production of abnormal thyroid stimulator.

Administration of iodide in normal persons has two effects: decreased oxidation and organification of iodide, and decreased hormone release from thyroglobulin. In Graves' disease this effect is exaggerated: serum thyroxine decreases nearly to normal levels and stabilizes at this range. Like the abnormal response to T3 suppression, sensitivity to iodide frequently persists after the patient becomes euthyroid; indeed, euthyroid patients with Graves' disease may become hypothyroid after small pharmacologic doses of iodide (Braverman *et al.*, 1969). It is interesting that similar responses to both T3 and iodide may be observed in Hashimoto's disease; a relationship between these two conditions has been postulated, but not proved (Fatourechi *et al.*, 1971).

Hypothyroidism and Myxedema

Hypothyroidism refers to inadequate delivery of hormone to peripheral tissues; myxedema refers to severe deficiency with deposition of mucopolysaccharide in subcutaneous tissues of the face, tongue, and larynx.

Hypothyroidism may develop during fetal life, infancy, childhood, or adult life. Thyroid hormone is essential for growth and maturation; a deficiency causes cretinism, manifested by developmental failure of the brain and skeletal system. Various grades of cretinism occur, depending upon time of onset, completeness of the deficiency, and therapy. During fetal development, placental transfer of thyroxine is insufficient to meet needs for growth; fortunately, total absence of fetal thyroid is rare, and hypothyroidism at birth is unusual in the U.S.A. After birth the infant is deprived of maternal hormone, and hypothyroidism may develop either during the first two weeks of life or later, depending upon the amount of thyroid tissue present. DIAGNOSIS MUST NOT BE DEFERRED UNTIL THE CLASSIC FEATURES OF INFANTILE HYPOTHYROIDISM APPEAR, but should be suspected in infants with feeding problems, difficulty in nursing, attacks of cyanosis, or failure to thrive. Delay in bone maturation, decreased serum thyroxine, and decreased T3 resin uptake will confirm the clinical impression. Cretinism may be due to: (1) failure in anatomic development of the thyroid, (2) endemic iodine deficiency, or (3) dyshormonogenesis. In the United States about 70 per cent of cases fall into the first category, which includes partial deficiency as well as athyreosis. With failure of thyroid development, there is usually sufficient hormone for normal intrauterine development; diagnosis and therapy begun early in postnatal life generally prevent irreversible damage. Although cretinism is rare, early diagnosis is essential to prevention of irreversible damage. Endemic cretinism is not found in the United States but occurs in areas with severe iodine deficiency and endemic goiter, such as Switzerland, the Andes, India, and Africa. Even with early therapy, such infants seldom can be brought to normalcy because of insufficient hormone during intrauterine life.

Adult hypothyroidism in the United States is usually due to primary atrophy. The etiology is unknown, although Hashimoto's thyroiditis may progress to atrophy and hypothyroidism. The high titers of thyroid antibodies found in about 70 per cent of patients with Hashimoto's thyroiditis and in about 20 per cent of patients with primary hypothyroidism are consistent with such a relationship. Atrophy may also follow subacute thyroiditis or Graves' disease. The second most common cause of adult hypothyroidism is iatrogenic, following surgery or RAI therapy of Graves' disease. Incidence of hypothyroidism following RAI therapy is about 40 per cent after one year, with progressive increase to about 70 per cent after 10 years: presumably, all these patients eventually become hypothyroid (Goldsmith, 1972). Drug-induced hypothyroidism (e.g., propylthiouracil) is rare, since these agents ordinarily are not used on a continuing basis. Less common causes for primary hypothyroidism include thyroiditis, inborn errors of metabolism (may not appear until adult life), iodine deficiency (rare in U.S.), and dietary goitrogens.

Secondary hypothyroidism due to pituitary failure may be difficult to distinguish from primary hypothyroidism. The former condition typically is characterized by panhypopituitarism, although isolated deficiency of TSH may occur. However, primary hypothyroidism *per se* may impair pituitary function, causing abnormal response to metyrapone and/or decreased growth hormone (Lessoff *et al.*, 1969). With secondary hypothyroidism, serum TSH is decreased (rather than high); the diagnosis may be confirmed by normal response of RAI and serum thyroxine to exogenous TSH.

Hypothalamic hypothyroidism is usually associated with deficiencies of other hypothalamic releasing factors and pituitary tropic hormones. Other symptoms related to hypothalamic damage may include: abnormal temperature and appetite regulation, somnolence, and abnormal water balance (lack of ADH may cause diabetes insipidus and hypernatremia). Surprisingly, the pituitary cells retain capacity to secrete TSH, and exogenous TRF causes a normal rise in serum levels of this tropic hormone (Gorman and McConahey, 1970).

Advanced hypothyroidism is usually easily diagnosed. However, diagnosis of slight hypothyroidism may be difficult, since there appears to be a continuum between patients who are clinically hypothyroid and patients who are euthyroid with decreased thyroid reserve. Patients with damaged thyroid glands and primary hypothyroidism almost invariably have elevated serum TSH and decreased free thyroxine. However, some individuals with diffuse thyroid disease remain clinically euthyroid, with normal levels of free thyroxine in serum. In such patients, serum TSH may be either normal or increased. The response of RAI and serum thyroxine to exogenous TSH may be used to evaluate "thyroid reserve." Decreased thyroid reserve is considered present in a euthyroid patient if:

1. Serum TSH is normal, but exogenous TSH fails to produce an increase in RAI uptake and serum thyroxine.* This may occur in patients with multinodular goiter, as well as following surgery, RAI therapy, or thyroiditis. In such patients the thyroid gland is responding maximally to a normal level of TSH.
2. Serum TSH is increased and exogenous TSH fails to produce an increase in RAI uptake or serum thyroxine. Presumably such patients are borderline hypothyroid with a slight decrease in free hormone, causing the rise in endogenous TSH.
3. Serum TSH is increased and exogenous TSH produces an increase in RAI and/or serum thyroxine. This is uncommon and may represent a developmental stage at which thyroid reserve is still present, but the damaged gland requires an increased stimulus to maintain normal levels of free hormone (Nelson *et al.*, 1972).

Clinical symptoms of hypothyroidism may be caused by:

1. Failure of the thyroid gland *per se*, or primary hypothyroidism. This may be goitrous ("compensatory" goiter; inborn error of metabolism; Hashimoto's disease) or nongoitrous (primary myxedema; postoperative myxedema; myxedema following RAI therapy). Serum TSH is high, and increases even further in response to exogenous TRF.
2. Failure of pituitary TSH, or secondary hypothyroidism. Causes include pituitary tumor, pituitary infarct, or granulomatous disease involving the pituitary. Serum TSH is low and does not respond to exogenous TRF.
3. Failure of hypothalamic TRF or "hypothalamic hypothyroidism" (Shenkman *et al.*, 1972). Serum TSH is low, but increases in response to exogenous TRF.
4. Failure of end-organ response. This condition is rare, and reported cases are not always well documented. Findings include normal serum thyroxine, free thyroxine, and triiodothyronine; decreased basal metabolic rate; and clinical hypothyroidism which responds to exogenous hormone.

Several varieties of thyroid dyshormonogenesis have been described. These vary from clinically severe (cretinism and congenital goiter) to moderate (adult hypothyroidism and goiter) or mild (euthyroidism and variable degrees of compensatory goiter formation).

Reported biochemical lesions include the following:

1. Failure of iodide trapping; the same effect may be produced by perchlorate or thiocyanate administration.
2. Failure of iodide oxidation and organification, with defective binding of iodide to thyroglobulin tyrosine; the same effect may be produced by thiouracil, para-aminobenzoic acid, and other goitrogenic agents.
3. Impaired coupling of MIT and DIT.
4. Lack of iodotyrosine deiodinase, causing iodine deficiency as a result of loss of MIT and DIT in urine.
5. Production and release of abnormal, metabolically hypoactive, iodinated proteins.

In the first type of defect, ^{131}I uptake is very low and the ratio of ^{131}I in saliva and serum close to one. Large doses of iodide may bring about improvement in thyroid status and regression in size of the gland.

With the second defect, ^{131}I uptake may be normal, but the radioactivity is discharged by perchlorate, which blocks the trapping mechanism and releases first pool iodide which has

*Occasionally there may be dissociation between iodide trapping and hormone release.

not been oxidized and incorporated in thyroglobulin tyrosine. A positive perchlorate discharge test is also found during therapy with thiouracil-type drugs, and in about 50 per cent of patients with autoimmune thyroiditis.

With defective coupling of MIT and DIT, ^{131}I uptake is increased because of high levels of TSH. The PBI may be decreased, or it may be elevated because of escape of MIT and DIT into plasma. The T3 resin uptake, the BEI, and serum thyroxine are decreased. On biopsy the gland is hyperplastic, and there is an abnormally high ratio of iodotyrosines to iodothyronines.

Deficiency of iodotyrosine deiodinase results in severe iodine deficiency owing to loss of MIT and DIT in the urine. ^{131}I uptake is high, followed by rapid disappearance of ^{131}I from the thyroid. Urine chromatography shows ^{131}I incorporated into MIT and DIT.

Abnormal iodinated proteins may be produced and released in some cases of autoimmune thyroiditis, thyroid carcinoma, euthyroid nodular goiter, toxic nodular goiter, and Graves' disease. In addition, a group of patients with primary dyshormonogenesis has been recognized with abnormal iodoprotein production. The abnormal iodinated proteins cause a high PBI, but the BEI, serum thyroxine, and T3 resin uptake are decreased. Since the abnormal iodinated proteins are metabolically inactive, TSH levels are high and the RAI is markedly increased. Biopsy reveals hyperplastic thyroid tissue.

Laboratory Measurements of Thyroid Function

"Thyroid function tests are . . . being ordered by . . . physicians with increasing frequency and fewer indications. . . . Diagnosis is no longer a systematic exercise in deductive logic but a rapid reflex arc that begins with a few perfunctory observations . . . and ends with a profound list of entries in the . . . order book. Since they do not know what they are ordering, physicians . . . have difficulty interpreting (laboratory) results. . . . This often . . . (means) still further thyroid function tests. Finally, the puzzled physician telephones a thyroidologist. . . . The patient . . . usually is found to be euthyroid. . . . It is not surprising that, after . . . such an experience, many patients . . . wonder about the benefits of . . . 'scientific medicine'". (Becker and Hurley, 1972).

During the past few years a large number of "thyroid function tests" have been developed; however, each measures a different aspect of thyroid physiology, and most are subject to interferences unrelated to "thyroid function" *per se*. Intelligent selection and interpretation of these measurements requires an understanding of: (1) normal thyroid physiology; (2) thyroid pathophysiology; and (3) currently available methods and their limitations.

The classification and abbreviations in Table 11-21 are based on recommendations of the American Thyroid Association (Solomon *et al.*, 1972).

Table 11-21. CLASSIFICATION OF "THYROID FUNCTION TESTS"

	ABBREVIATIONS
Measurements of thyroid hormones	
Protein-bound iodine	PBI
Butanol-extractable iodine	BEI
Thyroxine iodine–chromatographic	T4I (C)
Thyroxine–chromatographic	T4 (C)
Thyroxine–displacement	T4 (D)
Thyroxine–radioimmunoassay	T4 (RIA)
Triiodothyronine–displacement	T3 (D)
Triiodothyronine–radioimmunoassay	T3 (RIA)
Estimates of the inverse of unoccupied thyroxine-binding sites	
Per cent free thyroxine	%FT4
Per cent free triiodothyronine	%FT3
Resin triiodothyronine uptake	RT3U
Resin thyroxine uptake	RT4U
Indicators of free hormone concentration	
Free thyroxine	FT4
Free triiodothyronine	FT3
Thyroxine-resin T3 index	T4-RT3
Thyroxine-resin T4 index	T4-RT4
Thyroxine-displacement "normalized" by addition of patient serum to assay (also referred to as T4N–normalized serum thyroxine)	T4 (D) (S) or T_4N
Thyroxine-binding proteins	
Thyroxine-binding globulin capacity	TBG_{cap}
Thyroxine-binding prealbumin capacity	$TBPA_{cap}$
Tropic hormone measurements	
Thyroid-stimulating hormone	TSH
Long-acting thyroid stimulator	LATS
Antibody studies	
Tanned red cell agglutination	
Latex particle agglutination	
Complement fixing antibodies	
RAI uptake studies	
RAI uptake with measurements at 2 and 24 hours	
Thyroid scan	
T3 suppression test	
TSH stimulation test	
T3 withdrawal test	
Perchlorate discharge test	
Measurements of target organ response	
Basal metabolic rate	
Photomotogram	

Measurements of Thyroid Hormones

Measurement of serum protein-bound iodine (PBI) became widely accepted during the early 1950's, and until the early 1960's provided the best available estimate of serum thyroxine. The procedure, based on catalytic effect of iodide on a mixture of arsenious acid and ceric ammonium sulfate, is sensitive and can be standardized against an aqueous solution of inorganic iodine. Precision is good, with a S.D. of about 0.5 μg./dl.; agreement between different laboratories is excellent, with a generally accepted normal range of 4.0–8.0 μg./dl. Diagnostic accuracy of the PBI is in the 90 per cent range, substantially better than the previously used BMR.

Limitations of the PBI as a "thyroid function test" are widely recognized, and include:

1. Mercurial diuretics and gold therapy may inhibit iodine catalysis in the arsenious acid ceric ammonium sulfate system; however, this is not a problem with the alkaline ash procedure.

2. The PBI is invalidated by "contamination" from a wide range of iodinated materials; following ingestion or injection, these may remain bound to serum protein for months, or even years (Table 11–22).

3. The PBI—and other measurements of serum hormone—may be invalidated by increase or decrease in TBG binding capacity.

4. The PBI—and other measurements of serum hormone—may be invalidated by an increase or decrease in the T4:T3 ratio.

"False high" PBI results frequently are due to endogenous or exogenous iodine contamination. Endogenous contamination may be due to: release of MIT, DIT, or abnormal iodinated proteins in: (1) thyroiditis; (2) inborn errors of metabolism; or (3) some patients with thyroid carcinoma. Exogenous contamination is far more frequent (Table 11–22): it is often difficult to judge whether a "high" PBI is

Table 11–22. IODINE-CONTAINING COMPOUNDS WHICH MAY CAUSE DECREASED RAI UPTAKE AND INCREASED PBI

COMPOUND	APPROXIMATE DURATION OF EFFECT*	COMPOUND	APPROXIMATE DURATION OF EFFECT*
Iodine antiseptics		Amebicides	
Tincture of iodine	1– 4 weeks	Diodoquin	2– 4 weeks
Betadine	1– 4 weeks	Entero-Vioform	2– 4 months
Topical preparations		*Iodinated radioisotopes used for diagnosis*	
Cosmetics	1– 4 weeks	RISA	1– 8 weeks
Suntan preparations	1– 4 weeks	Rose bengal ^{131}I	1– 8 weeks
Antidandruff medications	1– 4 weeks	*Radiographic contrast media*	
Proprietary medications		Cholecystography	
Cough syrups and lozenges	1– 4 weeks	Biligrafin	3 weeks
Cod liver oil products	1– 4 weeks	Orabilex	8 weeks
Toothpastes containing iodine	1– 4 weeks	Oragrafin	8 weeks
Multivitamin preparations	1– 4 weeks	Cholegrafin	1– 4 months
Miscellaneous		Telepaque	1– 4 months
Potassium iodide (large doses)	1– 6 weeks	Priodax	4–12 months
Foods or drugs colored red	1– 4 weeks	Teridax	1–30 years
with erythrosine (tetraiodo-		Pyelography	
fluorescein)		Hypaque	1 week
Iodinated penicillin	1– 4 weeks	Diodrast	2 weeks
Iodothiouracil (antithyroid drug)	1– 4 weeks	Hippuran	2 weeks
DOPA (used in treatment of	1– 4 weeks	Miokon	2 weeks
Parkinson's disease)		Neo-Iopax	2 weeks
BSP (some lots)	1– 4 weeks	Pyelombrine	2 weeks
Metrecal	1– 4 weeks	Renografin	2 weeks
Choloxin (dextrothyroxine)	1– 4 weeks	Skiodan	2 weeks
Indwelling venous or arterial	1– 4 weeks	Urokon	4 weeks
catheters		Bronchography-myelography	
Bromides	1– 4 weeks	Dionosil	1– 5 months
Barium (used for gastro-	0– 6 days	Lipiodol (myelogram)	1–30 years
intestinal radiography)		Lipiodol (bronchogram)	1– 5 years
Antiparasitic drugs		Pantopaque	1–30 years
Trichomonacides (vaginal suppositories)		Salpingography	
Vioform	1– 3 weeks	Salpix	1– 5 months
Floraquin	1– 2 weeks		

*Varies in different patients

clinically significant, or whether a "normal" PBI is masking hypothyroidism. The problems caused by iodine interference were recognized early and led to development of more specific methods for measuring thyroid hormone in serum.

Measurement of butanol-extractable iodine (BEI), introduced during the early 1950's, eliminates endogenous contamination (MIT, DIT, thyroglobulin), as well as inorganic iodide interference. However, this procedure never became popular, since it is time-consuming, technically difficult, and does not solve the most common problem—interference from organic iodides (Table 11–22).

The first important improvement was the chromatographic thyroxine, or "T4 by column." This new measurement was developed during the early 1960's; by 1966 an automated version had become widely available and largely replaced the PBI. In analogy to the PBI, many laboratories report the T4 by column as thyroxine iodine: this may be multiplied by 1.5 to obtain serum thyroxine. The abbreviation T4I(C) is recommended for T4 by column reported as thyroxine iodine (normal range about 3.2 to 7.2 μg./dl.); the abbreviation T4(C) is recommended for T4 by column reported as serum thyroxine (normal range about 5.0 to 11.0 μg./dl.).

In the T4 by column procedure, both T3 and T4 are absorbed on resin, and both are eluted together by a series of buffers with decreasing pH. Thus, despite its name, the "T4-by-column" measures both T3 and T4. Two of the column fractions are collected and analyzed for iodine: if the second fraction contains more than 15 per cent of the iodine, contamination is suspected. Thyroxine in the two eluates may be analyzed by: the arsenious acid–ceric ammonium sulfate system as for PBI, or reaction of eluate with bromine, which enables thyroxine to catalyze the ceric-arsenite reaction.

The following types of iodine contamination are eliminated: (1) endogenous contamination, including MIT, DIT, and abnormal iodinated protein; (2) exogenous iodide contamination; and (3) exogenous iodine contamination from a number of radiographic contrast media, including: Cholografin, Dionosil (low levels), Hippuran, Hypaque, Miokon, Orabilex (low levels), Oragrafin, Pantopaque, Renografin, Salpix, Skiodan, and Urokon. Although this method does not completely solve the problem of iodine contamination, much of the interference is either eliminated or detected—a great improvement over the PBI!

In 1964 Murphy and Pattee described a radioisotopic procedure utilizing competitive protein-binding technique for the assay of serum thyroxine (Table 11–11). This method, unaffected by contamination with iodine (organic or inorganic, as well as mercury) has gained widespread acceptance. The principles involved in this technique are as follows:

1. The patient's serum is extracted with ethanol to denature the serum proteins, including TBG. The total amount of thyroxine in the serum extract is left in the free state.
2. ^{125}I-thyroxine bound to TBG is added to the dried ethanol extract of the patient's serum which contains free T_4, thus redissolving the patient's serum thyroxine.
3. An equilibrium is established in which a proportionate amount of the radioactive T4 is displaced from TBG by the patient's T4. The controlling factor in this equilibrium is the amount of patient T4 available.

$$TBG \cdot T4^* + T4 \rightleftarrows TBG \cdot T4^* + TBG \cdot T4 + T4^* + T4$$

$T4^*$ = radioactive thyroxine
T4 = unlabeled thyroxine

The amount of $T4^*$ released is proportional to the amount of T4 competing for the available binding sites on TBG.

4. An anion exchange resin sponge is added to absorb the unbound T4 (both patient's and T4 radioactive).
5. Total radioactivity added to each test is determined by means of a scintillation counter.
6. The sponge is removed and washed and a second count is taken on the sponge. Only T4 radioactivity not attached to TBG will be present after this washing.
7. A per cent uptake on the resin sponge is calculated as follows:

$$\frac{\text{Sponge count}}{\text{Total count}} = \text{Per cent uptake}$$

The percentage is compared to a standard curve to determine the quantity of T4 present in the patient's serum. The normal ranges can either be expressed as T4 iodine (3.9–7.7 μg./dl.) or as serum thyroxine (5.9–11.8 μg./dl.). Serum thyroxine iodine is a calculated value obtained by multiplying serum thyroxine by 0.653 (the proportion of iodine in T4 or thyroxine).

Problems with iodine contamination are completely eliminated using "T4 by displacement," or T4(D), also called "T4 by competitive protein binding" or "Murphy-Pattee thyroxine." This radiochemical procedure, developed during the middle 1960's, measures ability of T4 extracted from patient sera to displace ^{125}I-labeled thyroxine from reagent TBG. The technique requires careful attention to detail; pitfalls include:

1. Ethanol extraction of thyroxine from patient sera varies in efficiency (usually 75 to 85 per cent) and should be checked by recovery studies.
2. Standard curves must be checked with each run.
3. Some commercial kits include shortcuts

which degrade precision and accuracy (Becker and Hurley, 1972, Murray *et al.*, 1970).

4. Inter-laboratory agreement may be poor, possibly related to the fact that some laboratories correct results for recovery while others do not, and some multiply T4 values by 65 per cent (T4 is 65 per cent iodine by weight) to report results as "thyroxine iodine."

Although T4(D) appears to be gradually replacing other estimates of serum thyroxine, standards for reagent purity, methodology, and technique are urgently needed so that agreement between laboratories may become comparable to the "first generation" PBI, as well as the "second generation" T4(C).

None of the methods for measuring serum thyroxine can give clinically useful results if the T4:T3 ratio is markedly abnormal. Although serum T3 concentration is relatively low, it is estimated that over half the total thyroid hormonal effect is due to T3 (Sterling *et al.*, 1971). Normal T4(D) is about 5 to 11 μg./dl.; normal T3 is about 0.2 to 0.3 μg./dl. (200–300 ng./dl.); normal T4:T3 ratio is about 20:1 (Gharib and Wahner, 1972).

In Graves' disease and toxic nodular goiter, if serum T4 is elevated, serum T3 is elevated also, and there is no need for the latter measurement. In primary hypothyroidism, serum T3 is either low or normal and again there is no need for this measurement.

However, if clinical findings suggest hyperthyroidism but serum T4 is normal, T3 measurements may be helpful. Such patients may have T3 hyperthyroidism (a variant of Graves' disease) or a toxic goiter producing T3 rather than T4. Laboratory findings typically include: abnormal T3 suppression test, elevated serum T3, increased basal metabolic rate, and normal serum T4 and T3 resin uptake.

Clinical and laboratory findings similar to endogenous T3 hyperthyroidism may occur in factitious hyperthyroidism caused by T3 ingestion; however, such cases usually are characterized by a very low RAI, decreased serum thyroxine, and decreased T3 resin uptake.

Serum T3 measurement may also be helpful in patients who are clinically euthyroid but have decreased serum T4: in some such patients euthyroidism is maintained by increased T3. Cases of this type have been reported following ^{131}I therapy, with Hashimoto's thyroiditis (? related to increased TSH), with iodide deficiency (? compensatory mechanism), and as a premonitary sign of thyrotoxicosis.

Two methods for serum T3 measurement are available: a T3 by displacement method, or T3(D); and T3 by radioimmunoassay, or T3(RIA). The T3(D) procedure requires removal of T4 and T3 by cation exchange chromatography, followed by separation of T4 from T3 by paper chromatography, and quantitation of T3 by competitive protein binding (displacement). Although technically difficult and rather time-consuming, no special reagents (antisera to T3) are required. The T3(RIA) is less time-consuming but requires special reagents which are not widely available.

Radioimmunoassays

With respect to clinical endocrinology, radioimmunoassays are used to measure TSH, T3, HGH, LH, FSH, progesterone, cortisol, 11-desoxycortisol, testosterone, estradiol, aldosterone, renin activity, insulin, and parathormone. Any radioimmunoassay (RIA) requires an antiserum to the hormone. Only hormones of molecular weight over 10,000 are good antigens; however, smaller hormones can act as haptens when conjugated to large protein molecules, and antisera to such conjugates show specificity to the haptens. Commonly used protein molecules include bovine serum albumin, human serum albumin, and thyroglobulin. A radioimmunoassay also requires labeled hormone of high specific activity: tritium, ^{125}I, and ^{131}I are most commonly used.

After these reagents have been prepared, the first step is to incubate known amounts of antiserum, labeled or "hot" hormone, and "cold" hormone (patient serum). The cold hormone competes with hot hormone for binding sites on the antibody. The second step is to separate antibody-bound hormone from free hormone using:

1. Double antibody technique – a second antibody is added which is specific for the first antibody, causing precipitation of antibody-bound hormone.
2. Solid phase absorption of free hormone on Florisil or charcoal.
3. Solid phase absorption of antibody.
4. Precipitation of antibody by ammonium sulfate.

A standard curve is drawn, relating the amount of cold hormone added to the percentage of hot hormone bound by antibody. As cold hormone increases, less hot hormone is bound by the antibody. On the basis of this standard curve, the amount of cold hormone in a given sample can be calculated.

Although radioimmunoassays have revolutionized clinical endocrinology, the technique is not entirely free from pitfalls. Certain commercial antisera have less than optimal titer, specificity, and avidity. Specificity is defined as the ability of an assay system to measure the desired substance without interference from other compounds in serum or plasma. Since FSH, LH, and TSH are all glycoproteins and have a portion of their molecules which is similar, tests for specificity of TSH antisera must include addition of LH and FSH to determine if they inhibit TSH binding. If they do, it must be established whether inhibition is due to immunologic cross reactivity, or to TSH contamination of the LH and FSH. Most of the steroid hormone assays lack complete specificity, and organic solvent extraction followed by chromatography often is necessary.

It is not always easy to obtain radioactive hormones of high purity and high specific activity. The hormone preparation *per se* may be impure, or iodination may be incomplete, with free radioactive iodine present.

When setting up a radioimmunoassay, precision and accuracy must be checked with special care. If the procedure involves an extraction, recovery must be checked on a regular basis. Even if no extractions are involved, recovery studies should be performed by adding known amounts of hormone to a constant volume of plasma or serum: a plot of quantity added against quantity measured should give a straight line of slope 1.0 passing through the X,Y intercept at zero. A quality control program is essential, with pools used to determine day-to-day variability in high, low, and normal ranges; and it is essential that each laboratory establish its own normal range, rather than using published results. Sources of antisera and radioimmunoassay materials are presented in detail in a recent article by Skelley *et al.* (1973). There is evidence that the normal range for serum T3 may vary in different parts of the U.S.A., possibly due to variations in iodine intake. (A low intake seems to be associated with a higher normal range for serum T3.)

Estimates of the Inverse of Unoccupied Thyroxine-Binding Sites

None of the methods for measuring "total hormone" (thyroxine and/or triiodothyronine) can be clinically useful if there is a marked change in amount of binding capacity of thyroxine-binding globulin (TBG). Normally about 99.98 per cent of thyroxine is bound to TBG, thyroxine-binding prealbumin, and albumin. The bound thyroxine exists in equilibrium with free thyroxine (about 0.02 per cent of thyroxine) and unsaturated thyroxine-binding globulin (UTBG). Normal total thyroxine is about 8 μg./dl.; total TBG about 24 μg./dl.; UTBG about 16 μg./dl.; free thyroxine about 0.002 μg./dl. (2 ng./dl.). Thus, about two-thirds of the TBG is unsaturated and available for binding free hormone. If we do not consider binding by TBPA and albumin, the relationship between bound thyroxine (TBG-T4), free thyroxine (FT4), and unsaturated TBG (UTBG) may be expressed in the equation:

$$\text{TBG} \cdot \text{T4} \rightleftharpoons \text{FT4} + \text{UTBG}$$

hence:

$$\frac{(\text{TBG} \cdot \text{T4})}{(\text{UTBG})\ (\text{FT4})} = \text{K}$$

and:

$$\frac{(\text{TBG} \cdot \text{T4})}{(\text{UTBG})}\ \frac{1}{\text{K}} = \text{FT4}$$

but TBG · T4 = T4

(where T4 = total serum thyroxine)

Therefore:

$$\text{FT4} = \frac{1}{\text{K}}\ \frac{\text{T4}}{\text{UTBG}}$$

$$\text{If } \%\text{FT4} = \frac{\text{FT4}}{\text{TBG} \cdot \text{T4}} \times 100 \text{ then:}$$

$$\%\text{FT4} = \frac{1}{\text{K}}\ \frac{\text{T4}}{\text{UTBG}} \cdot \frac{1}{\text{T4}} = \frac{1}{\text{K}}\ \frac{100}{\text{UTBG}}$$

Let us assume a TBG of 24 μg./dl., a T4 of 8 μg./dl., a UTBG of 16 μg./dl., and K = (4 ng./dl.,)$^{-1}$, then $\frac{1}{K} = 4$ ng./dl. and:

$$\text{FT4} = \frac{1}{\text{K}}\ \frac{\text{T4}}{\text{UTBG}}$$

$$\text{FT4} = 4 \text{ ng./dl.}\ \frac{8\ \mu\text{g./dl.}}{16\ \mu\text{g./dl.}} = 4 \text{ ng./dl.} \times 0.5$$

$$\text{FT4} = 2 \text{ ng./dl.}$$

$$\%\text{FT4} = \frac{1}{\text{K}} \times \frac{100}{\text{UTBG}} = 4 \text{ ng./dl.} \times \frac{100}{16\ \mu\text{g./dl.}} = 4 \text{ ng./dl.} \times \frac{100}{16\ \mu\text{g./dl.}}$$

$$\%\text{FT4} = \frac{400 \text{ ng./dl.}}{16000 \text{ ng./dl.}} = 0.025\%$$

Causes for decreased UTBG are listed in Table 11–23. If TBG decreases to 12 μg./dl., initially UTBG will decrease to 4 μg./dl. and:

$$\text{FT4} = 4 \text{ ng./dl.} \times \frac{8\ \mu\text{g./dl.}}{4\ \mu\text{g./dl.}}$$

$$\text{FT4} = 4 \text{ ng./dl.} \times 2 = 8 \text{ ng./dl.}$$

Thus, there will be an increase in FT4 owing to the decrease in UTBG. The increased FT4 causes decreased TSH which, in turn, causes decreased T4 as needed to restore the ratio $\frac{\text{T4}}{\text{UTBG}}$ to its normal value of 0.5.

Since UTBG = TBG − T4, and TBG = 12, then at the new equilibrium:

$$0.5 = \frac{\text{T4}}{12 - \text{T4}}$$

$$6\text{–}0.5\ \text{T4} = \text{T4}$$

$$6 = 1.5\ \text{T4}$$

$$\text{T4} = 4\ \mu\text{g./dl.}$$

$$\text{and UTBG} = 8$$

At the new equilibrium, FT4 is restored to normal, while TBG, T4, and UTBG all are reduced to one-half their previous values.

Causes for increased UTBG are listed in Table 11–23. If TBG increases to 48 μg./dl., initially UTBG will increase to 40 μg./dl. and:

$$\text{FT4} = 4 \text{ ng./dl.} \times \frac{8\ \mu\text{g./dl.}}{40\ \mu\text{g./dl.}}$$

$$\text{FT4} = 4 \text{ ng./dl.} \times 0.2 = 0.8 \text{ ng./dl.}$$

Table 11-23. CAUSES FOR INCREASE OR DECREASE IN TBG- OR TBPA-BINDING CAPACITY

PROTEIN	INCREASE	DECREASE
TBG	Estrogens, including oral contraceptives	Androgens, including anabolic steroids
	Pregnancy	Active acromegaly
	Newborn infant (due to maternal estrogen)	
	Hepatic disease* Acute intermittent porphyria	Hepatic disease* Acute illness or surgical stress†
		Prednisone
		Nephrotic syndrome
	Perphenazine (Trilafon)	Diphenylhydantoin (Dilantin)‡
	Hypothyroidism	Hyperthyroidism
	Hereditary	Hereditary
TBPA	Androgens, including anabolic steroids	Acute illness or surgical stress
	Prednisone	Nephrotic syndrome
	Hepatic disease	Salicylates‡
		Hyperthyroidism

*May cause either increase or decrease in TBG (Inada and Sterling, 1967).
†May be due to inhibitor of T4 binding (Lutz *et al.*, 1972).
‡May be due to competition for T4 binding sites.

Thus, there will be a decrease in FT4 owing to the increase in UTBG. The decreased FT4 causes increased TSH which, in turn (assuming normal thyroid reserve), causes increased T4, as needed to restore the ratio $\frac{T4}{UTBG}$ to its normal value of 0.5. Since UTBG = TBG − T4 and TBG = 48, then:

$$0.5 = \frac{T4}{48 - T4}$$
$$24 - 0.5\ T4 = T4$$
$$24 = 1.5\ T4$$
$$T4 = 16$$
$$\text{and UTBG} = 32$$

At the new equilibrium FT4 is restored to normal, while TBG, T4, and UTBG are all stabilized at twice their original values. These relationships are shown graphically in Figure 11-24.

Three estimates of $\frac{1}{UTBG}$ are commonly used: per cent free thyroxine (%FT4), resin triiodothyronine uptake (RT3U), and resin thyroxine uptake (RT4U). At present, per cent free triiodothyronine (%FT3) remains a research procedure and is not widely available for clinical use.

Per cent free thyroxine may be measured by ultrafiltration, column chromatography, or dialysis. In the latter technique a small amount of radioactive T4 is added to serum and incubated with buffer. The added radioactive hormone (T4*) may either: bind to UTBG, giving T4* TBG, or remain unbound as FT4*. In this mixture containing:

T4 · TBG
FT4
T4* · TBG
FT4*
UTBG

the percentage of free radioactive hormone (FT4*) will be inversely proportional to UTBG. The free radioactive hormone is separated by dialysis or ultrafiltration, and the per cent free T4* calculated. Since only a small amount of T4* is added, it is assumed that per cent free T4* is identical to per cent free T4 (unlabeled hormone). This measurement may be subject to interference from heparin; a "false elevation" in per cent free thyroxine may be observed following heparin administration in clinically euthyroid patients. A less complex and time-consuming free T4 assay has been reported which makes this a more feasible assay (Wilson and Henry, 1971). McCullagh and Rosenbaum (1972) have confirmed the diagnostic value of the free thyroxine assay.

The resin triiodothyronine uptake (RT3U)

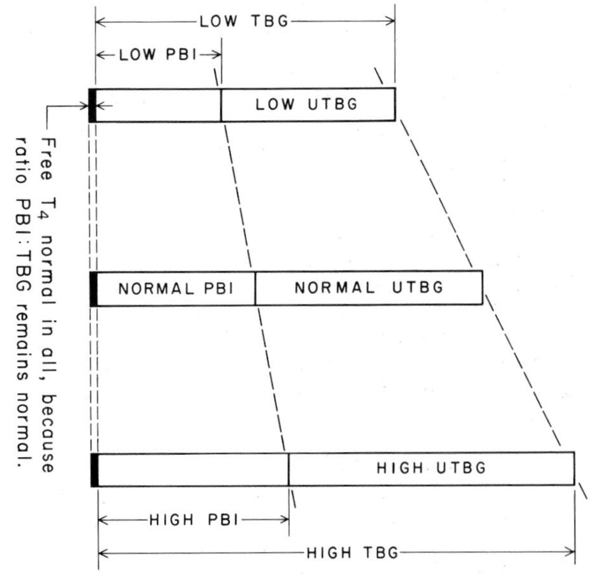

Figure 11-24. Effects of proportional changes in protein-bound iodine (PBI) and thyroxine-binding globulin (TBG) upon absolute concentrations of free T4 and unbound TBG (UTBG).

and resin thyroxine uptake (RT4U) also are inversely proportional to UTBG. In these procedures a small amount of radioactive T3 (RT3U) or radioactive T4 (RT4U) is added to serum and incubated with a resin sponge, which binds T3 and T4 more weakly than TBG.* The added radioactive hormone may either: bind to UTBG, or bind to the resin sponge. Amount of radioactivity bound to the resin sponge is inversely proportional to UTBG. There is close correlation between RT3U and %FT4, since both are proportional to $\frac{1}{UTBG}$. Results of RT3U and RT4U are very similar; as the former is more widely used, this discussion will use the abbreviation RT3U as referring to both procedures.

Compared with measurement of per cent free thyroxine, the RT3U is rapid and simple. At least eight commercial kits for T3 resin uptake are now available. Despite their seductive simplicity, such kits present pitfalls for the unwary:

1. Those commercial kits which appear most attractive in terms of speed and simplicity may have the poorest precision and diagnostic accuracy (Murray *et al.*, 1970).
2. There are no absolute standards; resin uptakes can be expressed only as a percentage or as the ratio of patient's serum to a control.
3. Normal range as given by the manufacturer may be incorrect.
4. Normal range and clinical significance may change abruptly when the manufacturer suddenly changes resin without altering the package insert or notifying users in advance.
5. Variations in technique may cause wide differences in normal range even between laboratories using "the same method."
6. Although the %FT4, RT3U, and RT4U are largely unaffected by iodine contamination, their diagnostic accuracy when used alone is less satisfactory than measurements of total hormone such as PBI, T4(C) and T4(D).
7. Some types of interference which apparently do not affect %FT4 may cause increased T3RU: barbiturates, anticoagulants (Warfarin), Butazolidin, pulmonary insufficiency with CO_2 retention, prolonged tachycardia, and sodium ipodate (Oragrafin), may cause "false high" results (not constant in all patients).

Indicators of Free Thyroxine and Free Hormone Concentration

In 1965 Clark and Horn utilized the close correlation between %FT4 and RT3U to propose the "free thyroxine index," also known as "T-7" and thyroxine-resin T3 index (T4-RT3). (The last name and abbreviation are recommended by the American Thyroid Association.) Multiplication of serum thyroxine times per cent free thyroxine gives absolute free thyroxine:

$$T4(C) \times \%FT4 = FT4 \text{ or:}$$
$$T4(D) \times \%FT4 = FT4$$

Multiplication of serum thyroxine by resin T3 uptake (RT3U) gives the thyroxine-resin T3 index (T4-RT3):

$$T4(C) \times RT3U = T4\text{-}RT3 \text{ or:}$$
$$T4(D) \times RT3U = T4\text{-}RT3$$

Close correlation between this index and FT4 has been confirmed in many different laboratories.

Other workers have pointed out that RT3U does not show exact correlation with %FT4 and have proposed mathematical transformations to provide improved agreement (Goolden *et al.*, 1967; Hamada *et al.*, 1970). It is not yet certain: whether clinical value of the improved correlation is worth potential confusion from "another thyroid function test," and which mathematical transformation should be used in association with: (1) which total hormone measurement, or (2) which RT3U or RT4U method.

Diagnostic accuracy of FT4 or T4-RT3 exceeds that of total hormone measurements and is far superior to RT3U alone. Either FT4 or T4-RT3 should be used whenever there is reason to suspect altered binding capacity of TBG and/or TBPA (Table 11–23), or whenever total hormone measurements do not correlate with clinical findings. Euthyroid patients with increased TBG typically have increased total hormone, decreased %FT4, decreased RT3U, normal FT4, and normal T4-RT3 (Fig. 11–24). Euthyroid patients with decreased TBG typically have decreased total hormone, increased %FT4, increased RT3U, normal FT4, and normal T4-RT3 (Fig. 11–24). In such cases reliance on total hormone measurements alone may prove misleading. The RT3U does NOT have good diagnostic accuracy when used alone, even if TBG is normal; hence, this measurement ordinarily is used only as a means for determining T4-RT3U.

In a few situations neither FT4 nor T4-RT3 correlates well with clinical status of the patient. Euthyroid "sick" patients frequently have increased FT4 and T4-RT3, without symptoms or signs of hyperthyroidism. Such patients may have an "inhibitor" which prevents hormone binding to TBG (Lutz *et al.*, 1972); the nature of this inhibitor is not known. It has been suggested that tissue response to free hormone may be decreased in acute illness, with concomitant "reset" of FT4

*Erythrocytes, charcoal, or Sephadex may be used in place of resin, since these also bind T4 more weakly than TBG.

receptors in the pituitary; at present this remains speculation rather than proven fact.

Decreased FT4 or T4-RT3 has been described in euthyroid patients during pregnancy; in some cases this may be related to decreased thyroid reserve, or to "lag" in response of the pituitary-thyroid axis to increased TBG.

During therapy for hypothyroidism the T4(D), FT4, and T4-RT3 are of limited value, since commercial thyroid preparations do not necessarily provide a "normal" T4:T3 ratio of 20:1. If this ratio is high, adequate replacement will cause a high serum thyroxine and a high RT3U. If this ratio is low, adequate replacement will be associated with a low serum thyroxine and a low RT3U.

The assay for T4(D) can be modified to "correct" for variations in TBG by adding a small amount of unextracted patient serum to the mixture of extracted patient T4, TBG, and radioactive T4. This modification was first described by Mincey *et al.* (1971) as the "effective thyroxine ratio" or ETR, with results reported as a ratio between patient serum and reference serum. Other workers used the same principle and reported results in μg./dl. as "normalized serum thyroxine" or T4N (Ashkar and Bezjian, 1972). Correlation with free thyroxine index appears excellent (Thorson *et al.*, 1972), and this principle may be applied to any competitive protein-binding method for T4 (Mincey, 1972). Since the procedure basically involves adding patient serum to a T4(D) assay, we will use the abbreviation T4(D) (S) since this corresponds to nomenclature recommended by the American Thyroid Association.

Usefulness of the T4(D) (S) is based on the fact that increased TBG normally is accompanied by increased T4 and increased UTBG, while decreased TBG normally is accompanied by decreased T4 and decreased UTBG (Fig. 11-24). With increased TBG the laboratory finding of increased T4 may be misleading, because FT4 is normal owing to a proportional increase in UTBG, with consequent decrease in %T4 and RT3U. Measurement of T4(D) involves alcoholic extraction of T4 from the patient's serum, and addition of this extract to TBG fully saturated with radioactive T4. With the T4(D) (S), untreated patient serum is added to each assay in addition to the alcoholic extract of T4 (and normal serum added to each standard at the same stage):

1. A patient with increased UTBG will have "less T4" owing to additional binding sites added to the reaction mixture.
2. A patient with normal UTBG will have "normal T4" since a "normal number" of binding sites are added to the reaction mixture.
3. A patient with decreased UTBG will have "more T4" owing to "fewer than normal" extra binding sites added to the reaction mixture.

Obviously the "normal serum" must be carefully controlled: variations in this critical component will cause invalid results. Provided UTBG in the "normal serum" is held constant, this procedure may obviate the need for routine measurements of RT3U or %FT4 in addition to T4(D).

Measurements of urinary thyroxine (Chan and Landon, 1972) and urinary triiodothyronine (Chan *et al.*, 1972) have been proposed as estimates of circulating "free" hormone, analogous to use of urinary cortisol as an estimate of unbound or free plasma cortisol. Normal excretion of thyroxine is about 4–12 μg./24 hr., while normal excretion of triiodothyronine is about 2–4 μg./24 hr. Additional experience is needed to determine whether these procedures offer any advantage over free thyroxine index or the recently introduced T4(D) (S).

Measurements of Thyroxine-binding Protein

Levels of thyroxine-binding globulin usually are expressed as maximal binding capacity for thyroxine. The recommended abbreviation is TBG_{cap} (Solomen *et al.*, 1972). If it is assumed that TBG has a single binding site per molecule, a molecular weight of 59,000, and a binding capacity of 20 μg./dl., the approximate concentration of TBG in plasma may be calculated as 1.5 mg./dl. However, it is more convenient to express results as TBG_{cap} rather than concentration of TBG *per se*.

TBG may be measured by a radiochemical electrophoretic procedure. An excess of "cold" T4 plus radioactive T4 is added to serum, displacing patient T4 from TBG. After saturating TBG, the cold and radioactive T4 bind to TBPA and to albumin. Electrophoresis is performed and TBG_{cap} expressed as the alpha globulin capacity to bind T4 (calculated from total T4 and relative amount of radioactive T4 in the alpha globulin region) (Wahner and Walser, 1972). Occasionally measurements of TBG are helpful as a check on the total thyroxine and resin uptake: any one of these three parameters can be estimated if the other two are known.

At present, measurements of TBPA appear to be of little clinical value and are primarily of research interest.

MEASUREMENT OF THYROID-STIMULATING HORMONES

Radioimmunoassays for human TSH were developed during the mid 1960's and are now established as clinically useful. As yet, these assays are rather insensitive in the normal range; definitive information on (a) TSH diurnal variation, and (b) TSH levels in nontoxic goiter must await improved sensitivity.

TSH measurements are of greatest value in primary hypothyroidism. Although increased TSH does not establish this diagnosis, a normal serum TSH virtually excludes primary hypothyroidism. Most asymptomatic patients with increased TSH probably have subclinical hypothyroidism; however, there is one report of hyperthyroidism with raised TSH due to a pituitary chromophobe adenoma (Hall, 1972). Recently Lemarchand-Beraud *et al.* (1972) have suggested that serum TSH may be slightly increased in liver disease; additional studies are needed to confirm this observation.

In early hypothyroidism with "high normal" serum TSH, the TSH response to TRF may be useful: following TRF, hypothyroid patients have an exaggerated and prolonged rise in TSH (Hall, 1972). In most cases the TSH stimulation test will also show decreased thyroid reserve. Subclinical hypothyroidism may occur in association with Hashimoto's disease, iodide deficiency goiter, iodide-induced goiter, and following treatment of Graves' disease by surgery or radioactive iodine.

An additional use for TSH measurements in hypothyroidism is evaluation of replacement therapy (Burger and Patel, 1972). When hypothyroid patients receive adequate exogenous hormone, their TSH levels become normal or undetectable: patients who remain clinically hypothyroid with increased serum TSH despite apparently adequate therapy may be failing to take the hormone regularly.

The finding of a normal or low TSH in a hypothyroid patient implies pituitary or hypothalamic hypothyroidism; however, present TSH measurements are not sufficiently sensitive to distinguish decreased levels from normal, and patients with pituitary hypothyroidism typically have levels in the "normal range." Administration of TRF provides a method for evaluating TSH reserve in suspected pituitary hypothyroidism: a normal TSH response to TRF is strong evidence against pituitary hypothyroidism. Following TRF, patients with hypothalamic disease characteristically show a delayed rise in TSH, with the one-hour level exceeding the 20-minute level (in normal individuals, the 20-minute TSH usually is about twice the one-hour TSH).

In hyperthyroidism TSH levels typically are "within normal limits," probably owing to insensitivity of the assay. However, there is some evidence that TSH assays may provide information in borderline hyperthyroidism. Normal subjects respond to intravenous injection of 200 μg. TRF with a rise in serum TSH; however, in hyperthyroid patients, elevated levels of free hormone, acting at the pituitary level, suppress this effect. Failure of response is also seen in some euthyroid subjects with thyroid adenomas, Graves' disease in remission, and some patients with ophthalmic Graves' disease (Hall, 1972). Failure of response to TRF may correlate with abnormal response to the T3 suppression test, although additional studies are needed (Hall, 1972).

Other thyroid stimulators include long-acting thyroid stimulator (LATS), human chorionic thyrotropin (HCT), and human molar thyrotropin (HMT). LATS is present in some patients with Graves' disease, as well as in some euthyroid relatives. During the late 1960's it appeared that LATS might be the cause of Graves' disease; however, this impression has proved to be an oversimplification, and the exact etiology of Graves' disease remains obscure. HCT can be extracted from human placenta; it has a molecular weight similar to TSH, but far less biologic activity. The physiologic role of HCT is not established. HMT has been extracted from hydatidiform moles and is detected in the serum of patients with hyperthyroidism due to presence of the mole; it has a molecular weight similar to albumin and may contain HCT as a subunit (Hall, 1972). The clinical significance of these "other thyroid stimulators" is not yet well established.

RADIOACTIVE IODINE UPTAKE AND RELATED MEASUREMENTS

When tracer amounts of ^{131}I are administered orally (1 to 5 μCi.), this isotope is rapidly absorbed and distributed within the total body iodide space of plasma plus extracellular fluid (about 35 per cent of body weight). The thyroid and kidney together clear ^{127}I and ^{131}I from plasma. With a high total body iodide, the tracer dose is relatively small in comparison with the iodide pool, and the per cent uptake by the thyroid will be low. Either increased dietary iodide or decreased glomerular filtration rate may cause increased total body iodide and low thyroid uptake of radioactive iodine (RAI). Conversely, decreased total body iodide will cause increased RAI uptake. The relationship between dietary iodine and ^{131}I uptake is shown in Figure 11–25. Obviously the RAI can be used to measure thyroid function only if total body iodide is "within normal limits." Variations in intrathyroidal iodide stores also affect the RAI: increased thyroid iodide causes decreased trapping, while decreased iodide stores cause increased trapping. In some cases, decreased intrathyroidal iodine may

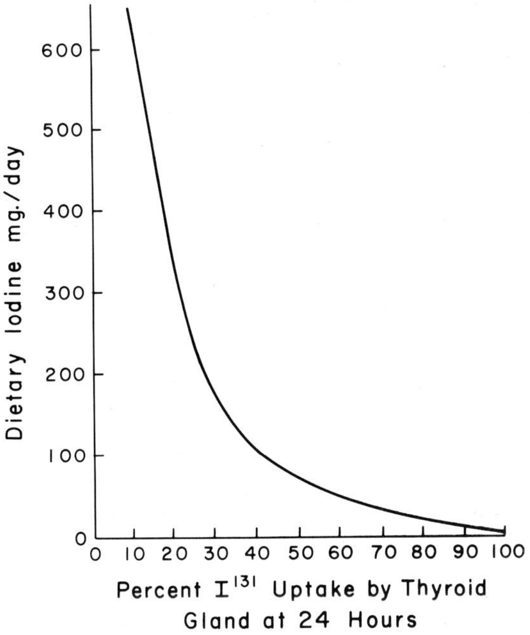

Figure 11-25. Relation of dietary iodine intake to RAI. (Modified from Means, DeGroot and Stanbury: The Thyroid and Its Diseases. New York, McGraw-Hill Book Co., Inc., 1963.)

develop because of thyroiditis and will cause a falsely high RAI.

During the 1950's thyroid uptake of radioactive iodine (RAI uptake) was a widely used "thyroid function test." Many workers noted that iodine contamination with elevated PBI was frequently associated with decreased RAI uptake. The reason for this was that iodinated substances such as radiographic contrast media typically are slowly deiodinated over weeks, months, or years, although a few materials, such as Teridax (used for cholecystography), are not physiologically deiodinated, and cause increased PBI with no change in RAI uptake. Thus, the finding of a low RAI and a high PBI is suggestive evidence of iodine contamination.

Today newer methods for serum thyroxine have eliminated the need to use RAI as a "check" on PBI contamination. And wide variations in iodide intake due to dietary supplements have led to shifts in the "normal range" for RAI (Ghahremani *et al.*, 1971). Reported "normal ranges" for thyroid ^{131}I uptake now include: 30 to 70 per cent (Dyrbye *et al.*, 1964); 15 to 45 per cent (Williams, 1968); and 5 to 30 per cent (Pittman *et al.*, 1969).

The tendency for this normal range to shift downward probably is related to increased use of iodine in food additives. Use of such additives varies in different regions; indeed a person may change from "normal" to "abnormal" on traveling to a nearby town (Pittman *et al.*, 1969). Thus, it may be difficult to accurately predict the "correct normal range" in a patient whose diet is not known or who travels extensively.

Variations in technique as well as variations in dietary iodine may cause marked differences in thyroid RAI uptake: "(due to) . . . variations in counting equipment . . . technique . . . and . . . standards . . . uptake ranges . . . (are) not comparable even between . . . laboratories . . . in the same city. . . . Over 300 laboratories (measured) thyroid uptake by their own "standardized" procedure in . . . specially prepared mannequins. . . . Only 15 . . . laboratories obtained results within 5 percentage points of the correct answer. . . . (This) problem is likely to become even worse" (Becker and Hurley, 1972).

Other variables which may affect thyroid RAI uptake include:

1. A variety of drugs which interfere with thyroid function may cause decreased RAI; immediately after such drugs are discontinued, a "rebound" with increased RAI may occur (Table 11–24).

2. Exogenous thyroid hormone causes a low RAI, while dyshormonogenesis (production of metabolically ineffective hormone) causes a high RAI.

3. With hyperthyroidism, iodide taken up may be rapidly discharged as thyroxine into the circulation; in such cases the RAI uptake may be increased at two or six hours and normal or low at 24 hours.

For the above reasons, results of thyroid RAI uptake frequently are difficult to interpret. The RAI uptake is NOT a suitable "screening test" for thyroid dysfunction. However, certain modifications of the RAI may be useful to evaluate:

1. Borderline hyperthyroidism with autonomous function of the thyroid gland (T3 suppression test).

2. Borderline hypothyroidism with decreased thyroid reserve (TSH stimulation test).

3. Defective oxidation and organification (perchlorate discharge test).

4. Thyroid function in patients on long-term replacement therapy (T3 withdrawal test).

5. Solitary thyroid nodules and ectopic thyroid tissue (thyroid scan).

As discussed in the section on Graves' disease, hyperthyroidism may be due to: Graves' disease, Hashimoto's disease, thyroid adenoma, autonomous nodule(s) in multiple colloid adenomatous goiter. Normally, administration of T3 (25 μg. three times daily for 6 days) causes a decrease in RAI to half its original level. However, the four conditions listed are characterized by autonomous thyroid function

Table 11-24. EXTRATHYROIDAL CAUSES FOR ABNORMAL THYROID FUNCTION

I. Block iodide trapping
   Chlorate
   Hypochlorite
   Iodate
   Nitrate
   Perchlorate
   Thiocyanate
II. Block oxidation and organification of iodide
   Amphenone
   Carbimazole
   Cobalt
   Iodide
   Methimazole
   Methylthiouracil
   Para-aminosalicylate
   Phenylbutazone
   Phenylindanedione (anticoagulant)
   Plants of genus Brassica, ingested directly (raw turnips) or as milk from cattle (reported as cause of goiter in children)
   Propylthiouracil
   Resorcinol
   Sulfonamides (rarely if ever cause goiter; may cause ↓ RAI during treatment, with ↑ RAI after drug is discontinued)
III. Block gastrointestinal reabsorption of thyroxine(?)
   Soybean milk formulas for infants
IV. Suppress TSH (?)
   ACTH, cortisone (do not cause goiter; may cause ↓ RAI during therapy)
V. Block thyroglobulin hydrolysis
   Iodide (in Graves' disease; rarely in euthyroid individuals)
VI. Mode of action not established (goiter not reported in humans, but may cause ↓ RAI, with ↑ RAI after drug is discontinued
   Acetazolamide (Diamox)
   Chlorpromazine
   Chlor-trimeton
   Brompheniramine maleate (Dimetane)
   Thiopental
   Tolbutamide

with loss of pituitary feedback control and an abnormal T3 suppression test. Especially in Graves' disease, autonomous function may appear *prior* to clinical hyperthyroidism and may persist after return to the euthyroid state. The T3 suppression test may be considered analogous to the dexamethasone test used for evaluation of hyperadrenalism.

Decreased thyroid reserve may occur in a wide variety of conditions, including: borderline hypothyroidism, multiple colloid adenomatous goiter, Hashimoto's disease and other types of thyroiditis, and following subtotal thyroidectomy or radioiodine therapy. Normally, daily injection of 10 units of TSH for 3 days will cause an increase in RAI to twice its original level. However, in the four conditions listed, the thyroid frequently is unable to respond to additional stimulation. The TSH stimulation test may be considered analogous to the ACTH stimulation test used for evaluation of hypoadrenalism.

Defective oxidation and organification of iodide may occur in Hashimoto's thyroiditis, or inborn errors of metabolism (may present with diffuse goiter at any age, with patient either euthyroid or hypothyroid), or following therapy with antithyroid drugs. If thyroid uptake is measured three hours after a trace dose of ^{131}I, and 1 gm. of potassium perchlorate is administered at this time, normal subjects will discharge less than 15 per cent of the three-hour uptake within one hour, while patients with defective oxidation and organification will discharge more than 15 per cent. This test is primarily useful for investigation of unusual problems and is NOT a "routine" procedure.

A frequent problem is evaluation of nongoitrous patients who have been on long-term thyroid hormone therapy for a questionable diagnosis of hypothyroidism. In such patients the TSH stimulation test sometimes is unreliable, and the T3 withdrawal test may be helpful. If fully suppressive doses of T3 are administered for 30 days, then discontinued for 10 days, a RAI uptake in the normal range, or a rise in PBI exceeding 1.0 μg./dl., suggests that pituitary-thyroid reserve probably is adequate to maintain normal hormone levels (Stein and Nicoloff, 1971).

Thyroid scan of a "solitary" nodule may reveal:

1. Multiple nodules, not detected on physical examination; these may vary from cold to hot, with a pattern of "patchy" uptake characteristic of benign multiple colloid adenomatous goiter.

2. A single hyperfunctioning "hot" nodule, with suppression of surrounding thyroid gland; such nodules are almost invariably benign.

3. A single "warm," "cool," or "cold" nodule, for which surgery may be indicated.

4. Ectopic thyroid tissue, either along the thyroglossal duct or substernally.

Thyroid scan is of greatest value in studying solitary thyroid nodules. It occasionally may be useful in differential diagnosis of hyperthyroidism in elderly patients (Graves' disease vs. autonomous nodule), or in detecting functional metastases from follicular carcinoma. Thyroid scanning is NOT indicated as a "routine" in all patients with an enlarged gland or clinical hyperthyroidism: it has been suggested that this procedure may be "performed . . . more frequently than is really useful" (Becker and Hurley, 1972).

Recently Ashkar and Smith (1971) have reported a thyroid evaluation method using pertechnetate Tc-99m with the Anger camera to view thyroid and cervical vessels, and measure the carotid-thyroid transit time

(CTTT). As an index of function in over 200 patients, the CTTT correlated well with other tests of thyroid function, with a CTTT less than 2.5 seconds in hyperthyroidism, more than 2.5 seconds in euthyroid subjects, and prolonged in hypothyroidism. Additional study is needed to evaluate the merits of this procedure which evaluates thyroid function and anatomy.

Estimates of Thyroid Hormone Effect on Target Organs

The two most frequently used tests of hormone effect on peripheral tissues are the basal metabolic rate (BMR) and Achilles tendon reflex test (photomotogram). Although increased cholesterol is characteristic of hypothyroidism, this measurement is NOT a useful "thyroid function test."

The basal metabolic rate (BMR) measures rate of oxygen consumption in the resting, fasting state. Under these conditions about 25 per cent of oxygen consumption comes from functional activity of organs (heart, liver, kidneys, and so forth), and perhaps 50 per cent from maintenance of tone in skeletal muscles.

A major problem is defining and obtaining a truly "basal state" in the individual patient. Hospitalization is sometimes recommended, but opinions differ as to whether this is essential. Measurement of the BMR during anesthesia or sedation has been proposed but is not widely accepted. Alternatively, several measurements of BMR may be performed to familiarize the patient with this procedure and the lowest value used for diagnosis. Although rate of oxygen consumption is decreased in hypothyroidism and increased in hyperthyroidism, many other variables are involved. Reported causes for increased BMR without thyroid disease include the following: anxiety, stress, and lack of sleep; food intake within 12 hours; congestive heart failure; increased cardiac workload due to anemia, polycythemia, or hypertension; dyspnea due to pulmonary disease; fever; neoplasms, especially leukemia, lymphoma, and pheochromocytoma; drugs, including caffeine, amphetamine, and epinephrine; and oxygen leak due to a perforated ear drum or defective apparatus.

An apparent decrease in BMR without thyroid disease may occur with the following: increased metabolically inactive tissue due to ascites, edema, or obesity; malnutrition; hypoadrenalism; eunuchoid states; and menopause; and in some normal individuals who have low BMR's without evidence of pathology.

It has been suggested that some patients with clinical hypothyroidism and normal circulating free hormone may have "decreased tissue response" to free T3 and T4: in such cases, all measurements except the BMR would be normal. However, this condition is extremely rare, if indeed it exists at all. The BMR also has been suggested as a method of following patients being treated with T3 or T4; however, it is of limited value in view of poor precision, a wide normal range (−20 to +20), and the many extrathyroidal variables. The BMR is NOT a suitable screening test for hyperthyroidism or hypothyroidism.

Duration of the Achilles tendon reflex may be measured by means of a photoelectric cell attached to an electrocardiograph. There is incomplete agreement as to which portion of the reflex should be measured, but the relaxation time and half-relaxation time are frequently used. Total duration of the reflex, as well as relaxation time, is increased in hypothyroidism. Diagnostic use of this procedure is largely limited to hypothyroidism, since there appears to be considerable overlap between normal and hyperthyroid patients (Gorman and McConahey, 1970 and Gross, 1971). Although the "photomotogram" is technically simple, it may be influenced by many extrathyroidal factors. Reported causes for a rapid reflex (short reflex time) include: catecholamines, such as adrenaline; insulin, including intravenous insulin and insulin coma; exercise; amphetamines; estrogens; and ACTH or cortisone.

Reported causes for a slow reflex (long reflex time) include: peripheral neuropathy due to diabetes, malignancy, generalized infection, collagen disease, pernicious anemia, sarcoidosis, sprue, vascular disease, or neurosyphilis; peripheral edema; adrenergic blocking agents, including reserpine and propranolol; procainamide or quinidine; parkinsonianism; increasing age; cooling of the lower extremities; postpartum state; glucose administration; and potassium administration or endogenous hyperkalemia (renal failure). Because of these exogenous factors, the photomotogram is of limited value and is not widely used at the present time.

Clinical Correlation

"Typical" laboratory results in various conditions are outlined in Table 11–25.

It may be necessary to evaluate thyroid function of a patient who is already on thyroid medication. Such individuals are placed on thyroid hormone, often because of a little obesity, a feeling of tiredness, or even dry skin and menstrual irregularities. They are receiving thyroid hormone in full suppressive doses or partial suppressive doses and the physician who encounters such a patient does not know

Table 11-25. TYPICAL RESULTS OF THYROID FUNCTION STUDIES IN VARIOUS CONDITIONS

DISEASE	T4 (D) or T4 (C)	TBG	%FT4 or RT3U	FT4 or T4-RT3	TSH	Response to TRF	RAI Uptake	COMMENTS
Hyperthyroidism								
Graves' disease (active)	↑	N or ↓	↑	↑	N (↓)	↓	↑	Abnormal T3 suppression test
Graves' disease (following surgery)	N	N	N	N	N	N or ↓	N	Abnormal T3 suppression test may persist
Graves' disease (following thiouracil)	N	N	N	N	N	N or ↓	Variable during during therapy, with rebound	Abnormal T3 suppression test may persist
Graves' disease (following RAI Therapy)	N	N	N	N	N	N or ↓	N or ↓	About 20%-50% hypothyroid after one year
Graves' disease (with incr. TBG)	↑	↑	N or ↑	N	N (↓)	↓	↑	Abnormal T3 suppression test
Graves' disease (with decr. TBG)	N	↓	↑	N	N (↓)	↓	↑	Abnormal T3 suppression test
Toxic nodular goiter	↑ or N	N	↑ or N	↑ or N	N	N or ↓	↑ or N	Abnormal T3 suppression test
Toxic adenoma	↑	N or ↓	↑	↑	N	N or ↓	↑ or N	Abnormal T3 suppression test
T3 thyrotoxicosis	N	N	N	N	N	–	N or ↑	Increased serum T3
Thyrotoxicosis factitia								
Due to T3	↓	N or ↓	↓	↓	N (↓)	–	↓	Increased serum T3
Due to T4	↑	N or ↓	↑	↑	N (↓)	–	↓	Present TSH methods cannot detect ↓ levels
Hypothyroidism								
Primary	↓	N or ↓	↓	↓	↑	↑	↓	Failure of response to TSH
Primary (with incr. TBG)	N	↑	↓	↓	↑	↑	↓	Physiologic increase in TBG due to pregnancy may unmask borderline hyperthyroidism
Primary (with decr. TBG)	↓	↓	↑	↓	↑	↑	↓	Causes for altered TBG listed in Table 11-23

(*Table 11-25 continues on the opposite page.*)

Table 11-25. TYPICAL RESULTS OF THYROID FUNCTION STUDIES IN VARIOUS CONDITIONS (*Continued*)

DISEASE	T4 (D) or T4 (C)	TBG	%FT4 or RT3U	FT4 or T4-RT3	TSH	Response to TRF	RAI Uptake	COMMENTS
Primary with T3 Rx (euthyroid)	↓	N	↓	↓	N	–	↓	Commercial desiccated thyroid may vary in T4:T3 ratio
Primary with T4 Rx (euthyroid)	↑	N	↑	↑	N	–	↓	
Pituitary (secondary)	↓	N	↓	↓	N (↓)	None	↓ or N	Normal TSH stimulation test; usually have lack of other pituitary hormones
Hypothalamic (Tertiary)	↓	N	↓	↓	N (↓)	Delayed rise in TSH	↓ or N	Hypothalamic symptoms and signs often present
Decreased thyroid reserve	N	N	N	N	N or ↑	N or ↑	N or ↓	Abnormal TSH stimulation test
Increased TBG (eumetabolic)	↑	↑	↓	N	N	N	N	Clinical significance of increased T4 (D) should be checked by FT4 or T4-RT3
Decreased TBG (eumetabolic)	↓	↓	↑	N	N	N	Variable	Nephrotic syndrome may mimic hypothyroidism
Dilantin therapy	↓ or N	N	N	↓ or N	N	–	N	See Larsen, P. R., *et al.*: J. Clin. Invest. *49*:1266, 1970.
Heparin therapy	N or ↑	N	↑	↑	N	–	N	See text for other drugs which influence RT3U
Hashimoto's thyroiditis	↑, N or ↓	N	↑, N or ↓	↑, N or ↓	N or ↑	–	N or ↓	Thyroglobulin antibodies present
Subacute thyroiditis	N or ↑	N	N or ↑	N or ↑	N	–	↓	Elevated ESR; needle biopsy may confirm diagnosis
Iodine excess	N (↑)	N	N (↑)	N (↑)	N	–	↓	Some iodinated compounds may interfere with T4 (C); ipodate may interfere with RT3U
Iodine deficiency (endemic goiter)	N or ↓	N	N or ↓	N or ↓	N or ↑	N or ↑	↑	Severe iodine deficiency causing decreased serum T4 is rare in U.S.A.

whether the patient is hypothyroid or not. Evaluation of thyroid function in such individuals can be achieved as follows: switch the patient from whatever thyroid medication he is taking to a maintenance dose of triiodothyronine (Cytomel), 75 μg. per day, which is the same employed in the suppression test. Cytomel (75 μg./day) is continued for four weeks or more. At that time Cytomel is withdrawn for 10 days, and even if the patient has no thyroid function, he will not develop signs and symptoms of hypothyroidism during that period in which he is off thyroid hormone or Cytomel in this situation. If the patient is normal or if there is enough thyroid function remaining to maintain normal circulating levels of hormone, the radioactive iodine uptake (RAI) will be greater than 16 per cent. In other words, it will rise to a normal value or above in about 95 per cent of normal patients. Serum hormone levels such as thyroxine or PBI will rise about 1 μg. per cent from the low value with Cytomel administration. Furthermore, immunoassayable TSH levels will be less than 15 μU./ml. In other words, TSH will be in the normal range.

Serum thyroxine by displacement (T4(D)) and "normalized serum thyroxine" probably are the best single measurements for assessment of thyroid function in the vast majority of patients. In those individuals who have alterations in thyroid-binding protein, either normalized serum thyroxine, free thyroxine assay (FT4), or free thyroxine index should be measured, rather than total hormone.

TSH levels when elevated confirm a diagnosis of primary hypothyroidism. The best single test for equivocal or borderline elevated values of serum thyroxine in evaluation of hyperfunction is the radioactive iodine uptake and scan, including suppression tests. The RAI suppression test requires 75 μg. of Cytomel each day for seven days; RAI is suppressed in normal subjects. Suppression of the baseline uptake to less than half the original occurs in normal subjects, but in hyperthyroidism regardless of whether it is Graves' disease or a thyroid nodule, no significant suppression will occur. Hence, patients with borderline elevated serum thyroxine or free thyroxine tests in which the diagnosis of hyperthyroidism is not established can be further evaluated with a suppression test to determine whether or not the gland is truly autonomous or if the elevation is consistent with hyperthyroidism.

In terms of monitoring treatment with thyroid preparations, the TSH level would appear to be the best single laboratory measurement, although the T4(D) test is acceptable if serum thyroid-binding proteins are not altered. Likewise, the serum thyroxine (T4(D)) or free thyroxine (FT4) may also provide laboratory assessment of replacement therapy effect, depending on the thyroid medication preparation, i.e., T4:T3 ratio.

REFERENCES

General

Alvioli, L.: Overview: Vitamin D. *In* International Symposium: Clinical Aspects of Metabolic Bone Disease. Amsterdam, Excerpta Medica, 1972.

Cantarow, A., and Schepartz, B.: Biochemistry. 4th ed. Philadelphia, W. B. Saunders Company, 1967.

DeLuca, H. F.: Vitamin D. New Eng. J. Med. *281*:1103, 1969.

Raisz, L. G.: A confusion of vitamin D's. New Eng. J. Med. 287:926, 1972.

Cyclic AMP

Broadus, A. E., Hardman, J. G., Kaminsky, N. I., *et al.*: Extracellular cyclic nucleotides. Ann. N.Y. Acad. Sci. In press.

Butcher, R. W., and Sutherland, E. W.: Adenosine 3′,5′-phosphate in biological materials. I. Purifications and properties of cyclic 3′,5′ nucleotide phosphodiesterase and use of this enzyme to characterize adenosine 3′,5′-phosphate in human urine. J. Biol. Chem. 237:1244, 1962.

Chase, L. R., Melson, G. L., and Aurbach, G. D.: Pseudohypoparathyroidism: Defective excretion of 3′,5′-AMP in response to parathyroid hormone. J. Clin. Invest. *48*: 1832, 1969.

Gilman, A. G.: A protein binding assay for adenosine 3′,5′-cyclic monophosphate. Proc. Nat. Acad. Sci. USA *67*:305, 1970.

Liddle, G. W., and Hardman, J. G.: Cyclic adenosine monophosphate as a mediator of hormone action. New Eng. J. Med. *285*:560, 1971.

Murad, F., and Pak, C. Y. C.: Urinary excretion of adenosine 3′,5′-monophosphate and guanosine 3′,5′-monophosphate. New Eng. J. Med. *286*:1382, 1972.

Rasmussen, H.: Ionic and hormonal control of calcium homeostasis. Amer. J. Med. *50*:567, 1971.

Rasmussen, H., Kurokawa, K., Mason, J., and Goodman, D. B. P.: Cyclic AMP, calcium and cell activation. *In* Talmage, R. V., and Munson, P. L. (eds.): Calcium, Parathyroid Hormone and the Calcitonins: Proceedings of the Fourth Parathyroid Conference. Amsterdam, Excerpta Medica, 1972.

Sutherland, E. W.: On the biological role of cyclic AMP. J.A.M.A. *214*:1281, 1970.

Sutherland, E. W.: Studies on the mechanism of hormone action. Science *177*:401, 1972.

Sutherland, E. W., Oye, I., and Butcher, R. W.: The action of epinephrine and the role of the adenyl cyclase system in hormone action. Recent Progr. Hormone Res. *21*:623, 1965.

Walsh, D. A., Krebs, E. G., Reiman, E. M., Brostrom, M. A., Corbin, J. D., Hickenbottom, J. P., Soderling, T. R., and Perkins, J. P.: The receptor protein for cyclic AMP in the control of glycogenolysis. *In* Greengard, P., and Costa, E. (eds.): Advances in Biochemical Psychopharmacology. Vol. 3. New York, Raven Press, 1970.

Hypothalamus and Pituitary

du Vigneaud, V., Ressler, C., Swan, J. M., Roberts, C. W., Katsoyannis, P. G., and Gordon, S.: The synthesis of an octapeptide amide with the hormonal activity of oxytocin. J. Amer. Chem. Soc. 75:4879–4880, 1953.

Fore, W., and Wynn, J.: The thyrotropin stimulation test. Amer. J. Med. *40*:90, 1966.

Gomez-Sanchez, C., and Kaplan, N. M.: Apparent inade-

quacy of L-Dopa stimulation as a clinical test of growth hormone release. J. Clin. Endocr. *34*:1105, 1972.
Guillemin, R., and Burgus, R.: The hormones of the hypothalamus. Sci. Amer. 227:24, 1972.
Katz, F. H.: Laboratory aids in the diagnosis of endocrine disorders. Med. Clin. N. Amer. *53*:79, 1969.
Liddle, G. W.: Preliminary characterization of some ectopic hormones. Vitamins Hormones (N.Y.) 26:293, 1968.
Moses, A. M., and Miller, M.: Urine and plasma osmolality in differentiation of polyuric states. Postgrad. Med. 52:187, 1972.
Moses, A. M., and Miller, M.: Urine and plasma osmolality in diagnosis and management of dilutional hyponatremia. Postgrad. Med. 52:232, 1972.
Northcutt, R. C., and Albert, A.: Laboratory tests for pituitary gonadotropins. J.A.M.A. *210*:2386, 1969.
Omenn, G. S.: Ectopic polypeptide hormone production by tumors. Ann. Intern. Med. 72:136, 1970.
Rabin, D., Spitz, I., Bercovici, B., Bell, J., Laufer, A., Benveniste, R., and Polishuk, W.: Isolated deficiency of follicle-stimulating hormone. New Eng. J. Med. 287:1313, 1972.
Reichlin, S.: Anterior pituitary—six glands and one. New Eng. J. Med. 287:1351, 1972.
Utiger, R.: Diabetes insipidus. J.A.M.A. *207*:1699, 1969.
VanderLaan, W. P., Parker, D. C., Rossman, L. G., and VanderLaan, E. F.: Implications of growth hormone release in sleep. Metabolism *19*:891, 1970.
Wolfsdorf, J., Farquhar, J. W., and Rigal, W. M.: Screening test for growth hormone deficiency in dwarfism. Lancet *2*:1271, 1967.

Adrenal Cortex

Biglieri, E. G., and Stockigt, J. R.: Primary aldosteronism. *In* Clinician-1 The Adrenal Gland, p. 58. Prepared for G. D. Searle & Co. by MEDCOM, Inc., 280 Park Avenue, New York, New York, 1971.
Bledsoe, T., and Longscope, C.: The gonads. *In* Harvey, A. M., Johns, R. J., Owens, A. H., Jr., and Ross, R. S. (eds.): The Principles and Practice of Medicine. 18th ed., 1972.
Bondy, P. K.: Adrenal masculinizing and feminizing syndromes. *In* Clinician-1 The Adrenal Gland, p. 94. Prepared for G. D. Searle & Co. by MEDCOM, Inc., 280 Park Avenue, New York, New York, 1971.
Bongiovanni, A. M., and Root, A. W.: The adrenogenital syndrome. New Eng. J. Med. *268*:1283, 1342, 1963.
Brown, R. D., and Strott, C. A.: Plasma deoxycorticosterone in man. J. Clin. Endocr. *32*:744, 1971.
Carey, R. M., Douglas, J. G., Schweikert, J. R., and Liddle, G. W.: The syndrome of essential hypertension and suppressed plasma renin activity. Arch. Intern. Med. *130*: 849, 1972.
Chattoraj, S. C.: Endocrinology. *In* Tietz, N. W. (ed.): Fundamentals of Clinical Chemistry. Philadelphia, W. B. Saunders Company, 1970.
Demetriou, J. A., and Austin, F. G.: Quantitation of plasma testosterone by improved competitive protein-binding technique. Clin. Chem. *16*:111, 1970.
Dorfman, R. I., and Ungar, R.: Metabolism of Steroid Hormones. New York, Academic Press, Inc., 1965.
Estep, H. L., Island, D. P., Ney, R. L., and Liddle, G. W.: Pituitary-adrenal dynamics during surgical stress. J. Clin. Endocr. *23*:419, 1964.
Ettinger, B., Goldfield, E. B., Burrill, K. C., Von Werder, K., and Forsham, P. H.: Plasma testosterone stimulation-suppression dynamics in hirsute women. Amer. J. Med. *54*:195, 1973.
Forsham, P. H.: The adrenals. *In* Williams, R. H. (ed.): Textbook of Endocrinology. 4th ed. Philadelphia, W. B. Saunders Company, 1969.
Gabrilove, J. L., Nicolis, G. L., and Kirschner, P. A.: Cushing's syndrome in association with carcinoid tumor. Ann. Surg. *169*:240, 1969.
Gunnels, J. C., Jr., Grim, C. E., Robinson, R. R., and Wilderman, N. M.: Plasma renin activity in healthy subjects and patients with hypertension. Arch. Intern. Med. *119*:232, 1967.
Horton, R., and Finck, E.: Diagnosis and localization in primary aldosteronism. Ann. Intern. Med. *76*:885, 1972.
Hsu, T. H., and Bledsoe, T.: Measurement of urinary free corticoids by competitive protein-binding radioassay in hypoadrenal states. J. Clin. Endocr. *30*:443, 1970.
Jubiz, W., Frailey, J., and Tyler, F. H.: A cause of apparently abnormal urinary 17-hydroxy corticosteroid responses to metyrapone in normal subjects. Clin. Chem. *16*:352, 1970.
Kaplan, N. M.: Assessment of pituitary ACTH secretory capacity with metopirone: 1. Interpretation. J. Clin. Endocr. *23*:945, 1963.
Kimberg, D. V.: Effects of vitamin D and steroid hormones on the active transport of calcium by the intestine. New Eng. J. Med. *280*:1396, 1969.
Kliman, B., and Peterson, R. E.: Double isotope derivatives assay of aldosterone in biological extracts. J. Biol. Chem. *235*:1639, 1960.
Krieger, D. T., Kolodny, H., and Krieger, H. P.: Methopyrapone tests in hypothalamic-pituitary disease. J. Clin. Endocr. *24*:1169, 1964.
Landau, R. L.: Tests of testicular function. J.A.M.A. *207*: 353, 1969.
Liddle, G. W.: Tests of pituitary suppressibility in Cushing's syndrome. J. Clin. Endocr. *20*:1539, 1960.
Liddle, G. W.: The physiology of adrenocortical function: A review of modern concepts. In Clinician-1 The Adrenal Gland, p. 7. Prepared for G. D. Searle & Co. by MEDCOM, Inc., 280 Park Avenue, New York, New York, 1971.
Liddle, G. W.: Adrenal cortex. *In* Beeson, P. B., and McDermott, W. (eds.): Cecil-Loeb Textbook of Medicine. 13th ed. Philadelphia, W. B. Saunders Company, 1971.
Lurie, A. O.: Plasma cortisol assay: Interference by spironolactone. J.A.M.A. *211*:1851, 1970.
Mattingly, D.: A simple fluorometric method for the estimation of free 11-hydroxycorticoids in human plasma. J. Clin. Path. *15*:374, 1962.
Migeon, C. J.: Adrenal androgens in man. Amer. J. Med. *53*:606, 1972.
Murphy, B. E. P.: Some studies of the protein-binding of steroids and their application to the routine micro and ultramicro measurement of various steroids in body fluids by competitive protein-binding radioassay. J. Clin. Endocr. *27*:973, 1967.
Spark, R. F., and Melby, J. C.: Hypertension and low plasma renin activity: Presumptive evidence for mineralocorticoid excess. Ann. Intern. Med. 75:831, 1971.
Stockigt, J. R., Noakes, C. A., Collins, R. D., Schambelan, M., and Biglieri, E. G.: Renal-vein renin in various forms of renal hypertension. Lancet *1*:1194, 1972.
Streeten, D. H. P.: Secondary aldosteronism. *In* Clinician-1 The Adrenal Gland, p. 76. Prepared for G. D. Searle & Co. by MEDCOM, Inc., 280 Park Avenue, New York, New York, 1971.
Thorn, G. W.: Adrenal cortical hypofunction. *In* Clinician-1 The Adrenal Gland, p. 22. Prepared for G. D. Searle & Co. by MEDCOM, Inc., 280 Park Avenue, New York, New York, 1971.
Tyler, F. H., and West, C. D.: Laboratory evaluation of disorders of the adrenal cortex. Amer. J. Med. *53*:664, 1972.
White, M. G.: Bartter's syndrome: A manifestation of renal tubular defects. Arch. Intern. Med. *129*:41, 1972.
Wolff, E., Glasser, M., Gordon, G. G., Olivo, J., and Southren, A. L.: Virilizing luteoma of pregnancy: Report of a case with measurements of testosterone and testosterone binding in plasma. Amer. J. Med. *54*:229, 1973.

Estrogen and Progesterone

Genazzani, A. R., Casoli, M., Aubert, M. L., Fioretti, P., and Felber, J. P.: Use of human-placental-lactogen radioimmunoassay to predict outcome in cases of threatened abortion. Lancet 2:1385, 1969.
Kankaanrinta, R.: On the pregnanediol excretion in the urine during the last trimester of normal and toxemic pregnancy. Scand. J. Clin. Lab. Invest. *15*:74, 1964.
Knox, B. S., and France, J. T.: Measurement of unconjugated 17 β-estradiol in plasma by competitive protein binding. Clin. Chem. *18*:212, 1972.

Magendantz, H. G., Klausner, D., Ryan, K. J., and Yen, S. S. C.: Estriol determinations in the management of high-risk pregnancies. Obstet. Gynec. *32*:610, 1968.
Manley, W. F. (ed.): Symposium on obstetric endocrinology. Clin. Obstet. Gynec. *8*:517, 1965.
Marais, W. D., and DuToit, F. E.: Clinicopathologic assessment of the value of urinary estriol assays during the third trimester of pregnancy. S. Afr. J. Gynec. *3*:41, 1965.
Mishell, D. R., Jr., Nakamura, R. M., Crosignani, P. G., Stone, S., Kharma, K., Nagata, Y., and Thorneycroft, I. H.: Serum gonadotropin and steroid patterns during the normal menstrual cycle. Amer. J. Obstet. Gynec. *111*:60, 1971.
Nesbitt, R. E. L., Jr., Aubry, R. H., Goldberg, E. M., and Jacobs, R. D.: Correlated hormone excretion patterns and cytohormonal variations in normal and complicated pregnancies. Amer. J. Obstet. Gynec. *93*:702, 1965.
Paulsen, C. A.: Estrogen Assays in Clinical Medicine. Seattle, University of Washington Press, 1963.
Yen, S. S. C., Vela, P., Rankin, J., and Littell, A. S.: Hormonal relationships during the menstrual cycle. J.A.M.A. *211*:1513, 1970.

Adrenal Medulla

Axelrod, J., and Weinshilboum, R.: Catecholamines. New Eng. J. Med. *287*:237, 1972.
Brown, J. J., Ruthven, C. R. J., and Sandler, M.: Diagnostic value of detailed metabolic pathway investigations in two cases of pheochromocytoma with minimal increase in total catecholamines output. J. Clin. Path. *19*:482, 1966.
Engelman, K., and Sjoerdsma, A.: The adrenal medulla: Catecholamines and pheochromocytoma. *In* Clinician-1 The Adrenal Gland, p. 110. Prepared for G. D. Searle & Co. by MEDCOM, Inc., 280 Park Avenue, New York, New York, 1971.
Gitlow, S. E., Mendlowitz, M., and Bertani, L. M.: The biochemical techniques for detecting and establishing the presence of a pheochromocytoma. Amer. J. Card. *26*:270, 1970.
Hunter, R. B., Marshall, T. D., and Oram, F. J.: Catecholamine excretion in cases of pheochromocytoma. Quart. J. Med. *32*:225, 1963.
Jacobs, S. L., Sobel, C., and Henry, R. J.: Excretion of 3-methoxy-4-hydroxymandelic acid and catecholamines in patients with pheochromocytoma. J. Clin. Endocr. *21*:315, 1961.
Molinoff, P. B., and Axelrod, J.: Biochemistry of catecholamines. Ann. Rev. Biochem. *40*:465, 1971.
Pickett, L. K., and Voorhess, M. L.: Neuroblastoma in childhood. Surg. Clin. N. Amer. *44*:1469, 1964.
Pisano, J. J., Crout, J. R., and Abraham, D.: Determination of 3-methoxy-4-hydroxymandelic acid in urine. Clin. Chim. Acta *7*:285, 1962.
Sandhu, R. S., and Freed, R. M.: Catecholamines and associated metabolites in human urine. *In* Cooper, G. R. and King, Jr., J. S. (eds.): Standard Methods of Clinical Chemistry. Vol. 7. New York, Academic Press, Inc., 1972.
Sunderman, F. W., Jr.: Measurements of vanilmandelic acid for the diagnosis of pheochromocytoma and neuroblastoma. Amer. J. Clin. Path. *42*:481, 1964.
Sweeley, V. C., and Williams, C. M.: Microanalytical determinations of urinary aeromatic acid by gas chromatography. Anal. Biochem. *2*:83, 1961.
Voorhess, M. L.: Urinary catecholamine excretion by healthy children. I. Daily excretion of dopamine, norepinephrine, epinephrine and 3-methoxy-4-hydroxymandelic acid. Pediatrics *39*:252, 1967.
Voorhess, M. L.: Adrenal medulla and sympathetic nervous tissue. *In* Barnett, H. L. (ed.): Pediatrics. 15th ed. New York, Appleton-Century-Crofts, Inc., 1972.
Voorhess, M. L., and Gardner, L. I.: Urinary excretion of norepinephrine, epinephrine and 3-methoxy-4-hydroxymandelic acid by children with neuroblastoma. J. Clin. Endocr. *21*:321, 1961.
Williams, C. M., and Greer, M.: Diagnosis of neuroblastoma by quantitative gas chromatographic analysis of urinary homovanillic and vanilmandelic acid. Clin. Chim. Acta *7*:880, 1962.
Williams, C. M., and Greer, M.: Homovanillic acid and vanilmandelic acid in diagnosis of neuroblastoma. J.A.M.A. *183*:836, 1963.
Williams, C. M., and Greer, M.: Gas chromatography of urinary vanilmandelic acid in pheochromocytoma. Clin. Chim. Acta *11*:495, 1965.

Thyroid

Ashkar, F. S., and Bezjian, A. A.: Use of normalized serum thyroxine (T4N). J.A.M.A. *221*:1483, 1972.
Ashkar, F. S., and Smith, E. M.: The dynamic thyroid study: A rapid evaluation of thyroid function and anatomy using ^{99m}Tc as pertechnetate. J.A.M.A. *217*:441, 1971.
Becker, D. V., and Hurley, J. R.: The impact of technology on clinical practice in Graves' disease. Mayo Clin. Proc. *47*:835, 1972.
Braverman, L. E., Woeber, K. A., and Ingbar, S. H.: Induction of myxedema by iodide in patients euthyroid after radioiodine or surgical treatment of diffuse toxic goiter. New Eng. J. Med. *281*:816, 1969.
Burger, H. G., and Patel, Y. C.: The value of serum thyrotrophin measurement in the diagnosis and management of hypothyroidism. Med. J. Aust. *2*:292, 1972.
Chan, V., Besser, G. M., Landon, J., and Ekins, R. P.: Urinary triiodothyronine excretion as index of thyroid function. Lancet *2*:253, 1972.
Chan, V., and Landon, J.: Urinary thyroxine excretion as index of thyroid function. Lancet *1*:4, 1972.
Christensen, L. K., Skovsted, L., and Hansen, J. M.: Protein-bound iodine during antithyroid treatment. Acta Med. Scand. *185*:483, 1969.
Clark, F., and Horn, D. B.: Assessment of thyroid function by the combined use of the serum protein-bound iodine and resin uptake of 131-triiodothyronine. J. Clin. Endocr. *25*:39, 1965.
DeGroot, L. J., Niepomniszcze, H., Nagasaka, A., and Hati, R.: Mechanism of thyroid hormone formation. Ann. Clin. Res. *4*:113, 1972.
Dyrbye, M. O., Peitersen, E., and Friis, T. H.: Diagnostic value of I^{131} in thyroid disorders. Acta Med. Scand. *176*:91, 1964.
Fatourechi, V., McConahey, W. M., and Woolner, L. B.: Hyperthyroidism associated with histologic Hashimoto's thyroiditis. Mayo Clin. Proc. *46*:682, 1971.
Ghahremani, G. G., Hoffer, P. B., Oppenheim, B. E., and Gottschalk, A.: New normal values for thyroid uptake of radioactive iodine. J.A.M.A. *217*:337, 1971.
Gharib, H., and Wahner, H. W.: Clinical experience with assays for triiodothyronine. Med. Clin. N. Amer. *56*:861, 1972.
Goldsmith, R. E.: Radioisotope therapy for Graves' disease. Mayo Clin. Proc. *47*:953, 1972.
Goolden, A. W. G., Gartside, J. M., and Sanderson, C.: Thyroid status in pregnancy and in women taking oral contraceptives. Lancet *1*:12, 1967.
Gorman, C. A., and McConahey, W. M.: Diagnosis of hyperthyroidism and hypothyroidism by laboratory methods. Med. Clin. N. Amer. *54*:1037, 1970.
Greer, M. A.: Factors regulating triiodothyronine (T3) and thyroxine (T4) in the blood. Mayo Clin. Proc. *47*:944, 1972.
Gross, M. A.: Achilles-reflex timing in diagnosis of thyroid status. New York J. Med. *71*:2283, 1971.
Hall, R.: The immunoassay of thyroid-stimulating hormone and its clinical applications. Clin. Endocr. *1*:115, 1972.
Hamada, S., Nakagawa, T., Mori, T., and Torizuka, K.: Re-evaluation of thyroxine binding and free thyroxine in human serum by paper electrophoresis and equilibrium dialysis and a new free thyroxine index. J. Clin. Endocr. *31*:166, 1970.
Hayles, A. B., and Cloutier, M. D.: Clinical hypothyroidism in the young. Med. Clin. N. Amer. *56*:871, 1972.
Henneman, G., and Bussemaker, J. K.: Thyroid suppression by triiodothyroxine before and after treatment for Graves' disease. Lancet *1*:588, 1969.
Hershman, J. M., and Pittman, J. A.: Control of thyrotropin secretion in man. New Eng. J. Med. *285*:997, 1971.
Hollander, C. S., Mitsuma, T., Nihei, N., Shenkman, L.,

Burday, S. Z., and Blum, M.: Clinical and laboratory observations in cases of triiodothyronine toxicosis confirmed by radioimmunoassay. Lancet *1*:609, 1972.

Inada, M., and Sterling, K.: Thyroxine turnover and transport in Laennec's cirrhosis of the liver. J. Clin. Invest. *46*:1275, 1967.

Lemarchand-Beraud, T., Griessen, M., and Scazziga, B. R.: Clinical significance of LATS and TSH in the blood. Ann. Clin. Res. *4*:121, 1972.

Lesoff, M. H., Lyne, C., Maisey, M. N., and Sturge, R. A.: Effect of thyroid failure on the pituitary-adrenal axis. Lancet *1*:642, 1969.

Lutz, J. H., Gregerman, R. I., Spaulding, S. W., Hornich, R. B., and Dawkins, A. T.: Thyroxine binding proteins, free thyroxine, and thyroxine turnover relationships during acute infectious illness in man. J. Clin. Endocr. *35*:230, 1972.

McConahey, W. M.: Hashimoto's thyroiditis. Med. Clin. N. Amer. *56*:885, 1972.

McCullagh, E. P., and Rosenbaum, H. M.: Diagnostic value of the absolute free thyroxine iodine test. Cleveland Clin. Quart. *39*:87, 1972.

Miller, J. M., and Block, M. A.: Functional autonomy in multinodular goiter. J.A.M.A. *214*:535, 1970.

Mincey, E. K.: Effective thyroxine ratio in assessment of thyroid function. J.A.M.A. *222*:1653, 1972.

Mincey, E. K., Thorson, S. C., and Brown, J. L.: A new in vitro blood test for determining thyroid status. Clin. Biochem. *4*:216, 1971.

Murphy, B. E. P., and Pattee, C. J.: Determination of thyroxine utilizing the property of protein-binding. J. Clin. Endocr. *24*:817, 1964.

Murray, I. P. C., Joasoo, A., and Parkin, J.: The assessment of thyroid function by in vitro techniques. Med. J. Aust. *2*:173, 1970.

Nelson, J. C., Johnson, D. E., and Odell, W. D.: Serum TSH levels and the thyroidal response to TSH stimulation in patients with thyroid disease. Ann. Intern. Med. *76*:47, 1972.

Pittman, J. A., Dailey, G. F., III, and Beschi, R. J.: Changing normal values for thyroidal radioiodine uptake. New Eng. J. Med. *280*:1431, 1969.

Ryness, J.: The measurement of serum thyroxine in children. J. Clin. Path. *25*:726, 1972.

Shenkman, L., Mitsuma, T., Suphavi, A., and Hollander, C. S.: Hypothalamic hypothyroidism. J.A.M.A. *222*:480, 1972.

Silverstein, G. E., and Burke, G.: Thyroid suppressibility and long-acting thyroid stimulators in thyrotoxicosis. Arch. Intern. Med. *126*:615, 1970.

Skelley, D. S., Brown, L. P., and Besch, P. K.: Radioimmunoassay. Clin. Chem. *19*:146, 1973.

Solomon, D. H., Benotti, J., DeGroot, L. J., Greer, M. A., Pileggi, V. J., Pittman, J. A., Robbins, J., Selenkow, H. A., Sterling, K., and Volpe, R.: A nomenclature for tests of thyroid hormones in serum. J. Clin. Endocr. *34*:884, 1972.

Solomon, D. H., and Chopra, I. J.: Graves' disease – 1972. Mayo Clin. Proc. *47*:803, 1972.

Stein, R. B., and Nicoloff, J. T.: Triiodothyronine withdrawal test – a test of thyroid-pituitary adequacy. J. Clin. Endocr. *32*:127, 1971.

Sterling, K., Brenner, M. A., and Newman, E. S.: Conversion of thyroxine to triiodothyronine in normal human subjects. Science *169*:1099, 1970.

Sterling, K., Brenner, M. A., Newman, E. S., Odell, W. D., and Bellabarba, D.: The significance of triiodothyronine (T3) in maintenance of euthyroid status after treatment of hypothyroidism. J. Clin. Endocr. *33*:729, 1971.

Thorson, S. C., Mincey, E. K., McIntosh, H. W., and Morrison, R. T.: Evaluation of a new in vitro blood test for determining thyroid status: The effective thyroxine ratio. Brit. Med. J. *1*:67, 1972.

Wahner, H. W., and Walser, A. H.: Measurements of thyroxine-plasma protein interactions. Med. Clin. N. Amer. *56*:849, 1972.

Wallack, M. S., Adelberg, H. M., and Nicoloff, J. T.: A thyroid suppression test using a single dose of L-thyroxine. New Eng. J. Med. *283*:402, 1970.

Werner, S. C., Wegelius, O., Fierer, J. A., and Hau, K. C.: Immunoglobulins (E,M,G) and complement in the connective tissues of the thyroid in Graves' disease. New Eng. J. Med. *287*:421, 1972.

Williams, E. S., Erkins, R. P., and Ellis, S. M.: Thyroid suppression test with serum thyroxine concentration as index of suppression. Brit. Med. J. *4*:338, 1969.

Williams, R. H. (ed.): Textbook of Endocrinology. 4th ed. Philadelphia, W. B. Saunders Company, 1968.

Wilson, F., and Henry, J. B.: Correspondence. Analytical Letters *4*:805, 1971.

Wolff, J.: Iodide goiter and the pharmacologic effects of excess iodide. Amer. J. Med. *47*:101, 1969.

Zacharewicz, F. A.: Management of single and multinodular goiter. Med. Clin. N. Amer. *52*:409, 1968.

Chapter 12

WATER, ELECTROLYTES, ACID-BASE, AND OXYGEN

by HARRY F. WEISBERG, M.D.

WATER

According to Gamble, the total body water (TBW) represents about 70 per cent of the total body weight. This is divided into the intracellular fluid (ICF), about 50 per cent of the total body weight, and the extracellular fluid (ECF), 20 per cent. The extracellular fluid is divided into the interstitial fluid (ISF), comprising about 15 per cent of the total body weight, and the intravascular fluid (IVF) or plasma volume (PV), which makes up about 5 per cent of the total body weight.

The TBW content of a person will vary inversely with the total fat content ("obesity"). An obese individual has less body water, resulting in a larger per cent daily turnover and, therefore, a smaller reserve to combat dehydration. In the usual clinical laboratory the TBW is not determined. In research laboratories the TBW is determined by measuring the volume of distribution of a substance that can penetrate all the cells of the body; e.g., heavy water (D_2O), tritiated water (HTO), or derivatives of antipyrine. The ECF can be determined by measuring the volume of distribution of a substance that does not penetrate the cell membrane (e.g., inulin, mannitol, sucrose, thiocyanate, sulfate, bromide, thiosulfate, sodium, and chloride). Low values for ECF result from the use of inulin, since it does not fully penetrate the interstices of connective tissue, and higher values probably result with chloride since it does enter some cells (e.g., gastric mucosa) and is more concentrated in the connective tissue than in free ECF. Since the ICF compartment is calculated by the difference, it is obvious that such values are subject to criticism.

The TBW is approximately 73 per cent of the body weight when computed on a fat-free or lean muscle mass basis. Because the fat content of the body varies from patient to patient and depends especially on the sex, the TBW ranges between 50 and 71 per cent of the total body weight in the adult male, with an average of about 60 per cent; in the adult female the range is 40 to 60 per cent of body weight, with an average of 50 per cent. In the newborn the TBW is much greater, ranging from 70 to 83 per cent, with an average of 77 per cent.

The average TBW of a young adult man has been given as 60 per cent of the body weight; the usual average for the ICF and ECF compartments are 45 and 15 per cent, respectively, of the body weight. The ICF water is computed as the difference between the TBW and the water held in the extracellular spaces. Radioactive tracer studies have shown that the value for the ICF compartment is too large, because the ECF compartment now includes more than the IVF and ISF previously included in this category. The plasma volume is 4.5 per cent of the body weight. The ISF compartment (12 per cent of the body weight) now also includes the lymph and a rapidly equilibrating phase of the connective tissue. The major portion of the connective tissue and cartilaginous tissue contains water equal to 4.5 per cent of the body weight. ECF water found in bone also equals 4.5 per cent of the body weight. The smallest amount of water (1.5 per cent of the body weight) is found in the transcellular compartment, which is formed by the transport activity of certain cells: gastrointestinal tract (e.g., salivary glands, pancreas, liver, and biliary tract, mucous membranes, and the intraluminal fluid), "epidermal" cells (e.g., skin and mucous membranes of the respiratory tract), kidneys, cerebrospinal fluid, humors of the eye, and endocrine secretions (e.g., thyroid and gonads).

Thus, the TBW still comprises 60 per cent of the body weight (adult male), but the new values for the ICF and ECF compartments are 33 and 27 per cent, respectively, of the body weight.

In addition, the water content changes with age, so that the average TBW in a geriatric male is 51 per cent, and in the geriatric female, 45 per cent of the total body weight.

The plasma volume is the only "compartment" of the body water that is easily determined; it is related to the weight of the individual. The average values for man, woman, and infant are 4.5, 4.3, and 4.1 per cent of body weight, respectively. A more accurate relationship pertains to the surface area of the individual. For men the plasma volume in milliliters is 1630 × m.^{2} (total blood volume is 2730 × m.^{2}) and in women the plasma volume is 1410 × m.^{2} (total blood volume is 2250 × m.^{2}). The plasma contains 92 to 95 per cent water, whereas the red blood cells contain about 70 to 75 per cent.

Water Balance

The normal adult who indulges in routine activities will have an intake and an output of water balanced in the range of 1500 to 3000 ml. per day. The mythical 70-kg. adult male may be in water balance with an intake of 2500 ml. This amounts to about 24 per cent of his extracellular fluid, which is contained in the interstitial and intravascular compartments. A normal intake will be maintained for the adult if he is supplied with 30 ml. of water per kg. of body weight. This will supply approximately 1 L. for loss owing to insensible perspiration and 1 L. for urine excretion. A minimum total water output for the average adult is about 1500 ml. per day; about 900 ml. are required for insensible perspiration and 600 ml. for minimum urine excretion.

One of the major sources of fluid loss from the body is via the gastrointestinal tract. Under normal circumstances only 50 to 200 ml. of water are lost in the semisolid feces. However, during the course of a day approximately 8 L. of fluid are secreted into the gastrointestinal tract via the juices from the salivary glands, bile, pancreas, and intestines. Approximately 8 L. must be reabsorbed, a volume approximately two to three times that of the normal plasma volume. The concentration of electrolytes will vary in the different secretions of the gastrointestinal tract. The gastric secretions are high in chloride and low in sodium content; the potassium concentration is about three times that found in plasma. Fluid obtained from the pancreatic or ileal regions of the intestinal tract has a high sodium and a relatively low chloride content, but the potassium concentration is again higher than that found in plasma. The bile secretion has a composition approximating that of the extracellular fluid, whereas juices from the jejunal region of the gastrointestinal tract have almost equal concentrations of sodium and chloride.

ELECTROLYTES

Electrolytes are usually determined in serum or plasma rather than in whole blood, since there is an unequal distribution of electrolytes between the serum component of the blood and the red blood cells. Any anemia or change in hematocrit reading will cause an alteration when the electrolytes in whole blood are determined, whereas the determination of the electrolyte in serum or plasma will remain constant no matter what the actual red blood cell count.

Describing electrolyte concentrations in the blood and other body tissues in terms of milligrams per 100 ml. (weight/volume) is not adequate for the proper understanding of the balance of the positively charged (cation) and negatively charged (anion) electrolytes present in the body. However, the anions and cations balance one another when expressed as milliequivalents per liter (reactants/volume)—the law of "electroneutrality" (Table 12–1).

Cations

SODIUM

Dietary sodium is usually obtained as sodium chloride, the amount ingested varying according to the taste of the individual. In the adult approximately 40 to 90 mEq. of sodium are excreted per liter of urine, or an average of approximately 110 mEq. per 24 hours. A reported normal range of urinary sodium excretion is 40 to 215 mEq. per day. In a young child the daily requirement for sodium is approximately 50 mEq. per day, and in infants of about one year the requirement is approximately 17 mEq. per day.

The daily adult exchange of sodium is about 3 to 6 per cent of the total sodium contained in the body, and about 4 per cent for a child. This exchange of sodium is brought about by ingestion via the gastrointestinal tract and the loss via urinary excretion and the sweat. In a fasting individual without any sodium intake the urinary loss of sodium will occur for the first two or three days and then drop to minimal values, provided no abnormal losses of water occur. When sodium is lost from the body, there

Table 12–1. REPRESENTATIVE NORMAL VENOUS PLASMA OR SERUM ELECTROLYTES*

ELECTROLYTE	EXPRESSED AS: "Weight"/Volume mg./100 ml. of plasma	"Reactants"/Volume mEq./L. of plasma	"Particles"/Volume mosmol./L. of plasma (or mmol./L. of plasma)
Cations			
Sodium	326.0	142	142
Potassium	20.0	5	5
Calcium	10.0	5	2.5
Magnesium	2.4	2	1
Total cations	358.4	154	150.5
Anions			
Bicarbonate	60.5†	26	26
Chloride	365.7	103	103
Phosphate	3.4	2	1
Sulfate	1.6	1	0.5
Organic acids	17.5	6	5.5
Proteinate	6500.0	16	2
Total anions	6948.7	154	138
Total electrolytes	7307.1	308	288.5

*Modified from Weisberg, H. F.: *Water, Electrolyte, and Acid-Base Balance.* 2nd ed. Baltimore, The Williams & Wilkins Company, 1962. Reproduced with permission of the publisher.
†Volumes per cent (ml. of carbon dioxide/100 ml.).

is also a loss of extracellular water to maintain a normal osmotic equilibrium.

Contrary to the belief that sodium is always extracellular and not found within the cells, it has been shown that sodium is present within the cells, the amount depending upon conditions existing in the extracellular compartment. Energy-producing reactions are necessary for the transfer of the sodium ion out of the cell. The amount of intracellular sodium is 10 to 35 mEq. per liter of cell water. The intracellular sodium acts as an additional buffer, protecting the pH of the extracellular fluid. In the adult there are about 1.09 gm. of sodium per kg. (fat free), and in the newborn the sodium content is 1.78 gm. per kg. of body weight. The average man contains about 65 gm. of sodium in his body; about 38 gm. are extracellular, 21 gm. are in the bones, and about 6 gm. are found within the cells.

If a patient is given 3 L. of isotonic saline in 24 hours, he will receive 465 mEq. of sodium (155 × 3)—an amount that exceeds the tolerance of a healthy adult on an average diet. If a healthy adult is given 3 L. of isotonic saline in 24 hours, and if this adult has been ingesting less than 250 mEq. of sodium per day, it will take him from 24 to 48 hours to excrete the excess sodium.

Following surgery, trauma, or shock, however, there is an absolute or relative decrease in extracellular fluid volume. Replacement of extracellular fluid is essential if water and electrolyte balance is to be maintained. The ideal replacement solution will have an electrolyte composition similar to that of normal plasma and will, therefore, have a sodium concentration of 140 mEq. per liter.

Plasma Sodium vs. Urine Sodium. Plasma sodium determinations are useful in detecting gross changes in water and salt balance but are of little help in detecting early or subtle changes. For example, in adrenal insufficiency, plasma sodium levels can remain normal until late in the course of the disease. The urinary excretion of sodium, on the other hand, is a more sensitive indicator of altered sodium balance.

In general, sodium excretion tends to reflect sodium intake and, on an average diet, urine sodium excretion will range between 80 and 180 mEq. per day. If sodium intake is reduced to less than 30 mEq. per day, urine excretion should fall below 15 mEq. per day. With adrenal insufficiency, however, there is inappropriate sodium excretion; and, alternatively, when adrenal aldosterone production is increased (as in shock, heart failure, or cirrhosis) sodium excretion is decreased.

The quickest method of determining sodium concentrations is with a flame photometer, using lithium as an internal standard. (See

Chapter 8.) The sodium of the blood is almost entirely in the plasma or serum fraction; the normal range for serum sodium is 135 to 147 mEq. per liter. Plasma sodium determination is preferred to eliminate platelet effects observed with serum (Whitfield, 1966).

POTASSIUM

On a normal average diet there is no deficiency of potassium, since this element is found in practically all foodstuffs. The adult takes in about 60 mEq. of potassium per 24 hours. Normally about 80 to 90 per cent of the potassium is excreted in the urine; the remainder is excreted in the feces and, to a small extent, in the sweat. In contrast to a fasting adult in whom sodium excretion will soon decrease, the excretion of potassium continues while the adult is fasting or on a diet adequate in calories but potassium free. About 50 to 60 mEq. of potassium are lost per day in the urine; this daily loss is more important in children. A reported normal range of urinary potassium excretion is 25 to 125 mEq. per day. The daily exchange of potassium in the adult is 1 to 2 per cent of the total body potassium content, whereas in a one year old child the exchange is 14 per cent of the total body potassium.

Potassium is the major cation found inside cells. The body content of potassium in the adult is 2.65 gm. per kg. (fat free) and 1.90 gm. per kg. in the newborn.

Recognition of Potassium Deficiency. Normal plasma potassium levels are commonly thought to lie between 3.8 and 5.0 mEq. per liter. Each individual's potassium concentration is constant, and almost all normal adults have plasma potassium values between 4.0 and 4.7 mEq. per liter. Values of 3.5 mEq. per liter are usually associated with potassium deficiency, not normality. Furthermore, retrospective studies have shown that the plasma potassium tends to fall 0.1 to 0.2 mEq. per day during the development of potassium deficiency. A falling trend is therefore indicative of potassium deficiency.

High Potassium. Levels above 5 mEq. per liter indicate hyperpotassemia but not necessarily excess total body potassium. When plasma levels rise above 6.5 mEq. per liter, cardiotoxicity may occur, and when levels reach 7.5 mEq. per liter cardiotoxicity is usually imminent.

Red Blood Cell Potassium, Hemolysis, and Plasma Potassium. On the average there are 90 mEq. of potassium per liter of red cells. Therefore, if blood with a 50 per cent hematocrit were hemolyzed, the potassium concentration would be about 45 mEq. per liter.

A unit of whole blood contains only 450 ml. of whole blood, or about 200 ml. of red cells. Thus, a unit of whole blood contains only 18 mEq. of potassium, and the potassium toxicity of hemolyzed blood has been greatly exaggerated.

When a blood specimen is visibly hemolyzed, the plasma hemoglobin concentration usually ranges between 100 and 200 mg. per 100 ml. A plasma hemoglobin of 200 mg. per 100 ml. would add about 0.5 mEq. of potassium per liter of plasma. Therefore, visible hemolysis will cause a false increase in plasma potassium levels.

The measurement of red blood cell potassium may be useful in the evaluation of potassium deficiency or potassium excess (Bugyi *et al.*, 1969).

Plasma Potassium and Blood pH. Plasma potassium rises about 0.6 mEq. per liter for each 0.1 unit fall in blood pH. If, for example, a patient had a pH of 7 and a plasma potassium of 4.5 mEq. per liter, the patient should be considered to have hypokalemia in spite of the normal plasma potassium. When the pH returns to normal (7.40), plasma potassium will be depressed about 2.4 mEq., going from the original level of 4.5 mEq. per liter to a new level of only 2.1 mEq. per liter. Such a patient should receive potassium before the plasma potassium falls. Another patient with a blood pH of 7 but a plasma potassium of 7 mEq. per liter should not receive potassium, because when the pH returns to normal the plasma potassium will fall to only about 4.6 mEq. per liter—a normal level.

Plasma vs. Serum. Potassium is released from leukocytes and platelets during clotting and retraction; therefore, serum potassium tends to be elevated with time. Plasma potassium, on the other hand, is stable. In patients with leukemia or thrombocythemia, serum potassium levels can be as much as 1 to 2 mEq. per liter too high 30 minutes after blood has clotted. Do not measure serum potassium; measure plasma potassium instead.

Urine Potassium and the Sodium: Potassium Ratio. The urinary excretion of potassium varies with diet but usually ranges between 40 and 80 mEq. per day. The usual ratio between urine sodium and urine potassium is about two parts sodium to one part potassium. With increased aldosterone excretion, however, the urinary sodium/potassium ratio may reverse itself. In Addison's disease, on the other hand, the sodium/potassium ratio will increase so that the urine may contain 10 parts sodium and only 1 part potassium.

Normal Values

Plasma: 3.8 to 5.0 mEq. per liter.

Urine: 40 to 80 mEq. per 24 hours (varies with diet).

Note. The plasma potassium concentration of infants is higher than that of children and adults. This difference usually disappears by three or four months of age.

Measurement. Potassium (like sodium) is best measured by emission flame photometry with lithium as an internal standard. (See Chapter 8.)

CALCIUM

The requirement for calcium varies from individual to individual and even in the same individual at various times. Factors that regulate the absorption and retention of calcium in normal individuals are: normal gastric acidity to allow for the absorption of soluble calcium salts, adequate supply of vitamin D to aid in absorption of calcium, normal fat digestion, a proper ratio of calcium and phosphorus in the diet, and a large enough intake to allow for precipitation of insoluble calcium salts in the intestine.

The urinary excretion of calcium accounts for 20 per cent of the calcium excreted and is influenced by the calcium intake, skeletal size, kidney regulation of anions and cations, and various endocrine factors. Approximately 80 per cent of the calcium excreted is via the feces as insoluble salts. An adult will be in calcium equilibrium when the intake is 10 mg. per kg. of body weight. An ample intake of calcium for an adult will be provided by two to three glasses of milk per day. Calcium is never completely absorbed from the gastrointestinal tract; calcium is also present in the gastrointestinal juices secreted into the gut. These juices contain 5 to 10 mg. of calcium per 100 ml. and therefore serve as an important factor in the reabsorption of calcium and in the adjustment of cell permeability. About 99 per cent of the body calcium is situated in the bones and teeth; the remainder is presumably present in the extracellular fluid and not within the cells. Small amounts of calcium are present within tissue cells outside the skeletal system. The body content of calcium in the adult is 20.1 gm. per kg. (fat free) and 9.2 gm. per kg. in the newborn.

All the calcium in the blood is present in the plasma. The normal range for total serum or plasma calcium is between 8.5 to 10.5 mg. per 100 ml. or 4.3 to 5.3 mEq. per liter. In infants, especially prematures, with adequate intake of vitamin D, the serum level of calcium may be as high as 12 to 13 mg. per 100 ml. The calcium present in serum is found in three major fractions: a portion bound to protein, a portion that is ionized, un-ionized complexes of calcium citrate, and so forth. (See Chapter 9.) Various formulas or nomograms have been described to calculate the ionized calcium. The best method, however, is the determination using an ion-specific electrode.

MAGNESIUM

The magnesium requirement during the growth period is less than 10 mg. per day. Magnesium is so widespread in foods that a magnesium deficiency is rarely seen in individuals who are partaking of their normal food intake. Approximately 60 per cent of the dietary magnesium is excreted via the feces and 40 per cent via the urine. Probably the same factors that control calcium absorption also govern the absorption of magnesium. The intermediary metabolism of magnesium resembles that of phosphorus; both are present in bone and within tissue cells. The body content of magnesium in the adult is 0.36 gm. per kg. (fat free) and 0.27 gm. per kg. in the newborn. Magnesium also governs neuromuscular irritability and is important for the coenzymes in the metabolism of carbohydrates and proteins.

Magnesium deficiency is known to occur in severe malabsorption states and after prolonged periods of intravenous therapy with magnesium-free solutions. Iatrogenic magnesium deficiency, however, is easily prevented by the routine use of solutions containing from 3 to 5 mEq. of magnesium per liter.

Excess magnesium acts as a sedative, and extreme excesses may cause cardiac arrest. Magnesium levels rise in uremia along with potassium.

The normal concentration is 1.6 to 2.1 mEq. per liter. The best method to determine magnesium (and total calcium) is by atomic absorption spectroscopy.

Anions

CHLORIDE

The urinary excretion of chloride suggests that most reported chloride requirements are too high. In the adult the daily exchange of chloride is about 2 to 7 per cent of the total body chloride, and in the child the daily turnover of chloride is about 4 per cent of the body content of chloride. Chloride losses usually follow those of sodium; however, the proportions will differ, since the loss of chloride can be compensated for by an increase of the serum bicarbonate. Such compensatory changes do not occur when sodium is lost and therefore there is loss of body water. Chloride losses will produce the same effects in intracellular and extracellular compartments as are seen with the loss of potassium. A deficiency of either chloride or potassium will lead to a deficit of the other.

Chloride plays an integral role in the buffering action when oxygen and carbon dioxide exchange in the erythrocytes – the "chloride shift." When blood is oxygenated, chloride travels from the red blood cells to the plasma, while bicarbonate leaves the plasma and enters the red blood cells. This shift in the ratio of cell chloride to plasma chloride also occurs when the blood becomes more alkaline; thus, venous blood will have a lower plasma chloride concentration in comparison to the oxygenated arterial blood. Water travels in the same direction as chloride; the erythrocytes become dehydrated when blood is oxygenated. Normal venous serum or plasma chloride concentration is 100 to 106 mEq. per liter in men and 102 to 108 mEq. per liter in women. By contrast the amount of chloride found within the cells may range up to about 25 mEq. per liter of cell water. The body content of chloride in the adult is 1.56 gm. per kg. (fat free) and 2.0 gm. per kg. in the newborn.

BICARBONATE

The concentration of bicarbonate in the blood plasma will vary with the pH according to the Henderson-Hasselbalch equation. Titration methods to determine bicarbonate are incorrect since they assume a normal pH to be present in the patient's blood; only if the titration is performed to have the endpoint at the actual pH of the patient's blood is the bicarbonate accurate. The total CO_2 content is essentially a measure of the bicarbonate (or combined CO_2) and of the dissolved CO_2 and carbonic acid (both comprising the free CO_2). Carbonic acid in the plasma represents the undissociated acid as well as the carbon dioxide dissolved in the plasma. The ratio of the dissolved carbon dioxide to the undissociated carbonic acid is about 700 to 1000:1.

In the past the bicarbonate concentration was reported in terms of the CO_2 combining capacity or combining power (Table 12–2). Many hospital laboratories list the term CO_2 to avoid confusion of the terms "carbon dioxide content," "carbon dioxide capacity," "carbon dioxide combining power," and "carbon dioxide combining capacity"; these terms do not have the same meaning. Since carbon dioxide, expressed as millimoles, represents the determination of bicarbonate, and 1 mEq. of bicarbonate will yield 1 mmol. of carbon dioxide, the two terms can be interchanged, so that CO_2 determinations are expressed as milliequivalents per liter or as millimoles per liter.

Table 12–2 compares the various CO_2 determinations and also lists the "CO_2" as determined by the Autoanalyzer technique. The original Autoanalyzer method was a true CO_2 combining power, with equilibration to P_{CO_2} of 40 mm. Hg but has been changed and erroneously called "CO_2 content." Determination of the CO_2 content is the technique to be preferred, since this represents the concentration of carbon dioxide in the blood at the partial pressure found in the patient's body. It is apparent that the closeness and overlap of values of the various CO_2 determinations have resulted in a mix-up of terms. The CO_2 content is the only determination which can be utilized in the Henderson-Hasselbalch equation.

True plasma is obtained by collecting blood anaerobically (syringe or Vacutainer), and if any equilibration or alteration in the partial pressure of carbon dioxide is necessary, the changes are made before the blood cells are separated from the plasma. Such true plasma will represent the buffering action of the plasma or serum and also of the red blood cells. By contrast, separated plasma is also obtained by anaerobic collection of the blood, but the blood cells are separated from the plasma before any equilibration or change in the partial pressure of CO_2 is made; such separated plasma will represent only the buffering action of the plasma or serum. A greater change in carbon dioxide concentration can be withstood by true plasma in comparison to separated plasma before any change in pH occurs. The CO_2 combining power is done on blood collected aerobically; if the cells are separated immediately after drawing, the CO_2 combining power will be the same as the CO_2 combining capacity – the longer the delay in separation, the greater the difference between the two.

The true bicarbonate of venous plasma is 24 to 28 mmol. per liter for men and 22 to 26 for women; however, the sum of chloride and bicarbonate will be the "same" in both sexes.

PHOSPHORUS

Phosphorus is present in practically all foods and is absorbed from the gastrointestinal tract more efficiently than calcium or magnesium. If the dietary intake of calcium from milk is sufficient to meet the minimum daily requirements, phosphorus requirements will also be satisfied. On an adult diet with less milk consumption, the intake of phosphorus usually exceeds that of calcium. About 10 to 20 per cent of the phosphorus is found in body tissues other than bone; it is the major anion found within the cells. Phosphorus of soft tissues seems to have priority over bone for necessary

Table 12–2. COMPARISON OF VARIOUS "CO_2" DETERMINATIONS*

FACTORS	CO_2 CONTENT (TOTAL) CO_2 CT	CO_2 CAPACITY (TOTAL) CO_2 CY	CO_2 COMBINING CAPACITY CO_2 CC	CO_2 COMBINING POWER CO_2 CP	CO_2 BY AUTO-ANALYZER† CO_2 A/A
Blood collection	Anaerobic	Anaerobic	Anaerobic	"Aerobic"	"Aerobic"
Type of plasma used	True	True	Separated	Separated	Separated
"CO_2" determined:					
Combined: $[HCO_3^-]$	Yes	Yes	Yes	Yes	Yes
Free: $[H_2CO_3]$ + [diss CO_2]	Yes	Yes	No	No	No
Equilibration with CO_2 gas to 40 mm. Hg‡	None	20° C.	20° C.; 37° C.	20° C.; 37° C.	None‖
Correction factors for free CO_2 (at 40 mm. Hg)	None§	None	−1.8‡; −1.2‡	−1.8‡; −1.2‡	None
"Normal" values:					
Arterial	25.2 (23–27)§	25.8 (24–28)	24.0 (22–26)	CP ≦ CC	(24–32)
Venous	27.0 (25–29)§	27.4 (25–29)	25.6 (24–28)	CP ≦ CC	

*Modified from Weisberg, H. F.: *Water, Electrolyte, and Acid-Base Balance.* 2nd ed. Baltimore, The Williams & Wilkins Company, 1962. Reproduced with permission of the publisher.

†Method does *not* employ plastic discs, etc., or alkalinization (Gambino).

‡Respective proportionality constants ("solubility") of CO_2 at 20° C. and 37° C. are 0.046 and 0.03 ml./mm. Hg.

§Result corrected to 37° C. Arterial P_{CO_2} at "40" and venous P_{CO_2} at "46" mm. Hg.

‖Original method (Skeggs) did equilibrate—CO_2 combining power.

If P_{CO_2} 40 mm.: $CT_a^{37°} = [CY^{20°} - 0.6] = [CC + 1.2] \geqq [CP + 1.2]$

$CT_v^{37°} = [CY^{20°} - 0.4] = [CC + 1.4] \geqq [CP + 1.4]$

If P_{CO_2} increased: CT > CC > CY ≷ CP. If P_{CO_2} decreased: CY > CC > CT ≷ CP.

metabolic processes. Of the phosphorus that is excreted from the body, about 40 per cent is excreted via the feces and 60 per cent via the urine. An average total of about 30 mEq. of phosphate calculated as phosphorus, or 0.93 gm., are excreted per day via the urine. Vitamin D has little effect on phosphorus absorption via the gastrointestinal tract; however, it does increase the rate of reabsorption via the renal tubules. Other factors affecting the urinary output of phosphorus (as for calcium) are intake, acid-base regulation, and endocrines.

The normal plasma phosphorus level is 1.7 to 2.4 mEq. per liter or 3 to 4 mg. per 100 ml. In children the level is higher, being 2.3 to 3.5 mEq. per liter or 4 to 6 mg. per 100 ml. The serum or plasma phosphorus is mainly in the form of inorganic phosphate. The serum phosphorus is high in hypoparathyroidism and low in hyperparathyroidism. In patients on prolonged milk and alkali intake the serum phosphorus may be normal or elevated, whereas the serum calcium is high. The phosphorus present within the cells is essentially present as organic combinations. It is the largest anion component found within the cells, about 80 mEq. per liter of cell water. The phosphorus content in the adult is about 11.6 gm. per kg. (fat free) and 5.4 gm. per kg. in the newborn.

Phosphorus is involved with calcium metabolism, but it is also related to the pituitary growth hormone. The serum level of phosphorus is elevated in children; this is presumably due to growth hormone activity. The serum phosphorus (in the absence of parathyroid or renal disease) is elevated in periods of active growth, as in children or in patients with excessive growth hormone activity (e.g., the active phases of gigantism or acromegaly). Conversely, the phosphorus level is decreased during active transfer of sugars from the blood to the cells. Glucose enters the cells as glucose-6-phosphoric acid, presumably in the form of the potassium salt of this strong acid.

This transfer of phosphorus with glucose has been shown to occur in the course of a glucose tolerance test. The phosphorus and potassium levels in the blood are virtual mirror images of the changing levels of glucose during the course of the tolerance test in a normal individual. In severe diabetes there is no drop of the phosphorus (and potassium) level correlating to the impaired passage of glucose into the cells. Minor impairment of the phosphorus change is seen in patients with relatively mild diabetes. The parenteral administration of hypertonic glucose with 40 units of regular insulin is of practical use in the temporary therapy of acute hyperkalemia if no vivodialysis apparatus is available.

SULFATE

The sulfate is usually expressed as inorganic sulfate (SO_4^{2-}); the concentration in the serum is 0.5 to 2 mg. per 100 ml. or 0.3 to 1.3 mEq. per liter. Since red cells contain sulfur-containing amino acids and proteins, the blood should be separated as soon as possible to avoid hemolysis; sulfate in whole blood is about twice that found in serum. The inorganic sulfate of the serum is increased early in renal insufficiency, even before other tests reveal any change in renal function. Increases have been noted in nephritis, 18 to 24 mg. of sulfate (SO_4^{2-}) per 100 ml. of serum. Any case of nitrogen retention in the blood is accompanied by an increase in the serum inorganic sulfate.

ORGANIC ACIDS

Ketone Bodies. The ketone bodies—betahydroxybutyric acid, acetoacetic acid, and acetone (Fig. 12–1)—are found in the blood in very low concentrations, namely, 2 to 4 mg. per 100 ml. or 0.2 to 0.4 mEq. per liter. Once the blood level exceeds 6 to 8 mg. per 100 ml. (0.6 to 0.8 mEq. per liter) expressed as acetone, the ketone bodies will be found in the urine. Under normal conditions the ketones present in the blood exert very little effect as part of the 6 mEq. per liter of organic acid anions. However, in diabetic acidosis, starvation acidosis, and other conditions, the greatly increased amounts of ketone bodies will depress the concentration of bicarbonate in the blood. In diabetes, elevations up to 300 to 400 mg. per 100 ml. may be seen. In normal urines up to 50 mg. per day are seen, while in diabetes 1 to 5 gm. per 100 ml. may be found; most of this is in the form of betahydroxybutyric acid. The test below may be used in distinguishing between true diabetic acidosis, in which the serum ketone bodies usually exceed 50 mg. per 100 ml. (5 mEq. per liter), and surgical conditions in the diabetic, in which the level rarely exceeds 20 mg. per 100 ml (2 mEq. per liter).

In conditions leading to moderate ketonemia, the quantity of ketone bodies excreted in the urine is only a small portion of the total ketone body production and utilization. Since there are renal threshold-like effects which vary between individuals, measurement of ketonemia, not ketonuria, is the preferred method of assessing the severity of ketosis.

The ketone bodies are themselves mildly toxic, tending to interfere with the excretion of uric acid and to produce mild central nervous system depression. More important, however, is their ability to ionize and to release hydrogen ions. Acidemia ensues as the H^+ (proton) load becomes more than the kidney tubules can handle, the plasma bicarbonate concentration falls, and the pH is depressed.

The relative proportions of the three ketone bodies in blood may differ; an average figure is 78 per cent betahydroxybutyric acid, 20 per cent acetoacetic acid, and 2 per cent acetone. The most commonly used methods for the determination of ketone bodies in serum or urine do not react with all ketone bodies.

Testing serially diluted plasma for ketones by simple "dip-sticks" gives a semiquantitative result (Dumm and Shipley, 1946). The last unquestionable positive dilution is the concentration in milliequivalents per liter (e.g., positive 1:7 and negative 1:8 equals 7 mEq. per liter).

Lactic Acid. The venous blood of normal individuals in a resting state usually contains 8 to 17 mg. of lactic acid per 100 ml. (or 0.9 to 1.9 mEq. per liter) of venous blood. Oliva

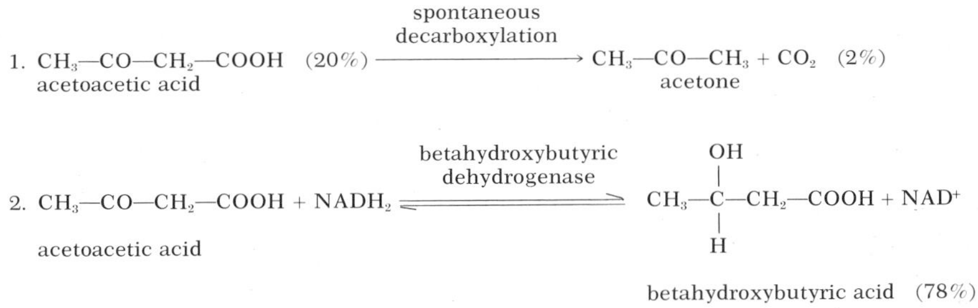

Figure 12–1. Acetoacetic acid builds up in the blood and is, in part, converted to acetone by spontaneous decarboxylation (1) and, in part, converted to betahydroxybutyric acid by betahydroxybutyric dehydrogenase (2).

(1970) has reviewed the physiologic factors influencing blood lactate levels. As the end-product of anaerobic glucose metabolism, lactate is formed by the reduction of pyruvic acid in the presence of $NADH_2$.

$$\underset{\text{pyruvic acid}}{CH_3\,\underset{\underset{O}{\|}}{C}\,COOH} + NADH_2 \rightleftharpoons \underset{\text{lactic acid}}{CH_3\,\underset{\underset{OH}{|}}{CH}\,COOH} + NAD$$

By the law of mass action, therefore:

$$(\text{lactate}) = (\text{pyruvate}) \times K\,\frac{(NADH_2)}{(NAD)}$$

Theoretically, then, an alteration in blood lactate concentration may be brought about in two ways: (1) by an alteration in pyruvate concentration; (2) by a change in the oxidation state of the tissues, which results in a change in the $(NADH_2)$:(NAD) ratio.

For example, the oral or intravenous administration of glucose will cause a rise in blood pyruvate, with a concomitant rise in blood lactate. Under these circumstances the lactate: pyruvate ratio remains constant and no "excess lactate" is produced.

Tissue hypoxia, on the other hand, will result in an increase in reduced $NADH_2$ and a consequent accumulation of lactic acid. The pyruvate level, under these conditions, remains constant, and the lactate produced is referred to as "excess lactate" (Huckabee, 1961). Although subject to certain theoretical objections (Oliva, 1970), this concept of excess lactate has proved to be useful clinically as a characteristic of conditions associated with tissue hypoxia.

In addition to these factors, lactate levels are influenced also by the rate of lactate utilization, principally in the liver. Experimental data suggest that normally the liver is able to take up all the lactate that is produced by extrahepatic tissues (Berry, 1967). With decreased hepatic blood flow, as in shock, the liver may instead contribute further to the increased lactate production.

In Oliva's review (1970), he divides the causes of lactic acidosis into two groups: those with and those without excess lactate production. Elevated lactate levels without excess lactate are seen in only a few clinical situations. The infusion of pyruvate or glucose will produce a small rise in lactate by elevating the blood pyruvate level. The infusion of bicarbonate produces a similar rise, but the mechanism is not known. Glycogen storage disease (glucose-6-phosphatase deficiency) is uniquely associated with a significant rise in both lactate and pyruvate, without any excess lactate.

Elevated lactate levels with an increase in excess lactate are much more important clinically. Physiologically, exercise causes a transient oxygen deficit and excess lactate production, although it is rarely, if ever, a cause of clinical lactic acidosis. In the clinical setting, the most important causes of excess lactate production, with consequent acidosis, are those associated with circulatory failure and shock: hemorrhage, gram-negative septicemia, and myocardial infarction or cardiac arrest. The degree of hyperlactatemia in such circumstances is thought by some to be of prognostic significance, those patients with higher levels having less chance of survival (Broder and Weil, 1964). Acute, severe hypoxemia may also result in lactic acidosis, although chronic hypoxemia, such as in chronic lung disease, does not.

Phenformin (DBI), an oral hypoglycemic agent, has been associated with lactic acidosis. This may be due to an impairment of aerobic glucose metabolism, with a consequent increase in anaerobic glucose utilization and lactate production.

Finally, a number of cases of "spontaneous" lactic acidosis have been reported (Huckabee, 1961). These patients, all of whom were already hospitalized for various reasons, developed hyperpnea, tachypnea, and stupor or coma without any fall in blood pressure or signs of poor peripheral perfusion. They are presumed to have had tissue hypoxia, although the reason could never be ascertained. Although survival could be prolonged for up to 13 days by the use of bicarbonate, the outcome was fatal in every case.

Lactate may be measured by either colorimetric or enzymatic methods. All these methods measure the lactate anion and thus represent the endogenous "lactic acid" which exists almost entirely as lactate anion at physiologic pH (Oliva, 1970). However, if exogenous lactate is administered in the form of sodium lactate, the laboratory procedure will determine the total lactate anion present, even though not all is due to the presence of lactic acid.

PROTEIN

Plasma proteins are usually considered as part of liver function, but it should not be forgotten that they function as anions, since at the pH of the blood the protein molecules (zwitterions) have a negative charge. The variations in plasma proteins do not have as great an effect on the concentration of bicarbonate as do the other anions. The amount of protein present in the blood will determine the amount of protein anions present; thus, the factor for conversion of protein to the electrolyte equivalent is grams of protein per 100 ml. times 2.43, which equals milliequivalents of proteinate per liter. The factor 2.43 is a good approximation of the equivalents of protein under normal conditions and normal pH. The isoelectric point of proteins varies and will affect the combining capacity of the carboxyl groups in the protein. Formulas 1, 2, and 3 give more accurate derivations for the milliequivalents of the protein fractions:

mEq. albumin/L. = (1)
0.125 (gm. alb./L.) (pH − 5.16)
mEq. globulin/L. = (2)
0.077 (gm. glob./L.) (pH − 4.89)
mEq. total protein/L. at pH 7.35 = (3)
(0.273 × gm. alb./L.) + (0.189 × gm. glob./L.).

Anion-Cation Electroneutrality

The original term "undetermined acids" was based on the sum of chloride and bicarbonate being subtracted from the sodium concentration (Hald *et al.*, 1947); the range of values was 0 to 8.5. Other names have since been used—undetermined anions, unmeasured anions, "R" fraction, organic acid accumulation, "lactic acid," anion gap, and electrolyte gap; potassium and/or calcium and magnesium have been added to the sodium cation, various "CO_2" tests have been substituted for bicarbonate, proteinate has been added to the anions, and the effect of pH on proteinate has been considered; and the reported normal ranges vary between −2 and +25. The usual electrolyte panel consists of sodium, potassium, chloride, and bicarbonate (i.e., "CO_2"). I prefer to utilize "total" anions and cations to check on the balance of electroneutrality, using the following formula:

$$[Na^+] + [K^+] + \text{"7"} :: [Cl^-] + [HCO_3^-] + \text{"25"} \quad (4)$$

If the sums are within 10 mEq. of each other, the anions and cations are in balance, considering the "assumed" values and the standard deviation inherent in each electrolyte determination; the value is reported as "cation balance" with normals of ±10. The value of "7" is based on assumed normal values for calcium and magnesium (Table 12–1), and the value of "25" is based on assumed normal values for sulfate, phosphate, organic acid anions, and proteinate (Table 12–1). The fact that the anion-cation balance is "normal" does not preclude abnormalities of the individual electrolytes. For example, a patient with hypopotassemic, hypochloremic alkalosis may have the following substitutions in Formula 4:

$$133 + 2 + \text{"7"} :: 82 + 32 + \text{"25"}$$
$$142 :: 139$$

The result is a normal "cation balance" of +3, yet the low chloride and especially the low potassium require institution of therapy by the physician.

If proteinate (the major portion of the assumed anions—16/25) is included in the calculation for "electroneutrality," the pH should be determined and Formula 4 is transformed to Formula 5:

$$[Na^+] + [K^+] + \text{"7"} :: [Cl^-] + [HCO_3^-] + [(pH - 5)\ TP] + \text{"9"} \quad (5)$$

The normal range can be reduced to ±5. The advantage of evaluating such anion-cation balance (Formula 4 or 5) is that the physician can be alerted to seek unsuspected causes of the abnormality (Table 12–3). A diabetic out of control may have the following substitutions in Formula 4 (normal ±10).

$$135 + 4 + \text{"7"} :: 95 + 10 + \text{"25"}$$
$$146 :: 130$$
$$\therefore \text{Cation balance} = +16$$

If the patient has a pH of 7.20 and a total protein of 5.5 gm./dl., Formula 5 (normal ±5) may be used.

Table 12–3. CAUSES FOR "CALCULATED IMBALANCE" OF ANION-CATION ELECTRONEUTRALITY*

- I. Calculated anions > cations
  - A. Lab "errors"
  - B. R_C^+ more than assumed "7"
    - 1. Hypercalcemia
    - 2. Hypermagnesemia
    - 3. Lithium toxicity
  - C. R_A- less than assumed "25"
    - 1. Proteinate ↓
      - a. Total protein ↓
      - b. A/G ratio ↓
      - c. pH ↓
- II. Calculated anions < cations
  - A. R_C^+ less than assumed "7"
    - 1. Hypocalcemia
    - 2. Hypomagnesemia
  - B. R_A- more than assumed "25"
    - 1. Proteinate ↑
      - a. Total protein ↑
      - b. A/G ratio ↑
      - c. pH ↑
    - 2. Sulfate and phosphate ↑
    - 3. Organic acid anions ↓
      - a. Ketones
      - b. Lactic acid
      - c. Citric acid
      - d. Unusual anions
        - (1) Protein metabolism (amino acids)
        - (2) Fat metabolism (fatty acids)
        - (3) Iatrogenic
        - (4) Toxicology

*Modified from Weisberg, H. F.: *Interpretation of Electrolyte and Acid-Base Imbalance.* 3rd ed. 2 Vols. 1971. (Mimeographed edition.)

135 + 4 + "7" :: 95 + 10 + [(7.20 − 5) 5.5] + 9
146 :: 126
∴ Cation balance = +20

Obviously, with either formula, the calculated cations are greater than the calculated anions. This can and should be expected by the physician, since ketones are increased in uncontrolled diabetes (see Table 12–3, II.B.3.a); the difference from normal is greater with Formula 5 since the proteinate is actually 12 (see Table 12–3, I.C.a and c) instead of the "assumed" 16 of the total "25."

OSMOLALITY

The physicochemical ("colligative") properties of solutions, e.g., osmotic pressure, vapor pressure, boiling point, and freezing point of the solvent, depend upon the *number* of particles in solution at a certain temperature, the nature of the particles being immaterial. Because one mole of a substance contains 6.023×10^{23} molecules, equimolecular concentrations of all substances which are present in solution in the molecular (undissociated) state exert the same osmotic pressure, and so forth. When one mole of nonelectrolyte is dissolved in 1 kg. of water, the osmotic pressure of the solution is *increased* 22.4 atm. (17,000 mm. Hg), the vapor pressure is *decreased* 0.3 mm. Hg (the vapor pressure of pure water is 17.5 mm. Hg at 20° C.), the boiling point is *increased* 0.52° C., and the freezing point is *decreased* 1.86° C.

An aqueous solution containing 180 gm. of glucose per liter of solution contains 1 mol. or 1 osmol. and has an *osmolarity* of 1. For more precise work in physical chemistry, *molal* solutions are used (e.g., 180 gm. of glucose or 1 osmol. dissolved in 1 kg. of solvent, e.g., water); such a solution has an *osmolality* of 1. More important for glucose is the fact that 180 gm. of glucose dissolved in 1 kg. of water (volume at 20° C. is about 1001.8 ml.) displaces water so that the final volume is about 1128 ml. The molarity of a solution (moles per liter of solution) will *vary* with the temperature because liquids expand and contract with changes in temperature; therefore, a specific temperature is inscribed, usually 20° C. The molality of a solution (moles per kilogram of solvent) and the mole fraction *do not vary* with temperature. The approved abbreviation for mole has been changed from M. to mol. and the *proper* abbreviations for osmole and milliosmole are osmol. and mosmol., respectively; older abbreviations were mosM. and mosm. for milliosmolar and milliosmolal, respectively, whereas mOsm. was the noncommitted type of abbreviation used by some authors.

As the solute concentration in an aqueous solution approaches 0, at 4° C. the molality and molarity approach each other. At the low solute concentrations and the relatively constant temperature occurring in body fluids, the difference between molar and molal concentrations is *negligible.* At room temperature the difference is only 0.18 per cent or an "error" of about 0.5 mosmol. for plasma determinations and about 2 mosmol. for normally concentrated urines; at 37° C. the "differences" would be about 1 mosmol. for plasma and 4 mosmol. for urine.

The theoretical concentration of the "electrolytes" in terms of milliosmoles is 288.5 per *liter of plasma* (Table 12–1), which becomes 308.8 when expressed per *liter (or kilogram) of plasma water.* Expressed as per liter of plasma water, the total electrolyte concentration is about 330 mEq., in contrast to 309 mosmol. per kg. (L.) of plasma water. The smaller total of the latter is due to lesser osmolar concentrations of multivalent ions (calcium, magnesium, phosphate, sulfate, some organic acids, and especially proteinate). *Actual* cryoscopic measurements with an osmometer yield values of about 285 mosmol. per kg. of plasma water (normal range 270 to 300). The discrepancy exists since osmolality is expressed in terms of the standard aqueous solution of pure sodium chloride, ignoring the interionic and other factors existing in the more complicated "solution" of plasma.

While the exact values for the intracellular osmole concentrations may vary, the *total will be equal* (317.2 mosmol. per kg. of water) to that of the interstitial compartment; but the intracellular and interstitial total is *less* than the intravascular value (318.7 mosmol. per kg. of plasma water). The respective concentrations are 285.5 and 286.8 when corrected for the "activity" of the electrolytes and other forces acting on the molecules and ions. The difference of 1.3 mosmol. in the corrected osmolality values is essentially due to the plasma proteins and accounts for the difference of 25 mm. Hg (the plasma colloid "oncotic" pressure). The "osmolality" is converted by Equation 6 into millimeters of mercury to express the "osmotic pressure."

$$\text{Osmotic pressure at 37° C.} = 19.3 \times (\text{mosmol./kg.})\ (\text{mm. Hg}) \quad (6)$$

Osmotic pressures can be obtained indirectly from concentration estimates using *conductivity meters* or *specific ion electrodes*; these techniques cannot be used to monitor osmotic pressures of solutions with more than one salt and/or significant amounts of nonelectrolytes. *"Membrane" osmometers* function on the basis of osmosis and are used primarily to determine number-average molecular weights in the range of 20,000 to 1,000,000, especially in polymer chemistry. In the *vapor pressure* method of osmometry, water vapor condenses on the sample, causing its temperature to rise; the measured change in the resistance of thermistors is directly proportional to the induced temperature change which, in turn, is directly proportional to the osmotic concentration. Calibration can be achieved with standards of saline, sucrose, or mannitol; measurements can be made at any convenient temperature, e.g., the plasma osmolality can be determined directly at 37° C.

Methods based on measuring the temperature effect (*cryoscopy* or *ebullioscopy osmometers* for freezing point or boiling point, respectively) are less sensitive than membrane osmometers; present instruments employ thermistors capable of detecting a change of ±0.001° C. Freezing point osmometers essentially monitor the temperature changes of a liquid sample while the solution is carried through a controlled freezing cycle. Since solvent crystallizes out during the freezing, the concentration of the solution changes. Therefore, prior calibration of the instrument is required, using standard solutions of known concentration of pure sodium chloride. Physiological solutions are relatively concentrated (plasma is about 0.15 molar concentration) and extrapolation to infinite dilution is often difficult or impossible to carry out with precision; but the measured results are correlated to much more complex (clinical) phenomena.

Simple substances such as sodium chloride have been described by the Debye-Hückel theory to have an activity less than their concentration. The *activity coefficient* for sodium chloride is 0.80 at 0.1 formal concentration, 0.90 at 0.01 formal, and 0.96 at 0.001 formal; only at *more dilute* solutions does the coefficient approach one. The presence of a "common ion" between two salts in a solution diminishes the dissociation. Thus, *osmolality is not necessarily a linear function of the amount of solutes*. The ionic activity of electrolytes (sodium, potassium, and chloride) in plasma is affected by the displacement of water by plasma proteins and by lipids. Plasma is not an "ideal" aqueous solution, and the sodium concentration is 0.14 to 0.15 formal. Thus, the activity coefficients in plasma are 0.75 to 0.80 for sodium, potassium, and chloride, and 0.50 for calcium.

True osmolality is a cardinal property of the solvent; it represents the effect of solutes on the vapor pressure of *any* solvent at *any* temperature. *Measured osmolality* is usually in terms of freezing-point depression because it is the most convenient, and *does* reflect changes in true osmolality. The *recorded osmolality* by cryoscopy determines changes in terms of *millidegrees* rather than milliosmoles, which would reflect the true osmolality only if the biologic specimens were pure watery solutions of sodium chloride. The *calculated osmolality* assumes that ideal conditions exist in the plasma or urine, with complete ionization, and so forth, and does *not* take into account the *unknown* solutes which are present in abnormal conditions.

The osmotic pressure exerted by the plasma nonelectrolytes can be neglected, except in cases of diabetes mellitus with *excess glucose* or uremia with *excess nonprotein nitrogenous* compounds. A normal blood glucose value of 100 mg. per 100 ml. equals 1 gm. per liter or 1/180 osmol., which equals 5.5 mosmol. per liter. However, a blood glucose concentration of 500 mg. per 100 ml. equals 27.5 mosmol. per liter. A normal serum urea nitrogen concentration of 15 mg. per 100 ml. equals 150 mg. per liter. Urea has a gram molecular weight of 60, of which only 28 is attributable to nitrogen ($NH_2CONH_2 = 2(14) + 4(1) + 1(12) + 1(16) = 60$). Thus, 0.15/28 osmol. equals 5.3 mosmol. per liter. If the serum urea nitrogen rises to 150 mg. per 100 ml. the concentration as mosmol. per liter would be 53.

Holmes (1962) utilizes a formula which considers the concentrations of urea nitrogen (UN) and blood glucose (BG) in milligrams per 100 ml. of plasma or serum.

$$\text{mosmol./kg.} = 1.86\ [Na^+] + \frac{BG}{18} + \frac{UN}{2.8} \quad (7)$$

Many variations of Formula 7 have been presented. A simplification that I use allows one to do the calculations mentally:

$$\text{mosmol./kg.} = 2\ [Na^+] + \frac{BG}{20} + \frac{UN}{3} \quad (8)$$

The calculated osmolality of plasma is usually *lower* than the determined osmolality, but the difference will vary with the particular formula used. Rubin *et al.* (1956) reported patients with various disease states in which the measured osmolality exceeded the calculated osmolality by 40 to 125 mosmol./kg.; 98 per cent of this group died within two weeks after the finding of the hyperosmolality. Mansberger *et al.* (1969) report this "difference" in osmolality or "osmolal discriminate" (mosm.-D) to return to normal in patients with hemorrhagic shock who survived, whereas in those who died the average difference persisted at about 29 mosmol. per kg.

Osmolal concentration is *not equivalent* to urine specific gravity, but in clinical circumstances, a *rough* approximation is 40 mosmol. for one "unit" of specific gravity; thus, specific gravity values of 1.010, 1.020, and 1.030 are roughly equivalent to 400, 800, and 1200 mosmol., respectively. Specific gravity and osmolality have been reported to have the following relationship.

$$\text{osmol./kg.} = 42.5 \pm 5\,(\text{Sp. Gr.} - 1.000) \quad (9)$$

Calculated values of urine osmolality are *higher* than the determined values, especially if the urines are alkaline; the solute "activities" are presumably less in alkaline urines in contrast to acid urines.

The volume of urine excreted per minute consists of the water required to excrete the urinary solutes as a solution isotonic with the plasma (osmolal clearance) and the excess of water (free water clearance) *per se.*

$$V = C_{osmol.} + C_{H_2O} \quad (10)$$

The formula of the *osmolal* (or osmolar) *clearance* ($C_{osmol.}$ or $C_{osm.}$) is similar to that of any urinary "clearance" formula:

$$C_{osmol.} = \frac{U_{osmol.}}{P_{osmol.}} V \quad (11)$$

The *free water clearance* (C_{H_2O}) is that amount of water excreted in the urine in *excess* of that needed to have the urine isosmotic with the plasma (U/P = 1). Substituting Equation 11 into Equation 10 results in Equation 12.

$$C_{H_2O} = V - C_{osmol.} = V\left[1 - \frac{U_{osmol.}}{P_{osmol.}}\right] \quad (12)$$

The free water clearance is a quantitative value of the diluting ability of the kidney (milliliters of *nonosmotically obligated* water excreted per minute).

In comparing healthy and diseased kidneys (e.g., right and left), the free water clearance should be factored by the nephron population of the appropriate kidney. Assuming that the glomerular filtration rate is directly proportional to the number of functioning nephrons in that kidney, one can obtain a percentage value of free water clearance per nephron for each kidney.

$$C_{H_2O}/\text{nephron} = \frac{C_{H_2O}}{GFR} \times 100 \quad (13)$$

When the urine is concentrated, the osmolal clearance (ml./min.) is greater than the urine volume (ml./min.), imparting a negative value to the free water clearance. Such a *"negative free water clearance"* can be regarded as the "medullary water reabsorption" during concentration or as the rate of "tubular water reabsorption" ($T^C_{H_2O}$) in excess of that which would result in urine isosmotic with plasma. The negative free water clearance is a quantitative value of the concentrating ability of the kidney (milliliters of nonosmotically obligated water *reabsorbed* per minute).

$$-C_{H_2O} = T^C_{H_2O} = C_{osmol.} - V = V\left[\frac{U_{osmol.}}{P_{osmol.}} - 1\right] \quad (14)$$

In moderate water diuresis C_{H_2O} may reach 10 to 15 ml./min. or up to 7 ml./m.^{2}/min. Under most conditions, $T^C_{H_2O}$ is about 1 ml./min., reaching a maximum rate of about 5 ml./min. with maximally concentrated urine during very high rates of solute excretion or up to 3.6 ml./m.^{2}/min. In maximally concentrated urines the $C_{osmol.}$ can reach about 6 ml./min. or up to 4.4 ml./m.^{2}/min.

The *U/P ratio* is a measure of how much of the filtered water has been removed in forming the final urine; for example, a high U/P creatinine ratio (e.g., 100) is seen in a concentrated urine, whereas a low U/P ratio (e.g., 5) is present in a dilute urine. The ratio of $U_{osmol.}/P_{osmol.}$ ranges from 0.2 to 4.7; in normal circumstances the ratio is above 1, whereas in intrinsic renal disease the ratio is about 1. After 14-hr. dehydration (overnight) the U/P osmolal ratio is above 3 in normal individuals. The U/P osmolal ratio is decreased in patients with severely impaired concentrating ability in whom the glomerular filtration rate is only slightly decreased; examples are medullary cystic disease, secondary amyloidosis of kidneys, hypercalcemia, potassium deficiency (except when caused by magnesium deficiency), and sickle cell anemia.

In familial nephrogenic diabetes insipidus, cystinosis, trauma to the head, and severe pyelonephritis, the U/P osmolal ratio is under 1. In diabetes insipidus the ratio will remain under 1 even with water deprivation, whereas in psychogenic diabetes insipidus the value will rise to 2 or 3 with water deprivation. In the inappropriate secretion of antidiuretic hormone syndrome, or ISADH, the plasma osmolality is decreased and the urine value increased, but the U/P ratio is still above 1. The classic features of the ISADH syndrome are hyponatremia, decreased plasma osmolality, U/P osmol. ratio above 1, high urinary sodium (>25 mEq./L.) not caused by renal or adrenal disease, absence of peripheral edema or dehydration, and a poor response to therapy with hypertonic saline. Such findings occur quite often in neurosurgical patients and as a manifestation of neurotoxicity of vincristine therapy of leukemia. Such "findings" may be seen as a complication of therapy with ethacrynic acid and furosemide diuretics.

In acute tubular necrosis the U/P osmol. ratio is equal to or less than 1; in contrast, acute oliguric failure due to glomerulonephritis is accompanied by a ratio greater than 1. In a study of circulatory shock with renal failure, urinary volume, urinary sodium concentration, and sodium clearance were unreliable indicators of the status of renal function, whereas the U/P osmol. ratio was a reliable prognosticator of renal injury at the time of shock; a ratio below 1.5 was presumptive evidence of progressive renal failure, whereas with a ratio above 1.5 the likelihood of pro-

Table 12–4. DIFFERENTIAL DIAGNOSIS OF OLIGURIA*†

	HYPOPERFUSION (Hypovolemic Kidney)	HYPERPERFUSION ("Conduit" Syndrome; Diffuse Nephron Disease)
Examples:	Shock	"Shock kidney"
	Congestive heart failure	Acute renal failure
	Hepatorenal syndrome	Acute tubular necrosis
	Nephrotic syndrome (especially with hypotension)	Chronic renal insufficiency (end stage)
	Acute glomerulonephritis	Severe transfusion reaction
	Acute urinary tract obstruction	Chronic urinary tract obstruction
FINDINGS:		
Urine sp. gr.	>1.020	<1.015
U/P ratio: Creatinine	>40	<15
Urea	>20	<5
Osmolal	>1.2	<1.1
Urine [Na] mEq./L.	<20	>30

*Modified from Weisberg, H. F.: *Osmolality*. ASCP Commission on Continuing Education Council on Clinical Chemistry, Check Sample CC-71, 1971.

†Most useful in absence of azotemia or urinary tract obstruction.

gressive renal failure was remote. Table 12–4 summarizes some reported laboratory findings to distinguish between the causes of oliguria.

The total solute output per day has a very definite relationship to the urine solute concentration and to the total urine volume. The usual adult intake of food results in an output of 1200 mosmol. of solutes. At normal concentrations of approximately 0.8 osmol. per liter as exemplified by urine with a specific gravity of 1.020, these solutes can be excreted in a daily urinary output of approximately 1500 ml. of fluid. Under fasting conditions the total output of solutes per day is 800 mosmol.; at a concentration seen in a specific gravity of 1.020 the amount of urine per day needed for such excretion will be 1000 ml. of fluid. The administration of 100 gm. of carbohydrate in the form of glucose to such fasting individuals will cut the solute load to 400 mosmol. per day and, under similar concentrations, will be excreted in a total volume of 500 ml. per day. The protein-free glomerular filtrate issuing from the proximal renal tubules has a solute concentration of approximately 0.3 osmol. per liter. This urine will have a specific gravity of about 1.008 to 1.010. The average maximal solute concentration in urine is 1.4 osmol. per liter, with a specific gravity of 1.035. Under these conditions a person with normal kidneys excreting 1200 mosmol. per day can, under average maximum urine concentration, excrete these solutes in approximately 750 ml. of fluid. The fasting patient with an excretion of 800 mosmol. per day who can concentrate maximally will accomplish this in a volume of 500 ml. of fluid. The fasting patient who is given 100 gm. of carbohydrate can excrete his 400-mosmol. load in a total volume of 250 ml. of fluid.

ACID-BASE EQUILIBRIUM

Acid-base balance can be described by the Henderson-Hasselbalch equation:

$$pH = pK + \log \frac{[\text{proton acceptor}]}{[\text{proton donor}]} \qquad (15)$$

The pK of an acid is measured at standardized conditions for dilute (ideal) aqueous solutions of the acid and its dissociated products (H^+ and anion$^-$). The cations of the blood are neither acid nor base; they are aprotic. The anions of the blood are potentional proton acceptors or conjugate bases, whereas carbonic acid and the blood organic acids are the proton donors. This scheme (based on Brønsted) is different from the old terminology in which the cations were called "bases" and the anions were called "acids." Although not intended to confuse the reader, Figure 12–2 shows the interrelationships of various terms that have been applied to different components of the plasma anions. Though *all* the anions are "conjugate bases" and can act as a base by accepting a proton, the "buffer" anions are the major buffers since their pK′ values are closer to the pH of blood (the pK′ values of the "fixed" anion systems are lower).

The blood pH is protected and controlled by the blood buffers – bicarbonate:carbonic acid system, hemoglobin, protein, and phosphate; of these the bicarbonate:carbonic acid system is the major buffer system, especially because of the action of the lungs in getting rid of carbon dioxide gas. Equation 15 can be rewritten to represent the system in the body:

$$pH = pK' + \log \frac{[HCO_3^-]}{[H_2CO_3]} \qquad (16)$$

The pK′ is the *apparent* acid constant, taking into consideration the activity of the hydrogen ion, the concentration of the acid, and the concentration of the conjugate base (anion). Thus, the pK for (molecular) carbonic acid in aqueous solution at 25° C. is 3.70, whereas the addition of CO_2 gas (and the hydration of CO_2 to carbonic acid) changes the pK to 6.35. The complete system in *plasma* at 37° C. has a pK′ of 6.10. pK by definition is the pH at which the concentration of proton donors (acid) over proton acceptors (base or salt) is equal. Therefore, it identifies the selection of a buffer in terms of optimal pH since buffers by definition function to resist a change in pH. Substituting values for arterial blood in Equation 16 results in the following data:

$$pH = 6.10 + \log \frac{24}{1.2}$$
$$= 6.10 + \log 20$$
$$= 6.10 + 1.30$$
$$= 7.40$$

The normal range of arterial blood is 7.35 to 7.45 (7.32 to 7.42 for venous blood); the pH range compatible with life is 6.80 to 7.80.

Figure 12–3 illustrates the fundamental chemical reactions involved in acid-base equilibrium. The metabolic activities of the tissues result in the formation of carbon dioxide and water, which are transferred to the interstitial fluid and intravascular fluid. A very small amount of free CO_2 is in equilibrium with its hydrated form $CO_2 \cdot H_2O$ or H_2CO_3; however, in the presence of carbonic anhydrase (C-A), within the membrane or cyto-

$[HCO_3^-]$ + $[Prot^-]$ + $[HPO_4^{2-}]$ + $[Cl^-]$ + $[SO_4^{2-}]$ + [Org. acids$^-$]

COMBINED CO_2
CO_2 combining capacity
CO_2 combining power

*Alkaline reserve**†
Available anion
Available "acid"
Gaseous "acid" (anion)
Volatile "acid" (anion)
"Base" bicarbonate

Fixed anions

Fixed (noncarbonic) "acids"
Nongaseous "acids" (anions)
Nonvolatile "acids" (anions)

$[HCO_3^-]$
Buffer base

[Buf⁻]
Nonbicarbonate buffer base

Alkaline reserve (Cummer)†
Labile anions
Buffer anions (also *Buf⁻*)
BUFFER BASE (B_B+) (B^-)‡
Equivalent to: Buffer cations
Body buffers (BB)

Fixed anions
Nonbuffer anions

TOTAL ANIONS§
Total "acids"

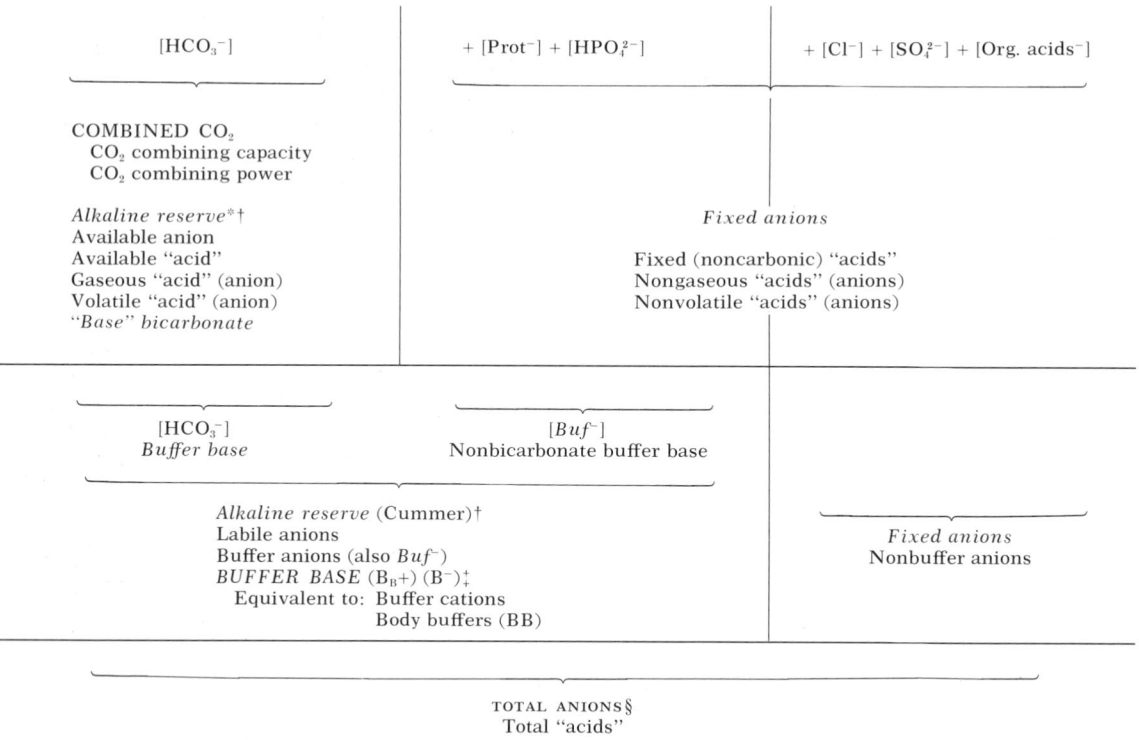

*Duplicated terms in italics.
†Additional "definitions" of *alkaline reserve:*
Total CO_2 content: combined CO_2 $[HCO_3^-]$ + free CO_2 $[H_2CO_3]$
CO_2 capacity: (combined CO_2 + free CO_2) at P_{CO_2} 40 mm. Hg
Portion of $[Na^+]$: *"base" bicarbonate* or bicarbonate-bound "base" or available alkali or available "base," or available cation.
Total cations or total "base" or fixed cations or fixed "base."
‡*Buffer base* of whole blood also includes buffer activity of hemoglobin, and so forth, of erythrocytes.
§Total anions minus those anions which have been determined equals RESIDUAL ANIONS or residual "acids."

Figure 12–2. Terms applied to various plasma anion fractions.

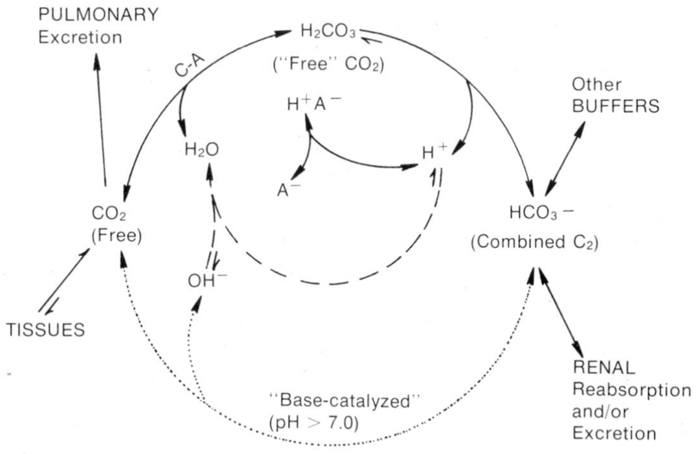

Figure 12–3. Fundamental chemical reactions in acid-base equilibrium.

plasm of the erythrocytes, the equilibrium is altered to favor the formation of carbonic acid (also a form of "free" CO_2). Carbonic acid does not exist as such but immediately dissociates into hydrogen ion and bicarbonate ion (combined CO_2). This bicarbonate ion is in equilibrium with bicarbonate derived from other buffer systems (Fig. 12–4), and the actual amount present in the blood is determined by renal reabsorption or excretion, and so forth. A very small amount of bicarbonate can be formed via the base-catalyzed reaction (CO_2 combines with OH^-) at the pH found within the body (Fig. 12–3). Even though the Henderson-Hasselbalch equation depicts carbonic acid as the denominator (Eq. 16), it is obvious from Figure 12–4 that the majority of hydrogen ions are derived from the organic acids (part of the fixed "non-buffer" anions). The 20:1 ratio for bicarbonate (combined CO_2) to carbonic acid (free CO_2, including CO_2 gas) is completely different from the 600,000:1 ratio of bicarbonate ion to hydrogen ion (Fig. 12–4).

Since it is not feasible to determine the

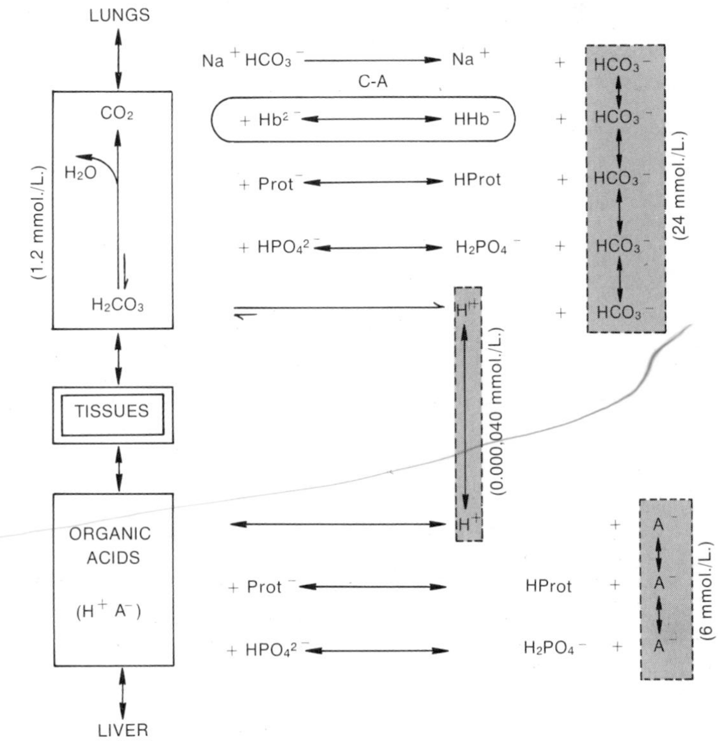

Figure 12–4. The role of three major "common ions" (shaded areas) in endogenous acid-base equilibrium.

"carbonic acid" concentration (which is in equilibrium with the tension or partial pressure of CO_2 gas) the denominator of Equation 16 can be replaced by the P_{CO_2} multiplied by the solubility coefficient. In a similar fashion the numerator can be expressed as the total CO_2 content less the "free" CO_2. Thus, Equation 16 can be rewritten as follows:

$$pH = 6.10 + \log \frac{\text{total } CO_2 \text{ CT} - (0.03 \times P_{CO_2})}{0.03 \times P_{CO_2}} \qquad (17)$$

With any two of the three unknowns, the third can be calculated or determined by special slide rules or it can be obtained from diagrams or nomograms.

Acid-base balance is described with a modified total CO_2 content-pH diagram (Fig. 12–5), based upon diagrams by Cullen and Jonas (1923) and Hastings *et al.* (1924–1925). It can be used for venous or arterial blood, has values for hydrogen ion concentration, and $[HCO_3^-]/[H_2CO_3]$ ratios corresponding to the pH values, and has the CO_2 isopleths (or isobars) in terms of P_{CO_2} and as carbonic acid. The carbon dioxide titration or buffer curve has a buffer slope (*in vitro*) of 28 slykes (assuming hemoglobin is 15 gm./100 ml.). My descriptive term for metabolic acid-base alterations is delta CO_2 content (ΔCT) as shown in Equation 18; normal values ±2.

$$\Delta CT = \left(\begin{matrix}\text{actual}\\ CO_2 \text{ content}\end{matrix}\right) - \left(\begin{matrix}\text{theoretical}\\ CO_2 \text{ content}\end{matrix}\right) \qquad (18)$$

The theoretical CO_2 content of arterial or venous blood can be determined from the intercept of the actual pH with the CO_2 buffer slope (Fig. 12–5) or from Equations 19 and 20:

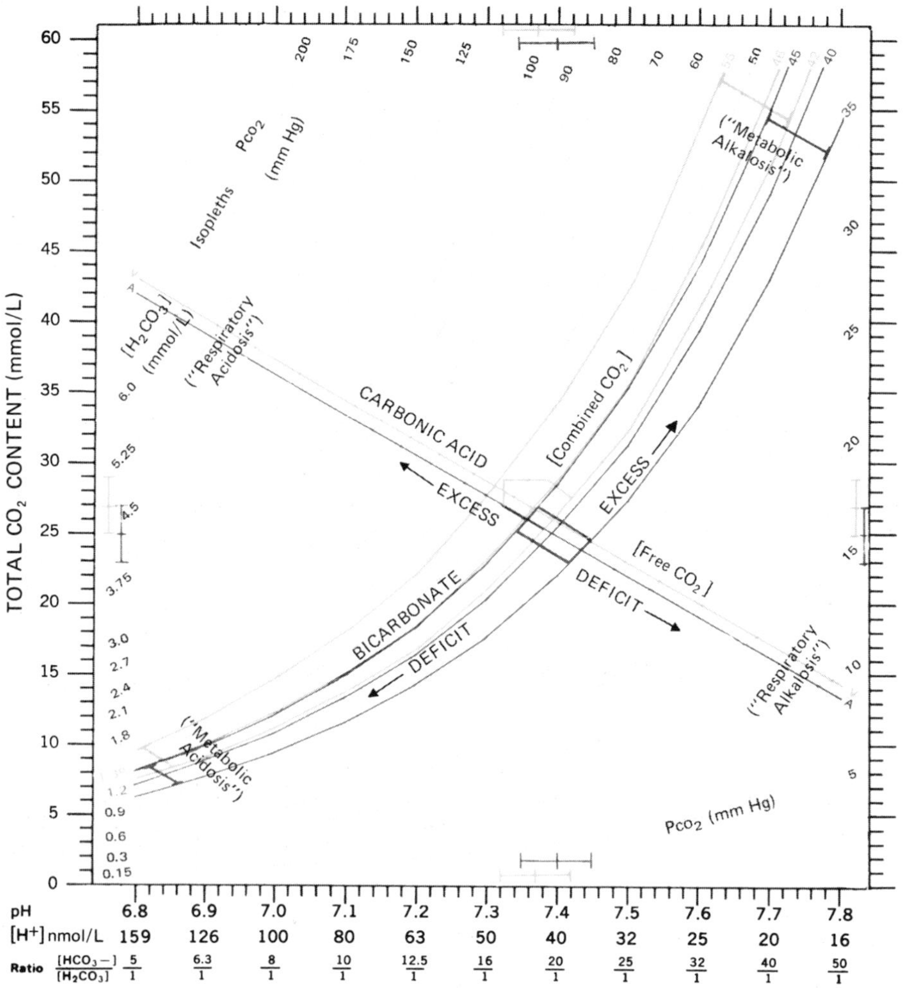

ACID-BASE EVALUATION DIAGRAM (1972)

Figure 12–5. Acid-base evaluation diagram.

$$\text{Theoretical } CO_2\ CT_a = 25 + 28\,(7.40 - pH) \quad (19)$$

$$\text{Theoretical } CO_2\ CT_v = 27 + 28\,(7.37 - pH) \quad (20)$$

A negative delta content signifies a bicarbonate (combined CO_2) deficit or metabolic acidosis and is equivalent to "base excess negative" or "base deficit" of Astrup *et al.* (1965); a positive ΔCT signifies bicarbonate excess or metabolic alkalosis and is equivalent to "base excess positive" or "base excess." Changes in the bicarbonate concentration may be substituted for the CO_2 content changes, but only when the P_{CO_2} value is normal.

Some authors state that the blood *in vivo* behaves as if it were diluted by the interstitial fluid into which bicarbonate, generated from blood carbon dioxide, diffuses. Thus, Severinghaus and Bradley (1969) use the one-third hemoglobin concentration for their calculations of the *in vivo* value for "base excess." Similarly, the delta content can be calculated on the basis of the extracellular fluid distribution (*in vivo*) by using Equations 21 and 22 to obtain the ECF theoretical value for substitution in Equation 18.

$$\text{Theoretical } ECF_{CO_2\ CT_a} = 25 + 12\,(7.40 - pH) \quad (21)$$

$$\text{Theoretical } ECF_{CO_2\ CT_v} = 27 + 12\,(7.37 - pH) \quad (22)$$

Such calculations can be avoided by use of Table 12–5, which gives various data correlated to pH values compatible with life; if necessary, the in-between value can be extrapolated.

Various volumes of distribution for water are used by different authors to calculate therapy for acid-base alterations; values of 40, 30, and 25 per cent volumes have been used. I use the following formula, based on an extracellular fluid value of 25 per cent; the answer is in milliliters of 1/6 molar solution for theoretical repair of the imbalance:

$$1.5 \times \text{kg.} \times \Delta CT = \text{ml. } 1/6 \text{ molar sol.} \quad (23)$$

If the answer is negative, bicarbonate deficit is present and should be treated with sodium lactate or bicarbonate, acetate, citrate, gluconate, and so forth, whereas a positive answer denotes bicarbonate excess, and ammonium chloride is used. The "base excess" value may be substituted for ΔCT. If 5 per cent sodium bicarbonate is used, the factor is 0.4 (instead of 1.5), and if 4.2 per cent sodium bicarbonate is used, the factor is 0.5; for 2.14 per cent ammonium chloride the factor is 0.6, whereas if a "gastric" solution is used (containing 70 mEq. of NH_4), the factor is 3.5. No matter what type of calculation, it is best to administer half the calculated volume and reevaluate the patient's condition before therapy is continued.

There is much confusion concerning use of the terms "acidosis" and "alkalosis." These terms had been reserved for the decrease or increase, respectively, of the alkaline reserve, but have also been used to represent a fall in pH (increased acidity) or a rise in pH (decreased acidity) of the blood. Others prefer to use the terms "acidemia" and "alkalemia" to represent the changes in blood pH, and use the terms "acidosis" and "alkalosis" to describe the overall physiological process or condition which tends to cause a deviation in pH without being dependent upon deviation of pH *per se*. A satisfactory compromise may be to use eu*pH*emia and eu*pH*uria to represent normal pH of blood and urine, respectively. A noted lexicographer (Schmidt, 1970) states that these terms "are compact, easily spelled, and easily pronounced." In a similar vein I propose the terms hypo*pH*emia to designate a decreased pH ("acidosis" and/or "acidemia") and hyper*pH*emia to represent an increased pH ("alkalosis" and/or "alkalemia").

In order to properly diagnose an acid-base imbalance one must know several bits of data. A pH determination will denote the presence of "eupHemia," "hypopHemia," or "hyperpHemia," and the determination of P_{CO_2} (or, multiplying P_{CO_2} by 0.03, "carbonic acid") will yield information concerning the respiratory component of the Henderson-Hasselbalch equation. Normal values (and ranges) of men and women for venous and arterial blood are given in Table 12–6. Lack of unanimity exists, however, regarding which test to use to determine the renal ("metabolic") component; various tests have been and are still being used.

The old term for measuring metabolic alterations was "alkaline reserve;" this was calculated by various tests. (See Figure 12–2.) I prefer to use *delta content* (ΔCT), utilizing Figure 12–5 or the Weisberg TRI-SLIDE™ calculator (data in Table 12–5); ΔCT and base excess have the "same" numerical and diagnostic values. *Base excess* is defined as the deviation of the buffer base from the "normal" buffer base; *buffer base* is the cation equivalent to the sum of buffer (or labile) anions—bicarbonate, proteinate, and phosphate in the plasma, and the oxyhemoglobin and other erythrocyte buffer anions. *Standard bicarbonate* is the concentration of bicarbonate in plasma separated from the cells, with the hemoglobin completely oxygenated at a P_{CO_2} of 40 mm. Hg at 38° C.; it is not influenced by the oxygen saturation of the original blood sample. Standard bicarbonate has recently been changed to *plasma bicarbonate at* P_{CO_2} *40*. In contrast to the standard bicarbonate, measured *in vitro*, the T_{40} *bicarbonate* has been introduced as the *in vivo* or extracellular fluid equivalent of the standard bicarbonate.

Table 12–5. VARIOUS DATA CORRELATED TO pH VALUES*
Theoretical values are from "normal" buffer slopes for carbon dioxide titration curves

pH	$[H^+]$ nmol./L.	Theoretical (*in vitro*) CO_2 CONTENT (mmol./L.) ART[a]	VEN[b]	Ratio: $[HCO_3^-]/[H_2CO_3]$	Theoretical (*in vivo*) $ECF_{CO_2\ CT}$ (mmol./L.) "Art"[c]	"Ven"[d]
7.80	15.9	13.8	15.0	50.0/1	20.2	21.8
7.78	16.6	14.4	15.5	47.9/1	20.4	22.1
7.76	17.4	14.9	16.1	45.7/1	20.7	22.3
7.74	18.2	15.5	16.6	43.6/1	20.9	22.6
7.72	19	16.0	17.2	41.6/1	21.2	22.8
7.70	20	16.6	17.8	40.0/1	21.4	23.0
7.68	21	17.2	18.3	38.0/1	21.6	23.3
7.66	22	17.7	18.9	36.3/1	21.9	23.5
7.64	23	18.3	19.4	34.7/1	22.1	23.8
7.62	24	18.8	20.0	33.1/1	22.4	24.0
7.60	25	19.4	20.6	31.6/1	22.6	24.2
7.58	26	20.0	21.1	30.2/1	22.8	24.5
7.56	28	20.5	21.7	28.8/1	23.1	24.7
7.54	29	21.1	22.2	27.5/1	23.3	25.0
7.52	30	21.6	22.8	26.3/1	23.6	25.2
7.50	32	22.2	23.4	25.1/1	23.8	25.4
7.48	33	22.8	23.9	24.0/1	24.0	25.7
7.46	35	23.3	24.5	22.9/1	24.3	25.9
7.44	36	23.9	25.0	21.9/1	24.5	26.2
7.42	38	24.4	25.6	20.9/1	24.8	26.4
7.40	40	25.0	26.2	20.0/1	25.0	26.6
7.38	42	25.6	26.7	19.0/1	25.2	26.9
7.36	44	26.1	27.3	18.2/1	25.5	27.1
7.34	46	26.7	27.8	17.4/1	25.7	27.4
7.32	48	27.2	28.4	16.6/1	26.0	27.6
7.30	50	27.8	29.0	15.8/1	26.2	27.8
7.28	53	28.4	29.5	15.2/1	26.4	28.1
7.26	55	28.9	30.1	14.4/1	26.7	28.3
7.24	58	29.5	30.6	13.8/1	26.9	28.6
7.22	60	30.0	31.2	13.2/1	27.2	28.8
7.20	63	30.6	31.8	12.6/1	27.4	29.0
7.18	66	31.2	32.3	12.0/1	27.6	29.3
7.16	70	31.7	32.9	11.5/1	27.9	29.5
7.14	73	32.3	33.4	11.0/1	28.1	29.8
7.12	76	32.8	34.0	10.5/1	28.4	30.0
7.10	80	33.4	34.6	10.0/1	28.6	30.2
7.08	83	34.0	35.1	9.5/1	28.8	30.5
7.06	87	34.5	35.7	9.1/1	29.1	30.7
7.04	91	35.1	36.2	8.7/1	29.3	31.0
7.02	96	35.6	36.8	8.3/1	29.6	31.2
7.00	100	36.2	37.4	8.0/1	29.8	31.4
6.98	105	36.8	37.9	7.6/1	30.0	31.7
6.96	110	37.3	38.5	7.3/1	30.3	31.9
6.94	115	37.9	39.0	6.9/1	30.5	32.2
6.92	120	38.4	39.6	6.6/1	30.8	32.4
6.90	126	39.0	40.2	6.3/1	31.0	32.6
6.88	132	39.6	40.7	6.0/1	31.2	32.9
6.86	138	40.1	41.3	5.8/1	31.5	33.1
6.84	145	40.7	41.8	5.5/1	31.7	33.4
6.82	152	41.2	42.4	5.3/1	32.0	33.6
6.80	159	41.8	43.0	5.0/1	32.2	33.8

*Based upon Weisberg TRI-SLIDE™ calculator for Henderson-Hasselbalch equation.
[a] Theoretical $CO_2\ CT_{art} = 25 + 28\ (7.40 - pH)$
[b] Theoretical $CO_2\ CT_{ven} = 27 + 28\ (7.37 - pH)$
[c] Theoretical $ECF_{CO_2\ CT_{art}} = 25 + 12\ (7.40 - pH)$
[d] Theoretical $ECF_{CO_2\ CT_{ven}} = 27 + 12\ (7.37 - pH)$

Table 12–6. NORMAL VALUES (AND RANGES) FOR ARTERIAL AND VENOUS BLOOD OF VARIOUS TESTS USED IN THE DIAGNOSIS OF IMBALANCE OF ACID-BASE AND BLOOD GASES

		VENOUS		ARTERIAL	
		Male	Female	Male	Female
pH		7.36 (7.31–7.41)	7.37 (7.32–7.42)	7.39 (7.34–7.44)	7.40 (7.35–7.45)
P_{CO_2}	mm. Hg	46 (42–55)	43 (39–52)	40 (35–45)	37 (32–42)
$[H_2CO_3]$	mmol./L.	1.38 (1.26–1.65)	1.29 (1.17–1.56)	1.20 (1.05–1.35)	1.11 (0.96–1.26)
$[HCO_3^-]$	mEq./L.	26 (24–28)	24 (22–26)	24 (22–26)	22 (20–24)
CO_2 CT	mmol./L.	27.4 (25–29)	25.3 (23–27)	25.2 (23–27)	23.1 (21–25)
ΔCT	mmol./L.	−2 to +2			
Base excess	mmol./L.			0 (−2.4 to +2.3)	−1 (−3.3 to +1.2)
Buffer base	mmol./L.			49 (46–52) Blood 43 (40–46) Plasma	
Standard bicarbonate	mEq./L.			24 (22–26)	
CO_2 capacity	mEq./L.	27.4 (25–29)		25.8 (24–28)	
P_{O_2}	mm. Hg	40 (30–50)		95 (75–100)	
O_2 saturation	%	75 (60–85)		97.5 (95–98)	

Bicarbonate Deficit

Other names for bicarbonate deficit are metabolic acidosis (or acidemia), primary alkali deficit, uncompensated alkali deficit, nonrespiratory acidosis (or acidemia), and "addition" (of acid salts) acidosis; it may be caused by excess production of organic acids (proton donors), administration of acidifying salts (proton donors), excess loss of bicarbonate (with cations), displacement of bicarbonate (by retained anions), and "dilution" acidosis. Examples of such alterations are given in Table 12–7.

For example, a 60-kg. woman with a history of diabetes enters the hospital with a CO_2 content of 10 mEq. per liter and a venous pH of 7.20. Plotting these two values on Figure 12–5 will yield a P_{CO_2} value of about 25 mm. Hg (or a carbonic acid concentration of 0.75 mmol. per liter). Subtracting 0.75 from 10 gives a true bicarbonate value of 9.25 mEq. per liter. The decreased P_{CO_2} (from 46 to 25) shows that partial compensation (hyperventilation as response to the low pH) has occurred (to line I in Figure 12–6); if no compensation had occurred, the P_{CO_2} would have been within the normal venous limits, e.g., P_{CO_2} 46 mm. Hg with pH 7.06 and CO_2 content 13.5 mmol. per liter. Reference to Table 12–5 gives a theoretical venous CO_2 content of 31.8 mmol. per liter for a pH of 7.20; substitution in Equation 20 gives the same theoretical value. Substituting values in Equation 18 gives

$$\Delta CT = 10 - 31.8 = -21.8$$

and substitution in Equation 23 gives

$$1.5 \times 60 \times (-21.8) = -1962 \text{ ml.}$$

as the volume of 1/6 molar solution of sodium bicarbonate, lactate, and so forth. If 5 per cent sodium bicarbonate were to be used in therapy, the theoretical volume would be 523 ml.:

$$0.4 \times 60 \times (-21.8) = -523$$

Neither calculated volume should be given; administration of such amounts of "conjugate base" would neutralize enough hydrogen ion so that the pH (assuming no change in P_{CO_2}) would become 7.55! Therefore, only half the calculated volumes should be given and the patient reevaluated in several hours.

Therapy should be directed toward the patient and not the numbers obtained from the laboratory. For example, suppose that the same patient is able to hyperventilate to about 13 mm. Hg with pH of 7.30 and CO_2 content of 7 mmol. per liter (again assuming no renal compensation). The theoretical content at 7.30 for venous blood is 29 (Table 12–5) and therefore the ΔCT is −22 (Formula 23). If therapy is directed to treat the ("same") $-\Delta CT$ while the pH is practically normal, the theoretical new pH value achieved would be about 7.72! Thus, the actual pH value takes precedence over the ΔCT (or base excess).

Table 12–7. CONDITIONS LEADING TO BICARBONATE (COMBINED CO_2) DEFICIT OR METABOLIC ACIDOSIS*

A. Excess production of organic acids (proton donors)
  1. Endocrine disorders
  2. Disturbances in food intake
  3. Impairment of liver function
  4. Violent exercise or convulsions
  5. Hypoxia (lactic acid acidosis)
  6. Shock
  7. Extracorporeal circulation
  8. Insulin hypoglycemia
  9. Fanconi syndrome
  10. Toxicology
    a. Salicylate intoxication (late stages)
    b. Methyl alcohol poisoning
    c. Ethylene glycol intoxication

B. Administration or absorption of acidifying salts (proton donors)
  1. Ammonium chloride
  2. Hydrochloric acid
  3. L-Lysine monohydrochloride
  4. Calcium chloride (oral)
  5. Ammonium mandelate
  6. Ureterosigmoidostomy

C. Excess loss of bicarbonate (with cations)
  1. Diarrhea
  2. Addison's disease
  3. Intestinal, pancreatic, or biliary drainage or fistula
  4. Renal tubular insufficiency
  5. Inhibition of carbonic anhydrase

D. Displacement of bicarbonate (by retained anions)

E. "Dilution" (or "expansion") acidosis

*Modified from Weisberg, H. F.: *Water, Electrolyte, and Acid-Base Balance.* 2nd ed. Baltimore, The Williams & Wilkins Company, 1962. Reproduced with permission of the publisher.

Carbonic Acid Excess

Synonyms used for carbonic acid excess are respiratory acidosis (or acidemia), primary carbon dioxide excess, uncompensated carbon dioxide excess, gaseous acidosis (or acidemia), nonmetabolic acidosis (or acidemia), hypoventilation, hypercapnia, and hypercarbia; it may be caused by groups of various diseases, listed in Table 12–8. An acute retention of carbon dioxide will result in increased P_{CO_2} values (of both arterial and venous blood),

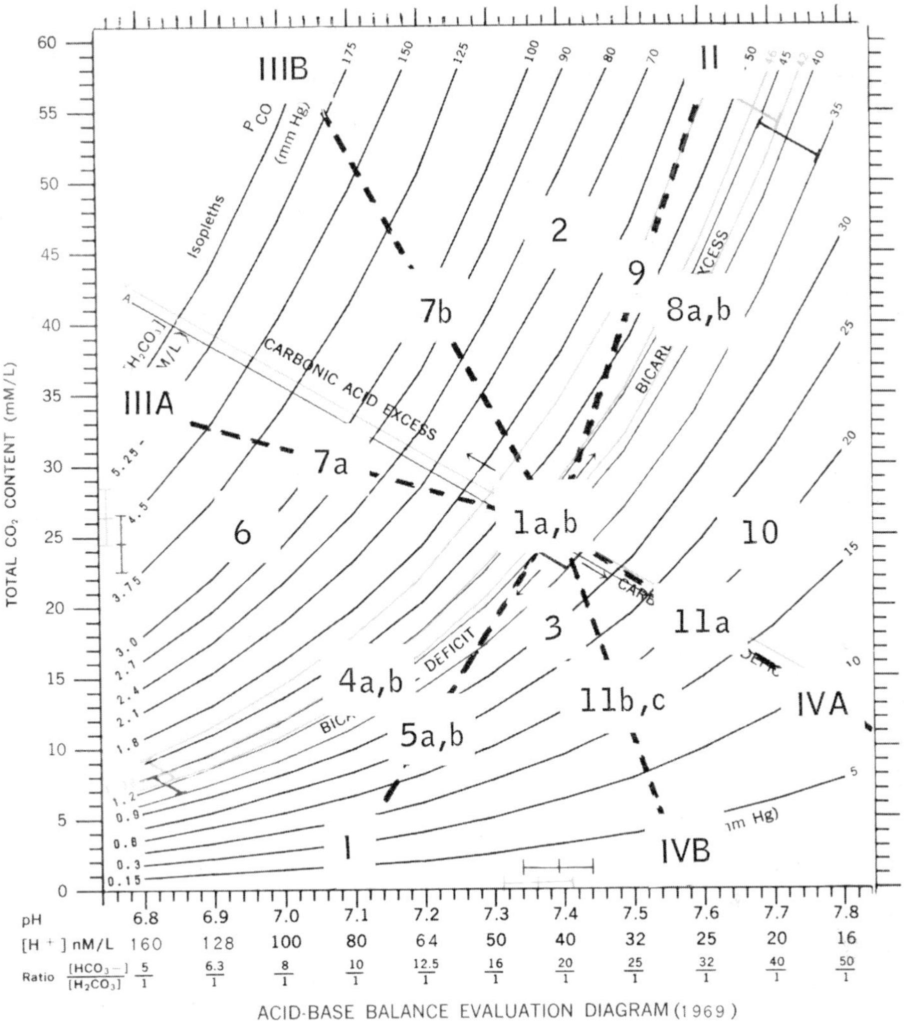

Figure 12–6. Acid-base diagram showing average compensation (dashed lines marked with Roman numerals). I, partially compensated metabolic acidosis; II, partially compensated metabolic alkalosis; IIIA, carbon dioxide titration curve of acute respiratory acidosis; IIIB, chronic respiratory acidosis; IVA, acute respiratory alkalosis; and IVB, chronic respiratory alkalosis. Areas with arabic numbers are explained in Table 12–11.

but the buffering of the carbon dioxide will not be along the *in vitro* slope (Fig. 12–5); but, as discussed previously, the entire extracellular fluid rather than only the intravascular fluid acts as the *in vivo* buffer and therefore will follow the slope of line IIIA in Figure 12–6.

With chronic carbonic acid excess (increased P_{CO_2}), renal reabsorption of bicarbonate is increased; in addition, there is an increased excretion of hydrogen ion by the kidneys. A patient with chronic emphysema may have an arterial carbon dioxide content of 35 mEq. per liter, pH of 7.30, and P_{CO_2} of 70 mm. Hg. Inspection of Figure 12–4 and Table 12–5 gives a theoretical content of 27.8 for arterial blood and, thus, the ΔCT is $35 - 27.8 = +7.2$ mmol. per liter. Respiratory disorders are treated primarily by directing therapy to the underlying disease process. Calculations to treat the positive ΔCT (or the positive base excess) would be contraindicated; similarly, trying to elevate the pH to normal levels with sodium bicarbonate would increase the amount of carbon dioxide (neutralization of hydrogen by bicarbonate will produce carbon dioxide and water) and thus put a greater demand on the already compromised pulmonary function of the patient. Figure 12–7 summarizes the pathophysiology and the differential diagnosis of the two types of acidosis (hypopHemia).

Table 12–8. CONDITIONS LEADING TO CARBONIC ACID (FREE CO_2) EXCESS OR RESPIRATORY ACIDOSIS*

A. Primary hypoventilation syndrome (respiratory center disease)

B. Respiratory center depression
   1. Alcohol
   2. Barbiturates
   3. Carbon dioxide
   4. Morphine
   5. Surgical anesthesia

C. Asphyxia

D. Pulmonary disease, e.g., alveolar hypoventilation, emphysema, COAD (chronic obstructive airway disease)

E. Cardiopulmonary syndrome of obesity

F. Cardiac disease

G. Musculoskeletal disease

H. Neuromuscular disease

*Modified from Weisberg, H. F.: *Water, Electrolyte, and Acid-Base Balance.* 2nd ed. Baltimore, The Williams & Wilkins Company, 1962. Reproduced with permission of the publisher.

Bicarbonate Excess

Synonyms for bicarbonate excess are metabolic alkalosis (or alkalemia), primary alkali excess, uncompensated alkali excess, and nonrespiratory alkalosis (or alkalemia); it may be caused by excess loss of hydrogen ion (with anions), administration of "alkaline" salts (proton acceptors), body deficit of potassium, increased reabsorption of bicarbonate (with sodium), "contraction" alkalosis, and x-ray, ultraviolet, or radium therapy. Examples of such alterations are given in Table 12–9.

Let us analyze the data of a patient with severe duodenal obstruction: sodium 135, potassium 3, chloride 50, CO_2 content 45, total protein 8, and pH 7.50. Substituting in Formula 5 gives the following cation balance.

$$135 + 3 + \text{“7”} :: 50 + 45 + [(7.50 - 5)\ 8] + \text{“9”}$$
$$145 :: 104 + (2.5 \times 8)$$
$$145 :: 124$$
$$\therefore \text{Cation balance} = +21$$

Instead of the unmeasured anions being 9, the "extra" cations (or anion "deficit") were due to the presence of 5 mEq. per liter of phosphate and sulfate and 16 mEq. per liter of ketone anions (and other organic acid anions). Despite

Condition	HypopHemia (blood pH *decreased*)	
Differential diagnosis	BICARBONATE DEFICIT ↓	CARBONIC ACID EXCESS ↓
Blood changes		
$[HCO_3^-]$	Decreased	Normal
Pco_2	Normal	Increased
$[H_2CO_3]$ (= 0.03 Pco_2)	Normal	Increased
pH	As $[HCO_3^-]/[H_2CO_3]$ ratio decreases, blood pH decreases	
COMPENSATORY MECHANISMS		
Primary	*Respiratory* (decrease of Pco_2) Low pH: Hyperventilation	*Renal* (increase of serum $[HCO_3^-]$) HCO_3^- reabsorption: Increased H^+ excretion: Increased NH_4^+ formation and excretion: Increased Titratable acidity: Increased Cation reabsorption: Increased
Secondary	*Renal* (increase of serum $[HCO_3^-]$) H^+ excretion: Increased NH_4^+ formation and excretion: Increased Titratable acidity: Increased Cation reabsorption: Increased HCO_3^- formation and reabsorption: Increased	*Respiratory* (decrease of Pco_2) Low pH: Hyperventilation High Pco_2: Hyperventilation
CO_2 Content	Decreased	"Increased"
Final result	As $[COH_3^-]/[H_2CO_3]$ ratio approaches normal 20/1 of arterial blood, pH approaches normal 7.4.	

Figure 12–7. Pathophysiology and differential diagnosis of hypopHemia (acidosis). Modified from Weisberg, H. F.: *Water, Electrolyte, and Acid-Base Balance.* 2nd ed. Baltimore, The Williams & Wilkins Company, 1962. Reproduced with permission of the publisher.

Table 12–9. CONDITIONS LEADING TO BICARBONATE (COMBINED CO_2) EXCESS OR METABOLIC ALKALOSIS*

A. Excess loss of hydrogen ion (with anions)
  1. Vomiting
  2. Gastric suction or lavage
  3. Diarrhea of pancreatic fibrosis
  4. Potassium deficit (see below)
  5. Therapy with diuretics
  6. Loss of less permeant anions
    a. Infusions or administration of sulfate, phosphate, nitrate, etc.
    b. Posthypercapnic (in presence of low chloride)
  7. Chloride depletion

B. Administration of "alkaline" salts (proton acceptors)

C. Body deficit of potassium
  1. Poor intake and/or absorption
  2. Loss of GI secretions
  3. Increased renal excretion
  4. Extensive burns
  5. Iatrogenic
    a. I.V. therapy without potassium
    b. Excess steroids
    c. Diuretics
    d. Laxatives and/or enemas

D. Increased reabsorption of bicarbonate (with sodium)
  1. ECF volume depletion
  2. Edema

E. "Contraction" alkalosis

F. X-ray, ultraviolet, or radium therapy ("acute radiation syndrome")

*Modified from Weisberg, H. F.: *Water, Electrolyte, and Acid-Base Balance.* 2nd ed. Baltimore, The Williams & Wilkins Company, 1962. Reproduced with permission of the publisher.

the increased keto- and organic acids (only the anions are increased since their accompanying hydrogen ions have been neutralized by the blood buffers), the pH is on the alkaline side because the ratio of bicarbonate to carbonic acid is increased!

Plotting the content of 45 and pH of 7.50 on Figure 12–4 gives a Pco_2 of approximately 57 mm. Hg (or $57 \times 0.03 = 1.71$ mmol. of carbonic acid); the actual bicarbonate, therefore, is $45 - 1.7 = 43.3$ mEq. per liter. From Table 12–5 the theoretical CO_2 content is 23.4, so that the $\Delta CT = 45 - 23.4 = +21.6$ mmol. per liter. This can be utilized in calculating the theoretical amount of ammonium chloride needed for acute reversal of the alkaline pH, again remembering the precautions of administering half the volume and later reevaluating the patient. This patient, exhibiting hypochloremic, hypopotassemic alkalosis, should be treated with potassium chloride (in addition to daily electrolyte needs).

Carbonic Acid Deficit

Synonyms for carbonic acid deficit are respiratory alkalosis (or alkalemia), primary carbon dioxide deficit, uncompensated carbon dioxide deficit, gaseous alkalosis (or alkalemia), nonmetabolic acidosis (or alkalemia), hyperventilation, hypocapnia, and hypocarbia. Examples of such alterations are given in Table 12–10.

A two year old child is admitted to the hospital because of severe hyperpnea, acetone aroma to breath, and a fever of 41° C. (106° F.). An electrolyte study reveals sodium 136, potassium 4, chloride 100, and carbon dioxide content 12; the "total" cations (136 + 4 + "7") equal 147 and the "total" anions (100 + 12 + "25") equal 137. The urine is found to contain a trace of sugar and moderately positive ketone bodies. The findings of hyperventilation, low carbon dioxide, glycosuria, and ketonuria can easily lead the physician to a diagnosis of diabetic acidosis. Therapy with insulin is contraindicated until a more definitive diagnosis can be made; in any child presenting with such signs and symptoms, the possibility of salicylate intoxication must be excluded. The whole blood pH is reported as 7.60, and a plasma salicylate is 60 mg. per 100 ml. Thus, the correct diagnosis is respiratory alkalosis owing to salicylate intoxication, which causes hyperpnea by stimulation of the respiratory center; the glycosuria and ketonuria are the result of depletion of liver glycogen by salicylates (uncoupling of oxidative phosphorylation, which also leads to the hyperpyrexia). At a later stage of salicylate intoxication there may be a shift

Table 12–10. CONDITIONS LEADING TO CARBONIC ACID (FREE CO_2) DEFICIT OR RESPIRATORY ALKALOSIS*

A. Respiratory center stimulation
  1. CNS disease
  2. Acidosis of respiratory center or surrounding CSF
  3. Drug toxicity
    a. Salicylate (early stages)
    b. Sulfanilamide (early stages)
    c. Quinine
  4. Hypoxia
  5. Fever
  6. High room and/or ambient temperature

B. "Hyperventilation syndrome"

C. Hepatic insufficiency and/or coma

D. Gram-negative bacteremia

*Modified from Weisberg, H. F.: *Water, Electrolyte, and Acid-Base Balance.* 2nd ed. Baltimore, The Williams & Wilkins Company, 1962. Reproduced with permission of the publisher.

of blood pH to the acid side (due to excess production and dissociation of lactic acid), which would complicate a differential diagnosis of diabetes and salicylism.

The greater amount of ketonuria, in contrast to the glycosuria, occurs in carbohydrate starvation, excess insulin (Somogyi effect), phenothiazine intoxication, and salicylate intoxication. The hyperpyrexia is an important factor in the morbidity of salicylism. In addition, the abnormal body temperature of the child will give rise to a spurious pH (as determined at 37° C.). Formula 24 gives the temperature correction for pH when measured in whole blood (WB).

$$\text{Corrected } pH_{WB} = pH_{37^\circ C.} - 0.0147\,(\text{Pt.} - 37^\circ\text{ C.}) \quad (24)$$

Thus, the pH of the child with fever was actually less than reported:

$$= 7.60 - 0.0147\,(41 - 37)$$

$$= 7.60 - 0.0688 = 7.53$$

Instead of the factor 0.0147 for whole blood, the factors for plasma and cerebrospinal fluid are 0.011 and 0.003, respectively. For practical purposes, for a patient who has a temperature of 36 to 38° C. (97 to 100° F.) no corrections are indicated. Corrections are necessary for P_{CO_2} and P_{O_2} when the patient's temperature is not near the 37° C. at which the instruments are used; nomograms are available for easy use (Greenburg and Moulder, 1965; Siggaard-Andersen, 1966; Severinghaus, 1965).

Figure 12–8 compares the pathophysiology and differential diagnosis of alkalosis.

Other Schemes

The acid-base evaluation diagram presented is only one of the more than 95 diagrams that have been developed in the past 60 years. The Davenport bicarbonate-pH diagram is very closely related to my modification. The log P_{CO_2}-pH nomogram of Astrup and Siggaard-Andersen is very popular; others that have their adherents are the P_{CO_2}-bicarbonate (Austin, 1965) and the Kintner nomogram.

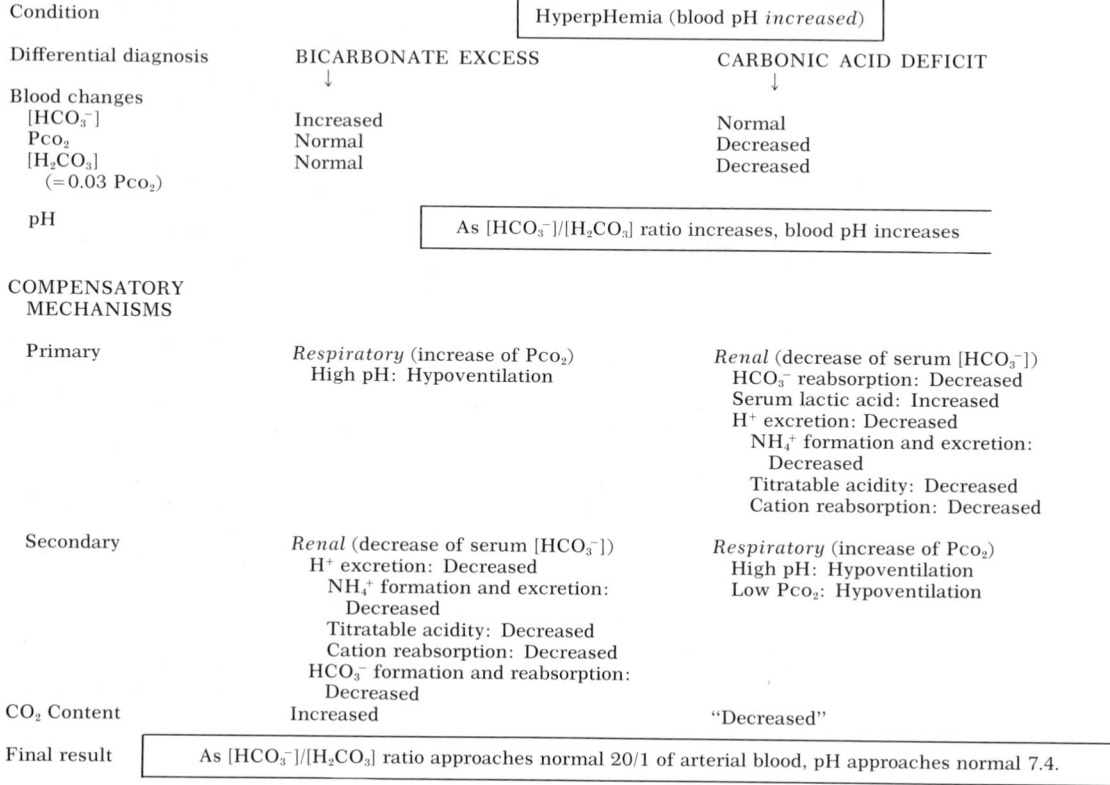

Condition	HyperpHemia (blood pH *increased*)	
Differential diagnosis	BICARBONATE EXCESS ↓	CARBONIC ACID DEFICIT ↓
Blood changes		
$[HCO_3^-]$	Increased	Normal
P_{CO_2}	Normal	Decreased
$[H_2CO_3]$ $(=0.03\ P_{CO_2})$	Normal	Decreased
pH	As $[HCO_3^-]/[H_2CO_3]$ ratio increases, blood pH increases	
COMPENSATORY MECHANISMS		
Primary	*Respiratory* (increase of P_{CO_2}) High pH: Hypoventilation	*Renal* (decrease of serum $[HCO_3^-]$) HCO_3^- reabsorption: Decreased Serum lactic acid: Increased H^+ excretion: Decreased NH_4^+ formation and excretion: Decreased Titratable acidity: Decreased Cation reabsorption: Decreased
Secondary	*Renal* (decrease of serum $[HCO_3^-]$) H^+ excretion: Decreased NH_4^+ formation and excretion: Decreased Titratable acidity: Decreased Cation reabsorption: Decreased HCO_3^- formation and reabsorption: Decreased	*Respiratory* (increase of P_{CO_2}) High pH: Hypoventilation Low P_{CO_2}: Hypoventilation
CO_2 Content	Increased	"Decreased"
Final result	As $[HCO_3^-]/[H_2CO_3]$ ratio approaches normal 20/1 of arterial blood, pH approaches normal 7.4.	

Figure 12–8. Pathophysiology and differential diagnosis of hyperpHemia (alkalosis). (Modified from Weisberg, H. F.: *Water, Electrolyte, and Acid-Base Balance.* 2nd ed. Baltimore, The Williams & Wilkins Company, 1962. Reproduced with permission of the publisher.)

A review of the differential diagnosis of acid-base imbalance is presented in Table 12–11; the numbers in the first column refer to the numbered areas in Figure 12–6. The pH determination can only distinguish the conditions of eupHemia, hypopHemia, and hyperpHemia; with each of these three categories the Pco_2 may be normal (as in uncompensated "metabolic" disorders) or elevated (hypoventilation, primary in respiratory acidosis or secondary compensation in metabolic alkalosis) or decreased (hyperventilation, primary in respiratory acidosis or secondary compensation in metabolic alkalosis).

In most circumstances the CO_2 content (or bicarbonate concentration) will parallel the ΔCT (or base excess). However, in examples No. 6 and 7a of Table 12–11 and Figure 12–6, these values are different and thus aid in distinguishing between acute respiratory acidosis and the combined respiratory and metabolic acidosis; the ΔCT is useful to distinguish between acute (No. 7a) and chronic (No. 7b) respiratory acidosis. In a similar fashion one can use the CO_2 content and ΔCT to distinguish between acute respiratory alkalosis (No. 11a) and the combined respiratory and metabolic alkalosis (No. 10); the ΔCT is useful to differentiate acute (No. 11a) and chronic (No. 11b) respiratory alkalosis. Table 12–11 also describes changes in Po_2, which are discussed in the next section.

OXYGEN

The important blood gases are carbon dioxide and oxygen; these gases are carried in the blood as the "free" gas and in a "combined" form. As described in Table 12–2 and Figure 12–3, carbon dioxide is combined as the bicarbonate ion, and the free form is essentially dissolved CO_2 gas and carbonic acid. The free form of oxygen is the dissolved gas, whereas the combined form is oxyhemoglobin (HbO_2^{2-}). Table 12–12 shows the effect of altered partial pressures of the two major blood gases on pulmonary ventilation and on cellular metabolism.

The term *anoxia* means without oxygen but has been accepted, as has *anemia* (literally without blood), to represent *anoxemia*—a "deficiency" of oxygen in the blood; the preferred term for decreased oxygen is *hypoxia.* Confusion exists with the term *asphyxia,* literally without a pulse, which should be used for the presence of hypoxia and an elevated Pco_2; thus, asphyxia often follows hypoxia. Oxygen is not as soluble as carbon dioxide in blood plasma at 38° C.; in contrast to the solubility of 0.03 ml. CO_2 per mm. Hg of Pco_2, the value for oxygen is 0.003 ml. per mm. Hg of Po_2. The *oxygen capacity* (volumes per cent or ml./dl.) is that amount of oxygen which can be combined with hemoglobin at full saturation, there being no difference between arterial and venous blood. The maximum amount of oxygen which can combine with 1 gm. hemoglobin is reported as 1.34 ml. (ranging to 1.39 ml./gm.) at full saturation. The *oxygen content* of blood varies with the Po_2 in a nonlinear fashion and is the sum of the "free" dissolved oxygen and the "combined" oxygen as oxyhemoglobin. The *per cent saturation* is the content divided by capacity, times 100. The partial pressure of oxygen (Po_2) is also called the "tension" (both expressed in terms of millimeters of mercury). Figure 12–9 demonstrates the sigmoid-shaped curve of the dissociation of oxyhemoglobin—the relationship of per cent saturation vs. Po_2—under normal conditions. The P_{50} (or T_{50} as used in Europe) is that pressure of oxygen at pH 7.40 and 38° C. at which the hemoglobin is 50 per cent saturated. The P_{50} is on the steepest part of the curve (Fig. 12–9), so that small shifts of the oxyhemoglobin dissociation curve to the left or right are easily detected by measuring the oxygen pressure changes; the normal P_{50} is about 26 mm. Hg. The P_{50} value has also been called the "unloading" tension.

The cause of a left or right shift of the oxyhemoglobin dissociation curve has been found to be due to the effects of the intraerythrocyte concentration of organic phosphates, of which 2,3-diphosphoglycerate (2,3-DPG) is the most physiologically active. 2,3-DPG is produced by DPG mutase as part of the Embden-Meyerhof pathway. (See page 203.)

Oxygen is bound to hemoglobin in a stepwise manner referred to as heme-heme interaction. Each heme molecule binds one oxygen molecule which, in turn, facilitates the next heme to oxygen binding. 2,3-DPG inhibits heme-heme interaction and can be said to have decreased the avidity of hemoglobin for oxygen.

Oxygen delivery to the tissues is known to depend upon a sufficient gradient between the Po_2 of tissues and the Po_2 of plasma. If hemoglobin is 100 per cent saturated at a low Po_2, a left-shifted oxyhemoglobin dissociation curve, unloading of oxygen to the tissues is compromised.

Decreased avidity of hemoglobin for oxygen, a right shift of the oxyhemoglobin dissociation curve, is of significant advantage to a patient who suffers from an inability to achieve a high arterial Po_2, as in severe anemias, or has an increased demand for oxygen, as in thyrotoxicosis. In these situations a high avidity of heme for oxygen would seriously impair oxygen delivery to the tissues, whereas a decrease in avidity of heme for oxygen facilitates oxygen

Table 12–11. DIFFERENTIAL DIAGNOSIS OF ACID-BASE EQUILIBRIUM*
(ARTERIAL VALUES FOR P_{O_2})

No.	pH	P_{CO_2}	CO_2 CT or $[HCO_3^-]$	ΔCT or BE	P_{O_2}†	COMMENTS
	Eu*pH*emia					
1a	N	N	N	N	N	Normal *blood* "gases" (Hemic hypoxia) (Ischemic hypoxia) (Histotoxic hypoxia)
1b	N	N	N	N	↓	$\dot{V}/\dot{Q}$ inequality Shunts
2	N	↑	↑	↑	↓	Respiratory acidosis, compensated; see Nos. 6 and 7 Hypoventilation‡ (Shunts)§ ($\dot{V}/\dot{Q}$ inequality)§ (Metabolic alkalosis, compensated)‖; see Nos. 8, 9, and 10
3	N	↓	↓	↓	↑ N	Respiratory alkalosis, compensated; see Nos. 10 and 11 (Metabolic acidosis, compensated); see Nos. 4, 5, and 6
	Hypo*pH*emia					
4a	↓	N	↓	↓	N	Metabolic acidosis, uncompensated (Hemic hypoxia) (Ischemic hypoxia) (Histotoxic hypoxia)
4b	↓	N	↓	↓	↓	$\dot{V}/\dot{Q}$ inequality Shunts
5a	↓	↓	↓	↓	↑ N	Metabolic acidosis, partial compensation (by hyperventilation)

*Arrows show direction and not extent of change; N = normal.
†(Excluding errors) any "low" P_{O_2} may become "normal" or "increased" due to:
Hyperventilation
O_2 Therapy
Increased concentration (100% should produce P_{aO_2} >600)
Increased pressure (hyperbaric chamber)
‡P_{O_2} usually <50.
§If present in addition to hypoventilation, P_{O_2} will be lowered further.
‖P_{O_2} usually >50.

(*Table 12-11 continues on the opposite page.*)

Table 12–11. DIFFERENTIAL DIAGNOSIS OF ACID-BASE EQUILIBRIUM (ARTERIAL VALUES FOR Po_2) *(Continued)*

No.	pH	Pco_2	CO_2 CT or $[HCO_3^-]$	ΔCT or BE	Po_2†	COMMENTS
5b	↓	↓	↓	↓	N ↓	Metabolic acidosis and shock; see No. 11c
6	↓	↑	N	↓	N ↓	Respiratory acidosis and metabolic acidosis
7a	↓	↑	↑	↓ N	↓	Respiratory acidosis, acute
7b	↓	↑	↑	↑	↓	Respiratory acidosis, chronic
	Hyper*pH*emia					
8a	↑	N	↑	↑	N	Metabolic alkalosis, uncompensated (Hemic hypoxia) (Ischemic hypoxia) (Histotoxic hypoxia)
8b	↑	N	↑	↑	↓	$\dot{V}/\dot{Q}$ inequality Shunts
9	↑	↑	↑	↑	↓	Metabolic alkalosis, partial compensation (by hypoventilation)
10	↑	↓	N	↑	N ↑	Respiratory alkalosis and metabolic alkalosis
11a	↑	↓	↓	N	↑ N	Respiratory alkalosis, acute¶
11b	↑	↓	↓	↓	↑	Respiratory alkalosis, chronic Impaired diffusion
11c	↑	↓	↓	↓	↓	Decreased ambient O_2 (Impaired diffusion) (Shunt) ($\dot{V}/\dot{Q}$ inequality) "Inappropriate pulmonary ventilation in acutely ill patient" e.g., Myocardial infarct Pulmonary embolus Shock Later pH ↓ ; see No. 5b

¶Also transient hyperventilation in response to arterial puncture.

Table 12–12. EFFECT OF ALTERED PARTIAL PRESSURE OF BLOOD GASES ON PULMONARY VENTILATION AND CELLULAR METABOLISM

GAS PRESSURE CHANGE		EFFECT ON	
Pco_2	Po_2	Pulmonary Ventilation	Cellular Metabolism (O_2 Uptake)
↑	↓	Stimulation	Depression
↓	↑	Depression	Stimulation

delivery to the tissues. This latter phenomenon is achieved by increasing the intraerythrocyte levels of 2,3-DPG. (See page 203.)

The principle of the Po_2 polarographic electrode is different from the pH (glass membrane sensitive to hydrogen ion) and Pco_2 (modified pH) electrodes. A voltage is applied across a platinum cathode and silver anode in dilute potassium chloride solution, all of which are separated from the blood by a membrane which is permeable to oxygen molecules. The reactions that occur are summarized in the equations shown at the top of page 801.

Normal values for Po_2 and per cent saturation for arterial and venous blood were given in Table 12–6. The Po_2 normally decreases with age; for each year, the Po_2 is decreased by approximately 0.3 mm. Hg. Oxygen therapy should be instituted in an individual with normal circulation and normal concentration of hemoglobin if the arterial oxygen saturation falls to about 80 per cent, or a Po_2 of about 45 mm. Hg; loss of consciousness occurs at arterial values of 40 per cent saturation or Po_2 of about 20 mm. Hg. Prognosis for life is poor if the individual has an arterial Po_2 of less than 20 mm. Hg, and yet survival has been reported in patients who had arterial Po_2 values of 7.5 mm. Hg or venous Po_2 values of 2 mm. Hg.

The venous Po_2 value is of little use if the patient is actively moving about or exercising; however, during resting conditions the venous Po_2 is a good guide to the state of tissue oxygenation. The venous oxygen saturation cor-

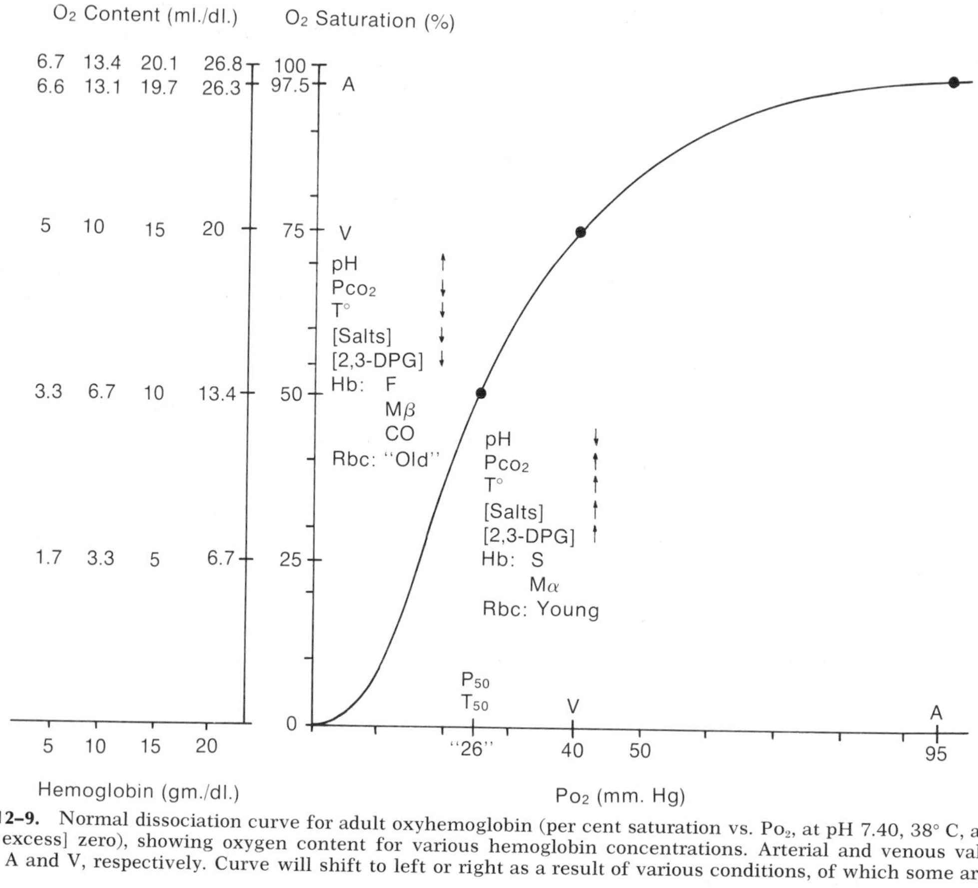

Figure 12–9. Normal dissociation curve for adult oxyhemoglobin (per cent saturation vs. Po_2, at pH 7.40, 38° C, and ΔCT [or base excess] zero), showing oxygen content for various hemoglobin concentrations. Arterial and venous values are noted by A and V, respectively. Curve will shift to left or right as a result of various conditions, of which some are listed.

(25)

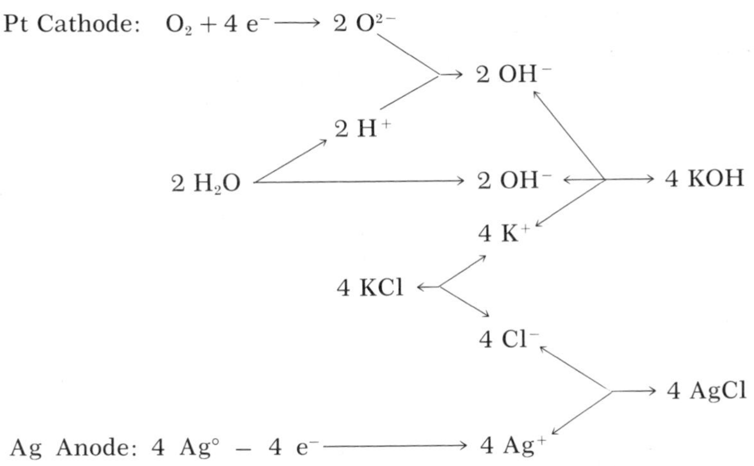

(26)

relates well with the arterial lactic acid concentration. Figure 12–9 lists some conditions which affect the oxyhemoglobin dissociation curve. Temperature, pH, and ΔCT (or base excess) alter the position but not the shape of the curve; corrections should be made for such differences (Severinghaus, 1965; Kelman and Nunn, 1966; Astrup *et al.*, 1965). Table 12–13 summarizes the spurious results that arise from lack of "corrections."

For a valid interpretation of Po_2 values one should study both the arterial and venous blood. The arterial-venous oxygen saturation difference is 25 per cent, and the oxygen content difference is 5 ml./dl. (Fig. 12–9). These differences are "constant" even if the oxyhemoglobin curve has been shifted by pH, anemia, and so forth. The *Bohr effect* has been extended to state that, at a given value for Po_2, the oxygen content (or per cent saturation) will be affected in a direct relationship by changes in pH and indirectly by changes in Pco_2 and ΔCT (or base excess); this can be represented as Equation 27.

$$\underset{\text{(at given } Po_2\text{)}}{O_2 \text{ content or \% sat.}} \; \alpha \; \frac{(\text{pH})}{(Pco_2)\,(\Delta CT)} \qquad (27)$$

The *Haldane effect* states that, at a given Pco_2, the carbon dioxide content will be affected inversely by changes in Po_2 (or oxygen

Table 12–13. RELATIONSHIP OF LABORATORY VALUES (*IN VITRO*) COMPARED TO ACTUAL UNDER BODY CONDITIONS (*IN VIVO*)*

	PATIENT HAS ALTERED			
	TEMPERATURE		ACID-BASE	
DETERMINATION	Fever	Hypothermia	Hypophemia (Acidosis) *or* +ΔCT (BE)	Hyperphemia (Alkalosis) *or* −ΔCT (BE)
pH	↑	↓		
Pco_2	↓	↑		
CO_2 content	↓	↑		
ΔCT (or base excess)	=	=		
Po_2	↓	↑	↓	↑
O_2 saturation	↑	↓	↑	↓

* ↑ Determined higher than actual.
↓ Determined lower than actual.
= Determined same as actual.

content or per cent saturation) as expressed in Equation 28.

$$\underset{\text{(at given } Pco_2)}{CO_2 \text{ content}} \; \alpha \; \frac{1}{Po_2} \quad (28)$$

The *Root effect* states that the oxygen capacity will be affected directly by changes in pH and indirectly by Pco_2 changes (Equation 29).

$$O_2 \text{ capacity} \; \alpha \; \frac{pH}{Pco_2} \quad (29)$$

Hypoxia can be caused by many conditions, but not all cases will result in decreased arterial Po_2! *Anoxic* hypoxia is characterized by decreased arterial values for Po_2, per cent saturation, and oxygen content; the "lack of oxygen" may be due to a decrease of the ambient oxygen supply or to pulmonary disease. The three additional causes of hypoxia—*hemic, ischemic,* and *histotoxic*—have *normal* arterial values for Po_2 and oxygen saturation; however, the venous values are abnormal. Thus, a blood specimen may be normal in all respects pertaining to acid-base and oxygen values and yet hypoxia may be present (No. 1a in Table 12–11 and Figure 12–6); similarly metabolic acidosis (No. 4a) or metabolic alkalosis (No. 8a) may be present in the presence of a *normal* arterial Po_2.

Four types of pulmonary impairment may be present—hypoventilation, alveolar-capillary block (or impaired diffusion), uneven ratio of circulation (perfusion) to ventilation of the lungs ($\dot{V}/\dot{Q}$ inequality), and venous-arterial shunts (anatomic and/or physiological). In the presence of shunts or $\dot{V}/\dot{Q}$ inequality, the arterial Po_2 (and oxygen saturation) is decreased, with a normal Pco_2 even though the pH may be normal (No. 1b), decreased (No. 4b), or increased (No. 8b).

Study of Table 12–11 and Figure 12–6 will reveal the various combinations possible in Po_2 values with respect to acid-base imbalance. Hypoventilation is the major cause of respiratory acidosis—rise of Pco_2—and a decreased Po_2 (Nos. 2, 6, and 7), whereas hyperventilation will result in respiratory alkalosis, with a decreased Pco_2 and an increased Po_2 (Nos. 3, 10, and 11a and b). Endogenous or assisted hyperventilation and oxygen therapy (increased concentrations or pressures) will increase a "low" Po_2 to normal or elevated values. Section No. 11c is most important in clinical medicine for, despite the hyperventilation which decreases the Pco_2, the Po_2 values are low when it would be expected to find elevated Po_2 values resulting from the hyperventilation; with the presence of shock, infarction, and so forth, the pH may shift from the alkaline side (due to hyperventilation) to the acid side of the normal 7.40. In histotoxic hypoxia the venous oxygen saturation may be above 90 per cent, since the tissues are unable to utilize the oxygen; the venous Po_2, therefore, is also above the usual venous range of normal.

REFERENCES

Andersen, O. S., Astrup, P., Campbell, E. J. M., Chinard, F. P., Nahas, G. G., and Winters, R. W.: Report of *ad hoc* committee on acid-base terminology. Ann. N.Y. Acad. Sci. *133*:251, 1966.

Armstrong, B. W., Mohler, J. G., Jung, R. C., and Remmers, J.: The in-vivo carbon-dioxide titration curve. Lancet *1*:759, 1966.

Astrup, P., Engel, K., Severinghaus, J. W., and Munson, E.: The influence of temperature and pH on the dissociation curve of oxyhemoglobin of human blood. Scand. J. Clin. Lab. Invest. *17*:515, 1965.

Astrup, P., Jørgensen, K., Siggaard-Andersen, O., and Engel, K.: The acid-base metabolism. A new approach. Lancet *1*:1035, 1960.

Austin, W. H.: Acid-base balance. A review of current approaches and techniques. Amer. Heart J. *69*:691, 1965.

Berry, M. N.: The liver and lactic acidosis. Proc. Roy. Soc. Med. *60*:1260, 1967.

Boyd, D. R., Addis, H. M., Chilimindris, C., Lowe, R. J., Folk, F. A., and Baker, R. J.: Utilization of osmometry in critically ill surgical patients. Arch. Surg. *102*:363, 1971.

Broder, G., and Weil, M. H.: Excess lactate. An index of reversibility of shock in human patients. Science *143*: 1457, 1964.

Bugyi, H. I., Magnier, E., Joseph, W., and Frank, G.: A method for measurement of sodium and potassium in erythrocytes and whole blood. Clin. Chem. *15*:712, 1969.

Collier, C. R., Hackney, J. D., and Mohler, J. G.: Use of extracellular base excess in diagnosis of acid-base disorders. A conceptual approach. Chest *61*(Feb. Suppl.):6S, 1972.

Cullen, G. E., and Jonas, L.: The effect of insulin treatment on the hydrogen ion concentration and alkali reserve of the blood in diabetic acidosis. J. Biol. Chem. 57:541, 1923.

Davenport, H. W.: *The ABC of Acid-Base Chemistry.* 5th ed. Chicago, University of Chicago Press, 1969.

Dumm, R. M., and Shipley, R. A.: The simple estimation of blood ketones in diabetic acidosis. J. Lab. Clin. Med. *31*:1162, 1946.

Finch, C. A., and Lenfant, C.: Oxygen transport in man. New Eng. J. Med. *286*:407, 1972.

Fleischer, W. R., and Gambino, S. R.: *Blood pH, Pco_2, Po_2, and Oxygen Saturation.* 4th ed. Chicago, ASCP Commission on Continuing Education, 1972.

Gambino, S. R.: Simpler graph for use in determining oxygen saturation of blood by means of spectrophotometry. Amer. J. Clin. Path. *43*:599, 1965.

Gambino, S. R.: pH and Pco_2. *In* Meites, S. (ed.): *Standard Methods of Clinical Chemistry.* Vol. 5. New York, Academic Press, Inc., 1965, pp. 169–198.

Gambino, S. R.: Oxygen, partial pressure (Po_2) electrode method. *In* MacDonald, R. P. (ed.): *Standard Methods of Clinical Chemistry,* Vol. 6. New York, Academic Press, Inc., 1970, pp. 171–182.

Gambino, S. R., Astrup, P., Bates, R. G., Campbell, E. J. M., Chinard, F. P., Nahas, G. G., Siggaard-Andersen, O., and Winters, R. W.: Report of the *ad hoc* committee on acid-base methodology. Ann. N.Y. Acad. Sci. *133*:259, 1966.

Greenburg, A. G., and Moulder, P. V.: Temperature coefficients for Pco_2 and pH in whole blood. Arch. Surg. *91*:867, 1965.

Hald, P. M., Heinsen, A. J., and Peters, J. P.: The estimation of serum sodium from bicarbonate plus chloride. J. Clin. Invest. *26*:983, 1947.

Hamilton, L. H.: Respiratory and blood gas analysis. *In*

Stefanini, M. (ed.): *Progress in Clinical Pathology.* Vol. 2. New York, Grune & Stratton, 1969, pp. 284–340.
Hastings, A. B., Neill, J. M., Morgan, H. J., and Binger, C. A. L.: Blood reaction and blood gases in pneumonia. J. Clin. Invest. *1*:25, 1924–1925.
Holmes, J. H.: Measurement of osmolality in serum, urine, and other biologic fluids by the freezing point determination. *In Pre-Workshop Manual on Urinalysis and Renal Function Studies.* Chicago, ASCP Commission on Continuing Education, 1962.
Huckabee, W. E.: Abnormal resting blood lactate. II. Lactic acidosis. Amer. J. Med. *30*:840, 1961.
Hutter, A. M., Jr., and Moss, A. J.: Central venous oxygen saturation. J.A.M.A. *212*:299, 1970.
Johnson, R. B., Jr., and Hoch, H.: Osmolality of serum and urine. *In* Meites, S. (ed.): *Standard Methods of Clinical Chemistry.* Vol. 5. New York, Academic Press, Inc., 1965, pp. 159–168.
Jones, L. W., and Weil, M. H.: Water, creatinine and sodium excretion following circulatory shock with renal failure. Amer. J. Med. *51*:314, 1971.
Kaitz, A. L., and London, A. M.: Osmolar urinary concentrating ability and pyelonephritis in hospitalized patients. Amer. J. Med. Sci. *248*:7, 1964.
Kelman, G. R., and Nunn, J. F.: Nomograms for correction of blood P_{O_2}, P_{CO_2}, pH and base excess for time and temperature. J. Appl. Physiol. *21*:1484, 1966.
Kintner, E. P.: A new approach to an old concept. Amer. J. Clin. Path. *47*:614, 1967.
Mansberger, A. R., Jr., Boyd, D. R., Cowley, R. A., and Buxton, R. W.: Refractometry and osmometry in clinical surgery. Ann. Surg. *169*:672, 1969.
Maxwell, M. H., and Kleeman, C. R. (eds.): *Clinical Disorders of Fluid and Electrolyte Metabolism.* 2nd ed. New York, McGraw-Hill Book Co., Inc., 1972.
Nunn, J. F.: *Applied Respiratory Physiology.* New York, Appleton-Century-Crofts, Inc., 1969.
Oliva, P. B.: Lactic acidosis. Amer. J. Med. *48*:209, 1970.
Retzlaff, J. A., Tauxe, W. N., Kiely, J. M., and Stroebel, C. F.: Erythrocyte volume, plasma volume, and lean body mass in adult men and women. Blood *33*:649, 1969.
Rubin, A. L., Braverman, W. S., Dexter, R. L., Vanamee, P., and Roberts, K.: The relationship between plasma osmolality and concentration in disease states. Clin. Res. Proc. *4*:129, 1956.
Schmidt, J. E.: Medical Lexicographer: Normal pH. Mod. Med., June 29, 1970, p. 119.
Severinghaus, J. W.: Blood gas concentrations. *In* Fenn, W. O., and Rahn, H. (eds.): *Handbook of Physiology.* Section 3, Respiration, Vol. II. Washington, D.C., American Physiological Society, p. 1475, 1965.
Severinghaus, J. W., and Bradley, A. F.: *Blood Gas Electrodes or What the Instructions Didn't Say.* Published by authors, 1969.
Siggaard-Andersen, O.: *The Acid-Base Status of the Blood.* 2nd ed. Baltimore, The Williams & Wilkins Company, 1964.
Siggaard-Andersen, O.: Titratable acid or base of body fluids. Ann. N.Y. Acad. Sci. *133*:41, 1966.
Siggaard-Andersen, O., Engel, K., Jørgensen, K., and Astrup, P.: A micro method for determination of pH, carbon dioxide tension, base excess and standard bicarbonate in capillary blood. Scand. J. Clin. Lab. Invest. *12*:172, 1960.
Skeggs, L. T., Jr.: An automatic method for the determination of carbon dioxide in blood plasma. Bull. Reg. Med. Technol. *30*:1, 1960.
Sorbini, C. A., Grassi, V., Solinas, E., and Muieson, G.: Arterial oxygen tension in relation to age in healthy subjects. Respiration *25*:3, 1968.
Weisberg, H. F.: A better understanding of anion-cation ("acid-base") balance. Surg. Clin. N. Amer. *39*:93, 1959.
Weisberg, H. F.: *Water, Electrolyte, and Acid-Base Balance.* 2nd ed. Baltimore, The Williams & Wilkins Company, 1962.
Weisberg, H. F.: Parenteral fluid therapy in adults. *In* Conn, H. F. (ed.): *Current Therapy 1969.* Philadelphia, W. B. Saunders Company, 1969, pp. 414–425.
Weisberg, H. F.: *Interpretation of Electrolyte and Acid-Base Imbalance.* 3rd ed. 1971. (Mimeographed edition.)
Weisberg, H. F.: Osmolality. ASCP Commission on Continuing Education Council on Clinical Chemistry, Check Sample CC-71, 1971, pp. 1–49.
Weisberg, H. F.: Antics with acid-base semantics. Lab. Med. 3:11–13; 32–35, 1972.
Whitfield, J. B.: Spurious hyperkalemia and hyponatremia in a patient with thrombocythaemia. J. Clin. Path. *19*:496, 1966.
Winters, R. W.: Terminology of acid-base disorders. Ann. N.Y. Acad. Sci. *133*:211, 1966.

Chapter 13

TESTS OF HEPATIC FUNCTION

by HYMAN J. ZIMMERMAN, M.D.

The liver is a complex organ which performs many metabolic functions. More than 100 tests of hepatic functions have been based on the hundreds of reactions that have been shown to occur in the liver. Many of these have been abandoned after early study. A few have been found to be clinically useful. In Table 13–1 is shown a classification of the types of functions performed by the liver and of the types of tests that have been based on these functions.

Classic experiments in hepatic physiology have shown that removal of large portions of the liver of normal animals may leave some types of hepatic function unimpaired. This has led many authors to emphasize the great reserve power of the liver and to suggest that mild hepatic disease will not be exposed by tests of hepatic function. The relevance of such experiments to clinical problems, however, may be questioned. Diffuse though mild disease, such as viral hepatitis or early cirrhosis of the liver, produces impairment of many tests of hepatic function, with the severity of disease reflected in the degree of hepatic dysfunction. Disturbed hepatic function does not necessarily mean hepatic disease, since some nonhepatic diseases also may produce impairment of liver function. Nevertheless the occurrence of abnormal hepatic function can usually be found to have a rational basis when considered in the light of the clinical problem.

No one test of liver function is sufficient for clinical analysis of most problems. From the many tests that have been devised, a group of procedures that are most applicable to the particular clinical problem should be selected. In the following pages the physiologic basis for hepatic function testing is discussed, a

Table 13–1. CLASSIFICATION OF TYPES OF HEPATIC FUNCTION AND RELATED TESTS

FUNCTION	TEST	COMMENT
Bilirubin	Serum bilirubin level and partition (direct and indirect fraction)	Very useful
	Urine bilirubin	Very useful
	Urine urobilinogen	Very useful
	Fecal urobilinogen	Useful
Carbohydrate metabolism	Glucose, Fructose, Lactate } tolerance tests	Not usually applied to the study of liver disease
	Galactose tolerance	Some value in differential diagnosis of jaundice (Used rarely)
	Epinephrine, Glucagon tolerances	Helpful in the diagnosis of glycogen storage disease but not generally in other hepatic disease

(Table 13–1 continues on the opposite page.)

Table 13–1. CLASSIFICATION OF TYPES OF HEPATIC FUNCTION AND RELATED TESTS *(Continued)*

FUNCTION	TEST	COMMENT
Protein metabolism	Serum protein level	Useful in detecting hepatic and nonhepatic diseases
	Albumin, globulin, gamma globulin level; electrophoretic analysis	
	Flocculation and turbidometric tests	Useful in detecting hepatic and nonhepatic diseases; less widely used than before
	Serum mucoprotein levels	Not widely used
	Serum haptoglobin level	May be of value
	Amino acid levels in blood and urine	Of research rather than ordinary clinical value
	Blood ammonia levels	Useful in understanding, diagnosis, and treatment of hepatic coma
	Blood urea levels	Of clinical interest; late and insensitive reflection of liver damage
Lipid metabolism	Plasma or serum cholesterol level	Definite but limited usefulness
	Plasma or serum cholesterol ester level	Little clinical value
	Bile acids levels and fractionation	Of research interest; use limited by technical difficulties
Foreign substance excretion	(Dye excretion tests)	
	Rose bengal	Old test; revived as radioactive rose bengal test (see text)
	Sulfobromphthalein (BSP)	Most sensitive measure of hepatic function, also useful for hepatic blood flow studies
	Indocyanine green	Used for research and for hepatic blood flow studies; little use for clinical liver function testing as yet
Detoxification and synthesis	Hippuric acid excretion	Formerly widely used, now largely abandoned
	Prothrombin time and response to vitamin K administration	Useful
	Plasma levels of other coagulation factors	Of interest, but clinical usefulness as measure of liver function limited by time-consuming nature of assays
Serum enzyme levels	Alkaline phosphatase, Transaminases	Very useful and widely used in study of liver disease
	Cholinesterase (see Chapter 14 for large number of other serum enzymes)	Not widely used
Levels of serum "metals" and electrolytes	Serum iron and iron-binding capacity	Helpful in the diagnosis of hemochromatosis; limited usefulness in differential diagnosis of jaundice
	Serum ceruloplasmin and copper levels	Helpful in the diagnosis of hepatolenticular degeneration
	Serum zinc levels	Abnormal in "alcoholic" cirrhosis; clinical applicability not adequately studied
Vitamin metabolism	Serum vitamin A levels	Not useful
	Serum vitamin B_{12} levels and tolerance tests	Proposed for differential diagnosis of jaundice; questionable value. May prove to be useful

number of individual tests of liver function are analyzed, the batteries of tests that are considered useful are presented, and the results in various diseases are illustrated.

BILIRUBIN METABOLISM

Knowledge of bilirubin metabolism is essential for the proper understanding of hepatic disease. Bilirubin is a product of hemoglobin, from which it is formed in the cells of the reticuloendothelial system. Here the protoporphyrin is separated from the iron and globin portions of the molecule, and the ring is opened to form bilirubin (Fig. 13–1). Approximately 85 per cent of the bilirubin is derived from senescent erythrocytes. Most of the remainder is produced by intracorpuscular degradation of hemoglobulin in the bone marrow (erythropoietic component). Very small amounts are derived from the degradation of nonhemoglobin, heme-containing proteins (catalase, cytochromes, tryptophan pyrrolase, myoglobin) and, perhaps, from "shunting" of heme precursors directly to bilirubin products. The bilirubin is transported through the blood (bound to albumin) to the liver. Transport of bilirubin from sinusoidal blood into the hepatocyte depends on mechanisms which are currently under intensive study. It involves dissociation of bilirubin from albumin and is facilitated by or depends on specific transport proteins described by Arias and his associates (1969). In the liver bilirubin is conjugated with glucuronic acid* to form the diglucuronide (Fig. 13–2), which is excreted by the liver into the duodenum. In the intestines bacterial enzyme action converts bilirubin, through a group of intermediate compounds, to several related compounds collectively referred to as "urobilinogen" (Fig. 13–1). A portion (estimated to be 10 per cent or more) of the uro-

*A fraction of the bilirubin excreted by the liver is conjugated with other groups. The conjugates of bilirubin that are formed differ in different series and are modified by disease.

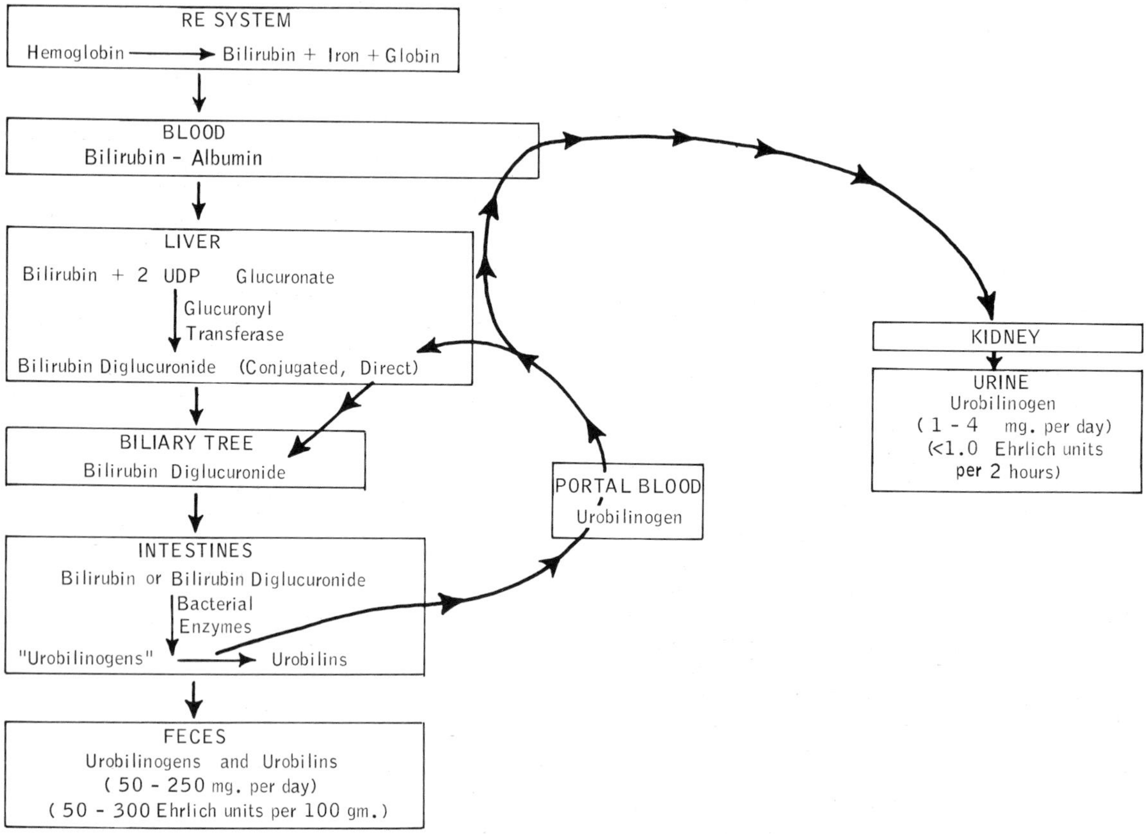

Figure 13–1. Approximately 80% of bilirubin derives in the RE system from effete erythrocytes. The remainder includes bilirubin formed from non-hemoglobin heme compounds (e.g., catalase, perioxidase) and that formed by breakdown of erythrocyte precursors (e.g., normoblasts) within the bone marrow.

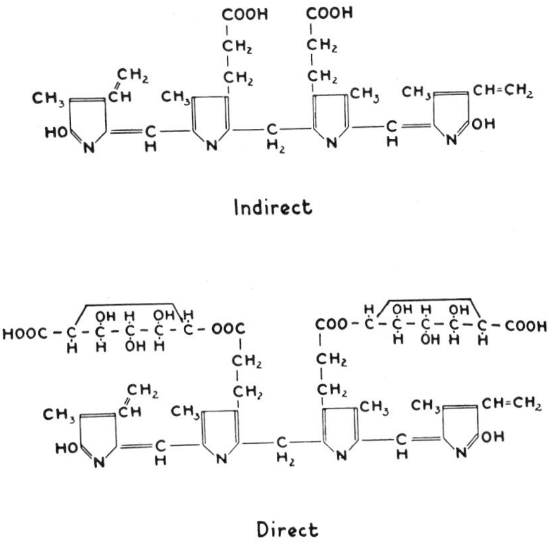

Figure 13–2. The structure of indirect and direct bilirubin. Note that direct bilirubin is bilirubin diglucuronide and that indirect is unconjugated bilirubin. Conversion of bilirubin to the diglucuronide is catalyzed by glucuronyl transferase. (This schematic representation of bilirubin as a linear tetrapyrrole is the conventional model, although a ring-shaped structure is more accurate).

bilinogen is reabsorbed into the blood and reexcreted by the liver. Normally, small amounts (1 to 4 mg. per 24 hr.) are excreted in the urine. When the Watson "2-hour method" is used, normal individuals have less than 1 Ehrlich unit per 2-hour specimen. Fecal urobilinogen levels in normals range from 50 to 250 mg. per day or 300 Ehrlich units per 100 gm. Some of the urobilinogen is oxidized to urobilin in the intestines or later in the feces. Measurement of fecal urobilinogen usually includes the sum of urobilinogens and urobilins. The metabolism of bilirubin is summarized in Figure 13–1.

Determination of the level of serum bilirubin was first performed by van den Bergh and Müller, who found that bilirubin in normal serum reacted with the Ehrlich diazo reagent (diazotized sulfanilic acid) only when alcohol was added. Their observation that bile pigment in human bile reacted with the diazo reagent without the addition of alcohol led to the recognition that some change in bilirubin had been effected by the liver. Van den Bergh called the form of bilirubin that reacted with the diazo reagent without the addition of alcohol "direct" and the variety that reacted only in the presence of alcohol "indirect." Serum from patients with jaundice owing to excessive hemolysis gave the indirect reaction, while in the serum of patients with jaundice owing to obstruction of the biliary tree the increased serum bilirubin levels gave the direct reaction. The response of the serum to the van den Bergh test has been the basis for several classifications of jaundice. The physiochemical reasons for the different types of response have been clarified only during the past several years.

The properties of indirect and of direct bilirubin are summarized in Table 13–2. It is clear that indirect bilirubin is "free" or unconjugated bilirubin en route to the liver from the reticuloendothelial system, where it has been formed. The unconjugated bilirubin is nonpolar and therefore not soluble in water. Consequently it will react with the diazo reagent only in the presence of an agent (alcohol) in which it and the diazo reagent are soluble. The nonpolar nature of unconjugated bilirubin is also the basis for the failure of indirect bilirubin to appear in the urine in more than trace amounts. Unconjugated bilirubin is so tightly bound that it cannot be filtered at the glomerulus, and there appears to be no known tubular secretion of bilirubin. Accordingly, unconjugated bilirubin is not excreted in the urine. Direct (conjugated) bilirubin is a polar compound. It is therefore soluble in water solution, reacting directly with the diazo reagent, and able to appear in the urine when the blood levels are increased. Conjugated bilirubin is, in part, not protein bound; hence, it can be filtered at the glomerulus and excreted in the urine.

Reports of a few years ago that a monoglucuronide of bilirubin could be formed have been challenged by some authors, who have suggested that apparent monoglucuronide is a chemical illusion produced by mixtures of unconjugated bilirubin and bilirubin diglucuronide. Recent studies again support the view that monoglucuronides of bilirubin are formed.

Qualitative analysis of serum bilirubin according to the type of van den Bergh reaction as indirect or direct has long been replaced by quantitative determination of the amount of direct and of total bilirubin, the difference being presumed to represent indirect bilirubin.

Table 13–2. COMPARISON OF PROPERTIES OF DIRECT AND INDIRECT BILIRUBIN

	DIRECT (CONJUGATED)	INDIRECT (UNCONJUGATED)
Structure	Bilirubin diglucuronide	Bilirubin
Type of compound		
Solubility	Polar	Nonpolar
Water	+	−
Alcohol	+	+
Van den Bergh reaction	Direct	Indirect
Affinity for brain tissue	Low	High*
Presence in urine of patients with jaundice	+	−

*Kernicterus (deposition of bilirubin in brain tissue occurs only in association with very high levels of unconjugated bilirubin.

A commonly used method, that of Malloy and Evelyn (1937), has been replaced in many laboratories by the modification of Ducci and Watson (1945) or by the method of Jendrassik. In the Ducci and Watson method the amount of bilirubin that has reacted with the diazo reagent at the end of 1 minute is determined. This "1-minute" bilirubin presumably represents the "prompt, direct reacting" bilirubin of van den Bergh. The total bilirubin is measured 15 minutes after the addition of methyl alcohol. The difference between the total and 1-minute bilirubin is the indirect bilirubin. Other methods are available but are employed much less extensively than that of Malloy and Evelyn or a modification of it.

The level of bilirubin in the serum of normals in our laboratory is less than 1 mg. per 100 ml. This is almost entirely unconjugated bilirubin. In some laboratories the normal upper limit is reported to be as high as 1.5 mg. The upper limit of normal for conjugated bilirubin varies from 0.2 to 0.4 mg. in different laboratories. Levels of total serum bilirubin above 2.5 mg. per 100 ml. usually produce jaundice.

Jaundice has been classified by various authors according to pathophysiology, etiology, or both. The classification of McNee (1923) was based on etiology, and that of Rich (1930) was based on mechanisms. The classification of Ducci (1947) was based on both. An understanding of jaundice may be facilitated by a consideration of each of these classifications.

McNee proposed that jaundice be categorized as hemolytic, toxic and infectious, and obstructive. Others have substituted the term "hepatocellular" or "hepatogenous" for the "toxic and infectious" category. This classification has no place for constitutional hepatic dysfunction and for the jaundice that, although due to hepatic disease, may simulate obstructive jaundice (intrahepatic cholestasis, cholangiolitic hepatitis, hepatocanalicular jaundice). These defects are remedied by the rational classification of Ducci, which includes the categories of McNee.

Rich, on the basis of presumed pathophysiologic mechanisms, divided jaundice into "retention" and "regurgitation" types. *Retention jaundice* referred to hyperbilirubinemia in which there is retention of indirect bilirubin because it has not been converted to direct bilirubin and excreted by the liver. This category included hemolytic jaundice and would also have included the jaundice resulting from defective ability to conjugate bilirubin or clear it from the blood had these categories been recognized at the time of the studies by Rich.

Regurgitation jaundice referred to the hyperbilirubinemia in which levels of direct as well as indirect bilirubin were elevated. The elevated level of direct bilirubin was attributed to *regurgitation* of bilirubin into the blood after it had been acted on by the liver and excreted into a nonpatent biliary tree. The regurgitation type, in the classification of Rich, also referred to the usual form of hepatocellular jaundice, since it also is characterized by elevated levels of direct bilirubin. The classification of Rich clearly is the forerunner of the current one that will be presented below, namely, the classification of jaundice into the two categories of *unconjugated* and *conjugated* hyperbilirubinemia.

The classification of Ducci retains the categories of McNee and the principles of the Rich classification. It is based on the presumed site of the physiologic or anatomic abnormality. The categories are prehepatic, hepatic, and posthepatic jaundice.

Prehepatic jaundice is that variety of jaundice in which the increased serum bilirubin is mainly unconjugated (indirect). In *hepatic* and *posthepatic* jaundice, much of the elevated bilirubin is conjugated, i.e., it has traversed the liver cell, been conjugated with glucuronate, and been returned to the blood. *Posthepatic* jaundice refers to the jaundice caused by obstruction of the biliary tree, while *hepatic* jaundice refers to the jaundice produced by hepatic disease.

Attractive and useful as the Ducci classification has been, it contains the anomaly of including as "prehepatic" the jaundice due to hemolysis, which is truly *prehepatic,* with the jaundice due to *hepatic* defects in bilirubin uptake, which is therefore better dubbed hepatic.

The currently employed classification of jaundice (Table 13–3, Fig. 13–2) is rational and simple. Hyperbilirubinemia is classified as *unconjugated* and *conjugated.* The unconjugated category includes those forms of jaundice in which at least 80 per cent of the serum bilirubin is indirect. This may be prehepatic, in which excess bilirubin production (hemolysis) is responsible, or hepatic, in which either removal of bilirubin from the blood or conjugation of bilirubin by the liver is defective. The *conjugated* category also includes two groups, namely, hepatic, which includes a variety of genetic and acquired defects of the liver, and posthepatic, which refers to anatomic obstruction of the extrahepatic biliary tree.

The *prehepatic* type of unconjugated hyperbilirubinemia commonly referred to as hemolytic jaundice occurs because excessively rapid destruction of erythrocytes results in the production of bilirubin at a rate exceeding the ability of the liver to conjugate and excrete it. It may result from any of the genetic or acquired types of hemolytic disease. The hyperbilirubinemia, accordingly, is largely the indirect type. The increased production of

Table 13–3. RECOMMENDED CLASSIFICATION OF JAUNDICE

CLASSIFICATION	PHYSIOLOGIC DEFECT	EXAMPLES OF ETIOLOGY
Unconjugated		
Prehepatic	Excessive production of bilirubin	Hemolysis
Hepatic	Defective transport of bilirubin from sinusoidal blood into hepatocyte	Gilbert's syndrome
	Defective conjugation of bilirubin	Crigler-Najjar syndrome Neonatal jaundice
Conjugated Hyperbilirubinemia		
Hepatic		
Hepatocellular	Hepatocellular damage	Viral or toxic hepatitis Cirrhosis
Hepatocanalicular*	Hepatic disease with defective secretion of bilirubin into canaliculus	Primary biliary cirrhosis Some forms of drug jaundice (e.g., chlorpromazine)
Posthepatic	Mechanical obstruction of biliary tree	Carcinoma of pancreas or common duct stones

*Also referred to as intrahepatic cholestases.

bilirubin usually results in an increase in the amount of fecal urobilinogen, a characteristic of hemolytic jaundice. Often there is also an increase in the urine content of urobilinogen. Presumably this results from the reabsorption from the intestines of greater amounts of urobilinogen than can be reexcreted by the liver. Bilirubin does not appear in the urine in hemolytic jaundice, since the elevated level of blood bilirubin consists largely of the unconjugated type.

The *hepatic* type of unconjugated hyperbilirubinemia includes the Gilbert syndrome (constitutional hepatic dysfunction) and the Crigler-Najjar syndrome (constitutional hyperbilirubinemia with kernicterus). The Gilbert syndrome is a mild condition which appears to result from a genetic defect in the transport of bilirubin from sinusoidal blood into the hepatocyte. (The Gilbert syndrome probably includes several different conditions, all of which present a similar benign syndrome of mild unconjugated hyperbilirubinemia.) The Crigler-Najjar syndrome is a severe disease with marked hyperbilirubinemia that results from a genetic deficiency of the hepatic microsomal enzyme, glucuronyl transferase, which is needed for the conjugation of bilirubin. Another form of glucuronyl transferase deficiency, which is a clinically much more benign syndrome, has been described. Hepatic unconjugated hyperbilirubinemia resembles that of hemolytic (prehepatic) hyperbilirubinemia in that it is largely unconjugated. The fecal and urine urobilinogen content in the hepatic type of *unconjugated* hyperbilirubinemia, in contrast to that in the prehepatic type, is normal or reduced, since the rate of bilirubin entry into the duodenum is depressed rather than increased.

Posthepatic jaundice, commonly called obstructive jaundice, usually is the result of obstruction of the common bile or hepatic duct by carcinoma of the head of the pancreas, papilla of Vater, or common duct, by choledocholithiasis, or by pancreatitis. Rarely diseased lymph nodes surrounding the duct or neoplastic invasion of the *porta hepatis* may produce obstructive jaundice. Obstruction of the biliary tree produces jaundice by preventing the entry into the duodenum of bilirubin that has been conjugated. The bilirubin is "regurgitated" into the blood, raising the serum level of direct reacting bilirubin, which then appears in the urine. The exclusion of bilirubin from the duodenum results in clay-colored feces and very low levels of urobilinogen in the feces and urine.

Hepatic conjugated hyperbilirubinemia can be divided into two subcategories: the hepatocellular and hepatocanalicular types. *Hepatocellular jaundice* is equivalent to the "toxic and infectious" category of the McNee classification. *Hepatocanalicular jaundice* closely resembles obstructive jaundice in its clinical and biochemical features. This is also commonly referred to as *intrahepatic cholestasis.*

The hepatocellular type of hepatic jaundice results from injury to the parenchyma (viral hepatitis, toxic hepatitis, cirrhosis). Hepatic damage theoretically might be expected to produce an unconjugated hyperbilirubinemia because of (theoretically) impaired conjugating ability. Indeed, late in convalescence the jaundice may be of the unconjugated type. During the more deeply jaundiced phase of hepatitis, however, there are features similar to those of obstructive jaundice. Thus, in hepatitis there is a distinct increase in the direct-reacting bilirubin fraction with bilirubin in the urine. The degree of exclusion of bilirubin from the duodenum, however, is much less marked than in obstructive jaundice. Stools usually are only somewhat lighter than normal but may be clay colored. The urobilinogen content of the stool is usually decreased, but rarely to the levels characteristic of obstructive jaundice. Even though amounts of bilirubin entering the duodenum are less than normal, liver damage prevents adequate hepatic clearing from the blood of the urobilinogen reabsorbed from the duodenum. Urine urobilinogen, therefore, is often increased in some stages of hepatocellular jaundice (Fig. 13–3 D).

It has been presumed, therefore, that in hepatitis, as in obstructive jaundice, much of the bilirubin presented to the liver cell is conjugated and excreted into the canaliculi but regurgitates back into the blood, perhaps because of necrotic cells or increased permeability of the canaliculi. It is more probable that some other mechanism is responsible, perhaps impaired synthesis of bile acids, necessary to permit adequate transport of bile into the canaliculus.

The hepatocanalicular type of hepatic jaundice simulates obstructive jaundice very closely (Fig. 13–3 E). It has also been called "cholangiolitic," a term based on the theory that jaundice occurs because bilirubin regurgitates into the blood through inflammatory defects in the cholangioles. It is better called *intrahepatic cholestasis*, a term that describes

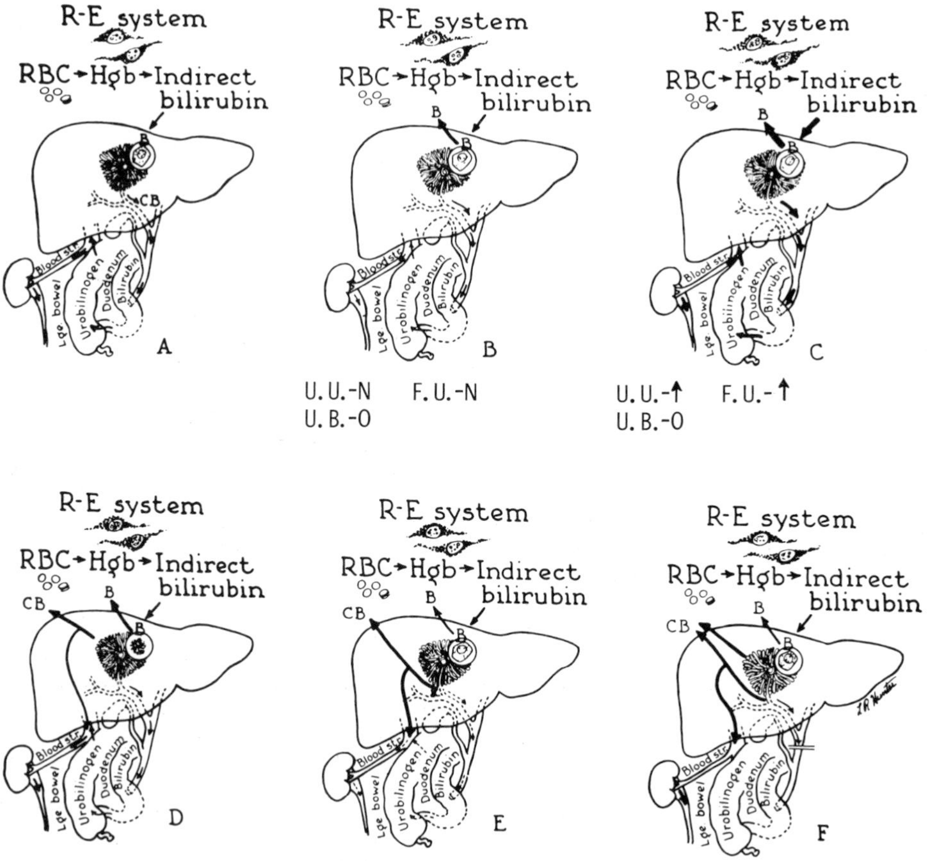

Figure 13–3. Diagrammatic representation of (A) normal bilirubin metabolism and the type of defect in (B) Gilbert or Crigler-Najjar syndrome, (C) hemolytic jaundice, (D) hepatocellular jaundice, (E) hepatocanalicular jaundice (intrahepatic cholestasis), and (F) posthepatic jaundice. In the diagrams, B represents unconjugated and CB conjugated bilirubin; U.U. represents urine urobilinogen, U.B. urine bilirubin, and F.U. fecal urobilinogen. N represents normal; + indicates present; 0 indicates absent; number of upward or downward-directed arrows indicates increase or decrease, respectively.

Table 13–4. SOME DIFFERENTIAL FEATURES OF VARIOUS TYPES OF JAUNDICE

TYPE OF HYPERBILIRUBINEMIA	CAUSE	SERUM BILIRUBIN (RATIO, DIRECT/TOTAL)	URINE		FECAL UROBILINOGEN
			BILIRUBIN	UROBILINOGEN	
Unconjugated					
Prehepatic	Hemolytic states	< 0.2	–	↑ or N	↑
Hepatic	Gilbert syndrome Crigler-Najjar syndrome	< 0.2	0	N or ↓	↓ or N
Conjugated					
Hepatic					
Hepatocellular	Hepatitis (viral, toxic) Cirrhosis Other causes of hepatic necrosis	0.3–0.6	+	↑ or N†	N or ↓
Hepatocanalicular	Intrahepatic cholestasis induced by some drugs Primary biliary cirrhosis Several forms of familial jaundice*	> 0.5	+	N, ↑ or ↓	↓
Posthepatic	Obstruction of biliary tree by carcinoma, calculus or other lesion	> 0.5	+	↓ or N	↓

*The Dubin-Johnson syndrome is a genetic disorder characterized by a black pigment in the hepatocytes and a special form of "dissociated" intrahepatic cholestasis in which there is defective excretion of bilirubin into the canaliculus but other components of bile apparently are normally excreted, thus differing from other forms of hepatic canalicular jaundice. The Rotor syndrome resembles the Dubin-Johnson syndrome in some but not all features. Other familial forms of hepatocanalicular jaundice include "benign intermittent juvenile cholestatic jaundice" and cholestatic jaundice of pregnancy.

†In hepatitis depends on the stage of the disease (Fig. 13–4).

the fact that bile flow into the duodenum is inhibited by intrahepatic disease. This type of jaundice is seen most commonly with certain drug reactions (chlorpromazine, organic arsenicals, methyltestosterone); it is thought to occur occasionally as a result of viral hepatitis or it may be "idiopathic."

Tests

Determination of the total serum bilirubin level is useful in measuring the depth and progress of jaundice. Determination of the direct and indirect fraction has been of some value in the differential diagnosis of jaundice. When the direct fraction is less than 20 per cent of the total bilirubin value, the jaundice is considered to be a manifestation of unconjugated hyperbilirubinemia—either owing to hemolysis or to one of the types of constitutional hyperbilirubinemia (Table 13–4). Little specific aid in the distinction of hepatic from posthepatic causes of conjugated hyperbilirubinemic jaundice can be obtained from the relative levels of direct and indirect bilirubin. The direct fraction may constitute more than 50 per cent of the total bilirubin in either hepatic or posthepatic jaundice. Levels of the direct fraction that constitute between 20 and 50 per cent of the total bilirubin are infrequent in posthepatic jaundice and are more characteristic of hepatic jaundice.

Testing for urine bilirubin (urine "bile") is useful in the differential diagnosis of jaundice. The presence of bilirubin in the urine of a patient with jaundice shows that the hyperbilirubinemia is of the conjugated type, i.e., hepatic or posthepatic. Bilirubin may also be present in the urine of patients without jaundice, as in early or anicteric hepatitis, in metastatic carcinoma, or in early obstruction of the biliary tree.

Decreased *fecal urobilinogen* is characteristic of obstructive (posthepatic) jaundice but may also be found in patients with hepatocellular jaundice. An extremely low level (below 5 mg. or 5 Ehrlich units per day) of stool urobilinogen is strong evidence that the jaundice is posthepatic. An increased level of fecal urobilinogen (above 250 mg. or 300 Ehrlich units per day) is evidence of hemolysis. When fecal urobilinogen levels are being determined as measures of hemolysis, they should be correlated with the degree of anemia. (See Chapter 4.)

Urine urobilinogen levels are decreased in posthepatic jaundice and in some phases of hepatic jaundice. Increased levels are observed usually in hemolytic jaundice and with subsiding hepatitis. Increased levels may also be a sensitive measure of hepatic damage even in the absence of jaundice, as in some patients with cirrhosis of the liver, metastatic carcinoma, or congestive heart failure.

Studies of urine and stool pigments are extremely useful to the clinician, but there are several pitfalls in the application of bile pigment study to the analysis of jaundice. Very low levels of urobilinogen in the stool are characteristic of obstructive jaundice but may also occur in patients who have received "broad-spectrum" antibiotics. These agents suppress the intestinal bacteria which convert bilirubin to urobilinogen. On the other hand, normal levels of fecal urobilinogen and even increased levels of urine urobilinogen may be found in patients with incomplete obstructive jaundice. During the course of viral hepatitis (Fig. 13–4), urobilinogen and bilirubin content of the urine may be characteristic of hepatocellular jaundice (phases a and c) and of obstructive jaundice (phase b) and may even simulate hemolytic icterus (phase d). Hemolytic icterus may be complicated by hepatic necrosis (as in sickle cell anemia) and thus by hepatocellular jaundice or by pigment stones obstructing the common duct and producing posthepatic jaundice.

Other tests based on bilirubin metabolism have been devised but have found little clinical application. The *bilirubin tolerance test* consists of administering a known amount of bilirubin and observing the rate of disappearance from the blood. This test is a sensitive measure of hepatic function but has not been adopted widely because it is laborious and expensive. The *urobilinogen tolerance test* consists of the measurement of urine urobilinogen excretion after the intravenous administration of stercobilin. This test is also too complicated for general use.

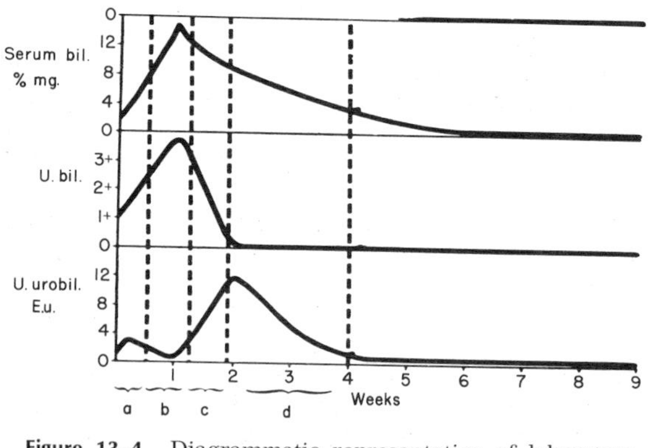

Figure 13–4. Diagrammatic representation of laboratory abnormalities during the course of viral hepatitis. Note that early in the course (phase *a*) there is presence of bilirubin and increased amounts of urobilinogen in the urine with elevated serum bilirubin levels. This is followed by the phase (*b*) of deepening jaundice with decreased urine urobilinogen and increased urine bilirubin, after which there is an increase in urine urobilinogen (phase *c*) as the serum and urine bilirubin begin to decrease. In phase *d* bilirubin often disappears from the urine, but serum bilirubin levels are still distinctly elevated. Most patients show or are observed only in phases *c* and *d*, but some show this complete pattern. (Modified from Watson and Hoffbauer: Ann. Int. Med., 25:195, 1947.)

METABOLIC TESTS

A number of hepatic function tests have been based on the role of the liver in carbohydrate, protein, and fat metabolism. Those tests related to carbohydrate metabolism have been least useful and those related to protein metabolism most useful. Only one commonly used test of hepatic function relates to lipid metabolism.

Carbohydrate Metabolism

Patients with hepatic disease may have hypoglycemia; diminished tolerance for administered glucose, galactose, fructose, or lactate; and decreased hepatic glycogen stores, the last being measured by the blood sugar response to administered epinephrine or glucagon.

Hypoglycemia occurs regularly in hepatectomized animals, occasionally in patients with acute hepatic necrosis, but rarely in patients with chronic liver disease. It has been described in biliary cirrhosis, in primary or metastatic carcinoma of the liver, and in the hepatic congestion of heart failure. Hypoglycemia is particularly characteristic of two peculiar forms of fatty livers, one associated with a febrile state in children referred to as *Reye's syndrome* and the other, the rare *fatty liver of pregnancy.* The incidence of hypoglycemia in hepatic disease, however, is low. The hypoglycemia that occurs in alcoholic patients results from acute direct and indirect effects of alcohol, not from the liver disease of alcoholism.

Glucose tolerance is characteristically abnormal in patients with cirrhosis of the liver. There is a rapid rise of the blood sugar value to abnormal levels and a slow return to normal. This pattern in patients with liver disease can be distinguished from that of diabetes mellitus by the normal or low fasting blood sugar in liver disease and the occurrence of subnormal values by the fifth hour after the glucose has been given. Although the oral or intravenous glucose tolerance test is of interest in the study of patients with hepatic disease, it is of little specific value in diagnosis in these patients.

The *galactose tolerance test* has been applied to the study of liver disease for many years. The normal liver is able to convert galactose to glucose, which is stored as glycogen. In patients with hepatic disease this ability is defective. Administration of galactose results in persistence of abnormal blood levels for several hours and in urinary excretion of abnormal amounts of galactose. This test yields abnormal results in patients with hepatocellular jaundice but normal results in patients with obstructive jaundice of brief duration (less than three weeks). Although formerly recommended by some authors for the differential diagnosis of jaundice, this test was never widely employed and today is used in few centers.

The *fructose tolerance test,* based on a principle similar to that of galactose tolerance, has found no clinical application. Elevated blood levels of lactic acid have been described in patients with severe liver disease. This observation and a *lactic acid tolerance test* have been described as tests of hepatic function but also have not been applied extensively to clinical problems.

The *epinephrine tolerance test* has been used to estimate hepatic glycogen stores by observing the blood sugar response to a standard dose of epinephrine. Normal individuals show a blood sugar rise of 40 to 60 mg. per 100 ml. within 1 hour after the epinephrine has been given. Patients with hepatic disease (cirrhosis, hepatitis) and patients with genetic deficiency in glycogenolytic enzymes (glycogen storage disease) show a subnormal response. The test has not been applied widely to the diagnosis of liver disease but has been useful in clinical research and for the diagnosis of glycogen storage disease. The *glucagon tolerance test,* a recent modification of this test, has involved the use of glucagon, instead of or combined with epinephrine, to produce glycogenolysis. In either epinephrine or glucagon tolerance tests the subject should receive a high-carbohydrate diet for three days before the test.

Lipid Metabolism

The liver is importantly involved in many phases of lipid metabolism, including the synthesis, esterification, and excretion of cholesterol. Only the determination of the free and esterified *cholesterol* levels of the serum has been applied intensively to the study of hepatic disease. In normal individuals (in the United States) the serum cholesterol level ranges between 150 and 250 mg. per 100 ml. with approximately 70 per cent (100 to 170 mg. per 100 ml.) esterified. In general, the cholesterol level is normal or depressed in hepatocellular jaundice and elevated in obstructive jaundice. In patients with hepatitis the total cholesterol level may be mildly depressed or normal, but the level of esterified cholesterol is usually moderately decreased. In severe hepatitis or cirrhosis the serum cholesterol (total and esterified) levels may be markedly depressed. In patients with obstructive jaundice or intrahepatic cholestasis the blood cholesterol level is usually elevated to levels of 250 to 500 mg. per 100 ml. Greater elevations occur occasionally but are more characteristic of hepatocanalicular jaundice (intrahepatic cholestasis) than of posthepatic jaundice. In "primary biliary cirrhosis," levels up to 1800 mg. per 100 ml. may be observed. It is generally stated that patients with obstructive jaundice usually have a normal (2/3) cholesterol-ester/total cholesterol ratio. Strictly speaking, this is not true. Although the degree of depression of the ratio is characteristically less than that seen in hepatic disease, moderate degrees are regularly seen. Determination of the cholesterol level is widely used in the diagnosis of hepatic disease, but determination of the ester fraction is of little diagnostic value.

Abnormal values of other plasma lipids occur in patients with hepatic and biliary tract disease. Increased plasma levels of triglycerides are observed in patients with obstructive jaundice, in alcoholic patients with hemolytic anemia, hyperlipemia, and fatty liver (Zieve's syndrome) and in those with pancreatitis. Plasma levels of free fatty acids are increased in patients with all forms of parenchymatous hepatic disease. Plasma levels of phospholipids are increased in obstructive jaundice and in biliary cirrhosis. While measurement of the several lipid fractions has been of investigative interest, it has been too time consuming and complex for routine clinical application.

Bile acids are formed from cholesterol in the liver. Normally they include dihydroxy and trihydroxy "cholic acids" and are excreted as conjugates of glycine (glycocholic acid) and taurine (taurocholic acid). The simple and qualitative methods used in the past (Hay's and Pettenkofer's tests) have shown increased blood and urine levels of bile acids in patients with obstructive jaundice. The lack of satisfactory quantitation and the demonstration that bile acids may also be found in the urine of patients with hepatocellular jaundice prevented the clinical application of these procedures. Quantitative methods have been applied recently to the study of patients with hepatobiliary disease and have yielded characteristic patterns. The methods for the measurement of total serum bile acid levels and of the ratio of the dihydroxy to the trihydroxy acids, however, are too difficult and time consuming for clinical application.

The *cinnamic acid* tolerance test is an interesting test of hepatic function that couples two reactions known to occur in the liver.

These are fatty acid oxidation and conjugation. The normal liver oxidizes (beta oxidation) cinnamic acid to benzoic acid, which in turn is conjugated with glycine to form hippuric acid. Abnormal hepatic function is reflected in the decreased excretion of hippuric acid. Although this test has found no clinical application, it is cited here as an interesting approach to the measurement of hepatic function.

Protein Metabolism

Amino acid metabolism, urea synthesis, and protein metabolism occur in the liver. Evidence of defects in each of these areas may be observed in patients with hepatic disease. These include abnormal plasma levels of amino acids, proteins, urea, and ammonia, and abnormal urine levels of amino acids. Several measures of hepatic function have been based on these phenomena.

Serum Protein Levels. A number of plasma proteins are formed in the liver. These include albumin, fibrinogen, and some of the alpha and beta globulins. Accordingly, changes in the plasma (or serum) proteins form the basis for important laboratory aids to the diagnosis of hepatic disease. Depression of serum albumin is characteristic of chronic hepatic disease. For reasons that are not clear, the *serum globulin* level is often elevated in patients with chronic hepatic disease (cirrhosis), representing mainly the gamma globulin fractions and reflecting, at least in part, immune responses to disease.

The procedures used to evaluate serum protein changes in patients with liver disease include determination of serum albumin and globulin levels, serum electrophoresis, and several turbidometric ("flocculation") tests. The turbidometric tests reflect largely changes of the gamma globulin and albumin levels.

The *serum albumin* level is considered a reliable index of severity and prognosis in patients with chronic hepatic disease. In patients with cirrhosis there is a positive correlation between the degree of hypoalbuminemia and the severity of the ascites. Patients who show a rise of the albumin level have a more favorable prognosis than those whose levels remain low. In patients with acute hepatic disease (viral or toxic hepatitis) serum albumin levels are usually normal or only mildly depressed. Those who develop subacute hepatic necrosis ("subacute yellow atrophy") frequently have moderate to marked hypoalbuminemia.

The total serum globulin level is often elevated in patients with cirrhosis. The degree of elevation is usually moderate in Laennec's and in biliary cirrhosis, with levels of 3 to 4 gm. per 100 ml. In active postnecrotic cirrhosis and in chronic active hepatitis elevations also may be moderate but at times are marked, with values in the range of 6 to 9 gm. per 100 ml. occasionally observed. Levels in patients with acute hepatitis are usually normal or only mildly elevated but in occasional patients may exceed levels of 4 gm. per 100 ml. In patients with obstructive jaundice the globulin level is usually normal, although it may be elevated.

Serum electrophoresis (see Protein Electrophoresis, Chapter 9) is useful to demonstrate the globulin fraction which is elevated. In Laennec's and postnecrotic cirrhosis it reveals that the hyperglobulinemia represents largely gamma globulin elevation. In biliary cirrhosis the alpha-2, beta, and gamma fractions show an increase, while in obstructive jaundice the gamma globulin level is usually normal but the alpha-2 and beta fractions are increased. The serum protein abnormalities in patients with hepatic disease are listed in Table 13–5.

The *total serum protein* level in patients with cirrhosis is occasionally low, often normal, and at times even elevated. Reversal of the "A/G ratio" has been emphasized in this

Table 13–5. ABNORMALITIES OF SERUM PROTEINS IN LIVER DISEASE (MAGNITUDE OF CHANGE INDICATED BY NUMBER OF ARROWS)

	ACUTE HEPATITIS	CIRRHOSIS (LAENNEC'S)	CIRRHOSIS (POST-NECROTIC)*	CIRRHOSIS (BILIARY)	OBSTRUCTIVE JAUNDICE	PRIMARY‡ OR METASTATIC CARCINOMA
Albumin	N or ↓	↓ ↓	↓ ↓	↓	N or ↓	↓
Globulin	N or ↑	↑	↑	↑	N	N
Alpha-1†						
Alpha-2		N	N	↑	↑	↑ ↑
Beta	↑	↑	↑	↑ ↑ ↑	↑ ↑	N
Gamma	↑	↑ ↑	↑ ↑ ↑	↑	N	N

*Includes chronic active hepatitis.

†A majority of patients with primary carcinoma have the abnormal protein alpha beta globulin in their serum (see text).

‡Values not sufficiently consistent to be useful in study of hepatic disease.

Table 13–6. LIST OF SOME FLOCCULATION TESTS INCLUDING SERUM PROTEIN ABNORMALITIES THAT THEY REFLECT*

	PRECIPITATING REAGENT	PROTEIN FRACTIONS PRODUCING ABNORMALITY	ALBUMIN† INHIBITION
Cephalin flocculation	Cephalin-cholesterol emulsion	γ	+
Thymol turbidity	Supersaturated solution thymol	γ (β)	(+)‡
Colloidal gold	Colloidal gold	γ	+
Zinc sulfate turbidity	$ZnSO_4$	γ	(+)
Takata-Ara	$HgCl_2$	γ (β)	+
Cadmium sulfate	$CdSO_4$	γ ($\alpha\beta$)	+

*Modified from Maclagan, N. F., *et al.:* J. Clin. Path. 5:1, 1952.
†Indicates that addition of albumin *in vitro* can convert a positive to a negative result.
‡(+) Indicates that addition of albumin is less effective in decreasing the degree of abnormal results.

and in other hyperglobulinemic diseases. Reference to the A/G ratio, however, is needlessly awkward and imprecise. A low A/G ratio may occur because there is either hyperglobulinemia or hypoalbuminemia or both. The term should be abandoned and the depression or elevation of the respective protein values described.

Flocculation Tests. A large number of tests which reflect abnormality of plasma proteins have been developed. These reactions, which have been called the "flocculation tests," "globulin reactions," or tests of the "serum colloidal stability," have been very useful to the clinician. In Table 13–6 are listed a few of these procedures with an indication of the presumed related protein abnormalities.

These tests have in common the tendency to be abnormal in patients with intrinsic hepatic disease (hepatitis, cirrhosis) and to be normal in patients with obstructive jaundice. Indeed, serum from patients with obstructive jaundice has the property of inhibiting the flocculation or turbidity tests when mixed with serum that gives a positive reaction. The responsible factor for this inhibition may be a phospholipid. In patients with various systemic diseases characterized by hyperglobulinemia (Table 13–7), the flocculation tests also may yield abnormal results. The various tests differ in the relative incidence of abnormality in various diseases. Of greatest application and interest (in the United States) are the cephalin-cholesterol flocculation and thymol turbidity tests. In the European literature there are more references to the use of other flocculation tests.

The *cephalin-cholesterol flocculation* test is positive in approximately 90 per cent of patients with hepatitis and in approximately 60 per cent of patients with cirrhosis (Fig. 13–5). It depends on hypergammaglobulinemia and the degree of inhibition produced by the serum albumin. Albumin decrease contributes to a "positive" cephalin-cholesterol flocculation. It has been stated that a qualitative change in the albumin molecule also contributes to a positive cephalin flocculation result.

The *thymol turbidity* test also depends on the degree of elevation of gamma globulin. The beta globulin fraction has also been considered to play a role, since the precipitate is a thymol-globulin lipid complex. The degree of turbidity has been expressed in arbitrary units (Maclagan units), which may be determined by visual comparison with a turbidity standard or by use of a spectrophotometer. In our laboratory normal individuals have values below 4 units; in some laboratories values as high as 5 or even 6 units have been considered normal.

Table 13–7. CLASSIFICATION OF DISEASES ASSOCIATED WITH HYPERGLOBULINEMIA

I. Infections (especially chronic)
   A. Bacterial (subacute bacterial endocarditis, chronic suppurative infections, granulomatous infections)
   B. Spirochetal (syphilis)
   C. Viral (lymphogranuloma venereum, psittacosis)
   D. Fungal (histoplasmosis, coccidioidomycosis)
   E. Protozoal (leishmaniasis, malaria)
   F. Helminthic
II. Liver disease (cirrhosis, chronic hepatitis)
III. Collagen disease (rheumatoid arthritis, lupus erythematosis, polyarteritis nodosa, scleroderma)
IV. Neoplastic (multiple myeloma, macroglobulinemia, lymphomas, and leukemia, but rarely in carcinoma except for bronchogenic carcinoma)
V. Miscellaneous (sarcoidosis)

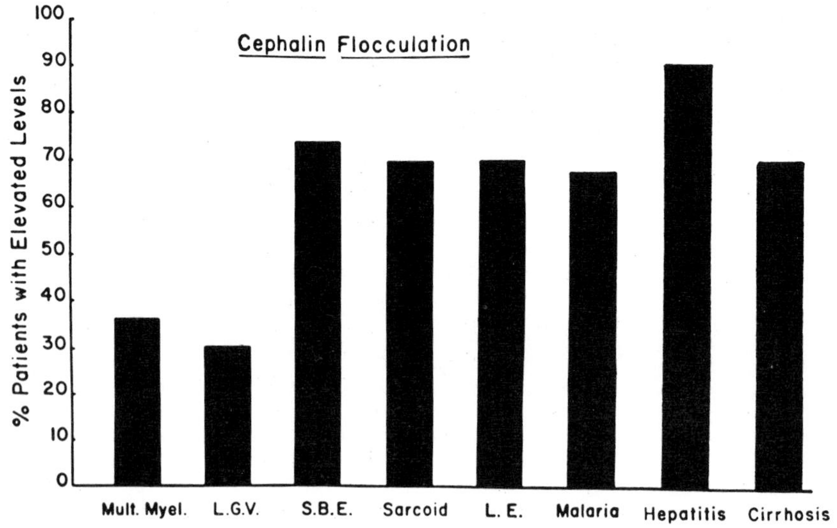

Figure 13–5. Incidence of abnormal cephalin flocculation results in various hyperglobulinemic diseases and in hepatitis and cirrhosis.

Elevated levels are observed in approximately 80 to 90 per cent of patients with acute viral hepatitis and in 20 to 70 per cent of patients with cirrhosis, depending on the stage and type (Fig. 13–6). During the course of viral hepatitis the thymol turbidity becomes abnormal a few days after the cephalin flocculation test but may remain abnormal after the latter has already become normal.

Abnormal values for the thymol turbidity and cephalin flocculation tests occur in a number of other hyperglobulinemic diseases (Figs. 13–5 and 13–6). Technical "false-positive" results may be obtained with sera that have a high lipid content. In fact, the thymol turbidity test has been applied to the estimation of fat absorption by observing changes after ingestion of a fat-containing meal.

The variety of hyperglobulinemic diseases that may yield abnormal values for the flocculation tests has led a number of workers to consider them too nonspecific for clinical application and to suggest that the introduction of the clinically useful enzyme tests has made the flocculation procedures obsolete. Nevertheless, the tests provide useful information and are still employed in some laboratories.

Turbidimetric Estimation of Gamma Globulin Levels. There are several turbidimetric procedures in which the turbidity produced correlates quantitatively with the gamma globulin concentration of the serum. Some of these tests

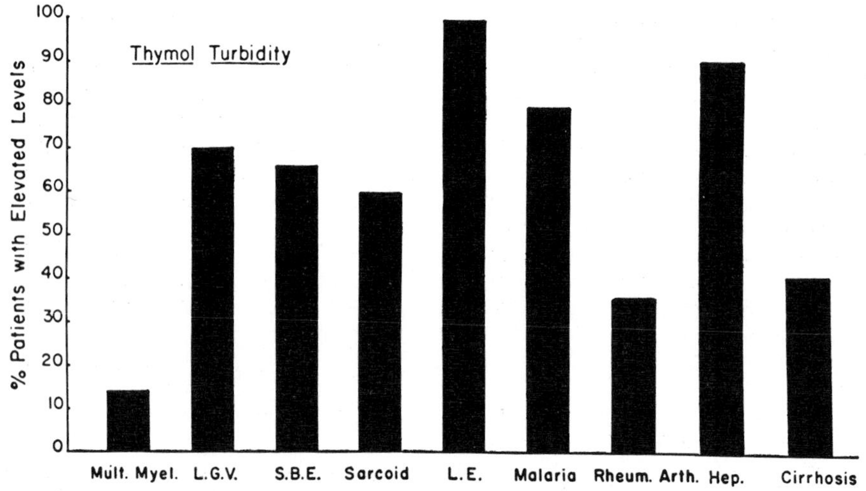

Figure 13–6. Incidence of abnormal thymol turbidity results in various hyperglobulinemic diseases and in hepatitis ("Hep.") and cirrhosis.

depend on the tendency for gamma globulin to be precipitated by low concentrations of metallic or other ions in solutions of low total ionic strength or by high concentrations of salts. One of these, the zinc sulfate turbidity test (Kunkel test), has been applied to the distinction of hepatocellular from obstructive jaundice and in following the levels of gamma globulin in cirrhosis and other hyperglobulinemic diseases. Most laboratories today, however, choose to measure gamma globulin electrophoretically.

Mucoprotein Determinations. Determination of the serum mucoprotein level has been employed in the study of patients with hepatic disease. It has been observed that patients with intrinsic hepatic disease (hepatitis or cirrhosis) have low levels of this group of proteins, presumably because their synthesis by the liver is depressed. Since the patients with obstructive jaundice have been found to have normal or elevated serum mucoprotein levels, this determination has been offered to assist in the differential diagnosis of jaundice but has not been adopted widely.

Haptoglobin levels of the serum also may be abnormal in patients with hepatic disease. Haptoglobins have the chemical characteristics of mucoproteins and migrate with the alpha-2 globulins, but the usual method for serum mucoprotein determination does not measure the haptoglobins. Haptoglobin levels, however, like those of mucoproteins, are high in patients with obstructive jaundice but low in those with hepatocellular disease. Accordingly, the measurement of the serum haptoglobin level has been suggested as an aid to the differential diagnosis of jaundice, but thus far this procedure is only of research interest and not of clinical value.

Alpha-fetoprotein is an alpha globulin which, when present in the serum of adults, is virtually diagnostic of primary carcinoma of the liver (hepatocellular type). It is synthesized only by embryonal liver cells and is found normally only in the serum of the fetus and newborn infant. Studies during the past few years have demonstrated that it is found in the serum of most (30 to 80 per cent) patients with hepatocellular carcinoma and in some children with very undifferentiated teratoblastoma of the ovary or testes. A positive result in any other clinical setting is extremely rare. Accordingly, testing for the alpha-fetoprotein (by immunochemical methods) is being widely employed for the diagnosis of primary carcinoma of the liver.

Aminoaciduria. It has been known for a long time that patients with acute hepatic necrosis ("acute yellow atrophy") have leucine and tyrosine crystals in the urine. These amino acids represent, at least in part, products of autolyzed hepatic tissue. Other amino acids are found in the urine of patients with severe cirrhosis or hepatitis (toxic or viral). This aminoaciduria reflects the elevated levels of blood amino acids that result from impaired amino acid metabolism by the liver as well as from the release from necrotic tissue already described. (See Chapter 2.)

These observations may be applied to the study of hepatic disease. Demonstration of aminoaciduria by paper chromatography is preferable to and more reliable than the laborious search for characteristic tyrosine and leucine crystals. Amino acid content of the blood and urine, however, has found less routine than research application. Tests of hepatic function that have been based on the impaired ability of the damaged liver to metabolize amino acids include the *tyrosine tolerance,* the *methionine tolerance,* the *glycine tolerance,* and the *protein hydrolysate tolerance* tests. Each of these procedures may reveal a defect in the disappearance of administered amino acids from the blood of patients with hepatic disease, but they have not been applied extensively to the study of clinical problems.

Blood Ammonia Determination. A relationship between elevated levels of blood ammonia and liver disease has been recognized for the past 30 years and suspected for over 60 years. It is uncertain whether ammonia, as measured in the blood, represents this substance as such or is ammonia released from some bound state by chemical manipulation.* At any rate, the amount of ammonia released from blood or plasma by treatment with alkali has been shown to be relatable to the severity of the liver disease.

A variety of methods are available for ammonia determination. A simple and widely used method is that of Seligson (1951), which uses whole blood. By the method of Seligson, as modified by Bessman (1959), the normal levels are under 100 μg. per 100 ml. of whole blood.

Studies have shown conclusively that the major source of blood ammonia is the gastrointestinal tract, although a minor contribution is made by the kidney. Bacteria, particularly those in the area of the cecum, release ammonia from nitrogen-containing foods. This ammonia, as well as ammonia ingested as ammonium salts or released from urea by bacterial or other urease, is absorbed into the portal vein. The liver normally removes most

*Almost all the blood "ammonia" is present as NH_4^+ ion rather than NH_3 at the pH of normal blood. Alkalosis increases the levels of free NH_3 by its effect on the equilibrium

$$NH_4^+ \rightleftharpoons NH_3 + H^+$$

This has a bearing on the effect of alkalosis on the neurotoxicity of hyperammonemia, since free NH_3 crosses cell membranes more readily than does NH_4^+ ion.

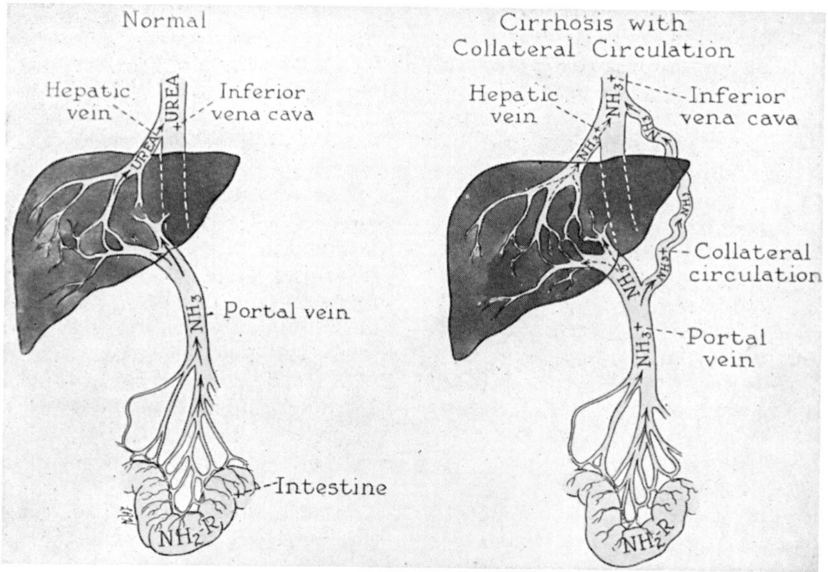

Figure 13–7. Pictorial representation of intestinal formation of ammonia in normal and cirrhotic individuals and of the role of the normal liver in removing ammonia brought to it by the portal blood. Figure also shows the production of elevated plasma ammonia levels by "shunting" of blood through the collateral circulation or by impaired hepatic parenchymal function.

of the ammonia from the portal vein blood, converting it to urea. Little ammonia escapes from the liver into the hepatic vein to be carried to the systemic circulation.

Elevated blood ammonia levels in patients with hepatic disease appear to depend on two mechanisms, "shunting" of portal blood past the liver and impaired parenchymal function (Fig. 13–7). In patients with cirrhosis and extensive collateral portal circulation, elevation of the ammonia levels has been ascribed largely to the shunting of portal blood past the liver. Hepatic vein catheterization studies have shown that patients with severe hepatitis or cirrhosis remove less than normal amounts of ammonia from the portal blood, perhaps as a manifestation of defective urea synthesis.

Elevated ammonia levels are seen in impending or fully developed hepatic coma owing to cirrhosis or severe hepatitis and occasionally in severe heart failure, azotemia, cor pulmonale, and erythroblastosis fetalis. They have also been described in animals and humans with Eck fistulae and in animals in shock.

The use of the blood ammonia determination has been of assistance in the recognition of impending or established hepatic coma. As much or more, however, can be learned by proper clinical appraisal of the patient or by use of electroencephalography. Blood ammonia determination may be useful for monitoring the efficacy of treatment of hepatic coma. An additional application has been suggested: In patients with cirrhosis and hemorrhage from esophageal varices or from any other source in the esophagus, stomach, or small intestine, blood ammonia levels are elevated; whereas in noncirrhotic patients with gastrointestinal bleeding the ammonia levels are usually normal. Combining the ammonia level with the determination of sulfobromphthalein excretion is of assistance in recognizing gastrointestinal bleeding in cirrhotic patients. Measuring the plasma ammonia level after a standard dose of an ammonium salt has been recommended as an aid in estimating the patency of a portocaval shunt.

Steigmann *et al.* (1963) and others have shown that the level of cerebrospinal fluid (CSF) glutamine correlates well with the degree of hepatic encephalopathy. Glutamine is synthesized in brain tissue from ammonia and glutamic acid. As more and more glutamic acid is diverted toward the synthesis of glutamine, intermediates of oxidative metabolism such as α-ketoglutaric acid are depleted. Depletion of these intermediary metabolites of cerebral metabolism is thought to be one of the etiologic factors in hepatic encephalopathy. Normal values for CSF glutamine are less than 12 mg. per 100 ml.

FOREIGN SUBSTANCE EXCRETION

It has been recognized for many years that the abstraction of foreign dyes from the blood by the liver can be applied to the testing of hepatic function. The three dyes of greatest interest for this purpose are rose bengal, sulfobromphthalein (BSP) and indocyanine green. The BSP excretion test is a standard and widely used test of hepatic function. The place of the rose bengal (radioactive) and of the indocyanine green excretion tests in clinical medicine remains to be crystallized. Hepatic extraction of dye from blood perfusing the liver also has been used to measure hepatic blood flow. The technique, which is used primarily as a research tool, involves hepatic vein catheterization, measurement of the fraction of dye extracted per unit volume of blood, and application of the Fick principle.

Rose Bengal Excretion

Rose bengal excretion was the first test of liver function based on the elimination of dyes by the liver that received significant clinical application. In this test the dye was administered parenterally, and either excretion of the dye into the duodenum or retention in the blood was measured. For technical reasons this procedure was considered inferior to the bromsulfalein test and abandoned. Rose bengal excretion has been recently revived with the introduction of rose bengal "tagged" with ^{131}I. The rate of accumulation of the radioactivity over the liver and its rate of disappearance from the liver have been used to help to detect hepatic disease. This procedure has been adapted to the differential diagnosis of jaundice but has not been applied to an extent sufficient to appraise its clinical usefulness. The available data suggest that it may be of help in distinguishing hepatocellular from obstructive jaundice but is of little assistance in distinguishing intrahepatic cholestasis from extrahepatic obstruction. The use of rose bengal and other radioactive substances for scanning of the liver surface is discussed elsewhere in this chapter.

Sulfobromphthalein (BSP) Excretion

The BSP excretion test is one of the most widely used measures of hepatic function. It is also the most sensitive test of liver function. Normal results with this procedure can, for practical purposes, be considered to exclude active parenchymal hepatic disease.

Dye is administered intravenously and the disappearance from the blood is determined. The BSP is almost completely cleared from the blood by the normal liver. (In hepatectomized animals less than 20 per cent of the dye may be removed by extrahepatic tissue.) The two factors involved in BSP excretion by the liver are normal hepatic function and an adequate hepatic circulation.

Excretion of BSP by the liver involves three steps: The dye is (1) transferred from the blood to the hepatic parenchymal cell; (2) it is stored there briefly and conjugated with glutathione; and (3) the conjugate* is excreted by active transport into the bile. Refined techniques are available for the measurement of clearance from the blood and excretion into the bile and for the estimation of storage capacity. Excretion into the bile is the rate-limiting step for which a transport maximum (Tm) has been defined. These measurements and the determination of blood levels of conjugated and unconjugated BSP are research tools useful for unraveling the relative roles of hepatic uptake, conjugation (and storage), and biliary excretion in the clearance of BSP; but they are too elaborate for ordinary clinical use. Simplified techniques have been used to demonstrate defective transport of conjugated BSP into the bile in the Dubin-Johnson syndrome and in individuals with impaired hepatic function induced by methyltestosterone and other C-17 alkylated steroids.

Several standardized tests have been based on the ability of the liver to remove BSP from the blood. In the most widely used procedure a dose of 5 mg. per kg. of body weight is administered intravenously, and a blood specimen is obtained 45 minutes later. (In the original method, the dose of BSP was 2 mg. per kg., and the specimen was drawn at 30 minutes.) The dye level at 45 minutes is expressed as the per cent of dye "retained," i.e., not excreted. A level of 10 mg. per 100 ml. is considered to represent 100 per cent retention.

The determination of the rate of disappearance (percentage disappearance rate [PDR]) by obtaining multiple serum samples after administration of the dye provides a greater degree of accuracy than does the single specimen method but is too elaborate for routine clinical application.

Normal individuals have less than 5 per cent retention at 45 minutes. Abnormal degrees of retention occur in patients with obstructive or hepatocellular jaundice. It is therefore of little diagnostic value to perform the BSP excretion test in patients with jaundice that may be either hepatocellular or obstructive. It is our practice to perform BSP excretion in such patients only when the bilirubin level is below 4 mg. per 100 ml. Although there is evidence that in hepatocellular jaundice the BSP retention at any particular degree of hyperbilirubinemia is greater than in obstructive jaun-

*A small fraction (10 to 20 per cent) of the dye is excreted in the unconjugated form.

dice, this is of no value in the differential diagnosis of jaundice. The estimation of the amount of BSP retained in the blood may be interfered with by high levels of bilirubin if the estimation is done by visual colorimetry or with a photoelectric colorimeter in which specific filters are used. On the other hand, if a spectrophotometer that can establish a precise wavelength is used, BSP levels can be estimated quite satisfactorily in the presence of hyperbilirubinemia. As indicated previously, this is of little diagnostic value. In hemolytic jaundice BSP excretion is usually normal.

Abnormal results are also observed in patients who are not jaundiced if there is parenchymal hepatic disease, biliary tract disease, or extrahepatic disease (Table 13–8).

Excretion of BSP is regularly impaired in patients with disease of the hepatic parenchyma. In Laennec's cirrhosis normal excretion is rarely found. Retention may be slight (5 to 15 per cent) when the degree of cirrhosis is slight or marked (15 to 50 per cent) or when there is severe and "active" disease. When there is ascites or portal hypertension owing to Laennec's cirrhosis, there is a high degree of BSP retention. In postnecrotic cirrhosis, impaired BSP excretion is also frequent, although patients with "healed" postnecrotic cirrhosis, even with severe portal hypertension, may occasionally have normal parenchymal function as measured by BSP excretion.

In fatty metamorphosis of the liver BSP "retention" is frequent and, in general, parallels in degree the intensity of the fatty metamorphosis. Indeed, impaired BSP excretion may be the only abnormal hepatic function in such patients.

Table 13–8. DISEASES CHARACTERIZED BY ABNORMAL BSP EXCRETION

I. Parenchymal hepatic disease
  A. Cirrhosis
  B. Fatty metamorphosis
  C. Viral hepatitis
  D. Toxic hepatic injury
  E. Infectious mononucleosis
II. Biliary tract disease
  A. Common bile duct obstruction (with or without jaundice)
  B. Cholelithiasis and cholecystitis
III. Extrahepatic disease
  A. Circulatory
    1. Congestive heart failure
    2. Hepatic vein occlusion (Chiari's syndrome)
    3. ? Shock
    4. Spinal cord injuries
  B. Systemic disease producing infiltrative lesions of liver
    1. Metastatic carcinoma
    2. Lymphomas and leukemias
    3. Granulomatous disease (tuberculosis, histoplasmosis, sarcoidosis)
    4. Amyloidosis
  C. Nonspecific (fever, chronic and debilitating diseases)

In patients with viral hepatitis BSP excretion is, of course, abnormal during the icteric phase. It remains abnormal, however, after jaundice has subsided and may be abnormal before jaundice has appeared. Similarly, in patients with toxic hepatitis, BSP retention is regularly present. Most patients with infectious mononucleosis (with or without jaundice) have impaired BSP excretion.

In patients with biliary tract obstruction, even when incomplete and producing no jaundice, BSP excretion is usually impaired. Dye excretion is also abnormal in patients with cholecystitis and cholelithiasis.

Patients with nonhepatic disease may also have impaired BSP excretion. In heart failure the BSP retention, which is regularly found, is proportional in degree to the severity of the heart failure, especially as reflected in the degree of venous pressure elevation. In hepatic vein occlusion (Chiari's syndrome) the mechanisms are similar to those of heart failure. Impaired hepatic blood flow and hepatic cell anoxia appear to contribute to the dysfunction. Shock may result in a minimal to moderate degree of BSP excretion. The impairment of BSP excretion observed in paraplegic patients has been ascribed to alterations in hepatic blood flow.

Certain extrahepatic diseases impair liver function by producing infiltrative lesions in the liver. These include metastatic carcinoma, the lymphomas and leukemia, the systemic granulomatous diseases (disseminated tuberculosis, histoplasmosis, coccidioidomycosis, sarcoidosis), and amyloidosis. In metastatic carcinoma, with enough involvement to produce hepatomegaly, there is a 90 per cent incidence of impaired BSP excretion ranging in degree from 5 to 50 per cent retention. In the other diseases cited, the degree of retention is less.

Other nonhepatic diseases lead to impaired BSP excretion by different mechanisms. Febrile illnesses with fever of more than 103° F. usually produce some abnormality of this function. Certain chronic and "debilitating" diseases, such as rheumatoid arthritis, may also lead to moderate impairment of this function.

It is apparent that the BSP excretion test is of greatest value in the patient with little or no jaundice. A normal result is extremely helpful in excluding hepatic parenchymal disease. Patients with gastrointestinal hemorrhage owing to a peptic ulcer usually have normal or minimally abnormal BSP excretion (less than 20 per cent retention), although in about 5 per cent of patients in this category it may be greater. Patients with esophageal varices owing to cirrhosis almost always have moderate to marked degrees of BSP retention (15 to 50 per cent), with the occasional exception in postnecrotic cirrhosis referred to previously. This test is also useful in measuring the severity of liver disease and in assessing the completeness of recovery (e.g., in hepatitis). It is of aid in detecting hepatic damage in patients who have been exposed to hepatotoxins. It is of help in the recognition of metastatic carcinoma. Pitfalls in the application of this test lie in its great sensitivity and, accordingly, in the large number of extrahepatic causes of abnormal values. The extrahepatic causes of impaired BSP excretion do not pose a diagnostic problem if clinical appraisal of the patient is properly done. Conversely, some forms of intrinsic hepatic disease may be associated, though infrequently, with normal BSP excretion. These include occasional instances of hemochromatosis, polycystic disease of the liver, amyloidosis, and inactive postnecrotic cirrhosis. An additional source of error in interpreting results of the BSP test is the interference with excretion of the dye induced by some gallbladder dyes. Accordingly, an unexpectedly abnormal value within 24 hours of a cholecystogram should not be accepted until confirmed by repetition at another time. An extremely rare* but serious complication of BSP administration is anaphylactic (or anaphylactoid) shock. Concern over this reaction has led to some decrease in use of this test.

Indocyanine Green Excretion

Indocyanine green (ICG) excretion has been utilized as a test of hepatic function during the past few years. Excretion of this dye by the liver does not appear to involve conjugation. Furthermore, there is virtually no extrahepatic removal from the blood of ICG, which is removed almost exclusively by the liver. Accordingly, this dye has been studied as a possible substitute for BSP. Results of the ICG excretion test in the dose ordinarily used (0.5 mg./kg.) are comparable to those of the BSP test in patients with severe hepatic disease, but the BSP test appears to be a more sensitive indicator of mild hepatic abnormality than does the ICG. Although ICG has been found to be a very useful dye for hepatic blood flow studies, its eventual role in clinical liver function testing remains to be determined.

DETOXIFICATION AND SYNTHESIS

A number of conjugating reactions occur in the liver. The conjugation of bilirubin with glucuronide to convert the indirect to the direct bilirubin has been discussed. Steroid hormones are metabolized by the liver, and metabolites are excreted as conjugates of glucuronide and other substances. Similarly certain foreign substances are conjugated in the liver and, if toxic, converted to nontoxic products.

*Approximately 1 in 100,000 patients in the experience of the author.

Hippuric Acid Excretion

One conjugating mechanism that has been applied as a measure of liver function is the synthesis of hippuric acid in the liver by the conjugation of benzoic acid with glycine. The test consists of administering a standard amount of benzoic acid orally or sodium benzoate intravenously and determining the amount of hippuric acid excreted in a specific period of time. The ability to synthesize hippuric acid depends not only on the conjugating enzyme systems of the liver but also on the availability of glycine stores in the liver. Furthermore, the hippuric acid formed is measured by its concentration in the urine. This depends, therefore, on renal function, which must be intact to use hippuric acid excretion as a reflection of hepatic function. Excretion of hippuric acid after a standard dose of benzoic acid has been found to be decreased in patients with intrinsic hepatic disease, such as cirrhosis or severe hepatitis. It has been advocated for use in the differential diagnosis of jaundice, since in early obstructive jaundice excretion of hippuric acid is generally normal. Although formerly popular, this test has fallen into disuse. In the opinion of the author it is mainly of historic interest.

Prothrombin Level and Vitamin K Response

It has been known for a long time that patients with severe hepatic disease as well as those with obstructive jaundice may have coagulation defects. It was observed in 1940 that vitamin K deficiency results in hypoprothrombinemia and that vitamin K, which is fat soluble, requires bile salts for absorption. This led to the recognition that bleeding tendencies in obstructive jaundice could be improved by the parenteral administration of vitamin K. The hypoprothrombinemia of obstructive jaundice was then considered to be due to vitamin K deficiency resulting from lack of absorption. The hypoprothrombinemia of the patient with parenchymatous hepatic disease was not restored to normal by parenteral administration of vitamin K.

On this basis a test of hepatic function was devised. Administration of a standard dose of vitamin K to a patient with obstructive jaundice usually restores prolonged prothrombin time to normal, whereas it fails to do so in patients with the hypoprothrombinemia of intrinsic hepatic diseases. This test has been considered to be of some value for the differential diagnosis of jaundice. In a patient with deep jaundice the restoration of an abnormal prothrombin time to normal by vitamin K administration may be considered good evidence that jaundice is obstructive. Lack of improvement of the marked prolongation of the prothrombin time may be considered good evidence that the jaundice is hepatocellular. There are several pitfalls to the application of this procedure. Patients with obstructive jaundice may have only a mildly prolonged prothrombin time; the difference after administration of vitamin K, therefore, may be insufficient to provide a conclusive answer. Furthermore, in intrinsic hepatic disease (even with deep jaundice), parenchymal dysfunction at times may be relatively slight, and the response of the hypoprothrombinemia may be similar to that of obstructive jaundice. This is particularly characteristic of patients whose hepatic disease simulates obstructive jaundice in other respects ("intrahepatic cholestasis" and "cholangiolitic hepatitis").

The degree of hypoprothrombinemia in patients with parenchymal hepatic disease is a useful measure of the severity of the hepatic injury. In patients with acute hepatitis, marked prolongation of the prothrombin "time" is an ominous sign and may herald a fatal outcome. In cirrhosis it is also a reflection of severely impaired parenchymal function.

It has been recognized recently that coagulation defects in patients with hepatic disease or even with obstructive jaundice may include factors other than prothrombin deficiency (Table 13–9). The normal liver synthesizes factors of the "prothrombin complex" (II, VII, IX and X), factor V, fibrinogen and probably factor XIIIa, the fibrin-stabilizing factor. The prolonged prothrombin time (one-stage method) frequently observed in parenchymal hepatic disease probably reflects depression of all the factors of the prothrombin complex. Measurable deficiency of factor V, however, is found only in association with severe liver disease. Deficiency of fibrinogen synthesis is a preterminal event and of little clinical significance.

Table 13–9. CLOTTING ABNORMALITIES IN PATIENTS WITH LIVER DISEASE

Deficiency of plasma factors	
Prothrombin	
Factors VII	Measured by one-stage prothrombin time
IX	Measured by one-stage prothrombin time
X	Measured by one-stage prothrombin time
V	Measured by one-stage prothrombin time
Fibrinogen	
(XIIIa)	
Thrombocytopenia (as result of hypersplenism)	
Decreased platelet adhesiveness	
Disseminated intravascular coagulation	
Fibrinolysins	

Excess fibrinolysis, either as a direct reflection of liver disease, or more probably as the result of the disseminated intravascular coagulation syndrome (D.I.C.) may be responsible for a hemorrhagic tendency in patients with terminal cirrhosis. Thrombocytopenia secondary to hypersplenism and decreased platelet adhesiveness also contribute to hypocoagulability of the blood. In spite of these difficulties response of the prothrombin time to parenteral vitamin K may be a useful ancillary measure in the differential diagnosis of jaundice.

ENZYME LEVELS OF BLOOD*

A large number of enzymes are found in normal serum or plasma, to which they gain access from the tissues. The characteristically abnormal serum enzyme levels produced by various diseases and the general aspects of serum enzymology are considered in Chapter 14. The present discussion describes the type of change in serum enzyme levels caused by hepatic disease and deals with the clinical usefulness of a few enzyme tests for the diagnosis of disease of the liver and biliary tree.

Serum enzymes can be arranged into four categories according to the changes in their levels produced by obstructive jaundice and acute hepatitis (Table 13–10). *Group I* includes enzymes the levels of which are higher in obstructive jaundice than they are in acute hepatitis. The prototype of this group is alkaline phosphatase (Alk. phosph.). This category also includes leucine aminopeptidase (LAP), 5′-nucleotidase (5′-N), and glutamyl transpeptidase (Gl TP). *Group II* includes enzymes the levels of which are much higher in acute hepatitis than in obstructive jaundice. The best known members of this group are the glutamic oxaloacetic (GOT)† and the glutamic pyruvic (GPT)‡ transaminases. Ornithine carbamoyl transferase (OCT), isocitric dehydrogenase (ICD), aldolase (Ald.), sorbitol dehydrogenase (Sorb. D.), and a number of other enzymes are also in this category. In *Group III* are enzymes the levels of which are elevated

*References relevant to this section will be found at the end of Chapter 14.

†Also referred to as aspartate aminotransferase.

‡Also referred to as alanine aminotransferase.

Table 13–10. CATEGORIES OF SERUM ENZYMES ACCORDING TO THEIR BEHAVIOR IN HEPATITIS AND OBSTRUCTIVE JAUNDICE

GROUP	CHARACTERISTICS	PROTOTYPE	OTHER ENZYMES IN GROUP
I	Higher in obstructive jaundice than in hepatitis	Alk. phosph.	LAP, 5′-N, GTP
II	Higher in hepatitis than in obstructive jaundice	GOT, GPT	OCT, ICD, Sorb. D., Ald.
III	Normal or only slightly elevated in hepatitis and obstructive jaundice	LDH, CPK	Lipase Lecithinase Amylase
IV	Depressed in hepatitis and normal in obstructive jaundice	Cholinesterase	Cholesterol esterase

only slightly or not at all in hepatitis and in obstructive jaundice. This group includes lactic dehydrogenase (LDH), creatine phosphokinase (CPK), lipase, lecithinase, and a number of other enzymes. A fourth main type of serum enzyme response to hepatic disease (*Group IV*) is seen with cholinesterase, the levels of which are *decreased* in acute hepatitis and normal or only slightly decreased in obstructive jaundice.

The selection of the serum enzyme tests for the diagnosis of hepatic and biliary disease has been based on sufficient experience in correlating the serum levels with other measures of hepatic function and disease to assure adequate sensitivity and specificity, and on the technical ease of performing the procedure. These considerations have led to the widespread adoption of alkaline phosphatase, glutamic oxaloacetic transaminase, and glutamic pyruvic transaminase measurement for the diagnosis of hepatic and related disease. These virtually routine hepatic tests are discussed in the following pages. The levels of other serum enzymes in hepatic and other types of disease are considered in Chapter 14.

Alkaline Phosphatase

Alkaline phosphatase, the first serum enzyme to be studied in hepatic disease, has been extensively applied to the differential diagnosis of jaundice. Early interest in this enzyme focused on the elevated levels seen in patients with osteoblastic bone disease, presumably as a reflection of increased activity of the osteoblasts, which are rich in phosphatase. This was soon followed, however, by the observation that values of alkaline phosphatase were also increased in patients with obstructive (posthepatic) jaundice. When the obstruction is complete, the serum enzyme activity is almost always increased, with levels often above 25 Bodansky units (normal, 1 to 4 B.U.). Levels below 25 units, however, may be observed in patients with obstructive jaundice, especially when the obstruction is incomplete. Biliary obstruction resulting from carcinoma produces higher values than those observed in patients with gallstones producing obstruction. One variety of obstructive jaundice with normal alkaline phosphatase levels in the serum is that seen in infants with congenital atresia of the extrahepatic biliary tree. In these patients the serum alkaline phosphatase level is not elevated unless bony lesions of hepatic rickets develop. In contrast, infants with intrahepatic biliary atresia show striking elevations of serum alkaline phosphatase values (Table 13–11).

Elevated levels of serum alkaline phosphatase also occur in hepatocellular jaundice. Approximately 90 per cent of patients with viral hepatitis or with toxic hepatocellular jaundice have elevated serum alkaline phosphatase values. Almost all these have values below 15 Bodansky units (B.U.), and in most the value is below 10 units. Approximately 5 per cent of patients with hepatocellular jaundice may have levels of 15 to 25 units. In otherwise characteristic viral hepatitis it is rare to have alkaline phosphatase levels above 25 units. In jaundiced patients with higher levels posthepatic jaundice should be considered.

Occasional patients with hepatic disease may present a laboratory and clinical picture simulating obstructive jaundice. This has been called "intrahepatic cholestasis" or *hepatocanalicular jaundice* (Table 13–4). Although it has been considered to be a form of viral hepatitis ("cholangiolitic hepatitis"),* it is usually idiopathic or a manifestation of drug-induced hepatic injury. Drugs particularly likely to produce hepatocanalicular jaundice are chlorpromazine or organic arsenicals. Patients with intrahepatic cholestasis have values of alkaline phosphatase at least as high as those observed in patients with posthepatic jaundice.

*A poor term since it implies the etiology to be viral hepatitis, which is probably rarely true, and suggests that cholangiolar inflammation is the pertinent lesion, also untrue.

Table 13–11. ALKALINE PHOSPHATASE VALUES IN HEPATOBILIARY DISEASE

DISEASE	INCIDENCE ALK. PHOSPH. ELEVATION	USUAL RANGE OF VALUES	INCIDENCE OF VALUE >20 B.U.
1. Jaundiced states			
Hepatic jaundice			
Hepatocellular	80-100%	5-15 B.U.	5%
Hepatocanalicular	100%	15-70 B.U.	30%
Posthepatic			
Obstruction due to neoplasm	95-100%	15-40 B.U.	80%
Obstruction due to gallstone	95-100%	10-25 B.U.	40%
Congenital atresia of bile ducts	100%		
Intrahepatic	20- 30%	50-70 B.U.	100%
Extrahepatic		N-15 B.U.	0
2. Jaundice absent or present			
Infectious mononucleosis	60- 70%	5-40 B.U.	20%
Cirrhosis, Laennec's	40%	5-15 B.U.	5%
Cirrhosis, postnecrotic	50%	5-35 B.U.	15%
Cirrhosis, biliary, primary	100%	15-100 B.U.	50%
3. No jaundice			
Space-occupying lesions			
Carcinoma	80%	5-70 B.U.	20%
Tuberculosis	50%	5-50 B.U.	10%
Sarcoidosis	40%	5-18 B.U.	15%
Amyloidosis	Frequent	5-100 B.U.	–
Stone in common duct or in one hepatic duct	Frequent	5-90 B.U.	–

The serum alkaline phosphatase level is of value in the differentiation of hepatocellular from obstructive jaundice with several qualifying considerations. As stated previously, levels in the "obstructive" jaundice range may occur in intrinsic hepatic disease, and levels in the "hepatocellular" range may be seen in patients with incomplete biliary obstruction. When taken with other measures of liver disease and clinical features, it is a useful diagnostic aid.

Serum alkaline phosphatase elevation may also occur in nonjaundiced patients with hepatobiliary disease. In patients with "space-occupying" lesions of the liver, such as granulomatous disease, metastatic or primary carcinoma of the liver, liver abscess, and amyloidosis, the degree of alkaline phosphatase elevation may at times be striking (50 to 100 B.U.), with little or no rise in the serum bilirubin values. This pattern of hepatic dysfunction is useful in the recognition of these "space-occupying" lesions, particularly in the recognition of metastasis to the liver in patients with carcinomatosis (Table 13–11).

There is another type of disease associated with normal or only slightly elevated serum bilirubin levels but with distinctly increased alkaline phosphatase levels. This is occlusion of one hepatic duct or incomplete occlusion of the common bile or hepatic duct. This condition should be kept in mind, particularly in dealing with patients with cholelithiasis who develop this "dissociated" pattern of hepatic dysfunction.

Levels of alkaline phosphatase in Laennec's cirrhosis are usually normal or only mildly elevated. In postnecrotic cirrhosis the levels are generally somewhat higher. In biliary cirrhosis elevated levels of alkaline phosphatase are regularly seen. In obstructive biliary cirrhosis the elevations are modest, usually under 15 B.U., except during bouts of ascending cholangitis. In patients with primary biliary cirrhosis, alkaline phosphatase levels in the range already described for "cholangiolitic hepatitis" may be seen.

The basis for elevated serum levels of alkaline phosphatase in patients with hepatobiliary disease is obscure. Impaired hepatic excretion of enzyme formed in bone or liver or both was considered formerly to be the mechanism. Increased formation of alkaline phosphatase by hepatic parenchymal or ductal cells, perhaps supplemented by impaired excretion, is the apparent mechanism.

Transaminase

Enzymes that catalyze the reversible transfer of an alpha amino group from an amino acid to an alpha keto acid (Fig. 13–8) were first demonstrated in animal tissue by Braunshtein

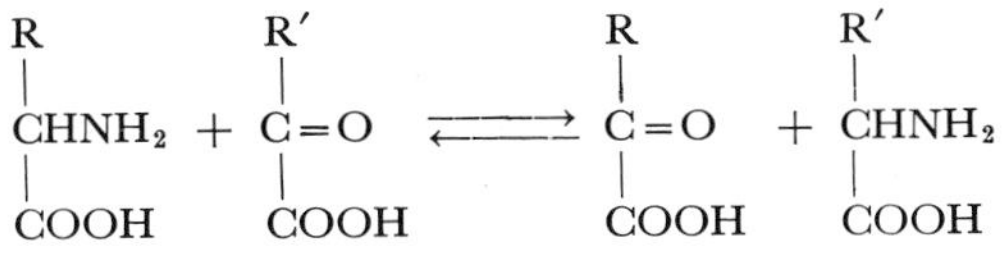

$$
\begin{array}{ccccccc}
\text{R} & & \text{R}' & & \text{R} & & \text{R}' \\
| & & | & & | & & | \\
\text{CHNH}_2 & + & \text{C}=\text{O} & \rightleftharpoons & \text{C}=\text{O} & + & \text{CHNH}_2 \\
| & & | & & | & & | \\
\text{COOH} & & \text{COOH} & & \text{COOH} & & \text{COOH}
\end{array}
$$

Figure 13–8. Prototype of transamination reactions.

and Kritzmann in 1937. These authors called the enzymes *aminopherases*. Although a large number of substrate-specific transaminases have been demonstrated in various animal tissues, only two have been described in the serum, *glutamic oxaloacetic transaminase* (GOT) and *glutamic pyruvic transaminase* (GPT). Abnormal levels of GOT are seen in patients with hepatic disease, myocardial and skeletal muscle necrosis, and other diseases to be described. Glutamic pyruvic transaminase (GPT) elevations are absent or slight in disease that does not involve the liver primarily or secondarily.

Glutamic Oxaloacetic Transaminase. Glutamic oxaloacetic transaminase (GOT) is an enzyme that catalyzes the reversible transfer of the amino group from glutamic to oxaloacetic acid (Fig. 13–9). It has been demonstrated in the serum and tissues of all animals studied. In man it is found in cardiac, hepatic, skeletal muscle, renal, and cerebral tissue in decreasing concentrations. The recognition of the high myocardial content of this enzyme led to the observation, in 1953, that patients with acute myocardial infarction had elevated levels in the serum for a few days after the infarction. Shortly thereafter studies in several laboratories showed high serum levels of this enzyme in patients and animals with acute hepatic necrosis.

The activity of this serum enzyme was first demonstrated by a chromatographic technique, which was too laborious for routine use. The methods that have been used for routine determination have included the spectrophoto-

GLUTAMIC OXALOACETIC TRANSAMINASE

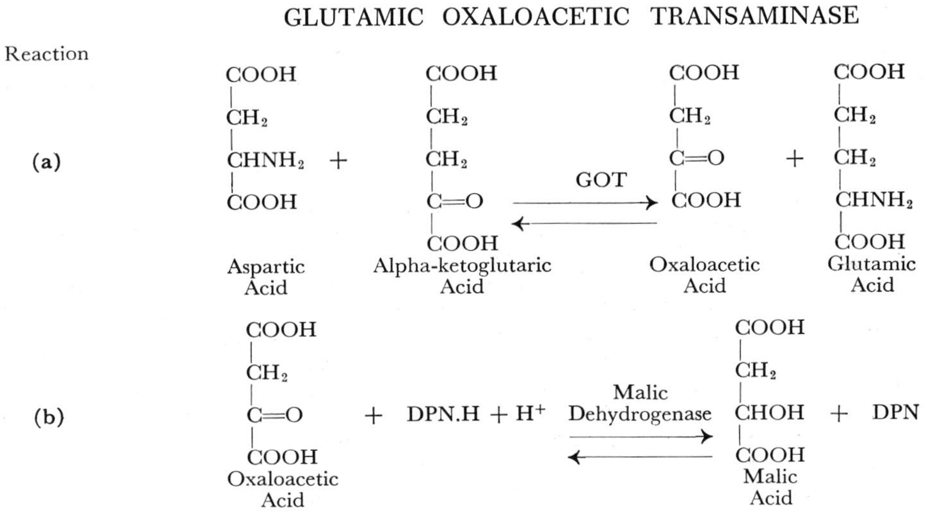

Figure 13–9. Reaction catalyzed by GOT, principles of assay methods, and conditions in which increased serum levels are observed.

Method of assay is based on measurement of rate of formation of product (oxaloacetic acid) of the reaction. This may be done (1) indirectly, by the coupled reaction (b) in which the rate of DPNH oxidation, in the presence of added malic dehydrogenase is a measure of oxaloacetic acid formed (method of Karmen), or (2) directly, by one of several colorimetric methods that depend on the formation of the dinitrophenylhydrazone of oxaloacetate or its decarboxylation product (pyruvate) or other colorimetric reactions.

Conditions in which abnormal serum levels of enzyme are observed include the following:

    A. *Hepatic Disease*
        Hepatic necrosis
            Hepatitis (infectious, toxic), infectious mononucleosis
            Cirrhosis
            Hematogenous tuberculosis
            Hepatic congestion
        Metastatic carcinoma
        Obstructive jaundice
    B. *Other Disease*
        Myocardial infarction
        Skeletal muscle necrosis
        Hemolysis (slight)
        Pancreatitis (acute)
        Renal necrosis
        Cerebral necrosis

metric procedure of Karmen (1955) and several simplified colorimetric procedures (Fig. 13–9 and Chapter 14). Most laboratories express the value in "Karmen units." The normal range is 6 to 40 units per ml. of serum. Conversion of these units to International milli-units may be accomplished by dividing the value by a factor (1.95).

The range of values of GOT in patients with various types of hepatic disease and in myocardial infarction is shown in Figure 13–10. Striking elevations (300 to 4000 units per ml.) are observed in the serum of patients with acute hepatic necrosis (viral hepatitis, carbon tetrachloride poisoning). Patients with posthepatic jaundice and intrahepatic cholestasis have more modest elevations (usually less than 300 units per ml.). In patients with cirrhosis of the liver there is a 60 to 70 per cent incidence of elevated GOT levels (also below 300 units per ml.).

Approximately half the patients with metastatic carcinoma have elevated serum GOT levels, usually in the same range as patients with cirrhosis and posthepatic jaundice. Less frequently such moderately elevated GOT levels are observed in patients with lymphoma and leukemia. In 80 per cent of patients with infectious mononucleosis moderate (100 to 600 units) GOT elevations are observed. Patients with myocardial infarction usually show GOT levels of less than 400 units. The incidence and significance of GOT elevations in patients with this and other nonhepatic conditions are discussed in Chapter 14.

Glutamic Pyruvic Transaminase. This enzyme catalyzes the reversible transfer of an amino group from glutamic to pyruvic acid (Fig. 13–11). It also has been found to be widely distributed in humans. The high hepatic content compared to the relatively low concentration in myocardial and other tissues has led to the application of GPT determination to the study of hepatic disease.

The methods used for determination of this enzyme in the serum are similar to those used

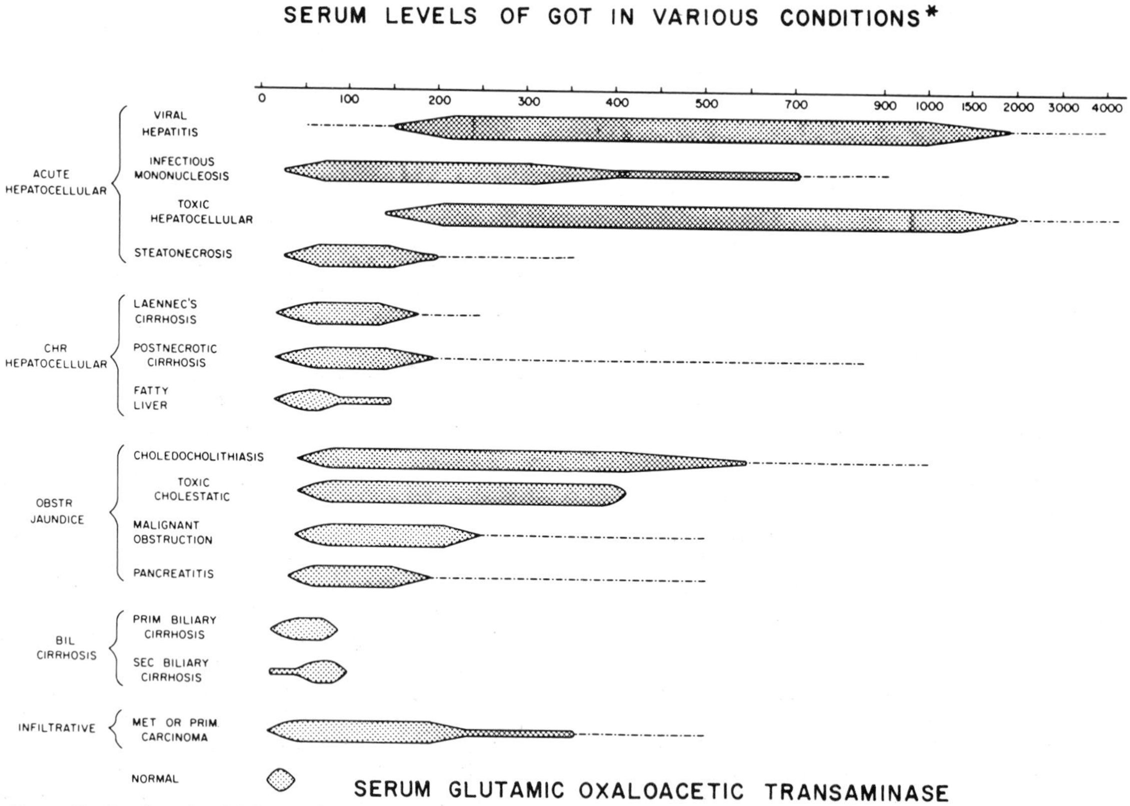

Figure 13–10. Levels of GOT in "Karmen units" observed in patients with various types of liver disease. "Toxic" hepatocellular refers to some types of drug (e.g., halothane) toxicity or CCl_4 poisoning. Steatonecrosis refers to "alcoholic hepatitis." Values shown for postnecrotic cirrhosis are also characteristic of chronic active hepatitis. Toxic cholestatic jaundice refers to drug-induced or other acute intrahepatic cholestasis. "Prim" biliary cirrhosis also is called "chronic intrahepatic cholestasis." "Sec" biliary cirrhosis refers to the cirrhosis that follows prolonged obstruction of the common bile or hepatic duct. "Met" refers to metastatic and "prim" refers to primary carcinoma of the liver, respectively. From Zimmerman, H. J. and Seeff, L. B.: Enzymes in Hepatic Disease. In Diagnostic Enzymology. Coodley, E. L. (Ed.) Lea and Febiger, Philadelphia, 1970 (with permission).

GLUTAMIC PYRUVIC TRANSAMINASE

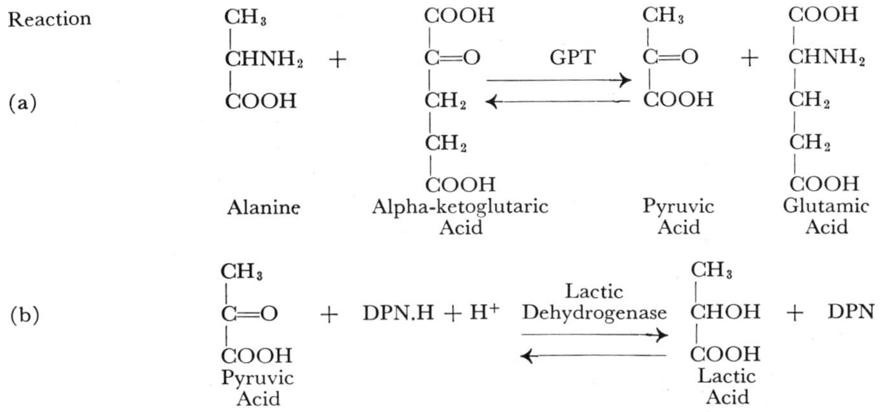

Figure 13–11. Reaction catalyzed by GPT, principles of assay methods, and conditions in which increased serum levels are observed.

Method of assay is based on measurement of rate of formation of product (pyruvic acid) of reaction. This may be done (1) indirectly by the coupled reaction (b) in which the rate of DPNH oxidation, in the presence of added lactic dehydrogenase, is a measure of pyruvic acid formed (method of Karmen), or (2) directly, by one of several colorimetric methods that depend on formation of the dinitrophenylhydrazone of pyruvate.

Conditions in which abnormal serum levels of enzyme are observed, arranged in the order of decreasing levels:

A. *Hepatic Disease Abnormalities*
   - Hepatic necrosis; e.g., hepatitis (infectious, toxic), infectious mononucleosis, cirrhosis
   - Obstructive jaundice
   - Metastatic carcinoma
   - Hepatic congestion (centrilobular liver cell necrosis) secondary to heart failure or hepatic vein thrombosis

B. *Other Abnormalities (Slight)*
   - Myocardial infarction
   - Acute pancreatitis

for GOT assay. Both spectrophotometric and colorimetric methods have been employed. The normal range for this enzyme in Karmen units is almost the same as that for the GOT (6 to 36 units per ml.).

Patients with viral hepatitis and other forms of hepatic necrosis usually show striking elevations of the serum GPT level (500 to 4000 units). Values of GPT are modestly elevated (300 units) in most patients with posthepatic jaundice, intrahepatic cholestasis, metastatic carcinoma, cirrhosis or alcoholic steatonecrosis (alcoholic hepatitis). Values for GPT are as high or higher than those of GOT in most patients with viral hepatitis, posthepatic jaundice, or intrahepatic cholestasis, while they are much lower than the respective values for GOT in patients with cirrhosis or metastatic carcinoma. Levels of GPT are normal or only minimally elevated in patients with myocardial infarction (Fig. 13–12).

Clinical Value of Transaminase Determination. The determination of the serum transaminase is of distinct clinical aid. Differentiation of hepatic (hepatocellular) from posthepatic jaundice is facilitated by determining the GOT or GPT values, since levels above 300 units per ml. are rare in patients with posthepatic jaundice. In the hepatocanalicular type of hepatic jaundice (intrahepatic cholestasis) the GOT (or GPT) levels are like those of posthepatic jaundice. Likewise in cirrhosis of the liver, even with deep jaundice, the moderate GOT level and the lower GPT level are in contrast with the high levels of both transaminases observed in acute viral hepatitis. Determination of GOT, GPT, or both is useful in the early recognition of viral or toxic hepatitis and is, therefore, helpful in studying patients exposed to hepatotoxic drugs. Elevations of the GPT level appear to reflect acute hepatic disease somewhat more specifically than is true of the GOT values. The level of either enzyme, particularly the GOT, may be elevated in patients with extrahepatic disease. (See Chapter 14.)

The levels of alkaline phosphatase, GOT, and GPT are individually helpful in the differential diagnosis of hepatic disease. Their diagnostic usefulness may be enhanced by observing the patterns of abnormality obtained by measuring all three, especially when combined with lactic dehydrogenase levels. (See Chapter 14.) In Figure 13–13 are shown diagrammatically the patterns obtained with a variety of hepatic lesions. The very high values for GOT and GPT and relatively slightly elevated ones for alkaline phosphatase observed in acute hepatitis and other necroinflammatory diseases of the

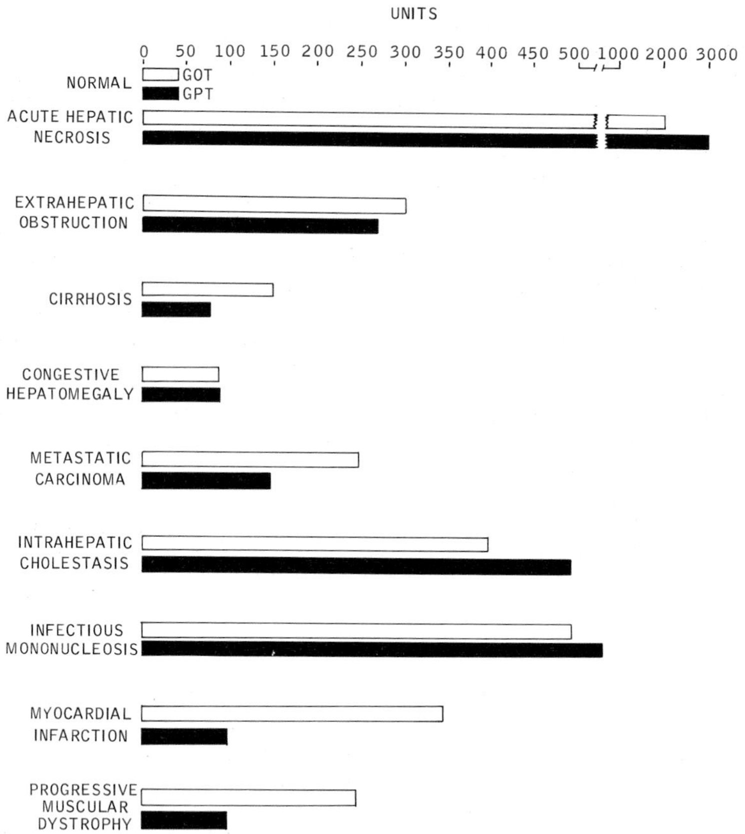

Figure 13–12. Relative levels of glutamic oxaloacetic transaminase and glutamic pyruvic transaminase in patients with hepatic, biliary, and other diseases.

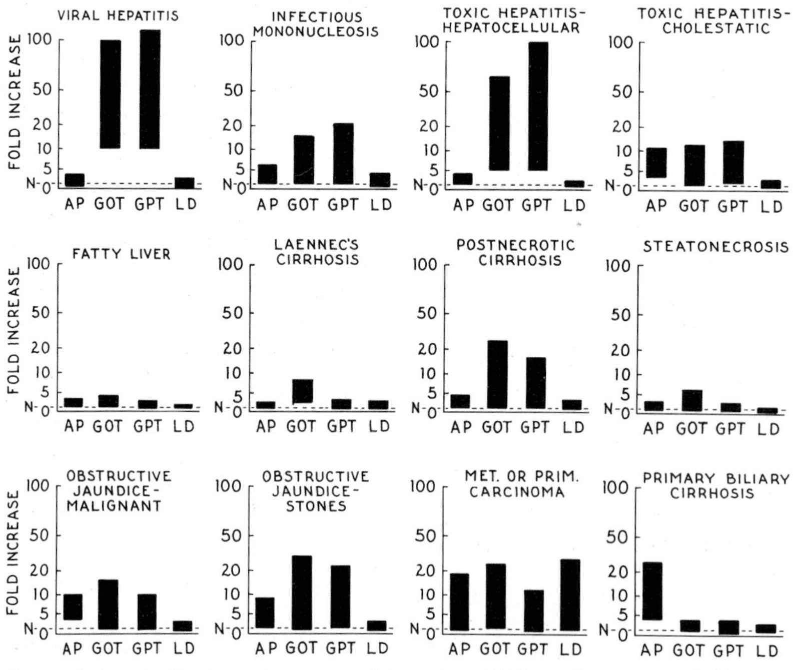

Figure 13–13. Patterns of abnormality in various types of hepatic and biliary disease provided by levels of alkaline phosphatase (AP), glutamic oxaloacetic transaminase (GOT), glutamic pyruvic transaminase (GPT), and lactic dehydrogenase (LD).

liver differ sharply from the lower transaminase and higher alkaline phosphatase values of obstructive jaundice. The pattern of the "incomplete" obstructive jaundice of choledocholithiasis overlaps with that of hepatitis, while the patterns of acute hepatocanalicular jaundice or of biliary cirrhosis simulate that of posthepatic jaundice.

The patterns in cirrhosis are characteristically different. In Laennec's cirrhosis, GOT elevations are slight, GPT values even lower, and lactic dehydrogenase (LD) and alkaline phosphatase values very slightly elevated or normal. In inactive postnecrotic cirrhosis, the values resemble those of Laennec's cirrhosis; but in active postnecrotic cirrhosis and chronic active hepatitis, the GOT values may be as low as those of Laennec's cirrhosis or as high as those of hepatitis, and the values of the two transaminases may be approximately equally elevated. The pattern of metastatic or primary carcinoma of the liver is distinctive in that the transaminase levels resemble those of Laennec's cirrhosis, while the LD and alkaline phosphatase levels are much higher. (See Chapter 14 for LD values in carcinomatosis.)

The various patterns are not necessarily pathognomonic of the respective entity, since overlapping of values and patterns may be observed. Nevertheless, when taken with other diagnostic measures they may be of great diagnostic assistance.

SERUM "METALS"

Abnormal levels of certain metallic substances are found in patients with some hepatic diseases. Elevated serum *iron* levels and reduced iron-binding capacity are observed in patients with hemochromatosis and transfusion hemosiderosis and may be of aid in diagnosis. Acute elevations of serum iron levels are observed in viral hepatitis and in other patients with acute hepatic necrosis. It has been observed that patients with obstructive jaundice usually have normal serum iron levels. This has led to the application by European and South American workers of the serum iron level determination to the differential diagnosis of jaundice. This application, however, has not been adopted widely in this country.

Elevated blood levels of "free" *copper* and increased amounts of tissue copper have been observed in patients with Wilson's disease (hepatolenticular degeneration). The increased levels of free copper are associated, in most patients with this disease, with decreased levels of ceruloplasmin, a copper-carrying protein that is also an enzyme (copper oxidase). Diagnosis of Wilson's disease is aided by the demonstration of depressed levels of ceruloplasmin in the plasma. Increased levels of serum and tissue copper are also observed in primary biliary cirrhosis.

Abnormal levels of other metallic ions of the blood have been described in patients with chronic hepatic disease. Depressed serum levels of *zinc* have been reported in patients with "alcoholic cirrhosis." The significance of this observation remains to be determined. Lower than normal serum *magnesium* levels have been reported in alcoholic patients with delirium tremens and with cirrhosis. Among the factors considered responsible is malnutrition. In cirrhotics with ascites the *hyponatremia* commonly observed is considered to be a manifestation of water retention, not sodium loss. *Hypokalemia* is frequent in patients with hepatic coma.

LIVER FUNCTION TESTS BASED ON ROLE OF LIVER IN VITAMIN ECONOMY

Deficiency in a number of vitamins is prone to occur in the malnourished alcoholic patient. Accordingly, in alcoholic cirrhosis evidence of beriberi, pellagra, and scurvy may be observed. In addition, abnormal levels of vitamins A and B_{12} have been described in patients with hepatic disease.

Depressed plasma levels of vitamin A are characteristic of patients with parenchymal hepatic disease. The observation that patients with early obstructive jaundice usually have normal levels has led to the application of vitamin A level determination to the differential diagnosis of jaundice. The dependence of the absorption of this fat-soluble vitamin on an adequate concentration of bile salts in the duodenum, however, also leads to depressed levels in obstructive jaundice; accordingly, this determination is of little value in the differential diagnosis of jaundice.

Vitamin B_{12} is stored in the liver. In patients with acute viral hepatitis very high plasma levels of this vitamin are observed, presumably resulting from release by necrotic hepatic cells. Somewhat elevated levels are observed in cirrhosis also. A test of hepatic function based on the estimation of the hepatic "uptake" of an oral dose of vitamin B_{12} labeled with radioactive cobalt has been described. The clinical value of these determinations remains to be confirmed by adequate trial.

LIVER BIOPSY

In considering the laboratory approach to the diagnosis of hepatic disease, reference should be made to needle biopsy of the liver. This procedure, which has been widely used during the last decade, is of assistance in the diagnosis of hepatic and nonhepatic disease.

It is particularly useful in the differential diagnosis of hepatomegaly. It may be helpful in defining the specific cause of hepatocellular jaundice (e.g., hepatitis or cirrhosis). The application of needle biopsy to the differentiation of hepatic from posthepatic jaundice, however, is limited. The procedure is hazardous in patients with complete obstruction of the common bile duct. Furthermore, in those instances in which the differential diagnosis is difficult on clinical and biochemical grounds, the histologic distinction is also difficult. Liver biopsy may be of assistance in the diagnosis of the cause of ascites and in the differential diagnosis of gastrointestinal hemorrhage. Of interest has been the usefulness of this procedure in the diagnosis of systemic diseases that produce recognizable lesions in the liver (Table 13–12). The indications and contraindications are also shown in Table 13–12.

RADIOISOTOPES IN DIAGNOSIS OF HEPATIC DISEASE

A variety of radioisotopic substances have been applied to the study of hepatic disease. Radioactive (I^{131}) rose bengal, the most widely used, has been employed as a test of hepatic function, as a means of measuring hepatic blood flow, and for scintillation scanning of the liver. Other isotopic compounds that have been used include ^{60}Co- or ^{58}Co-labeled cyanocobalamin and radioactive molybdate (^{99}Mo), proposed for measurement of hepatic function, and ^{51}Cr-labeled chromic phosphate, ^{131}I-labeled albumin, radioactive colloidal gold (^{198}Au or ^{199}Au, and, most recently, technetium-99m proposed as measures of hepatic blood flow. The only regular clinical application of radioisotopes to the study of hepatic disease is scintillation scanning. (See Chapter 7.)

Photoscanning (scintiscanning, scintillation scanning, liver scanning) of the liver provides a simple means for visualizing the configuration and size of the liver and for demonstrating "space-occupying" masses in the liver. The scan is a pattern of the radioactivity concentrated in the liver. Areas within its boundaries that fail to accumulate radioactivity ("cold" areas) represent pathologic processes. The requirements for photoscanning include a scintillation counter and an appropriate isotopic substance which is concentrated by normal liver tissue. Two types of radioactive substances are available for photoscanning the liver. One group consists of agents removed from the blood by the parenchymal cells in which they concentrate. The other group consists of radioactive colloids that are removed from the blood by the reticuloendothelial cells in which they accumulate. Radioactive rose bengal is the prototype of the agents which are removed from the blood by the parenchymal cells of the liver, while the radioactive colloidal gold (^{198}Au) is a prototype of the agents removed by the reticuloendothelial cells of the liver (and other organs).

Radioactive rose bengal, accordingly, does not accumulate as well in the liver of patients with severe parenchymal hepatic disease (e.g., cirrhosis) as does the radioactive gold. Either the rose bengal or radioactive gold is suitable for the diagnosis of space-occupying masses in the liver with an otherwise normal parenchyma; but the radioactive gold is much more suitable for scintiscanning in patients with cirrhosis. Furthermore, radioactive gold provides a sharper outline of the liver and also outlines the spleen. Scanning with an appropriate scintiscanner of the patient in the supine and lateral positions is performed at suitable intervals after the intravenous administration of 150 mc. of radioactive rose bengal or of colloidal ^{198}Au. When rose bengal is used, the scans are performed 20 minutes and 1 hour after the injection. When radioactive gold is used, the scan is performed 2 hours after the administration. The recently introduced use of technetium-99m colloids for scintiscanning has provided sharper images requiring less time for scanning. Interpretation of the resulting scans (Fig. 13–14) can be

Table 13–12. INDICATIONS AND CONTRAINDICATIONS FOR LIVER BIOPSY

I. Possible applications
   A. Distinction of cause of hepatomegaly, jaundice, ascites, gastrointestinal bleeding or of abnormal liver function or serum enzyme values
   B. Establishment of precise diagnosis in patients with probable hepatic disease, e.g., chronic hepatitis, cirrhosis, fatty liver, or carcinoma (metastatic or primary)
   C. Recognition of systemic disease, e.g., hematogenous tuberculosis, sarcoidoses, amyloidoses and lymphoma (may be helpful in "staging" in known Hodgkin's disease)
   D. Evaluation of response to therapy of acute or chronic liver disease

II. Relative contraindications
   A. Clotting defects (abnormal bleeding time, coagulation time, or partial thromboplastin time), prothrombin time (>5 seconds greater than control) or history of recent hemorrhagic tendency
   B. Firm clinical diagnosis of posthepatic jaundice
   C. Severe anemia
   D. Uncooperative or unduly apprehensive patient
   E. Bacterial infection in area to be traversed by biopsy needle, e.g., right lower lobe pneumonia

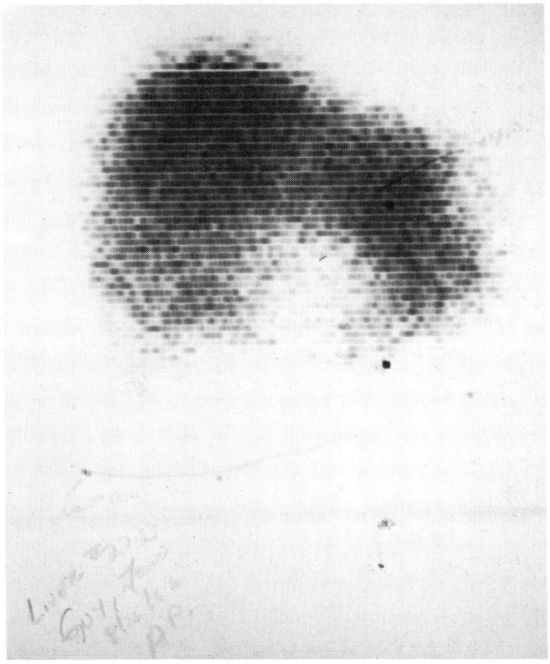

Figure 13–14. Scintiscan of liver containing metastatic carcinoma. Dark areas show uptake by normal parenchyma. Light area surrounded by dark is site of metastasis.

facilitated by superimposing them on the abdominal roentgenogram and by comparing them with the physical findings at the bedside.

Scintiscanning is an important diagnostic measure for the study of hepatic disease. It is useful for the detection of masses in the liver, such as metastatic carcinoma, hepatoma, cysts, or abscesses (Fig. 13–14). In a patient suspected of having one of these lesions or with unexplained hepatomegaly, the scan may confirm the diagnosis or indicate the site for biopsy if a carcinoma is suspected. Recognition of a single mass in the liver is possible if it exceeds 2 cm. in diameter. Smaller masses cannot be recognized. Even larger masses, if multiple, may escape identification, since multiple infiltrative masses and cirrhosis may give a similar pattern. Conversely, the scan of a coarse nodular (postnecrotic) cirrhosis may be mistaken for that of multiple infiltrative masses.

Scanning of the liver is also useful in defining hepatic size, contours, and extent. This is especially important in patients who are extremely obese, in those with marked ascites, and in those with an abnormal contour of the right leaflet of the diaphragm observed on chest roentgenography.

SEROLOGIC TESTS

Several serologic tests that may be of assistance in the diagnosis of hepatic disease have been introduced recently. The most important is the one used to detect the presence of the HAA (hepatitis-associated antigen) in the blood. This substance, also called the Australia (Au) or serum hepatitis (SH) antigen, is a low density lipoprotein which is found in the blood of a majority of patients with acute virus B hepatitis (also called "serum," "long-incubation type," or MS-2 hepatitis). The HAA is now widely believed to be a fragment, perhaps the coat, of the agent responsible for virus B hepatitis. It is found in asymptomatic carriers of virus B and in a significant proportion of patients with chronic viral hepatitis. Recent attention has focused on the presence of HAA in the blood of patients with hepatocellular carcinoma, an observation which has led to a reconsideration of the possible role of viral hepatitis in the etiology of carcinoma of the liver. The HAA is not found in the blood of patients with virus A hepatitis (infectious, short-incubation type, MS-1 hepatitis).

A variety of immunologic techniques have been introduced to detect the HAA and the corresponding antibody. These include immunodiffusion in agar gel, counterimmunoelectrophoresis, complement fixation, hemagglutination-inhibition, radioimmunoassay and others. Radioimmunoassay seems to be the most sensitive method and is likely to achieve the greatest popularity (Chapter 23).

Testing for HBAg has been most widely applied to the detection of the hepatitis carrier state among blood donors. It is also useful for the identification of virus B hepatitis and for its distinction from other forms of acute liver disease (p. 1230).

Table 13–13. APPLICATION OF LIVER FUNCTION TESTING

I. Diagnosis
  A. Recognition of presence or absence of hepatic disease
  B. Differential diagnosis
    1. Hepatomegaly
    2. Jaundice
    3. Ascites
    4. Gastrointestinal hemorrhage
  C. Testing for hepatotoxicity of drugs or industrial hepatotoxins
  D. Recognition of nonhepatic disease, e.g., hematogenous tuberculosis, sarcoidosis, amyloidosis, and infectious mononucleosis
II. Estimating severity in known hepatic disease
  A. Monitoring convalescence (hepatitis, cirrhosis)
  B. Preoperative evaluation
    1. In patients with recent hepatic disease
    2. In patients with extrahepatic disease that may affect liver status and function, e.g., hyperthyroidism, cholelithiasis, ulcerative colitis

A recent serologic test of considerable interest is the antimitochondrial "antibody" test. Almost all patients (90 per cent) with primary biliary cirrhosis have been found to have in their serum a protein which behaves like an "antibody" against a component of the inner cristae of mitochondria. The test antigen-system utilized to demonstrate this serologic substance can be any tissue rich in mitochondria (rat stomach, thyroid, kidney), and the test is performed by demonstrating deposition of fluorescinated gamma globulin on the tissue. The chief usefulness of the procedure is in the exclusion of surgical obstruction of the biliary tree as a cause of a chronic cholestatic syndrome. It is also of considerable interest as a tool for study of the syndromes of chronic intrahepatic cholestasis (Lam *et al.*, 1972) (p. 1231).

CLINICAL APPLICATION OF LIVER FUNCTION TESTS

Some of the clinical applications of liver function tests are listed in Table 13–13. They are useful for the diagnosis of hepatic disease and specifically for the differential diagnosis of jaundice, hepatomegaly, ascites, and gastrointestinal hemorrhage. Systematic monitoring of selected tests of hepatic function is necessary in testing for the hepatotoxicity of new drugs or of industrial exposure to chemicals. Characteristic patterns of abnormality are observed in extrahepatic diseases and assist in their recognition. Estimation of the severity of known hepatic disease and response to treatment is facilitated by testing of liver function.

A large number of tests of hepatic function have been described or mentioned in the preceding material. Only some of these are readily applicable to clinical problems. A "battery" of tests, which we use regularly in the diagnosis of hepatic disease, is shown in Table 13–14. In patients with jaundice whose serum bilirubin level is greater than 4 mg. per 100 ml., the BSP excretion test is not peformed, since it adds no useful information to that obtained by other procedures. With this group of procedures, patterns of hepatic dysfunction are observed that are useful in the differential diagnosis of jaundice (Table 13–15), hepatomegaly (Table 13–16), ascites (Table 13–17), and gastrointestinal hemorrhage (Table 13–18) and that are even helpful in the recognition of extrahepatic disease (Table 13–19). The patterns shown represent those most frequently observed in each instance. Exceptions occur, and the patterns should be regarded only as guides.

HEPATIC FUNCTION IN NONHEPATIC DISEASE

Abnormal results with one or more tests of hepatic function may be obtained in patients with a variety of extrahepatic diseases. These have been considered at times to reflect on the value and specificity of liver function testing. Even in nonhepatic disease, however, fairly consistent patterns of hepatic function may be observed. In Table 13–19 is shown a classi-

Table 13–14. PROCEDURES USEFUL IN THE DIAGNOSIS OF HEPATIC DISEASE*

Serum bilirubin (total, direct, and indirect)
Urine bilirubin (qualitative)
Urine urobilinogen (2- or 24-hour urine)
Stool urobilinogen (24- or 72-hour specimen)
BSP excretion (in the nonjaundiced patient)
Serum protein determination (albumin, globulin)
  Electrophoresis and gamma globulin estimation preferred with total serum protein
Flocculation tests
  Cephalin cholesterol
  Thymol turbidity
Serum cholesterol (total)
Serum alkaline phosphatase
GOT, GPT
Liver biopsy
Scintiscanning
Special tests
  Hepatitis-associated antigen
  α-fetoprotein
  Antimitochondrial antibody

*From H. J. Zimmerman: Liver function tests. Modern Treatment, *1*:490, 1964.

Table 13–15. LABORATORY APPROACH TO DIFFERENTIAL DIAGNOSIS OF JAUNDICE*

TYPE OF HYPER-BILIRUBINEMIA	CAUSES	BILIRUBIN TESTS				FLOCCULATION TESTS			SERUM ENZYMES†		
		Serum Bilir. D/T Rates	Urine Bil.	Urine Urob.	Feces Urob.	T.T.	C.F.	Chol. Level	A.P.	GOT	GPT
Unconjugated											
Prehepatic	Hemolysis	<0.2	0	↑	↑↑	N	N	N	N	N	N
Hepatic	Crigler-Najjar syndrome Gilbert syndrome	<0.2	0	N	N, ↑	N	N	N	N	N	N
Conjugated											
Hepatic											
Hepatocellular	Viral, toxic hepatitis	0.4–0.6	+	↑	N	↑↑↑	+	N(↓)	↑↑	↑↑↑↑	↑↑↑↑
	Cirrhosis and other chronic forms of parenchymal injury	0.4–0.6	+	↑	N	↑	+	N(↓)	↑↑	↑↑↑↑	↑↑↑↑
Hepato-canalicular	Cholestatic forms of drug jaundice	0.4–0.6	+	(↓)N(↑)	(↓)	N(↑)	N(+)	↑↑↑	↑↑↑	↑↑	↑↑
	Primary biliary cirrhosis	0.4–0.6	+	N(↑)	(↓)	N(↑)	N(+)	↑↑↑↑	↑↑↑↑	↑↑	↑↑
Posthepatic	Carcinoma of pancreas or bile ducts	0.4–0.6	+	↓	↓↓↓↓	N	N	↑↑	↑↑↑	↑↑	↑↑
	Choledocholithiasis	0.4–0.6	+	(↓)N, ↑	↓↓	N(↑)	N(+)	↑	↑↑	↑↑	↑↑

*Number of arrows indicates direction, degree, and incidence of abnormal results. N indicates normal.
†See Figures 13–10 and 13–11.
↓↓↓↓, ↑↑↑↑ Almost all patients show abnormality, many to marked degree.
↑↑↑ Almost all patients show abnormality, usually to moderate degree.
↓↓, ↑↑ Many patients show abnormality, usually slight to moderate.
↓, ↑ Many patients show abnormality, usually slight.
(↓),(↑) Slight abnormality in some of the patients.

Table 13–16. LABORATORY AIDS TO THE DIFFERENTIAL DIAGNOSIS OF HEPATOMEGALY

	BSP	T.T.	C.F.	BIL.	ALB.	GLOB.	ALK. PHOSPH.	GOT	GPT	LDH
Hepatitis	↑↑↑	↑↑↑	+	↑↑	N, ↓	↑, N	↑	↑↑↑↑	↑↑↑↑	↑
Cirrhosis	↑↑↑	↑	+	↑	↓	↑	↑	↑↑	↑	↑
Metastatic carcinoma	↑	N	N	N	N, ↓	N	↑↑↑	↑↑	↑	↑↑↑
Infectious mononucleosis	↑	↑	+	↑	N	N, ↑	↑↑	↑↑	↑↑	↑↑
Extrahepatic disease	See Table 13-19.									

*No grading of the degree or incidence of abnormality has been included.

Table 13–17. LABORATORY AIDS IN THE DIAGNOSIS OF ASCITES*

	BSP	T.T.	C.F.	BIL.	ALB.	GLOB.	ALK. PHOSPH.	GOT	GPT	LD
Cirrhosis	↑↑↑	↑	+	↑	↓	↑	↑	↑	↑	N, ↑
Carcinomatosis	↑, N†	N		N	N, ↓	N	↑↑↑	↑	↑	↑↑↑
Tuberculosis	↑, N†	↑	+	N	N, ↓	↑	↑↑	↑	↑	↑
Heart failure	↑↑	N	0	↑	N, ↓	N	↑	↑-↑↑	↑-↑↑	↑-↑↑

*Transaminases (GOT, GPT) add little to this differential diagnosis.
†Degree of abnormality depends on presence of lesions in liver; results will be normal if only peritoneum is involved.

Table 13–18. LABORATORY AIDS TO THE DIFFERENTIAL DIAGNOSIS OF GASTROINTESTINAL HEMORRHAGE

	BSP	T.T.	C.F.	BIL.	ALB.	GLOB.	NH_3	GOT	GPT
Peptic ulcer	N	N	N	N	N	N	N	N	N
Alcoholic gastritis*	N, ↑	N, ↑	N, +	N, ↑	N, ↓	N, ↑	N, ↑	N, ↑	N
Esophageal varices									
Intrahepatic portal block (cirrhosis)	↑	↑ ,N	+	↑	↓	↑	↑	↑	–
Extrahepatic portal block	N	N	N	N	N	N	↑	N	N

*Results of liver functions depend on degree of liver disease present.

Table 13–19. LIVER FUNCTION IN NONHEPATIC DISEASE

I. Abnormality of a number of different types of function similar to intrinsic hepatic disease (BSP, T.T., C.F., bilirubin, proteins), e.g., pneumococcal pneumonia and infectious mononucleosis
II. Dissociated patterns
  A. Disproportionately abnormal BSP excretion*
  B. Disproportionately abnormal BSP and alkaline phosphatase*
  C. Disproportionately abnormal flocculation test values and globulin (gamma) increase*
III. Combinations of dissociated patterns (IIB + IIC)
  A. Hyperglobulinemic diseases with space-occupying lesions, e.g., tuberculosis or sarcoidosis with granulomas in the liver
  B. Subacute bacterial endocarditis plus heart failure
IV. Diseases with normal hepatic function, e.g., peptic ulcer, chronic nephritis

*Compared to other test of liver function.

Table 13–20. SOME COMMON PITFALLS IN APPLICATION OF LIVER FUNCTION TESTS

1. Dependence on results of one test rather than patterns of dysfunction to detect abnormality
2. Assumption that normal results signify no parenchymal disease (e.g., values for GOT normal in 25 per cent and for GPT normal in 50 per cent of patients with Laennec's cirrhosis)
3. Assumption that abnormal values for "liver function" tests mean only liver disease
4. Failure to recognize acute jaundice as
  a. *Hepatocellular* because GOT and GPT values are unexpectedly low (below 300 Karmen units in 20 per cent of patients with acute viral hepatitis) or because alk. phosph. values are unexpectedly high (above 15 Bodansky units in 5 per cent of patients with acute hepatitis)
  b. *Obstructive* because values for GOT and GPT are unexpectedly high (above 300 units in 15 per cent of patients with choledocholithiasis) or because values for alk. phosph. are unexpectedly low (below 15 Bodansky units in 30 per cent of patients with choledocholithiasis)
5. Failure to reconcile results of tests with clinical features

fication of nonhepatic diseases in terms of the type of hepatic dysfunction observed and the presumed basis for it. Understanding of these patterns should make it possible to avoid confusing hepatic with nonhepatic disease and to assist in the diagnosis of disease in each category.

CONCLUSIONS

The foregoing discussion has attempted to review the basis for liver function testing and has listed a large number of laboratory procedures for this purpose. A small group of useful tests has been selected from this group and their applications in a clinical setting has been considered.

It should be recalled that there are a number of pitfalls in the application of the tests to the diagnosis and management of hepatic disease (Table 13–20). Correlation of laboratory results with clinical features should obviate most of these potential difficulties.

REFERENCES

Liver Function (General)

Gabrieli, E. R., Kawasaki, H., Orfanas, A., and Sinka, S. O.: Computer-oriented laboratory testing of hepatic status. *In* Popper and Schaffner, F. (eds.): *Progress in Liver Diseases.* Vol. III. New York, Grune & Stratton, 1970.

Hargreaves, T.: *The Liver and Bile Metabolism.* New York, Appleton-Century Crofts, 1968.

Kew, M. C., Dos Santos, H. A., and Sherlock, S.: Diagnosis of primary cancer of the liver. Brit. Med. J. *4*:408, 1971.

Reinhold, J. G.: Chemical evaluation of the functions of the liver. Clin. Chem. *1*:351, 1955.

Schiff, L.: *Diseases of the Liver.* 4th ed. Philadelphia, J. B. Lippincott Co., 1969.

Sherlock, S.: *Diseases of the Liver.* 4th ed. Philadelphia, F. A. Davis Co., 1968.

Tingstrom, B.: The discriminatory ability of a galactose-tolerance test and some other tests in the diagnosis of cirrhosis of the liver, hepatitis, and biliary obstruction.

Zimmerman, H. J.: The differential diagnosis of jaundice. Med. C. N. Amer. *52*:1417, 1968.

Bilirubin Metabolism and Jaundice

Arias, I. M., Gartner, L. M., Cohen, M., *et al.*: Chronic nonhemolytic unconjugated hyperbilirubinemia with glucuronyl transferase deficiency. Clinical, biochemical, pharmacologic and genetic evidence for heterogeneity. Amer. J. Med. *47*:395, 1969.

Billing, B. H.: The enigma of bilirubin conjugation. Gastroenterology *60*:258, 1971.

Bernstein, R. B.: Comparison of serum clearance and urinary excretion of mesobilirubinogen-H^3 in control subjects with liver disease. Gastroenterology *61*:733, 1971.

Ducci, H.: Contribution of the laboratory to the differential diagnosis of jaundice. J.A.M.A. *135*:694, 1947.

Ducci, H., and Watson, C. J.: The quantitative determination of bilirubin with special reference to the prompt-reacting and chloroform-soluble types. J. Lab. Clin. Med. *34*:145, 1949.

Fleischner, G., and Arias, I. M.: Recent advances in bilirubin formation, transport, metabolism and excretion. Amer. J. Med. *49*:576, 1970.

Israels, L. G.: The bilirubin shunt and shunt hyperbilirubinemia. *In* Popper, H., and Schaffner, F.: *Progress in Liver Diseases.* Vol. III. New York, Grune & Stratton, 1970.

Jendrassik, L., and Grof, P.: Vereinfachte photometrische Methoden zur Bestimmung des Blutbilirubins. Bioch. Ztschr. *297*:81, 1938.

Malloy, H. T., and Evelyn, K. A.: The determination of bilirubin with the photoelectric colorimeter. J. Bioch. Chem. *119*:481, 1937.

McNee, J. W.: Jaundice. A review of recent works. Quart. J. Med. *16*:390, 1923.

Michaelsson, M.: Bilirubin determination in serum and urine. Scand. J. Clin. Lab. Invest. *13*(Suppl. 56):5, 1961.

Poland, R. L., and Odell, G. B.: Physiologic jaundice; the enterohepatic circulation of bilirubin. New Eng. J. Med. *284*:1, 1971.

Rich, A. R.: Pathogenesis of forms of jaundice. Bull. Johns Hopkins Hosp. *47*:338, 1930.

Schmid, R.: Hyperbilirubinemia. *In* Stanbury, J. B., Wyngaarden, J. B., and Fredrickson, D. S. (eds.): *The Metabolic Basis of Inherited Disease.* 3rd ed. New York, McGraw-Hill Book Co., 1972.

Thompson, R. P. H.: Recent advances in jaundice; physiology. Brit. Med. J. *1*:223, 1970.

Watson, C. J.: The importance of the fractional serum bilirubin determination in clinical medicine. Ann. Intern. Med. *45*:351, 1956.

Serum Proteins and Flocculation Tests

Hobbs, J. R.: Serum proteins in liver disease. Proc. Roy. Soc. Med. *60*:1250, 1967.

Maclagan, N. F., Martin, N. H., and Lunnon, J. B.: The mechanism and interrelationships of the flocculation tests. J. Clin. Path. *5*:1, 1952.

Osserman, E. F., and Takatsuki, K.: The plasma proteins in liver disease. Med. C. N. Amer. *47*:679, 1963.

Owen, J. A., Padangi, R., and Smith, H.: Serum haptoglobins and other tests in the diagnosis of hepatobiliary disease. Clin. Sci. *21*:189, 1961.

Purves, L. R., Bersohn, I., and Geddes, E. W.: Serum alpha-feta-protein and primary cancer of the liver in man. Cancer *25*:1261, 1970.

Smith, J. B.: Alpha-feta-protein occurrence in certain malignant diseases and review of clinical applications. Med. C. N. Amer. *54*:797, 1970.

Steigmann, F., Kazemi, F., Dubin, A., and Kissane, J.: Cerebrospinal fluid glutamine in the diagnosis of hepatic coma. Amer. J. Gastroenterol. *40*:378, 1963.

Blood Ammonia Levels

Bessman, S. P.: Blood ammonia. *In* Sabotka, H., and Stewart, C. P. (eds.) Advances in Clinical Chemistry. Vol. 2. New York, Academic Press, Inc., 1959.

Gabuzda, G. J.: Ammonium metabolism and hepatic coma. Gastroenterology *53*:806, 1967.

Summerskill, W. H. J., and Wolpert, E.: Ammonia metabolism in the gut. Amer. J. Clin. Nutr. *23*:633, 1970.

Walker, C. O., Schenker, S.: Pathogenesis of hepatic encephalopathy. Amer. J. Clin. Nutr. *23*:619, 1970.

Galactose Tolerance

Tengstrom, B.: An intravenous galactose tolerance test and its use in hepatobiliary diseases. Acta Med. Scand. *183*:31, 1968.

Dye Excretion Tests

Jablonski, P., and Owen, J. A.: The clinical chemistry of bromsulfophthalein and other cholephilic dyes. *In* Bodansky, O., and Stewart, C. P. (eds.). *Advances in Clinical Chemistry.* Vol. 12. New York, Academic Press, Inc., 1969.

Javitt, N.: Clinical and experimental aspects of sulfabromophthalein and related compounds. *In* Popper, H., and Schaffner, F.: *Progress in Liver Diseases.* Vol. III. New York, Grune & Stratton, 1970. *In* Sabotka, H., and Stewart,

C. P. (eds.). *Advances in Clinical Chemistry.* Vol. 12. New York, Academic Press, Inc., 1969.

Leevy, C. M., Smith, F., Longueville, J., *et al.*: Indocyanine green clearance as a test for hepatic function; evaluation by dichromatic or densitometry. J.A.M.A. *200*:236, 1967.

Radioisotopic Tests

Bekerman, C., and Gottschalk, A.: Diagnostic significance of the relative uptake of liver compared with spleen in ^{99m}Tc-sulfur colloid scintiphotography. J. Nuclear Med. *12*:237, 1971.

Cantor, R. E., Cohn, E. M., Park, C. H., and Shapiro, B.: Comparative liver scanning; technetium sulfide Tc^{99m} vs. gold Au^{198}. J.A.M.A. *211*:1677, 1970.

Ghadimi, H., and Sakk-Kortusk, A.: Evaluation of the radioactive rose-bengal test for the differential diagnosis of obstructive jaundice in infants. New Eng. J. Med. *96*:351, 1961.

Rossi, P., and Gould, H. R.: Angiography and scanning in liver disease. Radiology *96*:553, 1970.

Wilson, F. E., Preston, D. F., and Overholt, E. L.: Detection of hepatic neoplasm; hepatic scanning combined with liver-function studies. J.A.M.A. *209*:676, 1969.

Australia Antigen and Other Serologic Tests

Blumberg, B. S., London, W. T., and Sutnick, A. I.: Practical applications of the Australia antigen test. Postgrad. Med. *50*:70, 1971.

Coussart, Y. E.: Australia antigen and hepatitis. A review. J. Clin. Path. *24*:394, 1971.

Lam, K., Mistilis, S. P., and Perrott, N.: Positive tissue antibody tests in patients with prolonged extra-hepatic biliary obstruction. New Eng. J. Med. *286*:1400, 1972.

Sherlock, S.: The immunology of liver disease. Amer. J. Med. *49*:693, 1970.

Walker, J. G.: Immunological tests in liver disease. Ann. Clin. Biochem. *7*:93, 1970.

Vitamin B_{12} Levels in Liver Disease

Rachmilewitz, M., and Eliakim, M.: Serum B_{12}—a diagnostic test in liver disease. Israel J. Med. Sci. *4*:47, 1968.

Transaminases and Alkaline Phosphatase

See references for Chapter 14.

Chapter 14

SERUM ENZYME DETERMINATIONS AS AN AID TO DIAGNOSIS

by HYMAN J. ZIMMERMAN, M.D., and JOHN BERNARD HENRY, M.D.

Enzymes, organic catalysts that are responsible for most of the chemical reactions of the body, are found in all tissues. Some have been identified in the plasma (or serum), to which they gain access from injured cells or even perhaps from intact cells. Interest of clinicians in serum enzymes began about four decades ago with the demonstration of the usefulness of alkaline phosphatase levels in the diagnosis of osseous and hepatobiliary disease, of acid phosphatase levels in the diagnosis of carcinoma of prostate, and of amylase and lipase levels for the diagnosis of pancreatic disease. Despite the clinical usefulness of these parameters of disease and the demonstration, during the next 25 years, of a number of other enzymes in the serum, clinical interest in serum enzymology remained relatively dormant until 1953. The demonstration in that year of a transaminase (glutamic oxalacetic transaminase) in the serum of normals and the subsequent observations that increased levels of this enzyme were helpful in the diagnosis of cardiac and hepatic disease led to a marked intensification of interest in serum enzymology.

By now, more than 50 enzymes have been identified in the serum (Tables 14–1 and 14–2). The levels of many enzymes have been studied extensively in a variety of conditions (Table 14–1). Some serum enzyme tests have been applied so widely to clinical problems as to be considered routine laboratory procedures (Table 14–2, Group A). Others (Table 14–2, Group B), though clearly shown also to reflect various diseases reliably, are performed in relatively few clinical laboratories because the assay is technically difficult or because the information provided is considered to add too little to that provided by the enzymes in Group A. Others are of investigative rather than regular clinical interest (Group C) or of importance only in special clinical situations (Group D). A fifth group (Group E) includes enzymes that have not been studied sufficiently to assess their clinical usefulness. In Table 14–1 are shown the main conditions in which abnormal values of the enzymes listed are found.

The usefulness of several serum enzymes (alkaline phosphatase, glutamic oxalacetic transaminase, glutamic pyruvic transaminase) in the diagnosis of hepatic disease and of several other enzymes (amylase, lipase) in the diagnosis of pancreatic disease is considered in the chapters devoted to liver function (Chapter 13) and pancreatic function (Chapter 15). In this chapter the more general aspects of serum enzymology are considered. The principles of the methods for measuring enzyme activity are discussed, the possible factors responsible for abnormal values are analyzed, and special attention is devoted to a few of the enzymes found in the serum. Brief reference is made to enzymes of other body fluids and to the clinical significance of enzymes in the formed elements of the blood.

PRINCIPLES OF ENZYME DETERMINATIONS

Because they exist in very small amounts in biologic fluids and are so similar chemically,

Table 14–1. CLASSIFICATION OF ENZYMES DEMONSTRATED IN SERUM WITH TYPE AND DEGREE* OF ABNORMALITY IN DISEASE

TYPE OF ENZYME	CONDITION†								
	HEPATITIS	INF. MONO.	CIRRHOSIS	MET. CA.	OBST. JAUNDICE	HEART FAILURE	MYOCARD. INFARCT.	PROG. MUSC. DYST.	COMMENTS OR OTHER ABNORMALITIES
I. Carbohydrate metabolism									
A. Glycolytic									
1. Phosphoglucomutase	↑ ↑		N	↑	↑				
2. Phosphohexoisomerase (PHI)	↑ ↑ ↑	↑ ↑	↑	↑	↑	↑	↑ ↑	↑	Fig. 14-7
3. Fructose 1, 6-diphosphate aldolase (Ald.)	↑ ↑ ↑	↑	↑	↑	N or ↑	↑	↑ ↑	↑ ↑ ↑	Figs. 14-7, 14-8 Table 14-11
4. Fructose-P-aldolase	↑ ↑ ↑			N	N		N	N	
5. Lactic dehydrogenase (LD)	↑	↑ ↑	↑	↑ ↑	N or ↑	↑	↑ ↑	↑ ↑	
6. Pyruvate kinase (PK)	↑ ↑			↑ ↑					
7. Enolase	↑						↑		Fig. 14-7
8. Triose-P-isomerase				↑					
9. Glyceraldehyde 3-P-dehydrogenase	↑	↑							
B. Hexose monophosphate shunt (pentose phosphate pathway)									
1. Glucose-6-phosphate dehydrogenase (G-6-PD)	N		N		N		↑ ↑		Fig. 14-10
2. 6-P-Gluconic dehydrogenase (6-P-GD)	↑	↑							
3. 5-Phosphoriboisomerase	N		↑ ↑	↑ ↑	↑				
4. Transketolase	↑								
C. Citric acid cycle									
1. Malic dehydrogenase (MD)	↑ ↑ ↑	↑	↑	↑	↑	↑	↑ ↑		
2. Isocitric dehydrogenase (ICD)	↑ ↑ ↑	↑	N or ↑	↑ ↑	N or ↑	↑	N	N	Fig. 14–9
3. Fumarase	↑		↑						
D. Other									
1. Amylase	N	N	N or ↓	N	N	N	N	N	Chapter 15
2. β-Glucuronidase	↑ ↑						N or ↑		Ca, Pregnancy
3. Sorbitol dehydrogenase (Sorb. D.)	↑ ↑ ↑	↑	↑	N or ↑	N or ↑		N	N	Fig. 14-13
II. Esterases									
A. Lipid									
1. Lipase	N	N	N	N	N	N	N	N	Chapter 15
2. Aliesterase	N	N	N	N	N	N	N	N	Acute panc.
3. Cholesterol esterase	↓		↓	N or ↓	N				
4. Lipoprotein lipase (LPP)	↑ ↑		↑ ↑		↓				
5. Lecithinase	N		N	N	N				Acute panc.
B. Nonlipid									
1. Cholinesterase (pseudo)	↓	↓	↓		N or ↑	N or ↑		N	Fig. 14-11
2. Phosphatases									
a. Alkaline phosphatase (Alk. phosph.)	↑	↑	↑	↑ ↑	↑ ↑ ↑	↑	N	N	Increase in bone disease. Table 14-7
b. Acid phosphatase (Acid phosph.)	N	N	N	N	N	N	N	N	Ca. of prostate
c. 5′-Nucleotidase (5′-N)	↑		↑	↑ ↑	↑ ↑ ↑				Normal in bone disease.
d. Adenosine triphosphatase (ATPase)	↑		↑	↑	↑ ↑				Elevated in bone disease.
3. Deoxyribonuclease I (DNAse)	↑	+			N			N	Acute hemorrhagic pancreatitis
4. Ribonuclease (RNase)	N		N	N	N	↑	↑		Uremia, myeloma
5. Adenosine deaminase	↑ ↑	↑ ↑ ↑	↑ ↑	↑ ↑ ↑		↑ ↑	N		Leukemia
III. Protein and amino acid enzymes									
A. Proteolytic enzymes (trypsin)									Acute pancreatitis.
B. Peptidases									
1. Leucine aminopeptidase (LAP)	↑	↑ ↑ ↑	↑	↑ ↑	↑ ↑ ↑	↑ ↑	N	N	Pregnancy Ca. of pancreas Pancreatitis
2. Aminotripeptidase	↑ ↑	↑ ↑	↑	↑ ↑	↑ ↑				
3. γ-Glutamyl transpeptidase (Gl. TP)	↑		↑	↑ ↑ ↑	↑ ↑	↑	↑ ↑		
C. Pepsinogen									Duod. ulcer
D. Amino acid substrate									
1. Transaminases									
a. Glutamic oxalacetic transaminase (GOT)	↑ ↑ ↑	↑ ↑	↑	↑	↑	↑	↑ ↑	↑ ↑	Table 14-10 Fig. 14-6

* ↑ -slight increase
↑ ↑ -moderate increase
↑ ↑ ↑ -marked increase
N-no change

†Inf. Mono – infectious mononucleosis
Met. Ca. – metastatic carcinoma
Obst. Jaundice – obstructive jaundice
Prog. Musc. Dyst. – progressive muscular dystrophy
Myocard. Infarct. – myocardial infarction

(Table 14–1 continues on the opposite page.)

Table 14–1. CLASSIFICATION OF ENZYMES DEMONSTRATED IN SERUM WITH TYPE AND DEGREE* OF ABNORMALITY IN DISEASE (*Continued*)

	CONDITION†								
TYPE OF ENZYME	HEPATITIS	INF. MONO.	CIRRHOSIS	MET. CA.	OBST. JAUNDICE	HART FAILURE	MYOCARD. INFARCT.	PROG. MUSC. DYST.	OTHER ABNORMALITIES
b. Glutamic pyruvic transaminase (GPT)	↑↑↑	↑↑	↑	↑	↑	↑	N or ↑	↑↑	Chapter 13
c. Glutamic dehydrogenase (Gl. D)	↑↑	N	N or ↑	N	N	N	N	N	
2. Urea cycle									
a. Ornithine carbamyl transferase (OCT)	↑↑↑		↑	↑↑					Acute cholecytisis. Fig. 14-12
b. Arginase	↑↑		↑						
IV. Other enzymes									
A. Glutathione reductase (GR)	↑↑		↑	↑↑			↑		
B. Ceruloplasmin	↑↑		↑	↑↑	↑↑				Wilson's dis.
C. Creatine phosphokinase (CPK)	N		N	N	N	N	↑↑↑	↑↑↑	Dermatomyositis Fig. 14-13
D. Benzidine oxidase	↑		↑	↑↑↑	↑↑	↑	↑↑↑		
E. Hydroxybutyrate dehydrogenase (HBD)	↑	↑	±	↑	±	↑	↑↑↑	±	Isoenzyme of LD.
F. Guanase	↑↑↑	↑	↑	↑	↑				

enzymes are measured by their activity rather than their concentration. Enzyme activity is expressed in units that usually represent one of the following: (1) increase in concentration of one of the products, (2) decrease in concentration of substrate, or (3) rate of change in concentration of coenzyme as a measure of rate of reaction.

Although a great deal of confusion has resulted from the lack of uniform terminology in the expression of units, attention has been directed to this problem and recommendations have been made recently by the Commission on Enzymes of the International Union of Biochemistry. (Tables 14–3 and 14–4).

An enzyme may be considered as follows:

$$\text{Holoenzyme} = \text{apoenzyme} + \text{coenzyme}$$

Apoenzyme is the protein portion subject to denaturation, as are all proteins. This denatura-

Table 14–2. CATEGORIZATION OF SERUM ENZYMES ACCORDING TO CLINICAL USEFULNESS

GROUP	ENZYMES*
A. Routinely employed in most hospitals	Alk. phosph., acid phosph., lipase, amylase, GOT, GPT, LD, CPK
B. Clinically useful, but employed much less widely than enzymes in Group A	Pseudocholinesterase, LAP, 5′N, GLTP, Ald., PHI, ICD, OCT, HBD, Sorb.D.
C. Primarily of investigative interest; employed for routine clinical purposes in few or no hospitals	α-lecithinase, LPP, aliesterase, fructose-6-P aldolase, MD, B-glucuronidase, Gl. D, GITP, guanase, GR
D. Employed only in special circumstances	Ceruloplasmin (for diagnosis of Wilson's disease): pseudocholinesterase (to study patients with insecticide poisoning and patients with prolonged apnea after muscle relaxants), muramidase in patients with leukemia
E. Data too scanty to evaluate prospective usefulness or indicative of no clinical utility	ATPases (alk. and acid), heroin esterase, procaine esterase; DNAses (I and II), cholesterol esterase, glucokinase, phosphoglucomutase, triose-P-isomerase, glyceraldehyde-3-P dehydrogenase, phosphoglycerate dehydrogenase, enolase, 3-P-glyceric acid kinase, pyruvate kinase, malic enzyme, fumarase, succinic dehydrogenase, G-6-PD, 6-PGD, 5-P-riboisomerase, transketolase, tripeptidase, dipeptidases, oxytocinase, amine oxidases, arginase, adenosine deaminase, benzidine oxidase

*See Table 14-1 for meaning of abbreviations.

Table 14–3. CLASSIFICATION OF ENZYMES WITH EXAMPLES

- Oxidoreductases
  - Oxidases
    - Cytochrome oxidase
  - Dehydrogenases
    - Lactate dehydrogenase
    - Malate dehydrogenase
    - Isocitrate dehydrogenase
    - Glucose-6-phosphate dehydrogenase
    - Glutamate dehydrogenase
    - Hydroxybutyrate dehydrogenase
- Transferases
  - Glutamic oxalacetic transaminase
  - Glutamic pyruvic transaminase
  - Galactose-1-phosphate uridyl transferase
  - Transketolase (glycolaldehyde transferase)
  - Ornithine carbamoyltransferase
- Hydrolases
  - Esterases
    - Phosphatases, acid and alkaline
    - Cholinesterase
    - Lipase
  - Peptidases
    - Leucine aminopeptidase
    - Trypsin
    - Pepsin
  - Glycosidases
    - Amylase
    - Amylo-l-6-glucosidase
    - Glucosidase
    - Galactosidase
- Lyases
  - Aldolase
  - Glutamate decarboxylase
  - Pyruvate decarboxylase
  - Tryptophan decarboxylase
- Isomerases
  - Glucose phosphate isomerase
  - Ribose phosphate isomerase

tion, due to physical and chemical agents, is associated with a loss of enzyme activity.

Coenzyme is the dialyzable portion and a type of substrate essential for catalytic activity. It is tightly bound to enzyme and is not a protein. An example of a coenzyme is DPN (diphosphopyridine nucleotide), which is also termed NAD (nicotinamide adenine dinucleotide).

Activators are substances which modify reactions catalyzed—metal ions such as zinc and magnesium, for example.

Enzymes display specificity with regard to substrate (substance which is acted on) and effect (chemical action). Lactic dehydrogenase catalyzes the following reaction:

$$\text{Lactic acid} + \text{NAD} \rightleftarrows \text{pyruvic acid} + \text{NADH}_2$$

It catalyzes both the forward and reverse reactions as indicated. It acts virtually only on L-lactic acid and pyruvic acid as substrates and catalyzes the reversible transfer of hydrogen ion (H^+) between lactic acid and NAD. Other enzymes are required for the decarboxylation or amination of pyruvic acid.

Many chemical and physical agents exert a marked influence on enzymes. Temperature and hydrogen ion concentration are probably the two best-studied agents. Inactivation of most enzymes will occur in the neighborhood of 65° C. Freezing, however, does not usually destroy enzymes. For each 10° C. rise in temperature, several enzymes will demonstrate a twofold increase in activity, but the increase in denaturation is even greater. Hence, the temperature activity curve for an enzyme will show a maximum, depending on the opposed activating and denaturing effects of rising temperature.

A bell-shaped curve will also often describe the optimum pH for an enzyme (Fig. 14–1). This may also reflect the cumulative effects of hydrogen ion concentration on activation and denaturation of enzyme protein.

Although an enzyme reaction represents very complex mechanisms that are not fully understood, it can be stated that an enzyme reversibly forms a transitory complex with its substrate. Functional groups of coenzymes or prosthetic groups or both may play a role in the formation of the enzyme-substrate complex. The enzyme-substrate complex decomposes to enzyme and product. The enzyme

Table 14–4. CONVERSION OF CLINICAL ENZYME VALUES TO STANDARD UNITS

*Standard units:**

1 standard unit = the amount of enzyme that catalyzes the conversion of 1 micromole (microequivalent) of substrate or coenzyme per minute under the defined conditions of the test (temperature with optimal pH and substrate concentration). Activity may be expressed in milliunits, microunits, etc. per milliliter of sample.

1 unit = 1 micromole per minute (μ mol./min.)

1 milliunit (mU.) = 1 millimicromole per minute (mμmol./min.)

1 microunit (μU.) = 1 micromicromole per minute ($\mu\mu$mol./min.)

Example:

Lactic dehydrogenase 25° C.

O. D. unit = O. D. of (.001)/min./ml.

$$\text{Standard unit} = \frac{\text{O.D.}}{6.25} \times \frac{3.0}{0.2} = \text{O.D./min.} \times 2.4$$

Standard unit = difference of 5 min. lines on graph = $\text{O.D.}_5 \times 0.48 = \text{O.D.} \times \frac{1}{2}$

Example: Test gave O.D. = 0.020/min. for 0.2 ml. sample

Old method: O.D. = 20 × 5 = 100 O.D. units

Standard method: 0.020 × 2.4 = 0.048 units, or 48 mU.

Normal range:

80 to 120 O.D. units

40 to 60 standard milliunits (mU.)/ml.

*Also called "International Unit."

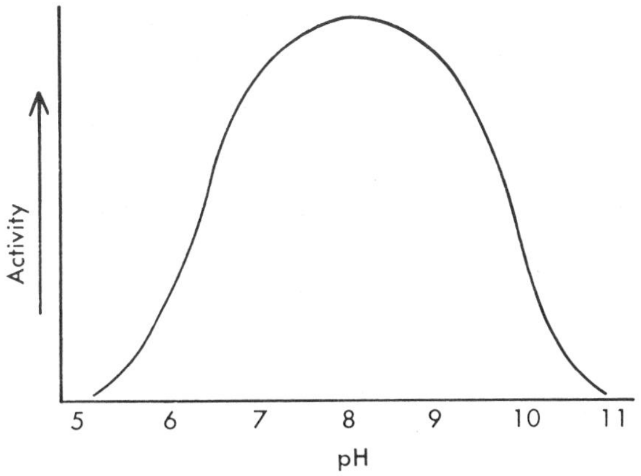

Figure 14–1. Typical curve of activity versus pH for an enzymatic reaction. (From Henry, J. B.: Postgrad. Med. *33*:A–66, 1963.)

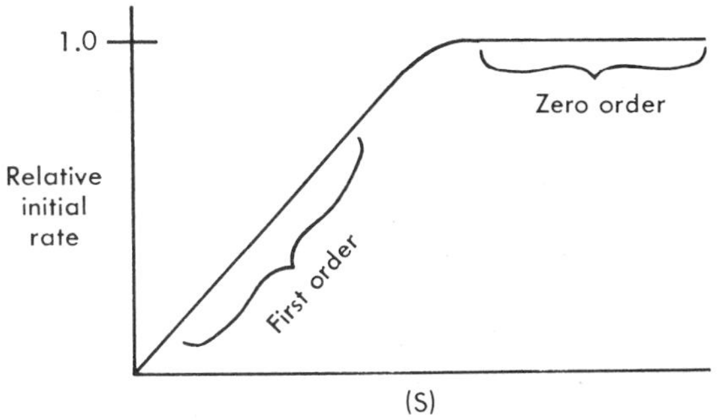

Figure 14–2. Relative rate of reaction expressed as function of substrate concentration (*S*). (From Henry, J. B.: Postgrad. Med. *33*:A–66, 1963.)

is not altered in the overall reaction. The Michaelis-Menten hypothesis describes this sequence of events as shown at the bottom of this page.

In addition to a high substrate concentration, with the important assumption of an intermediate enzyme-substrate complex, this theory further states that the rate of conversion of the substrate to the products of the reaction is determined by the rate of conversion of the enzyme-substrate complex to reaction products and the enzyme.

Units of enzyme activity are best expressed in terms of rate of the catalyzed reaction. The rate of reaction can be considered graphically (Figs. 14–2 and 14–3). In Figure 14–2, the relative rate of reaction is expressed as a function of substrate concentration [S]. At low concentration, the rate is first order* with respect to [S]. The rate is zero order,* independent of [S], at a high concentration. In measuring enzyme activity, one should use this part of the curve.

In an enzyme assay, one may measure activity as $\triangle P$ or $-\triangle S$ depending on which is more convenient analytically (Fig. 14–3). Often the product or substrate may be colored and, if so, may be quantitatively determined by colorimetry or spectrophotometry. The concentration of coenzyme (e.g., NAD [DPN] with virtually no absorption at 340 mμ; $NADH_2$ [DPNH] with maximal absorption at 340 mμ) can be measured spectrophotometrically as in the lactate dehydrogenase assay.

An enzyme exerts maximal influence when substrate concentration is highest and product concentration nil. This is most likely to be the case at the beginning of the reaction, when the rate is described as zero order with respect to substrate, followed by a progressive decrease in reaction velocity as equilibrium is reached. Zero-order reaction rate simply means in this case that the rate is constant and independent of substrate and product concentrations. If reaction is zero order, concentration of product will rise linearly with respect to time (Fig. 14–3 *a*). Ideally, enzyme assays are performed under conditions which permit reaction to approach zero order with respect to product and substrate during the entire measuring period. Multiple determinations of substrate or product concentration against time are recorded in the assay.

*A first-order enzyme reaction is one in which the rate of reaction is determined by the concentration of substrate as well as enzyme. Accordingly, the reaction rate changes continuously with time as the substrate is consumed, and measurement of enzyme activity is difficult. In zero-order enzyme reaction, the rate of reaction is linear with time, independent of the concentration of substrate and directly proportional to the concentration of enzyme (Fig. 14–4). The greater ease of measuring enzyme activity in a zero order, than in a first-order reaction, is shown in Figure 14–5.

$$\text{Enzyme (E)} + \text{substrate (S)} \underset{k_2}{\overset{k_1}{\rightleftarrows}} \text{enzyme-substrate complex (ES)}$$

$$\downarrow k_3$$

$$\text{products (P)} + \text{enzyme (E)}$$

$(k_1, k_2, k_3 = \text{rate constants})$

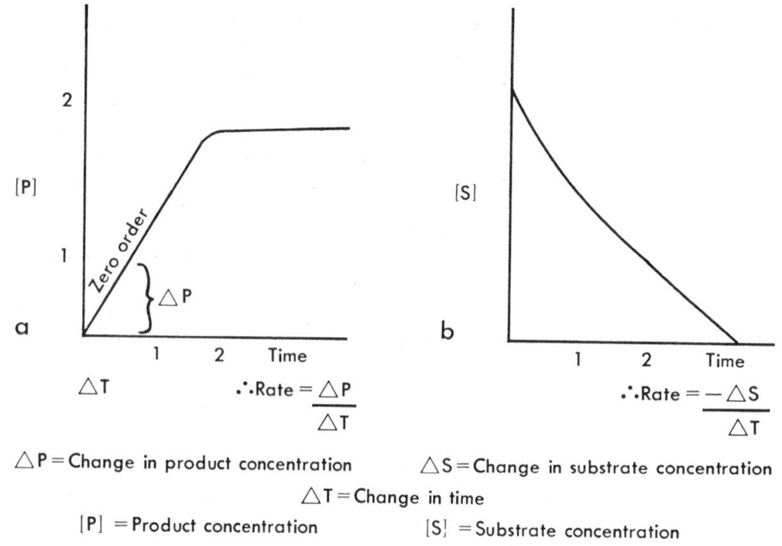

Figure 14–3. Rate of product formation (*a*) and substrate disappearance (*b*). (From Henry, J. B.: Postgrad. Med. *33*:A–68, 1963.)

To be valid, an enzyme assay must be so designed that the enzyme concentration is the only limiting factor; i.e., the result reflects the amount of enzyme and is not influenced by other substances present. This is illustrated graphically in Figure 14–4. The rate of product formation increases proportionately with enzyme concentration, e.g., one unit of product formed per minute per each 0.1 ml. of serum. Ultimately, the concentration of enzyme exceeds the amount of substrate available; i.e., substrate concentration becomes a limiting factor and proportionality is no longer present. At this point, the assay is no longer a reflection of enzyme activity.

Figure 14–5 illustrates potential hazards of utilizing a single determination. With a single or one-point (E) measuring system, three different reaction rates would have given the same apparent activity.

An assay system must progress in a zero-order reaction during its entire period of observation if the measurement is to reflect true enzyme activity. Performance of multiple determinations has the advantage of permitting assessment of kinetics and confirmation of zero-order reaction.

Multiple-point measurements of the concentration of products per unit time permit the recognition of rapid attainment of equilibrium and substrate exhaustion with samples of biologic fluids containing very high concen-

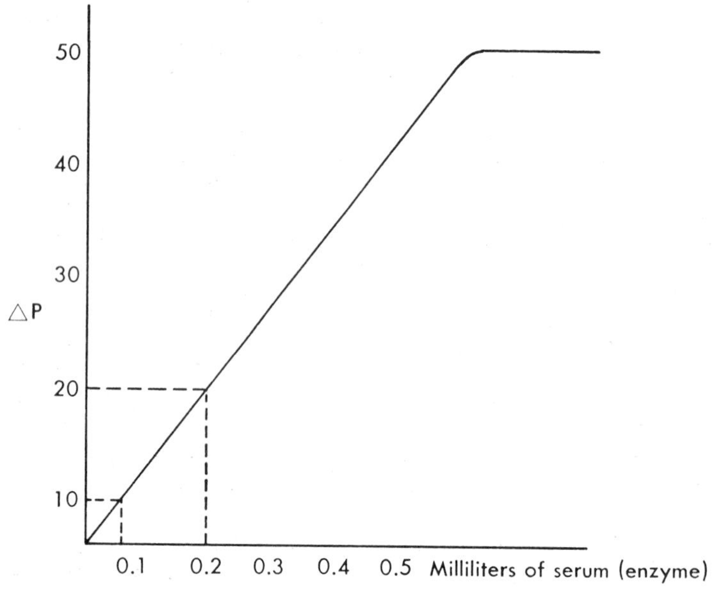

Figure 14–4. Change in product concentration (ΔP) as a function of enzyme concentration. The abscissa represents increments of serum added to reaction mixture. (From Henry, J. B.: Postgrad. Med. *33*:A–70, 1963.)

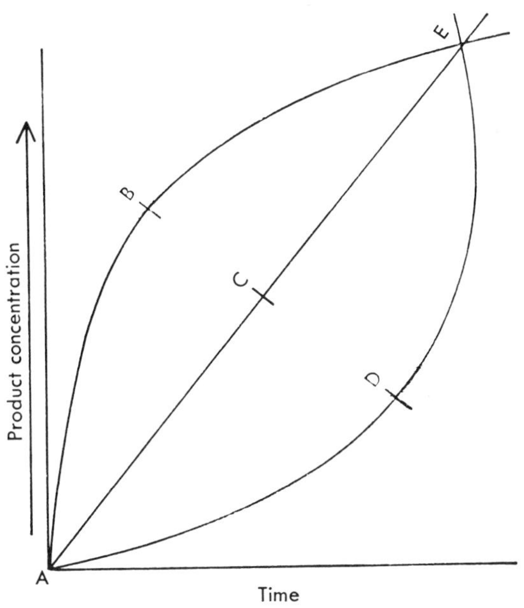

Figure 14–5. Illustration of potential hazards of using a single determination in enzyme assays. Line *ACE* is a zero-order reaction that permits accurate determination of enzyme activity for the entire reaction time. Curve *ABE* shows initial zero-order reaction of high rate followed by falling off of rate of reaction. This is possibly due to exhaustion of substrate prior to termination of assay at point *E*. Curve *ADE* reveals an initial lag phase which masks true activity. (From Henry, J. B.: Postgrad. Med. 33:A–72, 1963.)

trations of enzyme. In such instances it is preferable to use a smaller volume of sample rather than to make dilutions of sample in repeat assays. In the lactic dehydrogenase assay, we often employ a sample of 0.01 ml. rather than 0.1 ml. of the serum when very high concentrations of enzyme activities are suspected.

Numerous pitfalls are encountered in enzyme assays in the clinical laboratory. Hemolysis may be associated with the release of enzymes from red blood cells into the serum, causing falsely high serum values. Plasma may be used interchangeably with serum, although the effect of various anticoagulants should be considered and investigated in specific enzyme determinations. Lactescence, or milky serum, may result in variable absorbance readings in spectrophotometric assays. Most enzymes in biologic fluids are quite stable at 6° C. for at least 24 hours and at room temperature for lesser periods. For prolonged storage, temperatures of –20° C. or lower* must be used in order to assure preservation of enzyme activity. Heat lability must be considered with respect to each enzyme to be assayed as well as other components in the entire enzyme system, especially coenzymes and substrates. Accuracy in timing each assay and use of meticulously clean glassware are essential.

Enzyme assays requiring kinetic measurements in the ultraviolet wavelength region pose new problems for many clinical laboratories. Most of these procedures depend on the changes in absorption at 340 mμ (nm.) of pyridine nucleotides (NAD → $NADH_2$). Owing to the increasing number of nucleotide-dependent enzymes of clinical importance, the ability to work in the 340 nm range is becoming more important. Indeed, a spectrophotometer which measures accurately in the ultraviolet range is virtually essential in clinical enzymology.

A review of the lactic dehydrogenase determination underscores salient features of clinical enzyme assays. In the pH range 7 to 8, the equilibrium favors reduction of pyruvate to lactate, whereas the reverse reaction is favored in the pH range 9 to 10. Wacker, Ulmer, and Vallee (1956) have reported a lactic dehydrogenase assay incorporating a buffer at pH 8.8, lactate as the substrate, and NAD as the coenzyme. The addition of serum provides enzyme, and the assay is conducted at 25° C. Spectrophotometric measurements of absorbance (optical density) are made each minute for 5 minutes at wavelength 340 mμ. Lactate is oxidized to pyruvate with conversion of coenzyme (NAD) to reduced coenzyme ($NADH_2$). The multiple measurements at 1-minute intervals provide an assessment of adherence to zero-order reaction. One unit of activity represents a change in absorbance of 0.001 optical density units per ml. of serum per minute at 25° C.

Cabaud and Wroblewski (1958) reported a colorimetric assay for lactic dehydrogenase in which the substrate pyruvic acid is converted to lactic acid. Pyruvic acid reacts with 2,4-dinitrophenylhydrazine to form a colored hydrazone. The amount of pyruvate remaining after the incubation is inversely proportional to the amount of lactic dehydrogenase present in the reaction.

To insure accuracy and precision in clinical enzyme determinations, one must be aware of the pitfalls and informed regarding the principles of enzyme assays. A quality control program for clinical enzyme assays should include the following: (1) adherence to zero-order kinetics, (2) proportionality studies with increments of sample, (3) use of pooled frozen serum or stable reference materials (lyophilized) as control solutions, and (4) replicate measurements to evaluate precision of assay.

PRINCIPLES OF DIAGNOSTIC SERUM ENZYMOLOGY

All the serum enzymes have their origin in cells. Some enzymes are found in many tis-

*Some enzymes (e.g., CPK) do not remain reliably preserved at –20° C. and must be kept at –70° C. to retain activity.

sues (e.g., lactic dehydrogenase, aldolase, phosphohexoisomerase, malic dehydrogenase). Other enzymes are uniquely concentrated in one or two tissues. For example, ornithine carbamyl transferase and sorbitol dehydrogenase are found almost exclusively in the liver; significant amounts of creatine phosphokinase are found only in skeletal muscle, myocardium, and brain. Increase in the serum levels of an enzyme which is ubiquitous in its distribution, however, is a less specific biochemical clue to the site of injury. In order to enhance the diagnostic value of serum enzymology, attention has been directed to the different molecular forms of a given enzyme (isoenzyme) that may be found in different tissues. Some of the enzymes for which multiple molecular forms have been identified are listed in Table 14–5. Isoenzymes of amylase, alkaline phosphatase, acid phosphatase, glutamic oxalacetic transaminase, leucine aminopeptidase, lactic dehydrogenase, malic dehydrogenase, isocritic dehydrogenase, creatine phosphokinase and cholinesterase, and other enzymes have been demonstrated in different tissues and are of interest to the biochemist, physiologist, geneticist, and clinical investigator. Only the isoenzymes of the lactic dehydrogenase and of the alkaline phosphatase of the serum, however, have been of important clinical relevance. These are discussed and the types of methods available for their demonstration are listed in a subsequent portion of this chapter. Some enzymes are found in the cytoplasm of cells and reach the plasma with relatively slight injury (lactic dehydrogenase, aldolase). Enzymes that are found only in mitochondria (e.g., glutamic dehydrogenase) gain entry to the serum as the result of sufficient injury to those organelles. At present, the efforts to define the organelle injury by correlation of the intracellular source of the enzyme with the serum levels are of investigative rather than clinical interest.

Table 14–5. SOME ENZYMES* FOR WHICH ISOENZYME FORMS HAVE BEEN DEMONSTRATED

α-Glycerophosphate dehydrogenase
LD
MD
ICD
G-6-PD
6-PGD
Peroxidase
GOT
CPK
Phosphoglucomutase
Esterases
Acetylcholinesterase
Cholinesterase
Alk. phosph.
Acid phosph.
5′-N
LAP
Ceruloplasmin
RNAse
Amylase
γ-Glutamyl transpeptidase

*See Table 14-1 for meaning of abbreviations.

The use of serum enzymes as diagnostic aids has been largely empirical; but the values observed in clinical and experimental circumstances permit speculative analysis of the factors that lead to abnormal levels in diseased subjects (Table 14–6). The serum levels of a particular enzyme may be increased in diseases that lead to increased rates of release from tissue, increased amount available for release, or decreased rate of disposition. The levels of an enzyme may be decreased in disease that interferes with its production.

Increased rate of release is clearly responsible for the high serum levels of hepatic, pancreatic, and myocardial enzymes in diseases that produce necrosis of the respective tissue. The pattern of abnormality of serum enzyme values that results depends on the normal enzyme content of the tissue involved, on the extent and type of necrosis, and on other poorly understood factors. Thus, high serum levels of a number of digestive enzymes are found in acute pancreatitis, and a number of enzymes of intermediary metabolism are found in myocardial infarction or acute hepatitis. Although these enzymes are richly concentrated in both liver and myocardium, higher levels are produced by hepatitis than by myocardial infarction, presumably because the necrosis and degeneration of hepatitis is diffuse and that of infarction, discrete.

High serum levels of enzymes* in which liver is uniquely rich (GPT, OCT, Sorb. D.) are produced almost exclusively by acute hepatic disease. The minimal degree of elevation of serum ICD levels in myocardial infarction, despite the rich myocardial content of this enzyme, has been attributed to the rapid removal of this enzyme from the circulation. The relatively slight increase of LD levels in hepatic necrosis, despite the high hepatic content of this enzyme, remains to be explained adequately. Conceivably, it may relate to the simultaneous release of an inhibitor of LD.

Increased rate of release of enzyme into the circulation may occur even without apparent tissue necrosis. Increased permeability of cell membranes seems to account for the elevated serum levels of aldolase, CPK, and other enzymes in progressive muscular dystrophy.

*See Table 14–1 for meaning of abbreviations.

Table 14–6. HYPOTHETICAL MECHANISMS FOR ABNORMAL SERUM ENZYME LEVELS

MECHANISM	EXAMPLE	ENZYMES	COMMENTS
I. Increased serum levels			
A. Increased release			
1. Necrosis	Myocardial infarction	GOT, LD, Ald., MD, GR, CPK, HBD, RNase, and others	
	Acute hepatitis	GOT, GPT, OCT, ICD, Sorb. D, Gl. D, LD, Ald., PHI, MD, GR, Alk. phosph., LAP, and others	Increased levels of some enzymes (Alk. phosph.) may represent increased production as well as release from necrotic cells and decreased excretion
	Acute pancreatitis	Amylase, lipase, lecithinase, trypsin, DNAse I	
2. Increased permeability; cell membranes without necrosis	Progressive muscular dystrophy, delirum tremens, dermatomyositis	CPK, Ald., LD, PHI, MD, GOT, GPT	
B. Increased tissue source of enzymes; Increased release from tissue or both	Neoplastic disease (carcinoma, lymphoma), granulocytic leukemia	LD, Ald., PHI, MD, GR, glucuronidase	
	Megaloblastic Anemia	LD, Ald., PHI, MD	May be result of increased numbers of megaloblasts, increased intramedullary destruction, or both
	Osteoblastic lesions (Paget's disease, osteogenic sarcoma, healing fractures, rickets, etc.)	Alk. phosph., ATPase	
	Peptic ulcer	Pepsinogen	
C. Impaired excretion of enzyme	Uremia	Amylase	Elevated amylase levels secondary to renal failure rare and of uncertain origin
	Obstructive jaundice	Alk. phosph., LAP, 5-N, GITP	Increased production main factor in increased levels of alk. phosph. in obstructive jaundice.
II. Decreased serum levels			
D. Decreased formation			
1. Genetic	Hypophosphatasia	Alk. phosph.	
	Wilson's disease	Ceruloplasmin	
	Acholinesterasemia	Pseudocholinesterase	
2. Acquired	Hepatitis	Pseudocholinesterase	
	Starvation	Amylase	
B. Enzyme inhibition	Insecticide poisoning	Pseudocholinesterase	
C. Lack of cofactors	Pregnancy	GOT	Pyridoxine deficiency or defective pyridoxine metabolism
	Cirrhosis		

The high serum levels of CPK, GOT, aldolase, PHI, LD, and MD in patients with delirium tremens or alcoholic myopathy, but without recognizable liver disease, also may depend upon increased permeability of skeletal muscle membrane.

An increase in the tissue source of enzymes because of increased rate of production per cell or increase in the number of cells may be responsible for increased serum levels. This seems to be the mechanism for the increased levels of pepsinogen, alkaline phosphatase, and acid phosphatase in patients with peptic ulcer, osteoblastic bone lesions, and prostatic carcinoma, respectively. The serum levels of glycolytic and other enzymes associated with neoplastic diseases seem to reflect the total mass of tumor. There is evidence that the increased alkaline phosphatase levels of the serum in obstructive jaundice are primarily the result of increased hepatic production of the enzyme, although decreased biliary excretion may play a role.

Impaired disposition of serum enzymes has been considered to contribute to the increased levels of AP and GOT in biliary obstruction and for increased amylase levels in renal failure. Evidence for this thesis remains insufficient.

Abnormally low levels of some serum enzymes are also observed, presumably as the result of decreased synthesis. Levels of cholinesterase and cholesterol esterase may be low in hepatic disease; levels of amylase are low in chronic hepatic or pancreatic disease or in starvation; levels of pepsinogen are low in gastric mucosal atrophy; levels of alkaline phosphatase are low in hypophosphatasia; and levels of ceruloplasmin are low in Wilson's disease.

The selection of serum enzyme tests for clinical use has depended on historical circumstance, the experience gained in correlating the values with other measures of disease, and the technical ease of performing the respective procedure. A serum enzyme, the diagnostic value of which has been established for a clinical setting, is not likely to be supplanted by a subsequently discovered one, unless the diagnostic usefulness of the more recent candidate is far superior to that of its predecessor. Alkaline phosphatase, a time-honored aid for the diagnosis of hepatobiliary disease, has not been replaced by leucine aminopeptidase,* or 5′-nucleotidase,* despite recent reports of the diagnostic advantages of the latter two enzymes. Ornithine carbamyl transferase* and sorbitol dehydrogenase,* more recent arrivals than GPT to the serum enzyme scene, have not replaced the latter as measures of hepatic disease, despite reports of somewhat greater specificity.

*See later section of chapter for description of these enzymes.

The serum enzymes discussed in detail below are those which have been of the greatest clinical usefulness or interest in the past or which hold the most promise. Particular attention is given to the phosphatases, transaminases, lactic dehydrogenase and its isoenzymes, and cholinesterase. Many of the other serum enzymes are described, and their clinical relevance is discussed briefly.

Phosphatases

The phosphatases of the blood, more properly called phosphomonoesterases, include two main types. The "alkaline phosphatase" has a pH optimum of approximately 9, while the "acid phosphatase" has its optimal activity at a pH of approximately 5. Although there is evidence that alkaline and acid phosphatases each include several different enzymes (isoenzymes), it has been convenient for clinical purposes to consider each a single enzyme.

Alkaline Phosphatase. The application of alkaline phosphatase determination to the study of hepatic disease is discussed in Chapter 13. The demonstration that bone is rich in alkaline phosphatase and that normal plasma (or serum) contains the same or a similar enzyme led to the study of serum alkaline phosphatase levels in patients with diseases of bone. Elevated levels of the enzyme occur in patients with bone diseases characterized by increased osteoblastic activity (Table 14–7). These include osteitis deformans, rickets, osteomalacia, hyperparathyroidism, healing fractures, and osteoblastic bone tumors, both primary and secondary. Growing children and pregnant women in the third trimester have "physiologically" elevated serum alkaline phosphatase levels.

Lower than normal levels are observed in

Table 14–7. CONDITIONS IN WHICH THE SERUM ALKALINE PHOSPHATASE LEVEL IS INCREASED*

HEPATOBILIARY DISEASE		BONE DISEASE		OTHER CONDITIONS	
Obstructive jaundice	↑ ↑ ↑	Osteitis deformans	↑ ↑ ↑	Healing fractures	↑
Biliary cirrhosis	↑ ↑ ↑	Rickets	↑ ↑	Normal growth	↑
Cholangiolitic hepatitis	↑ ↑ ↑	Osteomalacia	↑ ↑	Pregnancy (last trimester)	↑
Intrahepatic cholestasis	↑ ↑	Hyperparathyroidism	↑ ↑		
Space-occupying lesions (granuloma, abscess, metastatic carcinoma)	↑ ↑	Metastatic bone disease	↑ ↑		
Viral hepatitis	↑	Osteogenic sarcoma	↑ ↑ ↑		
Infectious mononucleosis	↑ ↑				
Cirrhosis, Laennec's	↑				

*Degree of increase indicated by number of arrows.
Depressed values: hypophosphatasia, malnutrition.

Table 14–8. CHARACTERISTICS OF ISOENZYME OF ALKALINE PHOSPHATASE

	INHIBITION* BY		
SOURCE OF ENZYME	Phenylalanine (%)	Heat or Urea (%)	ORDER ANODAL MIGRATION
Liver	10	60	1
Bone	10	90	2
Intestine	75	60	4
Placenta	80	0	3
Regan (carcinoma)	80	0	3

*Approximate figures.

patients with hypophosphatasia (an inborn error of metabolism), and in malnourished patients.

The alkaline phosphatase determination is useful in the recognition of diseases of bone, especially osteitis deformans, hyperparathyroidism, and bone neoplasms. Hepatic disease as a cause of serum alkaline phosphatase elevation usually can be distinguished by other laboratory procedures and clinical features. The increased levels of this enzyme in normal, growing children should be kept in mind when attempting to apply the serum alkaline phosphatase levels to diagnosis.

Isoenzymes of Alkaline Phosphatase. Studies of the properties of alkaline phosphatase isolated from various tissues (liver, bone, spleen, kidney, intestine) indicate that each differs from the others. Total serum alkaline phosphatase in normals consists of isoenzymes contributed by liver, bone, and, in some individuals, intestine. During the last trimester of pregnancy 40 to 65 per cent of the serum alkaline phosphatase derives from placenta. Isoenzymes from these four sources have been distinguished from each other by electrophoretic analysis, differential inhibition by chemicals and heat, and immunochemically, although there are also differences in substrate dependence and reaction kinetics.

The degrees of inhibition of isoenzymes of hepatic, osseous, intestinal, and placental origin produced by heating to 56° C. for 15 minutes, exposure to 3 M urea for 18 minutes, incubation with 5×10^{-3} M phenylalanine, and the relative electrophoretic migration of these isoenzymes are shown in Table 14–8. (Note that the Regan isoenzyme, found in the serum of about 5 per cent of patients with carcinomas of various types, resembles the placental alkaline phosphatase). These properties are helpful in identifying placental and intestinal alkaline phosphatase (both phenylalanine-inhibited) and in distinguishing them from hepatic and bone isoenzymes. Distinction of hepatic from osseous alkaline phosphatase is aided by heat or urea inhibition, but the overlapping effects lead to imprecision. Nevertheless, the susceptibility of the osseous isoenzyme to heat inactivation has been applied quite widely to distinguish it from the hepatic isoenzyme. Electrophoretic analysis of alkaline phosphatase isoenzymes will also, in most instances, permit identification of the main isoenzyme contributing to an elevated alkaline phosphatase level, although quantitation of the fractions is prevented by the lack of distinct separation of the two rapidly moving isoenzymes (hepatic and osseous). None of the methods employed is reliable in distinguishing between hepatocellular and posthepatic jaundice as a cause of elevated alkaline phosphatase levels, although an isoenzyme which migrates more slowly than any of the others has been described in the serum of patients with posthepatic jaundice. Regular clinical application of alkaline phosphatase isoenzymology, however, must await improved means of quantitation of the individual isoenzymes and extensive testing of quantitative values in clinical circumstances.

Study of placental alkaline phosphatase has yielded interesting data. It appears in plasma at the beginning of the second trimester of pregnancy, rises to a maximum during the third trimester, when it contributes 40 to 65 per cent of alkaline phosphatase activity, and then declines to normal during the first postpartum month.

Acid Phosphatase. This enzyme, first demonstrated in the urine in 1925, was found to be much more prevalent in male than in female urine. It was soon shown that prostatic tissue contains this enzyme in high concentration. Another acid phosphatase, which differs from that found in the prostate (Table 14–9), is present in erythrocytes and platelets. The methods used for determination of acid phosphatase are similar to and include the same substrates as those used for alkaline phosphatase assay.

Elevated serum levels of acid phosphatase are seen in patients with prostatic carcinoma that has metastasized. One-half to three-fourths of patients with carcinoma of the prostate that has extended beyond the capsule have elevated acid phosphatase levels. Patients with prostatic carcinoma still confined within the capsule usually have normal serum levels of this enzyme. However, patients with benign prostatic hypertrophy may have slight elevations of the serum acid phosphatase level after vigorous prostatic "massage." Since other tissues, such as erythrocytes, may also release acid phosphatase into the serum, minor elevations of enzyme levels may reflect such an origin rather than the prostate. Accordingly, efforts have been made to distinguish "prostatic" acid phosphatase from the isoenzymes that are of erythrocyte and other origin. The efforts to distinguish "prostatic" acid phosphatase from erythrocyte acid phosphatase have been based on the differential effect of various substrates and various inhibitors on enzymes from these two sources (Table 14–9). Such efforts have been considered not to be necessary when the apparently specific method of Bodansky (beta-glycerophosphate as substrate) is used. When the King-Armstrong method (phenylphosphate as substrate) is used, and particularly when the acid phosphatase levels are only slightly elevated, the use of inhibitors may be of assistance. The inhibition of prostatic acid phosphatase by tartrate and the lack of inhibition by cupric ion, compared to the lack of inhibition of erythrocyte acid phosphatase by tartrate and the inhibition by cupric ion, are the properties most commonly utilized (Table 14–9).

Elevations of the serum acid phosphatase using the method of Bodansky (β-glycerophosphate as substrate) usually reflect carcinoma of the prostate (as discussed previously), especially if the levels exceed 5 Bodansky units. When the method of Gutman (phenylphosphate as substrate) or the King-Armstrong method is used, other diseases may yield abnormal levels occasionally. Such elevations are frequent in Gaucher's disease and occasional in osteitis deformans.

Table 14–9. EFFECT OF INHIBITORS ON ACID PHOSPHATASE OF PROSTATE AND OTHER TISSUES*

INHIBITOR	INHIBITION OF PROSTATIC PHOSPHATASE	INHIBITION OF ERYTHROCYTE PHOSPHATASE
Ethyl alcohol 40%	+	−
L(+)–Tartaric acid acid 0.02 M	+	−
Formaldehyde 2%	−	+
Cupric sulfate 0.001 M	−	+

*+represents marked inhibition
−represents minimal inhibition

Acid phosphatase determination has been useful in detecting metastases from carcinoma of the prostate. As a diagnostic clue to the presence of resectable carcinoma of the prostate, however, it is of no value.

Transaminases

The application of the serum transaminases to the study of hepatic disease and the principles of assay for these enzymes are discussed in Chapter 13. Glutamic oxalacetic transaminase (GOT) levels of the serum are elevated in patients with hepatobiliary disease, cardiovascular disease, muscle disease, and some miscellaneous conditions. Glutamic pyruvic transaminase (GPT) levels are elevated in the serum of patients with hepatic disease. In other conditions elevations are negligible unless there is hepatic involvement.

Glutamic Oxalacetic Transaminase.* This enzyme is elevated in diseases involving the tissues that are rich in it. In Table 14–10 are also shown the tissues with the highest GOT concentration, the categories of disease that may show abnormal levels, and the range of values seen in many of these conditions. The GOT levels in patients with disease of the liver are discussed in Chapter 13.

Extensive studies have shown that 92 to 98 per cent of patients with acute myocardial infarction have elevated serum GOT levels, which are usually four to 10 times the upper limit of normal. These usually develop within 12 hours of the time of infarction and reach the peak by the second day; the values usually return to normal by the fifth day after infarction (Fig. 14–6). Secondary rises may reflect extension or recurrence of myocardial infarction. Experimental work with animals suggests that the degree of rise of serum GOT is related to the extent of myocardial necrosis.

In patients with electrocardiographic and clinical criteria of "coronary insufficiency" rather than myocardial infarction, elevated serum GOT levels may occur. It is not clear whether this represents myocardial necrosis which has not been recognizable by other means or "leakage" of the enzyme into the serum even without frank myocardial necrosis.

Mild elevations of the serum GOT levels have been reported in some patients with pulmonary infarction. The incidence has varied from 0 to 30 per cent, and the elevations are slight to moderate. Animal studies have also

*Currently accepted nomenclature for the glutamic oxalacetic transaminase (GOT), is *aspartate transaminase* or aspartate *aminotransferase*. The term GOT is used throughout this chapter, since it is still the one that is understood most widely.

yielded inconclusive results on the occurrence of elevated serum GOT levels in experimental pulmonary infarction. The incidence of increased values in humans is low, the degree

Table 14–10. TISSUES RICH IN GOT AND CONDITIONS IN WHICH THE SERUM ENZYME IS ABNORMAL*

	Usual Values (Karmen units)
A. Tissue content of GOT (descending order of concentration)	
1. cardiac	
2. hepatic	
3. skeletal muscle	
4. kidney	
5. brain	
6. pancreas	
7. spleen	
8. lung	
9. serum	
B. Conditions in which serum GOT is elevated	
1. *Cardiac disease*	
myocardial infarction	40–400 μ
pericarditis	< 100 μ
cardiac arrhythmias	< 200 μ
acute rheumatic fever (?)	< 100 μ
postcardiac surgery and catheterization	< 100 μ
heart failure	< 200 μ
2. *Hepatic disease*	
acute hepatitis (viral, toxic)	500–4000
infectious mononucleosis	50–800
cirrhosis	< 200 μ
hepatic congestion	< 200 μ
space-occupying lesions (granuloma, metastatic carcinoma)	< 300 μ
obstructive jaundice	< 300 μ
3. *Other diseases*	
shock	40–2000
pulmonary infarction	< 100 μ
acute pancreatitis	40–1500
renal infarction (experimental animals)	< 300
cerebral necrosis	< 100
dermatomyositis	< 300
progressive muscular dystrophy	< 300
delirium tremens	< 100
hemolysis (slight)	< 100
gangrene (slight)	< 100
C. Conditions in which serum GOT is depressed	
1. Pregnancy (abnormal pyridoxal metabolism)	0–6

*In acute hepatitis, values above 300 units are usual and above 500 are frequent. In all the other conditions shown the levels are usually below this value, although higher values are occasionally observed in infectious mononucleosis and shock. Almost all patients with acute myocardial infarction have elevated values during the first few days. In the other cardiac diseases listed, elevations are less frequent and usually are slight.

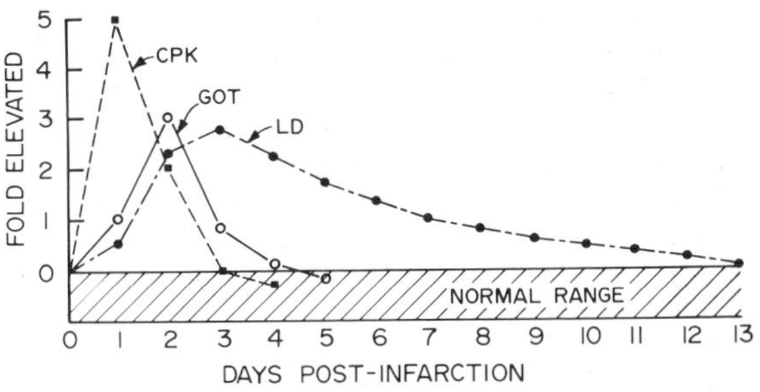

Figure 14–6. GOT, GPT, and CPK levels after myocardial infarction (means of values for 200 patients). Note that the CPK rise is earliest, the LD rise is latest, and the LD elevations are present longer than those of CPK and GOT.

of abnormality slight, and the rise delayed for three to five days after the onset of pain.

In patients with congestive heart failure and in those with marked tachycardia, mild to moderate degrees of GOT elevation may occur. These have been attributed to the hepatic necrosis secondary to hepatic congestion. Patients with pericarditis have also been reported to have a 50 per cent incidence of slightly elevated GOT levels. The incidence and mechanism of occurrence of elevated enzyme levels in patients with rheumatic fever are not clear. Slight serum GOT elevations have been reported after cardiac catheterization and mitral commissurotomy.

Glutamic oxalacetic transaminase determination is not necessary for the diagnosis of myocardial infarction in most patients with classic clinical and electrocardiographic evidence of this condition. This determination is of value in patients whose electrocardiographic changes are insufficiently helpful, e.g., those with left bundle branch block or Wolff-Parkinson-White syndrome or in those with electrocardiographic abnormalities remaining from previous infarction, which may obscure acute changes. Determination of this serum enzyme is also of value in recognizing the recurrence or extension of an infarction during convalescence. Normal values obtained at the proper time are of value in excluding a diagnosis of myocardial infarction.

Patients with disease or injury producing inflammation or destruction of skeletal muscle may also have elevated serum GOT levels. Patients with progressive muscular dystrophy, dermatomyositis, and trichinosis may have elevated levels, while those with amyotrophic lateral sclerosis, myasthenia gravis, and nerve section do not. Gangrene of the extremities and surgical or other trauma may produce slight GOT elevations. In less than 50 per cent of patients with cerebrovascular accidents serum GOT elevations may be found.

Elevated serum GOT levels in patients with hepatic disease are discussed in Chapter 13. In acute pancreatitis, both normal and elevated

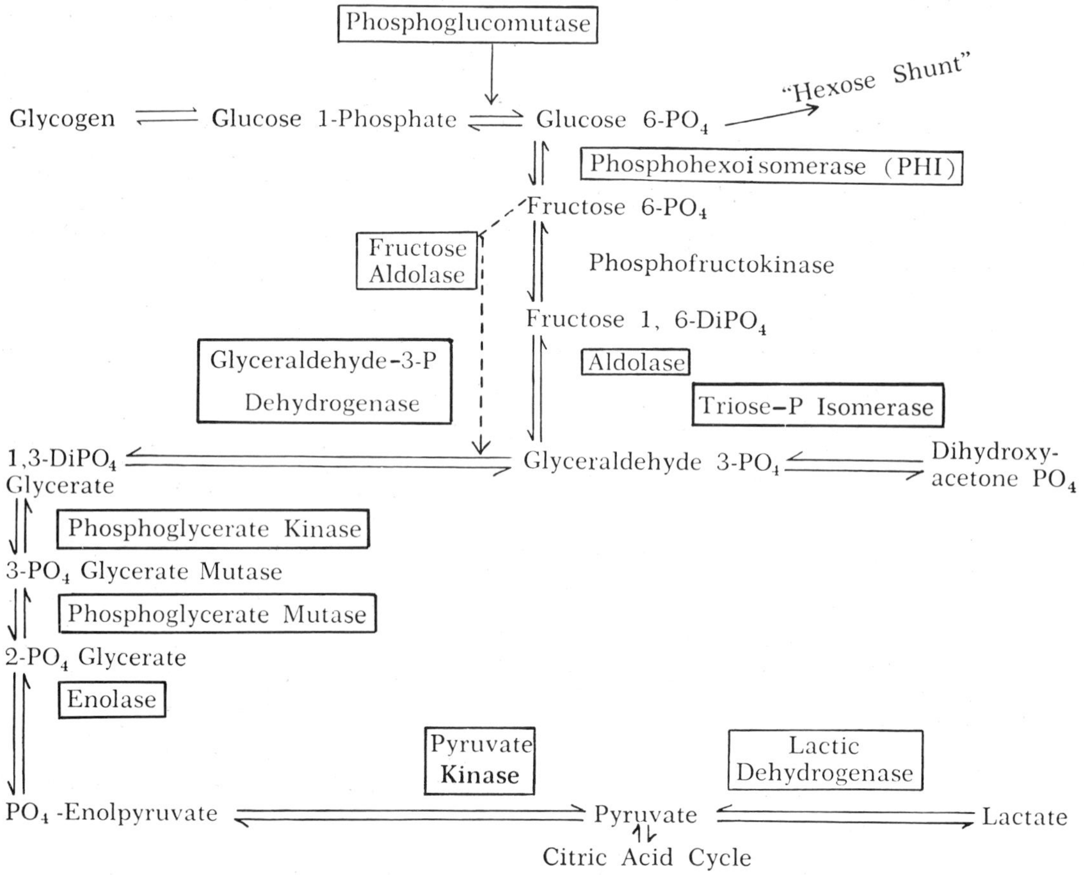

Figure 14–7. Scheme of glycolytic pathway of carbohydrate metabolism. Enzymes demonstrated in human serum are shown in boxes.

levels have been reported. It has been suggested that obstruction of the biliary tree by the edematous pancreas and the presence of associated hepatic disease or of delirium tremens may contribute to the elevated GOT levels in these patients.

Glutamic Pyruvic Transaminase (GPT).* This enzyme is also discussed in Chapter 13. In patients with myocardial infarction elevations of the serum levels of GPT are slight or absent. Heart failure or shock with the attendant hepatic necrosis may lead to elevated GPT levels. The chief application of determination of this serum enzyme is in the diagnosis of hepatobiliary disease.

Glycolytic Enzymes

The glycolytic pathway, which is found in virtually all tissues, includes a number of enzymes (Fig. 14–7). Almost all these have been demonstrated in the serum. In patients with extensive carcinoma elevated levels of several of these enzymes (phosphohexoisomerase, aldolase, and lactic dehydrogenase) have been observed. These elevations have served as a guide to chemotherapy, particularly in carcinoma of the breast and prostate.

Elevated levels of these enzymes also have been observed in patients with megaloblastic and hemolytic anemias and in granulocytic and acute leukemias but not in patients with chronic lymphocytic leukemia, aplastic anemia, or iron deficiency anemia. The most extensively studied of the glycolytic enzymes in the serum are lactic dehydrogenase (LD), aldolase (Ald.) and phosphohexoisomerase (PHI). The serum levels of all three are elevated to approximately the same degree in patients with extensive carcinomatosis, megaloblastic anemia, granulocytic leukemia, infectious mononucleosis, hemolytic states, and myocardial infarction (Table 14–11). Levels of PHI seem to reflect carcinomatosis more sensitively, and those of LD seem to be a more sensitive reflection of megaloblastic anemia than do those of the other two. Aldolase is the most sensitive of the three as a reflector of muscle diseases (progressive muscular dystrophy, trichinosis, and dermatomyositis). Levels of Ald. and PHI are much more strikingly elevated than those of LD in patients with hepatic necrosis. Indeed, the very insensitivity of the serum LD level to parenchymal hepatic damage coupled with its sensitivity as a measure of carcinomatosis enhances its usefulness for the recognition of metastatic or primary carcinoma of the liver. Other glycolytic enzymes have not been studied sufficiently to delineate their value in clinical circumstances.

Phosphohexoisomerase (PHI). This glycolytic enzyme catalyzes the conversion of glucose-6-phosphate to fructose-6-phosphate (Fig. 14–7). First studied in the serum of tumorous rats by Warburg and Christian, PHI levels of the serum have been investigated in patients with carcinoma and other diseases during the past few years.

The activity of PHI is assayed by using glucose-6-phosphate as substrate. The rate of formation of fructose-6-phosphate using the Seliwanoff reaction (resorcinol) is a measure of PHI activity.

Phosphohexoisomerase levels have been used as an index of metastases in patients with carcinoma of the breast and prostate and to monitor the response to therapy. Other diseases in which elevations are observed are listed in Tables 14–1 and 14–11. Determination of this serum enzyme, however, has not been applied extensively to clinical medicine.

Aldolase. This glycolytic enzyme catalyzes the cleavage of fructose-1-6-diphosphate into two triose molecules (glyceraldehyde phosphate and dihydroxyacetone phosphate) (Fig. 14–7). Several methods have been devised for this assay, based on the rate at which the trioses are formed. One involves measuring the colored dinitrophenylhydrazone.

Serum aldolase levels are elevated in skeletal muscle disease, carcinomatosis, granulocytic leukemia, megaloblastic anemia, hepatitis, other types of hepatic necrosis, and the other conditions that are listed in Figure 14–8 and Tables 14–1 and 14–11. The aldolase levels reflect particularly sensitively progressive muscular dystrophy and inflammatory muscle disease (dermatomyositis, trichinosis), in which strikingly elevated values can be seen. Patients destined to develop progressive muscular dystrophy usually have elevated aldolase levels

Table 14–11. RELATIVE SENSITIVITY OF GLYCOLYTIC ENZYME LEVELS TO VARIOUS TYPES OF DISEASES

	LD	ALD.	PHI
Myocardial infarction	↑↑	↑↑	↑↑
Pulmonary infarction	↑	↑	↑
Carcinoma, granulocytic leukemia	↑↑	↑↑	↑↑↑
Megaloblastic anemia	↑↑↑	↑↑	↑↑
Hepatic necrosis	↑ or N	↑↑↑	↑↑↑
Muscle disease	↑↑	↑↑↑↑	↑↑

*The currently accepted term for glutamic pyruvic transaminase is *alanine transaminase* or *alanine aminotransferase*.

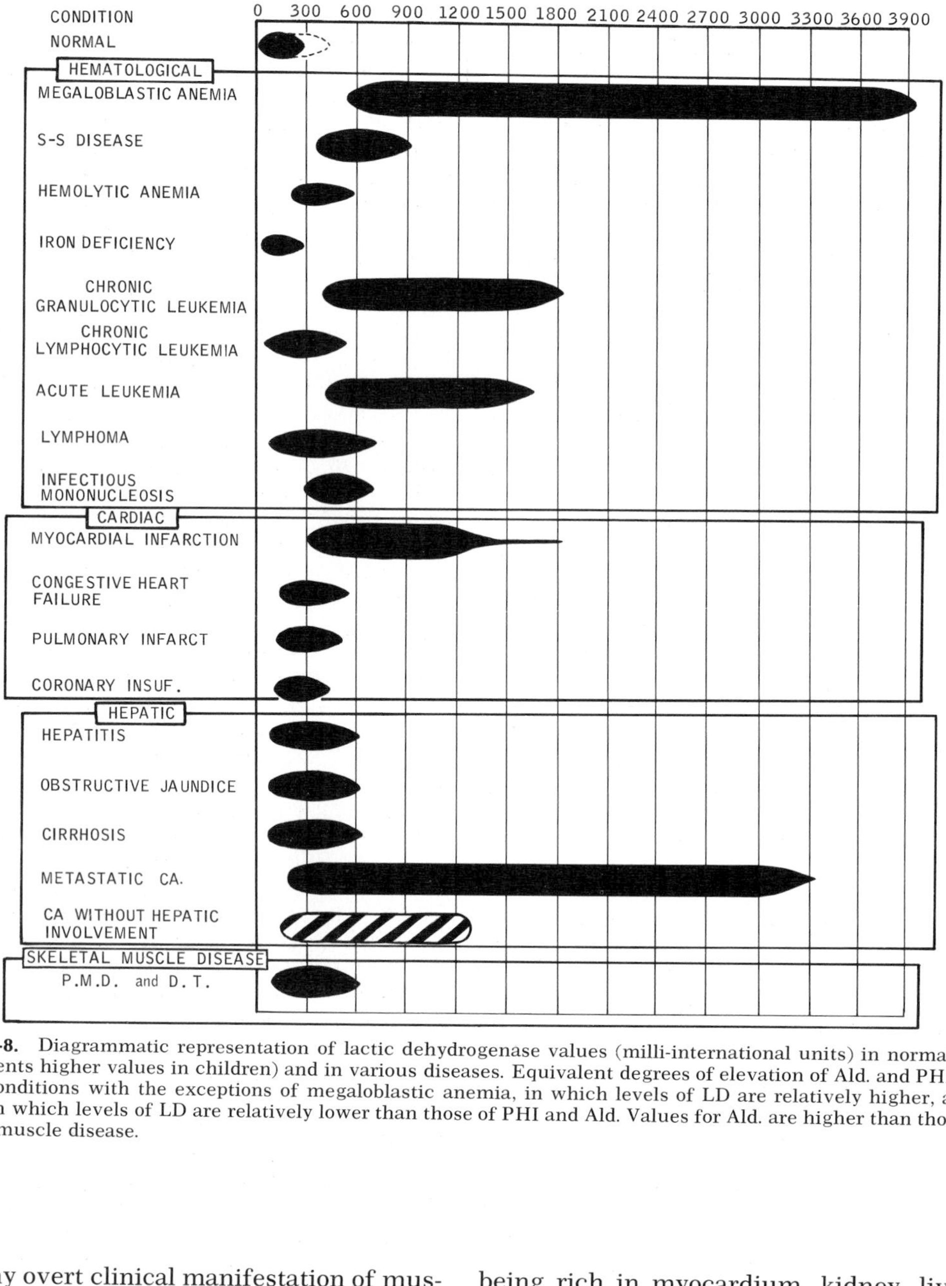

Figure 14–8. Diagrammatic representation of lactic dehydrogenase values (milli-international units) in normals (dotted line represents higher values in children) and in various diseases. Equivalent degrees of elevation of Ald. and PHI occur in all these conditions with the exceptions of megaloblastic anemia, in which levels of LD are relatively higher, and acute hepatitis, in which levels of LD are relatively lower than those of PHI and Ald. Values for Ald. are higher than those of PHI and LD in muscle disease.

before any overt clinical manifestation of muscle disease. The chief clinical application of aldolase assay in the United States has been in the study of muscle disease. In other parts of the world and in a few laboratories in the United States, aldolase levels are employed as sensitive measures of hepatic disease and in the study of neoplastic disease.

Lactic Dehydrogenase (LD)

This enzyme catalyzes the reversible oxidation of lactic to pyruvic acid (Fig. 14–7). It is widely distributed in mammalian tissues, being rich in myocardium, kidney, liver, and muscle.

Methods. Spectrophotometric and colorimetric methods have been applied to the assay of this enzyme. In the spectrophotometric method, the rate of change in concentration of DPNH is determined. The reaction may be measured by following the disappearance of DPNH (pyruvate + DPNH $\xrightarrow{\text{LD}}$ lactate + DPN) at a pH of 7.4 or by following the appearance of DPNH (lactate + DPN $\xrightarrow{\text{LD}}$ pyruvate + DPNH) at a pH of 8.8 or higher. The results have been expressed as units or as micromols of DPNH altered.

Elevated serum levels of LD are observed in a variety of conditions (Fig. 14–8). The highest values (two- to fortyfold elevations) are seen in patients with megaloblastic anemia, in those with extensive carcinomatosis, and in those with severe shock and anoxia. Moderate elevations (two- to fourfold) occur in patients with myocardial infarction, pulmonary infarction, granulocytic or acute leukemia, hemolytic anemia, infectious mononucleosis, and in patients with progressive muscular dystrophy. Relatively slight elevations occur in patients with hepatitis, obstructive jaundice, or cirrhosis, but higher values occur in those with delirium tremens. Patients with chronic renal disease, especially those with nephrotic syndrome or hemolytic anemia, also have increased values. In patients with myxedema, the LD values are also regularly elevated.

The pattern of elevated serum LD levels in patients with myocardial infarction is quite characteristic. High levels are observed in almost all patients within 24 hours of the apparent onset of infarction. Although the degree of elevation is not so striking as that of GOT, the elevated levels persist longer (10 to 14 days). The characteristically prolonged period of elevated LD values and briefer period of elevated GOT values provides a pattern that may be useful in the recognition of myocardial infarction (Fig. 14–6).

Most patients with pulmonary infarction have elevated levels of LD, usually within 24 hours of the onset of pain. The pattern of normal GOT and elevated LD levels within one to two days after an episode of chest pain provides suggestive evidence for pulmonary infarction.

Almost all patients with megaloblastic anemia have elevated LD levels. Often the values are strikingly increased. Possible factors in the production of the high values include the large number of megaloblasts, presumably rich in LD, and the intramedullary destruction of these cells. As the anemia responds to treatment, the LD levels return to normal. Hemolytic anemias yield slightly elevated levels. Patients with aplastic and iron deficiency anemias usually have normal values.

Patients with granulocytic and acute leukemia have moderately elevated LD levels. In lymphocytic leukemia, the values are usually normal, unless there is an associated hemolytic state. In patients with lymphosarcoma and Hodgkin's disease, LD levels are normal or moderately elevated, depending on the total mass of tumor and the presence of hemolysis.

Patients and animals with small, localized carcinomas usually have normal serum levels of LD, while those with distant metastases or even local extension have increased levels. The highest values occur in patients with metastases to the liver, although increased levels are also found in some patients with only extrahepatic metastases or extension.

The serum LD level does not provide a sensitive measure of hepatic disease. Patients with viral hepatitis have slightly elevated (one- to twofold) values. In patients with infectious mononucleosis, LD levels are usually somewhat higher, perhaps released from the aggregates of immature mononuclear cells throughout the body. Only slightly increased values are seen in patients with obstructive jaundice and in those with cirrhosis. Interestingly, almost all patients with delirium tremens have increased values, perhaps of skeletal muscle origin, since, like the elevated LD levels of progressive muscular dystrophy, they are accompanied by increased serum levels of creatine phosphokinase (see later).

The large number of conditions in which elevated LD levels are seen detracts somewhat from the diagnostic usefulness of its measurement. The LD level is clinically useful in the recognition of myocardial infarction and pulmonary infarction. It is often a somewhat superfluous clue to extensive carcinomatosis, but it may be used to monitor the course of cancer chemotherapy, since response to therapy is often mirrored by decreasing serum levels. Other clinical applications entail analysis of the clinical problem in the light of conditions known to cause elevated LD levels.

Isoenzymes of Lactic Dehydrogenase. The lactic dehydrogenase of human serum has been found to be separable into five different components by appropriate electrophoretic techniques. Each of these isoenzymes is distinguishable from the others by serologic, electrophoretic, and various other chemical procedures (Table 14–12). Indeed, the great current interest in isoenzymology derives from the observations on the multiple molecular forms of lactic dehydrogenase. The isoenzymes of LD are designated in ordinary usage according to their electrophoretic mobility. The fraction with the greatest mobility (anodic) is called LD_1, the one with least anodic mobility is called LD_5, and the other three are designated accordingly as LD_2, LD_3 and LD_4, respectively.

The five LD isoenzymes have the same molecular weight (135,000) but differ in the charge that they carry. Each isoenzyme is a tetramer made up of four subunits, each of 34,000 molecular weight. There are two types of these subunits, designated A and B, respectively. The five isoenzymes of LD consist of the five possible combinations of monomers A and B (Table 14–13).

Tissue lactic dehydrogenase consists of the five isoenzymes in varying proportions, and the LD activity of each tissue has a characteristic isoenzyme composition (Table 14–13). Thus, the LD of myocardium, erythrocytes,

Table 14–12. PRINCIPLES OF SOME OF THE TECHNIQUES EMPLOYED TO MEASURE ISOENZYMES OF LACTIC DEHYDROGENASE

METHOD	COMMENT	CLINICAL APPLICABILITY
I. Physical		
A. Electrophoretic	Demonstrates the five isoenzymes	Somewhat cumbersome and not sufficiently quantitative, but clinically useful
B. Selective absorption on DEAE cellulose	Selective absorption of fast ($LD_{1,2}$) isoenzymes, leaving slow ($LD_{3,4,5}$)	Remains to be demonstrated
C. Solvent precipitation techniques in which acetone or chloroform is used	Selective precipitation of slow isoenzymes, leaving fast in supernatant	Remains to be demonstrated
D. Heat denaturation at 65° C. for 30 minutes	Destroys activity of all isoenzymes except most rapid (LD_1)	Useful in the diagnosis of myocardial infarction
II. Chemical		
A. Substrate-product relationship		
1. Measurement of ability to dehydrogenate α-hydroxybutyrate dehydrogenase (HBD) activity	1. HBD activity is largely equivalent to LD_1 activity	1. Suitable for demonstrations of approximate LD_1 activity
2. Relative inhibition by various concentrations of pyruvate or lactate	2. Individual isoenzymes show different degrees of inhibition by high pyruvate concentration	2. Of theoretical interest, but no clinical applicability as yet
B. Coenzyme affinity Measurement of relative activity isoenzymes with DPN and its analogues	Each isoenzyme shows characteristic rates of activity with various analogues of DPN	Extremely useful research tool. Remains to be clinically applicable
C. Differential chemical inhibition of LD activity	Individual isoenzymes are characteristically and differentially inhibited by several chemical agents (urea, sulfate, oxamate, chloroform)	No clinical application as yet

and kidney consists largely of the fastest moving isoenzymes (LD_1 and LD_2).

In liver and skeletal muscle, the principal isoenzymes are LD_4 and LD_5. A number of tissues (spleen, pancreas, thyroid, adrenals, and lymph nodes) consist mainly of LD_3. The relative concentration of the several isoenzymes in normal serum is LD_2, LD_1, LD_3, LD_4, and LD_5, in descending order. Normal serum LD has been presumed to derive mainly from erythrocytes.

Studies of the isoenzyme composition of the elevated serum LD levels of various diseases have revealed abnormal patterns that reflect the tissues involved (Table 14–14). In acute myocardial infarction, the elevated serum LD levels consist largely of LD_1 and LD_2, the isoenzymes in which myocardium is par-

Table 14–13. NOMENCLATURE, COMPOSITION, ISOENZYMES, AND TISSUE SOURCE OF LACTIC DEHYDROGENASE FOUND IN HUMAN SERUM BY ELECTROPHORETIC TECHNIQUES

NOMENCLATURE OF ISOENZYME STARTING WITH MOST ANODIC	COMPOSITION PROPORTION OF MONOMERS* IN EACH ISOENZYME	RELATIVE CONTENT† OF ISOENZYME					
		MYOCARDIUM	LIVER	SKELETAL MUSCLE	BRAIN	KIDNEY	RBC
1	AAAA	++++	±	±	++	+	+++
2	AAAB	++++	±	±	++	+	+++
3	AABB	+	+	+	++	++	+
4	ABBB	±	++	++	++	++	±
5	BBBB	±	++++	++++	±	++	±

**A* refers to monomer H (myocardial). *B* refers to monomer M (skeletal muscle).
†Content graded from ±, which represents almost no activity, to ++++, which represents high activity.

Table 14–14. RELATIVE DEGREE OF INCREASE OF LACTIC DEHYDROGENASE AND PATTERN OF ABNORMALITY OF ISOENZYME IN VARIOUS DISEASES

		ISOZYME FRACTION MOST ABNORMAL				
	RELATIVE DEGREE	MOST ANODIC (+)				(−)
DISEASE	INCREASE TOTAL LD ACTIVITY	LD_1	LD_2	LD_3	LD_4	LD_5
Myocardial infarction	↑ ↑	X	X			
Pulmonary infarction*	↑				X	X
Congestive heart failure	↑				X	X
Viral hepatitis	↑				X	X
Toxic hepatitis	↑				X	X
Cirrhosis	↑				X	X
Leukemia, granulocytic	↑ ↑		X	X		
Pancreatitis	↑		X	X		
Carcinomatosis (extensive)	↑ ↑ ↑		X	X		
Megaloblastic anemia	↑ ↑ ↑ ↑	X	X			
Hemolytic anemia	↑	X	X			
Muscular dystrophy†	↑	X	X			

*In pulmonary infarction, LD_3 may be elevated.
†In muscular dystrophy, LD_1 and LD_2 are elevated only in a relative sense because LD_4 and LD_5 are depressed.

ticularly rich, whereas in acute viral hepatitis, the serum LD shows a higher proportion of LD_4 and LD_5 than does the normal. Some of the isoenzyme patterns observed in other diseases are indicated in Table 14–14. The determination of the LD isoenzyme "profile" for the analysis of clinical problems, however, is still an investigative procedure and is not ready for routine diagnostic application. Quantitation of the isoenzymes is difficult and the techniques are too awkward for use in the study of large numbers of sera. Measurement of LD_1, the myocardial isoenzyme, however, may be accomplished by techniques that are as simple as the measurement of total LD activity. Isoenzyme LD_1 resists denaturation at 65° C. for 30 minutes, while the activity of the other four isoenzymes is destroyed under these conditions. Accordingly, the relative amounts of LD_1 can be estimated by comparing the heat-stable LD to the total LD activity. A number of clinical laboratories determine "heat-stable" LD as a relatively routine aid in the diagnosis of acute myocardial infarction. An estimate of the serum level of LD_1 can also be obtained by measuring the level of α-hydroxybutyrate dehydrogenase (HBD). At one time considered to be the activity of a separate enzyme, HBD activity is now recognized to represent that of isoenzymes of LD (largely LD_1, with smaller amounts of other isoenzymes). The measurement of HBD activity is accomplished by a technique similar to that for measuring LD. Measurement of HBD is much less widely employed than that of heat-stable LD for clinical purposes. Indeed, the only routine application of LD isoenzymology to clinical problems is the measurement of heat-stable LD in the diagnosis of myocardial infarction, although some laboratories do employ electrophoretic analysis.

"Citric Acid Cycle" Enzymes

Several of the enzymes identified in the serum have been considered to be citric acid cycle enzymes (Fig. 14–9) released into the blood. Although they are shown as such in this discussion, this is an oversimplification for convenience. Enzymes of the citric acid cycle are located in the mitochondria, and are less likely to enter the blood than the cytoplasmic enzymes. Furthermore, the isocitric dehydrogenase (ICD) found in the serum requires TPN as the coenzyme, while the mitochondrial ICD is a DPN-linked enzyme. Malic

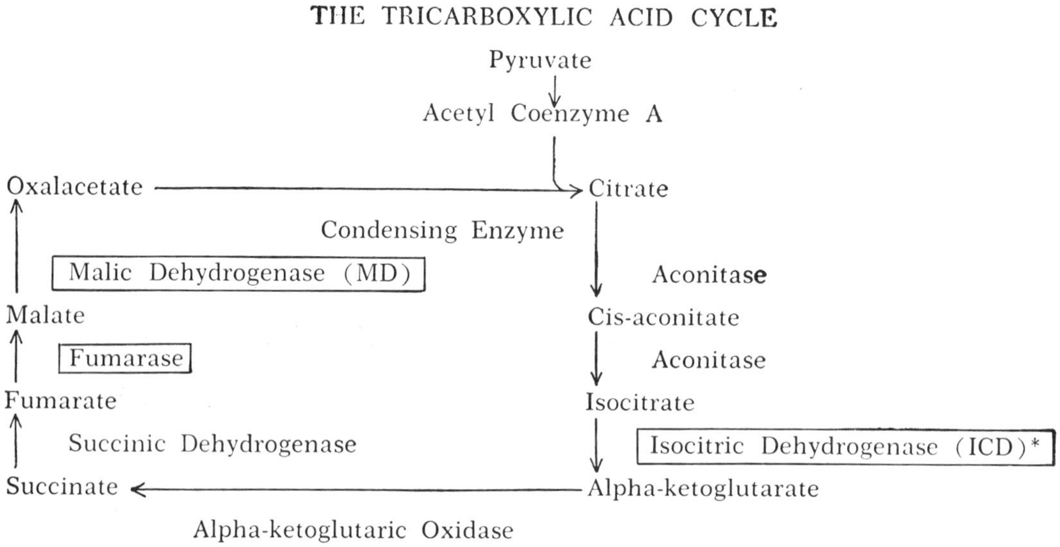

*Strictly speaking, the ICD of the serum differs from that of the citric acid cycle. The ICD demonstrated in the serum is TPN-linked, while that of the citric acid cycle is DPN-linked.

Figure 14–9. The tricarboxylic acid cycle. Scheme of citric acid cycle pathway of carbohydrate metabolism. Enzymes demonstrated in human serum are shown in boxes.

dehydrogenase activity has been demonstrated in the cytoplasm and mitochondria. Fumarase appears to be a mitochondrial enzyme.

Isocitric Dehydrogenase (ICD). ICD catalyzes the conversion of isocitric acid to alpha-ketoglutarate. The serum levels have been reported to be increased up to fortyfold in patients with viral hepatitis. Values are moderately elevated in patients with cirrhosis, obstructive jaundice, and metastatic carcinoma of the liver. Carcinoma, even without metastatic involvement, megaloblastic anemia, and congestive heart failure are also associated with mildly elevated levels of this enzyme. Levels have been reported to be normal in patients with myocardial infarction. While ICD levels are sensitive reflections of acute hepatic necrosis, this serum enzyme test has not been widely adopted. It is not so sensitive, and is no more specific a test of acute hepatic injury than is GPT. It is likely that this procedure will continue to be of investigative interest rather than a clinical tool.

Malate Dehydrogenase (MD). This enzyme catalyzes the reversible oxidation of malate to oxaloacetate. Elevated values have been observed in patients with myocardial infarction, hepatic necrosis, hemolytic syndromes, megaloblastic anemia, and neoplastic disease. In general, the abnormalities of this enzyme appear to parallel those observed with the glycolytic enzymes, but the degree of abnormality is usually less. This enzyme test is also of investigative rather than clinical usefulness.

Hexose "Shunt" Enzymes

Several of the enzymes of the hexose monophosphate shunt have been demonstrated in the serum (Fig. 14–10). Reports have appeared on the occurrence of elevated serum levels of glucose-6-phosphate dehydrogenase and of 6-phosphogluconic dehydrogenase in patients with hepatic disease. 5-P-ribosisomerase and transketolase have also been reported to be found in the serum; but the clinical significance and applicability of assay of these serum enzymes remain to be established. See Tables 14–1 and 14–2.

Cholinesterase

The cholinesterase of the serum (SChE) has been referred to as pseudocholinesterase to distinguish it from the true cholinesterase (AcChE) of the erythrocytes and nerve tissue. The tissue enzyme acts optimally on acetylcholine and on acetylbetamethyl choline, while the serum enzyme hydrolyzes acetylcholine and other cholinesters even more rapidly (Fig. 14–11; Table 14–15). Alkylphosphates are potent inhibitors of both serum and tissue cholinesterases. Simplified electrometric, manometric, and colorimetric methods have been devised for cholinesterase assay.

Levels of SChE are characteristically depressed in patients with parenchymatous liver

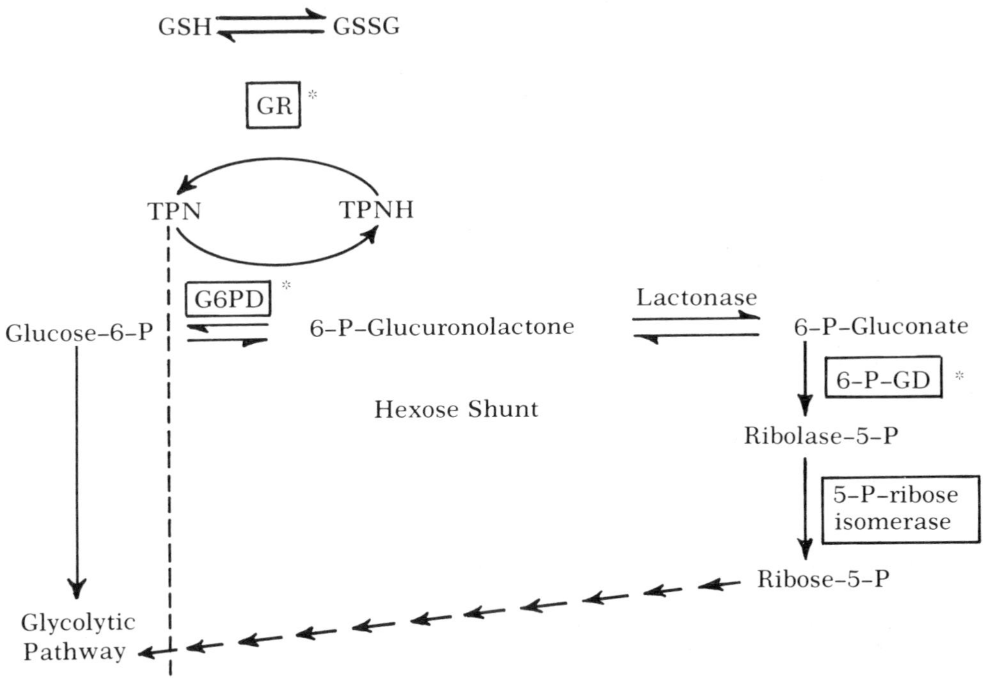

Figure 14–10. Initial reactions of hexose monophosphate shunt showing the rate of generation of TPNH in maintaining reduced glutathione. Enzymes in boxes (GR, G6PD, 6-P-GD, 5-P-ribose isomerase) may be found in serum. Transketolase (not shown) also reported in serum. *Assays performed most frequently on hemolysates of erythrocytes. (After Carson and Frischer, 1966.)

disease, including viral hepatitis, cirrhosis, metastatic carcinoma, the hepatic congestion of heart failure, and amebic hepatitis and abscess. In acute hepatitis, levels of the enzyme are lowest at the peak of the disease. Since, with recovery, the SChE level returns to normal, it has been suggested that the enzyme level may serve as an index of recovery and prognosis. In cirrhosis with jaundice, ascites, or other evidence of parenchymal insufficiency, SChE levels are usually depressed. In cirrhotics without these manifestations,

$$RCOCH_2CH_2N^+ (CH_3)_3Cl^- + H_2O \xrightarrow{ChE} RCOOH + HOCH_2CH_2N^+ (CH_3)_3Cl^-$$

R = CH_3 optimally for acetylcholinesterase.
R = CH_3 and many other alkyl or aryl groups for cholinesterase.

Method of assay is based on pH change (electrometric titration) that results from acid liberated.

Tissue content: acetylcholinesterase, RBC, nerve cells, synapses, and motor end plates. *Cholinesterase (pseudo):* serum or plasma, pancreas, and liver.

Conditions characterized by abnormal levels:

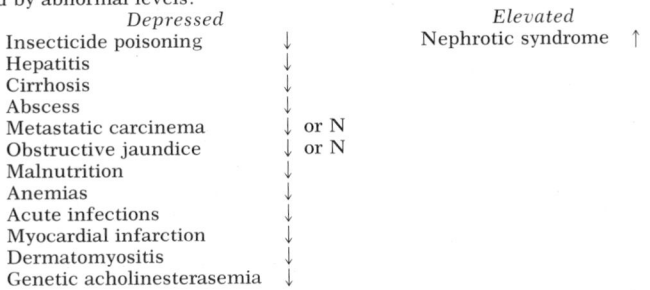

Depressed		*Elevated*	
Insecticide poisoning	↓	Nephrotic syndrome	↑
Hepatitis	↓		
Cirrhosis	↓		
Abscess	↓		
Metastatic carcinema	↓ or N		
Obstructive jaundice	↓ or N		
Malnutrition	↓		
Anemias	↓		
Acute infections	↓		
Myocardial infarction	↓		
Dermatomyositis	↓		
Genetic acholinesterasemia	↓		

Figure 14–11. Reaction catalyzed by cholinesterases (ChE), principle of assay, and list of conditions that cause decreased (↓) or increased (↑) serum levels.

Table 14–15. SUBSTRATE RELATIONSHIP OF BLOOD CHOLINESTERASES

ENZYME	SOURCE IN BLOOD	SUBSTRATES HYDROLYZED				KINETICS WITH ACETYLCHOLINE	
		Acetyl-choline	Acetylbeta-methylcholine	Butyryl-choline	Benzoyl-choline	Optimal concentration	Inhibition by excess
Acetylcholinesterase (true cholinesterase)	RBC	+	+	−	−	3×10^{-3}	+
Cholinesterase (pseudocholinesterase)	Plasma or serum	+	−	+	+	2×10^{-2}	−

the enzyme levels may be normal. Persistent depression of the SChE level in cirrhotics has been considered a poor prognostic sign.

In patients with obstructive jaundice, SChE levels are often normal. After prolonged obstruction, or when there is cholangitis, the level of SChE may be low.

Low values are also observed in patients with malnutrition, acute infections, anemias, myocardial infarction, and dermatomyositis (Fig. 14–11). In these nonhepatic diseases and in hepatic disease, the SChE level is depressed in those patients who also have a low serum level of albumin. Accordingly, it has been suggested that the low SChE level reflects impaired hepatic protein synthesis. Some support for this concept is derived from the observation that patients with the nephrotic syndrome, in whom the rate of albumin synthesis is increased, may have increased SChE levels, even though serum albumin levels are low.

As a measure of hepatic function and status, the serum cholinesterase determination is not employed widely. It is not sufficiently consistent to be useful in the differential diagnosis of jaundice. As an index of parenchymal function during the course of hepatic disease, it appears to add little to more commonly used laboratory measurements.

Assay of serum cholinesterase has found several applications other than in the diagnosis of hepatic disease. The organophosphorous insecticides are potent inhibitors of the cholinesterases. Depression of the acetylcholinesterase of the tissue (reflected in levels of erythrocyte, AcChE) and of the pseudocholinesterase of the serum (SChE) occurs. Serum ChE, which is depressed before erythrocyte AcChE, is a sensitive measure of overexposure to these agents. Severe exposure is usually reflected in depression of both erythrocyte AcChE and serum ChE. Serum levels appear to return to normal earlier than do the erythrocyte values.

The genetic control of SChE activity has been of great theoretical interest and is of some practical importance. At least two forms of SChE have been recognized. One has been called "normal" and the other "atypical." The genes controlling their synthesis are allelic to each other. Individuals homozygous for the "atypical" gene can be distinguished readily from the homozygous normal. The homozygous abnormal has very low SChE levels and the abnormal SChE is not inhibited by dibucaine. The homozygous normal has much higher levels of SChE activity, inhibitable by dibucaine, while the heterozygote has intermediate levels and response to the inhibitors. Not only is hereditary hypocholinesterasemia an interesting genetic state to study, it is also of clinical importance in regard to the administration of muscle relaxants (succinylcholine). Homozygous abnormals may develop prolonged apnea after they receive succinylcholine. Accordingly, patients who become apneic under these circumstances should have their SChE studied. Indeed, it has been proposed that one of the simple screening methods for SChE be performed prior to administration of an acetylcholine antagonist in order to exclude subjects who should not receive the agent.

Ornithine Carbamyl Transferase (OCT)

This enzyme, which catalyzes the reversible conversion of ornithine to citrulline (Fig. 14–12), is intimately involved in urea synthesis. It is found almost exclusively in the liver. The intestine has an OCT content of about 1 per cent that of the liver. There is virtually no activity in other tissues. Serum levels are very low in normal individuals, but are markedly elevated (ten- to two hundredfold) in those with acute viral hepatitis and other forms of hepatic necrosis. Relatively slight elevations occur in obstructive jaundice, cirrhosis, metastatic carcinoma, heart failure, delirium tremens, cholecystitis, and intestinal infarction. Indeed, serum OCT activity appears to be quite a specific and sensitive measure of hepatocellular injury. The first methods proposed for measurement of OCT activity did not lend themselves to routine assay. The recent introduction of a simplified colorimetric meth-

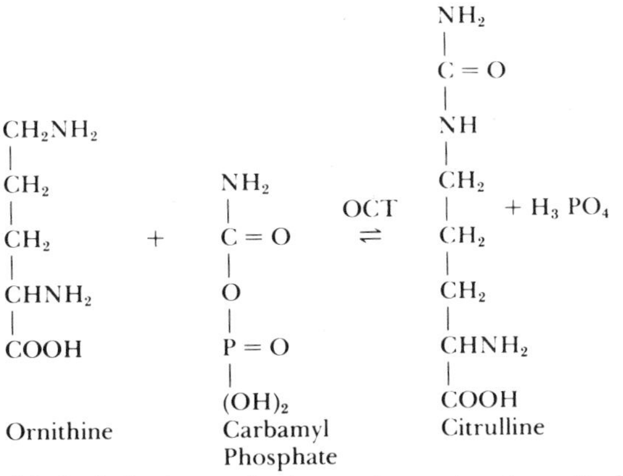

Methods for assay: In the most recent and practical method, citrulline formed is measured colorimetrically. Older methods were too cumbersome for clinical use.

Elevated levels reflect acute hepatic injury (hepatitis, toxic hepatic necrosis) sensitively and specifically. Levels are only slightly elevated in chronic hepatic disease and in obstructive jaundice.

Figure 14–12. Reaction catalyzed by ornithine carbamyl transferase (OCT), principle of assay, and clinical significance of abnormal values.

od, has made OCT measurement a practical routine procedure. Nevertheless, it is performed in relatively few centers.

Sorbitol Dehydrogenase (Sorb. D.)

Sorbitol dehydrogenase, which catalyzes the reaction shown in Figure 14–13, resembles OCT in that it is restricted to the liver. Accordingly, elevated values are to be expected only in those conditions that lead to hepatic injury. Normal serum has negligible activity. The highest values are observed in patients with acute hepatitis or carbon tetrachloride poisoning or other forms of acute hepatic necrosis. Most of the studies of this serum enzyme have been largely investigative, however, and the likelihood that it will replace or routinely supplement the established enzyme tests remains to be seen.

Leucine Aminopeptidase (LAP)

A number of peptidases have been identified in the serum of patients with various diseases. One of these, leucine aminopeptidase (LAP, naphthylamidase*), has been studied more extensively than the others. Elevated levels of this serum enzyme have been reported in most types of hepatobiliary diseases. These include hepatitis, cirrhosis, obstructive jaundice, metastatic carcinoma of the liver, and pancreatitis. Patients with carcinoma of the pancreas have increased levels only if obstructive jaundice or metastases of the liver have developed. The occurrence of elevated values during the last trimester of pregnancy remains to be explained.

The serum values for this enzyme in patients with hepatobiliary diseases appear to parallel those of alkaline phosphatase, with the highest levels in obstructive biliary disease and only moderately elevated levels in hepatocellular injury. Values for LAP, however, are normal in patients with bone disease. This has led to the suggestion that distinction between osseous and hepatobiliary disease as a cause of elevated alkaline phosphatase levels can be provided by assay of LAP activity. Differentiation between the high alkaline phosphatase levels of hepatobiliary disease and those of osseous disease, however, can usually be resolved by clinical

*Recent usage has favored the term "naphthylamidase" rather than LAP, since the enzyme is usually assayed by employing an acyl-β-naphthylamide as substrate.

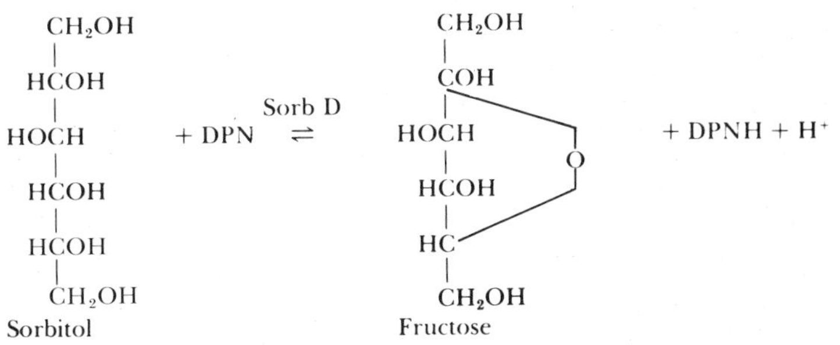

Figure 14–13. Reaction catalyzed by sorbitol dehydrogenase (Sorb D), principle of method of assay, and conditions in which abnormal values are found.

Method of assay depends on measuring the rate of reduction of coenzyme (DPN), which is measured spectrophotometrically.

Abnormal levels	
Acute hepatitis	$\uparrow\uparrow\uparrow$
Cirrhosis	$\uparrow$ or N
Obstructive jaundice	$\uparrow$

and other criteria; LAP determination has enjoyed a limited popularity.

5′-Nucleotidase (5′-N)

A serum esterase that has been the subject of a number of recent reports is 5′-nucleotidase. Introduced as a measure for the differentiation of obstructive from hepatocellular jaundice and of hepatobiliary from osseous disease, 5′-N has been the subject of a number of studies. The effects of disease on serum levels of 5′-N are similar to those of LAP. The highest values are observed in patients with obstructive jaundice, intrahepatic cholestasis, and infiltrative lesions of the liver. Relatively slightly elevated levels are observed in patients with hepatocellular disease. Values in patients with osseous disease, like those of LAP, are normal. Measurement of 5′-N also has been proposed as a diagnostic aid, more specific than alkaline phosphatase, in patients with hepatobiliary disease. In our experience this enzyme test has been less sensitive than alkaline phosphatase as a measure of obstructive biliary disease. Furthermore, as indicated above, distinction of hepatobiliary from bone disease is rarely a sufficiently knotty problem to warrant inclusion of 5′-N, LAP, or γ-glutamyl transpeptidase (Gl. TP) in the enzymologic diagnostic armamentarium.

Creatine Phosphokinase (CPK)

This enzyme also referred to as a creatine kinase and ATP creatine phospherase, catalyzes the reversible reaction shown in Figure 14–14. Its concentration in skeletal muscle and myocardium is very high. Appreciable amounts are found in the brain. Tiny amounts are found in a few other organs. None is found in the liver. Many studies have shown that CPK values are high in patients with myocardial infarction, progressive muscular dystrophy, alcoholic myopathy, and delirium tremens, but normal in patients with hepatitis and other forms of liver disease. The high values in patients with hypothyroidism have been attributed to the muscle changes in this condition. Although CPK is found almost exclusively in myocardium, muscle, and brain, and early reports suggested it to be an almost specific index of injury of myocardium and muscle, more recent reports indicate that inexplicably high serum CPK values can occur in patients with pulmonary infarction and pulmonary edema. Other causes of CPK elevation include exercise, intramuscular injections and occasionally acute psychotic reactions. Further studies are required to define the degree of specificity of high serum CPK values. At present, it should be regarded as a useful but not completely specific adjunct in the diagnosis of myocardial and muscle disease.

$$\text{Creatine-P} + \text{ADP} \overset{\text{CPK}}{\rightleftharpoons} \text{Creatine} + \text{ATP}$$

Method of assay: Several are available. One depends on measuring creatine-P formed by measuring phosphorus after liberating it. Another involves several coupled reactions in which ADP formed is utilized to convert phosphoenolpyruvate to pyruvate in the presence of pyruvate kinase. Pyruvate formed is measured by following disappearance of DPNH (at 340 mμ) under influence of added lactic dehydrogenase.

Conditions characterized by increased levels:
Progressive muscular dystrophy
Dermatomyositis
Myocardial infarction
Delirium tremens
Crush syndrome
Hypothyroidism

Figure 14–14. Reaction catalyzed by creatine phosphokinase (CPK), principle of assay, and significance of abnormal serum levels.

Other Serum Enzymes

Many other enzymes have been demonstrated in the serum (Table 14–1). These are too numerous for individual description in this discussion, but there are a few that warrant special mention. These include guanase, an enzyme that has been reported to reflect, sensitively and specifically, hepatic disease; beta glucuronidase, considered a biochemical clue to neoplastic, hepatic, and other diseases; alcohol dehydrogenase, proposed as a measure of hepatic disease; plasma pepsinogen, an enzyme precursor that reflects function and disease of the stomach (high levels in patients with peptic ulcer, low levels in patients with pernicious anemia); and ceruloplasmin, a copper-carrying protein that is also an enzyme and the serum levels of which are depressed in patients with hepatolenticular degeneration (Wilson's disease). Ceruloplasmin measurement is useful in the diagnosis of Wilson's disease. The practical role that the other enzymes cited and others listed in Tables 14–1 and 14–2 may play in clinical medicine remains to be demonstrated.

CLINICAL APPLICATION OF SERUM ENZYME ASSAY

Serum enzymology provides aid in making the diagnosis, monitoring the course, and demonstrating subclinical evidence of disease. Diseases that are characterized by distinctly abnormal values of one or more enzymes (Table 14–16) can be readily distinguished

Table 14–16. ABNORMAL LEVELS OF SOME SERUM ENZYMES IN VARIOUS PATHOLOGIC PROCESSES*

			NECROSIS OF				NEOPLASTIC DISEASE†	
ENZYME	OSTEO-BLASTIC ACTIVITY	BILIARY OBSTRUCTION	LIVER	HEART	SKELETAL MUSCLE	PANCREAS	NEOPLASTIC GROWTH	HEPATIC METASTASES
Alk. phosph.	1-4+	4+	+	–	–	–	–	1-4+
Acid phosph.	–	–	–	–	–	–	+(prostate)	
LAP	–	4+	+	–	–	–	–	1-4+
5′-N	–	4+	+	–	–	–	–	1-4+
Gl. TP	–	4+	+	+	–	–	+	1-4+
GOT	–	+	4+	2+	1+	±	–	2+
GPT	–	+	4+	±	±	±	–	1+
Sorb. D.	–	+	4+	–	–	–	–	1+
ICD	–	+	4+	–	–	–		1+
LD	–	+	+	2+	2+	±	3+	3+
HBD	–	±	±	2+	±	±	+	+
MD	–	+	2+	2+	2+	±	2+	2+
Ald.	–	+	3+	2+	4+	±	3+	3+
PHI	–	+	3+	2+	2+	±	3+	3+
CPK	–	–	–	4+	4+	–	–	–
Amylase	–	±	–	–	–	4+	–	–
Lipase	–	±	–	–	–	4+	–	–

*1-4+ represents grades of elevated values; – represents normal values.
†Includes granulocytic leukemia.

from clinically similar states in which abnormal values for the respective enzymes do not occur. The diagnostic circumstances that are most clearly aided by serum enzymology are the distinction of myocardial infarction from other causes of chest pain, the differential diagnosis of hepatobiliary and muscle disease, the diagnosis of pancreatitis, and the recognition of metastases of neoplastic disease to bone or liver (Table 14–17).

The diagnostic application of serum enzyme assays is based on the accumulated clinical experience and experimental data that permit formulation of factors that lead to abnormal enzyme levels (Table 14–6) and correlation of particular serum enzymes with the nature of the pathologic process and the organ involved (Table 14–16). This type of assessment serves to epitomize most of the foregoing material. It permits selection of the enzyme tests most likely to be of diagnostic value and of the clinical circumstances most likely to be benefited by current knowledge of serum enzymology. Some disease processes are characterized by abnormal values of one or more enzymes (Table 14–16). Thus, osteoblastic lesions lead to elevations of alkaline phosphatase values that range from slight to marked. Obstruction of the biliary tree (or intrahepatic cholestasis) leads to markedly elevated values of alkaline phosphatase, LAP, 5′-N, Gl. TP; relatively slightly elevated values of transaminases, OCT, Sorb. D., ICD, LD, HBD, MD, Ald. and PHI; and normal values for CPK. Hepatic necrosis leads to lesser values of alkaline phosphatase, LAP, 5′-N, and Gl. TP but very high values of GOT, GPT, OCT, Sorb. D., ICD, MD, Ald., and PHI and normal values for CPK. In myocardial necrosis, moderately elevated levels of GOT, LD, HBD, MD, Ald., PHI, and

Table 14–17. PATTERNS OF ABNORMAL SERUM ENZYME VALUES IN SEVERAL CLINICAL SETTINGS*

		GOT	GPT	LD	LD (HEAT STABLE) (HBD)	CPK	ALD.	ALK. PHOSPH.
CHEST PAIN AND RELATED CIRCUMSTANCES	MI†	↑↑	±	↑↑	↑↑	↑↑↑	↑↑	N
	PI†	±	±	↑↑	±	±	↑↑	N
	CHF†	±	±		±	±	↑	↑
	Shock	↑↑	↑	↑↑	±	±	↑↑	N
MUSCLE DISEASE	Progressive muscular dystrophy, Trichinosis, Dermatomyositis, Polymyositis, Delirium tremens	↑↑	↑	↑↑	↑	↑↑↑	↑↑↑	N
	Neurogenic muscle disease	N	N	N	N	N	N	N
JAUNDICE (SEE CHAPTER 13)	Acute hepatitis	↑↑↑↑	↑↑↑↑	↑	±	N	↑↑	↑
	Cirrhosis (Laennec's)	↑	±	±	±	±	±	↑
	Obstructive jaundice	↑↑	↑↑	↑	±	±	↑	↑↑↑
NEOPLASTIC DISEASE	Localized carcinoma of small size	N	N	N	N	N	N	N
	Extensive carcinoma without hepatic or bone metastases	N	N	↑↑	±	±	↑↑	N
	Carcinoma with metastases to liver or hepatoma	↑↑	↑	↑↑	±	±	↑↑	↑↑↑
	Carcinoma with osteoblastic metastases to bone	N	N	↑↑	±	±	↑↑	↑↑↑
	Leukemia (granulocytic or acute)	N	N	↑↑	±	±	↑↑	N
	Leukemia (chronic lymphatic)	N	N	N	N	N	N	N
ANEMIA	Megaloblastic	N	N	↑↑↑↑	↑	N	↑↑↑	N
	Iron deficiency	N	N	N	N	N	N	N
	Hemolytic	N	N	↑↑	↑	N	↑↑	N

*Number of arrows indicates magnitude of increase; N indicates no change.
†MI = myocardial infarction.
PI = pulmonary infarction.
CHF = heart failure.

CPK are noted. Skeletal muscle disease of the progressively degenerative or inflammatory type (progressive muscular dystrophy, dermatomyositis, trichinosis) leads to striking elevations of CPK and aldolase levels; moderate elevations of LD, PHI, and MD values; slight elevations of the GOT level and even lesser values of GPT; and normal levels of the other enzymes listed in Table 14–16. Neoplastic disease is characterized by increased values of LD, Ald., PHI, MD, with the increase seemingly dependent on the tumor having reached sufficient total mass. Reports of Gl. TP suggest that this enzyme is also increased in the serum of patients with carcinomatosis. Metastatic carcinoma of the liver leads to moderate or marked elevations of alkaline phosphatase, LAP, 5′-N, and Gl. TP and to slightly or moderately elevated values of GOT and GPT. These abnormalities are also seen with other space-occupying lesions of the liver (granuloma, abscess, amyloidosis). The pattern of serum enzyme abnormality of hepatic metastases also includes increased values of enzymes that reflect neoplastic growth. Metastases to various sites from prostatic carcinoma lead to high acid phosphatase levels. Metastases of carcinoma to the bone, if osteoblastic, lead to high alkaline phosphatase levels but to normal values of GOT and GPT.

Monitoring the course of disease by serial determinations of serum enzyme levels is useful in the management of hepatitis, in the chemotherapy of neoplastic disease, and in the recognition of recurrent infarction or other complications during the convalescence from acute myocardial infarction. Detection of subclinical disease by serum enzyme assay is exemplified by the use of serum aldolase or CPK levels to recognize individuals destined to develop progressive muscular dystrophy, or the employment of GOT, GPT, and alkaline phosphatase to monitor patients exposed to known or potentially hepatotoxic agents. In Table 14–17 are shown the patterns of abnormality obtained in various clinical circumstances utilizing a small panel of enzyme tests.

Serum Enzymes in Myocardial Infarction

Serum enzyme analysis has become as routine a measure as electrocardiography in the diagnostic approach to patients suspected of having sustained a myocardial infarction. Of the large number of enzymes released to the blood from infarcted myocardium (Tables 14–6, 14–16), only a few have been regularly applied to the diagnosis of infarction (Table 14–17). Most extensively employed are the GOT and LD, each of which yields abnormal values in almost all patients (92 to 98 per cent) with proven infarction. The degrees, onset, and duration of rise of each are characteristic. The GOT value increases by four- to tenfold and the LD by two- to fourfold. The values for each become abnormal by 12 to 24 hours after the bout of chest pain. The GOT value returns to normal in three to five days, and the LD in 10 to 14 days. Distinction is usually readily made from pulmonary infarction, which is characterized by elevated LD levels and usually by normal GOT values. In a small proportion of patients with pulmonary embolism, slightly elevated values for GOT occur by three or four days after the bout of chest pain.

Refinement of diagnoses can be provided by measuring the heat-stable LD or the HBD level. Both are alternative techniques for measuring the isoenzyme of LD that is relatively specific for myocardium. The other techniques cited previously in this chapter for demonstrating the myocardial isoenzyme are more cumbersome and no more helpful than either of these. A fourth diagnostic enzymologic measure of mounting popularity for the clinical recognition of myocardial infarction is the serum CPK level. The incidence of elevated CPK values in this condition is approximately equal to that of GOT and LD. The significance of high CPK values is somewhat more specific (see section on CPK).

The complication of myocardial infarction by shock leads to higher values of GOT and LD and to abnormal levels of enzymes that reflect hepatic injury (GPT, ICD). Indeed, shock of any origin, or severe anoxia, leads to high levels of a large number of enzymes presumably released from the liver.

As discussed in the section devoted to GOT, most instances of myocardial infarction can be diagnosed without dependence on serum enzyme levels. Enzymologic assistance is of most value when the diagnosis is obscured by atypical clinical or electrocardiographic features or by residual electrocardiographic abnormalities of a previous infarction. Perhaps the most important aspect of serum enzyme measurement in patients with chest pain is the value of normal enzyme levels in excluding the diagnosis of myocardial infarction. If the GOT and LD remain normal in three successive daily determinations after the bout of chest pain, the diagnosis of infarction is virtually excluded. In patients whose clinical diagnosis would otherwise be that of coronary insufficiency or angina pectoris, a pattern of transiently elevated enzyme levels (GOT, LD, CPK) should be regarded as evidence of an overlooked infarction. The values for GOT, CPK, and LD in other forms of heart disease are discussed in the sections devoted to the respective enzymes.

Serum Enzymes in Liver Disease

The enzymologic approach to liver disease is discussed in Chapter 13. It remains to be proved that employment of the apparently liver-specific OCT, Sorb. D., or guanase or of the isoenzymes of LD will add a significant measure of sensitivity or specificity to that provided by the simple panel of GOT and GPT. Similarly, the distinction of the elevated alkaline phosphatase levels of hepatobiliary disease from those caused by osteoblastic lesions offers little difficulty if consideration is given to other laboratory measurements and clinical features of hepatic and biliary tract disease. Accordingly, little additional benefit is obtained by performing the leucine aminopeptidase, glutamyl transpeptidase, or 5′-nucleotidase, the levels of which parallel those of alkaline phosphatase in hepatobiliary disease but are normal in diseases of bone. Studies of isoenzymes of alkaline phosphatase by electrophoretic, kinetic, or other techniques for the purpose of distinguishing bone from hepatic phosphatase seem at present to be of greater theoretical interest than clinical benefit. Cholinesterase levels, at one time considered a valuable enzymologic tool for the management of hepatic disease, have been supplanted by the more readily measurable, more sensitive, and more specific transaminases.

Enzyme analysis in hepatobiliary disease is useful in differential diagnosis, as discussed in Chapter 13. Monitoring the course of serum enzyme levels is helpful in following the course of acute or chronic hepatitis or of active postnecrotic cirrhosis. For this purpose GOT and GPT assays may be employed. Monitoring of patients exposed to possible hepatotoxins is usefully accomplished by a simple panel consisting of alkaline phosphatase, GOT, and GPT. If evidence of mitochondrial injury is sought, glutamic dehydrogenase levels also may be measured.

Muscle Disease

Measurement of serum enzyme levels has become a major component of the diagnostic approach to muscle disease. The enzymes that have been studied most extensively are Ald., GOT, LD, and CPK. The last named is the most reliable measure of skeletal muscle disease, since, as discussed previously, elevated values are relatively specific for disease of striated muscle (skeletal muscle and myocardium). Aldolase levels appear to be as sensitive to disease of muscle, although somewhat less specific.

Elevated levels of these enzymes occur in patients with dystrophic or myositic processes. In the progressive muscular dystrophies, especially the Duchenne type, the values are particularly high. Moderate or marked elevations are seen in dermatomyositis, in polymyositis, in scleroderma with an associated myositis, and in trichinosis. Slightly or moderately increased levels of these enzymes are also observed in myotonic dystrophy, in myotonia congenita, in the crush syndrome, and in McArdle's disease. High values of these and other enzymes occur in patients with delirium tremens, irrespective of associated hepatic disease, and may arise in muscle. The muscle involvement of myxedema appears to be responsible for the elevated serum enzyme levels seen in this condition. Strenuous muscle activity in untrained individuals also leads to increased levels of these enzymes. Serum enzyme levels are normal in patients with neurogenic muscle disease. Disease of the upper motor neuron, the anterior horn cell, or the peripheral nerve does not lead to elevated values.

For the clinical application to the diagnosis of muscle disease, both Ald. and CPK should be measured. If values of both are abnormal, the results can be interpreted with greater confidence. These tests are of help in recognizing early muscular dystrophy before clinical manifestations appear and may be useful clues to the carrier female. They are also of value in the differential diagnosis of the other muscular diseases cited and in following the course of inflammatory disease of the muscle.

Neoplastic Disease

A large number of studies have demonstrated high serum levels of glycolytic and other enzymes (Table 14-16) in the serum of animals and humans with a variety of carcinomas and other neoplastic lesions. In general, the levels of enzymes studied are normal in patients with small localized tumors; increased values are seen when the local tumor has become large, has extended to surrounding tissue, or has reached distant metastatic sites. Data from several laboratories indicate that the serum levels of these enzymes reflect and are proportional to the total mass of tumor rather than the involvement of tissue at specific metastatic sites. Measurement of levels of any of the glycolytic or other enzymes that are elevated in patients with carcinomatosis fails to provide a means of detecting early neoplasms that are resectable; however, perhaps the search for such an enzymologic clue should continue to be pursued. Patterns of serum enzyme abnormality are of value in supporting the diagnosis of carcinomatosis, and the monitoring of serum enzyme levels is useful in following the response to chemotherapy of patients with inoperable neoplasms.

Increased levels of the same enzymes are observed in patients with Hodgkin's disease, lymphosarcoma, and granulocytic and acute leukemia. Adequate response to chemotherapy is reflected in decreasing values. The values are normal in patients with chronic lymphocytic leukemia and in most patients with multiple myeloma.

The enzymes that have been most extensively studied in neoplastic states and that can be used to monitor the course of widespread neoplastic disease are lactic dehydrogenase, phosphohexoisomerase, and aldolase; however, the others listed in Table 14-17 also reflect the process.

ENZYMES OF THE FORMED ELEMENTS OF THE BLOOD

During the past few years, considerable attention has been devoted to the metabolic activity and enzyme content of erythrocytes and leukocytes. The extensive studies related to the employment of these elements as *in vitro* metabolic models and to the factors involved in blood preservation are beyond the scope of this discussion. This section attempts to summarize some of the studies of erythrocyte enzymes that have unraveled several genetic hemolytic syndromes (Table 14-18) and the studies of erythrocyte and leukocyte enzymes that have been useful in the diag-

Table 14–18. DISEASES IN WHICH DIAGNOSIS CAN BE ESTABLISHED BY ANALYSIS OF ENZYME* ACTIVITY OF FORMED ELEMENT OF BLOOD

CONDITION	FORMED ELEMENT UTILIZED FOR ENZYME ASSAY	ENZYME ASSAY	COMMENT
Hemolytic Anemias			
G-6-PD deficiency	RBC	G-6-PD	There are several varieties of this condition.
6-PGD deficiency	RBC	6-PGD	Status equivocal
GR deficiency	RBC	GR	Rare
GSH peroxidase deficiency	RBC	GSH-Px	Few cases
GSH synthetase deficiency	RBC	GSH	Content of GSH measured; enzyme not assayed, but deficiency inferred
Hexokinase deficiency	RBC	HK	Several forms described
PHI deficiency	RBC, WBC	PHI	Rare
Phosphofructokinase (PFK) deficiency	RBC	PFK	Two forms described, one with hemolytic anemia only, the other with hemolytic anemia and Type VII glycogenosis (muscle)
Familial spherocytic anemia	RBC	Ald	Relationship of depression of erythrocyte Ald. content to hemolytic anemia uncertain.
Triosephosphate isomerase (TPI)	RBC, WBC	TPI	Hemolytic anemia accompanied by severe neuromuscular disease also presumed to be due to the demonstrated TPI deficiency in several tissues
2-3 Diphosphoglycerate mutase (2-3 DPGM) deficiency	RBC	2-3 DPGM	Status of syndrome equivocal
Phosphoglycerate kinase (PGK) deficiency	RBC RBC, WBC	PGK	Two forms described, one with hemolytic anemia only and the defect found only in the RBC, the other with neurologic defect as well and enzyme deficiency demonstrable in RBC and WBC
Pyruvate kinase (PK) deficiency	RBC	PK	Well-established defect with a spectrum of clinical syndromes reported
ATPase deficiency	RBC	ATPase	Relationship between ATPase deficiency and hemolysis remains to be clarified

*See Table 14–1 or text for meaning of abbreviations.

nosis of several genetic and acquired systemic conditions (Table 14–19).

Hemolytic Anemia Associated with Deficiency of Erythrocyte Enzymes*

Genetic defects in erythrocyte metabolism have been found to be responsible for at least 14 forms of hemolytic anemia (Table 14–18). Some of the demonstrated or assumed enzymatic defects relate to the hexose monophosphate shunt (G-6-PD, 6-PGD, GR, GSH-synthetase, GSH-peroxidase), and some of the enzymatic defects relate to the anaerobic glycolytic pathway (HK, PHI, PFK, Ald., TPI, 2-3DPGM, PGK, PK, and ATPase). The hemolytic syndromes associated with these enzymatic defects are listed in Table 14–18.

*Also see Chapter 4, pp. 202–206.

Table 14–19. SYSTEMIC DISEASES IN WHICH DIAGNOSIS CAN BE ESTABLISHED BY ANALYSIS OF ENZYME ACTIVITY OF FORMED ELEMENT OF BLOOD

CONDITION	FORMED ELEMENT	ENZYME ASSAY
Genetic		
Methemoglobinemia	RBC	DPNH-methemoglobin reductase
Acatalasemia	RBC	Catalase
Galactosemia		Gal-1-P-uridyl transferase
Glycogenosis (Type III)	WBC	Amylo-1-6-glucosidase
(Type IV)	WBC	Phosphorylase
(Type VII)	RBC	PFK
Hypophosphatasia	WBC	Alk. phosph.
Lipid storage diseases*		
Gaucher's	WBC	β-Glucosidase
Niemann-Pick	WBC	Sphyngomyelinase
Krabbes' leukodystrophy (globoid)	WBC	β-Galactosidase
Metachromatic leukodystrophy	WBC	Sulfatidase
Fabry's disease	WBC	α-Galactosidase
Tay-Sachs disease	WBC	Hexosaminidase
Acquired		
Thiamine deficiency	RBC	Transketolase
Pyridoxine deficiency	RBC	GPT
Hyperthyroidism	RBC	Carbonic anhydrase
Leukemia, granulocytic	WBC	Alk. phosph.
Lead poisoning	RBC	δ-Aminolevulinic acid dehydrase

*Also see Figure 9–61, p. 632.

Hemolytic Anemia Secondary to G-6-PD Deficiency. Deficiency of erythrocyte G-6-PD activity has been estimated to involve 2 to 3 per cent of the world population and to be responsible for almost one-third of the cases of chronic or recurrent nonspherocytic hemolytic anemia. The defect is sex-linked and appears in a number of genetic variants. The first to be recognized is the relatively mild condition observed almost exclusively in blacks and characterized by deficient concentration of G-6-PD in erythrocytes but normal concentration in leukocytes and platelets. These individuals develop hemolysis on exposure to a number of drugs, including primaquine, sulfonamides, and other agents, and to other stresses, including various infections. A more severe form of G-6-PD deficiency, characterized by G-6-PD deficiency in leukocytes and erythrocytes, by more severe anemia, and by sensitivity to fava beans and to various drugs, is seen in Caucasians, particularly Sephardic Jews, other ethnic groups of the Mediterranean littoral, American Indians, and Orientals. Studies of the various forms of G-6-PD deficiency have shown, not only differences in the severity of the clinical illness and the degree of depression of enzyme levels of erythrocytes and leukocytes, but also that there are different molecular variants (isoenzymes) of G-6-PD. The mechanism whereby G-6-PD deficiency permits drug-induced hemolysis remains incompletely understood but is indirectly related to the inability to maintain adequate levels of reduced glutathione in the erythrocyte on exposure to offending agents.

Assay of G-6-PD activity has become a routine procedure in patients with hemolytic anemia, especially if it occurs after administration of a drug or during an acute illness. A precise assay of G-6-PD activity of hemolysate involves measuring the rate at which TPN is reduced in the presence of glucose-6-phosphate. Simplified assays suitable for screening large populations are available.

Deficiency of 6-PGD. Decreased erythrocyte levels of 6-PGD have been reported, but the role of this abnormality in inducing susceptibility to hemolysis remains to be proved. The principle of assay of 6-PGD activity of erythrocytes is similar to that of G-6-PD.

Hemolytic Anemia Secondary to Deficiency of Glutathione Reductase (GR), Glutathione Peroxidase (GSH-Px) or Glutathione Synthetase

A few instances of mild hemolytic anemia have been reported in patients with genetic deficiency in erythrocyte levels of GR. Some have been instances of chronic hemolysis and others of hemolytic anemia after exposure to drugs (primaquine). Thus far, the condition appears to be rare and primarily of genetic interest. Almost complete absence of glutathione from erythrocytes as a genetic abnormality has been found to occur in several genera. The deficiency of glutathione in these individuals appears to be transmitted as an autosomal recessive and presumably results from subnormal glutathione synthetase activity. The erythrocytes of patients with GSH deficiency, like those of patients with G-6-PD and GR deficiency, are susceptible to drug-induced hemolysis. A similar syndrome has been attributed to deficiency of GSH-Px, the enzyme presumed to be mainly responsible for destroying H_2O_2 in human erythrocytes.

Hemolytic Anemias Secondary to Deficiency in Glycolytic Enzymes

Pyruvate kinase (PK) deficiency is the most frequent and important form of hemolytic anemia due to deficiency of glycolytic enzymes in the erythrocyte. It is transmitted as an autosomal recessive and characterized by a nonspherocytic, chronic hemolytic anemia. The hemolysis is attributable to the inability of the PK deficient erythrocyte to maintain normal ATP levels and the resulting membrane defect. Enzyme activity of the erythrocyte can be assayed by measuring the ability of hemolysate to form pyruvate from ADP and phosphoenol pyruvate.

Similar syndromes appear to result from deficient erythrocyte content of hexokinase, phosphohexoisomerase, phosphofructokinase, triose phosphate isomerase, 2-3 diphosphoglycerate mutase, phosphoglycerate kinase, and ATPase (Table 14–18). These are rare and, at present, of little clinical importance (see p. 206).

Systemic Diseases Reflected in Abnormal Erythrocyte and Leukocyte Enzymes

Several genetic diseases are reflected by abnormal levels of enzymes in the erythrocytes (Table 14–19). Acatalasia, also called Takahara's disease or oral gangrene, is a condition characterized by marked deficiency in the concentration of catalase in the tissues and in the erythrocytes. Deficiency of catalase, an enzyme which destroys hydrogen peroxide ($2\,H_2O_2 \xrightarrow{\text{catalase}} 2\,H_2O + O_2$), leads to the accumulation of hydrogen peroxide when it is produced in excess. This is often asymptomatic and becomes of clinical importance only in some patients with oral sepsis, in whose oral cavities peroxide formed by bacteria can accumulate and lead to gangrene. It is a self-limiting state which disappears after the teeth are lost. Transmitted as an autosomal recessive, the condition is of greater genetic interest than clinical importance. Homozygous abnormals who have almost no catalase in the erythrocytes can be distinguished from the heterozygotes whose values are midway between the homozygote abnormal and normal. Hereditary methemoglobinemia secondary to deficiency of erythrocyte diaphorase is a rare oligosymptomatic condition which is transmitted as an autosomal recessive. The methemoglobinemia, which leads to cyanosis, is the result of deficiency of DPNH-methemoglobin reductase (diaphorase).

Glycogenosis of types III, IV, and VII and hypophosphatasia can be identified by measuring the leukocyte content of the relevant enzyme. Confirmation of the diagnosis of type IV glycogenosis, which is due to *hepatophosphorylase* deficiency, can be obtained by measuring the phosphorylase activity of leukocytes. Type III glycogenosis, which is a manifestation of deficiency of the glycogen *debrancher* enzyme (amylo-1-6-glucosidase), can also be diagnosed by measuring the leukocyte content of that enzyme. Type VII glycogenosis, which is associated with a hemolytic anemia, can be identified by demonstrating deficient phosphofructokinase activity in the erythrocytes. *Hypophosphatasia* is characterized by a genetic deficiency of alkaline phosphatase content of tissues and blood. Measurement of alkaline phosphatase levels of the leukocytes can in the proper clinical setting assist in establishing the diagnosis.

Galactosemia is an inborn error of metabolism characterized by a specific defect in the utilization of galactose which results in widespread tissue damage. The defect has been found to be deficiency of the enzyme phosphogalactose-uridyl-transferase. The resulting accumulation of galactose-1-phosphate is considered responsible for the development of cataracts, liver disease, renal disease, and other abnormalities. The hereditary enzyme deficiency can be demonstrated by studying the erythrocyte. The ability of hemolysate to catalyze the conversion of galactose-1-phosphate to UDP-galactose in the presence of UDP-glucose is measured by following the disappearance of UDP-glucose. The test, which can be readily performed, yields very low values in patients with galactosemia, who are homozygous for the abnormal gene. Heterozygote carriers can usually be identified by this test, which yields values intermediate between the normal and the homozygous abnormal.

A number of lipid storage diseases can be identified by demonstrating deficient activity of the related enzyme in circulating leukocytes (Table 14–19). Several acquired diseases can also be identified by studying enzyme activity of the formed elements. Thiamine deficiency can be confirmed by demonstrating depressed transketolase activity of hemolysate. Pyridoxine deficiency can be demonstrated by measuring the GPT activity of erythrocytes before and after incubation with pyridoxal-5-phosphate. Abnormal levels of cholinesterase, carbonic anhydrase, and several other enzymes have been demonstrated in the erythrocytes of patients with a variety of acquired systemic diseases, but these are of pathophysiological rather than diagnostic importance. The recent description of depressed erythrocyte levels of δ-aminolevulinic acid dehydrase as a measure of blood levels of lead suggests that measurement of this enzyme may be useful in the diagnosis of lead poisoning. Measurement of leukocyte alkaline phosphatase helps in distinguishing granulocytic leukemia from leukemoid states. Alkaline phosphatase levels are very low in the leukocytes of granulocytic leukemia, but they are normal or elevated in patients with nonleukemic leukocytosis.

ENZYME CONCENTRATIONS IN OTHER BODY FLUIDS

Measurement of enzyme activity in serous effusions, gastrointestinal juices, cerebrospinal fluid, and urine has been applied to the diagnosis of various diseases. Localized release of enzyme from neoplastic cells has been considered responsible for the high levels of LD (and other glycolytic enzymes) in malignant pleural and peritoneal effusions, in the gastric juice of patients with carcinoma of the stomach and in the urine of patients with renal carcinoma. The glucuronidase in the urine of patients with carcinoma of the bladder and in the vaginal fluid of patients with carcinoma of the cervix may also be considered to be enzyme shed by neoplastic cells.

Determination of levels of LD in serous cavity effusions has been proposed as a method of demonstrating neoplastic involvement of serosal surfaces. In such circumstances, the serous fluid usually shows higher levels of LD than does the serum. High levels of LD, however, are also found in patients with inflammatory and hemorrhagic effusions. Accordingly, measurements of enzyme content of serous effusions appear to be of limited clinical value. Measurement of LD levels of gastric juice or urine to detect renal or gastric carcinoma, respectively, or of glucuronidase in the urine or vaginal fluid to detect carcinoma of the bladder or cervix, respectively, remains to be proven of clinical value.

The demonstration of a high amylase value in pleural or ascitic fluid is useful in making the diagnosis of pancreatitis. The demonstration of increased levels of amylase in the urine is also a useful supplement to the measurement of serum levels of the enzyme in the diagnosis of pancreatitis. (See Chapter 15.)

Measurement of urinary levels of lactic dehydrogenase, alkaline phosphatase, muramidase (lysozyme), catalase, β-glucuronidase, and pepsinogen has been proposed for the diagnosis or monitoring of a number of conditions. Increased levels of lactic dehydrogenase, alkaline phosphatase, and β-glucuronidase are frequent in patients with carcinoma of the urinary tract, but may also be caused by hematuria, urinary tract infection, or glomerulonephritis and are, accordingly, too nonspecific to be clinically useful. Catalase may be found in the urine when there is bacteriuria, pyuria, or hematuria. Muramidase activity of the urine may be very high in patients with monocytic or monomyelocytic leukemia. For monitoring the course of the disease, however, serum levels of this enzyme are probably more useful. Urinary (and plasma) pepsinogen values are increased in patients with peptic ulcer and low in those with pernicious anemia. These observations are of pathophysiological interest rather than clinical value.

Increased levels of β-glucuronidase and 6-phosphogluconate dehydrogenase have been demonstrated in the vaginal fluid of a high proportion of patients with carcinoma of the uterus, especially the cervix. However, the normal values found in some patients with cancer, and the elevated values found in some patients with benign conditions prevent useful application of assay of vaginal fluid enzyme activity for the recognition of carcinoma. Measurement of tartrate inhibitable acid phosphatase in vaginal fluid is a useful procedure for the diagnosis of rape, since this isoenzyme is of prostatic origin and therefore high in semen.

Cerebrospinal fluid enzyme levels are relatively independent of the serum levels. Increased spinal fluid levels of glutamic oxaloacetic transaminase, lactic dehydrogenase, ribonuclease, and glutathione reductase have been described in patients with various diseases of the central nervous system. The levels of one or more of these enzymes are increased in patients with cerebrovascular hemorrhage, thrombosis or embolism, meningitis, and neoplasms of the central nervous system. The clinical application and value of spinal fluid enzyme determinations remain to be established. (Also see Chapter 25, p. 1264.)

REFERENCES

General

Abderhalden, R.: *Clinical Enzymology*. Princeton, N.J., D. Van Nostrand Co., 1961.
Baron, D. N.: The clinical significance of serum enzyme estimations. Abstr. Wrld. Med. *40*:377, 1967.
Bergmeyer, H. U. (ed.): *Methods of Enzymatic Analysis*. New York, Academic Press, Inc., 1963.
Bodansky, O.: Diagnostic applications of enzyme in medicine: General enzymological aspects. Amer. J. Med. 27:861, 1959.
Cabaud, P. G., and Wroblewski, F.: Colorimetric measurement of lactic dehydrogenase activity of body fluids. Amer. J. Clin. Path. 30:234, 1958.
Cohen, L.: Serum enzyme determinations: Their reliability and value. Med. Clin. N. Amer. 53:115, 1969.
Coodley, E. L. (ed.): *Diagnostic Enzymology*. Philadelphia, Lea & Febiger, 1970.
Greenberg, D. N., and Harper, H. A. (eds.): *Enzymes in Health and Disease*. Springfield, Illinois, Charles C Thomas, 1960.
Henly, K. S., Schmidt, E., and Schmidt, F. W.: *Enzymes in Serum*. Springfield, Illinois, Charles C Thomas, 1966.
Henry, J. B. (ed.): *Clinical Enzymology: Pre-Workshop and Technical Manuals*. Chicago, American Society of Clinical Pathologists, 1964.
Hess, B.: *Enzymes in Blood Plasma*. New York, Academic Press, Inc., 1963.
King, E. J.: Editorial. Amer. J. Med. 27:849, 1959.
Kontinnen, A.: Serum enzymes as indicators of hepatic disease. Scand. J. Gastroent. 6:667, 1971.
Lawrence, S. H.: *The Zymogram in Clinical Medicine*. Springfield, Illinois, Charles C Thomas, 1964.
Mullen, D. P.: *Studies in Clinical Enzymology*. St. Louis, The C. V. Mosby Co., 1969.
Report of the Commission on Enzymes of the International Union of Biochemistry. New York, The Macmillan Company, 1961.
Wacker, W. E. C., Ulmer, D. D., and Vallee, B. L.: Metalloenzymes and myocardial infarction. New Eng. J. Med. 255:449, 1956.
Warburg, O., and Christian, W.: Gärunopfermente im blutserum von tumorratten. Biochem. Ztschr. *314*:399, 1943.
West, M., Eshchar, J., and Zimmerman, H. J.: Serum enzymology in the diagnosis of myocardial infarction and related cardiovascular conditions. Med. Clin. N. Amer. *50*:171, 1966.
White, L. (ed.): Enzymes in blood. Ann. N.Y. Acad. Med. 75:1, 1958.
Wilkinson, J. H.: *Isoenzymes*. Philadelphia, J. B. Lippincott Co., 1966.
Wroblewski, F.: Increasing clinical significance of alterations in enzymes of body fluids. Ann. Intern. Med. *50*:62, 1959.

Phosphatases

Fishman, W. H. (ed.): *The Phosphohydrolases: Their Biology, Biochemistry and Clinical Enzymology*. New York, N.Y. Academy of Science, 1969.
Gutman, A. B.: Serum alkaline phosphatase activity in diseases of the skeletal and hepatobiliary systems. Amer. J. Med. 27:875, 1959.
Kaplan, M. M.: Alkaline phosphatase. New Eng. J. Med. *286*:200, 1972.
Woodard, H. Q.: The clinical significance of serum acid phosphatase. Amer. J. Med. 27:902, 1959.

Cholinesterase

Juul, P., and Leopold, I. H.: Human plasma cholinesterase isoenzymes. Clin. Chim. Acta *19*:205, 1968.
Vorhaus, L. J., and Kark, R. M.: Serum cholinesterase in health and disease. Amer. J. Med. *14*:707, 1953.

Transaminases

Clermont, R. J., and Chalmers, T. C.: The transaminase tests in liver disease. Medicine *46*:197, 1967.
DeRitis, F., Coltori, M., and Giusti, C.: Diagnostic value and pathogenic significance of transaminase activity changes in viral hepatitis. Minerva Med. *47*:101, 1956.
Wroblewski, F.: Clinical significance of alterations in transaminase activities of serum and other body fluids. Advances Clin. Chem. *1*:313, 1958.

Enzymes of Erythrocytes and Leukocytes

Brady, R. O., Johnson, W. G., and Uhlendorf, B. W.: Identification of heterozygous carriers of lipid storage diseases: Current status and clinical applications. Amer. J. Med. *51*:423, 1971.
Carson, P. E., and Frischer, H.: Glucose-6-phosphate dehydrogenase deficiency and related disorders of the pentose phosphate pathway. Amer. J. Med. *41*:744, 1966.
Jaffe, E. R.: Hereditary hemolytic disorders and enzymatic deficiencies of human erythrocytes. Blood *35*:116, 1970.
Stanbury, J. B., Wyngaarden, J. B., and Fredrickson, D. S.: *The Metabolic Basis of Inherited Disease*. 3rd ed., New York, McGraw-Hill Book Co., Inc., 1972.
Weisberg, J. B., Lipschutz, F., and Oski, F. A.: δ-Aminolevulinic acid dehydratase activity in circulating blood cells: A sensitive laboratory test for the detection of childhood lead poisoning, New Eng. J. Med. *284*:565, 1971.

Chapter 15

LABORATORY EVALUATION OF PANCREATIC DISORDERS

by MYRTON F. BEELER, M.D., and WEI T. WU, Ph.D.

Of the various developmental, inflammatory, neoplastic, degenerative, and infiltrative processes which may affect the pancreas, the most serious and therefore the most important from a diagnostic and prognostic point of view are acute pancreatic necrosis, chronic pancreatitis, and pancreatic carcinoma in adults, and cystic fibrosis of the pancreas (mucoviscidosis) in children. The first of these generally requires rapid differential diagnosis because of the similarity of its symptoms to those of an acute abdominal condition requiring surgery. The second is a common cause of the malabsorption syndrome. (See Chapter 17, "The Examination of Feces.") The third may also cause this syndrome. However, especially when situated in the body and tail of the gland, it often gains an ineradicable foothold before its presence is detected. Fibrocystic disease is also commonly associated with malabsorption, as well as with chronic lung disease.

Laboratory diagnosis of pancreatic disease is generally approached through analysis of blood serum, urine, duodenal contents, peritoneal fluid, and feces for pancreatic digestive enzymes or bicarbonate; or through quantitative analyses of substances whose digestion and absorption from the gut depend upon integrity of pancreatic secretion (Howat, 1972). Assay of substances whose concentration in blood is secondarily altered by pancreatic disease (such as serum calcium) may also be helpful.

AMYLASE

Alpha amylase (α, 1,4-glucan 4-glucanohydrolase) is an enzyme which acts on starch to split α 1,4 glucosidic bonds (except for that of maltose) randomly. Chlorides activate the reaction. Pancreatic and salivary amylases are both alpha amylases. (Beta amylases are of plant origin.) Amylase was first shown to be present in pancreatic juice in 1845 by Bouchardat, and in blood by Magendie in 1847. It is reported to have a molecular weight of 45,000 and an optimum pH of 6.9. In humans it is normally present in pancreas (approximately 200 mg. per kg.), salivary glands, liver, muscle, adipose tissue, saliva, blood, urine, feces, milk, and semen.

Isoenzyme fractionation has not yet been found to be useful clinically, although three peaks have been found by DEAE-cellulose column chromatography of human pancreatic drainage, and isoelectric *focusing* has been reported to have detected isoenzymes of crystalline amylase (Berndt *et al.*, 1970).

Little is known about the normal mechanism of entrance of pancreatic enzymes, such as amylase, into blood, where normally the pancreatic enzyme appears to account for less than 25 per cent of serum amylase activity. Increased serum activity in acute pancreatitis presumably results from escape of enzymes into the interstitial tissue and peritoneal cavity, with increased absorption through the lymphatics and veins. Blood amylase is excreted by the kidney, and renal clearance has been estimated as 1 to 3 ml. per minute, appearing to be constant over a wide range of urine flow; therefore, increased release into the blood is followed by increased excretion in the urine.

Amylase is first detectable in serum of infants between the ages of one and two months, and by one year of age, low normal adult levels are reached.

Methodology

Somogyi's saccharogenic amylase method (Somogyi, 1938) is a single endpoint method. In its original form it employs no buffer for pH control, and the color reagent does not always react stoichiometrically with liberated reducing compounds of different chain length. Also, it is difficult for inexperienced persons to perform reproducibly. It is not, therefore, an accurate method. However, it serves as the reference method for his iodometric method and the many modifications of it. Most clinicians are familiar with the normal range when expressed in Somogyi units (the amount of enzyme in 100 ml. of serum which produces reducing substances equivalent to 1 mg. of glucose from starch substrate in 30 minutes at 40° C. under the conditions specified in his test). Therefore, it is still taken to be the reference method by many in this country. We prefer the modification of Henry and Chiamori (1960), which incorporates use of phosphate buffer, pH 7.0. In our hands the use of buffer yielded higher values with commercial control material than did the original method, although Henry and Chiamori reported a normal range (95 per cent limits) for adult serum from males of 38–118 units/100 ml. and from adult females of 46–141 units. This is slightly lower than the normal range reported by Somogyi, who did not describe how he determined it, and did not separate male from female values.

We recommend Somogyi's amyloclastic manual method or the automated saccharogenic method of Wu and Beeler (Wu and Beeler, 1972) for routine diagnostic use. We do not recommend use of the many modifications of the amyloclastic method based on photometric examination of the starch-iodine complex, chiefly because of their liability to false elevations, often unrecognized as artefact, especially when applied to urine. Most of the interference appears to result from the presence of radiographic contrast media in urine. Another drawback is lack of reproducibility of the starch substrates used in the modified methods. Insufficient attention may have been paid to this point by some of the several investigators who, in recent years, have been reporting preliminary results with photometric amylase methods employing dyes such as Remazol Brilliant Blue, R-amylose, Cibachron Blue-amylose (Klein *et al.*, 1966), Brilliant Red M-2BS-amylopectin, and Reactone Red 2B-amylopectin. Otherwise, these procedures show considerable promise for the future. "No quick and easy way to determine amylase has yet been found" (Koch and Tonks, 1971).

Diagnostic Application of Amylase Determination

Acute Pancreatitis. Acute pancreatic necrosis (acute hemorrhagic pancreatitis) is a serious disease with a mortality rate greater than 50 per cent. It is known to have a significantly high coincidence with gallstones, alcoholism, trauma (including abdominal surgery), infection (5 per cent of mumps) and various disorders of metabolism, including hyperlipemia, uremia, and hyperparathyroidism. Recently, it has been described as a complication of renal transplantation.

Etiology and pathogenesis are still in doubt. The most popular hypothesis is that ductal obstruction, whether from gallstones, pancreatic stones, sphincter or duct spasms, epithelial proliferation, edema, or parasites, presumably coupled with strong stimulus to secretion, increase intraductal pressure to the point of acinar or ductal rupture, with leakage of pancreatic digestive enzymes into the interstitial tissue. The enzymes somehow become activated and initiate the necrosis. There is an alternate hypothesis which states that increased intraduodenal pressure rather than obstruction of the ducts is the cause. It is possible that vascular spasm secondary to the inflammatory process, with resultant ischemia, plays an aggravating role. Activation of enzymes by reflux of bile in patients with an anatomic arrangement which would permit this has also been suggested as a possible etiologic mechanism. Hemorrhage of various degree is usually present, presumably caused by necrosis of blood vessels attacked by elastase and other proteolytic enzymes. Lipase causes fat necrosis, not only in the pancreas but in the surrounding fat, the mesentery and omentum, and, rarely, even subcutaneously. Shock may result from decreased vascular tone leading to hypotension and may be partly attributable to activation of kallikrein (another proteolytic enzyme present in pancreas) and subsequent elaboration of bradykinin-like polypeptides by the action of kallikrein on circulating alpha-2 globulin. Complications include abscess and pseudocyst formation.

Clinically the diagnostic problem is differentiation from an acute surgical abdominal emergency; the prognostic problem is distinguishing this serious disease (acute hemorrhagic pancreatitis), carrying a mortality rate greater than 50 per cent, from the much more common (about 75 per cent of cases), milder, edematous form of acute pancreatitis, carrying a mortality rate of about 5 per cent.

The serum amylase test has been widely used in the diagnosis of acute pancreatitis. However, results can be within the normal range, or borderline in occasional patients with very little functioning pancreatic tissue left, as may occur in overwhelming acute pancreatic necrosis. Activity may, on the other hand, be elevated, even to very high values—to 500 or even 1000 Somogyi units—in the absence of pancreatitis, as in patients with intestinal obstruction, strangulation, or perforation, following upper abdominal surgery, with ruptured ectopic pregnancy, with mumps, with renal insufficiency, or following morphine administration. The latter suggests the desirability of drawing blood for the determination before administration of opiates.

Serum amylase activity rises within a few hours of onset in patients with acute pancreatitis, but not proportionately to severity of the disease. Values over five times the upper limit of normal are highly suggestive of the diagnosis. Activity usually returns to normal in two to five days in patients with the milder edematous forms of the disease. Elevated values persisting longer than this suggest continuing necrosis or possible pseudocyst formation. The urine amylase activity rises promptly, often within several hours of the rise in serum activity. Urine activity may remain abnormal after the serum activity has returned to the normal range. Values of 1000 units per hour or higher are seen, almost exclusively, in patients with acute pancreatitis (Bockus, 1965).

Although amylase activity of peritoneal fluid may be elevated in patients with perforated ulcer, intestinal strangulation, and ectopic pregnancy, values over 5000 units suggest a diagnosis of acute pancreatic necrosis.

Chronic Pancreatitis. "Chronic pancreatitis" is a term used in pathology to refer to perilobular and interacinar fibrosis, with variable parenchymal atrophy, and might well be termed "cirrhosis of the pancreas." Ductal pathology may include dilatation and epithelial hyperplasia and metaplasia and presence of calculi. There may be interstitial lymphocytic infiltration. The changes sometimes result from clinically recurrent bouts of relapsing acute pancreatitis, sometimes from continuous pancreatitis, but they may have a clinically insidious onset. It has been claimed that alcoholic pancreatitis is more often relapsing than is the pancreatitis associated with gallstones. When damage is sufficiently extensive, malabsorption supervenes. This syndrome and its differential diagnosis are considered in the chapter on the examination of feces (Chapter 17). Diagnosis, as in the case of acute pancreatitis, depends in part on determination of amylase activity in serum and urine.

The urinary output of amylase (units per hour), has been claimed to be more sensitive a test in patients with mild attacks of pancreatitis (Gambill and Mason, 1963), and to remain elevated longer after an attack.

An analysis of laboratory results on 149 patients at Ochsner Foundation Hospital (Beeler, 1970) known to have, or suspected of having, pancreatitis (either acute or chronic) yields the following data: of 221 serum amylase determinations on these patients, 100 (45 per cent) were above 150 Somogyi units. Of 72 urine amylase determinations, 32 (44 per cent) were above 250 Somogyi units/hour.

Of course, relative sensitivity depends, in part, upon the value chosen for the upper limit of normal. Gambill and Mason took the upper limit of normal for serum to be 320 units (Smith and Roe units, comparable to Somogyi units); for urine, 300 Somogyi units/hour.

At Charity Hospital of Louisiana in New Orleans, 1-hour urinary amylase activity (based on a 2-hour collection) (urine assayed by the original Somogyi saccharogenic method) was calculated for 42 apparently healthy men and women by Gilchrist (1967) in an unpublished study. From his data, average activity was 130 units per hour; the standard deviation, 56. Taking the average plus two standard deviations as an approximation of the upper limit of normal, we obtain the value, 242 units/hour. Three standard deviations would be 298 units, a figure almost identical to that of Gambill and Mason. Calculated similarly, the upper limit of normal for serum amylase activity is approximately 150 units, considerably lower than their upper limit. Thus, the upper limits of normal chosen by Gambill and Mason might have caused the urine test to appear relatively more sensitive than it is.

However, our experience at Ochsner Clinic (where we used Somogyi's amyloclastic method) was similar to theirs in at least one respect: we frequently observed elevated urinary values in the presence of normal serum values in patients suspected of having, or known to have, pancreatitis. Sometimes the discrepancy was strikingly in favor of the urinary assay. For example, we have seen urine activity as high as 1377 units/hour when the serum activity was only 145 units. More often, of course, both were elevated. We have also seen elevated serum amylase activity in the presence of normal urine activity on a few occasions, but have not had an opportunity to investigate the reason for this type of discrepancy. Some patients may have had retention as a result of renal disease. Conceivably there were one or two patients with undiagnosed macroamylasemia (in which case, the large molecule does not pass freely into the urine—see later). The possibility remains that some of the patients may have had pancreatitis, although in none of the patients on whom the test was performed (it was performed in most) was the serum lipase elevated.

In 1964, Wilding, Cooke, and Nicholson

reported what appears to be the first documented instance of hyperamylasemia due to the formation of an amylase-globulin complex. Berk and associates (1967) reported three similar cases characterized by a persistent elevation of serum enzyme activity not accompanied by hyperamylasuria. The term "macroamylasemia" was coined at that time to describe this peculiar condition. One year later Levitt and Cooperband (1968) reported persistent hyperamylasemia with low renal clearance of amylase in a patient who was found to have an abnormally large amylase (11S), probably resulting from the binding by an abnormal 11S immunoglobulin (IgA), postulated to be the result of an autoimmune reaction. The patient had a syndrome consisting of intestinal mucosal disease (villous atrophy), malabsorption, and a large serum amylase molecule.

Today, hyperamylasemia resulting from protein binding is an accepted clinical entity, which has been associated with malabsorption and/or the effects of alcoholism (Berk *et al.*, 1970). However, to date there is no concrete evidence to correlate macroamylasemia directly with any single disease state.

It has been suggested that macroamylase might be a polymer of amylase similar to that of *Bacillus subtilis* (Stein and Fischer, 1960), but there is no experimental evidence to support this in man. It is now clear that the large amylolytic enzyme found in patients with macroamylasemia is not homogeneous (Take *et al.*, 1970) and is felt by many investigators to be of at least two distinct types: One form can be dissociated at pH 3.4 into normal size amylase and has an 11S IgA as the binding protein. The other cannot be dissociated by lowering the pH and is not precipitable with antiserums against immunoglobulins. The heterogeneity of properties of macroamylase in the various cases reported makes it obvious that there may be several types of complexes. Take *et al.* (1970) suggest that the amylase in some cases of macroamylasemia may be a complex of normal size amylase bound to glycoprotein(s). Another consideration is that even though the macroamylase complex is not precipitated by specific antiserum to immunoglobulins (second category of macroamylase complex), it might simply be that the amylase masks the antigenic determinants of the immunoglobulins, as suggested by Wilding *et al.* Scattered reports now indicate that the binding protein can be IgG, as identified by electrophoretic, solubility, and immunochemical criteria (Hansen *et al.*, 1972).

Most investigators have employed either gel filtration or ultracentrifugation in studying the properties of these macromolecules. Their molecular weights have been estimated to range from 150,000 to greater than 1 million. Cross-linked dextran gel (Sephadex G-200) has been the most popular matrix for fractionation of serums suspected of having a macroamylase. However, because of the tendency of molecular complex dissociation, gel filtration cannot be used to determine the relative amounts of bound versus free amylase which exist in the serum in vivo. To date the best measurement of normal-sized amylase present in the serum (as might be performed in a clinical laboratory) is the ratio of the renal clearance of amylase to the renal clearance of creatine (Cam/Ccr), which averages 2.3 per cent in normal subjects (Levitt *et al.*, 1969).

Recently a microcolumn chromatographic procedure has been worked out as a reliable screening procedure for macroamylasemia (Fridhandler *et al.*, 1971). Using this method, investigators have found a small but significant number of individuals who possess macroamylasemia in the face of normal total serum amylase activity (Barrows *et al.*, 1972).

As previously stated, only 44 per cent of 72 urine amylase determinations yielded elevated results, while 45 per cent of 221 serum amylase determinations yielded results higher than normal. The highest urine amylase we encountered was 7129 units/hour in a patient whose serum amylase was 620 units (and whose serum lipase exhibited only borderline elevation). The highest serum amylase we encountered was one of 1684 units (urinary assay not performed). The highest assay result we have seen for any material was an activity of 160,000 units/100 ml. in fluid from a pancreatic cyst.

Carcinoma of the Pancreas. Malignant tumors of the pancreas are usually adenocarcinomas arising from the ducts. Most occur in the head of the gland, where they may obstruct the pancreatic or bile ducts, causing hyperbilirubinemia (in less than half of the patients) or the malabsorption syndrome late in their course. Carcinomas of the body and tail of the pancreas are even more insidious, presenting an area of real laboratory diagnostic impotence. In any case, surgery carries a high mortality rate and results in only a very small five-year salvage rate. Serum amylase may be elevated, but is of little diagnostic assistance.

Miscellaneous Disorders. Casey and associates (1971) studied the correlation of serum amylase activity determined by an automated amyloclastic method with 28 other serum constituents and with disease in 17,431 consecutive hospitalized patients. Amylase activity was found to be closely related to albumin and calcium concentrations. Low values were found in patients with diabetes mellitus and with serum protein loss in congestive heart failure, gastrointestinal cancer, fracture, pleurisy, and intestinal obstruction; high values occurred in those who had had gynecologic surgery for conditions other than cancer and in those with cataracts.

LIPASE

Lipase is an esterase acting on ester linkages in triglycerides. Bile salts and calcium enhance activity. The latter presumably acts by precipitating products of the reaction as calcium soaps.

Lipase occurs predominantly in the pancreas and, for this reason, its diagnostic possibilities have been intriguing. According to Abderhalden (1961), the mucosa of the stomach and small bowel may produce a small amount of lipase, and there are conflicting but predominant reports that there is normally a small amount of lipase activity in serum. Also present in serum is a true esterase (aliesterase) which cleaves ester linkages of short-chain fatty acids, unlike lipase, which acts more specifically on long-chain glycerol-ester linkages of fatty acids. Esterase is found in the liver as well as the pancreas and is inhibited by sodium taurocholate, which activates lipase. These enzymes are unrelated to the lipoprotein lipase which is activated by heparin.

Methodology

The classic method for serum lipase determination is that of Cherry and Crandall (1932), using olive oil as substrate, overnight incubation (24 hours), and titration of the liberated fatty acids with sodium hydroxide, using phenolphthalein as indicator. Henry and his associates (1957) have slightly modified the method, titrating with either a pH meter or with thymolphthalein as an indicator, and shortening the incubation time to 16 hours (after which they state there is little increase in value). They point out that incubation time can be shortened to 4 hours and the final result multiplied by 2 to approximate the 16-hour value (reaction does not follow zero order kinetics). Normal range of values is up to 1.5 units. Tietz and Fiereck (1966) reduced the incubation time to 3 hours.

The patient with acute pancreatitis presents as a medical emergency. If there is a surgically correctable abdominal catastrophe present, there is no time to be lost. If the diagnosis is acute pancreatic necrosis, surgical intervention may worsen the prognosis. The classic serum lipase assay may be too slow to provide diagnostic help when it is most needed. For this reason, at Ochsner Clinic we turned to a rapid (20-minute incubation) specific turbidimetric method described by Vogel and Zieve in 1963. The method is simple as well as rapid, but unfortunately may yield spuriously high results in the presence of jaundice. This may be avoided by absorption of the interfering pigments onto DEAE-cellulose; but the procedure loses much of its attractiveness in the process. Values above 10 units are doubtful; above 19 units, definitely abnormal. An additional problem has been the fact that the substrate (preparation of which requires meticulous adherence to directions) is not very stable, and that, in less than expert hands, precision of the procedure is poor. We have not set up this procedure at Charity Hospital, where we continue to use a modification of the method of Cherry and Crandall.

Diagnostic Application of Serum Lipase Determination

Acute Pancreatitis. Serum lipase activity rises more slowly than serum amylase activity in patients with acute pancreatitis, sometimes as late as 24 to 48 hours after onset, often peaking on the fourth day. It may remain elevated longer than the serum amylase. Although it is a less sensitive test than the serum amylase, it provides confirmatory evidence for the diagnosis when positive. Elevation in patients with mumps strongly suggests significant pancreatic as well as salivary gland involvement by the disease.

Chronic Pancreatitis. Of the 149 Ochsner patients already referred to, only 28 (16 per cent) had lipase activity above 10 Vogel-Zieve units (serum amylase, 45 per cent; urine amylase, 44 per cent). Furthermore, in only one of the instances in which the serum lipase was elevated was there normal serum and urine amylase activity, whereas the reverse occurred frequently. Also, in only three instances was the result higher than three times the upper limit of normal (161, 109, and 50 Vogel-Zieve units, respectively). Therefore, it seems to us that the serum lipase determination is of relatively little value in the diagnosis of chronic pancreatitis.

We also studied the urine lipase in some of these patients (70 determinations on 48 patients). Eight of these were above 10 units VZ/hour, 17 were above 5 units/hour; in 12 of these 17 cases, serum lipase results were also available, and of these, only three were elevated. In some instances, serum amylase and urine amylase were also normal. One patient, with urine amylase 7129 units/hour, serum amylase 620 units/100 ml., and serum lipase 12 units, had a urine lipase of 7.8 units/hour; another, with urine amylase 360 units/hour, serum amylase 200 units/100 ml., had a urine lipase of 30.6 units/hour; still another, with serum amylase 89 units/100 ml., urine amylase

203 units/hour, and serum lipase 50.5 units, had only 4.3 units urine lipase/hour.

Since we do not have an adequate series of urine lipase values on healthy patients, and since we have not studied the reported presence of inhibitors of lipase in the urine, we are not able to interpret this data definitively. It seems to suggest that the urine lipase determination (at least by the turbidimetric method) adds little or nothing to our diagnostic armamentarium.

Pancreatic Carcinoma. It has been claimed that serum lipase is elevated more often in patients with pancreatic carcinoma than is serum amylase, although not with sufficient frequency to make it of much value diagnostically.

SECRETIN TEST

A double lumen tube, providing for separate aspiration of gastric and duodenal contents, is passed into the duodenum, using fluoroscopic guidance and maintaining constant aspiration of gastric contents. Duodenal contents are aspirated until clear. The patient is then given intravenously one unit of secretin per kg. of body weight, and pancreatic secretion entering the duodenum is collected for 80 minutes (Levine, 1972). The aspirate is examined for volume, bicarbonate content, and amylase activity.

The test is not used for the diagnosis of acute pancreatic necrosis (it would be hazardous, among other reasons). According to Dreiling (1953), patients with chronic pancreatitis are unable to secrete juice of high bicarbonate content. The lower limit of normal in their series was 90 mEq. bicarbonate per liter, and only 4 per cent of patients with chronic pancreatitis showed values above this.

As in the case of chronic pancreatitis, the secretin test may be helpful in diagnosis of pancreatic carcinoma, depending on site and extent of pancreatic duct obstruction. Tumors of the head of the pancreas tend to depress the overall volume flow, only 5 per cent of the patients in the series of Dreiling (1953), falling above the lower limit of normal of 2 ml. per kg. of body weight per 80 minutes. On the other hand, almost half the patients with carcinoma of the body of the pancreas exhibited normal volume flow, and almost all did when the lesion was in the tail. Patients with obstructive ductal lesions may exhibit elevation of serum amylase during and following the test; normally there is no elevation of serum amylase activity. The pattern of increased volume with decreased bicarbonate and normal amylase has been seen in hemochromatosis. Rarely, an increase in the amylase with normal bicarbonate concentration and volume flow has been noted in patients with nutritional and metabolic pancreatic fibrosis, as well as in pancreatitis associated with inflammatory disease of the intestines. In some patients with pancreatic ductal obstruction, levels may rise.

Tumors of the head of the pancreas associated with jaundice must be differentiated from nonsurgical cholestatic liver disease; from carcinoma, obstructing stone, or other obstructing pathologic lesions of the common bile duct; and from ampullary carcinoma.

Duodenal aspirate containing cholesterol crystals or calcium bilirubinate pigment and pus, especially when associated with a normal secretin test, suggests gallstone etiology. However, a duodenal aspirate containing calcium bilirubinate pigment is not specific for cholelithiasis. Unremittent jaundice, acholic duodenal fluid and stools, consistently negative urine urobilinogen tests, and less than 5 mg. fecal urobilinogen per 24 hours, associated with a normal secretin test, suggest carcinoma of the common duct or gallbladder. Intermittent jaundice and presence of blood in the aspirate suggest carcinoma of the duodenal papilla, especially when associated with an abnormal secretin test. Cytologic examination of aspirate may be helpful in the diagnosis of carcinoma, as are the results of enzyme and volume outputs (Levine, 1972).

Because of discomfort and possible hazard to the patient, this test should be among the last to be used in an attempt to diagnose chronic pancreatitis or pancreatic carcinoma, although, clearly, it is less of an ordeal than is an exploratory laparotomy.

MISCELLANEOUS LABORATORY TESTS IN ACUTE PANCREATITIS

There is usually leukocytosis in patients with acute pancreatitis, white blood cell counts sometimes reaching $30,000/mm.^3$ There may also be signs of hemoconcentration. Serum levels of lecithinase A, trypsin, and deoxyribonuclease activity are also elevated, but these determinations have not gained popularity. Lecithinase A may be the enzyme primarily responsible for pancreatic necrosis. An assay suitable for clinical use has been described (Zieve and Vogel, 1961). A falling serum calcium points to the more serious form of pancreatitis, as does turbidity of the serum. The falling calcium presumably results from formation of calcium soaps of the fatty acids liberated by the action of pancreatic lipase. Hyperbilirubinemia occurs in many patients, not only those with gallstones but those in whom the pancreatitis appears to be related to alcoholism. The reason is not well understood. Results of other liver function tests may also be abnormal. Transient hyperglycemia may also occur.

MISCELLANEOUS LABORATORY TESTS IN CHRONIC PANCREATITIS AND PANCREATIC CARCINOMA

Malabsorption is discussed in Chapter 17, The Examination of Feces. Since it may be caused by inadequacy of pancreatic secretion, and may result from chronic pancreatitis or pancreatic carcinoma, various tests for malabsorption, such as the serum carotenoid level, the glucose tolerance test, the ^{131}I-labeled triolein absorption test (Calkins, 1966), the starch tolerance test, and the three-day fecal fat determination may be useful diagnostically, as may gross and microscopic examination of stools. Although these tests are discussed in greater detail elsewhere, it should be stated that the ^{131}I triolein test yields many false positive and false negative results, which has prompted most gastroenterologists to abandon this test (Levine, 1972). Only about one-third of patients with pancreatic carcinoma are reported to have abnormal starch tolerance test results. A similar percentage have abnormal ^{131}I triolein test results. A larger percentage may have a "flat" glucose tolerance curve; but this is very nonspecific, diagnostically. The D-xylose test, discussed in Chapter 17 (The Examination of Feces), while potentially a very useful test for distinguishing malabsorption caused by pancreatic disease from that caused by intestinal disorders, is, in legal status, doubtful.

SWEAT ELECTROLYTES BY PILOCARPINE IONTOPHORESIS

Pilocarpine is iontophoresed into the skin to stimulate locally increased sweat gland secretion. The resulting sweat is absorbed by filter paper, diluted with distilled water, and analyzed for sodium and chloride content. The method is painless and reliable. Total body sweating in patients with cystic fibrosis is hazardous, and a number of deaths from the procedure have been recorded. Cellulose sponges have been used successfully in place of filter paper, although we have found that use of a syringe to express the sweat from the cellulose sponge is inefficient and necessitates use of ultramicro techniques, whereas the present method is suitable to micro techniques. Potentiometric methods are also available.

Diagnostic Application of Sweat Testing

Fibrocystic Disease (Mucoviscidosis). This is a familial, Mendelian recessive disease characterized by abnormal secretion by the various exocrine glands of the body, including pancreas, salivary glands, peritracheal, peribronchial, and peribronchiolar glands, lacrimal glands, sweat glands, mucosal glands of the small bowel, and even the bile ducts.

Involvement of the intestinal glands may result in presence of meconium ileus at birth. Chronic lung disease and malabsorption resulting from pancreatic involvement are the major clinical problems of those who survive beyond infancy. The histologic appearance of the pancreas is one of dilatation of ducts and acini, with plugging by acidophilic material and flattening of the lining epithelial cells. There may be an increased amount of fibrous tissue present.

Laboratory diagnosis depends largely on demonstration of increased sodium and chloride in the sweat, found in about 99 per cent of patients. Screening tests for sweat chloride have also been used and depend on hand imprints on silver nitrate-containing agar or paper. The sweat chloride precipitates with silver, and the intensity of the print is roughly proportional to the sweat chloride concentration. We believe that a careful history and physical are better screening procedures, and that the definitive sweat test should be applied only when indicated. In children, chloride concentrations over 60 mEq. per liter of sweat are diagnostic. Levels between 50 and 60 mEq. per liter are suggestive in the absence of adrenal insufficiency. Sodium concentrations are usually about 10 to 20 mEq. per liter higher than chloride.

Sweat electrolytes in about half of a group of premenopausal adult women have been shown to undergo cyclic fluctuation, reaching a peak chloride concentration most commonly five to 10 days prior to the onset of menses. Peak values were slightly under 65 mEq. per liter. Men showed random fluctuations up to just under 70 mEq. per liter. For this reason, interpretation of values in adults must be approached with caution.

Normal Values in Children

Chloride	*Sodium*
Below 50 mEq. per liter: normal	Below 70 mEq. per liter: normal
50 to 60 mEq. per liter: equivocal	70 to 90 mEq. per liter: equivocal
Over 60 mEq. per liter: abnormal	Over 90 mEq. per liter: abnormal

PROTEOLYTIC ENZYMES IN FECES

Trypsin and chymotrypsin are nearly always present in grossly measurable quantities in the stools of normal young children. There is frequently much less activity detectable, however, in the adult stool, except when there is rapid transit through the gastrointestinal tract. The enzymes are apparently partially destroyed by bacteria within the gastrointestinal tract, and activity is seldom detectable at all by the cruder tests when there is constipation. The simpler tests are therefore not very useful for adults. On the other hand, many bacteria produce proteolytic enzymes which may give positive tests in the absence of pancreatogenous enzymes. For this reason, results must be interpreted with caution in children also. In spite of these drawbacks, the tests have gained wide popularity.

A number of methods have been devised for detecting and measuring proteolytic enzyme activity in stools and duodenal fluid. These include tests based on ability of stool solutions to digest such substrates as serum proteins, hemoglobin, casein, and gelatin. The methods lack specificity and precision. One has been widely used as a screening test for fibrocystic disease of the pancreas. It depends on the ability of stool suspension to digest the gelatin emulsion on x-ray film.

Serial dilutions are made of stool with barbital buffer pH 8. Strips of x-ray film are partially immersed in them and are incubated for 1 hour at 37° C. Proteolytic activity is indicated by digestion and removal of the opaque emulsion from the film.

METHODS AND METHODOLOGY DISCUSSION

Amylase Determination (Serum, Urine, Duodenal Aspirate, Peritoneal Fluid)*

PRINCIPLE. Amylase present in serum is permitted to act on starch substrate of known concentration at 40° C. The reaction is followed by periodically transferring aliquots of the starch solution to an iodine solution and observing the color; first blue, then purple, then reddish brown. The endpoint is taken to be the tube showing the last trace of purple in the developing red-brown of the erythrodextrin mixture.

PROCEDURE

1. Remove starch solution from refrigerator and mix well.
2. Flame mouth of flask and pour out about 6 ml. of starch solution.
3. Transfer 4 ml. of starch solution (containing 3 mg. starch) to a test tube and incubate in 40° C. water bath for 5 minutes.
4. While incubating, transfer 0.5 ml. of dilute iodine solution to each of the nine test tubes (7 mm. inside diameter).
5. Add 1 ml. serum (or urine or diluted duodenal or peritoneal aspirate) to starch solution and start stopwatch. Mix well and return to water bath.
6. After 1 minute, transfer 0.5 ml. of the starch-serum mixture to the first iodine tube, noting color immediately before a "daylight" lamp.
7. If the color is dark blue, wait 2 more minutes and try a second sample.
8. If the sample is blue, double the waiting period and continue in this manner until the first purple is obtained.
9. Judging from the time of appearance of the first purple, take subsequent samples until the endpoint is reached (a barely perceptible tint of purple in the red-brown). It may be helpful to go past the endpoint in order to be sure it has been reached. With experience, one learns to judge the shade of purple signaling the halfway point.
10. If endpoint is reached before 8 minutes, dilute serum appropriately with 0.5 per cent (w./v.) sodium chloride and repeat the test, using 0.3-ml. aliquots of iodine rather than the 0.5-ml. aliquots called for with undiluted serum. (This balance is important.)
11. Occasional urine-starch incubates cause fading of the iodine solution when aliquots are added. The cause in most or all cases is the presence in urine of Telapaque, Agrafin, or other radiopaque media. Color can be restored for a long enough time to read the endpoint by judicious addition of extra iodine to the urine-starch-iodine mixture. Alternatively, one can dilute out the interference and still have an endpoint, although this results in a rather lengthy test. The interference has not been encountered in serum determinations.

CALCULATION

$$\frac{1600}{\text{time in minutes}} = \text{Somogyi units of amylase activity}$$

EXPLANATION. Somogyi arbitrarily defined these units to correspond with those of his saccharogenic method. The Somogyi unit may be defined as the amount of reducing substance produced by incubation of serum with buffered starch substrate for 30 minutes at 40° C. It is expressed as milligrams of glucose equivalent per 100 ml. of serum. It would be appropriate to check the factor for the brand of starch used, although Somogyi noted it to be relatively constant over many years when cornstarch was used.

REAGENTS

1. Iodine solution (stock). Dissolve 2.5 gm. potassium iodide and 1.27 gm. resublimed iodine in distilled water and dilute to 100 ml.

*Somogyi, M.: J. Biol. Chem., *125*:399, 1938.

2. Iodine solution (working). Dilute 2 ml. stock iodine solution to 100 ml. with 2 per cent (w./v.) potassium iodide.

3. Dry starch (can be purchased prepared from Dade Reagents, Inc., Miami, Florida). Suspend 100 gm. Argo corstarch in 1 liter of approximately 0.01 normal HCl and agitate frequently for 1 hour. Let stand (may take several hours to settle out) and decant HCl. Add 1 liter of approximately 0.05 per cent NaCl and let stand until starch settles out. Decant. Repeat wash with 0.05 per cent NaCl. Decant and spread starch out on evaporating dishes. Blot surface with coarse filter paper to absorb moisture. Spread out on filter paper to dry in air overnight. When thoroughly dry, transfer to brown, stoppered bottle.

4. *Starch solution.* A. Grind 10 gm. washed starch in mortar with 50 ml. water; add to 400 ml. boiling distilled water in a beaker with constant stirring. Wash mortar with 50 ml. distilled water and add to contents of beaker. Boil with stirring for 1 minute. Add 5 ml. 25 per cent NaCl and heat for 30 minutes in boiling water bath with inverted beaker over mouth of flask. Let settle in refrigerator overnight. Centrifuge at 3000 r.p.m. for 30 minutes. Decant and save supernatant.

B. Dilute supernatant fluid to proper volume (see below) with NaCl and buffer solution. Distribute in Erlenmeyer flasks stoppered with gauze-covered cotton. Autoclave. Keep in refrigerator, sterile.

Determining proper final dilution for starch (75 mg. starch per 100 ml., 250 mg. NaCl per 100 ml.):

1. Hydrolyze aliquot of starch solution: Into a 25 × 200 mm. NPN tube, place 5 ml. starch solution, 1 ml. 3.6 N HCl; stopper with one-hole rubber stopper fitted with two-foot glass tube to act as reflux condenser, immerse in boiling water bath for 2 hours and 30 minutes. (This converts the starch to glucose.) Neutralize with NaOH (phenol red indicator, red to yellow). This requires approximately 6 ml. of 20 per cent NaOH.

2. Dilute to 25 ml. with distilled water and determine the glucose content. We prefer the automated ferricyanide reduction method. To convert answer from glucose to starch, results must be multiplied by 0.9 to correct for equivalent weight of starch compared with that of glucose.

3. Calculate proper dilution of starch solution (75 mg. starch and 250 mg. NaCl per 100 ml.) and buffer 0.012 M pH 6.8.

This is easy once the principle is understood. If one dilutes 75 ml. of the stock starch solution to the same number of milliliters as the numerical value of its concentration (in mg./dl.) one will always end with a working solution containing 75 mg. starch/dl. For example, if the stock starch solution contains 434 mg./dl., then:

$$\frac{75 \text{ ml. stock starch solution}}{434 \text{ ml. working starch solution}} \times \frac{434 \text{ mg. starch}}{100 \text{ ml. stock starch solution}} = \frac{75 \text{ mg. starch}}{100 \text{ ml.}}$$

Let C = starch content of stock starch solution (mg./100 ml.)

Then,

$$A = \frac{C}{2} - 75 = \text{ml. 0.25 per cent NaCl needed}$$

$$B = \frac{C}{2} \div 2 = \text{ml. mixed buffer needed}$$

$$C = \frac{C}{2} \div 2 = \text{ml. 0.5 per cent NaCl needed}$$

$$D = 75 = \text{ml. stock starch solution needed}$$

EXAMPLE:

Stock starch solution contains 434 mg./dl.

$$A = \frac{434}{2} - 75 = 142 \text{ ml. 0.25 per cent NaCl}$$

$$B = \frac{C}{2} \div 2 = 109 \text{ ml. mixed buffer needed}$$

$$C = \frac{C}{2} \div 2 = 109 \text{ ml. 0.5 per cent NaCl needed}$$

$$D = 75 \text{ ml. stock starch solution needed}$$

C. Reagents for preparation of starch solution:

1. HCl, 3.6 N.
2. HCl, 0.01 N.
3. NaCl, 25 per cent (w./v.).
4. NaCl, 0.5 per cent (w./v.).
5. NaCl, 0.25 per cent (w./v.).
6. NaCl, 0.05 per cent (w./v.).
7. NaOH, 20 per cent (w./v.).
8. Phenol red indicator.
9. 0.05 M phosphate buffer: KH_2PO_4, 3.6280 gm. per 500 ml. water; K_2HPO_4, 3.6448 gm. per 500 ml. water. Mix in equal proportions.
10. Reagents for glucose determination.

DISCUSSION. The usual methods of assay involve incubation with starch and measurement of decreased viscosity or turbidity, or appearance of reducing substances produced, or of loss of capacity to give a blue starch color with iodine.

Starch itself is a mixture of polysaccharides. When treated with boiling water, part (the unbranched chains) dissolves and part (the branched chains) is relatively insoluble. Iodine and amylose will combine by secondary coordinate valences to form a blue-black color.

Amylase first acts on amylose to split the more central linkages, forming a mixture of smaller dextrins and some maltose. Gradually the dextrins are also converted to maltose.

In 1938 Somogyi described two methods of assay: A saccharogenic method, based on determination of reducing substances formed by incubation with starch substrate, and an amyloclastic method, based on disappearance of the blue color given by iodine and amylose. Units for the two methods were made to correspond numerically, the former being the reference method.

Somogyi's methods appear to be commonly used clinically for determination of amylase activity. Other methods in common usage include those of Smith and Roe (1949), Van Loon *et al.* (1952), Peralta and Reinhold (1955), Gomori (1957), Caraway (1959), and Rice (1959); for all of these methods, the numerical values of the units correspond closely with those of the reference methods. Many of them are photometric adaptations of Somogyi's amyloclastic technique.

Because the chief value of the amylase determination clinically has been in the diagnosis of acute pancreatitis, it is generally offered as an emergency procedure for use at night and on weekends, and it is often performed by relatively poorly trained personnel. Consequently the rapidity and simplicity of the amyloclastic method cause us to regard it as the method of choice.

Performance of Somogyi's amyloclastic method presents no particular problems. Serum is preferred to plasma, as oxalated or citrated plasma is said to show levels 10 to 15 per cent lower than heparinized plasma or serum. Hemolysis may result in artefactually elevated values because of interference with the endpoint.

As in any enzyme determination, careful attention should be paid to control of temperature. A pH change, such as might result from improper cleaning of glassware, will alter results, usually downward. Soap may cause an apparent increase in activity. Serum chloride, calcium, bilirubin, urea, and alcohol levels have been said not to affect results.

Obviously contamination with saliva resulting from improper pipetting, coughing, sneezing, and even talking may cause apparent elevation of serum activity.

According to Somogyi, one should be able easily to reproduce results within 1 minute, and we have found this to be true in our laboratory. On serum diluted 1:1, the calculated amylase activities at an endpoint of 12 and 13 minutes are 266 and 246 units, respectively, a difference of no clinical significance. For this reason we presently see no great advantage to the increased precision resulting from the many photometric adaptations of the procedure. In addition, they may yield artificially high results in some circumstances because of fading of the color caused by albumin or radiographic contrast media. Although in perhaps 10 or 15 per cent of urine samples assayed by this amyloclastic method (but virtually never in serum samples) there will be an immediate disappearance of the starch-iodine color upon addition of urine starch incubate to the iodine, the color can be temporarily reestablished by addition of a second aliquot of iodine. Also, diluting the urine with saline obviates the effect, so that these materials can be analyzed by a slight modification of the usual method. Heating urines to boiling for an hour does remove amyloclastic activity when assayed by the Somogyi method. Variations in serum albumin content do not cause difficulty with Somogyi's amyloclastic technique.

Preparation of the starch substrate is tedious. In our laboratory Argo cornstarch has been consistently satisfactory. Reif and Nabseth (1962) have confirmed Somogyi's finding that cornstarch, not soluble starch, must be used to prepare a standard substrate. They proposed a simplified method for standardizing the starch but stated that the determination of glucose equivalence is preferable. The starch is stable for several months if kept sterile in the refrigerator. Commercially prepared starch substrate is available. We have tested one lot and found it to be satisfactory.

In 1960 Somogyi published some modifications of his method and recommended that dilute sodium hydroxide be used for washing the starch, as washing with dilute hydrochloric acid causes slight hydrolysis.

The original report of the Commission on Enzymes of the International Union of Biochemistry included a recommended International Enzyme Unit. Whenever practicable, enzyme concentration units were to be defined as micromoles (or microequivalents) of substrate transformed per minute per milliliter of sample at 25° C. under optimum conditions of pH and substrate concentration. When this resulted in an inconvenient value, usage of milliunits or kilounits was recommended.

Subsequently, use of 30° C. has been recommended, apparently because it is closer to room or cuvette temperature in many laboratories throughout the world than was 25° C. Choice of 37° C. (body temperature) might have seemed more reasonable, but significant heat inactivation of some enzymes (alkaline phosphatase) is apparently a problem at this temperature. This is not true, of course, with amylase.

Multiplying Somogyi units by 1.85 would give an international milliunit (millimicromoles of glucose equivalent substances formed per minute per milliliter of sample at 40° C.). Until conditions for each enzyme measurement are more specifically defined, however, we do not recommend adoption of these units.

Automated Amylase Assay (Wu and Beeler, 1972)*

PRINCIPLE. Amylase present in serum, urine, peritoneal fluid, or duodenal content is allowed to act on a buffered starch solution at 50° C. for 30 minutes. After incubation the enzyme reaction is stopped by addition of sulfuric acid. Reducing substances present in the original serum before incubation and those present in the incubation mixture after incubation are determined by the standard Technicon N2b automated method for serum glucose. The difference in reducing power (as glucose) is used for calculation of amylase activity in unknowns.

PROCEDURE

1. Pipette into a 12-ml. conical centrifuge tube (or a 13 × 100 test tube) exactly 1 ml. of starch solution. (Always mix well, then pour small amount of substrate from the storage flask into a small container from which to pipette. Use a magnetic stirrer to maintain homogeneity of the substrate while pipetting.)
2. Add 0.5 ml. of serum. Mix.
3. Place the tube in a 50 ± 0.5° C. water bath.
4. After exactly 30 minutes remove tube from the water bath, and immediately add 0.1 ml. of 3 N H_2SO_4. Mix.
5. Centrifuge for 2 or 3 minutes in a table model clinical centrifuge (2000 to 3000 r.p.m.).
6. Decant clear supernatant into AutoAnalyzer plastic sample cup and analyze for reducing power as glucose.
7. The glucose concentration of the same serum is determined separately on the same AutoAnalyzer.
8. Moni-trol I and Moni-trol II (or equivalents) are run as "standards." Reference serum of known amylase activity is also analyzed as control sample.

EQUIPMENT

1. 12-ml. conical centrifuge tubes or other tubes of suitable size.
2. Water bath. 50 ± 0.5° C.
3. Clinical centrifuge.
4. Hotplate-magnetic stirrer.
5. Pipettes: 0.5 ml. TC
   1.0 ml. Ostwald
   0.1 ml. or 0.2 ml. measuring (or microburette)

REAGENTS

1. Starch substrate (Somogyi):
   a. To 1.50 gm. of treated cornstarch* add approximately 10 ml. of phosphate buffer (0.10 M, pH 7.0. Dissolve 4.55 gm. KH_2PO_4, 9.35 gm. Na_2HPO_4, and 2.5 gm. NaCl in distilled water and dilute to 1 liter. Mix.)
   b. The starch paste prepared in "a" is added slowly to a beaker containing approximately 70 ml. of phosphate buffer which has been brought up to its boiling temperature on a hotplate-stirrer (i.e., S/P S9302-5 Therm-O-Swirl) with continuous stirring.
   c. Use a few ml. of cold buffer solution to wash down the remaining starch from the beaker into hot substrate.
   d. Boil substrate gently with stirring for 2 to 3 minutes.
   e. Transfer substrate into a 100-ml. volumetric flask. Cool the contents to room temperature. Fill to mark with cold boiled buffer.
   f. Put a magnetic stirring bar into the flask. Stir the substrate for a few minutes before use.
   g. Stopper and store in refrigerator at 2 to 4° C., taking care not to contaminate unnecessarily.
   h. Under normal conditions, the substrate is good for at least 2 weeks.
2. 3 N H_2SO_4.

CALCULATIONS

$$\text{Amylase activity of unknown (Somogyi units/dl.)} = (I - 0.3125\ C) \times F$$

where I = reducing power after incubation (as mg./dl.)
C = glucose concentration before incubation (as mg./dl.)
F = factor (see below)

$$F = \frac{F_1 + F_2}{2}$$

*Wu, W. T., and Beeler, M. F.: Amer. J. Clin. Path. 57:497, 1972.

*Treatment of cornstarch (Somogyi, 1960).
1. Heat approximately 1800 ml. of 0.25 per cent NaOH in a 2-liter beaker to 50 to 55° C.
2. Discontinue heating.
3. With stirring, add approximately 200 gm. cornstarch (Argo). Stir for 1 to 2 hours on a magnetic stirrer.
4. Let settle overnight.
5. Decant.
6. Suspend starch in distilled water, agitate for 1 hour.
7. Settle overnight.
8. Decant, wash with distilled water until the washings are no longer alkaline.
9. Let dry at room temperature.
10. Transfer to suitable container.

$$\text{where } F_1 = \frac{\text{labeled amylase activity of Moni-trol I}}{I_I - 0.3125^* C_I}$$

$$F_2 = \frac{\text{labeled amylase activity of Moni-trol II}}{I_{II} - 0.3125^* C_{II}}$$

Sample calculation:

	REDUCING POWER (AS GLUCOSE mg./dl.)		
	Before Incubation	After Incubation†	LABELED AMYLASE
Moni-trol I	102	60	95
Moni-trol II	250	138	200
Unknown	104	52	?

$$F_1 = \frac{95}{60 - (102 \times 0.3125^*)} = \frac{95}{28.1} = 3.38$$

$$F_2 = \frac{200}{138 - (250 \times 0.3125^*)} = \frac{200}{59.9} = 3.34$$

therefore,

$$f = \frac{3.34 + 3.38}{2} = 3.36$$

Amylase activity of unknown

$$= [52 - (104 \times 0.3125)] \times F$$
$$= (52 - 32.5) \times 3.36$$
$$= 29.5 \times 3.36$$
$$= 66$$

DISCUSSION. Starch substrate may be pipetted into a number of tubes before starting the analysis. No warming of the substrate is necessary.

It is good practice to add unknowns to substrate tubes at a fixed time interval. For instance, add unknowns No. 1 and No. 2 into respective substrate tubes within the first minute, No. 3 and No. 4 the second minute. As soon as Nos. 1 and 2 tubes are placed in water bath, a clock with a second hand is started. After 30 minutes, Nos. 1 and 2 tubes are removed from the water bath, and 0.1 ml. of 3 N H_2SO_4 is quickly added to them. Tubes Nos. 3 and 4 are treated similarly during the second minute, and so on. An 0.2-ml. pipette or a microburette is recommended for addition of sulfuric acid.

F values should fall between 3 and 4, and should remain fairly constant from day to day. Any sudden change in F value is indicative of contamination of the starch substrate. If the substrate is kept stoppered and in the refrigerator, we have found it to be unchanged even after 5 months.

*A dilution factor: $\frac{0.5 \text{ ml.}}{1 \text{ ml.} + 0.5 \text{ ml.} + 0.1 \text{ ml.}}$

†This figure, in most cases, is lower than that listed under "before incubation." The lower value is due to dilutions by substrate and sulfuric acid.

It is essential to use more than the normal number of glucose standards for construction of the calibration curve. Recommended glucose standard solutions: 20, 40, 80, 100, 125, 150, 200, 250, and 300 mg./dl.

The upper limit of linearity for this method has been found to be 450 Somogyi units per dl. Serum containing more than 450 units per dl. should be rerun after diluting with the buffer solution used to make substrate.

Under carefully controlled conditions (two analysts, one instrument, different days, different substrates, different Moni-trol lots, different reagent lots), the coefficient of variation for this method has been found to be better than 4 per cent.

Enza-trol or other commercially available enzyme controls may be used instead of Moni-trol I and II.

Normal values: Sera from 106 male and 101 female blood bank donors have been analyzed to establish normal values. The mean for males is 99 units/dl. (S.D. 34) and for females it is 79 units/dl. (S.D. 30). The medians are 100 and 77 for males and females, respectively.

Table 15–1 converts glucose concentration prior to incubation as read from AA chart according to the expression in the calculation formula "0.3125 C." Proposed NORMAL VALUES are:

Males —40–180 Somogyi units/dl.
Females—30–160 Somogyi units/dl.

The method is satisfactory for urine and other fluid amylase assays. In these cases, however, a blank is incubated with buffer alone, along with the unknown, then analyzed for reducing substances, along with the unknown. Calculations are then (U-B) × F = Somogyi units/dl., where U = the unknown, B = blank. It may be desirable to set up two assays; one on the original fluid, one on urine diluted 1 to 10, or more (depending on expected activity).

Lipase Determination (Serum, Urine) (Vogel and Zieve, 1963)

PRINCIPLE. Lipase activity of serum is determined by the decrease in absorbance of purified, buffered (pH 9.1) olive oil emulsion when incubated at room temperature (23° C.) for 20 minutes with diluted serum. Absorbance is measured at 650 mμ. Units are equivalent to change in absorbance (O.D.) × 1000.

PROCEDURE

1. To 0.8 ml. of buffer diluent add 0.2 ml. of serum and mix well.
2. Start timing clock. Add 0.2 ml. of diluted serum to 4 ml. of substrate. Mix five times by inversion. Transfer mixture immediately to a 1-cm. 3-ml. Beckman cuvette.

Table 15–1. VALUES OF "0.3125 C" CORRESPONDING TO GLUCOSE CONCENTRATION OF UNKNOWN PRIOR TO INCUBATION, AS READ FROM CHART RECORDING

mg. glucose/dl. as read from AA chart prior to incubation	0	1	2	3	4	5	6	7	8	9
20	6.3	6.6	6.9	7.2	7.5	7.8	8.1	8.4	8.8	9.1
30	9.4	9.7	10.0	10.3	10.6	10.9	11.3	11.6	11.9	12.2
40	12.5	12.8	13.1	13.4	13.8	14.1	14.4	14.7	15.0	15.3
50	15.6	15.9	16.3	16.6	16.9	17.2	17.5	17.8	18.1	18.4
60	18.8	19.1	19.4	19.7	20.0	20.3	20.6	20.9	21.3	21.6
70	21.9	22.2	22.5	22.8	23.1	23.4	23.8	24.1	24.4	24.7
80	25.0	25.3	25.6	25.9	26.3	26.6	26.9	27.2	27.5	27.8
90	28.1	28.4	28.8	29.1	29.4	29.7	30.0	30.3	30.6	30.9
100	31.3	31.6	31.9	32.2	32.5	32.8	33.1	33.4	33.8	34.1
110	34.4	34.7	35.0	35.3	35.6	35.9	36.3	36.6	36.9	37.2
120	37.5	37.8	38.1	38.4	38.8	39.1	39.4	39.7	40.0	40.3
130	40.6	40.9	41.3	41.6	41.9	42.2	42.5	42.8	43.1	43.4
140	43.8	44.1	44.4	44.7	45.0	45.3	45.6	45.9	46.3	46.6
150	46.9	47.2	47.5	47.8	48.1	48.4	48.8	49.1	49.4	49.7
160	50.0	50.3	50.6	50.9	51.3	51.6	51.9	52.2	52.5	52.8
170	53.1	53.4	53.8	54.1	54.4	54.7	55.0	55.3	55.6	55.9
180	56.3	56.6	56.9	57.2	57.5	57.8	58.1	58.4	58.8	59.1
190	59.4	59.7	60.0	60.3	60.6	60.9	61.3	61.6	61.9	62.2
200	62.5	62.8	63.1	63.4	63.8	64.1	64.4	64.7	65.0	65.3
210	65.6	65.9	66.3	66.6	66.9	67.2	67.5	67.8	68.1	68.4
220	68.8	69.1	69.4	69.7	70.0	70.3	70.6	70.9	71.3	71.6
230	71.9	72.2	72.5	72.8	73.1	73.4	73.8	74.1	74.4	74.7
240	75.0	75.3	75.6	75.9	76.3	76.6	76.9	77.2	77.5	77.8
250	78.1	78.4	78.8	79.1	79.4	79.7	80.0	80.3	80.6	80.9
260	81.3	81.6	81.9	82.2	82.5	82.8	83.1	83.4	83.8	84.1
270	84.4	84.7	85.0	85.3	85.6	85.9	86.3	86.6	86.9	87.2
280	87.5	87.8	88.1	88.4	88.8	89.1	89.4	89.7	90.0	90.3
290	90.6	90.9	91.3	91.6	91.9	92.2	92.5	92.8	93.1	93.4

To use: Find glucose concentration (as read from glucose chart recording) along ordinate and abscissa, follow across and down to read the value of the expression, in the calculation formula "0.3125 C."

3. Let stand at room temperature (23° C.) for 20 minutes and again determine absorbance.

Reagents

1. Tris buffer (0.05 M, pH 9.1). Dissolve 6.057 gm. tris-(hydroxymethyl)-aminomethane in about 980 ml. of water and adjust to pH 9.1 with 1 N HCl. Bring to a volume of 1 liter.

2. Buffer diluent. Dissolve 3.5 gm. sodium deoxycholate in above buffer and make up 1 liter with distilled water. Readjust to pH 9.1 if necessary.

3. Purified olive oil. Pass U.S.P. olive oil through alumina to remove free fatty acids. Collect nearly colorless effluent after a few hours. (Add reagent aluminum oxide to a 2 × 32 cm. chromatographic tube fitted with a coarse, brieted disk. Pour in double this amount of olive oil. Let filter.)

4. Stock olive oil solution (10 per cent v./v.). Dissolve 10 gm. of treated olive oil in reagent grade acetone to volume of 100 ml.

5. Olive oil solution (1 per cent, v./v.). Dilute 10 ml. of stock solution to 100 ml. with acetone.

6. Triglyceride substrate (0.05 per cent, v./v.) (available commercially). Set metal top of homogenizer, containing 100 ml. of buffer diluent, in vigorously boiling steam bath. When temperature reaches 92° C., remove from bath

and place on base connected to Powerstat variable voltage transformer set at 35 volts. Add 4 ml. of the 1 per cent olive oil solution at once, drop by drop over a 2-minute interval. Then run homogenizer uncovered at 110 volts for 10 minutes. Transfer to a reagent bottle. Our reagent has had an absorbance of about 0.650 at 650 nm. when measured against the buffer diluent. It has a pearly opalescence. At room temperature there is a tendency for a rim of olive oil to form on the bottle. The reagent should be shaken vigorously prior to use. It appears to be stable over a period of four to five days at room temperature. If absorbance is less than 0.600, it may be increased by reheating and remixing in the blender.

CALCULATIONS. Absorbance at time 0 minus absorbance at 20 minutes × 1000 = units of lipase activity.

DISCUSSION. Values up to 10 units are normal, values above 15 units are definitely abnormal, values from 11 to 15 units are doubtful. This method has the great advantage of speed and simplicity. The high pH is said to be optimum for lipase activity in the pancreatitis sera studied. It is above the optimum for lipase activity of normal serum. The reaction is nonlinear and, therefore, the technique should be adhered to rigidly. Unfortunately this procedure may give spuriously elevated results in the presence of jaundice. In 1966 Zieve and Doizaki published a procedure for eliminating effects of bilirubin on this lipase procedure. Although what some authorities consider the limited usefulness of the serum lipase measurement seems hardly to justify the extra trouble involved, others place great emphasis on lipase assays. Hence, for the purpose, clean commercial DEAE-cellulose with 0.5 sodium hydroxide, wash with distilled water, methanol, and chloroform (the last two alternately four times), and then air dry. Suspend 3 gm. in 75 ml. ice-cold 0.1 molar Tris buffer (pH 8.8). Pipette 4 ml. aliquots into centrifuge tube and spin in the cold at 3000 r.p.m. for 10 minutes. Discard supernatant and wash residue three times with cold buffer, spinning each time. Loosen final compacted residue with a stirring rod. Add 0.5 ml. serum and 1 ml. cold buffer, spinning each time. Combine washings with original supernatant and bring final volume to 5 ml. Final dilution is 1:10. Use 0.4 ml. of final dilution for assay.

Sweat Electrolytes by Pilocarpine Iontophoresis (Gibson and Cooke, 1959)

PRINCIPLE. Pilocarpine iontophoresed into the skin stimulates locally increased sweat gland secretion. The resulting sweat is absorbed by filter paper, diluted with distilled water, and analyzed for sodium and chloride content.

PROCEDURE

1. Transfer a salt-free filter paper disc, 2.5 cm. in diameter, to a weighing bottle, using dry, clean forceps, and weigh on an analytical balance to the nearest 0.1 gm. (S and S No. 589 Green Ribbon is satisfactory.)
2. Tape a 2 × 2 inch gauze square to each of the two electrodes of the iontophoresis unit. The metal must not be able to come in contact with the patient's skin, or pain and a burn may result.
3. Saturate the gauze covering the positive electrode with pilocarpine solution and apply to the patient's forearm, halfway between wrist and elbow.
4. Saturate the gauze covering the negative electrode with bicarbonate solution and apply to the extensor surface of the forearm directly opposite the other electrode.
5. Press electrode firmly, wiping the skin around the electrode thoroughly.
6. Place rubber strap around forearm to hold electrodes in place.
7. Turn iontophoretic unit on. (We have been satisfied with the Alloyd Iontophoresor. Other instruments are available.)
8. Adjust rheostat to 2.5 milliamps.
9. Allow to run for 10 to 12 minutes unless the patient complains of discomfort or pain, in which case double check to be sure that the gauze completely covers the electrodes and that the electrodes are in firm contact with the skin. Burns can be caused by incomplete saturation of the gauze with the solutions or by inadequate electrode contact caused by loose application as well as by direct contact of metal of electrode with skin.
10. Remove electrodes and thoroughly wash with distilled water, drying with 4 × 4 inch gauze squares previously determined to have a low NaCl content.
11. Using dry, clean forceps, remove filter paper discs from weighing jar and place over reddened area of patient's forearm where positive electrode had been.
12. Cover filter paper with Parafilm.
13. Tape each edge of Parafilm with waterproof adhesive tape, making sure that the seal is airtight.
14. Leave in place for 1 hour.
15. Remove tape and Parafilm carefully, transfer filter paper with dry, clean forceps to weighing jar without delay to avoid evaporation, and send to laboratory.
16. Reweigh jar to nearest 0.1 gm. Satisfactory collection requires at least a 100 mg. increase in weight. Further procedure will depend on chloride and sodium method.
17. Add distilled water equivalent to 1:40 dilution and let stand with intermittent swirling for at least 5 minutes.

18. Determine chloride on 1-ml. aliquot. Depending on result, add appropriate amount of lithium nitrate solution to remainder of sample and determine sodium content by flame photometry.

CALCULATIONS. Calculate milliequivalents of chloride per liter of sweat. Using the Schales method, titrate 1 ml. aliquot of diluted sweat and 1 ml. aliquot of standard (10 mEq. of chloride per liter) correcting for chloride dilution:

Chloride (mEq. per liter of sweat) =

$$400 \times \frac{\text{ml. of unknown titration}}{\text{ml. of standard titration}}$$

REAGENTS

1. Pilocarpine solution (1.5 per cent, w./v.). Dissolve one-quarter grain (0.016 gm.) pilocarpine hydrochloride tablet in 3.2 ml. of distilled water. Prepare fresh for each test. Add bicarbonate solution.

Secretin Test (Dreiling and Hollander, 1948)

PRINCIPLE. A double lumen tube, providing for separate aspiration of gastric and duodenal contents, is passed into the duodenum, using fluoroscopic guidance and maintaining constant aspiration of gastric contents. Duodenal contents are aspirated until clear. The patient is then given secretin (one unit per kg.) intravenously, and the pancreatic secretion entering the duodenum is collected for 80 minutes. The aspirate is examined for volume, bicarbonate content, and amylase activity.

PROCEDURE

1. After a 12-hour fast, pass a radiopaque double lumen tube, under fluoroscopic guidance, through the mouth to beyond the ampulla of Vater.

2. Maintain constant suction on both gastric and duodenal outlets with a negative pressure of 25 to 40 mm. of mercury. Gastric content must be completely and continuously removed to prevent contamination of duodenal aspirate.

3. When duodenal aspirate is clear and alkaline (determined by pHydrion paper), collect aspirate for a controlled period of 20 minutes.

4. Perform intradermal skin test with secretin for sensitivity. (Do not use in patients with atopic asthma.)

5. If no hypersensitivity is present, inject 1.0 clinical units of secretin per kg. of body weight intravenously.

6. Collect duodenal aspirate for 80 minutes, fractionally, at 20-minute intervals.

7. Clear tube between fractions by injecting air.

8. Place containers with duodenal aspirate in ice.

9. Transport to laboratory for analysis for volume, bicarbonate content, amylase activity, and pH. (Drop of pH below 7 indicates contamination by gastric juice and invalidates other results.) Microscopic examination may be performed to note presence or absence of cholesterol crystals, calcium bilirubinate pigment, and parasites. Cytologic study may also be performed.

10. Draw blood samples at 1, 4, and 24 hours following the injection of secretin for determination of serum amylase.

A number of technical problems may complicate the procedure. Incomplete gastric drainage may lead to inactivation of enzymes by contamination with gastric content. This may also alter bicarbonate content. Secretion can be lost by regurgitation into stomach (signaled by sudden increase in volume, pH, and appearance of bile in gastric aspirate) or by passage into jejunum, especially in uncooperative patients.

According to Dreiling and Hollander (1950), the lower limit of normal for volume is 2 ml. per kg. of body weight; the lower limit of normal for maximum bicarbonate is 90 mEq. per liter; and the lower limit of normal for total amylase is 6 units per kg. of body weight.

Stool Proteolytic Activity (Johnstone, 1952)

PRINCIPLE. Normal adults usually contain the equivalent of 20 or more μg. of trypsin and 74 or more μg. of chymotrypsin per gm. of feces. Patients with exocrine insufficiency of the pancreas generally have values far below these. The correlation with chymotrypsin activity is better than that with trypsin. Because of the specificity, the test is useful for differential diagnosis of malassimilation disorders.

PROCEDURE

1. Collect a random stool specimen and perform test within a few hours of collection. If this is impossible, freeze the stool for storage.

2. Make a 1:6 (v./v.) dilution of stool by mixing well 1 ml. of stool with 5 ml. of buffer in a 16 × 125 mm. test tube.

3. Label twelve 13 × 100 mm. test tubes with numbers 1 through 12.

4. Place 1 ml. of buffer solution in each of tubes 2 through 12, leaving tube 1 empty.

5. Place 1 ml. (each) of the 1:6 dilution of stool in tubes 1 and 2.

6. Mix tube 2 (1:12 dilution) and transfer 1 ml. of mixture to tube 3 (1:24 dilution).

7. Repeat step 6, transferring 1 ml. from 3 to 4, 4 to 5, etc., to produce dilutions of 1:48, 1:96, 1:192, etc.

8. Add strip of x-ray film to each tube and

to one extra tube (13) with 1 ml. buffer alone, as a control.

9. Incubate for 1 hour at 37° C.

10. Remove strips and wash for about 5 seconds in running tap water (without rubbing the surface).

Complete digestion is indicated by the complete clarity of the portion of the film submerged in the solutions. Stools of most normal children will show complete digestion at dilutions of 1:96 or higher. In cystic fibrosis of the pancreas, the test is usually negative or positive only in lower dilutions. It is very rarely positive in dilutions as high as 1:96, even when gelatinase-producing bacteria are present. The test is invalid in children over four years of age.

REAGENTS

1. Barbital buffer. Dissolve 20.6 gm. of sodium barbital (sodium diethylbarbiturate) in 1 liter of distilled water. Bring the solution to pH 8, using 0.1 N HCl (requires approximately three parts of 0.1 N HCl for each seven parts of barbital solution).

2. Undeveloped x-ray film of a type found to give expected results with positive and negative controls. Cut in strips about 5 mm. wide and slightly longer than test tubes (over 100 mm.). (Dupont Cronex II is satisfactory.)

REFERENCES

Abderhalden, R.: *Clinical Enzymology.* Princeton, New Jersey, D. Van Nostrand Co., Inc., 1961.

Barrows, D., Berk, J. E., and Fridhandler, L.: Macroamylasemia: Survey of prevalence in a mixed population. New Eng. J. Med. *286*:1352, 1972.

Beeler, M. F.: Amylase and lipase. Check Sample Program, Council on Clinical Chemistry, Commission on Continuing Education, American Society of Clinical Pathologists, 1970.

Berk, J. E., Kizu, H., Take, S., and Fridhandler, L.: Macroamylasemia: Clinical and laboratory features. Amer. J. Gastroent. *53*:211, 1970a.

Berk, J. E., Kizu, H., Take, S., and Fridhandler, L.: Macroamylasemia: Serum and urine amylase characteristics. Amer. J. Gastroent. *53*:223, 1970b.

Berk, J. E., Kizu, H., Wilding, P., and Searcy, R. L.: Macroamylasemia: A newly recognized cause for elevated serum amylase activity. New Eng. J. Med. *277*:941, 1967.

Berndt, W., Kolhoff, H., and Standt, U. Characterization and separation by isoelectric focusing of pancreatic alpha-amylases of various species into isoenzymes. Science Tools, The LKB Instrument Journal *17*:45, 1970.

Bockus, H. L., Lopusniak, M. S., and Tachidjean, V.: *In* Bockus, H. L.: Gastroenterology. 2nd ed. Volume III, Chapter 123, pp. 892–931. Philadelphia, W. B. Saunders Company, 1965.

Calkins, W. G.: The starch tolerance test in pancreatic disease. Arch. Intern. Med. *118*:103, 1966.

Caraway, W. T.: A stable starch substrate for the determination of amylase in serum and other body fluids. Amer. J. Clin. Path. *32*:97, 1959.

Casey, A. E., Gilbert, F. E., Gravlee, J. F., and Downey, E. L.: Disease and chemical syndromes associated with serum levels of glucosyl transferases. Alabama J. Med. Sci. *8*:322, 1971.

Cherry, I. S., and Crandall, L. A., Jr.: The specificity of pancreatic lipase: Its appearance in the blood after pancreatic injury. Amer. J. Physiol. *100*:266, 1932.

Davis, J., Berk, J. E., Take, S., and Fridhandler, L.: Electrophoretic characteristics of macroamylasemic serum. Clin. Chim. Acta *35*:305, 1971.

Dreiling, D. A.: Studies in pancreatic function. V. The use of the secretin test in the diagnosis of pancreatitis and in the demonstration of pancreatic insufficiencies in gastrointestinal disorders. Gastroenterology *24*:540, 1953.

Dreiling, D. A., and Hollander, F.: Studies in pancreatic function. I. Preliminary series of clinical studies with the secretin test. Gastroenterology *11*:714, 1948.

Dreiling, D. A., and Hollander, F.: Studies in pancreatic function. II. A statistical study of pancreatic secretion following secretin in patients without pancreatic disease. Gastroenterology *15*:620, 1950.

Fridhandler, L., Berk, J. E., and Ueda, M.: Macroamylasemia: Rapid detection method. Clin. Chem. *17*:423, 1971.

Gambill, E. E., and Mason, H. L.: One-hour value for urine amylase in 96 patients with pancreatitis. J.A.M.A. *186*:24, 1963.

Gibson, L. E., and Cooke, R. E.: A test for concentration of electrolytes in sweat in cystic fibrosis of the pancreas utilizing pilocarpine by iontophoresis. Pediatrics *23*:545, 1959.

Gilchrist, T.: Personal communication, 1967.

Gomori, G.: Assay of serum amylase with small amounts of serum. Amer. J. Clin. Path. *27*:714, 1957.

Hansen, H. R., Van Kley, H., and Knight, W. A., Jr.: Macroamylasemia due to binding by protein. Amer. J. Med. *52*:712, 1972.

Henry, R. J., and Chiamori, N.: Study of the saccharogenic method for the determination of serum and urine amylase. Clin. Chem. *6*:434, 1960.

Henry, R. J., Sobel, C., and Berkman, S.: On the determination of "pancreatitis lipase" in serum. Clin. Chem. *3*:77, 1957.

Howat, H. T.: The exocrine pancreas. *In* Clinics in Gastroenterology. Philadelphia, W. B. Saunders Company, 1972.

Johnstone, D. E.: Studies on cystic fibrosis of the pancreas. Amer. J. Dis. Child. *84*:191, 1952.

Klein, B., Foreman, J. A., and Searcy, R. L.: New chromogenic substrate for determination of serum amylase activity. Clin. Chem. *16*:32, 1970.

Koch, P., and Tonks, D. B.: A comparison of various methods for assaying amylase activity. Presented at the Joint Meeting of the American Association of Clinical Chemists and the Canadian Society of Clinical Chemists, Seattle, Washington, 1971.

Levine, R. A.: Personal communication, 1972.

Levitt, M. D., and Cooperband, S. R.: Hyperamylasemia from the binding of serum amylase by an 11S IgA globulin. New Eng. J. Med., *278*(9):474, 1968.

Levitt, M. D., Duane, W., and Cooperband, S. R.: Study of macroamylase complexes. J. Lab. Clin. Med. *80*:414, 1972.

Levitt, M. D., Rapoport, M., and Cooperband, S. R.: The renal clearance of amylase in renal insufficiency, acute pancreatitis and macroamylasemia. Ann. Intern. Med. *71*:919, 1969.

Peralta, O., and Reinhold, J. G.: Rapid estimation of amylase activity of serum by turbidimetry. Clin. Chem. *1*:157, 1955.

Reif, A. E., and Nabseth, D. C.: Serum amylase determination by Somogyi's amyloclastic method with use of a photometric end point. Clin. Chem. *8*:113, 1962.

Rice, E. W.: Improved spectrophotometric determination of amylase with a new stable starch substrate solution. Clin. Chem. *5*:592, 1959.

Smith, B. W., and Roe, J. H.: A photometric method for the determination of α-amylase in blood and urine, with use of the starch-iodine color. J. Biol. Chem. *179*:53, 1949.

Somogyi, M.: Micromethods for the estimation of diastase. J. Biol. Chem. *125*:399, 1938.

Somogyi, M.: Modification of two methods for the assay of amylase. Clin. Chem. *6*:23, 1960.

Stein, E. A., and Fischer, E. H.: Bacillus subtilis α-amylase, a zinc-protein complex. Biochim. Biophys. Acta *39*:287, 1960.

Take, S., Fridhandler, L., and Berk, J. E.: Macroamylasemia: Possible role of polysaccharide in composition of macroamylase. Clin. Chim. Acta 27:369, 1970.

Tietz, N. W., and Fiereck, E. A.: A specific method for serum lipase determination. Clin. Chim. Acta *13*:352, 1966.

Ueda, M., Berk, J. E., Fridhandler, L., and Davis, J.: Ultracentrifugal characteristics of macroamylasemic serum. Clin. Chim. Acta 35:299, 1971.

Van Loon, E. J., Likins, M. R., and Seger, A. J.: Photometric method for blood amylase by use of a starch-iodine color. Amer. J. Clin. Path. 22:1134, 1952.

Vogel, W. C., and Zieve, L.: A rapid and sensitive turbidimetric method for serum lipase based upon differences between the lipases of normal and pancreatitis serum. Clin. Chem. *9*:168, 1963.

Wilding, P., Cooke, W. T., and Nicholson, G. I.: Globulin-bound amylase. A cause of persistently elevated levels in serum. Ann. Intern. Med. *60*:1053, 1964.

Wu, W. T., and Beeler, M. F.: A simplified semi-automatic saccharogenic method for serum amylase assay. Amer. J. Clin. Path. 57:497, 1972.

Zieve, L., and Doizaki, W. M.: Influence of jaundice on turbidimetric measurement of serum lipolytic activity. J. Lab. Clin. Med. 67:127, 1966.

Zieve, L., and Vogel, W. C.: Measurement of lecithinase A in serum and other body fluids. J. Lab. Clin. Med. 57:586, 1961.

Chapter 16

EXAMINATION OF GASTRIC AND DUODENAL CONTENTS

by DONALD C. CANNON, M.D., Ph.D.

EXAMINATION OF GASTRIC CONTENTS

Although it is true that analysis of gastric secretion has not fulfilled some of the previous claims and expectations, this procedure maintains an important role in clinical diagnosis and in the evaluation of therapy. As with most other laboratory examinations, information derived from gastric analysis is by itself seldom of pathognomonic significance but rather must be interpreted in light of the patient's history and with the results of other pertinent clinical, roentgenologic, and laboratory examinations. For example, anacidity does not invariably indicate pernicious anemia, although it is true that adult patients with pernicious anemia invariably have anacidity. Studies of peripheral blood and bone marrow, a thorough neurological examination, and perhaps an investigation of intrinsic factor activity may be necessary to substantiate or eliminate the diagnosis of pernicious anemia. Furthermore, in interpreting the results of gastric analysis, it must be kept in mind that there exists no sharply delineated normal range such as one is accustomed to use as a reference point for many laboratory measurements in chemistry, hematology, or serology. It is indeed only at the extremes of gastric secretion—anacidity or the marked hypersecretion such as is seen in the Zollinger-Ellison syndrome or in some cases of duodenal ulcer—that one can say with certainty that an underlying disease exists.

Considering both its limitations and its value, it is probable that properly performed gastric analyses are done too infrequently at the present time. Among the factors that have contributed to this situation is the fact that many of the previously held beliefs regarding gastric secretion have been disproved by newer tests and better controlled surveys, thus adding a note of bewilderment and pessimism in the mind of the physician confronted with a patient having gastrointestinal complaints. For example, studies using the augmented histamine test have disproved the notion engendered by the older and now obsolete tests—standard histamine, alcohol stimulation, or various test meals—that anacidity is frequently a variant of normal. Anacidity, furthermore, is no longer considered to be a reliable screening test for gastric carcinoma, since most afflicted individuals do not have gastric anacidity; when it occurs it is usually only in the more advanced cases. Gastroscopy, roentgenography, and gastric cytology are far more useful in establishing the diagnosis of probable gastric carcinoma than is gastric analysis. Even in the diagnosis of duodenal ulcer, the hypersecretory state that was once considered typical for the disease does not occur in most affected patients. An element of confusion has perhaps been added by the fact that the physicochemical basis for the older concept of "free," "combined," and "total" acid has now been shown to be untenable.

The properly performed gastric analysis requires a relatively large investment of time by the physician who must perform the intubation and supervise the collection of samples. Although in itself a benign procedure, intubation is apt to be an unpleasant experience for the patient, not a few of whom submit to the procedure with reluctance. In view of these facts and the inherent limitations of the information to be gained, it is essential that there be a definite indication for performing routine gastric analysis. In general there are four clear-cut indications:

1. To determine whether or not the patient

can secrete any gastric acid. The finding of anacidity is of major importance in three situations: the patient with macrocytic anemia, neurologic disorders, or other signs and symptoms of pernicious anemia; the patient suspected of having pernicious anemia who has been treated with vitamin B_{12} before the diagnosis was unequivocally established; and the exclusion of simple peptic ulceration in a patient with a suspicious ulcerating lesion of the stomach.

2. To measure the amount of acid produced by a patient with symptoms of peptic ulcer, particularly a patient with suspected duodenal or postoperative stomal ulcer who has no roentgenographically demonstrable lesion.

3. To reveal the hypersecretory state characteristic of the Zollinger-Ellison syndrome.

4. To determine the completeness of vagotomy by the insulin test.

In addition, gastric analysis is considered by some to be helpful for judging the efficacy of surgical, medical, or roentgen therapy for peptic ulcer and for determining the proper type of surgical procedure to be performed in the patient with peptic ulcer.

Physiology of Gastric Secretion

Gastric secretion has three major physiological functions—the initiation of protein digestion, the physical and chemical preparation of ingested food resulting in an optimal mixture for subsequent digestion in the small intestine, and the secretion of intrinsic factor which promotes vitamin B_{12} absorption in the ileum. The first of these functions is not absolutely essential to the welfare of the human body as shown by the fact that individuals with anacidity of long duration and therefore with failure of gastric protein digestion can exist free of gastrointestinal complaints and in good nutritional status.

Gastric secretion is classically considered to occur in three phases, although present information clearly demonstrates an interrelationship among these various phases. The cephalic or neurogenic phase consists of stimuli that are transmitted by the vagus nerves. This phase consists of anticipatory stimuli which arise from visual or olfactory perceptions associated with the ingestion of food and psychogenic stimuli which are derived from mental processes not related to the ingestion of food. Vagal impulses directly stimulate the parietal cells to secrete acid but also stimulate the antral mucosa to secrete gastrin into the blood. The polypeptide hormone, gastrin, is the most powerful known stimulus to gastric secretion, being several hundred times as potent in this respect as histamine. Its elaboration and secretion is the paramount feature of the second or gastric phase of secretion. In addition to vagal stimulation gastrin is released by distention of the antrum with food or fluid and by contact of protein and protein breakdown products, the so-called secretagogues, with the antral mucosa. Secretagogues probably also act to stimulate the parietal and chief cells directly. The gastric phase is thus diminished but not abolished by vagotomy. The intestinal phase is quantitatively the least important phase of gastric secretion and is presumably mediated by humoral substances secreted into the blood by the duodenum in response to the entry of digestive products. It is probable that gastrin, formed by the duodenum, is the major humoral agent in this phase. Gastrin or a very similar substance has also been isolated from nonbeta-cell adenomas of the pancreas associated with the hypersecretory state of the Zollinger-Ellison syndrome.

Various mechanisms serve to inhibit gastric secretion. Particularly important is the inhibition of gastrin secretion which occurs when the acidity of antral contents falls below a pH of about 1.5. An additional effect of high acidity of antral contents has been postulated to be the secretion of an inhibitory hormone by the antrum. A variety of inhibitory and neural reflex mechanisms have also been postulated to originate in the duodenum. It appears well established that an inhibitory hormone, enterogastrone, is liberated into the blood following contact of fatty acid breakdown products with the duodenal mucosa. Psychic mechanisms are not without participation in the inhibition of gastric secretion as shown by the diminished secretion reported in patients suffering from chronic depression.

Composition of Gastric Secretion

Gastric secretion is a complex solution the synthesis of which is not completely understood. Although the cells which secrete hydrochloric acid, pepsin, and mucus have been clearly identified, the varying concentration of inorganic ions in particular remains the object of speculation. The most widely popularized theory is the two component hypothesis of Hollander (1952), which states that gastric secretion is composed of a parietal or acid component of fixed composition and a nonparietal or alkaline component consisting of a mixture of several secretions in varying proportions (Table 16–1). According to this theory, the variations in electrolyte concentrations are a reflection of the degree of dilution and neutralization of the parietal component by the alkaline component. Although it has served as

Table 16–1. THE CONCENTRATION OF ELECTROLYTES IN GASTRIC SECRETION (mEq. per liter)*

ION	COMPONENT	
	Parietal	Nonparietal
Hydrogen	160	–
Sodium	–	160
Potassium	10	10
Calcium	–	4
Chloride	170	125
Bicarbonate	–	45
Phosphate	–	6

*From the data of Hunt (1959) as interpreted by Sparberg, M., and Kirsner, J. B.

a useful concept, the two component hypothesis fails to explain some of the more important facts regarding the composition of gastric secretion. The following are components of gastric secretion:

Hydrochloric Acid. It is a remarkable biochemical feat that the stomach can secrete hydrogen ions at a concentration of more than one million times the plasma concentration – a concentration of about 160 mEq. per liter prior to dilution with the other secretory components. Hydrochloric acid is secreted by the parietal cells which are located in the isthmus and neck of the gastric glands of the fundus and body of the stomach but not those at either anatomical extreme – the narrow rim of cardia or the pylorus and antrum. The major importance of hydrochloric acid to digestion is to provide the high acidity necessary for the activation of pepsin from pepsinogen but also to a limited extent to partially hydrolyze polypeptides and disaccharides directly. As a result of the ease of measurement and relatively good correlation with disease states, the determination of gastric acidity is the most commonly used clinical index of gastric secretory activity.

Digestive Enzymes. The major digestive enzyme of gastric secretion is pepsin, which is elaborated by the chief or peptic cells located at the base of the gastric glands of the body and fundus. Pepsin is secreted as the zymogen, pepsinogen, which is activated by gastric acid at an optimal pH of 1.6 to 2.4. Pepsin catalyzes the degradation of proteins to proteoses and peptones but does not liberate free amino acids, this being the function of the more potent proteases in the secretions of the pancreas and small intestine. A small amount of pepsinogen enters the blood, presumably by direct absorption from the peptic cells, and is secreted in the urine as uropepsinogen. It has recently been shown that gastric proteolytic activity is shared by several enzymes. At least one of these, gastricsin, has a higher pH optimum (approximately 3.2) than pepsin. Gastricsin apparently arises from the same zymogen precursor as pepsin, and its concentration in gastric secretion is about one-third that of pepsin. The significance of multiple gastric proteolytic enzymes is not yet known.

Other digestive enzymes include rennin and gastric lipase. Rennin has weak proteolytic activity and is best known for its ability to coagulate caseinogen in milk. Its high pH optimum (approximately 5 to 6) would seem to obviate any important contribution to gastric digestion. Gastric lipase, similarly, has a high pH optimum and appears to be of no importance to digestion.

Mucus. Gastric mucus is a chemically complex mixture of mucoproteins and mucopolysaccharides, the physiological significance of which is poorly understood. Attempts have been made to correlate alterations or deficiencies in gastric mucus with the occurrence of peptic ulcer, but such studies are inconclusive. Mucus is secreted by specialized cells of the gland necks in the fundus and body of the stomach, by cells of the surface epithelium, and by the acinar cells of the cardia, antrum, and pylorus. Mucus secretion is probably stimulated largely by mechanical and chemical stimuli and is inhibited by adrenal corticosteroids.

Electrolytes. Gastric secretion contains all the electrolytes found in other body fluids in a combined osmolar concentration equal to or slightly greater than plasma. The individual electrolytes vary widely in concentration, and with the exception of hydrogen ion, such variations have no known clinical significance. The concentration of electrolytes in the parietal and nonparietal components is shown in Table 16–1.

Nondigestive Enzymes. Using the technique of intragastric neutralization, various enzymes have been described in gastric secretion including lactic dehydrogenase, glutamic pyruvic transaminase, isocitric dehydrogenase, leucine amino peptidase, glutamic oxalacetic transaminase, beta-glucuronidase, alkaline phosphatase, and ribonuclease. These enzymes are doubtless the result of active gastric metabolism and have no function in digestion, particularly since all are inactivated by gastric acid except perhaps ribonuclease. Attempts have been made to correlate the levels of lactic dehydrogenase and beta-glucuronidase with gastric malignancy, but the results are equivocal (Piper *et al.*, 1963).

Serum Proteins. Small amounts of serum albumin and gamma globulin are normally present in gastric secretion. Their presence can usually be detected only in the anacid stomach or by use of intragastric neutralization. Albumin may be increased in the gastric secretion in cases of giant hypertrophic gastritis or Menetrier's disease, in carcinoma, and in benign peptic ulcer.

Miscellaneous Substances. The most important component in this group and probably in the gastric secretion as a whole is intrinsic factor, which is elaborated and secreted by the gastric mucosa. It is a mucoprotein with molecular weight of about 17,000. The manner in which intrinsic factor promotes vitamin B_{12} absorption in the ileum is uncertain but it has been convincingly shown to involve a complex between the two substances.

In approximately 80 per cent of individuals, those possessing the dominant secretor gene in homozygous or heterozygous state, the water-soluble blood group specific substances are present in the gastric secretion. This is of no particular significance to gastric secretion, since in these individuals the group specific substances are present in all body fluids.

Nomenclature of Gastric Secretion

At present the nomenclature relating to the measurement of gastric secretion is in a state of transition. As previously mentioned, the concept underlying the older terminology has recently been justifiably challenged on the grounds that it lacks physicochemical validity. Nevertheless, such terms as "free acid," "combined acid," "total acid," and "clinical units" continue in common but hopefully diminishing usage. For this reason the intended meaning of these terms will be reviewed.

It was previously believed that the hydrochloric acid in gastric secretion existed in two distinct phases, the relative amounts of which depended on the pH of the secretion. At high pH values, generally taken to be greater than 3.0 or 3.5, the acid supposedly existed almost exclusively as a mixture of organic salts formed from combination of the acid with proteins and peptones in the gastric secretion. This phase, the "combined acid," was a direct reflection of the buffering capacity of the gastric secretion. Only when the buffering capacity was exceeded could the hydrochloric acid supposedly exist as ions in solution or as "free acid." Acidity was measured in "clinical units" or "degrees of acidity" which were equal to the number of milliliters of 0.1 N NaOH required to titrate 100 ml. of gastric secretion to the endpoint of Topfer's reagent (pH 2.8 to 3.5) for "free acid" or to the endpoint of phenolphthalein (pH 8.2 to 10) for "total acid."

The older concept of gastric acidity was supported by titration curves obtained from the neutralization of gastric acid with sodium hydroxide. Such curves were similar to the titration curve of an aqueous solution of hydrochloric acid at pH values below about 2.8, but above this pH the curves resembled more closely those of a buffer mixture composed of a weak acid and its salt. As pointed out by Bock (1962), however, such studies failed to take into account the buffering effect of the various test meals then in use as gastric stimulants, an effect which could prove considerable. It has, in fact, now been shown that the titration curve of gastric secretion collected after histamine or Histalog stimulation rather closely resembles that of a solution of pure hydrochloric acid although a slight buffering effect is evident at high pH values, generally above pH 4.0 (Moore and Scarlata, 1965). It is clearly apparent from such studies that a significant amount of "free" hydrochloric acid is present in gastric secretion at pH values greater than 3.5.

It is therefore recommended that the older terms of "free," "combined," and "total" acid be avoided entirely. Gastric secretion can best be described in terms of three measurements to be performed on each sample of gastric secretion:

1. *Volume* in milliliters.
2. *Titratable acidity* expressed in milliequivalents per liter. This is determined by titration of a suitable aliquot of gastric secretion with 0.1 N NaOH to neutrality (pH of 7.0 or 7.4 as preferred by some). The endpoint should be measured electrometrically with a suitable pH meter. If a pH meter is not available the endpoint can be determined colorimetrically with phenol red (color change of yellow to red in the pH range of 6.8 to 8.4).
3. The *pH* measured electrometrically.

The *acid output* in milliequivalents for each sample can be calculated by multiplying its volume in milliliters by the titratable acidity and dividing by 1000. In addition to reporting the measured *volume, titratable acidity,* and *pH* and the calculated *acid output* for each individual sample, the *total volume* and *total acid output* will usually be reported for a given test by adding the individual sample values. Thus, for the study of basal secretion, a 1-hour collection is generally employed consisting of four individually segregated 15-minute samples. The *basal acid output* in milliequivalents per hour is reported as the sum of the acid outputs for the four samples.

The *maximal acid output* is the milliequivalents of acid secreted in the hour following injection of histamine in the augmented or maximal histamine test. This is not to be confused with the *maximal histamine response,* which was defined by Kay (1953) as the output of acid in milliequivalents in the period from

15 to 45 minutes after histamine injection. Since these terms are easily confused, the term *maximal histamine response* is best avoided.

The *peak acid output* is defined as the greatest acid output in any two successive 15-minute periods in the augmented histamine test (Baron, 1963).

Various terms have been employed to qualitatively describe the results of gastric secretion tests. Most of these terms originated in relation to the older concepts of gastric acid and therefore must be redefined or discarded. Some useful terms have been given different definitions by different investigators. Only with the anticipation of vociferous objection can any definition of these terms be attempted.

Anacidity was previously defined as the absence of "free" acid, usually taken to mean a failure of the gastric secretory pH to fall below 3.5. Most investigators now define *anacidity* as a failure of the pH to fall below either 6.0 or 7.0 in the augmented histamine or Histalog tests. It is the most reasonable compromise between clinical usefulness and strict physicochemical definition to define *anacidity* as a failure of the pH to fall below 6.0 following augmented or maximal histamine or Histalog stimulation. The reason for choosing 6.0 is that *anacidity* so defined will apply to virtually all adult patients with pernicious anemia. Some of these patients, however, will secrete gastric juice with pH values a fraction of pH unit below strict neutrality, pH 7.0, at some time during the maximal histamine test (Callender *et al.*, 1960).

Achlorhydria is used synonymously with anacidity by some investigators but is defined differently by others. Some define *achlorhydria* as a gastric secretion with pH persistently above 3.5 and with failure of the pH to fall more than one unit with maximal histamine stimulation (Callender *et al.*, 1960). *Hypochlorhydria,* on the other hand, has been used to refer to gastric juice with a pH persistently above 3.5 but falling more than one pH unit with maximal histamine stimulation. This fine distinction does not appear justified on clinical grounds. Furthermore, since pH 3.5 has been shown to have neither a unique physicochemical significance nor any particular clinical usefulness, the terms *achlorhydria* and *hypochlorhydria* should probably be avoided entirely.

Hyposecretion and hypersecretion are relative terms referring to the secretion of acid in amounts less than or greater than normal. Since the normal range for gastric secretion is not sharply delineated from that of pathological states, these two terms, though admittedly useful clinically upon occasion, do not admit to strict definitions.

Gastric Intubation

The general procedure of intubation should be carefully explained to the patient in order to obtain the fullest possible cooperation and to avoid undue apprehension. The best recovery of gastric secretion will be obtained with the patient in a sitting position. Towels or a large apron should be provided to protect clothing. The bedfast patient should lie on his left side with his head elevated approximately 45 degrees. For intubation, a Levin tube, usually number 14F or 16F, may be passed through the nose, or a Rehfuss or similar tube may be passed through the mouth. Whether to use oral or nasal intubation depends largely on the preference of the individual examiner. It is likely that less difficulty will be encountered with nasal intubation if the patient has a hyperactive gag reflex. It is essential for the tube to have a radiopaque tip so that it can be adjusted fluoroscopically.

Many recommend preliminary chilling of the tube with ice in the belief that nausea during intubation is diminished. For oral intubation the patient is instructed to open his mouth and project his chin slightly forward and upward. The tip of the tube is placed on the superior aspect of the posterior portion of the tongue and pushed gently to the posterior pharynx, avoiding the uvula as much as possible. After the patient has closed his mouth gently on the tube he should be encouraged to alternate swallowing and deep oral breathing, the tube being pushed intermittently to its destination as he swallows. It is common for gastric tubes to be calibrated with several measurements, one of which is likely to be 55 cm., which corresponds to the approximate distance from the mouth to the antrum. It is imperative, however, for the position of the tube to be adjusted fluoroscopically so that the tip lies in the most dependent portion of the stomach, which will usually be the antrum if the patient is sitting and in the middle of the greater curvature if he is lying on his left side. Placement of the gastric tube on the basis of measurement, clinical judgment, or trial aspiration will be unsuitable for maximal aspiration in at least half of the intubation attempts. Following correct positioning, the tube should be directed lateral to the third molar tooth and can be maintained in position by taping to the patient's face.

The principles of nasal intubation are similar to those of oral intubation. With the patient's chin elevated, the tube is directed slightly upward and then pushed gently posteriorly into the nasopharynx and esophagus. Some recommend preliminary spraying of the nasopharynx with a local anesthetic, although this should rarely be necessary.

If gastric secretion is to be collected over a period of time, as in the basal 1-hour secretion or the augmented histamine test, continuous aspiration should be employed, since intermittent withdrawal of secretion has been shown to result in significantly lower recovery volumes (Kay, 1953). Continuous aspiration can be performed either with a syringe or by mechanical means. In one study in which isotopically (^{131}I) labeled human serum albumin was instilled into the esophagus during gastric intubation in order to simulate gastric secretion, significantly greater recovery was achieved with continuous aspiration with a glass syringe than with suction apparatus (Johnston and McCraw, 1958). After brief instruction, the patient can usually be depended upon to operate the syringe successfully. It is important to caution the patient to expectorate all saliva and nasorespiratory secretions while aspiration is in progress.

Gastric intubation is usually contraindicated for patients with esophageal varices, diverticula, stenosis, or malignant neoplasms of the esophagus, aortic aneurysm, recent severe gastric hemorrhage, congestive heart failure, or pregnancy.

Physical Examination of Gastric Contents

Secretion from the normal fasting stomach is a pale gray, translucent, slightly viscous fluid with a faintly pungent odor. The fasting volume varies up to about 50 ml. Following a 12-hour fast the presence of food particles is distinctly abnormal and indicates delayed gastric emptying, often the result of pyloric obstruction.

Bile. Yellow to green coloration is the result of bile, which is occasionally regurgitated in the normal stomach and frequently accompanies excessive gagging during intubation. Large amounts of bile may be present with obstructing lesions of the small intestine distal to the ampulla of Vater.

Mucus. The mucus normally present is largely responsible for the viscosity of gastric secretion. In addition to mucus of gastric origin, important contributions of mucus result from swallowed saliva and nasorespiratory secretions and to a minor degree from the reflux of duodenal contents. The latter is identified by its bile staining. Saliva is identified by its frothy flocculent nature, which causes it to float on the surface of the gastric secretion. Nasorespiratory mucus is highly tenacious and may contain dust particles.

Blood. Flecks or streaks of blood are commonly seen as a result of minor trauma during intubation. Blood of greater amount and longer duration in the acid-secreting stomach will be brown and granular, the so-called "coffee-ground" appearance. Such quantities of blood may be from a gastric lesion such as gastritis, ulcer, or carcinoma or may be swallowed from the mouth, nasopharynx, or lungs. The presence of significant quantities of blood should be confirmed by the orthotolidine (Hematest) or guaiac tests.

pH. pH should be measured electrometrically with a reliable pH meter. There may be occasions when a rapid bedside estimate is indicated, in which case the use of pH indicator paper is permissible if due regard is given the inherent inaccuracies.

Microscopic Examination of Gastric Contents

A variety of structures may be recognized on microscopic examination. Components which may be present in the normal stomach include erythrocytes, leukocytes, epithelial cells, yeast, bacteria, and particles of mucus. Cellular elements are usually in various stages of autolysis, and their specific identity may be difficult.

As noted previously, small numbers of erythrocytes are of no consequence.

Leukocytes may be of gastric origin or may be from swallowed secretions. Small numbers of leukocytes are present in normal gastric secretion. Increased numbers may result from inflammation of the gastric mucosa, mouth, paranasal sinuses, nasorespiratory tract or, less commonly, from the pancreas, biliary tract, or duodenum.

Epithelial cells will be found in small numbers as a result of desquamation from various mucosal surfaces. Squamous cells may be dislodged from the mouth, nose, pharynx, or esophagus during intubation and may even appear in small clumps. Gastritis may result in a significant increase in columnar epithelial cells, but this is usually not a helpful criterion.

As a result of the high acid secretion and perhaps other secretory factors inimical to the survival of bacteria, the normal stomach does not have an established microbiological flora. Although bacteria and yeasts can be regularly cultured from gastric secretion, these usually reflect the flora of the mouth and nasorespiratory tract from the swallowing of secretions. These same bacteria probably do exist as an established flora in the anacid stomach. Yeasts may be present in large numbers in retention of gastric contents, such as occurs with pyloric obstruction.

In the past, considerable interest has focused on the Boas-Oppler bacillus, a species of lactobacillus. These large, nonmotile, gram-positive bacilli commonly occur in chains or clumps. Although once attributed special significance in the diagnosis of gastric carcinoma, their proliferation is probably the result of retention of gastric contents, with decreased or absent hydrochloric acid which yields a favorable fermentative environment.

Protozoan and metazoan parasites occur rarely and then usually with reflux of duodenal content. *Giardia lamblia* trophozoites or cysts, strongyloides larvae, or ascaris or hookworm ova may be found.

Tests of Gastric Function

Basal Gastric Secretion. Basal gastric secretion represents the response of the stomach to endogenous stimuli which are continually present in the interdigestive or fasting state. These endogenous stimuli include psychoneurogenic influences mediated by the vagus nerves and hormonal stimuli, such as gastrin and perhaps adrenocorticosteroids. For clinical validity it is essential that basal physiological and environmental conditions be maintained as much as possible during collection of the secretion. Minimum requirements include the following: (1) the patient must be in the fasting state and free from the sight or odor of food. (2) All medications influencing gastric secretion must be withheld for 24 hours. The most obvious medications in this regard include antacids and antisecretory (anticholinergic) drugs and also such secretory stimulants as reserpine, alcohol, adrenergic blocking agents, and adrenocorticosteroids. (3) The patient should be removed from environmental situations evoking untoward psychological reactions such as fear, anger, or depression.

The 1-hour morning aspiration is now the standard method of measuring basal secretion, having replaced the cumbersome and inherently less precise 12-hour nocturnal aspiration.

TECHNIQUE

1. Following a 12-hour overnight fast, the patient is intubated. Water may be taken until 8 hours prior to intubation.

2. The residual volume of gastric secretion is measured and qualitatively examined.

3. Continuous aspiration is begun, preferably manually with a syringe. The aspirate should be segregated into 15-minute samples. Usually the first one or two samples are discarded to allow for adjustment of the patient to the intubation procedure. Subsequent to this adjustment period, four 15-minute samples are taken.

4. If the basal secretion study is to be followed by the augmented histamine test, a suitable dose of antihistamine should be administered parenterally 30 minutes before completing the collection of basal secretion.

5. For each 15-minute sample, the volume, pH, and titratable acidity are measured and the acid output calculated. The sum of the acid outputs in the four samples, expressed in milliequivalents, represents the 1-hour basal acid output.

CLINICAL EVALUATION. The mean basal acid output reported for normal males ranges from 1.3 to 4.0 mEq. per hour in various series. This variation among series is a reflection, in part at least, of different collection techniques and in methods of measuring titratable acid. Lower values occur in females and with aging. Somewhat lower than normal values are reported in most large series for gastric carcinoma and benign gastric ulcer and distinctly higher values for duodenal ulcer or jejunal ulcer following partial gastrectomy with gastrojejunostomy (Table 16–2). Extremely high acid output is present in patients with the Zollinger-Ellison syndrome. In 25 such patients reviewed by Ellison and Wilson (1964), the 1-hour basal acid output varied from 11 to greater than 80 mEq. A high ratio of basal acid output to maximal acid output is of even greater significance, however, in the diagnosis of the Zollinger-Ellison syndrome.

It is important to emphasize that no pathognomonic range exists for any of the disease states listed, with the possible exception of the very high acid output found in patients with the Zollinger-Ellison syndrome. For example, in the series of 20 normal individuals reported by Marks *et al.* (1962), the acid output in normal individuals ranged from 0 to 13.8 mEq. per hour. Nevertheless, a basal acid output greater than 10 mEq. per hour is found

Table 16–2. BASAL AND MAXIMAL ACID OUTPUT IN VARIOUS CONDITIONS*

CONDITION	SEX	NUMBER OF PATIENTS	ACID OUTPUT (mEq./hour) Basal	Maximal
Controls	Male	35	4.2	22.6
	Female	26	1.8	15.2
Medical students	Male	145	5.3	26.7
	Female	16	3.3	21.4
Duodenal ulcer	Male	256	7.1	35.2
	Female	64	4.2	25.7
Gastric ulcer	Male	117	2.9	19.6
	Female	43	1.6	13.1
Gastric carcinoma	Male	74	1.5	6.7
	Female	32	0.7	3.0
Jejunal ulcer	Male†	10	7.9	25.1
	Female	4	5.5	16.4
	Male‡	4	9.1	36.1

*From Marks, I. N., *et al.*: S. Afr. J. Surg. *1*:53, 1963.
†Following partial gastrectomy with gastrojejunostomy.
‡Following gastroenterostomy alone.

in only about 4 per cent of normal individuals but about 13 to 19 per cent of duodenal ulcer patients (Marks, 1961).

The volume of gastric secretion in the basal hour, which ranges from about 50 to 100 ml., has by itself little diagnostic significance.

Augmented Histamine Test. Histamine is a powerful stimulant to gastric secretion and for several decades has been used clinically in gastric function tests. Earlier studies, including the "standard histamine test," utilized small doses of histamine and consequently resulted rather frequently in the incorrect diagnosis of anacidity. The augmented, or maximal, histamine test was introduced by Kay (1953), who showed that a dose of histamine acid phosphate of 0.04 mg. per kg. of body weight resulted in an acid output which did not increase further with larger doses of histamine. Since all parietal cells capable of secreting hydrochloric acid are presumably stimulated by the augmented histamine test, this test is sometimes used to estimate the number of functioning parietal cells, or what is sometimes termed the "total functioning parietal cell mass." The augmented histamine test or the analogous maximal Histalog test is now established as the *sine qua non* for the diagnosis of anacidity.

The untoward systemic effects of histamine are largely prevented by a previous injection of antihistamine which does not interfere significantly with the stimulatory effect on gastric secretion. Side effects were recorded in one series of 166 patients and, although frequent, were for the most part relatively mild clinically (Callender *et al.*, 1960). A decrease in blood pressure lasting from 30 to 45 minutes occurred in 61 per cent of the patients. The fall in blood pressure varied from 3 to 65 mm. systolic with a mean of 19 mm. and from 3 to 40 mm. diastolic with a mean of 13 mm. Hypotension necessitated discontinuation of the test in only one patient, however. In contrast, a slight rise in blood pressure occurred in 12 per cent. Other side effects of less significance were as follows: subjective feeling of warmth usually lasting approximately 30 minutes, 95 per cent; increased pulse rate (mean increase of 11 per minute with a maximum of 52 per minute), 70 per cent; drowsiness attributable to administration of antihistamine, 61 per cent; decreased pulse rate, 16 per cent; generalized patchy erythema, 12 per cent; headache, 7 per cent; lacrimation and nasal obstruction, 6 per cent.

A history of bronchial asthma or urticaria, the presence of severe cardiac, pulmonary, or renal disease, and paroxysmal hypertension or other possible signs and symptoms of pheochromocytoma are contraindications to the performance of this test.

TECHNIQUE

1. Following a 12-hour fast, basal secretion is collected for 1 hour as previously described.
2. Thirty minutes before completion of the basal secretion collection, a suitable dose of antihistamine is administered intramuscularly, e.g., 10 mg. chlorpheniramine maleate (Chlor-Trimeton), 50 mg. pyrilamine maleate (Neo-Antergan), or 50 mg. diphenhydramine hydrochloride (Benadryl).
3. After the conclusion of the basal secretion study, histamine acid phosphate is administered subcutaneously in a dose of 0.04 mg. per kg. body weight.
4. Gastric contents are then collected in 15-minute samples for 1 hour.
5. The volume, pH, and titratable acidity are measured for each sample and the acid output is calculated. From these the 1-hour or maximal acid output in milliequivalents is calculated.

CLINICAL EVALUATION. The maximum rate of acid secretion is characteristically attained within 15 minutes after histamine injection and is maintained for approximately 30 minutes. By 60 minutes after histamine injection acid secretion usually will have fallen to basal levels. The maximum acid output, representing the sum of the acid outputs for the four 15-minute posthistamine samples, is the most generally accepted expression of gastric acid secretion. Values for various conditions are listed in Table 16–2.

As in the case of basal acid secretion, the extended range of the maximal acid output for normal individuals obviates strict diagnostic categorization. Thus, in the series of Marks *et al.* (1962), the range for maximal acid output in normal males was 4.9 to 38.9 mEq. per hour. Some generalizations are useful, however. A maximal acid output of greater than 40 mEq. per hour is found in about 40 per cent of males with duodenal ulcer but only rarely in normal individuals (Marks, 1961). In addition to the marked hypersecretion, patients with the Zollinger-Ellison syndrome have a high ratio of basal to maximal acid output. Ratios greater than 60 per cent are strongly indicative of this disorder, while ratios of between 40 to 60 per cent are suggestive. The maximal acid output is not of great help in distinguishing benign gastric ulcer from gastric carcinoma unless anacidity is found, in which case benign peptic ulceration can be excluded.

Anacidity in the augmented histamine test is most commonly found in adults with pernicious anemia or gastric carcinoma. Nevertheless, it has been reported in a variety of other conditions, including hypochromic anemia, rheumatoid arthritis, steatorrhea, aplastic anemia, myxedema, nutritional megaloblastic anemia, and the asymptomatic relatives of patients with pernicious anemia. Such cases are uncommon, as indicated by the series of Card *et al.* (1955) in which, of 500 consecutive patients subjected to the maximal histamine test, all patients with anacidity proved to have pernicious anemia. Pernicious anemia in adults is virtually always accompanied by anacidity, but this does not hold true for the rare cases of juvenile pernicious anemia, in which normal acid secretion may be present. In a series of 30 patients with classic pernicious anemia reported by Callender *et al.* (1960) the pH of the gastric contents remained above 6.0 in all samples during both the basal and augmented histamine studies. Furthermore, following histamine stimulation, the pH actually increased from basal levels in 25 of the 30 patients, failed to show any change in three, and fell slightly to acid levels in two. In neither of the two cases did the pH fall more than a fraction of one unit.

Anacidity with gastric carcinoma is the exception rather than the rule. In one series, 10 of 38 males and six of 14 females with gastric carcinoma had anacidity in the augmented histamine test (Marks *et al.*, 1962).

Data from the basal and augmented histamine tests have been used by some physicians as an aid in determining which surgical procedure should be employed in the treatment of peptic ulcer. It has been suggested that an increased functioning parietal cell mass evidenced by an elevated maximal acid output indicates the need for gastric resection. On the other hand, elevated basal secretion with normal or only slightly elevated maximal secretion has been interpreted as an indication for vagotomy with drainage procedure. These are by no means universally accepted dictums.

Acid secretion is not expressed solely in terms of pH and maximal acid output by all workers. The *maximal histamine response*, which is the acid output in the interval from 15 to 45 minutes after histamine, was proposed on the basis of its high reproducibility (Kay, 1953). More recently, the similar concept of peak acid output has been used to represent the greatest acid output in any two successive 15-minute posthistamine samples. In about one-half of the cases, the peak acid output will occur in the period from 15 to 45 minutes after histamine (Baron, 1963). The peak acid output does not occur at the same interval in repeated tests on the same patient, but its value is the most reproducible measurement of acid secretion in the augmented histamine test. Some confusion has been introduced by the fact that the peak acid output is reported in milliequivalents per hour by doubling the peak half-hour value.

Histamine Infusion Test. The use of a slow intravenous infusion of histamine has recently been introduced to allow measurement of acid output in a sustained steady state. The dose rate of histamine which is employed elicits a maximal acid response in the sense that no further increase in acid output occurs if the dose rate of histamine is increased above the recommended level.

The infusion test has several distinct advantages. The attainment of a steady state circumvents the need for evaluating a secretory cycle including both basal levels and the peak acid output as is done in the augmented histamine test. Also, the greater acid output achieved in the sustained steady state facilitates the detection of low levels of acid output. The results of the infusion test are highly reproducible in a given patient. Furthermore, the slow intravenous infusion of histamine results in fewer and less severe side effects than when histamine is administered by a single subcutaneous injection.

TECHNIQUE (Lawrie *et al.*, 1964)

1. Following a 12-hour overnight fast the patient is intubated.
2. A basal hour collection is obtained.
3. Thirty minutes before completion of the basal hour, a suitable dose of antihistamine is administered intramuscularly.
4. Upon completion of the basal hour, an intravenous infusion of histamine in physiologic saline is begun with a suitable infusion apparatus such as the Palmer slow-injection pump. The dose rate is adjusted to deliver 0.04 mg. of histamine phosphate per kg. body weight per hour.
5. The infusion is continued until four 15-minute steady state samples have been collected. The initiation of the steady state is evident from the plateau reached in volume output and usually requires about 30 to 45 minutes to obtain after the start of the infusion.
6. Each sample of the basal hour and steady state is analyzed for volume, pH, and titratable acidity.

CLINICAL EVALUATION. The rate of acid output in the steady state of the infusion test is somewhat greater than the maximum rate that can be attained in the augmented histamine test. The acid output of the steady state hour compares most closely with the figure obtained by multiplying by four the acid output of the peak 15-minute sample in the augmented histamine test. In 45 patients on whom both tests were performed, the steady state hour of the infusion test was greater than the number obtained by multiplying by four the peak 15-minute sample of the augmented histamine test by a mean difference of 3.70 ± 1.05 mEq. (Lawrie *et al.*, 1964). Acid outputs for normal individuals and duodenal ulcer patients are shown in Table 16–3.

Table 16–3. ACID OUTPUT IN THE HISTAMINE INFUSION TEST*

CONDITION	SEX	NUMBER OF SUBJECTS	ACID OUTPUT (mEq./hr. ± 1 S.D.)
Normal	Male	26	24.0 ± 7.9
Normal	Female	23	21.0 ± 4.2
Duodenal ulcer	Male	107	42.3 ± 13.1

*From Lawrie, J. H., and Forrest, A. P. M.: Postgrad. Med. *41*:408, 1965.

Histalog Test. Histalog (3-B-aminoethyl pyrazole dihydrochloride, betazole), an analogue of histamine, is frequently used in place of histamine as a stimulus in gastric secretory studies. Histalog has the distinct advantage that side effects are minimal or absent; thus, premedication with antihistamines can be omitted. Results of Histalog stimulation are as reproducible as those of the augmented histamine test.

The dose of Histalog which gives maximal acid response, the augmented Histalog dosage, has been determined to be 1.7 mg. per kg. of body weight injected intramuscularly (Zaterka and Neves, 1964). The test is performed in the same manner as the augmented histamine test except that (1) prior administration of an antihistamine is omitted, and (2) eight instead of four 15-minute post-Histalog samples are collected.

The acid secretory response to Histalog is similar to that of histamine but has a distinctly greater latency period and longer duration of action. Whereas the peak secretion is regularly attained in the second or third 15-minute period in the augmented histamine test, it is not reached until sometime in the second to fifth 15-minute period in the augmented Histalog test. The peak secretory rate may last for 45 to 90 minutes in the augmented Histalog test. The peak 30-minute acid output is comparable in the two tests, being approximately 12 to 14 mEq. in normal subjects.

Insulin Hypoglycemia Test. Hypoglycemia resulting from the administration of insulin is a potent stimulus to gastric acid secretion. The major component of this stimulus is transmitted by the vagus nerves and can be abolished by vagotomy. The hypoglycemic response is complex, however, and probably consists of three phases. For about 30 minutes after insulin injection there is a slight depression of gastric secretion, the mechanism of which has not been explained. The predominant effect during the remainder of the first 2 hours consists of marked enhancement of gastric secretion. It is believed that this results from stimulation of the anterior hypothalamus by the hypoglycemia and subsequent transmission of this stimulus to the vagal centers of the brain. The final effect, which is manifested after 2 hours, also stimulates gastric secretion but presumably by a humoral mechanism. This late effect may result from initial stimulation of the posterior hypothalamus, with secondary neurohumoral stimulation of the anterior pituitary to release adrenocorticotropic hormone. The adrenocortical hormones which are thereby released probably act directly on the parietal cells, since this late effect of insulin hypoglycemia may be clearly manifested after complete vagotomy.

TECHNIQUE (Modified from Hollander, 1948)

1. After a 12-hour overnight fast the patient is intubated. A 2-hour basal secretion is obtained in 15-minute samples.
2. Blood samples for glucose determinations are obtained upon completion of the basal secretion study and at 30, 60, and 90 minutes after insulin injection.
3. Insulin is administered intravenously either at a fixed dosage of 15 or 20 units or at a calculated dosage of 0.20 units per kg. of body weight. It is essential that a 50-ml. syringe filled with 50 per cent (w./v.) glucose solution be readily available to counteract any serious hypoglycemic effects.
4. Gastric secretion is collected in 15-minute samples for 2 hours after insulin.
5. For each basal and postinsulin gastric sample, the volume and titratable acidity are determined, and the acid output is calculated.

CLINICAL EVALUATION. The insulin test is valid only if the blood glucose falls below 50 mg. per 100 ml. at some point in the test, which will usually be 30 minutes after insulin administration. The test is furthermore valid only for the stomach, which has been shown to be capable of secreting hydrochloric acid. Therefore, if no acid is present in either the basal or postinsulin periods, it is necessary to perform an augmented histamine test in an attempt to evoke acid secretion. If the stomach is truly anacid, no conclusion can be drawn regarding the completeness of vagotomy, but the question of simple peptic ulceration is then effectively excluded.

There is no clear delineation of normal from abnormal results in the insulin test. Nevertheless, several generalizations can be made. The patient can be considered to be completely vagotomized if the acid output in the greater of the two postinsulin hours is less than the greater of the two basal hours. Incomplete vagotomy is likely if the acid output in the 2-hour postinsulin period exceeds that of the 2-hour basal period by more than 0.5 mEq. (Stempien, 1962). Incomplete vagotomy is also suggested by an acid output of greater than 2 mEq. in either basal hour.

The time of increased acid output in the insulin test appears to be of some prognostic significance in incompletely vagotomized patients. Bell *et al.* (1965) reported the clinical course of 42 patients shown to be incompletely vagotomized by the insulin test. Of 28 patients giving an elevated acid output in the first postinsulin hour, 10 eventually developed recurrent peptic ulceration. In contrast, ulceration recurred in only one of the remaining 14 patients who showed an elevated acid output in the second postinsulin hour.

Gastrin Secretory Test. Purified gastrin prepared from the gastric antra of swine has been used in clinical studies of gastric secretion. The results of gastric secretory tests using gastrin as the stimulus have proved highly reproducible, and, unlike histamine, significant side effects have not been reported. Analogous to the optimal doses of histamine or Histalog required for maximal acid output, optimal doses of gastrin have been reported as 2 μg. per kg. of body weight for subcutaneous administration and 50 μg. for a single intravenous injection (Makhlouf *et al.*, 1964a). With the maximal subcutaneous dose of gastrin, the secretory response is somewhat slower than with histamine, but the peak acid output is approximately 10 per cent greater and is maintained for a longer period of time (Makhlouf *et al.*, 1964b). Most subjects will show a maximum acid output beginning about 20 minutes after gastrin injection and will maintain this level of acid output for 20 to 40 minutes. The response is much more rapid following intravenous administration, with peak levels occurring in 5 to 10 minutes.

Pentagastrin is a synthetic pentapeptide related to the active nucleus of gastrin. Studies thus far indicate that intravenous infusion of pentagastrin is a safe and reproducible method of gastric stimulation which is more potent than histamine and free of side effects (Konturek and Lankosz, 1967).

Twelve-Hour Nocturnal Aspiration. This method of determining basal gastric secretion continues to be used, although the much less complicated 1-hour morning basal collection has been shown to give qualitatively comparable results (Levin *et al.*, 1951). The 12-hour collection has no proven superiority over the 1-hour morning collection. It has been claimed to be more representative of basal gastric secretory activity by allowing freer expression of the normal fluctuations in gastric secretion, but this theoretical advantage is probably largely offset by the mechanical difficulties attendant upon the prolonged aspiration. Other disadvantages of the 12-hour nocturnal aspiration include the following: (1) Hospitalization is required, whereas the 1-hour morning basal collection followed by the augmented histamine test may be performed on an outpatient basis. (2) The test requires continual attention to proper functioning of the suction pump, including intermittent flushing with air. (3) The swallowing of saliva and nasorespiratory secretions cannot be avoided. (4) The test unduly extends for the patient the discomfort which is attendant upon any intubation procedure.

TECHNIQUE (Levin *et al.*, 1948)

1. For 24 hours prior to the start of aspiration, all medication influencing gastric secretion is withheld.

2. The usual diet is allowed until 12:30 P.M. on the day of the test, and normal activity is conducted until 5:30 P.M. At this time the patient is hospitalized and given a clear liquid meal. Food and water are subsequently withheld.

3. At 8:00 P.M., nasogastric intubation is performed and the stomach emptied completely. Continuous aspiration is begun.

4. At 8:30 P.M. and continuing for the next 12 hours the gastric secretion is collected by continuous aspiration. Hourly samples are segregated. Suction should be frequently interrupted and the tubing flushed with air.

5. For each hourly sample, the volume and titratable acidity are measured and the acid output calculated. Samples contaminated with bile are discarded. The total acid output and volume are also reported.

CLINICAL EVALUATION. Levin *et al.* (1948) studied 21 normal males and 12 normal females and found a mean 12-hour nocturnal volume of 643 ml. and 460 ml., respectively. In contrast, the mean volume was 1004 ml. in 32 duodenal ulcer patients. The secretory volumes were not significantly different from normal in patients with gastric ulcer (623 ml.) or gastric carcinoma (436 ml.).

The total acid output for the 12 hours is about 15 to 30 mEq. for normal individuals.

The 12-hour nocturnal aspiration has been thought to have special usefulness in the diagnosis of the Zollinger-Ellison syndrome, but the 1-hour basal test combined with the augmented histamine test is probably superior in distinguishing this entity from other hypersecretory states such as duodenal ulcer. Overnight secretion was studied in 55 patients of the series collected by Ellison and Wilson (1964). Total secretory volumes ranged from 250 ml. to greater than 4000 ml. In 85 per cent of the patients, the volume exceeded 1 liter, 49 per cent exceeded 2 liters, 22 per cent exceeded 3 liters, and 14 per cent exceeded 4 liters. Data on acid output were available on 54 patients. In 74 per cent of these the acid output exceeded 100 mEq., and in 35 per cent it exceeded 300 mEq. In view of the normal range reported for the 12-hour nocturnal aspiration, it may be concluded that the Zollinger-Ellison syndrome is to be considered probable if the total volume exceeds 2 liters and the acid output 100 mEq.

Tubeless Gastric Analysis. The tubeless gastric analysis is an indirect method for detecting gastric acid secretion and has as its only significant advantage the elimination of gastric intubation. The method utilizes a carboxylic cation exchange resin, the hydrogen ions of which have been replaced by those of an indicator cation. After ingestion the indicator cations are in turn released from the resin by hydrogen ions if acid is present in the gastric secretion. The indicator cations which are released are subsequently absorbed in the small intestine and eventually excreted in the urine. The measurement of the quantity of indicator cations in the urine is thus an indication of gastric acidity.

Initially quininium was used as the indicator but was later replaced by the dye azure A. Azure A has the advantage that its excretion can be estimated by direct visual inspection.

A variety of stimulants to gastric secretion have been recommended for use in this test, including oral caffeine sodium benzoate, Histalog, or alcohol and parenterally administered histamine or Histalog. Orally administered caffeine sodium benzoate and Histalog are the ones most commonly used.

The test reagents and comparator block are now commercially available as a complete kit (Diagnex Blue Test, Squibb).

TECHNIQUE (Segal, 1960)

1. Upon rising, the patient urinates and discards the urine. No food is ingested until completion of the test.

2. The gastric stimulant, either 500 mg. caffeine sodium benzoate or 50 mg. Histalog is taken with a glass of water. Alternatively, histamine or Histalog can be administered subcutaneously.

3. One hour later the patient urinates and again discards the sample. Immediately thereafter, 2 gm. of azuresin (U.S.P. granules) are ingested with one-half glass of water.

4. Two hours later the patient again urinates and saves the entire sample. The urine sample is diluted to 300 ml. with water, and a 10 ml. aliquot is placed in each of three test tubes.

5. Two of the tubes serve as color controls, and to each of these approximately 300 mg. of L-ascorbic acid is added. This reduces the azure A to a colorless form.

6. The tubes are then placed in a comparator block containing azure A standards of 0.3 mg. per 300 ml. and 0.6 mg. per 300 ml. If the color of the test urine is more intense than that of the 0.6 mg. standard, the test is completed and the patient is presumed to secrete hydrochloric acid.

7. If the color of the test urine is less than that of the 0.6 mg. standard, a drop of a solution containing 195 mg. $CuSO_4 \cdot 5H_2O$ in 100 ml. of 18 per cent HCl (Diagnex Blue reagent, Squibb) is added to each of the three urine tubes. All three tubes are placed in a boiling water bath for 10 minutes.

8. After cooling at room temperature for 2 hours, the color development is again compared to the standard solutions. The results are reported as less than 0.3 mg., 0.3 to 0.6 mg., or greater than 0.6 mg.

CLINICAL EVALUATION. The tubeless gastric analysis is strictly a qualitative test. An excretion of greater than 0.6 mg. azure A in 2 hours is considered to be indicative of hydrochloric acid secretion, while values less than 0.3 mg. are considered presumptive evidence of anacidity. Values between 0.3 and 0.6 mg. represent borderline secretion.

Considerable difference of opinion exists regarding the reliability of the tubeless gastric analysis. Much of the reported variation in false positives and false negatives is the result of differences in the standard of comparison for the tubeless analysis, different methods of gastric stimulation, and problems in the definition of anacidity. Marks and Shay (1960) compared the results of the azure A tubeless gastric analysis following caffeine sodium benzoate with those of the augmented histamine test in 85 selected patients. Defining anacidity as a failure of the pH to fall below 6.0 in the augmented histamine test, they found one of the 85 patients to show a false positive tubeless analysis result and 14 to show a false negative result. Most of the false negative results occurred in patients with greatly diminished secretion.

Histalog given orally appears to be a more effective gastric stimulant than caffeine sodium benzoate. Segal *et al.* (1959) administered the tubeless analysis following stimulation with 50 mg. of oral Histalog in 149 patients who were anacid according to the results with 500 mg. caffeine sodium benzoate stimulation. They found that 51 per cent of these patients secreted detectable acid with the Histalog stimulus.

The tubeless gastric analysis is considered unreliable in patients with previous subtotal gastrectomy, gastroenterostomy, or pyloroplasty. These conditions have been reported as causing both false positive and false negative results, both due to the rapid transit of the resin through the stomach. False positive results in the case are caused by release of the azure A by cations in the small intestinal secretion such as sodium, magnesium, potassium, and calcium. It is recommended that oral administration of salts containing barium, iron, calcium, magnesium, or aluminum be discontinued for 48 hours prior to testing. A single case of diverticulosis of the small intestine has been reported as causing false positive results, probably as a result of altered bacterial flora (Forster, 1961). Other conditions which make the tubeless analysis unreliable are malabsorption syndromes, severe diarrhea, pyloric obstruction, severe hepatic or renal disease, marked dehydration, and urinary retention.

Some recommend repeating the tubeless gastric analysis following apparent negative or borderline results. It is advisable that five days be allowed to elapse before repeating the test in order to allow for delayed excretion of the azure A.

Miscellaneous Studies

Mycobacterial Culture. Aspiration of gastric contents for mycobacterial culture is indicated in patients who are suspected of having pulmonary tuberculosis but who are unable to produce adequate sputum samples. The procedure is particularly indicated for young children, since it is not until the age of about seven years that children can effectively expectorate pulmonary secretions. It is essential that the gastric content be collected in the early morning prior to eating or drinking and preferably immediately upon awakening before increased motor activity of the stomach has largely emptied its contents. Since gastric acidity is inimical to the survival of *Mycobacterium tuberculosis*, as well as to most other bacteria, it is important that specimens be submitted immediately for decontamination and culture. Acid-fast stains on gastric contents are considered unreliable by many investigators because of the frequent presence of saprophytic acid-fast organisms originating in the mouth.

Exfoliative Cytology of the Stomach. Gastric cytology, gastroscopy, and roentgenography are at present the most useful procedures for investigating lesions of the stomach for possible malignancy. To a large extent the three procedures complement one another, but in the final analysis the most discriminating information is provided by exfoliative cytology. Multiple techniques for obtaining specimens have been reported, including simple aspiration of gastric content, the use of abrasive balloons or brushes, and gastric lavage with saline, buffered salt solutions, or solutions of papain or chymotrypsin. Chymotrypsin is believed to facilitate the exfoliation of cells by liquefying the mucous coating. Accuracies of greater than 90 per cent have been reported for exfoliative cytology in the diagnosis of gastric carcinoma.

Recently Introduced Procedures in Gastric Analysis

Determination of Hydrogen Ion Concentration from Electrode pH Measurements. Moore and Scarlata (1965) have recommended, on the basis of both practicality and accuracy, the determination of hydrogen ion concentration from electrode pH measurements. This method utilizes the interrelationships between pH, hydrogen ion activity (a_{H+}), the hydrogen ion activity coefficient (γ_{H+}), and hydrogen ion concentration (c_{H+}) represented by the two equations:

$$pH = -\log_{10} a_{H+}$$
$$\gamma_{H+}\, c_{H+} = a_{H+}$$

The activity coefficient is a function of both total ionic strength and pH. Since the ionic strength of gastric juice is largely determined by the concentration of major cations, sodium, potassium, and hydrogen, it has been possible to tabulate the activity coefficients and therefore the concentration of hydrogen ions for various concentrations of sodium and potassium at a given pH. This method thus requires precise measurement of pH with a glass electrode and determination of the sum of potassium and sodium. This approach has not been widely accepted and does not appear to provide any additional information which is of unique clinical value.

Electrophoresis of Gastric Secretion. Electrophoresis of gastric secretion reveals distinct bands of albumin and gamma globulin (Cohen *et al.*, 1962), multiple bands composed largely of mucopolysaccharides, and perhaps a band of pepsin (Glass, 1961). Electrophoresis has proved helpful in detecting the marked loss of albumin into the gastric contents which occurs in Menetrier's disease (giant hypertrophic gastritis with hypoproteinemia). Losses of albumin have also been described in benign gastric ulcer and gastric carcinoma. This technique requires special attention to the collection of samples, intragastric neutralization usually being necessary to avoid autodigestion of proteins. Electrophoresis of gastric content requires further evaluation, but studies thus far do not indicate the likelihood of adoption of this technically involved, time-consuming procedure for routine clinical use.

Determinations of Intrinsic Factor. Until recently intrinsic factor activity could be determined only by *in vivo* methods, such as the Schilling test, which measure the absorption of cobalt^{60}-labeled vitamin B_{12}. Several *in vitro* methods for assaying intrinsic factor have now been reported which utilize various immunological methods and such techniques as starch-gel or paper electrophoresis, column chromatography, or charcoal absorption. None of these methods has as yet received general acceptance, but it is anticipated that in the near future *in vitro* assays for intrinsic factor will become established as an important supplement to gastric analysis in selected cases.

Determination of Plasma Gastrin. Although not an integral part of gastric analysis *per se*, radioimmunoassay of plasma or serum gastrin is now available as a sensitive (5 pg. per ml.) and specific clinical laboratory determination. The assay is a valuable adjunct in diagnosis of the Zollinger-Ellison syndrome and pernicious anemia, both of which are associated with marked elevations of gastrin. The two diseases are readily distinguished on the basis of concomitant gastric acid secretion studies and by the fact that intragastric installation of dilute hydrochloric acid results in a precipitous decrease in plasma gastrin in pernicious anemia, whereas no appreciable change occurs in the Zollinger-Ellison syndrome (Yalow and Berson, 1970). In general in normal individuals, fasting plasma gastrin levels, which range up to approximately 300 pg. per ml., are inversely related to the rate of gastric acid secretion. Plasma gastrin concentrations in duodenal ulcer patients do not differ from those of normal individuals, while small increases are associated with gastric ulcers and with aging (Trudeau and McGuigan, 1971).

Tests of Gastric Function No Longer Recommended for Routine Clinical Use

Determination of Organic Acids. Small quantities of organic acids are occasionally present in the gastric content either as a result of ingestion with food or more importantly as a result of putrefaction. Putrefaction is apt to occur only in the stomach with the combination of retained contents and diminished acid secretion. Under these circumstances lactic acid is more commonly present, but acetic or butyric acid may be detected upon occasion. Lactic acid can be determined by several methods which have in common color development with ferric chloride. Lactic acid in increased amounts was formerly considered an important indication of gastric obstruction, particularly due to carcinoma, but this information can now be gained by far more discriminating clinical tests.

Determination of Peptic Activity. Pepsin is the most important digestive enzyme in gastric secretion. Detailed methods of analysis have been described based on the digestion of protein substrates such as egg albumin or hemoglobin. The peptic activity of gastric juice closely parallels the level of acid secretion and has not been shown to add significant additional clinical information. Although formerly a common procedure, this analysis is no longer indicated for routine clinical use.

Determination of Rennin. Rennin, which is derived from renninogen in the presence of hydrochloric acid, can be detected by incubation of an aliquot of gastric juice with fresh milk, which results in coagulation of the milk. The level of rennin activity has no special clinical significance. Deficiencies parallel those of pepsin and hydrochloric acid, and routine clinical determinations are therefore not indicated.

Determination of "Free," "Combined," and "Total" Acidity. As previously discussed, these older concepts of gastric acid are no longer tenable. Detailed methodology is given in previous editions of this book, to which the reader is referred for purposes of historical completeness.

Test Meals. A variety of substances have been used in the past to stimulate gastric secretion, including test meals ingested by the patient, ethyl alcohol (50 ml. of a 7 per cent [v/v] solution) or caffeine (0.2 gm. in 200 ml. of water) introduced through a gastric tube, or plain water. The most common test meal has been Ewald's test breakfast, which consists of two slices of bread without butter or eight arrowroot cookies and 350 ml. of water or unsweetened tea. Among other test meals used on occasion was Riegal's test meal, consisting of 400 ml. of bouillon, 200 gm. of broiled beefsteak, and 150 gm. of mashed potatoes.

Although it is true that test meals are more physiologic gastric stimulants than histamine or Histalog, they share with alcohol and caffeine the disadvantage that the stimulus is submaximal. A further disadvantage of the test meals is the fact that the acid output cannot be reliably quantitated, because of the buffering effect of the test meal itself. In view of these facts and particularly the need for confirming the diagnosis of anacidity with the augmented histamine or Histalog test, the test meals and other submaximal stimulants are now largely considered to be obsolete.

Fractional Gastric Analysis. The fractional gastric analysis was designed to measure the free acid present at varying times after a test meal stimulus. Following an overnight fast the patient is intubated and then given a test meal such as the Ewald test breakfast. After ingestion of the test meal, 10 ml. aliquots of gastric contents are removed at 15-minute intervals for a period of 2 hours. Each aliquot is grossly examined and its free acid determined by titration.

The fractional gastric analysis was originally intended only to be a qualitative test. Some feel that it gives useful information regarding the chymification and emptying functions of the stomach in addition to the acid concentration.

The information to be gained, however, is not adequate justification for the continued clinical use of this test.

Tetracycline Fluorescence. It has recently been found that the gastric sediment from patients with carcinoma of the stomach shows strong autofluorescence following prolonged administration of tetracycline or one of its derivatives. The test has resulted in many false positive as well as false negative results and is distinctly inferior to good cytological techniques.

EXAMINATION OF DUODENAL CONTENTS

The duodenal contents are composed of exocrine pancreatic secretion, bile, and the succus entericus or secretion of the intestine itself mixed with gastric secretion which may contain partially liquefied and digested food particles. Clinical examinations are usually performed in the fasting state, and samples are collected in such a manner that gastric secretion is effectively excluded.

Pancreatic Exocrine Secretion

Pancreatic exocrine secretion probably exceeds 1500 ml. per day in the normal adult and is thus the major contributor to duodenal contents from the standpoint of volume. It is a colorless, clear, nonviscid, highly alkaline solution with a pH of approximately 8.0. The secretion consists of 1 to 2 per cent organic material, mostly enzymes or their precursors including trypsinogen, chymotrypsinogen, amylase, lipase, lecithinase, elastase, collagenase, leucine aminopeptidase, and various esterases. The secretion contains about 1 per cent inorganic material, with sodium the major cation and bicarbonate the major anion. Compared with serum, sodium and potassium are present in about the same concentrations while calcium and magnesium are present in lower concentrations. The bicarbonate concentration varies directly with the rate of pancreatic secretion from about 25 to 150 mEq. per liter, while chloride varies inversely with the rate of secretion, so that the sum of these two ions remains approximately constant.

Pancreatic exocrine secretion occurs in response to both vagal and hormonal stimuli. The vagal component is relatively slight and results in a small volume of secretion which is rich in enzymes. Two hormones, secretin and pancreozymin, which are elaborated in the duodenal mucosa, are potent stimuli to pancreatic secretion. They are released into the blood following the entry of peptones, amino acids, or fluid into the duodenum. Acid by itself can apparently stimulate the release of secretin. Secretin results in a copious flow of pancreatic secretion which is low in enzyme content and high in bicarbonate. Pancreozymin, on the other hand, stimulates the pancreas to secrete enzymes and consequently results in degranulation of the acinar cells. Investigations over the past several decades have established useful clinical tests using these two hormones.

Bile

Approximately 500 to 1000 ml. of bile enters the duodenum daily. Bile is yellow to brown or green and usually alkaline, with a pH of 7.0 to 8.5. In addition to the bile salts, chiefly sodium glycocholate and taurocholate, bile contains the bilirubin pigments, cholesterol, phospholipids, and various inorganic salts. The only enzyme present in significant amount is alkaline phosphatase, which has no function in digestion. Bile flow is enhanced by two substances which have been termed choleretics and cholagogues. Choleretics are substances, such as bile salts and secretin, which increase the secretion of bile by the hepatic cells. Cholagogues, on the other hand, increase bile flow by causing contraction of the gallbladder and relaxation of the sphincter of the common bile duct. Magnesium sulfate and the hormone cholecystokinin are included in this category. Cholecystokinin is secreted by the duodenum in response to the entry of acid, fats, or partially digested protein, and perhaps also in response to nervous reflex mechanisms. This hormone is of some importance in clinical laboratory tests for the collection of stimulated bile and also for the reason that it is commonly present as an impurity in preparations of pancreozymin.

Succus Entericus

The duodenal secretion, as the pancreatic secretion, contains a variety of digestive enzymes which are capable of breaking down fats, proteins, and carbohydrates. Unlike the pancreatic secretion, however, the enzymatic activity of the succus entericus is considered to be relatively weak. The daily volume of duodenal secretion is not known but it is mildly alkaline with a pH of about 7.6. Various disease states of the small intestine are not reflected in abnormalities of the succus entericus.

Duodenal Intubation

Duodenal intubation is usually performed in the fasting state by a double-lumened tube, such as the Diamond, Lagerlöf, or Dreiling tubes. This allows simultaneous collection of gastric and duodenal contents and largely eliminates entrance of gastric secretion into the duodenum. This same result has been achieved with a variety of other techniques, each of which has its advocates, such as the use of two separate tubes or a three-lumened tube, one lumen of which is used to inflate one or more balloons for sealing the duodenum from the stomach. It is essential for the tube to be equipped with a radiopaque tip so that its position may be verified fluoroscopically.

A rapid method of intubation has been described by Raskin *et al.* (1958): Following an overnight fast, a sedative dose of pentobarbital is administered parenterally. A double-lumen Diamond tube is inserted into the mouth and passed a distance of 45 cm., which brings the tip approximately to the cardia. The patient is then placed in a left lateral decubitus position on a table, the cephalic end of which is elevated 16 inches. The tube is then slowly swallowed for another 15 cm., which results in its being positioned along the greater curvature. The patient then sits on the edge of the examining table with his body bent forward at the waist as far as possible. Several deep inspirations will assist entrance of the tube into the antrum. Peristalsis will move the tube into the duodenum if the patient lies in the right lateral decubitus position with his feet elevated for about 5 minutes. Finally the patient lies on his back for another 5 minutes while the tube is slowly advanced another 10 to 15 cm. The tube is adjusted with fluoroscopic visualization so that its tip is located in the middle of the third portion of the duodenum. Proper location of the tube can be maintained by taping it to the patient's face. This entire procedure can usually be completed in about 15 minutes in contrast to the 1 or 2 hours required for many other methods of intubation.

Secretions are collected with continuous suction by a vacuum pump or other suitable apparatus to obtain a pressure of at least 25 mm. Hg. During aspiration the patient may lie either on his back or right side. The duodenal aspirate can be collected in suitable containers, such as centrifuge tubes, which can be placed as a trap in the suction line. This will facilitate the frequent changing of containers which is required. The character of the aspirate may be continuously monitored by placing a section of glass tubing in the duodenal tube just before the collection container. The gastric aspirate is discarded.

In addition to the conditions which are contraindications for gastric intubation, duodenal intubation should not be performed as a general rule on patients with acute cholecystitis or acute pancreatitis.

Physical Examination of Duodenal Contents

In the fasting state the residual content of the duodenum varies up to 20 ml. The fluid may be slightly turbid as a result of mixture with gastric secretion; normal duodenal fluid from which gastric juice is excluded is transparent or slightly translucent, pearly gray, and moderately viscid. Bile staining is usually absent, but its presence is of no significance. Slight blood streaking may result from the intubation procedure. Larger amounts of blood suggest neoplasm involving usually the ampulla of Vater. The presence of food particles is distinctly abnormal and usually indicates either intestinal obstruction or a duodenal diverticulum. Sediment or flocculent debris may be seen in inflammation of the duodenal mucosa, pancreas, or biliary tract.

Microscopic Examination of Duodenal Contents

For maximum preservation of cellular elements, the duodenal secretion should be collected in containers chilled in an ice bath and should be examined as soon as possible. Following centrifugation, a drop of sediment may be examined unstained. A few leukocytes or epithelial cells are normal. Increased numbers of polymorphonuclear leukocytes and exfoliated epithelial cells, with or without masses of bacteria, enmeshed in mucus may be found in inflammation of the duodenum, bile ducts, or pancreas. The presence of bile staining may prove of some help in differentiating inflammatory conditions of the biliary tract. Rarely, parasites such as the larvae of *Strongyloides stercoralis*, cysts or trophozooites of *Giardia lamblia* or *Entamoeba histolytica*, or the ova of Necator, Ancylostoma, or Ascaris may be found.

Bacteriologic Examination of Duodenal Contents

Normally the duodenal content is nearly sterile, largely as a result of the bactericidal effect of gastric acid. Elaborate mechanisms have been devised for the collection of culture specimens from the duodenum, but these are not indicated for routine clinical use. One of these utilizes a gelatin cap to cover the sterilized duodenal tube, the cap being forced off after the tube is in place. Although seldom indicated, bacterial cultures can be removed from the aspirate of residual duodenal content or following stimulation of pancreatic or biliary secretion.

Chemical Examination of Duodenal Contents

The most important electrolyte in the duodenal contents is bicarbonate, but its measurement is indicated only in tests of pancreatic function, such as the secretin test. Chloride is infrequently determined and provides no useful information.

The determination of amylase, lipase, or trypsin activity in the pancreatic secretion following secretin or pancreozymin stimulation is an important index of pancreatic exocrine function. Variations in the three enzyme levels usually parallel one another so that only one of the determinations is indicated. Amylase is the most commonly measured and has the advantage of greatest stability. Determination of lipase and trypsin, in addition to amylase, is occasionally helpful in infants with suspected cystic fibrosis or with diarrhea or steatorrhea of unknown etiology. Methods for determining either serum amylase or lipase may be easily adapted to duodenal content following an appropriate initial dilution. The Somogyi method for serum amylase, for example, may be adapted to duodenal content by eliminating the initial protein precipitation and substituting a 1:50 or 1:250 dilution of duodenal fluid for the sample (Dreiling, 1955). Trypsin activity may be determined by testing for digestion of the gelatin coating on x-ray film as is done for fecal trypsin. As in the case of fecal trypsin determination, false positive tests may occur as a result of bacterial gelatinase.

Determination of bilirubin and urobilinogen in duodenal contents yields no information that cannot be deduced from measurements of serum bilirubin, urine bilirubin or urobilinogen, or fecal urobilinogen.

Provocative Tests of Pancreatic Secretion

The most important of these are the secretin and pancreozymin tests, which are discussed in Chapter 15.

EXAMINATION OF STIMULATED BILE

Since bile flow into the duodenum is intermittent in the fasting state, it is usually necessary to induce bile flow with a suitable stimulant if examination of bile is indicated. Although secretin is a potent choleretic agent, the increased bile production by the liver is stored in the gallbladder if the cystic duct is patent. In the presence of normal gallbladder function, secretion may result in a decrease or even disappearance of bile flow into the duodenum. Pancreozymin, on the other hand, will usually result in abundant bile flow as a result of its content of cholecystokinin. Magnesium sulfate, olive oil, and purified cholecystokinin have all been used to stimulate bile flow. Magnesium sulfate functions as an active cholagogue when applied topically to the duodenal mucosa but not when administered orally. Olive oil is probably an even more potent cholagogue but has the disadvantage that the oil interferes with subsequent microscopic examination of the bile. Commercial preparations of cholecystokinin have been used clinically but have no significant advantage over the other more readily available substances.

Technique (Lyon, 1919)

1. Duodenal intubation is performed and the position of the tube confirmed fluoroscopically. The test may be performed following the secretin test for pancreatic function.
2. Following aspiration of the residual duodenal content slowly introduce 50 to 100 ml. of a sterile 25 per cent saturated solution of magnesium sulfate through the duodenal tube.
3. After a minute or so, aspirate the magnesium sulfate and duodenal content. The collections are pooled and discarded until yellow bile first appears in quantity; this usually requires about 2 to 10 minutes.
4. Three fractions of bile are subsequently collected in separate containers. The first of these to appear, the "A" bile, is light yellow and watery. After 1 to 3 minutes, it will normally give way abruptly to a viscid deep yellow-brown bile, the "B" bile. Eventually the bile again becomes pale yellow and watery heralding the appearance of the "C" bile.
5. If no "B" bile appears after 15 to 20 minutes, stimulation with magnesium sulfate and the entire collection may be repeated one or two times.

Clinical Evaluation. "A" bile will usually amount to 5 to 20 ml. and originates in the common duct. "B" bile is the result of concentration and probably comes solely from the gallbladder under normal circumstances. Approximately 30 to 75 ml. of "B" bile will normally be recovered. It may be absent in advanced cholecystitis, cholelithiasis with obstruction of the cystic duct, or recent cholecystectomy. Absence of "B" bile is not proof of gallbladder disease, and this finding should be confirmed with cholecystography and other examinations. On the other hand, it has been demonstrated that "B" bile can be obtained following cholecystectomy or in cases of congenital absence of the gallbladder. This is probably the result of other portions of the extrahepatic ducts assuming the function of bile concentration. This explanation is supported by the observation that usually a year or more is required for "B" bile to reappear following cholecystectomy. The hepatic ducts and intrahepatic radicles are presumed to be the source of "C" bile.

Inflammation of the biliary tract may be evidenced by the presence of flocculent debris, which will be found to consist of bile-stained epithelial cells, and leukocytes in a mucous network, often with clumps of bacteria. The finding of bile sand, often in deep red-brown bile, is highly suggestive of cholelithiasis or calculus elsewhere in the biliary tract.

The importance of microscopic examination of bile for crystals, particularly the transparent rectangular or rhomboidal crystals of cholesterol or the amorphous yellow to orange masses of calcium bilirubinate is to be emphasized. Bockus *et al.* (1931) found that the presence of either or both of these crystals was associated with calculi in approximately 90 per cent of patients.

Culture of stimulated bile is occasionally informative. As a consequence of the circumstances of the collection, interpretation is frequently difficult and depends on quantitative as well as qualitative evaluation of cultures. The coliform organisms (*Escherichia coli* and the Klebsiella-Aerobacter group) staphylococci, beta-hemolytic or anaerobic streptococci, enterococci, and various species of Salmonella may be found in cases of acute or chronic cholecystitis and cholangitis.

REFERENCES

Baron, J. H.: Studies of basal and peak acid output with an augmented histamine test. Gut *4*:136, 1963.

Bell, P. R. F., Checketts, R. G., Johnston, D., and Duthie, H. L.: Augmented histamine response after incomplete vagotomy. Lancet 2:978, 1965.

Bock, O. A. A.: The concepts of "free acid" and "total acid" of the gastric juice. Lancet 2:1101, 1962.

Bockus, H. L., Shay, H., Willard, J. H., and Pessel, J. F.: Comparison of biliary drainage and cholecystography in gallstone diagnosis with especial reference to bile microscopy. J.A.M.A. *96*:311, 1931.

Callender, S. T., Retief, F. P., and Witts, L. J.: The augmented histamine test with special reference to achlorhydria. Gut *1*:326, 1960.

Card, W. I., Marks, I. N., and Sircus, W.: Observations on achlorhydria. J. Physiol. (London) *130*:18, 1955.

Cohen, N., Horowitz, M. I., and Hollander, F.: Serum albumin and gammaglobulin in normal human gastric juice. Proc. Soc. Exp. Biol. Med. *109*:463, 1962.

Dreiling, D. A.: The technique of the secretin test: Normal ranges. J. Mount Sinai Hosp., N.Y. *21*:363, 1955.

Ellison, E. H., and Wilson, S. D.: The Zollinger-Ellison syndrome: Re-appraisal and evaluation of 260 registered cases. Ann. Surg. *160*:512, 1964.

Forster, G. M.: An unusual false-positive response to the azuresin test. J.A.M.A. *176*:619, 1961.

Glass, G. B. J.: Paper electrophoresis of gastric juice in health and disease. Amer. J. Dig. Dis., *6*:1131, 1961.

Hollander, F.: Laboratory procedures in the study of vagotomy (with particular reference to the insulin test). Gastroenterology *11*:419, 1948.

Hollander, F.: Gastric secretion of electrolytes. Fed. Proc. *11*:706, 1952.

Hunt, J. N.: Gastric emptying and secretion in man. Physiol. Rev. *39*:491, 1959.

Johnston, D. H., and McCraw, B. H.: Gastric analysis – evaluation of collection techniques. Gastroenterology *35*:512, 1958.

Kay, A. W.: Effect of large doses of histamine on gastric secretion of HCl, an augmented histamine test. Brit. Med. J. 2:77, 1953.

Konturek, S. J., and Lankosz, J.: Pentapeptide infusion test. Scand. J. Gastroent. 2:112, 1967.

Lawrie, J. H., and Forrest, A. P. M.: The measurement of gastric acid. Postgrad. Med. J. *41*:408, 1965.

Lawrie, J. H., Smith, G. M. R., and Forrest, A. P. M.: The histamine-infusion test. Lancet 2:270, 1964.

Levin, E., Kirsner, J. B., and Palmer, W. L.: A simple measure of gastric secretion in man: Comparison of one hour basal secretion, histamine-secretion and twelve hour nocturnal gastric secretion. Gastroenterology *19*:88, 1951.

Levin, E., Kirsner, J. B., Palmer, W. L., and Butler, C.: The variability and periodicity of the nocturnal gastric secretion in normal individuals. Gastroenterology *10*:939, 1948.

Lyon, B. B. V.: Diagnosis and treatment of diseases of the gallbladder and biliary ducts, preliminary report on a new method., J.A.M.A. *73*:980, 1919.

Makhlouf, G. M., McManus, J. P. A., and Card, W. I.: Dose-response curves for the effect of gastrin II on acid gastric secretion in man. Gut *5*:379, 1964a.

Makhlouf, G. M., McManus, J. P. A., and Card, W. I.: The action of gastrin II on gastric-acid secretion in man. Comparison of the "maximal" secretory response to gastrin II and histamine. Lancet 2:485, 1964b.

Marks, I. N.: The augmented histamine test. Gastroenterology *41*:599, 1961.

Marks, I. N., Bank, S., Louw, J. H., and van Embden, B. H.: The augmented histamine test, an analysis of 672 consecutive tests. S. Afr. Med. J. *36*:807, 1962.

Marks, I. N., Bank, S., Moshal, M. G., and Louw, J. H.: The augmented histamine test, a review of 615 cases of gastroduodenal disease. S. Afr. J. Surg. *1*:53, 1963.

Marks, I. N., and Shay, H.: Augmented histamine test, Ewald test meal, and Diagnex test, comparison of results. Amer. J. Dig. Dis. *5*:1, 1960.

Moore, E. W., and Scarlata, R. W.: The determination of gastric acidity by the glass electrode. Gastroenterology *49*:178, 1965.

Piper, D. W., Macoun, M. L., Broderick, F. L., Fenton, B. H., and Builder, J. E.: The diagnosis of gastric carcinoma by the estimation of enzyme activity in gastric juice. Gastroenterology *45*:614, 1963.

Raskin, H. F., Wenger, J., Sklar, M., Pleticka, S., and Yarema, W.: The diagnosis of cancer of the pancreas, biliary tract, and duodenum by combined cytologic and secretory methods. 1. Exfoliative cytology and a description of a rapid method of duodenal intubation. Gastroenterology *34*:996, 1958.

Segal, H. L.: Clinical measurement of gastric secretion: Significance and limitations. Ann. Intern. Med. *53*:445, 1960.

Segal, H. L., Rumbold, J. C., Friedman, B. L., and Finigan, M. M.: Detection of achlorhydria by tubeless gastric analysis with betazole hydrochloride as the gastric stimulant. New Eng. J. Med. *261*:544, 1959.

Sparberg, M., and Kirsner, J. B.: Gastric secretory activity with reference to HCl, clinical interpretations. Arch. Intern. Med. (Chicago) *114*:508, 1964.

Stempien, S. J.: Insulin gastric analysis: technic and interpretations. Amer. J. Dig. Dis. *7*:138, 1962.

Trudeau, W. L., and McGuigan, J. E.: Relations between serum gastrin levels and rates of gastric hydrochloric acid secretion. New Eng. J. Med. *284*:408, 1971.

Yalow, R. S., and Berson, S. A.: Radioimmunoassay of gastrin. Gastroenterology *58*:1, 1970.

Zaterka, S., and Neves, D. P.: Maximal gastric secretion in human subjects after Histalog stimulation. Comparison with augmented histamine test. Gastroenterology *47*:251, 1964.

Chapter 17

THE EXAMINATION OF FECES

by MYRTON F. BEELER, M.D., and YUAN S. KAO, M.D.

Examination of stools is sometimes approached with reluctance because of the offensive nature of the material, yet simple observation may yield important diagnostic clues. Testing for occult blood may lead to early detection of carcinoma, and quantitative determination of fat is the definitive test for steatorrhea. In addition, bacteriologic and parasitologic examinations are often diagnostically helpful.

The average healthy adult defecates at frequencies varying from three times a day to three times a week. The common pattern is once a day. The stool tends to be soft and bulky on a diet high in vegetables, and small and dry on a diet high in meat. Two-thirds of the weight of the average stool is attributable to its water content and one-third is attributable to bacteria, indigestible material such as cellulose, undigested or unabsorbed food, gastrointestinal secretions, and desquamated cells. The normal brown color is of still undetermined origin. The odor results largely from indole and skatole, produced by bacteria from tryptophan.

SPECIMEN COLLECTION

Uninstructed patients sometimes exhibit considerable ingenuity in collecting stool specimens, but a few simple instructions are likely to produce more satisfactory specimens. A scoured, well-rinsed bedpan is a convenient collection container. If the patient does not own one, a carefully cleaned, rinsed, and boiled glass jar of suitable size is a satisfactory alternative. Patients should be warned against passing urine at the same time into the bedpan or container because, among other things, urine has a harmful effect on protozoa. Tongue depressors or pieces of cardboard are reasonably convenient instruments for transferring the stool from bedpan to transport vessel, for which plastic, cardboard, and glass containers are available. We prefer 2-oz. ointment jars with screw caps because they are odor free, leak proof, and easy to transport. Patients should be instructed not to contaminate the outside of the container and not to overfill the container. Gas, which frequently accumulates, should be released gradually by careful loosening of the cap. Failure to observe this simple precaution, especially in the case of an overfilled container, can result in an explosive release of contents.

Fecal matter left on the physician's gloved finger at the time of a rectal examination may be transferred to a piece of filter paper for inspection and testing for occult blood.

Because of wide variation in bowel habits, intestinal transit time, and bulk of stool, special consideration must be given to methods of timed stool collection. Unlike the urinary bladder and collection of timed urine specimens, for which the bladder can be emptied before and at the end of the collection period, the gastrointestinal tract cannot be emptied completely at will. Therefore, the amount of stool collected in a 24-hour period usually correlates very poorly with the amount of food ingested over a similar period of time. For determining the 24-hour fecal excretion of any substance, stools should be collected over a period of at least three days, and calculations should be based on the entire specimen divided by the number of days of collection. The accuracy of this method can be enhanced somewhat by having the patient ingest carmine dye (0.3 gm.) and charcoal (1 gm.) at the beginning and the end of a collecting period, respectively, collecting the stools from the beginning of the appearance of the dye to the beginning of the appearance of the charcoal. However, *Salmonella cubana* outbreaks in Massachusetts and California were traced to carmine dye (Lang *et al.*, 1967). Another method of signaling the collection period involves use of inert, nonabsorbable stool markers. These are taken in divided, uniform doses for several days prior to the beginning of the collection, continuing through the collection period. The concentration of the material found in the stool specimen is then used to determine the quantity of stool containing one day's ingestion of the material as an indication of the 24-hour output. For this purpose, chromium sesquioxide (Cr_2O_3) has been used and its concentration in the feces determined chemically (Rose, 1964). The substitution of radioactive chromium isotopes has made it possible to determine concentration by measurement of radioactivity of the stool (Spencer, 1969). Zirconium-95 oxide has been used in a similar manner (McDougall, 1964; Weber *et al.*, 1969). The latter methods as presently used are too time-consuming for routine determinations, but they may lead to future modifications permitting analysis of random specimens instead of the three-day collections now generally required.

INSPECTION OF FECES

Inspection of the feces is important, for it may lead to a diagnosis of parasitic infestation, obstructive jaundice, diarrhea, malabsorption, rectosigmoidal obstruction, dysentery or ulcerative colitis, or gastrointestinal tract bleeding.

The quantity, form, consistency, and color of the stool should be noted. Normally, 100 to 200 gm. of stool is passed per day. When there is diarrhea, the stool is watery. Passage of large amounts of mushy, foul-smelling, gray stool which floats in the water is characteristic of steatorrhea. Constipation may be associated with passage of little, firm, spherical masses of stool (scybala). Constipation most often results from the irritable colon syndrome of patients with anxiety, or from overuse of laxatives. In such patients, repeated tests for occult (hidden) blood are called for to detect more serious organic problems, such as carcinoma, which may also, of course, afflict those patients.

A narrow, ribbon-like stool suggests the possibility of spastic bowel or rectal narrowing or stricture. Clay color suggests diminution or absence of bile or presence of barium sulfate. Blood, especially when originating from the lower gut, may cause the stool to be red; beets in the diet may mimic this, as may bromsulphalein. Bleeding from the upper gastrointestinal tract is more likely to cause the stool to be black and of a tarry consistency. Bismuth, iron, and charcoal may also color the stool black. Standing in air for a time may cause the stool to darken on the surface. Green stools may result from ingestion of spinach and other green vegetables or calomel, or may result from the presence of biliverdin, seen in patients taking antibiotics orally. It is not unusual to see seeds and vegetable skins. Parasites are considered in Chapter 19.

MUCUS

Presence of recognizable mucus in a stool specimen is abnormal and should be reported. Translucent gelatinous mucus clinging to the surface of the formed stool suggests spastic constipation or mucous colitis. It is seen in stools of emotionally disturbed patients and may result from excessive straining. Bloody mucus clinging to the fecal mass suggests neoplasm or inflammatory processes of the rectal canal. Mucus associated with pus and blood is found in stool of patients with ulcerative colitis, bacillary dysentery, ulcerating carcinoma of the colon and, more rarely, acute diverticulitis or intestinal tuberculosis. Patients with villous adenoma of the colon may pass copious quantities of mucus, aggregating up to 3 or 4 liters in 24 hours. They frequently develop severe dehydration and electrolyte disturbances, especially hypokalemia (Wells *et al.*, 1962) (Fig. 17–1).

PUS

Patients with chronic ulcerative colitis and chronic bacillary dysentery frequently pass large quantities of pus with the stool, for the recognition of which, microscopic examination is required. This also occurs in patients with localized abscesses or fistulas communicating with the sigmoid rectum or anus. Large amounts of pus seldom accompany the stools of patients with amebic colitis (Bockus, 1964); therefore, its presence is evidence against this diagnosis. No inflammatory exudate is seen in the watery stools of patients with viral gastroenteritis (Fig. 17–1).

BLOOD

Bleeding into the gastrointestinal tract may be acute or chronic, massive or slight, obvious or occult, and may originate anywhere from the gingiva to the rectum. It should never be ignored, although often it results from minor pathology, such as hemorrhoids and anal fissures. Of one group of patients with significant gastrointestinal bleeding, 18 per cent were found to have malignant tumors, 30 per cent benign peptic ulcer. Slightly over 50 per cent had their bleeding source in the esophagus, stomach, or duodenum; 45 per cent in the colon and rectum (Thompson and McGuffin, 1949). Bleeding from the jejunum and ileum was seen in very few of the patients (Fig. 17–2).

Drugs, particularly salicylates, steroids, rauwolfia derivatives, indomethacin, and colchicine, have been shown to be associated with increased gastrointestinal blood loss in normal subjects and even more pronounced increases in blood loss in patients with gastrointestinal tract pathology (Bockus, 1964). This effect may even follow parenteral administration of the drugs (Grossman *et al.*, 1961; Matsumoto and Grossman, 1959). Apparent fecal peroxidase activity has also been shown to increase with use of carmine as a stool marker (Kirschen *et al.*, 1942) and occasionally with massive iron therapy. The latter, however, may result from actual bleeding secondary to gastrointestinal irritation produced by some iron compounds (Blumgart, 1963; Brayshaw *et al.*, 1963).

Loss of more than 50 to 75 ml. of blood from the upper gastrointestinal tract generally imparts a dark red to black color and a tarry consistency to the stool (Daniel and Egan, 1939). Persistence of a tarry appearance for two or three days suggests loss of at least 1000 ml. of blood. Following this amount of bleeding, occult blood may persist for five to 12 days (Schiff *et al.*, 1942). Somewhat smaller quantities entering the lower gastrointestinal tract may produce similar appearing stools, or may appear as bright red blood. Such stools should be considered grossly bloody only after verification with chemical tests to avoid confusion with coloring from dietary substances or medications. Smaller increases in blood content may not alter appearance of the stool. Such stools are said to contain "occult blood," detection of which can be most useful in uncovering or localizing disease. This is especially important because over half of all cancers (excluding skin) are those of the gastrointestinal tract; and early diagnosis and treatment of patients with colonic cancer results in a relatively good prognosis for survival (Greegor, 1971) (Figs. 17–2 and 17–3).

Methodology for Blood in Feces

The commonly applied tests depend on determination of peroxidase activity as an indication of hemoglobin content. Reagents used include guaiac, benzidine, ortho-tolidine, and ortho-dianisidine. Peroxidases (including

Figure 17–1.

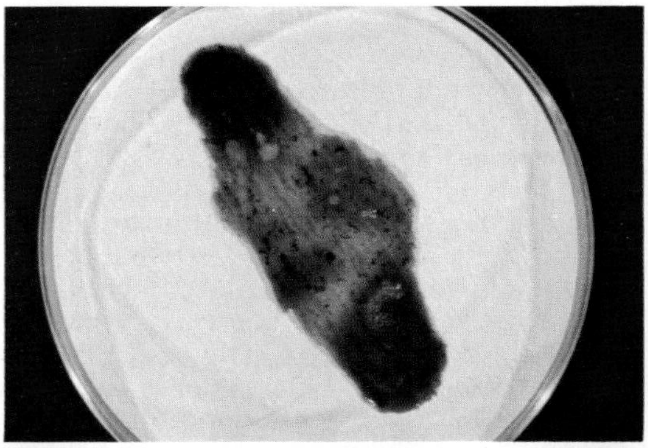

Figure 17–2.

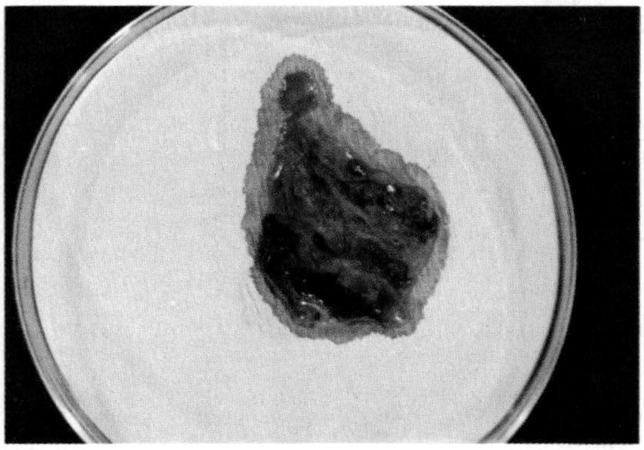

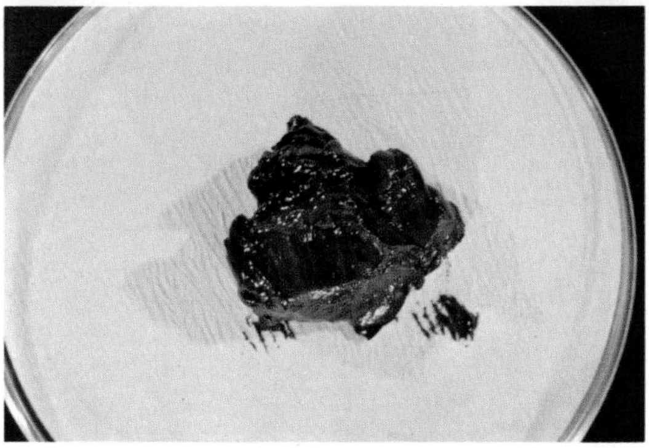

Figure 17–3.

Figure 17–1. Mucus, blood and pus.
Figure 17–2. Bloody stool.
Figure 17–3. Tarry stool.

hemoglobin, which can act as either a catalase or a peroxidase) catalyze oxidation of the test substances by peroxide, causing development of various shades and intensities of blue, depending on reagent, concentration of hemoglobin or other peroxidases, presence of other coloring matter, and presence (or absence) of inhibitors. The reagents differ chiefly in sensitivity. Ortho-tolidine is one to ten times more sensitive than benzidine; benzidine, ten to a thousand times more sensitive than guaiac, depending to some extent on the technique used (Hoerr *et al.*, 1949). The more sensitive reagents can be adapted to provide a less sensitive test by manipulation of techniques. Commercial preparations, such as Hematest (for examination of urine) and Occultest (for examination of feces), manufactured by the Ames Company, Inc., incorporate orthotolidine and have sensitivities intended to be consistent with the uses for which they are designed. According to Peranio and Bruger (1951), the amount of blood which must be ingested to yield a positive reaction in normal subjects on a meat- and fish-free diet is as follows:

Guaiac	20.0 ml.
Benzidine	3.5 ml.
Ortho-tolidine	1.0 ml.

On an unrestricted diet, however, normal subjects have a faintly positive guaiac test result after ingestion of only 2 to 3 ml. of blood. On the other hand, Mendeloff (1953) states that the guaiac test cannot be relied upon consistently to detect single blood losses in the stomach of less than 25 ml.

The usefulness of peroxidase tests is somewhat limited by lack of specificity and accuracy. Dietary meat contains hemoglobin and myoglobin as well as other enzymes which may give positive tests for as long as four days after ingestion. Three days of abstinence from meat prior to collection of the specimen is usually adequate to eliminate this problem, but this is so cumbersome clinically that we prefer to use tests of lower sensitivity that do not require a meat-free diet. A small amount of activity may also be contributed by dietary plant substances and by the bacterial flora of the intestinal tract. Modifications of the tests intended to destroy plant peroxidases by boiling have been shown also to destroy varying amounts of activity due to hemoglobin and are therefore not recommended (Hepler *et al.*, 1953).

The amount of peroxidase activity associated with heme moiety of hemoglobin in the stool produced by a given amount of bleeding varies with the location of the bleeding and the intestinal transit time. Other factors may include the level of digestive enzyme activity and the bacterial flora of the gastrointestinal tract. Although most of the hemoglobin entering the gastrointestinal tract reaches the stool in the form of hematin, which has peroxidase activity, a large amount of activity may be lost through further degradation to inactive materials. One group found an eighty- to one hundred twentyfold decrease in the peroxidase activity of blood passing through the gastrointestinal tract as compared to blood added directly to the feces (Ebaugh *et al.*, 1958). Furthermore, because of inhibiting substances in the stool, similar loss of activity may be found by adding blood to feces, as compared with adding similar quantities of blood to water. Ebaugh and associates (1958) suggest that this inhibition results from masking of indicator color by added color from the feces. Another factor may be competition for nascent oxygen by reducing substances in the feces.

Finally, techniques for measuring peroxidase activity are subject to considerable experimental error, particularly when large numbers of stool specimens must be screened by mass production methods. Specimens show marked variability in consistency and in their tendency to disperse in suspensions. This leads to inconsistencies in amount of aliquot used and in the portion of the aliquot actually available to react in suspension. Filter paper techniques are also limited in reproducibility by the tendency for liquid stools to be absorbed into the substance of the paper.

Further errors result from inaccurate measurement of reagents, inaccurate timing of the reaction, and variable interpretation of the color developed. Inconsistencies may also arise from sampling because of incomplete mixing of blood with the stool. Blood arising in the upper gastrointestinal tract is relatively uniformly mixed throughout the specimen, but blood from the lower gastrointestinal tract is likely to be segmental in distribution within the stool, or it may only coat the surface. Anorectal blood frequently produces red streaking of the surface. The presence of such focally distributed blood should be reported after chemical verification. In routine testing for occult blood, an attempt is made to use an aliquot from the center of the formed stool.

Partly because of the importance of these screening tests, numerous modifications have been developed based on the same fundamental processes in efforts to improve test precision and specificity and diagnostic accuracy. However, because of the many variable factors discussed, high degrees of precision specificity and accuracy cannot be achieved, even with elaborate techniques; and these, in any case, render the tests useless for screening purposes.

The guaiac method to be described represents a compromise suitable for routine screening and does not require a meat-free diet. It will detect 0.5 to 1.0 mg. of hemoglobin per ml. of aqueous solution. If one substitutes 0.2 per cent ortho-tolidine for guaiac and 0.3 per cent hydrogen peroxide for 3 per cent hydrogen peroxide in the same procedure, one obtains approximately the same sensitivity. We have found the Occultest and Hematest techniques to be capable of detecting as little as 0.1 mg. of hemoglobin per ml. of aqueous solution. They gave an unacceptable number of false positive reactions when patients were on a regular diet (Goldman *et al.*, 1964; Blumgart, 1963). Paradoxically, however, the Hematest sometimes gave only a trace or 1+ reaction with tarry stools. We believe this resulted from improper mixing of hematin with reagent, probably because of the tarry consistency of the stools, since emulsification of the stool (not recommended by the manufacturer) obviates the problem.

We advise use of a saturated solution of guaiac because of the tendency of some strongly positive reactions to fade with the weaker solutions available commercially. Addition of extra powdered guaiac will restore the coloring in these cases. The problem may be overcome by observing for maximal color development.

As blood traverses the gut, it is broken down into its constituents which may have decreased or no peroxidase activity. The actual form of hemoglobin most commonly found in the colon is hematin, which has much less peroxidase activity than heme. A source of hemorrhage in the upper gastrointestinal system or an increased transit time through the bowel will therefore decrease the peroxidase activity of hemoglobin.

Difficulties arise with the peroxidase method, since other constituents of feces have peroxidase activity. Foremost among these are the myoglobin and hemoglobin in fish and meat and plant peroxidases in such vegetables as horseradish and turnips. Bacteria in the bowel also possess peroxidases and can falsely elevate peroxidase activity. To further complicate interpretation, the normal individual loses 2.0 to 2.5 ml. of blood into the gastrointestinal tract daily (Ebaugh *et al.*, 1958; Roche *et al.*, 1957). Various chromogens are also present in feces which are known to interfere with color development in the tests, and orally administered iron will give falsely positive tests if guaiac is used as a reagent. This last problem does not arise with the other reagents available.

In the patient with severe gastrointestinal hemorrhage, the diagnostic problems are not such as to need a very sensitive test to detect blood in feces. The real benefit of these tests is as a screening procedure for hemorrhage from colonic carcinoma and other occult sources of hemorrhage. To be valid, the test employed must be repeated at least three and preferably six times with the patient on a diet free of the exogenous sources of peroxidase activity. This regimen is usually unacceptable to the patient, so that positive tests on a normal diet must be repeated following a three- or four-day period of abstinence from meat, fish, and vegetable sources of peroxidase activity. Only after this regimen can a positive series of tests be considered an indication for further evaluation of the patient.

Several different screening tests are available commercially: "Hematest" and "Occultest" by Ames Company, employing ortho-tolidine; "Hemoccult" by Smith, Kline and French, employing guaiac-impregnated filter paper; and several others, using benzidine or tablets impregnated with guaiac. The major disadvantage of tests employing ortho-tolidine, benzidine, and some guaiac tablets is that they give false positives in the presence of normal peroxidase activity in stool. "Hemoccult," employing guaiac-impregnated filter paper is of lower sensitivity and begins to turn positive in the presence of about 5.0 mg. of hemoglobin per gm. of stool. This is the upper limit of normal peroxidase activity of stool and represents a significant improvement in methodology, as false positives can be kept to about 1 per cent (Ostrow *et al.*, 1972). The "Hemoccult" test also has the advantage of being so simple and esthetically acceptable that specimens can be collected at home and mailed for evaluation.

Quantitative methods have been developed for study of gastrointestinal bleeding by use of radioactive chromium-51 (Spencer, 1969; Fall *et al.*, 1971). These methods have greater specificity than peroxidase tests. Furthermore, they can be combined with other techniques to determine the location of bleeding, when present. As they involve considerable time, effort, and expense, their use should be reserved for patients presenting special diagnostic problems.

The procedures are based on ability of radioactive chromium to be bound to red blood cells and on the fact that radioactive chromium is not reabsorbed from the gastrointestinal tract but is excreted in the feces, where it can be measured by gamma-ray spectrometry. For this purpose a sample of blood is withdrawn from the patient, mixed with citrate solution containing (^{51}Cr) chromium as sodium chromate, and then reinjected into the patient. Most of the sodium chromate is bound to the red blood cells and remains so bound until they are destroyed or lost through hemorrhage. Subsequently stools contain quantities of chromium-51 quantitatively related to the blood content. Gamma ray activity of the stool specimen is determined and the blood loss is calculated from comparison with activity of patient's blood. Bleeding source may be localized by similarly examining fluid for blood removed from various levels of the gastrointestinal tract through a Miller-Abbot tube or by use of an umbilical tape attached to a small bag of mercury in a lead sinker, swallowed by the patient, located by fluoroscope, then withdrawn and examined for blood staining.

STEATORRHEA

Pathological increase in stool fat is referred to as "steatorrhea." Normal individuals on a normal fat intake excrete daily up to 5 gm. of lipid (measured as fatty acids) in their feces (Frazer, 1955). While the source of fecal lipid is largely dietary, gastrointestinal excretions, cellular desquamation, and bacterial metabolism also contribute (Frazer and Sammons, 1956). Lipids are normally present as soaps and triglycerides. In addition, lipoids are present, including higher alcohols, paraffins, and vegetable carotenoids. Although diet has some effect on it, the pattern of lipids excreted may be very different from that of the diet, and the quantity of fat ingested by the normal individual has a relatively small effect on his total output of fat. According to one study, the fecal lipid is equal to a constant (2.93 gm.) plus 2.1 per cent of the dietary fat intake. On a fat-free diet, the output of fat normally varies from 1 to 4 gm. per day (Wollaeger *et al.*, 1947).

The stools in severe cases of steatorrhea are generally fluid, semifluid, or soft and pasty and bulky, pale, and foul smelling. They may be foamy and may tend to float on water.

THE MALABSORPTION SYNDROME

The malabsorption syndromes, of which steatorrhea is often a major feature, result from impaired digestion or assimilation of foodstuffs by the small bowel.

Maldigestion generally results from pancreatic disease (see Chapter 15), such as chronic pancreatitis, carcinoma of the pancreas, and fibrocystic disease of the pancreas, and subsequent lack of pancreatic digestive enzymes. Generally there is associated steatorrhea, evidenced by presence of undigested meat fibers in the feces, and with a relative increase in neutral fats (triglycerides) in the stool.

Hepatogenous maldigestion results from interference with bile flow. Loss of bile salts interferes with emulsification, diminishing the surface area available for lipolytic action. In addition, there is loss of bile salt activation of lipase activity. The diseases with which this syndrome is associated are discussed in Chapter 13. The patients are usually jaundiced, pass dark urine, and have other signs of liver disease. Hepatogenous steatorrhea may coexist with pancreatic steatorrhea, as when there is a neoplasm obstructing the ampulla of Vater.

Enterogenous malabsorption, in which intestinal assimilation is impaired, results from such conditions as gluten-induced enteropathy (celiac disease and nontropical sprue), tropical sprue, protein-losing enteropathy, hypogammaglobulinemia, a-beta-lipoproteinemia, lymphangiectasis, intestinal lipodystrophy (Whipple's disease), amyloidosis, lymphoma, vasculitis, surgical loss of functional bowel, diverticulosis, intestinal blind loops, and hormonal disorders. Significant malabsorption may also occur in acute diarrheal syndromes.

Patients with malabsorption, regardless of etiology, are liable to develop deficiencies of fat soluble vitamins. Primary and secondary alterations of bowel mucosa may also result in deficiency of water soluble vitamins. In addition, these patients are liable to lose weight because of large caloric loss and to have other evidence of nutritional deficiencies, such as hypoprothrombinemia, glossitis, anemia, edema, ascites, and osteomalacia.

Laboratory Diagnosis

Screening tests are available for detection of steatorrhea, such as determination of serum carotene, which tends, along with fat soluble vitamin A, to be lower than normal; microscopic examination of the stool for fat globules and undigested meat fibers; and measurement of serum turbidity at timed intervals following a fat meal. In patients with steatorrhea, there is less than a normal increase in serum turbidity. Definitive diagnosis depends upon quantitative demonstration of increased fecal lipid (Frazer, 1955; Pimparker *et al.*, 1961).

When the diagnosis of malabsorption has been established, differential diagnosis becomes important for determining treatment. The usual problem is differentiation of pancreatogenous from enterogenous malabsorption. In children the definitive test for mucoviscidosis, the main cause of pancreatic malabsorption is the sweat electrolyte determination described in Chapter 15. This test should be used whenever clinical evidence warrants it, although screening tests based on absent stool trypsin and on semiquantitative demonstrations of increased sweat chloride have been applied. One of the most valuable of the differential diagnostic tests, for adults especially, has been the D-xylose absorption test (Benson *et al.*, 1957; Santiago-Borrero *et al.*,

1971). In this procedure, a 25-gm. dose of the pentose sugar in water is administered orally, and the amount excreted in the urine over a 5-hour period is determined. If the amount excreted is less than 3 gm., the diagnosis is most likely enterogenous malabsorption, as pancreatic enzymes are not required for absorption of D-xylose. Poor kidney function may also result in low excretion, and for this reason blood levels should also be determined. High blood values coupled with low urine values suggest renal disease.*

There is no fully satisfactory alternative test, although isotopic techniques (see Chapter 7) are of some use, and starch tolerance tests have been used by some workers for this purpose. In the latter, absorption of starch is followed by serial blood glucose determinations. The rise in blood glucose is compared with that following a glucose tolerance test. Theoretically, if the patient lacks pancreatic amylase, the glucose tolerance will result in higher values than the starch tolerance test. The quantitative specific stool trypsin and chymotrypsin assays may be helpful (Haverback *et al.*, 1963; Johnstone, 1952); as may the Schilling test for vitamin B_{12} (see Chapter 7), which tends to be abnormal in patients with enterogenous steatorrhea. Probably the best present alternative laboratory diagnostic aid, although unpleasant for the patient, is duodenal intubation, as described in Chapter 15.

Fecal Fat Determinations. The amount of fat in the feces may be expressed as per cent by weight of wet stool, per cent by weight of dry stool, per cent of ingested fat retained (absorbed), and weight per 24-hour stool collection. Because of wide variation in water content of the stool, wet weight concentrations are the least informative. Dry weight concentrations are only slightly less variable because of the effect of diet on bulk. Total output of fat per 24 hours, based on analysis of at least a three-day stool collection, is the most reliable measurement. For this purpose, the patient is placed on a standard diet containing 100 gm. of fat per day. In infants and children, for whom the standard 100-gm. diet cannot be used, "per cent coefficient of fat retention" is the more useful expression. This is the difference between fecal fat and ingested fat expressed as a percentage of the ingested fat $\left(\frac{\text{dietary fat-fecal fat}}{\text{dietary fat}} \times 100\right)$. The coefficient of fat retention of normal children and adults is 95 per cent or higher, although in premature infants it may be much lower than this. A low value, otherwise, is indicative of steatorrhea. A number of methods are available for the measurement of fat content of stools. These include microscopic examination, gravimetric procedures, titrimetric procedures, radioisotope tagging techniques, and an electrical capacitance technique.

Microscopic Examination (Pihl and Hepler, 1953; Drummey *et al.*, 1961). The crudest technique is microscopic examination using Sudan III, Sudan IV, or oil red O stains. The procedure has been widely employed for screening because of its simplicity. In our experience, results have correlated well with quantitative measurements when aliquots of the same homogenized stool have been analyzed. For this purpose, a small aliquot of stool suspension is placed on a slide and mixed with 2 drops of 95 per cent ethanol, followed by addition of 2 drops of saturated ethanolic solution of Sudan III, with mixing. It is then coverslipped. Under these conditions fatty acids are present as lightly staining flakes or as needle-like crystals which do not stain and which, therefore, may be missed. Soaps, also, do not stain, but appear as well-defined amorphous flakes or as rounded masses or coarse crystals. Neutral fats, however, appear as large orange or red droplets. When 60 or more stained droplets of neutral fats per high-power field are seen, one may be reasonably certain that the patient has steatorrhea. Caution is advisable in interpretation, as mineral oil or castor oil may mimic neutral fat. The procedure is then repeated, adding several drops of 36 per cent (v./v.) acetic acid to the stool mixture and warming the slide several times over a flame until slight boiling occurs. This converts neutral fats and soaps to fatty acids and melts the fatty acids, causing them to form droplets which stain strongly with Sudan III. The slide is then examined while warm. After this procedure, presence of up to 100 stained droplets per high-power field is considered normal. Patients with pancreatogenous steatorrhea are likely to show greater increases in neutral fat; the ones with enterogenous steatorrhea are likely to show greater increases in fatty acids and soaps. Use of oil red O has been advocated by some because it permits substitution of isopropanol for ethanol.

Gravimetric Methods. A weighed aliquot of feces, either as homogenized wet specimen or as dried specimen, is extracted with an organic solvent, such as xylene or petroleum ether. The extract is evaporated to dryness and the

*Unfortunately the test cannot presently be used routinely in the United States because the Food and Drug Administration has defined D-xylose to be a new drug and, therefore, experimental. As of the date of this writing, no one has sponsored the drug. Because prolonged D-xylose administration to small rodents has been shown to be cataractogenic, it is possible, even though the cataracts are reversible, that the drug may never be cleared for routine human use. The only known human side effects are nausea, vomiting, and diarrhea, and these are generally no more severe than similar side effects observed in glucose tolerance tests.

residue is weighed. The weight is taken to represent the amount of fat present in the specimen. There have been many modifications of this general procedure (Webb, 1959), the chief differences among them being the spectrum of lipids and lipoids included in the measurement.

Isotopic Techniques (Rufin *et al.*, 1961). Recently there has been much interest in radioactive isotope techniques, in which oleic acid or triglycerides are labeled with ^{131}I and given orally to the patients. Subsequently, the blood is examined for ^{131}I by gamma spectrography. Slightly better correlation has been found with the chemical test if the iodine remaining in the stool is measured rather than that in the blood. The difference between the absorption rate of ^{131}I-labeled triglyceride and that of similarly labeled oleic acid has been interpreted as a measure of enzyme activity in the gastrointestinal tract and has been applied in the differential diagnosis of pancreatogenous and enterogenous steatorrhea. However, as neutral fat may be broken down in the absence of pancreatic lipase by bacterial lipase, the test is of limited diagnostic capability.

These methods frequently give conflicting results (Spencer, 1969) and have been criticized because of the questionable stability of the bonding between the iodine and the fat molecule; as Tuna and associates (1963) and others have shown, many commercially available preparations are contaminated by radioactive free fatty acids, fatty acid esters, and other substances, because the blood level of radioactivity depends upon multiple factors, including gastric emptying, hydrolysis, absorption, metabolism, and storage (which may differ from that of nonradioactive lipids); and because the rate of absorption is measured, rather than the total absorption.

Electrical Capacitance Method (Wolochow, 1965). A rapid method for quantitative determination of fecal fat has been described in which electrical capacitance is used. For this purpose an aliquot of fecal suspension is extracted with solvent consisting chiefly of chlorinated benzenes. The extract is filtered, and its electrical capacitance is measured and compared with standards of triolein similarly treated. Because of its speed and relative simplicity, this method may gradually replace the method of Van de Kamer, with which it correlates reasonably well.

Titrimetric Method of Van de Kamer (Van de Kamer *et al.*, 1949; Jover and Gordon, 1962). Fats and fatty acids are converted to soap by boiling with alcoholic potassium hydroxide. After cooling, excess hydrochloric acid is added to convert soaps to fatty acids. These are extracted with petroleum ether. An aliquot is evaporated, taken up in neutral alcohol, and titrated with sodium hydroxide. Fats are calculated as fatty acids.

Intestinal Disaccharidase Deficiency. Many of the conditions causing malabsorption listed previously may also be associated with intolerance for disaccharides, in which disaccharide absorption is diminished because of deficient disaccharidase activity in the small intestinal mucosa. These acquired (secondary) lactase deficiencies are usually transient. Permanent intolerance results from primary disaccharidase deficiency, possibly resulting from a genetically determined enzyme defect or from environmental factors, or both (Cook and Kajubi, 1966; Keusch *et al.*, 1969; Davis and Bolin, 1967). Lactose intolerance is by far the most common of these disorders. Unhydrolized disaccharides are fermented by intestinal bacteria producing gas and lactic acid. The osmotic effect of the lactose and its metabolites and irritation of the bowel by the lactic acid produced often result in diarrhea. Primary sucrase and maltase intolerance, although rarely seen, have been reported (Weijers *et al.*, 1961; Anderson *et al.*, 1963).

Laboratory Diagnosis. The stools are usually acid (pH 5.5 or below). The lactic acid content of the stools (in the case of lactase deficiency) is usually greater than 100 mg./24 hr. The most consistent test result is sugar content higher than 250 mg./100 ml. of stool (lactose, glucose, and galactose) (Anderson *et al.*, 1966). Stool can be analyzed for sugars by chromatography or by one of the semiquantitative, nonspecific tests for urinary sugars adapted for stool analysis. The Clinitest tablet is suitable for the purpose (Kerry and Anderson, 1964). Abnormally high results with this test are common, however, in normal infants between the ages of 3 and 7 days (Davison and Mullinger, 1970).

Definitive diagnosis depends on demonstrating low lactase activity in small bowel biopsy material; normal intestinal sucrase and maltase activity; intolerance to orally administered lactose; and a flat lactose test curve (Newcomer and McGill, 1967; Basford and Henry, 1967) (Table 17–1).

Glucose-Galactose Malabsorption. Primary glucose-galactose malabsorption is a rare hereditary disorder of active absorption of glucose and galactose from the small intestine. Recent studies suggest an autosomal recessive mode of inheritance (Melin and Meeuwisse, 1969; Lebenthal *et al.*, 1971). Symptoms and signs are similar to those seen in patients with disaccharide malabsorption, diarrhea being the main problem. Stools are watery, always contain several grams per 100 ml. of glucose and galactose. Fructose absorption is normal in this disorder (Linqvist and Meeuwisse, 1963).

Table 17–1. BLOOD GLUCOSE RISE OVER FASTING LEVEL (mg./dl.)

CARBOHYDRATE INGESTION	BLOOD GLUCOSE RISE		
	Normal	Lactose Intolerance	Idiopathic Sprue
Lactose, 50 gm.	14–62 (35)*	2–11 (6)	0–19 (9)
Glucose, 25 gm. Galactose, 25 gm.	25–66 (49)	20–71 (40)	24–34 (28)
Maltose, 50 gm.	(28–80) (52)	57–92 (74.5)	19 (one case)

*Figures in parentheses are average values. (From Basford, R. L., and Henry, J. B.: Postgrad. Med. *41*:A70, 1967.)

Laboratory Tests. Diagnostic laboratory tests for this disorder include identification of glucose and galactose in the stools, using glucose oxidase, galactose oxidase, or chromatography, and oral glucose tolerance tests and oral galactose tolerance tests, in which a flat curve is expected. Fructose tolerance tests should also be performed, results of which should be normal. A flat glucose tolerance curve alone does not, of course, indicate the presence of this disorder. Many variables affect blood glucose levels. Flat glucose tolerance curves are normal in newborn babies. Furthermore, blood glucose levels are affected by oral fructose loading (Meeuwisse and Melin, 1969; Meeuwisse and Linqvist, 1970). If oral sugar tolerance tests yield equivocal results, intubation and perfusion of a segment of the small intestine may be indicated to establish the diagnosis (Kaijser and Öckerman, 1970).

Miscellaneous Procedures

In addition to the diagnostic tests already described, a number of other procedures are available that are of lesser usefulness or are of interest primarily for research or other purposes. These include tests for nitrogen, porphyrins, phosphorus, sodium, calcium, magnesium, and chloride. Nitrogen determinations have been used for diagnosing pancreatic insufficiency syndromes, as fecal nitrogen is increased in these conditions as a result of impaired protein digestion. However, fecal nitrogen content also varies markedly with bacterial flora, and the clinical usefulness of the assay is therefore limited. Fecal calcium tends to vary with diet and with the serum calcium and is seldom determined except in special balance studies. Assay of other stool electrolytes has not proved clinically useful.

Stool urobilinogen determinations are occasionally useful for confirming a diagnosis of complete obstruction to bile flow (seen in carcinoma only). Urobilinogen concentration is increased in a number of conditions, but the urine test is usually preferred in these cases because of greater simplicity (see Chapter 2).

METHODOLOGY

Guaiac Test for Occult Blood

REAGENTS

1. 1:60 (w./v.) solution of gum guaiac in 95 per cent (v./v.) ethyl alcohol or, preferably, a saturated solution.
2. Glacial acetic acid.
3. 3 per cent (v./v.) hydrogen peroxide.

PROCEDURE

1. Place about 0.5 gm. of feces in a 10 × 100 mm. test tube.
2. Add about 2 ml. of tap water and mix with applicator sticks.
3. Add 0.5 ml. of glacial acetic acid and mix well.
4. Add about 2 ml. of the gum guaiac solution and mix well.
5. Add about 2 ml. of hydrogen peroxide and mix; start timer.
6. Observe for 2 minutes and record the maximal color development during that time as trace, 1+, 2+, 3+, or 4+, depending on the intensity of the blue color. Strongly positive reactions will fade rapidly and should be read according to maximal color development rather than the appearance at the end of the time period.
7. Reagents should be checked daily by testing a sample known to contain blood.

Hemoccult Slide Test for Occult Blood*

PROCEDURE

1. Collect a very small stool specimen on tip of wooden applicator.
2. Apply thin smear of specimen inside the circle.
3. Close cover; dispose of applicator.
4. Allow specimen to dry (important that specimen dry completely).
5. Open perforated window in back of slide.
6. Apply two or three drops of developing solution to slide opposite specimen.
7. Read results after 30 seconds.

Positive: Trace of blue indicates test is positive for occult blood.

Negative: No detectable blue anywhere on slide indicates test is negative for occult blood.

*Smith, Kline & French, Philadelphia.

D-Xylose Absorption Test (Roe and Rice, 1948)

PRINCIPLE. D-Xylose, 25 gm., is administered orally. Blood level is determined 2 hours later; urine excretion over a 5-hour postadministration period is also determined. Absorption proceeds normally even in presence of pancreatic steatorrhea. It is impaired in patients with enterogenous steatorrhea. Chemical determination depends on dehydration of pentose to furfural in the presence of acid, followed by condensation of furfural with p-bromoaniline to form a colored compound.

At 70° C. about 9 per cent of the available pentose is converted to furfural, but at this temperature very little furfural is formed from other precursors. p-Bromoaniline is used because it does not form any appreciable color with other substances; and thiourea, which is an antioxidant, also helps to prevent the formation of interfering colored compounds.

REAGENTS

1. Stock D-xylose standard solution (2 mg. per ml.). Place 0.500 gm. Pfanstiehl D-xylose in a 250-ml. volumetric flask. Add sufficient saturated benzoic acid solution to dissolve the D-xylose and dilute to the mark with saturated benzoic acid. Keep in refrigerator.

2. Working D-xylose standard (0.1 mg. per ml.). Transfer 10 ml. of stock standard to a 200 ml. volumetric flask and dilute to the mark with saturated benzoic acid solution. Keep in refrigerator.

3. Somogyi deproteinizing reagents (same as those used in Somogyi-Nelson blood glucose):

a. $ZnSO_4 \cdot 7\ H_2O$, 10.5 gm.; distilled water, 1000 ml.

b. $Ba\ (OH)_2 \cdot 8\ H_2O$, 9.5 gm.; distilled water, 1000 ml.

To adjust the solutions, remove 100 ml. from each. Using these solutions, titrate 10 ml. of the $ZnSO_4$ solution with the $Ba(OH)_2$ solution. Use 1 drop of 1 per cent alcoholic phenolphthalein as the indicator and the first faint pink as the endpoint. Dilute the remaining 900 ml. of the stronger solution so that 10 ml. of the $ZnSO_4$ requires 10 ml. (± 0.05 ml.) of the $Ba(OH)_2$ solution to neutralize it. Supernates using these solutions should be crystal clear.

4. Glacial acetic acid saturated with thiourea (Matheson, Coleman, and Bell); use approximately 4 gm. thiourea per 100 ml. glacial acetic acid. Keep 250 ml. on hand. It is stable.

5. D-Xylose color reagent. Make fresh just before use. Add 4 gm. p-bromoaniline (Eastman No. 473) to 200 ml. glacial acetic acid saturated with thiourea. This is enough for one complete set.

PROCEDURE. *Bedside*

1. Patient allowed nothing by mouth after midnight on the day of the test.

2. Between 8:00 and 9:00 A.M., have patient void. Discard urine.

3. Give patient 25 gm. of D-xylose dissolved in 250 ml. (8 oz.) of tap water. Follow immediately with an additional 250 ml. of tap water. Note time.

4. Exactly 2 hours following administration of D-xylose, draw 3 ml. of oxalated venous blood. This should be sent to the laboratory immediately.

5. Patient allowed no further fluid or food and is kept on bed rest or in a chair until completion of the test. Patient may experience a mild diarrhea later in the day from the D-xylose.

6. Save all urine voided during the test. Five hours after the test was started have the patient void. Add this urine to the rest. Send pooled urine to the laboratory immediately.

Laboratory

1. Prepare appropriate quantity of D-xylose color reagent.

2. Prepare a protein-free supernate 1:10 as follows: 1 ml. whole blood, 4.5 ml. $ZnSO_4$, 4.5 ml. $Ba(OH)_2$. Shake and centrifuge at 200 r.p.m. for 10 minutes.

3. Measure the volume of urine and prepare 1:50, 1:100, and 1:250 dilutions with distilled water.

4. Set up five sets of photometer tubes, three tubes in each set. Mark sets of three as follows: "standard," "1:50," "1:100," and "1:250."

5. Into each tube of the standard set pipette 2 ml. of the D-xylose working standard.

6. Into the other sets pipette 2 ml. of each of the dilutions of urine.

7. Set up a water bath at 70° C. It must be large enough to hold 10 photometer tubes. When the bath is at 70° C., pipette 10 ml. of the D-xylose color reagent into all 15 tubes. Mix all tubes and place the first two tubes of each set in the water bath. Maintaining bath at 70° C., heat tubes for 10 minutes. Cool tubes in running water to room temperature and replace in rack.

8. Place the rack containing the heated tubes and the unheated tubes in a dark place.

9. At the end of 70 minutes, read each set of tubes in the photometer, using the unheated tube of each set for the blank, with a 515 nm. filter.

10. Record average absorbance for each set and calculate results.

CALCULATIONS. *Abbreviations:* CS = concentration of standard (0.1 mg./ml.); AU = absorbance of unknown; AS = absorbance of standard.

Blood. Shown below.

Urine. Use the AU which most closely approaches the AS in the calculation shown at the top of the opposite page.

Blood

$$\frac{\text{CS} \times \text{AU}}{\text{AS}} = \frac{\text{mg. D-xylose}}{\text{aliquot (i.e., ml. supernate)}}$$

$$\frac{\text{mg. D-xylose}}{\text{aliquot}} \times \frac{\text{10 ml. supernatant}}{\text{1 ml. whole blood}} \times \frac{\text{100 ml. whole blood}}{\text{100 ml. whole blood}} = \frac{\text{mg. D-xylose}}{\text{100 ml. whole blood}}$$

Simplified

$$\frac{\text{AU}}{\text{AS}} \times 100 = \text{mg. D-xylose/100 ml. blood}$$

Urine

$$\frac{\text{CS} \times \text{AU}}{\text{AS}} = \frac{\text{mg. D-xylose}}{\text{aliquot (i.e., ml. dilute urine)}}$$

$$\frac{\text{mg. D-xylose}}{\text{aliquot}} \times \frac{\text{50, 100, or 250 ml. dil. urine}}{\text{ml. urine}} \times \frac{\text{ml. urine}}{\text{total urine vol.}} = \frac{\text{mg. D-xylose}}{\text{total urine vol.}}$$

Simplified:

$$\frac{0.1 \times \text{AU}}{\text{AS}} \times \text{volume (ml.) of urine dilution} \times \text{total volume (ml.) urine} = \frac{\text{mg. D-xylose}}{\text{per 5-hr. urine}}$$

INTERPRETATION

D-XYLOSE	2-HR. BLOOD (mg./dl.)	5-HR. URINE (gm.)
Normal	36 ± 16	6.5 ± 1.2
Sprue, untreated	12 ± 5	1.3 ± 0.7
Sprue, remission	19 ± 11	3.0 ± 1.2

Fecal Fat

Titrimetric Method of Van de Kamer (Van de Kamer et al., 1949)

PRINCIPLE. Fats and fatty acids are converted to soap by boiling with alcoholic potassium hydroxide. After cooling, excess hydrochloric acid is added to convert soaps to fatty acids. These are extracted with petroleum ether. An aliquot is evaporated, taken up in neutral alcohol, and titrated with sodium hydroxide. Fats are calculated as fatty acids.

PROCEDURE. All refluxing, evaporating, blending, and transferring of fecal emulsion should be done in a motorized hood. Ground glass joints are used throughout.

1. Weigh container in which stool is to be homogenized (paint can, blender, etc.) before use.
2. Blend, adding water to bring the consistency to that of ice cream mix.*
3. Reweigh container and contents.
4. Weigh 125-ml. flask with ground glass stopper.
5. Transfer (using open [broken] tip, 10-ml. serologic pipette, and rubber bulb) about 8 to 10 ml. of emulsion to weighed flask.
6. Reweigh flask, stopper, and contents.
7. Repeat steps 4 to 6 with a second flask.
8. Add 10 ml. 6 N KOH to each flask, using graduated cylinder.
9. Add 40 ml. ethanol with 0.4 per cent isoamyl alcohol to each flask, using graduated cylinder.
10. Add five glass beads to each flask.
11. Remove stopper from first flask, place on hot plate and couple to reflux condenser.
12. Reflux for 20 to 30 minutes.
13. Remove flask from condenser, replace stopper, place in ice bath. Place a strip of paper between the stopper and flask neck to prevent formation of a vacuum in the flask as it cools.
14. Connect second flask to condenser and reflux for 20 to 30 minutes.
15. When first flask has cooled to room temperature or below, add 17 ml. 6.8 N HCl, using graduated cylinder, and restopper (without paper).
16. When flask is again cold, add 50 ml. petroleum ether, using a rubber bulb and a 50-ml. transfer pipette.
17. Stopper and shake vigorously for 90 to 120 seconds by the clock.
18. When the upper petroleum ether has separated, transfer 25 ml. of this layer, using a rubber bulb and a 25-ml. transfer pipette, to a 125-ml. Erlenmeyer flask.
19. Connect flask (containing 25-ml. aliquot

*It has been suggested (Jover and Gordon, 1962) that coarse silica be added to the specimen (when using the paint can method) to hasten homogenization and dispersion of the feces. Cellulose gum is also added to stabilize the mixture. Ethanol is also added before blending.

of petroleum ether) to distilling apparatus. (Apparatus is a safety measure to minimize fire and explosion hazard from evaporated petroleum ether.) Place flask in 56° C. water bath. Evaporate almost to dryness.

20. Remove from bath, add 10 ml. ethanol, using a serologic pipette, rinsing down the sides of the flask with the alcohol.

21. Add 3 drops of 1 per cent alcoholic phenolphthalein indicator.

22. Titrate with standard NaOH to deep pink endpoint.

23. Repeat steps 13 and 15 to 22, inclusive, with second flask.

REAGENTS

1. KOH, aqueous 6 N (33 per cent w./v.).
2. Ethanol 95 per cent with 0.4 per cent isoamyl alcohol.
3. HCl 6.8 N (25 per cent w./v.).
4. Petroleum ether, B.P. 40 to 60° C. (approximately).
5. Ethanol 95 per cent, neutral.
6. One per cent alcoholic solution of phenolphthalein in dropper bottle.
7. Standard aqueous NaOH, approximately 0.1000 N.

EQUIPMENT

1. Hood.
2. Electric hot plate (about 500 watts).
3. Two ring stands – one burette clamp and one condenser clamp.
4. Ice bath.
5. Waring Blender, Osterizer, or equivalent.
6. Two-kg. platform balance and weights.
7. Glass beads.
8. Rubber bulb (or Propipette).
9. Two 125-ml. flasks, ground glass neck 24/40 (A. H. Thomas No. 5343). Two stoppers, ground glass (A. H. Thomas No. 9314-J).
10. One 50-ml. burette.
11. Two 125-ml. Erlenmeyer flasks.
12. One 25-ml. volumetric pipette and one 50-ml. volumetric pipette.
13. One 10-ml. serologic pipette with tip broken off (to transfer the fecal emulsion of step 5).
14. Two 10-ml. serologic pipettes.
15. One 50-ml. graduated cylinder and one 25-ml. graduated cylinder.
16. One distilling head (Claisen) with West condenser and ground glass joints 24/40 (Corning Cat. No. 3560).
17. One distilling tube with suction tube and ground glass joints 24/40 (Corning Cat. No. 9420).

CALCULATION

1. Calculate the total weight of the emulsion from steps 1 and 3.
2. Calculate the weights of aliquots in each flask from steps 4, 6, and 7.
3. Calculate ml. standard NaOH used to titrate the fatty acids in flasks from step 22.
4. Using the formula, calculate the $\frac{\text{gm. fatty acids}}{\text{24 hr.}}$ for each flask.
5. Average results and report as $\frac{\text{gm. total fat}}{\text{24 hr.}}$.

(In this method the gm. total fat is calculated as fatty acid.)

FORMULA. Shown at the bottom of this page.

EXPLANATION. Assumed average molecular weight of fatty acids is 284. When 50 ml. extract is made, 25 ml. is evaporated. A further correction is made for the partition of fatty acids between emulsion and petroleum ether.

NORMALS

Adults:

Fat intake gm./24 hr.	Fatty acids excreted gm./24 hr.	Per cent of intake excreted/24 hr.
50	2–3	4–6
100	4–5	4–5

Children: 5 per cent or less of daily dietary intake.

$$\frac{\text{gm. fatty acids}}{\text{24 hr.}} = \frac{\text{ml. NaOH used} \times \text{normality NaOH used} \times \text{gm. fecal emulsion} \times 0.5907}{\text{gm. of aliquot of emulsion taken} \times \text{number of days of collection}}$$

$$\frac{\text{gm. fatty acids}}{\text{24 hr.}} = \frac{\text{ml. NaOH used} \times \text{normality NaOH used}}{\text{25 ml. petroleum ether extract}} \times \frac{\text{50 ml. petroleum ether extract}}{\text{gm. aliquot of emulsion taken}} \times \frac{\text{gm. total fecal emulsion}}{\text{number of days of collection}} \times \frac{\text{1.04 gm. fatty acids (total)}}{\text{1.00 gm. fatty acids (extract)}} \times \frac{\text{284 gm. fatty acids}}{\text{1000 ml. NaOH}}$$

Fecal Reducing Substances

Clinitest for Reducing Substances in Stool (Kerry and Anderson, 1964)

PROCEDURE. Add 1 volume of stool to 2 volumes of distilled water and mix thoroughly. Transfer 15 drops of this suspension to a clean test tube and add a Clinitest tablet. The reaction and interpretation of results are described in the chapter on urinalysis.

INTERPRETATION. Presence of 0.25 gm./dl. reducing substance or less is considered normal; from 0.25 gm./dl. to 0.5 gm./dl. is regarded as suspicious; greater than 0.5 gm./dl. is interpreted as indicating abnormal amounts of sugar. Sucrose, of course, is not a reducing sugar and will not react in this test. However, in the case of sucrose intolerance, little sucrose but large amounts of glucose and fructose are found in the stool, presumably due to hydrolysis of sucrose by intestinal bacteria, so that the test is positive nonetheless.

Oral Lactose Tolerance Test (Basford and Henry, 1967). Following overnight fast, administer orally 50 gm. lactose dissolved in 400 ml. of water. Draw fasting blood and blood samples at 1, 2, and 3 hours after ingestion, as for a glucose tolerance test. Also collect a 5-hour stool specimen, examining and recording appearance, consistency, and pH.

Patients with lactase deficiency exhibit a peak rise less than 20 mg./dl. reducing substances expressed as glucose. In all persons with flat tolerance curves, the test should be repeated within two days and the less abnormal of the two curves used for interpretation. A control test may be performed, using 25 gm. glucose and 25 gm. galactose if the lactose test indicates malabsorption. Some investigators use a 100-gm. dose which has been reported by some to yield more definitive results. It may cause symptoms in cases of mild lactase deficiency. In children the dosage of lactose or other sugars is 2 gm./kg. of body weight.

Assay of Intestinal Disaccharidases (Dahlquist, 1968)

PRINCIPLE. Homogenized intestinal mucosa is incubated with disaccharides substrate; the enzyme is then inactivated, and the amount of liberated glucose is estimated photometrically by a second incubation step, using glucose oxidase, peroxidase, and a chromogen (Table 17–2).

METHODS. Preparation of intestinal homogenate. (Weigh and record specimen. Do not wash with water, as this may alter enzyme activity [Antonowicz *et al.*, 1970].) When a whole piece of intestine is available:

1. Scrape off the mucosa with a piece of glass.
2. Add four parts of distilled water.
3. Homogenize with an ultra-Turrax homogenizer.
4. Chill the mucosa and water well with crushed ice for at least 5 minutes before and during homogenization.
5. Centrifuge at 2000 to 4000 r.p.m. for 10 minutes in order to remove layer cell debris.

When only a very small amount of mucosa is available:

1. For 10 to 20 mg. of mucosa, add 0.5 ml. water.
2. Homogenize in a glass pestle homogenizer of Potter and Elvehjem, or in some similar type, for 1 to 2 minutes with motor giving speed of 200 to 300 r.p.m.
3. Chill the tube with its contents (including the pestle) with crushed ice for at least 5 minutes prior to homogenization and then during the whole homogenization procedure.

REAGENTS

1. Substrate. Maltose, sucrose, trehalose, lactose, and isomaltose are available commercially. Impurity of substrate will be revealed by a high blank reading in the assay procedure.
2. Buffer (sodium maleate buffer [0.1 M, pH 6.0]). Dissolve 1.16 gm. maleic acid in 15.3 ml. 1 N NaOH and dilute with distilled water

Table 17–2. DISACCHARIDASE ACTIVITIES AT THE LIGAMENT OF TREITZ IN 100 HEALTHY SUBJECTS*

DISACCHARIDASE	NO. OF SUBJECTS	ACTIVITY (WET WT.)					ACTIVITY (PROTEIN)				
		Mean	SD	SEM	Range	C†	Mean	SD	SEM	Range	C†
		(units/gm.)				(%)	(units/gm.)				(%)
Lactase	100	3.3	2.0	0.2	0–11.1	60.6	29.0	18.6	1.9	0– 82.8	64.1
Normal	94	3.5	1.9	0.2	0.7–11.1	54.2	30.9	17.6	1.8	3.0– 82.8	56.9
Deficient	6	0.2	0.2	0.07	0– 0.5	100.0	1.3	1.4	0.6	0– 4.1	108.0
Sucrase	100	5.9	2.3	0.2	1.2–14.0	39.0	51.3	22.9	2.3	4.6–121.0	44.6
Maltase	100	22.3	7.2	0.7	6.5–39.1	32.2	195.2	78.1	7.8	27.7–446.5	40.0
Isomaltase	14	7.2	2.6	0.7	3.0–12.1	36.1	67.3	19.4	5.2	28.5–103.0	28.8

*From Newcomer, A. D., and McGill, D. B.: Gastroenterology *53*:884, 1967.
†C, coefficient of variation (standard deviation:mean).

to 100 ml. Measure this pH and adjust, if necessary, to 6.0.

3. Substrate-buffer-solution. An 0.056 M solution of the appropriate disaccharide in 0.1 M sodium maleate buffer, pH 6.0. Substrate-buffer solutions are stored frozen in small aliquots.

4. Glucose oxidase reagents:

Stock solutions

a. Tris buffer (0.5 M, pH 7.0). Dissolve 61 gm. Tris in 85 ml. 5 N HCl and dilute with water to 1000 ml. Measure the pH and adjust, if necessary, to 7.0.

b. Peroxidase solution. Dissolve 10 mg. peroxidase (grade D, Worthington Biochemical Co., Freehold, N.J.) in water to 10 ml. Store frozen in small aliquots.

c. Detergent solution. Dissolve 20 gm. Triton X-100 (Rohm & Haas Co., Philadelphia, Pa.) in 80 gm. 95 per cent ethanol.

d. O-Dianisidine solution. Dissolve 100 mg. o-dianisidine (technical, Eastman, Rochester, N.Y.) in ethanol to 10 ml. Store in dark; discard when it becomes brown by oxidation.

Tris-glucose oxidase reagent (TGO-reagent)

Dissolve 2 mg. glucose oxidase 130,000 (Fermco Laboratories, Chicago, Illinois, 60680) in 100 ml. 0.5 M Tris buffer. Add 1.0 ml. o-dianisidine solution, 1.0 ml. detergent solution, and 0.5 ml. peroxidase solution. Mix well. This is stable for several days if stored in refrigerator. TGO reagent will interrupt disaccharidase activity.

Standard glucose solutions

Prepare solutions of glucose in distilled water containing:

a. 100 mg./ml.
b. 300 mg./ml.
c. 500 mg./ml.

Store frozen in small aliquots.

METHOD. The enzyme preparation should be diluted to contain a suitable activity of the disaccharidase to be assayed. If 1 molecule of glucose is formed per substrate molecule hydrolyzed, the diluted solution should contain somewhat less than 0.10 unit/ml.; if 2 molecules of glucose are formed, it should contain a little less than 0.05 unit/ml. When homogenates of peroral biopsy specimens are analyzed and have been prepared as described above, suitable dilutions for the different activities usually are about the following:

Maltase	1:50
Isomaltase	1:20
Sucrase (invertase)	1:10
Trehalase	1:5
Lactase	1:5
Cellobiase	1:2

The readings obtained with the incubated samples should not exceed the highest point of the standard curve. If they do, the enzyme must be further diluted and a new incubation performed.

1. Transfer to a conical test tube 100 μl. diluted enzyme solution.

2. Incubate in a 37° C. water bath for a few minutes to bring to temperature.

3. Add 100 μl. of substrate-buffer solution and mix. The reaction is started at this point.

4. Incubate for exactly 60 minutes.

5. Add 3.0 ml. TGO reagent. Mix well. This will immediately interrupt the disaccharidase reaction.

6. Let stand in the water bath at 37° C. for 60 minutes for development of color.

Blank

1. Transfer to a conical test tube, in order: 100 μl. diluted enzyme solution, 3 ml. TGO reagent, 100 μl. substrate-buffer solution.

2. Mix.

3. Incubate in 37° C. water bath for 60 minutes.

Reagent Blank

1. To a conical test tube add: 200 μl. distilled water, 3 ml. TGO reagent.

2. Mix.

3. Incubate in 37° C. water bath for 60 minutes.

After the development of color, measure in a spectrophotometer at 420 nm. against the reagent blank.

CALCULATION. 1 unit of enzyme hydrolyzes 1 μmol. disaccharide per minute. The disaccharidase activity per milliliter enzyme preparation is then calculated by the formula

$$10 \times \frac{a}{180} \times \frac{1}{60} \times \frac{1}{n} \times d \quad \text{or} \quad \frac{a \cdot d}{n \times 1080} \text{ units/ml.}$$

where:

a = μg. glucose liberated in 60 minutes (sample and blank).
d = dilution factor for the enzyme solution of which 100 μl. are used.
n = number of glucose molecules per molecules of disaccharide (for maltose, isomaltose, trehalose, and cellobiose, n = 2; for sucrose and lactose, n = 1).
180 = molecular weight of glucose
10 = factor to convert 0.1 ml. to 1.0 ml.

METHOD FOR ASSAY WITH A FINAL VOLUME OF 320 MICROLITERS. When limited amounts of material are available, as in the analysis of peroral biopsy specimens, amounts are employed which give a final volume of 320 μl.

In this procedure, special ultramicro test tubes are used. The tubes of the standard series will contain 2, 6, and 10 mg. glucose, respectively. All volumes in the procedure described above (I) are reduced tenfold. A spectrophotometer with an ultramicro cuvette is used for the readings. The disaccharidase activity is calculated in the following way (for symbols, see above).

$$100 \times \frac{a}{180} \times \frac{1}{60} \times \frac{1}{n} \times d \text{ or } \frac{a \cdot d}{n \cdot 108} \text{ units/ml.}$$

The disaccharidase unit is defined as the activity hydrolyzing μmol. of disaccharide per minute under the conditions used, i.e., temperature 37° C., substrate concentration 0.028 M, pH 6.0.

The disaccharidase unit is finally converted and expressed as units per gram (wet weight) or units per gram of protein. In the latter instance, protein content of the homogenate is measured.

DISCUSSION. These assay methods are performed in two separate incubation steps. Although accurate and sensitive, they are somewhat laborious and time-consuming. The one-stage ultramicro method is convenient and can be used for tiny tissue specimens obtained from peroral biopsy. However, maltase activity with this method was found to be 40 per cent lower than when measured with the micro method (Messer and Dahlquist, 1966).

Urobilinogen Method (Watson et al., 1944)

PROCEDURE

1. Weigh 10 gm. of feces in a 500-ml. Erlenmeyer flask.
2. Emulsify with 190 ml. of distilled water.
3. Add 100 ml. 20 per cent (w./v.) ferrous sulfate and 100 ml. 10 per cent (w./v.) sodium hydroxide.
4. Mix, stopper, and store in dark for 1 to 3 hours.
5. Filter and assay filtrate as by quantitative urine method.

CALCULATIONS. Calculate urobilinogen in filtrate (mg./100 ml.). Multiply by 40 (to correct for dilution). Report as mg. per 100 gm.

NOTE: The ferrous sulfate reduces urobilin (oxidized urobilinogen) back to urobilinogen. Further dilution of filtrate may be necessary when urobilinogen is present in high concentrations.

NORMAL RANGE. 75 to 350 mg. urobilinogen per 100 gm. of stool.

REFERENCES

Anderson, C. M., Messer, M., Townley, R. R. W., and Freeman, M.: Intestinal sucrase and isomaltase deficiency in two siblings. Pediatrics *31*:1003, 1963.

Anderson, C. M., Burke, V., Messer, M., and Kerry, K. R.: Sugar intolerance and celiac disease. Lancet *1*:1322, 1966.

Antonowicz, I., Ishida, S., Khaw, K. T., *et al.*: Effect of tissue preparation on determinations of disaccharidase activities in intestinal mucosa. Pediatrics *45*:104, 1970.

Basford, R. L., and Henry, J. B.: Lactose intolerance in the adult. Postgrad. Med. *41*:A70, 1967.

Benson, J. A., Jr., Culver, P. M., Ragland, S., *et al.*: The D-xylose absorption test in malabsorption syndromes. New Eng. J. Med. *256*:335, 1957.

Blumgart, L. H.: Faecal occult blood and ferrous fumarate. Brit. Med. J. *2*:1572, 1963.

Brayshaw, J. R., Harris, F., and McCurdy, P. R., *et al.*: The effect of oral iron therapy on stool guaiac and orthotolidine reactions. Ann. Intern. Med. *59*:172, 1963.

Bockus, H. L.: Gastroenterology. 2nd ed. Philadelphia, W. B. Saunders Company, 1964.

Cook, G. C., and Kajubi, S. K.: Tribal incidence of lactase deficiency in Uganda. Lancet *1*:725, 1966.

Dahlquist, A.: Assay of intestinal disaccharidases. Anal. Biochem. *22*:99, 1968.

Daniel, S. A., Jr., and Egan, S.: The quantity of blood required to produce a tarry stool. J.A.M.A. *113*:2232, 1939.

Davis, A. E., and Bolin, T.: Lactose intolerance in Asians. Nature (London) *216*:1244, 1967.

Davison, A. G. F., and Mullinger, M.: Reducing substances in neonatal stool detected by Clinitest. Pediatrics *46*:632, 1970.

Drummey, G. D., Benson, J. A., and Jones, G. M.: Microscopical examination of the stool for steatorrhea. New Eng. J. Med. *264*:85, 1961.

Ebaugh, F. G., Jr., Clements, T., Jr., Rodan, G., *et al.*: Quantitative measurement of gastrointestinal blood loss. Amer. J. Med. *25*:169, 1958.

Frazer, A. C.: Steatorrhea. Brit. Med. J. *2*:805, 1955.

Frazer, A. C., and Sammons, H. G.: Fat synthesis by intestinal bacteria. Clin. Chem. *2*:272, 1956.

Fall, D. J., Kuiper, D. H., and Pollard, H. M.: Use of isotopes in determining occult blood. Cancer *28*:135, 1971.

Goldman, P., Paver, W. K., and Corbett, W. H.: The detection of occult blood in the feces. Med. J. Aust. *1*:755, 1964.

Greegor, D. H.: Detection of silent colon cancer in routine examination. CA *19*:330, 1969.

Greegor, D. H.: Occult blood testing for detection of asymptomatic colon cancer. Cancer *28*:131, 1971.

Grossman, M. I., Matsumoto, K. K., and Lichter, R. J.: Fecal blood loss produced by oral and intravenous administration of various salicylates. Gastroenterology *40*:383, 1961.

Haverback, B. J., Dyce, B. J., Gutentag, P. J., *et al.*: Measurement of trypsin and chymotrypsin in stool. Gastroenterology *44*:588, 1963.

Hepler, O. E., Wong, P., and Pihl, H. D.: Comparison of tests for occult blood in feces. Amer. J. Clin. Path. *23*:1263, 1953.

Hoerr, S. O., Bliss, W. R., and Kauffman, J.: Clinical evaluation of various tests for occult blood in the feces. J.A.M.A. *141*:1213, 1949.

Johnstone, D. E.: Studies on cystic fibrosis of the pancreas. Amer. J. Dis. Child. *84*:191, 1952.

Jover, A., and Gordon, R. S., Jr.: Procedure for quantitative analysis of feces with special reference to fecal fatty acids. J. Lab. Clin. Med. *59*:878, 1962.

Kaijser, K., and Öckerman, P. A.: Diagnostic problems in glucose-galactose malabsorption. A case report. Acta Paediat. Scand. *59*:214, 1970.

Keusch, G., Troncale, T. J., Miller, L. H., *et al.*: Acquired lactose malabsorption in Thai children. Pediatrics *43*:540, 1969.

Kerry, K. R., and Anderson, C. M.: A ward test for sugar in faeces. Lancet *1*:981, 1964.

Kirschen, M., Sorter, H., and Necheles, M.: Occult blood, with note on the use of carmine for marking of stools. Amer. J. Dig. Dis. *9*:154, 1942.

Lang, D. J., Kunz, L. J., Martin, A. R., *et al.*: Carmine as a source of nosocomial salmonellosis. New Eng. J. Med. *276*:829, 1967.

Lebenthal, E., Garti, R., Mathoth, Y., *et al.*: Glucose-galactose malabsorption in an oriental-Iraqui Jewish family. J. Pediat. *78*:844, 1971.

Linqvist, B., and Meeuwisse, G. W.: Intestinal transport of monosaccharides in generalized and selective malabsorption. Acta Paediat. Scand. *146*(Suppl.):110, 1963.

McDougall, L. G.: Estimation of fat absorption from random stool specimens, measurement by zirconium-95 and iodine-131. Amer. J. Dis. Child. *108*:139, 1964.

Matsumoto, K. K., and Grossman, M. T.: Quantitative measurement of gastrointestinal blood loss during ingestion of aspirin. Proc. Soc. Exp. Biol. *102*:517, 1959.

Meeuwisse, G. W., and Melin, K.: Glucose-galactose malabsorption, a clinical study of 6 cases. Acta Paediat. Scand. *188*(Suppl.):3, 1969.
Meeuwisse, G. W., and Linqvist, B.: Glucose-galactose malabsorption – studies on the intermediate carbohydrate metabolism. Acta Paediat Scand. *59*:74, 1970.
Melin, K., and Meeuwisse, G. W.: Glucose-galactose malabsorption. A genetic study. Acta Paediat. Scand. *188*(Suppl.): 19, 1969.
Mendeloff, A. I.: Selection of a screening procedure for detection of occult blood in feces. J.A.M.A. *152*:798, 1953.
Messer, M., and Dahlqvist, A.: A one-step ultramicro method for the assay of intestinal disaccharidases. Anal. Biochem. *14*:376, 1966.
Newcomer, A. D., and McGill, D. B.: Disaccharidase activity in the small intestine: Prevalence of lactase deficiency in 100 healthy subjects. Gastroenterology *53*:881, 1967.
Ostrow, J. D., Mulvansy, C. A., and Hansell, J. R.: Sensitivity and reproducibility of guaiac Hematest, and Hemoccult test for fecal occult blood. Ann. Intern. Med. *76*:860, 1972.
Peranio, A., and Bruger, M.: The detection of occult blood in the feces including observation on the ingestion of iron and whole blood. J. Lab. Clin. Med. *38*:433, 1951.
Pihl, H. D., and Hepler, P. E.: Stains for fat in feces. Amer. J. Clin. Path. *23*:1273, 1953.
Pimparker, B. D., Tulsky, E. G., Kalser, M. H., *et al.*: Correlation of radioactive and chemical fecal fat determination in malabsorption syndrome. Amer. J. Med. *30*:910, 1961.
Roche, M., Perez-Gimenez, M. E., Layrisse, M., and DiPrisco, E.: Study of urinary and fecal excretion of radioactive chromium Cr^{51} in man. Its use in the measurement of intestinal blood loss associated with hookworm infection. J. Clin. Invest. *36*:1183, 1957.
Roe, J. H., and Rice, E. W.: Photometric method for determination of free pentose in animal tissue. J. Biol. Chem. *173*:507, 1948.
Rose, G. A.: Experiences with the use of interrupted carmine red and continuous chromium sesquioxide marking of human feces with reference to calcium, phosphorus, and magnesium. Gut *5*:274, 1964.
Rufin, F., Blahd, W. H., Nordyke, R. A., *et al.*: Reliability of I^{131}-triolein test in the detection of steatorrhea. Gastroenterology *41*:220, 1961.
Santiago-Borrero, P. J., Santini, R., Jr., and Maldonado, N.: The xylose excretion test in normal children and in pediatric patients with tropical sprue. Pediatrics *48*:59, 1971.
Schiff, L., Stevens, R. J., Shapiro, N., *et al.*: Observation on the oral administration of citrated blood in man: The effects on the stool. Amer. J. Med. Sci. *203*:409, 1942.
Spencer, R. P.: Use of radioisotopes in evaluation of the gastrointestinal canal. *In* Behrens, C. F., King, E. R., and Carpender, J. W. J.: Atomic Medicine. 5th ed. Baltimore, The Williams & Wilkins Co., 1969, pp. 672–694.
Thompson, H. L., and McGuffin, D. W.: Melena, a study of underlying causes. J.A.M.A. *141*:1208, 1949.
Tuna, N., Mangold, H. K., and Mosser, D. G.: Re-evaluation of the I^{131}-triolein absorption test. J. Lab. Clin. Med. *61*:620, 1963.
Van de Kamer, J. H., ten Bokkel Huinink, H., and Weyers, H. A.: Rapid method for the determination of fat in feces. J. Biol. Chem. *177*:347, 1949.
Watson, C. J., Schwartz, S., Sbarov, V., *et al.*: Studies of urobilinogen. V. A simple method for the quantitative recording of the Ehrlich reaction as carried out with urine and feces. Amer. J. Clin. Path. *14*:605, 1944.
Webb, R. L.: Determination of fecal lipids. Amer. J. Med. Tech. *25*:179, 1959.
Weber, P. M., O'Reilly, S., Pollycove, M., *et al.*: Gastrointestinal absorption of copper. Studies with ^{64}Cu, ^{95}Zr. A wholebody counter and the scintillation camera. J. Nucl. Med. *10*:591, 1969.
Weijers, H. A., Van de Kamer, J. H., and Ijsseling, J.: Diarrhea caused by deficiency of sugar splitting enzyme. Acta Paediat. *50*:55, 1961.
Wells, C. L., Moran, T. J., and Cooper, W. M.: Villous tumors of the rectosigmoid colon with severe electrolyte imbalance, a cause of unexplained morbidity and sudden mortality. Amer. J. Clin. Path. *37*:507, 1962.
Wollaeger, E. E., Comfort, M. W., and Osterberg, A. E.: Total solids, fat and nitrogen in the feces. III. A study of normal person taking a test diet containing a moderate amount of fat, comparison with result obtained with normal person taking a diet containing a large amount of fat. Gastroenterology *9*:272, 1947.
Wolochow, D. A.: A rapid method for quantitative determination of fecal fat based on the principle of electrical capacitance. J. Lab. Clin. Med. *65*:334, 1965.

Chapter 18

MEDICAL MICROBIOLOGY

by JAMES G. SHAFFER, Sc.D., and MILTON GOLDIN, Ph.D.

Medical microbiology, like all the divisions of the clinical laboratory, has undergone remarkable changes in recent years. These changes have resulted from the effects of a variety of developments that range all the way from the changes in microbial disease wrought by the introduction of modern medical and public health measures to the introduction of new techniques, reagents, and specialized media.

In Chapter 22, Hospital Epidemiology, there is a discussion of the changes in the patient population of the hospital that have resulted from the introduction of many lifesaving and preventive methods in medicine and public health and the impact of these changes on the problems of infection control in the hospital. To a great extent these alterations mirror the situation in the general population. The use of antibiotics and vaccines and the application of sound principles of environmental sanitation and preventive medicine have conspired to relegate most of the acute, fulminating, and highly contagious bacterial diseases to a position of rather minor importance. The bacteriologic issue with these diseases was relatively simple; e.g., in lobar pneumonia, clinical evidence coupled with a gram-stained sputum was more often than not diagnostic, and much the same situation, with some variations, was true with streptococcal infections and diphtheria.

Today the microbiologic aspects of disease are likely to be merely a part of a complex circumstance in which a series of events or an involved set of simultaneously existing facets may allow any one of a considerable group of microbial agents to enter the picture, not as primary causative agents, but as secondary contributors to the patient's total syndrome. This makes the interpretation of cultures more difficult than was the case in the past. It requires that those responsible for the operation of a clinical microbiologic laboratory be thoroughly familiar with the most modern aspects of microbial disease.

It is no longer possible to classify microorganisms that are associated with man as either pathogens or nonpathogens. The determination of a causative role often depends on the circumstances in which an organism occurs rather than on its nature. Microbial agents that were formerly considered to be seldom, if ever, associated with disease are being consistently identified with clinical syndromes. Many of these are members of the so-called normal flora, and some are organisms that for one reason or another were little known in the past. A number of factors are responsible for this. First, as a result of the fact that life is being prolonged, individuals are developing susceptibility to microbial disease that did not exist, at least to the same extent, in the past. Persons with metabolic problems, debilitated individuals, and those on steroid therapy or other therapy that depresses the normal immune mechanism are prone to microbial disease, presumably because the host offers the agent an opportunity for excessive propagation. In some cases one suspects that the organisms have always had the potential but were masked by the presence of other organisms that are now being eliminated, either by antibiotics or other means of control. Second, the extensive use of antibiotics has resulted in changes in the types of certain organisms, notably *Staphylococcus aureus*, to the extent that these organisms have taken on new importance. In the case of *S. aureus*, it appears that the extensive use of antibiotics allowed those that were, for one reason or another, able to resist the effects of these agents the opportunity to become widely distributed in the population. Another outgrowth of the effects of the use of antibiotics was to reveal more clearly the importance of the aftereffects of microbial infection. The outstanding example of this is rheumatic fever and glomerulonephritis, which are well-recognized sequelae of streptococcal infection.

The classic view of the host-parasite relationship as it applies to microbial disease needs some modification for the present and future understanding of the disease process. The contagiousness of microbial agents no longer occupies the major position it once did, and the needs for isolation and quarantine are not so great. The types of organisms involved most frequently are ubiquitous in their distribution, either as a part of the normal human body flora or in the environment. Although transmission of such organisms from person to person and from the environment to an individual is a part of the epidemiology of microbial disease, it does not have the critical implication that existed when the acute, fulminating microbial diseases were prominent. The conversion of infection into disease is a complex process that depends on a number of determinants which exist or pre-existed in the host, into which a certain number of a given microorganism are introduced at an appropriate time. Indeed, the organism may already be present in the host when the circumstances become such as to allow an opportunity for excessive propagation. It is to be suspected that the characteristics of the organism, although important, are not so important as the host. Although these complex determinants apply also to the acute, fulminating microbial diseases, as has eloquently been pointed out by Dubos, their importance becomes greater in the more chronic conditions that are presently more common.

It is probably not surprising to find that the more chronic microbial diseases do not respond to treatment so dramatically as the acute conditions. There are probably several reasons for this. Antibiotics notoriously exert their maximum effects on actively propagating bacteria, and this situation is much more likely to exist in an acute, fulminating disease; in chronic disease there is much more chance for the infection to be walled off by a tissue response or to reside in an area where adequate levels of an antibiotic are difficult to obtain; the organisms involved are less sensitive to the commonly used antibiotics.

One also finds a less direct correlation between *in vitro* susceptibility test results and the result of clinical use of antibiotics in certain types of low-grade chronic disease. Discrepancies occur with some frequency in urinary tract infections and in gastrointestinal conditions, especially where members of the genus *Salmonella* are involved. More will be said about this in the section on antibiotic susceptibility testing.

The epidemiology of certain infectious processes has changed over the years. Such changes have been mediated, not only by medical and public health practices, but also by technologic developments. One example of this seems to be the effects on the distribution of *Salmonella* that have occurred as a result of the widespread use of powdered eggs and the mass production, packaging, and distribution of frozen poultry. Salmonellosis no longer has quite the kind of seasonal variation it once had. Sporadic cases and outbreaks may occur year round. The occurrence of outbreaks of disease caused by enteropathogenic *E. coli* perhaps represents another instance where a combination of factors has allowed an organism to emerge as a recognized epidemiologic entity. No doubt this group of organisms does not represent a new variant, having probably been in existence for a long time. One could visualize that the combination of crowded nurseries, some laxity in techniques, and other unrecognized factors has conspired to reveal this organism as a pathogenic entity.

The appearance of resistant variants of the classic bacterial species requires constant surveillance and evaluation. The recent history of *Staphylococcus aureus* has been well documented. It would appear that, after several years of increasing resistance to certain antibiotics, there was a downward trend. This trend seemed to correlate with the development of penicillins that were not subject to the effects of penicillinase.

Mention has already been made of certain bacteria, some of which have been known for a long time, but which now are assuming increased importance. These include *Serratia, Flavobacterium, Listeria,* and the *Mima-Herellea* group. Increasing numbers of reports of the involvement of these bacteria in disease processes make it imperative that laboratories be equipped to isolate and identify them. With the identification of *Mycoplasma pneumoniae* and its role in primary atypical pneumonia, there arises the question as to what other members of this genus may have roles in human disease. There is also a need to define more clearly the possible relations or differences between mycoplasma, PPLO (pleuropneumonia-like organisms), and the L-forms that are a part of some sort of bacterial life cycle.

The so-called atypical acid-fast bacteria represent another relatively new complication. Laboratories must be alert to their presence and must be capable of identifying them according to group. These may be organisms that have existed for a long time, or variants that have emerged as a result of new means of therapy. Whatever their origin, their potential in human disease needs to be defined. At the present time this definition hinges on relating their presence to the clinical condition of the patient. Further study of the relationship between these organisms and the other mycobacteria, both classically recognized pathogens and essentially nonpathogenic species, is necessary.

GENERAL METHODS

Speed and accuracy have always been of great importance in the clinical bacteriology laboratory, and the advent of numerous specific chemotherapeutic and antibiotic drugs has served to re-emphasize this need. Improved methods for the isolation and identification of microorganisms are constantly being developed, and it is imperative that medical bacteriologists constantly reevaluate their techniques with the view of adapting new equipment and media to their own routines. Fortunately, improved media both for routine and special purposes are now available in dehydrated form or already prepared in tubes or plates and can be obtained from several commercial sources. It is no longer necessary, and in most cases is not desirable, to go through the time-consuming procedure of preparing media from basic ingredients.

In some cases the direct gram-stained smear may permit tentative identification of an organism, but most often culture on appropriate media is essential for both the tentative and final identifications. To that end, appropriate inoculations on certain basic media have to be made. In order to choose the proper procedure, the nature and source of the material to be cultured must be known, and some information about the condition of the patient should be available. The latter will help to select the suitable type of examination and the most direct approach for the isolation and identification of the offending microorganism.

There are points in the operation of a diagnostic microbiologic laboratory that cannot be overemphasized. Proper collection of material for examination and its transport to the laboratory are of utmost importance. No matter how good the methods used in the laboratory, it is not possible to get satisfactory results with specimens that are collected improperly or delayed unduly in arriving at the laboratory. Under no circumstances should a specimen arriving at the laboratory with any of the infectious material on the outside of the container be accepted, because there may be potentially serious consequences to those handling the specimen. Thus, there should be complete understanding and free exchange of information between the physician and those examining the material in the laboratory both before and during the course of the procedure.

In the laboratory the proper operation depends upon the availability of proper materials. In the actual operation it is, of course, essential to adequately organize, standardize, and develop the technique of preparation, staining, and culturing specimens. Accuracy, speed, and efficiency are to be emphasized. The prompt recording and reporting of results are important. When possible, interim reports can be of great assistance.

In smaller laboratories, physicians' offices, and clinics where space, time, and personnel are limited, it is possible to accomplish a great deal with simple methods and a minimum of material. In larger laboratories more extensive procedures can be made available and more extensive service offered. The size of the laboratory does not necessarily determine the amount or quality of the services rendered, for experience, organization, and ingenuity can accomplish a great deal.

GENERAL TECHNIQUES OF MICROBIOLOGIC EXAMINATIONS

Sterilization

There are four general methods of achieving sterilization, each of which has its special advantages, depending on the material and its projected use. These are moist heat (autoclaving or inspissating), dry heat (oven), filtration, and use of chemical agents.

Moist heat sterilizing is most frequently accomplished by using steam under pressure in an autoclave. Many types and sizes of autoclaves are used: horizontal or vertical, single or double wall, gas or electrically heated, or operated on a steam line (Fig. 18–1). The standard autoclaving procedure requires a pressure of 15 p.s.i. and a temperature of 121° C. for 15 minutes for most materials. In manually operated autoclaves it is imperative that all the air be allowed to escape before closing the escape valve, since air-steam mixtures will not produce the required temperature even though the pressure is the required 15 p.s.i. When large quantities of material are being autoclaved, it may be necessary to sterilize for more than 15 minutes to insure proper sterility. One can use indicators of various types that are designed to record the temperature reached inside the loads being sterilized.

Most routine media and solutions used in the laboratory may be sterilized by autoclaving. However, certain media containing carbohydrates, serum, or egg, and solutions of vitamins or other growth factors may be damaged by the autoclave temperature. Such materials may be sterilized by filtration or inspissation.

Glassware may be sterilized in the autoclave, but it is then necessary to provide some means

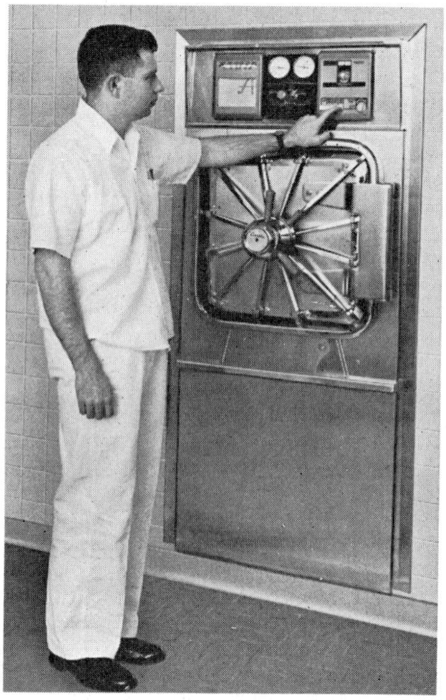

Figure 18–1. Modern laboratory autoclave with automatic controls. (Courtesy of the Castle Company, Rochester, New York.)

of drying. Most double wall autoclaves can be run under vacuum and evacuated after the sterilization is complete in order to remove moisture.

Dry heat sterilization is accomplished in an oven, operated by either gas or electricity. Such sterilization requires a higher temperature and a longer time than autoclaving. A good standard to use is 160° C. for 2 hours. This temperature will not char paper, cotton, or gauze. In packing material in an oven for sterilization, it is important to leave adequate space on the shelves to allow for free circulation of air. If this is not done, the material on the lower shelves closest to the source of heat will get too hot, while the upper shelves may not reach the required temperature.

Test tubes, pipettes, Petri dishes, flasks, syringes, and needles should be sterilized in dry heat, since it is desirable that these materials be dry for use and for storage. Rubber goods and certain other materials are adversely affected and must not be sterilized in an oven.

Handling Contaminated Materials

The problem of disposal of contaminated glassware, media, swabs, and specimen cartons in a laboratory is of considerable importance in order to avoid spread of infectious material throughout the laboratory area and its surroundings and to avoid cross-contamination of media, which may result in serious errors. Porcelain or stainless steel containers with snug-fitting tops are needed for the discard of contaminated glassware. Butcher pans, which can be obtained from restaurant supply houses, are quite good. For pipettes one can use cylindrical jars or rectangular pans containing disinfectant. These items should be placed conveniently to provide ready access. Once an item is discarded, it should never be removed from the discard pan until the pan and its contents have been autoclaved. After autoclaving, the glassware can be removed and washed. Bags of autoclavable plastic are now available and are very convenient for disposal of contaminated material.

Specimen cartons, applicators, tongue depressors, cotton, and similar materials should be autoclaved as soon as possible rather than incinerated before they are discarded.

Preparation and Sterilization of Media

The principles of preparing, dispensing, and sterilizing media are essentially the same, whether one uses the dehydrated form or starts from the beginning and adds the various ingredients separately. All the basic media contain a peptone and certain salts to which may be added growth promoting substances or agar, depending on the need. Since numerous peptones of superior quality are now available commercially, it is no longer necessary to prepare infusions and extracts.

Instructions for reconstituting dehydrated media are given on the label of each bottle, and it is only necessary to weigh out the required amount of the powder and to add distilled water. It is important to use a flask of sufficient size to allow adequate stirring or shaking to dissolve the medium. For example, if one is making 1 liter of medium, it is desirable to use a 2-liter flask. If the medium does not contain agar, it may dissolve without heating, but all media containing agar require the application of heat to raise the temperature to boiling. This heating should never be done over an open flame, because there is danger of scorching the medium or breaking the flask. The flask should be placed in a boiling water bath and stirred or shaken thoroughly at frequent intervals until the agar is melted. One can determine when the agar is melted by inspecting the sides of the flask during shaking. If flecks of agar can be seen, the agar is obviously not melted and heating should be continued. These media should be dispensed into appropriate containers while still hot, else they will solidify. If prolonged heating is used, volume may be decreased owing to evaporation and it may be necessary to add distilled water to replace the loss.

Except under special circumstances, no pH adjustment is necessary with dehydrated media. When this is necessary or when one starts with basic ingredients, relatively simple methods of adjustment are available.

The methods of dispensing the dissolved media into tubes or flasks depends on the type of medium and the purpose for which it is to be used. Fluid media (e.g., infusion broth) may be pipetted into tubes using a serologic pipette or an automatic pipette calibrated to deliver the desired amount. It is not necessary to use sterile tubes for this purpose, although at times this has considerable advantage, especially in handling material that needs to be inspissated. One may use specially constructed flasks with delivery tubes at the bottom to which is attached a standard glass filling device.

Media containing sufficient agar to be solid on cooling (1.5 per cent or more) are used ordinarily for agar slants or Petri dishes. For slants the medium is dispensed into test tubes, autoclaved in the vertical position, and then cooled in a slanted position. The amount of medium per tube is determined by the length of slant and butt desired. To pour Petri plates, the agar medium must first be sterilized in flasks or tubes and then poured to a depth of about 3 mm. into sterile plates. The melted agar is cooled to 50 to 55° C. before pouring the plates to prevent condensation of moisture on the walls of the container. Semisolid media (0.1 to 0.5 per cent agar) are tubed and sterilized in the same manner as fluid media.

It is often necessary to add carbohydrates or other substances to media for special studies. In some instances these materials can be weighed and dissolved in the medium before sterilization, but in other cases heat may adversely affect the substance and it must be added aseptically to the sterilized base. For carbohydrate fermentation tests it is necessary to use a base medium free of carbohydrate to which the desired carbohydrate, such as dextrose or maltose, is then added to produce a 0.5 to 1.0 per cent concentration. It is convenient to add the desired carbohydrate aseptically (using a filtered 10 to 20 per cent solution) to a previously sterilized base medium. Such base media containing an indicator (bromthymol blue, bromcresol purple, or phenol red) are readily available. The indicator changes color when acid is produced by bacteria.

To detect gas production, one can place an inverted vial or Durham tube (3 by 20 mm.) in the medium. When autoclaved, this vial fills with medium. Gas production is indicated when a bubble of gas appears in the vial after bacterial propagation. If one uses semisolid agar (0.3 to 0.5 per cent agar), the vial is unnecessary, because gas production will be revealed by bubbles in the medium.

There are now available sterile discs of dehydrated fermentation media, which, when added aseptically to tubes with sterile distilled water, provide a medium for fermentation tests. There are also discs containing various carbohydrates that may be added to a suitable base in the same manner or may be placed on agar plates. These materials seem ideally suited for use in smaller laboratories.

For sterilization of media, in most cases autoclaving at 15 p.s.i. for 15 minutes is satisfactory. If the medium is in screw-cap tubes, the caps should be left loose before autoclaving and tightened after removal from the autoclave. Some carbohydrates and other materials are changed or destroyed by the high temperatures. Inspissation should be used with all media containing ingredients that would be adversely affected by autoclaving.

pH Determination. Determination of the pH after growth of a culture can be done by taking aliquots and testing them in a potentiometer. Proper precautions must be taken when testing cultures of pathogenic bacteria. A simpler method is the spot plate procedure. One loopful of culture is placed in the concave depression of a white porcelain plate. One drop of indicator solution is mixed and the pH estimated by noting the resulting color and comparing it to the color chart for the indicator used. Another procedure is to add 1 or more drops of indicator solution to 1.0-ml. aliquots of the culture that have been transferred to small test tubes. The same amount of indicator solution is added to 1.0-ml. volumes of standard buffer solutions in similar tubes. The standard tube most closely matching the unknown is determined by visual examination.

In the case of the *Clostridia* it is best to read the pH after growth by the spot plate procedure just described, because many strains will destroy the indicator in the media rapidly and thus give erroneous results.

Preparation of Blood and Chocolate Agar. Media containing whole blood are the most commonly employed in the diagnostic laboratory. The type of blood, the agar base, and the technique of preparation are very important for the proper isolation of microorganisms.

There seems to be general agreement that defibrinated sheep blood is the most desirable for use in making blood and chocolate agar. Certain laboratories may have difficulty in obtaining sheep blood and may find it necessary to use human, rabbit, or horse blood. The advantages of sheep blood are consistency in the hemolysis seen with the streptococci, staphylococci, *Listeria*, etc., and its ability to support propagation of a wide variety of organisms. Also *Hemophilus hemolyticus*, the colonies of which resemble beta hemolytic streptococci, is inhibited.

The blood should not be more than a few days old and preferably defibrinated. If the blood is too old, the red cells are likely to be fragile and may hemolyze, making the blood agar unsuitable for use.

There are several good blood agar bases that can be obtained commercially.

To make blood agar, the sterile blood agar base contained in a flask is melted in a boiling water bath and cooled to 50 to 55° C. Blood is then added to the melted agar (5 ml. of blood per 100 ml. of medium) and thoroughly mixed by rotating the flask. After it is mixed, the agar is carefully poured into sterile Petri dishes to a depth of one-eighth to one-fourth inch. The depth to which the plate is poured is of considerable importance, since one is often interested in the presence or absence of hemolysis. If the agar is too thick, the hemolysis may be missed. Too vigorous shaking should be avoided, since air bubbles may make the agar rough. Air bubbles that do appear in the plates may be removed by passing a Bunsen flame quickly over the surface before the agar has set. Some workers prefer to place a layer of plain agar over the bottom of the plate and superimpose a thin layer of 10 per cent blood agar over this.

To make chocolate agar, the flask containing the medium with blood added is placed in a water bath at 70° C. and shaken gently until it has attained a definite chocolate color. This takes usually about 5 minutes. Excessive heating should be avoided. The agar should then be cooled to 50 to 55° C., supplements such as Isovitalex* or various antibiotics such as bacitracin added, if desired, and poured into Petri dishes.

Blood and chocolate agar plates can be stored in the refrigerator for several days, but should not be used if there is evidence of excessive drying or if the blood has darkened or otherwise changed its appearance. All blood and chocolate agar plates should be incubated overnight and checked for sterility before use.

Preparation of Coagulated Serum or Egg Media. The preparation of Loeffler's serum medium and coagulated egg media requires special technique. The ingredients are mixed thoroughly, avoiding bubbles, and tubed in the same manner as for other media. Because these media coagulate on heating, they must be slanted during heating. They are coagulated on the first day and are then heated in the inspissator on the two succeeding days for 1 hour each day.

An autoclave can be used with this type of medium, but special procedures are necessary. Layers of tubes should be placed in an enamel pan in a slanted position with several thicknesses of newspaper or similar material beneath the bottom layer of tubes, between the layers of tubes, and above the top layer to prevent too rapid heating or cooling. Not more than two layers of tubes should be used, for otherwise the insulating effect may prevent sufficient heating of both layers. Some workers use other materials but paper serves well. The autoclave is first brought up to 15 p.s.i. without releasing the air from the inner chamber. After about 15 minutes the air is slowly released, maintaining the pressure at 15 p.s.i. until the air has all been replaced with steam and the temperature has reached 121° C. This temperature is then maintained for 15 minutes and the pressure allowed to fall slowly. If these media are made in screw-cap tubes, the tubes may be stored at 4° C. for long periods of time.

*Bioquest, Cockeysville, Maryland.

Quality Control in Clinical Microbiology

Quality control is firmly established in most branches of the clinical laboratory, but presents certain difficulties in the microbiology laboratory. Microbiology is essentially qualitative in nature rather than quantitative and adequate reference material has not always been readily available. Reference bacteria with reproducible reactions are now available in the form of dried discs or lyophilized cultures and are very useful.* Cultures are also obtainable from the American Type Culture Collection, Rockville, Maryland, and other type culture collections. Proficiency surveys in microbiology such as those conducted by the American Society of Clinical Pathologists and the College of American Pathologists and state and federal agencies are of inestimable value in pinpointing areas of deficiency.

It should also be remembered that there are no "normal" values in microbiology, either in terms of numbers or types of organisms present in many types of cultures. Thus, there is really no such thing as a normal throat or stool culture. In some specimens, such as in cerebrospinal fluid, the presence of any microorganism should be viewed with great suspicion. In others, such as the urine, there are certain rough quantitative guidelines that one may use. It is imperative that the medical microbiologist recognize all the facets of the significance or lack of significance in various cultural situations.

The following represents only a partial list of areas that should be monitored and controlled in a systematic fashion. All checks should be recorded in writing, and any dis-

*Roche Diagnostics; Difco; Hyland Laboratories.

crepancies from acceptable standards should be reported promptly to the responsible individual and steps taken to correct them.

1. Collection and transmission of specimens; types of containers; adequacy of sample, and so forth.
2. Methodology of processing specimens.
3. Reporting and interpretation of results.
4. Culture media, both dehydrated and prepared, before and after sterilization.
5. Reagents.
6. Staining procedures.
7. Antimicrobial susceptibility test methods (p. 1008).
8. Safety precautions—disinfection, decontamination, safety hoods, air filters, and so forth.
9. Hospital infection surveillance program (see Chapter 22).
10. Autoclaves and adequacy of sterilization procedures.
11. Equipment—microscopes, incubators, water baths, refrigerators, freezers, and so forth.

It is obvious that each quality control program must be established individually, since laboratories vary so widely in their physical facilities and personnel. Detailed discussion of this subject is beyond the scope of this chapter. Much useful material will be found in Bartlett *et al.*, 1968; Russell *et al.*, 1969; Glaser *et al.*, 1971; and Vera, 1971.

Methods of Examination of Specimens

The examination of specimens received in the microbiology laboratory involves two general types of procedure. First, they may be examined by direct smear, stained or unstained, and, second, they may be cultured on appropriate media.

When certain specimens are being submitted for bacteriologic or mycologic examination, properly prepared and stained preparations may give excellent leads as to what media to inoculate or what further examination can be done. A preliminary report on such observations may, as in the case of spinal fluid, urethral smears, and sputum, be of great value to the physician in the management of the patient.

Clean slides must be used to make smears, and the slide must be marked adequately for identification and for delineation of the area in which the smear is to be placed. A slide may be divided into several sections with a marking pencil and several smears placed on the same slide, provided they are all to be stained identically.

One or two inoculating loopfuls of the material to be smeared are spread evenly over the designated area of the slide and allowed to dry. The dried smear is then passed rapidly through a flame to heat-fix the material to the slide.

There are several staining procedures used in bacteriologic work, the most common and useful being that of Gram or one of its many modifications. Loefflers' methylene blue, the acid-fast stain, spore stains, capsule stains, and flagella stains may be useful for special purposes. Organisms of known staining characteristics should be included as a staining control.

Gram staining is most likely to yield valuable information and should be done in all cases when staining is indicated. It is also used routinely for the examination of cultures to determine purity and for purposes of identification. Two of the best modifications of the Gram stain follow:

Hucker's Modification of Gram's Stain

SOLUTIONS

1. Ammonium oxalate crystal violet:

Solution A:

Crystal violet (certified)	2 gm.
Ethyl alcohol (95 per cent)	20 ml.

Solution B:

Ammonium oxalate	0.8 gm.
Distilled water	80 ml.

Mix solution A and B, store for 24 hr., and filter through paper.

2. Iodine solution (mordant):

Iodine	1 gm.
Potassium iodide	2 gm.
Distilled water	300 ml.

Grind iodine and potassium iodide in mortar, adding water a few milliliters at a time until dissolved. Store in dark bottle.

3. Counterstain:

Safranine O (2.5 per cent solution in 95 per cent ethyl alcohol)	10 ml.
Distilled water	100 ml.

PROCEDURE. After the smear has been dried and heat-fixed, proceed as follows:

1. Stain smears 1 minute with the crystal violet solution.
2. Wash briefly in tap water.
3. Add iodine solution and let stand for 1 minute.
4. Wash in tap water.
5. Decolorize until the solvent flows colorlessly from the slide. Wash briefly with acetone, or a mixture of equal parts of acetone and alcohol.
6. Counterstain 10 seconds with safranine.
7. Wash in tap water.
8. Dry and examine.

RESULTS. Gram-positive organisms stain blue; gram-negative, red.

Burke's Modification. This modification of the

Gram stain has the advantage that all solutions are aqueous and the decolorization is more vigorous, resulting in easier differentiation of the organisms in thick preparations.

SOLUTIONS

1. Alkaline crystal violet:

Solution A:

Crystal violet	1 gm.
Distilled water	100 ml.

Solution B:

$NaHCO_3$	5 gm.
Distilled water	100 ml.
Add Merthiolate (1:20,000)	

2. Iodine solution:

Iodine	1 gm.
KI	2 gm.
Distilled water	200 ml.

3. Decolorizing solution:

Ether	1 volume
Acetone	3 volumes

4. Counterstain:

Safranine O (85 per cent dye content)	0.5 gm.
Distilled water	100 ml.

PROCEDURE

1. Flood slide with solution A. Then add 3 to 5 drops of solution B, depending on the size of the flooded area, and allow to stand 1 minute. Wash well with water.
2. Cover with iodine solution and let stand 1 minute or longer.
3. Rinse with water.
4. Decolorize at once with the ether-acetone mixture, adding it to the slide drop by drop until no more color comes off in the drippings. Care must be taken to avoid excessive decolorization.
5. Wash with water.
6. Counterstain 10 to 15 seconds with the safranine O.
7. Wash in tap water.
8. Dry and examine.

RESULTS. Gram-positive organisms stain blue; gram-negative, red.

Spore Stain (Schaeffer and Fulton's Method). Malachite green (5 per cent) in distilled water. When freshly prepared allow to stand one-half hour and filter.

Safranine (0.5 per cent) in distilled water.

Flood the fixed smear with malachite green and steam gently over the flame for one-half minute. Wash thoroughly with water. Stain with safranine for one-half minute. Wash, blot, dry, and examine. Spores stain green; bacilli, red.

Spore Stain (Bartholomew and Mittwer's Method)

PROCEDURE

1. Fix the smear by passing through flame.
2. Stain 10 minutes with saturated aqueous malachite green (@ 7.6 per cent) without heat.
3. Rinse about 10 seconds with tap water.
4. Counterstain 15 seconds in 0.25 per cent aqueous safranine.
5. Rinse and dry.

RESULT. Spores stain green; rest of cell, red.

Capsule Stain (Hiss)

SOLUTION

Basic fuchsin (90 per cent dye content)	0.15 to 0.3 gm.
Crystal violet (85 per cent dye content)	0.05 to 0.1 gm.
Distilled water	100 ml.

PROCEDURE

1. Grow organisms in ascitic fluid or serum medium, or mix with drop of serum and prepare smears from this mixture.
2. Dry smears in air and fix with heat.
3. Stain with one of the above solutions a few seconds by gently heating until stain rises.
4. Wash off with 20 per cent aqueous $CuSO_4 \cdot 5\ H_2O$.
5. Blot dry and examine.

RESULT. Capsules stain faint blue; cells, dark purple.

Capsule Stain (Muir's Method)

MORDANT

Tannic acid	2 parts
Saturated aqueous solution of mercuric chloride	2 parts
Saturated aqueous solution of potassium alum	5 parts

PROCEDURE

1. Prepare an even thin film of the bacteria. Allow to dry with heating. Cover the film or smear with a strip of filter paper cut to the shape and size of the slide and flood with Ziehl-Neelsen carbolfuchsin. Warm with a flame until it just steams for 30 seconds.
2. Rinse gently with alcohol, then with water.
3. Add the mordant for 15 to 30 seconds and wash well with water.
4. Decolorize with alcohol until faintly pink.
5. Wash with water.
6. Counterstain with methylene blue for 30 seconds.
7. Allow to dry in air and examine.

RESULT. Cells are stained red and capsule is stained blue.

Flagella Stain (Leifson)*

SOLUTION

$KAl(SO_4)_2 \cdot 12\ H_2O$ or $NH_4Al(SO_4)_2 \cdot 12\ H_2O$ sat. aqueous solution	20 ml.
Tannic acid (20 per cent aqueous)	10 ml.
Distilled water	40 ml.
Ethyl alcohol, 95 per cent	15 ml.
Basic fuchsin (saturated solution in 95 per cent ethyl alcohol)	3 ml.

*This stain is available commercially in powder form.

Mix ingredients in order named. Keep in tightly stoppered bottle.

PROCEDURE

1. Prepare slides by cleaning in dichromate cleaning solution, wash in water, rinse in alcohol, wipe with clean piece of cheesecloth. Pass slides through a flame several times.

2. Flood slides with solution and allow to stand 10 minutes at room temperature in warm weather or in an incubator in cold weather.

3. Wash with tap water.

4. Dry and examine.

RESULT. Flagella are stained red, except those bacteria that have extremely delicate flagella.

Stain for Spirochetes (Fontana)

PREPARATION OF AMMONIACAL SILVER NITRATE. Dissolve 5 gm. of $AgNO_3$ in 100 ml. of distilled water. Remove a few milliliters, and to the rest of the solution add drop by drop a concentrated ammonia solution until the sepia precipitate which forms redissolves. Then add drop by drop enough $AgNO_3$ solution to produce a slight cloud which persists after shaking. The solution should remain in good condition for several months.

STAINING SCHEDULE

1. Prepare smear, and fix with heat.

2. Pour on a solution of 5 per cent tannic acid in 1 per cent phenol, and allow to steam 30 seconds.

3. Wash 30 seconds in running water.

4. Cover with a drop of the above ammoniacal silver nitrate, heat gently over a flame, and allow it to stand 20 to 30 seconds after steaming begins.

5. Wash in tap water.

6. Blot dry, and examine.

RESULT. Spirochetes stain dark brown or black in a dark maroon field.

Fluorescence Microscopy

The development of techniques for conjugating antibodies with fluorescein and the application of these techniques to identification of specific microorganisms introduced a valuable tool in the clinical microbiology laboratory. Thus, it is desirable at this point to describe a broad outline of fluorescent antibody (FA) techniques. In some cases, FA techniques completely replace time-consuming cultural methods; in other cases preliminary identification of microorganisms may be followed by cultural confirmation. It is probable that FA techniques will replace some of the older serologic methods of making final identification of bacteria. A great deal of investigative work is in progress in various laboratories, which will no doubt elucidate the role that FA techniques may play in clinical microbiologic work. Clinical microbiologists should be prepared to adapt these methods to their routine procedures at the earliest possible moment, since these FA techniques offer the opportunity to speed up microbiologic diagnosis.

The basic principle on which FA techniques depend is the nature of the combination of specific antibody with antigen. In the direct method the antibody coats the antigen (bacteria and protozoa, for example) and cannot easily be removed. If such an antibody has been rendered fluorescent by conjugation with fluorescein and all the nonantibody globulin is removed by washing, all that is left is that which is attached to the antigen. Thus, if the antigen is a bacterial cell and is viewed with an appropriate optical system, the fluorescent outline of the bacterial cell can be seen easily. The specificity of the test, as in any serologic procedure, depends on the purity of the antibody in the conjugated serum. To produce such a specific serum, one can immunize an appropriate animal with an organism (antigen) and absorb the serum to remove all but the specific, identifying antibody. For example, an animal may be given a series of inoculations with a suspension of group A *Streptococcus pyogenes,* and by appropriate absorption the cross-reacting antibodies can be removed. The absorbed serum then contains specific group A antibodies and when conjugated with fluorescein can be used to identify these organisms in smears.

An indirect FA technique may also be used. The basic principle of this method is as follows: The specific antiserum is not labeled with fluorescein. It is allowed to react with the antigen and the nonantibody globulin is washed off. If one is using a rabbit antiserum, the antigen is now coated with rabbit serum globulin. Treatment of this preparation with fluorescein-labeled antirabbit globulin results in a specific combination of this labeled antibody with the rabbit globulin already specifically attached to the antigen. When the nonantibody globulin is washed off, the antigen now can be seen as in the case of the direct technique. This indirect method has the advantage of reducing the number of labeled antiserums needed, since, if all diagnostic antiserums were produced in the rabbit, one would need only a fluorescein-labeled antirabbit globulin. Such a serum can be produced by inoculation of rabbit globulin into a sheep or other suitable animal. The indirect technique can be used for the detection of antibody in the serum of patients by combining such serum with specific organisms, such as *Toxoplasma,* and then using a fluorescein-labeled antihuman globulin serum.

An inhibition method has been used also for the purpose of checking the specificity of the reactions with a given antigen-antibody

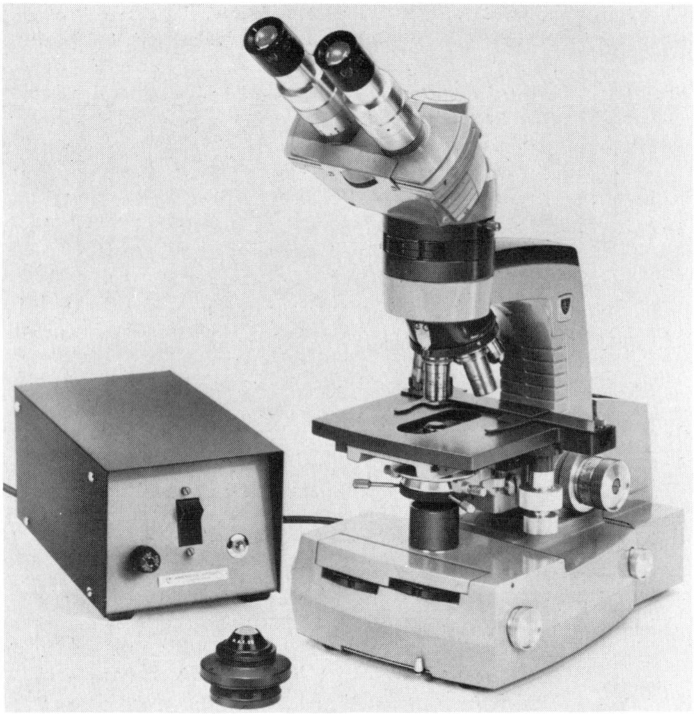

Figure 18–2. Fluorescence microscope with power supply. (Courtesy of American Optical Co., Buffalo, New York.)

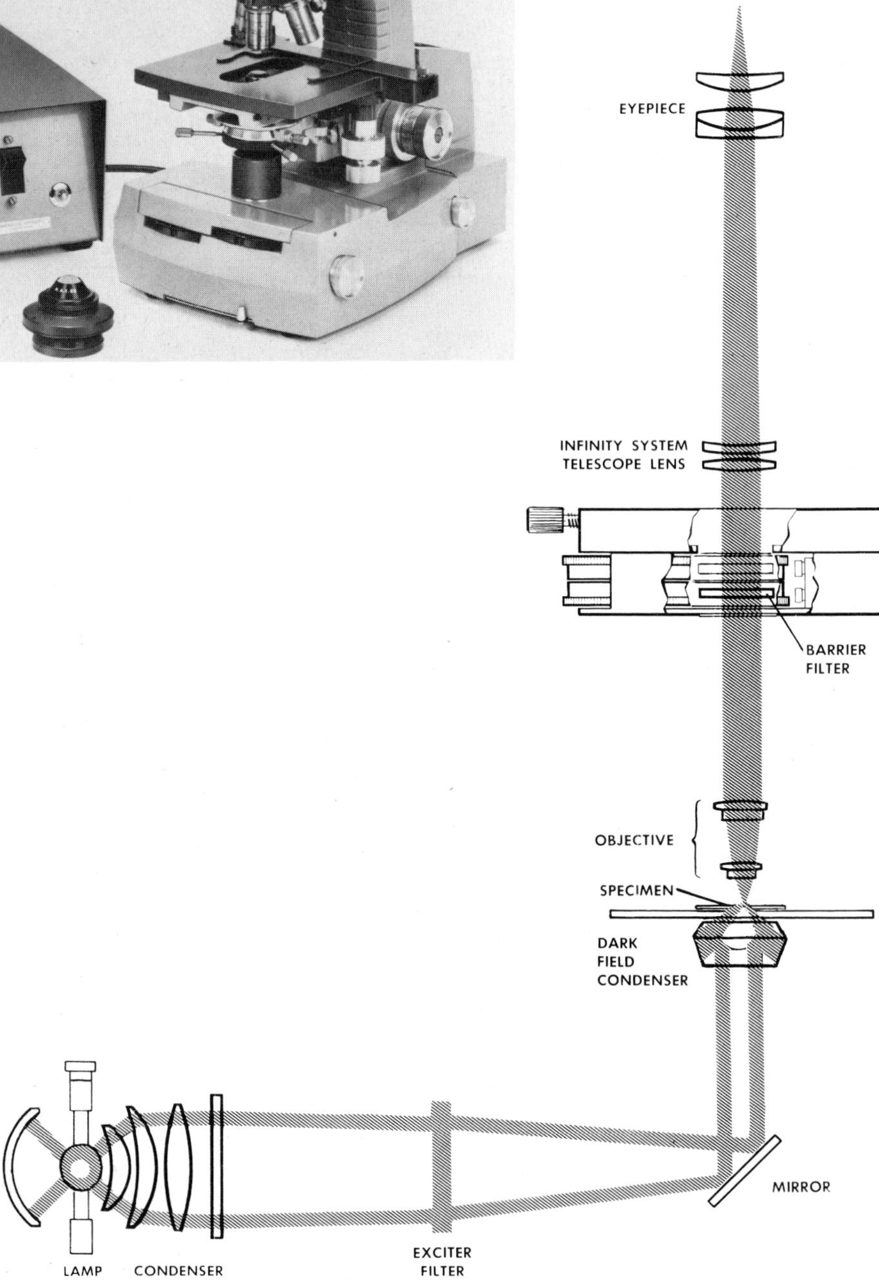

Figure 18–3. Path of light in fluorescence microscopy. (Courtesy of American Optical Company, Buffalo, New York.)

system. There is also a complement staining method, which, although rather complex, may be quite useful in certain types of work.

Use of Fluorescence Microscopy As a Diagnostic Technique in Bacteriology. Prior to the introduction of fluorescein isothiocyanate the conversion of amino fluorescein to fluorescein isocyanate for labeling serum globulin was a task that presented a major obstacle to many laboratories. This conversion required the use of phosgene gas, an extremely toxic reagent, and therefore the number of laboratories with facilities necessary for preparing labeled antiserums was limited. In addition to the toxicity of phosgene gas, the fluorescein isocyanate was unstable and had to be prepared immediately before mixing with the serum globulin to be conjugated. However, with the introduction of fluorescein isothiocyanate a stable reagent became available that greatly simplified the entire procedure for conjugating this derivative of fluorescein to serum globulin.

Essentially the procedure being used at present by most workers involves using half-saturated ammonium sulfate for repeated precipitation of serum globulin, which contains the antibodies. The precipitate is then dialyzed to remove the ammonium sulfate. The concentration of the precipitated globulin is usually adjusted to a concentration of about 1.0 per cent, and a calculated amount (0.05 mg. per mg. of protein) of fluorescein isothiocyanate is added. This step is carried out at 5° C., and the globulin-fluorescein isothiocyanate mixture is gently shaken for about 18 hours at 5° C.

After this, the preparation is usually adsorbed with an anionic resin to remove materials that are responsible for certain non-specific staining. If the preparation is adsorbed, a period of 1 to 2 hours at 5° C. usually suffices, after which the material is placed in a cheesecloth bag and centrifuged to collect the adsorbed conjugate.

The next step in the labeling procedure is another period of dialysis to remove the unconjugated fluorescein isothiocyanate. Dialysis is conducted at 5° C. in buffered saline until the dialysate no longer fluoresces when exposed to the beam of a Wood's light. After dialysis the conjugated globulin is centrifuged to remove any precipitate. Merthiolate is added as a preservative to give a final concentration of 1:10,000. The conjugated globulin is now ready for use. Small aliquots may be kept at 5° C. for immediate use, but the bulk of the conjugate should be kept frozen. Slow dissociation of the conjugate may occur when it is stored for long periods of time.

A second important consideration in this technique is the light source, microscope, and various heat-absorbing, exciter, and barrier filter combinations. Although fluorescence microscopy with a brightfield microscope can be used for certain preparations, it is advisable to use a darkfield condenser for routine work. One of two major types of condensers, cardioid or paraboloid, may be used for this purpose. The immersion oil used for these darkfield condensers should be of a very low fluorescence type.

Most light systems in use at present employ a mercury lamp or carbon arc varying in power from 100 to 1000 watts. A number of light units are available commercially, and a great deal of care should be exercised in the selection of a particular unit. The more expensive units feature a closed system and can be set up more permanently than the less expensive types, which use a separate light housing from which an open beam of light must be focused onto a mirror beneath the microscope condenser. This type frequently requires realignment of the light beam and produces a considerable amount of "stray" light, which can be disconcerting to the observer.

A heat-absorbing filter is incorporated into the system to remove light near and beyond 600 mμ. This is necessary to prevent such light from cracking or breaking the primary filter. The primary or exciting light filter usually passes light from 300 to 425 mμ, depending upon the particular filter employed, and the barrier or ocular filter is usually one that will pass light of wavelengths above 400 mμ. The combinations of exciter and barrier filters used for virus and tissue section work are usually different from those for bacteria; hence, the various systems should be studied to find the one most suitable for the specimens to be studied routinely (Figs. 18–2 and 18–3).

The three major techniques now in use are essentially as follows: In the direct method smears of the material to be examined may be fixed with heat or methanol or, in some cases, fixation is not necessary. Then the smear is flooded with the conjugated globulin reagent containing a specific antibody. This complex is usually incubated for 30 to 60 minutes at 37° C. in a moist chamber. Following this the smear is washed twice, the first time in buffered saline for 5 to 10 minutes and then in tap water for another 5 to 10 minutes. This washing is for the purpose of removing all uncombined conjugated globulin. A small drop of buffered glycerol is placed on the smear and a coverslip is added. The smear is then ready for examination.

In the indirect method the smear is treated with unlabeled antiserum exactly as in the direct test. This is the primary combining reaction. After this smear has been incubated and washed, fluorescein-labeled antiglobulin homologous to the globulin of the animal species whose serum is used in the primary reaction (e.g., if rabbit serum was the primary reagent, use labeled sheep antirabbit globulin) is added and the smear incubated and washed again as in the primary reaction. The smear is then mounted in buffered glycerol and examined.

The inhibition test is used as a control for the specificity of a reaction. In this test, duplicate smears are used. One smear is treated with a mixture of unlabeled homologous antiserum and labeled homologous antiserum. The second smear is stained with a mixture of unlabeled normal serum and labeled homologous antiserum. Staining is carried out as in the direct test. When the stained smears are examined, the first preparation (unlabeled homologous antiserum plus labeled homologous antiserum of the same species) should not fluoresce, but the second smear (stained with normal serum and labeled homologous antiserum of the same species) should fluoresce. This technique may also be used to detect antibody in unknown (patient's) serum. It requires a great deal of standardization, and before one attempts to use this method it should be thoroughly understood. The overall technique is too lengthy for this presentation. It is to be suspected that the direct and indirect methods will be much more useful in the clinical laboratory.

As FA work progresses, the new applications

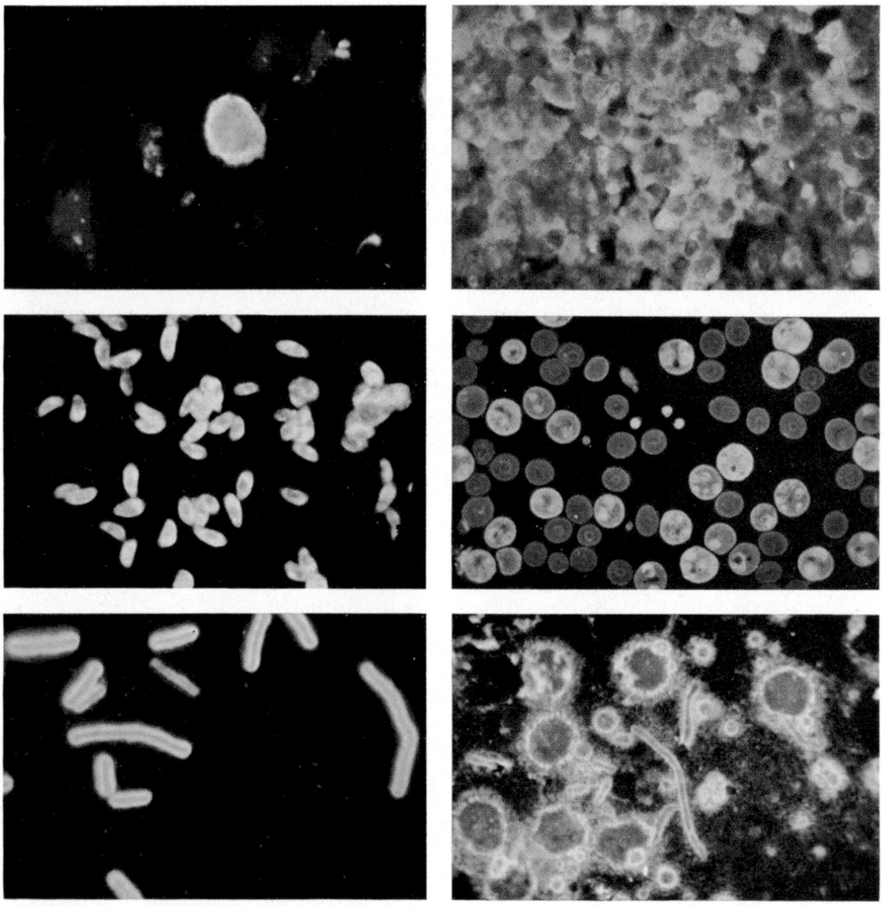

Figure 18–4. *A*, Fluorescent antibody staining* of microorganisms. *1*, *Entamoeba histolytica* in dried smear from culture (× 1050). *2*, *Toxoplasma gondii* in spleen of infected mouse. Tissue fixed in alcoholacetic acid and embedded in paraffin (× 1050). *3*, *Toxoplasma gondii* in peritoneal exudate of infected mouse (× 1050). *4*, *Plasmodium berghei*, a parasite of rodents, as seen in rat blood during preliminary studies of human malaria. *5*, *Bacillus anthracis* is an impression smear from the liver of a mouse. Homologous antibody was prepared by injecting whole encapsulated antigen. Note both encapsulated and stripped forms (× 600). *6*, *Pasteurella pestis* in smear of fluid aspirated from bubo of a fatal case of plague. Homologous antibody prepared by injecting whole-cell antigen. Note bizarre forms of plague bacilli and specifically stained soluble antigen surrounding tissue cells (× 1050). (From W. B. Cherry, M. Goldman, and T. R. Carski: Fluorescent Antibody Techniques. U.S. Department of Health, Education, and Welfare, 1960.)

*By the direct method.

(*Figure 18–4 continued on the opposite page.*)

of this technique that will no doubt evolve will make possible changes and refinements of present techniques. Detection of antigen in tissues has been reported as well as the successful demonstration of antibody. Streptococci have been detected in smears made from throat swabs from patients with acute streptococcal pharyngitis, and a rapid method for detecting human influenza virus infection utilizing nasal smears has been described. Fluorescent antibody studies have been extended to include members of the following genera of bacteria: *Leptospira, Hemophilus, Streptococcus, Salmonella, Treponema, Pasteurella, Yersinia, Escherichia,* and many others. The technique has also been used in the detection of numerous viruses, fungi, and protozoa. These cited cases represent but a few adaptations of fluorescence microscopy as a tool for studying and identifying microorganisms (Fig. 18–4).

Aerobic Culture Methods

The most frequently used item of equipment in the bacteriology laboratory is the inoculating loop. This can be made of platinum wire, nichrome wire, or other similar material and inserted in a holder. One should also have a straight wire for stab inoculations and for picking isolated colonies from streaked plates.

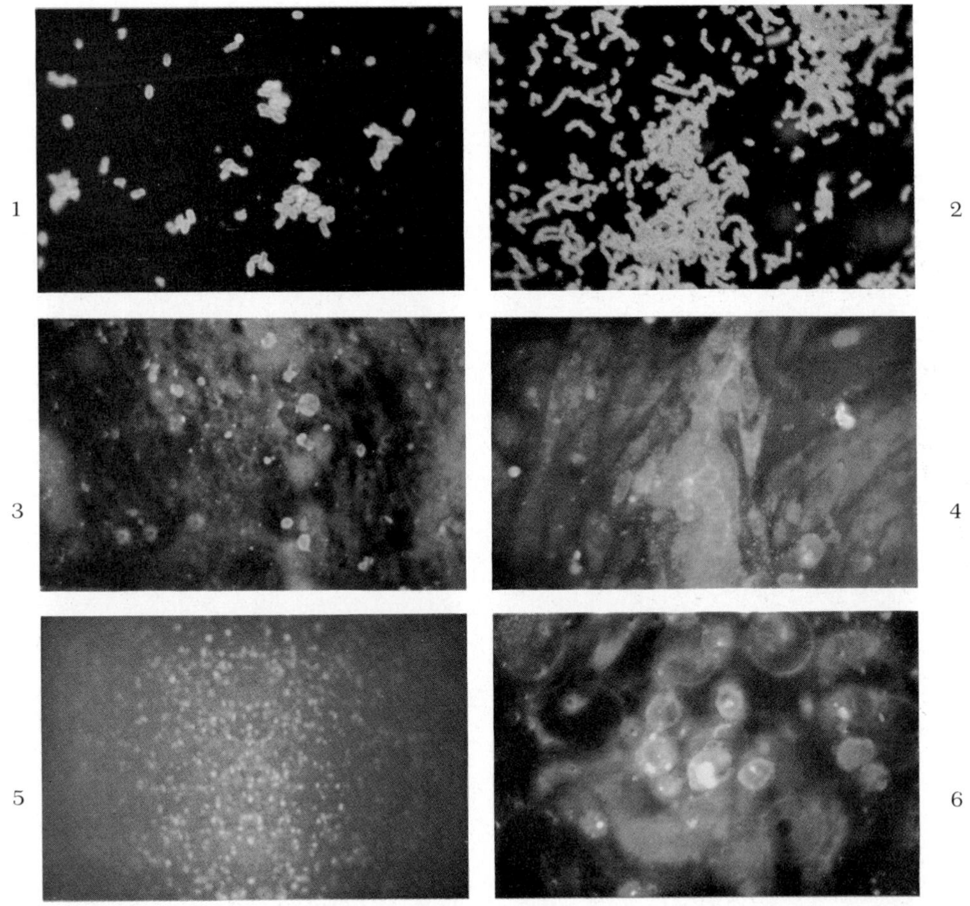

Figure 18–4. *B,* Fluorescent antibody staining* of microorganisms. *1, Escherichia coli* in feces from a case of infantile diarrhea. Stained with pooled antibodies for enteropathogenic types of *E. coli* (× 600). *2,* Group B streptococci in pure culture (× 600). *3,* Rabies virus in impression smear of the brain of a mouse infected with street virus. Note the large aggregates of stained antigen (Negri bodies) and the numerous smaller particles that stain (× 210). *4,* Simian foamy agent in a culture of monkey-kidney tissue on a coverslip. Two days after inoculation. Note stained antigen in nuclei of the multinucleated cells whose formation was induced by the infection (× 210). *5, Rickettsia prowazekii* (epidemic typhus) in a smear of egg yolk sac. Stained with homologous antibody (× 210). *6,* Polio virus type I in monkey-kidney tissue cultures, 12 hours post-inoculation. Stained by complement method, using antipolio monkey serum and guinea pig complement followed by labeled anti-guinea pig complement (× 210). (From W. B. Cherry, M. Goldman, and T. R. Carski: Fluorescent Antibody Techniques. U.S. Department of Health, Education, and Welfare, 1960.)

*By the direct method except for polio virus in 6.

Numerous types, most of which are satisfactory, are available at low cost from commercial sources.

The isolation of bacteria from specimens submitted to the laboratory is almost invariably accomplished by streaking on the surface of an agar plate. The purpose of streaking is to spread an inoculum so as to insure the appearance of isolated colonies on incubation. Most such isolated colonies will be pure cultures of an organism and may be picked for the next step—identification. The characteristics and the cellular morphology will also assist in final identification. It is therefore imperative that a suitable streaking technique be used.

A recommended technique is as follows: With a sterile inoculating loop place two loopfuls of the material near the edge of the plate. The loop should then be sterilized in the flame and allowed to cool. It should then be applied to the material on the plate and streaked, using a gentle pressure in the manner illustrated in Figure 18–5.

The streaked plates are incubated in an inverted position, media side up, at 37° C. and examined at 24- and 48-hour intervals. The various colonies should be observed carefully

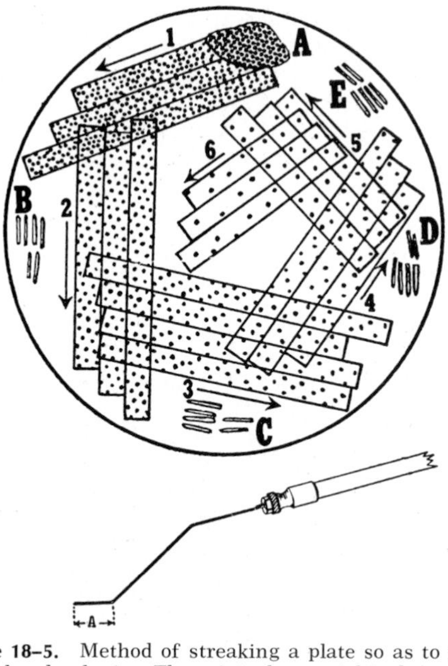

Figure 18–5. Method of streaking a plate so as to secure well-isolated colonies. The original material is deposited at *A*. The wire is afterward sterilized in the Bunsen flame. The material is then streaked with the flat part of the wire at 1, 2, 3, 4, 5, and 6, the wire being thrust into the agar to remove excess organisms, as at *B*, *C*, *D*, and *E*, after each series of parallel strokings. Isolated colonies are almost invariably found at the areas numbered 4, 5, and 6. The wire used in streaking is shown below the plate. The flat portion at *A* is brought into contact with the agar from tip to "heel." (From Frobisher, M., Jr.: Fundamentals of Bacteriology. 4th edition.)

and individual ones fished for gram stain and for transfer to appropriate media for further study. Fishing of colonies may be done with a loop if the colony is well separated from other colonies, but it may be better to use a straight wire for this, especially if the colonies are close together. It is essential that gram stains be done on all colonies to study staining characteristics, morphology, and purity.

Pour plates are sometimes used on certain types of specimens, e.g., urine or blood. The pour plate is made by placing a measured amount of the material in a sterile Petri plate and pouring in melted agar (cooled to 50° C.). The plate is then rotated to mix the material thoroughly throughout the medium. After solidifying at room temperature, the plate is inverted, incubated at 37° C., and examined for colonies. This technique has the advantage of giving quantitative bacterial counts. For heavily contaminated specimens, dilution must be done.

Agar slants are used frequently for maintenance of cultures or for certain biochemical studies. The slant is inoculated from a colony picked from a plate or from a broth culture. A loop is used to transfer the inoculum to the slant and is streaked over the entire slant. Slants are used only with pure cultures and are not for isolation. It is sometimes necessary to stab into the butt of a slant, as with Kligler's iron agar for enteric organisms. This is done with a straight wire, stabbing carefully in a straight line into the center of the tube. The stab should never be made completely to the bottom of the tube. Slants are examined after 24 and 48 hours of incubation, and gram stains are made to check purity of the culture.

Semisolid media are used for motility or biochemical studies and are stabbed with a straight wire. The stab is not extended to the bottom of the tube. Motility is read by examining for migration of growth away from the stab line; thus, it is important that the stab be made with care.

Broth media (e.g., infusion and extract media) are used for maintenance of cultures and other studies (such as carbohydrate fermentation). They are inoculated by transfer from colonies or other growth with a loop or wire. Propagation of bacteria in such media is indicated by the development of cloudiness. It is important to ascertain growth in fermentation media, since failure of growth results in no change of the indicator and may lead to false negative interpretation. Gram stains should be done on all broth cultures to determine the purity of the culture and to make sure no contamination has occurred.

For short-term storage of cultures one should use broth or agar slant cultures, since Petri dishes tend to dry out unless sealed with a rubber or plastic band.

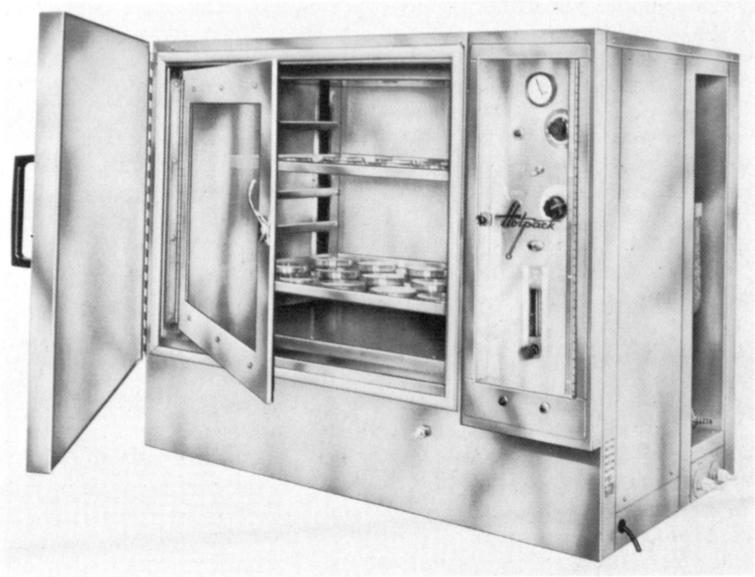

Figure 18–6. Carbon dioxide incubator. (Courtesy of Hotpack Company, Philadelphia, Pennsylvania.)

Incubation in an Atmosphere of Increased Carbon Dioxide. To obtain an atmosphere of increased carbon dioxide for assistance in the culture of numerous organisms, the simplest and probably most useful method is to use the candle jar. This is simply a jar or can with a tightly fitting top into which Petri dishes can be placed along with a smokeless candle. The candle is lit and the lid sealed tightly with plasticine or tape. When the candle burns out, the atmosphere contains approximately 3 to 5 per cent carbon dioxide. Modified Brewer jars containing disposable envelopes which generate CO_2 can also be used.* There are now available carbon dioxide incubators which automatically control the carbon dioxide content of the environment. These are very useful, particularly in the larger laboratories (Fig. 18–6).

Anaerobic Culture Methods

Most of the recognized pathogenic bacteria are aerobic or facultatively anaerobic and propagate well in an atmosphere free of oxygen; others are microaerophilic, preferring reduced oxygen concentrations.

Many pathogenic and nonpathogenic bacteria are incapable of propagation in the presence of oxygen and require a low oxidation-reduction potential. These are classified as obligate anaerobic bacteria (Fig. 18–7).

All specimens for anaerobic studies must be cultured as soon as possible after collection to avoid loss of viability. Collection in prereduced tubes or in Stuart's transport medium is recommended if a delay is unavoidable. Special methods are necessary for the isolation and study of anaerobic bacteria. The techniques are essentially of three types: the use of media containing reducing substances that eliminate oxygen from the medium; the use of media and methods by which oxygen can be excluded from the medium; and the use of anaerobic jars, plates, and incubators from which oxygen can be removed and replaced with hydrogen or nitrogen.

One of the most useful media for anaerobic

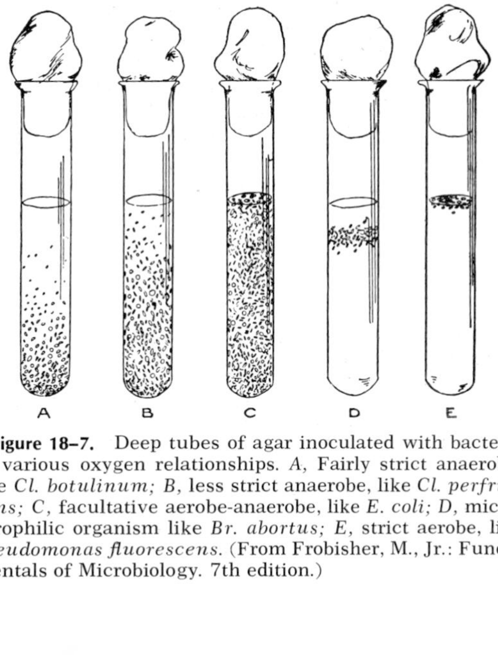

Figure 18–7. Deep tubes of agar inoculated with bacteria of various oxygen relationships. *A,* Fairly strict anaerobe, like *Cl. botulinum; B,* less strict anaerobe, like *Cl. perfringens; C,* facultative aerobe-anaerobe, like *E. coli; D,* microaerophilic organism like *Br. abortus; E,* strict aerobe, like *Pseudomonas fluorescens.* (From Frobisher, M., Jr.: Fundamentals of Microbiology. 7th edition.)

*Bioquest, Cockeysville, Maryland.

culture is Brewer's fluid thioglycollate medium. This medium contains sodium thioglycollate, which absorbs oxygen from the medium. It also contains a low concentration of agar, which limits convection, thus reducing the absorption of oxygen from air. Cysteine or reduced iron filings may also be used with or in place of the sodium thioglycollate. Other useful media are cooked meat and litmus milk, both of which can be obtained in dehydrated form. Before use these media should be heated in a boiling water bath for 10 to 15 minutes to drive off dissolved oxygen.

Fluid media serve well for study and identification of anaerobic bacteria but are not generally satisfactory for isolation of cultures from lesions. For isolation it is desirable to streak plates of blood agar, infusion agar, or thioglycollate agar. Such plates are then placed in an anaerobic jar or other special container and the oxygen removed. The Brewer anaerobic jar, the top of which contains an electrically heated platinum coil, is satisfactory for this purpose. The air is exhausted from the jar and replaced with hydrogen, exhausted again, and refilled with hydrogen. Then the jar is connected with electric current, which heats the platinum coil. This catalyzes the reaction between hydrogen and oxygen to form water, thus removing all remaining oxygen.

There are now available certain modifications of the Brewer, and the McIntosh and Fildes anaerobic jars which do not require the use of this platinum coil. These jars have certain advantages in routine use and are considerably less hazardous (Figs. 18-8 and 18-9).

Also recently developed are envelopes which will generate hydrogen or hydrogen plus carbon dioxide when water is added. Thus, it is no longer necessary to use tanks of these gases.

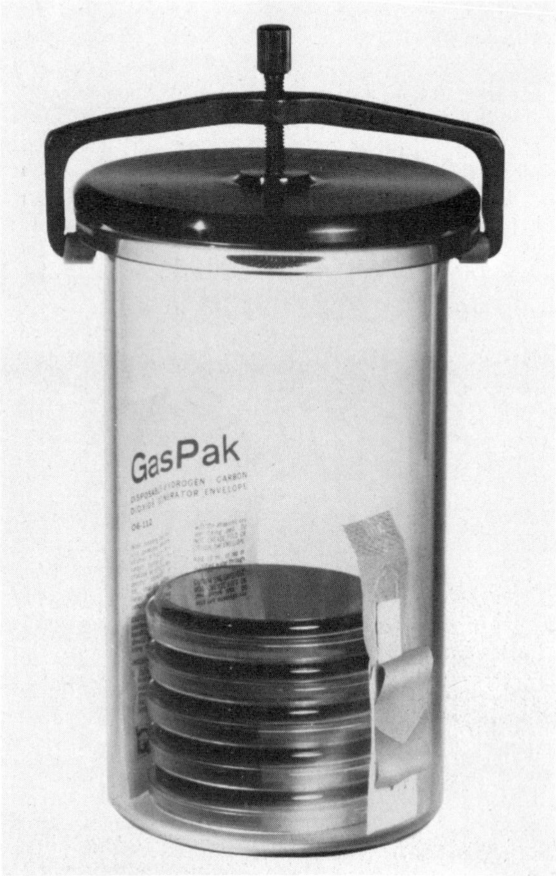

Figure 18-9. GasPak anaerobic system. (Courtesy of Bioquest, Cockeysville, Maryland.)

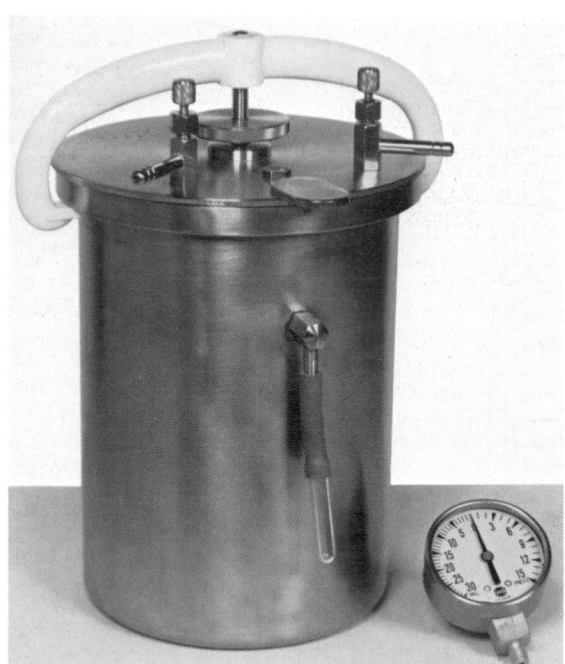

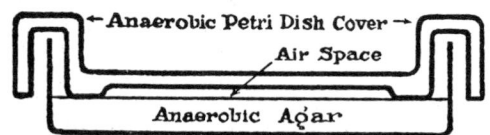

Figure 18-8. *A*, Stainless steel anaerobic jar. (Courtesy of Torsion Balance Company, Clifton, New Jersey.) *B*, Cross-section showing use of Brewer anaerobic Petri dish cover.

PREREDUCED MEDIUM TECHNIQUE

The media used in this method are tubed under oxygen-free gas by use of recessed butyl rubber stoppers. Since they are not exposed to air, a low oxidation-reduction potential can be maintained. This technique is beginning to become more widely established since it appears to be the most practical and reliable one for isolation of anaerobic bacteria. Prereduced media are now available commercially or can be prepared in the laboratory using equipment designed for this purpose.* Details of this method are beyond the scope of this book, but can be found in the texts of Smith and Holdeman (1968) and Shapton and Board (1971).

Visual evidence of adequate anaerobic conditions can be obtained by the use of the following anaerobic indicator solutions: (1) 0.1 N NaOH, 6 ml.; distilled water to 100 ml. (2) Methylene blue, 0.5 per cent, 3 ml.; distilled water to 100 ml. (3) Glucose, 6 gm.; distilled water to 100 ml. Place equal volumes of each solution in test tube. Add one small thymol crystal. Boil until colorless. Place in anaerobic jar. Solution remains colorless if anaerobic conditions are maintained. Disposable anaerobic indicators are also available.†

One of the problems most frequently encountered with the anaerobes is that of spreading overgrowth. Various methods of avoiding this are available, such as use of chloral hydrate, increased agar (4 per cent), and certain antibiotics (polymyxin B, neomycin, and similar substances).

Most of the pathogenic anaerobes, such as *Cl. tetani, Cl. perfringens,* and *Cl. botulinum,* produce spores that are resistant to heat of a degree capable of destroying all vegetative bacteria. It is often possible in attempting to culture these anaerobes from feces, suspected food, or wound swabs to inoculate fluid thioglycollate, cooked meat or infusion broth, or deep agar shake tubes. The culture is then put in a water bath at 75° C. for 10 to 15 minutes. This will destroy all vegetative forms (aerobic or anaerobic), and the spores will generate at incubator temperature and grow out. This may be more successful than attempts at plating.

Choice of Media

One of the problems in all laboratories is the choice of media for particular purposes. Practically, particularly in small laboratories, it is desirable to limit the number of media and to choose those that offer the greatest usefulness. Once media are chosen, it is important that the technologist become thoroughly familiar with each. This is best accomplished by constant use and careful observation. Changes in media should be made when improved formulas become available but should be done with care. Cultures on new medium should be run alongside the old for a time in order to decide whether or not the new medium offers advantages in the particular laboratory.

Media may be divided into categories as follows: isolation media, enrichment media, media for maintenance, identifying or differentiating media (such as carbohydrate fermentation, hemolysis, or indole production), and media for storage.

Isolation media are used to streak out specimens, such as urine or feces. They may be used for general isolation or for the selective isolation of a particular organism or group of organisms.

To be used for general isolation, a medium has to be capable of supporting a large variety of pathogenic and nonpathogenic bacteria. Blood and chocolate agar are such media and find wide usage in routine isolation work. Special media are designed for isolation of certain bacteria when their presence is suspected; they may be used by larger laboratories, but for most laboratories blood and chocolate agar, used either under atmospheric conditions or in the CO_2 jar, should serve very well. These general isolation media are satisfactory with such specimens as spinal fluid, urine, and throat swabs in which the number of types of bacteria is not excessive, but when one deals with fecal cultures it becomes necessary to use selective media.

Selective media incorporate substances inhibitory to propagation of a group of bacteria but allow other groups to grow. Thus, for enteric culture, the media routinely used contain certain dyes and other ingredients, which inhibit gram-positive organisms and allow the gram-negative enteric bacilli to propagate. If, on the other hand, one wishes to isolate enterococci or staphylococci in enteric work, one can incorporate substances, such as phenylethyl alcohol or certain antibiotics in blood agar, which inhibit the gram-negative bacilli.

Enrichment media may be used to good advantage, particularly in enteric cultures. Such media are designed to enhance the propagation of certain organisms without favoring others. They are routinely used in the isolation of *Salmonella* from feces.

Identification media are of various types and range from the fluid base with specific carbohydrates added, through semisolid motility media and urea media for aid in identifying members of the genus *Proteus,* to the more complex media, such as Kligler's or triple sugar iron medium for aid in differentiation among the Enterobacteriaceae.

Maintenance media may be of various types. Infusion broth is satisfactory for many of the

*Bellco Glass, Inc., Vineland, New Jersey; Robbins Laboratories, Chapel Hill, North Carolina.
†Bioquest, Cockeysville, Md.

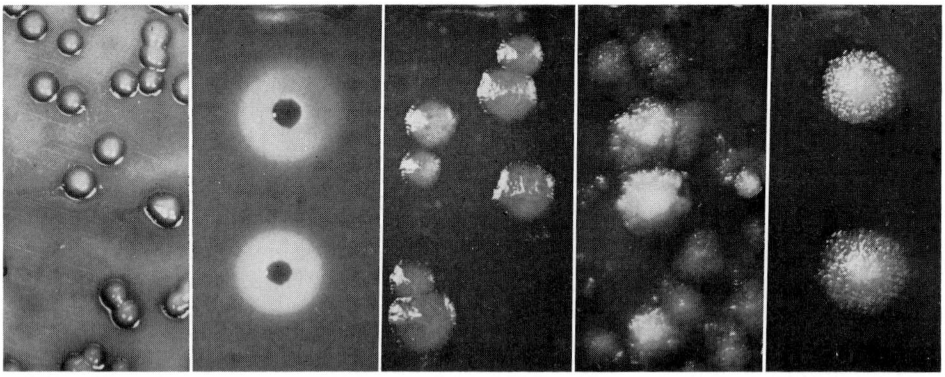

Figure 18–10. Morphologic types of bacterial colonies. *Left* to *right*, the raised, smooth, viscous colonies of the gonococcus on chocolate agar; β-hemolytic streptococcus colonies on blood agar showing the cleared zones of hemolysis and the slightly matted, slightly irregular edge of the typical colony; colonies of the typhoid bacillus on nutrient agar showing the typical irregular edge (maple leaf appearance) and irregular but smooth surface; colonies of the tubercle bacillus on Löwenstein's medium showing the characteristic roughened appearance; and colonies of the anthrax bacillus on nutrient agar in the typically rough, virulent form. (From Burrows, W.: Textbook of Microbiology, 19th ed.)

less fastidious organisms, as are infusion agar slants. For some organisms one needs an enriched medium, and blood or chocolate agar slants can be used. Certain organisms, e.g., *Diplococcus pneumoniae,* produce considerable amounts of acid from dextrose and tend to autolyze. In these cases a medium with only a little fermentable carbohydrate is advisable, else the culture may be lost. In general, cultures are best maintained by lyophilization.

Aside from these general statements, the experienced bacteriologist must be guided in the choice of media for use in any instance by the type of specimen, the nature of the suspected clinical condition, and the results of a preliminary examination of the specimen, such as gram stain.

In the section to follow there will be presented a set of procedures and certain alternatives for differentiating specimens of different types. First, there will be a list of the normal and abnormal microorganisms commonly found in the particular material or area involved, and then the routine of isolation, identification, and reporting of findings will be described. In a later section the primary identifying characteristics of the various organisms will be given. The procedures to be described represent an attempt to strike some balance between the purely academic or scientific and the practical approach that so often is necessary in smaller institutions.

The methods included here are obviously not the only ones that are appropriate. They have been used by the authors or are recommended by responsible workers. Each individual laboratory may make improvements and modifications of recommended techniques to fit its own special situation.

SPECIFIC METHODS FOR MICROBIOLOGIC EXAMINATION OF SPECIMENS

Mouth, Sputum, and Bronchial Secretions

MOUTH

Many organisms can be isolated from cultures taken from the normal mouth, and almost all organisms might conceivably be found there at one time or another. Some are found more frequently than others. There are spirochetes demonstrable in scrapings from the base of the teeth, and lactobacilli, microaerophilic actinomyces, staphylococci, and a few other organisms may be found almost routinely in the mouth. The protozoa, *Entamoeba gingivalis* and *Trichomonas tenax,* sometime occur in the mouth and can be demonstrated in scrapings from the teeth. *E. gingivalis* may be associated with gingivitis, but its etiologic significance is not fully established.

In the mouth, organisms that may be of definite pathogenic significance include: anaerobic streptococci, *Staphylococcus, M. tuberculosis,* Vincent's organisms, *Treponema pallidum,* various viruses, and fungi. For methods of isolation and identification see sections on the various specific organisms.

Lesions in the mouth may result from a variety of circumstances. In some cases culture may reveal heavy bacterial or fungal contamination, but the presence of the microbial agents is secondary to other processes. An example of this is the occurrence of lesions in the mouth that exist in patients with leukemia. Trench mouth (Vincent's disease), thrush (moniliasis), herpetic stomatitis, syphilis, and certain abscesses are conditions in which microbial agents are of primary importance. Diagnosis of trench mouth depends on direct smear and gram stain of material collected by vigorously swabbing the typical dirty appearing membrane. Demonstration of spirillae and fusiform bacteria in significant numbers in the smear is diagnostic. In thrush one may demonstrate typical budding yeasts by gram stain of a direct smear, but cultural confirmation is necessary. Syphilitic chancre in the mouth may occur in a variety of sites and may be grossly atypical. The lesion may not have the raised, indurated appearance of the classic hard chancre. Indication for darkfield examination of such lesions will usually come from the case history.

Thus, the bacteriologic examination of lesions of the mouth will be determined by the clinical picture of the lesion and the history of the case as taken by the physician.

SPUTUM

Organisms Normal to the Sputum. Sputum is frequently a more or less purulent exudate containing material from the lungs. "Normal" organisms are those picked up during passage through the nasopharynx.

The following organisms may be found in the sputum and are of possible pathogenic significance: *Diplococcus pneumoniae, Staphylococcus aureus, Streptococcus pyogenes, Klebsiella pneumoniae, Hemophilus influenzae,* and *Mycobacterium tuberculosis.* Less commonly isolated organisms include *Actinomyces, Nocardia asteroides, Histoplasma capsulatum, Coccidioides immitis, Mycoplasma pneumoniae* (Eaton agent) and such parasites as *Strongyloides stercoralis, Ascaris lumbricoides,* and *Trichomonas hominis.*

Collection of Sputum. The technique of collection of sputum is important not only to assist in the proper examination but also to avoid contamination of the outside of containers and of the surroundings and to prevent undue risk to those handling the material. Wide-mouth bottles with screw caps are best, but waxed paper cartons with tightly fitting tops may be used. Ideally the containers should be sterile, but this is not absolutely essential provided they have not been used previously or, in the case of glass bottles, have been thoroughly cleaned and dried. The patient should be carefully instructed about the proper procedure before collection.

It is important to distinguish sputum from saliva and postnasal discharges, and care should be taken to insure that only sputum is collected. It is desirable to rinse the mouth well before collection and then to raise the sputum by coughing. If difficulty is encountered in raising sputum, it sometimes helps to have the patient lie a few minutes with head and shoulders below the chest or to use heated aerosols. Since infants and small children tend to swallow sputum and cannot be induced to cough so readily as adults, it is frequently necessary to perform gastric, bronchial, or laryngeal washings. This is particularly useful in cases of suspected tuberculosis.

There are some who believe that routine expectorated sputum cultures are worthless and should be replaced with specimens collected by bronchoscopy, transtracheal aspiration, or bronchial brushing techniques.

Early morning collection of sputum and immediate transport to the laboratory is to be recommended. Collection over a 24- to 72-hour period is sometimes desirable for tuberculosis, but this is not suitable for routine bacterial examination.

The procedure for examination of sputum in the laboratory depends on the suspected condition. It is always desirable to make direct smears and stains. In acute bacterial pneumonias such smears often reveal large numbers of organisms, such as *D. pneumoniae* and *Staphylococcus.* In certain other types of pneumonia (e.g., viral) bacteria may be very sparse. Prompt reporting of such findings may be of great value to the physician in guiding therapy.

To make smears one should pick material from the more purulent portion of the sputum, flecks of mucus, and especially any blood-tinged material. Care must be used in examining gram stains of such preparations, since the morphologic appearance of an organism may be misleading. For example, staphylococci quite frequently are seen in pairs and may be mistakenly reported as resembling *D. pneumoniae.* It is also important to report on cytologic components of the material, especially pus cells, and to note the presence of ingested bacteria.

Some of the material similar to that used for staining should be used for culture. Preliminary digestion of the sputum with pancreatin, trypsin, dithiothreitol* or other mucolytic substances increases the chances of isolating significant pathogenic bacteria. Since most of the bacteria found in acute pneumonia grow well on blood agar, this is the medium of choice. The various gram-positive cocci, *Staphylococcus, Streptococcus,* and *Diplococcus,* found in such conditions produce characteristic colonies on this medium, and tentative identification can be made after from 18 to 24 hours' incubation. If the gram stain has shown small gram-

*Sputolysin, Calbiochem, Los Angeles, California.

negative bacilli, one may wish, especially in children, to inoculate a chocolate agar plate (*H. influenzae*) or, if the bacilli are larger, an E.M.B. plate (*K. pneumoniae*).

The inoculated plates should be incubated 18 to 24 hours and examined. Typical colonies should be picked and stained with the gram stain. Tentative identification can often be made at this point, and a report on findings should be made. Further study of the isolated organisms depends on the tentative identification. It may be desirable to do antimicrobial susceptibility tests, especially if such organisms as *S. aureus* or *K. pneumoniae* are isolated in significant numbers.

Examination of Sputum for Acid-fast Organisms. In suspected cases of tuberculosis special staining and cultural procedures are necessary. Since *M. tuberculosis* and other acid-fast organisms cannot be stained by gram stain, it is necessary to use one of several acid-fast staining procedures. Smears are prepared in the same manner as for the gram stain. One must, however, use only new slides. The stain should be dropped on the slide from bottles; immersion of the slide in Coplin jars is not recommended. The slide should be heat fixed gently; too much heat will distort the acid-fast organisms.

The following acid-fast staining techniques may be used:

Ziehl-Neelsen Method

SOLUTIONS

1. Carbolfuchsin stain:

Solution A:

Basic fuchsin (90 per cent dye content)	0.3 gm.
Ethyl alcohol (95 per cent)	10.0 ml.

Solution B:

Phenol (melted crystals)	5.0 gm.
Distilled water	95.0 ml.

Mix solutions A and B. Let stand for several days before use.

2. Loeffler's alkaline methylene blue:

Solution A:

Methylene blue (90 per cent dye content)	0.3 gm.
Ethyl alcohol (95 per cent)	30.0 ml.

Solution B:

Dilute KOH (0.01 per cent by weight)	100 ml.

Mix solutions A and B.

PROCEDURE

1. Stain smears 3 to 5 minutes with the carbolfuchsin, applying enough heat for gentle steaming. Do not allow to evaporate; add more stain as needed. Cool.
2. Rinse in water.
3. Decolorize in 95 per cent ethyl alcohol that contains 3 per cent by volume of concentrated HCl, until no more stain comes off.
4. Wash in tap water.
5. Counterstain with the methylene blue solution for 30 seconds.
6. Wash, dry, and examine.

RESULTS. Acid-fast organisms stain red; others, blue.

Kinyoun Acid-fast Stain

Basic fuchsin	4 gm.
Phenol, liquefied	8 ml.
Ethyl alcohol	20 ml.
Distilled water	100 ml.

Dissolve the fuchsin in the alcohol and add the water slowly while shaking. Add phenol.

Fix slide gently with heat. Stain for 3 to 4 minutes without heating. Wash, decolorize, and counterstain as per the Ziehl-Neelsen method. If desired, one drop of Tergitol 7* may be added to every 30 ml. of stain. This accelerates the staining time to 1 minute.

Another technique for staining acid-fast bacilli that is becoming more widely used is the fluorescent auramine procedure. This is described on page 941.

The finding of acid-fast organisms in sputum and gastric washings does not establish the diagnosis, although it is highly suggestive. Nonpathogenic acid-fast organisms do occur in these areas (*M. smegmatis* and *M. phlei,* for example) and can be differentiated only by culture or animal inoculation. Thus, the reports on the stained smear of necessity should read "acid-fast organisms seen" or "no acid-fast organisms seen."

Concentration techniques may be used routinely to prepare samples for culture and animal inoculation. In addition, acid-fast stains on smears from concentrates may reveal organisms when stains on the direct smear are negative.

Concentration of the sputum is accomplished by liquefaction, using one of several reagents. This not only liquefies but also destroys bacteria other than the acid-fast organisms so that they do not overgrow the culture or adversely affect the inoculated animal.

Techniques of Digestion and Decontamination

Sodium Hydroxide Method

1. Place 2 to 4 ml. of sputum in a suitable test tube, preferably a pointed centrifuge tube, and add an equal volume of 2 to 4 per cent NaOH or Hank's digestion solution (NaOH 40 gm., potassium alum 2 gm., bromthymol blue 0.004 per cent, distilled water to 1000 ml.).
2. Shake for 5 to 10 minutes or until liquefaction has occurred. The shortest time is most desirable, since on longer exposure the alkali may adversely affect acid-fast bacteria.
3. After liquefaction, centrifuge at 3000 r.p.m. for 15 to 30 minutes.

---

*Union Carbon and Carbide Co., New York, New York.

4. Aseptically remove the supernatant fluid to a disinfectant solution.

5. Add 1 drop of phenol red indicator to the sediment.

6. Neutralize by adding 2 N HCl drop by drop to a faint pink endpoint. This is an important step and must be done carefully.

The concentrate is then used to make smears for acid-fast staining, to inoculate special media (Löwenstein-Jensen or Petragnani's, for example), or to inoculate guinea pigs. Penicillin (50 to 100 units) may be added to the concentrate to help inhibit the growth of contaminating organisms.

Acetyl-Cysteine Method

1. Prepare the necessary volume of digestant as shown in Table 18–1. The solution should be used within 24 hours.

2. Transfer no more than 10 ml. of sputum to a sterile 50-ml. screw-cap centrifuge tube.

3. Add a volume of digestant equal to the sputum volume. Mix well on a test tube mixer (Vortex) for 5 to 30 seconds.

4. Let stand 15 minutes at room temperature to effect decontamination.

5. Fill tube within one-half inch of top with sterile M/15 phosphate buffer pH 6.8.

6. Centrifuge at 3000 r.p.m. for 15 minutes.

7. Decant supernatant fluid into splash can containing disinfectant, being careful to retain sediment.

8. To remaining sediment, add 1 to 2 ml. of sterile 0.2 per cent bovine albumin, fraction V in saline, pH 7.0. Make a tenfold dilution of the digested sputum in sterile saline and water. Inoculate TB media with both dilutions.

9. Use undiluted sediment for acid-fast stains.

TSP-Z (Trisodium-Phosphate Zephiran) Method

I. Dissolve 1000 gm. of trisodium phosphate $\cdot 12H_2O$ in 4,000 ml. of hot distilled water. Add 7.4 ml. of 17 per cent aqueous benzalkonium chloride concentrate.*

II. M/15 phosphate buffer, pH 6.6

A. Sodium monohydrogen phosphate (anhydrous)	9.47 gm.
Distilled water	1000 ml.
B. Potassium dihydrophosphate	9.08 gm.
Distilled water	1000 ml.

Mix 625 ml. of B with 375 ml. of A. Adjust the pH to 6.6 if required; dispense in small volumes in appropriate containers and autoclave at 121° C. for 15 minutes.

1. Mix equal volumes of specimen and trisodium phosphate-benzalkonium chloride in a 50 ml. centrifuge tube and shake.

2. Allow the mixture to stand at room temperature for 20 to 30 minutes.

3. Centrifuge at 3000 r.p.m. for 20 minutes.

*Zephiran, Winthrop Laboratories, New York.

Table 18–1. PREPARATION OF 0.5 PER CENT N-ACETYL-L-CYSTEINE-SODIUM HYDROXIDE DIGESTANT

REAGENT	VOLUME OF DIGESTANT NEEDED (ML.)				
	50	100	200	500	1000
NaOH (4 per cent) ml.	25	50	100	250	500
0.1 M (2.94 per cent) sodium citrate $2H_2O$, ml.	25	50	100	250	500
N-acetyl-l-cysteine powder, gm.	0.25	0.5	1.0	2.5	5.0

4. Decant the supernatant fluid into a disinfectant.

5. Resuspend the sediment in 10 to 20 ml. sterile phosphate buffer and recentrifuge for 20 minutes.

6. Again decant the supernatant fluid and inoculate the sediment to egg media. If non-egg media such as 7H 10 agar are used, residual benzalkonium chloride may inhibit the growth of mycobacteria. This inhibitory effect may be neutralized by adding 10 mg. per cent of lecithin to the sterile buffer.

The media is inoculated from the sediment and incubated at 35° C. The addition of 5 to 10 per cent CO_2 stimulates growth on egg media and is essential for growth on Middlebrook 7H 10 agar. The media should be incubated with the slant face horizontal for the first 24 hours to avoid settling of the entire inoculum into the point of the slant. Since nonpathogenic acid-fast bacteria grow faster than the pathogens, the appearance of colonies of acid-fast bacteria in the first 3 to 8 days of incubation probably indicates this type of organism. The pathogenic acid-fast organisms may produce visible colonies in 10 to 14 days, but often this takes 4 to 6 weeks. For descriptions of the type of growth and cell morphology, see section on basic characteristics of species (p. 999).

Fluorochrome Staining of Tubercle Bacilli. Fluorescence microscopy for the detection of acid-fast bacilli in smears has been used for many years. The present renewal of interest in this method stems from the widespread use of the fluorescent antibody techniques, which has made effective equipment available in many laboratories.

The identification of acid-fast bacilli in clinical specimens by classic methods is one of the most tedious tasks confronting the bacteriologist. With the fluorescent auramine technique, specimens may be screened more rapidly with less eye fatigue and provide a substantially greater yield of positive results than the carbolfuchsin techniques. It is especially recommended for laboratories that handle a considerable volume of clinical specimens and in which an adequate fluorescent light source is available.

REAGENTS

Auramine O (C.I. 41000)	1.5 gm.
Rhodamine B (C.I. 749)	0.75 gm.
Glycerol	75 ml.
Phenol	10 ml.
Distilled water	50 ml.

Combine dyes with phenol and half the water and mix well in a magnetic stirrer. Add the glycerol and the remainder of the water and mix well; filter through glass wool and store at room temperature in a dark glass bottle.

Decolorizer: Concentrated HCl, 0.5 per cent in 70 per cent ethanol.

Counterstain: Potassium permanganate ($KMnO_4$) 0.5 gm. in 100 ml. distilled water.

PROCEDURE

1. Make smears on clean individual slides and label with diamond point pencil. Allow to dry at room temperature and heat fix.
2. Flood with staining solution for 15 minutes at 37° C. or 30 minutes at room temperature. Do not allow stain to dry during this period.
3. Rinse with water. Decolorize for 2 to 3 minutes, depending on the thickness of the smear.
4. Rinse. Counterstain with $KMnO_4$ for 2 to 3 minutes. Rinse with water and allow to dry. Examine.

A fluorescent microscope apparatus with a darkfield condenser, 200 watt arc lamp, blue exciter filter (BG-12 or equivalent), and orange barrier filter (EK-15 or equivalent) is used. Slides are examined with the 20×, NA 0.50, and the 50× oil, NA 0.90, objectives and, if required, the 95× objective, NA 1.25. It is of prime importance that the microscope and condenser be properly aligned.

Under low power, tubercle bacilli appear as self-luminous, golden-yellow rods. Fluorescent artifacts may present a problem, but with experience, these can readily be differentiated from true bacilli. Slides may be prepared in duplicate and a Ziehl-Neelsen stain done on positive auramine slides for confirmation. While it is possible to stain Ziehl-Neelsen slides with auramine-rhodamine, the reverse procedure is often unsuccessful.

The auramine technique is also recommended for tissue sections and is reported to increase the yield of positive findings as much as 20 per cent over classic methods.

Animal Inoculation. Animal inoculation no longer occupies the position it once did in the laboratory diagnosis of tuberculosis. Cultural methods have superseded this procedure and are generally considered to be superior. Inoculation of animals is still used, however, to aid in the final identification of acid-fast bacteria in cases in which the cultural and morphologic nature of an organism is doubtful. The guinea pig is the animal of choice when working with the human and bovine strains of *M. tuberculosis.* When organisms from cultures are used, the guinea pig should be inoculated with 0.1 mg. (moist weight) of the culture into the groin by the subcutaneous route. Two guinea pigs should be used for each culture tested. The animals should be tested with 1 mg. of old tuberculin, and only negative reactors should be used. After inoculation the guinea pigs should be checked every 10 days and the site of inoculation palpated. Developing local lesions are an indication of the eventual result. After 4 weeks the animals should be tuberculin tested with 1 mg. of old tuberculin. A positive reaction is indicative of a positive result and one animal should be sacrificed for more extensive examination. The second animal should be held an additional 2 weeks. If the tuberculin test is negative the animals should be held an additional 2 to 3 weeks before sacrificing. At necropsy a search should be made of the local lymph nodes, spleen, and liver for necrotic caseous lesions. Presence of such foci constitutes evidence of infection which can be confirmed by acid-fast stains or smears and cultural or histological examination.

Cough Plates. The cough plate is used in the culture of *Bordetella pertussis* from cases of whooping cough. The plate is made with Bordet-Gengou medium (glycerin-potato agar containing 20 per cent blood and 0.3 to 1 unit of penicillin per ml.). The plate is held a few inches in front of the mouth of a child suspected of having whooping cough, and the child is encouraged to cough on the plate. The plate is incubated at 35° C. for 2 to 4 days and checked for the appearance of typical hemolytic, half-pearl colonies of *B. pertussis.* Some workers prefer to use a nasopharyngeal swab which is streaked on Bordet-Gengou agar plates. This is considered to be superior to the cough method for isolating *B. pertussis.* FA techniques are also very useful.

THROAT, NASOPHARYNX, AND SINUS DRAINAGE CULTURES

Organisms normal to the throat and nasopharynx include: *Streptococcus viridans, Hemophilus hemolyticus, Staphylococcus epidermidis, Neisseria catarrhalis,* diphtheroids, *E. coli, Enterobacter-Klebsiella,* nonhemolytic streptococci, *Proteus* sp., and *Actinomyces naeslundii.*

Organisms that may be of pathogenic importance include: *Diplococcus pneumoniae*, *Streptococcus pyogenes* (Group A and possibly B, C, and G), *Staphylococcus aureus*, *Neisseria meningitidis*, *Hemophilus influenzae*, *Bordetella pertussis*, *Corynebacterium diphtheriae*, *Candida albicans*, *Actinomyces israelii*, and *Borrelia vincentii*.

In evaluating cultures from the throat or nasopharynx, it is important to remember that an unusual predominance of a particular organism, even though it may be considered a normal inhabitant, may have some significance and such a finding should be reported. The list of organisms above is not a complete one, and a given situation might cause a so-called normal inhabitant to exert a deleterious effect. One cannot tell whether the predominance of one organism represents a cause or a result of some process.

Collection and Examination of Specimens. Throat and nasopharyngeal cultures are collected with cotton swabs. Dacron, rayon, or alginate is preferred by some. To collect the culture, insert the swab through the mouth, being careful not to touch the tongue, cheek, or other oral surface. The tongue may be depressed with a tongue depressor. Any obvious lesions (abscesses, follicles, or plaques) in the throat or tonsillar surfaces or any visible crypts should be explored vigorously with the swab, rotating it and getting beneath the surface. It is not sufficient simply to pass the rotating swab gently over the surface. If no obvious lesions are present, the swab should be vigorously rotated over tonsillar and other surfaces, especially any inflamed areas. In these cases it is well to obtain material from the nasopharyngeal area, which is behind and above the uvula. For this purpose a swab made with a bent wire, which may be inserted well up into the nasopharyngeal region, has definite advantages.

The nasopharyngeal swab has the advantage of avoiding much contamination with the normal flora and is particularly useful in cases of suspected whooping cough. Cultures taken from the upper nasopharynx have been found particularly successful in our experience with children. For this purpose a very thin swab on a flexible aluminum or copper wire (19-gauge) is inserted through the previously cleared nasal passage, being careful to avoid touching the sides. It is inserted until it meets definite resistance and there gently rotated. Such swabs may yield nearly pure cultures or organisms in cases of bronchial pneumonia and meningococcal infection and may be very useful in whooping cough. It cannot be too strongly emphasized that care in the collection and handling of swabs will be most rewarding in terms of results.

It is imperative that swabs not be allowed to dry out before transfer to culture media. This can be avoided by transporting the specimen to the laboratory immediately and inoculating the media, by inoculating the media at the bedside, or by using the Culturette swab (Fig. 18–11). Dacron strips and swabs are available for *Str. pyogenes* cultures. Stuart's transport medium can also be used for this purpose.

Blood agar is the medium of choice in most cases for inoculation of throat and nasopharyngeal swabs. Other, special media may and should be used in certain cases. *H. influenzae* and *N. meningitidis* propagate better on chocolate agar under CO_2. When diphtheria is suspected, special methods should be used (see p. 947).

Recently, emphasis has been placed on the need for detecting the presence of *Str. pyogenes*, Group A, in patients with sore throats. This is particularly important to physicians in deciding the course of antibiotic therapy. The implications of this organism in the causation of rheumatic fever make adequate treatment

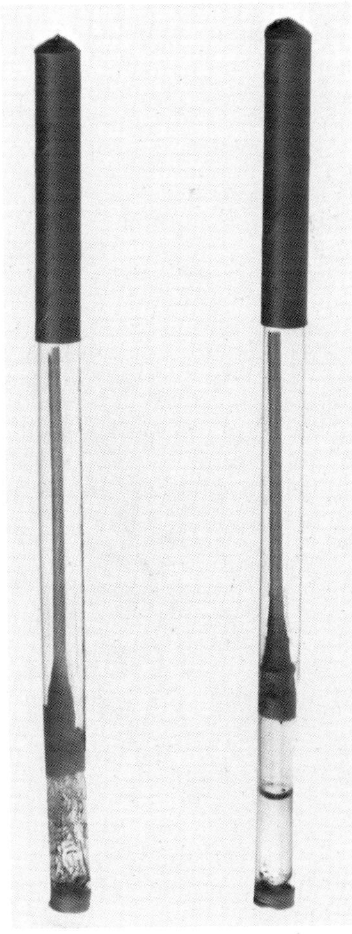

Figure 18–11. Culturette swab. The glass ampule containing preserving fluid (*right*) is broken by squeezing after the specimen is obtained, thus keeping the swab moist.

essential. A number of laboratories offer special services to physicians designed specifically to culture group A streptococci. In some cases the physician is furnished with a Dacron swab in a foil envelope so that the swab sealed in the envelope can be mailed to the laboratory for culture. Another system is to supply the physician with a vial of Stuart's transport medium or equivalent with an appropriate swab. The culture can be taken in the office and transported to the laboratory within 24 to 48 hours.

The FA technique is frequently used for rapid identification of *Str. pyogenes*. It is particularly applicable where large numbers of specimens are processed (Truant *et al.*, 1965).

When a direct smear is to be examined, it is advisable to collect two swabs, one of which is smeared over a marked area on a clean, dry slide. In most cases the smear should be gram stained, but special stains may be desired, especially in cases of suspected diphtheria or Vincent's infection. The results of examining direct smears should never be considered definitive but may be used to guide cultural procedures. Any reports made from such an examination must be descriptive and tentative.

The streaking of plates with swabs may be done in several ways, the primary goals being to obtain representative growth of the organism and to provide isolated colonies for study. One may rub the swab back and forth over one-fourth to one-third of the agar plate with continuous rotation. This may be followed by streaking with the inoculating loop at a 90° angle to the swab streaks, crossing over the swabbed area each time and covering all the rest of the plate. Another method is to emulsify the swab with broth before streaking on the plate. When bedside inoculation of media can be done, the first method may be used, but when some time elapses between collection and inoculation, emulsification is probably best to avoid drying.

The inoculated plates are incubated at 35° C. and examined after 24 hours, at which time the colonies are studied carefully. Incubation in an atmosphere of 10 per cent CO_2 enhances growth of *N. meningitidis* and certain other organisms. Colony size, color, shape, effect on blood, and gram stain are guides to tentative identification of the organisms present and will suggest means of final identification. The use of a hand lens or other magnifier is recommended, since colonies of some organisms (e.g., *H. influenzae*) may be very small. A tentative report of the findings should be made, and the plates may be reincubated for another 24 hours.

When diphtheria is suspected, special methods are indicated. It is necessary to rule out Vincent's disease and moniliasis and to differentiate between diphtheria and follicular tonsillitis (*Str. pyogenes*). The membranous lesion or follicles must be explored with the swabs vigorously enough to break the surface. At least two and preferably three swabs should be taken.

The first swab should be smeared on two clean slides and one stained with gram stain. In Vincent's infection one will see numerous spirillae (*B. vincentii*) and fusiform bacilli (large, curved, gram-negative bacilli) with tapering ends. Such a finding is highly suggestive (Fig. 18–12). The second slide should be stained with either Albert's or Loeffler's alkaline methylene blue. The FA technique can also be used.

Albert's Stain

SOLUTION

Toluidine blue	0.15 gm.
Methyl green	0.20 gm.
Acetic acid (glacial)	1.0 ml.
Ethyl alcohol (95 per cent)	2.0 ml.
Distilled water	100 ml.

PROCEDURE

1. Make smears as usual and fix with heat.
2. Stain 5 minutes in the staining solution.
3. Drain without washing.
4. Cover for 1 minute in a modified Lugol's solution (iodine, 2 gm.; KI, 3 gm.; distilled water, 300 ml.).
5. Wash briefly in tap water.
6. Dry and examine.

RESULTS. Metachromatic granules stain black; bars of diphtheria cells stain dark green or black; bodies of cells stain light green.

To stain with Loeffler's alkaline methylene blue, cover the fixed slide with the stain for 30

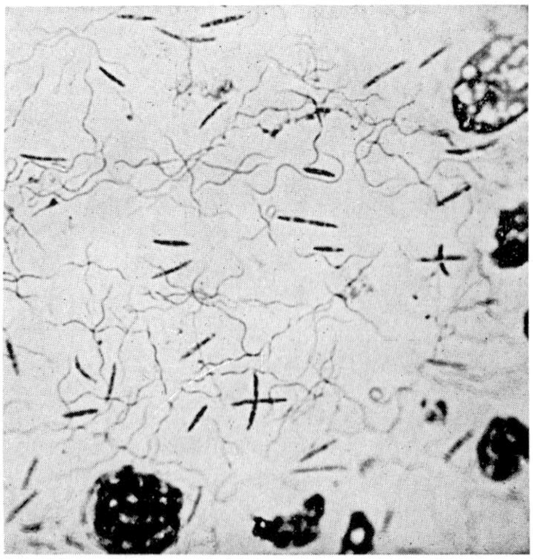

Figure 18–12. *Borrelia vincentii* and fusiform bacilli from the throat of a patient with Vincent's angina (× 1200).

to 60 seconds, wash in water, dry, and examine. The metachromatic granules stain dark blue to violet.

For morphologic descriptions of *C. diphtheriae* refer to the section describing the various species of microorganisms (p. 987). One must examine these direct smears carefully and interpret the findings with caution. Failure to see typical *C. diphtheriae* does not rule out their presence in the throat. Positive findings must be correlated with clinical findings, since there are nontoxigenic *C. diphtheriae* that are morphologically and culturally typical. This does not negate the value of the direct smear but does imply caution.

Three media should be inoculated in cases of suspected diphtheria: Loeffler's serum or Pai's slant, a tellurite agar plate, and a blood agar plate. There are several suitable tellurite media, among them Mueller's tellurite medium, Tinsdale's medium, and chocolate blood tellurite medium. If two swabs are available, one should be streaked over the entire Loeffler's or Pai's slant and on the surface of the tellurite agar. The other swab should be streaked on the blood agar plate. All media should be incubated at 35° C.

Pai's Egg Medium

Infusion broth (1 per cent dextrose)	30 ml.
Whole, mixed eggs	70 ml.
Glycerol, C. P.	8 ml.

Mix, tube, slant, inspissate.

Tellurite Serum Agar (Perry and Petran)

Meat infusion agar	1000 ml.
Serum, horse	50 ml.
Dextrose, 10 per cent solution	20 ml.
Potassium tellurite, 1 per cent solution (pH 9.5; filter)	10 ml.

Prepare the above stock solutions and sterilize. Melt agar and cool to 50° C. Add each of the other ingredients aseptically. Mix well and pour into Petri dishes.

Tinsdale's medium consists of a base medium containing proteose peptone No. 3, NaCl, and agar and an enrichment containing bovine serum, cystine, and potassium tellurite.* For use, 15 ml. of the rehydrated enrichment is added to 100 ml. of the base agar and dispensed in Petri dishes. Specimens are streaked on the plate and stabbed through the medium several times. *C. diphtheriae* produces smooth gray-black shiny convex surface colonies. *Gravis* and *mitis* biotypes produce dark brown halos after 24 hours of incubation. *Minimus* colonies produce smaller halos after 48 hours. Diphtheroids produce light gray to black colonies without halos.

Growth on the slant should be checked after 12 to 18 hours of incubation. More than 24 hours of incubation is not recommended, since overgrowth of other organisms may obscure *C. diphtheriae*. Smears are made from the growth on the slant stained with Albert's or Loeffler's stain and examined for the presence of morphologically typical *C. diphtheriae*.

The blood agar plate is examined after 24 hours for the typical small beta-hemolytic colonies of *Str. pyogenes*. The presence of numerous such colonies is suggestive of follicular tonsillitis, but one must still rule out *C. diphtheriae* because the two organisms may occur together in cases of diphtheria.

The tellurite plate is incubated for 48 hours and examined for the typical black or gray colonies of *C. diphtheriae*. Since certain other organisms, e.g., staphylococci, yeasts, and diphtheroids, may produce black colonies on this medium, it is necessary to do gram stains to determine the type of organisms present. It is well to be familiar with the differences between the microscopic appearance of *C. diphtheriae* on tellurite medium and a specimen yielding morphologically typical bacilli after growth on the Loeffler's slant. Another tellurite plate should be streaked from the growth on the Loeffler's medium. Likewise, failure to see typical organisms from Loeffler's, when suggestive colonies are found on the tellurite plate, should be followed by inoculation of a Loeffler's slant from the colony on the tellurite medium.

As indicated before, there are morphologically and culturally typical *C. diphtheriae* that do not produce toxin and are, consequently, nonpathogenic. Perhaps the simplest way to determine this is to grow a pure culture of the isolated organism on a Loeffler's slant for 24 to 48 hours and wash off the growth in 3 to 4 ml. of infusion broth. Add the broth to the slant and rotate vigorously between the hands. Inoculate 0.5 ml. of the suspended culture intraperitoneally into each of two guinea pigs, one of which has been protected by giving intraperitoneally 500 to 1000 units of diphtheria antitoxin a few hours previously. The unprotected guinea pig should die within 4 or 5 days, and the protected one should show no ill effects. The protected guinea pig should always be included to show that no toxic organisms other than *C. diphtheriae* are present. The toxicity test is not so important in clinically typical cases but is very important in following convalescents and in detecting carriers or doubtful cases. There are other techniques of toxicity testing, utilizing the skin of rabbits, day-old chicks, or agar diffusion methods (Bickham and Jones, 1972). For methods of examination of the throat and of the sputum for fungi and viruses see Chapters 20 and 21.

*Available commercially.

Cerebrospinal Fluid Cultures

Normally the cerebrospinal fluid is sterile. In meningitis, the following organisms may be found: *Neisseria meningitidis, Diplococcus pneumoniae, Haemophilus influenzae, Streptococcus pyogenes, Staphylococcus aureus, Mycobacterium tuberculosis, Listeria monocytogenes, Escherichia coli, Klebsiella pneumoniae,* and *Pseudomonas aeruginosa.* Under some conditions almost any other microorganism may be found in the spinal fluid.

Some of these organisms occur much more frequently in meningitis than others, and some have a definite age distribution. *Haemophilus influenzae* occurs most frequently in young children and seldom in adults. *Neisseria meningitidis* occurs frequently in children but also affects older age groups and may occur in epidemic form. Occasionally, as a result of injuries or for other reasons, bacteria of the normal flora may gain entry. Thus, any finding must be checked thoroughly before a final decision is made about its etiologic significance.

When cerebrospinal fluid is collected for bacteriologic examination, it must be transported to the laboratory immediately and examined at once. This is particularly important in meningococcal infection, since this organism tends to autolyze rapidly and thus may be missed. Speed is only slightly less important in other forms of meningitis, since the early initiation of appropriate treatment is of the greatest urgency.

In the bacteriologic examination of cerebrospinal fluid the gram-stained smear is extremely important. The specimen should be centrifuged at 2000 r.p.m. for 10 minutes and the sediment used for smear and culture. A loopful is spread on a clean slide, gram stained, and examined. The presence of gram-negative, bean-shaped, intra- or extracellular diplococci in indicative of *N. meningitidis.* Small gram-negative bacilli may indicate *H. influenzae,* especially in children. These can sometimes be difficult organisms to find, since one quite frequently finds strands of proteinaceous material in such preparations that are hard to distinguish from bacteria. These examinations require care and experience. The presence of gram-positive cocci indicates *Diplococcus, Streptococcus,* or *Staphylococcus,* and it is difficult to differentiate among them. Large gram-negative bacilli may be suggestive of *Escherichia* or *Enterobacter.* When present, these organisms are often filamentous and may be plentiful.

It is also important to note the relative number and types of cells present on the smear. In general, polymorphonuclear leukocytes are indicative of bacterial infection, but a predominance of lymphocytes points to viral involvement. The findings of this direct examination should be reported immediately.

For culture the media of choice are blood and chocolate agar, and it is well to inoculate each specimen on plates of both media if possible. *Neisseria meningitidis* and *H. influenzae* grow best on the chocolate agar. These plates should be incubated under 10 per cent CO_2. It is also desirable to inoculate a tube of fluid thioglycollate medium for possible anaerobic organisms.

Some workers recommend that enriched semisolid agar (ascitic fluid plus dextrose) be poured into the original tube containing the spinal fluid sediment after the other cultures have been made. Such a culture may be positive in cases in which no colonies appear on the agar plates.

The cultures are examined after 24 to 48 hours, and colonies are studied, picked, and gram stained. Further cultures for identification depend on these findings. Reports should be issued at this point, with any tentative or final identifications that can be made.

The examination of spinal fluid in cases of suspected tuberculous meningitis requires special comment. Since *M. tuberculosis* is usually not present in large numbers, it may be difficult to demonstrate. As much spinal fluid as possible should be obtained (10 ml. if possible). Several different specimens may be pooled if available. The fluid should be centrifuged and the sediment used to make smears for acid-fast stains or for cultures or guinea pig inoculation. The finding of acid-fast organisms on the stained smear is diagnostic. Several tubes of TB media should be inoculated and examined periodically for at least 8 weeks.

Not infrequently a pellicle will form in spinal fluid from patients with tuberculous meningitis if the specimen is allowed to stand in the collection tube in the refrigerator. This pellicle should be sedimented and examined carefully by smear and culture.

In the absence of positive findings on gram-stained smears in cases of suspected meningococcal or *H. influenzae* meningitis, one may do a ring precipitin test using specific antimeningococcal or anti-influenzal antiserum. Some of the spinal fluid is drawn up in a capillary tube, and then some of the antiserum is carefully drawn up so that the two are in contact. The capillary tube is then set in plasticine on the desk. If after 20 to 30 minutes a white ring forms at the juncture of spinal fluid and serum, the test is positive. This is the result of the presence of soluble bacterial antigens in the cerebrospinal fluid, and the test is fairly specific. Direct FA techniques can be used also; these are particularly valuable in cases where the patient has already been treated with antibiotics before the specimen was collected. Specific fluorescein-labeled antisera of high quality and adequate controls must, of course, be available. For mycologic and viral studies see Chapters 20 and 21.

Urine Cultures

Bacteria that may be found in urine include *E. coli, Klebsiella, Proteus, Pseudomonas aeruginosa, Streptococcus pyogenes, Staphylococcus aureus,* enterococci, *Mycobacterium tuberculosis, Salmonella sp., Serratia, Herellea,* and *Enterobacter*.

As it passes out through the urethra the urine may become contaminated with certain bacteria, especially *E. coli* and staphylococci. This is more likely to happen in the female. Consequently, the method of collection of urine for culture is important, and it is necessary to know how collection was accomplished in order to interpret results. In the past catheterization has been used most commonly, but in recent years, because of the real hazard of introducing organisms with the catheter and actually causing infection, use of midstream collection has increased. In the male one may collect the middle portion of the urine, allowing the first portion to wash out most of the contaminating organisms. In the female one needs to cleanse the area around the urethra prior to urination and then collect in the middle portion as in the male. Ten per cent aqueous green soap is recommended for this purpose. Bladder aspiration is occasionally used to avoid contamination. The use of a sterile, tightly sealed container is always necessary.

Once collected, the urine sample must be cultured promptly. No more than 1 hour should elapse between the time of collection and the time of culture. Refrigeration of the sample may be done if it is impossible to examine within this time. Preservatives can be useful. Boric acid or NaCl-polyvinylpyrrolidone (PVP) solution is effective in preventing overgrowth of saprophytes in urine that is delayed inordinately in transit to the laboratory.

The actual culture of the urine sample should include both a quantitative and qualitative technique. Since one deals with a wide variety of both gram-positive and gram-negative organisms, it is necessary to culture for both groups. Thus, the minimum should include inoculation of a portion of the urine on a blood agar plate, as well as a plate of E.M.B. or other medium specifically selective for gram-negative bacilli. One may also include a blood agar plate containing phenylethyl alcohol or Columbia CNA (colimycin-nalidixic acid) agar, both of which are selective for gram-positive bacteria.

An adequate quantitative urine culture can be done with a standard loop made to hold 0.01 ml. Such loops can be obtained from commercial sources. The following procedure has been found to suffice for routine purposes: Place a small drop of saline in the center of an agar plate. C.L.E.D. (cystine-lactose-electrolyte deficient) agar is excellent for this purpose since it inhibits the swarming of *Proteus* and allows good differentiation of colonies. Transfer 0.01 ml. of the urine to the drop of saline. Centrifugation of the urine prior to culture is not recommended. Using a bent wire with the bend about one-half inch from the end, streak the inoculum over the entire plate. The number of colonies appearing on the plate is then multiplied by 100 to estimate the number per milliliter of urine. In actual practice it has been found desirable to make a 1:10 dilution of the urine by adding 0.1 ml. of urine to 0.9 ml. of saline and streak out 0.01 ml. of this dilution on a second plate. This gives a better estimate with urine samples that contain greater numbers of bacteria. One multiplies the number of colonies on this plate by 1000.

The above technique can be used to provide a combined qualitative and quantitative urine culture. If 0.01 ml. of the specimen is streaked on the E.M.B. and phenylethyl alcohol or Columbia CNA plates, one can get a quantitative estimate of the numbers of certain specific organisms.

Greater accuracy can be obtained by making serial dilutions of the urine and doing pour plates, but the technique cannot easily be used extensively in routine laboratories. The technique outlined above provides a good estimate of the number of organisms in the urine and provides the physician with useful data that can be evaluated in relation to the patient's condition.

Kass and other investigators have shown that, in general, less than 10,000 bacteria per ml. of urine is insignificant, and 100,000 (10^5) or more is indicative of urinary tract infection. Counts between these figures are considered of variable significance, depending on the type of organism and the clinical picture presented by the patient. These criteria are valid *only* for properly collected specimens. Diuresis or indwelling catheter drainage may result in lower counts even in the presence of infection. Chemotherapy may result in lowered bacterial counts while the infection remains active. Quantitation alone is not enough. The type of organism is also important. Certainly the presence of 10,000 *S. aureus* per ml. in a urine culture would be viewed with more concern than would the same number of *E. coli*. Thus, the interpretation of the results of urine culture depends on the method of collection and delivery to the laboratory, the types and number of bacteria present, and an evaluation of these findings in relation to the patient's clinical picture.

Various rapid screening tests are now available. These are based on reduction of triphenyltetrazolium chloride, nitrate reduction or catalase activity. These may have some value in screening large numbers of urines for unsuspected infection but are not equivalent to a properly performed quantitative culture.

In suspected tuberculous infection of the urinary tract, examination of the sediment of centrifuged urine should be made. The morning collection of urine is advisable. Twenty-four-hour collection specimens are not suitable since they are invariably grossly contaminated. Smears of the sediment should be stained with an acid-fast stain or auramine-rhodamine. Since nonpathogenic acid-fast bacteria, such as *M. smegmatis,* may occur normally in the urinary tract, the demonstration of acid-fast organisms in stained smears should be interpreted with caution and must be confirmed by culture or animal inoculation.

Since the urine is usually contaminated with other bacteria, the urinary sediment should be digested as described for sputum in preparation for culture and animal inoculation. It is advisable to add penicillin or gentamicin to the sediment. Some prefer to add 2 ml. of tannic acid (5 per cent) per liter plus 2 to 3 drops of nitric acid (30 per cent). The specimen is allowed to stand in the refrigerator overnight. The sediment is then collected and treated as is sputum.

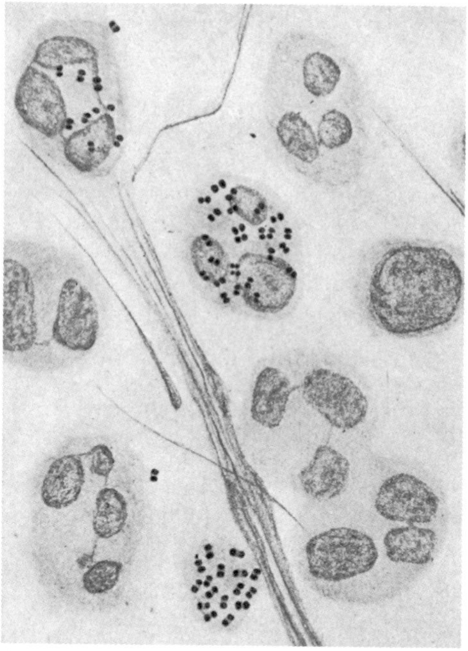

Figure 18–13. Gonococci in leukocytes in smear of pus from case of gonorrhea, stained with methylene blue. The long, fibrous objects are shreds of fibrin and mucus in the pus. Note that the gonococci are nearly all within the leukocytes. (From Frobisher, M., Jr.: Fundamentals of Microbiology. 8th edition.)

Urethral, Prostatic, and Vaginal Exudates

The normal flora of the urethral orifice of the male includes *E. coli,* diphtheroids, and *Staphylococcus epidermidis.* The prostate and its secretions are normally sterile. In the female the urethral and vaginal areas normally have a considerable microbial flora, which is largely dependent on the glycogen content of the vaginal epithelium. This may include Döderlein's bacillus (*Lactobacillus* sp.) in large numbers, the Coli-Enterobacter group, staphylococci, streptococci (aerobic and anaerobic), yeasts, *Bacteroides, Veillonella,* and *M. smegmatis.*

Pathogenic microorganisms of the region of the genital tract include: *Neisseria gonorrhoeae, Treponema pallidum, Hemophilus ducreyi* and *C. vaginale, Calymmatobacterium (Donovania) granulomatis, Streptococcus pyogenes* (groups B and D), anaerobic streptococci, *Staphylococcus aureus,* Mycoplasma, *Candida albicans* and various other yeasts, *Trichomonas vaginalis,* viruses of lymphogranuloma venereum and herpes.

The demonstration and identification of *N. gonorrhoeae* and *T. pallidum* as aids in the diagnosis of gonorrhea and syphilis are perhaps the most important procedures to carry out on urethral and vaginal exudates.

GONORRHEA AND NONSPECIFIC URETHRITIS

In the male acute gonorrhea manifests itself by a burning sensation accompanied by a purulent and rather continuous, brownish-tinged exudate. This exudate should be collected on an inoculating loop or cotton swab, gently smeared on a clean slide, and stained with the gram stain. The swab should be rolled on the slide rather than smeared to avoid disrupting the leukocytes. In gonorrhea the smear will reveal large numbers of pus cells with varying numbers of intra- and extracellular gram-negative, bean-shaped diplococci (Fig. 18–13). Such a finding can be considered diagnostic. It is important to point out that only a very few of the thousands of pus cells on the slide may contain bacteria, and sometimes it requires considerable search to find one. In chronic gonorrhea or in treated cases the number of bacteria may be small, and they may be mostly extracellular. In such cases culture from the anterior urethra is necessary. In homosexuals an additional culture specimen should be obtained from the anal canal and pharynx.

The Thayer-Martin (1966) selective medium is excellent for isolating gonococci from sites where this organism is outnumbered by other flora. Vancomycin, colistin, and nystatin* are added at a concentration of 3 μg., 7.5 μg., and 12.5 units per ml., respectively, to a conventional GC agar base.* Vials containing these antibiotics for this purpose are available commercially. Exudate taken with an inoculating loop or a swab should be promptly streaked over the entire warmed agar plate and the plate incubated under 10 per cent CO_2. For methods of identification see section on specific organisms (p. 957).

Since the infection tends to migrate up the urinary tract and may localize in the prostate, it may be necessary in chronic gonorrhea to examine the discharge resulting from prostatic massage. The discharge should be collected in a sterile container and examined immediately by a gram-stained smear and culture.

Not infrequently one encounters in the male a urethral discharge that is nongonorrheal in origin. These discharges usually occur in the morning and tend to be cloudy but not purulent or mucoid as in gonorrhea. Gram stains from discharges reveal large numbers of pus cells. Sometimes no bacteria are seen, or there may be sparse gram-positive cocci, usually *S. epidermidis*. Other specimens may have large numbers of small, gram-negative, pleomorphic bacilli, which vary in morphology from bacilli to cocci that occur in pairs. These organisms may be intra- and extracellular and, but for their size, might be confused with *N. gonorrhoeae*. Culture from such a discharge may reveal the presence of organisms in the *Mima* or *Hemophilus* groups. Mycoplasma may also be involved, especially T-stains (see p. 1003).

The diagnosis of gonorrhea in the female presents certain problems. The disease may be asymptomatic, or it may manifest itself only by an increased vaginal discharge. Swab specimens for smear and culture may be taken from the cervix, vagina, and urethra, as determined by the examining physician. For maximum yield, cultures of both the cervix and anal canal are recommended. Owing to the complex bacterial flora and the presence of epithelial cells, the examination of gram-stained smears from such material is difficult, and failure to find typical intra- and extracellular gram-negative diplococci cannot be considered final. This is especially true of chronic, longstanding infections. Thus, in the female, culture is a necessary adjunct in attempting to make a diagnosis. Swabs should be streaked over the surface of a Thayer-Martin plate and the plate incubated under enriched CO_2 (Fig. 18–14). FA by direct

*To suppress *Proteus*, trimethoprim lactate (5 μg./ml.) may be added. Pimarcin, 20 μg./ml. can be substituted for nystatin.

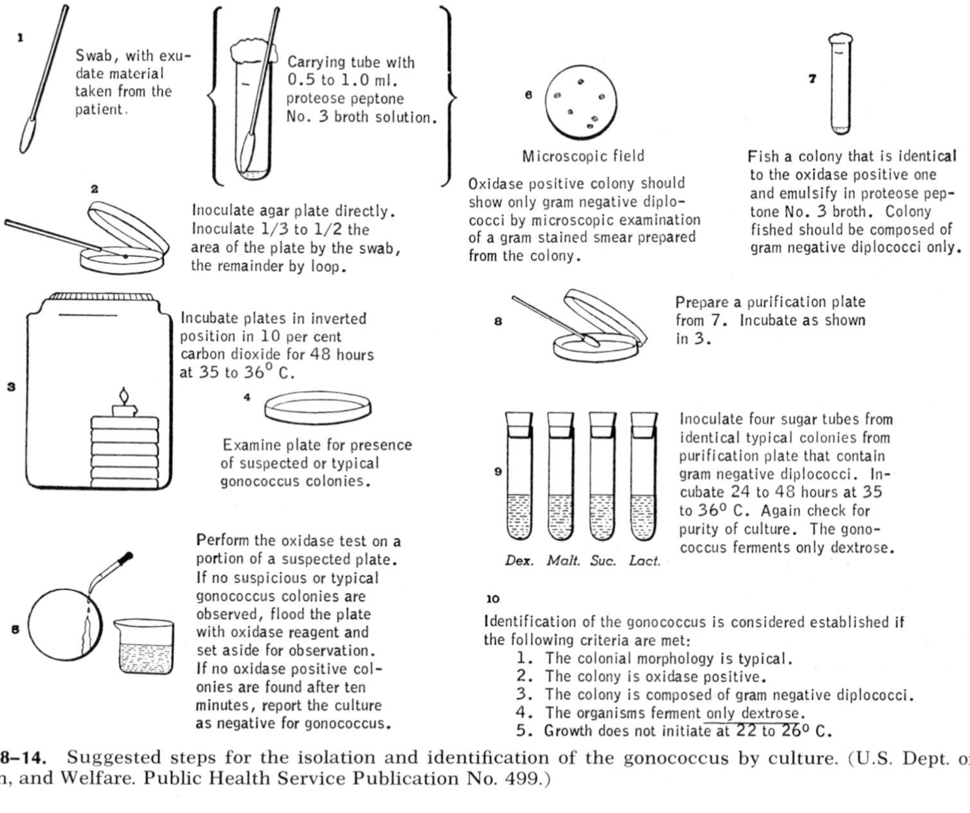

Figure 18–14. Suggested steps for the isolation and identification of the gonococcus by culture. (U.S. Dept. of Health, Education, and Welfare. Public Health Service Publication No. 499.)

or delayed techniques is not recommended for diagnosis or test of cure, except as an adjunct to culture.

The recently developed "Transgrow" medium is excellent for transport of specimens for gonococcus cultures. Viability of the cultures is retained for extended periods and growth of saprophytic bacteria is inhibited. The addition of trimethoprim is helpful in suppressing *Proteus* overgrowth. Stuart's transport medium or "Culturettes" are also useful for this purpose.

It is possible to culture urine sediments from either the male or the female. The urine should be the first morning specimen and should be sedimented and the sediment cultured immediately. Conjunctiva, joint fluid, skin lesions, and so forth, may also be cultured for gonococci.

If conditions other than gonorrhea are suspected, the cultural methods will depend on the clinical impression. Puerperal fever in the female is caused usually by aerobic or anaerobic streptococci (*Peptostreptococci*) or staphylococci. *Vibrio foetus* or *Listeria* may also be involved. Inoculation of swabs on blood agar or fluid thioglycollate and the use of anaerobic methods should reveal these organisms. An organism thought by many to be associated with leukorrhea, vaginitis, and cervicitis is known as *Corynebacterium (Hemophilus) vaginale*. This is a small, pleomorphic, gram-negative bacillus. On wet mounts of the discharge epithelial cells may be seen covered with such large masses of this organism as to obliterate the cell membrane—the so-called clue cell. Characteristically there is an almost complete absence of leukocytes in the preparation (Fig. 18–15). Cultures on rabbit blood agar under 10 per cent CO_2 show small, pinpoint, catalase-negative colonies. On human blood agar, colonies usually are beta hemolytic (Dunkelberg *et al.*, 1970).

SYPHILIS

Syphilis in the female frequently produces lesions in the cervix, vagina, and surrounding

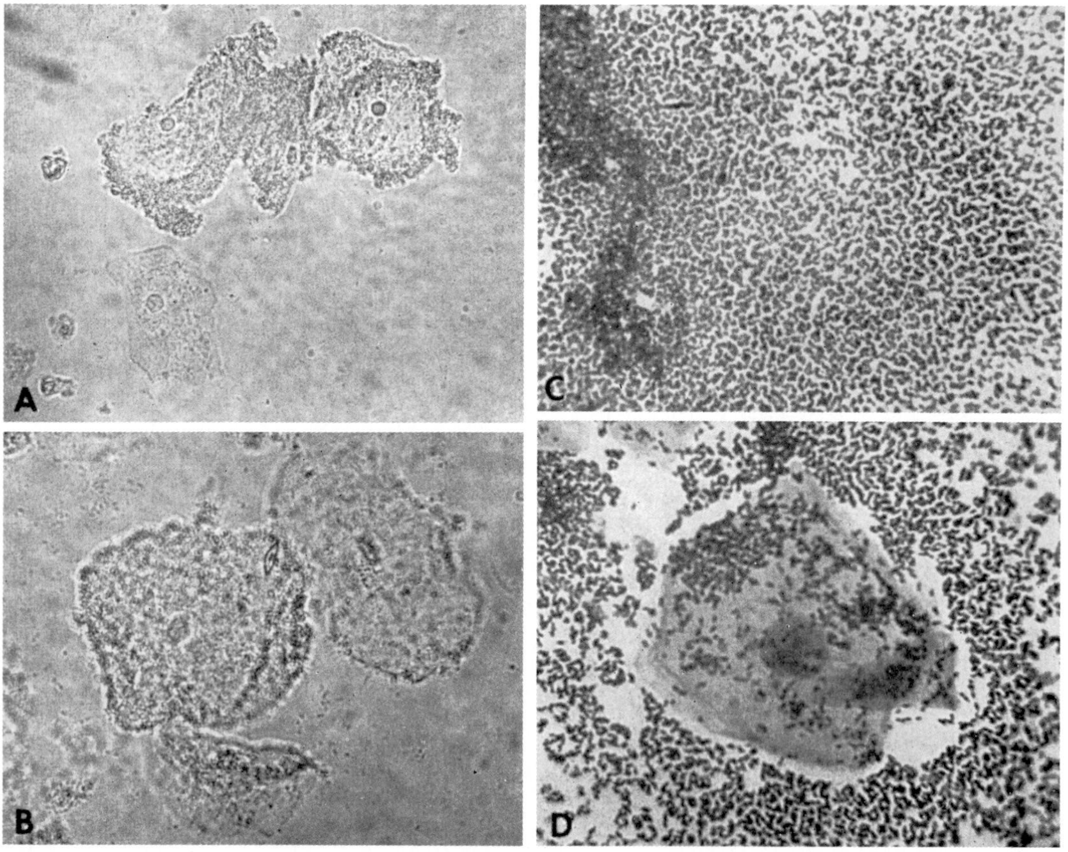

Figure 18–15. *A*, Wet mount showing involvement of epithelial cells with *H. vaginalis*, referred to as "clue cells." Uninvolved epithelial cell is seen in lower part of field. *B*, Higher magnification of epithelial "clue cells." *C*, *D*, Direct smears of vaginal discharge. Note large number of *H. vaginalis*. (From Gardner, H. L., and Dukes, C. D.: Amer. J. Obstet. Gynec., *69*:962, 1955.)

areas, and in the male the chancre may occur in the urethra or on the penis. The bacteriologic diagnosis of syphilis depends on demonstration of the spirochete *Treponema pallidum* by darkfield microscopy, fluorescent staining or silver impregnation staining. In exposed chancres material for examination is collected by first cleansing the surface and then grasping the lesion between thumb and forefinger and expressing the clear amber fluid by pressure. The operator should always wear rubber gloves and dispose of contaminated material in disinfectant solution. The expressed fluid may then be touched with a clean coverslip and the slip applied to a clean new microscope slide. Alternatively the fluid may be collected with a capillary pipette. The coverslip is sealed around the edge with petrolatum and the preparation promptly examined by darkfield microscopy. Considerable care and experience are required in making this examination. Sometimes nonpathogenic spirochetes are present. These are usually much less delicate than *T. pallidum*.

For cervical, vaginal, or other unexposed lesions it is necessary to visualize the lesion with a speculum or other instrument and to collect exudate with a Pasteur pipette or inoculating loop. This is placed on a slide and covered with a coverslip as just described.

Another condition occurring in the same region is soft chancre (chancroid), which is caused by *Hemophilus ducreyi*. Gram-stained smears from the lesion may reveal small gram-negative bacilli arranged in rows. Culture from the lesion may be made on enriched media or clotted rabbit blood but is frequently unsuccessful (see p. 982).

Granuloma inguinale is a granulomatous lesion, usually involving an inguinal lymph node. Stained aspirates from these lesions reveal gram-negative bacilli with large capsules (Donovan bodies). The causative agent (*Calymmatobacterium granulomatis*) is very difficult to culture.

For methods of diagnosing vaginal moniliasis and trichomoniasis see sections on mycology and parasitology.

Skin Lesions: Wounds, Boils, Furuncles, and Exudates

Normally the skin is contaminated with various saprophytic and potentially pathogenic bacteria. The microorganisms present on the skin and mucous surfaces at any time depend on the environment, the area of skin and its nature, and certain other unknown factors. Bacteria on the skin may be either "transient" or "resident"; the latter seem to be constantly present and consist primarily of gram-positive cocci.

When lesions occur in or upon the skin and microbiologic examination is required, certain basic principles should be observed. Material for smears and culture should be taken from an area as close to normal tissue as possible, that is, the edge or base of an ulcer or abscess after removal of pus or debris. In certain instances it is not profitable to culture pus or necrotic material. Pus may be completely sterile, even though the lesion from which it is derived may be caused by a specific bacterium. On the other hand, it may be heavily contaminated with saprophytic bacteria, and the culture may yield nothing but confusion. One should culture for anaerobic bacteria (*Bacteroides, Clostridium perfringens*, anaerobic streptococci, and so forth), especially in deep or penetrating wounds.

In certain conditions in which skin rashes occur, the causative organisms may sometimes be demonstrated in the lesions of the rash. In meningococcemia, incision of the bright red petechiae, followed by a gram-stained smear and culture on chocolate agar may reveal the typical gram-negative diplococci.

The most common cause of boils, furuncles, and carbuncles is *S. aureus*, although other organisms, such as *Str. pyogenes* and certain anaerobic organisms, may rarely be involved. Cultures from such lesions should be taken with care to avoid contamination with organisms from the skin surface. The area around and over the lesion should be thoroughly cleansed with alcohol and allowed to dry. Pus or other material in the lesion should be removed and a sterile swab used to explore the base of the lesion. More than one swab may be used, depending on the number of procedures to be done. The swab should be emulsified in a small amount of infusion broth. The broth suspension should be streaked on a blood agar plate and inoculated into a tube of fluid thioglycollate medium for detection of anaerobes. Also, when possible, one should streak a second blood agar plate and incubate in the anaerobic jar. A swab should be smeared on a slide and stained with gram stain. Such a stained smear may suggest the type of organism involved.

In superficial infections, such as impetigo or acne, the surface area should be cleansed thoroughly before cultures are taken. The surface of lesions should then be broken and material collected on swabs, as in boils and furuncles. Staphylococci, streptococci (aerobic and anaerobic), *Propionibacterium (Corynebacterium) acnes*, and certain anaerobic bacteria may be present in such conditions. It is not always easy or possible to assess the role of the isolated organisms in these conditions, especially in acne. In impetigo the causative agent is usually either *Str. pyogenes* or *S. aureus*.

Wound culture technique is determined in large measure by the existing situation. The site and method of taking material for culture are determined by the nature of the wound and whether evidence of obvious infection exists. Numerous organisms may be involved, depending on the amount of dirt and debris that may have been introduced. Wounds involving considerable trauma or penetrating wounds may contain anaerobes, such as *Cl. tetani* or *Cl. perfringens*. Thus, it is essential to do both aerobic and anaerobic cultures.

Recently, infection of surgical incisions with antibiotic-resistant *S. aureus* has become a serious problem. In certain areas, wound infection with *C. diphtheriae* is not uncommon. In such situations there may be membrane formation similar to that in the throat in classic diphtheria. Cultural techniques in this situation are similar to those described previously for diphtheria.

Infections of the Eye

Eye secretions may have certain of the normal skin inhabitants in small numbers, such as *Staph. epidermidis* and diphtheroids, but cultures from the normal eye, including the conjunctiva, should be relatively free of microorganisms.

The following organisms are of pathologic importance: *Diplococcus pneumoniae, Hemophilus aegyptius* (Koch-Weeks), *Klebsiella pneumoniae, Staphylococcus aureus, Moraxella lacunata* (Morax-Axenfeld), *Pseudomonas aeruginosa,* and *Neisseria gonorrhoeae.*

Eye infections are accompanied by inflammation (pink eye) and increased secretion of tears, which may become purulent. The most common bacteria involved are listed above, although the presence of any other bacteria in considerable numbers in infected eyes should be cause for suspicion.

Cultures from infected eyes should be taken by swabbing the inflamed area and streaking on blood or chocolate agar. Inoculation should also be made into infusion broth. At the same time smears should be made for staining by gram or Giemsa stain. Viral infections are common in some areas and must be considered.

Ear, Mastoid, Sinuses, and Antrum

A variety of organisms may be associated with lesions and abscesses in ear and in sinus infections, including *Pseudomonas aeruginosa,* members of the Coli-Enterobacter group, *Staphylococcus aureus,* diphtheroids, staphylococci, *Streptococcus pyogenes,* anaerobic streptococci, and alpha streptococci. Fungi may also be found in ear infections and must be considered.

The evaluation of cultural results from abscesses and lesions in the ear is not always easy and requires the same consideration as does the interpretation of cultures from other exposed areas where surface contamination and secondary growth of essentially nonpathogenic bacteria may occur. The presence of certain organisms may be the result rather than the cause of an infection. Nevertheless, it must be recognized that eradication of such organisms may be highly desirable.

In collecting material from sinus infections, one must take care to insure that the material actually comes from the sinuses and has not become contaminated from an outside source. The same general approach to culture should be followed in these situations as that described for the other areas.

Blood Culture Technique

Blood culture is one of the most important and critical procedures in clinical microbiology. When done properly, it can be of greatest assistance in diagnosis, but when poorly done, it can introduce confusion and misunderstanding. One of the best indications for blood culture is the presence of fever, especially if it is persistent. Numerous febrile conditions are accompanied by bacterial invasion of the blood, and the isolation of the organism has great diagnostic significance.

Organisms that may occur in the blood are as follows: *Neisseria meningitidis, Haemophilus influenzae, Diplococcus pneumoniae, Streptococcus pyogenes, Streptococcus viridans, Staphylococcus aureus, Brucella, Salmonella typhi,* other *Salmonella, Escherichia coli,* and *Histoplasma capsulatum.* There are occasions when such organisms as *Staphylococcus epidermidis,* certain anaerobic or microaerophilic bacteria, and others may be isolated in blood culture. These should not be written off as contaminants, even though the organism is generally considered a nonpathogen or a low grade pathogen, without proper evaluation of technique and repeat cultures when possible.

The time at which the blood culture is taken is important. It should always be taken before initiation of antibiotic therapy and, if possible, when the fever is rising. Once antibiotic therapy is started, the chances of obtaining a positive culture are greatly reduced. The stage of the disease may be important. For example, in typhoid fever the blood culture is most likely to be positive during the first two weeks of the disease. In some conditions, such as subacute bacterial endocarditis, repeated blood cultures should be done. This is also indicated in brucellosis, in which, at best, the organism is difficult to culture.

The actual procedure for blood culture can be divided into steps, each of which is of critical importance: preparation of the site for collection of blood, collection of blood, inoculation into media, incubation and examination of the blood culture, identification of cultured organisms, and reporting of results.

In preparation for taking a blood culture, the patient should be placed in a comfortable position with the vein accessible. As a rule, one of the veins in the antecubital fossa is used for puncture in adults. In small children and babies, blood may be collected from the jugular vein. This must be done by one experienced in such techniques. The skin over and surrounding the area of puncture should be cleansed thoroughly with alcohol or tincture of green soap to remove all oily deposits and then painted with disinfectant. Tincture of iodine (3 per cent iodine in 70 per cent ethyl alcohol) or PVP-iodine is recommended. The iodine should be left on for a few minutes and allowed to dry before the puncture is made. A tourniquet is applied to the arm and tightened to suppress venous flow of blood. The area should be wiped off with alcohol after the blood has been collected.

The materials for collection must be dry, i.e., sterilized with dry heat. There are a number of techniques for collection of blood that can be used, depending on the situation. The technique involving the least number of steps in collection and inoculation of appropriate media is the most desirable, since each step increases the possibility of contamination. One can obtain blood culture sets commercially at moderate cost. Each set consists of a rubber-capped vacuum bottle containing suitable medium and a sterile rubber tube with a needle at both ends. One needle is inserted into the vein and the other through the rubber cap into the bottle. The vacuum draws the blood into the bottle. When the proper amount of blood has entered, the rubber tube is pinched off, the tourniquet is removed, and the needle is removed from the vein. If the bottle contains 50 ml. of medium, one should collect no more than 5 ml. of blood. If one wishes to do an aerobic culture, a piece of sterile cotton is placed over the needle, and air is allowed to flow into the bottle. If anaerobic culture is to be done, the needle is removed from the bottle while the rubber tube remains pinched shut. Newly developed blood culture tubes require only the use of Vacutainer* needles to collect the specimens. These tubes are prereduced and support the growth of anaerobic bacteria very well.

If the blood is collected with a needle and syringe, one should collect 5 to 10 ml., release the tourniquet, and remove the needle. Immediately after collection the blood should be transferred directly into media or into a sterile flask or test tube containing 4 ml. of 2 per cent sodium citrate to prevent clotting. Once the medium is inoculated it should be incubated as soon as possible. If the blood is citrated, the tube or flask should be shaken gently and transported immediately to the laboratory for inoculation of media and pour-plates, if desired. Delays should be avoided, since antibody may adversely affect the organisms and citrate itself may be detrimental.

Sodium polyanethol sulfonate (Liquoid*) gives excellent results as an anticoagulant for blood cultures and is much less toxic than citrate. EDTA should not be used.

If the bottles and flasks are prepared in the laboratory, it is well to use a good aerobic broth, such as thiol or dextrose phosphate, as well as fluid thioglycollate medium or infusion broth plus cysteine for anaerobic culture. More satisfactory anaerobic blood cultures can be done by collecting the blood into a screw-cap bottle (without rubber diaphragm) of broth and incubating in an anaerobic jar or incubator. In most chronic or subacute conditions it is well to inoculate both types of media, since anaerobic streptococci, *Bacteroides*, and similar organisms will not grow aerobically.

In a number of conditions, such as subacute bacterial endocarditis and brucellosis, in which the number of organisms may be low, it may be desirable to culture more than 5 ml. of blood. In such instances it is better to inoculate several 50-ml. portions of media than to increase the amount of blood in each bottle. If one uses excessive blood, the natural inhibitory substances or antibodies present may prevent growth of bacteria that may be in the blood.

Some workers prefer to use a Castaneda bottle for blood culture. This is made by placing a layer of an agar medium (blood agar or infusion agar) on one side of a square or rectangular bottle, then adding aseptically 50 ml. of blood culture broth. After the blood is added, the bottle is tilted to bathe the agar, and colonies may then appear on this surface.

It is desirable to add 0.05 per cent p-aminobenzoic acid (PABA) to the blood culture medium to counteract sulfonamide drugs that may be in the blood of patients. Appropriate amounts of penicillinase may be added routinely or only in cases in which the patient

*Becton, Dickinson & Company, Rutherford, New Jersey.

*Hoffman-La Roche, Inc., Nutley, New Jersey.

has been treated with penicillin. This would not be effective when the new "semisynthetic" penicillins (oxacillin, methicillin, etc.) are used, since they are not neutralized by this enzyme.

The conditions of incubation are important. *Brucella abortus* grows only in an atmosphere containing 10 per cent CO_2 and *N. meningitidis* and *H. influenzae* grow better in 10 per cent CO_2. Such an atmosphere will not inhibit growth of any of the other organisms.

After inoculation the cultures should be shaken to distribute the blood throughout the medium before incubation at 35° C. Daily examinations should be made. Evidence of bacterial growth may appear as cloudiness in the broth above the settled red blood cells or as obvious changes in these cells, such as hemolysis. Some bacteria do not produce cloudiness, multiplying adjacent to the red blood cell layer (*Str. pyogenes*). When visible evidence of growth appears, samples should be removed for gram stain and subculture. With no visible evidence of growth, samples for gram stain and subculture should be taken at 24- to 48-hour intervals for 7 to 10 days and weekly thereafter.

To take a sample from the blood culture bottle, one should use a dry, sterile needle and syringe. The culture is shaken, and great care is used to sterilize the top before insertion of the needle. Routinely a drop should be smeared on a slide for gram stain and 1 or 2 drops streaked on a blood or chocolate agar plate. The plates should be incubated both aerobically and anaerobically. On the basis of the gram stain, other media may be inoculated. For example, in a patient with clinical signs of enteric fever, the presence of gram-negative bacilli suggests a *Salmonella* infection, and one should streak an E.M.B. plate or other enteric medium. The results of the preliminary finding should be reported as soon as possible.

The results of the gram stain and the type of growth in the blood culture will do much to determine the procedures for identification of the organism. Once growth has been detected and successful subcultures obtained, it is no longer necessary to hold the blood culture. How long negative cultures should be held is difficult to define. Growth is sometimes considerably delayed, and even in typhoid fever, cultures have become positive only after 14 to 21 days. In brucellosis it is desirable to hold cultures for 4 to 6 weeks before discarding. Most other blood cultures should be held at least 10 to 14 days. If space permits, nothing is lost by holding them longer. Progress reports on blood culture findings should be made as early as possible. Positive findings must be reported promptly and antibiotic susceptibility studies initiated when indicated.

Microbiologic Examination of the Feces

In this section the methods for bacteriologic examination will be described. For parasitologic examination of feces see Chapter 17, and for viral isolation see Chapter 21.

The lower portion of the intestinal tract represents a complex biologic system in which numerous species of microorganisms may normally be found. The flora may consist of vast numbers of the following organisms: *E. coli, Enterobacter, Proteus, Bacteroides, Staphylococcus,* enterococci, *Clostridium perfringens,* lactobacilli, vibrios, and yeasts.

A large portion of the feces, in fact, is made up of bacterial cells, most of which are dead. It is possible that bacteria that have not yet been isolated and identified are normally present in the digestive tract. Studies have indicated that the relative number of the various organisms of the normal flora fluctuates considerably from day to day. This probably depends on such things as diet and any other factors affecting the physiology and biochemistry of the intestine. Of the organisms most commonly cultured from the feces, *E. coli* normally predominates. *Bacteroides* and enterococci also occur in large numbers. A marked shift in the relative number of these bacteria in the stool flora may indicate an abnormal situation.

There are certain microorganisms that may be present in the intestinal tract and, although not normal inhabitants, appear to have little or no pathogenic potential. In addition, some of the organisms of the normal intestinal flora may produce disease under appropriate circumstances. For instance, it is likely that enterotoxin-producing strains of *S. aureus* are present frequently. Under special circumstances these organisms may produce severe disease. *Proteus morganii* has been suspected of contributing to diarrhea in children. Certain gram-positive organisms, such as staphylococci and possibly streptococci, have been suspected of playing a role in ulcerative colitis. These relationships are difficult to evaluate, and the whole subject of enteric disease needs much further study.

The microbiologic examination of feces involves several procedures: bacteriologic examination involving culture of specific recognized pathogens; examination for cysts and trophozoites of intestinal protozoa and ova, larvae, or other significant structures of intestinal helminths; examination for viruses; and cytologic descriptions of the feces in terms of cellular elements, undigested food particles, fatty acid crystals, blood cells, and yeasts. The presence of increased numbers of yeasts is not necessarily diagnostic in the ordinary sense but may be viewed as a reflection of conditions in the intestinal tract. Such examination often gives valuable leads about what cultural or other procedures might prove of value. For example, the presence of large numbers of pus cells might indicate a bacterial infectious process, and the presence of much undigested protein or fatty acid crystals may indicate faulty absorption.

Certain members of the normal flora of the intestine are capable of producing disease outside the digestive tract. *E. coli, Klebsiella, Proteus,* and *Enterobacter* are common causes of urinary tract infection. These organisms are not infrequently found in the blood as the terminal cause of death in carcinoma and other serious debilitating diseases.

Certain serotypes of *E. coli* can cause serious and sometimes fatal diarrhea in infants and children. Numerous outbreaks of diarrhea in nurseries have been caused by these strains.

In recent years there has been an increasing awareness of the occurrence of endotoxin shock. The organism most commonly associated with the clinical condition is *E. coli,* although other gram-negative bacilli are frequently involved. Occasionally other organisms, such as *Cl. perfringens,* anaerobic streptococci, and fungi, may play a role. The mechanism of bacterial shock involves the focal establishment of an organism, where it multiplies and releases endotoxin. The condition may develop in patients with prostatic infections, in the fetal membranes of pregnant females, or similar localized situations. The diagnosis is primarily a clinical one, but help can be given with direct smear and gram stain of material from the affected site and by culture. One of the requirements seems to be that the endotoxin-producing organism is able to multiply rapidly. As the bacteria reach the peak of their growth curve, endotoxin is released in large amount from the disintegrating bacterial cells and produces severe shock. The response in the walls of the blood vessels has been described as resembling the Shwartzman reaction.

The most common enteric bacterial pathogens are: *Salmonella,* including *S. typhi, Shigella,* enteropathogenic *E. coli, Vibrio cholerae,* and *S. aureus.*

COLLECTION OF SPECIMENS FROM THE INTESTINAL TRACT

A specimen of feces for examination should ideally be the first of the morning. When they can be examined immediately, the specimens can be collected in waxed paper cartons with tight-fitting tops. Collection may be made in bed pans and transferred to cartons. With infants, one may collect the feces from a diaper or use rectal swabs. In any case the specimen should be in the laboratory and ready for examination as soon as possible after collection. The use of barium or mineral oil should be avoided in patients whose stools are to be collected for microbiologic examination. The presence of these substances renders adequate stool examination impossible. If it is not possible to obtain fresh specimens, one can use certain preservatives. For bacterial culture one may emulsify a portion of the stool in buffered glycerol-saline which is made as follows:

Sodium chloride	4.2 gm.
Dipotassium phosphate, anhydrous	3.1 gm.
Monopotassium phosphate, anhydrous	1.0 gm.
Glycerol	300 ml.
Distilled water	700 ml.

Dispense in bottles and autoclave. It is desirable to add sufficient phenol red to the solution to give a pink color. If the phenol red changes to yellow, discard the bottles.

One may use rectal swabs for bacterial culture. This is quite useful in young children. An ordinary cotton swab is moistened in broth or peptone water and inserted through the anal orifice. Culturettes are convenient for this purpose (see p. 950). The swab may then be sent to the laboratory or streaked on plates of appropriate media at the bedside. Rather than use the plain swab, some prefer to place it in a lubricated rubber or plastic tube which is cut so as to have a tapered end. The rubber tube is inserted into the anus and the swab pushed through this. Some workers prefer to take the swab culture through the proctoscope.

The number of stool examinations necessary to diagnose or to rule out a given infection has been the subject of much study. It is difficult to establish a number in any given situation, and one should perhaps never set a maximum. The number of examinations depends on several circumstances. In general, though, for both bacterial and parasitologic examinations one should examine at least three specimens collected on successive or alternate days.

BACTERIOLOGIC EXAMINATION OF FECES

Since the feces normally contain a considerable number of different bacterial species, the isolation of any single species or group requires special techniques. The principles of fecal culture depend on the use of media designed either for enhancement or selection of particular organisms. Most of the well-recognized bacterial diseases of man (typhoid and paratyphoid fever, bacillary dysentery, Salmonella food poisoning, and Asiatic cholera) are caused by gram-negative enteric bacteria of the genera *Salmonella, Shigella,* and *Vibrio.* Sometimes other gram-negative enteric bacilli, such as *Proteus morganii,* enteropathogenic *E. coli,* Arizona, *Providencia,* and so forth, may be involved.

The numbers of any given pathogenic bacterium in the feces vary considerably, depending on the severity and type of infection and the stage of the disease. For example, in typhoid fever the number of *S. typhi* may be very small in the early stages but tends to increase greatly after the second week of the disease. In severe cases one may find a nearly pure culture of this organism in the stools. This may also occur with *V. cholerae* in cholera. In the carrier state the number of the organisms usually is quite small.

The enrichment media, such as GN broth, selenite F, and tetrathionate broth, are designed to assist in the isolation of *Salmonella* in cases in which few organisms are present. In these media *Salmonella* multiplies more rapidly than the other organisms during the first 12 to 18 hours of incubation at 35° C. Thus, if one inoculates from the fecal specimen into one of these media, incubates for from 12 to 18 hours, and then streaks from this onto the selective media, the chances of isolating these pathogens are increased.

Media for enteric bacterial pathogens can be divided into two groups: those that are selective and those that are differential. The most commonly used selective media are Salmonella Shigella (S.S.), X.L.D., brilliant green, bismuth sulfite, and Hektoen enteric (H.E.) agar. The most commonly used differential media are eosin methylene blue (E.M.B.), desoxycholate, Endo's and MacConkey's agar. It is not recommended that one use all these media, but it is well to choose one from each group. A good combination is X.L.D. or H.E. agar and E.M.B., although others may serve equally well, depending on experience and need (Table 18–2).

The routine procedure for fecal culture in the laboratory is as follows: Pick portions of the stool containing mucus or blood for inoculation of media. If the stool is liquid, it can be streaked directly on E.M.B. and X.L.D. or H.E. agar plates. Appropriate portions, particularly any blood or mucus, of formed or semiformed stools should be used to make a heavy suspension in infusion broth. At the same time a portion the size of a pea should be inoculated into a tube of enrichment broth and thoroughly emulsified. The enrichment broth should be incubated 12 to 18 hours at 35° C. and then streaked on the same plates, which should

Table 18–2. ENTERIC DIFFERENTIAL AND SELECTIVE MEDIA

MEDIUM	GRAM + BACTERIOSTATIC AGENT	FERMENTABLE CARBOHYDRATE	INDICATOR	COLONY COLOR: Fermenter	COLONY COLOR: Non-Fermenter
EMB agar*	Eosin Y Methylene blue	Lactose Sucrose	Eosin Y Methylene blue	Black with sheen	Colorless
Desoxycholate agar	Bile salts	Lactose	Neutral red	Red	Colorless
MacConkey agar	Crystal violet Bile salts	Lactose	Neutral red	Red	Colorless
XLD agar	Bile salts	Xylose Lactose Sucrose	Phenol red and H_2S indicator	Yellow	Pink to red
Bismuth sulfite	Brilliant green	Dextrose	Bismuth sulfite	†	†
Desoxycholate-citrate agar	Bile salts	Lactose	Neutral red	Red	Colorless
Hektoen enteric agar	Bile salts	Salicin Lactose Sucrose	Bromthymol blue and H_2S indicator	Yellow-orange	Green or blue-green
Salmonella-Shigella agar	Bile salts	Lactose	Neutral red	Red	Colorless

*Holt-Harris and Teague formulation.

†H_2S + Salmonellae produce black colonies; other organisms produce brown or greenish colonies.

be examined after 24 to 48 hours' incubation and suspicious colonies picked for further study.

BACTERIA OF CLINICAL SIGNIFICANCE

This section will present a brief résumé of the critical characteristics and possible clinical significance of the various groups of bacteria of medical importance. Descriptions will be given in both narrative and tabular form, with emphasis on the occurrence of the organism and a few of the specific characteristics that may be used to establish an identification. More detailed descriptions can be found in the references.

The Gram-positive Cocci

The first group of bacteria to be considered is that comprising the gram-positive cocci. The most important type species, their most important characteristics, and their occurrence are shown in Table 18–3.

As seen in this table, the disease-producing potential of the various members of the gram-positive cocci is large. A number of the more severe life-threatening diseases, such as lobar pneumonia and scarlet fever, have been relegated to minor roles largely as a result of the sensitivity of *Diplococcus* and *Streptococcus pyogenes* to penicillin and other antibiotics. However, these bacteria are still present in the population and account for a considerable morbidity. *Diplococcus pneumoniae* is a common cause of eye infections and mastoiditis and is the most common cause of meningitis in certain age groups. It may be found in 10 to 40 per cent of throat cultures from persons not on antibiotics. A high incidence of *Str. pyogenes,* group A, occurs in cultures from patients with mild to severe sore throats. This is a particularly important consideration, especially in children in whom there is the risk of the development of rheumatic fever or glomerulonephritis following streptococcal disease. This possibility also exists in adults, although to a lesser degree. A number of public health and hospital laboratories are now offering culture services specifically for group A streptococci to physicians in their surrounding area.

Staphylococcus aureus, with its wide potential and ubiquitous distribution, has assumed new importance, particularly in its role in hospital-acquired disease. Although the percentage of antibiotic-resistant *S. aureus* cultures seems to be decreasing, this is not to be interpreted as an indication of a reduction in the importance of the organism. Intensive study of this group of bacteria in recent years has revealed a multiplicity of phage types, and the observations of Cohen on antigenic structure have also revealed complex patterns which are not necessarily constant within phage types. Antimicrobial susceptibility, determined by utilizing a battery of antimicrobial agents, reveals variable patterns even within given phage types. It may also be noted that certain strains produce enterotoxin in varying amounts. Thus, it would appear that there are literally an infinite number of variants in what must be considered a group of bacteria designated as *S. aureus.* Certain phage types seem more prone to be associated with disease than other types, especially when these types are also resistant to antibiotics; but this is not a completely dependable criterion for determining disease-producing potential. Evidence obtained from extensive studies of the environment of hospitals seems to indicate that there are strains that readily adapt to existence in the environment and others that do not. Such adaptability does not necessarily relate to disease-producing potential.

Staphylococcus aureus is the most common cause of boils and carbuncles, as well as osteomyelitis, and when found in these circumstances its pathologic significance is unquestionable. It is also capable of causing a wide variety of diseases, such as pneumonia, endocarditis, septicemia, and impetigo. Staphylococcal impetigo occurs fairly frequently in newborn infants and causes considerable concern in hospital nurseries. Although outbreaks have occurred in nurseries where certain specific phage types have been primarily involved, a variety of types seem capable of causing this condition, especially in situations where the technique of caring for the infants is inadequate.

Staphylococcal enterocolitis (pseudomembranous enterocolitis) is an acute, fulminating process that results when, for reasons that are not clearly understood, *S. aureus* colonizes the intestinal mucosa. The rapidity with which this condition can develop is well illustrated by an example in which stool cultures done 36 to 72 hours before death failed to reveal the presence of *S. aureus.* A culture done 12 hours before death showed the presence of moderate numbers of the organism, and culture of the intestinal content at autopsy revealed a nearly pure culture. Although staphylococcal enterocolitis is most frequently a sequel to therapy with broad spectrum antibiotics, this is not the only circumstance in which it occurs. The condition has also been observed as a terminal event in patients in severe shock and in patients with intestinal hemorrhage. Thus, one suspects that this disease results when the physiologic circumstance in the patient is such as to allow *S. aureus,*

Table 18–3. CHARACTERISTICS OF THE GRAM-POSITIVE COCCI

SPECIES	DISEASES AND OCCURRENCE IN BODY	MORPHOLOGY AND GRAM STAIN	APPEARANCE ON BLOOD AGAR	PRIMARY DIFFERENTIATING CHARACTERISTIC
Diplococcus pneumoniae (pneumococcus)	Lobar pneumonia, eye infections, meningitis, otitis media, septicemia	Gram+, lance-shaped, encapsulated diplococcus	Small, shiny, transparent colonies, elevated in center. Alpha hemolytic	Optochin sensitive Bile soluble Quellung reaction
Streptococcus pyogenes (beta streptococcus)	Bronchopneumonia, follicular tonsillitis, nephritis, septicemia, scarlet fever, rheumatic fever, osteomyelitis, erysipelas	Gram+, spherical cocci, occurring in chains and pairs	Small colonies Beta hemolytic	May be grouped by Lancefield's technique
Streptococcus viridans group	Subacute bacterial endocarditis. Normal inhabitant of nasopharynx	Gram+, spherical cocci, occurring in chains and pairs	Small, raised convex, opaque colonies Alpha hemolytic	Optochin negative Not bile soluble
Streptococcus faecalis (enterococcus)	Urinary infections, septicemia (may be found in blood). Normal inhabitant of intestinal tract	Gram+, round cocci, occurring in chains and pairs	Small colonies. May be beta, alpha, or gamma hemolytic	Grows in media containing 6.5% NaCl; heat resistant; may be antibiotic resistant. Lancefield's group D
Streptococcus anhemolyticus (gamma streptococcus)	Nasopharynx, intestinal tract, sputum, wounds	Gram+, round cocci, occurring in chains and pairs	Small colonies No hemolysis	Primarily nonpathogenic
Staphylococcus aureus	Skin, nasopharynx. Boils, carbuncles, food poisoning, osteomyelitis, impetigo, septicemia, pneumonia	Gram+, round cocci, occurring in characteristic grapelike clusters	Large gold-pigmented colonies; usually beta hemolytic	Most pathogenic strains are coagulase, DNA, phosphatase, mannitol positive
Staphylococcus epidermidis	Skin and mucous membranes. Not generally pathogenic	Gram+, round cocci, occurring in characteristic grapelike clusters	Large, white, opaque colonies; usually nonhemolytic	Coagulase negative, DNA negative, phosphatase negative

either already present or introduced from the outside, the opportunity to invade the mucosa and to propagate without the usual inhibition provided by the regular bacterial flora or the normal tissue resistance of the host. When viewed in this way, the antibiotic is merely one of the contributing factors in the development of the condition. On suspicion with a patient on antibiotic therapy or in shock, etc., early diagnosis can be made by gram stain of either a fecal smear or material obtained by rectal swab. The presence of any significant number of typical staphylococci in such a preparation must always be viewed with suspicion. The time required for culture of such material may be too great to benefit the patient.

Certain other gram-positive cocci that are members of the normal flora are capable of causing problems under appropriate circumstances. *Streptococcus viridans* is involved in bacterial endocarditis and presents problems in isolation from the patient. It may require repeated blood culture with special procedures. *Streptococcus faecalis* is often found in urinary tract infections, especially in the catheterized patient. This organism may also be found associated with endocarditis and wound infection.

The medium of choice for isolation of the members of this group is blood agar, since some of the organisms are fastidious in their growth requirements and one of the important identifying and differentiating characteristics is their effect on blood. One may incorporate sodium azide, phenylethyl alcohol, gentamycin or other material to inhibit growth of gram-negative bacilli when this is needed. Specialized media for this group are also widely used; these will be described where appropriate.

Diplococcus pneumoniae (pneumococcus) contains many antigenic types, which are determined by differences in their polysaccharide capsule (Fig. 18-16). The pneumococcus is now generally considered to properly belong to the genus *Streptococcus*, rather than to the distinct genus *Diplococcus*. The latter name is still used here because it is more familiar. At one time it was very important to type these organisms (the quellung reaction), but since the advent of antibiotics, this has become less important in practice. Colonies of *D. pneumoniae* are small, moist, and 0.5 to 1.0 mm. in diameter and have a characteristic area of alpha (green) hemolysis surrounding them; they are indistinguishable from colonies of *Str. viridans* (Figs. 18-17, 18-18 and 18-19). It is also not possible to differentiate these organisms by gram stain.

The simplest way to differentiate between the organisms is to pick a colony, streak it heavily on one-fourth of a blood agar plate,

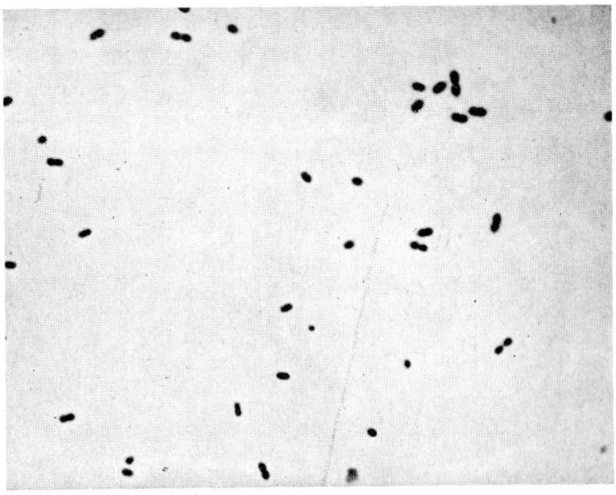

Figure 18-17. Pneumococcus, pure culture. Note the typical lanceolate shape and diplococcus arrangement. Fuchsin; × 1050. (From Burrows, W.: Textbook of Microbiology. 19th ed.)

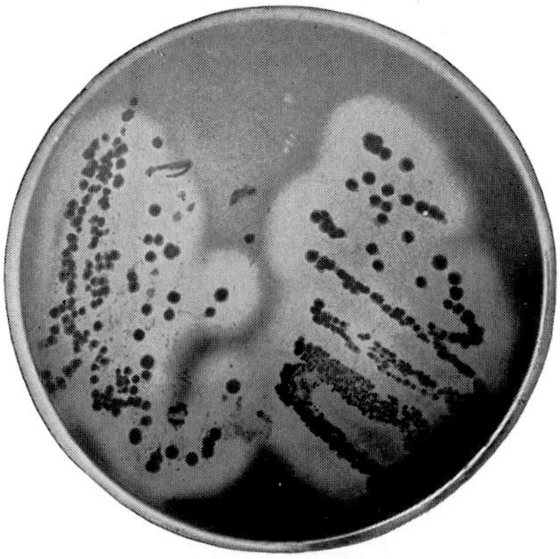

Figure 18-16. Blood agar culture of hemolytic *Staphylococcus aureus* (× 900).

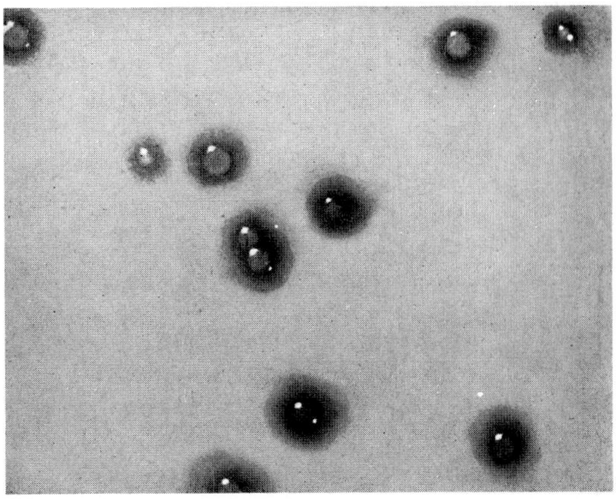

Figure 18-18. Colonies of the pneumococcus on blood agar. × 3. (From Burrows, W.: Textbook of Microbiology. 19th ed.)

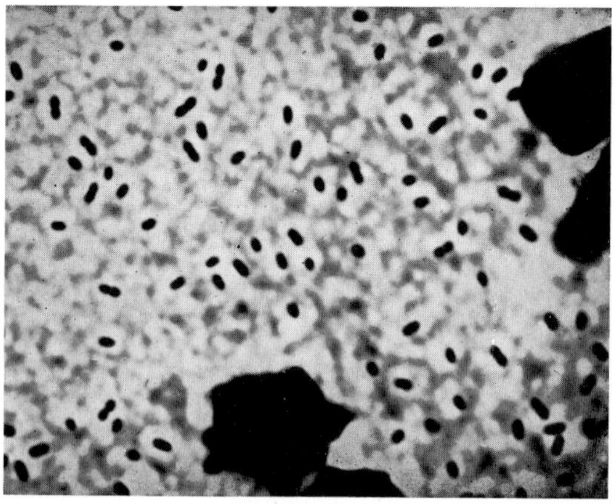

Figure 18–19. Pneumococcus in the peritoneal fluid of a mouse. Note the capsules. Fuchsin; × 2200 (From Burrows, W.: Textbook of Microbiology. 19th ed.)

and apply an optochin disc.* *Diplococcus pneumoniae* is inhibited by optochin (ethylhydrocupreine hydrochloride), and a zone of inhibition will be seen around the disc after incubation. Incubation under increased CO_2 may decrease the size of the zone of inhibition produced by the optochin disc. For this reason, it is preferable to incubate the plates in a room-air incubator. No zone of inhibition appears with *Str. viridans* or other alpha hemolytic streptococci. *Diplococcus pneumoniae* is also bile soluble and inulin positive, and these tests may be done if desired. White mice are highly susceptible to infection with *D. pneumoniae.* Virulent, smooth strains are encapsulated but change readily to the rough, nonencapsulated variants *in vitro.*

Bile Solubility Test for Pneumococci. Centrifuge the growth from a 5-ml. culture of the organism in dextrose broth and resuspend the growth in 0.5 M phosphate buffer, pH 7.6, containing 2 per cent sodium chloride and 0.05 per cent sodium desoxycholate. Incubate at 37° C. for 60 minutes and examine. Colonies of pneumococci lyse under these conditions. Some prefer to add a drop of 10 per cent aqueous sodium desoxycholate directly to the colony on the solid medium. Dissolution of the pneumococci is indicated by the disappearance of the colony.

Test for Catalase Production. Pour 1 ml. of H_2O_2 (10 volumes per cent) over the surface of a 24-hour agar slope culture. If catalase is present bubbles of oxygen will be released from the surface of the growth.

Alpha hemolytic *Str. faecalis* (enterococcus) is also difficult to differentiate from *D. pneumoniae* and *Str. viridans* on blood agar. *Streptococcus faecalis* will grow in medium containing 6.5 per cent NaCl and decarboxylate tyrosine; the others will not. Lancefield and FA grouping can be done as well.

A medium termed "SF broth" is useful for the differentiation of group D streptococci from other streptococci. *Streptococcus faecalis* grows in this medium and ferments dextrose, changing the color of the indicator from purple to yellow. *Streptococcus faecalis* will also resist heating at 60° C. for 30 minutes and grows on media containing bile salts and esculin. A simple and reliable differential test is based on the failure of 5 μg. methicillin sensitivity discs to inhibit enterococci on Mueller-Hinton agar. Other streptococci show inhibition zones of 10 mm. or more. Gamma-type streptococci colonies vary considerably in size and are gray and translucent. No hemolysis occurs. Anaerobic streptococci (*Peptostreptococcus*) are a particularly important group in septicemias following puerperal fever. Most are hemolytic and produce a foul odor. Micro-aerophilic streptococci are also occasionally encountered in wound infections and septic conditions. They correspond in their general biologic characteristics to the aerobic forms. Group B streptococci are particularly important in gynecologic infections. They characteristically hydrolyze sodium hippurate to benzoate. They may be beta hemolytic and sensitive to bacitracin, hence can be mistaken for group A strains.

Streptococcus pyogenes can be divided into numerous groups and types by the methods of Lancefield and others. Most of the human pathogens fall into Lancefield's group A, although a few are found in groups B, C, and G. The presence of small, hard white colonies 0.5 to 1 mm. in diameter surrounded by a clear zone of hemolysis that reveals gram-positive cocci tending to form chains is diagnostic of *Str. pyogenes* and can be so reported (Fig. 18–20). Microscopic examination of the hemolyzed zone reveals no intact erythrocytes. Various selective media for the isolation of beta hemolytic streptococci have been devised; these usually incorporate gentian violet or neomycin and nalidixic acid (30 μg. and 15 μg. per ml., respectively) in a conventional blood agar.

If cultures are inoculated by the pour plate method, the hemolytic zones of beta streptococci are clearer. One method is to add the inoculum to a tube containing 10 ml. of infusion broth. One or two loopfuls are transferred to a similar second tube, which is shaken vigorously. One milliliter is then pipetted into a tube containing 20 ml. of melted blood agar base which has been cooled to 45° C. One milliliter of sheep blood is then added and the mixture rotated and poured into a Petri dish. After solidification the dish is incubated for

*Available commercially.

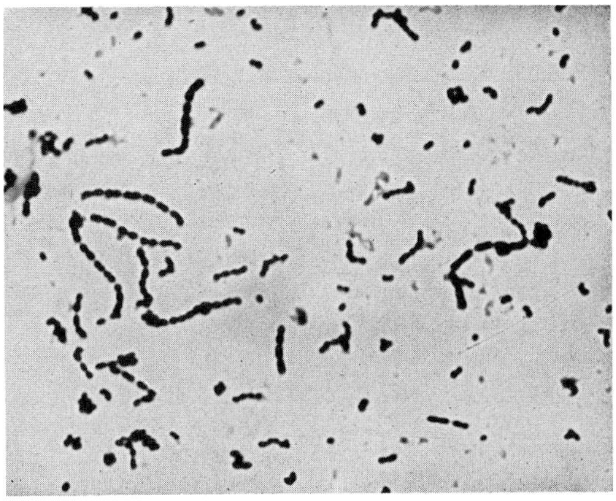

Figure 18–20. *Streptococcus pyogenes.* Note the tendency to diplococcus arrangement in the chains. Fuchsin; × 1050. (From Burrows, W.: Textbook of Microbiology. 19th ed.)

24 to 48 hours and examined for beta hemolytic colonies (Fig. 18–21).

It is important to determine the serologic group to which beta hemolytic streptococci belong, since the presence of group A streptococci may necessitate therapy, other groups usually being insignificant. A simple screening procedure that is reasonably accurate is to plate the streptococci on blood agar and to apply a bacitracin disc* to the inoculated surface. A definite zone of inhibition of growth around the disc indicates presumptively that the organism belongs to Lancefield group A. The FA procedure is also very useful for grouping.

Grouping of Beta Hemolytic Streptococci by the Precipitin Technique. Typing of streptococci can be done only in special laboratories. The determination of the type of a group A streptococcus is used primarily for epidemiologic and investigative studies and is rarely required in a clinical laboratory. However, the determination of the group to which a streptococcus belongs is an important procedure, particularly if it is Lancefield group A, to which most human pathogens belong.

*Available commercially.

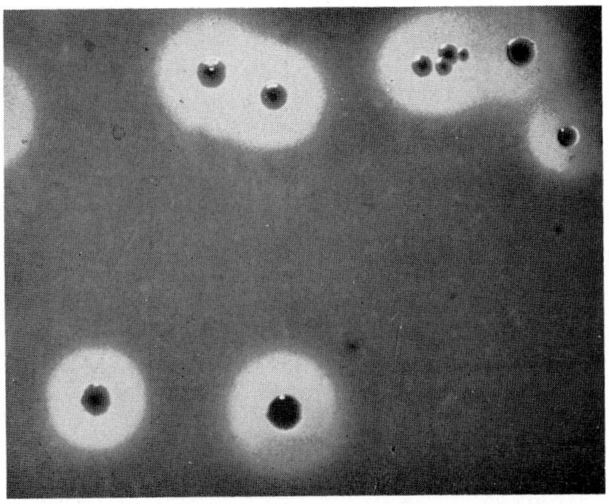

Figure 18–21. *Streptococcus pyogenes.* Pure culture on blood agar showing β hemolysis. × 5. (From Burrows, W.: Textbook of Microbiology. 19th ed.)

Preparation of Extract. It is necessary to bring about partial disintegration of the cell wall with the release of soluble carbohydrate ("C substance") in a form that retains its serologic reactivity. Several different methods are employed for this purpose, of which those of Lancefield, the autoclave method of Rantz and Randall, and the enzyme procedure of Maxted will be described briefly. More complete descriptions will be found in the references.

Lancefield Procedure. The organisms are grown for 18 to 24 hours in Todd-Hewitt broth, with 1 per cent additional glucose. The culture is centrifuged and the supernatant discarded, after which the sediment is discarded and one drop of 0.01 per cent phenol red is added to the clear supernatant fluid. Buffer (1 gm. sodium acid phosphate in 100 ml. 0.2 N NaOH) is added drop by drop until a pale pink color develops. Following another centrifugation, the clear supernatant fluid is used as the antigen for the precipitin test.

Autoclave Procedure (Rantz). The streptococci to be grouped are grown overnight in 50 ml. of trypticase soy or tryptose phosphate broth. The cultures are centrifuged and the sediment suspended in a small amount of sterile saline. The tube is then autoclaved at 15 p.s.i. for 15 minutes and the tube again centrifuged. The clear supernatant is used for the antigen.

Enzyme Procedure (Maxted). A loopful of growth of the streptococci to be grouped is placed in 0.25 ml. of the enzyme. The enzyme consists of a powerful proteolytic substance isolated from *Streptomyces albus*. Pronase B, an extract of *Streptomyces griseus*, is also effective. The tubes are placed in a water bath at 50° C. for 90 minutes. The clear solution contains the soluble antigen that is used in the test.

Ring Precipitin Technique

1. A capillary tube (1.0 to 1.5 mm. in diameter) is dipped into the streptococcus-grouping antiserum* and a column of 25 to 30 mm. is allowed to rise into the tube.

2. The excess serum is wiped from the outside of the capillary tube, which is then dipped into the previously prepared streptococcal extract. A column equal to the antiserum is allowed to enter into the capillary tube. Care

*Commercially available.

must be used to insure contact between the serum and antigen.

3. The tube containing the antiserum extract mixture is wiped, placed into a plasticine block, and incubated at room temperature. Microscopic precipitate appears within a few minutes and is complete in 30 minutes.

A control consisting of an extract of streptococci of a known group should be included. The procedure can be repeated with different dilutions of the antigen. If no reaction occurs, one may be dealing with streptococci of a different group or a prozone reaction may be occurring. To determine this, the extract should be diluted and retested with the antiserum.

Staphylococcus aureus is easily identified when it is typical, producing its gold pigment and usually having a zone of beta hemolysis surrounding the colonies. Some strains do not hemolyze all types of blood and this must be kept in mind. The most reliable indicator of pathogenicity in *S. aureus* is considered to be the coagulase test, but unfortunately, unless carefully standardized, the test is subject to many sources of error. This test may be done as follows:

1. Place 2 or 3 drops of an 18-hour broth culture of the *S. aureus* in a sterile test tube (10 by 100 mm.). One may use colonies from a plate by emulsifying a large loopful in 2 or 3 drops of broth.

2. Add 0.5 ml. of plasma (human or rabbit) and mix thoroughly by shaking. Desiccated or lyophilized plasma can be purchased for this purpose. Set up controls with known coagulase positive and negative strains in the same manner.

3. Place the tube in a water bath or incubator for 3 hours. Most positive strains will clot the plasma within 1 hour. Those not clotting at 3 hours are reexamined after incubation for an additional 18 hours. Any degree of clotting is considered positive.

Coagulase tests can also be done in plates containing fibrinogen (Bovine Fraction I) or plasma. Rabbit or human plasma (previously tested for suitability for coagulase tests) is mixed with sterile nutrient agar in a concentration of 12 to 15 per cent (v/v) at a temperature of 47° C. The mixture is poured into Petri dishes and allowed to solidify. Following spot inoculation, coagulase production is indicated by the development of opacity around the colonies after overnight incubation.

The slide test for coagulase is useful primarily as a screening procedure. Place a small drop of distilled water on a slide and emulsify organisms from a single colony in it. Then add a small drop of plasma or bovine fibrinogen which has been allowed to reach room temperature and mix thoroughly. If clumping of the organisms occurs in 5 to 15 seconds, the test is positive. If no clumping occurs, the organism should be tested by one of the other procedures. This test measures "bound" rather than "free" coagulase.

It has been found recently that estimation of deoxyribonuclease activity of staphylococci is considerably easier, more economical, and possibly a better indication of potential pathogenicity than is the coagulase test. Colonies are band streaked on a desoxyribonuclease test medium plate and incubated overnight at 35° C. It is then flooded with 1 N HCl. A clear zone around the colony streak indicates a positive reaction. Alternatively 0.1 per cent toluidine blue can be used; a bright pink zone around the colony is a positive reaction.

Another useful test is the estimation of phosphatase activity. This is accomplished by adding 0.01 per cent phenolphthalein phosphate to melted blood agar base. Swabs are plated in the usual way. After overnight incubation the plate is exposed to the fumes from a bottle of concentrated ammonia. Phosphatase positive colonies turn bright pink, while others remain unchanged. This test correlates very well with the coagulase and deoxyribonuclease activity.

Many other tests for determination of the potential virulence or pathogenicity of staphylococci are available. Most of these reactions are impractical for the clinical laboratory. Details of these reactions may be found in the references.

1. Egg yolk opacity test
2. Hyaluronidase production
3. Toxin production (plate or embryonated eggs)
4. Alpha hemolysin
5. Leukocidin production (Panton-Valentine factor)
6. Necrotoxin production
7. Virulence in rabbits or mice
8. Ammonium molybdate chemical test (A.M.C.)
9. Mercury sensitivity

Another reaction, particularly useful in identifying enterotoxigenic food poisoning strains of *S. aureus*, involves the capacity of the organisms to ferment mannitol anaerobically and to propagate in the presence of 7.5 per cent NaCl. These tests can be run simultaneously in mannitol-salt agar. Many other selective media have been devised—tellurite glycine, Baird-Parker, Medium 110, and so forth.

Staphylococcus aureus is antigenically rather heterogeneous, although certain definite antigen types have been described. A more workable classification is obtained by means of bacteriophage typing. This procedure has considerable usefulness in epidemiologic studies but should probably not be attempted in small laboratories and, at least at present, does not contribute greatly to diagnosis. All staphylococci that are coagulase negative may be considered as *S. epidermidis*. These are not typable with bacteriophage and are usually, but not always, nonpathogenic. Anaerobic staphylococci (*Peptococcus*) are primarily found in wound infections.

AUTOGENOUS VACCINES

Autogenous vaccines—those prepared from the bacterium isolated from the lesion—are sometimes resorted to in patients in whom antibiotic therapy has been ineffective or contraindicated. Best results are obtained in situations where staphylococci are involved.

Preparation of Vaccine. Examine gram stain of organisms cultured from the infected area. Select isolated colonies from culture plates and transfer to agar slants. After overnight incubation, add 2 or 3 ml. of sterile saline to the slants and suspend the growth with a wire loop. Filter through sterile glass wool into vaccine bottles containing glass beads.

The suspension is then standardized. Several methods can be used for this: counting chamber, the Coulter counter, photoelectric nephelometer, and others. The use of McFarland standards is simple and reasonably accurate for this purpose.

Prepare standards, if not already available, by adding the following to 10 uniform hard glass, screw-cap tubes:

Tube	1% H_2SO_4	1% $BaCl_2$	Density app. corresponding to bacterial suspension
1	9.9 ml.	0.1 ml.	300 million
2	9.8	0.2	600
3	9.7	0.3	900
4	9.6	0.4	1200
5	9.5	0.5	1500
6	9.4	0.6	1800
7	9.3	0.7	2100
8	9.2	0.8	2400
9	9.1	0.9	2700
10	9.0	1.0	3000

Place 1 ml. of the well-mixed bacterial suspension in a tube of the same diameter as the standard. A measured amount of sterile saline is then added slowly until the diluted vaccine matches the desired standard tube. The number of bacteria in 1 ml. of vaccine equals the number of the corresponding nephelometer tube times the dilution. For example, 1 ml. is diluted to 5 ml. to match tube No. 3. It therefore contains approximately 900 million × 5, or 4500 million bacteria per ml.

The vaccine is sterilized by heating in the water bath for 1 hour at 60° C. Tricresol (0.25 per cent), phenol (0.5 per cent) or Merthiolate (1:1000) are added as a preservative. The vaccine is then checked for sterility by culturing an aliquot in thioglycollate broth for one week. If sterile, it can then be released.

The Gram-negative Cocci

The gram-negative cocci of medical importance belong to the genera *Neisseria* and *Veillonella*. Two of the species, *N. gonorrhoeae* (gonococcus) and *N. meningitidis* (meningococcus), are well-recognized human pathogens.

Meningococcal meningitis is primarily an endemic disease that occurs as isolated cases in the general population. The disease is present in all age groups, with the highest incidence in the ages from birth through 14 years. Occasional explosive epidemics occur, especially in institutions or military establishments, where large numbers of susceptible individuals live in close contact. Carriers are probably responsible for transmission of the organism through the population, and carrier rates have been found to be quite variable in different groups. In epidemic times the carrier rate may be 50 to 60 per cent. It should be pointed out that even in an epidemic the number of persons developing sore throats, meningococcemia or meningitis is low by comparison with the number actually infected as indicated by positive nasopharyngeal cultures.

Although the clinical picture of meningococcal disease, especially in the younger age groups, may be highly suggestive, it is imperative that bacteriologic confirmation of the diagnosis be obtained at the earliest possible moment. The gram-stained smear from spinal fluid or from a petechial hemorrhage will in most cases reveal the presence of typical gram-negative diplococci. Culture of the spinal fluid, petechiae, nasopharynx, or blood may be done on appropriate media, but this requires time for incubation. Without the evidence supplied by the gram stain, the physician must treat the patient empirically until culture results are available.

The susceptibility of *N. meningitidis* to antibiotics, especially to the sulfonamides, has made prophylaxis a relatively simple matter for several years. Recently, there have appeared strains of group B *N. meningitidis* that are sufficiently resistant to the sulfonamides as to render prophylaxis and treatment with these drugs ineffectual. So far, the occurrence of these strains has been limited, but the implications are clear. It will be necessary in any epidemic or near epidemic situation, to determine whether or not one is dealing with a resistant organism.

Gonorrhea has increased markedly in incidence despite the fact that *N. gonorrhoeae* usually shows a high degree of susceptibility to penicillin and other antibiotics and that antibiotic therapy has generally been effective in the treatment of acute gonococcal disease. There are a number of possible explanations for this. Reporting of cases still leaves much to be desired. This does not allow for proper follow-up and location of contacts. Another important factor is the occurrence of asymptomatic infection in the female. The discovery of such individuals requires adequate epidemiologic follow-up of acute cases. Culture is an essential part of the diagnosis of gonorrhea in the chronically infected person, in asymptomatic cases, and in carriers. In the male with acute gonococcal urethritis the diagnosis can usually be made by direct smear and gram stain, but culture is also essential in the chronically infected male. Rectal and pharyngeal cultures in homosexuals on Thayer-Martin medium may yield positive cultures. Examination of urethral smears or smears from culture can also be done through the use of the FA procedure. (See p. 929.)

Certain problems may arise with the direct smear and gram stain. Occasionally staphylococci which have been overly destained may be mistaken for *N. gonorrhoeae*. Also, members of the *Mima-Herellea* group may occur in acute urethritis. The morphology of these organisms is sufficiently like that of *Neisseria*, especially in exudates and from growth on enriched media, as to be indistinguishable from it. The differentiation can be made by inoculation to unenriched extract agar or E.M.B. media. On these media, the *Mima-Herellea* group appear as bacilli and *N. gonorrhoeae* will not grow.

Neisseria catarrhalis, *N. sicca*, and the other so-called nonpathogenic *Neisseria* are widely distributed and must be differentiated from the recognized pathogens on cultural and morphologic grounds. *Neisseria catarrhalis* is found in over 90 per cent of throat cultures. It has been associated with certain catarrhal conditions, and when found to predominate in such circumstances must be viewed with suspicion.

Table 18–4 summarizes the most important characteristics of these species. It will be seen in the table that *N. meningitidis* and *N. gonorrhoeae* require enriched media and increased CO_2 for growth. The CO_2 is not so critical with *N. meningitidis* but should always be used. *Neisseria catarrhalis* and other nonpathogenic *Neisseria* grow well on ordinary agar. Anaerobic *Neisseria* are placed among the *Veillonella*.

The oxidase test is very useful in picking colonies of *Neisseria* in mixed cultures from vaginal and urethral smears. The test is performed as follows:

Oxidase Reagent

Di- (or tetra-) methyl paraphenylene diamine hydrochloride	1.0 gm.
Distilled water (fresh)	100.0 ml.

The test is performed by dropping the oxidase reagent on the colonies. Oxidase positive colonies become black rather rapidly. The reagent is quite unstable and must be made fresh every few days. Reagent droppers of oxidase* are stable and convenient (Fig. 18–22). Some prefer to use discs or paper strips impregnated with the reagent.

All *Neisseria* are oxidase positive, but there are certain other microorganisms that are also positive (certain of the gram-negative bacilli, yeasts, and fungi). Thus, it is necessary to do a gram stain of the colony to make sure it is a gram-negative diplococcus. Subculture and fermentation reactions can be made from the oxidase-positive colonies, provided sterile oxidase reagent has been used. It must be done immediately, since too long an exposure to the reagent will destroy the bacteria.

Neisseria meningitidis may be isolated from the spinal fluid, blood, throat, and nasopharynx or from the petechiae that may occur in the skin. This organism is divided into four antigenic groups. Final identification as *N. meningitidis* can be made by noting agglutination with a polyvalent antiserum, by capsular swelling (quellung reaction), or by FA. For epidemiologic purposes it is often desirable to determine the serotype, but species identification is usually enough for diagnosis (Fig. 18–23).

Neisseria gonorrhoeae is antigenically quite heterogeneous, but it is not likely to be confused with any other organism. Its morphology and culturally fastidious nature as well as clinical evidence usually leave little doubt about its identity (Figs. 18–24, 18–25, and 18–26). Carbohydrate fermentations are necessary for speciation. Morphologically similar organisms, which can be confused with gonococci, are occasionally encountered in the vagina or conjunctiva. These are either nonpathogenic *Neisseria* or members of the tribe *Mimeae* (see p. 980). Lactose fermenting species of *Neisseria*, called *N. lactamicus* are occasionally isolated.

Occasionally, the meningococcus has been isolated from endocervical infections, the gonococcus from the nasopharynx and cases of meningitis, and so forth. This points out the importance of careful cultural studies for differentiation in this group.

---

*Ceptiseal, Medical Supply Corp., Rockford, Illinois.

Table 18–4. CHARACTERISTICS OF THE GRAM-NEGATIVE COCCI

SPECIES	DISEASES AND OCCURRENCE IN BODY	MORPHOLOGY AND GRAM STAIN	MEDIUM OF CHOICE AND CONDITIONS FOR GROWTH	PRIMARY DIFFERENTIATING AND IDENTIFYING CHARACTERISTICS
Neisseria meningitidis (meningococcus)	Meningitis, meningococcemia, mild sore throat (may precede meningococcemia and meningitis)	Gram-negative, bean-shaped diplococci with adjacent sides flattened. May be seen in polymorphonuclear leukocytes in spinal fluid and in petechiae	Chocolate or blood agar. Growth greatly improved by 10% CO_2	Colonies 1 to 4 mm. in diameter, bluish white, opaque. Oxidase positive. Ferment dextrose and maltose, not sucrose. Agglutinated by polyvalent antiserum
Neisseria gonorrhoeae (gonococcus)	Acute urethritis in male and female, chronic infection of urogenital tract, gonococcal arthritis, ophthalmia neonatorum	Gram-negative, bean-shaped diplococci. Occur in polymorphonuclear leukocytes in urethral smears	GC medium (Thayer-Martin); Transgrow requires 10% CO_2	Colonies 1 to 4 mm. in diameter, oxidase positive. Ferment dextrose, not maltose or sucrose
Neisseria catarrhalis	Normal inhabitant of throat. May be found in catarrhal conditions in upper respiratory tract	Gram-negative, spherical diplococci with adjacent sides flattened	Grows well on most ordinary media	Colonies 1.5 to 5 mm. in diameter, oxidase positive. Do not ferment dextrose, maltose, or sucrose. Grow at room temperature.
Neisseria sicca	Normal inhabitant of respiratory tract	Gram-negative diplococci with adjacent sides flattened	Grows well on most ordinary media	Colonies dry, crumbling. Sometimes hemolytic, oxidase positive
Veillonella sp.	Digestive and vaginal tract. Occasionally pathogenic.	Gram-negative, minute, spherical diplococci	Weakly hemolytic on blood agar. Anaerobe	Acid and gas from dextrose. Nitrate positive

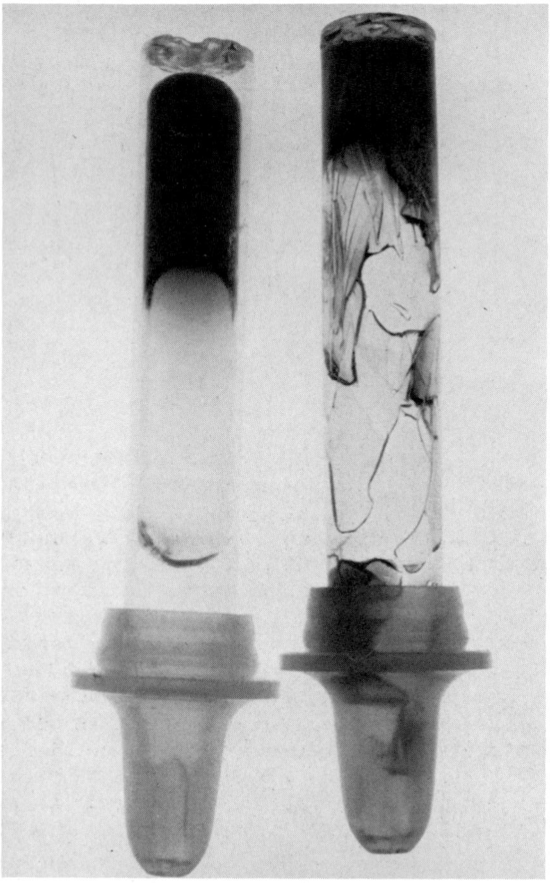

Figure 18–22. "Cepti-Seal" reagent droppers. Glass vial at right is crushed when reagent is needed. (Courtesy of Medical Supply Corp., Rockford, Ill.)

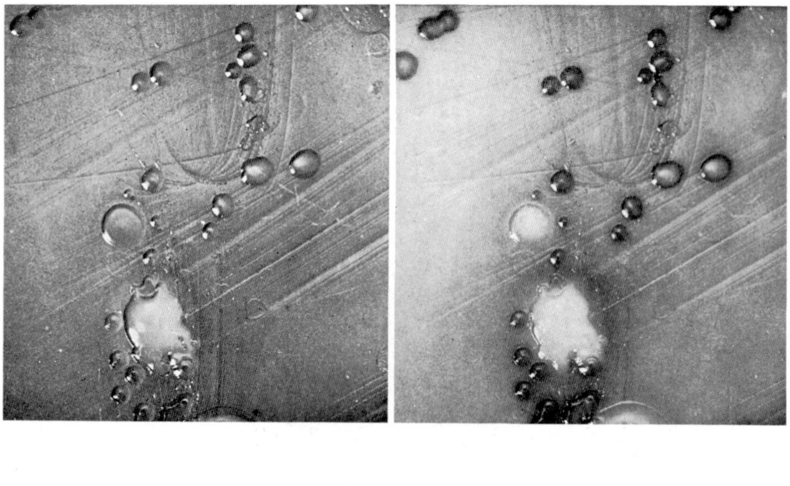

Figure 18–23. The oxidase test for the identification of meningococcus colonies. Mixed culture on blood agar. *Left,* colonies of meningococci and contaminants before the application of tetramethyl-*p*-phenylenediamine solution. *Right,* the same colonies after the application of the reagent. Note that the meningococcus colonies show the development of color first about the edges, and there is slight discoloration of the medium. × 5. (From Burrows, W.: Textbook of Microbiology. 19th ed.)

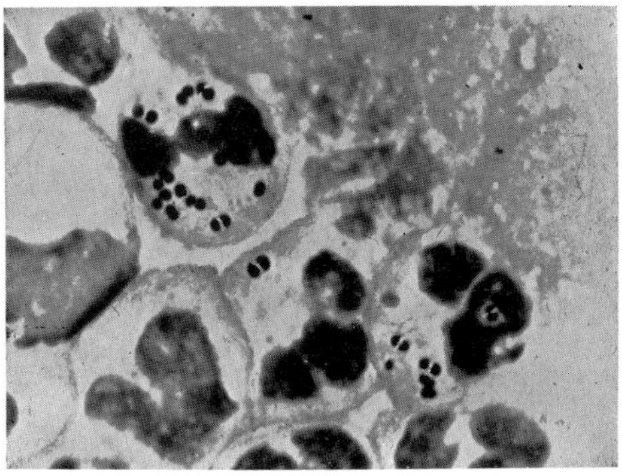

Figure 18–24. Meningococci in cerebrospinal fluid in a case of epidemic meningitis (× 1500).

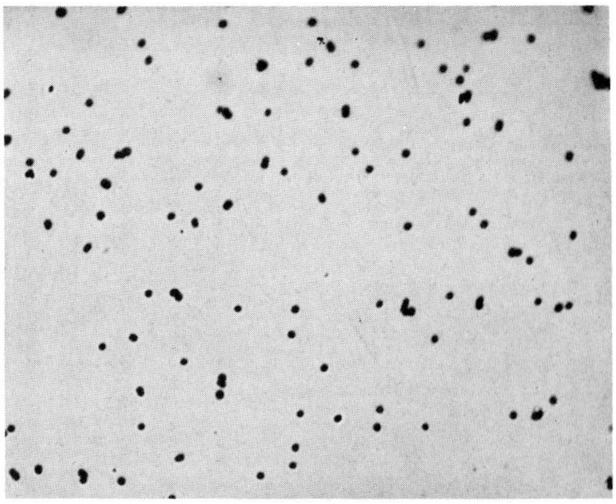

Figure 18–26. The gonococcus from pure culture. Fuchsin; × 1050. (From Burrows, W.: Textbook of Microbiology. 19th ed.)

The Gram-negative Enteric Bacilli

The Enterobacteria are a complex and often confusing group of bacteria comprised of a number of genera, the validity of which have been generally accepted. There are, however, many intermediates and the boundaries often become indistinct, leaving one with the impression that this is really a spectrum of organisms. Some of the genera have been studied extensively, especially *Salmonella*, with the result that a great many species have been described. In many cases these species differ only in minor ways, and the number is rather cumbersome. Numerous attempts at classification of this group have been made. Probably the most useful, at this time, is that of Ewing (1967), Table 18–5.

Table 18–6 shows the occurrence and pathogenic importance of the better known species of gram-negative enteric bacteria. It is beyond the scope of this book to discuss the more exact identification of species within these complex groups; such identifications are essential primarily for epidemiologic investigations. Indeed, for the purposes of clinical diagnosis it is, more often than not, unnecessary to carry the identification this far. For more detailed discussions, one may refer to the various textbooks and laboratory guides, some of which are listed in the references (Figs. 18–27 to 18–34).

The relative importance of the various members of the gram-negative enteric bacteria has changed remarkably in recent years. Various types of *Salmonella* have emerged as frequent causes of human disease. Although the number of cases of salmonellosis still shows a peak in the late summer and early fall, a consid-

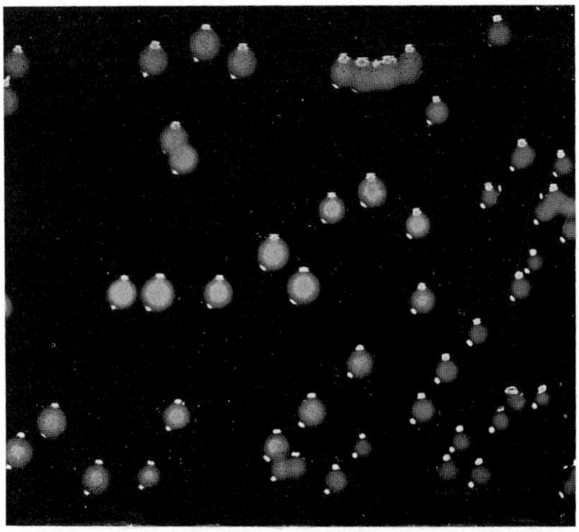

Figure 18–25. Colonies of the gonococcus on blood agar. × 6. (From Burrows, W.: Textbook of Microbiology. 19th ed.)

Table 18–5. THE TRIBES AND GENERA OF THE FAMILY ENTEROBACTERIACEAE

TRIBE	GENERA
Escherichieae	Escherichia (includes Alkalescens-Dispar) Shigella
Edwardsielleae	Edwardsiella
Salmonelleae	Salmonella Arizona Citrobacter (includes Bethesda-Ballerup and C. freundii)
Klebsielleae	Klebsiella Enterobacter Serratia
Proteae	Proteus Providencia

Table 18–6. THE GRAM-NEGATIVE ENTERIC BACTERIA

SPECIES	DISEASE IN MAN	SOURCE OF INFECTION	SOURCES OF CULTURE IN MAN
Salmonella typhi	Typhoid (enteric) fever	Human (man-to-man) cases and carriers	Blood culture (first 10–14 days) Stool culture (after 10–14 days) Urine culture (late in disease) Carrier (stool culture)
Salmonella choleraesuis	Septicemia, arthritis	Swine	Same as *Sal. typhi*
Salmonella enteriditis Serotype Enteriditis Serotype Typhimurium Serotype Dublin Other salmonellae; many serotypes	Enteric fever, gastroenteritis, septicemia, etc.	Primarily animal pathogens, but may establish carrier state in man	Same as *Sal. typhi* in enteric fever; otherwise stools, other organs, joints. Stool cultures: Seldom invade blood sufficiently for positive cultures
Shigella dysenteriae *Shigella sonnei* *Shigella flexneri* *Shigella boydii*	Bacillary dysentery (shigellosis)	Human (man-to-man) cases and carriers	Stool culture; rarely invade blood
Proteus morganii	Possible cause of diarrhea in infants and children	Probably human	Stool culture
Proteus vulgaris *Proteus mirabilis* *Proteus rettgeri* *Providencia*	Urinary tract infections, wound infections	Normal inhabitant of gastrointestinal tract; widely dispersed in nature	Urine, wound cultures
Escherichia coli	Urinary tract infections, terminal septicemia, infant diarrhea (enteropathogenic strains)	Normal inhabitant of lower gastrointestinal tract. Pathogenic strains probably of human origin	Urine culture; blood cultures in septicemia; stool cultures
Serratia marcescens	Chronic infections predominantly	Air and water. Usually nosocomial	Urine, sputum, etc.
Edwardsiella *Arizona* *Citrobacter*	Possible cause of diarrhea or urinary tract infection in some cases	Probably normal inhabitants of gastrointestinal tract	Stool culture; urine culture

erable number of cases occur throughout the year. Such diverse agents as carmine dye, powdered milk, powdered eggs, and frozen poultry have been identified with cases and outbreaks. Adequate stool culture of patients with clinically suggestive symptoms is very desirable, and it is often profitable to do cultures on the members of the family of any patient with a positive culture. *Salmonella* has shown considerable tendency to become re-

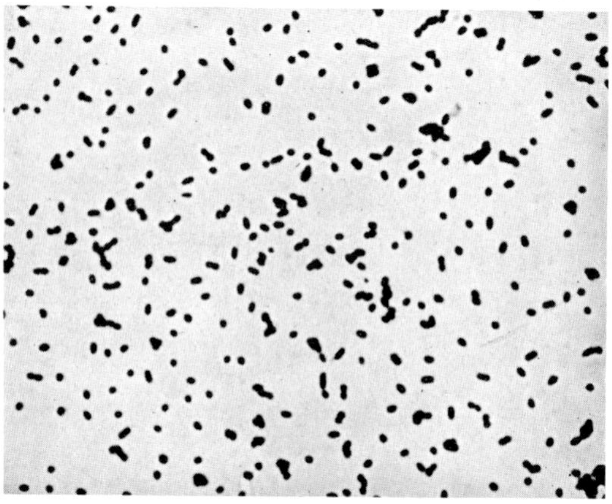

Figure 18–27. Coliform bacilli. Smear from a pure culture. Note the coccobacillary form. Fuchsin; × 1050. (From Burrows, W.: Textbook of Microbiology. 19th ed.)

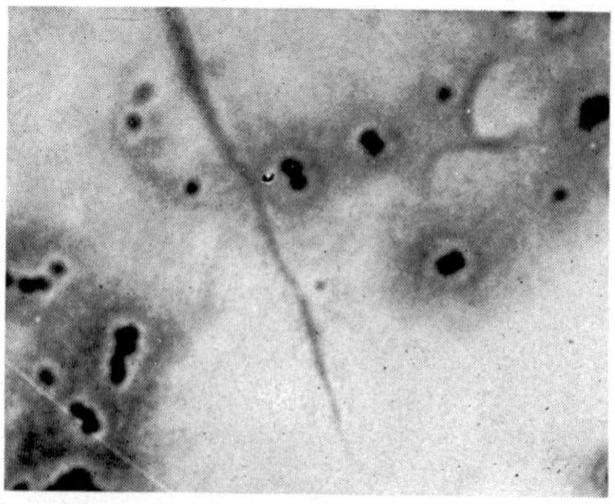

Figure 18–28. *Klebsiella pneumoniae* (Friedländer's bacillus) in pure culture on blood agar, showing capsules. Crystal violet; × 1200. (From Burrows, W.: Textbook of Microbiology. 19th ed.)

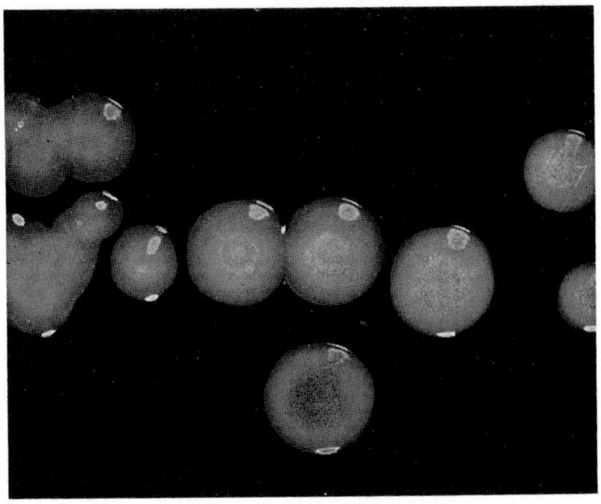

Figure 18–29. Colonies of Friedländer's bacillus on blood agar. Note the large size and mucoid appearance. × 3. (From Burrows, W.: Textbook of Microbiology. 19th ed.)

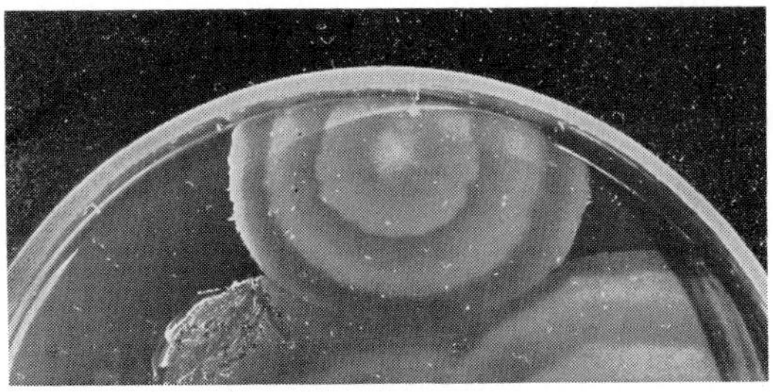

Figure 18–30. *Proteus vulgaris* colony on blood agar. Note the swarming exhibited as successive waves of growth.

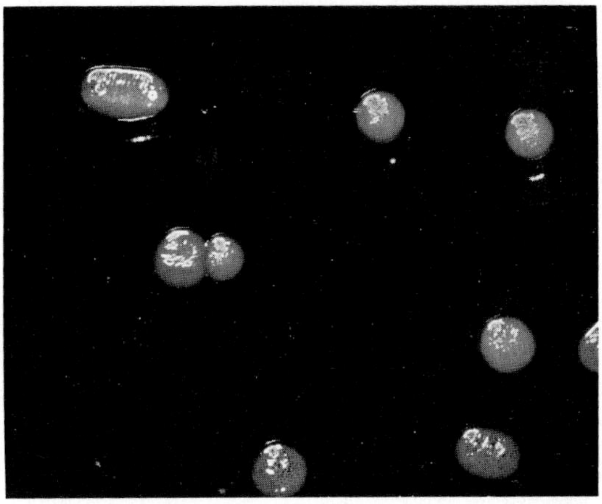

Figure 18–31. Colonies of *Salmonella typhimurium* on nutrient agar. Twenty-four-hour culture. × 3. (From Burrows, W.: Textbook of Microbiology. 19th ed.)

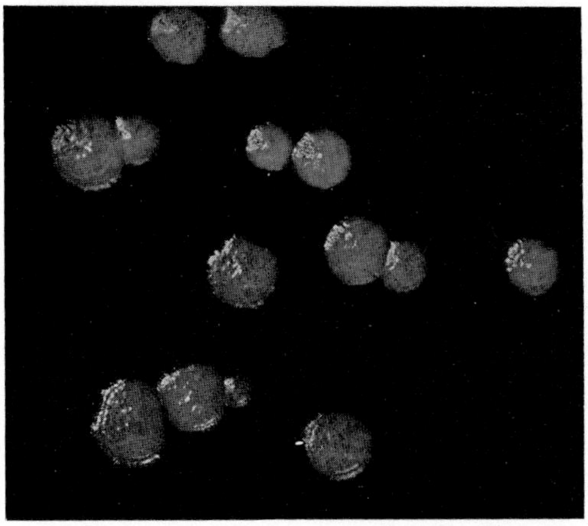

Figure 18–32. Colonies of typhoid bacillus on nutrient agar. Note the characteristic "maple-leaf" irregular margin and slightly roughened glistening surface. × 6. (From Burrows, W.: Textbook of Microbiology. 19th ed.)

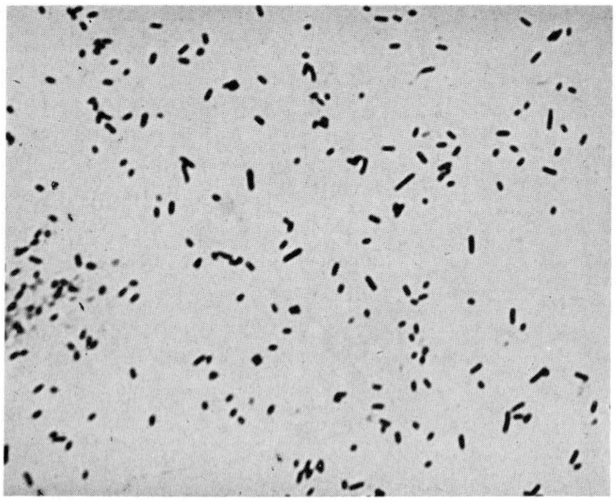

Figure 18–33. *Shigella flexneri.* Smear from a pure culture. Fuchsin; × 1050. (From Burrows, W.: Textbook of Microbiology. 19th ed.)

sistant to antibiotics in recent years. There is evidence to show that the organisms become resistant through some cellular transfer of material from resistant to sensitive organisms of different species, e.g., *E. coli* to *Salmonella* (Kabins and Cohen, 1966; Mitsuhashi, 1969). Thus, it is entirely likely that *Salmonella,* of which there are upwards of 1500 serotypes, may present even greater problems in the future.

The taxonomic scheme in current use recognizes three species of *Salmonella: S. choleraesuis, S. typhi* and *S. enteriditis.* The first two do not contain serotypes, but *S. enteriditis* contains over 1500. These serotypes are written in a capitalized nonitalicized form, e.g., *S. enteriditis* serotype Heidelberg.

Shigellosis remains a problem in areas of low economic standards and can cause serious epidemics, such as the recent outbreak due to *Sh. dysenteriae* (shiga) in Central America. It must be remembered that some strains are difficult to isolate on routine enteric media. Thus, repeated cultures are often necessary, and it is imperative to make certain that the stool specimen or rectal swab is transported to the laboratory immediately on collection and that the culture is inoculated at once. Some of the newer media have certain advantages over those that have been used in the past.

The occurrence of *Proteus, Escherichia, Enterobacter-Klebsiella, Citrobacter,* and certain other gram-negative bacilli in disease situations, including bacteremia, pneumonia, urinary tract disease, postsurgical wound infections, etc., has been the subject of considerable investigation, and the evidence indicates an increased incidence of clinical disease and nosocomial infections caused by these organisms. This began in the middle 1930's and has, to a degree, run parallel with the increasing use of antibiotics (Steinhauer *et al.,* 1966; Adler *et al.,* 1971). It is to be suspected that the importance of these organisms may increase further, since they tend to be relatively resistant to antibiotics and may certainly become more so in the future.

The *Serratia* group includes gelatin-liquefying and Voges-Proskauer-positive strains of

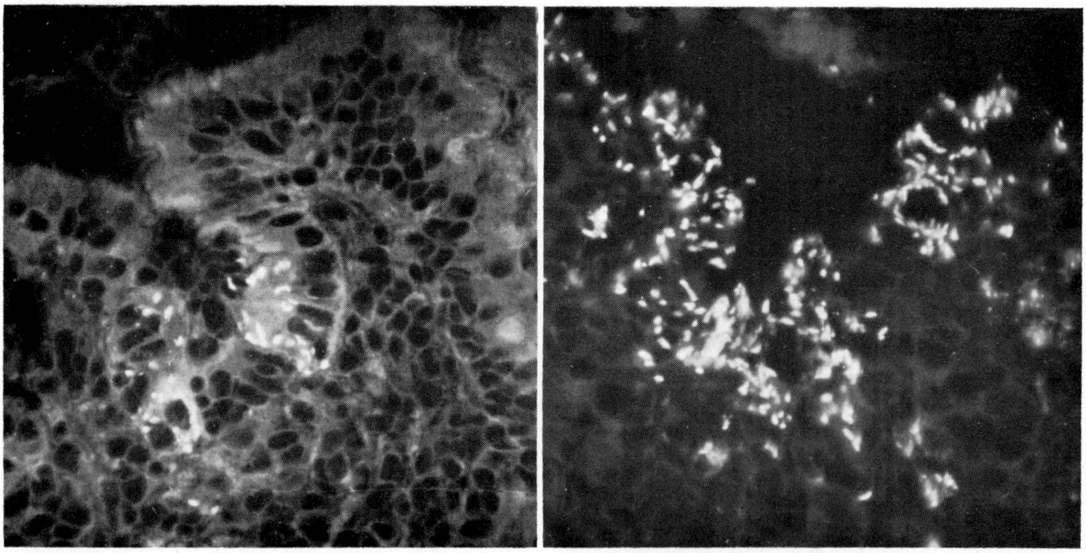

Figure 18–34. The pathogenesis of bacillary dysentery. *Left,* penetration of the ileal epithelium in the guinea pig at 12 hours by *Sh. flexneri* 2a; bacilli can be seen in the epithelial cells and some in the lamina propria. *Right,* small micro-ulcer in the colonic epithelium in the monkey 24 hours after infection; bacilli are present in the epithelial cells and in the lamina propria of the tubular glands of the colon. (Courtesy of Dr. E. H. LeBrec.) (Figure at right, also courtesy of Journal of Bacteriology.)

gram-negative bacilli. They are invariably deoxyribonuclease and O.N.P.G.* positive. Some, but not all, produce a distinct red pigment. They seem to be encountered more and more frequently in acute or chronic infections (Grieve and Goldin, 1966; Wilkowske *et al.*, 1970). Other related organisms, including *Klebsiella pneumoniae, Enterobacter aerogenes, E. cloacae* and *E. hafniae* are frequently encountered in a wide variety of infections. They are also increasingly important in nosocomial infections.

Erwinia is a diverse group of organisms, classified by some in the family Enterobacteriaceae, which are primarily plant pathogens. They have recently been incriminated in septicemias due to contaminated intravenous fluids and have been isolated from other infections in humans as well (Tilton *et al.*, 1971; Meyers *et al.*, 1972). They resemble *Enterobacter* except that most strains have a yellow pigment, are motile, and do not decarboxylate amino acids. The anaerogenic strains are classified as the *Herbicola-lathyri (Enterobacter agglomerans)* group.

The schemes for identification of the gram-negative enteric bacteria to be given here will emphasize generic identification and only proceed to species in certain special cases. Separation of the groups is determined primarily by fermentation of carbohydrates, decarboxylation of amino acids, and other biochemical and serological tests. Many species show definite patterns of susceptibility to antibiotics, and these can be helpful in their differentiation – e.g., *Citrobacter* and *Serratia* are resistant to cephalothin, *Enterobacter aerogenes* is resistant to ampicillin, and so forth. The majority of strains of enteric bacteria can be readily identified by techniques described later, but intermediate and aberrant strains are encountered with some frequency. These can present problems to inexperienced workers (Table 18–7).

The use of selective, inhibitory, and enrichment media for primary inoculation from a fecal culture has been discussed previously. The purpose is to inhibit gram-positive organisms and to separate the enteric bacilli on the basis of easily recognized cultural characteristics, i.e., lactose fermentation, lysine decarboxylation, etc. The colony characteristics of the different genera on commonly used selective media are described in Table 18–8.

Further identification is accomplished by transfer from the isolated colonies to triple sugar iron agar (T.S.I.) or an equivalent medium (Kligler's, etc.) and to urea. It is well to make separate transfers from several colonies of different types, if available. Urea medium is specific for the identification of *Proteus*, which breaks down the urea rapidly and renders the medium alkaline (red). Some workers add tryptophan to the urea medium to test for indole production simultaneously.

T.S.I. agar is a multipurpose medium designed to provide a tentative differentiation of the enteric bacilli. It contains lactose (1.0 per cent), sucrose (1.0 per cent), dextrose (0.1 per cent), and an iron salt. It is tubed as slants, with a deep butt and relatively short slant. The center of the colony from the original culture is touched with a straight wire and stabbed into the butt (be careful not to stab completely to the bottom of the tube). The wire is then streaked over the slant. Acid production is indicated by a change in the color of the medium from red to yellow. Gas production is shown by the appearance of the bubbles in the medium along and around the stab line. Fermentation of lactose is indicated by the development of acid and gas in the slant and butt. Fermentation of dextrose only is indicated by an acid butt, either with or without gas, and a slant that remains alkaline (red). The production of H_2S is indicated by the presence of blackening of the medium as a result of the formation of iron sulfide. T.S.I. slants should be read at 24 hours, since, on longer incubation, the reaction may revert to alkaline and the results may be quite confusing. The use of screw-cap tubes for T.S.I. slants should be avoided because their use may cause aberrant results.

In Table 18–9 are shown the characteristic reactions of the main groups on T.S.I. medium. Following the reading of the urea and T.S.I. results, one should do spot agglutinations with polyvalent antisera and send a preliminary report on the findings.

Other tube differential media that some find preferable are those of Freiwer and Shaugnessy, Kohn's two-tube medium, or Gillies' modification, and dulcitol-lactose-sucrose-iron motility medium. Lysine iron agar is also very useful in conjunction with these media in differentiating the various Enterobacteriaceae (Johnson *et al.*, 1966). Table 18–10 shows the reactions of enteric groups on this medium.

Further identification of the organism depends on biochemical studies and on specific agglutination. Antisera for the agglutination test are available commercially and the technique is simple. It can be done as follows: A loop of the growth from the T.S.I. slant is emulsified in a drop of saline on a clean slide. A drop of the antiserum is added and the mixture tilted back and forth for about 1 minute. In a positive test, clumped bacteria can be seen macroscopically. Weak reactions should be considered negative. A control with saline substituted for the antiserum is essential and the antiserum should be checked periodically

*Test for β-D-galactosidase.

Table 18–7. BIOCHEMICAL REACTIONS OF ENTEROBACTERIACEAE*

	Indole	M.R.	V.P.	Citrate	Motility	KCN	Urease	Phenylalanine	Malonate	Lactose	Sucrose	Mannitol	Dulcitol	Salicin	Lysine	Arginine	Ornithine
Escherichia	+	+	–	–	+/–	–	–	–	–	+	d	+	d	d	d	d	d
Shigella	+/–	+	–	–	–	–	–	–	–	–(1)	–(1)	+/–	d	–	–	–/(+)	d(1)
Edwardsiella	+	+	–	–	+	–	–	–	–	–	–	–	–	–	+	–	+
Salmonella	–	+	–	d	+	–	–	–	–	–	–	+	d(2)	–	+(2)	(+)	+(2)
Arizona	–	+	–	+	+	–	–	–	+	d	–	+	–	–	+	+/(+)	+
Citrobacter	–	+	–	+	+	+	–/w	–	d	d	d	+	d	d	–	d	d
Klebsiella	–/+	–	+	+	–	+	–/w	–	+	+	+	+	+/–	+	+	–	–
Enterbacter cloacae	–	–	+	+	+	+	–/w	–	+/–	+	+	+	+/–	+/(+)	–	+	+
E. aerogenes	–	–	+	+	+	+	–	–	+/–	+	+	+	–	+	+	–	+
E. hafniae (37° C.)	–	+/–	+/–	(+)/–	+	+	–	–	+/–	–/(+)	d	+	–	d	+	–	+
E. liquefaciens[3] (37° C.)	–	+/–	–/+	+	d	+	–/w	–	–	d	+	+	–	+	+/–	–	+
Serratia	–	–/+	+	+	+	+	w	–	–	–/(+)	+	+	–	+	+	–	+
Proteus vulgaris	+	+	–	d	+	+	+	+	–	–	+	–	–	d	–	–	–
P. mirabilis	–	+	–/+	+/(+)	+	+	+	+	–	–	d	–	–	d	–	–	+
P. morganii	+	+	–	–	+	+	+	+	–	–	–	–	–	–	–	–	+
P. rettgeri	+	+	–	+	+	+	+	+	–	–	d	+/–	–	d	–	–	–
Providencia	+	+	–	+	+	+	–	+	–	–	d	d	–	–	–	–	–

(1) *Sh. sonnei* ferments lactose and sucrose slowly and is ornithine +.
(2) *S. typhi* is ornithine and citrate neg.
S. paratyphi A is lysine neg. and citrate neg.
(3) Serratia liquefaciens

d – different biochemical types
(+) – delayed positive
w – weakly positive reactions

*Modified from *Differentiation of Enterobacteriaceae by Biochemical Methods.* Atlanta, Ga., National Center for Disease Control, 1970.

for specificity and reactivity with known cultures. For agglutination of possible *Shigella* cultures, the organisms should be boiled for 30 minutes to destroy heat labile K antigens. The use of six "H" sera (a, b, c, d, i and 1, 2, 3, 5) in conjunction with the O and Vi sera will allow satisfactory identification of most of the strains of *Salmonella* found in human disease (Silliker, 1965). Immunofluorescent techniques in which labeled globulin fractions of H and O antisera are used appear to offer a promising technique for serotyping these organisms.

Specific agglutination of suspected *Sal. typhi* requires special comment. Freshly isolated strains often have Vi antigen, and such organisms may not agglutinate with the *Sal. typhi* antiserum. Specific anti-Vi sera, if available, should be used. If such sera are not available, the Vi antigen can be destroyed by placing the suspension of the bacteria in a boiling water bath for 15 minutes. Following this, the organism should agglutinate with the routine anti-*Sal. typhi* O serum.

Exact identification of the species of organism may require further studies, since there are sometimes confusing cross-reactions in the agglutination tests, e.g., some of the Arizonae share antigens with some of the Salmonellae. This can be accomplished by doing biochemical studies and agglutinations with species-specific antisera. Bacteriophage suspensions spe-

Table 18–8. APPEARANCE OF COLONIES OF ENTERIC ORGANISMS ON SELECTIVE PLATING MEDIA

GROUP	E.M.B. AGAR	S.S. AGAR	BISMUTH SULFITE AGAR	X.L.D. AGAR	HEKTOEN ENTERIC AGAR
Escherichia coli	Flat, deep purple with metallic sheen	Inhibited; may develop as large opaque pink or red colonies	Inhibited; large, mucoid, glistening, brown	Inhibited; flat dry lemon-yellow colonies. Opaque yellow zone in surrounding agar	Inhibited, may be bright orange to salmon pink
Klebsiella-Enterobacter	Light blue, metallic sheen occasionally in depressed center	Inhibited; large white or cream colored; opaque	Inhibited; raised, mucoid, lenticular colonies	Raised, mucoid lemon-yellow colonies; opaque yellow zone in surrounding agar	Same as above
Salmonella typhi	Colorless, translucent	Colorless, but may have light tan, pinkish, or yellow appearance or have a yellow or tan center	Black with metallic surface surrounded by brownish black zone with metallic sheen. Subsurface colonies, no sheen	Flat red colonies with large, glossy black centers; red clear zone in surrounding agar	Blue to blue-green, varying in size. H_2S producers have black centers
Salmonella, Arizona, Edwardsiella	Colorless, translucent	Colonies sometimes larger than above; otherwise similar	Colonies similar to above but larger, tending toward a dark brown rather than black; usually lustrous	As above	Same as above
Proteus vulgaris and *mirabilis*	Colorless; may spread; fuzzy edges	Small, transparent colonies; may have fuzzy or veil-like edge. Sometimes show black centers	Some inhibited. Discrete green, some with dark centers	Appear like coliforms. Sometimes develop small black centers (*P. morganii* and *rettgeri*, same as *Shigella*)	Most strains inhibit H_2S. Producing strains similar to but smaller than *Salmonella.* Non H_2S producers resemble *Shigella*
Shigella	Small, round, translucent colorless	Colorless, transparent, 2 to 7 mm. *Sh. sonnei* may be large, flat, irregular	Inhibited, light or dark green smooth glistening colony, some ameboid in shape	Transparent red colonies surrounded by red clear zone in agar	Green; periphery of colonies often larger than central portion
Pseudomonas	Oval or lenticular, colorless, irregular edges, may be mucoid	Transparent grayish colonies usually rough with irregular edges	Greenish brown colonies, sometimes with darker centers	Amber-tinted, dry, rough-edged colonies; may resemble *Shigella*	Inhibited. When present, colonies small, flat green to brown
Alcaligenes faecalis	Colorless, small	Colorless, clear, transparent, small	Inhibited; dark green to black dry	Inhibited or same as *Shigella*	Inhibited; colonies small, brown

Table 18–9. REACTIONS OF ENTERIC BACILLI ON TRIPLE SUGAR IRON AGAR

GENERA AND SPECIES	SLANT	BUTT	GAS	H_2S
Escherichia	A	A	+	–
Shigella	Alk.	A	–	–
Salmonella typhi	Alk.	A	–	+
Other *Salmonella*	Alk.	A	+	++
Arizona	Alk.	A	+	++
Citrobacter	Alk.	A	+	++
Edwardsiella	Alk.	A	+	++
Klebsiella	A	A	++	–
Enterobacter	A	A	++	–
E. hafniae	Alk.	A	+	–
Serratia	Alk. or A	A	–	–
Proteus vulgaris	A	A	+	++
P. mirabilis	Alk.	A	+	++
P. morganii	Alk.	A	–	–
P. rettgeri	Alk.	A	–	–
Providencia	Alk.	A	+ or –	–

cific for *Salmonella* are available and may also be useful in identification. Where more complete identification is required it is desirable to send cultures to laboratories which specialize in these techniques. Some of the characteristic biochemical reactions of the members of this group of bacteria are shown in Table 18–7. As noted previously, variations from the listed reactions will occasionally be encountered.

The following section describes briefly some of the commonly used biochemical tests for differentiation of these organisms. Other reactions are described in the publications listed in the references.

Indole Production

Kovacs' Method

Paradimethylaminobenzaldehyde	5 gm.
Amyl or isoamyl alcohol	75 ml.
Hydrochloric acid, conc.	25 ml.

Add approximately 1 ml. of reagent to a 24- or (preferably) 48-hour peptone-water culture. Shake gently. The reagent rises to the surface. A cherry red color is a positive test for indole.

Oxalic Acid Paper Method. Prepare a saturated aqueous solution of oxalic acid (15 to 20 gm. per 100 ml.). Dip filter paper into this solution while warm, and dry thoroughly. Cut paper into strips 10 by 90 mm. With the paper strip form a loop under the cotton plug. Production of indole is shown by the development of a pink color on the paper during the growth of the culture.

Rapid Indole Test

Tryptone	2.0 gm.
Dibasic sodium phosphate (anhydrous)	0.2 gm.
Monobasic potassium phosphate (anhydrous)	0.1 gm.
Sodium chloride	0.8 gm.
Distilled water	100 ml.

The pH is adjusted to 7.0 to 7.2. The solution is autoclaved at 121° C. for 20 minutes and dispensed as needed with a sterile pipette. This solution should be diluted with an equal volume of normal saline before use.

To perform the test, dispense the diluted medium into tubes in 0.2-ml. amounts. Using a loop, inoculate with a generous amount of growth from the T.S.I. slant. Incubate 2 hours at 35° C., and then add 0.2 to 0.3 ml. of Kovacs' reagent. The change in color of the layer over the surface of the broth from yellow to red is a positive test.

Methyl Red Test

Methyl Red Solution

Methyl red	0.1 gm.
Ethyl alcohol (95 per cent)	300 ml.
Distilled water, to make	500 ml.

Table 18–10. REACTIONS OF ENTERIC GROUPS ON LYSINE IRON AGAR

SLANT	BUTT	H_2S	GAS	GROUP
Alk.	Alk. or N	–	– or +	*Escherichia*
Alk.	Acid	–	–	*Shigella*
Alk.	Alk. or N	+(–)	–	*Salmonella*
Alk.	Alk.	+ or –	–	*S. typhi*
Alk.	Acid	– or +	+ or –	*S. paratyphi A*
Alk.	Alk. or N	+(–)	–	*Arizona*
Alk.	Acid	+ or –	– or +	*Citrobacter*
Alk.	Alk.	+	– or +	*Edwardsiella*
Alk. or N	Alk. or N	–	+ or –	*Klebsiella, Enterobacter*
Alk. or N	Acid	–	+ or –	*E. cloacae*
Alk. or N	Alk. or N	–	–	*Serratia*
Red(Alk.)	Acid	–(+)	–	*Proteus, Providencia*

X = Symbols enclosed in parentheses indicate occasional reactions.
N = Neutral.
Red = Oxidative deamination of lysine.

Add 5 drops of the indicator solution to 5 ml. of a 2 to 3-day culture in MR-VP medium. A bright red color is positive; yellow is negative.

Voges-Proskauer Reaction

O'Meara Modification. To a 48-hour culture in MR-VP broth, add an equal amount of reagent (KOH, 40 gm.; creatine, 0.3 gm.; distilled water, 100 ml.). Leave at room temperature for 4 hours and shake. A positive reaction is indicated by production of a pink to red color.

Barritt Modification. Add 3 drops of 5 per cent alpha-naphthol in 95 per cent ethanol and 1 drop of 40 per cent KOH to 1 ml. of culture. Shake well. Production of a red color within 15 minutes is a positive reaction.

Urease

Rustigan and Stuart urea broth, or Christensen urea agar is inoculated with the organism to be tested. *Proteus* gives a red color in 2 to 4 hours. Other urease-positive organisms give an alkaline reaction much more slowly.

Rapid Urease Test

Urea	2.0 gm.
Monobasic potassium phosphate	0.1 gm.
Dibasic sodium phosphate	0.1 gm.
Sodium chloride	0.5 gm.
Ethyl alcohol	1.0 ml.
Distilled water	99 ml.

Adjust pH to 7.0 and add 0.5 ml. of a 0.2 per cent aqueous solution of phenol red. Sterilize by filtration.

To perform the test, dispense broth into tubes in 0.2-ml. amounts. Inoculate with a generous amount of growth from the T.S.I. slant. Incubate for 30 minutes at 35° C. A change in color from pale yellow to intense pink or fuchsia is a positive test.

Decarboxylase Reactions. Many organisms of the Enterobacteriaceae can be differentiated on the basis of their ability to attack various amino acids. Such reactions produce end products sufficiently alkaline to overcome any acid produced by fermentation of the small quantity of glucose incorporated in the basal medium. A positive reaction is indicated by an alkaline reaction (violet) and a negative by an acid reaction (yellow).

Moeller's Decarboxylase Basal Medium

Peptone (thiotone)	5.0 gm.
Beef extract	5.0 gm.
Pyridoxal	5.0 gm.
Glucose	0.5 gm.
Bromthymol blue, 0.2 per cent	5.0 ml.
Cresol red, 0.2 per cent	2.5 ml.
Distilled water	1000.0 ml.

Dissolve the solids in water by heating. Adjust the pH to 6.0, then add the indicator solution. Add amino acids as indicated below. Tube in small screw-cap tubes. Autoclave for 10 minutes at 121° C.

Add 10 gm. of l-lysine dihydrochloride, l-arginine monohydrochloride, or l-ornithine dihydrochloride per liter of basal medium. If dl-amino acids are used, use 20 rather than 10 gm. The pH may have to be readjusted after the addition of ornithine and prior to sterilization.

PROCEDURE

1. Inoculate the test medium as well as a control medium containing no amino acid with well-isolated colonies from an overnight growth on an agar plate or slant.
2. Overlay each tube with sterile mineral oil to exclude air.
3. Incubate at 35° C. for at least 18 hours. Delayed reactions may require 4 to 5 days' incubation. Purple in amino acid tubes indicates a positive reaction. The control tube must be yellow. Negative reactions may be reincubated up to 4 days if necessary.

Nitrate Reduction

Solution A:

Sulfanilic acid	8 gm.
5 N acetic acid	1000 ml.

Solution B:

Alpha naphthylamine	5 gm.
5 N acetic acid	1000 ml.

PROCEDURE

1. To 5 to 10 ml. of a culture grown in peptone broth containing 0.02 per cent potassium nitrate, add drop by drop 1 ml. of solution A followed by 1 ml. of solution B. If nitrite is present, a pink, red, or maroon color is produced.
2. If no color develops, this indicates the absence of nitrite and may mean one of two things: nitrate is not reduced, or both nitrate and nitrite have been reduced.
3. In order to determine definitely that the nitrate has not been reduced, the following procedure can be used:
   A. Add a small amount of zinc dust to the culture plus the nitrite reagents.
   B. If a red color develops, the zinc has reduced nitrate to nitrite. This indicates that nitrate was present and not reduced by bacterial action.
   C. If no red color develops, this indicates that the bacteria have reduced both nitrates and nitrites.

Tests for Hydrogen Sulfide Production

Lead Acetate Paper Method. Cut filter paper into 50- by 10-mm. strips and immerse them in a 5 per cent solution of lead acetate. Dry in air. Sterilize at 121° C. for 15 minutes.

Following inoculation of the liquid medium (which must contain available sulfur compounds) insert a strip of the sterilized paper between the plug and the glass, with the lower end above the liquid level. Incubate.

If H_2S is liberated, the lower portion of the paper will turn black. If, after incubation, there has been no color change, remove the plug and add 0.5 ml. of 2 N HCl, replace the paper, and plug without delay. The addition of the acid will liberate any dissolved sulfide, which will react with the lead to yield the black lead sulfide. This method is considered overly sensitive for the Enterobacteriaceae. The reaction of T.S.I. or Kligler's iron slants is more accurate with this group.

Gelatin Liquefaction. Place nutrient gelatin in tubes; inoculate and incubate at 20 to 22° C. for up to 30 days. Record time of liquefaction, if any. Another method is to streak cultures on a plate of nutrient agar containing 0.4 per cent gelatin. Incubate at 28° C. for two to 14 days, according to the rate of growth. Flood the plate with 8 to 10 ml. of a solution of 15 gm. of $HgCl_2$, 20 ml. concentrated HCl, and 100 ml. distilled water. A white opaque precipitate is formed with the unchanged gelatin; a liquefier is surrounded by a clear zone.

Phenylalanine Deamination. Streak surface of phenylalanine agar slant. Incubate overnight. Allow 4 to 5 drops of 10 per cent aqueous ferric chloride to run down over the growth on the slant. A dark green color on the agar slant and in the syneresis fluid is positive.

Rapid Paper Strip Method (Goldin and Glenn, 1962). Impregnate filter paper strips with 0.5 per cent l-phenylalanine in pH 7.4 phosphate buffer and dry overnight. Add a loopful of culture to a small amount of saline, place a phenylalanine strip into the suspension and incubate at 37° C. for 1 to 2 hours. Add 1 drop of 8 per cent $FeCl_3$ to the strip. A green color indicates a positive reaction.

Motility-indole-ornithine Medium (Ederer and Clark, 1970; modified).

Decarboxylase medium base	9.0 gm.
Tryptone	15.0 gm.
l-Tryptophan	1.0 gm.
l-Ornithine	5.0 gm.
Agar	3.5 gm.
Water	1000.0 ml.

Adjust pH to 6.5, dispense in small tubes, and autoclave 15 min. at 121° C. The medium is inoculated with a straight wire to the bottom of the tube. Oil overlay is unnecessary. After overnight incubation, motility is indicated by growth extending from the line of inoculation, ornithine decarboxylation by a purple color throughout the entire tube, and indole production by a red-to-pink color after the addition of a few drops of Kovacs' reagent.

Other reactions that are widely used in the identification of the enteric bacteria, besides carbohydrate fermentation, are:

Citrate
DNase
Indophenol oxidase
Malonate
Motility
Mucate
O.N.P.G. (β-galactosidase)
Potassium cyanide (KCN)
Tartrate

These will not be described here because of space limitations. Full discussions of these and other tests will be found in the references.

Over the past few years there have been developed a wide variety of substrate tablets and paper strips purported to simplify and expedite many of these biochemical reactions. Some of these may indeed be useful under some circumstances, but they should be used only after comparison with standard methods and with adequate controls.

In addition, many combinations of tests in kit form or in tubes have been marketed. Some of these may also prove useful, particularly for laboratories with limited facilities for enteric bacteriology. The results obtained by the use of these multitest kits should be compared with standard methods, and adequate controls must be used before any of these are adopted for routine use.

Identification of Enteropathogenic Types of Escherichia coli. Since the pioneer work of Kaufmann in 1943 on the antigenic analysis of *E. coli,* it has been found that certain serotypes are associated with diarrhea in infants and young children. Severe cases, both sporadic and epidemic, in which the etiology was formerly unknown have been proved to be caused by these serotypes. It has recently been shown that certain serotypes can cause severe diarrhea in adults as well. A water-borne outbreak due to *E. coli* O111 B_4 has also recently been documented. Consequently, it is essential to isolate and identify these organisms from clinical cases and from carriers.

Biochemical differences between the enteropathogenic strains and the normal types of *E. coli* are insufficient to differentiate them adequately from each other. Type differentiation thus depends entirely on their serological behavior.

E. coli possesses three types of antigens–O, K, and H. The O, or somatic, antigens are not inactivated by heat at 121° C. The K antigens, also somatic antigens, occur as capsules or envelopes which inhibit the O agglutination. This inhibitory effect is inactivated by heat at 100° C. The K antigens consist of three varieties known as L, A, and B. H antigens are the flagellar antigens found only in the motile strains.

In typing the enteropathogenic strains of *E. coli,* it is necessary to determine both the O antigen and the B variety of K antigen. The serotypes which most commonly are associated with diarrheal diseases are listed in Table 18–11.

PROCEDURE. Material for culture should be

Table 18–11. ENTEROPATHOGENIC STRAINS OF *ESCHERICHIA COLI* ANTIGENS

O (SOMATIC)	K (SHEATH ENVELOPE OR CAPSULAR)
26	B6
55	B5
86	B7
111	B4
112	B11
114	B90
119	B14
124	B17
125	B15
126	B16
127	B8
128	B12

collected before antibiotic therapy is instituted. If stools must be held for several hours before inoculation of media, they should be emulsified in buffered glycerol saline.

Specimens should be streaked onto E.M.B. or MacConkey's, and a blood agar plate. The blood agar is used because certain strains are inhibited on E.M.B. or MacConkey's agar and also because it is easier to avoid contaminants when picking colonies from this medium. Sorbitol agar may also be of assistance, since enteropathogenic strains of *E. coli* tend to be sorbitol negative. It is necessary, however, to use the other media, as well, since it has been found that sorbitol-positive strains of enteropathogenic *E. coli* are occasionally encountered. Sorbitol-negative strains should be checked with the acriflavine dye test. The test is done by suspending a colony in a drop of normal saline solution. Add 1 drop of neutral acriflavine (1:500 aqueous). Those that agglutinate within 1 minute may be discarded as negative.

After overnight incubation at 35° C., typical colonies of *E. coli* are picked to nutrient agar slants for serologic study. There are no distinct differences in colonial morphology between the pathogenic and nonpathogenic serotypes; hence, colonies must be picked at random. It has been noted, however, that enteropathogenic strains may give off a definite spermatic odor on first isolation and that when they are present they tend to predominate. The nutrient agar slants are incubated overnight and then tested for OB and O antigens. Colonies from blood or infusion agar may be typed directly from the plate, but this is not recommended for colonies from E.M.B. or MacConkey's agar, since the bile salts in the medium may cause confusing reactions.

Serologic Typing. In typing the enteropathogenic *E. coli*, the O antigen and the B variety of K antigen must be determined. Since the B antigen masks the O agglutinability of living cultures, the culture must be boiled before the O antigens can be determined. The OB antisera* contain the agglutinins for both the O and B antigens; the O antisera are used only after the B antigen has been destroyed by heating.

A drop of polyvalent OB antiserum is placed on a slide, and a small loopful of the culture from the agar slant is emulsified in the serum to give a homogenous suspension. The slide is then tilted back and forth for 1 to 2 minutes and agglutination observed macroscopically. The clumping must be rapid and strong; if it is not, it should be ignored. If positive, individual (specific) OB antisera are used. If strong agglutination occurs either in the polyvalent antisera or in any of the individual serotypes, a preliminary report that an enteropathogenic *E. coli* is present can be given and further serologic and biochemical tests done to confirm this and to determine the specific serotype.

If positive agglutination occurs in the OB antiserum, the O antigen must be determined. This can be done by first heating a saline suspension of the culture for 15 to 30 minutes in a boiling water bath and adding 0.5 per cent formalin. Serial dilutions of the specific antisera are then made in small test tubes so that a series of dilutions ranging from 1:20 to 1:2560 in 0.5 ml. of saline are prepared. These dilutions depend on the original titer of the antiserum. To each of these dilutions, 0.5 ml. of the suspension is added. The tubes are then incubated at 48 to 50° C. for 16 to 18 hours. Cultures showing agglutination in at least 1:160 or more are considered to have the same O antigen as the corresponding antiserum. If agglutination is not distinct except in low dilutions, this should be considered as negative for that particular O antigen. If strong agglutination occurs in more than one antiserum, this probably indicates a mixed culture, and the original agar slant should be streaked for purity and individual colonies retested.

It is also possible to test the O antigens by the slide test, but this should always be confirmed by the test tube procedure. The unboiled culture is tested on a slide with OB antisera and a boiled culture with O antisera. Agglutination in both antisera is strong evidence for the identification of that serotype.

If a strain of enteropathogenic *E. coli* is isolated, subcultures should be sent to a central public health laboratory for confirmation, together with pertinent information. This may help in tracing intra- and interhospital outbreaks. The final step in the identification is to

*Available commercially.

Table 18–12. OUTLINE OF PROCEDURE FOR EXAMINATION OF STOOL SPECIMENS IN CASES OF DIARRHEA IN INFANTS AND CHILDREN

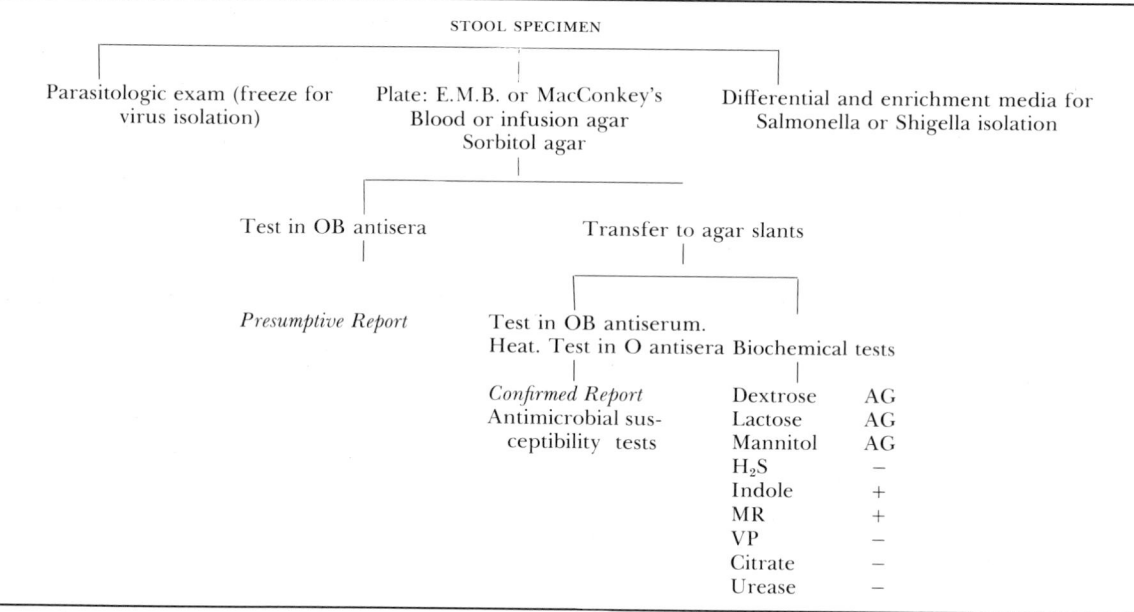

STOOL SPECIMEN

- Parasitologic exam (freeze for virus isolation)
- Plate: E.M.B. or MacConkey's Blood or infusion agar Sorbitol agar
  - Test in OB antisera
    - *Presumptive Report*
  - Transfer to agar slants
    - Test in OB antiserum. Heat. Test in O antisera
      - *Confirmed Report* Antimicrobial susceptibility tests
    - Biochemical tests
- Differential and enrichment media for Salmonella or Shigella isolation

Biochemical tests	
Dextrose	AG
Lactose	AG
Mannitol	AG
H_2S	–
Indole	+
MR	+
VP	–
Citrate	–
Urease	–

check the strain biochemically to make certain that it belongs to the *E. coli* group. See Table 18–12.

FA techniques are valuable in rapid examination of fecal specimens for enteropathogenic serotypes of *E. coli*, particularly in an epidemic situation. They are as yet, however, not a complete substitute for the cultural techniques described above. See Fried *et al.*, 1966.

The Nonfermentative Gram-negative Rods

Pseudomonas is present almost invariably on the surface of burns and may present serious problems, especially in patients who have sustained extensive burns. It also is a frequent contaminant in surgical wounds and occurs with some regularity in urinary tract infections. In the debilitated patient or the patient in shock, there is the danger of the development of *Pseudomonas* septicemia or pneumonia. Treatment of these infections is not easy, since the organism tends to be resistant to many of the commonly used antibiotics. It is essential that antibiotic susceptibility tests be done at the earliest possible time, although, as pointed out elsewhere, one must use caution in their interpretation.

Pseudomonas aeruginosa, the most commonly occurring species, is widely distributed in nature and is carried as a part of the normal flora of the gastrointestinal tract in the human. It may also be found as a part of the flora of the skin. It is capable of maintaining itself in the environment in areas of high moisture content. Drinking fountains, humidifiers, inhalation equipment, and mop closets are likely to be heavily colonized by this organism. In a dry environment it dies rapidly.

It is characterized by an almost complete lack of fermentative activity. It produces a pleasant, fruity odor and soluble pigments, which diffuse into the medium, giving a yellow-green color. Sabouraud's maltose agar is useful for enhancing pigment production (Fig. 18–35). Some *Pseudomonas* strains do not show any pigments and may be confused with other organisms. Methods that can be used to identify such strains are the following: (1) The *gluconate test* (Haynes) is based on the capacity of *Pseudomonas* to oxidize gluconate to ketogluconate. A gluconate substrate tablet* is placed in a test tube with 1 ml. of sterile water. A heavy suspension of the organism is made in the tube and incubated overnight at 35° C. A test for reducing sugar is then done, using Benedict's solution or a Clinitest tablet. A positive test is indicative of *Pseudomonas*. (2) The *cytochrome oxidase test* (Gaby) consists of adding 0.3 ml. of 1.0 per cent oxidase reagent (para-aminodimethylaniline oxalate) and 0.2 ml. of a 1.0 per cent

*Key Scientific Products Co., Los Angeles, California.

ethanol solution of alpha-naphthol to an overnight broth culture of the organism. The rapid appearance of a blue color after shaking the tube thoroughly indicates the presence of cytochrome oxidase, characteristic of *Pseudomonas*. Alternatively, a few drops of fresh 1 per cent tetramethyl-p-phenylenediamine dihydrochloride is placed on a square of Whatman No. 1 filter paper; the suspected colony is smeared with a loop on the reagent saturated paper. A positive reaction is recognized by a dark purple color developing in 5 to 10 seconds.

A simple selective medium for isolation of *Pseudomonas aeruginosa* is the modified cetrimide*-acetamide agar of Mossel and Indacochea (1971). This has given excellent results for the enumeration of *Pseudomonas* in contaminated materials.

A reliable technique for differentiating nonpigmented strains of *Pseudomonas aeruginosa* is the test for the presence of arginine dihydrolase (Taylor and Whitby). A medium consisting of peptone, 0.17 per cent; sodium chloride, 0.5 per cent; K_2HPO_4, 0.03 per cent; agar, 0.3 per cent; phenol red, 0.001 per cent; and l-arginine monohydrochloride, 1.0 per cent is dispensed in small screw-cap tubes and autoclaved at 15 p.s.i. for 20 minutes. The medium is inoculated by stabbing, the surface is covered with a 5-mm. layer of sterile liquid petrolatum, and the screw cap is tightened. After overnight incubation, the medium turns pink in a positive test. *Pseudomonas aeruginosa* is positive and *Alcaligenes*, *Herellea*, *Flavobacterium* and *Achromobacter* are negative.

Strains are occasionally isolated, particularly from children with cystic fibrosis of the pancreas, that have a distinctive slimy, mucoid capsule. The significance of this mucoid material is unknown (Doggett 1971) but is probably a mutation caused by host factors. There is evidence that these variants are more virulent than the nonmucoid strains.

*Cetyltrimethylammonium bromide.

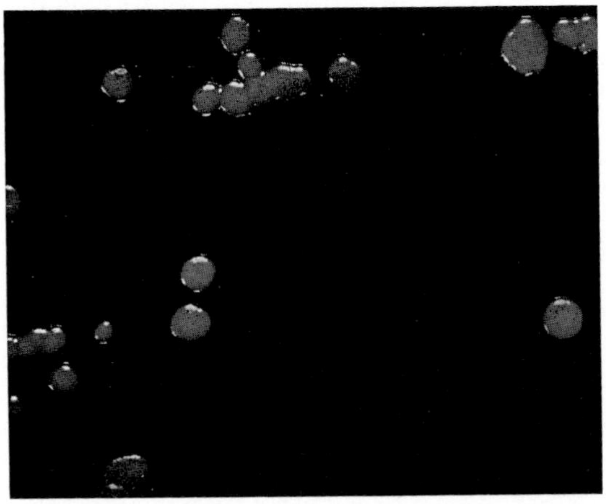

Figure 18–35. Colonies of *Pseudomonas* on nutrient agar; 24-hour culture; × 3. (From Burrows, W.: Textbook of Microbiology. 19th ed.)

Pseudomonas stutzeri, which is occasionally found in clinical material, is characterized by buff- or peach-colored dry colonies which resemble craters with elevated ridges. Bubbles of nitrogen gas appear in nitrate broth after 24-hour incubation. Gluconate is not oxidized, and the alkaline phosphatase is heat labile (von Graevinitz, 1965). *Pseudomonas pseudomallei*, an ubiquitous organism found in the damp soil of Southeast Asia, is the causative agent of melioidosis. This is a serious infectious disease which has occurred with increasing frequency in individuals returning to the United States from this area. Colonies are characteristically wrinkled, rough and corrugated on nutrient agar and bright red in color on MacConkey's agar. No green or blue pigment is produced; gluconate oxidation and growth on cetrimide agar is negative and oxidase is positive. It also oxidizes glucose and lactose and is resistant to colistin (Zierdt and Marsh, 1971). *Cultures of this organism must be handled with the greatest caution. Pseudomonas cepacia* (*P. kingii*, *P. multivorans*, EO-1) has been found in commercially packaged urinary catheter kits and germicidal solutions and has caused infections in debilitated individuals. It usually shows a yellow pigment on T.S.I. agar only and is resistant to the usual pseudomonad antimicrobial agents.

Speciation in this group is difficult, particularly because of the unsettled taxonomy. Table 18–13 shows some of the important characteristics of some of the more common species.

Alcaligenes faecalis is a normal inhabitant of the gastrointestinal tract but evidently does not have the ability of *Pseudomonas* to maintain itself in the environment. Isolation of this organism from sites other than the gastrointestinal tract, i.e., in blood culture, urine culture, or a surgical wound infection, must always be viewed with suspicion. It does not produce acid or gas from carbohydrates and characteristically turns litmus milk alkaline.

Aeromonas is a genus of the family Pseudomonadaceae, the members of which are primarily soil and water inhabitants. There is mounting evidence that they can be associated with human disease, especially gastroenteritis (von Graevinitz and Mensch, 1968). They characteristically ferment, rather than oxidize carbohydrates, with production of acid or acid and gas. They exhibit β-hemolysis on blood agar, produce gelatinase, lipase, and give a positive oxidase and extracellular desoxyribonuclease reaction.

Table 18–13. CHARACTERISTICS OF COMMON SPECIES OF PSEUDOMONAS

	P. aeruginosa	*P. fluorescens*	*P. cepacia*	*P. pseudomallei*	*P. stutzeri*	*P. maltophila*
Pigments, fluorescent	+	+	−	−	−	−
Pigments, phenazine	+	V	V	−	−	−
Poly-β-hydroxybutyrate	−	−	+	+	−	−
Denitrification	+	V	−	+	+	−
Growth at 4° C.	−	+	−	−	−	−
Growth at 41° C.	+	−	V	+	V	−
Extracellular hydrolase, gelatin	+	+	+	+	+	+
Extracellular hydrolase, starch	−	−	−	+	+	−
Arginine dihydrolase	+	+	−	+	−	−
Oxidase (Kovacs)	+	+	+	+	+	−
O.N.P.G.	−	−	+	−	−	+
DNAase	−	−	−	−	−	+
Polymyxin B susceptibility	+	+	−	+	+	+

V = Variable.

The Mima-Herellea Group. These poorly differentiated organisms are found normally in the mucosa of the nose and vagina, and the conjunctiva. The primary reservoir of these bacteria appears to be the skin. They have been found associated with disease in conjunctivitis, septicemia, meningitis, and urethritis. The urethritis, as has been pointed out before, may be confused with gonococcal urethritis. The closely related Morax-Axenfeld bacillus (*Moraxella lacunata*) is also associated with conjunctivitis.

Morphologically they are pleomorphic, short, plump, encapsulated gram-negative coccobacilli on primary isolation. They do not ferment carbohydrates and are nitrate negative. On T.S.I. slants they produce an alkaline reaction throughout the medium, thereby resembling *Pseudomonas* and *Alcaligenes*, with which they are frequently confused.

Mima polymorpha closely resembles the organism classified as *Acinetobacter wolffi*. The oxidase positive strains are now generally called *Moraxella osloensis*. *Herellea* resembles *A. anitratum*. Further work is required before an acceptable classification of this taxonomically perplexing group is universally adopted.

Flavobacterium is a slender gram-negative rod which produces a distinct pale yellow pigment. It is oxidase and catalase positive, peptonizes litmus milk, and acidifies dextrose and maltose slowly. It is urease, nitrate, citrate, and gelatin negative and does not grow at all on S.S. but slowly on MacConkey's agar. The reaction on Sellers' differential agar resembles that of *Mima polymorpha*. *F. meningosepticum* has been reported as a cause of meningitis in children. Other isolations from a variety of human infections have also been reported.

Chromobacterium is a motile rod producing a water-insoluble violet pigment. It is common in soil and water. Human infections have been reported, mainly from tropical areas.

The technique of Hugh and Leifson (1953) described below is very useful in differentiating organisms of this group.

DIFFERENTIATION OF OXIDATIVE AND FERMENTATIVE PRODUCTION OF ACID FROM CARBOHYDRATES
(Hugh and Leifson, 1953)

Peptone (casein hydrolysate)	2.0 gm.
NaCl	5.0 gm.
K_2HPO_4	0.3 gm.
Agar	3.0 gm.
Bromthymol blue (1 per cent aqueous)	3.0 ml.
Distilled water	1000 ml.

Dissolve the ingredients and adjust the pH, if necessary, to 7.1. Sterilize at 121° C. for 15 minutes.*

Prepare 10 per cent aqueous solutions of the carbohydrates to be tested and sterilize by Seitz filtration. Add 10 ml. of the carbohydrates aseptically to every 100 ml. of the sterile melted medium and dispense in 5-ml. amounts in sterile 150 by 13 mm. tubes.

Inoculate two tubes of each carbohydrate by stabbing with the organism to be tested. Cover the surface of one tube with sterile mineral oil.

Fermentative organisms produce acid throughout both tubes. Oxidative organisms produce acid in the open tube only. In the latter, acid appears first at the surface and then progressively toward the base. Slow oxidative reactions are sometimes preceded by a slight alkaline reaction. If organisms fail to grow, repeat the test using the basal medium enriched with 0.1 per cent yeast extract or 2 per cent horse serum.

A useful medium for differentiating and identifying the nonfermentative gram-negative bacilli is Sellers' (1964) differential agar. The medium (commercially available) is tubed, autoclaved, and cooled in long slants. Immediately before inoculating, 2 drops of sterile 50 per cent dextrose solution are added and allowed to run down the side of the tube opposite the slant. The tubes are inoculated by deep stab and streaking the slant. They are then incubated for 24 hours at 35° C. (Table 18–14).

*The base medium is available commercially.

Table 18–14. REACTIONS ON SELLERS' DIFFERENTIAL AGAR SLANTS

ORGANISM	SLANT COLOR	BUTT COLOR	BAND COLOR	FLUORESCENT SLANT	NITROGEN GAS
Pseudomonas aeruginosa	Green	Blue or no change	Sometimes blue	Yellow green	+
Herellea	Blue	No change	Yellow	None	None
Mima polymorpha	Blue	No change	None	None	None
Alcaligenes faecalis	Blue	Blue or no change	None	None	+

Table 18–15 summarizes some of the more common tests used in differentiating members of this group.

Hemophilus, Bordetella, Moraxella, and Calymmatobacterium (Donovania)

The species of gram-negative bacilli belonging to the genera *Hemophilus* and *Bordetella* are fastidious organisms requiring enriched media, usually factors contained in blood or potato (Figs 18–36, 18–37, and 18–38). Table 18–16 shows the medically important species of these genera.

Hemophilus influenzae and the closely related *Hemophilus parainfluenzae* occur normally in varying numbers of individuals as a part of the flora of the mucous surfaces of the throat and respiratory tract, respectively. Person-to-person transmission of these organisms apparently occurs throughout the population. When these organisms are found to predominate in inflammatory processes, one must suspect that they are playing a role in the disease process. *H. influenzae* may be the causative agent in bronchopneumonia, in which it may be secondary to a viral infection such as influenza. It is the most common cause of meningitis in children from three months to five years of age, occurring as a sporadic disease, not as an epidemic.

The need for "X" and "V" factors by the hemophilic bacteria is of considerable importance in diagnostic bacteriology. The "X factor" is heat stable and is associated with hemoglobin, and the "V factor" (nicotinamide adenine dinucleotide) is heat labile and associated with yeast and whole blood. Chocolate agar seems to make these factors more readily available; hence, it is a better medium than blood agar for these organisms.

Colonies of *H. influenzae* tend to be very small, and it may be necessary to examine the plates from spinal fluid and other cultures with a magnifying lens. Of considerable help in the successful isolation of *H. influenzae* is the "satellite phenomenon." This occurs when *H. influenzae* and *S. aureus* grow together on blood or chocolate agar. The colonies of *H. influenzae* close to the staphylococcus colonies become much larger, apparently owing to production of soluble growth factors which diffuse from the staphylococcus colonies. In practice, exudate from the throat or nasopharynx or the spinal fluid is first streaked over the plate, and then a streak of *S. aureus* is made across the plate. Sometimes this will produce positive cultures where, without the staphylococcus, no colonies of *H. influenzae* appear. Paper discs impregnated with "X" and "V" factors are now available and can be used instead of the *Staphylococcus* culture. Chocolate agar containing 300 μg. bacitracin/ml. makes an excellent selective medium for

Table 18–15. DIFFERENTIATION OF MIMA-HERELLEA GROUP FROM OTHER GRAM-NEGATIVE BACILLI

	DEXTROSE	LACTOSE	SUCROSE	LITMUS MILK	NITRATE	SIMMONS CITRATE	S.S. AGAR	MOTILITY
*Mima polymorpha**	–	–	–	NC	–	–	–	–
Herellea	Ox.	Ox.	–	NC/Coag.	–	+	–	–
Pseudomonas aeruginosa	Ox.	–	–	Alk., Pep.	+	+	+	+
Alcaligenes faecalis	–	–	–	Alk.	+	+	+	+
Enterobacteriaceae	Ferm.	Ferm./-	Ferm./-	Var.	+	±	±	±

NC = no change; Ox = oxidation; Coag. = coagulation; Alk. = alkaline; Pep. = peptonization; Ferm. = fermentation.
**M. polymorpha* var. *oxidans* and *Moraxella* sp. are oxidase positive.

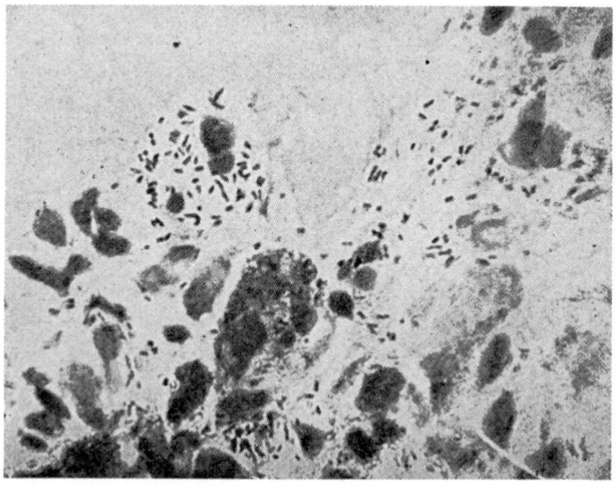

Figure 18-36. *Hemophilus influenzae* in spinal fluid in a case of meningitis (× 1000).

Hemophilus in material from the respiratory tract (Hovig and Aandahl, 1969).

There are at least six antigenic types of *H. influenzae* (a to f), determined by a specific capsular polysaccharide. Most of the pathogenic strains are type b. Typing can be accomplished by the Neufeld capsular swelling technique using specific antisera. Nontypable strains are probably avirulent.

Hemophilus aphrophilus is an organism which requires X factor but not V and is distinguished by distinctive quantitative growth in a CO_2 atmosphere and by serologic differences. Cases of brain abscesses, endocarditis, empyema, and so forth, have been reported to be caused by this organism. The source of these infections is unknown (Page and King, 1966; Sutter and Finegold, 1970). *Hemophilus aegyptius* (the Koch-Weeks bacillus), associated with acute conjunctivitis, is considered to be a variant of *H. influenzae.*

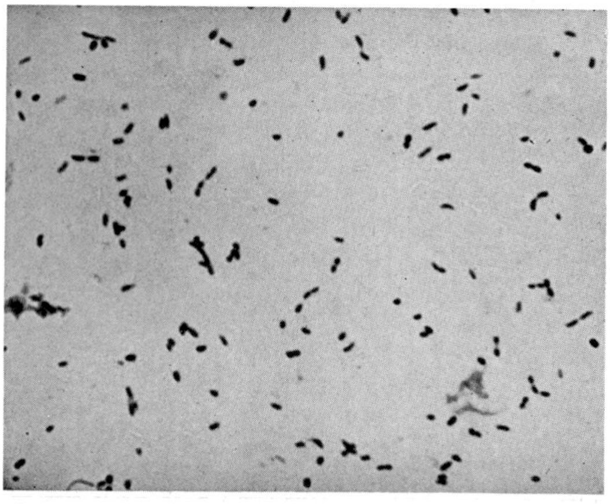

Figure 18-37. *Hemophilus influenzae,* pure culture. Note the variability from coccoid to bacillary form. Fuchsin; × 1050. (From Burrows, W.: Textbook of Microbiology. 19th ed.)

Hemophilus ducreyi is the causative agent of chancroid, which is an acute localized genital disease characterized clinically by necrotizing ulcerations at the site of inoculation. The lesions are commonly called "soft chancre." The organism can be demonstrated in pus aspirated from buboes and appears as typical streptobacilli distributed in clusters in leukocytes or in chain formation. Barritt's modification of Pappenheim's pyronine methyl green stain is highly recommended for this purpose. The stain is prepared as follows:

Methyl green, 1 per cent aqueous	100 ml.
Methanol, absolute	10 ml.
Pyronine	0.6 gm.
Phenol	1.0 gm.
Glycerol	20 ml.

The methyl green solution is first extracted with one-third volume of chloroform to remove methyl violet, which occurs as an impurity. The staining time is 30 to 60 seconds. Pus cells stain bluish green; the bacteria, brilliant red.

Cultures are done by adding the bubo pus aspirated under sterile conditions to agar slants containing 1 per cent rabbit blood. The technique of Borchardt and Hoke (1970) is very simple and efficient. The patient's blood is dispensed in 5-ml. amounts in sterile screw-capped tubes. After clotting, the serum is inactivated by heating in the water bath at 56° C. for 30 minutes. It is then cooled to room temperature, inoculated with the material from the lesion and incubated for 48 hours at 35° C. *Hemophilus ducreyi* can then be identified as gram-negative coccobacilli, 1–2 × 0.5 μ long in pairs and short chains and in the characteristic long parallel "school of fish" rows.

Granuloma venereum (inguinale) is a venereal disease probably caused by *Calymmatobacterium (Donovania) granulomatis.* The laboratory diagnosis depends primarily on the demonstration of the "Donovan body" (Fig. 18-39). The characteristic oval or bacilliform

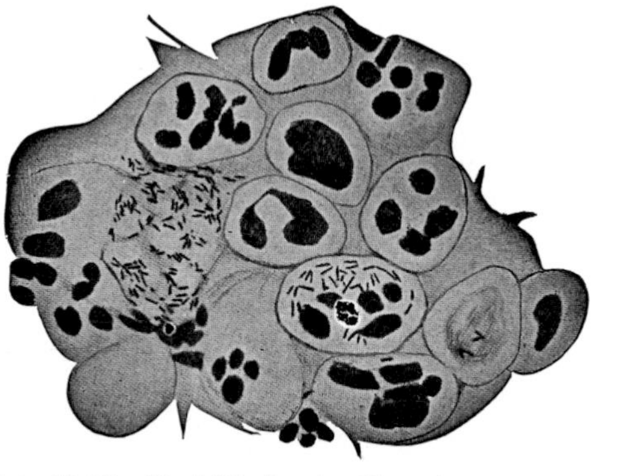

Figure 18-38. Koch-Weeks bacillus in conjunctivitis; × 900.

Table 18–16. CHARACTERISTICS OF HEMOPHILUS AND BORDETELLA

SPECIES	DISEASES IN MAN AND SITE	GROWTH REQUIREMENTS		MEDIUM OF CHOICE	HEMOLYSIS	REMARKS
		X Factor	V Factor			
Hemophilus influenzae (Pfeiffer's bacillus)	Bronchopneumonia, meningitis, conjunctivitis, throat infection	+	+	Chocolate or blood agar + 10% CO_2	Neg.	Exhibits satellite phenomenon with *Staphylococcus aureus*. Encapsulated, iridescent colonies
Hemophilus hemolyticus	Normal in nose and throat	+	+	Same as *H. influenzae*	Pos.	May be found in normal throat. Questionably pathogenic. Inhibited by sheep blood
Hemophilus ducreyi (Ducrey's bacillus)	Soft chancre (chancroid)	+	−	Clotted heated rabbit blood	Slight	Difficult to culture. Occurs as short chains
Hemophilus aegyptius (Koch-Weeks bacillus)	Acute conjunctivitis	+	+	Rabbit blood agar	Neg.	Agglutinates human red blood cells. Nonencapsulated. Satellitism
Bordetella pertussis	Whooping cough	−	−	Bordet-Gengou medium, charcoal agar	Pos.	Colonies are raised and white (half-pearl) and have a hazy zone of hemolysis
Bordetella parapertussis	Whooping cough (few cases)	−	−	Bordet-Gengou	Pos.	Grows readily on nutrient agar. Citrate positive
Bordetella bronchiseptica (*Alcaligenes*)	Rarely causes pneumonia. Whooping coughlike disease	−	−	Blood agar	Pos.	Classified as *Alcaligenes* by some. Urea positive
Moraxella lacunata (Morax-Axenfeld diplobacillus)	Angular conjunctivitis	−	−	Loeffler's medium	Variable	Diplobacilli. Liquefies coagulated serum. Related organism, *M. liquefaciens*, grows on blood agar
Calymmatobacterium granulomatis (*Donovania*)	Granuloma inguinale	−	−	Enriched heart infusion. Yolk sac of chick embryo	Neg.	Difficult to culture; stained smears (Wright's) from lesion show bacilli with large capsules (Donovan bodies)

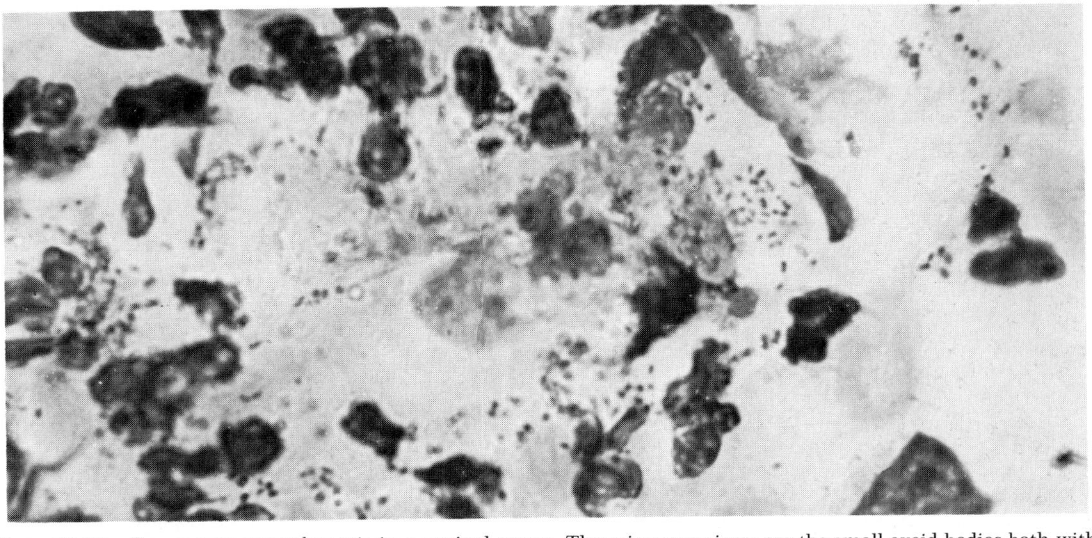

Figure 18–39. *Donovania granulomatis* in a vaginal smear. The microorganisms are the small ovoid bodies both within polymorphonuclear leucocytes and lying free. Wright's stain; × 1200. (From Burrows, W.: Textbook of Microbiology. 19th ed.)

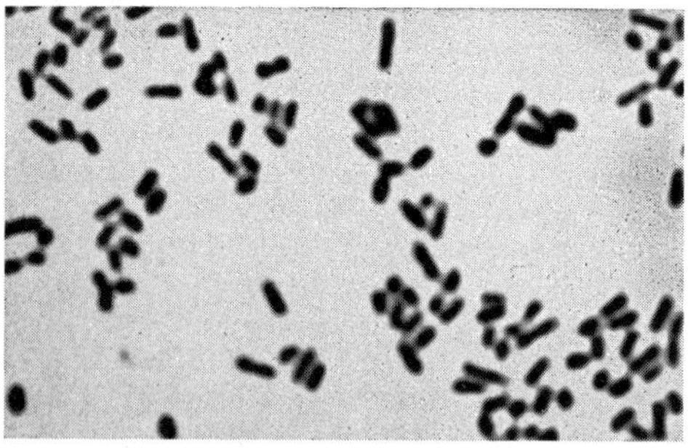

Figure 18–40. *Moraxella lacunata* (Morax-Axenfeld bacillus); pure culture. Gram stain; × 2400. (From Burrows, W.: Textbook of Microbiology. 19th ed.)

bodies surrounded by a dense capsule in large mononuclear cells are best demonstrated by spreading small pieces of clean granulation tissue and staining with Wright's, Giemsa, or 1 per cent pinacyanole stain. Cultures are generally not successful.

Moraxella lacunata is the cause of angular conjunctivitis. In smears of pus, the organisms appear as short, thick, gram-negative diplobacilli (Fig. 18–40). It appears to be closely related to the *Mima-Herellea* group.

The genus *Bordetella* includes *B. pertussis* and *parapertussis* and *B. bronchiseptica.* The latter organism has been placed in the genus *Alcaligenes* by some.

Mortality from whooping cough has decreased remarkably over the past 35 years. Well over half the deaths that do occur are in children under one year of age and about half the recognized infections occur in children under four years of age. The disease may occur in all age groups, however. Extensive use of vaccines has evidently been responsible for the reduction in mortality. The occurrence of mild cases, apparently modified by previous vaccination, has been noted. The diagnosis in such cases can be made only by culture of the organism. It would be difficult to determine how many unrecognized cases of whooping cough actually occur.

Bordetella pertussis, the causative agent of whooping cough, can be readily isolated, provided proper technique is employed (Figs. 18–41 and 18–42). Material collected from the trachea, bronchi, or nasopharynx by means of flexible wire swabs is much superior to the classic "cough plate" procedure. Specimens cultured on Bordet-Gengou agar containing penicillin (0.3 unit per ml.) and diamidinodiphenylamine dihydrochloride (2 μg. per ml.) reveal characteristic colonies in almost pure culture in 48 to 72 hours.* Adsorbed agglutinating antiserum (phase 1) for this organism is available and is useful in differentiating it from the closely related *B. parapertussis* and *B. bronchiseptica.* FA techniques are particularly useful in the diagnosis of pertussis, being more rapid and productive than cultural methods.

*Cephalexin, 40 μg./ml., is also excellent for this purpose.

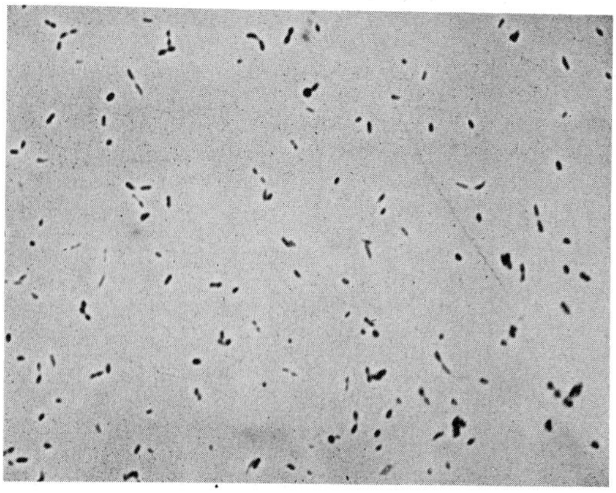

Figure 18–41. *Bordetella pertussis,* pure culture. Fuchsin; × 1050. (From Burrows, W.: Textbook of Microbiology. 19th ed.)

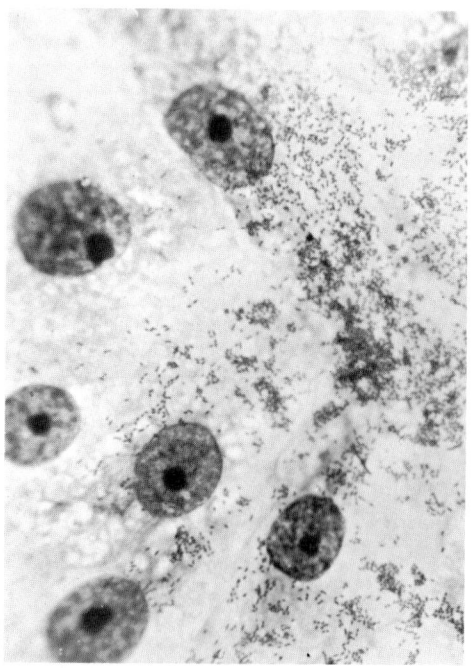

Figure 18–42. Monkey kidney tissue-cell culture infected with *Bordetella pertussis.* The large, dark, rounded objects are the nuclei of the tissue cells. The lighter cytoplasms, filling most of the picture, are crowded with myriads of the tiny bacilli. Note the ragged and vacuolated appearance of the infected and damaged cytoplasms. (About × 1400). (From Crawford and Fishel: J. Bact., 77:465, 1959.)

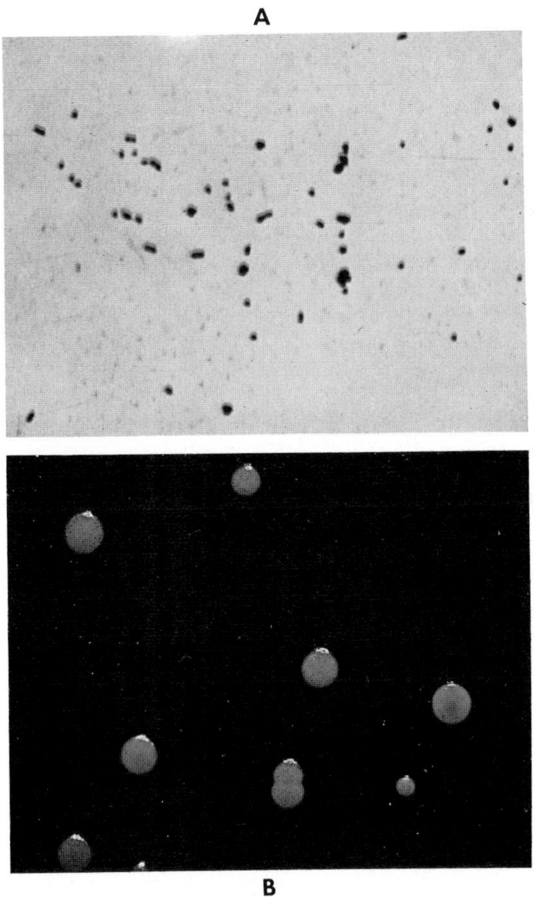

Figure 18–43. *Brucella melitensis,* pure culture. *A,* Note the coccobacillary appearance (Fuchsin; × 1050); *B,* on liver infusion agar (× 4). (From Burrows, W.: Textbook of Microbiology. 19th ed.)

Brucella, Yersinia, and Pasteurella

The *Brucella, Yersinia,* and *Pasteurella* are gram-negative bacilli that are primarily pathogens of animals but are transmissible to man either by direct contact or by means of arthropod vectors. *Brucella* produces undulant fever (brucellosis) in man, a disease that usually is chronic and presents serious diagnostic problems. The organisms tend to be disseminated in the tissues and can be cultured in the laboratory best by blood or sternal marrow culture. The organisms usually multiply slowly in blood culture, and it may be necessary to hold the cultures for 2 to 4 weeks before detectable growth occurs. There are three species of the genus: *Brucella abortus, B. melitensis,* and *B. suis.* All species grow well on tryptose or trypticase soy agar and on Albimi agar (Fig. 18–43). All strains grow better under 10 per cent CO_2, and *B. abortus* will not grow without it on primary isolation. The differentiation of the *Brucella* can be accomplished by means of the reactions shown in Tables 18–17 and 18–18. *Brucella abortus* and *suis* cannot be differentiated by using monospecific sera because they share identical antigens. Various serologic tests have been employed as aids in the diagnosis of brucellosis, but each has its disadvantages. This can also be said of skin testing with brucellergin.

Francisella (Pasteurella) tularensis is one of the most dangerous microorganisms to handle in the laboratory. It is highly infectious, and laboratory infections occur frequently. Patients with a history of exposure to wild

Table 18–17. CHARACTERISTICS OF BRUCELLACEAE

SPECIES	ANIMAL RESERVOIR	DISEASE IN MAN	MEDIUM OF CHOICE FOR ISOLATION	IDENTIFYING CHARACTERISTICS	REMARKS
Brucella abortus	Cattle, sometimes pigs or goats	Undulant fever (brucellosis)	Blood culture – 10% CO_2 Tryptose agar – 10% CO_2	Inhibited by thionine but not fuchsin. Requires CO_2; slow hydrolysis of urea. Colonies blue-gray, smooth, glistening	Causes abortion in cattle
Brucella melitensis	Goats, sometimes cattle or pigs	Same	Blood culture Tryptose agar	Not inhibited by thionine or fuchsin. Does not require CO_2	Causes abortion in goats
Brucella suis	Pigs, sometimes cattle or goats	Same	Blood culture Tryptose agar	Inhibited by fuchsin but not thionine. Rapidly hydrolyzes urea. Does not require CO_2	Causes abortion in pigs
Francisella tularensis	Rodents	Tularemia	Blood culture, glucose-cystine agar	Small, droplike colonies. Cells tend to show budding and filament formation	Absolute requirement for cystine
Yersinia pestis	Rodents (rats, ground squirrels)	Bubonic plague, "black plague" (pneumonia)	Infusion or blood agar	Organisms pleomorphic; bipolar staining. Colonies small dew-drop-like, nonhemolytic	Pathogens for mice and guinea pigs
Pasteurella multocida	Widely distributed in animals	Pneumonia, septicemia, meningitis	Rabbit blood agar	Bipolar staining. Encapsulated. Varies from mucoid to virulent iridescent phase. Grows on ordinary media and T.S.I. agar	Common in laboratory animals. Susceptible to penicillin

Table 18–18. DIFFERENTIATION OF BRUCELLA*

	CO_2 REQUIREMENT	H_2S PRODUCTION	GROWTH ON DYES: THIONINE 1:25,000	GROWTH ON DYES: BASIC FUCHSIN 1:50,000	AGGLUTINATION IN MONOSPECIFIC: ABORTUS SERA	AGGLUTINATION IN MONOSPECIFIC: MELITENSIS SERA
Brucella abortus	+	+ (3–4 days)	–	+	+	–
Brucella melitensis	–	–	–	+	–	+
Brucella suis	–	++ (3–4 days)	+	–	+	–

*There is considerable variation in these reactions, depending on the biotype.

rodents (rabbits, beavers) who have an initial skin lesion followed by fever may be suspected of having tularemia. The organism forms minute, mucoid, transparent colonies on Francis's glucose cystine-blood agar under 10 per cent CO_2 after 4 to 7 days at 35° C. A minute, pleomorphic, gram-negative coccobacillus with an absolute requirement for cystine that agglutinates with *F. tularensis* antiserum can be considered as a positive identification (Fig. 18–44). Agglutination tests are very useful in the diagnosis of this disease, and a skin test antigen (Foshay) has been prepared.

Yersinia (Pasteurella) pestis is the causative agent of plague (bubonic or pneumonic). Fortunately few cases of plague have occurred in man in recent years. The organism exists in the rodent population over a wide area of the western United States and causes widespread epidemics, especially in ground squirrels (sylvatic plague).

Bacteriologic diagnosis of plague is not difficult. Direct smear and gram stain from aspirates of buboes or sputum (pneumonic plague) may reveal gram-negative bacilli with bipolar granules in large numbers, which can be grown on trypticase soy agar plates (Fig. 18–45). The organism must be handled with extreme care in the laboratory. The use of FA techniques is of great aid in rapid identification of this organism.

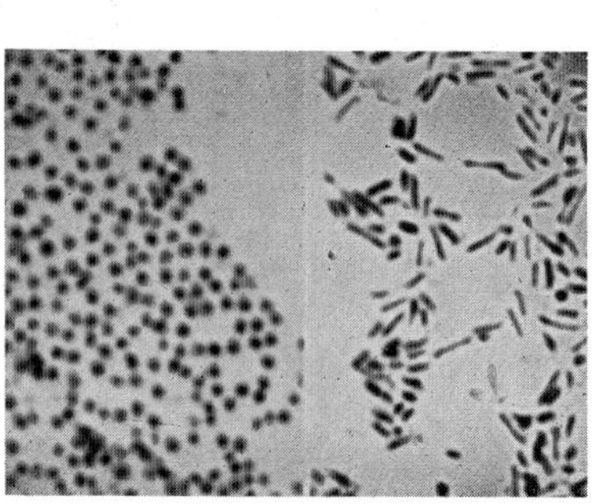

Figure 18–44. *Francisella tularensis.* Note change from coccoidal to bacillary form in 24 hours on fresh culture medium. (Francis.)

Yersinia enterocolitica, like the closely related *Y. pseudotuberculosis,* is chiefly important as an animal pathogen. Human infections are primarily acute mesenteric lymphadenitis, septicemia, and erythema nodosum. Morphologically the organism is a relatively large pleomorphic gram-negative coccobacillus. It produces an acid slant and butt on T.S.I. agar, is motile at room temperature, grows in KCN broth, and is Voges-Proskauer positive only at 22° C. Urease, ornithine, O.N.P.G., and nitrate are positive; arginine, lysine, phenylalanine, citrate, H_2S, and oxidase are negative. Acid, but no gas, is produced from glucose, sucrose, and mannitol, but not from lactose, rhamnose, and melibiose (Nilehn, 1969; Sonnenwirth and Weaver, 1970).

Members of the *Actinobacillus* group cause localized purulent lesions and septicemia in animals and man. They are small pleomorphic aerobic coccobacilli, which are difficult to distinguish from *H. aphrophilus.* They require either X or V factor and are catalase positive. Some strains of *A. actinomycetemcomitans* show distinctive star-like colony morphology (Page and King, 1966). This organism has been isolated from human cases of actinomycosis, either alone or in combination with *Actinomyces israelii.* (See p. 1120.)

Pasteurella multocida (septica) is an organism commonly found in a wide variety of animal species and has occasionally been isolated from man. It has been associated with cellulitis following an animal bite, bacteremia, pneumonia, arthritis and many other conditions. It grows well on blood agar, forming small, translucent colonies with a characteristic musty odor. Smears show it to be an ellipsoidal, gram-negative rod with a characteristic bipolar staining. It is H_2S, indole, and nitrate positive and produces acid but no gas in dextrose, sucrose, sorbitol, and galactose. An important differential point is that most strains

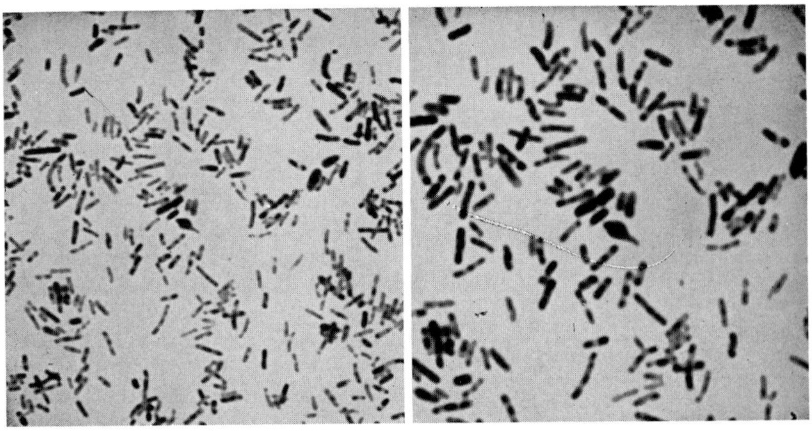

Figure 18–45. The plague bacillus. Smear from pure culture; fixed in methyl alcohol and stained with methylene blue to show bipolar staining. Note the involution forms present even at 24 hours' incubation. *Left,* × 1050; *right,* × 1800. (From Burrows, W.: Textbook of Microbiology. 19th ed.)

are sensitive to penicillin. Almost all strains are pathogenic for rabbits and mice (Fig. 18–46).

Streptobacillus moniliformis is a gram-negative, highly pleomorphic bacillus. It tends to occur in chains, requires media enriched with blood or serum, and may be cultured from lesions. The causative agent of one form of rat bite fever in man, it is primarily a pathogen of mice and rats and is transmitted to man accidentally.

The Gram-positive Aerobic Bacilli

CORYNEBACTERIUM DIPHTHERIAE AND DIPHTHEROIDS

Corynebacterium diphtheriae is the cause of diphtheria and is strictly a pathogen of man. It is a gram-positive bacillus that has characteristic cellular morphology. From the lesion or from observation of growth from Loeffler's or Pai's slants stained by Albert's technique or alkaline methylene blue, one sees considerable pleomorphism. Most cells are slender, slightly curved rods, which may have beads or bands of deep staining material (metachromatic granules). These cells tend to lie side by side in rafts or to form peculiar "Chinese letter" arrangements (Figs. 18–47, 18–48, and 18–49). Also there occur the so-called "snow shoe" forms. *Corynebacterium diphtheriae* occurs as four types – gravis, mitis, intermedius, and minimus – and the cellular morphology differs somewhat for each type.

As indicated in a previous section, the identification of *C. diphtheriae* depends to a considerable extent on the colony morphology on tellurite agar and the cellular morphology on Loeffler's or Pai's medium. Colonies of *C. diphtheriae* gravis tend to be large (3 to 5 mm.), with a wrinkled appearance and an ir-

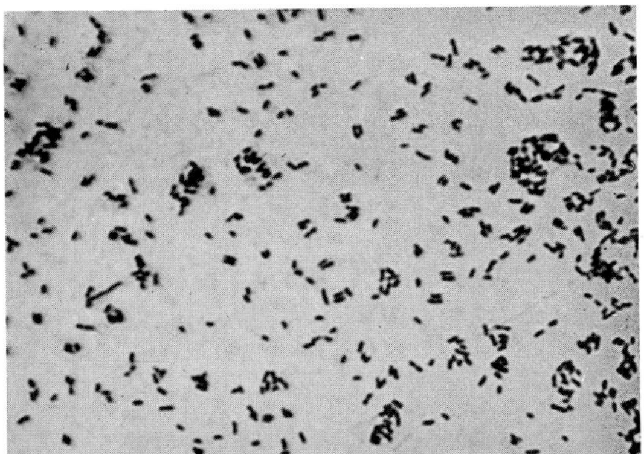

Figure 18–46. *Pasteurella multocida.* Smear from a pure culture. Fuchsin; × 1050. (From Burrows, W.: Textbook of Microbiology. 19th ed.)

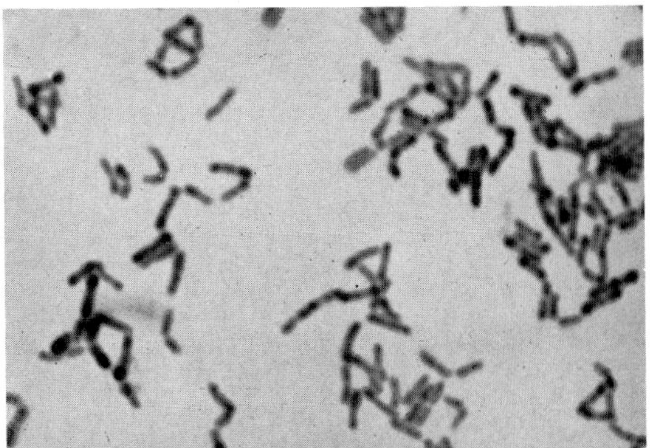

Figure 18–47. Metachromatic granules and bipolar staining in the diphtheria bacillus. Note the differences between these organisms and the plague bacilli. Methylene blue; × 1975. (From Burrows, W.: Textbook of Microbiology. 19th ed.)

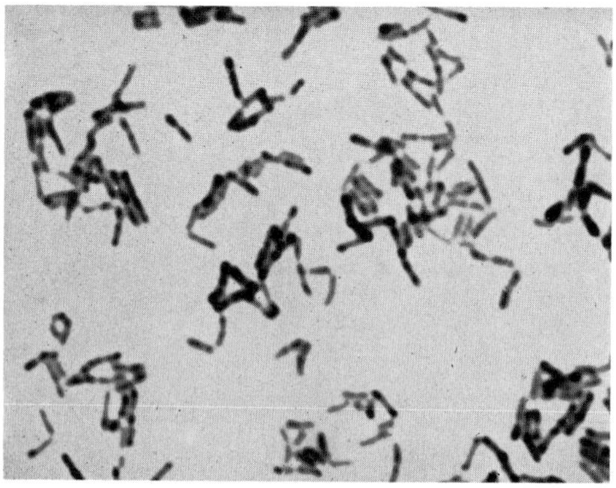

Figure 18-48. *C. diphtheriae,* gravis, pure culture on blood agar. Methylene blue stain. Note the bipolar staining and the club-shaped forms. The lightly stained cells with deeply stained areas are characteristic of gravis morphology. × 1200. (From Burrows, W.: Textbook of Microbiology. 19th ed.)

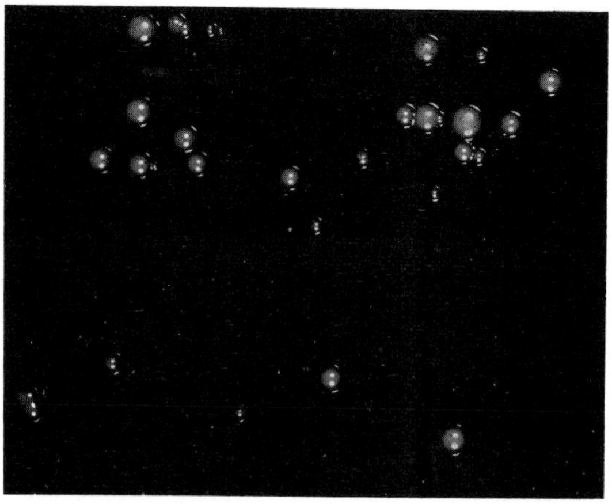

Figure 18-50. Colonies of *Corynebacterium diphtheriae* on blood agar. Note the smooth, raised translucent appearance and relatively small size. × 2. (From Burrows, W.: Textbook of Microbiology. 19th ed.)

regular edge. They are dark gray in color and may have a clear periphery. Mitis colonies tend to be smaller, dark gray, shiny, and buttery in consistency with a regular edge and a slightly raised center. Intermedius colonies are small, 0.5 to 1 mm. in diameter, with a dark gray or black center and a clear periphery. Minimus colonies are very small and are easily missed (Figs. 18-50 and 18-51).

The cells of *C. diphtheriae* gravis are less granular and banded than the others. There are usually some metachromatic granules, "snow shoe" forms, rafts, and "Chinese letters." In this regard gravis is most nearly like the diphtheroids. Mitis, intermedius, and minimus tend to be longer and more granular or banded.

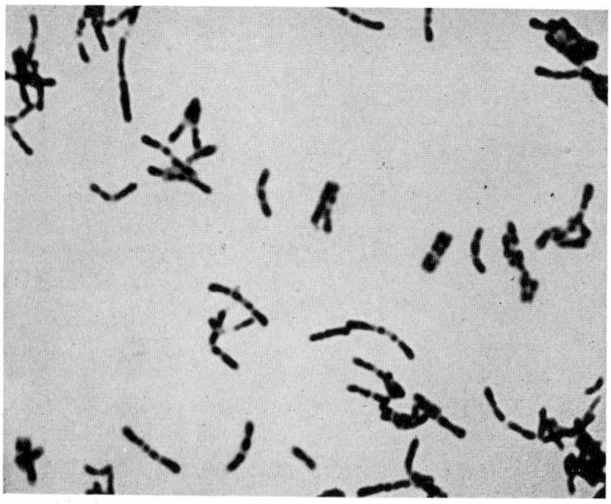

Figure 18-49. *C. diphtheriae,* intermedius, pure culture on blood agar. Methylene blue stain. Note the irregular staining and barred appearance characteristic of the intermedius variety. × 1200. (From Burrows, W.: Textbook of Microbiology. 19th ed.)

Corynebacterium diphtheriae does not invade the blood sufficiently to produce positive blood cultures. However, it can usually be isolated with ease from lesions in the throat or from the skin in cutaneous diphtheria. The organisms may disappear from the throat of a patient within one or two weeks after recovery, only to reappear at about the fifth or sixth week. It is therefore imperative that all convalescent patients be observed for six to eight weeks to be certain that they are not acting as carriers of the disease. Some individuals remain carriers for extended periods and present serious problems, because the carrier state is difficult to clear.

Diphtheroids comprise a large group of organisms that bear a close morphologic and cultural resemblance to *C. diphtheriae.* Most diphtheroids do not produce dark gray or black colonies on tellurite. Their colonies are usually smooth and glistening and are easily differentiated from the gravis strains of *C. diphtheriae.* This is an important point, since the cellular morphology of the diphtheroids is often similar to the gravis organism. The toxigenicity test is always the final test for virulence of a suspected *C. diphtheriae* (see p. 945). Occasionally this is the only certain means of differentiation, although some differences in biochemical activity exist between the gravis, mitis, intermedius, and minimus strains and the diphtheroids. Mitis strains tend to be hemolytic on blood agar and gravis ferments starch, while the diphtheroids are biochemically inactive. Gravis also tends to grow as a pellicle on the surface of fluid media.

The diphtheroids are widely distributed and constitute a major portion of the normal flora of the human skin along with *S. epidermidis.*

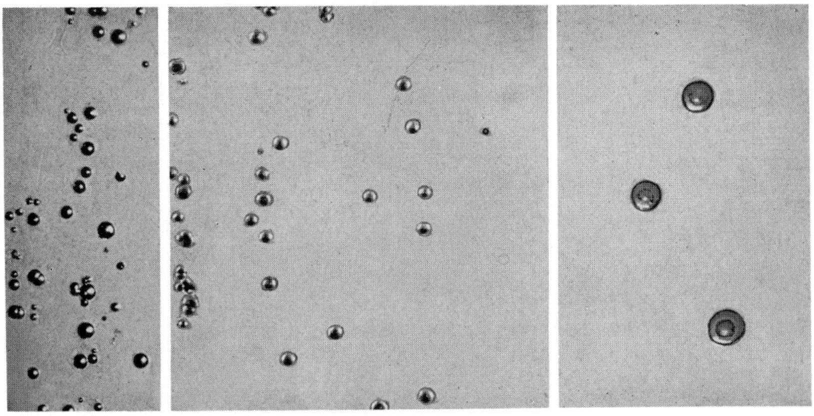

Figure 18–51. The varieties of the diphtheria bacillus on chocolate tellurite agar. *Left*, mitis type; note the characteristic raised, small black colony. *Center*, intermedius type; the lighter color, beginning radial striation, and small size are apparent. *Right*, gravis type; the gray color, larger size, raised center, and radial striation are evident. (From Burrows, W.: Textbook of Microbiology. 19th ed.)

They will be either aerobic or anaerobic. The aerobic species may be divided into two major groups—lipophilic and nonlipophilic. The lipophilic species form small colonies on ordinary culture media and the nonlipophilic species produce large colonies (Fig. 18–52).

Some anaerobic diphtheroids (*Propionibacterium*) resemble *Actinomyces israelii* culturally and morphologically. However, the diphtheroids grow more quickly than *Actinomyces*, are invariably catalase positive, produce acid, clot litmus milk, and do not ferment xylose, salicin, or raffinose. Their significance in human disease is not clearly understood.

The anaerobic diphtheroid *P. acnes* colonizes the deep sebaceous follicles that exist on the back and the nonbearded areas of the face.

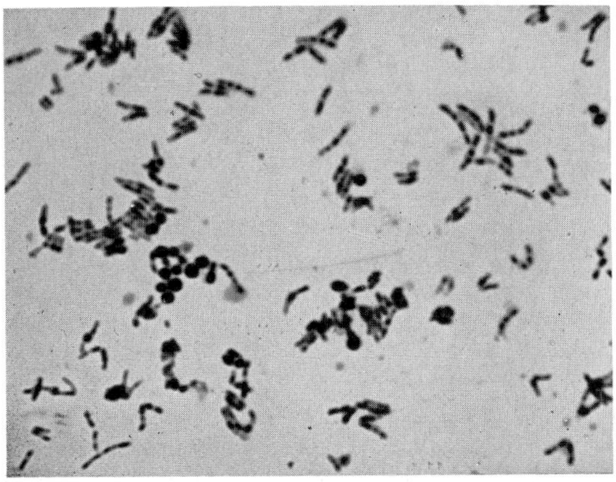

Figure 18–52. *Corynebacterium pseudodiphtheriticum.* Smear from pure culture stained with methylene blue. Note the irregular staining, club-shaped forms, and general close resemblance to *C. diphtheriae*. × 1050. (From Burrows, W.: Textbook of Microbiology. 19th ed.)

This species evidently contributes to certain pathologic conditions under proper circumstances and is certainly a secondary invader in acne vulgaris.

Trichomycosis axillaris is a superficial infection of the axillary or pubic hairs, characterized by soft pigmented nodules composed of minute bacteria-like organisms. These organisms have been classified as *Corynebacterium tenuis*, although other etiologic agents may be involved. Erythrasma is a superficial infection of the skin in the axillary and pubic areas. It is characterized by sharply circumscribed areas of reddish pigmentation with a nonvesiculated serpiginous erythematous border. The lesions give a coral-red fluorescence under the Wood's light. The etiologic agent appears in the scales as delicate, branching bacillary or coccobacillary forms (Fig. 18–53). Sarkany *et al.* (1962) have successfully isolated the organism on a bovine serum medium. Its taxonomic position remains in doubt, but most authorities classify it as *Corynebacterium minutissima*.

LISTERIA AND ERYSIPELOTHRIX

Listeria monocytogenes is found occasionally as the cause of meningitis (Lavetter *et al.*, 1971), septic perinatal infections, habitual abortions, and a wide variety of other infections in humans. It is probable that many human infections it causes are never diagnosed. Interestingly enough, this organism was at one time considered by many to be the specific etiologic agent of infectious mononucleosis. In the domestic rabbit it causes a severe purulent conjunctivitis when inoculated into the conjunctival sac (Anton's test). When the rabbit is inoculated intravenously or intraperitoneally, a severe monocytosis results. Morphologically

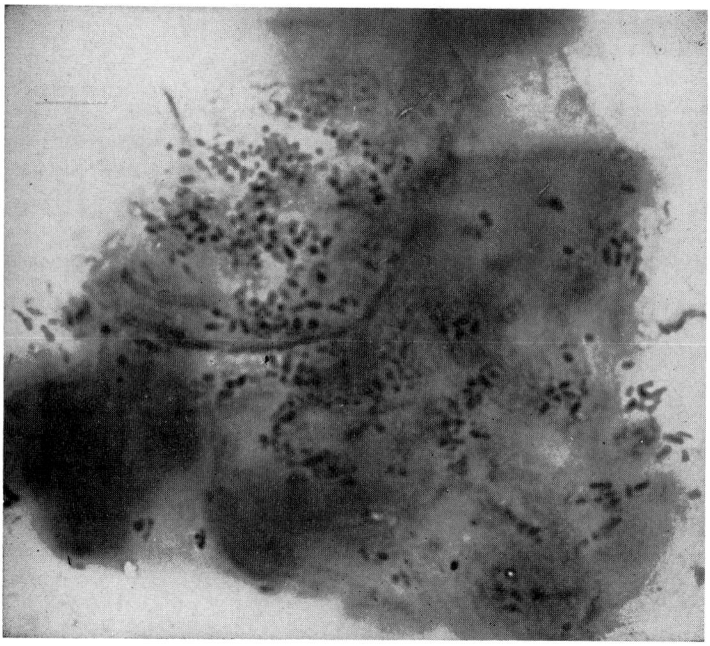

Figure 18–53. Erythrasma. Small bacillary forms (*Corynebacterium minutissimum*) seen in skin scrapings. × 1630. (Conant.)

L. monocytogenes is a gram-positive, motile bacillus that may resemble diphtheroids, or, when the rods are short, it may resemble *Str. pyogenes* (Fig. 18–54). The medium of choice is probably rabbit blood agar, and on this medium it produces a zone of beta hemolysis. Indeed, its colonies may be mistaken for *Str. pyogenes*, except that they tend to be larger and the hemolytic zone not so clear-cut. The single most important identifying feature of *L. monocytogenes* is its motility, which is readily demonstrable in semisolid agar at room temperature.

Erysipelothrix insidiosa (*rhusiopathiae*) is widely distributed in nature, causing erysipelas in swine and septicemia in mice. It may be isolated from infections in birds, turkeys, and ducks and causes erysipeloid in man, especially in fish handlers. It is a gram-positive bacillus that varies from a slender rod to short forms resembling cocci (Fig. 18–55). It grows on ordinary media and produces hemolysis on blood agar, which tends to be green at first, later changing to a slight but definite clear zone. Unlike *Listeria*, it is nonmotile and catalase and methyl red negative.

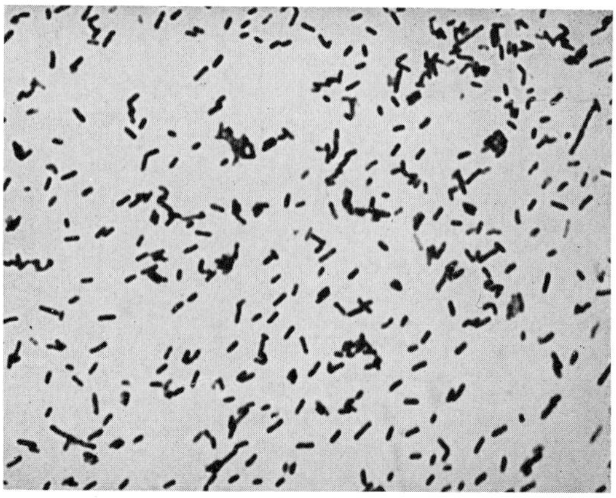

Figure 18–54. *Listeria monocytogenes.* Smear from a pure culture. Fuchsin; × 1050. (From Burrows, W.: Textbook of Microbiology. 19th ed.)

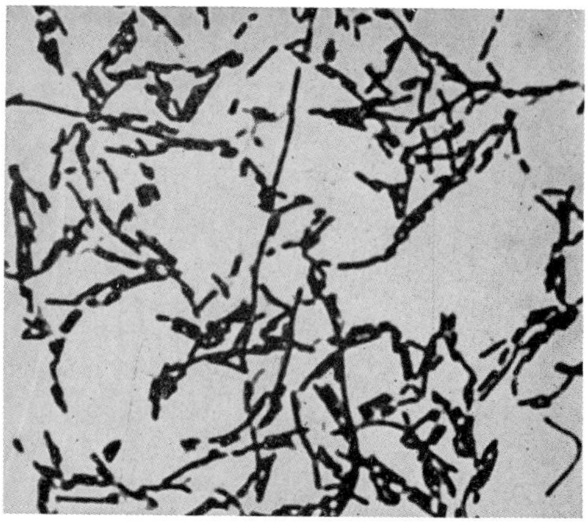

Figure 18–55. *Erysipelothrix rhusiopathiae.* Pure culture. Note the similarity of this microorganism to the actinomycetes; × 1000. (Kral.)

BACILLUS AND LACTOBACILLUS

The members of the genus *Bacillus* are gram-positive, spore-forming bacilli. There are two species of particular interest: *B. subtilis* and *B. anthracis*. *Bacillus anthracis* is the cause of anthrax in animals. It is transmissible to man and constitutes an occupational disease among those who handle animals, hides, and wool. In man the infection may appear as a skin lesion (malignant pustule), which usually remains localized but may progress to a rapidly fatal septicemia. Infection may occur by the respiratory route (wool sorter's disease), and when this occurs it often results in fatal septicemia.

The organism can frequently be demonstrated in gram-stained smears from the lesions and may be cultured on ordinary nutrient media. The colonies are rough and flat, with irregular edges approximately 3 mm. in diameter, and nonhemolytic. Gram stain reveals tangled coils of long parallel chains of large, square-ended rods. In culture the organisms are not capsulated, but capsules may be seen in smears from infected animals. It is nonmotile and produces central spores with no apparent swelling of the rods. No spore formation occurs in the infected animal but occurs readily on exposure to air (Figs. 18–56 and 18–57).

A reliable and simple test for the recognition of *B. anthracis* is the "perlschnurtest" or string-of-pearls test originally described by Jensen and Kleemeyer in 1953. The test is done as follows:

1. Prepare tryptose agar plates containing 0.5 unit of penicillin per ml. of medium.
2. Streak these plates with the suspected culture and incubate them for 3 to 6 hours at 37° C.

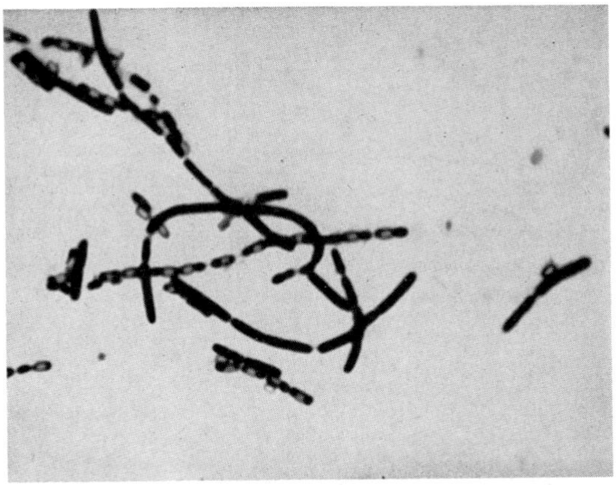

Figure 18–56. *Bacillus anthracis*, 48-hour culture. Crystal violet stain. The spores appear as unstained areas. Note the typical arrangement of the bacilli in coiled chains; × 1200. (From Burrows, W.: Textbook of Microbiology. 19th ed.)

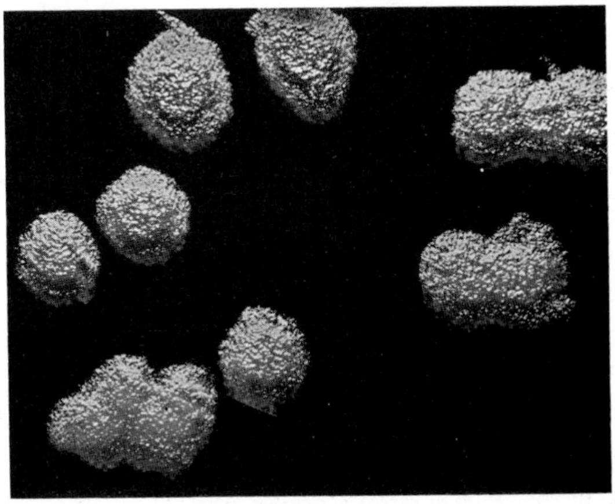

Figure 18–57. Colonies of *Bacillus anthracis* on nutrient agar. Twenty-four-hour culture. Note the large size and coarse texture suggestive of R variants; × 3. (From Burrows, W.: Textbook of Microbiology. 19th ed.)

3. Place a coverslip on the inoculated portion of the plate and examine it under oil immersion.
4. Within 3 to 6 hours *B. anthracis* cells swell up into round forms, giving the distinct appearance of a string of pearls. After 15 to 18 hours of incubation growth ceases. Other species of the genus *Bacillus* do not give this reaction.

Gamma phage and FA procedures are also very useful. The Ascoli test is done by preparing an extract of animal tissue or hide and layering it over anti-anthrax serum in a capillary tube. A ring of precipitate forms in a positive test.

Bacillus subtilis (the hay bacillus) and *B. cereus* are generally nonpathogenic organisms that are widely distributed in nature. They can be associated with infections occasionally, so their presence should not always be ignored (Pearson, 1970). Most of its importance lies in its close resemblance to *B. anthracis* (Figs. 18–58 and 18–59). It can be differentiated by inoculation of a broth suspension of the organism subcutaneously into a guinea pig. *Bacillus subtilis* does not produce disease, but *B. anthracis* will kill the guinea pig in from 36 to 48 hours.

The lactobacilli contain a number of species. Some are of considerable interest to the diagnostic bacteriologist. *Lactobacillus acidophilus* is probably identical with Döderlein's bacillus, which is a normal inhabitant of the vaginal tract and is usually present in large numbers. *Lactobacillus acidophilus* also occurs in large numbers in the intestinal tract of man and animals as a normal inhabitant. It is a rather large, gram-positive bacillus, occurring singly or in pairs. Colonies are small on ordinary media (Fig. 18–60).

Lactobacillus bifidus is closely related to

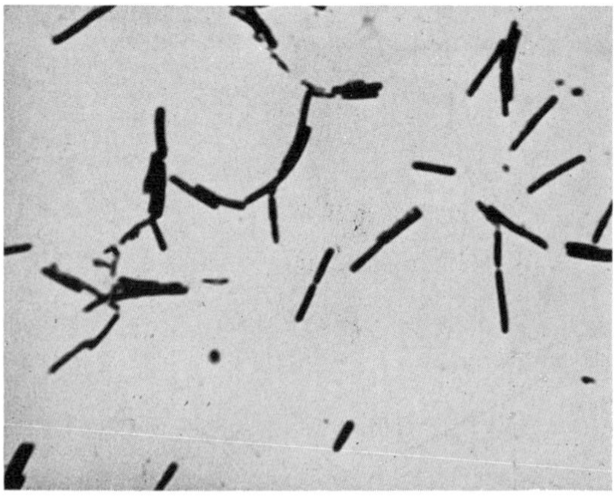

Figure 18–58. *Bacillus subtilis*, 24-hour culture. Crystal violet stain. No spores have formed as yet. Note the typical arrangement of the bacilli; × 1200. (From Burrows, W.: Textbook of Microbiology. 19th ed.)

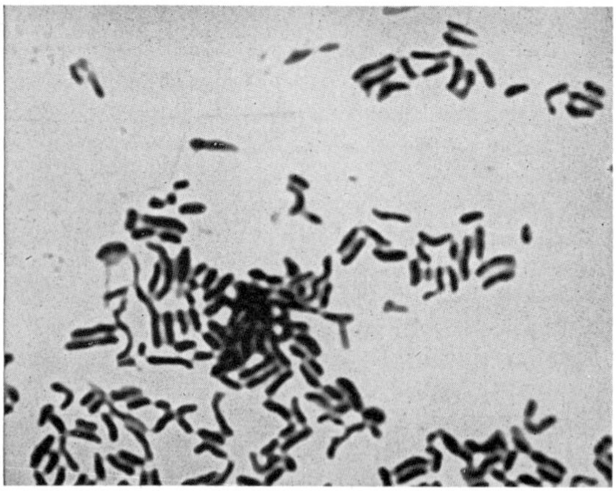

Figure 18–60. *Lactobacillus* sp. isolated from the mouth. Note the diplobacillary form and palisade arrangement of the cells; × 2500. (Harrison.)

L. acidophilus. It tends to appear early in the digestive tract of breast-fed infants and may comprise 90 per cent of the total flora. Cells of this organism exhibit an interesting type of bifurcation (Fig. 18–61). *Lactobacillus bulgaricus* is of interest, since it appears to be identical with or closely related to the Boas-Oppler bacillus, which was first seen in 1895 in the gastric juice of patients with gastric carcinoma.

Some strains of the lactobacilli are aerobic and facultatively anaerobic, some are microaerophilic, and some are anaerobic.

ANAEROBIC GRAM-POSITIVE BACILLI (CLOSTRIDIUM)

A number of species belonging to the genus *Clostridium* are pathogenic for man. These pathogenic clostridia all produce potent exotoxins, some of which are among the most toxic substances known to man. *Clostridium tetani* causes tetanus, *Cl. botulinum* causes botulism, and some species cause gas gangrene (*Cl. perfringens* [welchii] *Cl. septicum, Cl. novyi* [*oedematiens*], *Cl. histolyticum*).

None of these organisms is an active invader of tissue. *Clostridium tetani* and the gas gangrene organisms are usually introduced into wounds and multiply in necrotic tissue where anaerobic conditions exist. Usually culture from such wounds reveals that other anaerobic bacteria or aerobic bacteria are also present, and it is necessary to separately identify the various organisms. Thus, in diagnostic work it is best to streak the material on plates and to incubate anaerobically. The material submitted for culture is usually tissue that can be macerated for culture and gram stain.

Clostridium bolulinum probably does not multiply *in vivo.* It multiplies in food, *e.g.*, home-canned vegetables, producing its potent enterotoxin, which is then ingested by man or

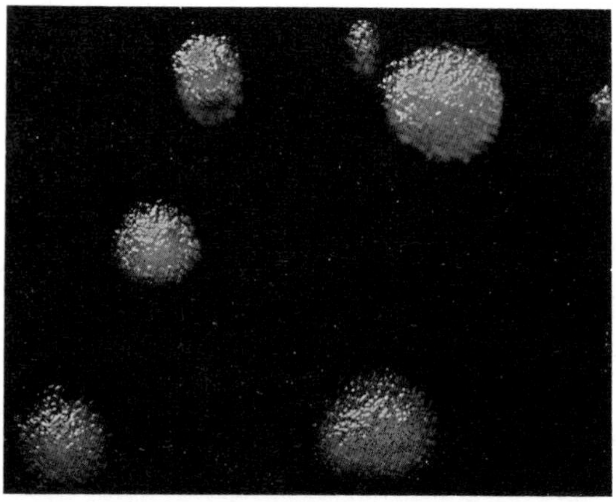

Figure 18–59. Colonies of *Bacillus subtilis* on nutrient agar. Twenty-four-hour culture. Note the resemblance to colonies of the anthrax bacillus; × 3. (From Burrows, W.: Textbook of Microbiology. 19th ed.)

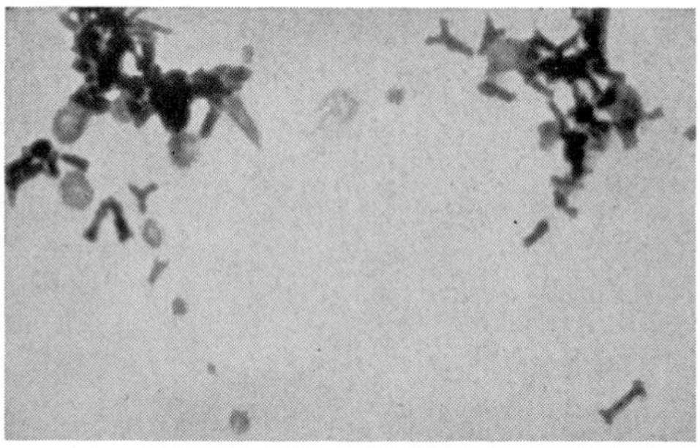

Figure 18–61. *Lactobacillus bifidus.* Note the Y-shaped forms. (Dack.)

animals. One may be able to demonstrate or to culture organisms from the suspected food or demonstrate the toxin by injection into mice with suitable controls of animals protected with antitoxin. Toxins A, B, and E are the most commonly found in human disease.

The clostridia are widely distributed in nature, especially in soil in areas where there are animals. These organisms (*Cl. tetani, Cl. perfringens*) are normal inhabitants of the intestinal tract of numerous animal species.

Gas gangrene is usually caused by *Cl. perfringens*, types A, D, or F, and *Cl. novyi*, types A and B. The disease is considered to be a histotoxic infection. The factors responsible are metabolites of the organisms—lecithinase, fibrinolysin, hyaluronidase, collagenase, and so forth. The identification of the clostridia depends on cellular morphology, spore formation, and cultural characteristics. (See Tables 18–19 and 18–20.) Determination of metabolic end products by gas chromatography has been shown to be very useful in identifying the various species of anaerobes. Details of this method can be found in Dowell and Thompson (1970). Since some of these organisms have a tendency to swarm in a thin film over a plate, it is well to use a cultural technique designed to prevent spreading. Sorbic acid, neomycin, chloral hydrate, sodium azide, and other substances are very useful in isolating clostridia from mixed cultures, and a wide variety of selective media are available (Smith and Holdeman, 1968). The plates should be incubated anaerobically for 48 hours or more, since colonies may develop slowly. Gram stain will show gram-positive rods that are likely to be quite variable morphologically but are fre-

Table 18–19. COLONY FORM, MORPHOLOGY, AND REACTIONS ON BLOOD AGAR OF SOME REPRESENTATIVE SPECIES OF CLOSTRIDIA*

SPECIES	COLONY FORM ON BLOOD AGAR**	HEMOLYSIS	VEGETATIVE MORPHOLOGY†	SPORES‡	PATHOGENICITY FOR GUINEA PIGS
Cl. perfringens	A	+	T, C	OE, R	+
Cl. butyricum	A	–	T	OE	–
Cl. botulinum (types B-E)	B, E	+	T	OE	+
Cl. histolyticum	C	+	S	OE	+
Cl. septicum	DG, F	+	S to T	OE, V	+
Cl. tertium	C	+	S	OT	–
Cl. sporogenes	D	+	S to T	OE	–
Cl. fallax	B	+	S to T, C	OE, R	+
Cl. tetanomorphum	E	V	S to T	ST	–
Cl. tetani	FG	+	S	ST	+

KEY

**Colony forms on blood agar:

A. Large, raised colonies; smooth to slightly ridged with entire to undulate margins, 2-4 mm.
B. Smaller colonies; smooth to irregular with entire undulate or serrate margins, 1-3 mm.
C. Minute colonies, raised, smooth to irregular; entire to irregular margins with short rhizoids, 0.2-1 mm.
D. Large colonies, raised; very irregular with wide-spreading, coarse rhizoids, 3-6 mm.
E. As D but smaller, finer rhizoids, 1-2 mm.
F. Irregular granular colonies with delicate spreading rhizoids to irregular rhizoid-like structures without a definite central colony.
G. Tendency to swarm.

†Vegetative morphology:
S—slender rods; T—thick rods; C—capsulated.

‡Spore morphology:
O—Oval; S—spherical; E—eccentric; T—terminal; R—rare; V—variable in size, shape, and position.

*Modified from Sterne, M., and vanHeyningen, W. E.: *In* Dubos, R. J., and Hirsch, J. G.: Bacterial and Mycotic Infections of Man. 4th Ed. Philadelphia, J. B. Lippincott Company, 1965.

Table 18–20. BIOCHEMICAL REACTIONS OF SOME REPRESENTATIVE SPECIES OF CLOSTRIDIA

SPECIES	MILK	H_2S	INDOLE	GELATIN LIQUE-FACTION	NITRATE REDUCTION	MOTIL-ITY	DEX-TROSE	MALTOSE	LACTOSE	SALICIN
Cl. perfringens	St.	V	−	+	+	−	+	+	+	V
Cl. butyricum	St.	−	−	−	−	+	+	+	+	+
Cl. botulinum (types B-E)	AD	−	−	+	−	+	+	+	−	+
Cl. histolyticum	CD	+	−	+	−	+	−	−	−	−
Cl. septicum	ACG	−	−	+	+	+	+	+	+	+
Cl. tertium	ACG	−	−	−	+	+	+	+	+	+
Cl. sporogenes	D	+	−	+	+	+	+	+	−	−
Cl. fallax	ACG	+	−	−	+	+	+	+	V	V
Cl. tetano-morphum	−	−	−	V	−	+	+	+	−	−
Cl. tetani	C	+	+	+	+	−	−	−	−	−

A = acid; C = clot; D = digestion; G = gas; St. = stormy fermentation; V = variable.

quently short and plump. *Clostridium tetani* is long and slightly curved, with a large characteristic terminal spore, giving it the appearance of a tennis racket. Other species have oval, subterminal spores (Figs. 18–62, 18–63, 18–64, and 18–65).

The gas gangrene group are highly saccharolytic and if inoculated into anaerobic litmus milk medium produce large amounts of gas, which results in a characteristic foamy appearance called "stormy fermentation" (Fig. 18–66).

These organisms tend to become gram negative in older cultures and this may be confusing. Space does not permit a more detailed discussion of these organisms; this can be found in the references.

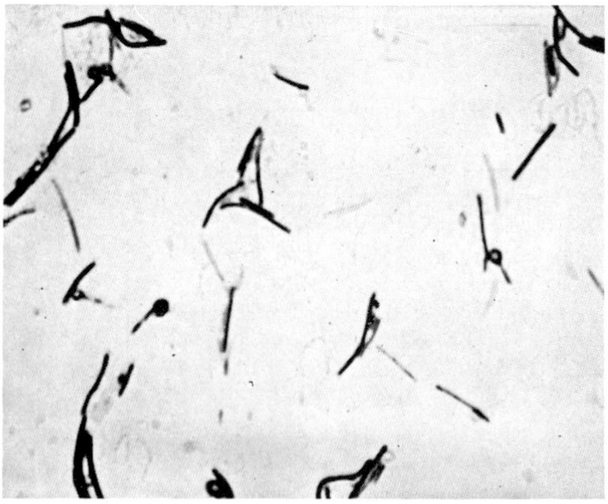

Figure 18–62. *Clostridium tetani* in pure culture. Young, actively growing culture showing beginning spore formation. Note the refractile, unstained spores; the drumstick appearance when these are attached to the cells; and the tendency of the vegetative cells to remain attached end to end. Fuchsin; × 1150. (From Burrows, W.: Textbook of Microbiology. 19th ed.)

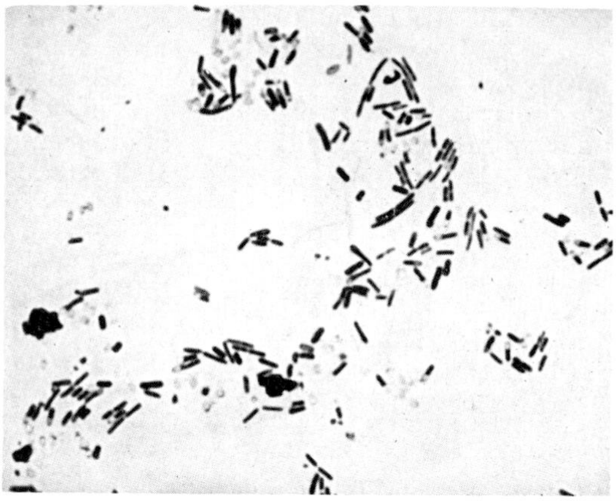

Figure 18–63. *Clostridium septicum* from pure culture. The tendency to form elongated vegetative cells is apparent. Fuchsin; × 1050. (From Burrows, W.: Textbook of Microbiology. 19th ed.)

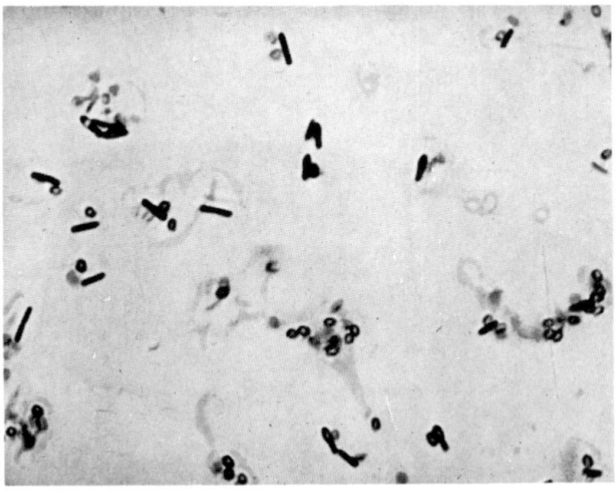

Figure 18–64. *Clostridium botulinum* type A from pure culture. Note the subterminal swollen spores and free unstained spores admixed with the vegetative cells. Fuchsin; × 1050. (From Burrows, W.: Textbook of Microbiology. 19th ed.)

Anaerobic Non-spore-forming Gram-negative Rods

The genus *Bacteroides* includes a number of species but is rather poorly classified. These are gram-negative, nonsporulating, anaerobic bacilli, which constitute a major portion of the normal microbiota of the gastrointestinal tract and can be found on the mucous surfaces of the nose and throat. Occasionally they are isolated in blood culture (Felner and Dowell, 1971) or from wounds and joint fluids.

They may be difficult to culture, requiring special media and prolonged incubation. They are oxygen sensitive, and most strains require 10 per cent CO_2. Most strains grow well in fluid thioglycollate medium but may require as much as 5 days to grow. Some do not grow well on the surface of agar plates (Fig. 18–67).

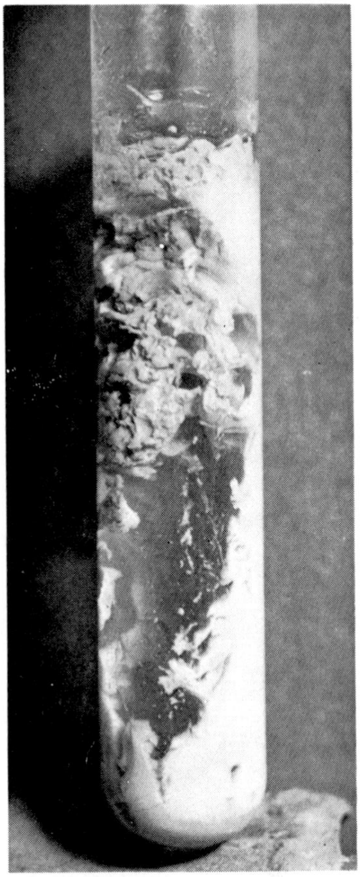

Figure 18–66. Tube of milk inoculated with *Clostridium perfringens* showing "stormy fermentation."

Fusobacterium fusiforme is probably a normal inhabitant of the respiratory tract. It is a large, gram-negative bacillus, occurring in pairs with blunt ends together and outer ends

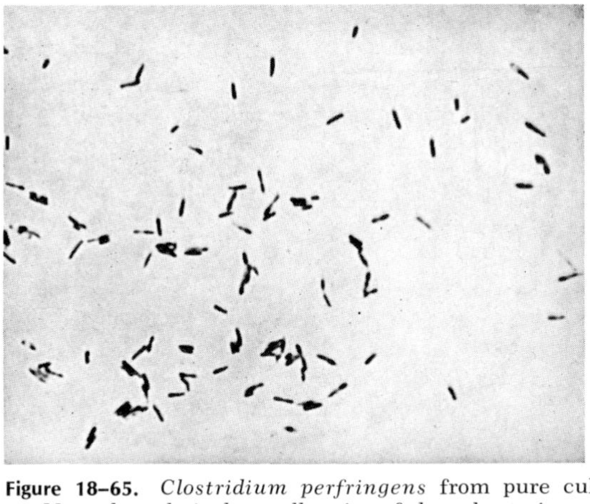

Figure 18–65. *Clostridium perfringens* from pure culture. Note the relatively smaller size of these bacteria and the central spores. Fuchsin; × 1050. (From Burrows, W.: Textbook of Microbiology. 19th ed.)

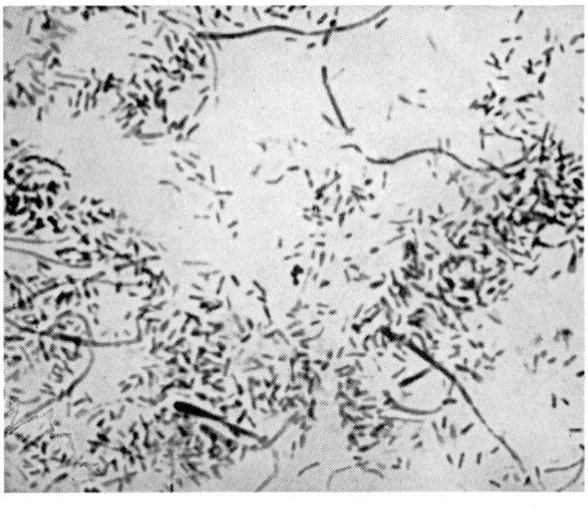

Figure 18–67. *Bacteroides fundiliformis.* The swollen and filamentous forms and poorly staining "ghost cells" are typical of the usual stained smear preparations; × 1000. (Dack.)

Table 18–21. MORPHOLOGICAL CHARACTERISTICS OF REPRESENTATIVE ANAEROBIC NON-SPORE-FORMING RODS*

SPECIES	GRAM STAIN	MORPHOLOGY Cellular	Colonial
Propionibacterium acnes	+	Pleomorphic rod; small, beaded, clubbed (thioglycollate, BAP)	"Dew-drop," white, convex, entire, opaque, glistening
Bacteroides fragilis	−	Regular rod with rounded ends; may be pleomorphic (BAP); commonly vacuolated (thioglycollate)	Mottled, circular, entire, glistening
B. variabilis	−	Small rod with rounded ends; vacuolated	Circular, entire, glistening, opaque with translucent edge
B. terebrans	−	Small rod with rounded ends; thin rods with rounded ends; filaments common, some chains	Circular, entire, translucent, raised to low convex
B. melaninogenicus	−	Coccoid rods (BAP); pleomorphic, vacuolated, degenerate rods (thioglycollate)	Black colonies on blood agar after incubation 4 to 5 days
Sphaerophorus necrophorus	−	Pleomorphic rods with rounded ends; spherules and round bodies	Umbonate, opaque with translucent edge, circular
Fusobacterium fusiforme	−	Thin rods with tapered ends; some or most cells filamentous (BAP, thioglycollate)	Circular, entire, glistening, mottled, low convex, translucent, often with greenish cast
F. girans	−	Small to medium spindles, usually in pairs	Low convex, slightly irregular, mottled, opaque

BAP = Blood agar plate.

*Modified from Dowell, V. R., Jr., and Hawkins, T. M.: Laboratory Methods in Anaerobic Bacteriology. Atlanta, Ga., Public Health Service Publication No. 1803, 1968.

pointed. It grows on ordinary agar media under anaerobic conditions. This organism is almost invariably present in considerable numbers along with a spirochete (*B. vincentii*) in Vincent's angina. It is not known whether the organism contributes in the causation of this condition. It is occasionally found in anaerobic wound infections. *Sphaerophorus necrophorus* is a pleomorphic rod which may also be associated with anaerobic infections (Table 18–21).

Vibrios, Spirillae, and the Spirochetes

The vibrios are a group of slightly curved, actively motile, gram-negative rods, which are aerobic or facultatively anaerobic. Most members of this genus are saprophytes, with the notable exceptions of *V. cholerae* and *V. El Tor*, the causative agents of Asiatic cholera. *Vibrio (Campylobacter) foetus*, which causes spontaneous abortion in cattle and sheep, is being reported with increasing frequency from human infections, including abortion, arthritis, and diarrhea. It is microaerophilic and requires enriched peptone media for its isolation. It reduces nitrates, is catalase and oxidase positive and is rather inert biochemically. *Vibrio parahemolyticus* is a halophilic organism found in sea water and fish. It has been incriminated as the cause of epidemics of gastroenteritis in the Orient (Fig. 18–68).

Comamonas terrigenea (*Vibrio percolans*) is a spirilliform bacterium that has been recovered from soil and water and occasionally in human infections. It is a motile, slightly curved rod with a polar tuft of flagella. It is catalase and oxidase positive and generally does not ferment or oxidize carbohydrates.

There are four genera of spiral bacteria in which there are a number of human pathogens. The genera are *Borrelia, Treponema, Leptospira,* and *Spirillum.* The important species are listed with certain of their important characteristics in Table 18–22. *Borrelia* and

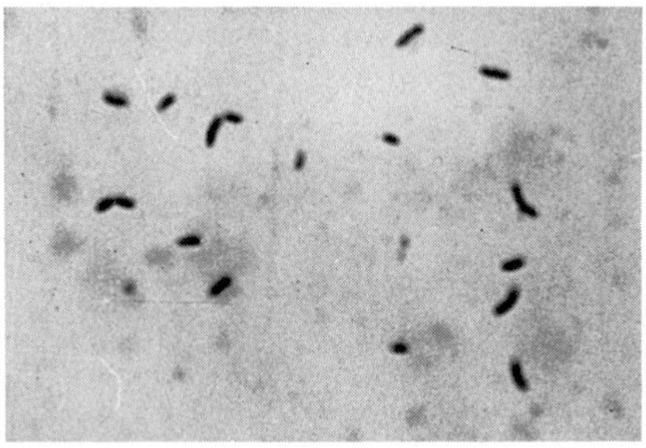

Figure 18–68. *Vibrio cholerae,* pure culture in peptone water. Gram stain; × 1200. (From Burrows, W.: Textbook of Microbiology. 19th ed.)

Table 18–22. CHARACTERISTICS OF THE SPIROCHETES AND SPIRILLA

SPECIES	DISEASE IN MAN	MODE OF TRANSMISSION	CULTIVATION	MORPHOLOGY	LABORATORY DIAGNOSIS	DISTRIBUTION
Borrelia recurrentis	European relapsing fever	Human body louse	Yes, special medium	Rather delicate, loose coils	Demonstration in blood smear stained by Giemsa. Mouse inoculation. Blood taken at onset of relapse	Europe
Borrelia novyi	American relapsing fever	Ticks	Same	Same	Same	American
Borrelia vincentii	Vincent's angina (trench mouth)	Probably contact	No	Same	Demonstration in smears from lesions together with fusiform bacilli	Worldwide
Treponema pallidum	Syphilis, bejel	Direct contact (venereal)	No	Delicate, tight coils	Darkfield examination of fluid from chancre or secondary rash. Serologic test. Fontana's stain	Worldwide
Treponema pertenue	Yaws	Contact (nonvenereal). Bite of flies	No	Same	Darkfield or Giemsa stain from lesion. Serologic test for syphilis	Mediterranean area, tropical Far East, Haiti, northern South America
Treponema carateum	Pinta (carate)	? insect vector	No	Same	Darkfield on early lesion. Serologic test for syphilis	Central and South America
Leptospira icterohaemorrhagiae	Weil's disease (infectious jaundice)	Rats to man	Yes, Fletcher's medium	Tight coils, hooked ends	Blood culture, inoculation of blood into guinea pig or weanling hamsters. Serologic tests on paired serums	Worldwide
Leptospira canicola	Canicola fever	Dogs to man	Same	Same	Same	Worldwide
Spirillum minus	Ratbite fever	Rat bite	No	Short, thick cells	Inoculation of blood into guinea pig or mouse. Demonstration in blood smear. Cultivation in peptone water (pH 8.5)	Japan, U.S.

Treponema are similar, being delicate, spiral organisms in which the 6 to 12 coils are rather loose; they tend to bend in the center. (See Fig. 18–69.)

In relapsing fever *Borrelia* appear in the blood at the onset of relapses and may be demonstrated in Giemsa-stained blood smears, where they appear as wavy, hair-like organisms. Blood can be inoculated into mice or rats. Large numbers appear in the blood after a few days. Mice often carry these organisms naturally, and great care must be exercised to make sure the mouse colony is free of the *Borrelia*. Culture of these organisms is difficult.

Treponema pallidum is best demonstrated by darkfield microscopy. In the absence of darkfield equipment one may stain smears from the aspirate of the chancre by Fontana stain. A delayed darkfield procedure using FA techniques has recently been reported. The India ink method to be described may also be used. No practical cultural methods are available (Fig. 18–70).

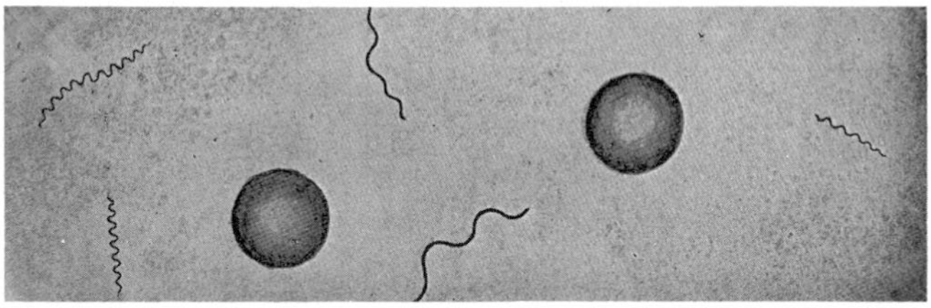

A B C

Figure 18–69. *A, Treponema pallidum; B, Borrelia refringens; C, Treponema microdentium.* Two erythrocytes (× 1200).

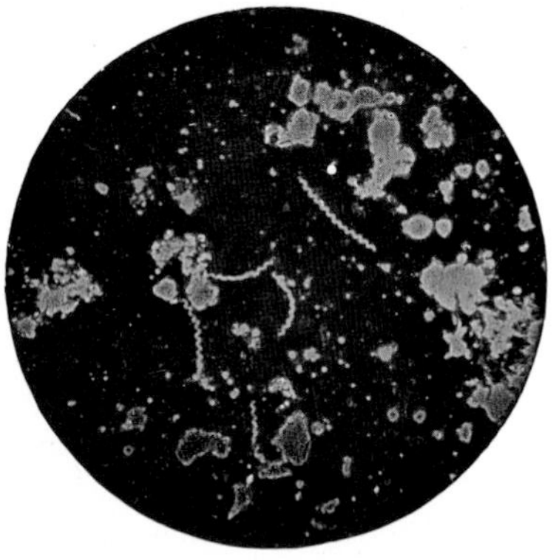

Figure 18–70. *Treponema pallidum* (× 1000); darkfield preparation.

Leptospira icterohaemorrhagiae, the causative agent of Weil's disease, is widely distributed in the infected individual and appears in the blood early in the disease. After 10 to 14 days the organisms are present in considerable numbers in the urine. These organisms are rather easily cultured in fairly simple medium containing rabbit serum, peptone, and Ringer's solution. Fletcher's medium is one of the most commonly used. It is prepared as follows:

1. Sterilize 1.76 liters of distilled water by autoclaving at 121° C. for 30 minutes.
2. Cool to room temperature and add 240 ml. of sterile normal rabbit serum.
3. Inactivate at 56° C. for 40 minutes.
4. Add 120 ml. of melted and cooled (not higher than 56° C.) 2.5 per cent meat extract agar at pH 7.4.
5. Dispense 5-ml. amounts in sterile 16 by 130 mm. screw-cap test tubes, or in 15-ml. amounts in sterile 25-ml. diaphragm-type, rubber-stoppered vaccine bottles.
6. Heat at 56° C. for 60 minutes on 2 successive days.

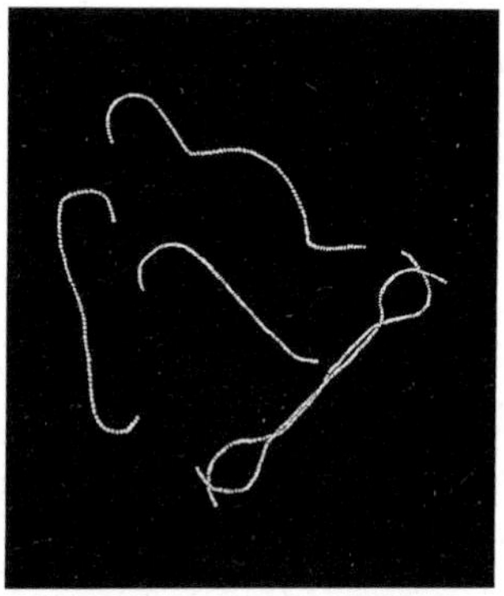

Figure 18–71. *Leptospira icterohaemorrhagiae.* Appearance of the organism in a darkfield preparation (about × 1000). (From Frobisher, M., Jr.: Fundamentals of Microbiology. 8th edition.)

Blood or urine may be inoculated intraperitoneally into a guinea pig, or into mice. The organisms can be demonstrated in the tissues at necropsy. *Leptospira* has tight coils and one or both ends are hooked. In darkfield preparations it is seen to rotate very rapidly (Fig. 18–71).

Patients with Weil's disease show striking antibody responses, and agglutination or complement fixation tests on acute and convalescent sera are useful in diagnosis. Antigens are available for testing antibody rises against the various other species of *Leptospira.*

In addition to Weil's disease members of the *Leptospira* are responsible for certain other diseases in various parts of the world, e.g., swamp fever in Europe (*L. grippotyphosa*) and swineherd's disease (*L. pomona*). There are a large number of serotypes of these organisms based on differences in agglutination–lysis and cross-absorption tests. The differentiation of these types is of considerable epidemiologic importance.

India Ink Method for Spirochetes. A relatively simple means of demonstrating spirochetes in blood or urine involves the use of India ink. It requires a good grade of ink.* A small drop of the India ink is mixed with 1 or 2 drops of the specimen. This mixture is then spread over the slide and allowed to dry. On examination with the oil-immersion lens the spirochetes appear white on a brown or black background. Some India inks contain wavy vegetable fibrils and bacteria that may be misleading, and exudates sometimes agglutinate the ink particles, making this type of preparation unsatisfactory.

The Acid-fast Bacilli (Mycobacteria)

A number of acid-fast bacteria are pathogenic for man. *Mycobacterium tuberculosis* (human) and *M. bovis* (bovine) have long been recognized for their role in human tuberculosis and have been studied extensively. In the last decade two new groups of acid-fast organisms, apparently capable of causing tuberculosis, have been recognized – the so-called "atypical" bacilli and *M. fortuitum.* These are large, acid-fast bacteria that are not pathogenic for rabbits and guinea pigs but usually are pathogenic for mice. Their pathogenicity is not yet completely understood. The avian strain, *M. avium,* has been reported in cases of chronic involvement of localized lymph nodes, but the extent of its pathogenicity in humans is not

*Not all India inks are suitable. It is advisable to select a bottle with a minimum amount of bacteria and to add phenol or tricresol as a preservative.

Table 18–23. CHARACTERISTICS OF THE MYCOBACTERIA

SPECIES	DISEASE IN MAN	TRANSMISSION	PATHOGENICITY FOR ANIMALS: GUINEA PIG	RABBIT	FOWL	CULTURAL CHARACTERISTICS
Mycobacterium tuberculosis (hominis)	Primarily pulmonary tuberculosis	Man to man	++++	+	0	Slow growth – 2-6 wks.; granular, wrinkled colonies; strict aerobe, grows on surface of liquid media
Mycobacterium bovis (bovine)	Tuberculosis of viscera or bone, sometimes pulmonary	Unpasteurized milk or milk products	++++	++++	0	Slow growth – 2-6 wks.; small, flat, smooth colonies; strict aerobe. Inhibited by glycerin above 0.25%
Mycobacterium ăvium	Mild chronic infection of submaxillary lymph nodes	?	0+	++	++++	Growth not so slow as human and bovine; smooth colonies. Optimal temp. 40° C. No pellicle in fluid medium
"Atypical" bacilli	Pulmonary or glandular tuberculosis, "swimming pool granuloma"	?	0	0	?	May be pathogenic for mice. Some species pigmented
Mycobacterium fortuitum	Nonpathogenic	Soil	0	0	0	Causes renal lesions in mice. Not photochromogenic; grows rapidly
Mycobacterium smegmatis		–	0	0	0	Grows rapidly. Normal inhabitant of human genitourinary tract
Mycobacterium phlei	Nonpathogenic	–	0	0	0	Widely distributed in nature. Timothy or "mist" bacillus. May be present in sputum or gastric washings. Grows rapidly
Mycobacterium leprae (Hansen's bacillus)	Leprosy	Probably man to man	0	0	0	Not cultivable; may be demonstrated by acid-fast stain of smears from lesions

clear. It does not appear to differ in any important respect from *M. intracellulare* (Battey).

In Table 18–23 are shown some of the important characteristics of the most important mycobacteria. Numerous similar organisms exist in nature and infect a number of warm- and cold-blooded animal species; many others are found in soil and water.

The diagnosis of tuberculosis depends on clinical, x-ray, and bacteriologic findings. Every effort must be made to demonstrate the organism in sputum, urine, or other material by acid-fast stain and cultures. In pulmonary tuberculosis the sputum, laryngeal and bronchial secretions, or gastric lavage are examined. The presence of acid-fast bacilli is highly suggestive, and when this is followed by a positive culture, it may be definitive. Acid-fast stains can be done on tissue smears and sections and may be very helpful. Mycobacterial phage typing has been developed and may be useful epidemiologically.

The human and bovine tubercle bacilli are slender, straight, or slightly curved rods, which occur singly or in clumps. They frequently have metachromatic granules (Much's granules) which may give them a beaded appearance, or they may be bipolar, giving the organism a dumbbell appearance. The nonpathogenic acid-fast bacilli tend to be less granular and are not so strongly acid-fast as the pathogens (Fig. 18–72). In culture the pathogens tend to be shorter and thicker than when seen in sputum, with less granulation. Culturally, the human and bovine bacilli grow best at 35° C.; the avian strain grows well at 42° C.; and many of the nonpathogens grow at much lower temperatures. At 35° C. the nonpathogens grow much more rapidly (sometimes in 2 to 3 days) and usually produce considerable pigment. Human tubercle bacilli are not inhibited by glycerol, whereas bovine strains are to a considerable extent. There are numerous special media on which these organisms can be cultured (Fig. 18–73). Some of the more commonly used media are described

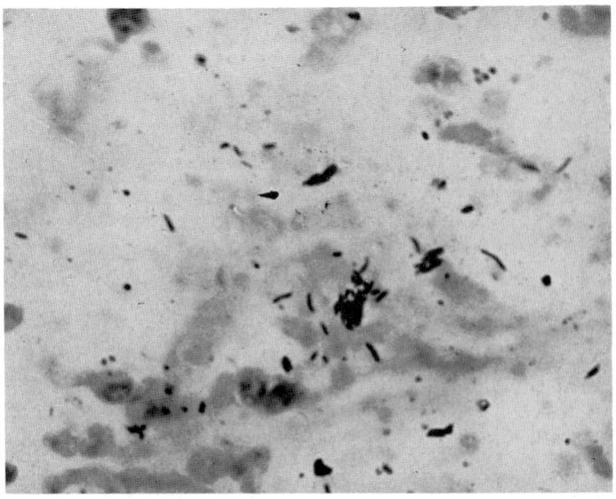

Figure 18–72. *Mycobacterium tuberculosis.* Acid-fast stained smear of tuberculous sputum. × 1050. (From Burrows, W.: Textbook of Microbiology. 19th ed.)

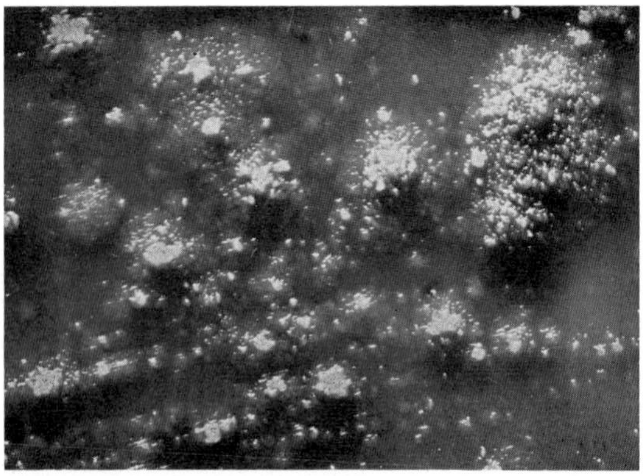

Figure 18–73. Colonies of the human variety of the tubercle bacillus, H-37 strain, on Löwenstein's medium, 5 weeks' incubation. × 3. (From Burrows, W.: Textbook of Microbiology. 19th ed.)

below. More complex media, such as Middlebrook 7H10, 7H11 or Peizer's, are best purchased in prepared form from reliable commercial sources. Media should be freshly prepared and controlled for contamination and growth-supporting properties before being put into routine use. In general, two or more media of different composition should be used for each specimen.

A.T.S. (American Trudeau Society) Medium

Egg yolk	500 ml.
Potato flour water (containing 2 per cent glycerol)	500 ml.

The potato flour water is made by adding 20 gm. potato flour to 500 ml. of 2 volumes per cent glycerol water in a flask. The mixture is heated to boiling with constant stirring and cooled to 50° C.

Egg yolk is obtained by carefully cleansing fresh eggs with wet gauze, rinsing them in alcohol, and separating the egg white and yolk. A proportion of one whole egg to 11 egg yolks is used, and 500 ml. of this combination is prepared.

The 500-ml. egg yolk mixture is poured into 500 ml. of potato flour water, and 20 ml. of 1 per cent malachite green in 50 per cent alcohol is added. All ingredients are thoroughly mixed and tubed. The tubes are slanted and inspissated for 60 minutes at 85° C.

Petragnani Medium (Modified)

Solution A:

Pasteurized, homogenized whole milk	275 ml.
Potato starch	20 gm.
Asparagin	1.9 gm.

These ingredients are blended in a suitable container to form a paste and then heated in a water bath at 56° C. for 1 hour; the mixture should be stirred frequently to maintain a uniformly smooth material.

Solution B:

Fresh whole eggs	10
Fresh egg yolks	3
Glycerol	30 ml.

Whole fluid from fresh eggs is collected as for Löwenstein's medium. Egg yolks are obtained by breaking the cleansed shells in the middle, parting the halves, separating the yolks from the whites, and pouring the yolks into the flask containing the whole egg fluid; the procedure must be carried out carefully to avoid contamination. Whites from the three eggs are discarded. Glycerol is added to the egg fluid, after which the mixture is homogenized thoroughly by shaking the flask.

Solution C:

Malachite green oxalate	2 per cent aqueous

Dissolve the dye in distilled water and sterilize in the autoclave at 15 p.s.i. for 15 minutes.

Combine solutions A and B, mix thoroughly until smooth and homogeneous, then filter through one layer of sterile gauze into a sterile graduated cylinder. Add aseptically 5 ml. of the sterile malachite green solution for each 100 ml. of medium. Mix the dye thoroughly with the medium, being careful to avoid bubble formation. After this the finished product is dispensed and sterilized as described for Löwenstein-Jensen medium.

Löwenstein-Jensen Medium (Modified)

Monopotassium phosphate	2.4 gm.
Magnesium sulfate (7 H_2O)	0.24 gm.
Magnesium citrate	0.6 gm.
Asparagin	3.6 gm.
Glycerol	12 ml.
Distilled water	600 ml.

Potato flour: Add 30 gm. of potato flour to the salt solution and autoclave the mixture at 121° C. for 30 minutes.

Homogenized whole egg mass: Use eggs not more than one week old. Clean the eggs by vigorous scrubbing in a 5 per cent soap-and-soda solution. Leave the eggs in the soap and soda solution for 30 minutes and then run cold water over them until the water becomes perfectly clear. Break the eggs into a sterile flask, homogenize completely by shaking, and filter through four layers of sterile gauze.

Malachite green stock solution:

Malachite green	2.0 gm.
Distilled water	100 ml.

Add 1 liter of homogenized whole egg mass to the flask of potato flour salt solution which has been cooled to room temperature. To this add 20 ml. of malachite green stock solution. Mix thoroughly and let stand for 1 hour at room temperature. If desired, 50 units of penicillin and 35 μg. of nalidixic acid per ml. may be added to the medium. These will help to reduce the contamination rate significantly.

Tube medium by use of sterile aspirator bottle and funnel with bell attachment or similar tubing device, using approximately 8 ml. for each 16- by 125-mm. test tube. Inspissate at 85° C. for 50 minutes. Check for sterility by incubating at 35° C. for 24 hours.

Tarshis Blood Medium

Plain agar	1.5 gm.
Glycerol	1.0 ml.
Human bank blood (with A.C.D. solution)	30.0 ml.
Distilled water	69.0 ml.
Penicillin	50–100 units/ml.

The final pH is 6.8.

Dissolve the agar in the glycerol water by heating. Autoclave at 15 p.s.i. for 15 minutes. Cool to 45° C., add penicillin and blood, mix well, and dispense in suitable sterile containers.

Kirschner's Medium

$Na_2HPO_4 \cdot 12\ H_2O$	19 gm.
KH_2PO_4	2.5 gm.
Magnesium sulfate	0.6 gm.
Sodium citrate	2.5 gm.
Asparagin	5 gm.
Glycerol	20 ml.
Phenol red (0.4 per cent)	3 ml.
Distilled water	1000 ml.

Dissolve the salts before adding glycerol. The pH is approximately 7.4 to 7.6. No adjustment of pH is necessary. Bottle 9-ml. amounts in 1-oz. bottles or tubes and autoclave at 10 p.s.i. for 10 minutes. Before use, add 1 ml. of sterile horse serum containing 100 units penicillin per ml. to each 9 ml. of medium.

Both clinicians and bacteriologists have now become more aware of the common occurrence of acid-fast bacilli that differ from the human strain of tubercle bacilli in several important respects. There seems little doubt that these organisms, the so-called "atypical", "unclassified" or "anonymous" mycobacteria, can cause tuberculosis-like disease in humans. In general, they have no or a low degree of virulence for guinea pigs and are usually resistant to isoniazid and para-aminosalicylic acid. A clear-cut classification of these organisms cannot be made until more is learned about them. The method of classification currently used, based on the recommendations of Runyon and others, is summarized in Table 18–24.

DIFFERENTIAL TESTS FOR MYCOBACTERIA

The following tests are those generally considered to be the most useful for classification of the mycobacteria. In each case it is obviously necessary to use adequate positive and negative control cultures. Other procedures are described by Kubica and Dye (1967) and Vestal (1969). However, it must be emphasized that unless physical facilities are available for carrying out these tests with safety, it is best to refer the cultures to specialized reference laboratories.

Niacin Test (Konno). Add 1 ml. of sterile distilled water to the slope of a culture showing luxuriant growth on egg medium or 7H10 agar plus 0.25 per cent l-asparagine. L-Aspartic acid also stimulates niacin production in this medium. Incubate at 37° C. for 2 hours with the tube lying flat. If the growth is confluent, puncture the surface so that the water comes in contact with the underlying medium. Add 0.5 ml. of the extract to a small screw-cap tube, add 0.5 ml. of aniline reagent (4 per cent in ethyl alcohol) and 0.5 ml. of cyanogen bromide (10 per cent aqueous). Shake gently. The presence of niacin is shown by the appearance of a yellow color almost immediately throughout the solution.

NOTE: The cyanogen bromide is highly toxic and should be handled in a safety hood. Discard into an alkaline germicidal solution.

The benzidine reaction is preferred by some because the color produced is easier to read and more stable than that produced in the aniline method. To the extract prepared as above, add 0.5 ml. of benzidine agent (3 per cent in 95 per cent alcohol) and 0.5 ml. of cyanogen bromide reagent. Shake gently. A red or pink precipitate is positive.

Paper strips are now available commercially and are generally satisfactory for this test provided the manufacturer's directions are followed closely and adequate controls are included.

Cording. Cord formation may be observed by inoculation of the organisms into a liquid medium (without wetting agent), such as the Proskauer and Beck medium with 5 per cent horse serum, or onto a clear solid medium such as oleic acid albumin agar. After good growth occurs, a small drop containing the organisms from the liquid medium is allowed to dry on a slide and a Ziehl-Neelsen stain is performed. Cords may be seen on low-power microscopic examination. Colonies on agar may be examined with a dissecting microscope using transmitted light. Growth of the bacilli in ropelike strands indicates cord formation. Only *M. tuberculosis*, *M. bovis*, and *M. ulcerans* will form cords.

Catalase. A few drops of a 1:1 mixture of 10 per cent Tween 80 and 30 per cent hydrogen peroxide* are added directly to the mycobacterial growth in plates or tubes. Catalase is de-

*Superoxol, Merck & Co., Inc., Rahway, New Jersey.

Table 18–24. DIFFERENTIATION OF ATYPICAL ACID-FAST BACTERIA

RUNYON GROUP	I	II	III	IV
FEATURES	PHOTOCHROMOGENS (*M. kansasii*, *M. balnei*)	SCOTOCHROMOGENS (*M. scrofulaceum*)	NONPHOTOCHROMOGENS OR BATTEY GROUP (*M. intracellulare*)	RAPID GROWERS
Associated with human disease	Yes	Abscesses or scrofula. Probably not otherwise important	Probably yes	Probably not except for *M. fortuitum*
Pigment	Buff in dark; yellow to orange in light	Yellow to orange in dark or light	Mostly nonchromogenic	Usually buff
Colony characteristics	Generally smooth or butyrous, rarely rough	Smooth, butyrous	Small spreading	Smooth or rough
Growth rate	30° C. 3 to 4 weeks 35° C. 2 to 3 weeks 45° C. 0	3 to 4 weeks 2 to 3 weeks 0	3 to 4 weeks 3 to 4 weeks 0	2 to 4 days 2 to 4 days 0 or 2 to 4 days
Microscopy	Larger than true tbc. Vacuolated and beaded	Larger than true tbc. Vacuolated and beaded	Pleomorphic	Pleomorphic
Cord formation	+ (loose cords)	−	−	+ and −
Arylsulfatase	−	−	−	+ (*M. fortuitum*)
Growth on MacConkey agar	−	−	−	+ (*M. fortuitum*)
Catalase reaction	++ (kansasii) + (balnei)	++	+	++
Tellurite reduction (3 days)	−	−	+	++
Drug resistance	Usually resistant to PAS. Variably to SM and INH	Resistant to antituberculous drugs	Resistant to antituberculous drugs	Resistant to antituberculous drugs
Guinea pig virulence	Subcutaneous usually without effect. Intracardial may be fatal in 3 weeks	−	−	−
Mouse virulence	Moderately pathogenic by I.V. or I.P. routes. Lesions in lung after 10 weeks	Generally not	+ and −	*M. fortuitum* said to be pathogenic

tected by formation of bubbles within 2 minutes. More precise methods are as follows:

1. Suspend one microspatula of bacilli in 0.5 to 1.0 ml. of M/15 phosphate buffer, pH 7.0.
2. Place tubes in 68° C. water bath for 20 minutes.
3. Cool tubes to room temperature. Add 0.5 to 1.0 ml. Tween 80-peroxide and observe for bubbling.

Semiquantitative Test. Inoculate surface of Löwenstein-Jensen medium in butt tubes. Incubate tubes for 2 weeks. Add 1 ml. of Tween 80-peroxide mixture. Leave in upright position for 5 minutes and measure the height of the column of bubbles above the surface of the medium. Most Group II, IV, and *M. kansasii* strains produce in excess of 50 mm. of bubbles.

Tween 80 Hydrolysis

Substrate:

M/15 phosphate buffer, pH 7.0	100 ml.
Tween 80	0.5 ml.
Neutral red, 0.5 per cent aq.	2.0 ml.

Dispense in 4-ml. amounts in screw-cap tubes and autoclave at 12° C. for 10 minutes. Should be light amber in color after sterilization.

PROCEDURE

1. Emulsify loopful of actively growing culture in the substrate.

2. Incubate at 37° C. up to 10 days.

A change in color from amber to red is a positive reaction. Most strains of *M. kansasii* are positive within 5 days. Clinically significant cultures of Group II and III are negative, while the clinically insignificant strains are positive.

Arylsulfatase Test (Wayne). Prepare commercial Wayne sulfatase agar as directed on the label in screw-cap tube slants. Inoculate slants with a loopful from an actively growing culture. Incubate 3 days at 37° C. Add a few drops of 2 N sodium carbonate solution. A color change to red or pink is positive.

Mycobacterium fortuitum gives a positive reaction. It can be readily differentiated from the avirulent *M. smegmatis,* which does not grow on MacConkey's agar.

Tellurite Reduction. Prepare Middlebrook 7H9 liquid with ACD and Tween 80 enrichment as per manufacturer's directions. Dispense in 5-ml. amounts in screw-cap tubes. Inoculate with a loopful of actively growing culture and incubate at 37° C. for 7 days. Add 2 drops of 0.2 per cent aqueous potassium tellurite solution and return to the incubator for 3 more days. A black or dark brown metallic precipitate is positive.

Mycobacterium intracellulare and most of the Group IV rapid growers are positive in 3 days.

OTHER MYCOBACTERIA

Leprosy (Hansen's disease) is primarily a tropical disease occurring in individuals living in rural areas. *Mycobacterium leprae* has been accepted as the etiological agent, although it has not been cultured successfully from leprous lesions. It has, however, been cultivated in the footpads of mice and recently in armadillos. Patients with leprosy have an altered immune response, possibly genetically determined. Bacteriologic diagnosis is made by finding acid-fast bacilli in scrapings of the nasal mucosa and in the tissue fluid expressed after superficial incisions of the skin from infected areas. The organisms are also found in the granulomatous lesions, being particularly numerous in the nodular form. They are distributed intracellularly for the most part, occurring in bundles arranged in parallel rows. Also useful is the skin test with lepromin (Mitsuda reaction). *Mycobacterium leprae* is not so strongly acid fast as *M. tuberculosis* and frequently shows distinct coarse beading (Fig. 18–74).

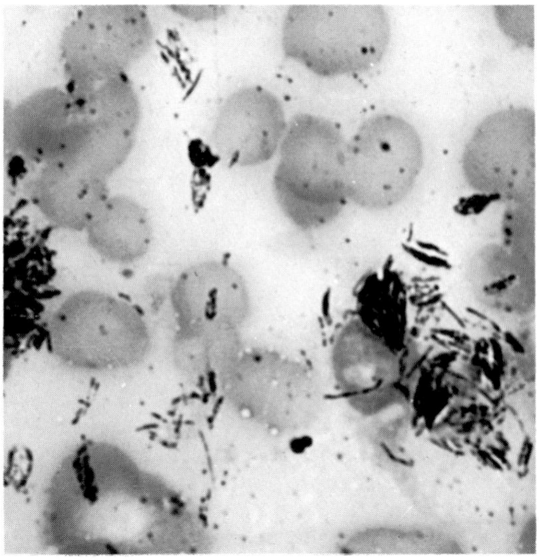

Figure 18–74. The leprosy bacillus. Acid-fast stained smear from a skin lesion. Note the characteristic tendency to parallel arrangement of the bacilli in packets. × 1800. (From Burrows, W.: Textbook of Microbiology. 19th ed.)

The causative agent of "rat leprosy," *Mycobacterium lepraemurium,* is similar to the leprosy bacillus. It is not pathogenic to man or other species of animals.

Mycobacterium paratuberculosis is the causative agent of a chronic enteritis in cattle and sheep called Johne's disease. It is not pathogenic to man. Other species have been isolated from many kinds of mammals and birds. Other mycobacteria are found in tuberculous-like lesions in a variety of poikilothermic vertebrates—*M. marinum* in fish, *M. ranae* in frogs, and so forth.

A number of acid-fast bacilli are found in dust, water, and soil. These are essentially avirulent but can be confused with other species of Mycobacteria. These include the well-known timothy hay bacillus, *M. phlei,* and *M. smegmatis.* The latter is also present in butter and smegma.

PPLO AND MYCOPLASMA

The causative agent of contagious bovine pleuropneumonia was first cultivated by Nocard and Roux in 1898. Similar organisms, which were subsequently isolated from other species of animals, were then called pleuropneumonia-like organisms or PPLO. Dienes and Edsall were the first to culture PPLO from human disease from an abscessed Bartholin's gland in 1937. Further studies showed that these organisms, now classified in the family *Mycoplasmataceae* of the order *Mycoplasmatales,* are widely distributed both as com-

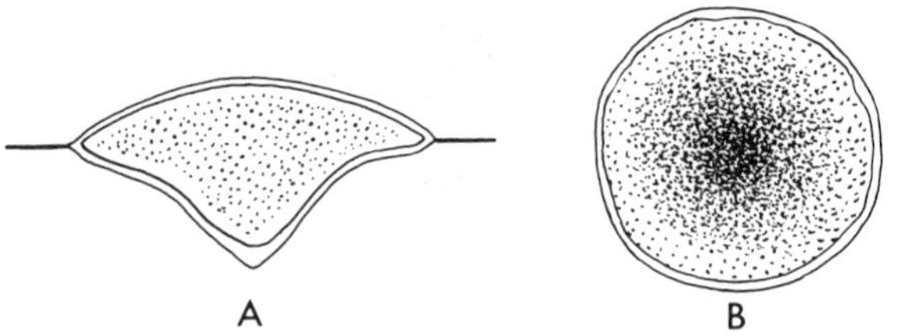

Figure 18–75. Non-Eaton agent Mycoplasma colony. *A*, Sagittal section; *B*, surface view of top. Colony size range, 10 to 200 μ.

mensals and pathogens in man and various animals. They are also present as common contaminants in tissue cultures, and saprophytic strains have been isolated from soil, sewage, plants, and insects.

Mycoplasmas are small (approx. 125 to 250 mμ) highly pleomorphic organisms enclosed in a thin semipermeable sheath rather than a rigid cell wall containing muramic acid. As a result, they are plastic and extremely fragile. They stain poorly or not at all with aniline dyes and best with Giemsa or Dienes stain (Fig. 18–75). They resemble in some ways the L forms of bacteria, which can be produced by the action of hypertonic salt solution or by penicillin, which inhibits the normal synthesis of the cell wall. Mycoplasmas, however, are genetically distinct and cannot be reverted back to the parent strain; thus, they are thought to be distinct entities. Unlike the viruses, they contain both DNA and RNA, are not dependent on the host cell for enzyme metabolites and are free-living.

Until recently the pathogenicity of mycoplasma for humans was controversial. Although they are frequently isolated from a variety of ill-defined urogenital and arthritic diseases, no direct causative relationship could be clearly established because similar strains were found in healthy individuals and antibody responses have been inconsistent. In contrast, the mycoplasmal etiology of a distinct form of primary atypical pneumoniae has been unequivocally established as the so-called Eaton agent (*Mycoplasma pneumoniae*). However, not all individuals suffering from this disease clinically called primary atypical pneumonia yield Eaton agent in their sputum, nor do all have elevated titers of cold agglutinins. The Eaton agent is the leading cause of pneumonia between infancy and early adulthood, and is particularly prevalent in military camps.

T, "tiny," strains (Shepard) are so called because of their extremely small size and characteristic colonial morphology. Their causative relationship to nongonococcal urethritis remains unproved as yet. *Mycoplasma hominis* type I has been associated with abscesses of the genital tract and exudative tonsillitis and pharyngitis. The other well-defined species of man appear to be ubiquitous saprophytes (Table 18–25). Reports relating mycoplasma to reproductive failure, rheumatoid arthritis, Reiter's syndrome, and so forth, must be looked upon with reservations until unequivocal proof is forthcoming.

Isolation of Mycoplasma. There is some question whether the routine culture of *Mycoplasma* from specimens is of any direct clinical value, since it is a slow procedure at best. In addition, because of their ubiquity, isolation of a strain from a specimen does not necessarily prove it is associated with the disease process. The demonstration of a fourfold increase in titer between the acute and convalescent phase serum samples may be more practical, at least in the case of Eaton agent pneumonia.

Specimens (sputum, throat swabs, urethral scrapings, and so forth) should be inoculated as soon as possible after collection on appropriate media. If plating will be delayed, the specimen should be collected in trypticase soy broth with 0.5 per cent bovine albumin and 500 units of penicillin/ml. added.

The isolation medium of choice is PPLO agar which is prepared as follows:

To 70 per cent heart infusion peptone agar,* 20 per cent noninactivated, gamma globulin-free horse serum and 10 per cent fresh yeast extract are added. Penicillin, 1000 U./ml., thallium acetate 1:2000 and amphotericin B, 5 μg./ml. are added if desired. For selective isolation of *M. pneumoniae*, methylene blue in a 0.002 per cent concentration may be added. Since some lots of agar may be inhibitory, it is necessary to check each lot for its growth-supportive ability. Prepared plates of this medium are available commercially and are preferable for those laboratories that

*PPLO agar base.

Table 18–25. MYCOPLASMAS OF HUMAN ORIGIN

SPECIES	USUAL HABITAT	CLINICAL MATERIAL FOR CULTURE
M. hominis, Types I and II	Respiratory and genitourinary tract	Urine, sputum, throat, prostatic secretions
M. salivarium	Oropharynx	Throat, sputum, teeth, gums
M. orale, Type I (*M. pharyngis*)	Oropharynx	Throat, sputum, bone marrow
M. orale, Type II	Oropharynx	Throat, sputum
M. fermentans	Genitourinary tract	Urine, prostatic secretions
M. pneumoniae	Respiratory tract, oral region	Sputum, bronchial layers, throat swabs
T-strains	Genitourinary tract	Prostatic secretions, urethral scrapings, urine

Table 18–26. DISTINGUISHING CHARACTERISTICS OF HUMAN MYCOPLASMA SPECIES*

SPECIES	COLONY MORPH.	PERIPHERY	AEROBIC GROWTH	REQ. FOR YEAST EXT.	GROWTH RATE	GLUCOSE FERM.	MANNOSE FERM.	G.P. RBC HEMOLYSIS	HEMADSORP-TION	TETRAZOLIUM REDUCTION
M. hominis, Type I	Fried egg	Smooth or foamy	+	0	Rapid	0	0	Slow	0	0
M. hominis, Type II	Fried egg	Smooth	+	0	Rapid	0	0	0	0	0
M. salivarium	Fried egg	Smooth	0	0	Rapid	0	0	0	0	0
M. orale	Fried egg	Small	+/−	+	Moderate	0	0	0	0	0
M. fermentans	Granular	None	+/−	0	Moderate	+	0	0	0	0
M. pneumoniae	Granular	None	+	+	Slow	+	+	Rapid	+	+
T-strains	Granular	None	0	0	Moderate	0	0	×	×	0

× = No data.
*Adapted from Hayflick, L., and Chanock, R. M.: Bact. Rev. *29*:186, 1965.

attempt to culture these organisms only occasionally.

In the attempted isolation of Mycoplasmas from material normally free of bacteria, such as blood or bone marrow, the antibiotics and thallium acetate should be omitted since they may possibly be inhibitory to the growth of some strains. Thallium acetate is inhibitory to T strains. Penicillin may induce L form transformation of bacteria present in the specimen, which can lead to confusing results.

Plates are incubated in an atmosphere of 95 per cent nitrogen and 5 per cent CO_2 at 35° C. Good results have been reported using 5 per cent CO_2 in air. The plates are incubated for at least 30 days before being reported as negative. The medium must be protected from drying during the long incubation period.

Mycoplasma colonies appear under the low power of the microscope as round and colorless, from 10 to 750 μ in diameter with dense centers and a less dense periphery, giving a characteristic "fried egg" appearance. This is absent with *M. pneumoniae* (Table 18–26 and Figs. 18–76 and 18–77).

Colonies may also be examined by the agar-block mount using the Dienes method.

Dienes Stain

Methylene blue	2.5 gm.
Azure II	1.25 gm.
Maltose	10 gm.
Sodium carbonate	0.25 gm.
Benzoic acid	0.20 gm.
Distilled water	100 ml.

1. Spread a drop of stain on a clean coverglass and allow to dry.
2. Cut out a small block of the agar containing a few *Mycoplasma* colonies and place, with colonies uppermost, on a clean glass slide.
3. Lay the coverglass, stain side down, on the agar block.
4. Seal preparation with Vaspar to prevent drying.
5. Examine under low power of the microscope.

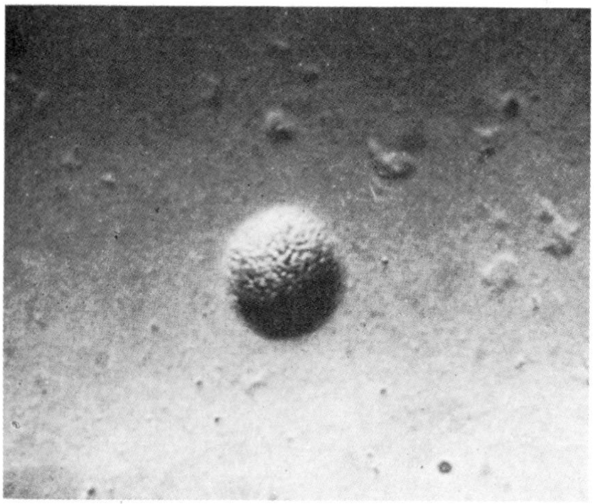

Figure 18–76. Colonies of *Mycoplasma pneumoniae* (Eaton agent). Note granular appearance. The organisms grew down into the agar beneath the surface colony. (From Chanock, Hayflick, and Barile: Proc. Nat. Acad. Sci., *48*:41, 1962.)

Mycoplasma colonies are distinct, with dense blue-stained centers and light blue peripheries.

Differentiation of Strains. Further identification of the various species of the mycoplasmas are made on the basis of their biochemical and serological reactions. These tests include requirements for yeast extract, fermentation of glucose, guinea pig red cell hemolysis and hemagglutination, tetrazolium reduction, arginine hydrolysis immunofluorescence, and others. The T strains are uniqely urease positive (Table 18–26). Of particular value for establishing the species identification of unknown strains is the recently developed paper-disc growth inhibition test. Multidiscs are prepared by dipping the end of each radial disc strip into a different specific antisera. Such rabbit antiserums, pretested and species specific, are available from several sources.* The impregnated discs are stable for one year when stored at –20° C. When a strain of mycoplasma is identified, a dry plate of PPLO agar is heavily inoculated by the agar block technique. The antiserum-impregnated multidisc is then placed onto the surface of the plate with sterile forceps. The plate is incubated for 7 days. A surrounding clear zone of inhibition identifies the species of the organism being tested (Fig. 18–78).

Further details concerning isolation and identification of Mycoplasma are given in more detail in Hayflick and Chanock (1965), Panos (1967), Sharp (1970), and Jansson (1971). These should be referred to before attempting to work with this group of organisms.

Much interest has been aroused by the numerous reports recently published concerning the isolation of cell-wall-defective (C.W.D.) variants from clinical material, particularly from patients treated with penicillin. The term C.W.D. may refer to either protoplasts, spheroplasts, transitional phase variants, or L-forms. Each of these terms refers to distinct phases and they should be clearly differentiated from one another. Their exact etiological relationship has not yet been clearly elucidated, but they appear to have at least an intrinsic pathogenic significance. Refer to Guze (1968) and McGee *et al.* (1971) for further details.

---

*Bioquest, Cockeysville, Maryland; Microbiological Associates, Bethesda, Maryland.

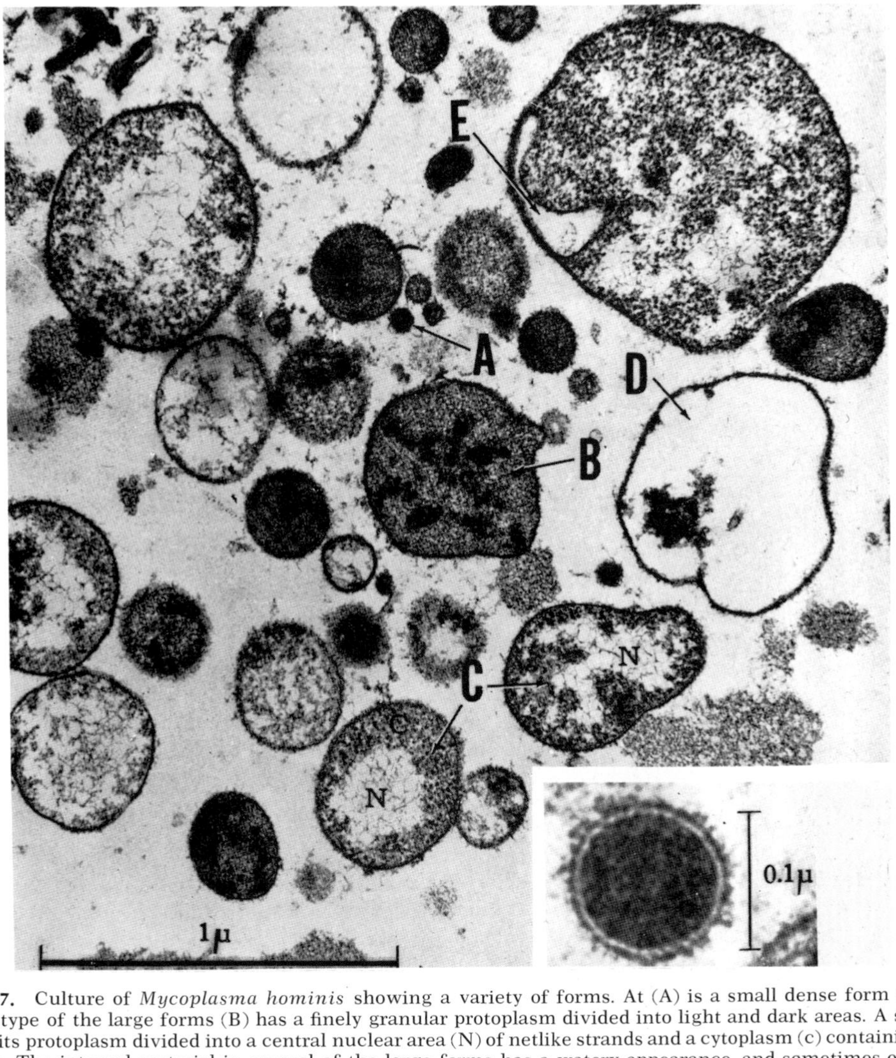

Figure 18–77. Culture of *Mycoplasma hominis* showing a variety of forms. At (A) is a small dense form ("elementary body"). One type of the large forms (B) has a finely granular protoplasm divided into light and dark areas. A second major type (C) has its protoplasm divided into a central nuclear area (N) of netlike strands and a cytoplasm (c) containing ribosome-like granules. The internal material in several of the large forms has a watery appearance, and sometimes only an empty plasma membrane is seen (D). One of the organisms in this field has a membrane-bound vacuole (E) at its periphery. × 53,000. Inset shows body similar to A at a higher magnification (× 200,000). (From Anderson and Barile: J. Bact., *90*:180, 1965.)

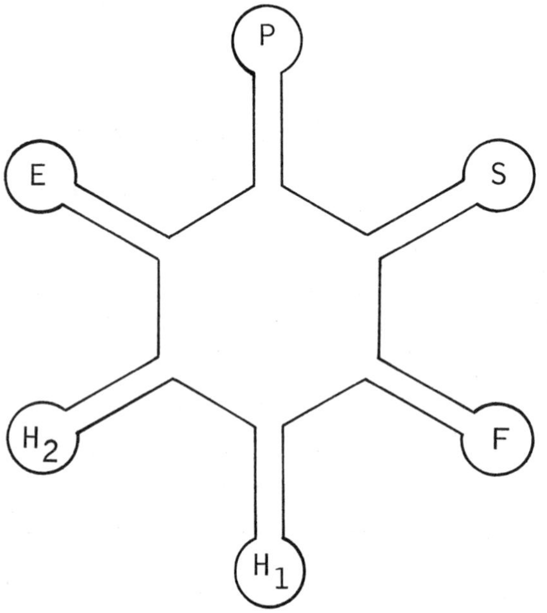

Figure 18–78. Serological identification of mycoplasma from human sources. E=Eaton agent *(Mycoplasma pneumoniae); P=M. pharyngis; S=M. salivarium; F=M. fermentans;* H_1=*M. hominis*, Type I; H_2=*M. hominis*, type II.

ANTIMICROBIAL SUSCEPTIBILITY TESTS

Chemotherapy, i.e., the destruction of microorganisms by drugs, was initiated by the pioneer studies of Ehrlich, which culminated in the development of salvarsan for the treatment of syphilis. The sulfonamides were introduced in 1935, following Domagk's work on the use of Prontosil, the active principle of which is sulfanilamide, in the treatment of streptococcal infections in mice. Since that time dozens of new sulfonamides have been synthesized with ever-increasing antibacterial activity and decreased toxicity.

The term "antibiotics" refers to substances elaborated by living microorganisms that have the capacity to inhibit the growth of other microorganisms. The story of the discovery of penicillin by Fleming in 1929, its application to the treatment of human disease, and the subsequent development of a host of new antibiotics is well known. Actually there is no clear-cut differentiation between the terms "antibiotic" and "chemotherapeutic agent," because some of the antibiotics originally isolated from natural sources have also been prepared synthetically. (A notable example of this is chloramphenicol.) Consequently the terms are used interchangeably.

The sulfonamides are primarily bacteriostatic substances. They are supposed to inhibit growth by competing with the microorganism for a special enzyme system associated with the essential metabolite, para-aminobenzoic acid (Wood-Fildes). Antibiotics exert their effect in three main ways: (1) by preventing synthesis of the cell wall during growth; (2) by inhibiting the synthesis of essential proteins; and (3) by affecting the permeability of the cell membrane. Antibiotics which inhibit protein synthesis (such as the tetracyclines) are generally bacteriostatic, while the others (i.e., penicillin) are bactericidal.

The tendency of many bacteria to become resistant to antibiotics has become a problem of ever-increasing importance, particularly with staphylococci and tubercle bacilli. These resistant strains have caused an alarming number of serious infections in and outside hospitals. This tends to emphasize that improper use of antibiotics can lead to serious consequences and, hence, the importance of selecting the correct antibiotic with the aid of susceptibility tests cannot be overemphasized.

The exact mechanism of the development of increased bacterial resistance is not clear. It is known that all bacterial populations are heterogeneous as regards their susceptibility to a given antibiotic. The resistant bacteria in a population may arise spontaneously as a result of mutation or perhaps by adaptation. In some instances resistance to an antibiotic is a function of the production of a specific enzyme that destroys the drug, e.g., penicillinase production by staphylococci. It is also possible that an organism actually can become dependent upon an antibiotic. Thus, it is clear how the continued usefulness of antimicrobial drugs depends to a great extent on our resourcefulness in meeting and counteracting the problems of drug resistance.

It has been shown recently that drug-resistant bacteria contain an extrachromosomal genetic element composed of DNA—the "R" factor. Resistance-determining sets of genes are attached to the R factor, which reproduces and transfers itself from cell to cell, thus transferring drug resistance to previously drug-sensitive strains on contact (Mitsuhashi, 1969). The transfer of antibiotic resistance among intestinal bacteria is a distinct possibility and may eventually involve an undue risk to public health. Intelligent and controlled use of antibiotics in animal nutrition and in the treatment of animal and human infections is obviously essential.

Many infections respond promptly to the empiric administration of one or another of the commonly used antibiotics, and susceptibility tests are unnecessary. However, when the diagnosis is uncertain, in cases that relapse, when the patients do not respond quickly to therapy, and when the disease is severe and fulminating, laboratory assistance is essential and may be lifesaving. The decisive factor involved in the choice of the proper antibiotic is the relative susceptibility of the invading bacterium. As used here, the terms "sensitivity" and "susceptibility" are synonymous. The term "antimicrobial susceptibility" is preferable to "sensitivity," since the latter term may be confused with the allergic or hypersensitivity reaction to antimicrobial agents occasionally encountered in patients.

The relationship between the results of *in vitro* susceptibility tests and response to treatment with drugs is not always direct. That is, the susceptibility test may indicate that an offending organism is susceptible to a given antibiotic, but the patient may not respond to treatment. Occasionally the opposite situation is observed: the *in vitro* test indicates resistance, but the clinical response is excellent. Infections of the urinary tract are particularly prone to show this lack of correlation, and a similar situation may be encountered in gastrointestinal infections involving some of the common pathogens of this tract. The frequency with which this situation occurs is difficult to determine, but it happens with sufficient regularity to cause occasional confusion and raise some question about the validity of susceptibility testing in some situations.

There are several possible explanations for the discrepancies just discussed. In the urinary tract, where mixed infection frequently occurs, the organism that is cultured, or may seem to predominate, may not be the one responsible for the clinical condition; thus, the susceptibility tests may not have been done on the critical organism. Certain investigators have reported the observation of organisms, such as *Proteus* and *Pseudomonas*, that exist in smooth and rough form in the urinary tract. The susceptibility of the two forms to antibiotics may be very different, so the results of the susceptibility test may be determined by the form that predominates on the culture. The colonies picked for testing may be all of one form. Another factor that may be important is the occurrence of L-forms, G-forms, spheroplasts, and mycoplasma. These structures tend to be resistant to certain antibiotics and may be contributing in some as yet unknown way to the propagation of some of the conditions that exist. There are certainly other factors that affect the effectiveness of antibiotic therapy, such as the location of the focus of infection, the ability to obtain adequate concentrations at such a site, chemical changes in the antibiotic as it is transported through the tissues, and the dose and route of administration. It must be remembered that *in vitro* testing of the antibiotic provides ready access of the antibiotic to the rapidly propagating microorganism. Thus, one has an ideal situation for the antibiotic to affect the organism, which may not be duplicable *in vivo.*

Choice of Method for Susceptibility Testing

The most widely used methods at the present time are the following:

Diffusion Methods. Paper discs or strips impregnated with known amounts of drugs are placed on the surface of Petri dishes seeded with the test organisms. Susceptibility is indicated by a zone of inhibited growth around the paper containing the drug.

Test Tube Dilution Methods. Tubes of a nutrient vehicle containing serial dilutions of the chemotherapeutic agent are inoculated with suspensions of the test organism. A measure of the susceptibility to the drug is manifest by failure of the organism to grow in a given dilution.

Agar Dilution Methods. Agar plates containing known amounts of drugs are streaked with the test organism, and inhibition of growth is noted.

Other Procedures. Susceptibility can also be shown by physical or chemical changes that accompany growth, such as shift in pH, reduction of hemoglobin, inhibition of hemolysis, and use of E_h indicators for detection of oxidation-reduction reactions.

The choice of the method used depends to a large extent on the facilities and experience of the laboratory personnel. It does not necessarily follow that a laborious technique, such as the tube-dilution method, is more accurate than a simpler technique, such as a diffusion method. By the tube method, gross errors can be obtained if the following factors are not taken into consideration and adequately controlled: the size of the inoculum, the solubility and stability of the antibiotic being tested, the composition of the culture medium used, and the growth requirements of the organisms being tested. On the other hand, the disc diffusion method gives results that are strictly qualitative. The size of the zone of inhibition depends on both the solubility and diffusibility of the antimicrobial agent and does not necessarily coincide with antibacterial activity.

The important factors in all antimicrobial susceptibility testing, regardless of the procedure used, are to make certain that the method is accurate and reproducible, that all steps are carried out precisely with adequate controls, and that the results are reported promptly.

There are many "short cuts" practiced in antimicrobial susceptibility testing that should be avoided if possible. In cases of life-threatening infections it might be advisable to attempt to determine the relative susceptibility of the invading organisms directly from the specimen. In general, however, there is no adequate substitute for culturing the specimen, determining the possible etiologic agent, and performing accurate susceptibility tests on those organisms for which such tests may be useful. Susceptibility tests to the following organisms are ordinarily unnecessary, since they have thus far shown little or no tendency to change in resistance: *Streptococcus pyogenes, Diplococcus pneumoniae,* and *Neisseria gonorrhoeae.* For organisms such as the following, susceptibility tests may be imperative: Coli-Enterobacter-Serratia group, *Proteus, Pseudomonas aeruginosa, Staphylococcus aureus,* and *Streptococcus faecalis.*

Procedures

SELECTION OF ANTIMICROBIAL AGENTS TO BE TESTED ROUTINELY

In order to simplify susceptibility tests, it is necessary to limit the number of agents that are tested routinely. In general, routine tests should include only one representative of each group of antimicrobials with closely related *in vitro* activity (Table 18–27). Tests should be limited to those agents which represent those currently utilized within the institution where the tests are performed and which are appropriate for use in the therapy of the specific pathogen under test. It is best to confer with the Infection or Therapeutic Committee of the institution or the clinicians concerned to arrive at a routine pattern agreeable to them. Additional drugs should be kept available for use for specific problems of the individual patient.

DISC DIFFUSION METHODS

Attempts made over the past few years by the Food and Drug Administration and other agencies to standardize diffusion methods has culminated in the development of a procedure based on that described by Bauer, Kirby *et al.* (1966). This represents at present the most completely described method for which well-documented interpretive standards have been developed. This procedure, together with rigid controls of the antimicrobial discs and interlaboratory quality controls, has been of great assistance in establishing a badly needed

Table 18–27. CLASSIFICATION OF CHEMOTHERAPEUTIC AGENTS

I. Polypeptides
   A. Gramicidin
   B. Bacitracin
   C. Polymyxin B
   D. Polymyxin E (Colistin)

II. Aminoglycosides
   A. Streptomycin
   B. Neomycin Group
      1. Neomycin
      2. Kanamycin
      3. Paromomycin
      4. Gentamicin
      5. Nebramycin

III. Chloramphenicol

IV. Tetracyclines
   A. Tetracycline
   B. Oxytetracycline
   C. Chlortetracycline
   D. Demeclocycline
   E. Doxycycline
   F. Methacycline
   G. Rolitetracycline

V. Macrolides
   A. Erythromycin
   B. Oleandomycin
   C. Triacetyloleandomycin

VI. Lincomycin, Clindamycin

VII. Novobiocin

VIII. Sulfonamides

IX. Nalidixic Acid

X. Nitrofurantoin

XI. Penicillins
   A. Penicillinase Sensitive Group
      1. Penicillin G
      2. Penicillin V
      3. Penicillin O
   B. Penicillinase Resistant Group
      1. Methicillin
      2. Cloxacillin
      3. Dicloxacillin
      4. Oxacillin
      5. Nafcillin
   C. Extended Spectrum Group
      1. Ampicillin
      2. Carbenicillin

XII. Cephalosporins
   A. Cephalothin
   B. Cephaloridine
   C. Cephaloglycin
   D. Cephalexin

XIII. Mandelamine

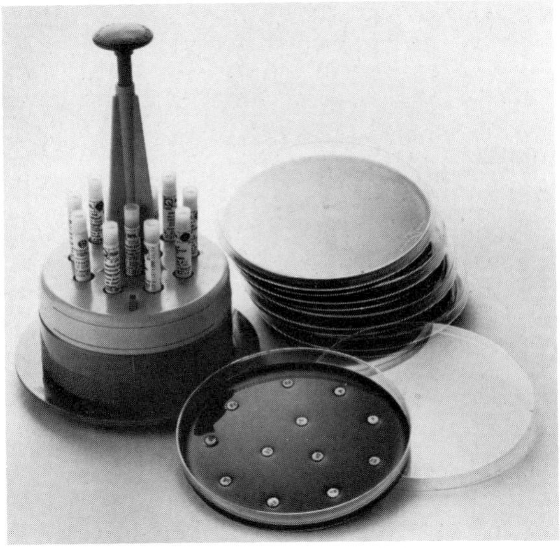

Figure 18–79. Disc dispenser for antimicrobial susceptibility testing with adapter for 150 mm. Petri dishes. (Courtesy of Bioquest, Cockeysville, Md.)

standardization of technique. The only generally acceptable alternative at this time is the agar overlay modification of Barry *et al.* (1970). These procedures are described in some detail in the following section. See also Ericsson and Sherris (1971) and Gavan *et al.* (1971).

STORAGE OF ANTIMICROBIAL SUSCEPTIBILITY TEST DISCS

Cartridges containing discs for susceptibility testing are generally supplied by the manufacturers in separate containers containing a desiccant. These containers should be kept refrigerated below 8° C. or frozen (−14° C. or less) until needed. They should be allowed to equilibrate to room temperature before being opened to avoid condensation of moisture. Discs containing antibiotics belonging to the penicillin and cephalosporin groups should be kept frozen except for one week's supply, which can be kept in the refrigerator. If a disc dispensing apparatus is used, it should be kept tightly sealed in a dust-free container (Fig. 18–79). Discs must be discarded on the expiration date on the label.

Bauer-Kirby Method for Determining Bacterial Antibiotic Susceptibility

1. A few (3 to 8) well-isolated colonies of the same morphologic type as the organism to be tested are transferred with a wire loop from the original culture plate to a test tube containing 4 ml. of tryptose phosphate or trypticase soy broth.

2. Incubate tubes 2 to 5 hours to produce a bacterial suspension of moderate cloudiness.

3. Dilute suspension, if necessary, with sterile saline or broth to a density equivalent to that of a standard prepared by adding 0.5 ml. of 1 per cent barium chloride to 99.5 of 1 per cent sulfuric acid (0.36 N). These standards should be replaced monthly.

4. For susceptibility plates, large (15 cm.) Petri dishes are used with Mueller-Hinton agar, pH 7.2 to 7.4 (4 mm. in depth). This will require from 70 to 75 ml. of agar. Fastidious organisms (*Hemophilus, Streptococcus,* etc.) may require the addition of 5 per cent blood. The large Petri dishes are spacious enough to accommodate 8 discs in an outer ring and 3 or 4 more in the center. It is advantageous to place antimicrobials which diffuse well in the outer circles and discs which produce smaller inhibition zones (such as vancomycin, polymyxin B, colistin or kanamycin) in the central area of the plate. High potency discs only are used. Small (100 mm.) Petri dishes may be used provided they are poured to a depth of 4 to 5 mm. and not more than 4 to 5 discs are used per plate.

5. Plates are dried for about 30 minutes before inoculation and should be used within 7 days of preparation.

6. The bacterial broth suspension is streaked evenly in three planes onto the surface of the medium with a sterile cotton swab. Surplus suspension is removed from the swab by rotating it against the side of the tube before the plates are seeded.

7. After the inoculum has dried (3 to 5 minutes), the appropriate discs are placed on the agar with flamed forceps or a disc applicator apparatus and gently pressed down to ensure contact. Since some diffusion of drug is almost instantaneous, a disc should not be moved once it has come in contact with the agar surface.

8. Plates are incubated within 30 minutes and held overnight (optimum 14 hours) at 35° C. Overlong incubation must be avoided.

9. Measure diameters of inhibition using sliding calipers, ruler, or template. A reading of 6 mm. indicates no zone. If necessary, zone diameters may be read after incubation for 6 to 8 hours provided distinct zones of inhibition have appeared.

10. The endpoint is taken as the area showing no visible growth that can be detected by the unaided eye. The sizes of the zones of inhibition are then interpreted by referring to Table 18–28.

In the case of sulfonamides, organisms must grow through several generations before inhibition takes effect. Slight growth (80 per cent or more inhibition) with sulfonamides is therefore disregarded; the margin of heavy growth is read to determine the zone size. Swarming

Table 18–28. ZONE SIZE INTERPRETATIVE CHART*

ANTIMICROBIAL AGENT		DISC POTENCY	INHIBITION ZONE DIAMETER (TO NEAREST MM.)		
			Resistant	Intermediate	Susceptible
Ampicillin	Gram negative and enterococci	10 μg.	11 or less	12–13	14 or more
	Staphylococci and penicillin-sensitive organisms		20 or less	21–28	29 or more
	Other organisms		11 or less	12–21	22 or more
Bacitracin		10 U.	8 or less	9–12	13 or more
Carbenicillin		50 μg.			
Pseudomonas sp.			12 or less	13–14	15 or more
E. coli and *Proteus*			17 or less	18–22	23 or more
Cephaloridine		30 μg.	11 or less	12–15	16 or more
Cephalothin		30 μg.	14 or less	15–17	18 or more
Chloramphenicol		30 μg.	12 or less	13–17	18 or more
Clindamycin		2 μg.	11 or less	12–15	16 or more
Colistin		10 μg.	8 or less	9–10	11 or more
Erythromycin		15 μg.	13 or less	14–17	18 or more
Gentamicin		10 μg.	12 or less	13–14	15 or more
Kanamycin		30 μg.	13 or less	14–17	18 or more
Lincomycin		2 μg.	9 or less	10–14	15 or more
Methicillin		5 μg.	9 or less	10–13	14 or more
Nafcillin and Oxacillin		1 μg.	10 or less	11–12	13 or more
Nalidixic acid†		30 μg.	13 or less	14–18	19 or more
Neomycin		30 μg.	12 or less	13–16	17 or more
Nitrofurantoin†		300 μg.	14 or less	15–18	19 or more
Novobiocin‡		30 μg.	17 or less	18–21	22 or more
Oleandomycin		15 μg.	11 or less	12–16	17 or more
Penicillin-G	Staphylococci	10 U.	20 or less	21–28	29 or more
	Other organisms§		11 or less	12–21	22 or more
Polymyxin B		300 U.	10 or less	11–14	15 or more
Streptomycin		10 μg.	11 or less	12–14	15 or more
Sulfonamides†‖		300 μg.	12 or less	13–16	17 or more
Tetracycline		30 μg.	14 or less	15–18	19 or more
Vancomycin		30 μg.	9 or less	10–11	12 or more

*As prepared by the National Committee for Clinical Laboratory Standards, Los Angeles, Calif., June, 1971.
†Urinary tract infections only.
‡Not applicable to blood-containing media.
§This category includes some organisms such as enterococci which may cause systemic infections treatable by high doses of penicillin G.
‖Any of the commercially available 250 or 300 μg. sulfonamide discs can be used with the same standards of zone interpretation.

(spreading) of *Proteus* species is not inhibited by all antibiotics; a veil of swarming into an inhibition zone should also be ignored. If colonies are seen within a zone of inhibition, the strain should be checked for purity and retested.

This method should not be applied to sulfonamide sensitivities of meningococci, gonococci or group A beta hemolytic streptococci. It is also not applicable to determine susceptibility of slow-growing CO_2-requiring organisms or slow-growing anaerobes such as *Bacteroides*, since the results cannot yet be properly interpreted.

QUALITY CONTROL FOR THE DISC ANTIMICROBIAL PROCEDURE

Standard control organisms of known susceptibility to the antimicrobial agents tested should be employed daily or each time the procedure is run. It is possible to use strains isolated from clinical specimens in the laboratory, provided their susceptibility pattern remains stable for extended periods. It is, however, preferable to employ the standard strains of *Staphylococcus aureus*, A.T.C.C. No. 25923, and *Escherichia coli*, A.T.C.C. No. 25922.*

To maintain these stock cultures, the organisms growing in vials containing 0.5 ml. of heat-inactivated fetal calf serum and 0.5 ml. of trypticase soy broth are frozen at −6° C. At the beginning of each week, a vial of each organism is thawed out, and the organisms are streaked on trypticase soy agar plates which are incubated overnight. Four to five isolated smooth colonies from the agar plates are picked into 4 ml. of trypticase soy broth, incubated 4 hours, the turbidity standardized if necessary, and susceptibility tests set up by the standard procedure.

Results of the susceptibility tests with the control strains should be recorded and the mean and standard deviations calculated for the various antimicrobial agents. Readings falling above or below the mean should be promptly investigated to determine which of the components of the test system is out of control. Readings which are consistently above or below the mean for all the agents suggest that the inoculum has been incorrectly standardized. Divergent readings between the aminoglycosides and tetracycline suggest that the pH of the medium is improper. Records of batch numbers of discs in current use should be kept in case deviant results requiring further study are obtained. If a disc gives a zone which is out of the acceptable range, it is best to discard the cartridge and to check the discs from a new cartridge prior to routine use. All tests done on a day when the results are out of control should not be reported.

The program outlined above should also be supplemented by external quality control and proficiency testing programs. Such programs, when used properly, are excellent for assuring improved performance. See Gaven *et al.* (1971), Russell *et al.* (1971) and Blazevic *et al.* (1972).

AGAR OVERLAY METHOD FOR DISC ANTIMICROBIAL SUSCEPTIBILITY TEST
(Barry *et al.*, 1970)

1. This technique is applicable only for rapidly growing bacteria and cannot be used when blood must be added to the agar medium. Select 5 to 10 colonies from an overnight culture and prepare a uniform, turbid suspension in 0.5 ml. of brain heart infusion broth in 13 × 100 mm. tubes.

2. Incubate the broth culture in a water bath at 37° C. for 4 to 8 hours.

3. Transfer a 0.001-ml. calibrated loopful of the well-mixed broth culture to 9.0 ml. of a 1.5 per cent sterile aqueous solution of agar (in 16 × 125 mm. screw-cap tubes) which has been melted and kept at 50° C. The caps are tightened after the agar is melted, and unused tubes are discarded at the end of the day to avoid changes in agar concentration due to evaporation.

4. Quickly mix this seeded agar by gentle inversion and then spread over the surface of a 150 × 15 mm. Petri dish containing Mueller-Hinton agar 4 mm. in depth. To facilitate this procedure, the plates are brought to room temperature before attempting to spread the thin layer of seeded agar. (If 90-mm. Petri dishes are used, seed 4 ml. of agar with 0.001-ml. loop.)

5. Allow the inoculated plates to stand 3 to 5 minutes undisturbed on a flat surface and then apply high concentration antimicrobial discs, gently pressing down on each with a sterile forceps to ensure complete contact with agar.

6. Invert the plates and incubate at 35° C. Steps 3 through 6 must be completed within 30 minutes.

7. After 16 to 18 hours' incubation, measure diameters of the zones of complete inhibition.

8. Results are reported by interpreting zone diameters according to the zone measuring chart, as for the Bauer-Kirby single disc susceptibility test (Table 18–28).

AGAR PLATE DILUTION METHOD

This method, in contrast to the disc procedure, is a quantitative one. It is particularly suitable for *N. gonorrhoeae* and *N. meningitidis*, but cannot be used for organisms that have a swarming tendency, such as *Proteus* or *Pseudomonas*.

Mueller-Hinton or trypticase soy agar is generally preferred. For fastidious organisms it is necessary to add 5 per cent blood. The agar is dispensed and sterilized in 18-ml. amounts for each 9-cm. plate. Serial dilutions of antibiotics of known potency are diluted in water as in the test tube procedure, using separate pipettes for each dilution. The first dilution usually contains 1000 U./ml., but other concentrations can be used as desired.

The agar is melted and cooled to 50° C. and 2 ml. of the required amount of drug is added to each agar tube, which is then mixed and poured into plates. The agar is allowed to solidify and dry before use. Such plates can be

*Available from the American Type Culture Collection, Rockville, Maryland.

stored in the refrigerator in sealed plastic bags without deterioration for up to 7 days.

The inoculum should be adjusted to contain 10^5 to 10^6 bacteria per ml. Spot inoculate the plates with a standardized loop calibrated to deliver 0.001 ml. Inoculate a plate without antibiotic at the same times as a control. The Steers inoculum replicator with a stainless steel head is very useful when large numbers of cultures are to be tested.

Incubate the plates at 35° C. overnight aerobically, under 10 per cent CO_2, or anaerobically, depending on the growth requirements of the organism being tested. The endpoint (M.I.C.) is the lowest concentration of antibiotic that completely inhibits growth.

Organisms of known susceptibility to the chemotherapeutic agent should be tested every week as a quality control check.

TEST TUBE DILUTION METHOD

1. Use stock antimicrobial solutions; stock crystalline drugs of known potency are available from commercial sources or from the various pharmaceutical manufacturers. Prepare stock solutions containing 1000 μg. or units per ml. in sterile distilled water. Solubilize with appropriate solvents, or by adjusting the pH if necessary. Sterilize if necessary by membrane filtration. These solutions can be frozen at −20° C. in individual tightly sealed containers for 6 to 8 weeks without loss of potency. They should be removed as required (never refrozen) and used within one day.

2. For each agent to be tested, prepare a series of 10 sterile 13 × 100 mm. test tubes in a rack. Further dilutions may be made for highly susceptible organisms if desired. Add to each of the last nine tubes in the series 0.5 ml. of broth. Trypticase soy, Mueller-Hinton, thioglycollate, or infusion broth enriched with ascitic fluid or rabbit blood may be used, depending on growth requirements of the organism being tested. Add 0.5 ml. of the working solution of the antibiotic, usually 100 U./ml. to the first two tubes. Mix, transfer 0.5 ml. from tube two to the next tube, and continue this process until tube nine. Discard 0.5 ml. from this tube. Tube ten serves as the culture control.

3. Prepare a 1:1000 dilution in broth of an overnight culture of the organisms to be tested, preferably in the logarithmic growth phase. For slow-growing or fastidious organisms, a 1:100 dilution should be used. Add 0.5 ml. of this dilution to each of the tubes in the series and shake. Incubate the titration overnight at 35° C. (Table 18–29; Fig. 18–80).

4. Examine the tubes macroscopically. The minimal inhibitory concentration (M.I.C.) is the highest dilution of the antibiotic in the last tube showing no visible growth, and is expressed in units or micrograms per milliliter. To determine the minimal bactericidal concentration, each of the clear tubes is subcultured to a suitable agar plate medium.

A strain of known M.I.C. should be run with each batch of tests as a control on the technique and reagents.

This technique must be modified for agents such as the sulfonamides, nalidixic acid and nitrofurantoin (Blair, 1970; Ericsson and Sherris, 1971). Possible synergistic combinations can be determined by mixing the stock solutions of the antimicrobial agents before diluting. There is some question, however, whether this procedure correlates well with the *in vivo* activity of combinations of chemotherapeutic agents.

Automated procedures for broth dilution techniques have recently been developed and appear to be practical for those laboratories which perform large numbers of these titrations. The procedure can also be done rapidly, using microtiter equipment.

Table 18–29. TEST TUBE DILUTION METHOD FOR ANTIMICROBIAL SUSCEPTIBILITY TESTS

TUBE NO.	BROTH ADDED (ml.)	ANTIMICROBIAL (ml.)	CULTURE INOCULUM (ml.)	ANTIMICROBIAL CONC. (U. or μg.)
1	0	0.5	0.5	100
2	0.5	0.5	0.5	50
3	0.5	0.5 from tube 2	0.5	25
4	0.5	0.5 from tube 3	0.5	12.5
5	0.5	0.5 from tube 4	0.5	6.25
6	0.5	0.5 from tube 5	0.5	3.12
7	0.5	0.5 from tube 6	0.5	1.56
8	0.5	0.5 from tube 7	0.5	0.78
9	0.5	0.5 from tube 8, discard 0.5	0.5	0.39
10	0.5	0	0.5	0

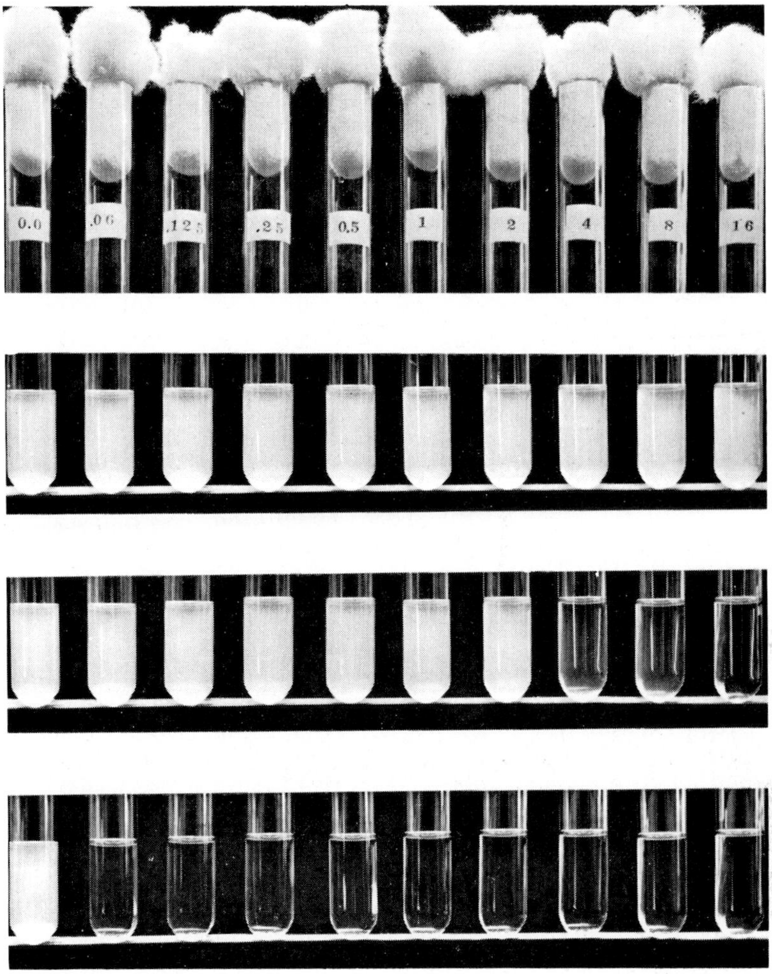

Figure 18–80. Testing susceptibility of a bacterium to chemotherapeutic agents by the tube dilution method. The top row of tubes of broth culture contain agent "A" in increasing amounts as shown by the figures on the tubes. The second row contains agent "B" in the same amounts, while the third row contains agent "C" in the same dilutions. All tubes were inoculated with organism "X" from the same culture at the same time and incubated together. Luxuriant growth, as shown by turbidity, has occurred even in the highest concentration of agent "A," showing that organism "X" is not affected by this drug. The drug of choice will be agent "C" which prevents growth of organism "X" even in the smallest concentration. Agent "B" is slightly effective. The tube at the left of each row is a control tube containing no inhibitory agent. (Courtesy of Abbott Laboratories, North Chicago, Illinois.)

Antimicrobial Levels in Body Fluids

The estimation of the amounts of a given antimicrobial agent in a body fluid is not so frequently required as in the past, since very large doses are usually given. Such determinations may be of considerable value when the patient has infection and renal shutdown. The methods briefly described can be readily adapted to the determination of other antibiotics, but it is necessary to standardize the technique for each different drug. Manufacturers of chemotherapeutic agents will provide assay procedures for their products on request. Detailed methods are described in the text of Grove and Randall (1955).

Penicillin (Method of Randall, Price and Webb). The test organism is *Bacillus subtilis*, N.R.R.L. strain 558.

PROCEDURE

1. Set up a series of nine small test tubes and add 0.5 ml. of Penassay broth to all but the first tube. Prepare serial dilutions of the fluid being tested (which must be sterile) by adding 0.5 ml. to tubes one and two; mix and transfer 0.5 ml. from tube two to tube three, and so on to tube nine. Discard 0.5 ml. from tube nine.
2. Prepare a standard for comparison by diluting penicillin of known potency (reference standard) to 1 unit per ml. in broth. Dilute this 1 unit standard exactly as for the body fluid in a second series of tubes, each containing 0.5 ml. of broth.
3. Add 1.5 ml. of a 1:100 dilution of an 18-hour culture of the test organism to all tubes. Incubate at 35° C. overnight.
4. The endpoint is the last tube in which no growth occurred. Determine the concentration of the unknown by comparing the endpoint with that of the standard. For example:

Tube No.	1	2	3	4	5	6	7	8	9
Standard	0	0	0	0	0	0	0	+	+
Serum A	0	0	0	0	+	+	+	+	+
Serum B	0	0	0	0	0	0	0	0	+

In this example the standard caused complete inhibition in the seventh tube. Since this represents 1 unit per ml., serum A contains 0.125 unit per ml. because it required a solution eight times as strong to cause complete inhibition. Serum B thus contains 2 units per ml.

To determine potencies lower than these, it is only necessary to vary the dilution series of both the standard and the unknown.

Streptomycin (Method of Price, Nielsen, and Welch). The test organism is *Bacillus circulans*, A.T.C.C. No. 9966.

PROCEDURE

1. Place 0.5 ml. of streptomycin assay broth in a series of small test tubes and make serial dilutions by halves as for penicillin.

2. Prepare a standard for comparison by diluting a streptomycin salt of known potency in broth to contain 10 μg. of the base per ml. Serially dilute this standard in the same manner as the body fluid.

3. To all tubes add 1.5 ml. of a 1:100 dilution of an overnight culture of the test organism in broth.

4. Incubate overnight at 35° C. and consider the last tube in which no growth occurred as the endpoint.

5. The interpretation is similar to that described for penicillin.

Determination of Penicillin Levels in Body Fluids by the Cylinder Plate Method. This method is not applicable to poorly diffusing antibiotics such as the polypeptides. For more details and for modifications for other antibiotics, refer to Grove and Randall (1955).

1. Prepare working solutions of penicillin in phosphate buffer pH 6.0 or 5 per cent sterile serum in concentrations of 0.25, 0.5, 1.0 and 2.0 u./ml.

2. Pour approximately 10 ml. of melted and cooled Penassay seed agar into each of 4 porcelain-topped Petri dishes. Add 0.2 ml. of a 24-hour Penassay broth culture of *Staphylococcus aureus*, A.T.C.C. No. 6538 P, to 100 ml. of melted and cooled Penassay base or yeast beef agar; mix thoroughly and pipette about 5 ml. to the surface of each seed plate and rotate to spread evenly.

3. Space evenly six sterile "penicylinders" (8 × 10 mm., porcelain or stainless steel) on the surface of each of three plates. Quickly pass the edge of each cylinder through a flame to heat before applying to make a closed seal with the agar. Place three cylinders spaced in a triangle on the fourth plate in the same manner.

4. Fill each of the cylinders on the plates containing the cylinders with one of the penicillin solutions so that on each of the three plates there will be a series from 0.1 to 1.5 units. Fill each of the three cylinders on the remaining plate with the fluid to be assayed. If the concentration of the antibiotic in the fluid is expected to be above the range of the standards, dilute accordingly. Incubate plates overnight.

5. After incubation, measure the zones of inhibition with calipers and, taking the average of each of the three cylinders of the same content, plot a standard curve on graph paper of the zone size against the concentration. Measure the zones of the cylinders of the fluid being assayed, take the average, and determine the content of the fluid on the curve. Report in units per milliliter of fluid.

Antibacterial Serum Level Determination (Schlichter; Dunlap, 1965). This test is useful for assessing the adequacy of antibiotic therapy, particularly in problem cases such as enterococcal subacute endocarditis or in patients with renal disease. It is equally valid when combinations of antibiotics are administered. This information, especially when combined with results of tube dilution susceptibility tests on the bacteria isolated from the patient, can be very useful to the clinician in planning subsequent therapy.

PROCEDURE

1. Inoculate a tube of Mueller-Hinton broth with the patient's isolate. Incubate at 35° C. for 6 hours. Set up two rows of 11 sterile plugged tubes. Pipette 0.5 ml. of sterile broth into each tube.

2. Collect 5 to 10 ml. of sterile blood from the patient at the desired intervals, preferably just before the next dose of drug. Separate the serum aseptically and add 0.5 ml. to tubes one and two. Dilute serially from tube two to tube ten, discarding 0.5 ml. from tube ten. Use separate pipette for each dilution. Tube eleven serves as the positive growth control.

3. Inoculate each tube of diluted serum and control in the first row with 1 drop (0.05 ml.) of a 1:1000 dilution of the 6-hour culture and inoculate the second row with a 1:100,000 dilution.

4. Incubate the tubes at 35° C. for 18 to 24 hours. Examine the tubes for turbidity. The bacteriostatic endpoint is considered to be the highest dilution of the serum in which no growth is visible. Subculture all tubes showing no visible growth to portions of a blood agar plate and incubate overnight. The bactericidal endpoint is considered to be the highest dilution showing no growth after subculture.

A bactericidal level of 1:2 or 1:4 is generally considered to be sufficient for therapeutic effectiveness in most cases. There is, however, some difference of opinion about this.

Susceptibility of Mycobacteria to Chemotherapeutic Agents

Testing of susceptibility of strains of Mycobacteria to the various drugs is a procedure which is very difficult to standardize. The drugs, when incorporated into different media, may change in their antimycobacterial activity and may vary in stability under different methods of sterilization and storage. Since the observed susceptibility result is based on a comparison of the amount of growth on drug-containing media as compared to drug-free controls, the inoculum must be of demonstrated uniformity.

The tests can be done by the direct method if acid-fast bacilli can be seen in a smear from the specimen or by the indirect method from a primary culture. In either case the procedures are subject to a wide range of error unless all parameters are carefully controlled. Serious consequences to the patient can result from an inaccurate susceptibility report. Consequently, it is felt that it is preferable to send cultures to a reference laboratory equipped for this purpose rather than attempt to do them if not fully equipped for this purpose.

Detailed descriptions of this methodology may be found in Kubica and Dye (1967), Vestal (1969), and Blair (1970).

REFERENCES

Adler, J. A., Burke, J. P., Martin, D. F., and Finland, M.: *Proteus* infections in a general hospital. Ann. Intern. Med. 75:517, 1971.

Alami, S. Y., and Riley, H. D.: Infections caused by Mimeae, with special reference to *Mima polymorpha*. Amer. J. Med. Sci. 252:527, 1966.

American Public Health Association: Diagnostic Procedures for Bacterial, Mycotic and Parasitic Infections. 5th ed. New York, American Public Health Association, 1970.

Bailey, W., and Scott, E. G.: Diagnostic Microbiology. 3rd ed. St. Louis, The C. V. Mosby Co., 1970.

Baillie, A., and Gilbert, R. J.: Automation, Mechanization and Data Handling in Microbiology. New York, Academic Press, Inc., 1970.

Barry, A. L., Garcia, F., and Thrupp, L. D.: An improved single disc method for testing the antibiotic susceptibility of rapidly growing pathogens. Amer. J. Clin. Path. 53:149, 1970.

Bartlett, R. O., Carrington, B. O., and Mielert, C.: Quality Control in Clinical Microbiology. Chicago, American Society of Clinical Pathologists, 1968.

Bauer, A. W., Kirby, W., Sherris, J. C., and Turck, M.: Antibiotic susceptibility testing by a standardized single disk method. Amer. J. Clin. Path. 45:493, 1966.

Bickham, S. T., and Jones, W. T.: Problems in the use of the *in vitro* toxigenicity test for *Corynebacterium diphtheriae*. Amer. J. Clin. Path. 57:244, 1972.

Blair, J. B. (ed.): Manual of Clinical Microbiology. Bethesda, Md., American Society of Microbiology, 1970.

Blazevic, D. J., *et al.*: Quality control testing of the disc antibiotic susceptibility test of Bauer-Kirby-Sherris-Turck. Amer. J. Clin. Path. 57:592, 1972.

Bokkenheuser, V.: *Vibrio foetus* in man: A serological test. Infect. Immun. 5:222, 1972.

Borchardt, K. A., and Hoke, A. W.: Simplified laboratory technique for diagnosis of chancroid. Arch. Derm. 102: 188, 1970.

Breed, R. S., Murray, E. G. D., and Smith, N. R.: Bergey's Manual of Determinative Bacteriology. 7th ed. Baltimore, The Williams & Wilkins Co., 1957.

Burrows, W.: Textbook of Microbiology. 19th ed. Philadelphia, W. B. Saunders Company, 1968.

Cherry, W. B.: Fluorescent antibody techniques in diagnostic bacteriology. Bact. Rev. 29:222, 1965.

Coons, A. H., Creech, H. J., and Jones, R. N.: Immunological properties of an antibody containing a fluorescent group. Proc. Soc. Exp. Biol. Med. 47:200, 1941.

Cowan, S. T., and Steel, K. J.: Manual for the Identification of Medical Bacteria. New York, Cambridge University Press, 1965.

Cruickshank, R.: Medical Microbiology. 11th ed. Baltimore, The Williams & Wilkins Co., 1965.

Doggett, R. G.: Incidence of mucoid *Pseudomonas aeruginosa* from clinical sources. Appl. Microbiol. 18:936, 1971.

Dolan, C. T., Brown, A. L., and Ritts, R. E., Jr.: Microbiological examination of postmortem tissues. Arch. Path. 92: 206, 1971.

Douglas, G. W., and Washington, J. A., II: Identification of Enterobacteriaceae in the Clinical Laboratory. Atlanta, Ga., National Center for Disease Control, 1969.

Dowell, V. R., Jr., and Hawkins, T. M.: Laboratory Methods in Anaerobic Bacteriology. Washington, D.C., U.S. Gov't. Printing Office, U.S. Public Health Service Publ. No. 1803, 1968.

Dowell, V. R., Jr., and Thompson, F. S.: Identification of Acid and Alcohol Products of Anaerobic Bacteria by Gas Liquid Chromatography. Atlanta, Ga., National Center for Disease Control, 1970.

Dubos, R. J., and Hirsch, J. G.: Bacterial and Mycotic Infections of Man. 4th ed. Philadelphia, J. B. Lippincott Co., 1965.

Dunkelberg, W. E., Jr., Skaggs, R., and Kellogg, D. S., Jr.: A study and new description of *Corynebacterium vaginale (Haemophilus vaginalis)*. Amer. J. Clin. Path. 53: 370, 1970.

Dunlap, S. G.: The serum-dilution bactericidal test for antibiotic effectiveness. Amer. J. Med. Tech. 31:69, 1965.

Ederer, G. M., and Clark, M.: Motility-indole-ornithine medium. Appl. Microbiol. 20:849, 1970.

Edmunds, P. N.: The biochemical, serological and hemagglutinating reactions of *Hemophilus vaginalis*. J. Path. Bact. 83:411, 1962.

Edwards, P. R., and Ewing, W. H.: Identification of Enterobacteriaceae. 3rd ed. Minneapolis, Burgess Publishing Co., 1972.

Ericsson, H. M., and Sherris, J.: Antibiotic sensitivity testing. Report of an international collaborative study. Acta Path. Microbiol. Scand. (Suppl.) 217:1971.

Ewing, W. H.: Enterobacteriaceae. Biochemical Methods for Group Differentiation. Atlanta, Ga., National Center for Disease Control, 1962.

Ewing, W. H.: Revised Definitions for the Family Enterobacteriaceae, Its Tribes and Genera. Atlanta, Ga., National Center for Disease Control, 1967.

Ewing, W. H., Davis, B. R., and Montague, T. S.: Studies on the Occurrence of *E. coli* Serotypes Associated with Diarrheal Disease. Atlanta, Ga., National Center for Disease Control, 1963.

Ewing, W. H., Johnson, J. G., and Davis, B. R.: The Occurrence of *Serratia marcescens* in Nosocomial Infections. Atlanta, Ga., National Center for Disease Control, 1962.

Felner, J. M., and Dowell, V. R., Jr.: *Bacteroides* bacteremia. Amer. J. Med. 50:787, 1971.

Fogan, L.: Atypical Mycobacteria: Their clinical, laboratory and epidemiological significance. Medicine 49:243, 1970.

Fried, M. A., *et al.*: *In vitro* comparison of fluorescent antibody technique with culture and slide agglutination for the detection of enteropathogenic *E. coli*. Amer. J. Med. Sci. 252:75, 1966.

Gardner, H., and Dukes, C. D.: *Hemophilus vaginalis* vaginitis. Amer. J. Obstet. Gynec. 69:962, 1955.

Gardner, P., *et al.*: Nonfermentative gram-negative bacilli of nosocomial interest. Amer. J. Med. 48:735, 1970.

Gavan, T. L., Cheatle, E. L., and McFadden, H. W.: Antimicrobial Sensitivity Testing, Chicago. American Society of Clinical Pathologists, 1971.

Glaser, L., Bosley, G. S., and Boring, J. R., III: A systematic program of quality control in clinical microbiology. Amer. J. Clin. Path. *56*:379, 1971.

Goldin, M., and Glenn, A.: A simple phenylalanine paper strip method for identification of *Proteus* strains. J. Bact. *84*:870, 1962.

Goldman, M.: Fluorescent Staining Methods. New York, Academic Press, Inc., 1968.

Graber, C. D.: Rapid Diagnostic Methods in Medical Microbiology. Baltimore, The Williams & Wilkins Co., 1970.

Gray, M. L., and Killinger, A. H.: *Listeria monocytogenes* and listeric infections. Bact. Rev. *30*:309, 1966.

Grieve, B., and Goldin, M.: The isolation of *Serratia marcescens* in a hospital laboratory. Amer. J. Med. Tech. *32*:131, 1966.

Grove, D. C., and Randall, W. A.: Assay Methods of Antibiotics. A Laboratory Manual. New York, Medical Encyclopedia, Inc., 1955.

Guze, L. B. (ed.): Microbial Protoplasts, Spheroplasts and L Forms. Baltimore, The Williams & Wilkins Co., 1968.

Hartman, P. A.: Miniaturized Microbiological Methods. New York, Academic Press, Inc., 1968.

Hayflick, L., and Chanock, R. M.: Mycoplasma species of man. Bact. Rev. *29*:186, 1965.

Hovig, B., and Aandahl, E. H.: A selective medium for the isolation of *Haemophilus* in material from the respiratory tract. Acta Path. Microbiol. Scand. *77*:676, 1969.

Hugh, R., and Leifson, E.: The taxonomic significance of fermentative versus oxidative metabolism of carbohydrates by various gram negative bacteria. J. Bact. *66*:24, 1953.

Jansson, E.: Isolation of fastidious Mycoplasma from human sources. J. Clin. Path. *24*:53, 1971.

Jensen, J., and Kleemeyer, H.: Die bakterielle Differentialdiagnose des Antrax mittels eines neuen spezifischen Tests "Perlschnurtest". Zbl. Bakt. *159*:494, 1953.

Johnson, J. B., Kunz, L. J., Barron, W., and Ewing, W. H.: Biochemical differentiation of the Enterobacteriaceae with the aid of lysine-iron-agar. Appl. Microb. *14*:212, 1966.

Kabins, S. A., and Cohen, S.: Resistance-transfer factor in Enterobacteriaceae. New Eng. J. Med. *275*:248, 1966.

Kilo, C., Hagemann, P. O., and Marzi, J.: Septic arthritis and bacteremia due to *Vibrio foetus*. Amer. J. Med. *38*:962, 1965.

Kletz, A. W.: Application of FA techniques to detection of *Clostridium perfringens*. Public Health Rep. *80*:305, 1965.

Kubica, G. P., and Dye, W. E.: Laboratory Methods for Clinical and Public Health Mycobacteriology. Washington, D.C., Gov't. Printing Office, U.S. Public Health Service Publ. No. 1547, 1967.

Kundsin, R. B. (ed.): Unusual isolates from clinical material. Ann. N.Y. Acad. Med. *174*:2, 1970.

Kuper, S. W. A., and May, J. R.: Detection of acid fast organisms in tissue sections by fluorescent microscopy. J. Path. Bact. *79*:59, 1960.

Lavetter, A., *et al.*: Meningitis due to *Listeria monocytogenes*. A review of 25 cases. New Eng. J. Med. *285*:598, 1971.

Lorian, V.: Antibiotics and Chemotherapeutic Agents. Clinical and Laboratory Practice. Springfield, Ill., Charles C Thomas, 1966.

Lorian, V.: The mode of action of antibiotics on gram-negative bacilli. Arch. Intern. Med. *128*:723, 1971.

Lubin, H., and Ewing, W. H.: Studies on the beta-D-galactosidase activities of Enterobacteriaceae. Public Health Lab. *22*:83, 1964.

McGee, A. Z., *et al.*: Wall defective microbial variants: Terminology and experimental design. J. Infect. Dis. *123*:433, 1971.

Meyers, B. R., *et al.*: Infections caused by microorganisms of genus *Erwinia*. Ann. Intern. Med. *76*:9, 1972.

Mitsuhashi, S.: The R factors. J. Infect. Dis. *119*:89, 1969.

Moeller, V.: Simplified tests for some amino acid decarboxylases and for the arginine dehydrolase system. Acta Path. Microbiol. Scand. *36*:158, 1955.

Moore, M. S., and Parsons, E. I.: A study of a modified Tinsdale's medium for the primary isolation of *Corynebacterium diphtheriae*. J. Infect. Dis. *102*:88, 1958.

Mossel, D. A. A., and Indacochea, L.: A new centrimide medium for the detection of *Pseudomonas aeruginosa*. J. Med. Microbiol. *4*:380, 1971.

Newton, B. A.: Mechanisms of antibiotic action. Ann. Rev. Microbiol. *19*:209, 1965.

Nilehn, B.: Studies on *Yersinia enterocolitica*. Acta Path. Microbiol. Scand. (Suppl.) *206*: 1971.

Page, M. I., and King, E. O.: Infection due to *Actinobacillus actinomycetemcomitans* and *Haemophilus aphrophilus*. New Eng. J. Med. *275*:181, 1966.

Panos, C.: A Microbial Enigma: Mycoplasma and Bacterial L Forms. Cleveland, World Publishing Co., 1967.

Parsons, E. I., Frobisher, M., Moore, M. S., and Aiken, M. A.: Rapid virulence test in the diagnosis of diphtheria. Proc. Soc. Exp. Biol. Med. *88*:368, 1955.

Pearson, H. E.: Human infections caused by organisms of the *Bacillus* species. Amer. J. Clin. Path. *53*:506, 1970.

Pien, F. D., Thompson, R. L., and Martin, W. J.: Clinical and bacteriologic studies of anaerobic gram positive cocci. Mayo Clin. Proc. *47*:251, 1972.

Prevot, A. R.: Manual for the Classification and Determination of the Anaerobic Bacteria. Philadelphia, Lea & Febiger, 1966.

Reinarz, J. A., and Sanford, J. P.: Human infections caused by non-group A or D streptococci. Medicine *44*:81, 1964.

Riemann, H.: Food-borne Infections and Intoxications. New York, Academic Press, Inc., 1969.

Rosebury, T.: Microorganisms Indigenous to Man. New York, McGraw-Hill Book Company, 1962.

Rosenstein, B. J.: Salmonellosis in infants and children. J. Pediat. *70*:1, 1967.

Rothberg, N. W., and Swartz, M. N.: Extracellular deoxyribonucleases in members of the family Enterobacteriaceae. J. Bact. *90*:294, 1965.

Russell, R. L., *et al.*: A quality control program in clinical microbiology. Amer. J. Clin. Path. *52*:489, 1971.

Sarkany, I., Taplin, D., and Blank, H.: Incidence and bacteriology of erythrasma. Arch. Derm. *85*:578, 1962.

Sellers, W.: Medium for differentiating the gram-negative nonfermenting bacilli of medical interest. J. Bact. *87*:46, 1964.

Shapton, D. A., and Board, R. G.: Isolation of Anaerobes. New York, Academic Press, Inc., 1971.

Sharp, J. T.: The Role of Mycoplasma and L Forms in Disease. Springfield, Ill., Charles C Thomas, 1970.

Silliker, J. H.: Polyvalent H agglutinations as a rapid means of screening non-lactose fermenting colonies for *Salmonella* organisms. Amer. J. Clin. Path. *43*:548, 1965.

Silver, H., Sonnenwirth, A. C., and Alex, N.: Modifications in the fluorescence microscopy technique as applied to identification of acid-fast bacilli in tissue and bacteriological material. J. Clin. Path. *19*:583, 1966.

Skerman, V. B. D.: A Guide to the Identification of the Genera of Bacteria. 2nd ed. Baltimore, The Williams & Wilkins Co., 1967.

Sonnenwirth, A. C., and Weaver, R. E.: *Yersinia enterocolitica*. New Eng. J. Med. *283*:1468, 1970.

Smith, D. T., Conant, N. F., and Overman, J. R.: Zinnser's Microbiology. 14th ed. New York, Appleton-Century-Crofts, Inc., 1968.

Smith, L. D. S., and Holdeman, L. V.: The Pathogenic Anaerobic Bacteria. Springfield, Ill., Charles C Thomas, 1968.

Smith, P. D.: The Biology of Mycoplasmas. New York, Academic Press, Inc., 1971.

Steinhauer, B. W., Eickhoff, T. C., Kislak, J. W., and Finland, M.: The *Klebsiella-Enterobacter-Serratia* division. Clinical and epidemiologic characteristics. Ann. Intern. Med. *65*:1180, 1966.

Stuart, R. D.: Transport media for specimens in public health bacteriology. Public Health Rep. *74*:431, 1959.

Sutter, V. L., and Finegold, S. M.: *Haemophilus aphrophilus* infections: Clinical and bacteriologic studies. Ann. N.Y. Acad. Sci. *174*:468, 1970.

Tennant, B. (ed.): Neonatal Enteric Infections Caused by *Escherichia coli*. Ann. N.Y. Acad. Sci. *176*, 1971.

Thayer, J. D., and Martin, J. E.: Improved medium selective for cultivation of *N. gonorrhoeae* and *N. meningitidis*. Public Health Rep. *81*:55, 1966.

Thomason, B. M., and Wells, J. G.: Preparation and testing of polyvalent conjugates for fluorescent-antibody detection of Salmonellae. Appl. Microbiol. *22*:876, 1971.

Tilton, R. C., Murphy, J. R., and van Soestberger, A.: *Erwinia* species from human sources. Amer. J. Clin. Path. *52*:187, 1971.

Tinsdale, G. F. W.: A new medium for the isolation and identification of *C. diphtheriae* based on the production of hydrogen sulfide. J. Path. Bact. *59*:461, 1947.

Traub, W. H., Raymond, E. A., and Linehan, J.: Identification of Enterobacteriaceae in the clinical microbiology laboratory. Appl. Microbiol. *20*:303, 1970.

Truant, J. P., Hadley, I. K., and Boyd, T. T.: A comparison of the immunofluorescence technique with conventional methods for the identification of Group A beta hemolytic streptococci. Henry Ford Hosp. Med. Bull. *13*:357, 1965.

U.S. Public Health Service: Management of Chancroid, Granuloma Inguinale and Lymphogranuloma Venereum in General Practice. Atlanta, Ga., National Center for Disease Control, U.S. Public Health Service Publication No. 255, 1964.

Vera, H. L.: Quality control in diagnostic microbiology. Health Lab. Sci. *8*:3, 1971.

Vestal, A. L.: Procedures for the Isolation and Identification of Mycobacteria. Atlanta, Ga., National Center for Disease Control, 1969.

Virginia Polytechnic Institute, Anaerobe Laboratory: Outline of Clinical Methods in Anaerobic Bacteriology. Blacksburg, Va., 1970.

von Graevinitz, A.: *Pseudomonas stutzeri* isolated from clinical specimens. Amer. J. Clin. Path. *43*:357, 1965.

von Graevinitz, A., and Mensch, A. H.: The genus *Aeromonas* in human bacteriology. New Eng. J. Med. *278*:245, 1968.

White, L. A., and Kellogg, D. S.: *Neisseria gonorrhoeae* identification in direct smears by a fluorescent antibody counterstain method. Appl. Microbiol. *13*:171, 1965.

Wiesner, P. J., *et al.*: Clinical spectrum of pharyngeal gonococcal infection. New Eng. J. Med. *288*:181, 1973.

Wilkowske, C. J., *et al.*: *Serratia marcescens.* Biochemical characteristics, antibiotic susceptibility patterns and clinical significance. J.A.M.A. *214*:2157, 1970.

Zierdt, C. H., and Marsh, H. H.: Identification of *Pseudomonas pseudomallei.* Amer. J. Clin. Path. *55*:596, 1971.

Chapter 19

MEDICAL PARASITOLOGY

by RUSSELL M. McQUAY, Ph.D.

Orientation of the subject matter in this chapter is basically from the parasite nomenclature or classification point of view. However, an integrated program established upon human organ system involvement for the various parasites appears in Table 18–9. There are no tissues exempt from parasitism, and frequently multiple parasitic infections may be observed in man, particularly in individuals who live or have lived in the tropics and subtropics. In these areas parasitic diseases abound and are among the most prevalent health problems.

General reference texts on medical parasitology are listed below and the reader will discover that photomicrographs in Spencer and Monroe, 1961, as well as the programmed text for self-instruction by Nice *et al.*, 1963 will be very useful tools for the laboratory. The pathologist is directed to detailed pathologic presentations in Ash and Spitz (1945), Edington and Gilles (1969), and Marcial-Rojas (1971).

Clinical diagnosis of endoparasitic and ectoparasitic infections, more frequently than not, depends upon the demonstration of parasite objects by laboratory methods. Recommended and alternate methods are presented.

MEDICAL PROTOZOOLOGY

The protozoa are single-cell organisms that are classified according to the type of motility they exhibit, e.g., Rhizopoda (Sarcodina), by ameboid activity; Mastigophora, by their flagella; Ciliata, by cilia; and the Sporozoa, by dissemination of spores. The disease-producing protozoa are presented in Table 19–1.

A number of protozoa are capable of living in the intestinal tract of man. None of these is a normal inhabitant, although most of them are considered nonpathogenic. The presence of large numbers of any one of these organisms in the stool of a patient may be viewed with some suspicion that the organism may be contributing to whatever clinical condition may exist. Most of the enteric protozoa have a worldwide distribution, and the percentage of any population harboring these organisms is determined by their living conditions, diet, and sanitary habits.

There are, in addition, several protozoa that live in the blood and tissues of man. All are pathogenic, producing such diseases as malaria, trypanosomiasis, and leishmaniasis. Their distribution is usually limited to areas where the proper arthropod vectors are present. They present serious problems in diagnosis, treatment, and prevention. In this section the fundamental characteristics of the parasitic protozoa will be related to diagnosis.

The Intestinal Amebae (Rhizopoda)

There are five well-recognized species of amebae, belonging to four genera, that may be found as single or mixed infections in the human digestive tract: *Entamoeba histolytica, Entamoeba coli, Endolimax nana, Iodamoeba bütschlii (williamsi),* and *Dientamoeba fragilis.* These amebae, with one exception, exist in three forms in the digestive tract of man. The *trophozoite* or vegetative stage multiplies by binary fission and moves about by means of pseudopods, which are quite characteristic in some of the species. The trophozoites ingest particles and contain these particles in vacuoles in their cytoplasm. In the *precyst* stage the trophozoite rounds up, the inclusions are extruded, and the cell wall thickens. The *cyst* is an extension of the precyst. The cell wall becomes fairly thick and resistant, and the nucleus may divide once or several times so that the cyst, depending on the species, may

Table 19–1. PROTOZOAN DISEASES IN MAN

PROTOZOA	DISEASE	GEOGRAPHICAL DISTRIBUTION	LENGTH OF PARASITE	SITE IN HOST	PORTAL OF ENTRY	SOURCE OF INFECTION FOR MAN	CLINICAL MANIFESTATIONS	LABORATORY FINDINGS	LABORATORY METHODS	ADDITIONAL INFORMATION
INTESTINAL										
Entamoeba histolytica (large race)	Amebic dysentery; Intestinal amebiasis	Cosmopolitan	Trophozoites, 12-40 μ Cysts, 10-16 μ	Colon	Mouth	Cysts in contaminated food or water; from stool	Asymptomatic to mild or severe gastrointestinal distress; dysentery	Cysts and/or trophozoites found in stool; same in diarrheic and purged stools	Direct smears: concentration; hematoxylin smears; culture	Strains may change from noninvasive to invasive within the host
	Amebic liver, lung and brain abscess; cutaneous amebiasis; hepatitis	Same	Trophozoites, 12 to 40 μ	Liver; lung; brain; skin	Mouth	Same	Symptoms depend on site of localization	Cysts or trophozoites may be in stool; x-ray; serologic tests; trophozoites in lesion.	Direct smears; hematoxylin smears; PVA smears; culture	Difficult to diagnose; depends on conditions
Entamoeba histolytica (small race) or *E. hartmanni*	Intestinal amebiasis	Same	Trophozoites, 5-12 μ; Cysts, 3-10 μ	Colon	Mouth	Same	Asymptomatic to chronic gastrointestinal disease; may be acute on occasion	Same	Same	Role of ameba often difficult to assess
Dientamoeba fragilis	*Dientamoeba* diarrhea (dientamebiasis)		Trophozoites, 5-12 μ; no cyst	Colon	Mouth	Trophozoites from stool; contaminated food or water	Abdominal discomfort; diarrhea	Trophozoites in stool	Same	No cystic stage observed; trophozoites may be found in tissues of appendix
Hartmanella (Acanthamoeba) castellani and *Naegleria* sp.	Primary amebic meningoencephalitis	Worldwide	8 × 40 μ	Meninges	Nose (nasal mucosa-olfactory bulb route)	Fresh water lakes, ponds, and streams	Rapidly fatal disease, headache, fever and stupor	Amebae in abscesses in brain	Special culture methods; microscopic examination body fluids and tissues	
Balantidium coli	Balantidiasis	Tropics; sometimes in temperate zones	50-100 μ	Colon	Mouth	Cysts from stools; contaminated food or water	Diarrhea; dysentery; sloughing of mucosa	Trophozoites and occasionally cysts, in stools	Same as for *E. histolytica* small race	Infection mainly from pig; cilia on trophozoites uniform length
Giardia lamblia	Giardiasis; flagellate diarrhea	Cosmopolitan	Trophozoites and cysts, 9 to 15 μ	Duodenum; upper small intestine	Mouth	Same	Asymptomatic; duodenitis; diarrhea	Stool: cysts and/or trophozoites in stools Duodenal drainage: trophozoites; no culture	Same, except for culture	Trophozoites may be in gallbladder; disease more common in children
Trichomonas vaginalis	Trichomoniasis	Same	Up to 27 μ	Vagina; urethra; prostate	Genital orifice	Trophozoites in vaginal and prostatic secretions	Vaginitis; urethritis	Trophozoites in vaginal and prostatic secretions; urine of males and females	Direct smear; concentration by centrifugation; culture	Treat both sexual partners and infected individuals
Isospora hominis	Isosporiasis	Same	Up to 33 μ	Ileum	Mouth	Spores from stool	Diarrhea; abdominal pain	Oocysts in stools	Direct smear; concentration	Self-limiting

(Table 19–1 continues on the following page.)

Table 19–1. PROTOZOAN DISEASES IN MAN *(Continued)*

PROTOZOA	DISEASE	GEOGRAPHICAL DISTRIBUTION	LENGTH OF PARASITE	SITE IN HOST	PORTAL OF ENTRY	SOURCE OF INFECTION FOR MAN	CLINICAL MANIFESTATIONS	LABORATORY FINDINGS	LABORATORY METHODS	ADDITIONAL INFORMATION
BLOOD AND TISSUE										
Toxoplasma gondii	Toxoplasmosis	Same	4-6 μ	All organs	(?)	Congenital; acquired – foods ?, droplet spray?; cat feces with oocysts	Asymptomatic; chorioretinitis; hydrocephalus; microcephalus; cerebral calcification, etc; convulsions; pneumonia	Organisms from tissues or biopsies; serologic tests	Methylene blue dye test; C-F; FA; animal inoculation	
Pneumocystis carinii	Interstitial pneumonia	Europe; U.S.A.	1-3 μ	Smooth muscle of lung, alveolar walls	Resp. (?)	No vector; direct transfer; highly contagious	Asphyxia; cyanosis; dyspnea	Uninucleated and multinucleated organisms; rosettes with eight spores	Chest x-ray clinical exam. (respiration)	
Plasmodium vivax	Benign tertian; vivax malaria	Tropics; subtropics; some in temperate zone	Variable, depending on stage	Intracellular: parenchymal cells of liver; within red blood cells	Skin	Bite of female *Anopheles* mosquito; blood transfusion	Paroxysm; fever, chill, and sweat; 48-hour cycle; enlarged spleen and liver	Characteristic morphology in blood smears taken at intervals	Stained thin and thick blood smears; serologic test	Some strains show relapses; may persist in liver cells
Plasmodium falciparum	Malignant tertian falciparum malaria; EA (estio-autumnal malaria); subtertian malaria	Tropics and subtropics	Same	Same	Same	Same	Paroxysm; 24- to 48-hour cycle; hemoglobinuria in blackwater fever	Same	Same	Does not persist in liver; no relapses; immediate treatment mandatory; ring forms and gametocytes found only in peripheral blood
Plasmodium malariae	Quartan malaria	Same	Same	Same	Same	Same	Paroxysm: 72-hour intervals	Same	Same	May persist in liver cells; relapses; do not use as blood donor
Plasmodium ovale	Ovale malaria	West and East Africa; Philippines	Same	Same	Same	Same	Paroxysm: 48-hour interval	Same	Same	Uncommon

Leishmania donovani	Kala-azar; visceral leishmaniasis	Same	2-3 μ		Intracellular; Reticulo-endothelial cells	Same	Bite of *Phlebotomus* fly	Enlarged liver and spleen; leukopenia	Liver aspiration; sternal puncture	Stained tissue smears; serologic tests; animal inoculation; culture media for blood and/or tissues	Flagellate forms in culture
Leishmania tropica	Cutaneous leishmaniasis; oriental sore	Africa; Asia; Mediterranean area	Same		Reticulo-endothelial cells in skin and mucosa	Same	Same	Lesions on skin with scarring	Skin scrapings	Same	Lasting immunity following infection; flagellate forms in culture
Leishmania braziliensis	Mucocutaneous leishmaniasis; American leishmaniasis; espundia; uta; Chiclero's disease	Central and South America	Same		Same	Same	Same	Primary lesion on skin-metastasize to become lesions on mouth and nose	Same	Same	Flagellate forms in culture
Trypanosoma gambiense and *rhodesiense*	African sleeping sickness; Gambian and Rhodesian trypanosomiasis	Africa		14-33 μ	Blood; skin lymph glands; brain; spinal fluid	Skin	Bite of tsetse fly (*Glossina*)	Fever; rash; headache; spleen and liver enlargement; enlargement of posterior cervical lymph nodes (Winterbottom's sign)	Blood smear; cerebrospinal fluid; gland puncture	Wet and stained blood smears; culture; concentration methods; serologic tests; animal inoc.	Trypanosomes multiply in the blood and are fairly numerous
Trypanosoma cruzi	South American trypanosomiasis; Chagas' disease	Central and South America		20 μ	Blood; skin tissues; cardiac muscle	Skin	Infective feces of reduviid bug (triatomid, cone-nose, kissing) into bite wound	Fever; spleen and liver enlargement; unilateral periorbital edema (Romaña's sign)	Leishmanial forms in heart muscle and other tissues; trypanosomal form in blood	Wet and stained blood smears; animal inoculation; culture; serologic tests; xenodiagnosis (laboratory-reared reduviid bugs)	"C" and "U" shapes to trypanosomal form; trypanosomes do not multiply in blood and are scanty

Table 19–2. DIFFERENTIAL CHARACTERISTICS OF THE INTESTINAL AMEBAE

ORGANISM	*Entamoeba histolytica* (large and small races)		*Entamoeba coli*		*Endolimax nana*		*Iodamoeba butschlii*		*Dientamoeba fragilis*
	TROPHOZOITES	CYSTS	TROPHOZOITES	CYSTS	TROPHOZOITES	CYSTS	TROPHOZOITES	CYSTS	TROPHOZOITES(only)
Size	6-40 μ: small race average 6-12 μ	3.5-15 μ; small race 3.5-10 μ	15-50 μ	10-30 μ	6-15 μ	5-14 μ	6-20 μ	5-20 μ	5-12 μ
Motility and pseudopodia; shape of cyst	Active, progressive and directional; fingerlike, rapidly extruded; small race usually not actively motile and rounded	Spherical	Sluggish; rarely progressive and directional; blunt	Spherical	Sluggish; hyaline; budding	Ovoid or spherical	Sluggish; hyaline, blunt, slowly extruded	Irregular	Active; hyaline, blunt, and leaflike
Unstained organism in saline	Motile or rounded; nucleus not visible; red blood cells visible; vacuoles seen	Nuclei (1 to 4) not visible; chromatoid matter refractile; glycogen refractile in young cysts	Motile or rounded; nucleus visible in endoplasm behind pseudopod; vacuoles seen	Nuclei (1 to 8) visible; chromatoid matter refractile; glycogen refractile in young cysts	Motile or rounded; nucleus not visible; vacuoles seen	Nuclei (1 to 4) not visible	Motile or rounded; nucleus not visible	Nucleus not visible; glycogen refractile	Motile or rounded; nuclei not seen
Unstained organism in phenol-alcohol-formalin (PAF) solution	Nonmotile, fixed as extended; nucleus visible	Nuclei visible; chromatoid matter refractile	Nonmotile, fixed as extended	(Same as in saline)	Nucleus not visible	Nuclei appear as punched-out holes; glycogen ball in young cysts	Nucleus not seen	Nucleus not visible; glycogen ball evident	Nuclei not seen
Iodine stained	Nucleus visible	Nuclei visible; chromatoids seldom seen; glycogen ball in young cysts	Nucleus visible	Nuclei visible; chromatoids seldom seen; glycogen ball	Nucleus not visible	Nuclei visible	Nucleus not visible	Nucleus not visible	Nuclei not visible
Hematoxylin stained (shows the most morphologic detail)	Nucleus visible; cytoplasm vacuolated	Nuclei visible; chromatoids stained; glycogen unstained	Nucleus visible; cytoplasm vacuolated	Nuclei visible; chromatoids stained; glycogen unstained	Nucleus visible; cytoplasm vacuolated	Nuclei visible; no chromatoids seen but baciliform bodies may be seen	Nucleus visible; cytoplasm vacuolated	Nucleus visible; volutin granules stained; glycogen ball unstained	Nucleus or nuclei seen; cytoplasm vacuolated
Inclusions	Red blood cells, in amebic dysentery; no bacteria when in fresh stool; no red blood cells in small race	None	Bacteria and food debris; no red blood cells	None	Bacteria and food debris; no red blood cells	None	Bacteria and food debris; no red blood cells	None	Bacteria and food debris; yeasts; no red blood cells
Chromatoid matter	None	Rods with rounded ends; irregular in small race	None	Bars with splinter ends; some comma or needle shaped	None	None	None	None	None
Glycogen	None	Diffuse in older cysts; mass in cysts with one or two nuclei	None	Diffuse in older cysts; mass in cysts with one or two nuclei	None	Diffuse; rarely as a mass in young cysts	None	Usually present as a well-defined mass	None
Nucleus	Single; ringlike; visible in stained preparations	One to four may be present	Single; ringlike; visible in all preparations	One to eight may be present	Single; visible with hematoxylin and other permanent stains only	One to four may be present	Single; same as *E. nana* trophozoite	Single	Single but more frequently two
Nuclear membrane	Delicate; beadlike chromatin dots	Same as trophozoite	Thick, coarse, irregular chromatin dots	Same as trophozoite	Chromatin seldom present	Same as trophozoite	Same as *E. nana*	Same as trophozoite	Delicate but no chromatin dots seen
Karyosome	Small and centrally located	Same as trophozoite	Large and eccentrically located	Same as trophozoite	Large, central or eccentric	Large, central or eccentric	Large, central or eccentric; surrounded with granules	Large, eccentric; chromatin dots on linin network	Four to six large fragments which may appear in a ringlike arrangement
Cytoplasm	Foamy; vacuolated	Delicate; nongranular	Coarse; vacuolated	Coarse	Smooth; often vacuolated	Smooth	Vacuolated	Smooth; vacuolated	Smooth; vacuolated

contain one to eight nuclei. These nuclei are much smaller than those in the trophozoite.

The differentiation of the species of protozoa depends on the size, type of pseudopod, and nuclear and cytoplasmic structure of the trophozoite and on the size and nuclear and cytoplasmic structure of the cysts and precysts. One must become thoroughly familiar with these features to do reliable parasitologic examinations (Fig. 19-3 and Table 19-2). A self-instructional course on the laboratory diagnosis of amebiasis is available (see amebiasis reference).

ENTAMOEBA HISTOLYTICA

Entamoeba histolytica (Tables 19-1, 19-2; Figs. 19-1, 19-3, 19-4, 19-6, 19-7) is the most pathogenic of the enteric amebae, although at times it may be a commensal. Some strains (Laredo, etc.) of this organism grow at room temperature and are apparently nonpathogenic. At times the pathogenic strains produce intestinal amebiasis, which may be seen as acute amebic dysentery in tropical areas and occasionally in temperate zones, and there is little question of direct etiologic significance in this condition. A varying percentage of various population groups in the temperate zones is infected with *E. histolytica*. Certain of these infections are asymptomatic and may remain so for extended periods. Others have an irregular course, with short bouts of diarrhea intermingled with periods of constipation. There may be selective dyspepsia to certain foods, such as milk and greasy foods, with considerable gas and abdominal discomfort. It is not easy to evaluate the role of *E. histolytica* in patients with these symptoms. It is highly desirable that, in patients with chronic gastrointestinal disease in whom *E. histolytica* is found, a complete workup be done to rule out such conditions as carcinoma and ulcerative colitis before attempting to determine the role of the amebae. The distribution of amebic lesions in the colon is shown in Fig. 19-2. The ripe cysts (quadrinucleated) are the infective forms. The life history of *E. histolytica* is shown in Figure 19-1. The differential diagnosis of the intestinal amebae is given in Table 19-2.

The trophozoite of *E. histolytica* (Figs. 19-4 *c, d*; 19-6) has certain diagnostic characteristics. The nucleus is round, with a delicate ring of chromatin around the periphery, which tends to be beaded. The chromatin ring may on occasion be heavier in some areas than in others. The nucleus has a small, delicate, centrally located karyosome. The nucleus is usually about one-third the diameter of the trophozoite. The cytoplasm is delicate and may appear foamy in stained preparations; there is a thin cell wall. This organism characteristically ingests red blood cells in amebic dysentery. In fresh, warm specimens the trophozoites send out clear, hyaline pseudopods, which tend to continue coming out in the same direction in an explosive manner, giving what has been termed unidirectional motion. In temporary wet mounts the nucleus is not visible in the unstained organism, except when fixed in phenol-alcohol-formalin (PAF) solution (Burrows, 1967; 1969). The size of *E. histolytica* trophozoites varies from 6 to 40 microns.

The precyst is usually round, and the cell wall is thicker than in the trophozoite. There is one typical nucleus. The ripe cyst of *E. histolytica* (Figs. 19-3 [*H* 1-4]; 19-4 *a, b*; 19-6) has a heavy cyst wall with a delicate, nongranular cytoplasm. Young cysts with one or two nuclei have a glycogen mass which is refractile in saline mounts, stains dark brown with iodine and is refractory to hematoxylin stain. Characteristically there appear rather large structures called chromatoidal bodies, which are cigar-shaped and stain black with hematoxylin but are refractile in unstained preparations. When found they are diagnostic, but they do not always occur. They tend to disappear as the stool ages.

There are characteristically four nuclei, but they are much smaller than the one in the trophozoite, although having the same structures. These nuclei cannot be seen in unstained cysts in temporary wet mounts unless fixed in the PAF solution mentioned above. The size of the cysts varies from 3.5 to 15.0 microns.

The variation in the size of the cysts and trophozoites of *E. histolytica* has led to an arbitrary classification into two races (Sapero *et al.*, 1942; Felsenfeld, 1945, 1965; Shaffer *et al.*, 1958; Faust, Russell and Jung, 1970; Hunter *et al.*, 1966; McQuay, 1967). The large race comprises those with average cyst sizes of 10 microns and over, and the small race those with average cyst sizes under 10 microns. Evidence indicates that the two races are different in certain fundamental respects. The large race is associated with the most severe pathologic lesions, i.e., acute amebic dysentery; liver, lung and brain abscess; and cutaneous amebiasis. The small race (Table 19-2; Figs. 19-4 *e-h*, and 19-6 *c, d*) tends to be found in persons with chronic gastrointestinal disease (Shaffer *et al.*, 1965) in which their role is difficult to evaluate; they have not been found in liver abscess or in other extraintestinal complications. They do not ingest red blood cells.

Some workers (Burrows, 1957) have described additional small amebae, which resemble the small race very closely and are termed *Entamoeba hartmanni*; they are said

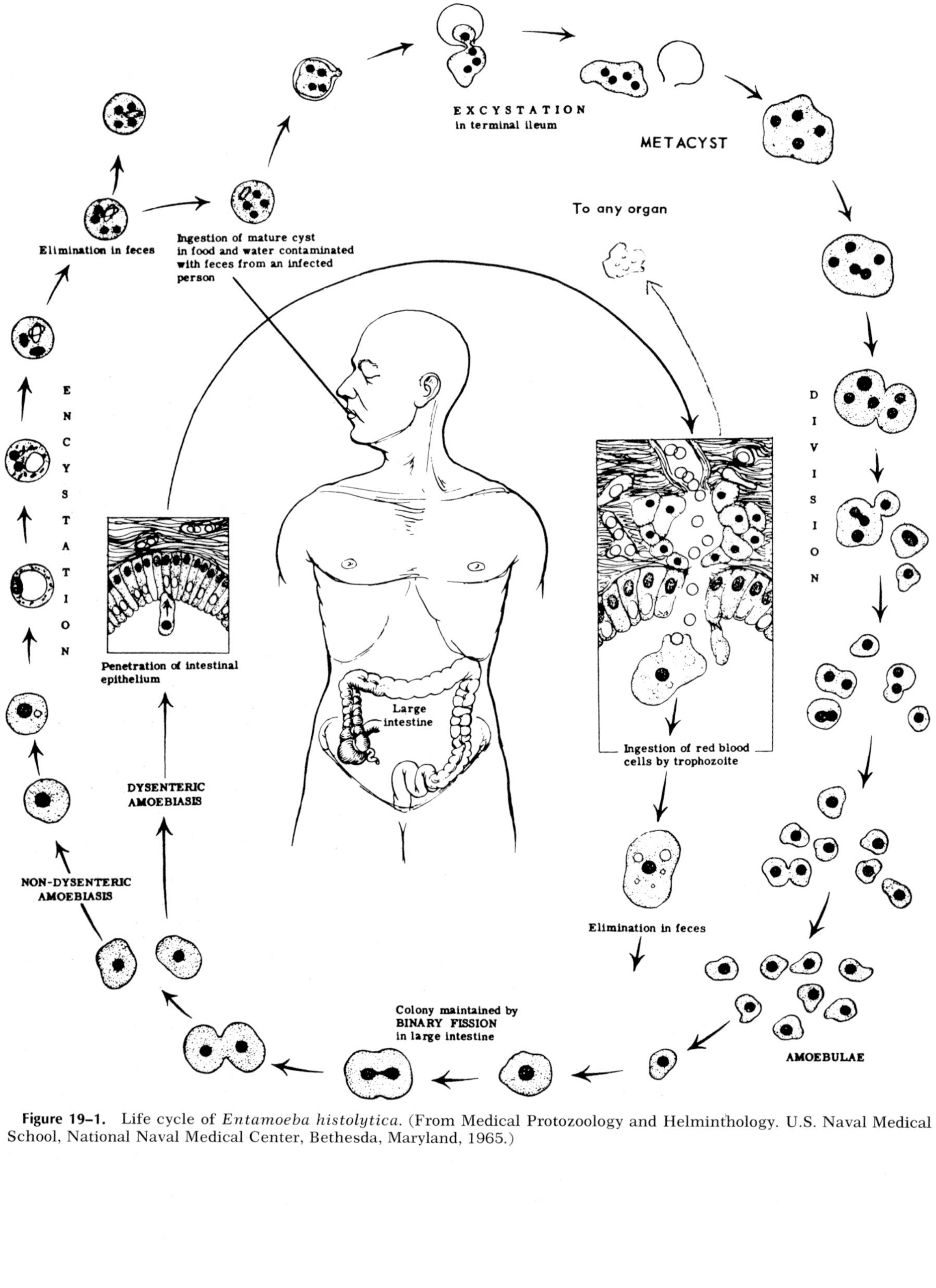

Figure 19–1. Life cycle of *Entamoeba histolytica*. (From Medical Protozoology and Helminthology. U.S. Naval Medical School, National Naval Medical Center, Bethesda, Maryland, 1965.)

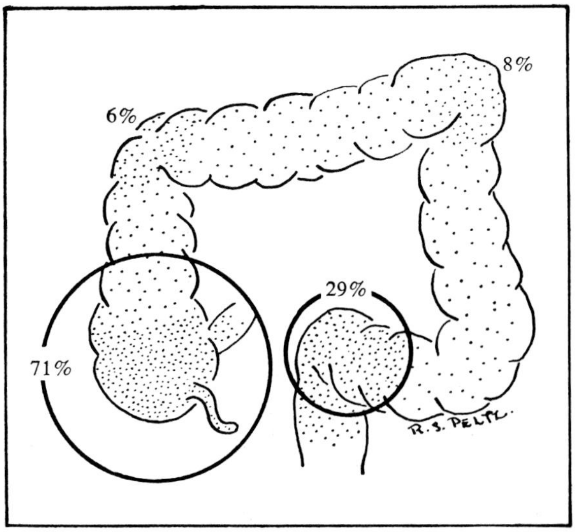

Figure 19–2. Distribution of amebic lesions in the colon. (From Sawitz, W. G.: Medical Parasitology. 2nd edition. New York, Blakiston Division, McGraw-Hill Book Company, 1956.)

to be nonpathogenic. Further study is needed to clarify the relationship between the large and small race *E. histolytica* (Figs. 19–4, 19–6) and *E. hartmanni.*

The laboratory diagnosis of acute amebic dysentery is usually not difficult. Examination of warm, freshly passed stool reveals characteristic trophozoites. On the other hand, in a chronic or asymptomatic case of amebiasis in which the stool may be formed, it is usual to find only the cysts in the stools. The cysts may be present in very small numbers and considerable searching is necessary. This is particularly true in small race infections, in which the cysts may be sparse. It is also important to emphasize that small race cysts are very difficult if not impossible to differentiate from *Endolimax nana* cysts in wet preparations (unstained or iodine stained). Thus, hematoxylin-stained preparations (Felsenfeld and Young, 1945) are very important for differential diagnosis, especially in mixed amebic and flagellate infections.

When purgation is employed for ameba studies, one may anticipate recovery of immature and mature cysts as well as trophozoites, while in ameba cultures only trophozoites multiply, although on rare occasions cysts are produced.

The number of positive findings depends on the care, diligence, experience, and motivation of the person doing the examinations. An experienced worker may be able to make a systematic search of a slide in 10 minutes, but the less experienced will need more time. The number of daily stool examinations for a given patient will be determined by the degree of suspicion that exists. One should never do less than three complete stool examinations, and six are recommended. It has been shown repeatedly that there is a direct relationship between the number of procedures done on a stool specimen and the percentage of positive findings of protozoa and helminths. This is particularly true in the case of the important pathogen *Entamoeba histolytica* (Fig. 19–5). Certain structures in the stool may be confusing (Fig. 19–97), and it is important to be thoroughly familiar with stool cytology (See later section on stool cytology and nonparasitic objects, p. 1034).

Culture Methods for Entamoeba histolytica and Certain Other Protozoa. Stool cultures for *E. histolytica* and certain other protozoa are time consuming but not difficult. When cultures are used properly, scanty infections may be revealed. Permanently stained preparations can be made from the cultures (with the PVA fixation method) and the trophozoites identified with reasonable ease in hematoxylin-stained preparations.

There are numerous media available for culture (Taylor and Baker, 1968). Several are described in this chapter (Boeck and Drbohlav, 1925—coagulated egg—and McQuay, 1956—charcoal). Alternate methods include Balamuth's (1946) liquid egg infusion medium and Cleveland and Collier's (1930) liver slant medium. The large race can be cultured in all these media relatively easily. The small race, which is difficult to culture in most media, can be grown in McQuay's medium.

Boeck-Drbohlav Locke Egg-serum Medium. This medium (Boeck and Drbohlav, 1925) may be employed for the initial cultivation of *Entamoeba histolytica* from various types of specimens and the following from feces: *E. coli, Endolimax nana, Dientamoeba fragilis, Chilomastix mesnili,* and *Trichomonas hominis.* For maintenance transfers are made every 48 hours except in the case of *E. coli,* which requires transfers every 72 hours. About 0.5 ml. of the fluid medium at the bottom of the tube is used for each transplant.

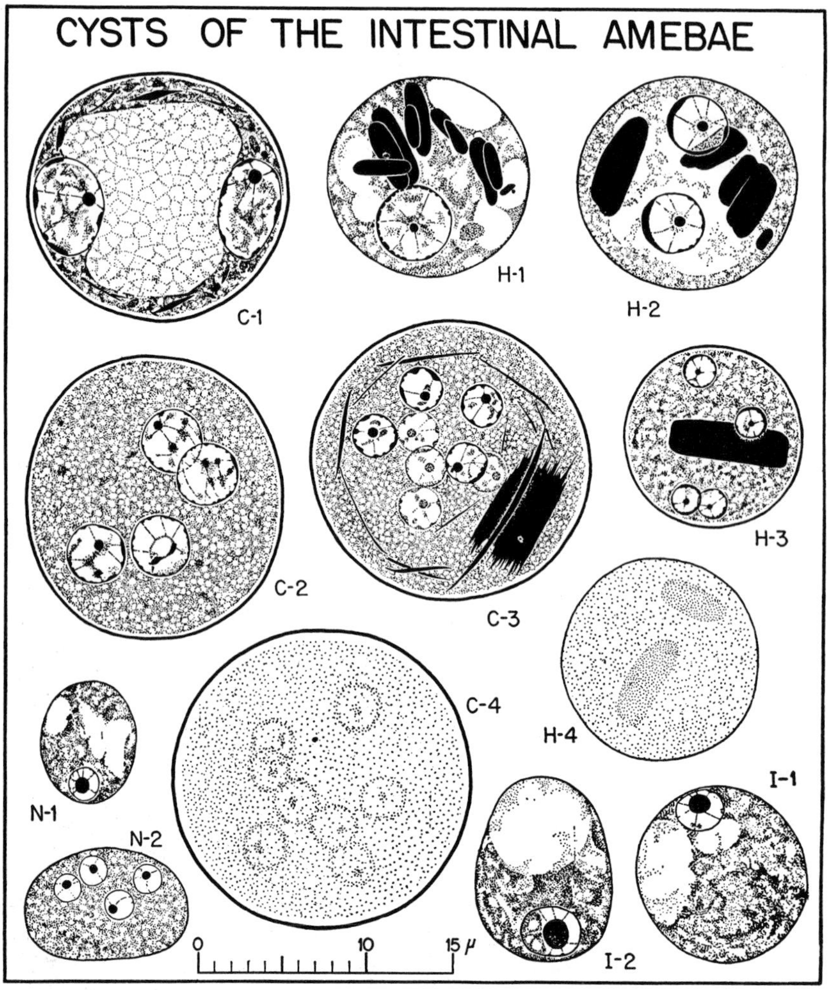

Figure 19–3. *C-1,* Iron-hematoxylin stained binucleate cyst of *Entamoeba coli. C-2,* Iron-hematoxylin stained quadrinucleate cyst of *E. coli. C-3,* Iron-hematoxylin stained mature cyst of *E. coli. H-1,* Iron-hematoxylin stained uninucleate cyst of *E. histolytica. H-2,* Iron-hematoxylin stained binucleate cyst of *E. histolytica. H-3,* Iron-hematoxylin stained mature cyst of *E. histolytica. N-1,* Iron-hematoxylin stained uninucleate cyst of *Endolimax nana. N-2,* Iron-hematoxylin stained mature cysts of *E. nana. I-1, I-2,* Iron-hematoxylin stained mature cysts of *Iodamoeba bütschlii. C-4,* Unstained mature cyst of *E. coli. H-4,* Unstained cyst of *E. histolytica.* (From Hunter, G. W., Frye, W. W., and Swartzwelder, J. C.: A Manual of Tropical Medicine. 4th ed.)

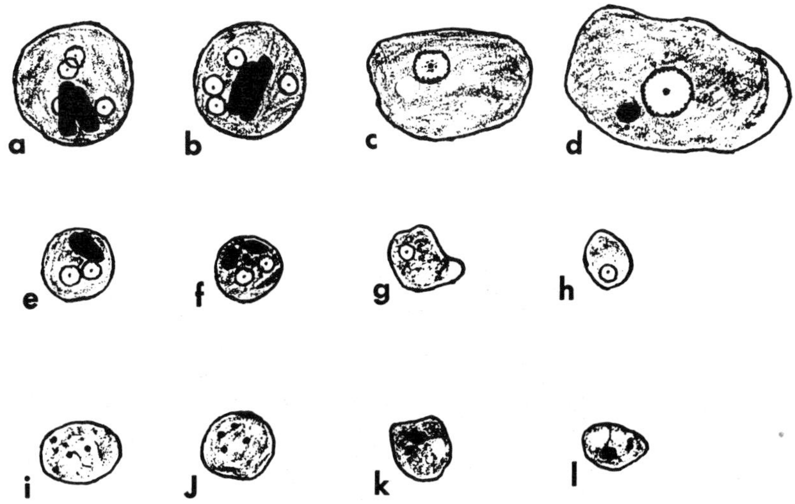

Figure 19–4. Camera lucida drawings of cysts and trophozoites of large and small race *Entamoeba histolytica* and *Endolimax nana:* (*a, b*) Large race cysts with four nuclei and chromatoid bars; (*c, d*) Large race trophozoites; (*e, f*) Small race cysts with two nuclei and chromatoid bars; (*g, h*) Small race trophozoites; (*i, j*) *Endolimax nana* cysts with four nuclei; (*k, l*) *Endolimax nana* trophozoites. × 2500.

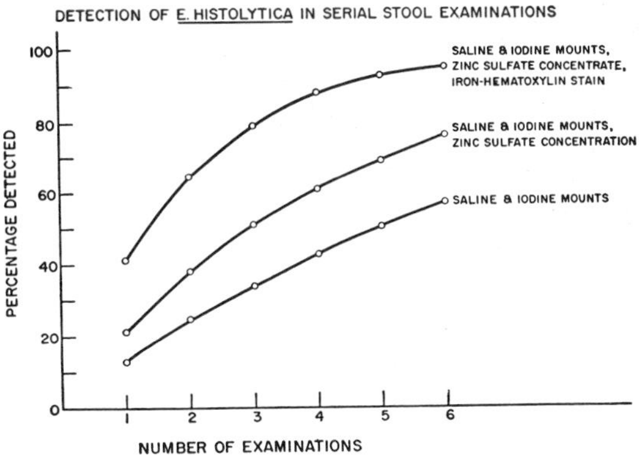

Figure 19–5. Probability of detecting *Entamoeba histolytica* by successive stool examinations in which various methods are used. (Adapted from Sawitz and Faust, 1942.)

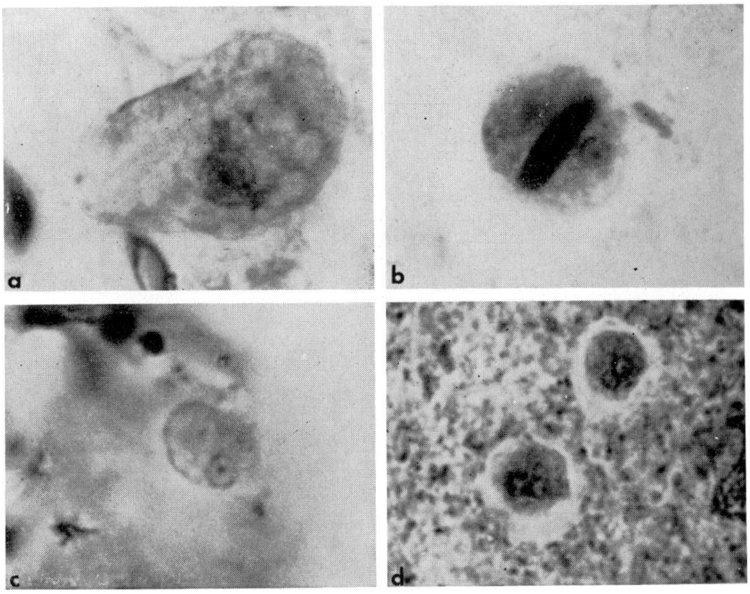

Figure 19–6. *Entamoeba histolytica:* large and small race trophozoites and cysts in fecal smears. (*a*) Large race trophozoite, showing the characteristic foamy cytoplasm and a typical nucleus with central karyosome. (*b*) Large race precyst with a single nucleus and typical large chromatoid bar. (*c*) Small race trophozoite. (*d*) Two small race cysts, each with two nuclei. Modified Mallory's phosphotungstic acid stain. × 2500.

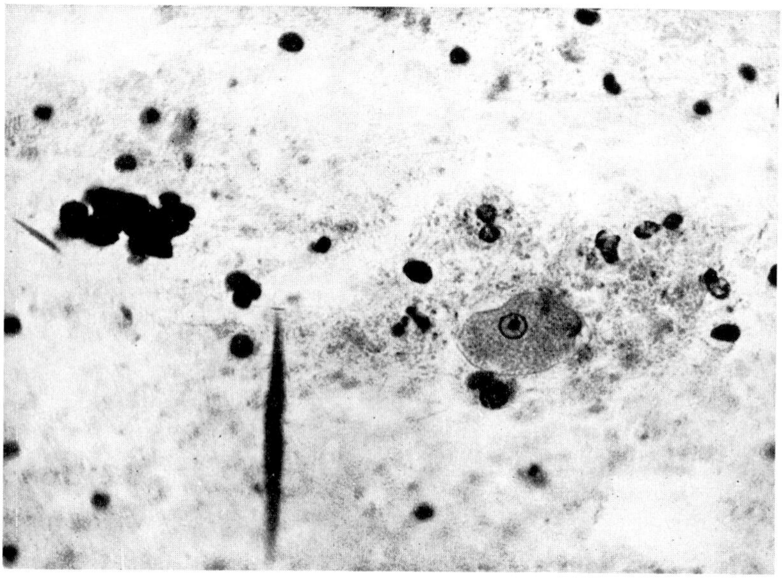

Figure 19–7. Early exudate in stool (iron-hematoxylin stain) showing trophozoite, clumped erythrocytes, pyknotic bodies, and Charcot-Leyden crystals. (From Hunter, G. W., Frye, W. W., and Swartzwelder, J. C.: A Manual of Tropical Medicine. 3rd edition.)

MATERIALS REQUIRED

1. Eggs
2. Sterile Ringer's solution

This is prepared according to the following formula:

NaCl	8.0 gm.
KCl	0.2 gm.
$CaCl_2$	0.2 gm.
$MgCl_2$	0.1 gm.
NaH_2PO_4	0.1 gm.
$NaHCO_3$	0.4 gm.
Distilled water	1000.0 ml.

It is then autoclaved at 15 p.s.i. for 20 minutes and allowed to cool.

3. Modified sterile Ringer's solution (serum-Ringer). Prepare by adding 0.25 gm. of Loeffler's dehydrated blood serum to 1000 ml. of Ringer's solution, which should be made up in addition to the Ringer's solution of step 2. Boil serum and Ringer's solution for 1 hour to facilitate solution of serum. Filter and autoclave for 20 minutes at 15 p.s.i. (Instead of the Loeffler's dehydrated blood serum, sterile human serum or sterile horse serum – inactivated and tricresol free – may be used, in which case the modified Ringer's solution should consist of 1 part serum to 8 parts of Ringer's solution. This solution is sterilized by passing through a Berkefeld filter and incubating at 37° C. to determine sterility before pouring onto egg slants.)

4. Sterile Chinese rice flour. The rice flour is sterilized by placing about 5 gm. in a test tube and plugging it with cotton. It is distributed evenly and loosely over the inner surface of

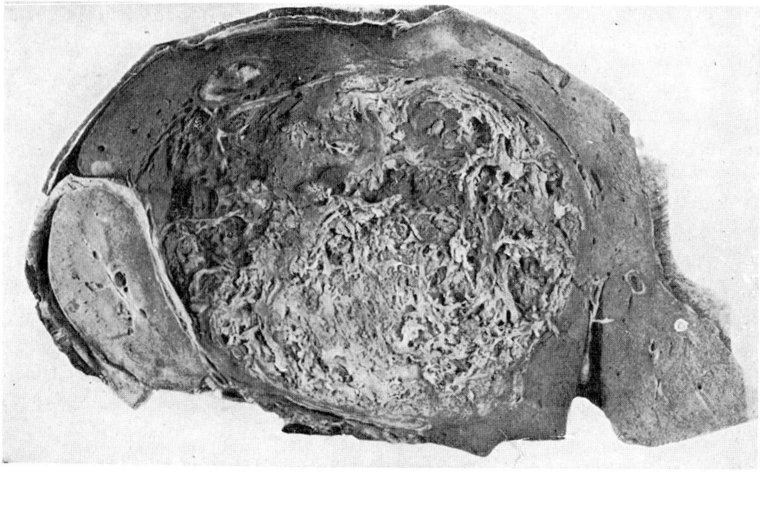

Figure 19–8. Amebic abscess of liver. (From Hunter, G. W., Frye, W. W., and Swartzwelder, J. C.: A Manual of Tropical Medicine. 4th edition.)

tube by shaking. Then it is sterilized in a horizontal position in dry heat at about 90° C. for 12 hours of intermittent sterilization; allow 4 hours for each period; flour remains white if not overheated.

TECHNIQUE

1. Wash four eggs thoroughly, rinse, and brush well with 70 per cent ethyl alcohol. Break into sterile Erlenmeyer flask containing glass beads and about 50 ml. of Ringer's solution. Emulsify completely by shaking. Place about 4 ml. of this material in each test tube and sterilize as follows (use autoclave as inspissator):

2. Place tubes in a preheated autoclave in such a position as to produce a slant of about 1 to 1½ inches. Close the door and vacuum exhaust valve, turn on the steam, and open the outside exhaust valve. When steam appears from this valve close it and allow the pressure to rise to 15 p.s.i.; then shut off steam and allow pressure to decline to zero; remove media from autoclave. Repeat on three successive days, storing media at room temperature between sterilizations.

3. To these sterile solid slants add enough modified Ringer's solution (about 5 or 6 ml.) to cover egg slant completely. Incubate at 37° C. for 24 hours to determine sterility before adding the sterile Chinese rice flour. Flour is added by taking up 0.25 ml. into a clean, sterile, dry wide bore, 1 ml. pipette and discharging it into the liquid medium by tapping the pipette against the inside wall of the tube. The tubes are again incubated at 37° C. for 24 hours to test for sterility.

Charcoal Medium for Amebae (McQuay, 1956). The charcoal diphasic medium (for the primary culture of feces) was developed for the growth of large and small races of *E. histolytica* as well as for the primary culture of *E. coli*, *E. nana*, *D. fragilis*, *I. bütschlii*, *C. mesnili*, and *T. hominis* and other flagellates and *B. coli*. Only *E. histolytica* (large and small races) and *T. hominis* have been maintained. *Giardia lamblia* has not as yet been grown *in vitro*. This medium is easily prepared, with the solid and liquid phases and the rice powder autoclavable separately.

In setting up cultures, emulsify a portion of stool about the size of a kidney bean in the liquid portion of the diphasic medium. Sample the stool from several areas, especially the moist areas and mucus, if present. Place the inoculated tube in the incubator at 37° C. for 48 hours (72 hours maximum), at which time the sediment from the bottom of the slant is examined for motile trophozoites. When trophozoites are demonstrated, the remainder of the sediment, or pooled sediment from the purged samples from the patient, may be placed in a vial containing 5.0 ml. PVA solution and processed for permanently stained preparations as directed on pages 1110–1113.

MATERIAL AND EQUIPMENT

1. Flasks, 3-liter Erlenmeyer.
2. Funnel, plastic, large.
3. Kelly bottles: (A) dispensing media—straight tubulation; (B) dispensing sterile buffered saline—bell attachment (several sterile).
4. Screw-cap tubes.
5. Rice powder, sterile.
6. Buffered saline, sterile, made as directed.
7. Ring stand.
8. Tripod with asbestos gauze.
9. Stirring rod.
10. Thermometer.
11. Media ingredients.

PROCEDURE

Charcoal Medium (diphasic). This diphasic medium has a solid phase (the slant) and a liquid phase (the sterile buffered saline overlay). Sterile rice powder must be added.

1. One liter of the charcoal agar for the *slants* is prepared as follows:*

Sodium phosphate, dibasic, ($Na_2HPO_4 \cdot 12\ H_2O$)	3.0 gm.
Potassium phosphate, monobasic (KH_2PO_4)	4.0 gm.
Sodium citrate ($Na_3C_6H_5O_7 \cdot 2\ H_2O$)	
Magnesium sulfate, crystals ($MgSO_4 \cdot 7\ H_2O$)	0.1 gm.
Ferric ammonium citrate (brown pearls, U.S.P.)	0.1 gm.
Asparagin	2.0 gm.
Tryptone	5.0 gm.
Glycerin (reagent grade)	10.0 ml.
Distilled water	1000.0 ml.

2. Stir these ingredients and use gentle heat for a few minutes to dissolve.

3. After this add the following:*

Agar agar (granular)	12.0 gm.
Norite A (Pfanstiehl Chem. Co.)	1.0 gm.

4. Stir these well and then add (keep flask a great distance from the flame while adding acetone) 25.0 ml. of a 1 per cent solution cholesterol in acetone (1 per cent solution 0.25 gm. to 25 ml. acetone). (Cholesterol, C.P., ash free, for Kline test—Pfanstiehl Chem. Co.)

5. Heat (be sure to use asbestos gauze) the entire charcoal agar to boiling in order to dissolve the agar. Employ frequent mixing to keep the agar from scorching and the charcoal in suspension.

6. Dispense the medium while hot in 2- to 3-ml. amounts into nonsterile tubes. Screw-cap the tubes loosely and autoclave for 15 minutes at 15 p.s.i. (250° F.).

7. *Immediately* upon removal of tubed me-

*One may substitute portion of the slant by obtaining commercially prepared product as follows: BBL 01-665 Hirsch charcoal medium modified to which the glycerol (glycerin of step 1) and cholesterol in acetone (of step 4) are added as directed. The slants are overlaid and sterile rice powder is added.

dia from the autoclave tighten the caps and make slants after resuspending the charcoal that has settled. *Note*: Make the slants entire, i.e., without butts.

8. Overlay the solidified slants completely with 3 to 5 ml. of sterile 0.5 per cent buffered saline with a pH of 7.4. Dispense the saline from sterile Kelly bottles with bell attachment. The slant should be covered with the buffered saline. This buffered saline is made by one of the following methods:

Quick method (using chemicals rather than M/15 solutions) for 3.5 liters of 0.5 per cent buffered saline pH 7.4. Use

27.0 gm. Na_2HPO_4 (anhydrous)
6.0 gm. KH_2PO_4 (anhydrous)
17.5 gm. NaCl
QS to 3.5 liters with distilled water

Long method (M/15 solution) to make 1 liter of 0.5 per cent buffered saline with pH of 7.4. Use

5.0 gm. NaCl
190.0 ml. M/15 KH_2PO_4 (solution A, below)
810.0 ml. M/15 Na_2PO_4 (solution B, below)

Solution A: To make M/15 KH_2PO_4, use 9.07 gm. KH_2PO_4 (anhydrous) Q.S. to 1 liter with distilled water.

Solution B: To make M/15 Na_2HPO_4, use (1) Na_2HPO_4 (anhydrous) 9.46 gm. Q.S. to 1 liter with distilled water, or (2) $Na_2HPO_4 \cdot 12\ H_2O$, 23.88 gm. Q.S. to 1 liter with distilled water.

9. A very small amount (a few grains to float on the surface of the saline overlay) of *sterile* rice powder (Bacto-Rice powder) is tapped into each tube. (The rice powder has been sterilized by autoclaving in screw-cap tube at 15 p.s.i. for 15 minutes and dried in an oven without scorching.)

10. Check the media for sterility by placing it in incubator overnight.

11. The diphasic medium will withstand prolonged storage in the refrigerator but must be brought to room temperature before use.

PROCTOSCOPY

Some workers have used proctoscopic aspirates with considerable success. This technique has been discussed in some detail by Shaffer *et al.*, 1965, p. 100. When done properly, proctoscopy reveals a higher percentage of positive findings than does stool examination.

Pathology of Intestinal and Extraintestinal Amebiasis. Many strains of *E. histolytica* produce primary intestinal lesions which initially are small and pinpoint. As the colony of trophozoites develops by multiplication in the tissues, a channel may be formed down to the muscularis mucosa. The lesion spreads to make a flask-shaped area of necrosis. In the lesion the amebae are more likely to be found at the margin near the normal tissue. Older lesions become complicated by secondary bacterial invasion. Lesions with shaggy, overhanging edges may develop. At times the amebae invade the submucosa and spread out radially. In more advanced involvements, one may see perforation of the intestinal wall. Some trophozoites may gain entrance into the circulatory system and thus develop in secondary, extraintestinal sites, such as the liver and brain. When they arrive in the liver, for example, the amebae produce areas of necrosis as parenchymal cells are destroyed. More detailed descriptions of the pathology of amebic infection can be found in the references (see Faust, Russell and Jung, 1970, pp. 150–158; Shaffer *et al.*, 1965, p. 11; Ash and Spitz, 1945, p. 78; Brown, 1969; Faust, Beaver, and Jung, 1968, p. 68; Manson-Bahr, 1966, pp. 426–427; Wilmot, 1962; Larsh, 1964, p. 23; Markell and Voge, 1971, p. 41; Hunter *et al.*, 1966, p. 291; Edington and Gilles, 1969, p. 60; and Marcial-Rojas, 1971. pp. 157–180).

The diagnosis of amebic liver abscess (Fig. 19–8) or brain abscess is largely clinical, although serologic tests and ameba cultures of specimens collected surgically may be of some assistance in extraintestinal amebiasis. In such abscesses the amebae are present in the tissues at the edge of the abscess and are only infrequently found in the pus in the center of the lesion. Thus, smears or sections made from tissue at the edge of the lesion should be examined and cultured for amebae. Proteolytic enzymes can be used to free the trophozoites for subsequent culturing in ameba media inoculated with *Clostridium perfringens*. Lung abscess sometimes results from extension of a liver abscess through the diaphragm. In such cases the amebae can be demonstrated in sputum or in aspirated material. Amebic peritonitis and involvement of other organs have been described.

Cutaneous amebiasis occurs most frequently in the perianal region or on the buttocks, and occasional cases have occurred on the abdomen as a result of the formation of a fistula from a liver abscess. Trophozoites can be demonstrated from the periphery of such lesions under the layer of overhanging skin. It may be noted that trophozoites and not cysts develop in the tissues.

OTHER INTESTINAL AMEBAE

Entamoeba coli. *Entamoeba coli* (Table 19–2; Fig. 19–3 [C1–4]) is a nonpathogenic ameba that occurs usually in a higher per cent of individuals than does *E. histolytica*. It is important from two standpoints: First, it is necessary that *E. coli* be differentiated from *E. histolytica* (Goldman, 1953), for it bears a considerable resemblance to the large race. Second, since this and other intestinal amebae are transmitted in the same manner as *E. histo-*

lytica, its presence in the stool increases the suspicion that *E. histolytica* might also be present.

The trophozoite of *Entamoeba coli* is generally larger than that of *E. histolytica*, varying from 15 to 50 microns in diameter. Its nucleus has a denser ring of intermittent chromatin around the edge, and its karyosome is larger, eccentric, and occasionally fragmented. The cytoplasm of *E. coli* is coarse and contains many vacuoles. It does not ingest red blood cells, but it may ingest bacteria. The cell wall tends to be thicker and its pseudopods are not so clear as those of *E. histolytica*. They are blunt and move sluggishly, providing a nondirectional movement.

The cyst may have one or more nuclei and chromatoid bars, but the bars are likely to be shorter and thicker and to have splintered ends. The cytoplasm is rather coarse. Young cysts have a large glycogen mass.

The ripe cyst of *E. coli* (Fig. 19–3) is usually larger (10 to 30 microns) than that of *E. histolytica* and usually has eight nuclei with eccentric karyosomes. Rarely, *E. coli* cysts may possess 16 or 32 nuclei. The cytoplasm again is coarse, and the cell wall is heavier than that of *E. histolytica*. At times some *E. coli* cysts fail to take up the hematoxylin stain when the phosphotungstic acid hematoxylin method (p. 1111) is employed. With experience the differentiation of *E. coli* from *E. histolytica* is not too difficult, especially with the cysts and precysts.

Endolimax nana. *Endolimax nana* (Table 19–2; Figs. 19–3 [N–1, N–2], 19–4 i–l) is a nonpathogen. It is a small ameba and may be confused easily with cysts and trophozoites of the small race of *E. histolytica* and small *D. fragilis* trophozoites. As mentioned previously, it is not easy to distinguish between these organisms in wet preparations.

Trophozoites are motile by means of clear, hyaline pseudopods and tend to be unidirectional but budding. In unstained preparations they have a greenish coloration. Their cytoplasm is smooth and the cell wall is thin. In permanently stained smears (Figs. 19–3 N–1; 19–4 *k,l*) the nucleus has a thin membrane and a large karyosome, which may fill a considerable part of the nucleus. There is a clear area between the karyosome and the nuclear wall, giving the appearance of a halo. The size of the trophozoite is 8 to 12 microns.

The cyst (Figs. 19–3, 19–4 i–j) tends to vary in shape from round to oval and has a smooth cytoplasm with a moderately thick cell wall. It varies from 5 to 10 microns in diameter. There are two to four small nuclei with the same structure as in the trophozoite. In hematoxylin-stained smears the cysts of *E. nana* are not too difficult to distinguish from those of the small race *E. histolytica*. The cysts do not have chromatoid bars but may contain bacilliform bodies that stain in the same manner. Young cysts may show a glycogen mass which does not stain with hematoxylin but does with iodine.

Iodamoeba bütschlii. *Iodamoeba bütschlii* (Table 19–2; Fig. 19–3 I–1, I–2), commonly called the "iodine cyst," is a nonpathogenic ameba characterized by a tendency to contain a large glycogen inclusion in the cyst, which is refractile in saline wet mounts, stains brown with iodine and is unstained in hematoxylin preparations. The glycogen inclusion, which must be differentiated from refractile chromatoidal material as observed in unstained *E. histolytica* cysts, may be so large as to push the nucleus to one side of the cell. The nucleus has a large karyosome, which may be central or eccentric, and one may see bands (lining network with scattered chromatin) connecting the karyosome with the thin nuclear wall. The trophozoite varies in size from 6 to 20 microns and their motility is similar to that seen in *E. coli* trophozoites. When stained with hematoxylin they resemble *E. nana*. The fully formed cyst has a heavy cyst wall; the glycogen inclusion may or may not be present and it has one or two nuclei. The cysts are 5 to 20 microns in diameter. Cysts and trophozoites show volutin granules.

Dientamoeba fragilis. *Dientamoeba fragilis* (Tables 19–1, 19–2; Fig. 19–9) is considered to be a pathogen producing dientamebiasis, with the capacity to invade the mucosa of the intestine and possibly the appendix (Burrows *et al.*, 1954). No cyst formation has been observed. The trophozoite of *D. fragilis* is small (5 to 12 microns). It is a delicate organism with a smooth cytoplasm and thin cell wall and may have one but more frequently two nuclei. When two nuclei are present, they are frequently arranged at opposite ends of an oval trophozoite. The nucleus has a beaded karyosome with the beads arranged in a rosette. This organism may be found in formed stools on occasions but is more frequently observed in mushy and/or liquid stools and in cultures from cases of diarrhea. Trophozoites move by extending angular pseudopodia, but when resting they are perfectly spherical and cystlike in their appearance.

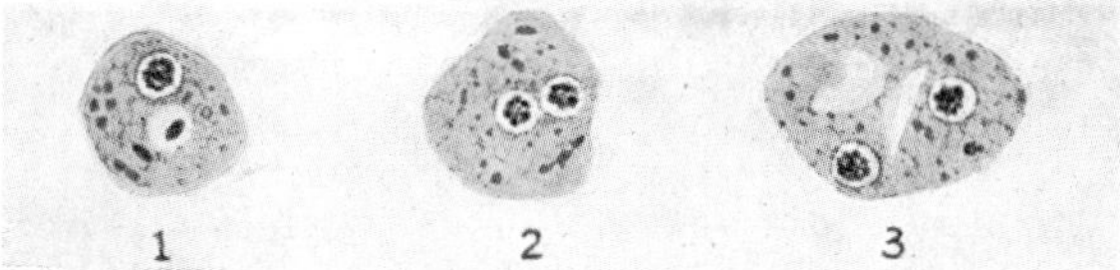

Figure 19–9. *Dientamoeba fragilis. 1,* Uninucleate amebae; *2, 3,* binucleate amebae. (After Dobell and O'Connor in Craig, C. F., Amebiasis and Amebic Dysentery. Springfield, Ill., Charles C Thomas.)

Miscellaneous Amebae

***Acanthamoeba castellanii (Hartmanella castellanii) and Naegleria* sp.** The free-living amebae, *A, castellanii* and *Naegleria* sp., once thought to be harmless, have been shown in recent years to produce a rapidly fatal amebic meningoencephalitis known as acanthamebiasis (Culbertson *et al.*, 1965; Patras and Andujar, 1966). Amebae occur in the pus and necrotic material covering the meninges and in the necrotic material of the brain. The portal of entry for the amebae is the nasal mucosa-olfactory bulb route. Culture methods for *A. castellanii* are available for body fluids and tissues. Animal inoculation of suspected materials is suggested.

STOOL CYTOLOGY AND NONPARASITIC OBJECTS

A myriad of nonparasitic objects (Fig. 19–97) appear in stool specimens. Among those which may be mistaken for amebae are yeast cells, macrophages, various white blood cells, epithelial cells, starch granules, and *Blastocystis hominis*. Once must learn to recognize these in various types of preparations as a prelude to parasite studies.

Yeast cells (Fig. 19–97 [7, 8]) have a thick wall, are refractile, and in hematoxylin-stained preparations appear to have a nucleus. Macrophages (Fig. 19–97 [2]) are likely to be troublesome, since they are motile and ingest red blood cells. Their nuclear structure, however, is quite different and can be used for differentiation, especially when stained with hematoxylin. In addition, they contain numerous foreign bodies. White blood cells, particularly polymorphonuclear leukocytes (pus cells) (Fig. 19–97 [3]), must not be mistakenly identified as amebic cysts since the former show nuclei which resemble those of *E. histolytica*. Plasma cells (Fig. 19–97 [5]) and epithelial cells (Fig. 19–97 [4])—both squamous and columnar—have a single nucleus and resemble amebic trophozoites.

The presence of certain structures in the stool, such as Charcot-Leyden (C-L) crystals (Figs. 19–7; 19–97 [11]), which are the crystalline remains of eosinophils, has been considered suggestive of *E. histolytica* infection. However, the structures occur also in the absence of amebae. Other crystals may be seen in stools. Refractile starch granules (Fig. 19–97 [28–31]) resemble amebic cysts when unstained, but iodine renders them blue, blue-black, or purple. Air bubbles (Fig. 19–97 [14]) and oil droplets (Fig. 19–97 [15]) must not be mistaken for amebic cysts.

Blastocystis hominis (Figs. 19–10, 19–11, 19–97 [6]) is a yeast-like organism that occurs frequently in the digestive tract of man. It is nonpathogenic but bears a close enough resemblance to protozoan cysts to cause some difficulty; therefore, it deserves special attention. It may be ovoid or spherical and 10 to 15 microns in diameter. The cytoplasm is hyaline and refractile and is enclosed in a membrane resembling a cyst wall. The outer wall of the cytoplasm is often differentiated, making the cell resemble a double-walled cyst. This outer layer contains granules and may have one or more structures resembling nuclei. The center portion of the cell is amorphous and resembles a large vacuole. One may also see dividing forms, which exhibit considerable variation in size and shape. One may destroy *B. hominis* by emulsifying the stool in water (Haakanson's phenomenon). In iodine-stained preparations the nuclei are stained and the central area may be brown. In hematoxylin-stained preparations the central area is gray and the periphery unstained except for the granules and nuclei. *Blastocystis hominis* may multiply in stool cultures for ameba studies.

The Intestinal Ciliates (Ciliata)

Balantidium coli. The most important ciliate that may be found in the human digestive tract is *Balantidium coli*. Balantidiasis may be asymptomatic, or it may produce severe diarrhea and dysentery indistinguishable clinically from acute amebic dysentery. Lesions may appear that are similar to those produced in amebiasis. Infection occurs through ingestion of cysts.

Balantidium coli (Table 19–1; Fig. 19–11 [10, 11]) is a large organism. Trophozoites vary

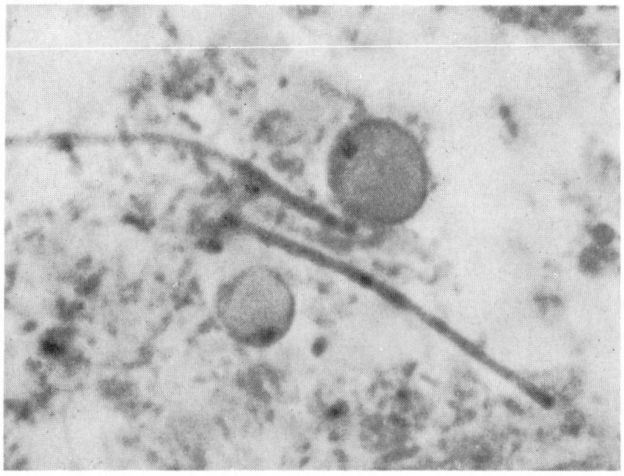

Figure 19–10. *Blastocystis hominis* in fecal smear showing the large, amorphous central area with nuclear staining material on the periphery of the cell. Modified Mallory's phosphotungstic acid stain. × 2500.

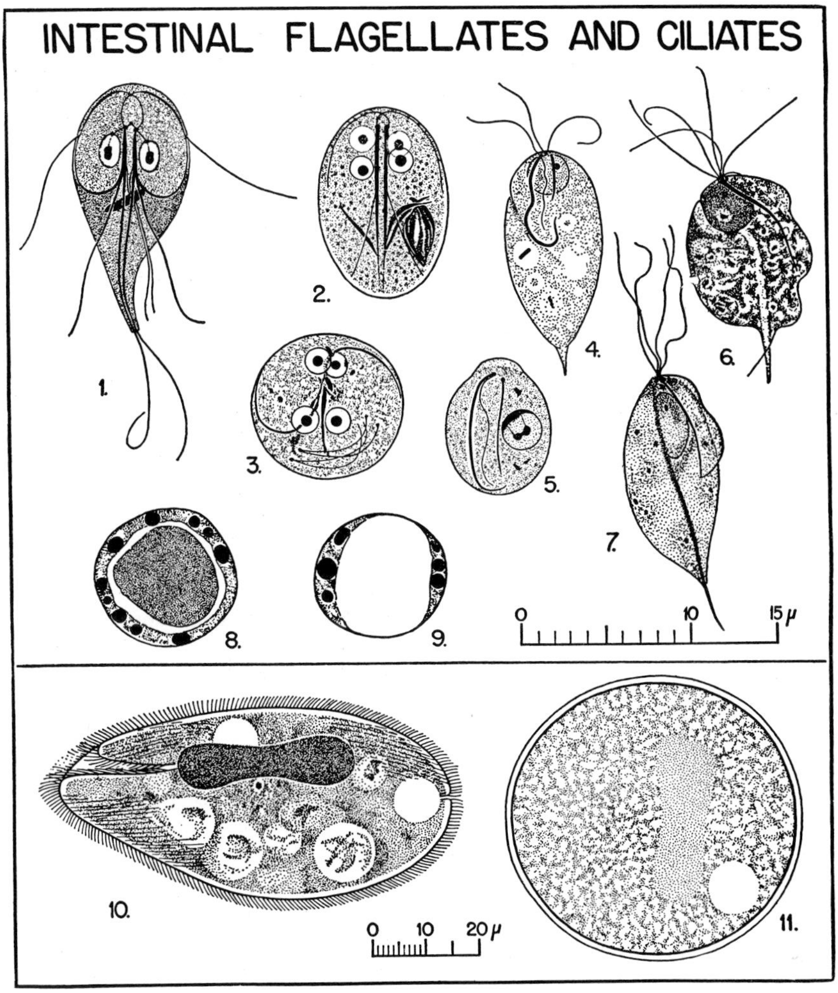

Figure 19–11. *1,* Iron-hematoxylin stained trophozoite of *Giardia lamblia. 2,* Iron-hematoxylin stained cyst of *G. lamblia. 3,* Iron-hematoxylin stained cyst of *G. lamblia,* end-view. *4,* Iron-hematoxylin stained trophozoite of *Chilomastix mesnili. 5,* Iron-hematoxylin stained cyst of *C. mesnili. 6,* Iron-hematoxylin stained trophozoite of *Trichomonas hominis. 7,* Iron-hematoxylin stained trophozoite of *T. vaginalis. 8,* Iron-hematoxylin stained *Blastocystis hominis. 9,* Unstained *B. hominis. 10,* Trophozoite of *Balantidium coli. 11,* Unstained cyst of *B. coli* (From Hunter, G. W., Frye, W. W., and Swartzwelder, J. C.: A Manual of Tropical Medicine. 4th edition.)

from 50 to 100 microns in length and from 40 to 60 microns in width and move by means of cilia, which are of uniform length and cover the entire organism. They exhibit a directional, tumbling motion. The organism is more pointed at the anterior end. *Balantidium coli* has two nuclei, a kidney-shaped macronucleus, and a small, spherical micronucleus.

Balantidium coli forms a cyst of 45 to 65 microns, which is round, with a thick cell wall having a double outline. Young cysts contain macro- and micronuclei and a single contractile vacuole, and one can often see movement inside the cyst wall.

The identification of *B. coli* trophozoites in a fecal preparation is not difficult, but it may require the examination of several samples with the low power lens to find the organism. It must be differentiated from ciliates which may be found as contaminants in stools. These ciliates have cilia of varying lengths on each trophozoite.

The Intestinal Flagellates (Mastigophora)

The flagellates are motile protozoa. The three most common species are *Giardia lamblia* (Fig. 19–11 [1–3]), *Chilomastix mesnili* (Fig. 19–11 [4–5]) and *Trichomonas hominis* (Fig. 19–11 [6], 19–12). Occasionally one may find *Embadomonas intestinalis* and *Enteromonas hominis.* With the exception of *Giardia lamblia,* these protozoa are all considered nonpathogens.

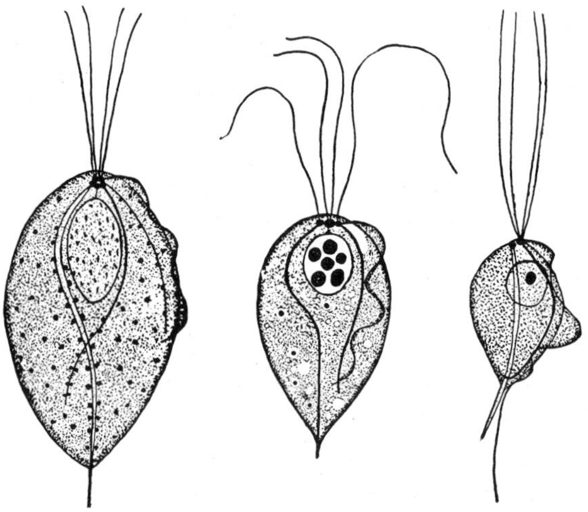

Figure 19–12. *Trichomonas vaginalis, Trichomonas tenax,* and *Trichomonas hominis.* × 2000. (Powell.)

Giardia lamblia. *Giardia lamblia* (Table 19–1; Fig. 19–11 [1–3]) trophozoite is a bilaterally symmetrical, pear-shaped organism with a broad, rounded anterior and a tapering posterior extremity. It is usually from 12 to 15 microns in length. There are a sucking disc, two nuclei, and fibrils across the two axostyles, which keep the organism rigid. Four pairs of flagella are present. Trophozoites are not usually found except in liquid stools of patients with diarrhea or upon purgation. When present they exhibit motility that resembles that of a leaf in a stream of water. When a purgative is used, some trophozoites become inactive.

Giardia lamblia produces giardiasis and lives high up in the intestinal tract; considerable evidence (mostly clinical) suggests that the trophozoites may be capable of producing inflammatory changes in the intestinal wall and diarrhea. Trophozoites of this parasite may be recovered in duodenal drainage or from the gallbladder. Proof of its primary role in gastrointestinal disease is available (Hoskin *et al.*, 1967; Moore *et al.*, 1969; Morbidity and Mortality, 1970).

Giardia lamblia forms a cyst, which is the most common structure present in stools. These are usually oval in shape. The cyst wall is smooth and well defined and the cytoplasm tends to shrink away from the wall. The cytoplasm is granular and contains two to four nuclei, which have a dense and comparatively large karyosome. Some of the structures of the trophozoite can be seen in the cyst, i.e., the axostyles, fibril, and the anterior and lateral flagella. The cyst is 9 to 12 microns in length. Sometimes the round cysts resemble and must be differentiated from those of small race *E. histolytica.* Young cysts may show a glycogen mass when stained with iodine. "Blue" *Giardia,* those staining blue with iodine, may be seen in stools. Routine *in vitro* culturing of *G. lamblia* is not feasible.

Chilomastix mesnili. *Chilomastix mesnili* is a small, nonpathogenic flagellate, which may be found as either the trophozoite or the cyst. The trophozoite is a small, pear-shaped organism 13 to 24 microns long (Fig. 19–11 [4]) and exhibits a spiral, jerking motion. The spiral groove is characteristic and there is no axostyle to keep the organism rigid. The cyst, which is also somewhat pear shaped, has a characteristic thickening at the narrow end. Internally there is an axoneme and a single, rather large nucleus. The cyst is 6.5 to 10 microns long (Fig. 19–11 [5]). In hematoxylin-stained preparations trophozoites and cysts resemble those of the small race of *E. histolytica.*

Trichomonas hominis. *Trichomonas hominis* is generally considered a nonpathogen, although it is occasionally found in considerable numbers in diarrheic stools. This organism does not form a cyst and accordingly is identified by finding the motile trophozoite in stool specimens. It is motile by means of a variable number of anterior flagella (three to five) and a single terminal flagellum. The terminal flagellum is an extension of an undulating membrane, which extends over most of the length of the organism. This undulating membrane can be seen under the microscope with reduced light and is diagnostic. The morphology of the organism is shown in Figs. 19–11 [6] and 19–12. A single nucleus and an axostyle which projects posteriorly are present. *Trichomonas hominis* may be cultured in several different media from feces. *Trichomonas vaginalis* may be present in situations in which stools have become contaminated by vaginal flow.

Other Trichomonads of Medical Importance

Trichomonas vaginalis. *Trichomonas vaginalis* (Table 19–1; Figs. 19–11 [7], 19–12) is frequently associated with persistent trichomonal vaginitis (trichomoniasis) and has been considered to have a causative role, especially by clinicians. The patient with *T. vaginalis* vaginitis presents signs of vaginal inflammation and complains of itching, burning, and discharge. The discharge exudes from the introitus and is frothy, creamy, yellowish, and acid and contains many vaginal epithelial cells, leukocytes, bacteria, and trichomonads. This is accompanied by inflammation over a considerable area. Infection in the urethra in the male also occurs and may be asymptomatic or symptomatic, resulting in some inflammation and discharge. The infection is probably transmitted by sexual contact.

In the female the diagnosis can usually be

made by collecting some of the frothy discharge with a speculum and emulsifying it in a drop of saline on a slide. A coverglass is applied and the preparation examined microscopically. Motile trichomonads (up to 27 microns in length) are easily seen when present. Specimens of vaginal discharge or material collected on a swab must be submitted to the laboratory in a small amount of saline (0.85 per cent NaCl) to prevent drying of the organisms. Dried smears on slides are unsatisfactory. *Trichomonas vaginalis* resembles *T. hominis* quite closely but is larger (Figs. 19–11 [6–7], 19–12). The organism can be cultured on special broth media (Kupferberg, 1955). *Trichomonas vaginalis* may occasionally be demonstrated with typical and atypical morphology in the urine of males and females.

Trichomonas tenax. *Trichomonas tenax* (a nonpathogen) is sometimes found in the mouth of individuals with oral disease or with poor dental hygiene (Fig. 19–12).

THE SYSTEMIC FLAGELLATES

A new nomenclature for the developmental stages of the hemoflagellates has been established (Hoare and Wallace, 1966) and is based upon the position of the flagellum (mastigote or whip) as follows: "amastigote" for the former "leishmanial stage" (no external flagellum is present); "promastigote" for the former "leptomonad stage" (flagellum arises from a kinetoplast in front of the nucleus and emerges at the anterior end); "epimastigote" for the former "crithidial stage" (flagellum arises from a juxtanuclear kinetoplast and emerges at the side of the body; an undulating membrane is present); "trypomastigote" for the former trypanosome stage (flagellum arises from a posterior kinetoplast and emerges from the side of the body; an undulating membrane is present). There are additional new terms which do not apply to medical parasitology. The older terminology has been retained for this edition.

Genus Leishmania

The several species that comprise this genus are apparently closely related to the trypanosomes.

They grow (as a flagellate form) at room temperature in sterile citrated blood placed in N.N.N. (Nicolle, Novy, McNeal) (Hunter *et al.*, 1966, p. 852) or Offutt's medium. Incubation for two to three weeks in the dark (in foil-wrapped tubes) is necessary before the cultures can be considered negative. Animal inoculation may be helpful.

Leishmania donovani. *Leishmania donovani* (Table 19–1; Figs. 19–13, 19–14, 19–15) is the cause of kala-azar, or visceral leishmaniasis, an important and common disease in India and certain other areas. When stained with Wright's stain, the Leishman-Donovan bodies are round or oval, light blue structures, 2 or 3 microns in diameter, with two distinct reddish purple chromatin masses, one large and pale (trophonucleus), the other small and deeply stained (blepharoplast) (Figs. 19–13, 19–15). A large vacuole is present. The parasites, which lie chiefly within endothelial cells, are especially abundant in the spleen and liver. Splenic, liver, and sternal punctures have been used for diagnosis but are not without danger (Figs. 19–14, 19–15). They may also be found, although with less certainty, in material obtained by puncture of superficial lymph nodes. Although they have been seen within endothelial leukocytes in the peripheral blood, particularly late in the disease, they are extremely difficult to find in ordinary blood films. The search may be greatly facilitated by concentrating the leukocytes. The leukocytes will form a whitish layer on top of the solidly packed erythrocytes. They should be skimmed off with a capillary pipette, spread on a slide, air dried, and stained with Wright's or fixed in methyl alcohol and stained with Giemsa's stain. Transfusion transmission of kala-azar is possible.

A leishmanin skin test (Montenegro reaction) is positive after recovery but not during active infection. A complement fixation and an agglutination test are available.

NAPIER'S SERUM TEST FOR KALA-AZAR. This is a nonspecific precipitin test. Place 1 ml. of clear serum in a small test tube. Add 1 drop of commercial formaldehyde and shake the tube thoroughly. In 3 to 20 minutes the serum will coagulate and become white and opalescent if it has been obtained from a patient who has untreated kala-azar. Normal serum remains clear and fluid. Serum of patients who have leprosy, tuberculosis, or malaria gives a somewhat similar but less pronounced reaction.

The fungus disease, histoplasmosis, may be confused with kala-azar; however, the latter disease probably does not occur in the United States, while the former occurs over a considerable area of the United States.

Other Species of Leishmania

Leishmania tropica. *Leishmania tropica* (Table 19–1) resembles the parasite just described. It is found lying intracellularly in granulation tissue in cases of Delhi boil or Oriental sore (cutaneous leishmaniasis). Infections with *L. tropica* provide the patient with a lasting

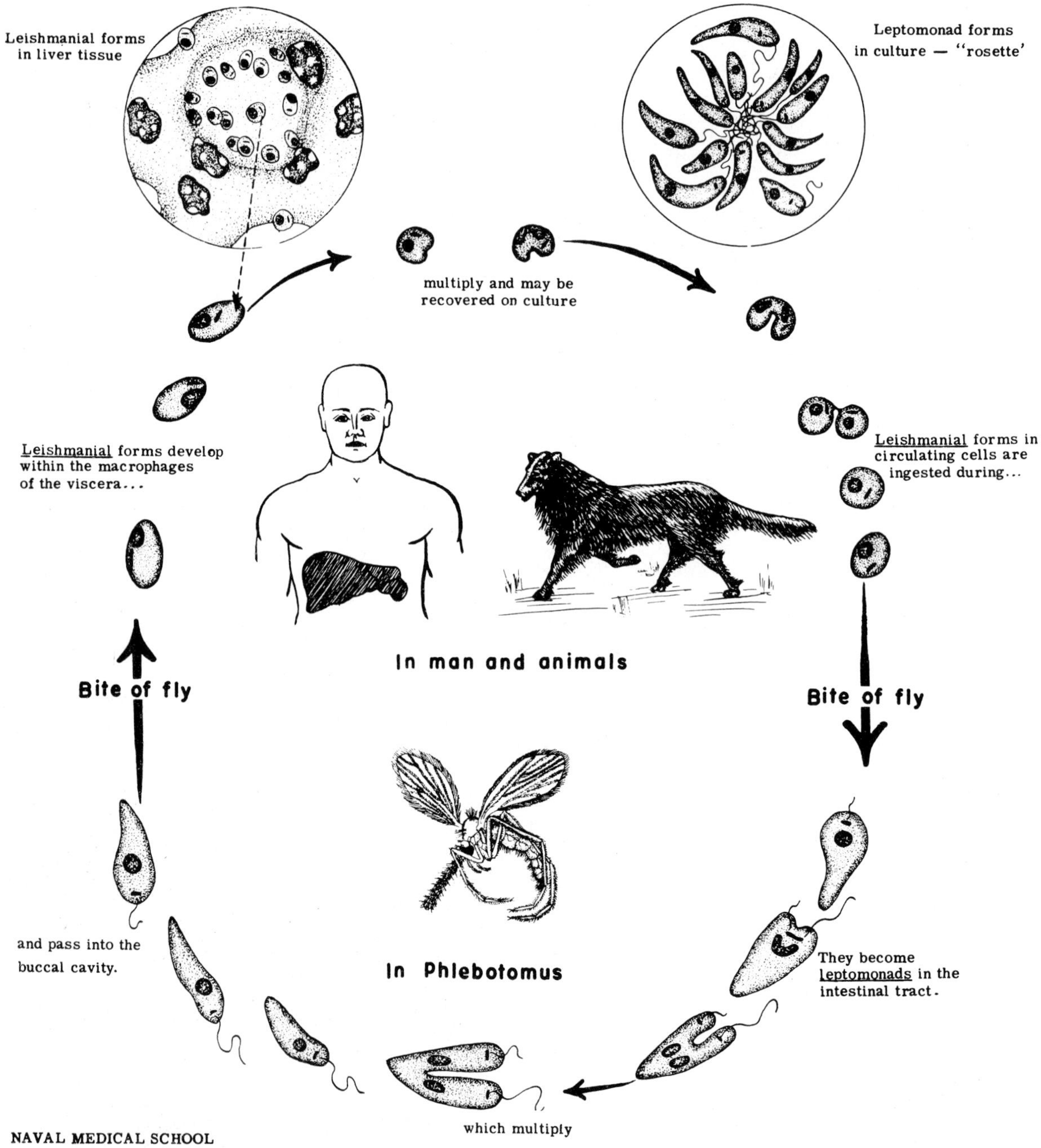
Leishmanial forms in liver tissue
Leptomonad forms in culture — "rosette'
multiply and may be recovered on culture
Leishmanial forms develop within the macrophages of the viscera...
Leishmanial forms in circulating cells are ingested during...
In man and animals
Bite of fly
Bite of fly
In Phlebotomus
They become leptomonads in the intestinal tract.
and pass into the buccal cavity.
which multiply
NAVAL MEDICAL SCHOOL

Figure 19–13. Life cycle of *Leishmania donovani.* (From Medical Protozoology and Helminthology. U.S. Naval Medical School, National Naval Medical Center, Bethesda, Maryland, 1965.)

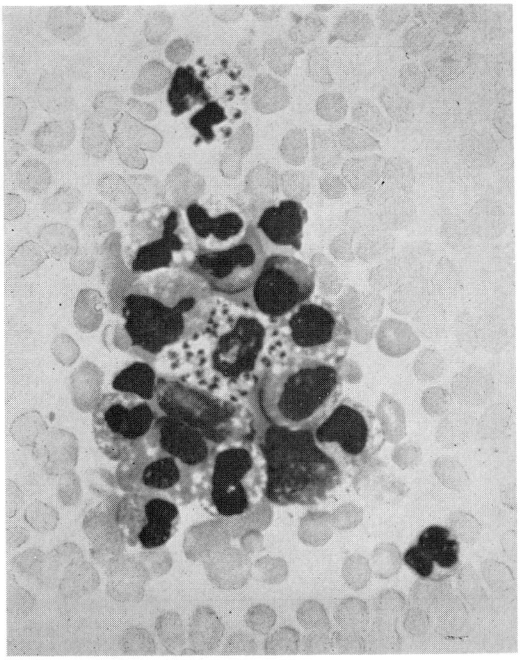

Figure 19–14. Smear from splenic pulp showing in the center a large mononuclear cell the cytoplasm of which is filled with Leishman-Donovan bodies. (A.F.I.P. No. 2186891.)

immunity, and in endemic areas children may be vaccinated. Stained smears may be made from the margins of the ulcer.

Leishmania braziliensis. A variety, sometimes described as a separate species, *Leishmania braziliensis* (Table 19–1), or *Leishmania tropica americana,* produces a disease known as American leishmaniasis, chiclero's disease, uta, or espundia. Organisms are recovered from primary ulcers or from the ulcers of espundia, a very chronic form of mucocutaneous leishmaniasis that occurs in South and Central America. A leishmanin skin test (Montenegro reaction) becomes positive early in *L. tropica* and *L. braziliensis* infections.

Genus Trypanosoma

Trypanosomes found in the blood plasma are easily recognized, but accurate determination of species is difficult and may be impossible on the basis of their shape alone. They are elongated, spindle-shaped bodies, the average length of different species varying from 10 to 70 microns. Along one side runs a delicate undulating membrane, the free edge of which appears to be somewhat longer than the attached edge, thus throwing it into folds. Near the middle is a comparatively pale-staining nucleus and near the posterior end is a smaller, more deeply staining chromatin mass, the blepharoplast. A number of coarse, deeply staining granules – chromatophores – may be scattered through the cytoplasm. A flagellum arises in the blepharoplast, passes along the free edge of the undulating membrane, and continues anteriorly as a free flagellum. These details of structure are shown in Figures 19–16 and 19–17.

At least three species of *Trypanosoma* are pathogenic for man. These are pathogenic to a variable degree for antelope and other game animals, which serve as reservoirs from which man may become infected through the agency of the insect host.

Trypanosoma gambiense and T. rhodesiense. *Trypanosoma gambiense* and *T. rhodesiense* trypanosomal forms (Table 19–1; Fig. 19–16) multiply by longitudinal binary fission in the peripheral blood. They can be seen in stained thin and thick films with a medium-power objective, but are best studied with an oil-immersion objective. Buffy coat preparations of citrated blood may aid recovery of organisms (see p. 1114). The parasites are more abundant in the fluid obtained by aspirating a lymph node with a large hypodermic needle. In the late stages of African trypanosomiasis (sleeping sickness) they can be found also in the cerebrospinal fluid. Diagnosis may rest upon culturing procedures (N.N.N. or Offutt's media), animal inoculation, or serologic testing. Trypanosomiasis is transmitted by a biting tsetse fly, *Glossina.* The chief difference between *T. rhodesiense* and *T. gambiense* is the situation of the nucleus close to, or even posterior to, the blepharoplast in the former.

Trypanosoma cruzi. *Trypanosoma cruzi*

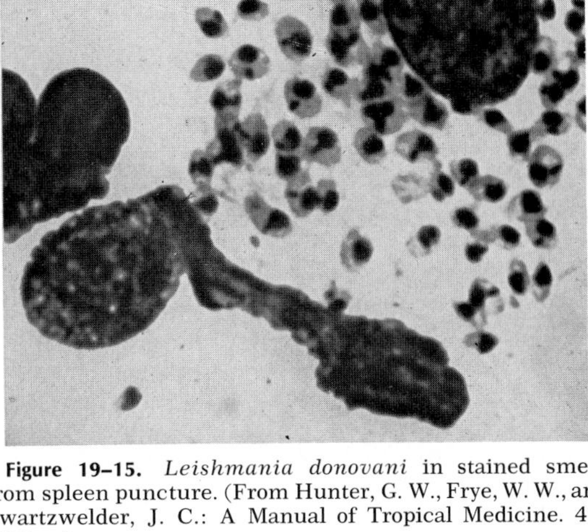

Figure 19–15. *Leishmania donovani* in stained smear from spleen puncture. (From Hunter, G. W., Frye, W. W., and Swartzwelder, J. C.: A Manual of Tropical Medicine. 4th edition.)

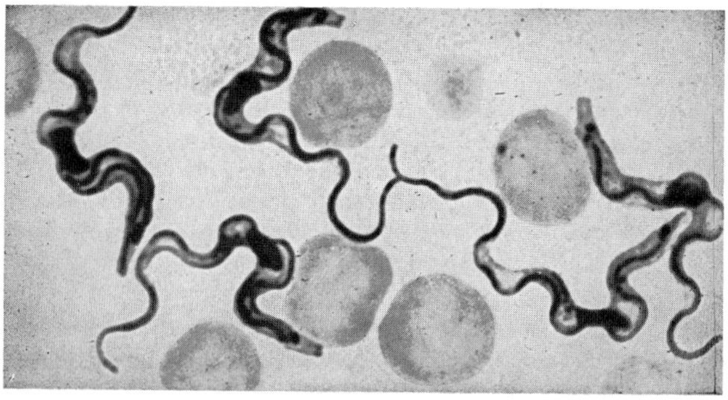

Figure 19–16. *Trypanosoma gambiense* in stained blood film; × about 2000. (Krall.)

(Table 19–1) is the cause of American trypanosomiasis or Chagas' disease. In the febrile stage of the disease the trypanosomal form of the organism is found in the peripheral blood as "C" and "U" shapes, but they do not multiply in this site as do the African species. Its average length is about 20 microns. Diagnosis is as outlined for the trypanosomes above, but xenodiagnosis, with laboratory-reared reduviid bugs, is helpful. The Machado-Guerreiro complement fixation test may be used. Transfusion infections have been recorded.

The life cycle (Fig. 19–17) is very complicated. In the vertebrate host multiplication takes place in the cardiac and other muscles and certain internal organs in which the parasites assume forms resembling *Leishmania donovani.* The early phase of the flagellated stage is passed into the blood plasma. The insect host by which the trypanosome is transmitted to man is a large reduviid bug belonging to the genus *Panstrongylus,* and others. Reduviid bugs are found also in the United States. Packchanian (1943) demonstrated that a Texan strain *T. cruzi* was capable of infecting man with a disease clinically identical with Chagas' disease.

In endemic zones in Central and South America another trypanosome, *T. rangeli,* has been found in humans, but no evidence of pathogenicity or clinical symptoms have been observed. There are no intracellular forms as in *T. cruzi.*

THE SPOROZOA

A number of protozoa of the group belonging to the Sporozoa are parasitic, and there are two genera that contain species parasitic in man. These are *Isospora* and *Plasmodium,* the latter containing the causative agents of malaria in man. Each of the sporozoa has a life cycle involving propagation by means of sporulation. In some the life cycle is quite complex, involving sexual and asexual reproductive cycles (*Plasmodium*) (Fig. 19–20).

Isospora hominis. *Isospora hominis* (Table 19–1; Fig. 19–18) is a coccidian that has been found in human feces. Apparently this parasite causes no particular disturbance, although a mucoid diarrhea and distress may develop. Diagnosis of isoporiasis depends on the recognition of oocysts in the feces. These are colorless, ovoid bodies, measuring about 14 by 33 microns. They have a clear-cut, definite wall, which usually consists of two or more layers. When they first pass out of the body, the protoplasm is unsegmented and appears as a rounded, granular mass that does not fill the cyst, as in Fig. 19–18 *a.*

Genus Plasmodium

Although malaria is now rare in the United States except in service men returned from Viet Nam, it is still a very important disease in much of the world and is responsible directly or indirectly for much debilitation and death. Drug-resistant strains of malaria, especially *P. falciparum,* may confront the clinician. In the U.S. we have "anophelism without malaria."

Four species of the protozoan *Plasmodium,* the generic name of the etiologic agent, are known, viz., *vivax, falciparum, malariae,* and *ovale* (Table 19–1; Figs. 19–19 through 25). *P. ovale* is encountered less frequently, as it is found only in East and West Africa and the Philippines. Simian species of *Plasmodium* have been recovered in man. Transmission from man to man is through the bite of certain species of infected female *Anopheles* mosquitoes; nevertheless, there are other means, such as congenital infection (McQuay *et al.,* 1967), use of contaminated needles by drug addicts, and particularly by blood transfusion. Non-mosquito-induced malaria develops from the introduction of the mature schizonts into the recipient's blood stream. Merozoites from within the transfused schizonts are freed and enter the recipient's erythrocytes to begin the

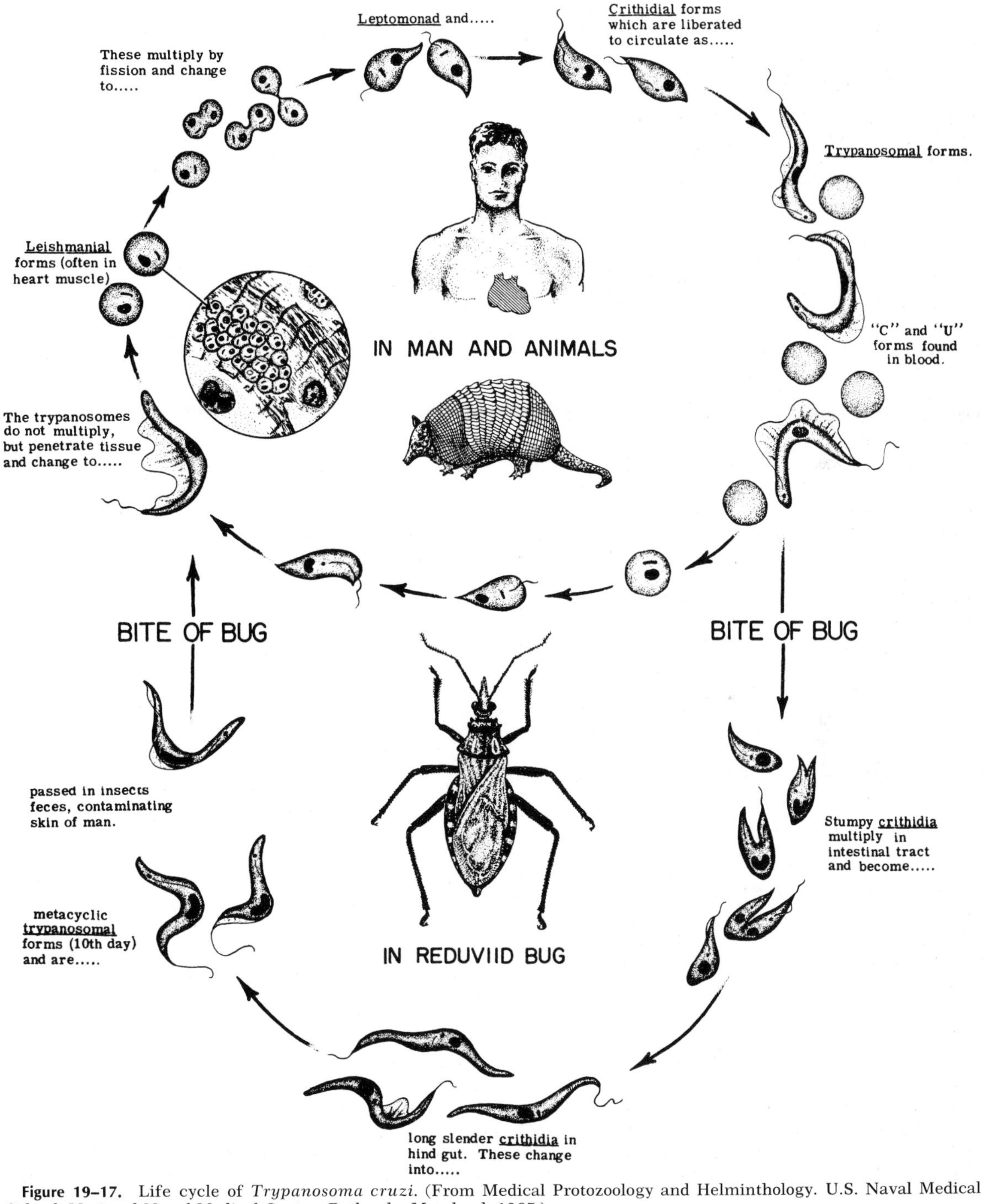
Leptomonad and.....
Crithidial forms which are liberated to circulate as.....
These multiply by fission and change to.....
Trypanosomal forms.
Leishmanial forms (often in heart muscle)
"C" and "U" forms found in blood.
IN MAN AND ANIMALS
The trypanosomes do not multiply, but penetrate tissue and change to.....
BITE OF BUG
BITE OF BUG
passed in insects feces, contaminating skin of man.
Stumpy crithidia multiply in intestinal tract and become.....
metacyclic trypanosomal forms (10th day) and are.....
IN REDUVIID BUG
long slender crithidia in hind gut. These change into.....

Figure 19–17. Life cycle of *Trypanosoma cruzi.* (From Medical Protozoology and Helminthology. U.S. Naval Medical School, National Naval Medical Center, Bethesda, Maryland, 1965.)

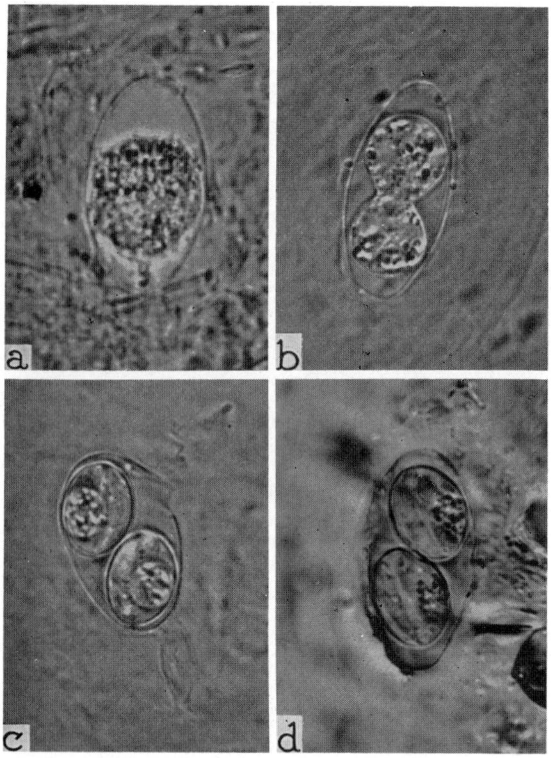

Figure 19–18. *Isospora hominis* (× 1000). *a*, Oocyst in stool at time of passage. *b*, Beginning formation of two sporocysts. *c*, Sporocysts formed (36 hours); large residual mass; sporozoites not completely formed; oocyst wall ruptured by pressure. *d*, Mature oocyst (56 hours). (From Magath: Amer. J. Trop. Med., March, 1935.)

asexual cycle. The disease, although generally referred to as malaria, may be specifically designated by the name of the etiologic agent (Table 19–3). Multiple infections are possible but do not occur regularly.

The life cycle of the malaria parasite in man is shown in Figure 19–20. Man is the intermediate host in whom the asexual cycle, schizogony, occurs, and the mosquito is the definitive host in which gametogony and sporogony take place.

Man becomes infected as sporozoites from infected mosquitoes are injected into the peripheral circulation during the bite. Pre-erythrocytic development takes place in the parenchymal cells of the liver during the following eight to 12 days, and there is a progressive development through several stages that eventually results in the development of numerous merozoites through schizogony (splitting). These merozoites initiate the erythrocytic cycle by rupturing from the cell and penetrating red cells or liver parenchymal cells (except for *P. falciparum*) to continue the exoerythrocytic phase. Both pre- and exoerythrocytic phases constitute tissue schizogony. Exoerythrocytic and erythrocytic development continue simultaneously in the body, except for *P. falciparum*, and the exoerythrocytic development may be responsible for relapse malaria.

Once the asexual phase of the cycle is begun in the red cells, the parasite develops, beginning with ring forms and progressing through the trophozoite to the early and mature schizonts. This process, known as erythrocytic schizogony, is a 48- to 72-hour process, depending upon the species, and begins with a primary splitting of the chromatin, continuing until merozoites are formed. These merozoites rupture from the mature schizonts and penetrate new red cells. This rupture of the red blood cells is associated with the chill and fever that characterize clinical malaria. After several asexual cycles some tend to become sexually differentiated forms, the male or microgametocyte and the female or macrogametocyte, while the majority continue the erythrocytic cycle. The gametocytes do not contribute to the production of symptoms and remain alive as long as the red cell lives, about 120 days. At times gametocytes will remain in the blood after treatment, especially when schizontocidal drugs are employed. The paroxysm, chill and fever, is somewhat characteristic and occurs every 72 hours with *P. malariae* infections but at 48-hour intervals with the other three species. Different broods of organisms may give irregular paroxysms, which may be quotidian rather than strictly tertian or quartan.

Only the gametocytes are infective for the mosquito. In the stomach of the female mosquito they mature as microgametes and macrogametes (gametogony). The microgametes exflagellate and fertilize the macrogamete to become a zygote. The zygote elongates and becomes actively motile and is called an ookinete. This form penetrates the stomach wall and rounds up on the outside of the wall to become an oocyst. As it matures to a sporocyst (sporogony), slender sporozoites develop,

Table 19–3. MALARIA CLASSIFICATION

Plasmodium	CLASSIC NOMENCLATURE	MODERN NOMENCLATURE
vivax	benign tertian malaria	vivax malaria
ovale	ovale malaria	ovale malaria
malariae	quartan malaria	malariae malaria or quartan malaria
falciparum	estivoautumnal (EA); subtertian malaria; malignant tertian	falciparum malaria

Table 19–4. MALARIA

TWO SEPARATE ENTITIES	
FALCIPARUM	VIVAX OR QUARTAN
Only cells containing young parasites (or gametocytes) seen in peripheral blood. Older stages in red cells adherent to endothelial lining, interfering with function (anoxia) of organism involved; hence, protean symptoms	All infected cells circulate freely and continually
Paroxysmal symptoms with schizogony; anemia from blood destruction	
Adequate treatment controls attack	
Cured because pre-erythrocytic stage is exhausted with primary attack	May relapse because pre-erythrocytic stage reseeds liver cells. Relapse of parasitism occurs when immunity decreases
Gametocytes appear late; persist some days	Gametocytes only with asexual forms

and these break out and migrate to the salivary glands where they are retained until the next blood meal, at which time they enter the blood of the new human host.

Differentiation of Species. Walker (1952) has given a concept of the basic facts of malaria that has an important bearing on the recognition of the species under the microscope as shown in Table 19–4.

Species diagnosis is important according to Walker to insure the immediate treatment of falciparum malaria (although strains resistant to certain drugs have recently been encountered), in which completely unpredictable symptoms may develop. Furthermore, in vivax malaria it is useful to be able to estimate from the observation of the developmental stage of the majority of the parasites when the next paroxysm may be expected.

Differential diagnosis of malaria may be made by examining either thin or thick films (see p. 1114) or saponin-treated whole blood (Keffer, 1966), but one must be cautious with scanty infections. Figures 19–19 and 19–21 through 19–24 show the parasites as they are seen within red cells in thin film preparations. Do not be misled by platelets on top of erythrocytes. Schüffner's granules on the red blood cell in *P. vivax* may be difficult to detect unless staining time in Giemsa's is extended from 40 minutes to $1\frac{1}{2}$ to 3 hours. The blood picture of the stages of the parasites found for *P. vivax*, *P. malariae*, and *P. ovale* changes as the disease progresses through each 48- or 72-hour cycle. Just prior to the paroxysm, most forms in the red blood cells are at the late schizont stage. After the paroxysm, most of the parasitized cells harbor the signet rings, while midway between paroxysms, older trophozoites and early schizonts tend to be the predominant forms.

In brief, thin film diagnosis of species is not too difficult and can be accomplished if the following criteria are employed:

	P. vivax	*P. malariae*	*P. falciparum*
Infected red cell			
Size	Increased	No change	No change
Shape	Irregular	No change	No change
Inclusions	Schüffner's granules	None	Maurer's spots
Parasite			
Hematin granules	Scanty	Abundant	None (except in gametocytes)
Forms seen	All (variety in one film)	All (variety in one film)	Ring forms and gametocytes (crescents) at times; or all forms in some fatal cases

Thick film diagnosis is a little more challenging, because the red cells are destroyed and the parasites are not spread out; however, more positive findings will be reported with thick films. For *P. vivax* the characteristic form for diagnosis is the trophozoite, which assumes a variety of shapes. The red blood cell, with its Schüffner's granules, has been destroyed. Matured schizonts show a cluster of 12 to 24 (av. 16) or more merozoites. *Plasmodium malariae* in thick films shows compact trophozoites with much hematin pigment. Mature schizonts have six to 12 merozoites. In the case of *P. falciparum*, the forms older than the signet rings leave the peripheral blood, except the gametocytes. Parasites that show purplish red chromatin and blue cytoplasm are stained properly. White cells can be used as a guide to staining (Fig. 19–25).

Blood from a suspected individual should be taken at six- to eight-hour intervals, and one need not necessarily wait until the rise in temperature before taking the blood. (For the technique of making and staining thin blood films, see below and Chapter 4, The Blood.) Thin and thick films can be made from the red cell layer collected immediately below the buffy coat in citrated or similarly treated blood. Serologic tests are available through each state health laboratory.

(Text continues on page 1050.)

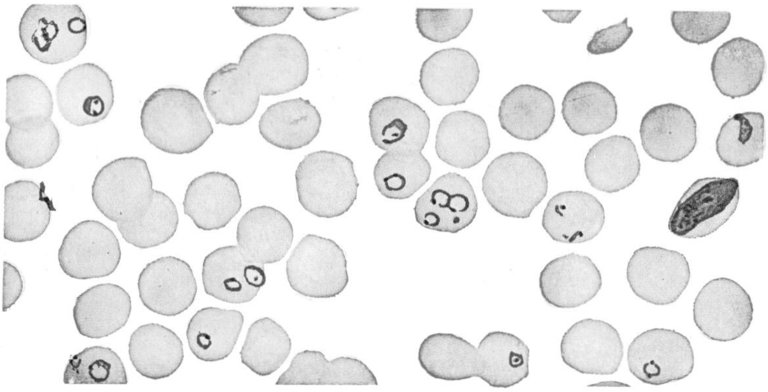

Estivo-autumnal malaria; exact reproduction of a portion of a field showing an exceptionally large number of parasites.

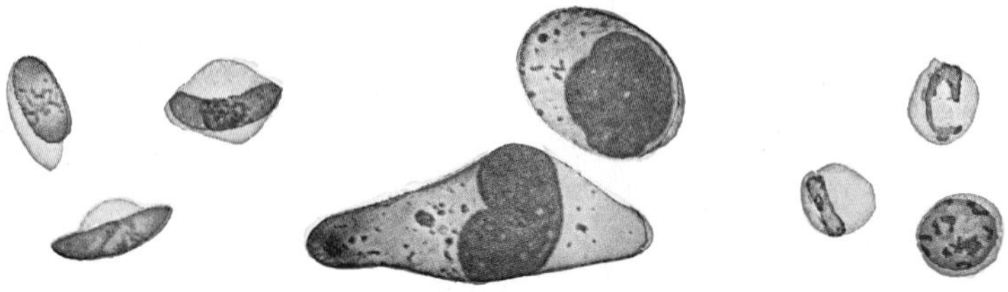

Estivo-autumnal gametocytes. Leukocytes with engulfed pigment. Quartan parasites.

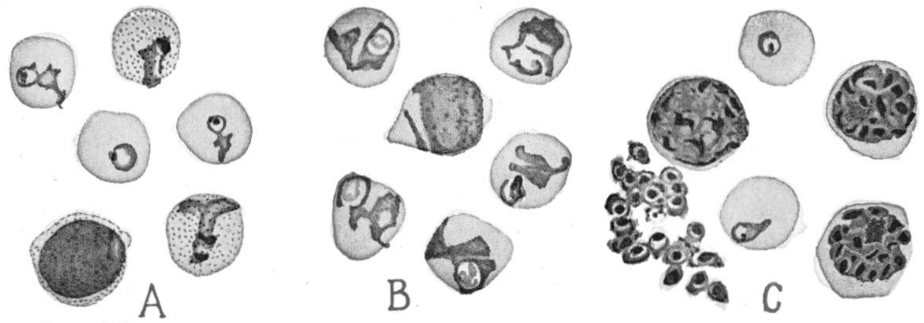

Figure 19–23. *Plasmodium falciparum.* *1,* Very young ring form trophozoite. 2, Double infection of single cell with young cyte from two slides. *B,* Twenty-four hours after chill; five half-grown parasites and one gametocyte. *C,* During chill; one presegmenter, two segmenters, a cluster of freshly liberated merozoites, and two very young parasites, from one slide. (J. W. Rennell, pinx.)

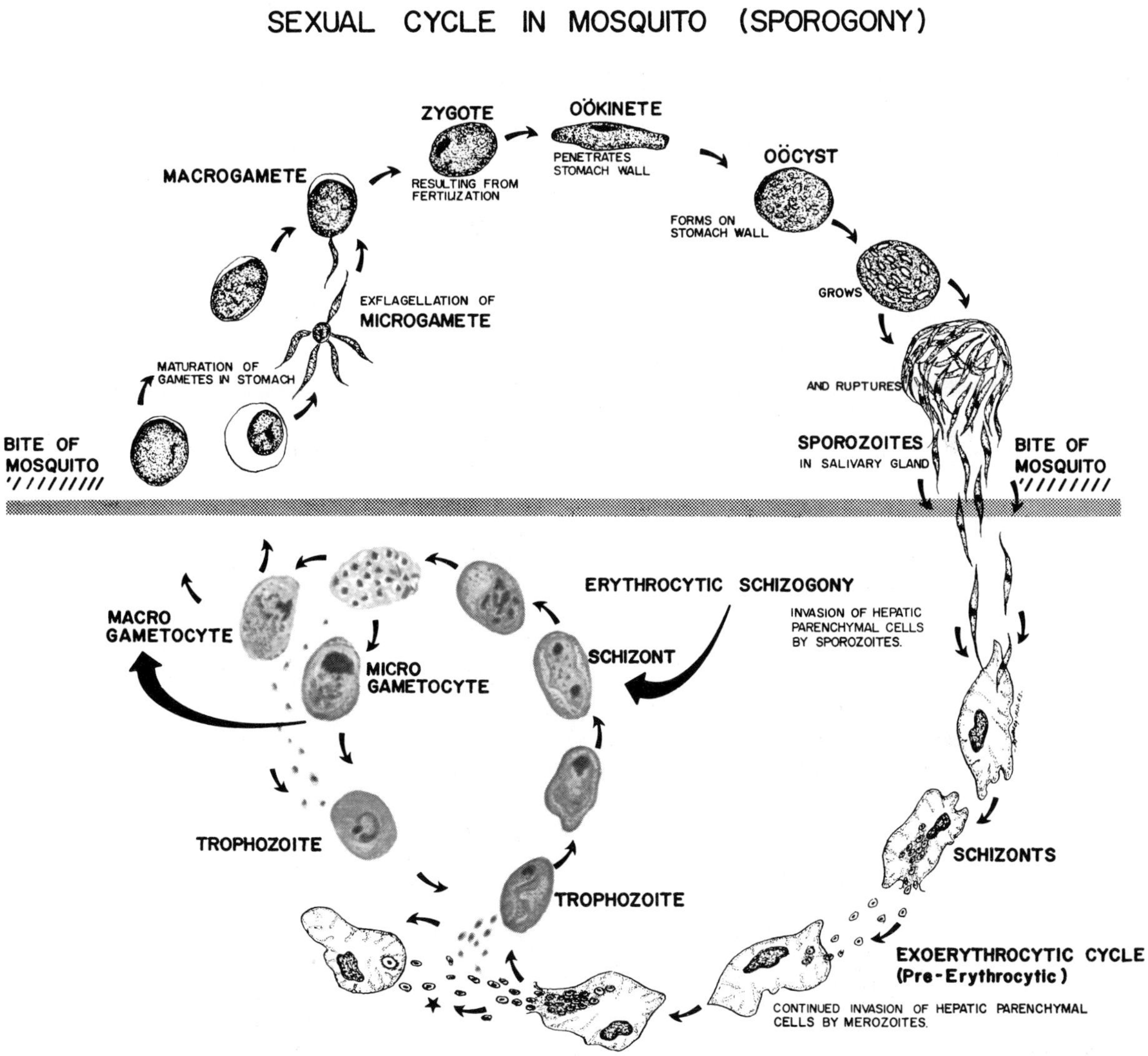

Figure 19–20. Life cycle of malarial parasites. *Note:* Exoerythrocytic cycle after invasion of red blood cells postulated in some human infections. (From Medical Protozoology and Helminthology. U.S. Naval Medical School, National Naval Medical Center, Bethesda, Maryland, 1965.)

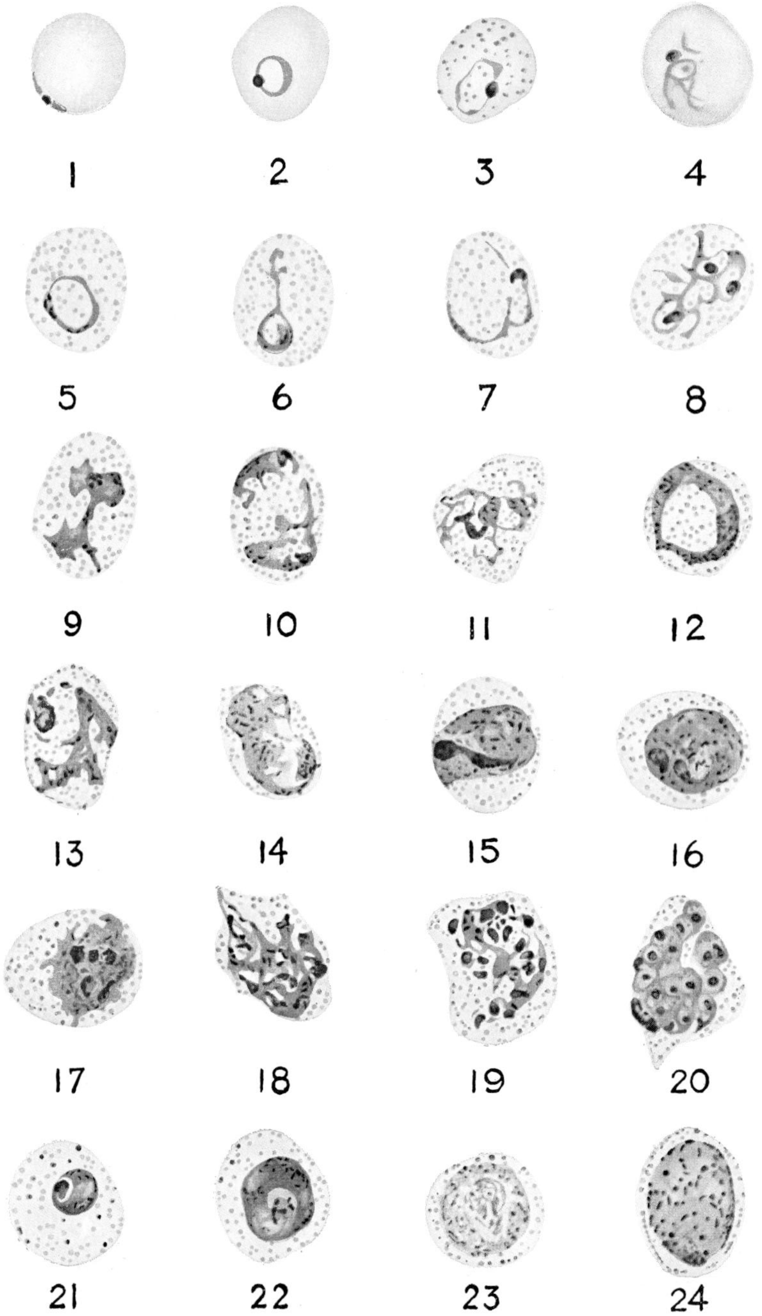

Figure 19–21. *Plasmodium vivax. 1.* Normal-size erythrocyte with marginal ring form trophozoite. *2.* Young signet-ring form of trophozoite in macrocyte. *3.* Slightly older ring form trophozoite in erythrocyte showing basophilic stippling. *4.* Polychromatophilic erythrocyte containing young tertian parasite with pseudopodia. *5.* Ring form of trophozoite showing pigment in cytoplasm of an enlarged cell containing Schüffner's stippling. This stippling does not appear in all cells containing the growing and older forms of *Plasmodium vivax,* but it can be found with any stage from the fairly young ring form onward. *6* and *7.* Very tenuous medium trophozoite forms. *8.* Three ameboid trophozoites with fused cytoplasm. *9, 11, 12,* and *13.* Older ameboid trophozoites in process of development. *10.* Two ameboid trophozoites in one cell. *14.* Mature trophozoite. *15.* Mature trophozoite with chromatin apparently in process of division. *16, 17, 18,* and *19.* Schizonts showing progressive steps in division (presegmenting schizonts). *20.* Mature schizont. *21* and *22.* Developing gametocytes. *23.* Mature microgametocyte. *24.* Mature macrogametocyte. (From Wilcox, Aimee: Manual for the Microscopical Diagnosis of Malaria in Man. Bulletin No. 180, National Institute of Health, 1942.)

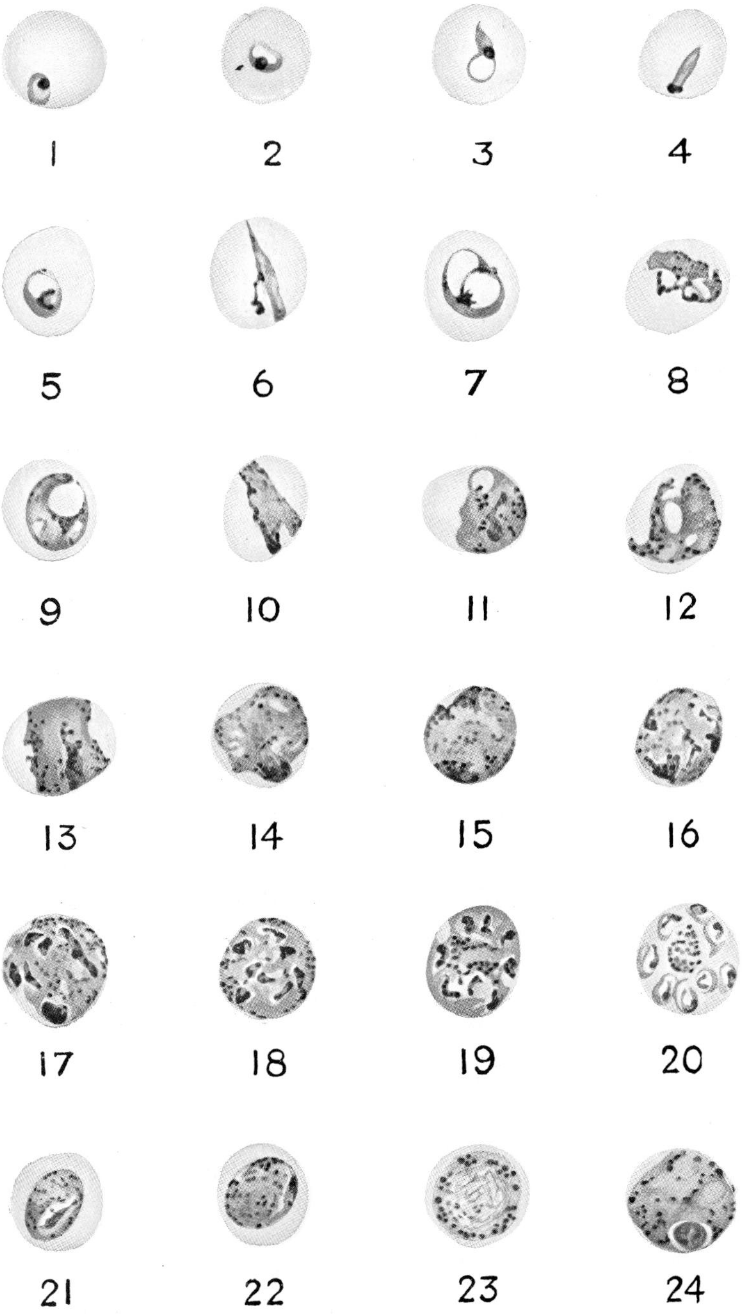

Figure 19–22. *Plasmodium malariae*. *1*. Young ring form trophozoite of quartan malaria. *2*, *3*, and *4*. Young trophozoite forms of the parasite showing gradual increase of chromatin and cytoplasm. *5*. Developing ring form of trophozoite showing pigment granule. *6*. Early band form of trophozoite–elongated chromatin, some pigment apparent. *7*, *8*, *9*, *10*, *11*, and *12*. Some forms which the developing trophozoite of quartan may take. *13* and *14*. Mature trophozoites–one a band form. *15*, *16*, *17*, *18*, and *19*. Phases in the development of the schizont (presegmenting schizonts). *20*. Mature schizont. *21*. Immature microgametocyte. *22*. Immature macrogametocyte. *23*. Mature microgametocyte. *24*. Mature macrogametocyte. (From Wilcox, Aimee: Manual for the Microscopical Diagnosis of Malaria in Man. Bulletin No. 180, National Institute of Health, 1942.)

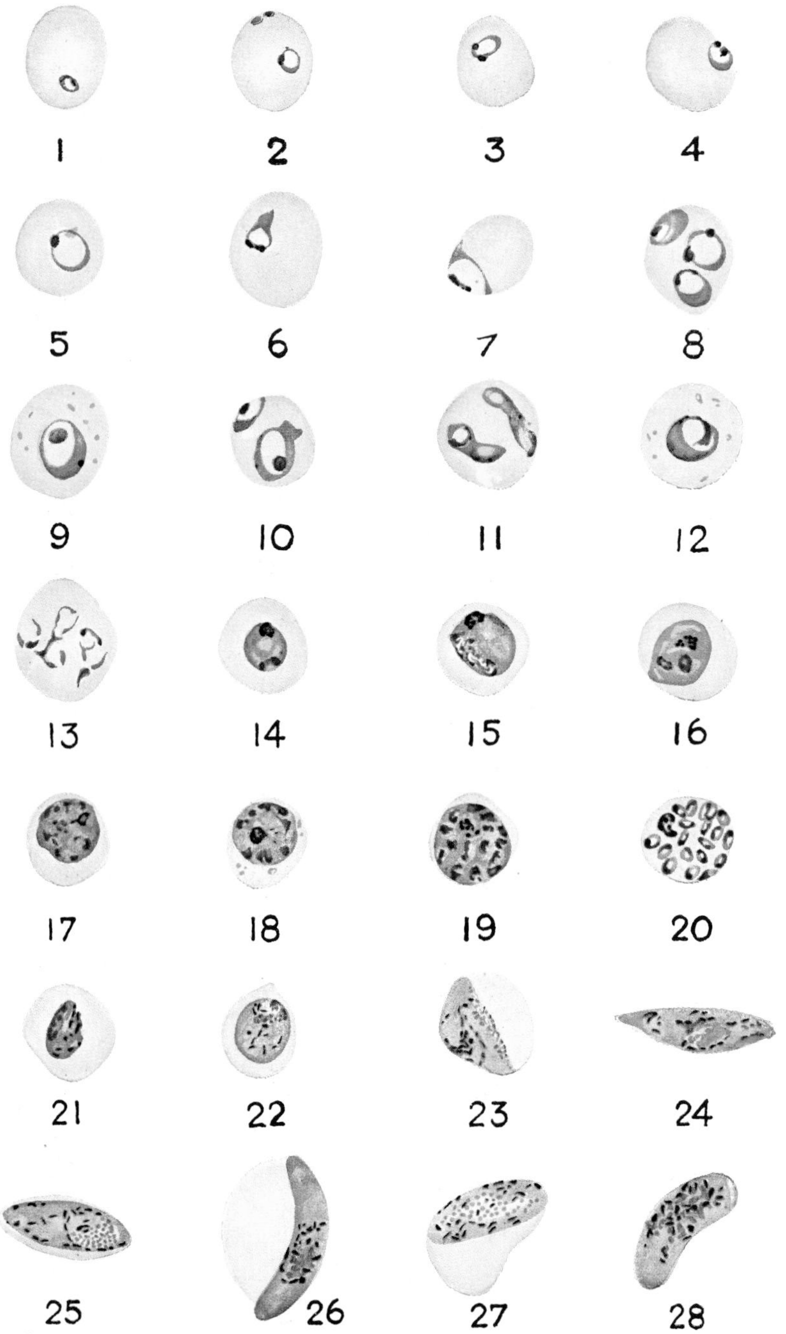

Figure 19–23. *Plasmodium falciparum. 1,* Very young ring form trophozoite. *2,* Double infection of single cell with young trophozoites, one a "marginal form," the other "signet ring" form. *3, 4,* Young trophozoites showing double chromatin dots. *5, 6, 7,* Developing trophozoite forms. *8,* Three medium trophozoites in one cell. *9,* Trophozoite showing pigment, in a cell containing Maurer's dots. *10, 11,* Two trophozoites in each of two cells, showing variation of forms which parasites may assume. *12,* Almost mature trophozoite showing haze of pigment throughout cytoplasm. Maurer's dots in the cell. *13,* Estivo-autumnal "slender forms." *14,* Mature trophozoite, showing clumped pigment. *15,* Parasite in the process of initial chromatin division. *16, 17, 18, 19,* Various phases of the development of the schizont (presegmenting schizonts). *20,* Mature schizont. *21, 22, 23, 24,* Successive forms in the development of the gametocyte – usually not found in the peripheral circulation. *25,* Immature macrogametocyte. *26,* Mature macrogametocyte. *27,* Immature microgametocyte. *28,* Mature microgametocyte. (Courtesy National Institutes of Health. U.S.P.H.S.)

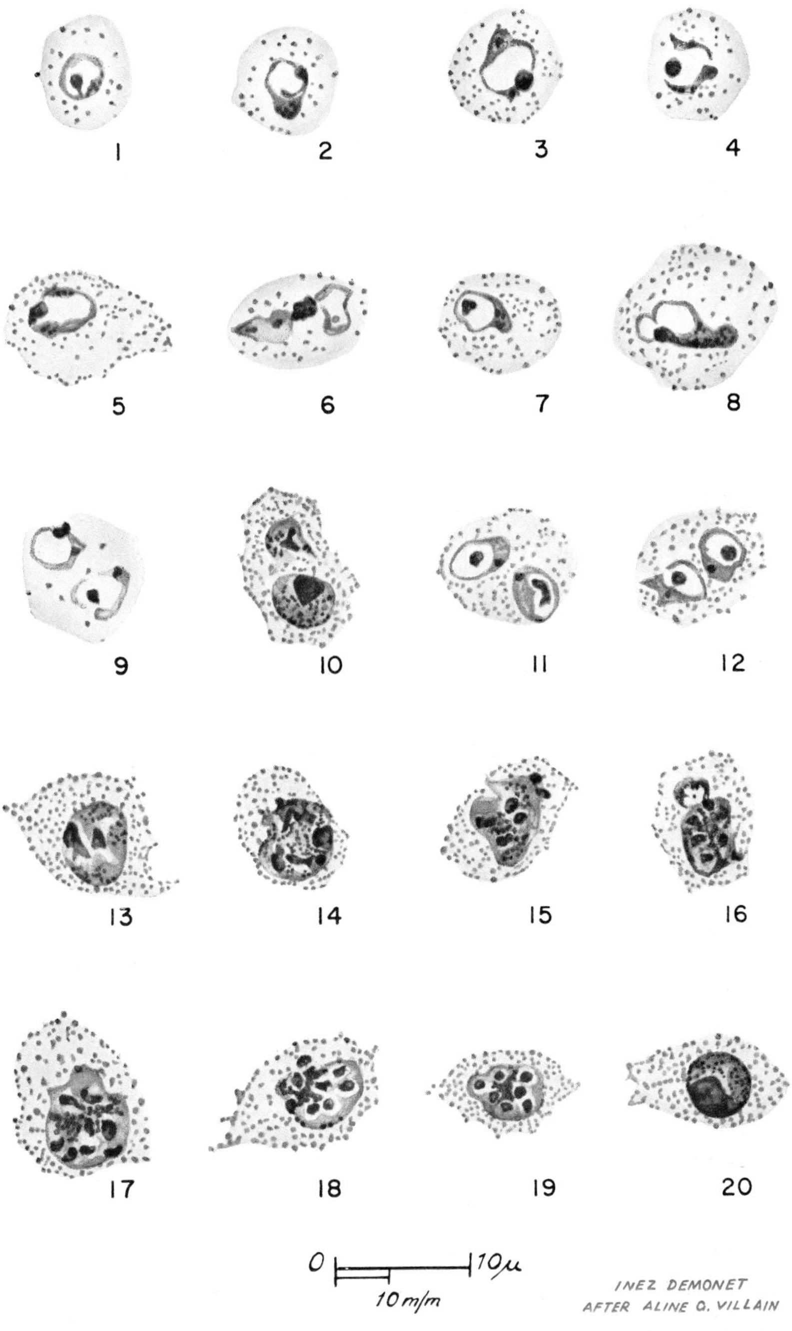

Figure 19–24. *Plasmodium ovale. 1,* Young ring-shaped trophozoite. *2, 3, 4, 5,* Older ring-shaped trophozoites. *6, 7, 8,* Older ameboid trophozoites. *9, 11, 12,* Doubly infected cells, trophozoites. *10,* Doubly infected cell, young gametocytes. *13,* First stage of the schizont. *14, 15, 16, 17, 18, 19,* Schizonts, progressive stages. *20,* Mature gametocyte.

Free translation of legend accompanying original plate in "Guide pratique d'examen microscopique du sang appliqué au diagnostic du paludisme" by Georges Villain. Reproduced with permission from "Biologie Medicale" supplement, 1935. (Courtesy of Aimee Wilcox, National Institutes of Health Bulletin No. 180, U.S.P.H.S.)

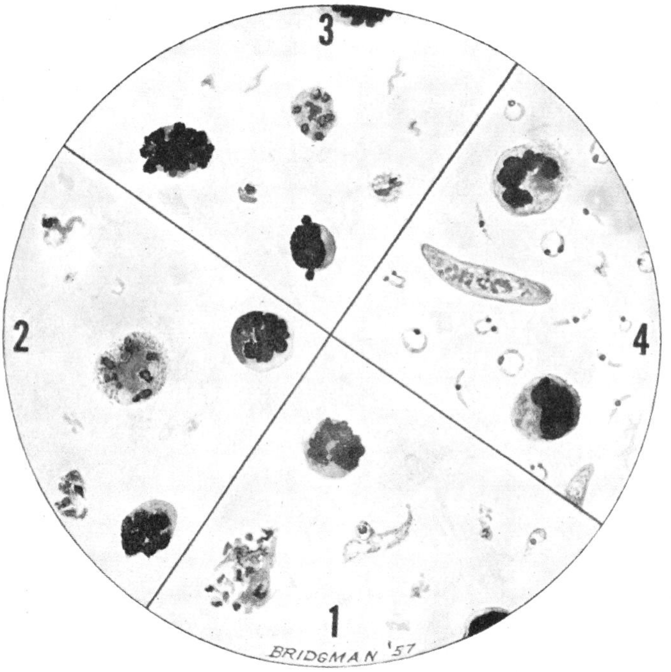

Figure 19–25. The human plasmodia as seen in thick film: *1, Plasmodium vivax:* young and older trophozoites and schizont; *2, P. ovale:* developing trophozoite and schizonts, one within a "ghost cell"; *3, P. malariae:* trophozoites and schizont; *4, P. falciparum:* young trophozoites and gametocyte. (From Markell, E. K., and Voge, M.: Medical Parasitology. 3rd ed.)

BABESIA sp.

Babesia sp. usually infects cattle, etc., but may produce the tick-borne disease babesiosis in man (Ristic *et al.*, 1971). The nonpigmented, pear-shaped organisms develop within the erythrocytes of the host and must be differentiated from malaria parasites.

TOXOPLASMA GONDII

Toxoplasma gondii (Table 19–1; Fig. 19–26) is the causative agent of toxoplasmosis in man and animals and is widespread in the population. Recently, the coccidian transmission of *Toxoplasma* has been presented by several authors (Sheffield and Melton, 1969; Frenkel *et al.*, 1969; Hutchison *et al.*, 1970; Weiland and Kuhn, 1970; Dubey *et al.*, 1970). In human adults the infection is usually acquired, asymptomatic, and unrecognized, although occasional symptomatic and fatal cases occur. In children the disease may produce a syndrome involving the central nervous system and the viscera. Congenital infection occurs and is manifest in the infant or young child as an encephalitis accompanied by such features as chorioretinitis, hydrocephalus or microcephaly, micro-ophthalmos, intracerebral calcification, and mental retardation. Convulsions may occur. In such cases parenchymal and reticulo-endothelial cells are generally affected, and lesions occur in the brain, spleen, kidneys, adrenals, and lymph nodes.

The clinical picture of acquired toxoplasmosis may resemble infectious mononucleosis, especially in a form of the disease characterized by enlarged lymph nodes (Siim, 1960). The similarity may be even more pronounced, since lymphocytes resembling those seen in infectious mononucleosis have been found

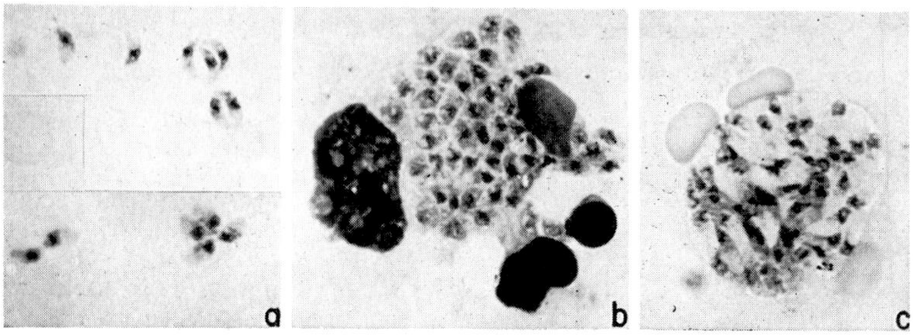

Figure 19–26. Toxoplasmata as seen (*a*) free in stained films of peritoneal exudate or tissue, (*b*) intracellularly, and (*c*) as pseudocyst in film of brain. Wright's stain (× 800) reduced from a photomicrograph with a magnification of 1000 diameters. (Courtesy of Dr. A. B. Sabin and J.A.M.A.)

(Couvreur and Desmonts, 1961). Retinal lesions may appear in toxoplasmosis in man.

Toxoplasma gondii, when it occurs in the free stage, is curved or crescent shaped, measuring 4 to 6 microns in length and 2 to 3 microns in width, with one extremity more rounded than the other. When stained by Wright's or Giemsa's method, the cytoplasm is blue and the nucleus is a red or purple, irregular structure occupying one-fifth to one-fourth of the cell. The nucleus lies near the rounded end of the organism. The cells tend to occur singly or in pairs (Fig. 19–26).

When *T. gondii* is found in the parenchymal or reticuloendothelial cells, the organisms lose their crescent shape and may be confused with the leishmanias. They occur singly or in clusters in these tissue cells. In certain instances, especially in the brain of mice, *T. gondii* occurs as clusters of organisms called pseudocysts.

The diagnosis of toxoplasmosis (Feldman, 1953) depends on demonstration of the organisms in blood, bone marrow, cerebrospinal fluid, or exudates from serous cavities by staining or by intracerebral or intraperitoneal inoculation of these materials into mice known to be free of *Toxoplasma* organisms.

Serologic tests are of value as presumptive evidence of toxoplasmosis. Complement fixation, the Sabin-Feldman methylene blue-dye test (a staining inhibition technique), a hemagglutination test, or fluorescent antibody techniques may be used (Goldman, 1957 a and b). Since few laboratories are equipped to do these tests, 10 ml. of blood should be collected aseptically and sent to an appropriate laboratory (usually the state health department laboratory). A second sample should be tested after a month to determine titer change. A rise in titer indicates active infection. It is not usually possible to demonstrate the organism in congenital cases; thus, it is usually necessary to do serial serologic tests on the blood of both the mother and the infant. Skin tests (toxoplasmin) may be of some value.

PNEUMOCYSTIS CARINII

Pneumocystis carinii is an unclassified protozoan believed to be responsible for an epidemic disease known as interstitial plasma-cell pneumonia (pneumocystic pneumonia), especially in newborn children. (Fig. 19–27). Several forms of the parasite have been described–isolated uninucleate forms, those with several nuclei, and those with a rosette of eight nuclei. The nuclei are about 1 to 3 microns in diameter and are rounded, ovoid, or crescent shaped. The rosettes are 8 microns in diameter. These organisms have blue cytoplasm and red nuclei when stained with Giemsa's stain. The disease is highly contagious and may result in sudden death. Complement fixation tests are available.

MEDICAL HELMINTHOLOGY

Two phyla of worms (helminths) are of medical importance: Nemathelminthes (roundworms) and Platyhelminthes (flatworms, viz., flukes and tapeworms). Some helminths are

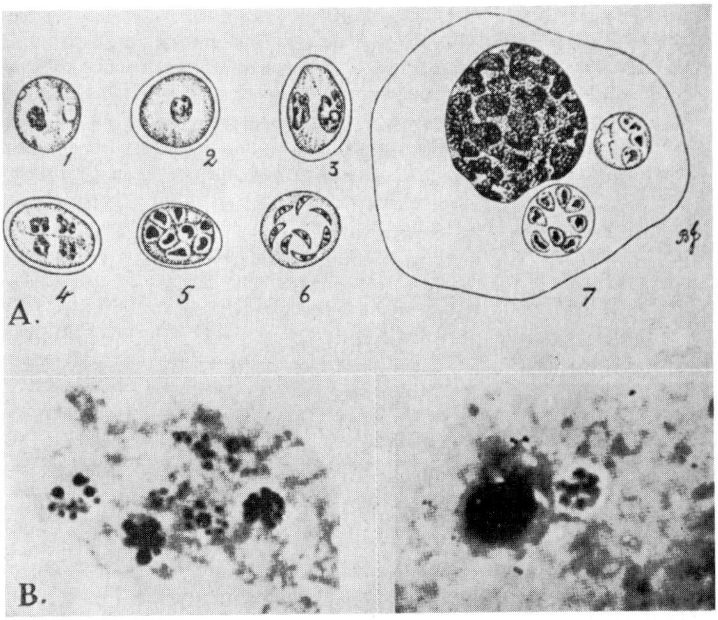

Figure 19–27. *Pneumocystis carinii. A,* From impression film of lung of infected dog. × 2000. (After Carini and Maciel, 1914, in Wenyon's Protozoölogy, courtesy of Baillière, Tindall & Cox, London); *B,* Gram-stained impression films of *P. carinii* from lung. × 1500. (After Westphal, courtesy Zeitschr. f. Tropen med. u. Parasitol. Hamburg.)

cosmopolitan but many are limited to well-defined geographic areas of the earth. Details of this distribution are available (Faust, Russell and Jung, 1970).

Diagnosis of these helminthic infections in the clinical laboratory is based upon the demonstration of the eggs, larvae, or other stages of the parasite in body fluids, stools, and tissues or in the environment. Nonparasitic objects (Fig. 19–97) which resemble helminths or portions of them or their eggs or larvae may be seen in stools. Many specimens for studies for helminth eggs or larvae are processed in much the same manner as for many of the protozoa, and where procedures equally apply they have been placed on pages 1110–1114. Unstained wet mounts are most desirable for locating and identifying helminth eggs and larva since iodine frequently overstains the eggs. Gross worm specimens should be submitted in saline, although specimens in formalin or alcohol may be suitable, except for tapeworms. The life cycles of the helminths may be quite complex, and one should know something of these life cycles to understand how the patient became infected, where the parasite migrates and settles down in the body, and what types of specimens are needed for laboratory examination and diagnosis. In order to explicate host determinations, the following definitions may be helpful: the *definitive host* harbors the adult or sexual stages of the parasite, whereas the *intermediate host* houses larval or asexual stages. Man is the definitive host in most helminthic infections with several notable exceptions, viz., echinococcosis (hydatid disease), sparganosis, and cysticercosis. The most important human helminths are presented in Table 19–5. Most helminthic infections provoke an eosinophilic response.

The Nematodes

Distinguishing features of the nematodes are as follows: cylindrical shape, nonsegmented body, separate sexes (dioecious), body cavity, complete alimentary tract (mouth, gut, and anus), tapered ends, and a cuticular covering. Generally the males are much smaller and more slender than the female worms and have curled posterior ends designed for copulation.

Several females of the nematodes are viviparous (*Trichinella spiralis, Dracunculus medinensis*) and ovoviviparous in the filarial worms, but generally oviparous females occur and produce eggs in quantities each day which are passed in the stool, a fact that makes diagnosis easier. Some of the common nematode eggs are seen in Figure 19–30. The reproductive organs are bilaterally symmetrical, tubular, and coiled within the body. An excretory system and a nervous system exist, but vascular and respiratory systems do not. Figure 19–28 shows the actual size relationships of the common adult nematodes. Figure 19–29 depicts the musculature types in cross section. The pathologist may be assisted in diagnosis of nematodes in tissue by knowing the three general types: polymyarian, meromyarian, and holomyarian. In the polymyarian type (Fig. 19–29 *A*), the cells are numerous and project well into the body cavity (*Ascaris*); in the meromyarian type (Fig. 19–29 *B*), the cells are few in number, two or three to a quarter section (*Enterobius* and the hookworms); and in the holomyarian type (Fig. 19–29 *C*), the cells are small and numerous and are closely packed in a narrow zone (*Trichuris, Trichinella,* and filarial worms), according to Belding, 1965.

Enterobius vermicularis. The seatworm or pinworm causing human enterobiasis or oxyuriasis is *Enterobius vermicularis* (*Oxyuris vermicularis*) (Table 19–5; Figs. 19–28, 19–31, and 19–70). This common helminth is widely distributed in families and in institutions. Broadly speaking, sanitation is not a primary factor in its dissemination; rather it is neglected individual hygiene that permits rapid spread of the infection. This infection occurs at all economic levels.

The female worm is distinctive in possessing a long, narrow, sharply pointed tail (Figs. 19–28, 19–31), the characteristic from which it gets the name pinworm. Females measure 8 to 13 mm. in length and 0.5 mm. in diameter; the male is 2 to 5 mm. in length and 0.5 mm. in diameter, with a ventrally curved posterior end. The immature worms (including larvae from broken egg shells) and adults are transparent when viewed microscopically and the former and the males must be differentiated from larvae of hookworm and *Strongyloides* (see below) and the free-living adults of the latter as seen in old stools or cultures.) The adults, which require only one month to reach sexual maturity, possess cephalic alae or wings as their anterior end (Fig. 19–28).

The site of predilection of the adult worms is the neighborhood of the cecum. The gravid female migrates to the anus where she crawls about on the perianal folds and deposits large numbers of eggs which are fully embryonated, are immediately infective, and only need to be swallowed (anus-to-mouth or by retrofection—that is, re-entry of hatched larvae into the rectum) for reinfection or to establish an infection in a new host.

Clinically the manifestations of enterobiasis are generally mild, but if larger numbers of worms are present, the effects are variable. Infected persons may be asymptomatic, or they may have combinations of *pruritus ani,* abdominal cramps, diarrhea, nervousness, and nocturia. Adult worms may be in ectopic sites, such as the female genitalia. When worms are

(Text continues on page 1060.)

Table 19–5. HELMINTH DISEASES IN MAN

PARASITE NAME	COMMON NAME AND DISEASE	GEOGRAPHICAL DISTRIBUTION	LENGTH OF PARASITE	SITE IN HOST	PORTAL OF ENTRY	SOURCE OF INFECTION; INTERMEDIATE HOST OR VECTOR	CLINICAL MANIFESTATIONS	LABORATORY FINDINGS	LABORATORY METHODS	ADDITIONAL INFORMATION
HELMINTHS: NEMATODES (ROUNDWORMS)										
Enterobius vermicularis	Pinworm; seatworm; oxyuris; oxyuriasis; enterobiasis; mistakenly called threadworm	Cosmopolitan	Male, 2-5 mm.; female, 8-13 mm.	Cecum; appendix; large intestine (attached)	Mouth; anus (retrofection)	Autoinfection—anus-to-mouth; eggs in environment; retrofection (re-enter body through the anus)	No symptoms; *pruritus ani;* abdominal cramps; diarrhea; nervous manifestations	Eggs 50 by 20 μ embryonated or unembryonated and/or adult females on perianum picked up on cellulose tape swabs; adult females on surface of stool; worms in purged stools; eggs rarely in urine or stools; x-sect. of adults in appendix	Cellulose tape technique	Transparent worms live about one year; tends to be family infection, check and treat *all;* take tapes upon arising—three days
Ascaris lumbricoides	Large roundworm (giant intestinal) ascariasis	Same	Adult: male, 10-30 cm.; female, 20-40 cm.; Larva: 0.2-2.1 mm.	Adult: small intestine; ectopic sites; Larva: lungs (adults in lumen)	Mouth	Embryonated eggs from soil into contaminated food or water	Pneumonitis (in early stages); allergic symptoms; abdominal pain or discomfort; intestinal blockage; nervous manifestations	Eggs average 60 by 40 μ, one-cell stage, fertile, infertile, or both, in stool; immature or mature worms passed; larvae in sputum (early in infection); adults, after therapy. Adults must be sexed	Direct smears; concentration methods; sedimentation; egg counts to determine worm burden	Worms live about one year; fever and/or some medicines cause worms to wander into peritoneum, bile duct, and elsewhere
Toxocara canis and *Toxocara cati*	Visceral larva migrans	Tropics and subtropics	Adult (in dogs and cats), 4-10 cm.; Larva, 0.3 mm.	Larvae in liver, brain, eye	Mouth	Same	Pneumonitis; eosinophilia; hepatomegaly	Larvae in tissues at biopsy or necropsy	Serologic tests	Pronounced eosinophilia; anemia; hyperglobulinemia
Trichuris (Trichocephalus) trichiura	Whipworm; trichocephaliasis; trichuriasis	Cosmopolitan	Male, 3.0-4.5 cm.; Female, 3.5-5.0 cm.	Ileum; cecum; large intestine (attached)	Mouth	Same	No symptoms; abdominal discomfort; anemia; bloody stools; prolapse of rectum; allergic symptoms; small hemorrhages	Eggs, (50 by 23 μ, one-cell stage) in stool; adults, after therapy	Direct smears; concentration methods; sedimentation; egg counts to determine worm burden	Worms live several years or longer; frequently coexist with *Ascaris*, since embryonated eggs are in soil
Necator americanus	New World (American) hookworm; uncinariasis; hookworm infection; hookworm disease	Tropics and subtropics	Adult, 7-11 mm.; Larva, 275 μ (rhab.)	Small intestine (attached)	Skin	Infective larvae (filariform) on surface of moist, sandy soil	Asymptomatic pneumonitis; anemia; growth retardation; gastrointestinal symptomatology; ground itch	Eggs (64-76 by 36-40μ, four- to eight-cell stage), rarely larvae, in stools; larvae in sputum early in infection; larvae in stool culture; adults, after therapy	Direct smears; concentration methods; sedimentation; stool cultures, smear, and charcoal plates; egg counts to determine burden	Adults live five to 14 years; all hookworm eggs similar; larvae to be differentiated from *S. stercoralis*
Ancylostoma duodenale	Old World hookworm; ancylostomiasis; hookworm infection; hookworm disease	Same	Adult, 8-13 mm.; Larva, 275 μ (rhab.)	Same	Same	Same	Same	Same, except eggs are 56-60 μ long and 36-40 μ in breadth	Same	Same, *Necator* adults with cutting plates; *Ancylostoma* with teeth

(Table 19–5 continues on the following page.)

Table 19–5. HELMINTH DISEASES IN MAN *(Continued)*

PARASITE NAME	COMMON NAME AND DISEASE	GEOGRAPHICAL DISTRIBUTION	LENGTH OF PARASITE	SITE IN HOST	PORTAL OF ENTRY	SOURCE OF INFECTION; INTERMEDIATE HOST OR VECTOR	CLINICAL MANIFESTATIONS	LABORATORY FINDINGS	LABORATORY METHODS	ADDITIONAL INFORMATION
Ancylostoma braziliensis	Cutaneous larva migrans; creeping eruption	Tropics and subtropics	Larva, to 0.3 mm. (adult in dogs and cats)	Intradermal	Skin	Infective larvae (filariform) of dog and cat hookworm in soil	Itch: serpiginous skin lesions; secondary bacterial infection	*None;* physical examination	*None*	Exposure on southern U. S. beaches and in shady, moist areas
Strongyloides stercoralis	Strongyloidiasis; Cochin China diarrhea; true threadworm	Tropics and subtropics	Parasitic female: 2.2 mm.; no males present; Larva, 225 by 16 μ (rhab.); Free-living adults, 0.7 mm.	Wall of small intestine, (embedded)	Same Bowel wall	Infective larvae, filariform, on surface of moist, sandy soil Infective larvae, filariform, invade bowel wall	Pneumonitis; duodenitis; watery diarrhea; abdominal discomfort; hepatitis; eosinophilia	Larvae (rhabditoid) in duodenal drainage, sputum, urine, aspirates from body cavities, and stool; eggs (70 by 40 μ) on surface of stool when free-living females develop on stool in moist container; eggs 50 by 30 μ in stool in severe diarrhea or strong purge	Direct smear; concentration; sedimentation; stool culture (larval and free-living forms); smear and charcoal plates	Adult parasitic female buried in intestinal mucosa lives long time; auto- or hyperinfection common; frequent in institutions for feebleminded
Trichinella spiralis	Trichinosis; trichiniasis; trichinelliasis; trichina worm	Cosmopolitan	Adult, 1.4-3.2 mm.; Larva, 0.8-1.0 mm.	Striated muscle	Mouth	Encapsulated larvae from infected raw or insufficiently cooked pork or pork products	Orbital edema; muscle pain; eosinophilia; gastrointestinal symptoms; painful respiration; myocardial damage	Adults or larvae in stools (diarrhea); larvae in blood; muscle biopsy (deltoid or other)	Skin test; serologic test; stool examination (direct and conc.); sed. from vol. laked blood; muscle (sect., pressing, digestion)	Adults live to six months; early in infection purge patient heavily to remove viviparous females
Wuchereria bancrofti	Bancroft's filariasis; wuchereriasis	Tropics	Adult: male, 2.5-4.0 cm.; female, 5-10 cm. Microfilariae: 244-296 μ	Lymphatics	Skin	Bite of infected mosquitoes (*Culex, Aedes, Anopheles*)	Fever; lymphangitis, lymphadenitis; blocked lymph nodes may cause elephantiasis	Sheathed microfilariae in blood – nocturnal periodicity; adults removed surgically	Stained thin and thick films; wet blood films; CSA (citrate-saponin-acid) method; Knott's conc.; heparinized prep.; serologic tests; skin test	Adults live for years, take one year to mature; take blood between 10 P.M. and 2 A.M. Microfilaria sheathed, no granules to tip of tail
Brugia (Wuchereria) malayi	Brug's filariasis; malayan filariasis	Malay Peninsula; Asia	Adult: male, 22 mm.; female, 5 cm. Microfilaria: 175-230 μ	Lymphatics	Skin	Same	Same	Same	Same	Same, except two cells in tip of tail in microfilaria
Loa loa	African eye worm; loaiasis	Central and West Africa	Adult, 30-70 mm. Microfilaria 250-300 μ	Eye; skin (subcutaneous)	Skin	Bite of fly (tabanid-*Chrysops*)	Callabar swellings (transient tumors); eosinophilia; allergic manifestations	Wet and stained blood smears diurnal (daytime *only*); surgical removal of adult from eye	Same	Microfilaria sheathed, row of granules to tip of tail
Acanthocheilonema (Dipetalonema) perstans	The persistent filaria	Tropical Africa; Brazil; Venezuela; West Irian	Adult, 45-80 mm. Microfilaria, 200 μ	Body cavities	Skin	Bite of *Culicoides* fly	Allergic state with eosinophilia	Wet and stained blood smears for microfilariae	Same	Unsheathed microfilaria with granules to tip of tail; nonperiodic
Acanthocheilonema streptocerca		Africa	Microfilaria, 180-240 μ	Skin	Skin	Same	Asymptomatic; cutaneous edema; elephantiasis?	Microfilariae from skin scrapings and biopsies of skin deep to dermal tissue	Saline preparation of biopsy material	Microfilaria unsheathed with crooked posterior end

Mansonella ozzardi	Ozzard's filariasis	Tropical America	Adult, 65-81 mm. Microfilaria, 185-200 μ	Body cavities	Skin	Same	Nonpathogenic; allergic state	Wet and stained blood smears for microfilariae	(Same as for *W. bancrofti*)	Unsheathed microfilaria with no granules in tip of tail; nonperiodic
Onchocerca volvulus	Onchocerciasis; blinding filariasis; the convoluted filaria	Mexico; Guatemala; Africa	Adult: male, 19-50 mm.; female, 35-50 cm.; both, 0.5 mm. or less in diameter Microfilaria: 150-287 μ or 285-368 μ	Subcutaneous	Skin	Bite of black fly *(Simulium)*	Subcutaneous fibrous nodules on head, trunk, arms, or hip; blindness when microfilariae in eye	Microfilariae from nodular fluid or adults and microfilariae from skin or nodule biopsy	Saline preparation of nodular fluid; serologic test	Microfilariae unsheathed but not in blood
Dracunculus medinensis	Dracontiasis; Guinea worm; medina worm	Africa; India; Near East; Brazil; East Indies	Adult: male, 2.0 cm. or less; female, 70-120 cm Larva: 500-700 μ	Same	Mouth	Ingestion of infected Cyclops	Inflammation; ulcers on legs and feet; anaphylactic symptoms	Adult under skin; larvae in blister on skin (at posterior end of female); x-ray of calcified worm	Saline preparation of material from blister	Worms take one year to mature; multiple worms common; boil or filter drinking water
Angiostrongylus cantonensis	Rat lung worm; cerebral angiostrongyliasis	Pacific, Thailand	?	Meninges	Mouth	Ingestion of snails or shrimps	Eosinophilic meningitis	Adult worm(s) at autopsy	Gross examination; histologic studies	
Capillaria philippinensis	Intestinal capillariasis	Pacific	?	Intestine	Mouth	Not known	Severe protein-losing enteropathy and malabsorption of fats and sugars; diarrhea	Eggs in stool (must be differentiated from *Trichuris*)	Stool direct smear; concentration method; sedimentation	
Anisakis sp.	Anisakiasis	Europe, Japan	10-25 mm.	Intestinal wall	Mouth	Ingestion of larvae in raw, smoked, or salted fish	Eosinophilic phlemonous enteritis	Identification of adult worm from tumor	Gross examination	G.I. lesion: eosinophilic granuloma or abscess containing adult worm
HELMINTHS: CESTODES (TAPEWORMS)										
Diphyllobothrium latum	Broad, fish tapeworm; diphyllobothriasis	Northern central U.S.A.; Canada; Europe; Russia; Japan; Israel	To 10 meters (4000 segments)	Small intestine	Mouth	Sparganum (plerocercoid) larva in raw or insufficiently cooked fresh-water fish	Asymptomatic; hyperchromic anemia (rare); digestive disturbances; loss of weight; toxemia	Immature, operculated eggs 45 by 70 μ in feces; chains of gravid segments passed; entire worm after therapy	Stool direct smear; concentration method; sedimentation; segment and scolex ident.	One worm as rule. Worm may break above gravid proglottids—reexamine stools over next four months; scolex is unarmed, spoon-shaped
Spirometra sp. (larval form)	Sparganosis	Orient; Africa; southern U.S.A.; South America	Varying sizes	Tissues; eye	Mouth or flesh application	Cyclops	Tissue: eosinophilic reaction Ocular: very serious	Identification of sparganum larva from tissues	Gross examination	White, ribbonlike; lateral slits at anterior end; also *Sparganum proliferum*
Taenia saginata	Beef tapeworm	Cosmopolitan	4-12 meters (1000 to 2000 segments)	Small intestine (attached)	Mouth	Ingestion of raw or insufficiently cooked beef containing *Cysticercus bovis*	Asymptomatic; diarrhea; increase in appetite; irritation of mucosa; obstruction; toxemia	Eggs 30-40 μ in feces; segments (single or chains) in feces; entire worm after therapy; Eggs morphologically identical to *T. solium*	Stool direct smear; concentration method; sedimentation; segment and scolex ident.	One worm as rule; reexamine stool after three months if scolex not recovered post therapy; scolex "unarmed"; segment (gravid) 15 or more branches one side

(Table 19–5 continues on the following page.)

Table 19–5. HELMINTH DISEASES IN MAN (*Continued*)

PARASITE NAME	COMMON NAME AND DISEASE	GEOGRAPHICAL DISTRIBUTION	LENGTH OF PARASITE	SITE IN HOST	PORTAL OF ENTRY	SOURCE OF INFECTION; INTERMEDIATE HOST OR VECTOR	CLINICAL MANIFESTATIONS	LABORATORY FINDINGS	LABORATORY METHODS	ADDITIONAL INFORMATION
Taenia solium (adult)	Pork tapeworm (adult)	Mexico; Central and South America; Europe	2-4 meters (less than 1000 segments)	Small intestine (attached)	Mouth	Ingestion of raw or insufficiently cooked pork containing *Cysticercus cellulosae*	Same	Same (eggs are morphologically identical to *T. saginata*)	Same	One worm as rule; reexamine as for above; scolex "armed"; segment (gravid) seven to 13 branches on one side
Cysticercus cellulosae	Bladderworm (larva)	Same	5 mm. by 8-10 mm.	Visceral organs; brain; eye	Anus-to-mouth; contaminated food; reverse peristalsis with eggs to stomach	Eggs of *T. solium*	Eye damage; epilepsy in brain involvement	Examination of larval form removed at surgery or necropsy	Serologic test; x-ray; skin test	Bladderworm possesses hooklets
Hymenolepis nana	Dwarf tapeworm; hymenolepiasis	Cosmopolitan	1-4.5 cm. long and 0.4-0.7 mm. wide (200 segments)	Adults and cysticercoid larvae in small intestine (adult attached)	Mouth	Anus-to-mouth infection; eggs in fecally contaminated food and water	Asymptomatic; toxemia; diarrhea; abdominal pain	Eggs 30-47 μ and sometimes adults in stool; worms after therapy	Same as for *D. latum*	Scolex is "armed"; multiple worms common
Hymenolepis diminuta	Rat tapeworm	Same	20-60 cm. by 4 mm. (over 1000 segments)	Small intestine (adult attached)	Mouth	Cysticercoid form from insects	Asymptomatic; emaciation	Eggs 56-80 μ by 24-40 μ; adult worm after therapy	Same	Scolex is "unarmed"
Dipylidium caninum	Dog tapeworm; dipylidiasis	Cosmopolitan	10-70 cm.	Small intestine	Mouth	Cysticercoid forms from insects	Asymptomatic	Eggs 36-60 μ (in packets); proglottids in feces; adult after therapy	Same	Gravid proglottids with twinned genitalia; scolex is "armed" (5 rows)
Echinococcus granulosus (cyst)	Unilocular hydatid disease; echinococcosis	Argentina; New Zealand; Australia; U.S.A.; Canada; Europe	Adult worm in *dogs*-2.5-5.0 mm.; cyst size depends on site	Bones; liver; lung; brain	Mouth	Eggs from dog feces in contaminated food or water; fondling of dogs; eggs in environment	Pressure; symptoms in various organs; allergic reactions	Skin test (Casoni); serologic test	Serologic test; x-ray; examination of fluid from hydatid for "hydatid sand"—mult. scolices 0.2-0.3 mm. (cyst may be sterile); sputum	Unilocular may be single or multiple; osseous hydatid in bones
Echinococcus multilocularis	Alveolar hydatid disease	Central Europe; Balkans; Siberia; Alaska; some islands of Japan	Adult worm in foxes, wolves, etc. 1.2-3.7 mm.	Liver and lungs (no capsulation)	Mouth	Eggs in contaminated food or water	Jaundice; ascites; splenomegaly	May be missed, possibly found by surgery; (skin test and serologic test not too reliable)	Serologic test (?); x-ray; examination of fluid from alveolar cysts for hydatid sand; sputum	Infection fatal
Multiceps multiceps	Coenurosis; coenurus disease	(?)	Adult worm in dogs	CNS; bladder-like coenurus	Same	Eggs from dog in contaminated food or water	?	Coenurus in CNS as bladderlike worm with multiple heads invaginated from wall into bladder cavity	Autopsy	Infection fatal (?)

HELMINTHS: TREMATODES (FLUKES)

Schistosoma mansoni	Manson's schistosomiasis; bilharzia; blood fluke	Brazil; Venezuela; Puerto Rico; Africa	Adults, 1-1.6 cm. long (males and females present)	Veins of large intestine; liver, and ectopic sites	Skin	Cercariae from fresh-water snails	Spleen and liver enlargement; intestinal fibrosis; chronic dysentery; urticaria; toxemia; cirrhosis of liver; variable symptoms when worms in ectopic sites	Mature, 150 by 60 μ, nonoperculated eggs (with miracidium) and conspicuous lateral spine in feces (occasionally in urine); eggs in pseudotubercles in tissues	Serologic tests; direct smear; concentration methods (some special); sedimentation with saline wash—(follow with egg hatching); rectal and liver biopsies (pressed and sectioned)	Worms may live 20 to 30 years; effects are cumulative; determine viability of eggs by egg hatch or viewing flame cells (solanocytes) in saline preparation
Schistosoma japonicum	Schistosomiasis japonica; bilharzia; blood fluke	Philippines; Japan; China; Formosa; Celebes	Adults, 2.2-2.6 cm. long (males and females present)	Veins of small intestine; liver, and ectopic sites	Same	Same	Same	Same, except egg with inconspicuous lateral spine; eggs 90 by 70 μ	Same	Same
Schistosoma haematobium	Urinary or vesical schistosomiasis; blood fluke; bilharzia	Africa; Israel; Greece; Spain; Portugal; India	Adults, 1-2 cm. long (males and females present)	Veins of urinary bladder	Same	Same	Chronic cystitis with secondary infection, also predisposition to cancer due to constant irritation; damage to genital organs; hematuria	Mature, nonoperculated eggs (with miracidium); eggs have terminal spine and are found in urine (occasionally feces); 150 by 60 μ	Urine (forced sample) concentration; sedimentation (24-hour sample; egg hatching from sediment; bladder biopsy; serologic test	Same
Clonorchis sinensis	Clonorchiasis; Chinese liver fluke	Orient	10-25 by 3-5 mm. (monecious)	Bile ducts	Mouth	Metacercariae from uncooked, salted, dried, or pickled fresh-water fish	Indigestion; diarrhea; hepatomegaly; edema	Mature, operculated eggs (29 by 16μ) in stool or duodenal drainage (shaped like an old-fashioned electric light bulb)	Direct smear; concentration methods; sedimentation	Egg must be differentiated from those of *Metagonimus*, *Heterophyes*, and *Opisthorchis*; hermaphroditic worms live many years
Fasciola hepatica	Sheep liver fluke; liver rot; fascioliasis	South America; U.S.A.; Europe; Africa	3 by 1.2 cm. (monecious)	Bile ducts	Mouth	Metacercariae on aquatic vegetation	Enlarged liver; mechanical and toxic irritation to the liver	Immature, operculated eggs (140 by 80 μ) in stool	Same	"Halzoun" in Lebanon and Syria—temporary attachment worms in respiratory area—worms in raw liver; false fascioliasis; hermaphroditic adult with cephalic cone
Fasciolopsis buski	Giant intestinal fluke; fasciolopsiasis	Far East; India; China; East Indies	2.0-7.5 cm. (monecious)	Small intestine	Mouth	Metacercariae on water nuts and vegetables	Diarrhea; edema; abdominal pain; toxemia; obstruction; ascites	Immature, operculated eggs (135 by 85 μ) in stool; adult after therapy	Same	Adult lacks cephalic cone; eggs similar to *F. hepatica*; hermaphroditic
Paragonimus westermani	Oriental lung fluke; paragonimiasis	Orient; Africa; South America	0.8-1.6 cm. in length, 0.4-0.8 cm. in width, 0.3-0.5 cm. thick (monecious)	Lungs	Mouth	Metacercariae from fresh-water crabs	Hemoptysis; cough; abdominal pain; fever; pneumonitis; chest pain; dyspnea	Immature, operculated eggs (85 by 50 μ) in sputum or stool	Same; stool and sputum	Spines cover adult worm (hermaphroditic)

MISCELLANEOUS FLUKES: *Heterophyes heterophyes, Metagonimus yokogawai, Opisthorchis viverrini, Opisthorchis felineus, Echinostoma revolutum.*

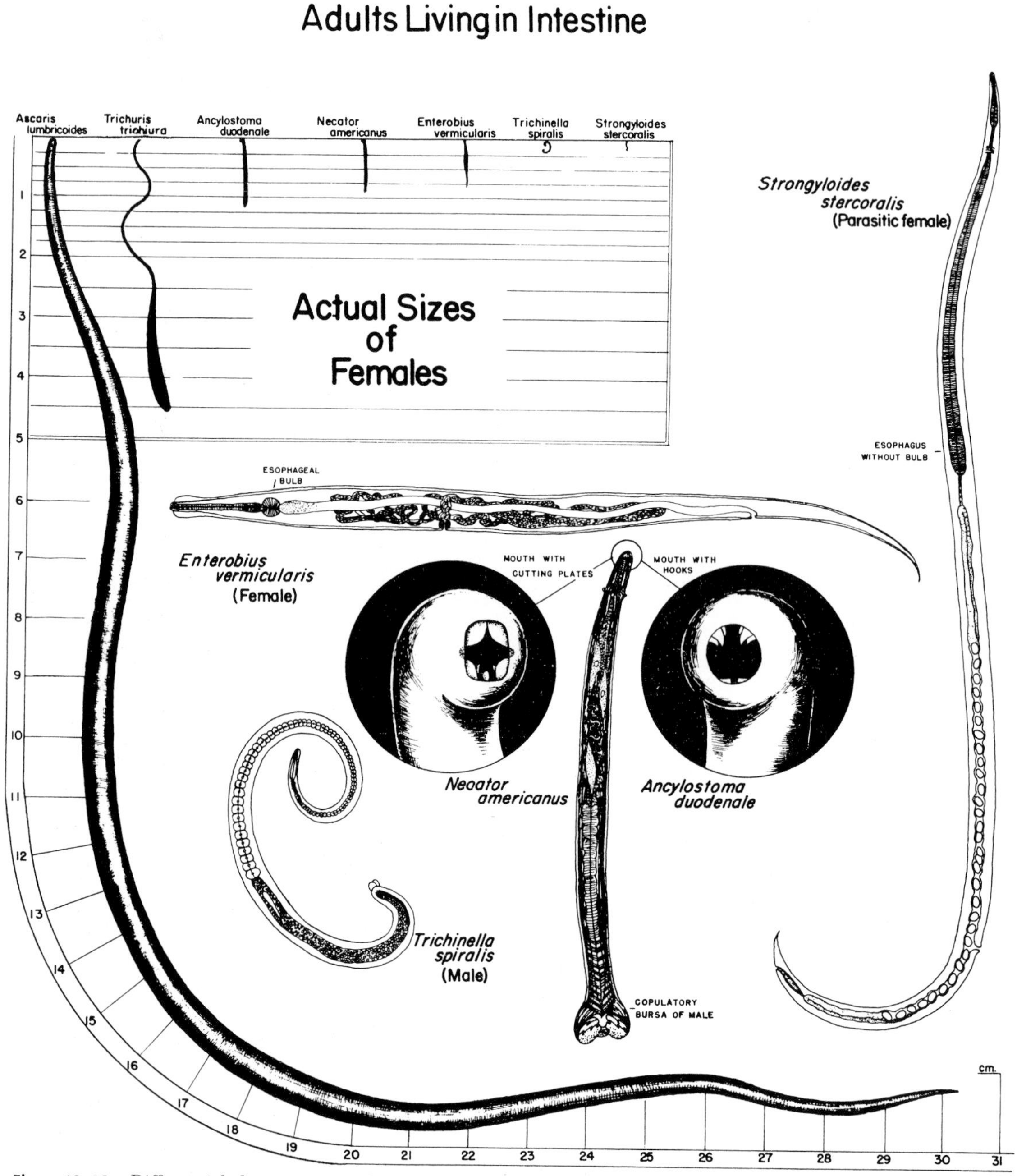

Figure 19–28. Differential characteristics of important human roundworms. (From Medical Protozoology and Helminthology. U.S. Naval Medical School, National Naval Medical Center, Bethesda, Maryland, 1965.)

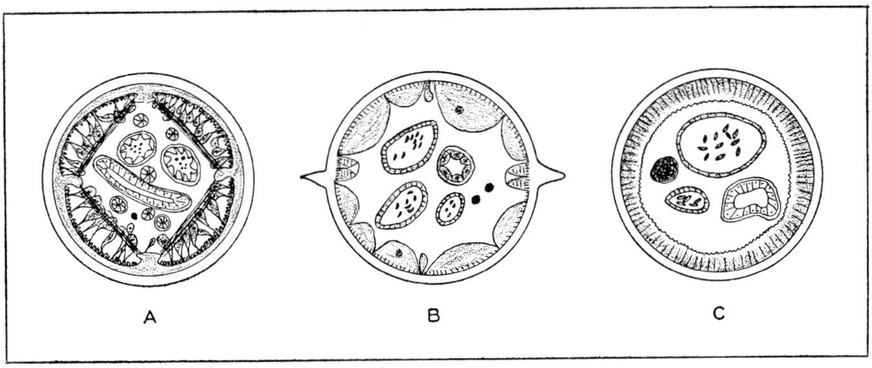

Figure 19–29. Musculature of nematodes. *A*, polymyarian type; *B*, meromyarian type; *C*, holomyarian type. (From Belding, D. L.: Textbook of Clinical Parasitology. New York, Appleton-Century-Crofts, 1942.)

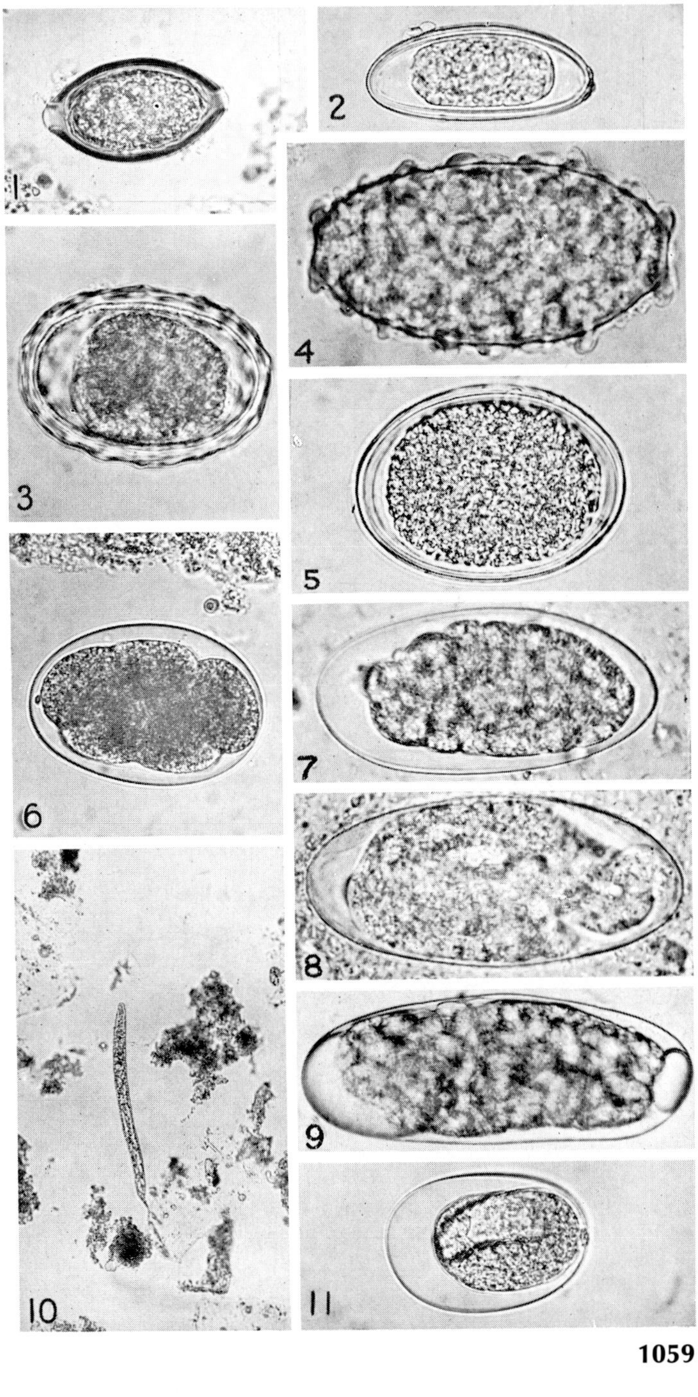

Figure 19–30. Some common nematode eggs. *1*, Whipworm, *Trichuris trichiura; 2*, pinworm, *Enterobius vermicularis; 3*, large roundworm, *Ascaris lumbricoides*, fertilized egg; *4*, *Ascaris*, unfertilized egg; *5*, *Ascaris*, decorticated egg; *6*, hookworm egg; *7*, immature egg of *Trichostrongylus orientalis; 8*, embryonated egg of *T. orientalis; 9*, egg of *Heterodera marioni*, a plant nematode which sometimes is found in stools; *10*, rhabditiform larva of *Strongyloides stercoralis*, the stage usually found in the stool; *11*, egg of *S. stercoralis*, rarely seen in the stool. All figures × 500 except *10*, × 75. (Nos. *5* and *6* courtesy of the Photographic Laboratory, AMSGS; photos by Milt Cheskis. Nos. *7*, *8*, and *9* courtesy of Dr. T. B. Magath, Mayo Clinic. All others courtesy of Dr. R. L. Roudabush, Ward's Natural Science Establishment, Rochester, N.Y.; photos by T. Romaniak.)

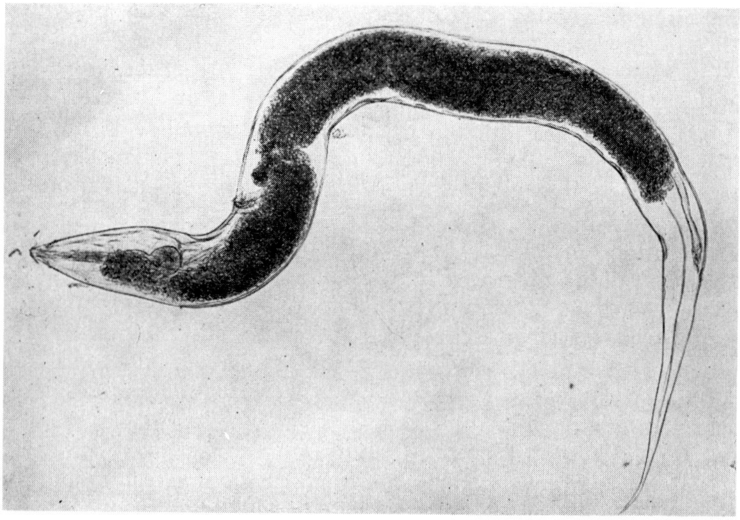

Figure 19–31. Adult female *E. vermicularis* showing cephalic alae, bulb behind esophagus, vulva, egg mass, anus, and pointed posterior end. (From Hunter, C. W., Frye, W. W., and Swartzwelder, J. C.: A Manual of Tropical Medicine, 4th ed.)

in the appendix they may be viewed in histologic sections showing crests (Fig. 19–32) and the meromyarian type of musculature (Fig. 19–29 *B*). Eggs may be recovered from the urine.

Occasionally females may be seen grossly on the perianal folds or on the surface of a stool or actively motile in a purged stool. Males are seen only after therapy, upon purgation, or at times with diarrhea. Immature worms may be demonstrated in purged stools.

Since eggs and/or hatched larvae and adults are seldom seen in feces, specific diagnosis rests upon the recovery of the eggs or adult females from the perianal region. Although there are numerous methods available, the best known is the Graham cellulose tape technique (Fig. 19–33). It is advisable for tape samples to be taken upon arising on three successive days from each member of the family. These tapes should be submitted to the laboratory. The egg has a thick hyaline shell with one flattened side and a larva within. There is a violet tint to the space surrounding the larva within the shell. Frequently the larva is slightly motile, although dead larvae or even empty egg shells may be found. The egg measures 50 to 60 microns in length and 20 to 30 microns in width (Figs. 19–30 [2], 19–34). The laboratory technologist should be cautioned about the infectiousness of the embryonated eggs on the cellulose tape preparations and/or in stools.

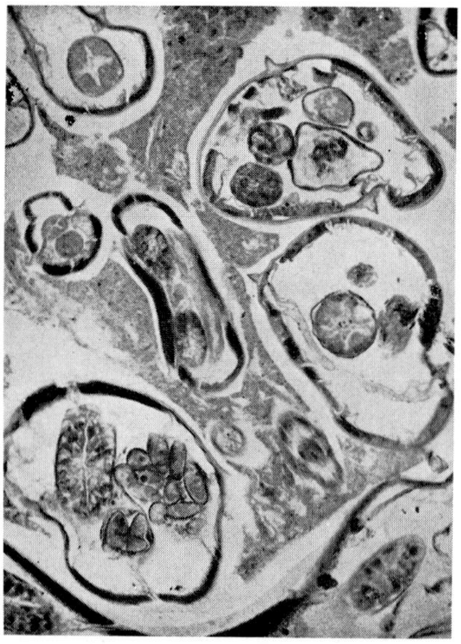

Figure 19–32. *Enterobius vermicularis* in lumen of appendix. Cross section of adult pinworms shows bilateral crests; one worm contains eggs. (From Hunter, G. W., Frye, W. W., and Swartzwelder, J. C.: A Manual of Tropical Medicine. 4th ed.)

CELLULOSE TAPE TECHNIQUE FOR PINWORMS AFTER GRAHAM, 1941. Follow the directions in Figure 19–33 or as described below:

1. Apply a strip of transparent cellulose tape 2½ to 3 inches in length on the upper side, beginning at one end, of a tongue blade. A small portion of the end on the opposite portion of the tongue blade should be folded on itself. This provides a nonsticky surface for handling the tape.
2. To obtain a sample, pull the folded tab so that the sticky side of the tape is freed, still leaving enough of it stuck to the tongue blade.
3. Carry the freed tape over the end of the blade so that the sticky side is out.
4. Hold the tongue depressor with the thumb and second finger and hold the tape to the tongue blade with the forefinger.
5. Press the sticky surface onto the right

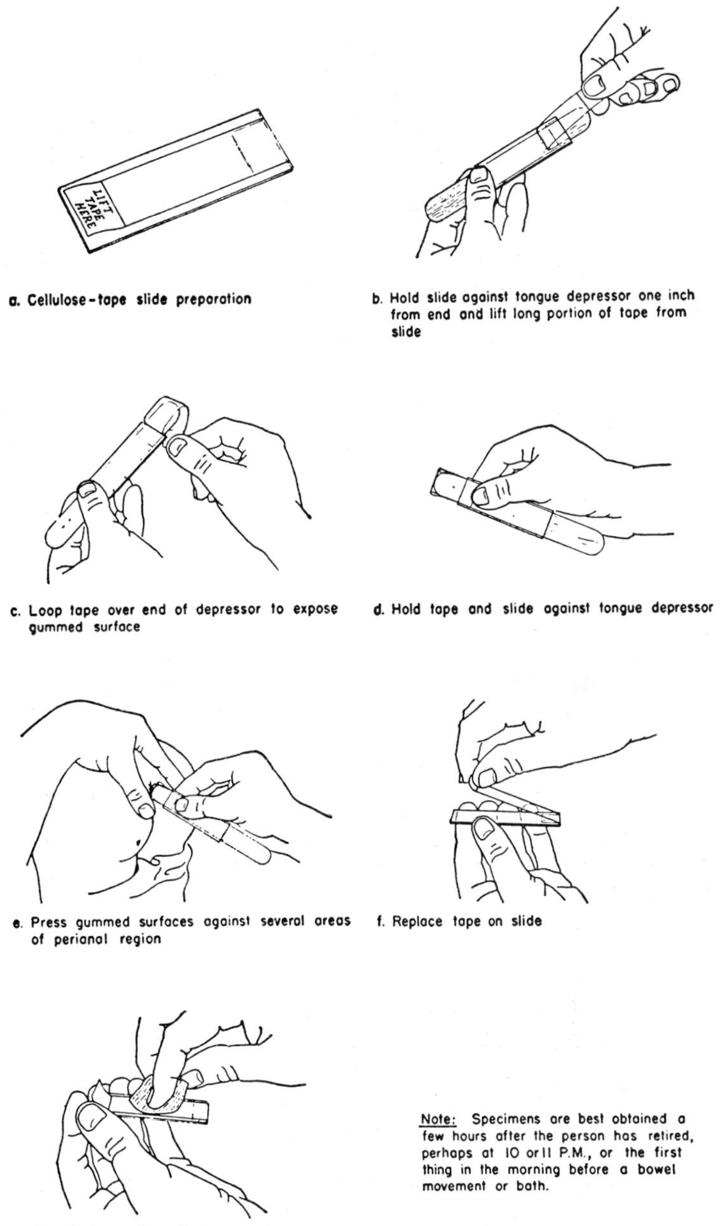

a. Cellulose-tape slide preparation

b. Hold slide against tongue depressor one inch from end and lift long portion of tape from slide

c. Loop tape over end of depressor to expose gummed surface

d. Hold tape and slide against tongue depressor

e. Press gummed surfaces against several areas of perianal region

f. Replace tape on slide

g. Smooth tape with cotton or gauze

Note: Specimens are best obtained a few hours after the person has retired, perhaps at 10 or 11 P.M., or the first thing in the morning before a bowel movement or bath.

Figure 19–33. Use of cellulose tape slide preparation for diagnosis of pinworm infections. (Adapted from Brook, Donaldson, and Mitchell, 1949.)

and left perianal folds but do not insert the blade into the rectum.

6. Replace the tape onto the tongue blade. (These blades can be carried or sent by mail to the laboratory.)

7. Transfer the tapes to microscope slides. (As a precaution, process these preparations over paper toweling which can be discarded later in disinfectant.)

8. Pull tape back from the slide, leaving a small portion attached.

9. Add a drop of toluene and replace the tape on the slide. (The toluene clears everything except the eggs and adults, if present.)

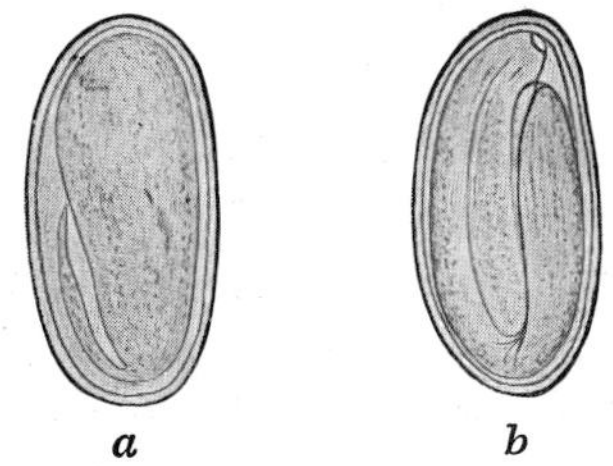

a *b*

Figure 19–34. Eggs of *Enterobius vermicularis. a,* Freshly deposited, with tadpole-like embryo; *b,* 12 hours after deposition, with nematode-like embryo (× 500). (After Fantham, Stephens, and Theobald.)

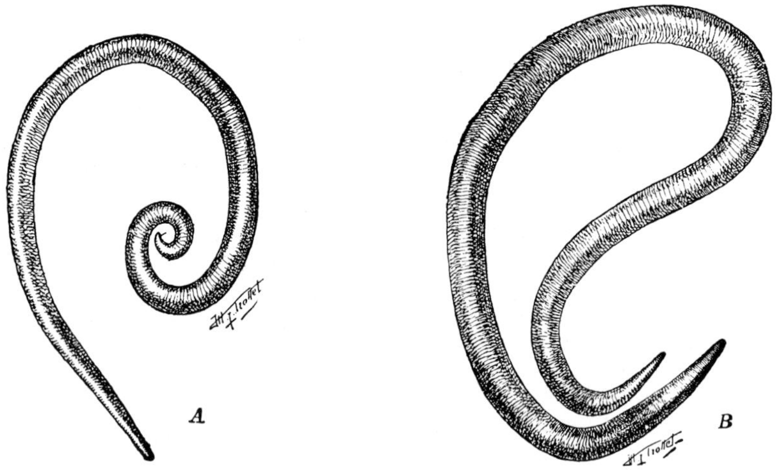

Figure 19–35. The common roundworm, *Ascaris lumbricoides,* natural size. *A,* Male; *B,* female. (After Brumpt.)

10. Smooth out the tape with a piece of gauze, which should be disinfected and discarded. Examine for the eggs and female adults under the low-power objective. In old or mailed-in specimens only empty egg shells may be seen. (Other helminth eggs, especially *Taenia,* may be seen on the cellulose tapes.)

Ascaris lumbricoides. *Ascaris lumbricoides* (Table 19–5; Figs. 19–28, 19–35, 19–71) is the intestinal roundworm that resides in the small intestine and causes ascariasis. The adult female worm measures 20 to 40 cm. in length (Figs. 19–28, 19–35 *B*) and is about 5 mm. thick or about the size of a lead pencil, with most of the worm given to reproductive organs; the males (Fig. 19–35 *A*), 10 to 30 cm. long, are more slender and have a ventrally curved tail. The worms become sexually mature in eight to 12 weeks and live for several years. The nearly opaque cuticle is pinkish white in color; however, after therapy the worms recovered may be brownish and the cuticle blistered. Never handle worms without plastic or rubber gloves. *Ascaris* worms, in spite of their size (even immature worms), have trilobate lips at their anterior end. A hand lens may assist in the detection of the lips. In cross sections polymyarian type musculature is observed (Fig. 19–29 *A*).

In bisexual infections the fertilized egg, which is unsegmented (Figs. 19–30 [3,5], 19–36), is broadly oval, measuring 45 to 75 microns in length by 35 to 50 microns in breadth. The thick shell has an outer albuminous covering, which is coarsely mammilated and is stained with bile to a golden brown or yellow color. Those fertilized eggs that have lost their albuminoid coat are denoted as decorticated (Fig. 19–30 [5]), and they must be differentiated from hookworm eggs. In all fertilized eggs there is a conspicuous, crescentic, clear space at each pole between the contents and the shell. Eggs may embryonate in 10 per cent formalin unless the formalin is preheated to 60° C. at the time of specimen fixation.

Unisexual infections are common, and when male worms only are present or passed it is obvious that no eggs could be recovered; but when only female worms are present or in early bisexual infections, only unfertilized eggs may be found (Figs. 19–30 [4], 19–37). There is much variation in unfertilized eggs, but they are longer and narrower than the fertile eggs and have a thinner shell. Internally there is a mass of coarse granules, which fill the shell. They may be decorticated. They may have light to heavy staining with bile. The inexperienced technician may overlook these eggs, since some are extremely irregular in outline and may show little likeness to fertilized *Ascaris* eggs.

Adult, fertilized female ascarids deposit about 200,000 eggs per day during the year or two of lifespan. Egg-counting methods (Beaver, 1950; Stoll, 1923; "Kato," reported by Komiya and Kobayashi, 1966) may be utilized to determine the worm burden. These eggs are noninfective in stool specimens and become infective for man only after a two-week or longer period of embryonation in the soil

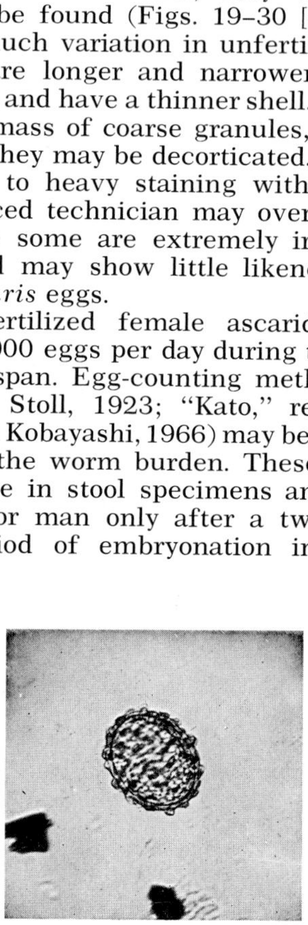

Figure 19–36. Egg of *Ascaris lumbricoides,* surface view (× 250).

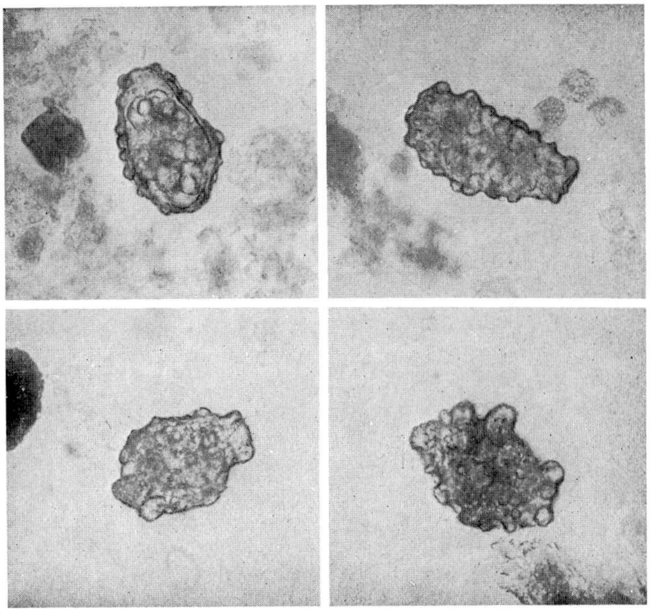

Figure 19–37. Unfertilized eggs of *Ascaris lumbricoides*, showing the great irregularity in shape. Some of these eggs are extremely difficult to identify (× 250).

where they remain infective for extended periods. *Ascaris* larvae may be seen in the sputum of infected individuals, especially during the *Ascaris* pneumonitis accompanying larval migration through the lungs (see p. 1000).

Ascaris worms may be passed spontaneously through the anus, mouth, or nose. Various conditions may cause them to ball up and cause bowel obstruction or wander to sites in the appendix, peritoneal cavity, and liver, where serious complications may ensue (Piggott *et al.*, 1970). For example, a patient with ascariasis and hookworm should be treated for the former first, as drugs used for hookworm may stimulate the ascarids to wander. Toxic manifestations may exist because of the presence of the adult worms. Eosinophilia may be present.

In most *Ascaris* infections eggs can be recovered from the stool by direct smears or concentration methods (see pp. 1110–1113, 1113–1114). In scanty infections the following sedimentation procedure is beneficial:

Sedimentation. This is a slow, natural (gravity) settling out of heavier parasite objects, with three or more alternate settlings and decantations of the supernatant. One of the simplest methods applicable to the recovery of all eggs, larvae, and cysts is this technique. There may be much confusing debris, however. Its value lies in the fact that, since a large sample of stool specimen is used, scanty infections (especially those involving helminths) can be detected by this method.

Material and Equipment

1. Tongue depressor.
2. Beakers, 250 ml.
3. Funnel, 50 mm. or larger.
4. Gauze (Brunswick), or gauze from a bolt.
5. Saline, normal (glycerin, 0.5 per cent solution may be used instead).
6. Glass, sedimentation (cone-shaped, 250 ml.). Polyethylene sedimentation units are available.
7. Pipette, capillary, with rubber bulb attached.
8. Slides, 2 by 3 inch.
9. Coverslips.

Technique

1. Place a sample of feces about the size of a plum, or larger, in about 100 ml. of normal saline or glycerinated water (to prevent hatching of the schistosome eggs). (The reduction in surface tension, resulting in a greater yield of eggs can be accomplished by using a 0.5 per cent solution of glycerin.)
2. Comminute the feces thoroughly, using a tongue blade.
3. Strain the suspension through four layers of dampened gauze into a 250-ml. sedimentation glass.
4. Allow the suspension to settle for 1 hour.
5. Carefully decant the supernatant.
6. Fill the sedimentation glass with saline to resuspend the sediment.
7. Repeat the washing and decanting until the supernatant is clear.
8. Decant carefully the last time.
9. Examine a portion of the bottom of the sediment under low power. Examine a second sample removed by spiraling upward through the sediment. Sediment may be refrigerated if the examination is delayed. (Viability of schistosome eggs, described later, may be determined by examining the miracidium

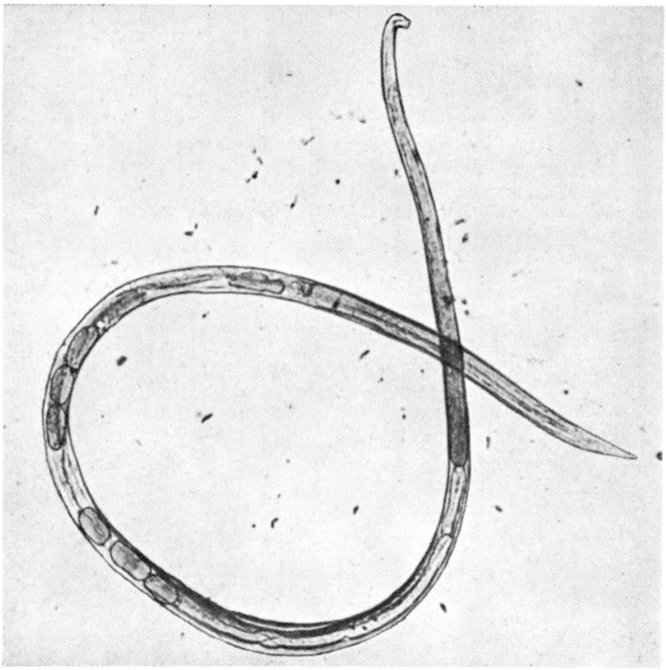

Figure 19–38. *Strongyloides stercoralis*, parasitic female. (From Markell, E. K., and Voge, M.: Medical Parasitology. 3rd ed.)

within the shell for flame cells and solenocytes or by employing an egg-hatching technique.)

Anisakis **sp.** Anisakiasis (Sindermann, 1970; Lab. Med., 1970) (Table 19–5) is a nematode disease of marine animals that can be transmitted to man upon ingestion of larvae in raw, "cold smoked," or "lightly salted" fish. The larvae invade the wall of the digestive tract and produce an eosinophilic phlegmonous enteritis.

Strongyloides stercoralis. *Strongyloides stercoralis* (Table 19–5; Figs. 19–28, 19–38, 19–72) is the true threadworm of man, producing Cochin-China diarrhea or strongyloidiasis, a condition that may be refractory to therapy. Outside of the endemic areas, which are the tropics and subtropics, strongyloidiasis may be observed to spread in mental institutions where dissemination of feces in moist surroundings permits development of the infective filariform larvae. The 2.2 mm. long parasitic females (Figs. 19–28, 19–38, 19–40, 19–72), which may be parthenogenetic and take about

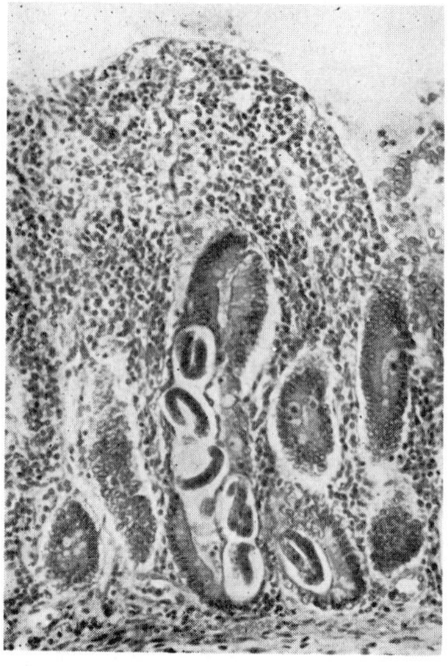

Figure 19–39

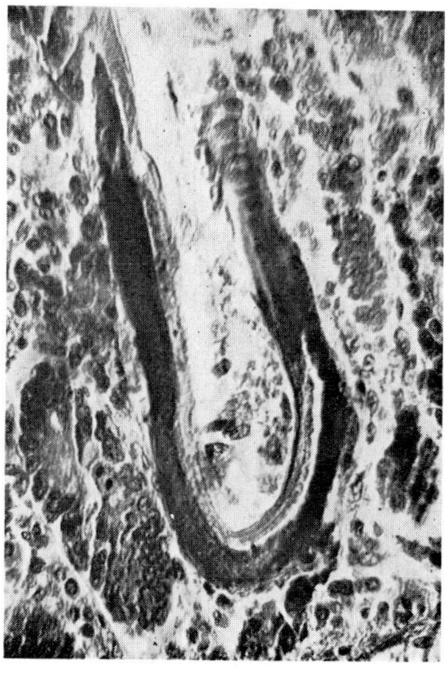

Figure 19–40

Figure 19–39. Embryonated eggs of *Strongyloides stercoralis* in mucosa of duodenum. (From Hunter, G. W., Frye, W. W., and Swartzwelder, J. C.: A Manual of Tropical Medicine. 4th ed.)

Figure 19–40. Portion of a parasitic adult female *S. stercoralis* in mucosa of small intestine. (From Hunter, G. W., Frye, W. W., and Swartzwelder, J. C.: A Manual of Tropical Medicine. 4th ed.)

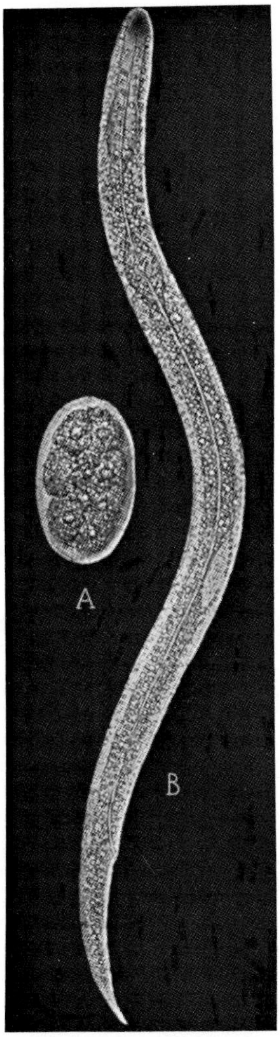

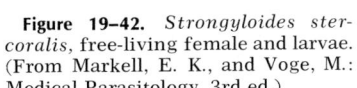

Figure 19–41. *A*, Egg of *Strongyloides stercoralis* (parasitic mother worm) found in stools in a case of chronic diarrhea; *B*, rhabditiform larva of *Strongyloides stercoralis* from the stools. (From W. S. Thayer: J. Exper. Med.)

one month to mature, are buried in the mucosa of the duodenum and much of the small intestine and cannot be seen with the unaided eye. They may live for a year or more. Since the eggs are deposited in the mucosa, they rarely are seen in the stool (Figs. 19–30 [11], 19–39, 19–41 *A*). The first larval stage, the noninfective rhabditiform larva (or rhabditoid) (Figs. 19-30 [10]), 19–41 *B*, 19–72) is observed. Actively motile larvae are usually seen in mushy or liquid stools, whereas nonmotile, often degenerated larvae may be recovered in dehydrated stools of infected persons. Inside the human host rhabditoids may become filariforms (see below). Once outside the host the rhabditoids may become either filariforms or free-living males or females. Eggs (50 by 30 microns) of *S. stercoralis* can be found in stools when the patient is diarrheic or strongly purged or when stools are submitted in a closed glass container (which serves as an artificial culture similar to the Petri dish smears described below) with sufficient moisture to allow rhabditiform larvae to develop into free-living adults, and the free-living females (Figs. 19–42, 19–72) (which are not to be confused with the parasitic females) to deposit eggs (70 by 40 microns) on the surface of the stool. In either case these eggs must be differentiated from those of hookworms. Larvae (rhabditoid) may be recovered from the stool by direct smears and concentration procedures (pp. 1110–1113, 1113–1114) or by sedimentation (p. 1063), as well as by special culture methods outlined below (p. 1067). (Filariform larvae, which develop rapidly from the rhabditoids, may be seen grossly if in large numbers, as they swarm in moisture of condensation in closed glass jars containing older stools. The fact that these filariform larvae are infective cannot be overemphasized.) Duodenal aspiration may be necessary to demonstrate the larvae. These must be differentiated from plant hairs (Fig. 19–97 [18]) as well as from filariform and rhabditoid larvae of the hookworms, *Rhabditis hominis* and *Trichostrongylus* sp. (Table 19–6). The rhabditiform larva measures 225 by 16 microns and possesses a conspicuous ovoidal, genital anlage (primordium) nearly midway and ventral in the body.

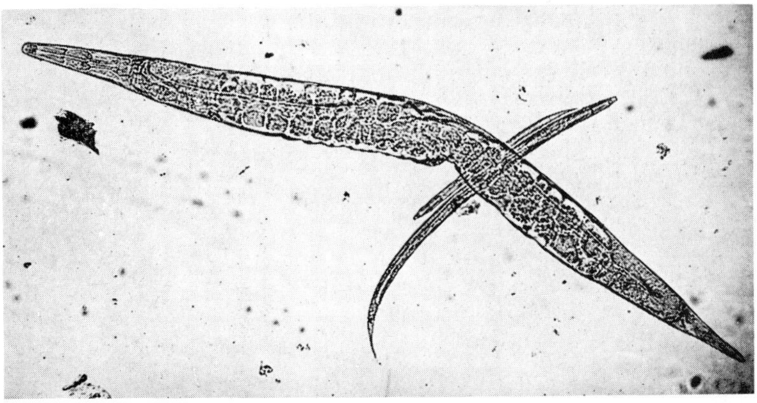

Figure 19–42. *Strongyloides stercoralis*, free-living female and larvae. (From Markell, E. K., and Voge, M.: Medical Parasitology. 3rd ed.)

Table 19–6. DIFFERENTIATION OF LARVAE OF HOOKWORM, *Strongyloides, Rhabditis,* AND *Trichostrongylus*

CATEGORY	*Strongyloides*	HOOKWORM	*Rhabditis hominis*	*Tricho-strongylus*
		RHABDITIFORM LARVAE		
Shape	Short, stout	Short, stout	Short, stout	Short, stout
Size (average)	225 × 16 microns	275 × 17 microns	240-300 × 12 microns	480 microns
Anterior	Short, narrow buccal cavity; esophagus near anterior tip	Long, narrow buccal cavity; esophagus distal from anterior tip	Long buccal cavity with thick cuticle	Long buccal cavity
Posterior	More blunt	Sharply pointed	Pointed	Bead-like swelling at tip
Genital anlage (primordium)	Conspicuous on ventral side halfway down midgut	Inconspicuous	Inconspicuous	Inconspicuous
Internal structures	Well developed for feeding	Well developed for feeding	Well developed for feeding	Well developed for feeding
		FILARIFORM LARVAE		
Shape	Long, slender	Long, slender	None	Long, slender
Size	700 microns	700 microns	None	690 microns
Anterior	Rounded	Rounded	None	Rounded
Posterior	Notched tail	Pointed tail	None	Bluntly rounded with a minute, sharp terminal process
Internal structures	One-half esophagus, one-half gut with line of demarcation; nonfeeding stage	Remnants of esophagus with gut; nonfeeding stage	None	Pseudofilariform type; nonfeeding stage

In addition, the buccal capsule is short, as evidenced by the close proximity of the esophagus to the anterior tip. The larvae are actively motile and have a snake-like, whipping motion. They must be slowed down with gentle heat, killed with formalin, or killed and stained with the iodine solution p. 1110) to see detailed morphology. Under favorable conditions these rhabditiform larvae, which pass out with the feces onto moist, warm soil, develop into free-living males or females or into the infective filariform stage.

Filariform larvae (Fig. 19–72), which are transparent like the other larvae, may develop also within the intestine from rhabditiform larvae, and autoinfection (hyperinfection) may take place as the larvae penetrate the mucosa. If these filariform larvae are in the stool or in cultures, they must be differentiated from the rhabditiform larvae and from the filariform larvae of the hookworm. They are characterized by a notched tail and a body that is nearly evenly divided into esophagus and gut, the latter being more granular and set off by a distinct line of demarcation. When in moist warm soil, the filariform larvae come to the surface, from which they penetrate the skin of the host. Subsequent to penetration they migrate to the lungs whence they are coughed up (may be observed in sputum) and swallowed to become parasitic females in the duodenum.

Diagnosis is based upon finding the migrating larvae in sputum, the distinctive rhabditiform in the feces or in duodenal contents. When an individual has a mixed infection of hookworm and *Strongyloides* there will be eggs of the former and rhabditoid larvae of the latter. Frequently the larvae are seen in the stool in a molting stage between the rhabditiform and filariform and cannot be specifically identified, but cultivation for 24 to 48 hours will produce transparent, free-living adults (Figs. 19–42, 19–72) and filariform larvae of *Strongyloides*, but only rhabditiform larvae will develop from the hookworm eggs. About eight days are required for the filariform larvae of hookworm to develop. The laboratory worker should be cautioned against self-contamination with stools or cultures containing filariform larvae of *Strongyloides*.

Clinically strongyloidiasis may be asymptomatic, or as the larvae pass through the lungs a pneumonitis may develop. An increase in eosinophils may be accompanied by abdominal pains and diarrhea. Where prolonged hyperinfection is present, liver function damage and cirrhosis may exist.

Cultures for Larvae of Hookworm and Strongyloides

PETRI DISH SMEARS

1. Cut a piece of filter paper so that a one-half inch space remains around it in the bottom of a Petri dish.
2. Smear feces on the filter paper or directly on the bottom of the dish with a tongue depressor in a thin layer and allow to dry slightly.
3. Layer a thin film of tap water over the surface of the feces and cover.
4. Culture at room temperature for 24 to 48 hours or longer.
5. Examine under the scanning lens of a microscope or dissecting scope. Handle the cultures wearing plastic or rubber gloves.
6. Transfer organisms to microslide, using a medicine dropper, and add coverslip.
7. Filariform larvae of *Strongyloides* have notched tails and appear in 24 to 48 hours. Free-living adults may be seen in 48 hours or more.
8. Filariform larvae of hookworm do not appear for eight days. However, the rhabditiform larvae may appear in 24 hours.

CHARCOAL CULTURE

1. Moisten 6 gm. of coarsely granular coconut charcoal (6-14 mesh, Fisher No. 5-685-B) with water and add about 1 gm. of feces and mix with a tongue depressor.
2. Place the charcoal in a Petri dish to form a cone of charcoal that will cover the bottom of the dish but will only remain in contact with an area about 2 inches in diameter on the center of the inside of the lid.
3. Incubate at room temperature for one to eight days. Keep moist.
4. Examine the droplets of the moisture of condensation under the scanning lens of a microscope by inverting the lid or examine the washings of the inside of the cover. Handle cultures wearing plastic or rubber gloves.
5. The filariform larvae of *S. stercoralis* have notched tails and appear in 24 to 48 hours, while the filariform of hookworm appear in about eight days. Sheathed larvae are difficult to classify. Rhabditiform larvae may appear in 24 hours at the bottom of the dish.

An alternate method is the Harada and Mori test tube method (Hsieh, 1961).

Trichuris (Trichocephalus) trichiura. *Trichuris trichiura (Trichocephalus trichiura)* (Table 19–5; Figs. 19–28, 19–43, 19–73) is commonly called the whipworm and causes trichuriasis (trichocephaliasis). The opaque adults (Figs. 19–28, 19–43, 19–73) are 3.5 to 5.0 cm. long with an attenuated, whip-like anterior end and a thicker posterior portion, which is bluntly rounded in the female (Figs. 19–28, 19–43 *A*, 19–73) and coiled like a watch spring in the male (Figs. 19–43 *B*, 19–73). The worms may be demonstrated following therapy and are pinkish white in color. In cross section they show a holomyarian musculature (Fig. 19–29 *C*). The noninfective, characteristic unsegmented eggs in stools (Figs. 19–31 [1], 19–45, 19–73) are football-shaped, with mucous plugs at either pole. They are golden brown, have a thick shell, and measure 50 to 54 microns long and about 23 microns wide. The eggs appear nearly spherical when viewed on end. They can be recovered from the stool by direct smears, concentration (pp. 1110–1113, 1113–1114), and sedimentation (p. 1063) methods. Eggs may embryonate in stored, formalin-fixed stools.

Embryonated eggs (Fig. 19–73) in the soil are infective when ingested by man, and larvae hatching from the eggs in the region of the duodenum merely descend to the large intestine, where they develop into adults in three months. The attenuated end is buried among villi and thereby "attached" and the thick end is free in the lumen of the colon. They may live several years or longer, during which time each female produces approximately 5000 eggs per day. Egg counts can be done to estimate the worm burden.

Large numbers of worms may cause symptoms, and cases of prolapsed rectum (Fig. 19–44), due to their presence have been reported.

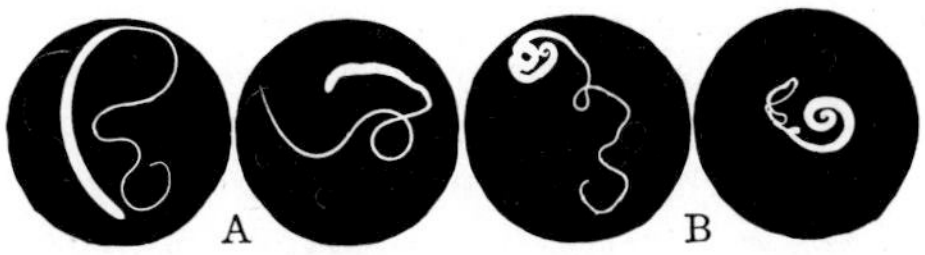

Figure 19–43. Whipworms (*Trichuris trichiura*). *A*, Females; *B*, males. The posterior portion of the male is usually coiled as is shown at the right. Photographs of mounted specimens. Natural size.

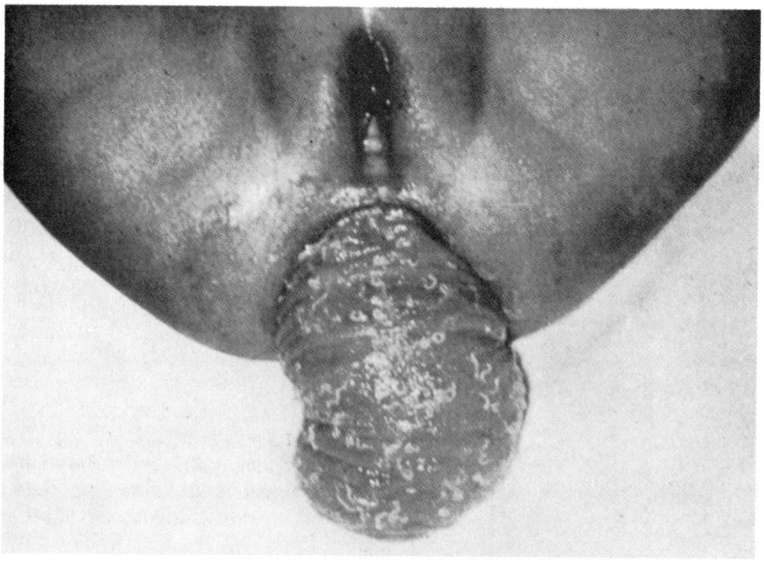

Figure 19–44. Prolapse of rectum in a Louisiana child, due to heavy infection with *Trichuris trichiura.* (Photo made by Drs. P. C. Beaver and R. V. Platou; copy to senior author through courtesy of Dr. J. C. Swartzwelder. From Hunter, G. W., Frye, W. W., and Swartzwelder, J. C.: A Manual of Tropical Medicine. 4th ed.)

A bloody diarrhea or constipation and abdominal pains may occur.

Capillaria philippinensis. In the Pacific a new, often fatal diarrheal disease, intestinal capillariasis, contingent upon the presence of the minute roundworm *C. philippinensis,* produces a severe protein-losing enteropathy and malabsorption of fats and sugars (Whalen *et al.,* 1969). The eggs appear in stools and must be differentiated from *Trichuris* (Chitwood *et al.,* 1968) (Table 19–5).

Trichostrongylus orientalis. A number of species of *Trichostrongylus* have been found in man, although they are primarily parasites of herbivorous animals. The larvae from the soil are ingested with contaminated food. The adults are small and live in the jejunum and upper ileum of man. Diagnosis is based upon finding the eggs (Fig. 19–30 [7,8]) in the feces by various techniques (see pp. 1063, 1110–1113, 1113–1114). They measure 75 to 91 microns in length and 39 to 47 microns in diameter. They resemble hookworm eggs in that they have a thin shell, but they are more nearly pointed at one end and are larger. They must be differentiated from eggs of *Strongyloides* and *Heterodera,* as well. The rhabditiform larva possesses a characteristic small knob at the tip of the tail (see Table 19–6). They may be found in feces or in cultures (see p. 1067). These worms are somewhat refractory to therapy, but they are essentially nonpathogenic.

Angiostrongylus cantonensis. Angiostrongyliasis has been observed in humans in the Pacific (Alicata and Jindrak, 1969). This rat-lung nematode produces eosinophilic meningitis in man.

Heterodera marioni. *Heterodera marioni* is a true parasite of plants, but man has been shown to harbor eggs of this organism, which are swallowed with parasitized vegetable tissues, such as onion roots. These noninfective eggs (Fig. 19–30 [9]) are passed in human feces and must be differentiated from hookworm, *Strongyloides* and *Trichostrongylus* eggs. They are 82 to 120 microns in length and 24 to 43 microns in breadth. They are elongated and ovoid with rounded ends and contain

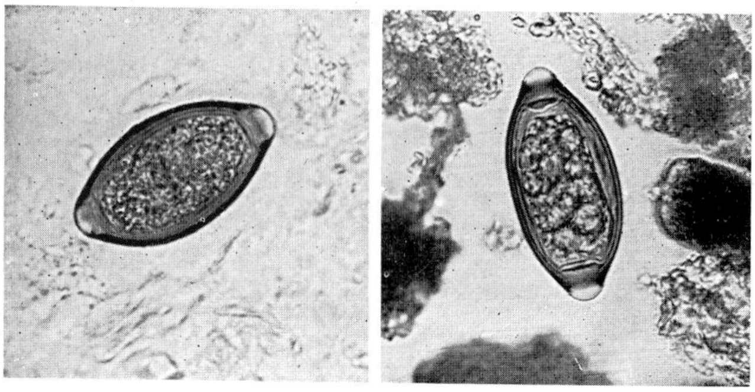

Figure 19–45. Eggs of *Trichuris trichiura* in feces (× 500).

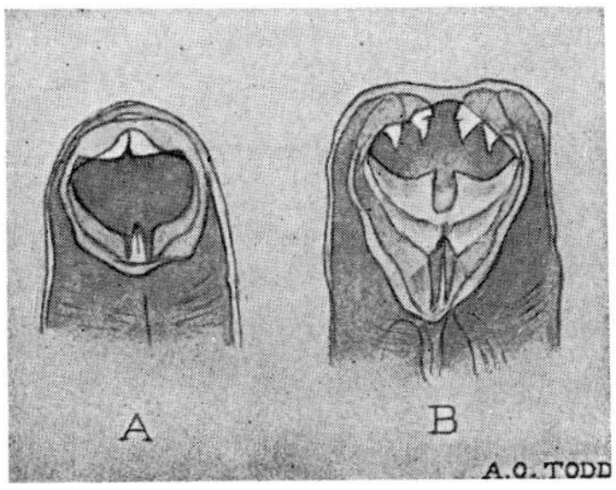

Figure 19–46. Heads of hookworms showing mouth parts. *A, Necator americanus; B, Ancylostoma duodenale.* Since the head of the hookworm is sharply curved backward, the upper part of the figure represents the ventral surface. (After E. R. Stitt.)

several globular masses in addition to the large, greenish granular mass. Embryonated eggs reveal a yellowish brown larva.

The Hookworms

Ancylostoma duodenale* and *Necator americanus. The hookworms *Ancylostoma duodenale* and *Necator americanus* (Table 19–5; Figs. 19–28, 19–46, 19–74) account for the diseases ancylostomiasis or uncinariasis and necatoriasis, respectively. *Ancylostoma duodenale* is called the Old World hookworm, while the latter is called the New World or American hookworm.

The adult hookworms, which take six weeks to mature but may live for many years, are small, cylindrical, pinkish white and opaque with a dorsal flexion and are attached to the mucosa of the small intestine. Adult worms are seen only after therapy. In cross section they show meromyarian musculature (Figs. 19–29 *B*, 19–47). The male worm measures 1.0 cm. in length and 0.5 mm. in width, while the female is slightly larger. *Ancylostoma* is larger than *Necator*. Males possess a fan-shaped bursa (Figs. 19–28, 19–74) at their posterior end. Spicules are separate in *Ancylostoma* but fused in *Necator*. The shape of the adults is of diagnostic importance, for although there is a curvature of the head in *Ancylostoma, Necator* shows a pronounced dorsal flexion, which is hooklike. The buccal capsule reveals diagnostic features. In *Necator* cutting plates are seen in contrast to teeth in *Ancylostoma* (Figs. 19–28, 19–46). Internal structures are seen only when a clearing agent is employed.

The eggs (Figs. 19–30 [6], 19–48, 19–74) of the two genera are identical except for a slight variation in size. *Ancylostoma* eggs are smaller than *Necator* eggs, which are 64 to 76 microns by 36 to 40 microns. These eggs, which possess a hyaline shell, are unsegmented or in the four-cell stage when passed in the fresh stool and are noninfective for man. Internal development is rapid from the four-cell stage through to the morula stage. Bacteria and debris may mask the shell by adhering to it. These must be differentiated from *Strongyloides stercoralis, Trichostrongylus* and *Heterodera* eggs. Occasionally larvae may be seen within the eggs, especially in stools that

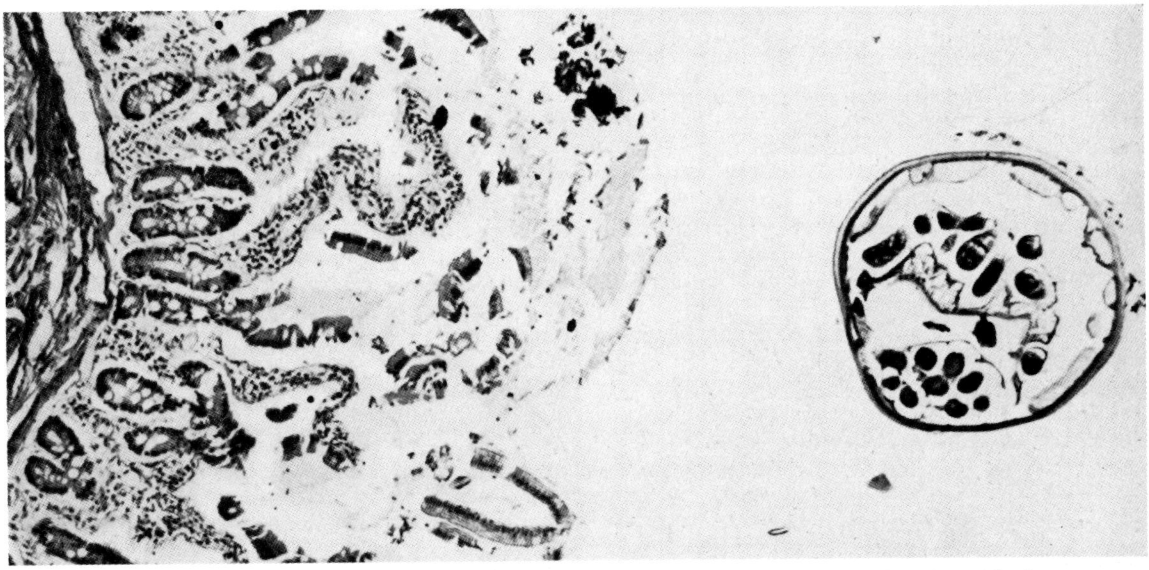

Figure 19–47. Cross section of hookworm showing meromyarial type of body musculature. In sections, hookworms may be confused with *Enterobius vermicularis,* and differentiation is made on the gross features of the worm and on differences in normal habitat. (From Ash, J. E., and Spitz, S.: Pathology of Tropical Diseases.)

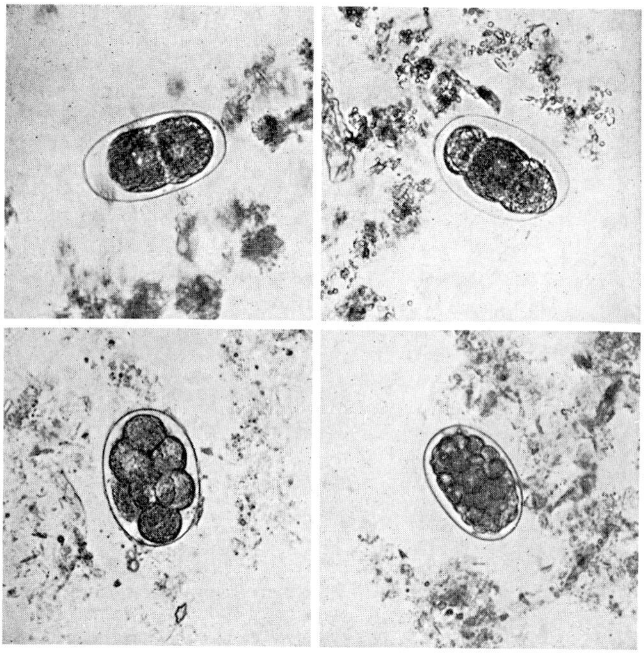

Figure 19–48. Eggs of *Necator americanus* in feces. The egg showing three cells is a lateral view of a four-cell stage (× 250).

have been standing without refrigeration for a few days, or that have not been fixed in 10 per cent formalin preheated to 60° C. Hookworm and *Strongyloides* may coexist in the patient. Eggs appear in the former and larvae in the latter. Hookworm eggs may be recovered by direct smears, concentration (pp. 1110–1113, 1113–1114), and sedimentation procedures (p. 1063).

The rhabditiform larvae (Fig. 19–74) (also noninfective), seen in specific cultures (p. 1067), have a long buccal cavity as evidenced by the position of the esophagus (Table 19–6). They must be differentiated from plant fibers (Fig. 19–97 [18]), rhabditoids of *Strongyloides, Rhabditis hominis,* and *Trichostrongylus* (Table 19–6) and from hookworm (Fig. 19–74) and *Strongyloides* filariforms (Fig. 19–72). Rhabditiform larvae may appear in cultures in a few days, but eight days are required for the filariforms. The laboratory worker should be cautious when handling culture containing the infective filariform larvae.

Patients with hookworm *infection* may show no symptoms, and few eggs are seen in the stool. Hookworm *disease,* on the other hand, is more serious and is established upon the presence of several hundred to a thousand worms, with accompanying symptomatology of cramps, diarrhea, and an associated blood loss (marked anemia). Egg counts (Beaver, 1950; Stoll, 1923; and "Kato," reported by Komiya and Kobayashi, 1966) can be done to estimate the worm burden. As the filariform larvae in the contaminated soil invade the skin, ground itch develops, and as they pass through the lungs, they provoke a pneumonitis. Hyperinfection (autoinfection) does not occur with hookworm. Even light infections should be treated, as the patient may be responsible for soil pollution.

Additional nematodes (filariae and *Trichinella*), which are in tissues, are discussed later in this chapter.

Miscellaneous Nematodes. Information on nematodes infrequently observed in man is available (Faust, 1949).

The Cestodes

The cestodes or tapeworms are common parasites of man. The adult tapeworms dwell in the small intestine and consist of a family of segments or proglottids, which are attached to the wall by means of suckers or, in some instances, by suckers and hooklets situated on the rostellum of the scolex or head (the holdfast). This chain of segments is called a strobila. Behind the scolex is the neck region from which the worm grows longer. Posterior to the neck one sees sets of immature, mature, and gravid segments, the latter being the oldest and displaying distinctive uterine designs. Segments are hermaphroditic. Eggs in the uterus generally are released by disintegration of the segment but in one genus (*Diphyllobothrium*) are expelled through a birth pore. All tapeworm eggs contain a hexacanth embryo, except those of *D. latum* (which are immature and operculated when recovered in feces). The hooklets in the cestode eggs function in the new host to permit the hatched embryo to penetrate and progress through tissues and have no relationship to the "armed" scolex (with hooks) of certain tapeworms.

Calcareous corpuscles (bodies) (Fig. 19–49) are characteristic of tapeworm tissue (McQuay *et al.*, 1966). They occur only in cestodes, but some cestodes in certain stages or at certain times may be without them. They may be destroyed by acid fixation.

Tapeworms, except for *H. nana*, utilize one or more intermediate hosts, in which the larval stage is found. Consumption of the specific larval stage results in infection in man.

Differentiating the tapeworms may be achieved by a study of their eggs (Fig. 19–50), gravid segments, and scolices (Fig. 19–51). To study the uterine design of the gravid segments of larger worms, press the segment between two wide glass slides and hold the segment against a good light source. One must be cautious, since *T. solium* eggs are infective for man. Segments, which may be passed singly or in chains, are frequently brought to

A

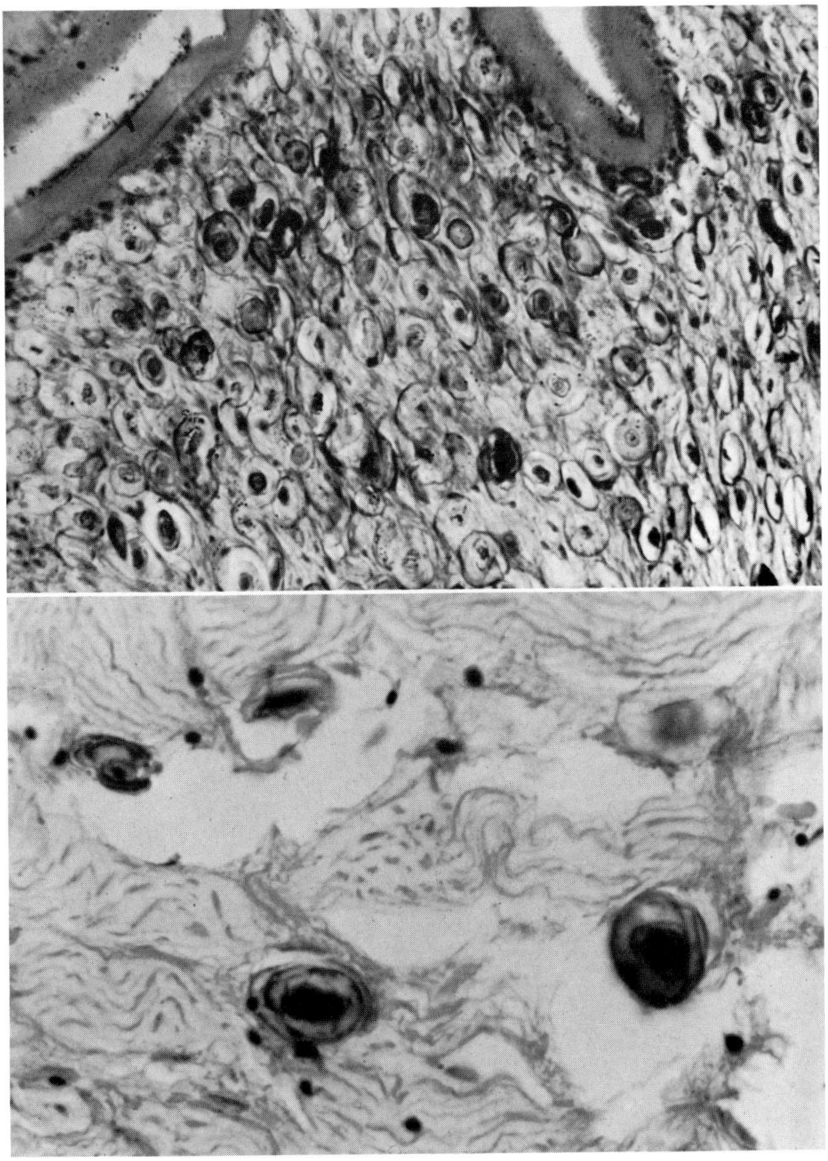

B

Figure 19–49. *A*, Cluster of calcareous corpuscles (bodies) in cestode tissue (*Cysticercus*). H & E, × 590. *B*, Isolated calcareous corpuscles in sparganum from human source. H & E, × 262.

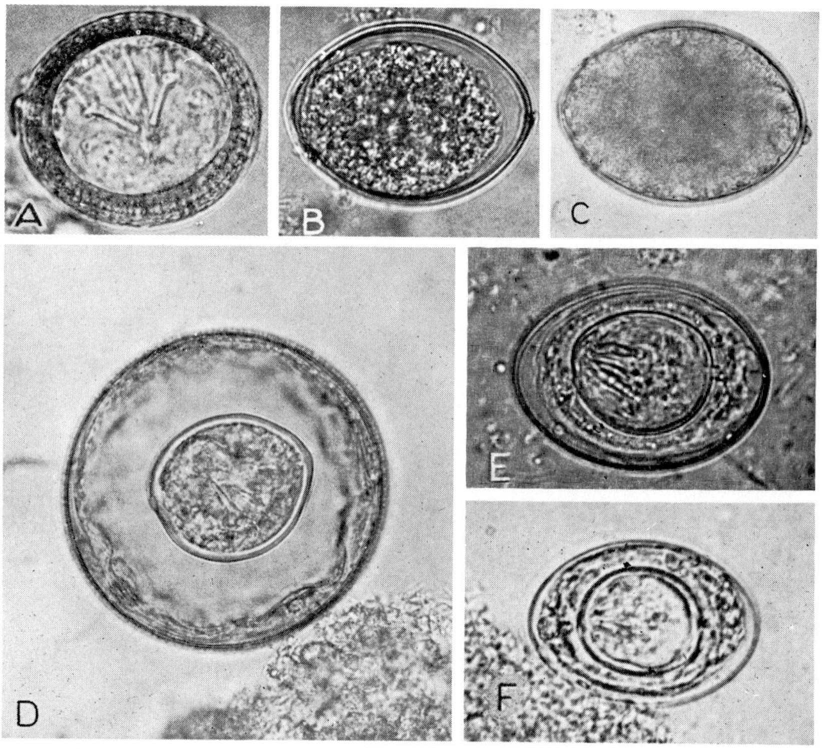

Figure 19–50. Some cestode eggs. *A*, Human tapeworm, *Taenia* sp. × 750. *B*, Broad tapeworm of man, *Diphyllobothrium latum.* × 500. *C*, Broad tapeworm of man, *Diphyllobothrium latum.* × 500. *D*, Rat tapeworm, *Hymenolepis diminuta.* × 650. *E*, Dwarf tapeworm, *Hymenolepis nana.* × 750. *F*, Dwarf tapeworm, *Hymenolepis nana* (note polar filaments). × 750. (Figs. *B* and *F* courtesy of Lt. L. W. Shatterly, School of Aviation Medicine, Gunter AFB, Alabama; all others courtesy of Dr. R. L. Roudabush, Ward's Natural Science Establishment, Rochester, New York; photos by T. Romaniak.)

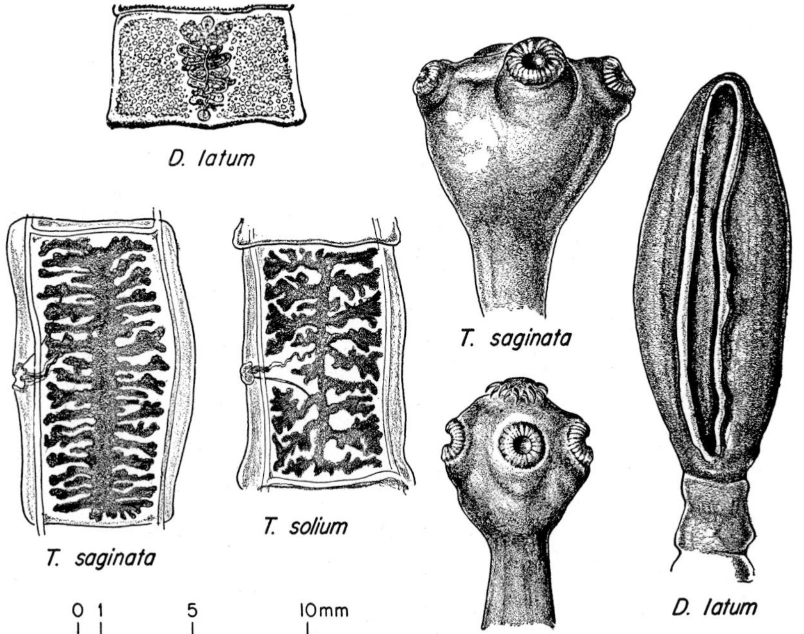

Figure 19–51. Scolices and gravid proglottids of some tapeworms of man. (From Mackie, T. T., Hunter, G. W., and Worth, C. B.: Manual of Tropical Medicine. 2nd ed.)

the physician. These should be placed in saline and sent to the laboratory for identification. Where chains of gravid segments break off there may be no eggs in the stool until mature segments become gravid. The scolex, however, remains attached to the intestinal wall and the worm continues to grow. Since the neck region behind the scolex is the source from which the worm grows, it is imperative to search for the head following therapy. The entire specimen should be submitted following therapy to the laboratory where a search should be made by straining the specimen through a special sieve. The eggs of all human tapeworms may be recovered from stools when mature worms are present by direct smear and concentration (pp. 1110–1113, 1113–1114) or sedimentation (p. 1063). *Taenia* sp. eggs may be recovered using the cellulose tape method (p. 1060).

If the patient has been prepared and managed properly for the removal of the larger tapeworms (*Taenia* and *D. latum*), the laboratory worker will have less searching through fecal specimens for the worm, especially the scolex, after treatment. A suggested routine is as follows:

1. Have patient consume large quantities of well-sugared drinks, unless contraindicated, during the week preceding therapy in an attempt to strengthen the worm and prevent breaking.
2. Patient should be on a low residue diet for several days prior to treatment; a liquid diet on the day before treatment is desired.
3. The evening of the day before treatment an oral purgative should be administered. The stool specimens may be collected and submitted to the laboratory, if desired.
4. No food is permitted on the morning of treatment. A cleansing saline enema should be given early in the day.
5. One hour after the enema, two 0.1-gm. tablets of quinacrine hydrochloride (Atabrine) are taken every 5 minutes until the entire dose is consumed (1.0 gm. for adults and smaller amounts for children). Tablets lost through vomiting may be replaced. Sodium bicarbonate administered with each dose may reduce nausea and vomiting.
6. A purgative is administered between 2 and 4 hours after the last tablets are given. All materials collected during the purge should be examined in the laboratory.

According to Dawson (1963) a Wood's ray lamp can be employed when Atabrine has been used to aid in the search for the scolex, which has become separated from the strobila. The acridine dye of the Atabrine will fluoresce.

If the scolex is not found, treat the patient again after one week or when and if segments are passed. If the scolex was retained, one may wish to wait three months to allow the worm to grow to maturity before specimens are examined to determine presence or absence of infection.

Recently Wittner and Tanowitz (1971) elaborated upon a new therapy for cestodes. Another new method utilizes Yomesan (Niclosamide 2,5-dichlor-4-nitrosalicylanilide) (See Marcial-Rojas, 1971, pp. 582–583). Apparently, the worm disintegrates *in situ*.

Taenia solium. *Taenia solium* (Table 19–5; Figs. 19–51, 19–75) is the pork tapeworm, occurring wherever man consumes raw or insufficiently cooked pork, but pork taeniasis is extremely rare in man in the United States. Infective cysticerci, *Cysticercus cellulosae* (Figs. 19–52, 19–75), which are small blad-

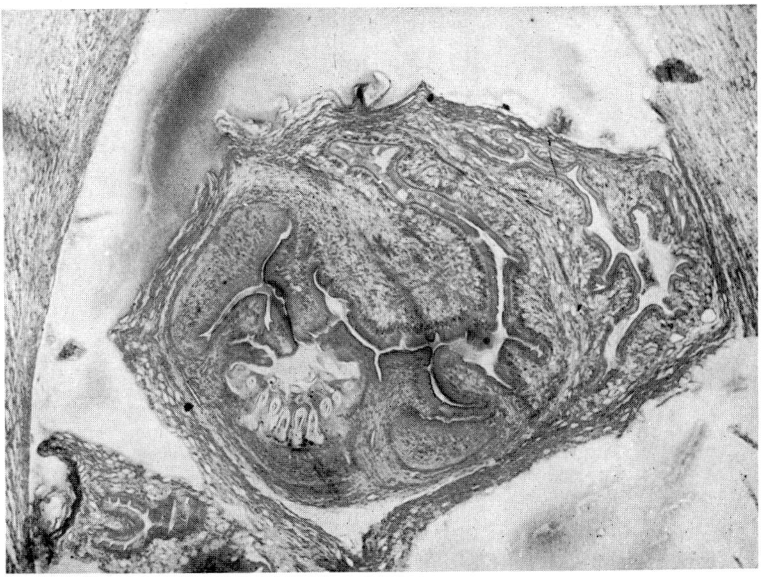

Figure 19–52. Cysticercus of *T. solium* in brain. Note slight tissue reaction of host, rostellar hooks, and laterally placed suckers of parasite. (From Hunter, G. W., Frye, W. W., and Swartzwelder, J. C.: A Manual of Tropical Medicine. 4th ed.)

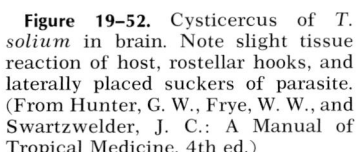

ders containing a scolex, are found in the pork. Man also may harbor the cysticerci (see section on cysticercosis, p. 1081). Extraordinary caution should be taken by the laboratory technologist in handling the adult worm or stools containing *Taenia* eggs, since the eggs of *T. solium* are immediately infective via the oral route.

The adult worm, which lives for many years, is 2 to 4 meters in length, and although numerous cysticerci may be swallowed, usually only one worm develops to maturity. The scolex (Figs. 19–51, 19–75) has four suckers and a rostellum with a double row of 25 to 30 hooklets; therefore, it is an "armed" scolex. The gravid segments (Figs. 19–51, 19–75) are longer than they are wide and contain a branched uterus. From the main uterine stem seven to 13 main branches arise on one side only. This number is of diagnostic importance, because it differentiates these segments from those of *T. saginata*. Species diagnosis cannot be made on the basis of eggs alone, because the eggs of the taenias are morphologically identical (Fig. 19–50 *A*) but physiologically different in that those of *T. solium* are immediately infective for man while those of *T. saginata* are for cattle. These eggs, which are 30 to 40 microns in diameter, are spherical with a thick, radially striated brown shell that contains a hexacanth onchosphere.

Adult worms may cause abdominal discomfort. Primary clinical concern occurs when cysticercosis is present.

Taenia saginata. *Taenia saginata*, the beef tapeworm of man, is commonly found in the United States. This worm, which may live for several years, may be 4 to 12 meters in length with as many as 2000 segments; thus, it is larger than *T. solium*. Usually only one worm develops to maturity even though many cysticerci may be consumed in raw or insufficiently cooked beef. The scolex (Fig. 19–51) has four suckers but is "unarmed" and about the size of a large pinhead. The gravid segments (Fig. 19–51) are longer than they are wide and are characterized by the presence of 15 to 30 main lateral branches on one side of the uterine stem (see *T. solium* for comparison). Individual gravid segments may be found on the surface of or in a stool or migrating from the anus. The eggs (30 to 40 microns) (Fig. 19–50 *A*) cannot be differentiated from those of *T. solium*. They are, however, infective for cattle but rarely for man (Faust, Russell and Jung, 1970, p. 536). In the musculature of cattle the larval stage (*C. bovis*) (similar to Fig. 19–52 but without hooklets) develops and serves as the source of infection for man. Beef taeniasis infections are generally subclinical.

Hymenolepis nana. The dwarf tapeworm, *Hymenolepis nana* (Table 19–5; Figs. 19–53, 19–76), differs from the larger tapeworms in that there may be hundreds of adult worms in a host, whereas only one of the other tapeworms of man develops to maturity.

The adult (Figs. 19–53, 19–76) is 1.0 to 4.5 cm. long and 0.4 to 0.7 mm. wide. The "armed" rostellum may be invaginated or evaginated and embraces 24 to 30 hooklets. Segments, which may number 200, are broader than long. Eggs escape only when the segments disintegrate. Characteristic eggs (30 to 47 microns) (Figs. 19–50 *E*, *F*, 19–76) are found by routine stool examination, but in light infections sedimentation is helpful. They are hyaline and nearly spherical and possess a thin outer shell and a hexacanth embryo. From each pole arise four to eight slender filaments or hair-like structures, which spread toward the center over the embryo. Considerable focusing may be necessary to locate these filaments. These eggs are immediately infective; thus, hyperinfection may occur by anus-to-mouth transfer

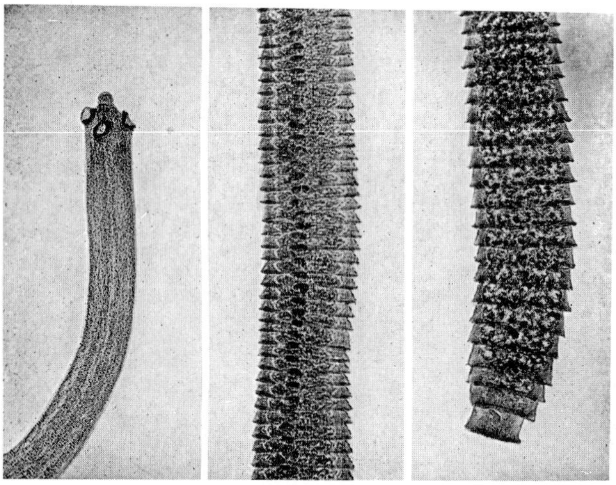

Figure 19–53. Dwarf tapeworm (*Hymenolepis nana*), head, middle segments, and terminal segments. Note the protruded rostellum and the three suckers. From stained and mounted specimens (× 30).

(as for *Enterobius vermicularis*). Since there is no need for an intermediate host, the laboratory worker is to be cautious in handling stools with *H. nana*. When swallowed, they hatch in the small intestine, and the onchospheres burrow into the villi where they become cysticercoid larvae which may be seen in histologic sections of the small intestine. These leave the villi and descend farther down the small intestine where they attach themselves and grow to maturity.

Few clinical signs appear in hymenolepiasis. In heavy infections there may be toxic manifestations. Children tend to be more heavily infected than adults, as in enterobiasis.

Hymenolepis diminuta. *Hymenolepis diminuta,* the rat tapeworm (Table 19–5), measures 20 to 60 cm. in length and about 4 mm. in width. The scolex is "unarmed" but there are four suckers. The distinctive eggs, which measure 56 to 80 microns by 24 to 40 microns (Fig. 19–50 *D*) may be observed in the stool. They are broadly oval and brown in color with a thick shell, possessing an outer thickening that is frequently striated. There are no polar filaments but there is an onchosphere. Unlike *H. nana,* eggs of *H. diminuta* are noninfective for man.

Dipylidium caninum. *Dipylidium caninum* (Table 19–5) or the dog tapeworm causes dipylidiasis particularly in children.

Diphyllobothrium latum. *Diphyllobothrium latum,* the broad fish tapeworm (Table 19–5; Figs. 19–51, 19–77) causes diphyllobothriasis in man. Man becomes infected upon consuming infected fresh-water fish, eaten raw or improperly cooked. The adult worms, which may live for many years, may reach a length of 10 meters with as many as 4000 segments, and generally only one worm develops, although multiple infections are known, in which case the worms are smaller. The "unarmed" scolex (Figs. 19–51, 19–77) is characteristically spoon-shaped and possesses two slit-like grooves, or bothria, which are placed laterally. The mature and gravid proglottids are broader than they are long, with a rosette-shaped uterus (Figs. 19–51, 19–77) which is centrally located. Single segments are seldom seen but chains may be passed. The uteri in the chain appear like a row of buttons. Thousands of eggs are liberated through a birth pore into the lumen of the intestine to be passed with the feces. These operculated eggs (Figs. 19–50 *B, C,* 19–77) with a mass of granules inside measure about 45 to 70 microns and are yellowish brown in color. Eggs in stools are immature and noninfective for man and must be differentiated from the larger operculated fluke eggs.

The patient may remain asymptomatic or have abdominal pain. Some have associated bothriocephalus anemia – macrocytic hyperchromic anemia. The worm absorbs vitamin B-12 from the host with subsequent interference with the erythrocyte maturing factor (EMF).

Miscellaneous Cestodes. Information on cestodes infrequently recovered from man is available (Faust, 1949).

The Trematodes

The trematodes or flukes are dorsoventrally flattened, unsegmented worms, which are leaf-like and hermaphroditic (monoecious) (except the schistosomes or blood flukes, which are diecious; i.e., there are males and females). All fluke eggs are operculated, except those of the three *Schistosoma* species, but none are infective for man.

Most adult species have two radially striated suckers, one oral and one ventral (the acetabulum). The digestive tract is incomplete, and most of the body is occupied by organs associated with the reproductive system. Thousands of eggs are found in the uterus. Adults are covered with spines, except *Clonorchis,* which is aspinose. Most flukes live many years. In general, trematode infections are more prevalent in the Orient, except for *S. mansoni* and *S. hematobium.*

Diagnosis of most fluke infections depends upon finding their eggs (Figs. 19–54, 19–78 through 19–80) in the feces. Techniques, such as the direct smears and concentration methods (pp. 1110–1113, 1113–1114), may be helpful but gravity sedimentation (p. 1063) is sometimes necessary. Egg-hatching procedure is beneficial in schistosomiasis. The life cycles are complex, with one or two intermediate hosts required, but the first host is always a snail.

Fasciolopsis buski. *Fasciolopsis buski* (Table 19–5) is the giant intestinal fluke of man and is found primarily in the duodenal region. Fasciolopsiasis in man results from the ingestion of metacercariae from aquatic plants. Bloody diarrhea, severe toxic or obstructive symptoms, or even death may occur in heavy infections. The adults (Fig. 19–55) are 2.0 to 7.5 cm. in length and 0.8 to 2.0 cm. in width and are covered with spines. They may be seen following therapy. The yellowish brown eggs (Fig. 19–54 *H*) have a thin shell, a small operculum, and granular contents. They measure 135 by 80 to 85 microns. They are difficult to differentiate from *F. hepatica.* The granules in the yolk cells of *F. buski* are evenly distributed throughout.

Echinostoma ilocanum. The *Echinostoma* are distinguished by possessing a horseshoe-shaped collar of spines on the dorsal and lateral sides of the oral sucker. The adults (Fig. 19–56) live in the small intestines, and they measure under 1.0 cm. in length and 0.2 cm. in width. Man develops echinostomiasis after consum-

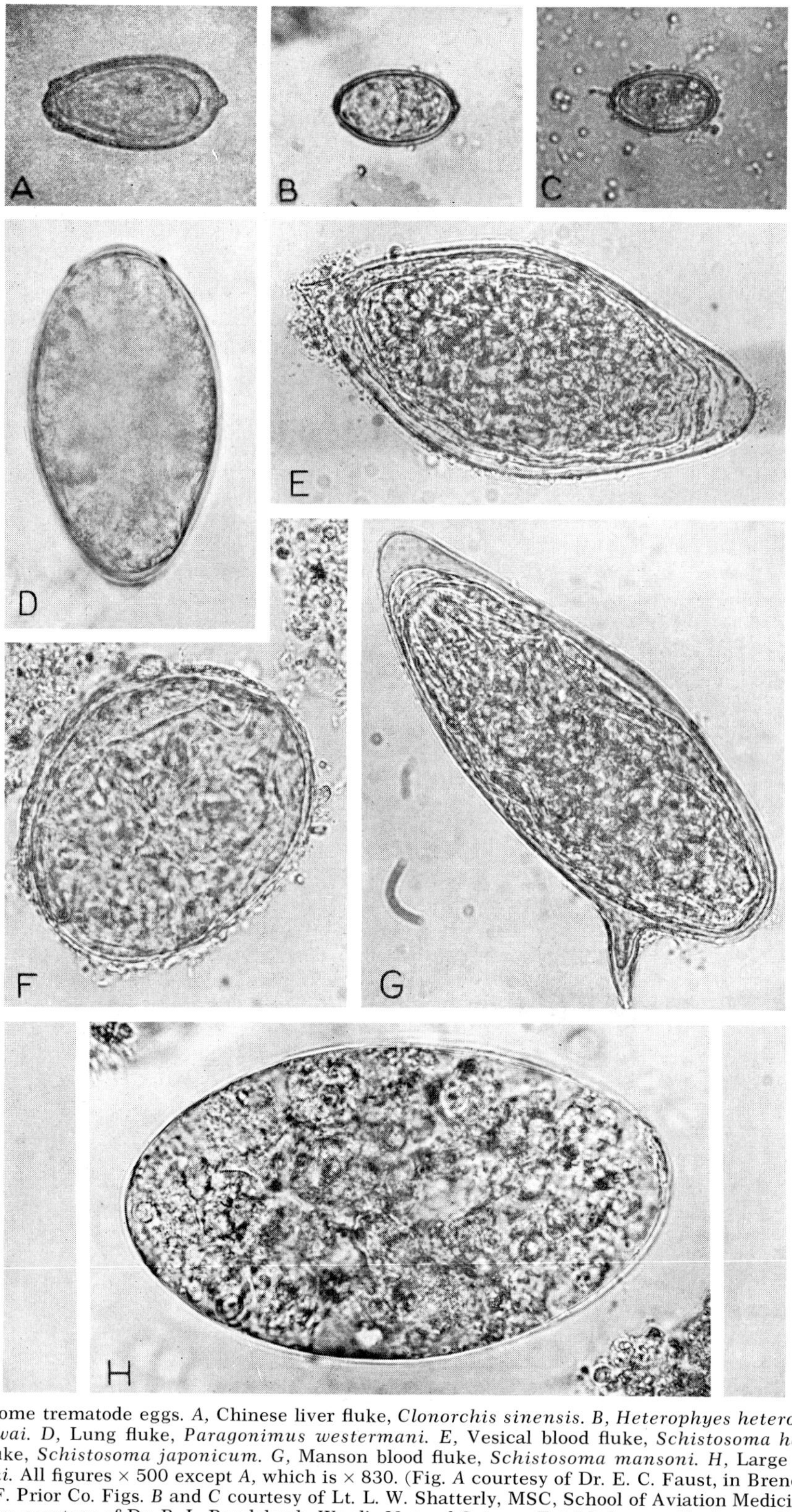

Figure 19–54. Some trematode eggs. *A*, Chinese liver fluke, *Clonorchis sinensis*. *B*, *Heterophyes heterophyes*. *C*, *Metagonimus yokogawai*. *D*, Lung fluke, *Paragonimus westermani*. *E*, Vesical blood fluke, *Schistosoma haematobium*. *F*, Oriental blood fluke, *Schistosoma japonicum*. *G*, Manson blood fluke, *Schistosoma mansoni*. *H*, Large intestinal fluke, *Fasciolopsis buski*. All figures × 500 except *A*, which is × 830. (Fig. *A* courtesy of Dr. E. C. Faust, in Brenemann: Practice of Pediatrics, W. F. Prior Co. Figs. *B* and *C* courtesy of Lt. L. W. Shatterly, MSC, School of Aviation Medicine, Gunter AFB, Alabama. All others courtesy of Dr. R. L. Roudabush, Ward's Natural Science Establishment, Rochester, New York; photos by T. Romaniak.)

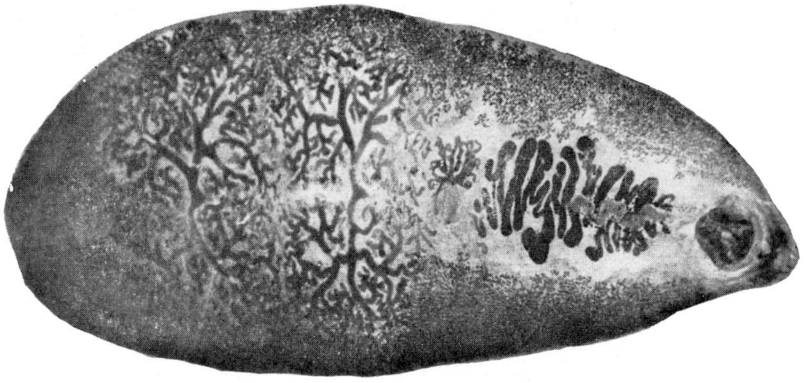

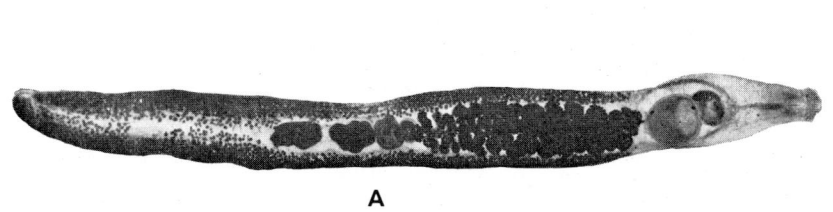

Figure 19–55. *Fasciolopsis buski.* (From Markell, E. K., and Voge, M.: Medical Parasitology. 3rd ed.)

ing raw fresh-water snails harboring metacercariae. Diagnosis is difficult, because the operculated eggs resemble those of other flukes (Fig. 19–54 *H*); however, adults can be diagnosed after therapy.

***Heterophyes heterophyes* and *Metagonimus yokogawai*.** The small, oval heterophyid worms are attached to the intestinal wall. *Metagonimus yokogawai* and *H. heterophyes* measure about 1.4 to 0.6 mm., and the latter possesses a genital sucker in addition to the oral and ventral suckers. Heterophyiasis and metagonimiasis in man are acquired through consumption of raw and pickled fish. The yellowish brown eggs (Fig. 19–54 *B, C*) contain a miracidium and an operculum, which is set on opercular shoulders that are thickened. The eggs measure 26.5 to 30 by 15 to 17 microns and must be differentiated from *Clonorchis sinensis*. *Heterophyes* eggs are widest at the middle and *Metagonimus* are widest below the middle.

***Clonorchis sinensis*.** *Clonorchis sinensis* (*Opisthorchis sinensis*) (Table 19–5; Fig. 19–78) is the Chinese liver fluke of man inhabiting the bile ducts, gallbladder, and pancreatic duct. The aspinose adult is 10 to 25 mm. in length and 3 to 5 mm. in width. The light yellowish brown eggs (Figs. 19–54 *A*, 19–78), which measure 29 by 16 microns and are bulb-shaped, are readily found in the feces. They have an operculum and opercular shoulders and an abopercular, comma-shaped thickening on the shell and a miracidium inside. These eggs must be differentiated from those of *Heterophyes* and *Metagonimus*. Man develops clonorchiasis upon consuming the metacercariae from raw or insufficiently cooked fresh-water fish. The adult worms may live for many years and may be seen only by surgical intervention or at autopsy. Other opisthorchids, such as *O. felineus* and *O. viverrini*, have also been found in man. Some persons are asymptomatic, while others develop cholangitis and biliary cirrhosis.

***Fasciola hepatica*.** *Fasciola hepatica* (Table 19–5; Fig. 19–57), the sheep liver fluke, is 3.0 cm. by 1.2 cm. and establishes itself in the bile ducts. The characteristic anterior end projects like a cone and is 3 to 4 mm. long. The eggs, which appear in the feces, are yellowish brown, oval, and operculated and measure about 130 to 140 by 76 to 90 microns but cannot be differentiated easily from those of *Fasciolopsis buski* (Fig. 19–54 *H*) and the echinostomes. The granules in the yolk cells are concentrated around the nuclei in *F. hepatica*. The spine-covered adult worms are seen only during surgery or at autopsy. Fascioliasis in man follows the consumption of

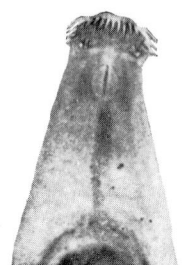

Figure 19–56. *A, Echinostoma* sp.; *B*, anterior end of *Echinostoma* showing circumoral spines. (From Markell, E. K., and Voge, M.: Medical Parasitology. 3rd ed.)

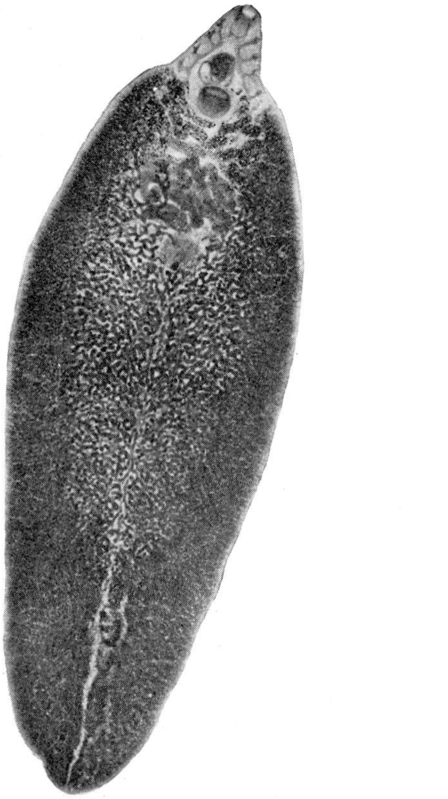

Figure 19–57. *Fasciola hepatica.* (From Markell, E. K., and Voge, M.: Medical Parasitology. 3rd ed.)

metacercariae on aquatic vegetation. Adults may cause necrosis of the liver or blockage of the ducts.

***Schistosoma mansoni* and *Schistosoma japonicum*.** *Schistosoma mansoni* and *S. japonicum* are blood flukes which produce intestinal schistosomiasis or intestinal bilharziasis. They are not endemic in the United States, but many individuals infected while in endemic zones (with Manson's schistosomiasis) now reside here, mainly in our larger cities. In the complex life cycles of the schistosomes (Fig. 19–79) the infective fork-tailed cercaria which emerges from the snail is attracted to the skin of man, the anterior portion penetrates the skin (the forked tail having dropped off) and is transported through the blood stream to develop into an adult (male or female) in specific sites for each species as follows: *S. japonicum,* superior mesenteric venules; *S. mansoni,* inferior mesenteric venules; and *S. haematobium* (see genitourinary tract parasites, next section), the vesical plexus. The first two species often get into the liver and ectopic sites.

The adult worms, which have minute spines (visible only by electron microscopy), exhibit slight morphologic differences for the three species and can be seen only at surgery or autopsy. They live for many, many years. *Schistosoma mansoni* (Table 19–5; Fig. 19–58) females are 1.6 cm. long (*S. japonicum,* 2.6 cm.) and reside in the gynecophoral canal of the male which is 1 cm. (*S. japonicum,* 2.2 cm.) in length. The flattened male curls himself ventrally around the female and in histologic sections appears as a C-shaped structure with the somewhat rounded female enclosed. Females produce few eggs (1–4/day/female for *S. mansoni* and 50–300/day/female for *S. japonicum*). The eggs are deposited into the lumina of the blood vessels, pass through the tissue barrier and into the lumen of the intestine to be passed out of the body in the feces. Diagnosis in the laboratory depends upon the recovery of the characteristic eggs (*S. mansoni* [Fig. 19–54 *G*]; *S. japonicum* [Figs. 19–54 *F*, 19–79]) from feces by special techniques (described below) and occasionally in urine or in rectal biopsies (discussed below) (Hernandez-Morales and Maldonado, 1946; Ottolina, 1947) or hepatic puncture (Kubasta, 1965). Pressed, fresh or salinized preparations of these biopsies can be examined as well as histologic sections of formalinized tissues.

The characteristic eggs of the schistosomes are large (*S. mansoni,* elongate, 112 to 162 by 60 to 70 microns; *S. japonicum,* more spherical, 74 to 106 by 55 to 80 microns), thick shelled, lightly bile-stained and contain a cili-

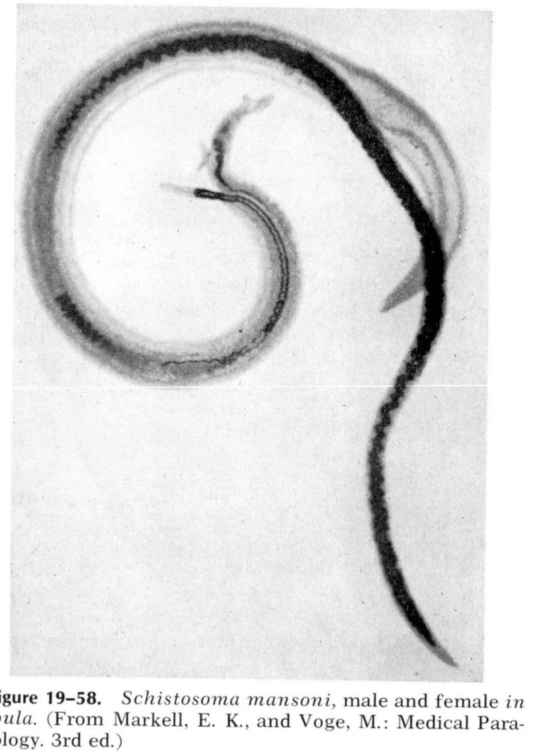

Figure 19–58. *Schistosoma mansoni,* male and female *in copula.* (From Markell, E. K., and Voge, M.: Medical Parasitology. 3rd ed.)

ated miracidium, although occasionally degenerated forms appear and are full of granules. The shell has a spine which is pronounced and lateral in *S. mansoni* and minute, inconspicuous and lateral in *S. japonicum*. Debris attached to the shell of the latter masks the spine, which fits snugly into the shell. Viable eggs can be detected by searching in a saline mount of feces (eggs are killed during most concentration techniques) for the four beating flame cells (solanocytes) within the captive miracidium. Viability may also be determined by utilizing an egg hatching technique (see below).

Clinically the manifestations of schistosomiasis are similar for all three species. The three stages include invasion and maturation of the worms, egg deposition and excretion, and tissue proliferation and repair. A dermatitis may accompany cercarial skin penetration. Later, fever and eosinophilia develop. Egg deposition results in abscess formation and enlargement of the liver and spleen. Urticaria and pulmonary signs diminish, but fever and eosinophilia increase. Tissue proliferation and repair set in with pseudotubercle formation and calcification. Intestinal and bladder walls thicken (in *S. haematobium*), and cirrhosis of the liver begins.

SCHISTOSOME TECHNIQUES

I. *Special Concentration* (p. 1113) *or Gravity Sedimentation* (p. 1063). These techniques may be necessary for diagnosis. Skin and serologic tests are available (state health department laboratory).

II. *Rectal Biopsy and Hepatic Biopsy*

A. *Pressed, fresh, unstained preparation (saline mount).* The advantage is that the entire biopsy specimen can be viewed and eggs or pseudotubercles can be seen more easily by low power examination than in histologic sections.

1. Rectal biopsy specimens are obtained from the first valve of Houston and placed in saline. Press the separate specimens between wide slides, examine under low power, and reexamine within five minutes after adding 1 or 2 drops of 10 per cent KOH.

2. Hepatic biopsies are treated as follows: Needle biopsy specimens 15 to 45 mm. in length are placed in saline. Press, as above, a series of 2 to 4 mm. length. When evidence of schistosomiasis is seen, fix remaining portion of specimen in formalin. If not seen, make additional studies or more needle biopsies.

B. *Histologic preparation (formalin-fixed).* It is important to point out that sections made from the biopsy specimen may bypass the eggs and/or pseudotubercles.

III. *Egg Hatching for Schistosoma Infections.* Utilizing this technique one can fulfill a twofold purpose, viz., determination of the viability of the eggs and revelation of infections which may be very light as evidenced by failures to detect eggs by other techniques. Follow the procedure for the sedimentation technique (p. 1063), and after the microscopic examination has been made, decant the saline and transfer the remainder of the sediment to one of the flask methods described below.

ERLENMEYER FLASK

1. Resuspend the sediment in a small quantity of chlorine-free water and pour it into a 500-ml. flask.

2. Fill the flask almost to the lip with chlorine-free water and darken the flask with aluminum foil so that only the top film is exposed to a bright light source directed toward the side of the flask at a distance of 6 to 12 inches.

3. After several hours the eggs will hatch, liberating the miracidia, which will swim to and collect in the neck of the flask. The miracidia are white against a dark background and swim rapidly in a straight course.

SIDE ARM HATCHING FLASK. The flask (after McMullen and Beaver, 1945; McQuay, 1967b) (Fig. 19–59) resembles a Florence flask, with a side arm emerging midway down the neck, protruding an inch or two, and bent upward and cut off even with the top of the flask. (Use the Corning flask No. 4920, bend tubulation upward and cut off excess.)

1. The fecal sediment is passed through the neck of the flask and settles to the bottom.

2. The flask is then partly filled with chlorine-free water up to the bottom of the side arm (at X).

3. Then the flask is completely filled to the top by adding the remainder of the water through the side arm (Y) so as to prevent debris from entering the arm.

4. The entire flask may be covered with foil, or it may have been painted with several coats of black enamel, except for the side arm.

5. Cover the flask neck opening with a small piece of foil to make the unit completely enclosed and dark, except for the side arm.

6. The side arm is exposed to a bright light source about 8 inches away. Miracidia, which are phototropic, will come to the side arm in a few hours and can be seen with the naked eye or a hand lens.

Paragonimus westermani. Lung fluke infection, or paragonimiasis, in man is caused by *Paragonimus westermani* (Table 19–5). The adult worms, which are seldom seen except

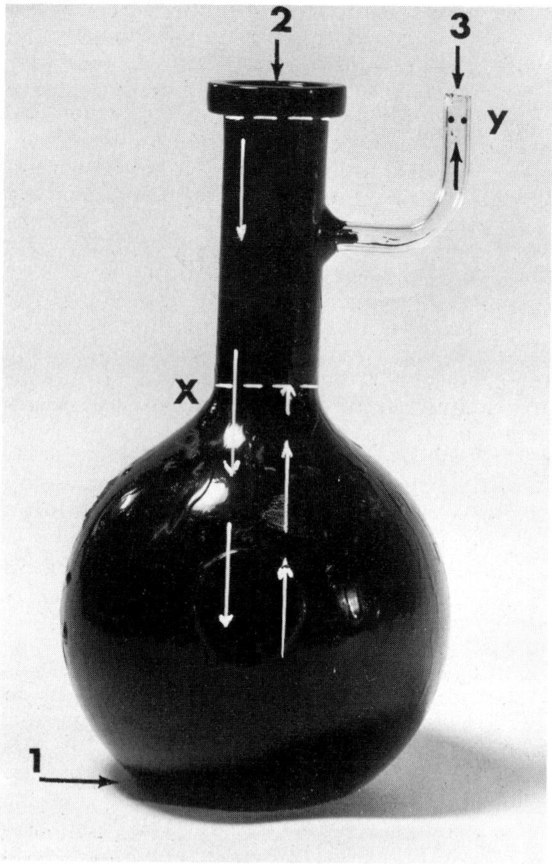

Figure 19–59. Side-arm hatching flask for *Schistosoma* eggs. See text for description. (After McMullen and Beaver.)

at autopsy, are reddish brown in color and thick-bodied, measuring 0.8 to 1.6 cm. in length, 0.4 to 0.8 cm. in width, and 0.3 to 0.5 cm. in thickness. They are covered with small spines. Their yellowish brown eggs (Figs. 19–54 *D*, 19–80) are thick shelled, operculated with a thickened opercular rim, and measure 80 to 120 by 48 to 60 microns. They may be seen in the sputum or in feces if the sputum is swallowed. Man becomes infected after ingesting raw or insufficiently cooked crabs or crayfish harboring the infective metacercariae, which migrate through the body to the lungs after they excyst (Fig. 19–80). The adult worms become encapsulated. Fever and eosinophilia are usually present. Patient may develop chronic cough with rusty brown sputum.

Examination of Sputum for Helminth Eggs and Larvae. Sputum is examined primarily for the eggs of *Paragonimus westermani*, and occasionally eggs of the blood flukes are coughed up. In some cases one can recover the larvae of *Strongyloides*, *Ascaris*, or hookworms from sputum. Hydatid cyst of the lung and amebic abscess in the lung may be diagnosed when the parasites are in the sputum.

Direct smear examination of the sputum may reveal the organisms mentioned above. Centrifugation of the sputum may be necessary in paragonimiasis as follows: Comminute sample with an equal amount of 3 per cent sodium hydroxide or full strength Clorox. Centrifuge at 3000 r.p.m. and examine the sediment.

Helminths Inhabiting the Genitourinary Tract

Two helminths are known to primarily inhabit the genitourinary tract. They are *Schistosoma haematobium* and the giant kidney worm, *Dioctophyma renale*, which is very rare in man. Their eggs may be recovered in urine. Microfilariae of *Wuchereria bancrofti* and *Strongyloides stercoralis* larvae may be recovered also.

URINE EXAMINATION

Techniques

Centrifugation

1. Collect the last 15 to 20 ml. of a forced, morning urine sample (which will contain a greater number of *S. haematobium* eggs) in a clean beaker.
2. Transfer to a 15-ml. centrifuge tube and centrifuge for 5 minutes at 2000 r.p.m.
3. Pour off the supernatant fluid. Transfer several drops of sediment to a slide for examination under low power.

Sedimentation

1. Collect a 24-hour sample of urine. (If urates have precipitated, place specimen in flask and immerse in warm water bath until urine is clear).
2. Transfer to a 1-liter graduated cylinder. Allow to settle one-half hour. Pour off supernatant and transfer sediment to 100-ml. graduated cylinder. Allow to settle one-half hour. Transfer sediment to a centrifuge tube, spin down for 5 minutes at 2000 r.p.m., and examine the sediment.

Hatching Technique for S. haematobium Eggs

1. Collect urine sediment as directed above.
2. Suspend in a clear test tube in 10 to 15 ml. of chlorine-free water.
3. Expose tube to a bright light source and examine for motile miracidia.

Schistosoma haematobium. Bilharziasis or urinary (vesical) schistosomiasis is caused by *Schistosoma haematobium* (Table 19–5), the blood fluke that inhabits the vesical plexus. The life history is similar to that of *S. japonicum* (Fig. 19–79). The male is 10 to 15 mm. long and 1 mm. broad; the female is 2 cm. long.

Their yellowish eggs (Fig. 19–54 *E*) are oval, elongated, house a ciliated miracidium, and possess a characteristic terminal spine. They measure 120 to 190 by 50 to 73 microns and may be recovered in urine and less commonly in feces. Daily egg output per female is only about 20 to 30 eggs. Degenerated eggs which are full of granules may be seen. Diagnosis may be made by observing the characteristic eggs in urine (using the technique above), by finding eggs in the bladder wall biopsy material, or by carrying out intradermal or certain serologic tests (available through each state health department laboratory). Bladder and genitourinary involvements lead to cancer in many patients.

Tissue-inhabiting Helminths

***Taenia solium* (Cysticercosis).** Cysticercosis is the disease in man caused by the larval stage, *Cysticercus cellulosae* (Table 19–5; Figs. 19–52, 19–75), of the tapeworm *Taenia solium*. Earlier in this chapter we learned that upon ingestion of the larval form, *C. cellulosae*, from pig, man develops the adult *T. solium* and thus becomes the definitive host. In cysticercosis man is the intermediate host, as he possesses the cysticercoid or larval stage. *Taenia solium* eggs are immediately infective and reach the mouth in contaminated food or water, from the anus via the fingers (if the adult worm is present), or directly from stools or the adult worm (in the laboratory). At times when the patient has the adult worm, eggs may be carried to the stomach by reverse peristalsis and progress as if they had been swallowed. Man may have either the worm alone or cysticercosis, but coexistence is also possible.

Eggs that are swallowed hatch in the vicinity of the duodenum where the onchospheres penetrate the intestinal wall and enter the blood. From the blood they may be carried to all parts of the body, especially the brain and the eye. The elongate, ovoid, fluid-filled bladder, 0.6 to 1.8 cm., develops in several months. Inside, a denser spot, the scolex, can be demonstrated. Specific diagnosis may be made following surgical removal of the cysticercus, which in serial section shows calcareous corpuscles (Fig. 19–49), hooklets, and suckers. A serologic test is available through each state health department laboratory.

The symptoms vary with the number of larvae and the organs or tissues involved. Death may result when larvae are in vital organs.

***Echinococcus granulosus* (Hydatid Disease).** Man is not the definitive host of *Echinococcus granulosus* (Table 19–5; Fig. 19–81). Dogs harbor the adult worm, usually in great numbers. Man, cattle, and sheep serve as intermediate hosts for the larval stage of hydatid cysts (Fig. 19–60), which cause echinococcosis or hydatid disease.

The adult worm, which is never found in man but is the smallest of the tapeworms, is 2.5 to 5.0 mm. long and is composed of a scolex and neck and immature, mature and gravid proglottids. The gravid segment contains many eggs, which resemble those of *Taenia*. Eggs from dog feces reach the digestive system of man where the hexacanth embryos are set free and find their way to the

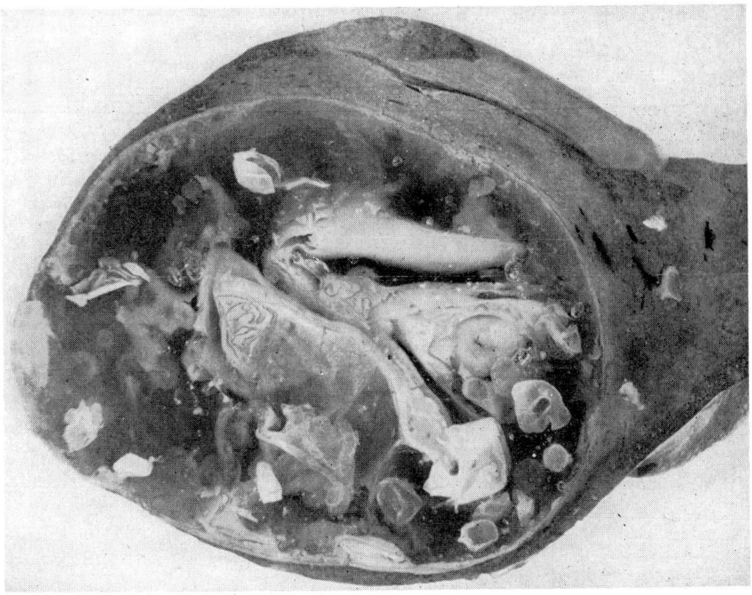

Figure 19–60. *Echinococcus granulosus,* section through unilocular hydatid cyst containing daughter cysts. (Courtesy of Ash and Spitz, Pathology of Tropical Diseases, Armed Forces Institute of Pathology, No. 31,977.)

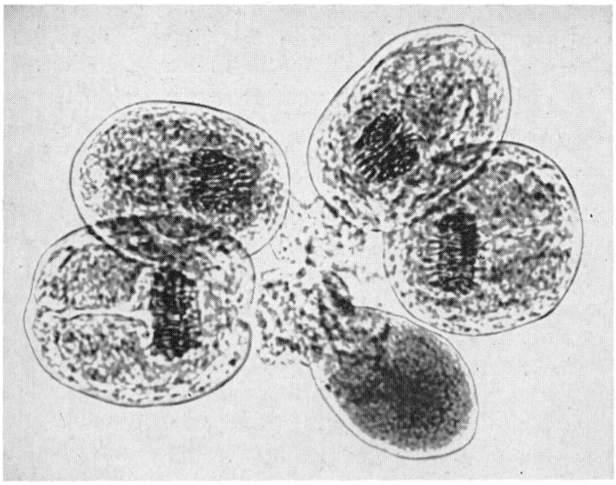

Figure 19–61. *Echinococcus granulosus*, hydatid sand. (From Markell, E. K., and Voge, M.: Medical Parasitology. 3rd ed.)

liver, lungs, or other organs in which they slowly develop into hydatid cysts, which vary considerably in size. From the inner germinal layer of the cyst wall brood capsules and daughter cysts bud. Within the former, scolices or "hydatid sand" (Figs. 19–61, 19–81) bud. Brood capsules with "hydatid sand" inside develop within the daughter cysts. This sand is composed of ovoid organisms, which are 0.2 to 0.3 mm. long and have four lateral suckers and an "armed" rostellum, which may be invaginated or evaginated. This type of hydatid is known as the unilocular cyst. Another type may occur—the osseous—which involves the bones. Some cysts may be sterile, i.e., without the "hydatid sand."

Laboratory diagnosis may be made by finding the scolices, hooklets, brood capsules, or daughter cysts in the cysts after surgical removal. Skin testing using a polyvalent antigen (the Casoni test), serologic tests available through each state health laboratory, and x-ray and photoscanning are also aids in diagnosis. Scolices and/or hooklets can be found in sputum if a lung cyst ruptures.

The slow-growing hydatid cysts cause clinical problems, depending upon their size and location in the body. If hydatid fluid is released from the cyst, the patient is apt to go into anaphylactic shock. Osseous hydatids may cause bone fractures.

Echinococcus multilocularis. Alveolar hydatid disease is caused by the multilocular hydatid cyst of *E. multilocularis* (Table 19–5) and may involve the liver and lung. No limiting cysts wall exists. Hepatomegaly and splenomegaly, icterus, and ascites characterize this disease, which is frequently fatal. Biopsy specimens are needed to make the diagnosis, as the Casoni test and serologic tests are not reliable. Adult worms are found in wolves, foxes, and so forth.

***Multiceps multiceps* (Coenurus Disease or Coenurosis).** *Multiceps multiceps* (Table 19–5) adult worms are found in dogs and the larval stage (coenurus), in cattle, sheep, and man.

Sparganosis (Table 19–5; Fig. 19–62). Man may acquire the sparganum, the larval stage of species of tapeworms related to the broad, fish tapeworm, by ingestion of the primary host, which is the infected fresh-water copepod *Diaptomus* (Swartzwelder *et al.*, 1964; McQuay *et al.*, 1966); by ingesting raw infected flesh of certain frogs, snakes, and birds; or by

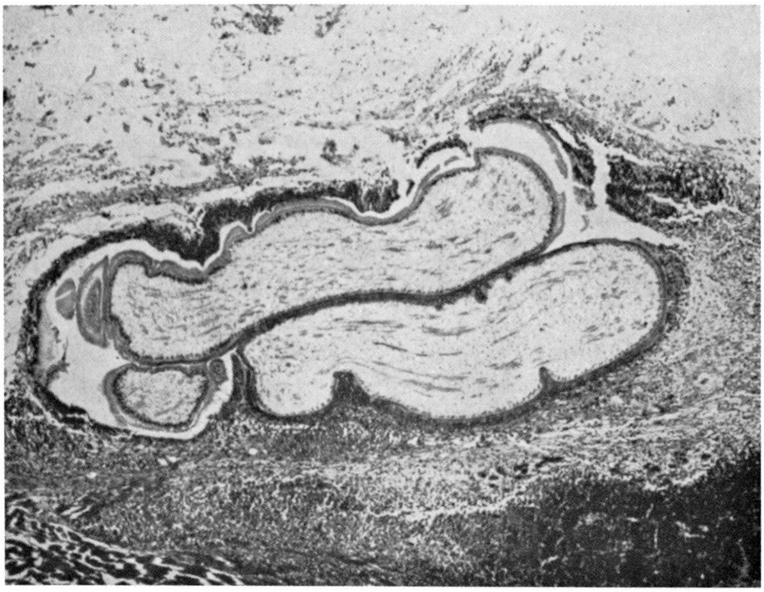

Figure 19–62. Sparganosis. Larva of *Diphyllobothrium mansonoides* in tissues shows surrounding inflammation and foreign body reaction. (From Hunter, G. W., Frye, W. W., and Swartzwelder, J. C.: A Manual of Tropical Medicine. 4th ed.)

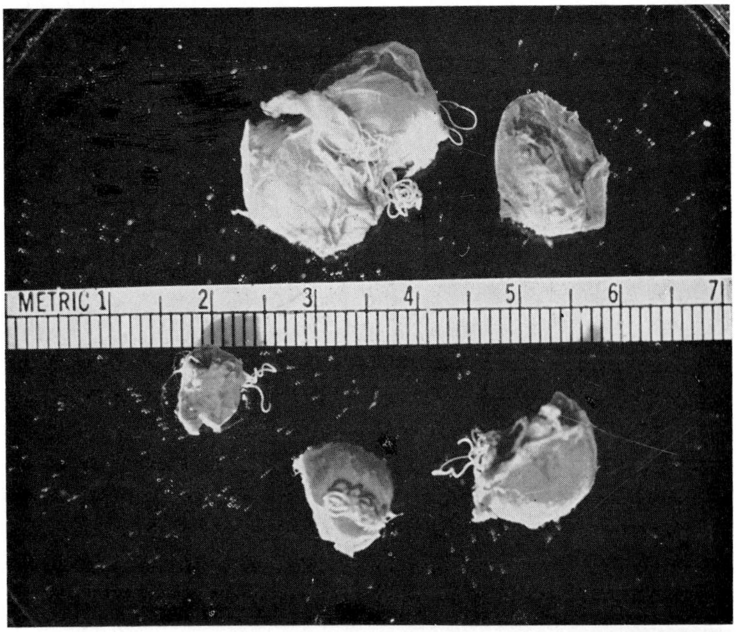

Figure 19–63. *Onchocerca volvulus* nodules. Portions of contained adult worms protruding. (From Markell, E. K., and Voge, M.: Medical Parasitology. 3rd ed.)

applying a poultice of infected flesh of frogs on open wounds or the eye.

The sparganum, which can be removed by surgery, is distinguished by its elongated ribbon shape with no transverse segmentation but with a pseudosucker. The living spargana elongate and contract like typical tapeworms. Skin test antigens are available. *Sparganum proliferum* is a proliferating larva (adult stage unknown) which may be in tissues of man, where it appears as an elongate mass with branched processes. Calcareous corpuscles (Fig. 19–49) are present in the sparganum upon microscopic study.

Onchocerciasis. Onchocerciasis is a disease in which the adult filarial parasite (the blinding filaria) *Onchocerca volvulus* (Table 19–5), is found in the skin and other tissue, where it may produce fibrous nodules. Within the nodule (Fig. 19–63) are the cream-white colored adults. The female may be 35 to 50 cm. long and 0.5 mm. or less in diameter, while the males are smaller. The microfilariae leave the nodule and migrate in the skin. They may migrate to the eye and cause permanent blindness. It is very important to emphasize that they do not appear in peripheral circulation. Specific diagnosis rests upon finding the characteristic unsheathed microfilariae (Fig. 19–64; Table 19–7) by means of scarification

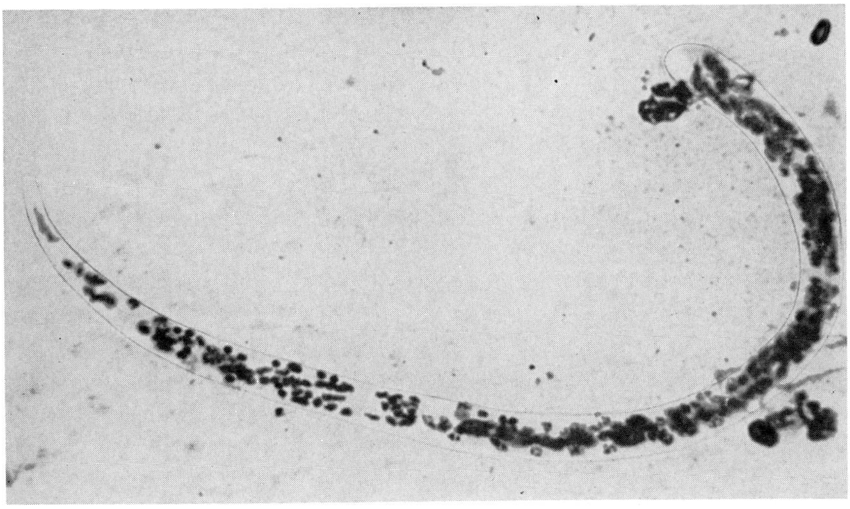

Figure 19–64. *Onchocerca volvulus*, microfilaria from scarification preparation. (From Markell, E. K., and Voge, M.: Medical Parasitology. 3rd ed.)

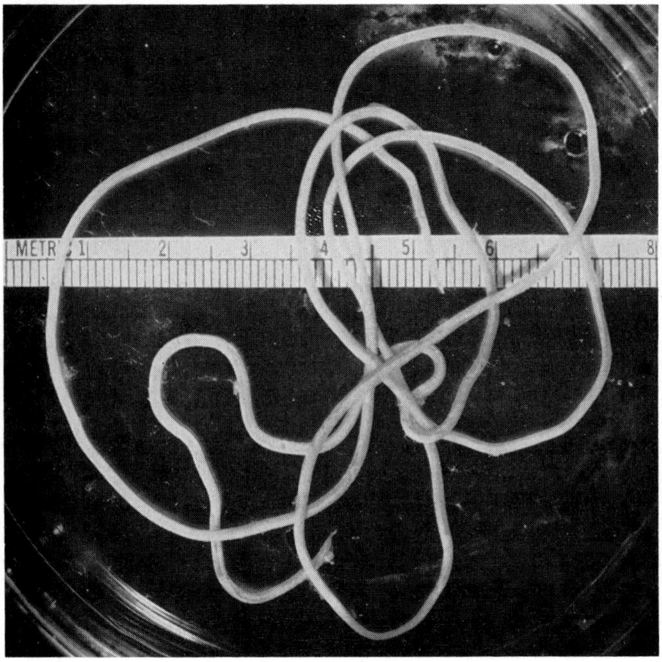

Figure 19–65. *Dracunculus medinensis*, female worm removed surgically. (From Markell, E. K., and Voge, M.: Medical Parasitology. 3rd ed.)

smears, skin snips placed in warm saline, or skin biopsy. The black fly *Simulium* is the vector.

Dracunculus medinensis. *Dracunculus medinensis* (Table 19–5) is the guinea worm of man, causing dracontiasis or dracunculosis. The worm (Fig. 19–65) is elongated and cylindrical, with males 2 cm. or less in length and females 70 to 120 cm. in length and 0.9 to 1.7 mm. in diameter. The viviparous, mature females develop in body cavities and migrate when gravid into subcutaneous tissues. The larvae (Fig. 19–66) are released from a blister formed on the skin and are discharged from the lesion into water in which copepods live. Man gets the infection by ingesting infected copepods. Larvae may be recovered from the ulcer, but adult worms are recovered by surgical intervention or by slowly winding them on sticks each day until they have been completely removed. Anaphylactic shock may develop if the worm is broken.

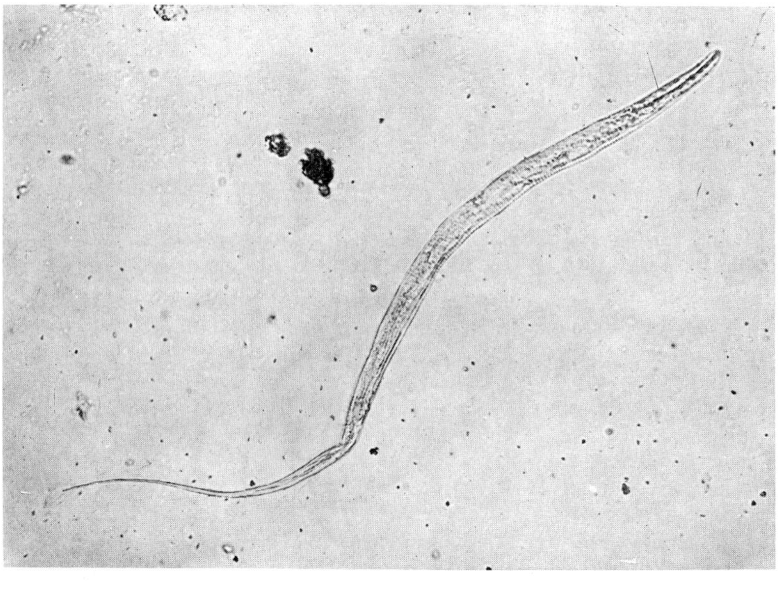

Figure 19–66. Larva of *D. medinensis* as discharged from cutaneous lesions; note long tapering tail. (From Mackie, T. T., Hunter, W. W., and Worth, C. B.: Manual of Tropical Medicine. 2nd ed.)

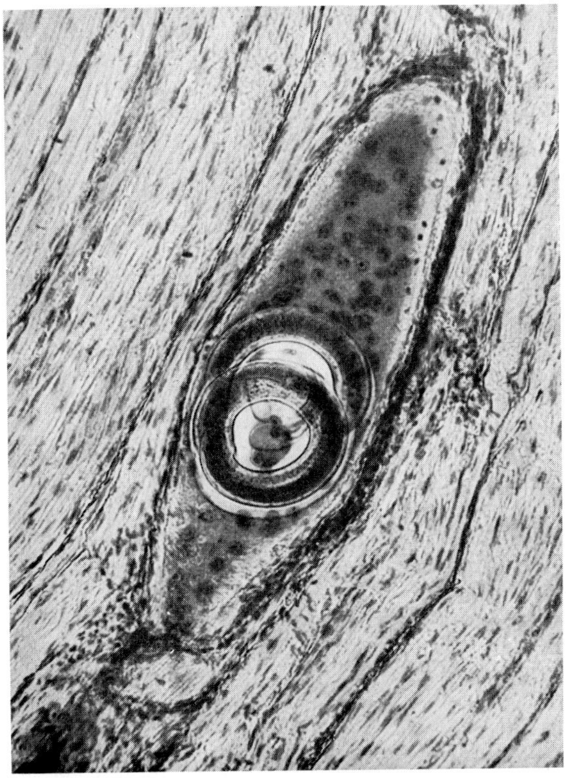

Figure 19–67. *Trichinella spiralis*, larva in muscle. (From Markell, E. K., and Voge, M.: Medical Parasitology. 3rd ed.)

Trichinella spiralis. *Trichinella spiralis* (Table 19–5; Fig. 19–67) is the trichina worm responsible for producing the disease known as trichinosis, trichiniasis, or trichinelliasis (Gould, 1970; 1971). The adult worms inhabit the small intestine where the viviparous females (Fig. 19–28) give birth to living larvae, which migrate to the skeletal muscles of the body after entering the circulatory system. The larvae coil themselves in the muscle fibers and become encapsulated (Fig. 19–67) and eventually the capsule becomes calcified.

Man becomes infected after the consumption of insufficiently cooked or raw pork or pork products or bear meat containing encapsulated larvae. Pigs and bears are infected from uncooked garbage. When the infected meat is ingested by humans, the ingested encapsulated larvae are released and penetrate into the mucosa of the intestine and there develop into adults in several days. The adult males (Fig. 19–28) measure 2 mm. or less, with a breadth of 0.04 mm., while the females are 2 to 4 mm. long and 0.06 mm. wide. Adults have the holomyarian muscular pattern in cross section. These adults may be observed microscopically in the stools of patients with diarrhea during the first few weeks of the infection. They live in the intestine about eight weeks before they die. When early trichinosis is highly suspected or diagnosed by the presence of maturing larvae or microscopic adults in diarrheic specimens, it is wise to purge the patient frequently, unless contraindicated, to remove as many worms as possible. This is done to prevent larvae from the female from reaching the circulatory system, from whence they go to the muscle, at which time severe symptomatology may begin.

The diagnosis in humans usually rests upon the history of having eaten improperly prepared pork and also upon clinical symptoms. During the first week intestinal invasion occurs, at which time vomiting, diarrhea, and abdominal pains are evident. As larvae penetrate the muscles, periorbital edema, fever, and a marked rise in eosinophils are noted. Larval encapsulation in the muscles follows. The patient may exhibit neurotoxic symptoms and myocarditis. The infection may prove fatal. Specific diagnosis may be made by muscle biopsy of skeletal muscles, such as the deltoid, biceps, or gastrocnemius. Skin tests and serologic tests are of distinct aid in diagnosis. Blood for serologic tests must be drawn before skin testing. Laking and centrifuging 25 ml. or more of whole blood may yield migrating larvae.

Muscle digestion methods are helpful for autopsy specimens, but will not detect larvae less than 21 days old; calcified larvae are frequently missed. Up to 200 gm. of ground-up diaphragm or other muscle tissue are digested in a liter of digestive fluid (pepsin, 5 gm.; HCl, 155.0 ml.; water q.s. to 1000 ml.). Place in an incubator at 37° C. for 12 to 18 hours. Discard supernatant. Screen (20 to 40 mesh) and resediment. Discard supernatant and examine sediment under a microscope. When alive, the larvae tighten and loosen their coils; when dead they appear as commas.

Larva Migrans

Larva migrans is the disease in which larvae of nematodes migrate without further development in unnatural hosts. In general there are two types of larva migrans – visceral and cutaneous – but they occur as a result of a variety of parasitic organisms. Cutaneous larva migrans, or "creeping eruption," is produced in the epidermis by filariform larvae of nonhuman hookworms, primarily from the dog and cat (*Ancylostoma braziliense*, *A. caninum*) (Table 19–5) and others. Diagnosis is based upon the observation of the characteristic tunnel-like lesions following exposure. Cutaneous and/or visceral larva migrans may be produced by nonhuman filarial worms (dog heartworm—*Dirofilaria*). Visceral larva migrans can be produced by the larvae of *Toxocara canis* (Table 19–5), dog and cat ascarids, reaching human visceral organs after the consumption of eggs from the soil. These larvae move very slowly through the organ tissues. Specific diagnosis is made by finding the larvae in biopsy materials. One may suspect this condition in a dirt-eating child with a history of contact with infected dogs or cats and manifesting hepatomegaly, chronic nonspecific pulmonary disease, and high eosinophilia. Serologic tests in which a purified worm antigen is used are available through each state health department laboratory. Finally, visceral and/or cutaneous larva migrans may be caused by immature spiruroid nematodes such as *Gnathostoma, Gongylonema, Thelazia,* and *Physaloptera*. These nonhuman nematode parasites are among those which produce the condition referred to as tropical eosinophila.

Blood Helminths

Flukes. Although the schistosomes (p. 1078) are blood flukes, with the adult worms living in the blood stream, laboratory diagnosis rests heavily upon the recovery of characteristic eggs in feces or urine, as the case may be.

Nematodes. The filariae are long thread-like nematodes that usually are diagnosed by the isolation of the microfilariae from peripheral blood. These microfilariae are noninfective for man, even by blood transfusion. Air-borne spores of helicosporus fungi superficially resembling microfilariae may be found on blood films (Norman and Donaldson, 1955). The adult filarial worms, which exhibit holomyarian type musculature in cross section, are found in various sites in the body (Table 19–7). There are no filarial infections endemic in the United States, but since the adult worms live for many years, infections acquired elsewhere persist. Figure 19–69 shows the differential features of the main species of microfilariae seen in man. Variability of periodicity of the microfilariae among some filarial species dictates blood collection time as indicated below. A non-species-specific serologic test is available through each state health department laboratory.

Wuchereria bancrofti. *Wuchereria bancrofti* (Table 19–5; Fig. 19–82) causes Bancroftian filariasis or wuchereriasis. This disease is widespread in the tropics. The adults are located in the lymphatics, where they are tightly coiled. Lymphangitis and lymphadenitis occur. Blockage of lymphatics causes elephantiasis in the lower extremities. Not all infected individuals exhibit elephantiasis, but many who do reveal no microfilariae in their peripheral blood. The males measure 2.5 to 4.0 cm. and the females 5 to 10 cm. in length. The females produce microfilariae 244 to 296 microns long that are sheathed (Figs. 19–68, 19–69, 19–82; Table 19–7); the sheath is actually the egg membrane. These microfilariae do not have nuclei to the tip of the tail. The adults require one year to mature, and at this time microfilariae appear. Therefore, the serologic test may be positive before microfilarial production begins.

The microfilariae of this species tend to exhibit nocturnal periodicity. That is to say, the greatest number of organisms may be recovered from the peripheral circulation at night, usually between 10:00 P.M. and 2:00 A.M. There is a nonperiodic type, however.

Table 19–7. DIFFERENTIAL CHARACTERISTICS OF FILARIAL WORMS IN MAN

FILARIA	GEOGRAPHICAL DISTRIBUTION	VECTOR	ADULT SITE IN BODY	PERIODICITY	MICROFILARIAE LOCATION	SHEATH	NUCLEUS
Wuchereria bancrofti	Tropical and subtropical areas	Mosquito	Lymphatic system, lower extremities	Nocturnal with most strains	Peripheral blood	Yes	No nuclei to the tip of tail
Brugia (Wuchereria) malayi	Southern Asia; East Indies	Mosquito	Lymphatic system, upper extremities	Nocturnal	Peripheral blood	Yes	Two nuclei to tip of tail
Loa loa	Africa	*Chrysops* fly	Wandering in subcutaneous tissues and across the eyeball	Diurnal (daytime)	Peripheral blood	Yes	Nuclei to the tip of the tail
Dipetalonema (Acanthocheilonema) perstans	Africa; South America	*Culicoides*	Body cavities; mesentery; perirenal and retroperitoneal tissues	None	Peripheral blood	No	Nuclei to the tip of tail
Mansonella ozzardi	South America	*Culicoides*	Body cavities; mesentery	None	Peripheral blood	No	No nuclei to tip of tail
Onchocerca volvulus	Africa; Central and South America	*Simulium*	Subcutaneous tissues	None	Lymph spaces of skin; subcutaneous nodules; rarely in peripheral blood	No	No nuclei to tip of tail

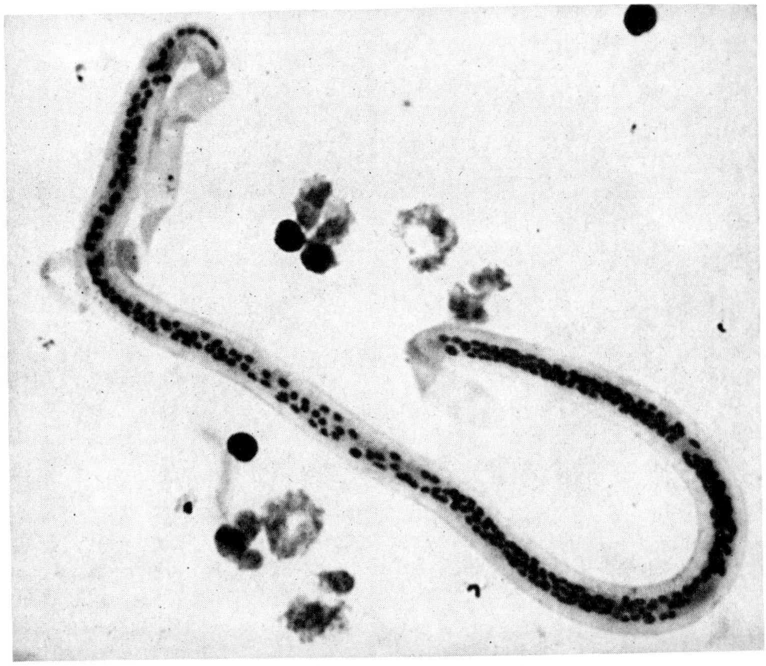

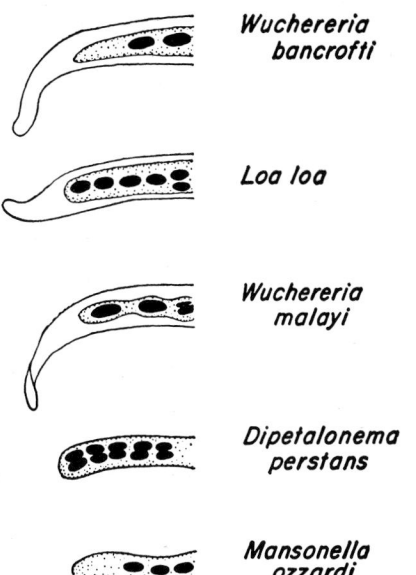

Figure 19-68. Microfilaria of *Wuchereria bancrofti* in thick blood film. (From Markell, E. K., and Voge, M.: Medical Parasitology. 3rd ed.)

Specific diagnosis may be made by finding the adult worm or microfilariae in material from biopsy or the microfilariae in peripheral blood in the resting patient, either in thick films or by concentration methods (see p. 1114). Serologic and skin tests are available also.

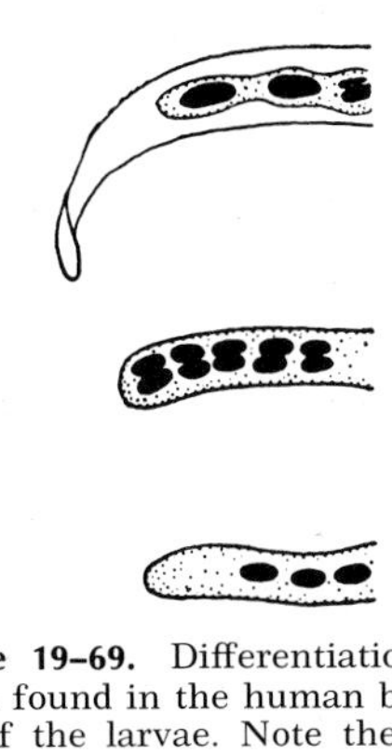

Figure 19-69. Differentiation of the species of microfilariae found in the human blood on the basis of posterior ends of the larvae. Note the distribution of nuclei, their presence or absence in the extreme caudal portion, and the presence or absence of a sheath. (From Markell, E. K., and Voge, M.: Medical Parasitology. 3rd ed.)

Brugia (Wuchereria) malayi. *Brugia malayi* (Table 19-5) is incriminated in the disease called Malayan filariasis. The adult worms are similar to *W. bancrofti,* but the sheathed microfilariae, 175 to 230 microns, that appear in peripheral blood do have body nuclei to the tip of the tail, with the two distal nuclei distinctly separated from the others (Fig. 19-69; Table 19-7). When elephantiasis occurs, it is in the upper extremities; otherwise, the infection resembles *W. bancrofti.* Mosquitoes are vectors, and the life history is similar to that shown in Figure 19-82.

Loa loa. Loiasis is caused by *Loa loa* (Table 19-5) which is commonly called the African eye worm. Males measure 30 mm. long, and the females are 70 mm. They live in subcutaneous tissues but migrate and produce raised areas called Calabar or "fugitive" swellings. As the worms pass across the bridge of the nose or in front of the eye, they cause much discomfort. The microfilariae (Fig. 19-69; Table 19-7) are found in the peripheral blood in the daytime only (diurnal [blood must be drawn between 10 A.M. and 2 P.M.]) as sheathed forms which possess a continuous row of nuclei to the tip of the tail. They measure 250 to 300 microns in length. Frequently it may be years after the Calabar swellings or the adults are observed before microfilariae are recovered. *Chrysops* flies are vectors.

Dipetalonema (Acanthocheilonema) perstans. Adults of the persistent filaria, *Acanthocheilonema perstans* or *Dipetalonema perstans* (Table 19-5), are found in various body cavities producing dipetalonemiasis. The microfilariae

(Text continues on page 1101.)

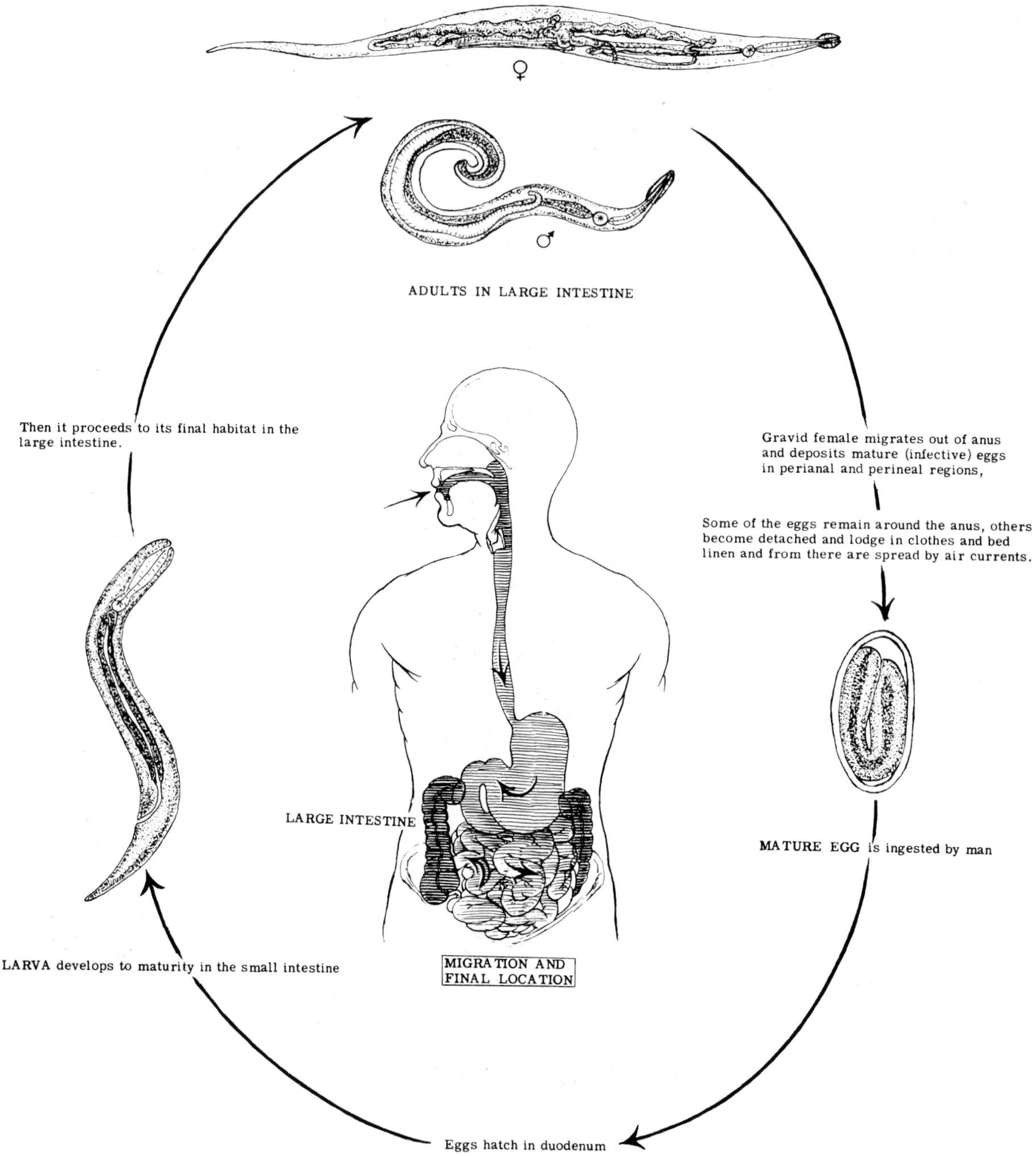
♀
♂
ADULTS IN LARGE INTESTINE
Gravid female migrates out of anus and deposits mature (infective) eggs in perianal and perineal regions,
Some of the eggs remain around the anus, others become detached and lodge in clothes and bed linen and from there are spread by air currents.
MATURE EGG is ingested by man
Eggs hatch in duodenum
LARVA develops to maturity in the small intestine
Then it proceeds to its final habitat in the large intestine.
LARGE INTESTINE
MIGRATION AND FINAL LOCATION

Figure 19–70. Life cycle of *Enterobius vermicularis.* (From Medical Protozoology and Helminthology. U.S. Naval Medical School, National Naval Medical Center, Bethesda, Maryland, 1965.)

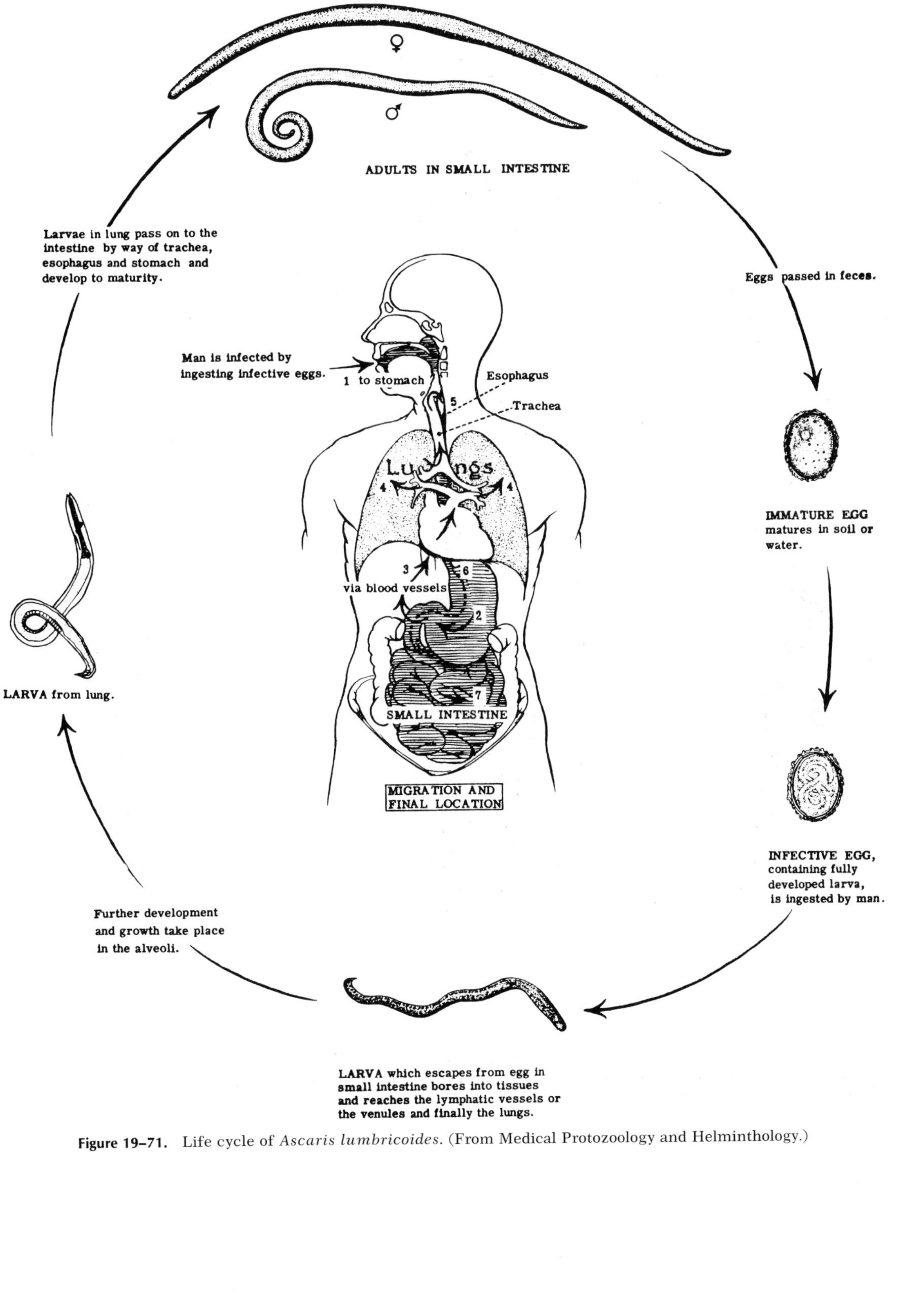
♀
♂
ADULTS IN SMALL INTESTINE
Eggs passed in feces.
IMMATURE EGG matures in soil or water.
INFECTIVE EGG, containing fully developed larva, is ingested by man.
LARVA which escapes from egg in small intestine bores into tissues and reaches the lymphatic vessels or the venules and finally the lungs.
Further development and growth take place in the alveoli.
LARVA from lung.
Larvae in lung pass on to the intestine by way of trachea, esophagus and stomach and develop to maturity.
Man is infected by ingesting infective eggs.
1 to stomach
Esophagus
5
Trachea
4
4
3
via blood vessels
6
2
7
SMALL INTESTINE
MIGRATION AND FINAL LOCATION

Figure 19–71. Life cycle of *Ascaris lumbricoides*. (From Medical Protozoology and Helminthology.)

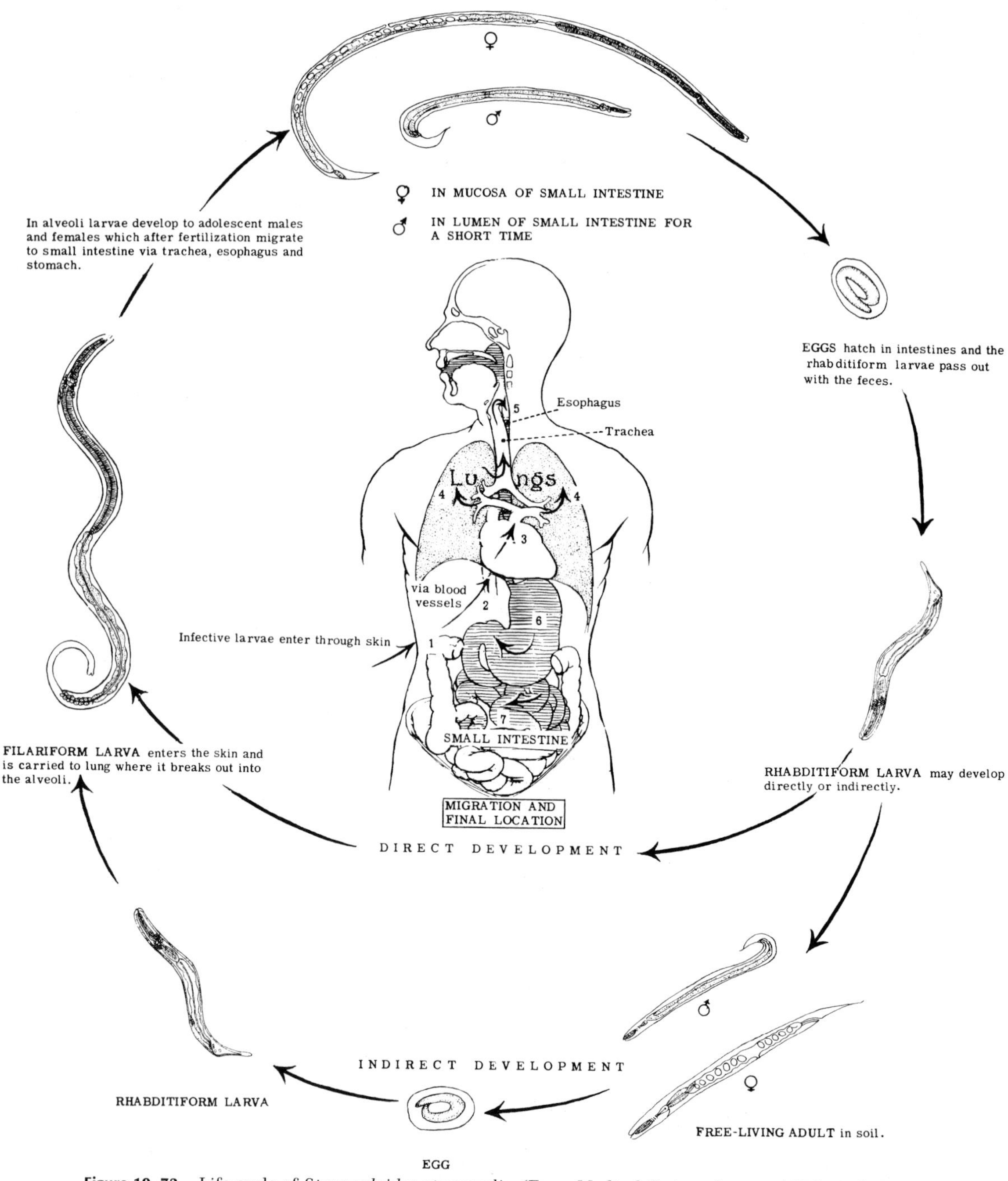

♀
♂
♀ IN MUCOSA OF SMALL INTESTINE
♂ IN LUMEN OF SMALL INTESTINE FOR A SHORT TIME
In alveoli larvae develop to adolescent males and females which after fertilization migrate to small intestine via trachea, esophagus and stomach.
EGGS hatch in intestines and the rhabditiform larvae pass out with the feces.
Esophagus
Trachea
Lungs
via blood vessels
Infective larvae enter through skin
SMALL INTESTINE
MIGRATION AND FINAL LOCATION
FILARIFORM LARVA enters the skin and is carried to lung where it breaks out into the alveoli.
RHABDITIFORM LARVA may develop directly or indirectly.
DIRECT DEVELOPMENT
INDIRECT DEVELOPMENT
RHABDITIFORM LARVA
FREE-LIVING ADULT in soil.
EGG

Figure 19–72. Life cycle of *Strongyloides stercoralis.* (From Medical Protozoology and Helminthology.)

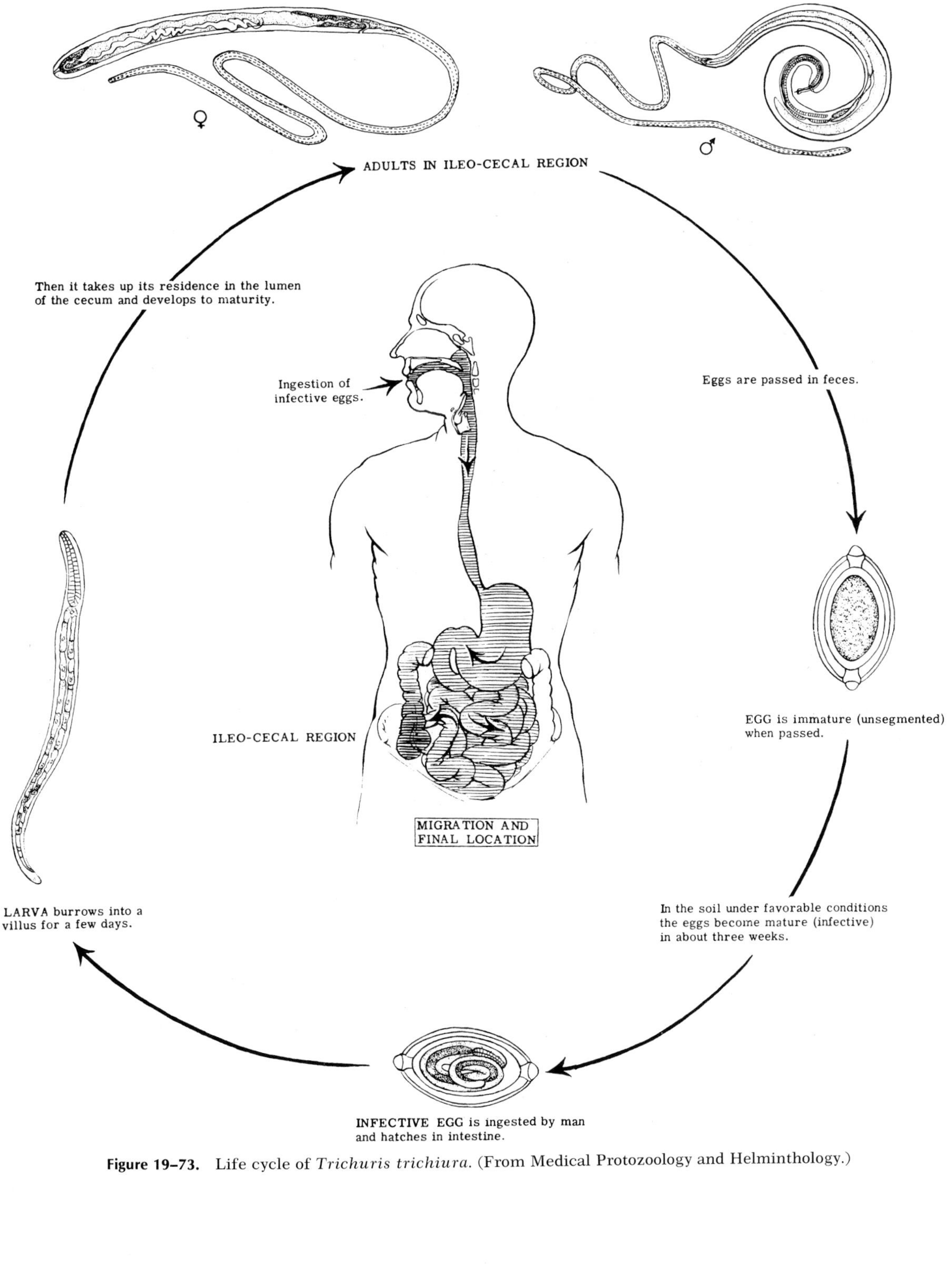
♀
♂
ADULTS IN ILEO-CECAL REGION
Eggs are passed in feces.
EGG is immature (unsegmented) when passed.
In the soil under favorable conditions the eggs become mature (infective) in about three weeks.
INFECTIVE EGG is ingested by man and hatches in intestine.
LARVA burrows into a villus for a few days.
Then it takes up its residence in the lumen of the cecum and develops to maturity.
Ingestion of infective eggs.
ILEO-CECAL REGION
MIGRATION AND FINAL LOCATION

Figure 19–73. Life cycle of *Trichuris trichiura.* (From Medical Protozoology and Helminthology.)

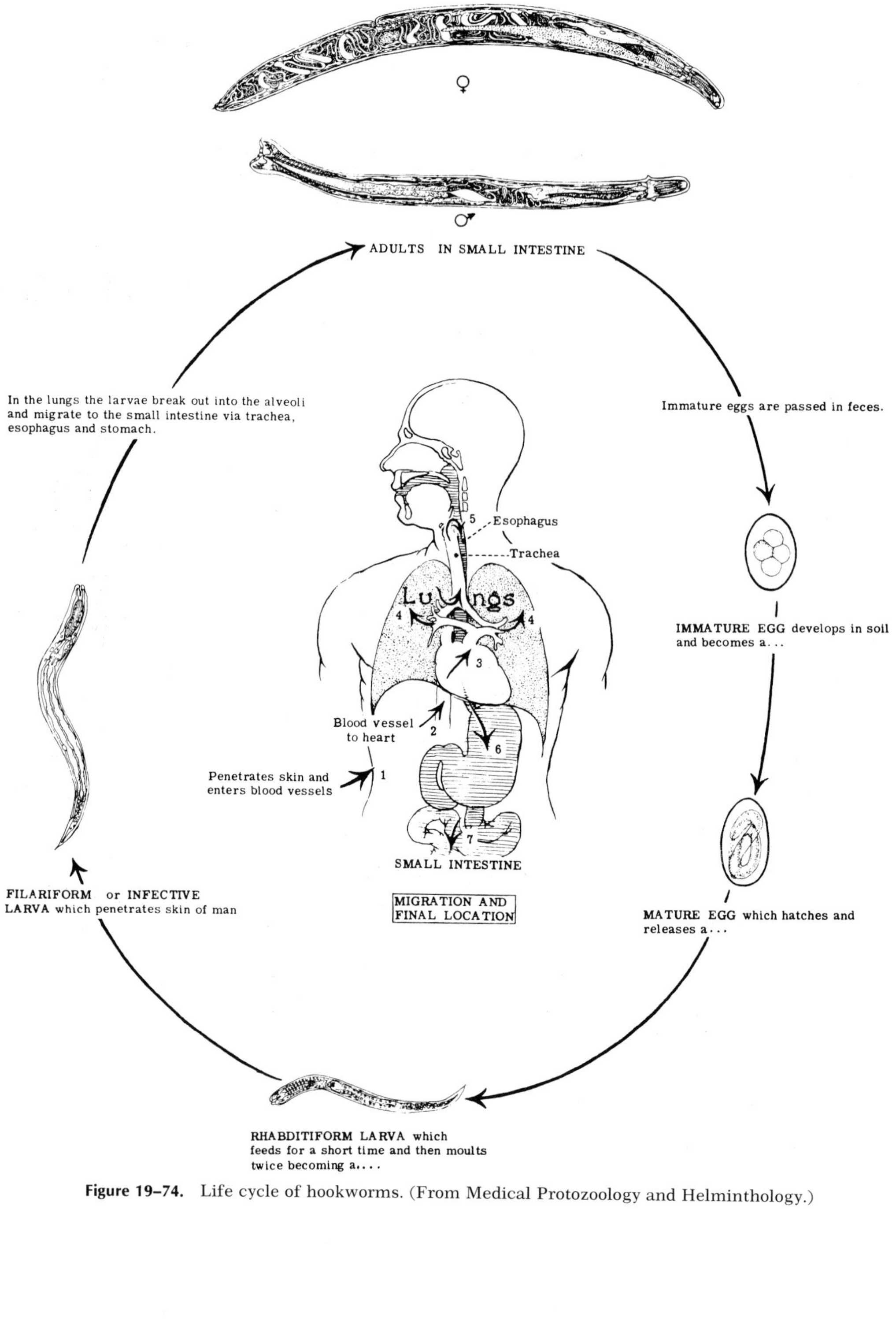
ADULTS IN SMALL INTESTINE
Immature eggs are passed in feces.
IMMATURE EGG develops in soil and becomes a...
MATURE EGG which hatches and releases a...
RHABDITIFORM LARVA which feeds for a short time and then moults twice becoming a....
FILARIFORM or INFECTIVE LARVA which penetrates skin of man
In the lungs the larvae break out into the alveoli and migrate to the small intestine via trachea, esophagus and stomach.
Esophagus
Trachea
Lungs
Blood vessel to heart
Penetrates skin and enters blood vessels
SMALL INTESTINE
MIGRATION AND FINAL LOCATION

Figure 19–74. Life cycle of hookworms. (From Medical Protozoology and Helminthology.)

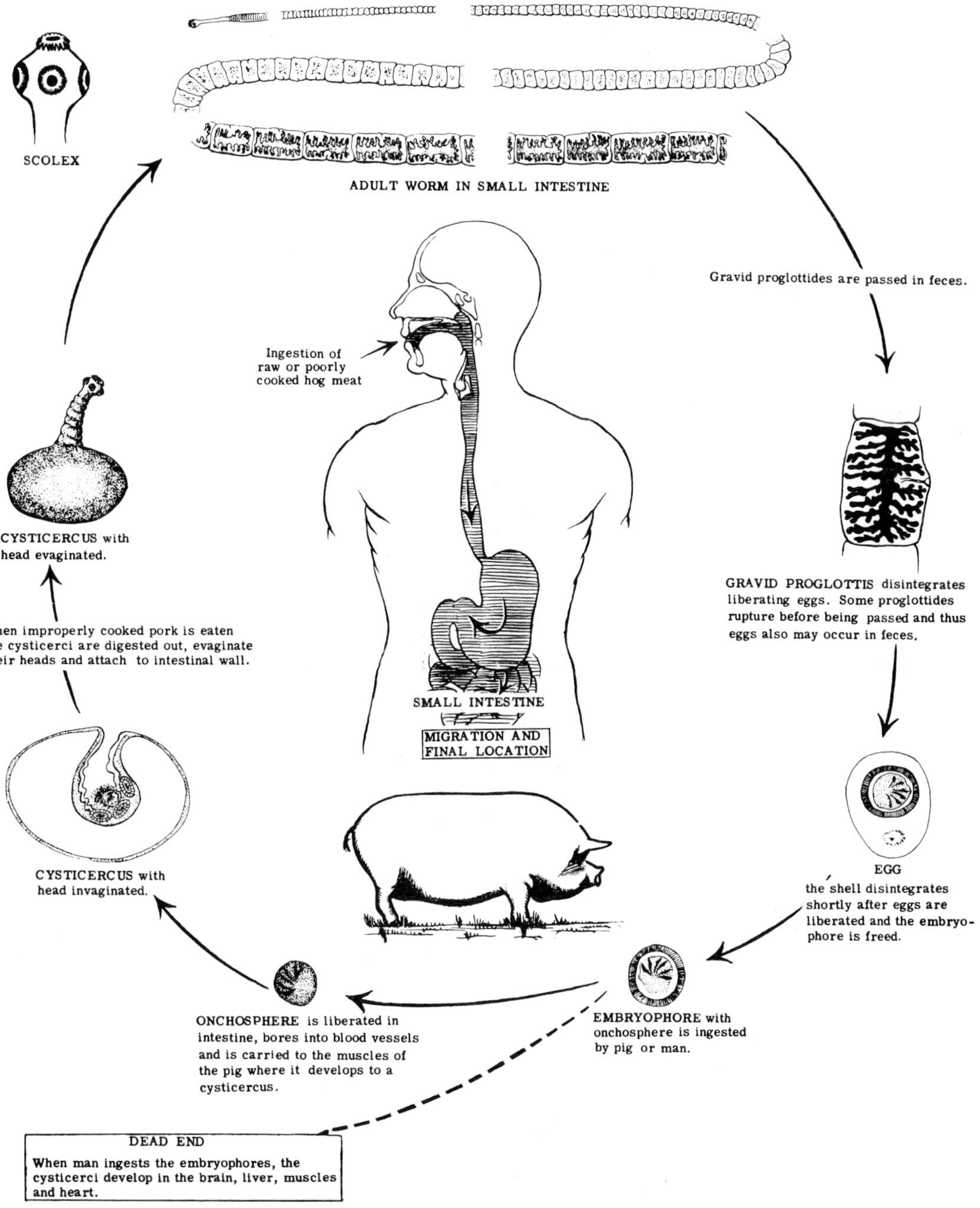
SCOLEX
ADULT WORM IN SMALL INTESTINE
Gravid proglottides are passed in feces.
Ingestion of raw or poorly cooked hog meat
CYSTICERCUS with head evaginated.
When improperly cooked pork is eaten the cysticerci are digested out, evaginate their heads and attach to intestinal wall.
SMALL INTESTINE
MIGRATION AND FINAL LOCATION
GRAVID PROGLOTTIS disintegrates liberating eggs. Some proglottides rupture before being passed and thus eggs also may occur in feces.
EGG
the shell disintegrates shortly after eggs are liberated and the embryophore is freed.
CYSTICERCUS with head invaginated.
ONCHOSPHERE is liberated in intestine, bores into blood vessels and is carried to the muscles of the pig where it develops to a cysticercus.
EMBRYOPHORE with onchosphere is ingested by pig or man.
DEAD END
When man ingests the embryophores, the cysticerci develop in the brain, liver, muscles and heart.

Figure 19–75. Life cycle of *Taenia solium*. (From Medical Protozoology and Helminthology.)

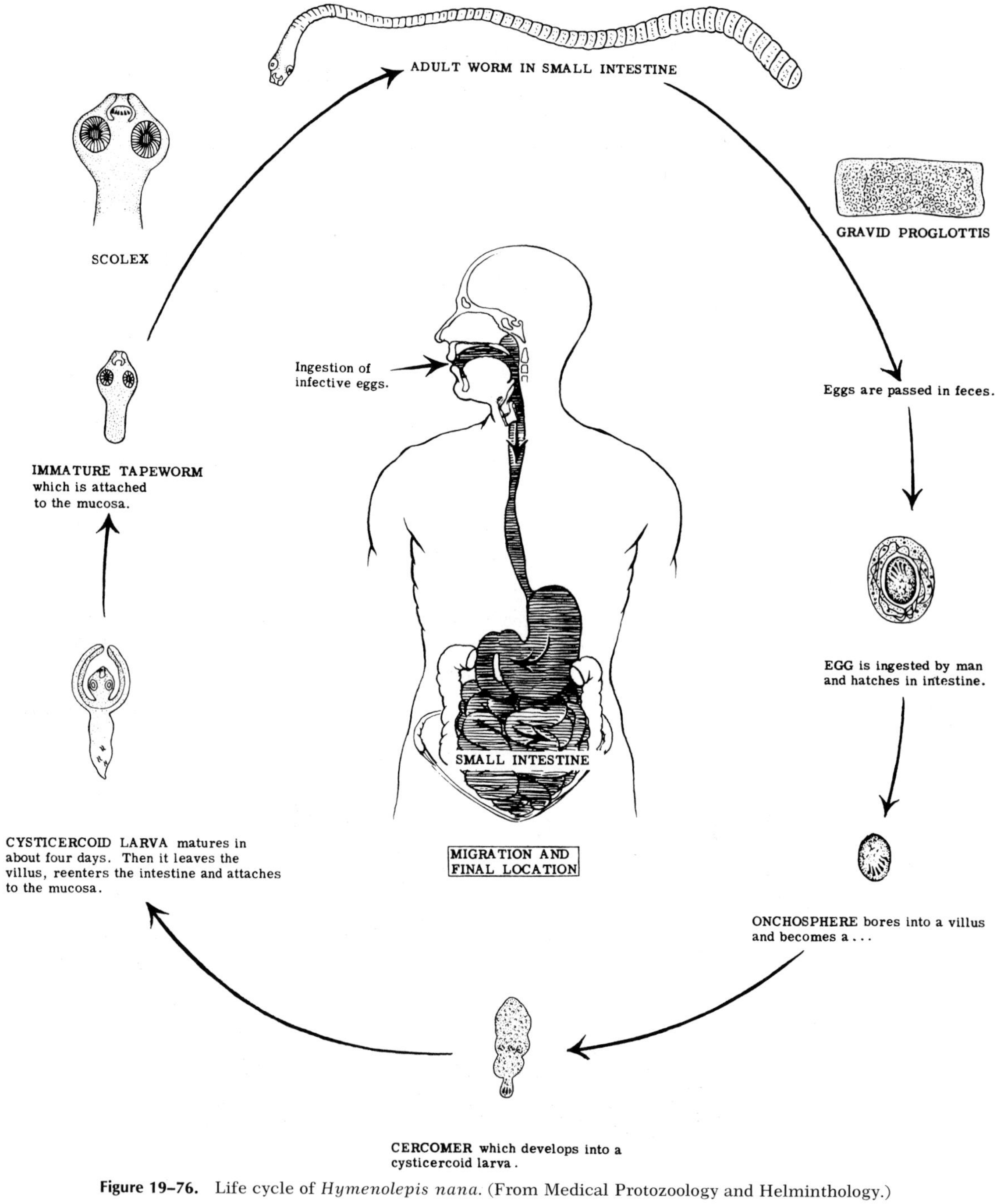

Figure 19–76. Life cycle of *Hymenolepis nana*. (From Medical Protozoology and Helminthology.)

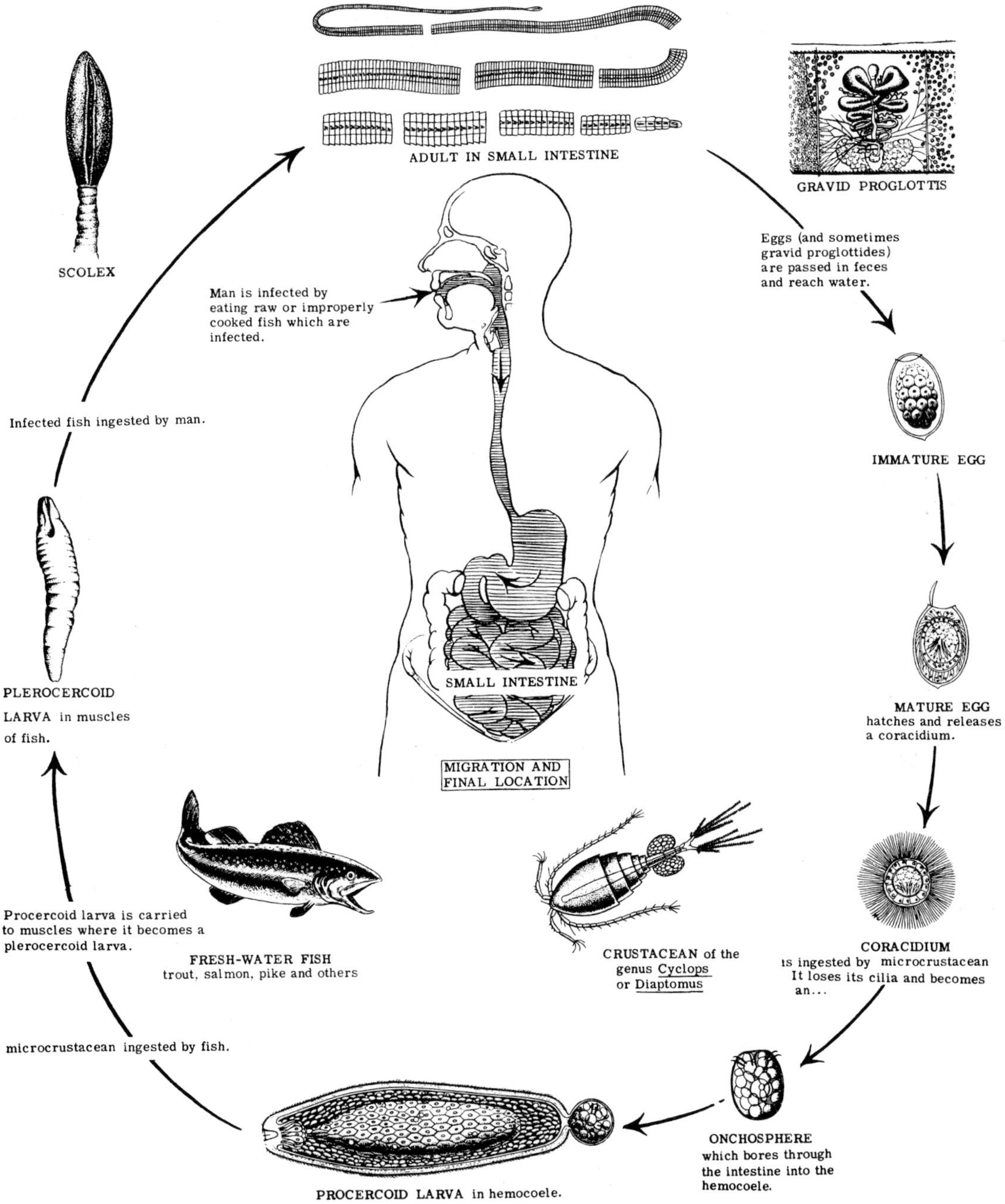

Figure 19–77. Life cycle of *Diphyllobothrium latum*. (From Medical Protozoology and Helminthology.)

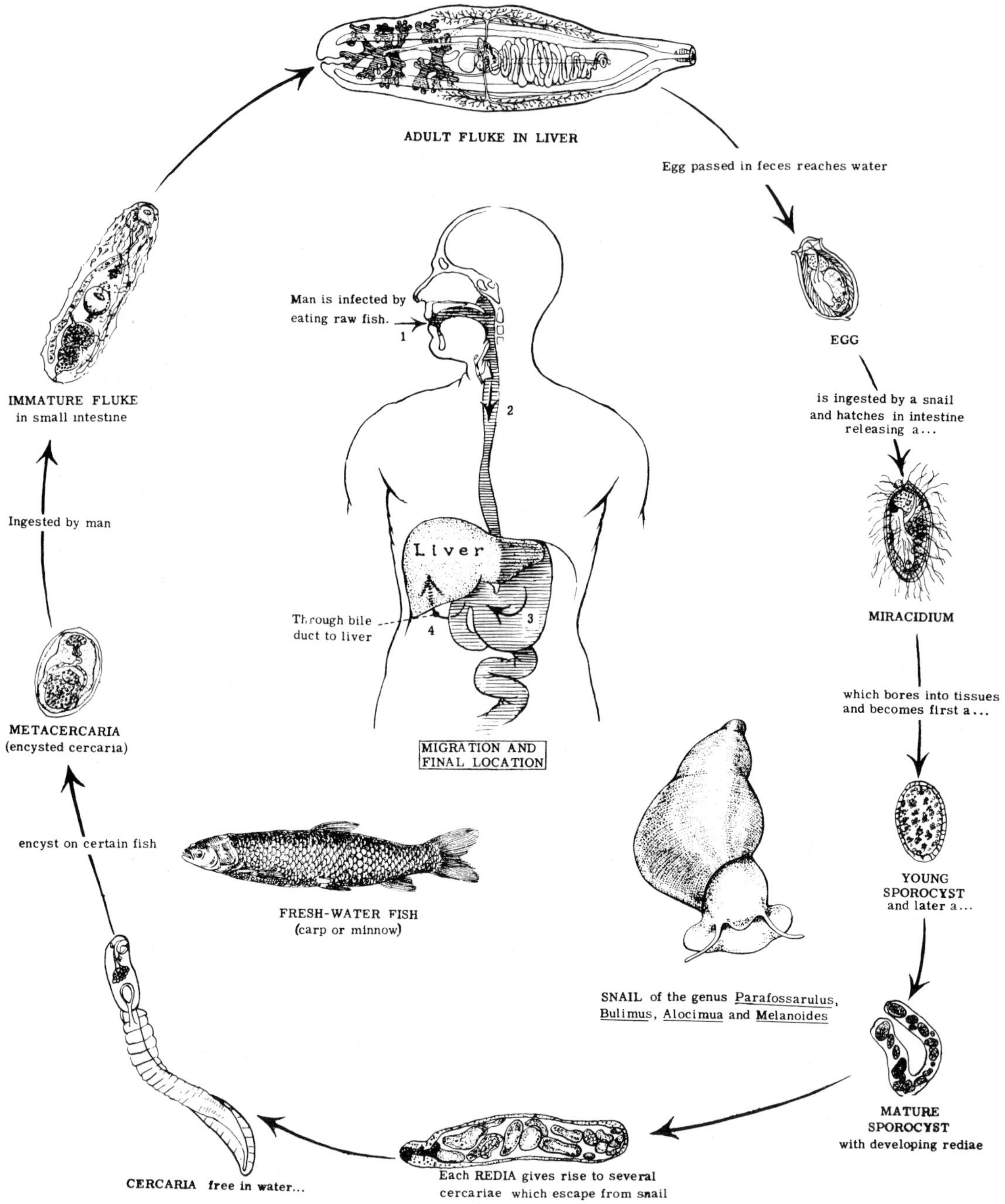
ADULT FLUKE IN LIVER
Egg passed in feces reaches water
EGG
is ingested by a snail and hatches in intestine releasing a...
MIRACIDIUM
which bores into tissues and becomes first a...
YOUNG SPOROCYST and later a...
MATURE SPOROCYST with developing rediae
Each REDIA gives rise to several cercariae which escape from snail
CERCARIA free in water...
encyst on certain fish
METACERCARIA (encysted cercaria)
Ingested by man
IMMATURE FLUKE in small intestine
Man is infected by eating raw fish.
1
2
3
4
Liver
Through bile duct to liver
MIGRATION AND FINAL LOCATION
FRESH-WATER FISH (carp or minnow)
SNAIL of the genus Parafossarulus, Bulimus, Alocimua and Melanoides

Figure 19–78. Life cycle of *Clonorchis sinensis.* (From Medical Protozoology and Helminthology.)

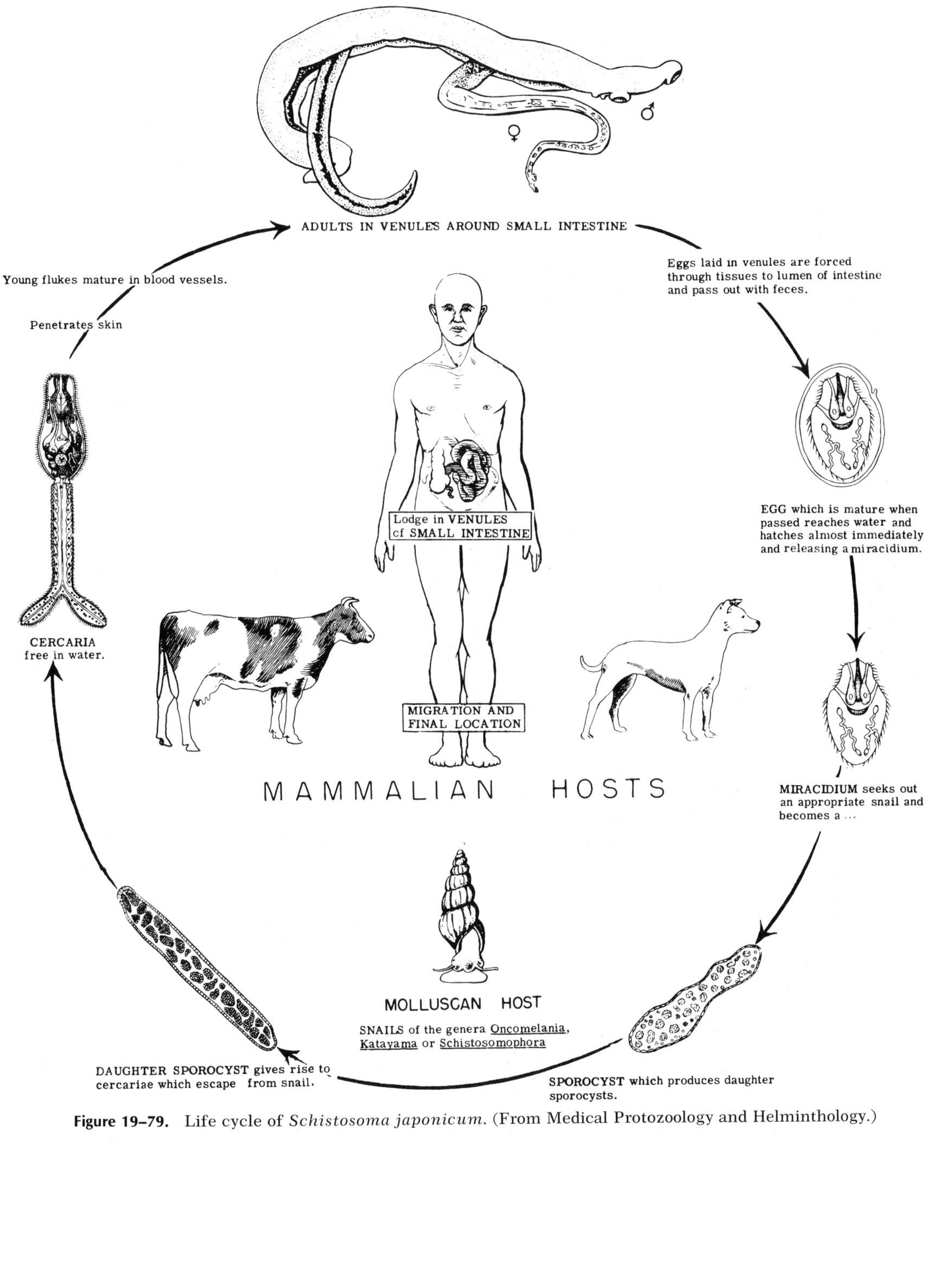
♀
♂
ADULTS IN VENULES AROUND SMALL INTESTINE
Eggs laid in venules are forced through tissues to lumen of intestine and pass out with feces.
EGG which is mature when passed reaches water and hatches almost immediately and releasing a miracidium.
MIRACIDIUM seeks out an appropriate snail and becomes a ...
SPOROCYST which produces daughter sporocysts.
MOLLUSCAN HOST
SNAILS of the genera Oncomelania, Katayama or Schistosomophora
DAUGHTER SPOROCYST gives rise to cercariae which escape from snail.
CERCARIA free in water.
Penetrates skin
Young flukes mature in blood vessels.
Lodge in VENULES of SMALL INTESTINE
MIGRATION AND FINAL LOCATION
MAMMALIAN HOSTS

Figure 19–79. Life cycle of *Schistosoma japonicum.* (From Medical Protozoology and Helminthology.)

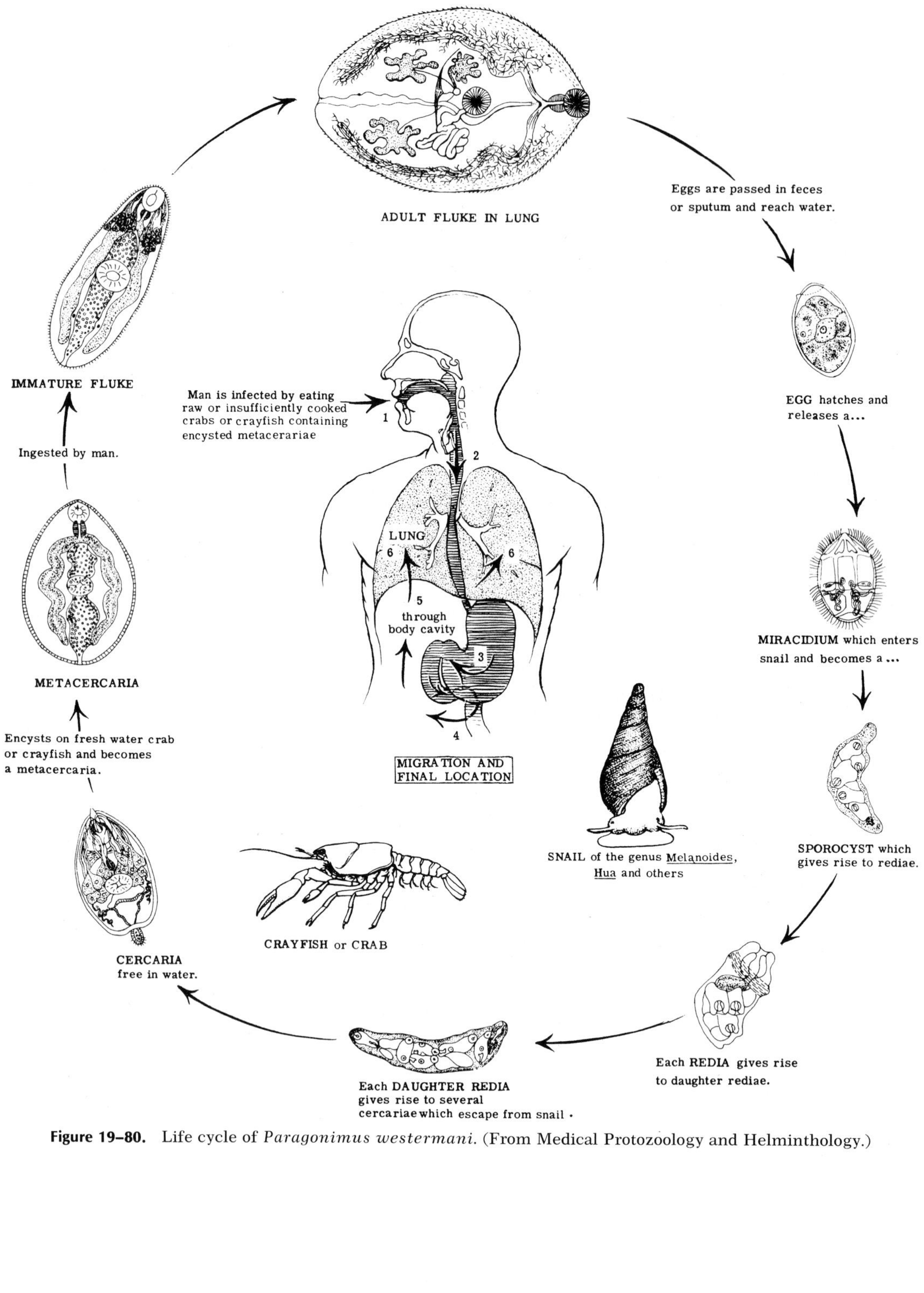
ADULT FLUKE IN LUNG
Eggs are passed in feces or sputum and reach water.
EGG hatches and releases a...
MIRACIDIUM which enters snail and becomes a ...
SPOROCYST which gives rise to rediae.
SNAIL of the genus Melanoides, Hua and others
Each REDIA gives rise to daughter rediae.
Each DAUGHTER REDIA gives rise to several cercariaewhich escape from snail .
CERCARIA free in water.
CRAYFISH or CRAB
Encysts on fresh water crab or crayfish and becomes a metacercaria.
METACERCARIA
Ingested by man.
IMMATURE FLUKE
Man is infected by eating raw or insufficiently cooked crabs or crayfish containing encysted metacerariae
1
2
LUNG
6
6
5
through body cavity
3
4
MIGRATION AND FINAL LOCATION

Figure 19–80. Life cycle of *Paragonimus westermani.* (From Medical Protozoology and Helminthology.)

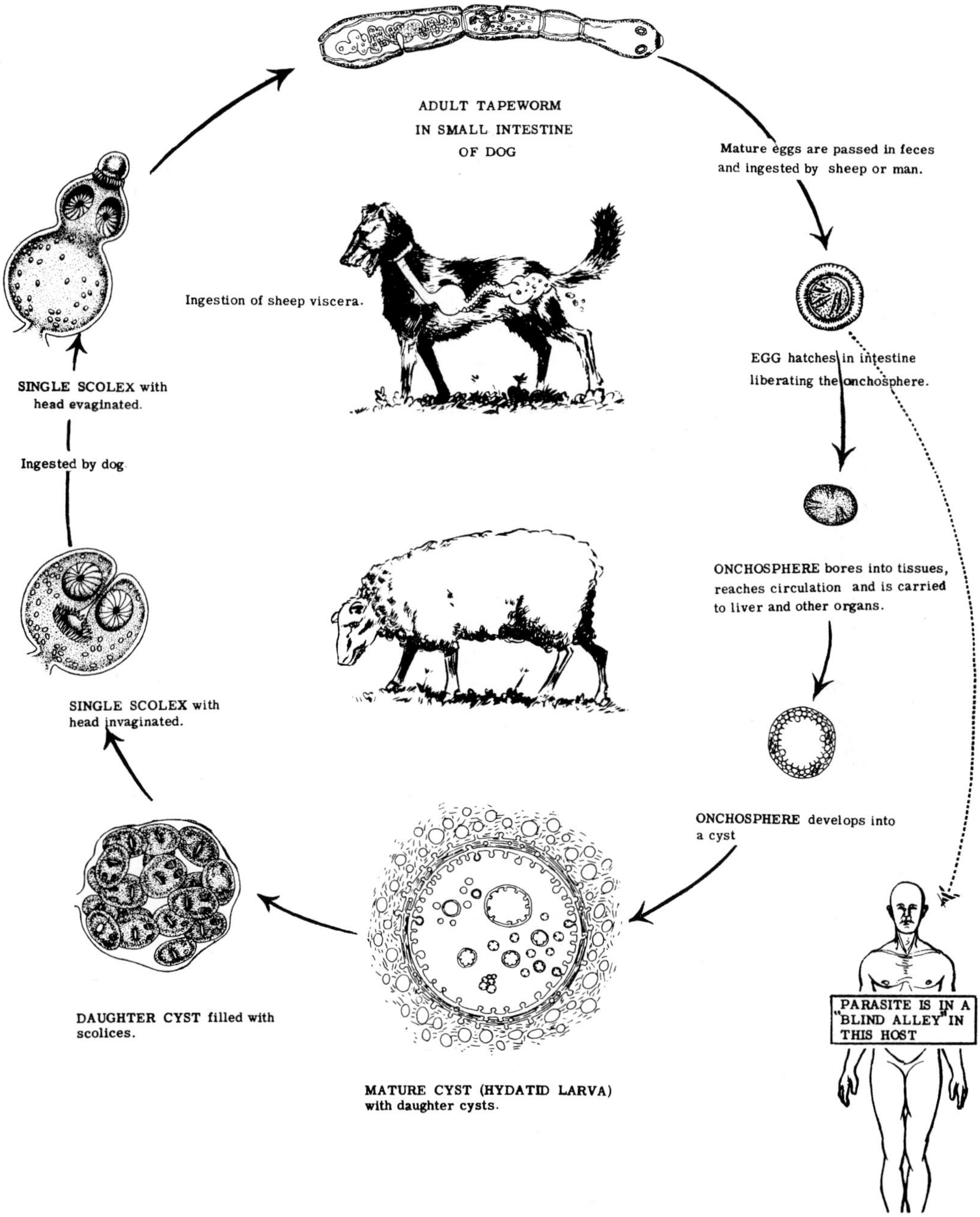
ADULT TAPEWORM
IN SMALL INTESTINE
OF DOG
Mature eggs are passed in feces
and ingested by sheep or man.
Ingestion of sheep viscera.
EGG hatches in intestine
liberating the onchosphere.
SINGLE SCOLEX with
head evaginated.
Ingested by dog
ONCHOSPHERE bores into tissues,
reaches circulation and is carried
to liver and other organs.
SINGLE SCOLEX with
head invaginated.
ONCHOSPHERE develops into
a cyst
PARASITE IS IN A
"BLIND ALLEY" IN
THIS HOST
DAUGHTER CYST filled with
scolices.
MATURE CYST (HYDATID LARVA)
with daughter cysts.

Figure 19–81. Life cycle of *Echinococcus granulosus.* (From Medical Protozoology and Helminthology.)

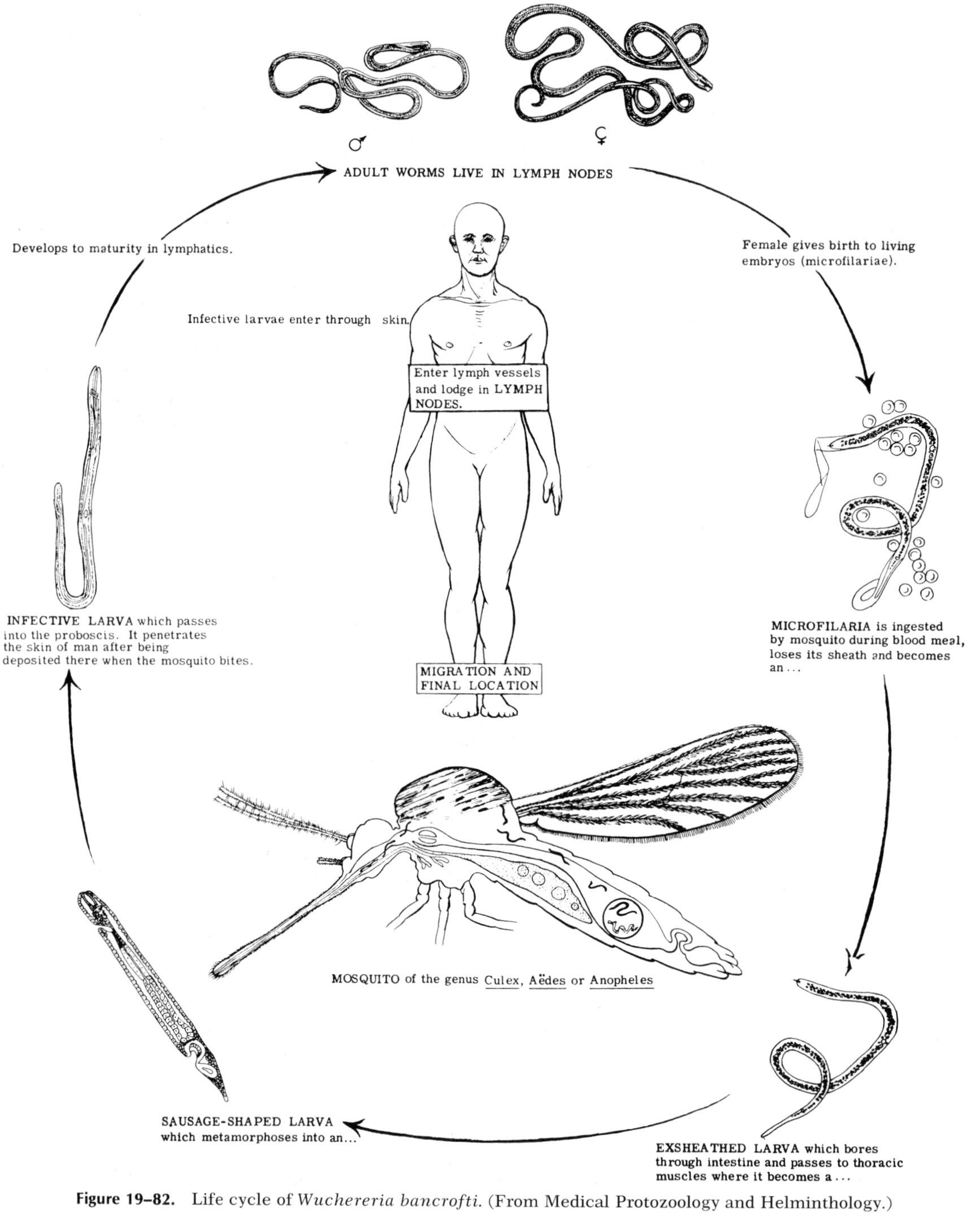

ADULT WORMS LIVE IN LYMPH NODES
Female gives birth to living embryos (microfilariae).
MICROFILARIA is ingested by mosquito during blood meal, loses its sheath and becomes an . . .
EXSHEATHED LARVA which bores through intestine and passes to thoracic muscles where it becomes a . . .
SAUSAGE-SHAPED LARVA which metamorphoses into an . . .
INFECTIVE LARVA which passes into the proboscis. It penetrates the skin of man after being deposited there when the mosquito bites.
Develops to maturity in lymphatics.
Infective larvae enter through skin.
Enter lymph vessels and lodge in LYMPH NODES.
MIGRATION AND FINAL LOCATION
MOSQUITO of the genus Culex, Aëdes or Anopheles

Figure 19–82. Life cycle of *Wuchereria bancrofti*. (From Medical Protozoology and Helminthology.)

(Fig. 19-69; Table 19-7), which show no periodicity and which are found unsheathed in peripheral blood, are about 200 microns long and 4.5 microns wide. They are characterized by having nuclei that extend to the tip of the tail. This parasite may produce symptoms (Adolph *et al.*, 1962) and is not as harmless as some suggest. This parasite and *Mansonella ozzardi*, below, are transmitted by the fly *Culicoides*.

Mansonella ozzardi. *Mansonella ozzardi* (Table 19-5) adults, 65 to 81 mm., also inhabit body cavities, and the unsheathed, nonperiodic microfilariae (Fig. 19-69; Table 19-7), which are characterized by the lack of nuclei to the tip of the tail, are found in peripheral blood, and measure 185 to 200 microns.

MEDICAL ENTOMOLOGY

Arthropods of Medical Importance

Arthropods are multicellular, segmented invertebrates that have a chitinous exoskeleton and paired articulated appendages. This is the largest phylum in the animal kingdom. Many species are of medical importance, for they may cause human disease (e.g., dermatosis, myiasis, injury to sense organs, allergy, injected or contact toxins or venoms, and nervous disorders), transmit pathogenic microorganisms to man as mechanical vectors, or act as biologic vectors when they serve as an essential host for a part of the life cycle of certain animal parasites (Table 19-8). Techniques for collecting, handling and examining arthropods may be found in many standard textbooks on medical parasitology and/or entomology, e.g., Medical Entomology (U.S. Naval Medical School, 1967), Herms and James, 1969 (see references at end of this chapter).

CLASS ARACHNIDA

This class is characterized by the following: forms with body divided into cephalothorax and abdomen; adults with four pairs of legs; absence of antennae and wings; and respiration by gills, booklungs, or tracheae or through cuticle. The most important members of this class are scorpions, spiders, ticks, and mites.

Table 19-8. DISEASES TRANSMITTED BY ARTHROPODS

VECTOR	DISEASE TRANSMITTED
CRUSTACEA	
Copepod—*Cyclops* and *Diaptomus*	*D. latum* infection; guinea worm *(D. medinensis)*
Crayfish and crabs	*P. westermani* infection
ARACHNIDA	
Mites	Tsutsugamushi fever (scrub typhus); rickettsial pox
Ticks	Tularemia; Russian spring-summer encephalitis; Q fever; Colorado tick fever; Rocky Mountain spotted fever, relapsing fever
INSECTA	
Lice	Epidemic typhus; relapsing fever; trench fever
Fleas	Plague; murine typhus; *Dipylidium caninum* infection
Bugs	Chagas's disease (American trypanosomiasis)
Beetles (some species)	*Hymenolepis diminuta* infection
Bloodsucking flies	
Phlebotomus (sand fly)	Leishmaniasis; pappataci fever; bartonellosis
Glossina (tsetse fly)	African trypanosomiasis
Simulium (black fly)	Onchocerciasis
Culicoides (midge, gnat)	*Dipetalonema (Acanthocheilonema) perstans* and *Mansonella ozzardi* infections
Chrysops (deer fly)	Loiasis; tularemia
Culex mosquito	Filariasis; viral encephalitides
Anopheles mosquito	Malaria; Bancroftian filariasis; Malayan filariasis
Aedes mosquito	Yellow fever; dengue; viral encephalitides; Bancroftian filariasis
Mansonia mosquito	Malayan filariasis

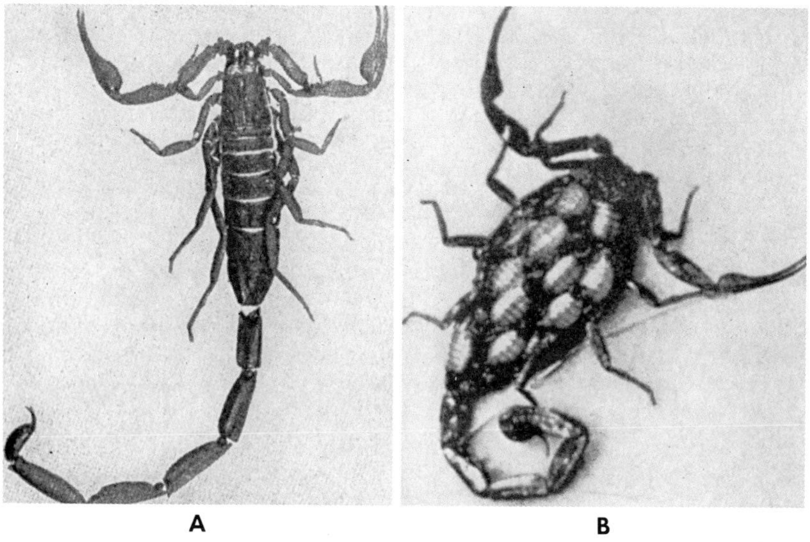

Figure 19–83. *A*, Male specimen of scorpion (*Centruroides*). × 1. (After C. C. Hoffmann, Anat. del Inst. de Biol., Mexico, from Faust, in Brennemann's Practice of Pediatrics; courtesy of W. F. Prior Company.) *B*, *Centruroides sculpturatus,* female with newly born young. × 1. (After Stahnke, Turtox News; courtesy of General Biological Supply House.)

Scorpions. Scorpions (Fig. 19–83) sting their prey and introduce neurotoxic venom by means of their caudal stinger. An ascending paralysis may be accompanied by respiratory failure, especially in children. The adult scorpions occur in and around houses in warm moist or dry areas and are nocturnal or hide themselves in dark places.

Spiders. The black widow spider, *Latrodectus mactans* (Fig. 19–84), is the best known of the poisonous spiders and is widely distributed throughout the western hemisphere.

The adult female is a lustrous black dorsally, and on the midventral surface is a diagnostic red spot, which usually resembles an hourglass.

The spider inhabits trash piles, outhouses, hollow stumps, lumber piles, cellars, and garages. The females are about 13 mm. in length, and the males, which differ in their color pattern from the females, are about half this size.

Arachnidism (Spider Poisoning). As the spider bites the human victim, the toxin is injected into the skin. Within 1 hour severe pain develops, with redness and swelling at the site of the bite. Abdominal cramps develop, followed by pains in the muscles of the legs, chest, and back. In time, marked board-like rigidity develops. These acute symptoms may persist for 12 to 48 hours. Accompanying the muscular rigidity one may observe excessive perspiration, nausea, vomiting, headache, elevated temperature and blood pressure, and leukocytosis. Some cases are fatal. Specific antivenin is available.

"Gangrenous spot," necrotic arachnidism, or loxoscelism in North America (Dillaha *et al.,* 1964) is produced by the bite of the brown recluse spider, *L. reclusa,* which has a characteristic dark brown "violin" marking on the cephalothorax. A gangrenous slough at the site of the bite and a severe systemic reaction occur. The former includes pain, bleb formation, erythema, ecchymosis, necrosis ending in an eschar, and ulceration. The systemic reac-

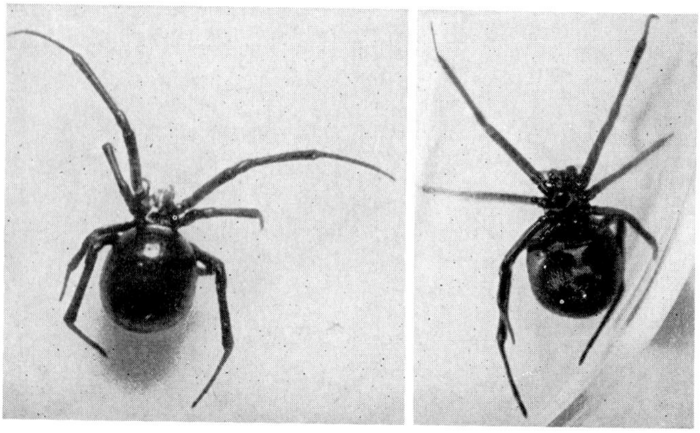

Figure 19–84. Black widow spiders, *Latrodectus mactans.*

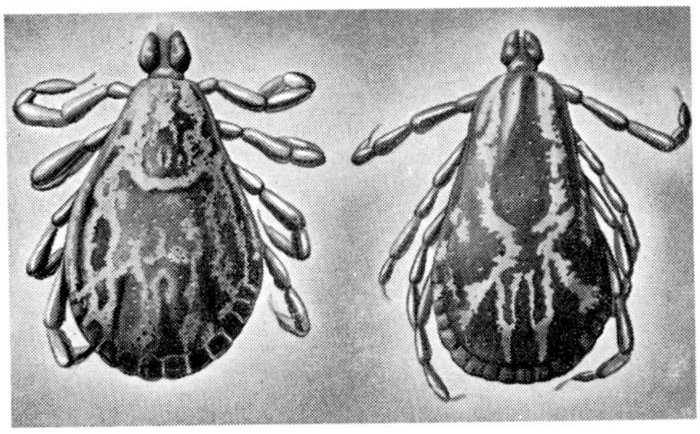

Figure 19–85. *Dermacentor andersoni* and *Dermacentor variabilis*; vectors of Rocky Mountain spotted fever rickettsiae. (Courtesy of Merck, Sharp & Dohme, Inc.)

tion may include fever, nausea, malaise, hemolysis, and thrombocytopenia. Deaths have been reported in small children.

Ticks. Ticks differ from mites in the following ways: they are larger; have no hairs; have a leathery integument; and have an exposed, armed hypostome and a pair of spiracles. There are soft-bodied ticks (Argasidae) (not pictured) and hard-bodied ticks (Ixodidae) (Fig. 19–85).

The soft-bodied ticks have no hard plate on the dorsum, the mouth parts are ventral to the anterior end, and the spiracles are behind the third pair of coxal segments. The hard-bodied ticks possess a dorsal plate, which is anterior only in the female but covers the entire dorsum in the male. The mouth parts extend beyond the anterior portion; and the spiracles are located behind the fourth pair of coxal segments.

Certain *Ornithodoros* species, soft-bodied ticks, are important vectors of endemic relapsing fever, and hard-bodied ticks may transmit rickettsiae, viruses, and bacteria. *Dermacentor andersoni,* a hard-bodied tick, is the chief vector of Rocky Mountain spotted fever.

Ticks may harm man by mechanical injury of their bites, by transmission of microorganisms, and by tick paralysis.

Tick Paralysis. This disease occurs mostly in young children and is characterized by an ascending flaccid paralysis. The tick is attached to the body, usually near the base of the brain or along the spinal column. The disease has a rapid onset and death may occur. Removal of the tick usually results in gradual recession of paralysis and abatement of symptoms.

Mites. Mites are microscopic in size and do not have a leathery integument. The hypostome, if present, is hidden and unarmed. On the cephalothorax of some mites spiracles are present. Mites serve as vectors of certain human diseases, but they may penetrate the skin directly, causing injury, as in scabies.

Sarcoptes scabiei, the itch mite (Figs. 19–86, 19–87, 19–88), is cosmopolitan in its distribution and causes a disease known as scabies or sarcoptic mange in man. A rare clinical form known as "Norwegian scabies," "scabies Crustosa," or "scabies keratotica" may be seen (Kurtin and Leider, 1968; Haydon and Caplan, 1971; Zakon and McQuay, 1972). The female is about 0.5 mm. in length, and the male is smaller. The male has pedunculated ambulacra on the fourth pair of legs and setae (bristles) on the third pair, whereas females have setae on the third as well as the fourth pairs. The adult females tunnel in the superficial layers of the skin (Fig. 19–88), producing lesions. These lesions are located in the soft folds of the body in areas such as the interdigital spaces, flexor surfaces of the wrists and forearms, popliteal folds, inguinal region, and the back, although any area except the head may

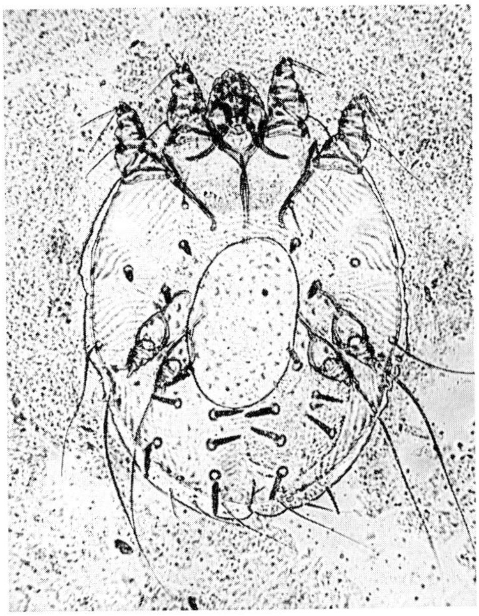

Figure 19–86. *Sarcoptes scabiei,* adult female. (From Markell, E. K., and Voge, M.: Medical Parasitology. 3rd ed.)

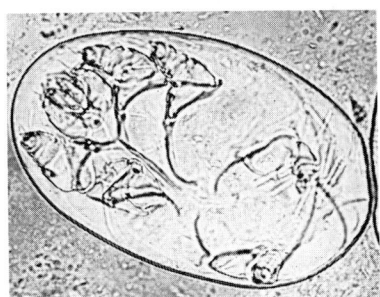

Figure 19–87. *Sarcoptes scabiei* egg containing fully developed larva. (From Markell, E. K., and Voge, M.: Medical Parasitology. 3rd ed.)

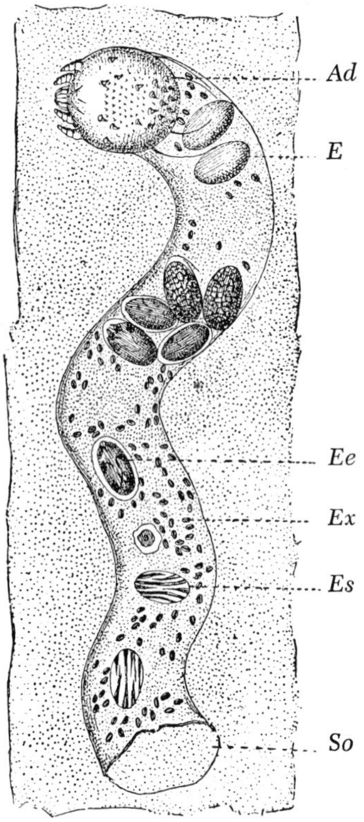

Figure 19–88. *Sarcoptes scabiei.* Diagram of a subcutaneous burrow; *Ad,* adult female; *E,* eggs; *Ee,* embryo egg; *Ex,* excrement; *Es,* egg shell; *So,* skin orifice. (After Railliet in Brumpt.)

be involved. An intense itching develops from the minute vesicles. Scratching introduces secondary bacterial invasion with scab formation. The parasite and its eggs may be removed from the tunnel by needle or skin scrapings, which are placed in 20 per cent potassium hydroxide for clearing and are examined under the low power field. Suspected areas may be examined by the use of hand lens before scrapings are made. In Norwegian scabies, eggs, six-legged larvae, and eight-legged nymphs, as well as males and females may be isolated.

Demodex folliculorum, the follicular mite (Fig. 19–89), parasitizes the hair follicles or sebaceous glands. In man it produces mild dermatitis, which may be evidenced by acne, blackheads, and keratosis. Material from the glands may be examined under the low power objective. The female is larger than the male, which measures 40 to 300 microns.

Trombiculid Mites. Eight-legged adults of the trombiculid mites do not parasitize man; however, the six-legged larvae attack man, producing a severe dermatitis (Fig. 19–90).

Eutrombicula alfreddugèsi is called the red bug, chigger, or harvest mite. These mites infect grasses and bushes, particularly berry

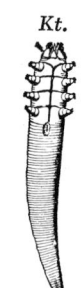

Figure 19–89. The "face insect," *Demodex folliculorum* (× 100); *Kt.,* biting jaws. (After R. Blanchard in Brumpt.)

bushes, and the larval forms attack man as he brushes against these infested objects. They burrow into the skin, causing intense itching.

Trombicula akamushi and other related species produce larvae that transmit tsutsugamushi fever or scrub typhus, a rickettsial disease.

CLASS INSECTA

Insects, also called hexapoda, are characterized by having a body divided into head, thorax, and abdomen. There are only three pairs of legs. Usually two pairs of wings are present, but there are some species without them.

Lice. Human lice are distinctively flattened dorsoventrally and are wingless, with piercing sucking mouth parts. The three species of lice that parasitize man are *Pediculus humanus* var. *capitis* (the head louse) (Fig. 19–91), *Pediculus humanus* var. *corporis* (the body louse) (Fig. 19–91), and *Phthirus pubis* (the pubic or crab louse) (Fig. 19–93).

The head louse lays its eggs or nits (Fig.

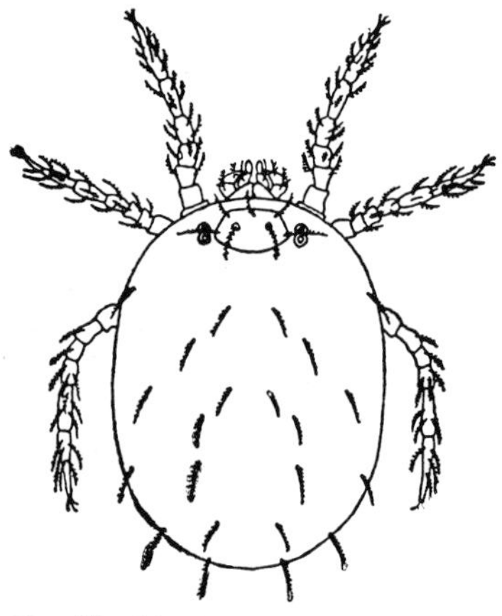

Figure 19–90. The North American chigger, *Trombicula irritans* (larva, × 100). (Ewing: A Manual of External Parasites. Springfield, Ill., Charles C Thomas.)

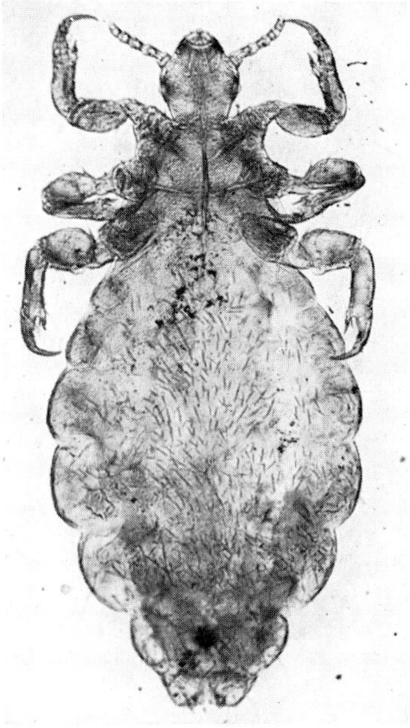

Figure 19–91. *Pediculus humanus.* (From Markell, E. K., and Voge, M.: Medical Parasitology. 3rd ed.)

19–92) on the hairs. Their claws are designed for clasping fine hairs of the head. The adults are 2 to 3 mm. long, with a pair of spiracles in each abdominal segment. The body louse lays its eggs in seams of woolen clothing and visits the host for a blood meal. The pubic or crab louse (Fig. 19–93), on the other hand, has claws designed for clasping the coarse hairs of the pubic region and axilla, the eyebrows, and the chest hairs. The adults are shorter and broader than *Pediculus,* the abdomen is more compressed, and the first abdominal segment has three pairs of spiracles.

When man is infested with body or head lice, the condition is referred to as pediculosis, which in sensitized individuals may be severe. Body lice are vectors of such diseases as epidemic typhus, trench fever, and relapsing fever, but pubic lice have not been incriminated.

Fleas. Fleas are bloodsucking, wingless, brown, laterally compressed ectoparasites with hind legs developed for jumping. The adults vary from 1.5 to 4 mm. in length (Fig. 19–94).

Salivary secretions of the flea may produce a lesion at the site of the bite. Certain species of fleas also serve as vectors of plague (*Xenopsylla cheopis,* the tropical rat flea) and endemic typhus and may mechanically spread bacterial and viral diseases.

A flea of tropical America and Africa, *Tunga penetrans* or the chigoe flea (Fig. 19–94) is exceptional in that it burrows into the skin of the feet producing tungiasis.

THE BUGS (HEMIPTERA)

Only two true bugs are of any medical importance, the bedbugs and the reduviids.

The bedbugs, *Cimex lectularius* (Fig. 19–95), frequently bite man, causing irritation. They infest houses, hotels, and tenement houses, hiding in furniture, floors, and walls during the day and coming out to feed at night. They are brown, flattened, oval insects without wings. The area of the bite may produce swelling, itching, and scratching and may produce secondary bacterial invasion. The bedbug may act as a mechanical transmitter of disease. However, there is no evidence of biologic transmission, although they have been observed experimentally as carriers of pathogenic organisms.

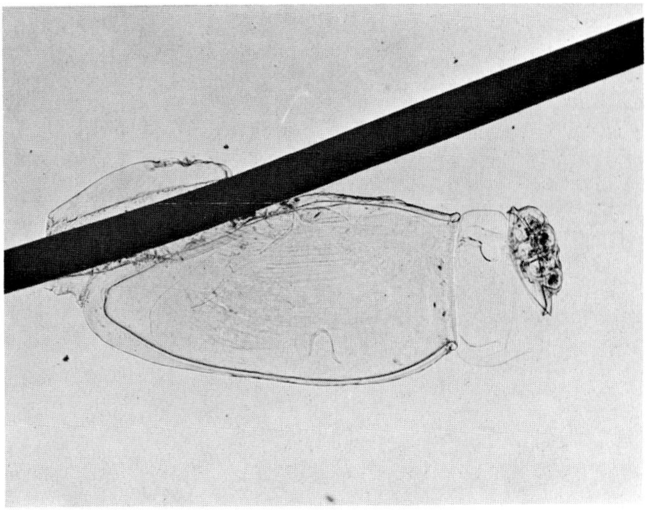

Figure 19–92. *Pediculus capitis.* Egg ("nit") attached to hair (× 60). (From Lynch, M. J., *et al.*: Medical Laboratory Technology and Clinical Pathology.)

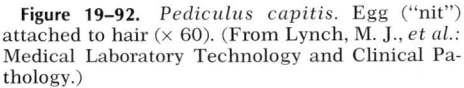

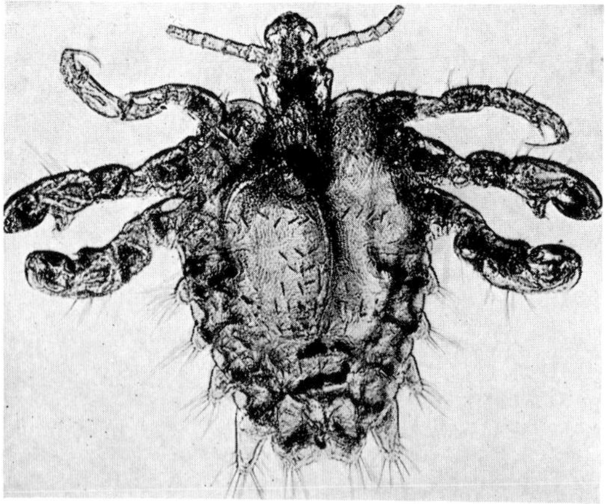

Figure 19–93. *Phthirus pubis.* (Courtesy of Army Medical Museum.)

The reduviid or kissing bugs or "cone-nose bugs" (Fig. 19–17) feed on blood, and certain species are responsible for the transmission of Chagas' disease, discussed earlier.

MOSQUITOES AND FLIES

The Diptera are the true flies and include mosquitoes and flies. They usually have two wings, with the halteres as the second pair. The mouth parts are adapted for sucking and in some instances for piercing.

Mosquitoes. Mosquitoes are flies that are slender and delicate. Those that suck blood play an important role in the transmission of human diseases, such as malaria, filariasis, dengue, yellow fever, and some of the encephalitides. The mosquitoes can be differentiated from other flies by the presence of scales on their wings and a proboscis, which is adapted for piercing and sucking. The antennae are long, with 15 joints.

Many species of the several genera of mosquitoes serve as vectors of human diseases. The genera incriminated are *Anopheles, Culex, Aedes,* and *Mansonia.* Differential diagnosis is based upon many varied morphologic structures, details of which can be found in textbooks or manuals on medical entomology.

The Bloodsucking Flies. Bloodsucking flies (see Table 19–8 and the appropriate life cycle figures) have blade-like cutting organs rather than the stylet of mosquitoes.

All bloodsucking flies, e.g., the stable fly *Stomoxys calcitrans,* as well as those listed in Table 19–8 are pests and may inflict painful wounds.

The Nonbloodsucking Flies. The non-bloodsucking flies are the filth flies, which have fleshy mouth parts adapted for sucking liquids. The adult flies may be mechanical transmitters of diseases such as enteric pathogens, tuberculosis, plague, tularemia, polio, anthrax, and brucellosis, but the larvae may invade the broken or unbroken skin or develop from ingested fly eggs to produce a condition known as myiasis.

Specific Myiasis. Eggs or larvae from certain filth flies are deposited on the tissues of the specific host, and the larva becomes parasitic as it invades the area. Examples of flies that produce this type of myiasis are the screwworm, *Calliphora (Cochliomyia) americana* and *C. macellaria;* the botfly, *Dermatobia hominis;* the sheep botfly, *Oestrus ovis;* the cattle botfly, *Hypoderma;* and *Gasterophilus.*

Semispecific Myiasis. Eggs or larvae of the semispecific flies are deposited in rotting vegetable matter or in open wounds and sores.

Accidental Myiasis. Eggs of the accidental myiasis-producing flies are laid in feces or decaying organic matter or on food. Man becomes infected by ingestion of the eggs or larvae or by contamination of wounds. Examples are *Musca domestica* and *Fannia.*

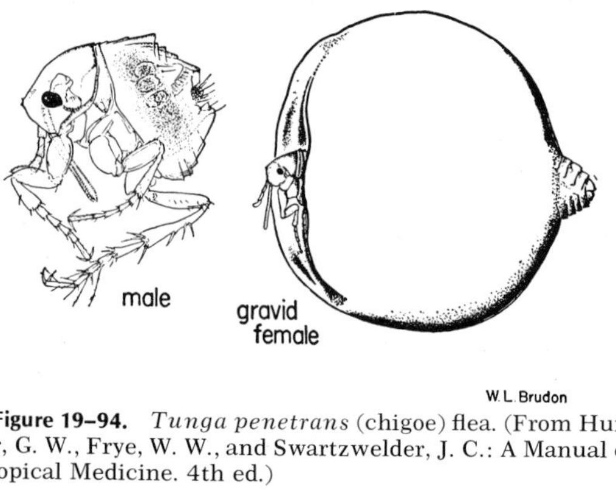

Figure 19–94. *Tunga penetrans* (chigoe) flea. (From Hunter, G. W., Frye, W. W., and Swartzwelder, J. C.: A Manual of Tropical Medicine. 4th ed.)

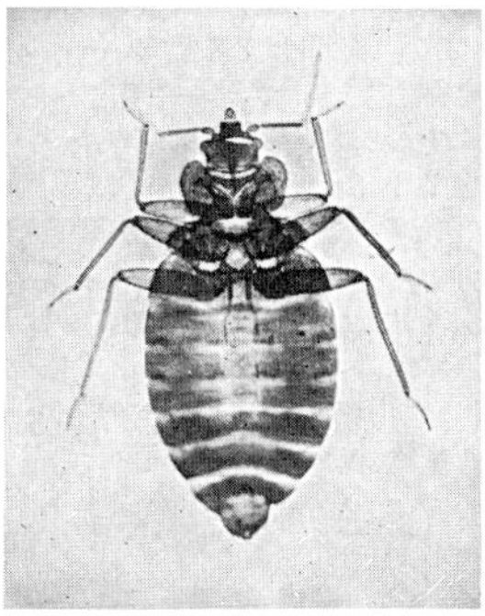

Figure 19–95. The common bedbug, *Cimex lectularius,* male (× 5). In the female the posterior end of the abdomen is more rounded. (Cleared with sodium hydroxide to bring out the structure more clearly.)

Table 19–9. ARRANGEMENT OF PARASITES BY THE HUMAN ORGAN SYSTEM INVOLVED

ORGAN SYSTEM	ORGANISM	DISEASE	REFERENCE PAGE(S)
*Muscle-Skeletal**			
Helminths	*Trichinella spiralis*	Trichinosis	1085
	Echinococcus granulosus (larva)	Echinococcosis, hydatid disease (osseous)	1081–1082
	Cysticercus cellulosae	Cysticercosis, bladderworm infection	1081
	Spirometra sp. (sparaganum larva)	Sparganosis	1082–1083
Gastrointestinal†			
Protozoa	*Entamoeba histolytica*	Amebiasis (various manifestations)	1025–1032
	Dientamoeba fragilis	Dientamebiasis (dientamoeba diarrhea)	1033
	Giardia lamblia	Giardiasis or lambliasis	1036
	Isospora hominis	Isosporiasis	1040
	Balantidium coli	Balantidiasis	1034–1035
Helminths‡	*Enterobius vermicularis*	Enterobiasis, pinworm infection	1052–1062
	Ascaris lumbricoides	Ascariasis, giant intestinal roundworm	1062–1063
	Strongyloides stercoralis	Strongyloidiasis, threadworm	1064–1067
	Necator americanus	Necatoriasis, American (New World) hookworm	1069–1070
	Ancylostoma duodenale	Ancylostomiasis, Old World hookworm	
	Trichostrongylus sp.	Trichostrongyliasis	1068
	Trichuris trichiura	Trichuriasis, whipworm	1067–1068
	Capillaria philippinensis	Intestinal capillariasis (G.I. symptoms)	1068
	Trichinella spiralis (adults)		1085
	Anisakis sp.	Anisakiasis	1064
	Diphyllobothrium latum	Diphyllobothriasis, broadfish tapeworm infection	1075
	Taenia saginata	Taeniasis saginata, beef tapeworm infection	1074
	Taenia solium	Taeniasis solium, pork tapeworm	1073–1074
	Hymenolepis nana	Hymenolepiasis, dwarf tapeworm infection	1074–1075
	Fasciolopsis buski	Fasciolopsiasis, giant intestinal fluke	1075
	Heterophyes heterophyes	Heterophyiasis	1077
	Metagonimus yokagawai	Metagonimiasis	
	Echinostoma sp.	Echinostomiasis	1075–1077
	Schistosoma mansoni	Bilharziasis (intestinal), intestinal schistosomiasis	1078–1080
	Schistosoma japonicum	Bilharziasis (intestinal), intestinal schistosomiasis	
	Schistosoma haematobium	(Occasionally in intestine)	1080–1081
Arthropods	Maggots (various filth, flies, etc.)	Intestinal myiasis	1106
Cardiovascular			
Protozoa	*Plasmodium vivax*	Malaria, benign tertian, vivax	1040–1050
	Plasmodium falciparum	Malaria, malignant tertian, subtertian E.A., falciparum	
	Plasmodium malariae	Malaria, quartan	
	Plasmodium ovale	Malaria, ovale	
	Trypanosoma gambiense	African trypanosomiasis, sleeping sickness	1039
	Trypanosoma rhodesiense	African trypanosomiasis, sleeping sickness	
	Trypanosoma cruzi	American trypanosomiasis, Chagas' disease	1039–1040
	Leishmania donovani	Leishmaniasis (visceral), kala-azar	1037
	Babesia sp.	Babesiosis	1050
Helminths	*Wuchereria bancrofti*	Filariasis (Bancroftian), wuchereriasis, elephantiasis	1086–1087
	Brugia malayi	Filariasis (Malayan, Brug's elephantiasis)	1087
	Loa loa	Filariasis, African eye worm, loiasis	1087
	Dipetalonema perstans	Filariasis (persistent), dipetalonemiasis	1087
	Mansonella ozzardi	Filariasis (Ozzard's), mansonelliasis	1101
	Cysticercus cellulosae	Cysticercosis (bladderworm)	1081
Respiratory			
Protozoa	*Entamoeba histolytica*	Amebiasis (extraintestinal) amebic abscess (lung)	1025–1032
	Pneumocystis carinii (a protozoan ?)	Pneumocystic pneumonia	1051

(Table 19–9 continues on the following page.)

Table 19–9. ARRANGEMENT OF PARASITES BY THE HUMAN ORGAN SYSTEM INVOLVED (*Continued*)

ORGAN SYSTEM	ORGANISM	DISEASE	REFERENCE PAGE(S)
Helminths	*Ascaris lumbricoides* (larvae)	*Ascaris* pneumonitis	1062–1063
	Toxocara sp. (larvae)	Visceral larva migrans (VLM)	1086
	Echinococcus sp. (larva)	Echinococcosis, hydatid disease (unilocular, alveolar or multilocular) in lung(s)	1081–1082
	Paragonimus westermani	Lung fluke (oriental), paragonimiasis	1080
Arthropods	Mites (various)	Acariasis (temporary) (asthmatic bronchitis)	1103–1104
Central Nervous System			
Protozoa	*Entamoeba histolytica*	Amebic abscess (brain)	1025–1032
	Hartmanella (Acanthamoeba) sp. and *Naegleria* sp.	Acanthamebiasis (amebic meningoencephalitis)	1034
	Toxoplasma gondii	Toxoplasmosis	1050–1051
	Plasmodium falciparum	Malaria (malignant tertian)	1040–1050
Helminths	*Cysticercus cellulosae*	Cysticercosis (brain)-(bladderworm)	1081
	Schistosoma japonicum	Ectopic schistosomiasis	1078–1080
	Schistosoma mansoni	Ectopic schistosomiasis	1078–1080
	Echinococcus sp. (larva)	Echinococcosis, hydatid disease (unilocular, alveolar or multilocular)	1081–1082
	Multiceps sp.	Coenurosis	1082
	Angiostrongylus cantonensis	Eosinophilic meningoencephalitis	1068
Genitourinary			
Protozoa	*Trichomonas vaginalis*	Trichomoniasis vaginalis	1036–1037
	Plasmodium falciparum	Malaria (blackwater fever)	1040–1050
Helminths	*Schistosoma haematobium*	Bilharziasis (urinary) or vesical schistosomiasis	1080–1081
	Dioctophyma renale	*Dioctophyma* infection	1080
	Echinococcus sp. (larva)	Echinococcosis, hydatid disease (kidney)-(unilocular alveolar or multilocular)	1081–1082
Liver			
Protozoa	*Entamoeba histolytica*	Amebic abscess, or amebic hepatitis	1025–1032
	Leishmania donovani	Leishmaniasis (visceral), Kala-azar	1037
Helminths	*Schistosoma japonicum*	Schistosomiasis, bilharziasis	1078–1080
	Schistosoma mansoni	Schistosomiasis, bilharziasis	1078–1080
	Echinococcus sp. (larva)	Echinococcosis, hydatid disease (unilocular, alveolar or multilocular)	1081–1082
	Capillaria hepatica	Capillariasis	1068
	Toxocara sp. (larvae)	Larva migrans (visceral) (VLM)	1085–1086
	Clonorchis sinensis	Chinese liver fluke	1077
	Fasciola hepatica	Sheep liver fluke, fascioliasis	1077–1078
	Ascaris lumbricoides	Ascariasis (adults in liver)	1062–1063
	Cysticercus cellulosae	Cysticercosis (bladderworm)	1081
Skin			
Protozoa	*Entamoeba histolytica*	*Amebiasis cutis*	1025–1032
	Leishmania tropica	Leishmaniasis (cutaneous), oriental sore	1037–1039
	Leishmania braziliense	Leishmaniasis (cutaneous–muco-cutaneous), American leishmaniasis, espundia, uta, chiclero's disease	1039
	Leishmania donovani	Leishmaniasis (visceral, may also be dermatologic)	1037
Helminths	*Necator americanus* (filariform larvae)	Ground itch	1069–1070
	Ancylostoma duodenale (filariform larvae)	Ground itch	1069–1070

(Table 19–9 continues on the following page.)

Table 19–9. ARRANGEMENT OF PARASITES BY THE HUMAN ORGAN SYSTEM INVOLVED (*Continued*)

ORGAN SYSTEM	ORGANISM	DISEASE	REFERENCE PAGE(S)
	Ancylostoma braziliense (filariform larvae)	Creeping eruption, cutaneous larva migrans (CLM)	1085–1086
	Onchocerca volvulus	Filariasis (blinding), onchocerciasis	1083–1084
	Loa loa	Filariasis (calabar swelling)	1087
	Dipetalonema perstans	Filariasis (calabar swelling)	–
	Acanthoceilonema streptocerca	Swellings(?), vesicular eruptions	–
	Dracunculus medinensis	Guinea worm infection, dracontiasis, dracunculosis	1084
	Spirometra sp. (sparganum larva)	Sparganosis	1082–1083
	Schistosoma sp. (human)	Urticaria	1078–1081
	Schistosoma sp. (avian)	Urticaria	–
Arthropods§	Scorpions	Venomous sting	1102
	Spiders		
	Latrodectus mactans (black widow spider)	Arachnidism	1102
	Loxosceles reclusus (brown recluse spider)	Necrotic arachnidism	1102–1103
	Ticks		
	Dermacentor, etc.	Tick paralysis, mechanical injury	
	Mites		1103
	Sarcoptes scabiei	Scabies, sarcoptic mange, dermatitis	
	Demodex folliculorum	Follicular mite	1103–1104
	Trombiculid mite (larva)	Chigger mite infestation, dermatitis	1104 1104
	Flies		
	(blood-sucking mosquitoes and flies)	Bite (painful), mosquito dermatitis	1106
	Flies, filth (many)	Myiasis	1106
	Lice		
	Pediculus humanus (varieties *corporis* and *capitis*)	Pediculosis (dermatitis)	1104–1105
	Phthirus pubis	Phthiriasis (pubic or crab louse)	1104–1105
	Fleas	Bite (painful) dermatitis, chigoe (tungiasis)	1105
	Bugs		
	Cimex lectularius	Dermatitis, bedbug bite (painful), psychosomatic reactions	1105
	Triatomid	Bite (painful), dermatitis	
	Wasps, bees and ants	Sting (painful), anaphylaxis in hypersensitized	–
	Caterpillars (urticating)	Blisters	–
	Beetles	Blisters	–
	Millipedes	Dermatitis	–
	Centipedes (some sp.)	Venomous bite, urticaria	–

*Nonpathogen: *Sarcocytis* sp. (a protozoan ?)

†Nonpathogens: *Trichomonas hominis; Enteromonas hominis; Embadomonas intestinalis; Chilomastix mesnili; Entamoeba coli; Entamoeba polecki; Endolimax nana; Iodamocha bütschlii.*

‡Miscellaneous tapeworms: *Hymenolepis diminuta* and *Dipylidium caninum*

§Many are mechanical (accidental) or biological (essential) vectors of parasitic, bacterial, rickettsial, and viral diseases.

TECHNICAL SECTION

In this section selected basic techniques employed in parasitologic studies will be presented. Some of the methods apply equally to the search for protozoa and the search for helminths. Other methods have been incorporated directly into the text, and many others may be found in the references. It is desirable to select those procedures that meet the needs of the individual laboratory (McQuay, 1966), but it should be emphasized that the parasitologic findings rest heavily upon the techniques selected and the skill with which the tests are performed. More cases of amebiasis, for example, will be diagnosed when purgation and cultures for amebae are employed (McQuay, 1967a). See Bodily *et al.*, 1970; CDC Laboratory Training Manual for Parasitology; Taylor and Baker, 1968; and Medical Protozoology and Helminthology (U.S. Naval Medical School), 1965, for additional procedures.

Feces

There are times when studies for eggs and parasites cannot be made (Table 19–10). It is suggested that stool examinations, including purgation, be done before admission to the hospital and particularly before medications of various types are administered.

Saline, Water, and Iodine Wet Mounts. Although macroscopic examination is efficacious for the recovery of such objects as nematode adults and tapeworm proglottids, the microscopic examination may reveal parasite objects and/or eggs. Saline wet mounts provide the examiner with preparations that are the best and easiest for the detection of the greatest variety of parasite objects. In them, trophozoites are frequently motile and cysts are alive and in their normal state. Certain helminth larvae may be motile and eggs may be demonstrated easily. In addition, abnormally seen objects such as erythrocytes, pus cells, macrophages, for example, may be detected in these wet mounts (Fig. 19–97). Search for parasite objects under low power and study them under high power magnification. Never use the oil immersion objective for wet mounts. Water mounts should be used only when the need arises to destroy *Blastocystis hominis,* which may be confused with amebic cysts.

Table 19–10. CONTRAINDICATIONS TO STOOL STUDIES FOR EGGS AND PARASITES

MATERIALS AND/OR DRUGS USED	REQUIRED INTERVAL (IN WEEKS) AFTER USE
Iron Bismuth Oil (castor or mineral) Particulate substances (Metamucil or others)	One
Barium Gallbladder dye Antibiotics Iodine preparations Antiamebic drugs Antimalarial drugs (certain)	Three

Iodine wet mounts provide the viewer with stained protozoan and helminth organisms in which additional morphologic characteristics may at times be seen.

IODINE SOLUTION (FOR PROTOZOA)

Potassium iodide (KI)	1.0 gm.
Iodine crystals	1.5 gm.
Distilled water	100.0 ml.

Store in a dark brown bottle.

TECHNIQUE

1. A random fleck of feces, with mucus or blood, if present, is obtained on the ends of two wooden applicator sticks.

2. Thoroughly comminute the sample initially in 1 drop of physiologic saline on a wide slide and emulsify some of the feces remaining on the sticks in a drop of iodine solution (for protozoa) on the same slide. The suspensions should be such that newspaper print is just legible through the préparation. For errors in preparation and diagnosis see Swartzwelder (1952).

Additional Wet Mount Procedures. Quensel's stain; Velat's stain (Velat *et al.,* 1950); and the Merthiolate-iodine-formaldehyde (M.I.F.) method (Sapero and Lawless, 1953; Blagg *et al.,* 1955) and Burrows (1967) phenol-alcohol-formalin (PAF) are useful. A dried, cellophane-covered smear for helminth eggs is the Kato thick-smear (Komiya and Kobayashi, 1966), which is reviewed by Faust, Beaver and Jung (1968, p. 401).

Sedimentation Procedure

For the sedimentation technique see pp. 1063, 1113.

Fixation Procedures

Schaudinn's Fixative. Fecal films must be fixed before permanent staining in Schaudinn's fixative, which is used primarily for the fixation of amebic and flagellate cysts in formed and semiformed stools. Schaudinn's working solution is unstable, so it must be made fresh daily. It contains 2.3 ml. of glacial acetic acid and 46.0 ml. of Schaudinn's stock solution (two parts saturated bichloride of mercury and one part of 95 per cent alcohol, kept in a dark brown bottle).

TECHNIQUE. On two narrow slides prepare fecal smears of moderate thickness with a sweeping stroke (Fig. 19–96). Remove any large particles and immerse immediately (slides must be back-to-back) in the fixative. The slides must remain in the fixative for at least 1 hour at room temperature, but overnight fixation is not harmful. Stain the slides with the phosphotungstic acid hematoxylin, or alternate method.

Polyvinyl Alcohol (PVA). This modified Schaudinn's fixative (Brooke and Goldman, 1949; Norman and Brooke, 1955) is designed for trophozoites in mushy and/or liquid stools. Permanent staining is required for microscopic

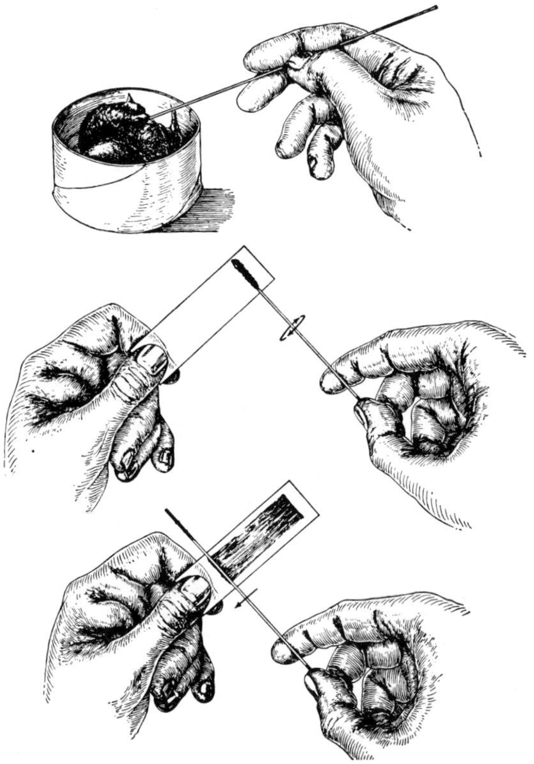

Figure 19–96. Preparation of fecal film for permanent staining. (From Markell, E. K., and Voge, M.: Medical Parasitology. 3rd ed.)

studies; therefore, direct wet mounts of the fixed specimen are unsatisfactory. A mixture of glacial acetic acid (5 ml.), glycerol (1.5 ml.) and Schaudinn's stock solution (93.5 ml.) are heated to 75° C. While mechanically stirring the mixture, slowly add 5 gm. of PVA powder. The solution should be clear and free of lumps before dispensing in 5-ml. amounts in screw-cap vials with a tight seal. Shelf-life is a few months or more. (The PVA powder and/or solution may be purchased from Delkote, Inc., Penns Grove, New Jersey. Specify Lot Rm-132 for use in the fixation of intestinal protozoa.)

TECHNIQUE

Microslide. A portion of mushy or liquid specimen is placed in the center of the slide and several drops of PVA solution added. After complete mixing, spread to make a smear of moderate thickness, dry these slides overnight in an incubator at 37° C., and stain with a permanent stain (the phosphotungstic acid hematoxylin below, or an alternate method). For better adhesion of the specimen to the slide, a thin film of stool known to be free of parasites may be placed on the slide prior to the addition of the specimen and the PVA solution.

Vials. Specimens placed in vials of PVA must be in 1:1 ratio, thoroughly emulsified, allowed to fix for 1 hr. or longer, spread and dried as for microslide preparations above. Sediment from positive ameba cultures may be fixed 1 hr. or more, centrifuged, and smears dried for future permanent staining.

Permanent Staining Procedures for Fecal Smears

Phosphotungstic Acid Hematoxylin Staining Method (Felsenfeld and Young, 1945). The phosphotungstic acid hematoxylin method is a good nuclear and yet a self-limiting stain (does not overstain and requires no decolorizing step).

PREPARATION OF THE STAIN. Dissolve 1 gm. of certified hematoxylin (for histologic staining) in 500 ml. boiling water. Dissolve 20 gm. phosphotungstic acid, C.P., in 200 ml. distilled water. Mix the cooled hematoxylin solution and the phosphotungstic acid solution by pouring into a brown storage bottle and then add 300 ml. distilled water. Add 100 ml. of freshly prepared 0.25 per cent aqueous solution of potassium permanganate, C.P. No ripening of the stain is necessary.

TECHNIQUE. Transfer slides (see fixation procedures for slides, above) from Schaudinn's fixative directly to the iodine alcohol (step 1, below) to prevent drying of the slides, and place any PVA smears (dried overnight at 37° C.) into the iodine alcohol.

1. Iodine alcohol (port wine color), 15 minutes.
2. 70 per cent alcohol, 5 minutes.
3. 70 per cent alcohol, 5 minutes.
4. Phosphotungstic acid hematoxylin stain, 2 hours (to overnight).
5. Running tap water (gentle stream) until blue, 5 minutes.
6. 70 per cent alcohol, 5 minutes.
7. 70 per cent alcohol, 5 minutes.
8. 95 per cent alcohol, 5 minutes.
9. 95 per cent alcohol, 5 minutes.
10. Absolute alcohol, 5 minutes.
11. Absolute alcohol, 5 minutes.
12. Xylol (water-free), 5 minutes.
13. Xylol (water-free), 5 minutes.
14. Mount with Permount or similar medium. (Do not permit slides to dry before mounting.) Remove any large particles which would interfere with the desired flatter mounting before adding Permount and No. 1 thin coverglass.
15. Begin examination of smear under oil immersion when Permount is "set," but to avoid lens contamination with Permount refrain from viewing marginal areas of the mount.

Iron Hematoxylin Stain (Heidenhain's) for Intestinal Protozoa

PREPARATION OF THE IRON HEMATOXYLIN STAIN

Hematoxylin crystals (Grubler)	1.0 gm.
Alcohol, 90 per cent	10.0 ml.
Distilled water	90.0 ml.

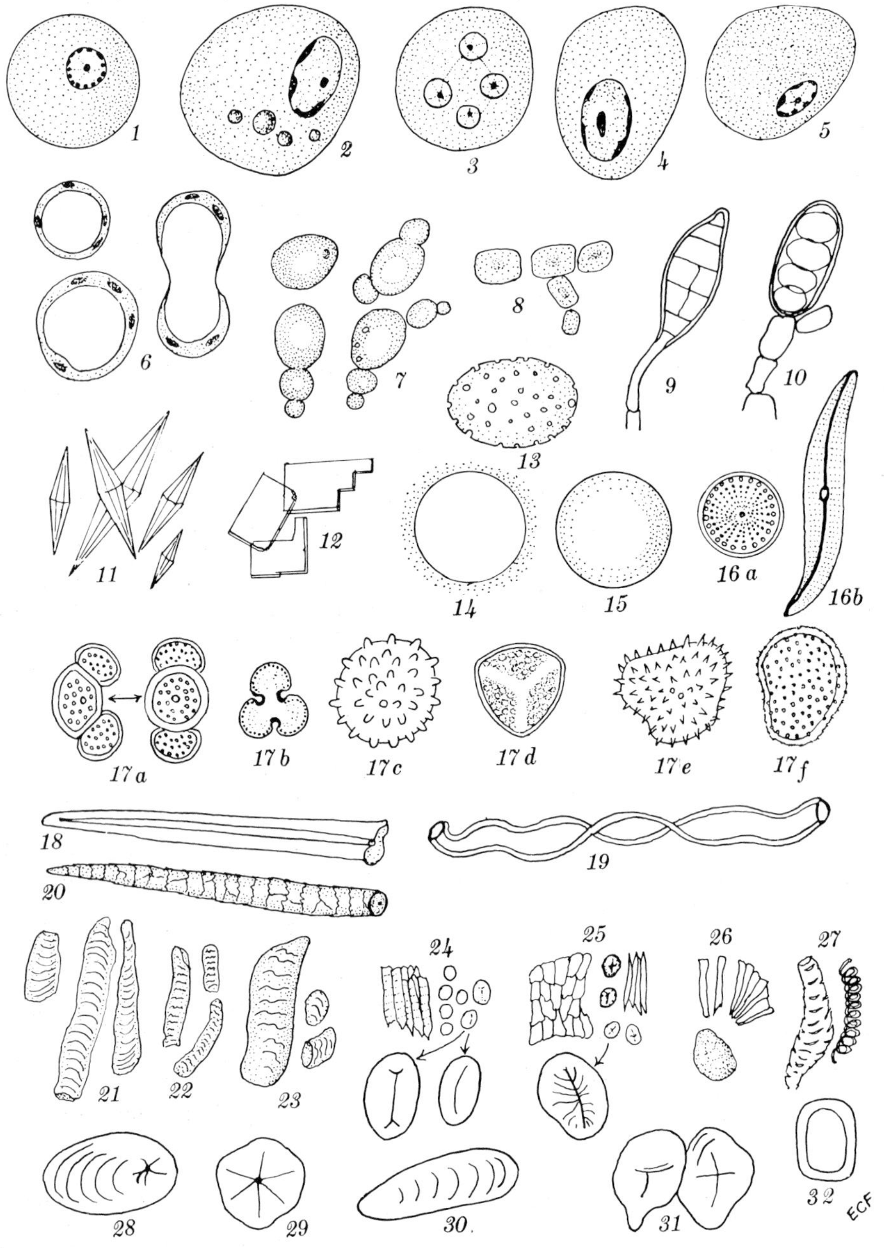

Figure 19–97.

1. Precyst of *Entamoeba histolytica,* for comparison with cellular exudate;
2. macrophage;
3. neutrophilic polymorphonuclear leukocyte;
4. squamous epithelial cell from aspirate of the rectum;
5. plasma cell from aspirate of the rectum;
6. *Blastocystis;*
7. yeast cells;
8. units from septate mycelium of *Monilia;*

9, 10. conidia respectively of the fungi *Alternaria* and *Helminthosporium;*

11. Charcot-Leyden crystals;
12. cholesterol crystals;
13. partly digested particle of casein;
14. air bubble;
15. oil droplet;

16*a*, 16*b*. diatoms;

17. pollen grains (*a*, pine; *b*, African violet; *c*, hibiscus; *d*, broom sage; *e*, ragweed; *f*, timothy grass);

(*Legend continues on the opposite page.*)

Dissolve the hematoxylin crystals in the alcohol using gentle heat and add the distilled water. Put the solution in a tightly stoppered flask and allow to ripen, preferably in the sun, for 10 days. Add 100 ml. of distilled water and the stain is ready for use.

MORDANT

Iron alum (violet crystals)	2.0 gm.
Distilled water	50.0 ml.

TECHNIQUE

1. Prepare smears of fecal sample and fix in Schaudinn's fixative.
2. Pass smears through 70 per cent alcohol, through 70 per cent alcohol containing enough iodine to produce a port wine color, and then through 70, 50, and 30 per cent alcohol, leaving in each for 5 minutes.
3. Place in distilled water for 10 minutes.
4. Place in mordant for 6 hours.
5. Rinse quickly with distilled water.
6. Place in staining solution for at least 6 hours or overnight.
7. Wash thoroughly with distilled water.
8. Place smears in a 1 per cent iron alum solution. This decolorizes the smear and should be continued until the nuclear detail of the amebae can be seen. This must be checked periodically by washing the slide with distilled water and checking under the microscope. Known positive slides must be run as controls to determine endpoint of decolorizing.
9. Wash smears in gently running water.
10. Dehydrate by placing smear in 70, 80, 95 per cent, and absolute alcohol, leaving in each for 5 minutes.
11. Clear in xylol and mount in Permount or similar medium.

This technique is time consuming and requires experience and skill but produces excellent permanent stains. All studies must be with oil immersion objective.

Alternate Permanent Staining Methods

Gomori's trichrome stain (Gomori, 1950) and Kohn's one-step method (Gleason and Healy, 1965) are alternate methods.

Concentration Techniques

Formalin-Ether Sedimentation (Ritchie, 1948)

TECHNIQUE

1. Feces about the size of a walnut is introduced into 12 ml. saline (or tap water). This sample may be placed in the refrigerator overnight if the test cannot be completed the day it is begun.
2. Strain about 10 ml. of the emulsion through four layers of wet gauze into a 15-ml. pointed centrifuge tube.
3. Centrifuge at 1500 to 2000 r.p.m. for 2 minutes. Decant supernatant.
4. Resuspend the sediment in fresh saline (or tap water). Centrifuge and decant as in step 3.
5. Add about 10 ml. of 10 per cent formalin to the sediment, mix thoroughly, and allow to stand 5 minutes.
6. Add 3 ml. of ether, close with a rubber stopper, and shake vigorously. Remove stopper.
7. Centrifuge at 1500 r.p.m. for 2 minutes. Four layers should result as follows: a small amount of sediment, a layer of formalin, a plug of fecal debris, and a layer of ether.
8. Free the plug of debris by ringing with an applicator stick, and carefully decant the top three layers. Remove the excess fecal debris by swabbing the inside of the tube with a cotton-tipped applicator.
9. Mix the sediment with a small amount of saline to prevent drying.
10. Examine as wet mount. Dilute as desired.

Zinc Sulfate Flotation (Faust et al., 1938; Faust, Beaver and Jung, 1968). This method depends upon the differences in specific gravity between the cysts and eggs on the one hand and the fecal debris on the other. If a zinc sulfate solution with a specific gravity of 1.18 is used, the cysts and eggs float while most of the debris sinks to the bottom. Trophozoites of the protozoa are destroyed and some of the cysts become distorted. The method is not satisfactory for most operculated helminth eggs. The zinc sulfate solution is made by dissolving 400 gm. of $ZnSO_4$ in 1000 ml. of water. Check the specific gravity with a hydrometer and adjust if necessary.

TECHNIQUE

1. Emulsify a pecan-size sample of feces in 10 ml. of distilled water in a test tube.
2. Filter the suspension through four layers of wet gauze to remove the large particles.
3. Centrifuge for approximately 2 minutes at 1800 r.p.m. and pour off the supernatant by inverting the test tube quickly.

Figure 19–97. *(Continued)*
18. plant hair;
19. fragment of cotton fiber;
20. mammalian hair;
21–32. food remnants (*21*, beef or pork muscle; *22*, crab meat; *23*, fish; *24*, wheat grain; *25*, corn kernel; *26*, string beans; *27*, conducting tubules of fibrovascular bundle; *28*, Irish potato starch grain; *29*, rice starch; *30*, plantain starch; *31*, sweet potato starch; *32*, woody cell wall). *1–12*, × 1125; *16a*, × 700; *16b*, × 200; *17–20*, × ca. 300; *21–27*, × ca. 240; *28–31*, × ca. 750; *32*, × 200. (From Faust, E. C., *et al.*: Animal Agents and Vectors of Human Disease. 3rd ed., Philadelphia, Lea & Febiger, 1968.)

4. Add approximately 2 ml. of water. Break up the sediment and fill the tube with water. Centrifuge and repeat these washings until the supernatant is fairly clear.

5. Add a small amount of the zinc sulfate and break up the sediment by tapping the tube. Fill the tube with zinc sulfate solution and centrifuge at 1800 r.p.m. (Do not disturb the film on the meniscus while transferring the tube from the centrifuge.)

6. With a wire loop (5 to 6 mm. in diameter) immediately, but carefully, remove a few loopfuls of a film to a microslide. Cover and examine. A second preparation may be put into iodine stain.

Alternate Concentration Methods

The acid-ether technique (Weller and Dammin, 1945), the acid-ether-xylol technique (Loughlin and Stoll, 1946), the Merthiolate-iodine-formaldehyde-concentration (M.I.F.C.) method (Blagg *et al.*, 1955) and the PAF sedimentation method (Burrows, 1967) are alternate methods.

Cultivation Techniques. The cultivation of protozoan parasites from the host's feces has been covered within this chapter (pp. 1027–1032). Cultures for *Strongyloides* and hookworm appear on p. 1067. Taylor and Baker, 1968, discuss *in vitro* cultivation of parasites in their book.

Blood

Thin and Thick Films. Thin film preparation is the same as outlined in the chapter on hematology. To demonstrate Schüffner's granules in *P. vivax* in thin film preparations, increase the staining time in freshly prepared Giemsa's stain from 40 minutes to 1½ to 3 hours. Thick film preparation for malaria and filariasis requires 1 to 3 small drops of blood to be spread (not stirred) quickly and evenly on a slide to about the size of a dime. Two thick films can be placed on one slide. Do not make them too thick or they will slough when dried. They must be thoroughly dried before laking and staining. To stain thick films, dip the dried films in methylene blue phosphate solution (see below) and rinse in two changes of distilled water. Place in freshly made Giemsa's for 8 to 10 minutes. Rinse in distilled water and air dry. In addition to fingertip blood, thin and thick smears for malarial studies may be made from the red cells directly below the buffy coat in centrifuged citrated or EDTA-treated blood. Microfilariae in thick films will be curled or coiled. Oil-immersion studies are necessary for malaria, but initial screening under low power is helpful in filariasis studies.

Alternate Staining Methods

An alternate method for malaria is Giemsa-Triton (X-100) (Melvin and Brooke, 1955). Alternates for filariasis are Bohmer's hematoxylin stain, hemalum stain, Delafield's hematoxylin method (Hunter *et al.*, 1966, p. 827), and a modified Papanicolaou smear by Harder and Watson (1964).

Concentration Techniques

Citrated Blood. The citrated blood method is useful for filariasis (buffy coat examination) and trypanosomiasis (plasma concentration) (Markell and Voge, 1971, p. 342). A saponin method for malaria has been described (Keffer, 1966).

Citrate-Saponin-Acid (CSA) for Filariasis. The CSA method (McQuay, 1970) is performed as follows:

REAGENTS

1. *Sodium Citrate Solution.** 2.0 per cent in 0.85 per cent saline solution.

2. *Saponin Solution.* 0.5 per cent in 0.85 per cent saline solution. (Saponin Powder Merck, purified B-0.6081). For convenience, place 0.25 gm. saponin powder into each of a desired number of 50-ml., plastic, graduated, conical tubes with screw caps (Falcon). Make fresh saponin as needed by adding 50 ml. of 0.85 per cent saline solution. Remove excess foam.

3. *Acetic Acid Solution.* 1.0 per cent.

4. *Methylene Blue Phosphate.* Methylene blue chloride 1 gm.; Na_2HPO_4 (anhydrous), 3 gm.; KH_2PO_4, 1 gm. Mix in a dry mortar; dissolve 1 gm. of mixture in 250 ml. distilled water.

5. *Giemsa Stain (aqueous).* Freshly made.

TECHNIQUE. The test is based upon the fact that many erythrocytes in a citrate-treated sample of blood are destroyed when subsequently treated with saponin, but the microfilariae remain actively motile and are easily demonstrated by concentration and in acid-treated permanently stained slides prepared from the sediment.

1. *Citrate Treatment.* Place 10 ml. of whole blood in a tube with 2 ml. freshly prepared sodium citrate.† Mix immediately and invert periodically to prevent clotting. Centrifuge for 10 min. at 1000 r.p.m. Aspirate and discard the plasma (top layer). Save packed erythrocytes and buffy coat for saponin treatment.

2. *Saponin Treatment.* Transfer all the packed cells (about 8 ml.) to 50 ml. freshly made saponin solution. Mix gently at intervals and let stand for 15 min. Centrifuge at 3500 r.p.m. for 10 min. Decant supernatant and discard. Spread several drops of the sediment collected over a small area of a narrow microslide and examine quickly under low power as

*EDTA (ethylene diaminetetraacetate) in purple-stoppered Vacutainer tubes may be substituted.

†Two EDTA Vacutainer tubes (purple-stoppered) may be substituted.

an uncovered wet mount. (The microfilariae will be actively motile.) Let slide air dry completely before permanent staining (below). (Microfilariae will be curved or coiled.) Examine rapidly the remaining sediment as wet mounts to detect the living organisms, but treat these preparations with acid *before* drying.

3. *Acid Treatment* ("Mini-Knott's"). To the several drops of sediment (wet mount) add two drops of 1 per cent acetic acid solution. Mix well with an applicator stick and spread over the slide surface. Allow slides to air dry. (Microfilariae will be killed and straightened.)

4. *Permanent Staining Treatment.* Dip the dried slides in methylene blue phosphate solution and rinse in two changes of distilled water. Place in Giemsa stain for 8 to 10 min. Rinse in distilled water and air dry. Screen dry slides for microfilariae under low power (16 mm.) with full lighting and study them under oil immersion.

Hemolyzed Blood. (Knott's method [1939], modified). The microfilariae are easier to demonstrate in preparations in which acetic acid (or formalin) is used and the red blood cells are hemolyzed. The microfilariae are concentrated in the sediment by centrifugation.

1. Obtain 1 to 2 ml. of blood and deliver it directly into a tube containing 10 ml. of 1 per cent acetic acid solution. Mix thoroughly to permit complete laking.
2. Centrifuge for 5 minutes at 1500 to 2000 r.p.m.
3. Decant supernatant.
4. Examine a small portion of the sediment as a wet mount.
5. Spread the remâinder of the sediment onto microslides to the approximate thickness of whole blood thick films (as for malaria) and allow them to dry thoroughly.
6. Stain with Giemsa stain, rinse in distilled water, and dry slides.
7. Screen the slides under low power with maximum lighting and turn to oil immersion when needed. (*Note:* The microfilariae will have been killed and straightened by the acid.)

REFERENCES

Adolph, P. E., Kagan, I. G., and McQuay, R. M.: Diagnosis and treatment of *Acanthocheilonema perstans* filariasis. Amer. J. Trop. Med. Hyg. *11*:76, 1962.

Alicata, J. E., and Jindrak, K.: Angiostrongylosis in the Pacific and Southeast Asia. Springfield, Illinois, Charles C Thomas, 1969.

Amebiasis: Laboratory Diagnosis. A Self-instructional Course. Washington, D.C., U.S. Department of Health, Education, and Welfare, Public Health Service Publ. No. 1187. Introd., Parts I, II, and III, Answer Booklets for Parts II and III, 1964.

Anisakis may infect man. Lab. Med. *1*(6):34, 1970.

Ash, J. E., and Spitz, S.: Pathology of Tropical Diseases: An Atlas. Philadelphia, W. B. Saunders Company, 1945.

Balamuth, W.: Improved egg yolk infusion for cultivation of *Entamoeba histolytica* and other intestinal protozoa. Amer. J. Clin. Path. *16*:380, 1946.

Beaver, P. C.: The standardization of fecal smears for estimating egg production and worm burden. J. Parasitol. *36*:451, 1950.

Belding, D. L.: Textbook of Parasitology. 3rd ed. New York, Appleton-Century-Crofts, Inc., 1965.

Blagg, W., Schloegel, E. L., Mansour, N. S., and Khalaf, G. L.: A new concentration technic for the demonstration of protozoa and helminth eggs in feces. Amer. J. Trop. Med. Hyg. *4*:23, 1955.

Bodily, H. L., *et al.*: Diagnostic Procedures for Bacterial, Mycotic and Parasitic Infections. 5th ed. New York, American Public Health Association, Inc., 1970.

Boeck, W. C., and Drbohlav, J.: The cultivation of *Entamoeba histolytica*. Amer. J. Hyg. 5:371, 1925.

Brooke, M. M., and Goldman, M.: Polyvinyl alcohol fixative as preservative and adhesive for protozoa in dysenteric stools and other liquid materials. J. Lab. Clin. Med. *34*: 1554, 1949.

Brooke, M. M., and Melvin, D. M.: Morphology of Diagnostic Stages of Intestinal Parasites of Man. Washington, D.C., U.S. Department of Health, Education, and Welfare, Publ. No. (HSM) 72-8116, 1969.

Brown, H. W.: Basic Clinical Parasitology. 3rd ed. New York, Meredith Corp., 1969.

Burrows, R. B.: *Endamoeba hartmanni.* Amer. J. Hyg. 65:172, 1957.

Burrows, R. B.: A new fixative and technic for the diagnosis of intestinal parasites. Amer. J. Clin. Path. *48*:342, 1967.

Burrows, R. B.: Other surface active agents for use with the PAF sedimentation technic for intestinal parasites. Amer. J. Clin. Path. *54*:155, 1969.

Burrows, R. B., Swerdlow, M. A., Frost, J. R., and Leeper, C. K.: Pathology of *Dientamoeba fragilis* infections of the appendix. Amer. J. Trop. Med. Hyg. 3:1033, 1954.

Cahill, K. M.: Tropical Diseases in Temperate Climates. Philadelphia, J. B. Lippincott Co., 1965.

Center for Disease Control (CDC): Laboratory Training Manual, Laboratory Diagnosis of Parasitic Disease. Microbiology Section, Laboratory Branch, U.S. Department of Health, Education, and Welfare, Public Health Service, Bureau of States Services, Atlanta,

Chatterjee, K. D.: Parasitology, Protozoology and Helminthology in Relation to Clinical Medicine. 7th ed., Calcutta, Sree Saraswaty Press, Ltd., 1969-70.

Chitwood, M. B., Valesquez, C., and Salazar, N. G.: *Capillaria philippinesis* sp. n. (Nematode: Trichinellidae) from the intestine of man in the Philippines. J. Parasitol. *54*:368-371, 1968.

Cleveland, L. R., and Collier, J.: Various improvements in the cultivation of *Entamoeba histolytica*. Amer. J. Hyg. *12*:606, 1930.

Couvreur, J., and Desmonts, G.: Toxoplasmose acquise et mononucleose infectieuse. Diagnostic différentiel et fréquence réspective. Nouvelle Rev. Franc. d'Hemat. *1*:345, 1961.

Culbertson, C. G., Ensminger, P. W., and Overton, W. M.: The isolation of additional strains of pathogenic *Hartmanella* species (*Acanthamoeba*): Proposed culture method for application to biological material. Amer. J. Clin. Path. *43*:383, 1965.

Dawes, B.: Advances in Parasitology. Vols. 1-8. New York, Academic Press, Inc., 1963-1970.

Dawson, J. B.: *Taenia in expulsis.* Lancet *1*:24, 1963.

Dillaha, C. J., Jansen, G. T., Honeycutt, W. M., and Hayden, C. R.: North American loxoscelism necrotic bite of the brown recluse spider. J.A.M.A. *188*:33, 1964.

Dubey, J. P., Miller, N. L., and Frenkel, J. K.: Characterization of the new form of *Toxoplasma gondii.* J. Parasit. *56*(3):447-456, 1970.

Edington, G. M., and Gilles, H. M.: Pathology in the Tropics. London, Edward Arnold Publishers, 1969.

Faust, E. C.: Human Helminthology. 3rd ed. Philadelphia, Lea & Febiger, 1949.

Faust, E. C., Beaver, P. C., and Jung, R. C.: Animal Agents and Vectors of Human Disease. 3rd ed. Philadelphia, Lea & Febiger, 1968.

Faust, E. C., D'Antoni, J. S., Odom, V., Miller, M. J., Peres, C., Sawitz, W., Thomen, L. F., Tobie, J., and Walker, J. H.: A critical study of clinical laboratory technics for the diagnosis of protozoan cysts and helminth eggs in feces. Amer. J. Trop. Med. *18*:169, 1938.

Faust, E. C., Russell, P. R., and Jung, R. C.: Craig and Faust's Clinical Parasitology. 8th ed. Philadelphia, Lea & Febiger, 1970.

Feldman, H. A.: The clinical manifestations and laboratory diagnosis of toxoplasmosis. Amer. J. Trop. Med. Hyg. 2:420, 1953.

Felsenfeld, O. F.: Significance of the small varieties of *Entamoeba histolytica*. Proc. Amer. Fed. Clin. Res. 2:58, 1945.

Felsenfeld, O. F.: Synopsis of Clinical Tropical Medicine: Pathogenesis, Clinical Picture, Diagnosis, Prognosis, and Therapy. St. Louis, The C. V. Mosby Co., 1965.

Felsenfeld, O. F., and Young, V. M.: An improved method for the examination of intestinal protozoa. Amer. J. Clin. Path. *9*:47, 1945.

Frenkel, J. K., Dubey, J. P., and Miller, N. L.: *Toxoplasma gondii:* Fecal forms separated from eggs of the nematode *Toxocara cati*. Science *164*:432–433, 1969.

Gleason, N. N., and Healy, G. R.: Modification and evaluation of Kohn's one-step staining technic for intestinal protozoa in feces or tissue. Amer. J. Clin. Path. *43*:494, 1965.

Goldman, M.: Cytochemical differentiation of *Entamoeba histolytica* and *Entamoeba coli* by means of fluorescent antibody. Amer. J. Hyg. *58*:319, 1953.

Goldman, M.: Staining *Toxoplasma gondii* with fluorescein labelled antibody. I. The reaction in smears of peritoneal exudate. J. Exper. Med. *105*:549, 1957a.

Goldman, M.: Staining *Toxoplasma gondii* with fluorescein labelled antibody. II. A new serologic test for antibodies to *Toxoplasma* based upon inhibition of specific staining. J. Exper. Med. *105*:557, 1957b.

Gomori, G.: A rapid one-step trichrome stain. Amer. J. Clin. Path. *20*:661, 1950.

Gould, S. E.: Trichinosis in Man and Animals. Springfield, Ill., Charles C Thomas, 1970.

Gould, S. E.: The story of trichinosis. Amer. J. Clin. Path. *55*:2–11, 1971.

Graham, C. F.: A device for the diagnosis of *Enterobius* infection. Amer. J. Trop. Med. *21*:159, 1941.

Harder, H. I., and Watson, D.: Human filariasis; identification of species on the basis of staining and other morphologic characteristics of microfilariae. Amer. J. Clin. Path. *42*:333, 1964.

Haydon, J. R., and Caplan, R. M.: Epidemic scabies. Arch. Derm. *103*:168–173, 1971.

Herms, W. B., and James, M. T.: Medical Entomology. 6th ed. New York, The Macmillan Co., 1969.

Hernandez-Morales, F., and Maldonado, J. F.: The diagnosis of schistosomiasis mansoni by a rectal biopsy technic. Amer. J. Trop. Med. *26*:811, 1946.

Hoare, C. A., and Wallace, F. G.: Developmental stages of trypanosomatid flagellates: A new terminology. (Correspondence.) Nature (London) *212*:1385–1386, 1966.

Hoskins, L. C., *et al.*: Clinical giardiasis and intestinal malabsorption. Gastroenterology *53*:265, 1967.

Hsieh, H. C.: Employment of a Test-tube Filter-paper Method for *Ancylostoma duodenale, Necator americanus* and *Strongyloides stercoralis*. WHO Mimeogr. Rept., 5 pp., 1961.

Hunter, G. W., Frye, W. W., and Swartzwelder, J. C.: Manual of Tropical Medicine. 4th ed. Philadelphia, W. B. Saunders Company, 1966.

Hutchison, W. M., Dunachie, J. F., Siim, J. C., and Work, K.: Coccidian-like nature of *Toxoplasma gondii*. Brit. Med. J. *1*:142–144, 1970.

Jeffrey, H. C., and Leach, R. M.: Atlas of Medical Helminthology and Protozoology. Baltimore, The Williams & Wilkins Co., 1966.

Keffer, J. H.: Malaria concentration method, comments on technique using saponin. Amer. J. Clin. Path. *46*:155–157, 1966, (Reprinted from Tech. Bull. Registry Med. Technol. *36*(6), 1966.)

Knott, J. I.: A method for making microfilarial surveys on day blood. Trans. Roy. Soc. Trop. Med. Hyg. *33*:191, 1939.

Komiya, Y., and Kobayashi, A.: Evaluation of Kato's thick smear technic with a cellophane cover for helminth eggs in feces. Jap. J. Med. Sci. Biol. *19*:59, 1966.

Kubasta, M.: Fresh tissue examination of liver biopsy specimens in *Schistosoma mansoni* infections. Amer. J. Clin. Path. *44*:283, 1965.

Kupferberg, A. B.: *Trichomonas vaginalis*: Nutritional requirements and diagnostic procedures. Int. Rec. Med. Gen. Prac. Clin. *168*:707, 1955.

Kurtin, S. B., and Leider, M.: Norwegian scabies – Report and lessons of a case. New Eng. J. Med. *278*:1099–1100, 1968.

Larsh, J. E.: Outline of Medical Parasitology. New York, Blakiston Division, McGraw-Hill Book Company, 1964.

Loughlin, E. H., and Stoll, N. R.: An efficient concentration method (AEX), for detecting helminth ova in feces. Amer. J. Trop. Med. *26*:517, 1946.

Manson-Bahr, P. H.: Manson's Tropical Diseases. 16th ed. Baltimore, The Williams & Wilkins Co., 1966.

Marcial-Rojas, R. A.: Pathology of Protozoal and Helminthic Diseases. Baltimore, The Williams & Wilkins Co., 1971.

Markell, E. K., and Voge, M.: Medical Parasitology. 3rd ed. Philadelphia, W. B. Saunders Company, 1971.

McMullen, D. B., and Beaver, P. C.: Studies on schistosome dermatitis; life cycles of three dermatitis-producing schistosomes from birds and discussion of subfamily Bilharziellinae (Trematoda; Schistosomatidae). Amer. J. Hyg. *42*:130, 1945.

McQuay, R. M.: Charcoal medium for growth and maintenance of large and small races of *Entamoeba histolytica*. Amer. J. Clin. Path. *26*:1137, 1956.

McQuay, R. M.: Good parasitologic examinations depend on proper procedures. Hosp. Topics *44*:85, 1966.

McQuay, R. M.: Parasitologic studies in a group of furloughed missionaries. I. Intestinal protozoa. Amer. J. Trop. Med. Hyg. *16*:154, 1967a.

McQuay, R. M.: Parasitologic studies in a group of furloughed missionaries. II. Helminth findings. Amer. J. Trop. Med. Hyg. *16*:161, 1967b.

McQuay, R. M.: Citrate-saponin-acid method for the recovery of microfilariae from blood. Amer. J. Clin. Path. *54*: 743, 1969.

McQuay, R. M., Silberman, S., Mudrik, P., and Keith, L. E.: Congenital malaria in Chicago. A case report and a review of published reports (U.S.A.). Amer. J. Trop. Med. *16*:258, 1967.

McQuay, R. M., Veiga, S., and Frumovitz, W. A.: Sparganosis in a Chicago resident originally from Arkansas: A case report. Amer. J. Clin. Path. *46*:645, 1966.

Medical Entomology, U.S. Naval Medical School, National Naval Medical Center, Bethesda, Maryland, 1967.

Medical Protozoology and Helminthology, U.S. Naval Medical School, National Naval Medical Center, Bethesda, Maryland, 1965.

Melvin, D. M., and Brooke, M. M.: Trition X-100 in Giemsa staining of blood parasites. Stain Tech. *30*:269, 1955.

Melvin, D. M., and Brooke, M. M.: Laboratory Procedures for the Diagnosis of Intestinal Parasites. Washington, D.C., U.S. Department of Health, Education and Welfare, Public Health Service Publ. No. 1969, 1969.

Moore, G. T., Cross, W. M., McGuire, D., Mollohan, C. S., Gleason, N. N., Healy, G. R., and Newton, L. H.: Epidemic giardiasis at a ski resort. New Engl. J. Med. *281*(8):402–407, 1969.

Morbidity and Mortality, Giardiasis in travelers. Weekly Report, Center for Disease Control *19*(47):455–459, 1970.

Mostofi, F. K.: Bilharziasis. New York, Springer-Verlag, Inc., 1967.

Nice, P. O., O'Connell, J. A., and Sykes, C. A.: Medical Parasitology: A Basic Systems Program. New York, Appleton-Century-Crofts, Inc., 1963.

Norman, L., and Brooke, M. M.: The effectiveness of the PVA-fixative technic in revealing intestinal amebae in diagnostic cultures. Amer. J. Trop. Hyg. *4*:479, 1955.

Norman, L., and Donaldson, A. W.: Spores of helicosporous

fungi resembling microfilariae in blood films. Amer. J. Trop. Med. Hyg. *4*(5):889–891, 1955.

Ottolina, C.: The rectoscopic biopsy by transparency. A new diagnostic method for *Schistosoma mansoni*. Amer. J. Trop. Med. 27:603, 1947.

Packchanian, A.: Infectivity of the Texas strain of *Trypanosoma cruzi* to man. Amer. J. Trop. Med. 23:309, 1943.

Patras, D., and Andujar, J. J.: Meningoencephalitis due to *Hartmanella* (*Acanthamoeba*). Amer. J. Clin. Path. *46*:226, 1966.

Piggott, J., Hansbarger, E. A., and Neafie, R. C.: Human ascariasis. Amer. J. Clin. Path. *53*:223, 1970.

Ristic, M., Conroy, J. D., Siwe, S., *et al.*: *Babesia* species isolated from a woman with clinical babesiosis. Amer. J. Trop. Med. Hyg. *20*:14–22, 1971.

Ritchie, L. S.: An ether sedimentation technic for routine stool examination. Bull. U.S. Army Med. Dept. *8*:326, 1948.

Sapero, J. J., Hakansson, E. G., and Louttit, C. M.: Occurrence of two significantly distinct races of *Entamoeba histolytica*. Amer. J. Trop. Med. 22:191, 1942.

Sapero, J. J., and Lawless, D. K.: The MIF stain-preservative technique for the identification of intestinal protozoa. Amer. J. Trop. Med. Hyg. 2:613, 1953.

Shaffer, J. G., Shlaes, W. H., Steigmann, F., Connor, P., Stahl, A., and Schneider, H.: Small race *Entamoeba histolytica*. Gastroenterology *34*:981, 1958.

Shaffer, J. G., Shlaes, W. H., and Radke, R. R.: Amebiasis: A Biomedical Problem. Springfield, Ill., Charles C Thomas, 1965.

Sheffield, H. G., and Melton, M. L.: *Toxoplasma gondii*: Transmission through feces in the absence of *Toxocara cati* eggs. Science *164*:431–432, 1969.

Siim, J. C.: Clinical and Diagnostic Aspects of Human Acquired Toxoplasmosis: Human Toxoplasmosis. Copenhagen, Ejnar Munksgaard, 1960.

Sindermann, C. J.: Disease of marine animals transmissible to man. Lab. Med. *1*(1):50, 1970.

Spencer, F. M., and Monroe, L. S.: The Color Atlas of Intestinal Parasites. Springfield, Ill., Charles C Thomas, 1961.

Stoll, N. R.: An effective method of counting hookworm eggs in feces. Amer. J. Hyg. *3*:59, 1923.

Swartzwelder, J. C.: Symposium on parasitology. 1. Laboratory diagnosis of amebiasis. Amer. J. Clin. Path. 22:379, 1952.

Swartzwelder, J. C., Beaver, P. C., and Hood, M. W.: Sparganosis in southern United States. Amer. J. Trop. Med. Hyg. *13*:43, 1964.

Taylor, A. E. R., and Baker, J. R.: The Cultivation of Parasites *in Vitro*. Oxford, Blackwell Scientific Publications, 1968.

Velat, C. A., Weinstein, P. P., and Otto, G. F.: A stain for the rapid differentiation of the trophozoites of the intestinal amoeba in fresh, wet preparations. Amer. J. Trop. Med. *30*:43, 1950.

Walker, A. J.: Laboratory diagnosis of malaria. Amer. J. Clin. Path. 22:495, 1952.

Weiland, G., and Kühn, D.: Experimentelle *Toxoplasma*–Infektionen bei der Katze. II. Entwicklungsstadien des Parasiten im Darm. (Experimental *Toxoplasma* infection in cats. II. Developmental stages of the parasite of the gut.) Reprinted from Berl. Münch. Tierärtzl. Wschr. *83*(7): 12 pp., 1970.

Weinman, D., and Ristic, M.: Infectious Blood Diseases of Man and Animals. Vols. I, II. New York, Academic Press, Inc., 1968.

Weller, T. H., and Dammin, G. J.: An improved method of examination of feces for diagnosis of intestinal schistosomiasis. Amer. J. Clin. Path. *15*:496, 1945.

Whalen, G. E., *et al.*: Intestinal capillariasis: A new disease in man. Lancet *1*:13, 1969.

Wilmot, A. J.: Clinical Amebiasis. Philadelphia, F. A. Davis Co., 1962.

Wittner, M., and Tanowitz, H.: Paromomycin therapy of human cestodiasis with special reference to hymenolepiasis. Amer. J. Trop. Med. Hyg. *20*:433–435, 1971.

Zakon, S. J., and McQuay, R. M.: Norwegian scabies in a male mongoloid: Report of a case and a review of the literature. Int. J. Derm. *11*:8–15, 1972.

Chapter 20

MEDICAL MYCOLOGY

by MILTON GOLDIN, Ph.D.

Many clinical pathologists and medical technologists become discouraged in their attempts to study fungi because of the unfamiliar nomenclature, the confusing synonymy and multiplicity of microscopic structures, and the widely held idea that mycologic techniques are difficult and complex. In actuality, once a few names and basic concepts are mastered, the identification of pathogenic fungi can become simpler and more rapid than that of bacteria.

In this chapter descriptions of the most important fungi are necessarily brief because of the limitations of space. More detailed descriptions may be found by consulting the references.

Fungi are heterotropic, eukaryotic, chlorophyll-free, thallophyllic organisms. They reproduce by spores, which germinate into long filaments called *hyphae.* As the hyphae continue to grow and branch, they develop into a mat of growth called the *mycelium* (pl. *mycelia*). From the mycelium, spores are produced in characteristic arrangements. These spores, when dispersed to new substrates, germinate and form new growths.

Reproduction of the pathogenic fungi is essentially asexual. The simplest type of reproduction is that characteristic of the *yeasts,* i.e., budding. A true yeast is a fungus that is unicellular and reproduces by budding.

Spores formed by budding are called *blastospores.* In certain fungi, e.g., *Candida,* the budding spores may elongate, remain attached to the parent cell, and form short abortive mycelia, the *pseudomycelia* or *pseudohyphae.* In other fungi, different types of spores are found. They may be thick-walled, unicellular, resting spores, the *chlamydospores,* or those produced by rectangular segmentation of the mycelium, the *arthrospores.* Those formed at the end of a specialized hypha, the *conidiophore,* are known as *conidia.* The conidia vary greatly in size and shape, and these differences help to identify many species (Fig. 20–1). Small conidia are known as *microconidia* and large, multicellular ones as *macroconidia* (micro- and macro-aleyrospores). Spindle-shaped macroconidia, such as those found in the genus *Microsporum,* are called *fuseaux* (Fig. 20–2).

Fungi are divided into four large classes:

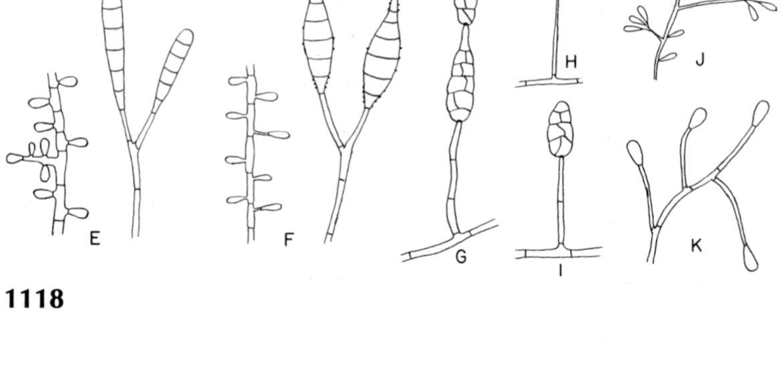

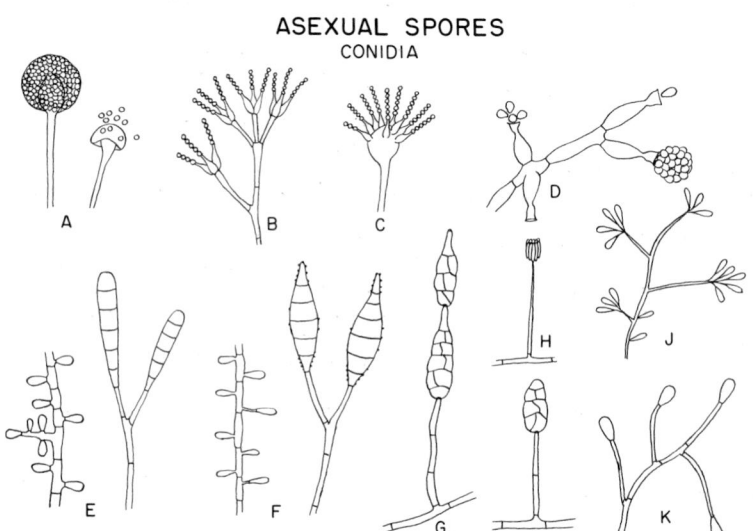

Figure 20–1. Various types of asexual spores (conidia). (From Conant, N. F., *et al.*: Manual of Clinical Mycology. 3rd ed.)

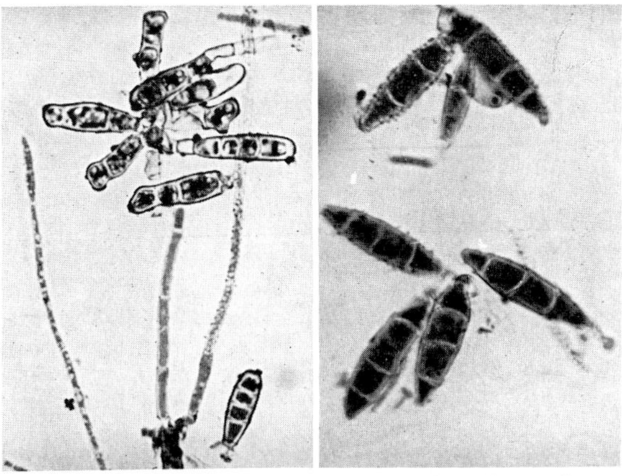

Figure 20–2. *Left,* blunt end fuseaux, *Epidermophyton floccosum.* Note the attachment to the mycelium. × 420. *Right,* pointed fuseaux, *Microsporum gypseum.* Mounted in Amann's lactophenol cotton blue solution; × 420. (From Burrows, W.: Textbook of Microbiology. 19th ed.)

Phycomycetes, Basidiomycetes, Ascomycetes, and Fungi Imperfecti (Deuteromyces). With few exceptions, all the pathogenic fungi belong to the latter class, which does not have a sexual stage. The demonstration of ascospores in some species of dermatophytes suggests that these fungi may belong to the class Ascomycetes. (See page 1130.)

Fungi associated with human disease can be divided into those affecting only the superficial keratinized layers of the skin—the *dermatophytes*; those capable of infecting the deeper tissues or organs within the body—the *deep* or *systemic* fungi; and those that are intermediate, i.e., capable of producing either superficial or deep infections (or both). Techniques of isolating and identifying these organisms depend on demonstrating them in tissue by direct examination and culturing them on media devised for that purpose (Table 20–1).

Table 20–1. SOURCE OF SPECIMENS AND MEDIA REQUIRED FOR DEMONSTRATION OF FUNGI FROM SPECIFIC TYPES OF INFECTIONS

DISEASE	TYPE OF SPECIMEN	ISOLATION MEDIUM
Superficial mycoses		
Tinea versicolor	Skin scrapings	None
Candidiasis (moniliasis)	Skin; vaginal discharge; mucocutaneous scrapings; etc.	Sabouraud's agar; E.M.B. (CO_2)
Onychomycosis (tinea unguium)	Nail scrapings	Cycloheximide agar; DTM
Tinea capitis	Plucked hair (preferably Wood's light positive)	Cycloheximide agar; DTM
Tinea corporis	Skin scrapings	Cycloheximide agar; DTM
Tinea pedis	Skin scrapings	Cycloheximide agar; DTM
Tinea cruris	Skin scrapings	Cycloheximide agar; DTM
Piedra	Hair	Sabouraud's agar
Trichomycosis axillaris	Hair	Ascitic fluid agar
Systemic mycoses		
Actinomycosis	Pus from draining sinus; sputum; aspirated fluid	Thioglycollate broth; infusion agar (anaerobic)
Blastomycosis, North or South American	Scrapings from edge of skin lesions; pus from abscesses; sputum	Brain-heart infusion blood agar plus antibiotics; cycloheximide agar
Candidiasis	Sputum; stools; urine; blood	Sabouraud's agar; E.M.B. (CO_2)
Chromomycosis	Scrapings from outgrowths; exudate	Cycloheximide agar, Sabhi
Coccidioidomycosis	Sputum; pus from draining sinuses; scrapings from skin lesions	Cycloheximide agar, Sabhi
Cryptococcosis	Spinal fluid; sputum; urine; pus from abscesses	Sabouraud's, brain-heart infusion agar (no antibiotics)
Geotrichosis	Sputum; bronchial washings; stools	Sabouraud's agar
Histoplasmosis	Blood, sternal marrow; sputum; skin scrapings; exudate from ulcers	Brain-heart infusion blood agar plus antibiotics; cycloheximide agar
Mycetoma	Pus from draining sinuses; biopsy specimens	Sabouraud's agar; brain-heart infusion agar; thioglycollate broth
Nocardiosis	Sputum; pus from abscesses; bronchial washings	Sabouraud's agar; infusion broth
Sporotrichosis	Pus from ulcers; aspirated fluid from abscesses	Cycloheximide, Sabouraud's agar
Aspergillosis, Mucormycosis, Phycomycosis	Sputum; bronchial washings; biopsy material	Sabouraud's agar

Success in identifying these organisms depends to a large extent on understanding the biology of the organisms and the nature of the disease in which they are involved. As in many other cases there must be a close association between the clinician and the laboratory as far as fungus diseases are concerned. The clinical impression should always be verified whenever possible by appropriate laboratory tests, a number of which are described in this chapter.

ACTINOMYCOSIS

The Actinomyces and Nocardia groups, strictly speaking, are not true fungi, since they are prokaryotic and belong to the class Schizomycetes, which includes the bacteria. However, they do differ in many respects from bacteria and may be thought of perhaps as transitional forms.

Actinomycosis in humans is caused by an obligate anaerobic organism known as *Actinomyces israelii (A. hominis)*. It can manifest itself in a variety of clinical conditions. Most commonly the cervicofacial area is involved, with swelling of the soft tissue of the face, neck, jaws, tongue, or other structures of this region and abscess formation and multiple draining sinuses. The thoracic form is found mostly in the lungs, with abscess cavitation resembling pulmonary tuberculosis. The organism may invade directly through the chest wall, forming numerous draining sinuses. Abdominal actinomycosis is a serious form, usually occurring by way of the cecum or appendix. A wide variety of symptoms may be produced, depending on the organ involved. Single or multiple sinuses may appear in the abdominal wall, and the infection may spread to the vertebral bodies.

In cattle, "lumpy jaw" is caused by *A. bovis*, which is morphologically similar to *A. israelii*. A facultative anaerobic microorganism which is a common nonpathogenic inhabitant of the human nasopharynx is known as *A. naeslundii. A. eriksonii (Bifidobacterium)* is an anaerobic species which is part of the indigenous oral flora. Anaerobic diphtheroid bacilli are sometimes confused with *A. israelii*. Thermophilic actinomycetes, growing between 40 and 56° C. have been associated with hypersensitivity pneumonitis and "farmer's lung." They have been isolated from the heating and humidification systems of homes and from decaying organic material. The important differential characteristics of these organisms are listed in Tables 20–2 and 20–3.

The disease occurs sporadically throughout the world. All races, both sexes, and all age groups may be affected. The organism is normally present around carious teeth, in dental plaques, and in tonsillar crypts. Trauma, dental defects, extractions, and other conditions which may set up anaerobic conditions predispose to invasion and infection. The infection may be transmitted from person to person by intimate contact, but this does not commonly occur. Animal actinomycosis is not transmissible to man.

Laboratory Diagnosis. Pus, material from draining sinuses, and sputum should be examined in the fresh state for the presence of "sulfur granules." These granules are lobulated masses composed of delicate, intertwined filaments about 1 micron in diameter, the ends of which are frequently surrounded by an eosinophilic sheath, giving a club-shaped appearance to the ends of the filaments. These club-shaped structures seem to be radiating from the center of the granule; hence, they have the name "ray" (actino-) fungus. Not all granules show these clubs, and similar granules may be seen in other conditions. The granules are gram positive and despite the name are usually not yellow in color but white (Fig. 20–3). In some cases the granules may not be present, but only short, branching, gram-positive filaments can be seen.

Culture. It is important to culture all material promptly, both aerobically and anaerobically, on suitable media. Material should be inoculated into Brewer's thioglycollate broth reinforced with 10 per cent horse meat infusion, and deep tubes of brain-heart infusion broth, streaked in duplicate on blood agar and brain-heart infusion agar plates, and incubated anaerobically.

In broth the organism grows as small, fuzzy, white colonies in four to six days at 37° C. On streaked plates the organisms appear as small (2 to 3 mm. in diameter) colonies that are white, rough or nodular, and adherent to the agar surface (Fig. 20–4). Smears show the colonies to consist of tangled masses of delicate branching hyphae and small, fragmented, diphtheroid-like, gram-positive rods (Fig. 20–5). No reliable immunologic test has been developed for this disease.

NOCARDIOSIS

Nocardiosis is a sporadic disease of man and animals that occurs in all parts of the world and is caused by several species of aerobic actinomycetes, most commonly *Nocardia asteroides*. It is usually a chronic suppurative granulomatous infection characterized by swelling, abscess formation, and multiple draining sinuses. A primary pulmo-

Table 20–2. MORPHOLOGIC CHARACTERISTICS OF *Actinomyces israelii, A. bovis, A. naeslundii,* AND ANAEROBIC DIPHTHEROIDS

MORPHOLOGY	*A. israelii*	*A. bovis*	*A. naeslundii*	ANAEROBIC DIPHTHEROIDS
Gross morphology on BHI agar with anaerobic incubation at 37° C. Colonies after 48 hours (× 100)	Colonies usually seen only microscopically as loose mass of long branching filaments on surface ("spider" colonies) and as small whitish granules with rough surface and fringed lace-like border. Smooth surfaced pinhead-size colonies with slightly fuzzy edges may occur ("S" forms)	Colonies usually pinhead in size, transparent; appear smooth, slightly convex with entire edge. Microscopically show a smooth but granular surface with a granular or denticulated edge. Some strains opaque and rough surfaced with irregular or fuzzy border. Rare strains microscopic in size, and appear as mycelial "spider" colonies.	Colonies similar to those of *A. bovis* or *A. israelii* "S" forms most common	Pinhead size, smooth, transparent glistening colonies with smooth edge
Colonies after 7 to 10 days	Raised, irregular to lobulated, with white glistening surfaces ("molar tooth" colonies). Tend to indent agar and are easily moved as a whole. Smooth-surfaced colonies, slightly convex with smooth edges, may occur in some "S" forms	Smooth, convex, cream to white, and shining, with entire border. Some strains show conical or irregular lumpy surface and scalloped borders. Rare strains produce typical "molar tooth" colony seen in "R" *A. israelii* strains	Colonies similar to those of *A. bovis* or *A. israelii* "S" forms most common	Smooth colonies which may show granular surface and entire, slightly granular edge
Growth in thioglycollate broth at 37° C.	Distinct colonies which are rough and lobulated or show fuzzy edges. Colonies do not break up when tube is shaken. Broth is clear. Smooth strains may appear more diffuse	Most strains produce a soft, diffuse growth. Others produce large lobulated breadcrumb colonies, which are easily broken up. Flaky or mucoid growth seen in some strains. Rare strains produce granular discrete colonies seen in "R" *A. israelii* strains	Rapid growth; usually more diffuse than *A. bovis.* Granular or floccose colonies may be present. Broth somewhat cloudy	Rapid growth; diffuse, and often pink colored. Tends to concentrate along side of tube. Colonies easily broken up. Broth cloudy
Microscopic morphology	Gram-positive rods and branched forms, 1 μ or less in diameter. Variations in diameter and clubbed ends are common. Long mycelial filaments occasionally seen. Nonbranching diphtheroid-like rods only may be formed by "S" forms	Gram-positive diphtheroid forms most common. Difficult to find branching. Some strains somewhat more filamentous. Rare "R" strains show long branching filaments	Similar to *A. bovis* or *A. israelii,* but more irregular forms. Gram-positive short mycelial forms with many branches. Some thick, very irregular forms, and few long mycelial elements, which vary in thickness. Some diphtheroid-like forms	Gram-positive bacillary or slightly branched organisms. X or Y shaped forms commonly occur

Table 20–3. PHYSIOLOGICAL CHARACTERISTICS OF *Actinomyces israelii, A. bovis, A. naeslundii,* AND ANAEROBIC DIPHTHEROIDS

	A. israelii	*A. bovis*	*A. naeslundii*	ANAEROBIC DIPHTHEROIDS
Maximum growth reached	3-7 days	2-3 days	1-2 days	3-4 days
O_2 requirements	Anaerobic (or microaerophilic) after first isolation	Anaerobic (or microaerophilic) after first isolation	Facultative, especially in presence of increased CO_2	Anaerobic or microaerophilic
Aerobic conditions	0 or 1+	0 or 1+	1+ to 2+	0 or 1+
Air + 10% CO_2 (candle jar)	0 or 1+	0 or 1+	4+	0 or 1+
Anaerobic conditions (N_2 + CO_2)	4+	4+	4+	4+
Catalase production	0	0	0	+
Starch hydrolysis	± or 0	4+	± or 0	0
Nitrate reduction	80% +	0	90% +	Usually +*
Indole formation	0	0	0	Usually +*
Gelatin liquefaction	0	0	0	+(may take 1-3 weeks)†
Litmus milk reactions	0 to 1+ acid. No coagulation. Slight reduction. No peptonization	0 to 1+ acid. No coagulation. Slight reduction. No peptonization	0 to 1+ acid with slight reduction, or acid and acid clot. No peptonization	Acid followed by peptonization (may take 1-3 weeks)†
Sugar fermentation (production of acid only)				
Glucose	+	+	+	+
Xylose	80% +	0	0	0
Mannitol	80% +	0	0	+
Raffinose	Variable	0	80% +	Variable
Starch	20% +	+	20% +	0
Glycerol	0	Occasionally +	0	+

*With *Corynebacterium (Proprionibacterium) acnes*, usually either nitrate or indole or both are produced.
†Several nonproteolytic species of anaerobic Corynebacteria have been reported, but these appear to be rare.

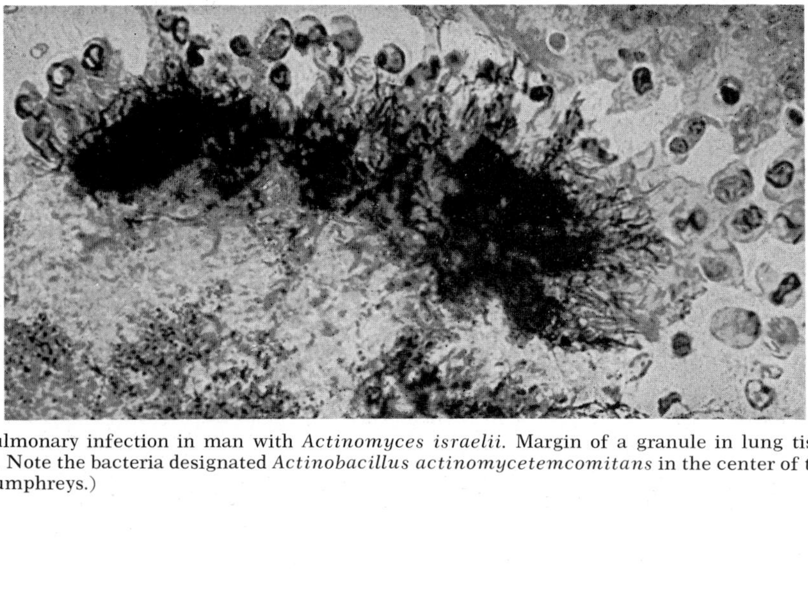

Figure 20–3. Pulmonary infection in man with *Actinomyces israelii.* Margin of a granule in lung tissue showing the ray-like structure. Note the bacteria designated *Actinobacillus actinomycetemcomitans* in the center of the granule. Gram stain; × 1000. (Humphreys.)

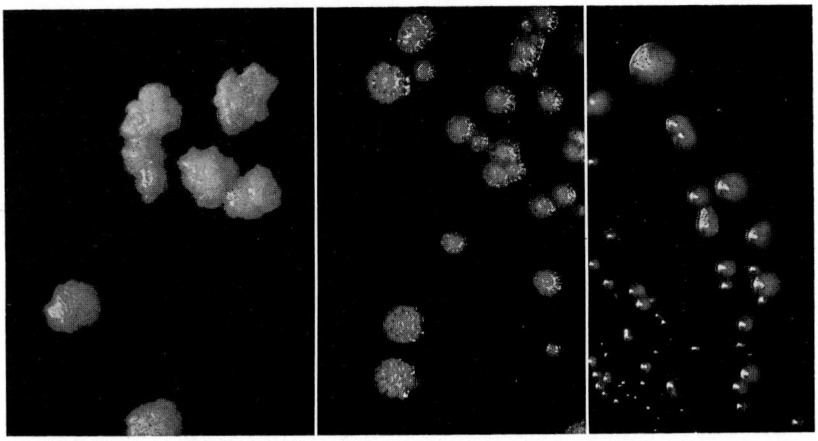

Figure 20–4. *Actinomyces israelii,* six-day growth on brain-heart infusion agar: *left* and *center,* rough type (× 3); right, smooth type (× 6). (Rosebury, Epps, and Clark.)

nary form also occurs, which occasionally may metastasize to other organs of the body. The pulmonary form may simulate tuberculosis clinically. The organisms are gram positive bacilliform filaments, and some strains are partially acid-fast and may be confused with *Mycobacterium tuberculosis* when seen on smears. The abdominal form may also be confused with tuberculosis. Since the treatment and control of these two diseases are entirely different, every effort must be made to differentiate the specific causative etiologic agent.

Infection of the subcutaneous tissue and bone (nocardial mycetoma) is more prevalent in tropical areas. The systemic form is world wide in distribution. In contradistinction to *Actinomyces israelii, Nocardia* is widely distributed in nature and infection is primarily exogenous in origin. The organism occurs in soil and may cause infection when introduced into tissues by injury or abrasions. Pulmonary infections presumably occur through inhalation of organisms suspended in dust. The differentiation between this organism and *Actinomyces* is summarized in Table 20–4.

Laboratory Diagnosis. Pus from a draining sinus or abscess should be examined for gram-positive, intertwining, branching filaments measuring approximately 1 micron in diameter or short, diphtheroid-like elements. Granules are rarely present except in mycetoma (see p. 1125). If present, they are not clubbed. When stained by the Ziehl-Neelsen method, some filaments appear to be acid fast. One per cent aqueous sulfuric acid should be used for decolorization rather than the 3 per cent HCl used for mycobacteria. Since this acid-fast property is only partial, the decolorization must not be prolonged (Fig. 20–6). The organism does not fluoresce when stained with auramine-rhodamine. (See page 941.)

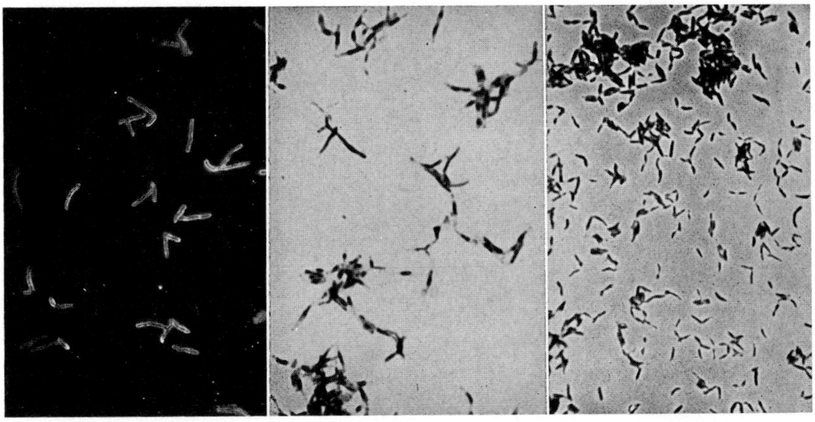

Figure 20–5. *Actinomyces israelii* from cultures. *Left,* darkfield. × 900. *Middle* and *right,* Gram stains of rough and smooth cultures respectively. × 1200. (Rosebury, Epps, and Clark.)

Table 20–4. DIFFERENTIATION BETWEEN ACTINOMYCES AND NOCARDIA

ACTINOMYCES	NOCARDIA
Obligate anaerobe	Aerobic
Not acid fast	Partially acid fast
Found only in human body	Found in many sources in nature (grasses, soil)
Infection primarily endogenous	Infection primarily exogenous
Sulfur granules commonly formed; clubs present	Sulfur granules not commonly produced; clubs absent
No growth on Sabouraud's agar	Grows well on Sabouraud's agar
Colonies not pigmented	Colonies frequently pigmented

Pus and sputum, when stained, show gram-positive or acid-fast filaments. The acid-fast varieties may be mistaken for tubercle bacilli in stained sputum smears. Since the pulmonary form of nocardiosis may clinically resemble tuberculosis, it is important to differentiate this organism culturally from *M. tuberculosis.* Since some strains of *Nocardia* cannot survive the acid or alkali concentration methods used for *M. tuberculosis,* it is essential to attempt to isolate these organisms before concentration is attempted. However, some strains survive digestion and grow on many of the routine culture media used for the isolation of *M. tuberculosis.* It is important not to mistake them for "atypical" mycobacteria, especially those in Runyon's group IV. (See page 1002.)

The organisms grow well on Sabouraud's or blood agar at 37° C. or at room temperature. Media containing antibiotics or cycloheximide should not be used. In contrast to *Actinomyces israelii, Nocardia* is aerobic. Colonies appear in four to eight days. They are raised, irregular, and usually wrinkled or granular and pigmented, ranging from light tan to orange to bright red in color. The pigment is best demonstrable on Czapek-Dox agar at room temperature. On fluid media, such as thioglycollate broth, the organisms grow in the form of a wrinkled surface pellicle, the media remaining clear. This is an important differential point between this organism and "atypical" tubercle bacilli.

Microscopically the colonies are composed of delicate, branching, intertwining filaments, which break up into bacillary forms of variable length. The organism is gram positive and may or may not be partially acid fast, depending on the species and the media in which it is grown. *Nocardia asteroides* is the most common species in the United States; *N. brasiliensis* is primarily involved in maduromycosis. No reliable diagnostic skin or serologic test is available for this disease at present.

MADUROMYCOSIS

Maduromycosis (madura foot, mycetoma) is a chronic, progressive infection affecting the

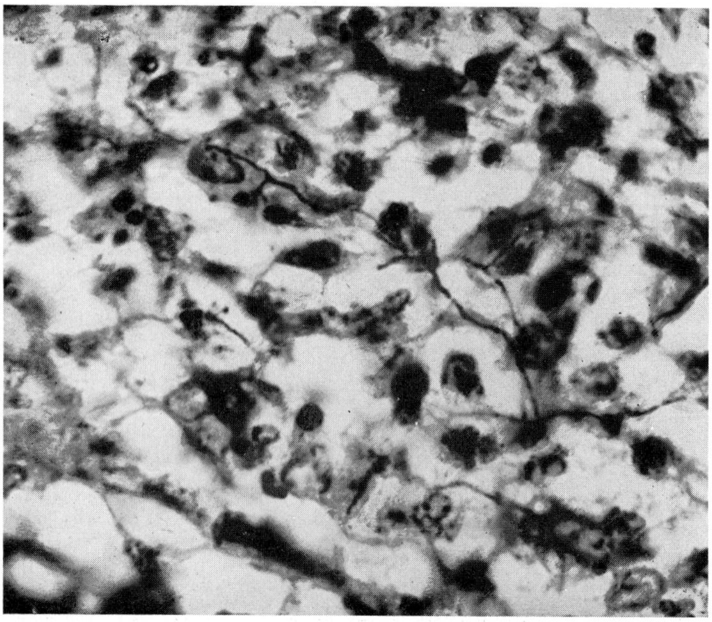

Figure 20–6. Nocardiosis. Delicate branching filaments in section of brain abscess stained by Gram's method. × 1300. (From Conant, N. F., *et al.:* Manual of Clinical Mycology. 3rd ed.)

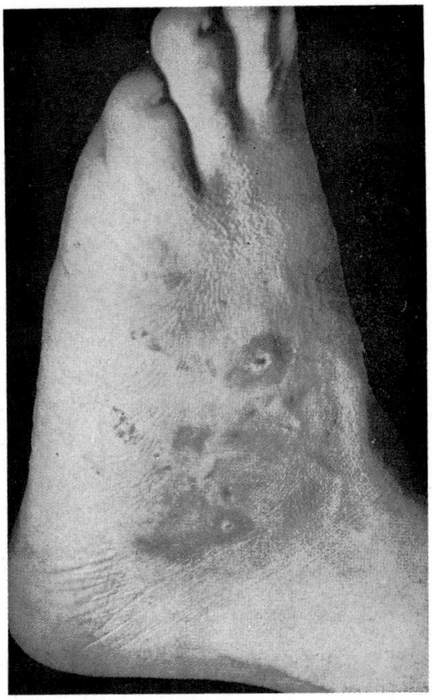

Figure 20–7. Maduromycosis of the foot caused by *Monosporium apiospermum.* Note the swelling of the foot and the multiple discharging sinuses. (From Conant, N. F., *et al.*: Manual of Clinical Mycology. 3rd ed.)

feet, hands, and rarely other parts of the body. It is characterized by severe tumefactions, abscess and sinus formation, and progressive enlargement and deformity of the infected area (Fig. 20–7). It occurs most commonly in the tropics and is exogenous in origin. Traumatic introduction of the etiologic agent from the environment is the most common source of infection.

The aerobic agents of actinomycotic mycetoma include *Streptomyces madurae, Str. pelletierii, Str. somaliensis, Nocardia brasiliensis*, and *N. caviae.*

The higher fungi include *Allescheria boydii* (Imperfect form–*Monosporum apiospermum), Cephalosporum falciforme, Madurella grisea, Madurella mycetomii, Phialophora jeanselmei,* and *Curvularia lunata.*

Diagnosis depends on direct examination of the granules from the pus, culture, and fungus stains such as periodic acid-Schiff (P.A.S.) or methenamine silver of biopsy material.

THE DERMATOPHYTES

Superficial infections of the skin caused by fungi (dermatophytosis, dermatomycosis) are exceedingly common; "athlete's foot" and ringworm of the scalp are particularly well known. Hypersensitivity to the fungi undoubtedly plays an important role in the pathogenesis of these diseases.

The fungi attack only the keratinized, dead layers of the skin, nails, and hair. A common lesion caused by these organisms is known as "ringworm" or tinea in which the lesion spreads in a circle about a healing, scaly, central portion. Clinically the dermatomycoses can be classified according to the area of the body involved. Tinea pedis, "athlete's foot," is a common infection producing a pruritic or vesicular maceration between the toes or on the plantar surfaces of the feet. Burning, itching, and pain may develop and pyogenic infections may be superimposed. Infections of the nails, tinea unguium or onycomycosis, may be caused by the same group of fungi as on the feet but may also be due to *Candida albicans.* These infections are difficult to diagnose clinically, since many other conditions can cause a similar picture. Ringworm of the scalp, tinea capitis, is frequently found in children and occasionally in adults. In this condition, the hair becomes brittle and breaks off a short distance from the surface of the scalp. Infection by *Microsporum canis* or *M. gypseum* can result in a boggy, tumor-like mass known as a kerion. *Trichophyton schoenleinii* causes a severe infection known as favus (tinea favosa), characterized by cuplike structures (scutula) formed by the infected hair follicles. Hairs infected by certain fungi may fluoresce when placed under a filtered ultraviolet light–the "Wood's" light (Table 20–5).

Infection of the bearded regions, tinea barbae, may resemble that due to pyogenic bacteria. Ringworm of the groin, tinea cruris ("jock itch"), is common in warm climates and in obese individuals. Ringworm of the body, tinea corporis, causes lesions that involve the glabrous skin anywhere on the body. The lesions advance slowly at the periphery and tend to heal in the center.

Table 20–5. WOOD'S LIGHT REACTIONS

SPECIES	FLUORESCENCE UNDER UV LIGHT	COLONIES UNDER UV LIGHT
Trichophyton rubrum	–	Light blue
T. mentagrophytes	–	Blue violet
T. verrucosum	–	Pink violet
T. tonsurans	–	Dark green
Microsporum audouini	+	Dull gray
M. canis	+	Bright blue and pink
M. gypseum	+/–	Dull brown
Epidermophyton floccosum	No hair infection	Dull olive

Miscellaneous Superficial Mycoses

Tinea versicolor (pityriasis versicolor) is a common disease of worldwide distribution characterized by diffuse brownish red scaly lesions on the chest and back. These lesions fluoresce under the Wood's light. The causative agent, previously known as *Malassezia furfur* appears to be identical with a lipophilic yeast-like organism called *Pityosporum orbiculare*. The laboratory diagnosis is readily made by mounting scrapings from the affected area of the skin in 10 per cent potassium hydroxide or by using the cellophane tape method (vide infra). The organisms are characteristically seen as thick-walled, round budding forms in clusters accompanied by fragments of mycelia (Fig. 20–8). Cultures are unnecessary in this condition.

Tinea nigra palmaris is a superficial infection of the epidermis that produces brown to black asymptomatic macules on the palms of the hands and occasionally on other parts of the body. It is reported most frequently in tropical areas. The causative agent is *Cladosporium werneckii*.

White piedra is a cosmopolitan disease characterized by the development of light colored, stony hard nodules along the hair shaft. The causative agent is *Trichosporon beigelii* or *Tr. cutaneum*. Black piedra is predominantly a tropical disease caused by *Piedraia hortai*. It causes dark nodules along the hair shaft.

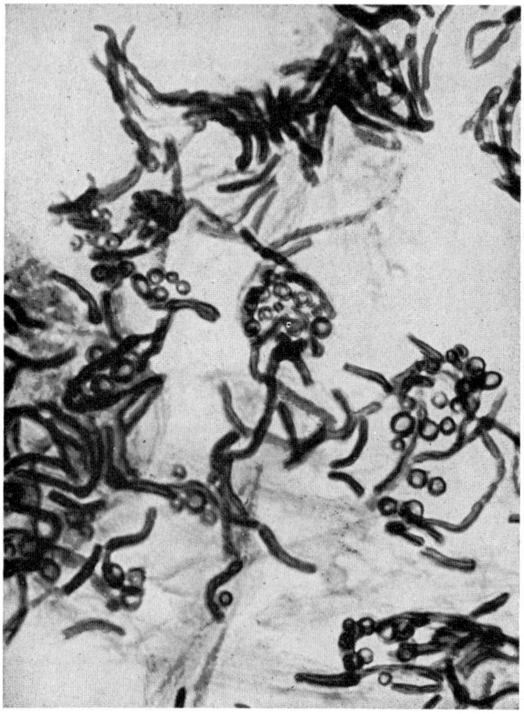

Figure 20–8. *Malassezia furfur*. Clusters of round budding cells and mycelial elements in skin. × 700. (From Conant, N. F., *et al.*: Manual of Clinical Mycology. 3rd ed.)

Otomycosis refers to fungus infection of the external ear, which is usually associated with a bacterial infection. Organisms involved include *Aspergillus niger, Absidia, Rhizopus,* and *Mucor*. Since these organisms are ubiquitous saprophytes, their etiologic relationship to this disease must be established by repeated examinations.

Mycotic keratitis is the term used for fungus infections of the cornea of the eye. A number of saprophytic fungi can secondarily invade the damaged cornea, most commonly *Aspergillus, Fusarium,* and *Cephalosporium*. Diagnosis is made by direct examination of scrapings from the ulcer and by culture.

Mycology of the Dermatophytes

Demonstration of the fungi in infected tissue can be accomplished readily. Hair, skin, or nail scrapings from infected areas are placed on a slide and a drop of 10 to 20 per cent potassium hydroxide added. Ten per cent tetramethyl ammonium hydroxide is excellent for this purpose. Dimethyl sulfoxide (40 per cent) added to a 20 per cent KOH solution permits quick examination without heating the preparation. A coverslip* is placed on top of the preparation, which is warmed gently and allowed to stand until clear. If the preparation is not to be examined until some time later, a solution of 5 per cent KOH and 25 per cent glycerol can be added under the coverslip. The preparation must not be allowed to dry out. When examined under the microscope with subdued light, fungi in skin or nails appear as refractile, branching fragments of hyphae (Fig. 20–9). In infected hair, in KOH preparations, the spores may be seen as dense clouds around the hair stub ("ectothrix") or as linear rows inside the hair shaft ("endothrix") (Fig. 20–10). Care must be taken to avoid confusing the so-called "mosaic" fungi or various artifacts with true fungi. The genus and species of the infecting fungi can be established only by culture.

A simple and practical method for demonstrating superficial fungi and bacteria from the skin is the vinyl tape method (Keddie *et al.*, 1961). Scotch tape (No. 681 or 800) is used to strip layers from the epidermis. The tape is mounted with the adhesive side toward the coverslip and stained by the P.A.S., Gram, or Giemsa method. Fungi and bacteria stain read-

*Plastic coverslips are superior to glass for this purpose.

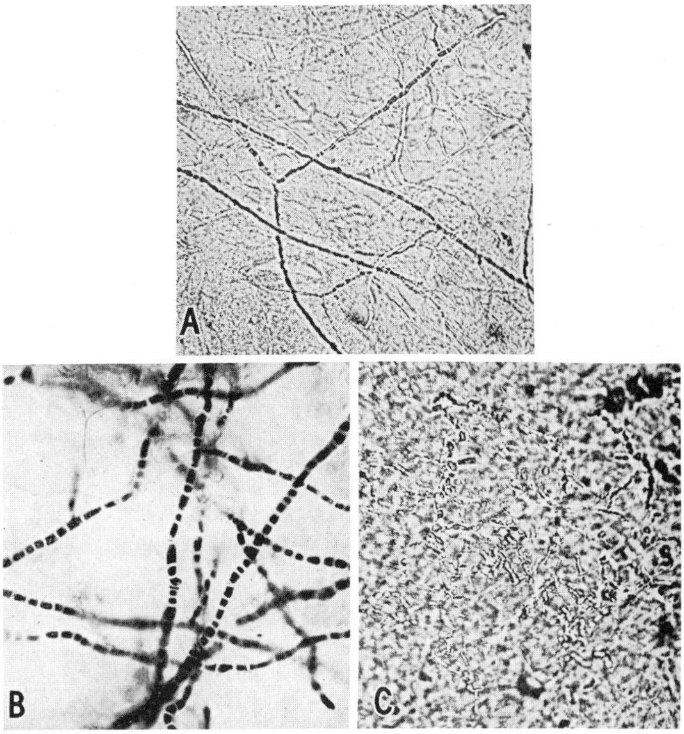

Figure 20–9. Infected skin. *A,* Branching hyphae that might yield in culture species of *Microsporum, Trichophyton,* or *Epidermophyton floccosum.* × 200. *B,* Typical close septate hyphae of *Trichophyton concentricum* in skin. × 450. *C,* Mosaic fungus, an artifact often seen in potassium hydroxide preparations of skin. × 200. (From Conant, N. F., *et al.*: Manual of Clinical Mycology. 3rd ed.)

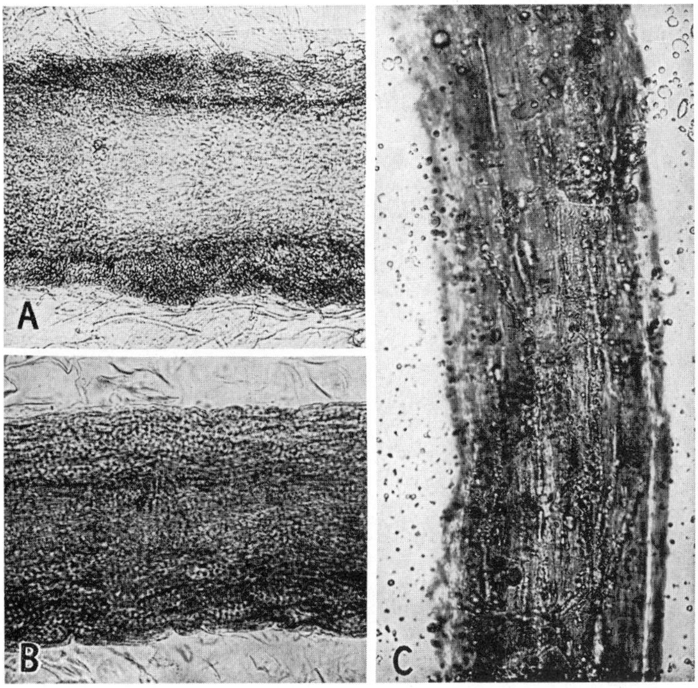

Figure 20–10. Infected hair. *A, Microsporum.* Small spores forming sheath around hair. × 110. *B, Trichophyton.* Parallel chains of arthrospores inside hair (endothrix). × 170. *C, Trichophyton.* Favus hair showing mycelial elements and numerous bubbles which are characteristic. × 220. (From Conant, N. F., *et al.*: Manual of Clinical Mycology. 3rd ed.)

ily with characteristic morphology. Portions of the tape can also be used for culture if desired. Acridine orange (A.O.) fluorescent staining is reported as useful for demonstrating fungi in fresh preparations and tissue sections (Chick, 1964). The material to be examined is placed on a slide with 2 to 3 drops of a solution made by adding 1 ml. of acridine orange 1:1000 to 9 ml. of 20 per cent potassium hydroxide. The preparation is carefully mixed, a coverslip added, and the preparation gently heated. It is then examined under the fluorescent microscope.

Cultures are made by inoculating various media, of which Sabouraud's, Littman's, or cycloheximide (Mycosel) agar is commonly used. Some laboratories prefer to use Emmons' modified Sabouraud agar (neopeptone, 10 gm.; dextrose, 20 gm.; agar, 20 gm.; pH 7.0). The addition of 10 mg. of thiamine per liter enhances the growth of some of the dermatophytes, particularly *Trichophyton verrucosum.* Yeast extract (0.5 per cent) added to Sabouraud's agar enhances growth and characteristic morphology. Ink blue agar (Wiegand, 1969) and Dermatophyte Test Medium* (DTM, Taplin *et al.,* 1969) are highly recommended for the original isolation of dermatophytes from clinical specimens. The marked change in color due to pH shift and the added antibiotics which suppress bacterial overgrowth make these media simple to use, particularly under suboptimal conditions. The latter medium has been used successfully in touch plates for culturing directly from the scalp lesions in tinea capitis. All the dermatophytes grow well at room temperature. They grow best at a pH of 6.8 to 7.0 but tolerate a wide range of pH levels.

Identification of the organisms is based on the gross appearance of the colonies, the rate of growth, pigment, nutritional patterns, and the microscopic appearance. These factors are markedly influenced by the composition of the medium in which the organism is grown. Three distinct types of colonies may develop—the yeast, the yeast-like, and the filamentous. Yeast colonies are smooth, moist, and soft. Under the microscope they contain only oval or round, budding cells. Yeast-like colonies are also soft and smooth but may be slightly granular. Under the microscope, pseudomycelia and budding cells are seen. Filamentous colonies show cotton-like growth projecting from the agar surface. The colonies show mycelia and various types of spore formation under the microscope (Fig. 20–11).

For examination of the colonies a straight or hooked wire is used to pick a fragment of the colony to a drop of Amann's lactophenol cotton blue* on a slide. The fragment is separated gently with teasing needles and a coverslip added. It is also possible to transfer growth from the colony to a slide with Scotch tape (No. 800), thus avoiding distortion of the fungus structures. Slight heating may help the stain to penetrate. The preparation is then examined for its characteristic microscopic appearance. Lactophenol cotton blue is also useful in examining scrapings from cases of erythrasma or tinea versicolor. If the skin scrapings are greasy or have a large amount of sebum, they should be washed with acetone or alcohol before the stain is added. Yeast-like colonies may be examined microscopically by suspending a loopful in a drop of water and covering with a coverslip.

Preparation of Permanent Lactophenol Cotton Blue Mounts for Fungi. Tease small portion of culture apart gently on a slide, add a drop of 95 per cent alcohol, and let dry. Add a small drop of lactophenol cotton blue and let it set for 3 minutes. Place clean coverslip on top and press gently to drive out air bubbles. Let dry for three weeks. Seal coverslip with a suitable agent (collodion or asphaltum). Such preparations remain usable for many years.

Cultural Characteristics of the Dermatophytes

The dermatophytes can be divided into those that are geophilic (soil inhabitants), i.e., *Microsporum gypseum;* zoophilic (primarily animal parasites), i.e., *M. canis;* and anthropophilic (primarily parasitic on man), i.e., *M. audouinii.* In general, infections caused by the geophilic and zoophilic species produce more severe reactions than do the anthropophilic.

Trichophyton species are the most common of the dermatophytes that cause infections of the skin, nails, and hair.

The fungus grows as cottony colonies, usually pigmented from light tan to red. The species are distinguished from each other by means of their colonial appearance, their predilection for particular tissues, nutritional requirements, the structure of the micro- and macroconidia, and the various shapes of the hyphae (Fig. 20–12). Common species are *T. mentagrophytes, T. rubrum, T. tonsurans, T. verrucosum, T. violaceum, T. schoenleinii, and T. megninii.*

Microsporum is primarily associated with

*Available commercially in prepared form.

*Phenol crystals, 20 gm.; glycerol, 40 ml.; lactic acid, 20 ml.; distilled water, 20 ml. Dissolve by heating gently. Add 0.05 gm. cotton blue (Poirrier's blue). Another excellent mounting fluid is Albert's (toluidine blue, 0.15 gm.; malachite green, 0.2 gm.; acetic acid, glacial, 1.0 ml.; 95 per cent alcohol, 2 ml.; and water, 110 ml.). This stock solution is diluted 1:2 with distilled water, and 10 per cent glycerol is added.

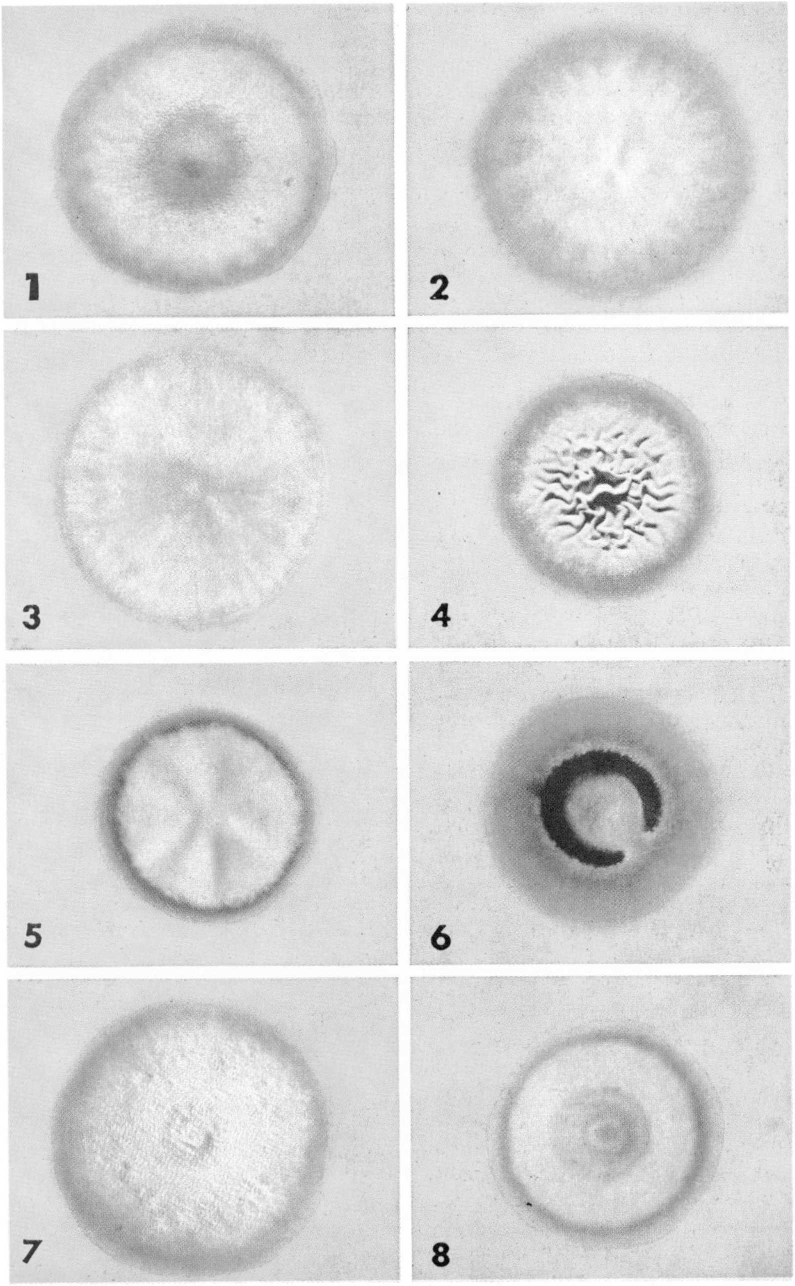

Figure 20–11. Colonies of some of the more common dermatophytes on Sabouraud's agar (× 3/4). *1, Microsporum audouinii. 2, Microsporum canis. 3, Microsporum gypseum. 4, Trichophyton schoenleinii. 5, Trichophyton rubrum. 6, Trichophyton violaceum. 7, Trichophyton mentagrophytes. 8, Epidermophyton floccosum.*

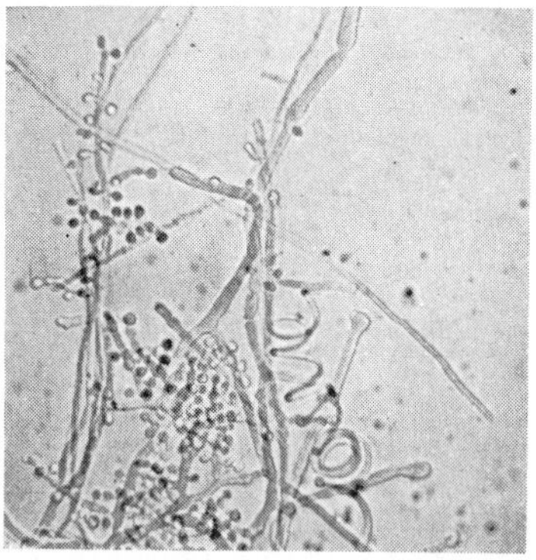

Figure 20–12. Culture of *Trichophyton mentagrophytes* (× 348). (From Lewis, G. M., and Hopper, M. E.: An Introduction to Medical Mycology. Year Book Medical Publishers, Inc., 1958.)

ectothrix infections of the hair and occasionally the skin. The colonies are slow growing, cottony to powdery, and light tan to brown in color. Under the microscope, the rough-walled, spindle-shaped macroconidia (fuseaux) are numerous and characteristic for *M. canis* and *M. gypseum*. *M. audouinii* grows slowly, giving rise to a light buff or orange velvety colony. Macroconidia are rarely seen on Sabouraud's agar. When present, they are thick walled and pleomorphic.

Epidermophyton is primarily associated with tinea cruris. Nails are rarely infected. It forms velvety to powdery, greenish yellow, round, rapidly growing colonies. Microscopically, oval or club-shaped multiseptate macroconidia are characteristic. There is only one species in this genus, *Epidermophyton floccosum (inguinale)* (Fig. 20–13; Tables 20–6 and 20–7).

Keratinomyces ajelloi is closely related to the genus *Trichophyton* and is able to infect skin and hair; it is essentially a soil inhabitant.

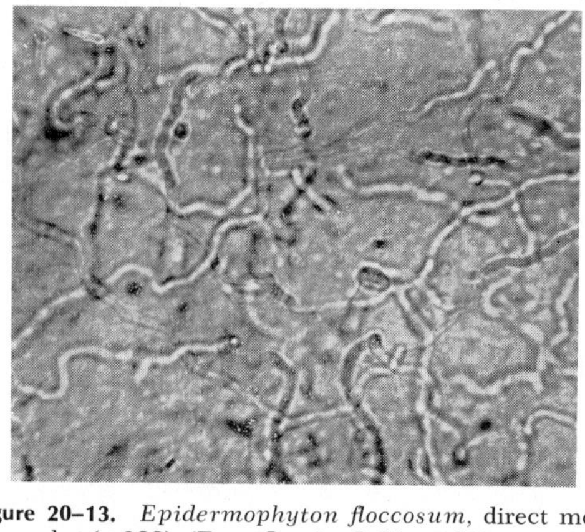

Figure 20–13. *Epidermophyton floccosum*, direct mount from scales (× 200). (From Lewis, G. M., and Hopper, M. E.: An Introduction to Medical Mycology. Year Book Medical Publishers, Inc., 1958.)

It produces characteristic smooth, cylindro-fusiform macroconidia.

The "perfect" or ascigerous forms of a number of dermatophytes have been discovered (Griffin, 1960; Stockdale, 1961). These forms are usually induced by growing the fungus on sterilized hair on the surface of sterilized, moist soil. Cleistothecia appear after two to eight weeks, developing asci which contain eight ascospores. Some of the dermatophytes that have been described are as follows:

IMPERFECT STATE	PERFECT STATE
Microsporum gypseum	*Nannizzia incurvata*
M. nanum	*N. obtusa*
M. cookei	*N. cajetani*
M. vanbreuseghemii	*N. grubyia*
Keratinomyces ajelloi	*Arthroderma uncinatum*
Trichophyton terrestre	*A. quadrifidium*
T. mentagrophytes	*A. benhamiae*

THE SUBCUTANEOUS AND SYSTEMIC FUNGI

Fungus diseases other than those infecting the skin and its appendages were at one time thought to be rare. It is now recognized, because of either improved diagnostic facilities or increasing incidence of infection, that many of these conditions are more widespread than heretofore realized. Also there is evidence that the more widespread use of antibiotics, steroids, cytotoxic drugs, and radiation predisposes to infection with these organisms.

It is important to realize that all the fungi to be described, with the exception of *Cryptococcus neoformans*, exist in two phases. In the body they are invariably in the form of yeast-like organisms; when cultured at room temperature, the organisms form mycelia and the colonies are usually cottony masses of entangled mycelia resembling those of the dermatophytes. When cultured on appropriate media at body temperature, the colonies are nonfilamentous and yeast-like. This is the so-called yeast-to-mycelia (Y→M) transformation. An understanding of this phenomenon is essential to those working with these organisms.

Techniques for Examining Specimens for Systemic Fungi

Examination of heat-fixed, stained films of pus are of little value in medical mycology. Preparations of material in 10 or 20 per cent potassium hydroxide, India ink, or lactophenol

Table 20–6. CULTURAL AND CLINICAL FEATURES OF THE COMMON DERMATOPHYTES

FUNGUS	COLONY APPEARANCE	MORPHOLOGY	CLINICAL FEATURES
Trichophyton mentagrophytes	White to tan; powdery or cottony	Coils; nodular bodies chlamydospores; microconidia in grape-like clusters	Ringworm of nails, skin; ectothrix infections of hair
T. rubrum	Cottony to velvety. Reddish to purple pigmentation reverse of colony	Numerous microconidia in clusters and singly along hyphae	Infections of skin and nails
T. tonsurans	Cream or yellow; folded, with central crater	Elongated microconidia along sides of hyphae	Endothrix infections of hair, skin, and nails
T. schoenleinii	Smooth, waxy to powdery, irregularly folded; brownish pigment	Hyphal swelling, "favic chandeliers"	Endothrix infection of hair (favus)
T. verrucosum	Growth slow, colony small; heaped and folded	Numerous chlamydospores at 37° C.; irregular mycelia	Ectothrix infection of hair
Microsporum audouinii	Velvety, radiating furrows; light orange pigment	Rare macroconidia; club-shaped microconidia	Human (anthropophilic) cause of epidemic tinea capitis in children
M. canis	Cottony white mycelia with bright orange on reverse of colony	Numerous large multicellular macroconidia (fuseaux)	Animal (zoophilic) species causes sporadic tinea capitis in children
M. gypseum	Powdery, rapidly growing; buff to brown	Many thin-walled, 4-6 septate, ellipsoidal macroconidia	As above. Has been isolated from soil
Epidermophyton floccosum	Velvety to powdery; radial furrows; surface greenish yellow in color	Broad, blunt to clavate macroconidia in clusters	Tinea cruris
Keratinomyces ajelloi	Powdery, fast growing; colorless or bluish black reverse of colony	Numerous long, slender macroconidia	Rare cause of tinea capitis in humans

cotton blue may be useful for demonstrating the etiologic agent.

Examinations of sections of tissue obtained at biopsy are important. The P.A.S., Gridley, mucicarmine, and methenamine silver stains are widely used for demonstration of fungi.

Cultures are done on a wide variety of media, of which Sabouraud's, Littman's ox-gall, cycloheximide, Sabhi, and cornmeal agars are commonly used. The dimorphic fungi are cultured both at 37° C. and room temperature; the monomorphic fungi, at room temperature only. Colonies are examined in KOH or lactophenol cotton blue as described under the dermatophytes. Points to be noted in identifying the fungus are colonial appearance, rate of growth, size, shape, septation, and color of the spores, and type of structure upon which spores are borne. Animal inoculations are also of considerable value in some cases. (See Table 20–8.)

Recent work has shown that the immunofluorescent (FA) procedure may prove useful for rapid diagnosis from clinical specimens and for speciation of the organisms. Further progress in this area may be expected. Serologic tests are of great help in the diagnosis of some of these diseases. Precipitin complement fixa-

Table 20–7. CHARACTERISTICS OF MACROCONIDIA OF DERMATOPHYTES

CHARACTERISTIC	*Microsporum*	*Trichophyton*	*Epidermophyton*
Frequency	Numerous, except *M. audouinii*	Common to rare	Numerous
No. of septae	1–15	2–8	2–4
Size	5–100/3–8 μ	20–50/4–8 μ	20–40/6–8 μ
Wall thickness	Variable	Variable	Thin
Wall surface	Rough	Smooth	Smooth
Manner of attachment	Single	Single	Groups of 2–3

Table 20–8. ANIMAL INOCULATION WITH PATHOGENIC FUNGI

ORGANISM	ANIMAL OF CHOICE	INOCULATION ROUTE	EXPOSURE INTERVAL	PATHOLOGIC FINDINGS	MICROSCOPIC FINDINGS
Nocardia asteroides	Guinea pig, mouse	Intraperitoneal (5% mucin)	8-10 days	Mesentery, peritoneum	Acid-fast branching filaments
*Cryptococcus neoformans**	Mouse	Intracerebral, intraperitoneal	1-2 weeks	Brain, peritoneum, spleen, gelatinous masses in mesentery	Budding encapsulated yeasts
Candida albicans	Rabbit	Intravenous	4-6 days	Abscesses in kidney	Thin-walled budding yeasts with or without pseudomycelia
*Blastomyces dermatitidis**	Mouse, guinea pig	Intraperitoneal (5% mucin + yeast phase)	1-2 weeks	Liver, spleen, lungs, lymph nodes, peritoneum	Single-budding cells with thick refractile walls
*Paracoccidioides brasiliensis**	Mouse, guinea pig	Intraperitoneal (5% mucin + yeast phase)	1-2 weeks	Spleen, liver, diaphragm, mesentery	As above, except many cells have multiple buds
*Histoplasma capsulatum**	Mouse	Intraperitoneal (5% mucin + yeast phase)	1-2 weeks	Mesentery, diaphragm, visceral organs	Small, oval budding cells
*Sporothrix schenckii**	Male mouse	Intratesticular	1-4 weeks	Peritonitis, orchitis	Cigar-shaped budding cells
Coccidioides immitis	Male mouse	Intratesticular, intraperitoneal	10-15 days	Orchitis, generalized infection	Double-walled spherical bodies containing endospores

*It is advisable to inoculate three to six mice and one to two guinea pigs. Mice should be killed and examined at two to three day intervals beginning two weeks after inoculation. Guinea pigs should be killed at the end of one week and at weekly intervals thereafter if death has not meanwhile ensued.

tion, agglutination, and newly developed immunoelectrophoretic methods (Gordon *et al.*, 1971) are used; these will be discussed briefly under the respective diseases.

North American Blastomycosis

North American blastomycosis (Gilchrist's disease) caused by *Blastomyces dermatitidis,* may occur as a chronic granulomatous infection of the skin and internal organs. The lungs, bones, and kidneys may be involved by spread from a cutaneous lesion or from a primary pulmonary focus (Fig. 20–14). The portal of entry of the systemic form is the respiratory tract. Bone and central nervous system involvement are common in the disseminated form.

The disease occurs sporadically, most cases occurring in central and southeastern United States and occasionally in Canda, Central America, and Africa. The reservoir is probably the soil, by inhalation of spore-laden dust. It is not transferable from man to man or animal to man. Individuals engaged in agricultural or outdoor occupations are more likely to become infected. Males are affected about seven times more frequently than females; two-thirds of the cases occur in individuals between the ages of 15 and 45.

Laboratory Diagnosis. Scrapings from lesions, sputum, and pus should be examined in 10 per cent potassium hydroxide. Characteristic thick-walled, double-contoured, single-budding yeast-like fungi 8 to 20 microns in diameter can be seen (Fig. 20–15). Hyphae are never seen in exudates or tissues. Material should be cultured on Sabouraud's, cycloheximide, and brain-heart infusion agar with antibiotics at room temperature and at 37° C. At room temperature after three or four days the colonies are first smooth and pasty but gradually become white and filamentous. Microscopic examination of the culture shows spherical or oval microconidia attached directly to the hyphae or at the end of short pedicles. At 37° C. the culture is slow growing, tan, heaped, and yeast-like. Microscopically the culture is composed of double-contoured, single-budding cells resembling those found in tissue.

Complement-fixing antibodies may be demonstrable in individuals with extensive or progressive disease but are usually unreliable. Since the sera may react with *Histoplasma capsulatum* antigens, the test should be done simultaneously with both. Patients with the local cutaneous form may have a negative re-

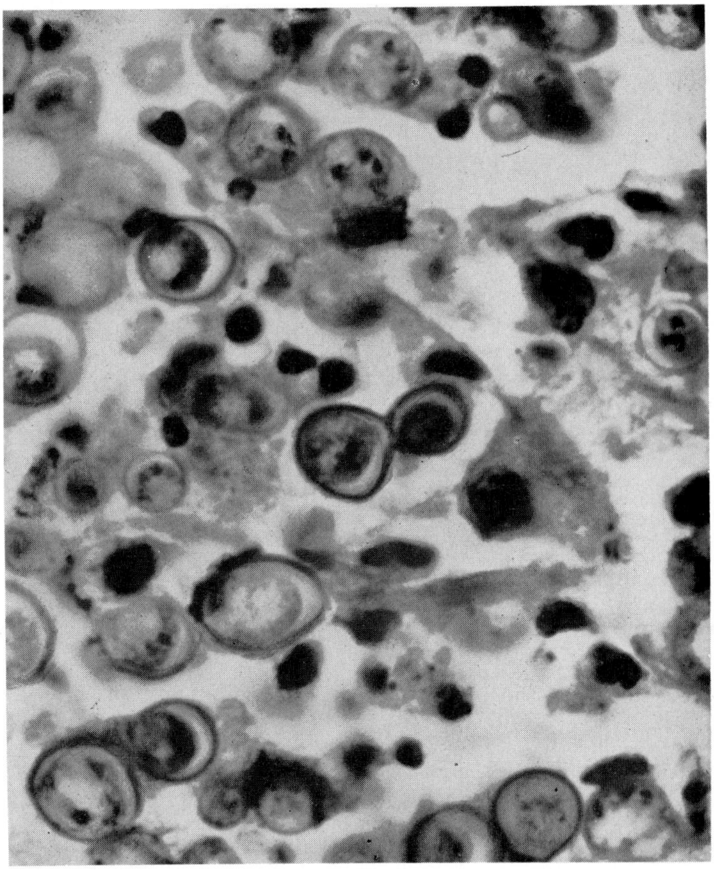

Figure 20–14. Blastomycosis of lung. Section of tissue showing budding forms. Periodic acid-Schiff stain. × 1500. (From Conant, N. F., *et al.*: Manual of Clinical Mycology. 3rd ed.)

action. Hypersensitivity to the skin test antigen, blastomycin, may occasionally be demonstrable, but blastomycin has such poor sensitivity and specificity that its use for diagnosis has generally been discontinued.

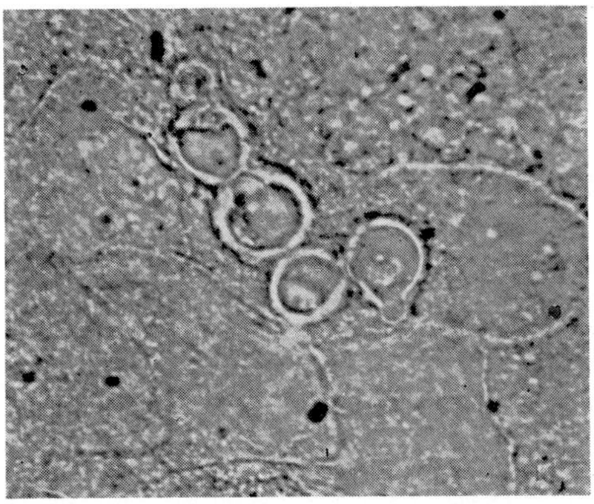

Figure 20–15. *Blastomyces dermatitidis*; direct mount of pus showing double-contoured budding cells (× 716). (From Lewis, G. M., and Hopper, M. E.: An Introduction to Medical Mycology. Year Book Medical Publishers, Inc., 1958.)

Coccidioidomycosis

Coccidioidomycosis (coccidioidal granuloma, valley fever), caused by *Coccidioides immitis,* is a highly infectious disease which results in a benign, self-limited respiratory infection, or, in a small percentage of cases (about 0.25 per cent) the primary disease may develop into a progressive disseminated infection involving the skin, viscera, bones, and central nervous system. The primary pulmonary disease may have minimal manifestations and is often overlooked. More severe cases show symptoms of chronic pulmonary disease. There may be many years between the primary infection and the disseminated form. Dissemination occurs most often in dark-skinned males. This disease is limited almost exclusively to the semiarid areas of the southwestern United States and parts of Central and South America. Humans apparently acquire the infection by inhaling dust contaminated with the infectious arthrospores or by introducing them into the skin following an injury. Laboratory workers may also become infected.

Laboratory Diagnosis. Pus, sputum, and pleural fluid should be examined as fresh

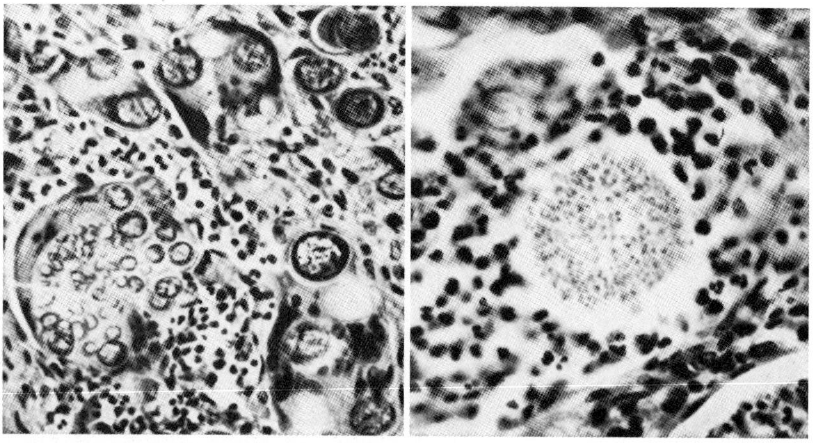

Figure 20–16. The chronic and acute types of lesion in coccidioidomycosis. *Left,* the chronic type of lesion showing many mature cells of *Coccidioides immitis.* × 475. *Right,* the active type of lesion showing a mass of spores beginning to spread in the tissue. Hematoxylin and eosin; × 710.

preparations. The thick-walled spherule, 30 to 200 microns in diameter, filled with numerous, small (2 to 5 microns in diameter) endospores, is characteristic (Fig. 20–16). Endospores are liberated by rupture of the cell wall, and "ghost" spherules may be present. Material should be cultured on Sabouraud's, Littman's, and cycloheximide agar and incubated at room temperature. Petri dishes should not be used. Colonies appear in three to four days, at first appearing moist, flat, and membranous and later developing cottony, aerial, buff-colored mycelia. Only the mycelial phase grows in culture ordinarily, but the tissue phase has been successfully obtained *in vitro.* Microscopically the cultures show thick, branching septate hyphae and numerous chains of rectangular or ellipsoidal, thick-walled arthrospores (Fig. 20–17). Typical spherules can be demonstrated by injecting a saline suspension of these spores intraperitoneally into mice. Recently, culture methods have been developed to produce spherules from the mycelial phase. *Note: The arthrospores are highly infectious and great care must be exercised in handling them and disposing of old cultures.*

In disseminated infections persistent precipitins and complement-fixing antibodies can be demonstrated. A progressive rise in titer is a grave prognostic sign. Sensitivity to the skin test antigen, coccidioidin, indicates past or present infection. It is frequently negative, however, during the disseminated stage of the disease.

A new technique, in which an immunodiffusion technique in agar gel is used, has been reported to be useful as a screening procedure for detecting serums which would be positive in the complement-fixation test (Huppert and Bailey, 1965). A fluorescent antibody inhibition test for *C. immitis* antibodies has also been reported (Kaplan *et al.,* 1966).

Cryptococcosis

Cryptococcosis (torulosis, European blastomycosis) is caused by a yeast known as *Cryptococcus neoformans* or *Torula histolytica.* The disease may involve the lungs, skin, bone and joints, or other parts of the body and has a marked predilection for the central nervous system. The primary infection may resemble a neoplasm or tuberculosis, and infection of the central nervous system may result in symptoms resembling those of bacterial meningitis. This type of infection generally terminates fatally unless treated (Fig. 20–18). Subclinical cryptococcosis is thought by some to be more prevalent than has previously been realized.

Cases of the disease occur sporadically throughout the world. They present a diagnostic challenge, because the symptoms may resemble those of tuberculosis, neoplasms, or brain tumors. It is thought that contaminated soil may be the source of infection from animals to man, but no evidence of direct transmission from man to man and animal to man has been reported. Recent work has shown that the organism abounds in pigeon excreta and that these may serve as reservoirs for infections (Walter and Atchison, 1966). In patients with pre-existing malignant disease, the organism may disseminate rapidly from a primary focus to other organs.

Laboratory Diagnosis. *Cryptococcus neoformans,* unlike the other systemic fungi, exists only in the form of oval or spherical, single or budding organisms, 5 to 20 microns in diameter, surrounded by a gelatinous, wide, re-

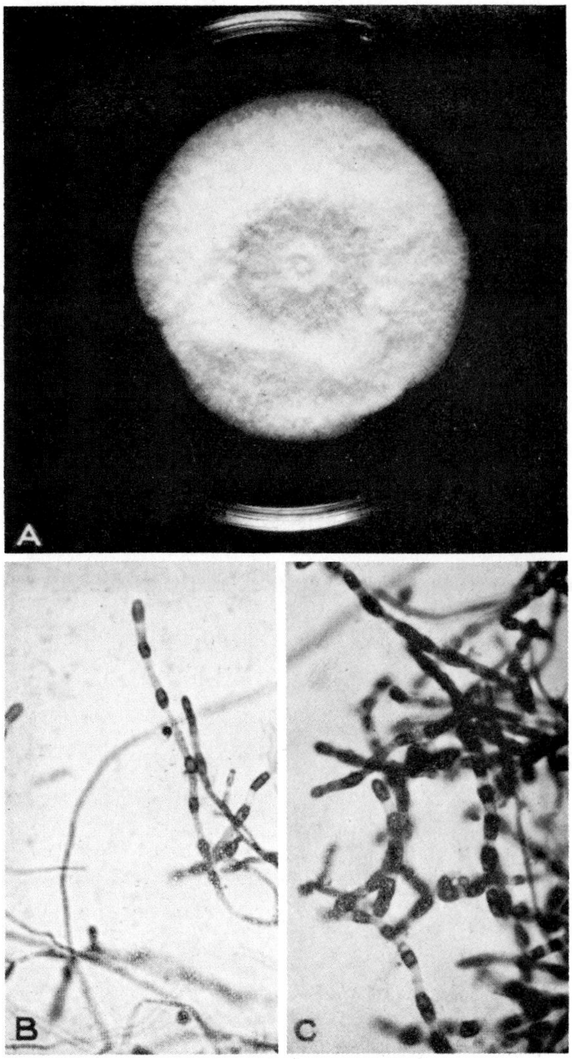

Figure 20–17. *Coccidioides immitis: A,* Culture on Sabouraud's glucose agar, 19 days, at room temperature. *B,* Arthrospore formation in young culture. × 580. *C,* Arthrospore formation in old culture. × 700. (From Conant, N. F., *et al.*: Manual of Clinical Mycology. 3rd ed.)

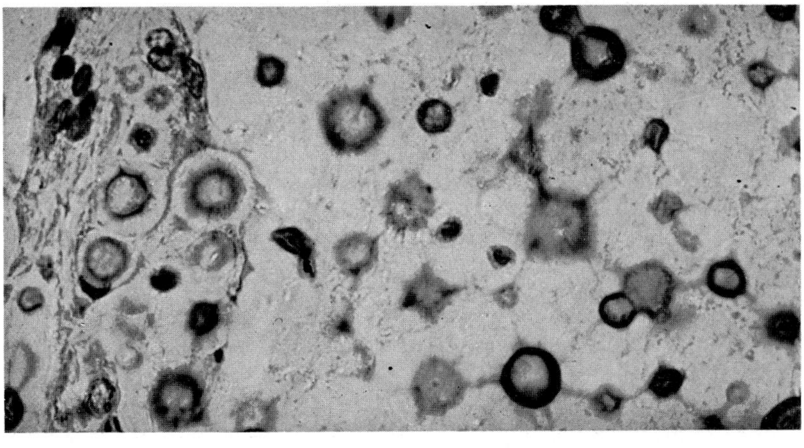

Figure 20–18. Cryptococcal meningitis. Growth of *Cryptococcus neoformans* in the cerebrospinal fluid. Note the budding cells, the stained capsules which give a double-contoured appearance, and the characteristic threads connecting the cells. Mucicarmine stain. × 950.

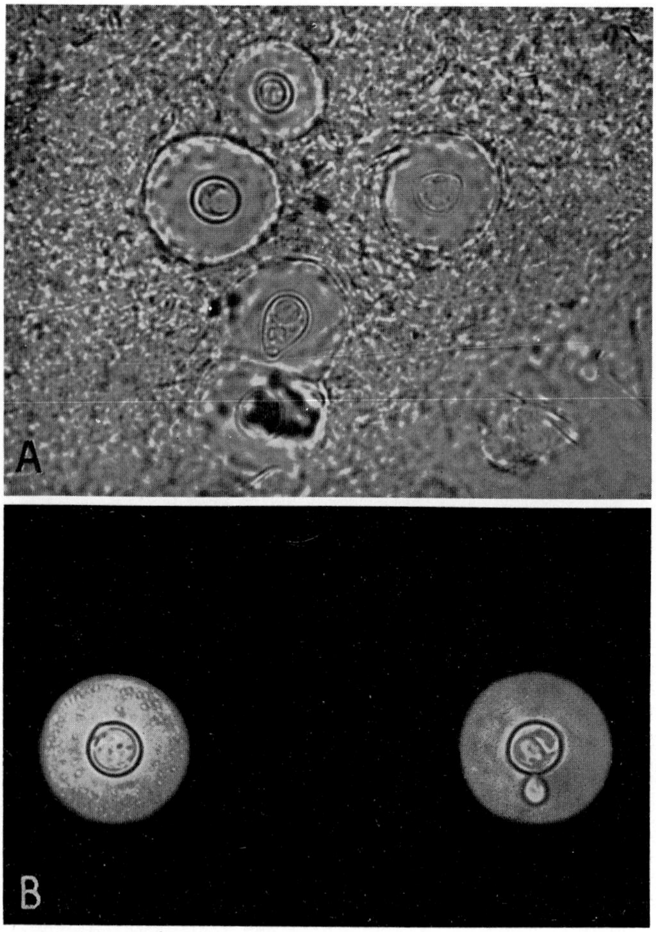

Figure 20–19. *Cryptococcus neoformans.* *A,* Pus containing the round, thick-walled budding fungus surrounded by capsule. × 850. *B,* India ink preparation of spinal fluid showing the budding fungus surrounded by capsule. × 821. (From Conant, N. F., *et al.*: Manual of Clinical Mycology. 3rd ed.)

fractive capsule. The presence of this capsule is pathognomonic for this organism (Fig. 20–19).

Pus from sputum or centrifuged spinal fluid should be examined unstained by placing a small amount on a slide and gently pressing to a thin film under a coverslip. The infection is often missed in spinal fluid examinations because the organisms are confused with lymphocytes. A turbid spinal fluid with an increase in lymphocytes and globulin and a decrease in glucose should be examined for fungi as well as bacteria. The material should also be mixed with a drop of India ink* or nigrosin; then a coverslip should be added and pressed down gently. The preparation should be examined with subdued light under the high dry objective. The characteristic encapsulated budding yeast is diagnostic.

Because the number of organisms may be small. large volumes of spinal fluid should be cultured. All material should be cultured on sheep blood and Sabouraud's agar with thiamine added at room temperature and at 37° C. Cycloheximide media is not satisfactory for this organism. A selective isolation medium has been described by Shields and Ajello (1966). This medium, which contains an extract of *Guizotia abyssinica* seeds, allows for direct isolation of *C. neoformans* from pigeon nests, pigeon droppings, and soil. Colonies on nonselective agar, both at room and incubator temperatures, are yeast-like and slimy, rapidly growing, cream to brown in color. Incubating the media under 10 per cent CO_2 at 36° C. enhances capsule formation.

Microscopically the typical encapsulated yeasts are seen. The size of the capsule varies with the strain and may be lost on primary culture. Intracerebral or intraperitoneal inoculation into mice results in the formation of gelatinous masses in the brain, lung, and abdomen from which the budding encapsulated yeast can be demonstrated. Criteria for identification of *C. neoformans* include capsule formation, ability to grow at 37° C., hydrolysis

*An excellent India ink preparation is made by mixing 15 ml. India ink ("Pelikan"), 30 ml. Merthiolate (1:1000 aq.), and 0.1 ml. Tween-80 (1:1000 aq.). Filter before use.

of urea, failure to form filaments on rice extract agar, lack of ascospore production, nonassimilation of lactose or potassium nitrate, and positive assimilation of dextrose, maltose, sucrose, and galactose.

Recently it has been shown (Hall *et al.*, 1972) that the oxidation-fermentation medium of Hugh and Leifson could be adapted for determining carbohydrate utilization in this group as well as in other yeasts. This method is considerably simpler and easier to interpret than the classic Wickerham or agar auxanogram procedures and should aid in the definitive characterization of the various yeasts associated with human disease (Table 20–9).

Serologic and skin tests are available for this disease at the present time only at specialized centers. Latex agglutination and complement fixation procedures have been developed that appear to be very promising (Goodman *et al.*, 1971) and will likely be in general use in the near future. In some patients, cryptococcal antigen or polysaccharide is also demonstrable. This is a very useful procedure, particularly in culturally negative patients.

Histoplasmosis

Histoplasmosis, (Darling's disease) caused by *Histoplasma capsulatum*, produces a wide variety of clinical manifestations. Respiratory infection may be mild or severe and is usually unapparent and self-limited. The progressive disseminated infection spreads to infect the reticuloendothelial system, causing fever, malaise, hepatomegaly, splenomegaly, anemia, and leukopenia. The symptoms that occur are related to the organs involved. Mucocutaneous lesions may also occur as manifestations of the systemic disease. The disease may closely resemble tuberculosis, other systemic mycoses, sarcoidosis, leukemia, Hodgkins' disease, or other lymphomas. In any patient with findings suggestive of these diseases, histoplasmosis should be considered.

The disease occurs throughout the world. There are areas of high endemicity in the United States, especially in the central Mississippi and Ohio River valleys. In some local areas as many as 80 per cent of the adult population react positively to the skin test antigen, histoplasmin. Infection occurs from the inhalation of infectious spores from exogenous sources. The organism has been isolated repeatedly from soil and fecal droppings around aviaries and chicken yards and from bats and feathers. There may be other, as yet unidentified, modes of infection.

A similar disease occurs in Africa and other parts of the world. The causative agent, *H. duboisii*, produces larger yeast cells *in vivo* than does *H. capsulatum*, but the mycelial phase cultures appear to be identical.

Laboratory Diagnosis. Smears made from bone marrow, lymph node biopsy specimens, and mucocutaneous lesions should be fixed with methyl alcohol and stained by Wright's or Giemsa's method. Acridine orange (A. O.) stain has been reported to be helpful in making a rapid diagnosis in liver biopsies and bone marrow aspirates. The fungus appears as small (1 to 4 microns), round or oval, yeast-like cells in the cytoplasm of histiocytes or lying free. They appear to have a clear halo surrounding a darker stained central area (Fig. 20–20). Direct mounts or KOH preparations are generally useless because of the intracellular localization of the organisms and their small size.

Sputum, gastric or bronchial washings, and pus should be cultured on Sabouraud's, cycloheximide, Sabhi or brain-heart infusion blood agar plus antibiotics at room and incubator temperatures. Recent work indicates that the

Table 20–9. DIFFERENTIAL CHARACTERISTICS OF YEASTS

	MICROSCOPIC MORPHOLOGY	CAPSULES	MYCELIUM	UREASE	GROWTH AT 37° C	GROWTH AT ROOM TEMP.	PIGMENT
Cryptococcus neoformans	Spherical, wide capsules	+	−	+	+	+	−
Cryptococcus sp.	Spherical or ellipsoidal	+	−	+	−	+	−
Rhodotorula sp.	Oval cells, single or short chains	−	−	+	−	+	Orange red
Trichosporon cutaneum	Round, oval to cylindrical; arthrospores	−	+	+	+	+	−
Torulopsis glabrata	Small, ovoid	−	−	−	+	+	−
Torulopsis pintolepsii	Small, ovoid	−	−	−	+	+	Buff

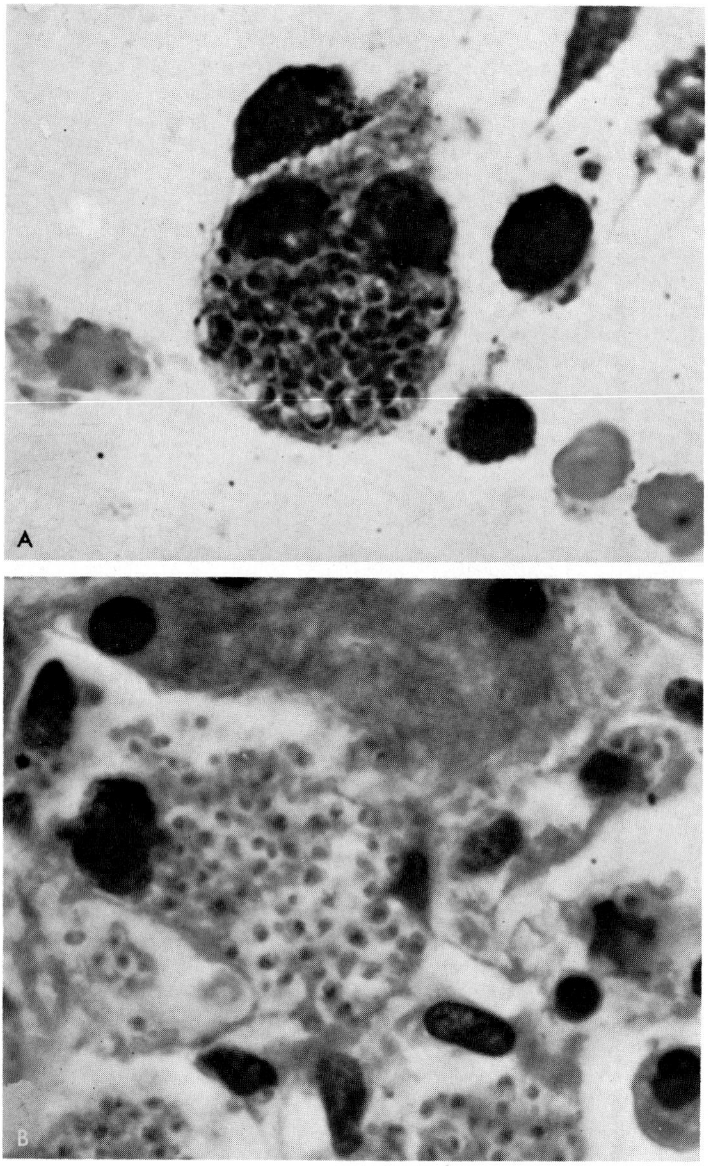

Figure 20–20. Histoplasmosis: *A*, Parasitized mononuclear cell in a peripheral blood smear. × 1300. *B*, *Histoplasma capsulatum* in macrophages in liver, × 1300. (From Conant, N. F., *et al.*: Manual of Clinical Mycology. 3rd ed.)

addition of 5-fluorocytosine* to the agar increases the chances of isolating *Histoplasma* by inhibiting the growth of *Candida* and other yeasts which are known to suppress this organism (Garrison *et al.*, 1971). In addition, bone marrow or blood should be inoculated into flasks of brain-heart infusion broth. All cultures should be held at least 30 days before discarding. Freshly expectorated sputum should be cultured, since the organism dies rapidly in sputum. Propylene glycol should not be used if induced sputum samples are collected for culture because it inhibits *Histoplasma*. Liquefaction of the sputum with pancreatin before plating on agar is reported to increase the percentage of positive isolates.

At 37° C. growth is slow (8 to 14 days), and the colonies are small, waxy, and membranous. Microscopically, small budding organisms resembling those seen in tissues and abortive hyphae are seen (Fig. 20–21). At room temperature (Fig. 20–22) white mycelial growth is produced after 14 to 18 days (Fig. 20–23), and microscopic examination shows the round, thick-walled, tuberculate chlamydospores (7 to 15 microns) that are diagnostic for *H. capsulatum* (Fig. 20–24). Repeated search for these

*Roche Laboratories, Nutley, New Jersey.

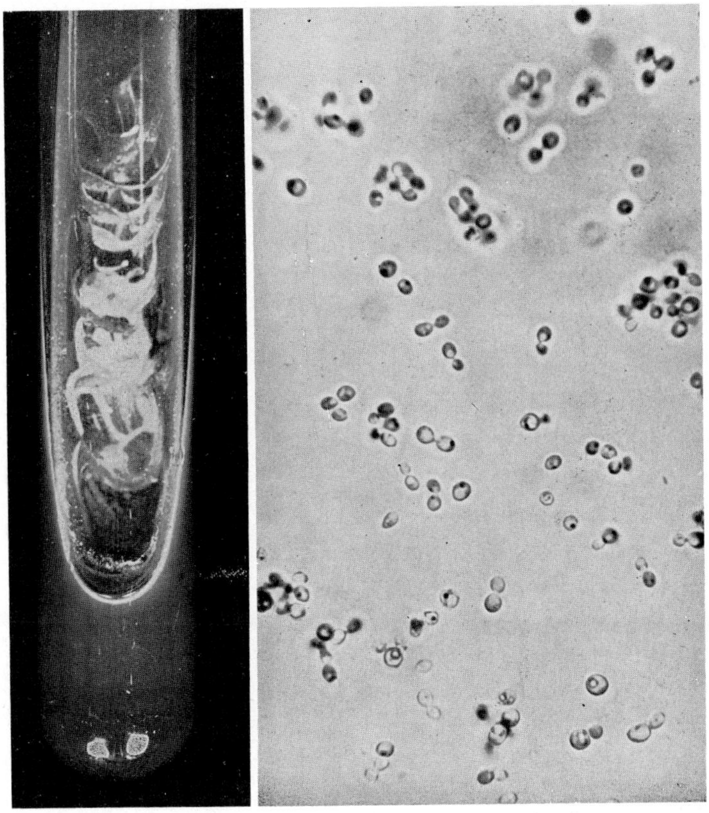

Figure 20–21. *Histoplasma capsulatum.* *A*, On blood agar six days at 37° C. *B*, From blood agar culture. × 700. (From Conant, N. F., *et al.*: Manual of Clinical Mycology. 3rd ed.)

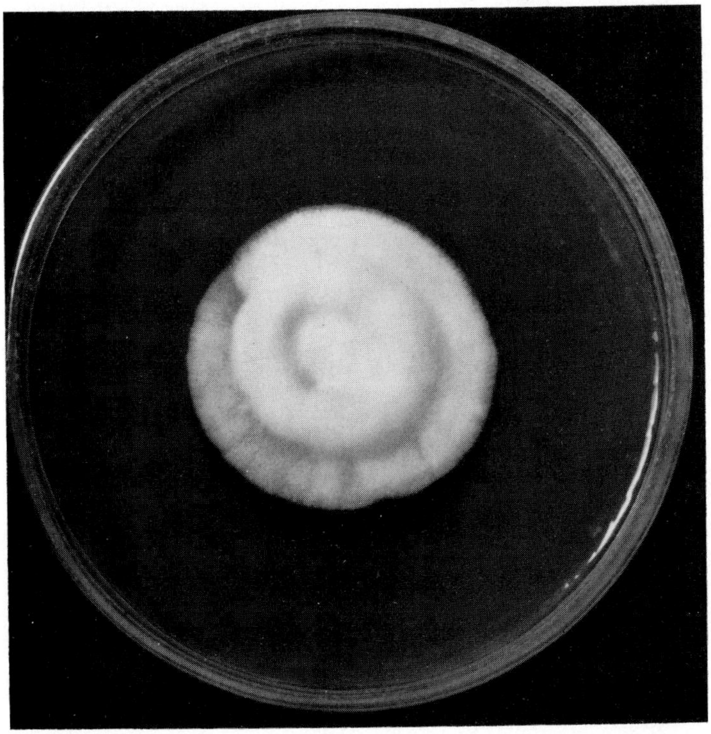

Figure 20–22. *Histoplasma capsulatum:* On Sabouraud's glucose agar, 23 days, at room temperature. (From Conant, N. F., *et al.*: Manual of Clinical Mycology. 3rd ed.)

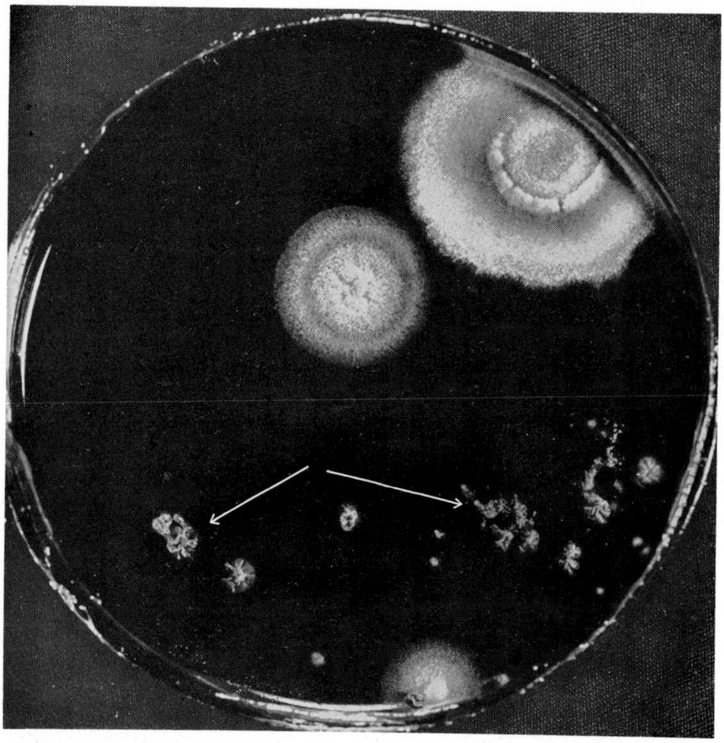

Figure 20–23. *Histoplasma capsulatum.* On brain-heart infusion glucose blood agar at room temperature. (From Conant, N. F., *et al.:* Manual of Clinical Mycology. 3rd ed.)

chlamydospores may be necessary, since they are occasionally few in number. They rarely grow on blood agar but can be demonstrated by transplanting the colonies to Sabouraud's agar. Intraperitoneal injection into mice sometimes gives a positive isolation when cultural procedures fail. It is important to demonstrate the dimorphism of the isolate to distinguish it from the morphologically similar soil saprophyte *Sepedonium* sp.

Complement-fixing antibodies, which react either with mycelial or yeast phase antigens of *H. capsulatum*, or with histoplasmin usually appear a few weeks after infection. Serial tests must be made throughout the course of the disease in order to demonstrate a rise in titer. Other serologic tests that are useful are the collodion particle, latex, and precipitin reactions in agar-gel. Positive skin tests to a standardized preparation of histoplasmin indicate past or present infection, although acutely ill patients may become anergic during the terminal stage. Also, in common with the other fungal skin test antigens, repeated skin tests may elevate titers of serologic tests to significant levels.

Sporotrichosis

Sporotrichosis, caused by *Sporothrix (Sporotrichum) schenckii*, is a subacute infection, which follows introduction of the fungus by trauma. From the initial lesion, which begins as a small, chancriform pustule, the regional lymphatics are invaded. The lymphatic vessels show cord-like thickening, and multiple abscesses appear along the course of the infected lymphatics. Occasionally, generalized infection may occur by way of the blood, with or without primary cutaneous lesions, and any organ or tissue of the body may be involved. An increased number of pulmonary infections without antecedent skin lesions have been reported in the last decade.

The disease occurs throughout the world, in both temperate and tropical zones, and the fungus is widely distributed in nature. Infections usually occur following injury to the skin with contaminated material. Farmers, horticulturists, and miners are most frequently infected.

Laboratory Diagnosis. The organisms are difficult to demonstrate in stained smears or sections because the number of yeast cells in the disease may be scanty. The presence of a characteristic asteroid body may suggest the diagnosis. Cultures are the most reliable procedure (Fig. 20–25). Pus from lesions or swabs from infected areas should be streaked on Sabouraud's or cycloheximide and brain-heart infusion agar at room temperature and at 37° C. At room temperature the colonies appear with moderate rapidity and are small, white to black, yeast-like, and without aerial mycelia. Micro-

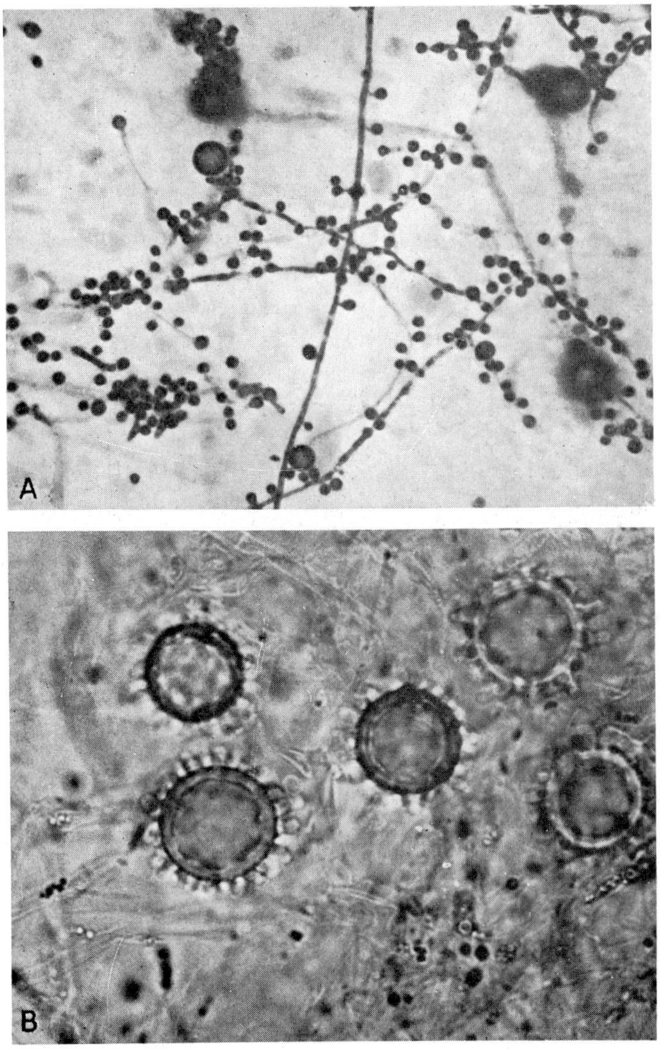

Figure 20–24. *Histoplasma capsulatum* from Sabouraud's glucose agar. *A*, Small, smooth, round to pyriform conidia. × 600. *B*, Large thick-walled, round, tuberculate chlamydospores. × 1150. (From Conant, N. F., *et al.*: Manual of Clinical Mycology. 3rd ed.)

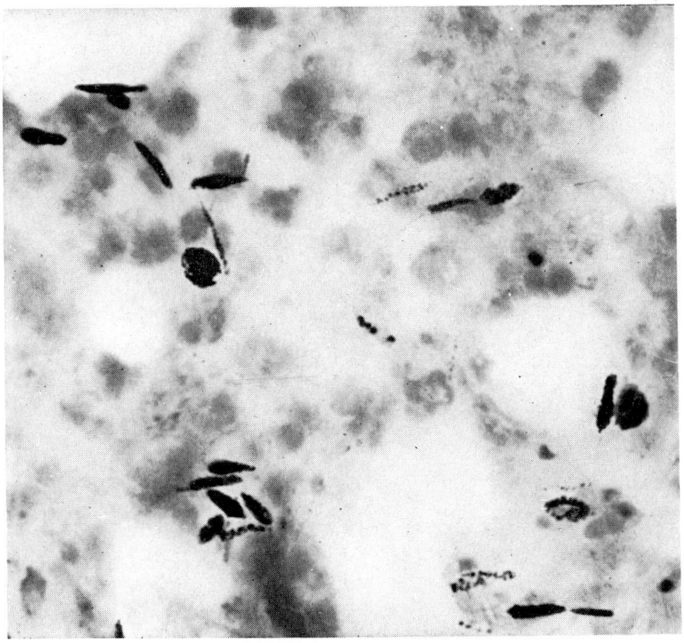

Figure 20–25. *Sporothrix schenckii.* Tissue forms in smear of pus from inoculated mouse. × 1100. (From Conant, N. F., *et al.*: Manual of Clinical Mycology. 3rd ed.)

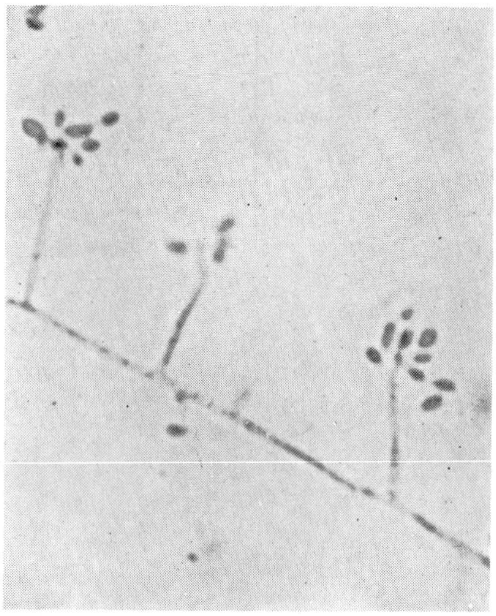

Figure 20–26. *Sporothrix schenckii,* culture showing clusters of spores on hyphae (× 1000). (From Lewis, G. M., and Hopper, M. E.: An Introduction to Medical Mycology. Year Book Medical Publishers, Inc., 1958.)

scopically the colony is composed of branching, septate hyphae upon which spherical or pyriform conidia are borne either directly or at the end of lateral branches in a characteristic rosette cluster (Fig. 20–26).

At 37° C. the colonies are grayish yellow, soft, and bacteria-like. Microscopically such colonies have a deep brown pigmentation and are composed of cigar-shaped, round, or oval (1 to 5 microns in diameter) conidia and small hyphal fragments. On media containing antibiotics, the dark pigmentation does not develop.

Several serologic techniques, such as whole yeast cell agglutination, complement fixation and immunodiffusion, are available at specialized centers. These may be useful as aids in the clinical diagnosis of this disease, particularly in extracutaneous infections (Roberts and Larsh, 1971).

Other Mycoses

Rhinosporidiosis is an infection characterized by polyps on the mucosa of the skin or mucous membranes, usually the nares, or on the face. The etiologic agent is *Rhinosporidium seeberi,* which has never been cultured. The disease occurs primarily in tropical areas, particularly in India and Ceylon.

Chromomycosis is a chronic granulomatous infection primarily involving the skin and subcutaneous tissues and characterized by formation of warty cutaneous nodules. Characteristic dark-brown, round, thick-walled cells are found in the infected tissues. Infections occur following abrasion to the skin which is contaminated with vegetable matter or soil containing the infectious fungi. The causative agents are distinguished by the types of conidiophores they form. The important etiologic agents are *Phialophora verrucosa, Cladosporium carrionii, Fonsecaea compactum (Hormodendrum compactum),* and *Fonsecaea pedrosoi.* This is also primarily a tropical and subtropical disease.

Paracoccidioidomycosis (South American blastomycosis, paracoccidioidal granuloma), which is a disease similar in many respects to North American blastomycosis, is caused by a closely related fungus known as *Paracoccidioides brasiliensis.* These infections occur almost exclusively in Latin America. The yeast phase cells can be differentiated from those of *Blastomyces dermatiditis* by their characteristic multiple buds (Fig. 20–27).

A related form found in the equatorial region of South America is known as lobomycosis. It produces a chronic infection of the skin resulting in keloids or fibrous tumors. Budding yeasts resembling *P. brasiliensis* can be seen in preparations from the lesions but cultures have been unsuccessful.

Dematiaceous (dark-pigmented) fungi may cause infection, usually by injury to the skin or inhalation of spores. These fungi are primarily various species of *Phialophora* and *Cladosporum.*

Aspergillus is ubiquitous in nature and is a common laboratory contaminant. Clinical infections in man are occasionally seen, particularly in patients receiving steroid hormones or

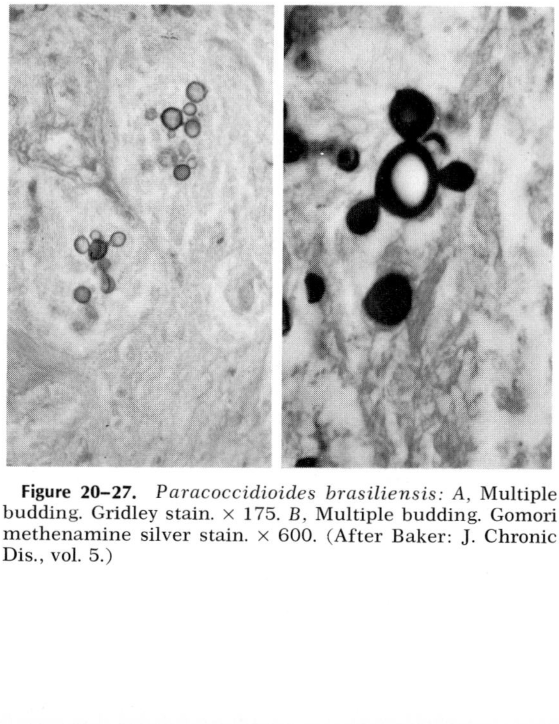

Figure 20–27. *Paracoccidioides brasiliensis: A,* Multiple budding. Gridley stain. × 175. *B,* Multiple budding. Gomori methenamine silver stain. × 600. (After Baker: J. Chronic Dis., vol. 5.)

antibiotics, those suffering with debilitating diseases, such as carcinoma or tuberculosis, and individuals exposed to grain or other material heavily contaminated with *Aspergillus* spores. Potent toxins (aflatoxins) may be produced in various foods. This can be a serious public health problem in animals and humans. Repeated isolation is necessary to establish this organism as the etiologic agent of the disease in question (Fig. 20–28). Precipitating antibodies against various extracts of *Aspergillus* may be found in the serum of patients, but show considerable cross-reactivity with other organisms. *Penicillium* (Fig. 20–29) is a very common contaminant and its relationship to disease is questionable.

Phycomycosis is a disease of ever-increasing incidence, found primarily in individuals who have metabolic disturbances or are on steroid, antibiotic or anticancer therapy. The pulmonary and central nervous systems are primarily involved, although it may also involve the gastrointestinal and urinary tracts. The disease may be rapidly fatal, and therapy is usually ineffective. Since many of these organisms are ubiquitous in nature, repeated isolation is required before etiologic significance can be established. At least five genera have been incriminated as pathogens in man–*Rhizopus*, *Mucor*, *Absidia*, *Mortierella*, and *Basidiobolus*. Identification of these genera is not difficult, but species identification can be done only by specialists. All these heterogeneous genera are characterized by their nonseptate, darkly pigmented mycelia, conidia born in sporangia, and ability to grow at 37° C. (Figs. 20–30, 20–31).

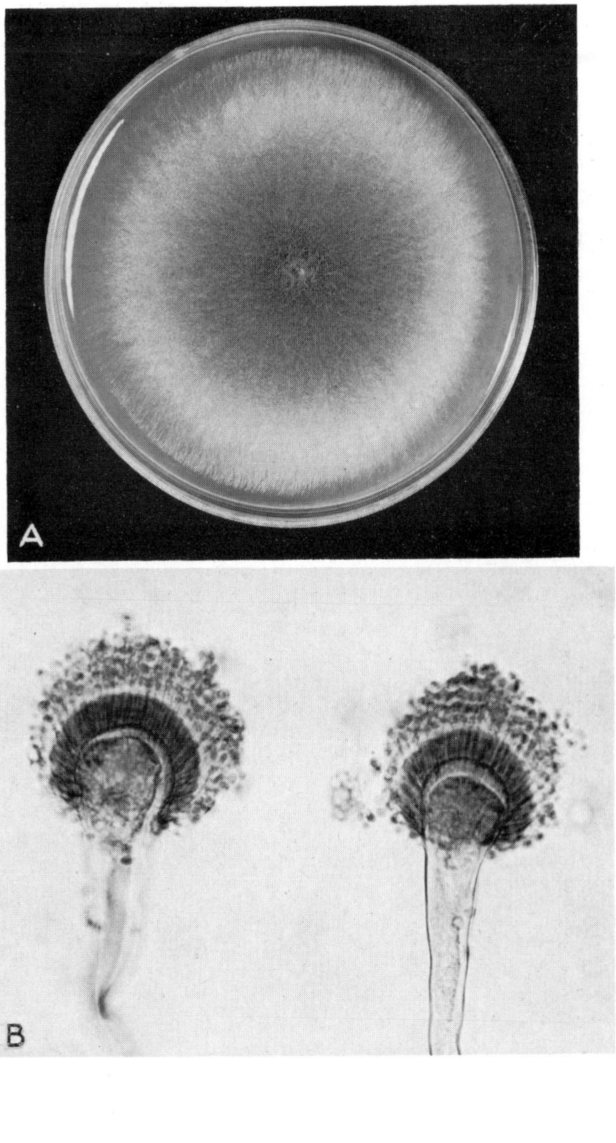

Figure 20–28. *Aspergillus fumigatus: A,* Culture on Sabouraud's glucose agar, six days, at room temperature. *B,* Conidiophores from Sabouraud's glucose agar. (× 825.) (From Conant, N. F., *et al.*: Manual of Clinical Mycology. 3rd ed.)

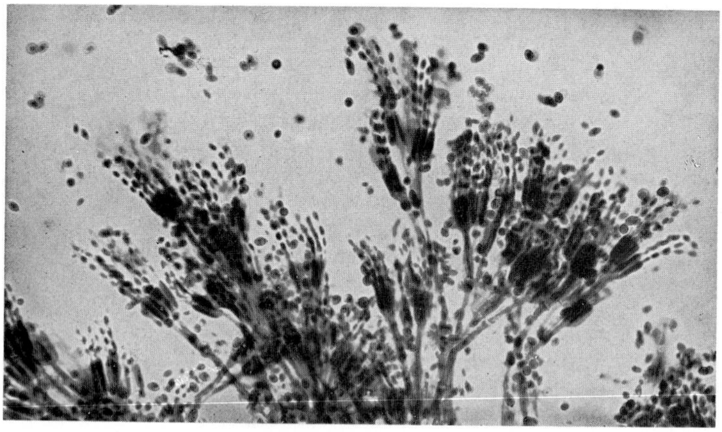

Figure 20–29. *Penicillium* sp. Note the characteristic finger-like verticillate branches and the terminal chains of conidia. × 440. (From Burrows, W.: Textbook of Microbiology. 19th ed.)

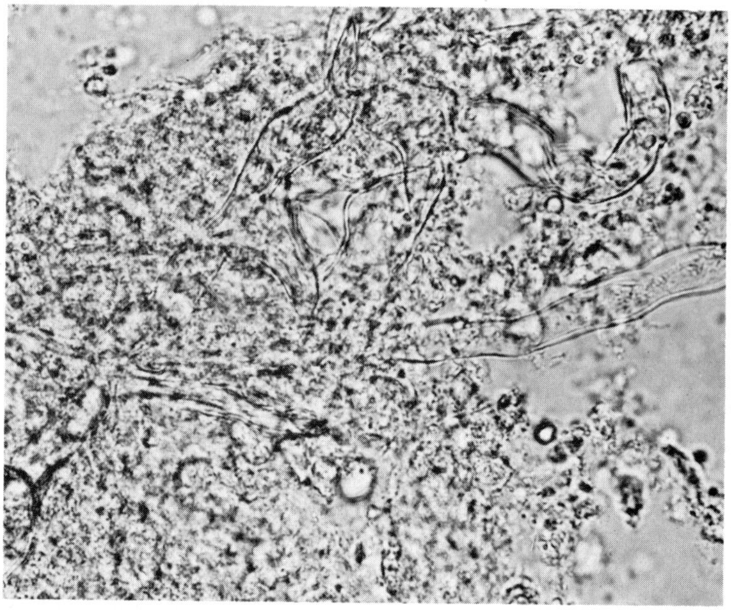

Figure 20–30. Phycomycosis. Wide, nonseptate hyphae in KOH preparation from lesion on palate. (After Smith et al. (eds.): Zinsser Microbiology, 14th ed. New York, Appleton-Century-Crofts, 1968.)

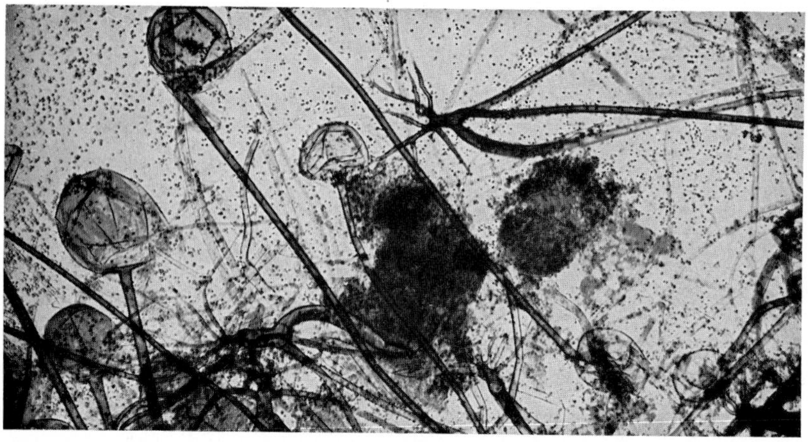

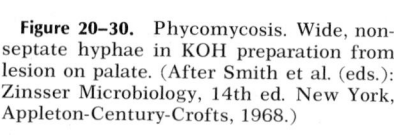

Figure 20–31. *Rhizopus* sp. mounted in lactophenol cotton blue. Note the single-celled (nonseptate) mycelium and ruptured, empty sporangia. The small oval bodies are free spores. The root-like structure at the base of the hyphae is the "hold-fast" by which the mold is attached to nutrient medium. × 80. (From Burrows, W.: Textbook of Microbiology. 19th ed.)

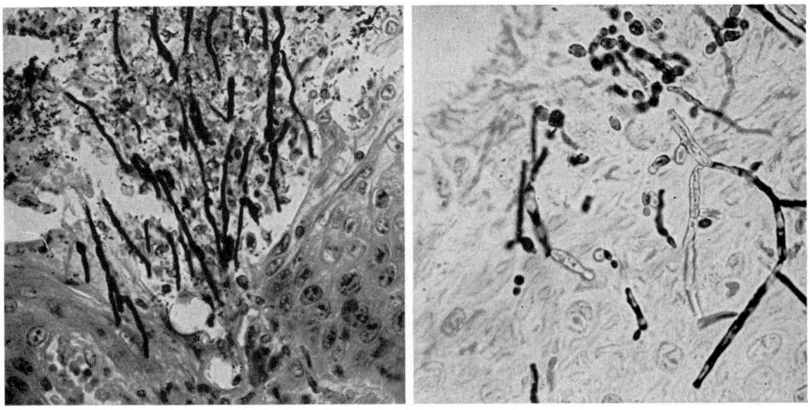

Figure 20–32. Moniliasis: invasion of the epithelial layer of the esophagus by *Candida albicans. Left,* beginning invasion of the superficial layer showing mycelium and yeast-like cells; note the gram-positive micrococci accompanying the fungus. × 600. *Right,* invasion of the deeper tissue showing both mycelium and yeast-like cells penetrating the epithelium. × 950.

THE INTERMEDIATE FUNGI

Certain fungi, notably the *Candida* group, may cause either superficial infections or widespread systemic disease and, hence, are classified as intermediate.

Candidiasis (Moniliasis)

Candida (Monilia) albicans can cause infection of the mouth, skin, nails, or vagina or a variety of systemic diseases. Oral infection, sometimes found in newborn infants, results in thick, creamy white patches known as thrush. Infection of the corners of the mouth is called perlèche. A common condition found most frequently in pregnant and diabetic women is a vulvovaginal infection known as vaginal moniliasis. Infections of the nails are known as onychia and of the cuticle as paronychia. Infection of the intertriginous areas of the body, i.e., the axilla, gluteal folds, and groin are known as "intertrigo." Candidids or monilids are sterile vesicular lesions which may be found in areas not contiguous to infected lesions. These probably represent localized dermal reactions to circulating antigens.

More serious infections are those involving the lungs – bronchopulmonary candidiasis – and those involving other organs of the body. Brain abscesses, endocarditis, and septicemia may be caused by this organism (Figs. 20–32, 20–33). Other species of *Candida* (e.g., *C. tropicalis, C. guillermondii*) have been isolated from endocarditis and other infections.

Candida albicans is frequently present on the skin, mucous membranes, and in the intestinal tract of normal individuals. Consequently

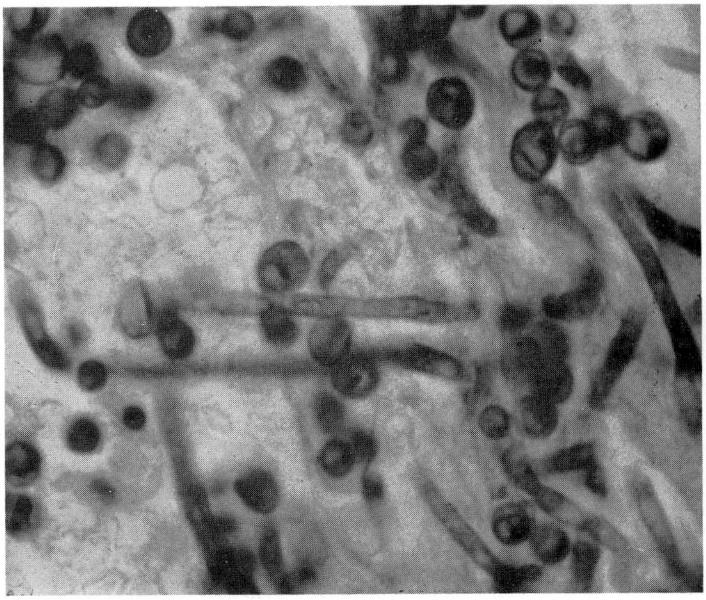

Figure 20–33. Candidiasis of brain. Growth of *Candida albicans* in ventricle in fatal meningitis. Periodic acid–Schiff stain. × 1200. (From Conant, N. F., *et al.:* Manual of Clinical Mycology. 3rd ed.)

infections are probably primarily endogenous in origin. Predisposing factors include diabetes, pregnancy, obesity, malignancies, endocrine diseases, and avitaminosis. Occupational conditions that cause maceration of the skin predispose to cutaneous infections. The incidence of severe or fatal cases has markedly increased because of the increased use of antibiotics; in these cases the organism proliferates abundantly to replace the normal bacterial flora (Seelig, 1966). Hypersensitivity undoubtedly plays an important role in the pathogenesis of the disease. The disease is worldwide in distribution.

Laboratory Diagnosis. *C. albicans* is the only consistently pathogenic species of the genus; hence, it is important to differentiate it from the other species. Skin and nail scrapings should be mounted on a slide with 10 per cent potassium hydroxide. Sputum, mucus, and pus should be crushed to a thin film and examined fresh. The material can also be stained by Gram's method or with methylene blue or lactophenol cotton blue. Candida appears in such preparations as small, oval, budding, yeast-like cells 3 to 6 microns in diameter; occasional fragments of hyphae can be seen. The organism stains intensely positive by Gram's method (Fig. 20–34). In tissues, clusters of pseudomycelia may be seen. These are distributed in a nondirectional manner rather than the directional alignment of hyphal elements of the phycomycetes.

Cultures should be inoculated on Sabouraud's, cycloheximide, or other selective media, a wide variety of which have been developed for this purpose. Phenol red agar base plus 0.2 per cent sulfadiazine serves as a simple but efficient selective medium for *C. albicans*. The organism grows rapidly and readily at either room or incubator temperature, appearing in two to four days as creamy, moist, flat colonies with a distinct yeasty odor (Fig. 20–35). On Levine's E.M.B. agar containing 0.1 mg. chlortetracycline per ml. incubated at 37° C. in a 10 per cent carbon dioxide atmosphere, colonies develop as a characteristic spidery or feathery growth. A related species,

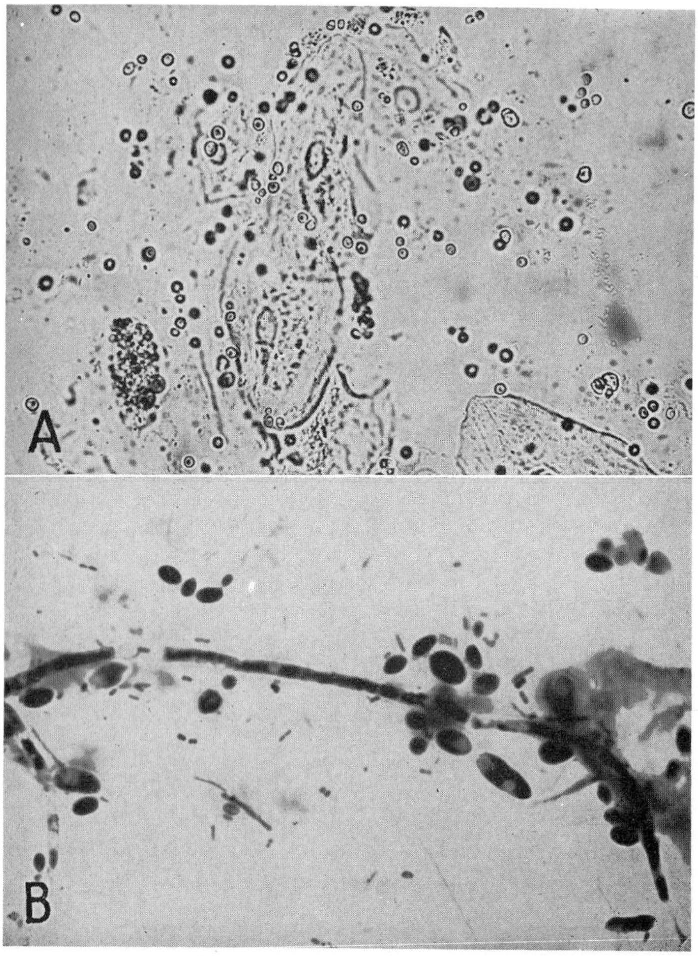

Figure 20–34. *A*, *Candida albicans* in sputum. Fresh preparation. × 300. *B*, Gram stained preparation. × 1350. (From Conant, N. F., *et al.*: Manual of Clinical Mycology. 3rd ed.)

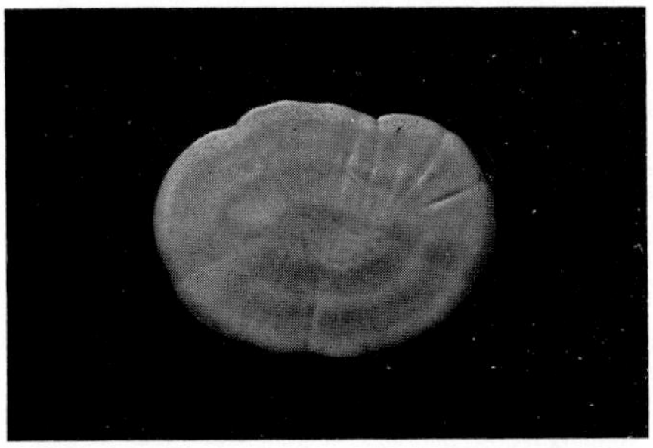

Figure 20–35. Giant colony of *Candida albicans* on Sabouraud's agar. Note the smooth, creamy growth characteristic of yeasts. × 3. (From Burrows, W.: Textbook of Microbiology. 19th ed.)

C. stellatoidea, which is occasionally found in vaginitis, produces star-like colonies on blood agar. It is thought by some that this organism represents only a morphologic variant of *C. albicans* rather than a distinct species. Microscopically clusters of oval, budding blastospores are seen, with occasional small fragments of mycelia.

To differentiate *C. albicans* from other species a simple procedure is as follows: A colony is picked, and deep cuts are made with a hooked wire into a plate of cornmeal, zein, or chlamydospore agar. We have found the dilute oxgall agar (Evron and Ganor, 1968; Fischer and Kane, 1968) excellent for this purpose. A sterile coverslip is placed over the streak. After 24 to 48 hours' incubation at room temperature, the preparation is examined with the low-power objective through the coverslip. Along the streak, *C. albicans* produces pseudomycelia-bearing clusters of blastospores and characteristic thick-walled round chlamydospores (Fig. 20–36).

An excellent medium for the demonstration of chlamydospores is Cream of Rice-Tween 80 agar, which is prepared as follows: one part of Cream of Rice is added to boiling tap water to which 1 per cent agar and one volume per cent Tween 80 are added. The medium is autoclaved and poured in plates. Zein agar is prepared as follows: Soak 40 gm. of zein in 1 liter of distilled water. Heat to 60° C. for 1 hour. Filter through gauze and coarse filter paper and make up to original volume. Add 15 gm. of agar, boil to dissolve, and autoclave at 121° C. for 15 minutes. Dispense as needed.

A rapid method has recently been developed which consists of inoculating a culture into sheep or human serum or egg white and incubating at 37° C. for 3 hours. Production of germ tubes is characteristic of *C. albicans.*

Many other procedures have been developed to differentiate the species of *Candida;* some of these are summarized in Table 20–10.

There have been many studies on the immunology of *C. albicans.* Immunodiffusion and agglutination tests may be of value in systemic infections (Taschdjian, 1972). Recent reports indicate that normal anti-Candida clumping activity is absent in the serum of individuals suffering from mucocutaneous or systemic candidiasis (Louria *et al.,* 1972).

Geotrichosis

Geotrichosis is an infection caused by a yeast-like organism known as *Geotrichum candidum.* This fungus resembles *C. albicans* in many respects and may cause oral, bronchopulmonary, or systemic infections. It can be found frequently in the mouth or intestinal tract of normal individuals. The filamentous type occurs as a contaminant of dairy products and in soil. Consequently the diagnosis of geotrichosis, like that of candidiasis, is justified only by repeated demonstrations of the organism and exclusion of other possible etiologic agents.

Fresh preparations or those mounted in 10 per cent potassium hydroxide or lactophenol cotton blue show oblong or rectangular arthrospores (4 to 8 microns) or larger spherical cells.

The organism grows rapidly on Sabouraud's agar at either room or incubator temperature.

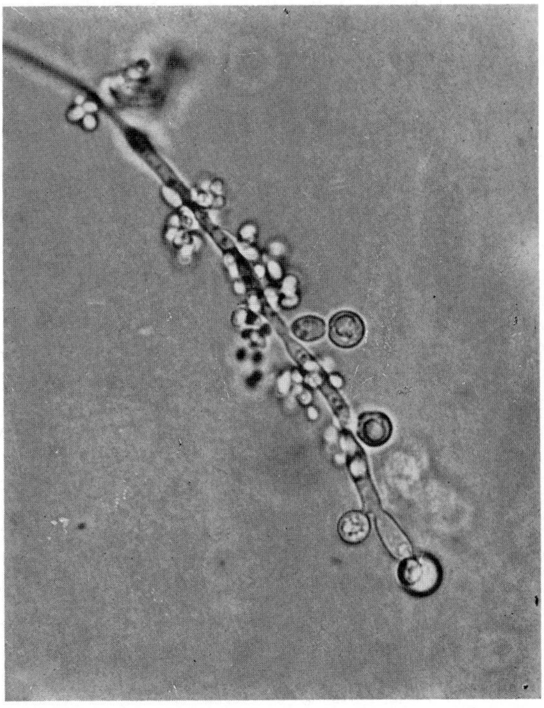

Figure 20–36. *Candida albicans*; terminal chlamydospores on cornmeal agar. (× 700.)

Table 20–10. IDENTIFICATION OF CANDIDA SPECIES

SPECIES	MORPHOLOGY ON CORNMEAL AGAR CUT-STREAK PLATES	GROWTH CHARACTERISTICS (SABOURAUD'S GLUCOSE BROTH)	CARBOHYDRATE FERMENTATION REACTIONS*			
			L	D	M	S
C. albicans	Branched tree-like mycelium with chlamydospores	No surface growth	O	AG	AG	A
C. stellatoidea	Mycelium with large ball-like clusters of blastospores	No surface growth	O	AG	AG	O
C. guillermondii	Well-developed mycelium; no chlamydospores	No surface growth	O	AG/O	O	O
C. krusei	Elongate cells forming a branched mycelium; "crossed sticks" at septa	Wide surface film	O	AG	O	O
C. parapsilosis	Well-developed mycelium; no chlamydospores	No surface growth	O	AG/A	O	O
C. pseudotropicalis	Poorly developed mycelium; no chlamydospores	No surface growth	AG	AG	O	AG
C. tropicalis	Blastospores anywhere along mycelium in irregular clusters; chlamydospores very rare	Narrow surface film with bubbles	O	AG	AG	AG

*L = lactose; D = dextrose; M = maltose; S = sucrose.

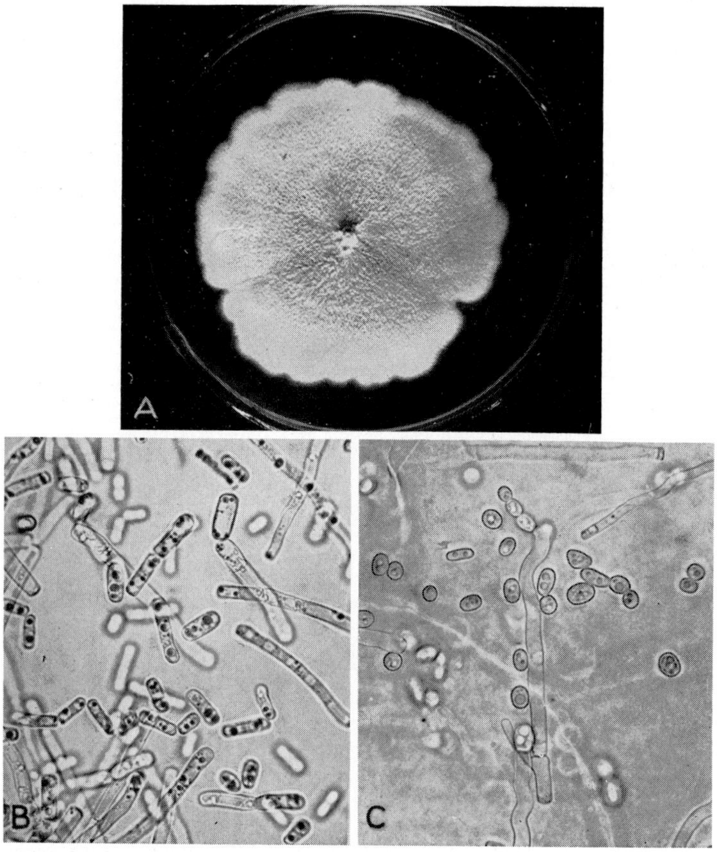

Figure 20–37. *Geotrichum candidum.* *A*, Colony on Sabouraud's glucose agar, 10 days, at room temperature. *B*, Elongate arthrospores. × 790. *C*, Rounded arthrospores. × 650.

The colony is large and mealy and grows mostly below the surface of the agar. There are deep, radial furrows, and older colonies may develop a coarse aerial mycelium. Microscopically hyphae segmenting into typical arthrospores and larger spherical cells are seen (Fig. 20–37). No serologic tests are available for the diagnosis of this disease.

Torulopsis glabrata is a common yeast-like organism in the gastrointestinal tract of man. Systemic infections involving this organism have been reported and are probably more frequent than has previously been suspected. It is frequently isolated from urine specimens, although it is probably not the causative agent of the urinary infection, except perhaps in a diabetic patient. The organism is an ovoid (2 to 3 × 4 to 5 microns) yeast lacking a true capsule and failing to produce hyphae *in vivo* and *in vitro* (Marks *et al.*, 1970).

The ubiquitous red-pigmented yeast *Rhodotorula* has been isolated in the terminal stages from patients with leukemia or carcinoma. It appears to have a very low degree of virulence (Louria *et al.*, 1967). Members of the *Trichosporon* group are the causative agent of white piedra and are rare opportunistic invaders of the skin or mucous membranes. The grow well at 37° C. and produce blastospores as well as arthrospores. *Saccharomyces*, an opportunistic ascosporogenous yeast, is occasionally isolated from human infections.

REFERENCES

Ajello, L.: Comparative ecology of respiratory mycotic disease agents. Bact. Rev. *31*:6, 1967.

Ajello, L. (ed.): Histoplasmosis. Proceedings of the Second National Conference. Springfield, Ill., Charles C Thomas, 1971.

Ajello, L., Georg, L. K., Kaplan, W., and Kaufman, L.: Laboratory Manual for Medical Mycology. Atlanta, Communicable Disease Center, 1963.

Alford, R. H., and Goodwin, R. A.: Patterns of immune response in chronic pulmonary histoplasmosis. J. Infect. Dis. *125*:269, 1972.

Baker, R. D. (ed.): Pathologic Anatomy of Mycoses. New York, Springer-Verlag, Inc., 1971.

Beneke, E. S., and Rogers, A. L.: Medical Mycology Manual. 3rd ed. Minneapolis, Burgess Publishing Co., 1971.

Blank, C. H., and Georg, L. K.: The use of fluorescent antibody methods for detection and identification of *Actinomyces* in clinical material. J. Lab. Clin. Med. *71*:283, 1968.

Brönnestam, R., and Hallberg, T.: Precipitins against an antigen extract of *Aspergillus fumigatus* in patients with aspergillosis or other pulmonary diseases. Acta Med. Scand. *177*:385, 1965.

Busey, J. F., and Hinton, P. F.: Precipitins in histoplasmosis. Amer. Rev. Resp. Dis. *92*:637, 1965.

Campbell, C. C.: Use and interpretation of serologic and skin tests in the respiratory mycoses: Current considerations. Dis. Chest *54*:49, 1968.

Carlisle, H. N., and Saslaw, S.: A histoplasmin-latex agglutination test. J. Lab. Clin. Med. *51*:793, 1958.

Chick, E. W.: Acridine orange fluorescent stain for fungi. Arch. Derm. *83*:659, 1964.

Conant, N. F., Smith, D. T., Baker, R. D., and Callaway, J. L.: Manual of Clinical Mycology. 3rd ed. Philadelphia, W. B. Saunders Company, 1971.

Curry, C. R., and Quie, P. G.: Fungal septicemia in patients receiving parenteral hyperalimentation. New Eng. J. Med. *285*:1221, 1971.

Dolan, C. T., and Woodward, M. R.: Identification of *Cryptococcus* species in the diagnostic laboratory. Amer. J. Clin. Path. *55*:591, 1971.

Emmons, C. W., Binford, C. H., and Utz, J. P.: Medical Mycology. 2nd ed. Philadelphia, Lea & Febiger, 1970.

Evron, R., and Ganor, S.: The use of sodium taurocholate medium for identifying *Candida albicans*. J. Invest. Derm. *51*:108, 1968.

Fetter, B. F., Klintworth, G. H., and Hendry, W. S.: Mycoses of the Central Nervous System. Baltimore, The Williams & Wilkins Company, 1967.

Fischer, J. B., and Kane, J.: Production of chlamydospores by *Candida albicans* cultivated on dilute oxgall agar. Mycopathologia *35*:223, 1968.

Garrison, R. G., *et al.*: A concentration and cultural method for the enhanced isolation of *Histoplasma capsulatum* from sputum. Health Lab. Sci. *8*:231, 1971.

Goldstein, E., and Hoeprich, I. D.: Problems in the diagnosis and treatment of systemic candidiasis. J. Infect. Dis. *125*: 190, 1972.

Goodman, J. S., Kaufman, L., and Koenig, M. G.: Diagnosis of cryptococcal meningitis. Value of immunologic detection of cryptococcal antigen. New Eng. J. Med. *285*:434, 1971.

Gordon, M. A.: Fluorescent staining of *Histoplasma capsulatum*. J. Bact. *77*:678, 1959.

Gordon, M. A., Almyre, G. C. H., and Fenton, J. W.: Diagnostic mycoserology by immunoelectrophoresis. Amer. J. Clin. Path. *56*:471, 1971.

Gorman, J. W.: Sabhi, a new culture medium for pathogenic fungi. Amer. J. Med. Tech. *33*:151, 1967.

Griffin, D. M.: Perfect stage of *Microsporum gypseum*. Nature (London) *186*:94, 1960.

Haley, L.: Diagnostic Medical Mycology. New York, Appleton-Century-Crofts, Inc., 1964.

Hall, C. T., Webb, C. D., and Papageorge, C.: Use of an oxidation-fermentation medium in the identification of yeasts. Pub. Health Rep. *87*:172, 1972.

Hazen, E. L., Gordon, M. A., and Reed, F. C.: Laboratory Identification of Pathogenic Fungi Simplified. 3rd ed. Springfield, Ill., Charles C Thomas, 1970.

Hosty, T. S., *et al.*: Prevalence of *Nocardia asteroides* in sputa examined by a tuberculosis diagnostic laboratory. J. Lab. Clin. Med. *58*:107, 1961.

Huppert, M., and Bailey, J. W.: The use of the immunodiffusion test in coccidioidomycosis. Amer. J. Clin. Path. *44*: 364, 1965.

Kahanpaa, A.: Bronchopulmonary occurrence of fungi in adults. Acta Path. Microbiol. Scand., Suppl. 227, 1972.

Kaplan, W., Huppert, M., Kraft, D. E., and Barley, J.: Fluorescent antibody inhibition test for *Coccidioides immitis* antibodies. Sabouraudia 5:1, 1966.

Keddie, F., Orr, A., and Liebis, D.: Direct staining on vinyl plastic tape; demonstration of the cutaneous flora of the epidermis by the strip method. Sabouraudia *1*:108, 1961.

Lopez, J. F., and Grocott, R. G.: Demonstration of *Histoplasma capsulatum* in peripheral blood by use of methenamine silver nitrate stain (Grocott's). Amer. J. Clin. Path. *50*:692, 1968.

Louria, D. B., *et al:* Fungemia caused by "nonpathogenic" yeasts. Arch. Intern. Med. *119*:247, 1967.

Louria, D. B., *et al.*: Anti-*Candida* factors in serum and their inhibitors. J. Infect. Dis. *125*:102, 1972.

Lynch, H. J., and Plexico, K. L.: A rapid method for screening sputums for *Histoplasma capsulatum* employing the fluorescent antibody technic. New Eng. J. Med. *28*:811, 1962.

Marks, M. I., *et al.*: *Torulopsis glabrata*—An opportunistic pathogen in man. New Eng. J. Med. *283*:1131, 1970.

McGinnis, M. R., and Hilger, A. E.: A key to the genera of medically important fungi. Mycopathologia *45*:269, 1971.

Rebell, G., and Taplin, D.: Dermatophytes. Their Recognition and Identification. 2nd ed. Coral Gables, Fla., University of Miami Press, 1970.
Roberts, G. O., and Larsh, H. W.: The serologic diagnosis of extracutaneous sporotrichosis. Amer. J. Clin. Path. *55*: 596, 1971.
Sanford, L. V., Mason, K. N., and Hathaway, B. M.: The concentration of sputum for fungus culture. Amer. J. Clin. Path. *44*:172, 1965.
Sawaki, Y., Huppert, M., Bailey, J. W., and Yagi, Y.: Patterns of human antibody reactions in coccidioidomycosis. J. Bact. *91*:422, 1966.
Schubert, J. H., and Wiggins, G. L.: The evaluation of serologic tests for histoplasmosis in relation to the clinical diagnosis. Amer. J. Hyg. *77*:240, 1963.
Seelig, M. S.: The role of antibiotics in the pathogenesis of *Candida* infection. Amer. J. Med. *40*:887, 1966.
Shields, A. B., and Ajello, L.: Medium for selective isolation of *Cryptococcus neoformans*. Science *151*:208, 1966.
Stockdale, P. M.: *Nannizzia incurvata gen. nov., sp. nov.,* a perfect state of *Microsporum gypseum* (Bodin). Sabouraudia *1*:41, 1961.
Taplin, D., Zaias, N., Rebell, G., and Blank, H.: Isolation and recognition of dermatophytes on a new culture medium (DTM). Arch. Derm. *99*:203, 1969.
Taschdjian, C. L., *et al.:* Serodiagnosis of Candidal infections. Amer. J. Clin. Path. *57*:195, 1972.
Vanek, J., Schwarz, J., and Hakim, S.: North American blastomycosis. A study of 10 cases. Amer. J. Clin. Path. *54*: 384, 1970.
Walter, J. W., and Atchison, R. W.: Epidemiological and immunological studies of *Cryptococcus neoformans*. J. Bact. *93*:82, 1966.
Wiegand, S. E.: Ink blue agar for recognition of dermatophytes. Bull. Path. *10*:68, 1969.
Wilson, J. W., and Plunkett, O. A.: The Fungus Diseases of Man. Berkeley, California, University of California Press, 1965.
Zaias, N., Taplin, D., and Rebell, G.: Mycetoma. Arch. Derm. *99*:215, 1969.

Chapter 21

LABORATORY DIAGNOSIS OF VIRAL, RICKETTSIAL, BEDSONIAL AND MYCOPLASMAL DISEASES*

by JESSE H. MARYMONT, JR., M.D.

More human diseases are caused by viruses than by any other single group of infectious agents. The common syndromes together with the viruses responsible for them are listed in Table 21-1. Most clinicians who care for patients with these illnesses and most pathologists responsible for the management of clinical laboratories know little about the techniques available for their definitive diagnoses. Moreover, only a handful of clinical laboratories do any diagnostic virology. There are many reasons given for this such as: too expensive; results take so long to obtain that they are of little value; and diagnosis makes little difference if no therapy is available. These statements are not true. Drugs have been developed that are of value in specific viral diseases, such as idoxuridine for herpes simplex encephalitis and amantadine for control of influenza; certainly more will become available in the future. Rapid diagnostic procedures that measure specific IgM antibodies or detect viral antigens by fluorescence microscopy have been developed. Such tests permit an etiologic diagnosis in only a few hours. These and other diagnostic procedures are not prohibitively expensive and should be done in clinical laboratories.

There are three basic methods for the laboratory diagnosis of a viral infection: (1) Microscopic examination of secretions or tissues for specific morphologic alterations; (2) demonstration of the presence of, or a rise in, the titer of a specific antibody; and (3) isolation and identification of the virus.

The first method has relatively few applications in the clinical laboratory, but on occasion may be of great value. For example, rapid differentiation of variola (smallpox) from the eruptions due to the herpesvirus group (herpes simplex and varicella-zoster) can be done by direct examination of smears from skin lesions. The elementary bodies characteristic of the poxviruses are easily distinguished from the giant cells and inclusions of herpes simplex or varicella-zoster infection. Other examples are the characteristic inclusions of congenital cytomegalovirus disease which may be found in the urinary sediment, and fluorescent antibody techniques for detection of Negri bodies in cases of suspected rabies.

Usually, but not always, serologic methods require two sera taken one to several weeks apart. Most viral illnesses are acute and of brief duration, and when it is necessary to show a fourfold rise in antibody titer, the diagnosis is retrospective. While it may have profound prognostic significance, such a diagnosis is established too late to guide or influence therapy. Several viruses can often produce a similar illness and the paired sera must be tested against a battery of antigens, a not inexpensive undertaking. These comments are not intended to minimize the importance of classic viral serology, but rather to indicate that the information may be expensive to obtain and relatively late in forthcoming. Since this information is not of immediate clinical value, the tests need not be done in the routine diagnostic laboratory. Public health facilities offer a variety of serologic procedures, and the

*Sections were reviewed by H. H. Marsh, III, M.D., R. Martins, M.D. and W. Walker, Ph.D. I am grateful for their suggestions.

Table 21–1. SYNDROMES AND THE VIRUSES WITH WHICH THEY ARE COMMONLY ASSOCIATED*

SYNDROME	VIRUS	SYNDROME	VIRUS
Neonatal jaundice, thrombocytopenia, hepatosplenomegaly, chorioretinitis	Cytomegalovirus Rubella virus Herpes simplex virus		Influenza virus Enterovirus Rhinovirus
Lymphadenopathy	Epstein-Barr virus or herpes-like virus Cytomegalovirus Cat scratch disease virus	Encephalitis and aseptic meningitis	Measles virus Mumps virus Poliovirus Echovirus Coxsackievirus Herpes simplex virus
Parotitis	Mumps virus Parainfluenza virus Lymphocytic choriomeningitis virus Enterovirus	Myocarditis	Coxsackie B virus Echovirus Mumps virus Measles virus
Rash	Varicella-zoster virus Herpes simplex virus Variola virus Vaccinia virus Rubella virus Coxsackievirus Echovirus Measles virus	Hepatitis	Cytomegalovirus Hepatitis-associated antigen Epstein-Barr virus
		Vaccine-associated disease	Measles virus Poliovirus Mumps virus Vaccinia virus Rubella virus Smallpox virus
Acute respiratory disease	Respiratory syncytial virus Parainfluenza virus Adenovirus		

*From Gershon, A. A.: Diagnostic Virology. Pediat. Clin. N. Amer. *18*:78, 1971.

clinical pathologist should be familiar with his local situation.

There are, however, a few serologic procedures of value when done on a single serum specimen. The mumps virus has two antigens, designated S (soluble) and V (viral). Antibodies develop earlier to the former, and an elevated S antibody titer with low or absent V antibody in the first few days of illness is presumptive evidence of mumps. Any titer in the rubella hemagglutination-inhibition test indicates previous disease (or vaccination), and hence immunity, and is significant in the pregnant woman exposed to German measles. Some of the arbovirus diseases are uncommon in this country, and an elevated titer on a single specimen from a sick patient is suggestive of the disease. Finally, one must mention tests that measure specific IgM antibodies. These have been developed for rubella and cytomegalovirus disease and are sometimes the only way to make a diagnosis rapidly. In the pregnant woman the availability of such a test for rubella may permit the decision to perform a therapeutic abortion while the surgery is still relatively simple. The diagnostic laboratory interested in viral serology should select procedures that give useful information from a single serum specimen.

Tissue culture systems have made virus isolation a relatively simple procedure. It is usually possible to determine the broad group to which an isolate belongs (i.e., adenovirus, herpesvirus or enterovirus) both quickly and easily but often more difficult and time consuming to make a specific identification (i.e., adenovirus type 5 or echovirus type 11). This is an obstacle to clinical diagnostic virology *only* if the information is essential to the clinician. A rapid presumptive report is preferable to a delayed definitive one. For example, report of an enterovirus in the spinal fluid of a patient in 48 hours or of a herpesvirus in the vagina of a pregnant woman near term in 24 hours is of great therapeutic value in contrast to a report of an adenovirus type 7 from an acute follicular conjunctivitis three weeks after submission of the specimen. Herrmann,* working at the Mayo Clinic, was able to give a presumptive identification of virus isolates within seven days in 73 per cent of his cases and in four days in almost 50 per cent, with a

*E. C. Herrmann, Jr., wrote many papers on diagnostic virology while at the Mayo Clinic. Some are provocative, but all are informative and should be read by those interested in establishing a diagnostic virology facility. Some are listed in the references of this chapter.

significant error of less than 5 per cent. Virus isolation, therefore, is a method that often will give valuable information while the patient is still ill.

SELECTION AND COLLECTION OF SPECIMENS*

Both the type of illness and its stage when the patient first seeks medical care (or the physician first considers the possibility of a viral etiology) determines the laboratory procedures and, therefore, the specimens to be obtained. As a general rule, virus isolation requires material gathered early in the course of illness, and demonstration of specific antibody is possible only later in the disease. These relationships are shown in Table 21–2.

There are some simple guidelines concerning specimens for virus isolation. Feces, throat swabs,† and spinal fluids should be obtained from all patients with aseptic meningitis or encephalitis. If mumps is suspected, urine may also be of value. Throat swabs are required from all patients with respiratory illnesses, and if an adenovirus or enterovirus is suspected, feces are obtained. Vesicle fluid and throat swabs are necessary from patients with vesicular lesions of the skin or mucous membranes. Urine, throat swabs, feces, and vesicle fluid (if available) are cultured from infants with congenital or neonatal illnesses suspected of having a viral etiology. The specimens desired are summarized in Table 21–3.

Feces are collected in 1-ounce, glass, screw-capped bottles and may be mailed without refrigeration. To prevent drying they should not be sent in cardboard containers. Remember that postal regulations require that all potentially infectious materials be shipped in double containers unless hermetically sealed.

Respiratory viruses are among the more labile responsible for disease, and correct handling of throat swabs and washings might be facilitated by a brief statement about how to avoid their inactivation. Most are damaged by an acid pH or by drying, and protein tends to serve as a stabilizer; therefore, throat swabs should immediately be thoroughly wrung out in a buffered, protein-containing solution. Any of the common bacteriologic broths such as trypticase soy or brain-heart infusion is entirely satisfactory. If throat washings are desired, 1 per cent skim milk is satisfactory and palatable; it is my personal opinion that authors who suggest gargling with bacteriologic media have never tasted it! If the laboratory does its own virus isolation, the throat swab media can contain antibiotics and an antimycotic and be kept stored frozen for months until ready for use. A satisfactory preparation is given in the section on reagents, p. 1158. It is left at room temperature for 30 to 60 minutes after wringing out the swab and then inoculated into tissue culture tubes. Liquid for throat washings should *never* contain antibiotics because of the risk of untoward reactions in those sensitive to them. If the specimen is to be mailed it should be both stored and shipped frozen at −50 to −70° C.; the ordinary −20° C. freezer is not satisfactory. In most laboratories dry ice will be used for both storage and shipment.

Spinal fluid (CSF) for virus isolation should be stored and shipped frozen with dry ice. Antibody levels on CSF are rarely useful, but if subacute sclerosing panencephalitis is suspected, high antibody levels against measles (rubeola) should be sought. CSF for this purpose need not be refrigerated.

Urine is usually not used for virus isolation, but if cytomegalovirus disease is suspected, 10 to 20 ml. should be collected and immedi-

Table 21–2. RELATION OF STAGE OF ILLNESS TO PRESENCE OF VIRUS IN TEST MATERIAL AND TO APPEARANCE OF ANTIBODY*

STAGE OF ILLNESS	VIRUS DEMONSTRABLE IN APPROPRIATE TEST MATERIAL	SPECIFIC ANTIBODY PRESENT IN SERUM
Incubation period	Rarely	–
Prodromal period	Rarely	–
Onset	Frequently	–
Acute phase	Frequently	Frequently or generally†
Recovery phase	Rarely	Generally
Convalescence	Very rarely	Usually

*From Lennette, E. H., and Schmidt, N. J. (eds.): Diagnostic Procedures for Viral and Rickettsial Infections. 4th ed. New York, American Public Health Association, 1969, p. 31.

†In certain widespread endemic diseases, antibody representing prior experience with the agent is generally encountered in acute-phase blood (e.g., influenza, herpes simplex). In other instances (Western equine encephalomyelitis, poliomyelitis), antibody is frequently present in acute-phase serum; antibody formation apparently is well under way by the time the acute-phase specimen is taken.

Whether antibody is encountered will also depend upon the type of antibody (neutralizing, CF, or HI), because of temporal differences in persistence after infection.

*Some of this material is from a draft of an informational guide, *Viral Laboratory Services of Public Health Laboratories in California*, and I am indebted to Dr. Edwin Lennette for permission to quote from it.

†Nasopharyngeal washings may be substituted for throat swabs.

Table 21–3. SPECIMENS TO BE COLLECTED FOR VIRUS ISOLATION FROM THE COMMON CLINICAL SYNDROMES

SYNDROME	FECES	THROAT SWABS	CSF	URINE	VESICLE FLUID
Meningitis* or Encephalitis					
Enterovirus	+	+	+		
Mumps		+	+	+	
Herpes simplex		+			+
Respiratory infection					
Adenovirus	+	+			
Influenza		+			
Parainfluenza		+			
Enterovirus	+	+			
Rhinovirus		+			
Resp. syncytial		+			
Skin and mucous membrane infection†					
Herpes simplex		+			+
Poxviruses		+			+
Varicella-zoster					+
Newborn and neonatal infections‡					
Herpes simplex		+			+
Cytomegalovirus		+		+	
Enterovirus	+	+			

*Lymphocytic choriomeningitis, arbovirus, and rabies infections are diagnosed serologically, not by routine virus isolation. Herpes simplex infection is usually diagnosed by brain biopsy.

†Herpangina is due to a coxsackievirus A that can be isolated only in suckling mice.

‡Rubella is a serologic diagnosis. Virus isolation is possible but difficult, and usually not required.

ately shipped *chilled on wet ice*. For other viruses urine should be sent frozen with dry ice.

Autopsy tissues in ½- to 1-inch cubes should be placed in individual screw-capped glass bottles and sent frozen. In cases of central nervous system disease, individual specimens from the temporal lobe cortex, midbrain, medulla, and spinal cord as well as a 2- to 3-inch segment of descending colon, tied off with contents for enteroviruses, should be sent.

Smears from possible smallpox victims are air dried. If lesions are vesicular the base of the vesicle is gently scraped, and if maculopapular a scalpel with a cutting edge is used; in either case epithelial cells are essential. Poxviruses withstand drying, and this material is highly infectious. If sent to a reference laboratory the package must be clearly labeled "Highly infectious material from suspected smallpox."

Viral antibodies are stable at 4° C., and sera to be kept in the laboratory for more than a few hours should be stored in the refrigerator. This is satisfactory for at least a month, and there is no good evidence that freezing is either necessary or beneficial. Serum should be removed from the clot before shipment, if possible, and need not be refrigerated during shipment.

TISSUE CULTURE TECHNIQUES*

Tissue culture remains an art in an era of scientific laboratory medicine, but fortunately the skills are fairly easily acquired and, since they are largely repetitive, an aide or laboratory assistant can be responsible for diagnostic cell cultures. There are a variety of cell culture techniques, but we shall be concerned only with monolayer cultures. These are prepared by dispersing tissue cells with a proteolytic enzyme such as trypsin, suspending them in growth medium (a liquid rich in nutrients), and then aliquoting them into tubes or bottles. The cells sink to the glass or plastic surface where they adhere and proliferate until a confluent cell sheet one cell in thickness develops. They then stop dividing as a result of a poorly understood phenomenon called contact inhibition, at which time maintenance medium (a liquid with only enough nutrients to keep the cells viable and slowly metabolizing and with no viral inhibitors) is substituted. On maintenance

*The chapter "Tissue Culture Technics for Diagnostic Virology" by N. J. Schmidt, in *Diagnostic Procedures for Viral and Rickettsial Infections*, 4th ed., American Public Health Association, New York, 1969, is a comprehensive source for specific details about all commonly used procedures. It served as a reference for some of the material in this section.

medium the cells are ready for virus isolation and remain satisfactory for this purpose for several weeks.

In this section we shall discuss the kinds of cells useful for diagnostic virology and the media required for their growth and maintenance. Preparation of specimens for inoculation into tissue culture and the common methods for recognition of the presence of an isolate will also be outlined.

Types of Cell Cultures

There are three basic types of cell cultures. *Primary cultures* are obtained directly from the parent tissue. The cells may be subcultured once, giving *secondary cultures* which are similar in microscopic appearance and viral sensitivity. For example, primary embryonic human kidney (EHK) cultures are prepared from fetuses of at least three months' gestation. With sterile technique the kidneys are removed and minced with scalpel or scissors, and the individual cells are dispersed with a trypsin solution. The cells are then suspended in growth medium and placed in tubes or bottles where a monolayer forms in four to six days. Although these primary cells are viable for several weeks, a pair of human kidneys supplies enough cells for hundreds of tubes, and since most laboratories cannot use that many at one time the bottle cultures can again be dispersed, the cells being placed in freezing medium and stored indefinitely in liquid nitrogen. When removed, they are suspended in growth medium and planted in tubes. The resultant monolayers of secondary cells are then used for virus isolation.

Primary (or secondary) cell cultures are among the most sensitive (and therefore desirable and satisfactory) for virus isolation. In addition to EHK, other primary cell cultures useful in diagnostic virology include those prepared from human amnion as well as rhesus and African green monkey kidney.

There are several *cell lines,* all with about the same viral spectrum and derived from human carcinomas, that are sometimes used in the clinical laboratory. The most popular are HeLa from a cervix carcinoma, KB from a carcinoma of the nasopharynx and HEp-2. These cells maintain some of their malignant characteristics in culture. They grow rapidly, are heteroploid, and can be passaged indefinitely; i.e., with proper care they are immortal. Most laboratories purchase a bottle of the desired strain which is periodically (every four to seven days) divided to produce both new tubes for virus isolation and bottles for continued laboratory propagation. Continuous cells do not have a wide range of viral sensitivity but are useful in specific situations.

Diploid cell strains are usually derived from embryonic human lung. Their initial preparation is similar to that described for primary EHK, but in contrast they maintain their diploid chromosome number on repeated passage. Unfortunately, however, they are mortal and usually die after 20 to 50 such passages. This problem is circumvented by periodically either buying or removing from liquid nitrogen previously frozen, low-passage cells. The diploid strains, in contrast to the other described, are connective tissue (fibroblast), not epithelial. They rival primary cells in sensitivity for virus isolation and are essential if certain agents such as cytomegalovirus (which will not grow in epithelial cultures) are to be isolated. A diploid cell strain is used in most diagnostic virus laboratories.

Selection of Cell Cultures

The success of the diagnostic virology laboratory is intimately related to the cell cultures used. The greater their number and variety the higher will be the virus isolation rate from clinical specimens, but financial considerations impose practical limitations.

Primary rhesus monkey kidney (RMK) cells have the widest spectrum of viral sensitivity and are the *best single cell culture available.** They are necessary for recovery of parainfluenza and mumps viruses and are highly satisfactory for most of the enteroviruses, adenoviruses, and influenza viruses. They cannot be depended upon for isolation of herpes simplex virus and most of the rhinoviruses.

The majority of clinical laboratories buy RMK tubes on a weekly or biweekly standing order basis. Cell suspensions are available for heavy users, and very large facilities buy and keep rhesus monkeys.

Primary embryonic human kidney cells are not satisfactory for parainfluenza or mumps virus isolation and this prevents their substitution for simian cells. They are, however, one of the best for both adenoviruses and herpes simplex virus and are satisfactory for many enteroviruses and rhinoviruses. They are unsatisfactory for respiratory syncytial virus, parainfluenza and influenza viruses, and cytomegalovirus. The laboratory that can readily obtain these from autopsy or abortion material should consider their use, but they are not worth purchasing in addition to RMK.

---

*Kidney cells from a variety of different monkey species are used in virology for specific purposes. While many have an approximately similar range of virus sensitivity, rhesus is generally preferred for routine diagnostic work.

Table 21–4. TISSUE CULTURE CELLS USEFUL IN DIAGNOSTIC VIROLOGY AND THE VIRUSES THAT CAN BE ISOLATED WITH THEM

VIRUS	PRIMARY RMK	PRIMARY EHK	DIPLOID HL	HUMAN CCL
Adenoviruses	+	++	+	+
Herpes simplex virus	0*	++	+	+
Echoviruses	++	+	+	0
Polioviruses	++	+	+	+
Coxsackieviruses A	0†	0	0	0
Coxsackieviruses B	++	+	0	+
Rhinoviruses	0‡	+	++	0
Parainfluenza viruses	++	0	0	0
Influenza viruses	+§	0	0	0
Mumps virus	++	0	0	0
Respiratory syncytial virus	+	0	++	++
Cytomegalovirus	0	0	++	0

RMK = rhesus monkey kidney; EHK = embryonic human kidney; HL = human lung; CCL = continuous cell line. A ++ means that the cell has maximum sensitivity for isolation of the virus, a + means that the cell is satisfactory for routine isolation, and an 0 means that the cell is not reliable for routine use. Viruses may be isolated in cells listed with an 0; however, this will be sporadic and unpredictable.

*Genital strains (type 2) of *H. hominis* may be isolated in primary RMK.

†Some coxsackieviruses A can be isolated in tissue culture, but many will be missed if suckling mice are not used.

‡A few rhinoviruses (designated M strains) can be isolated in primary RMK.

§Some strains of influenza A are isolated best in embryonated eggs. Influenza C is isolated only in eggs.

Diploid human lung cells are widely used and complement primary RMK. They are necessary for cytomegalovirus isolation, excellent for the rhinoviruses and respiratory syncytial virus, and satisfactory for many enteroviruses, adenoviruses, and herpes simplex virus. They are unsatisfactory for parainfluenza, influenza, and mumps virus isolation.

Continuous cell lines are excellent for respiratory syncytial virus. They are satisfactory for herpes simplex virus, some enteroviruses, and adenoviruses, but these and other commonly encountered agents can be isolated as well in one of the cells discussed previously.

In summary, at least two different cell cultures are necessary in the clinical laboratory, and the preferred are probably primary RMK and diploid human lung. Laboratories that use three cells commonly select one of the continuous cell lines in addition. Primary EHK are useful if the laboratory can obtain them from autopsy or abortion material. The virus sensitivity of the different cells is summarized in Table 21–4.

Media

There are a large number of different culture media available, but only a very few are required in the diagnostic laboratory. These can be purchased ready to use, as a concentrated (10×) solution, or as a powder that is mixed with water and then filter sterilized. The choice depends on the relative advantages of convenience versus cost, the latter being much cheaper than either of the former. Powdered media can be stored in a desiccator in the refrigerator for many months. Liquid media are stable for long periods of time when frozen at −20° C. In my laboratory we find it convenient to purchase the powder in preweighed packages for preparation of 10 liters of medium. Two are dissolved to make 2 L. of a 10× solution, filter sterilized, and frozen in 250 ml. aliquots. It is preferable to use pressure rather than suction filtration, and a membrane (millipore or nucleopore) rather than an asbestos pad (Seitz-type) filter. Asbestos pads may contribute undesirable inorganic ions and must be washed before use and then the first 100 ml. of filtered medium discarded. All media should be cultured routinely for sterility before use.

Hanks' and Earle's balanced salt solutions (BSS) serve as the base for almost all media and are used as general diluents in the virology laboratory. Both are similar in that the largest component is sodium chloride. They differ in buffering capacity, the latter being the stronger buffer and useful in maintenance medium where established cells produce large amounts of acid, and the former of value in growth medium where minimal acid is produced by developing cultures. The composition of each is shown in Table 21–5.

Phenol red, a nontoxic pH indicator in the range used in tissue culture work, is an integral part of most media. It is purple at a pH of 8.4 or greater, which is above that tolerated by

Table 21–5. COMPOSITION OF HANKS' AND EARLE'S BALANCED SALT SOLUTIONS*

COMPONENT	CONCENTRATION (GRAMS PER LITER) IN 1X SOLUTION	
	Hanks' BSS	Earle's BSS
NaCl	8.00	6.80
KCl	0.40	0.40
$CaCl_2$	0.14	0.20
$MgSO_4$-$7H_2O$	0.20	0.20
$Na_2HPO_4 \cdot 12H_2O$	0.12	–
NaH_2PO_4	–	0.125
KH_2PO_4	0.06	–
$NaHCO_3$	0.35†	2.20‡
Glucose	1.00	1.00
Phenol red, 1% solution	1.60 ml§	1.60 ml

*From Lennette, E. H., and Schmidt, N. J. (eds.): Diagnostic Procedures for Viral and Rickettsial Infections. 4th ed. New York, American Public Health Association, 1969, p. 93.

†Prepared as a 2.8 per cent stock solution and added at the time of use.

‡Prepared as an 8.8 per cent stock solution and added at the time of use.

§If a somewhat deeper red color is preferred, 2.0 ml may be used.

most cell cultures, yellow at a pH of 6.8 or below, and red in the physiological range.

Serum is almost always required in growth and usually in maintenance media. Fetal or agamma calf serum is free of most viral inhibitors and is preferable. If ordinary calf serum is used in growth medium, the cell sheet must be washed prior to addition of maintenance medium to remove these inhibitors. Chicken serum is usually free of inhibitors but is not so satisfactory for either growth or maintenance of cultures. Human serum is, of course, a rich source of viral antibodies. It can be used in growth medium, but washing of the cell sheets before use for virus isolation is mandatory. Sera are stable for months when stored frozen to protect labile components.

Bicarbonate ion is necessary for cell growth, and almost all media use a carbonic acid–sodium bicarbonate buffer system. Since the carbonic acid is volatile, cell cultures must be kept tightly sealed to avoid an undesirable rise in pH. For some tissue culture work in microtiter plates it is convenient not to need a closed system and this can be accomplished with nonvolatile HEPES buffer.* Leibovitz Medium No. 15 contains galactose instead of glucose and is useful when a low bicarbonate concentration is required, such as for isolation of some rhinoviruses.

Originally only biologic materials such as lactalbumin hydrolysate, yeast extract, and chick embryo extract, containing unknown concentrations of nutrients, were available for tissue culture work. They are still useful and are obtainable from many suppliers. Today, however, chemically defined media are readily available and enjoy great popularity, the most widely used being Medium 199 and two media devised by Eagle. Basal medium, Eagle (BME) contains all nutrients required for cell growth, while Eagle's minimum essential medium (MEM) contains these in optimum concentrations. The compositions of representative chemically defined media are shown in Table 21–6.

The choice of media and sera depends on personal preference and the tissue cultures used. MEM with Hanks' BSS base is excellent for growth of cell cultures, and with serum is satisfactory for all those usually employed in diagnostic virology. MEM with Earle's BSS will serve as the basis of a general maintenance medium. I personally prefer fetal bovine serum for both growth and maintenance. Although expensive, it is not necessary to wash cell cultures to remove viral inhibitors before using for isolation, as with human or calf serum.

*Calbiochem, P.O. Box 54282, Terminal Annex, Los Angeles, California.

Reagents

The selection of water for use in tissue culture work is important, and either deionized or double distilled (the second distillation being performed in a glass still) is recommended. We have always used liter bottles of sterile distilled water for intravenous use, an expensive but convenient and satisfactory source.

There are many satisfactory antibiotic combinations, but the simplest is penicillin G and streptomycin prepared in either sterile water or Hanks' BSS, frozen at a concentration of 25,000 U./ml. and μg./ml. respectively, and added to media at a final concentration of 1 per cent. These antibiotics are not toxic to tissue culture if used at moderately higher concentrations, and preparations from the pharmacy are satisfactory. They are stable for months when frozen.

Amphotericin B* for tissue culture use is a satisfactory antimycotic and is prepared in either sterile water or Hanks' BSS at a concentration of 100 μg./ml. and used in media at a final concentration of 1 per cent. If it does not readily go into solution, the pH should be adjusted to 7.3 to 7.4 with bicarbonate.

Sodium bicarbonate, 2.8 per cent for addition to growth medium and 8.8 per cent for maintenance medium, is prepared in water and filter sterilized. This is stored frozen.

*E. R. Squibb and Sons, New York, N. Y.

Table 21–6. COMPOSITION OF THREE SYNTHETIC MEDIA EMPLOYED IN DIAGNOSTIC VIROLOGY*

	CONCENTRATION (mg./L.)				CONCENTRATION (mg./L.)		
COMPONENTS	Medium #199	Eagle's Minimum Essential Medium	Leibovitz Medium #15 (L-15)	COMPONENTS	Medium #199	Eagle's Minimum Essential Medium	Leibovitz Medium #15 (L-15)
Amino acids				α-tocopherol phosphate	0.01		
L-alanine	50†		450†	calciferol	0.10		
L-arginine	70	105	500‡	menadione	0.01		
L-asparagine			250				
L-aspartic acid	60†			*Nucleic acid derivatives*			
L-cysteine	0.10		120‡	adenine	10		
L-cystine	20	24		guanine · HCl	0.3		
L-glutamic acid	150†			hypoxanthine	0.3		
L-glutamine	100	292	292	thymine	0.3		
glycine	50		200	uracil	0.3		
L-histidine	20	31	250‡	xanthine	0.3		
hydroxy-L-proline	10			adenylic acid	0.2		
L-isoleucine	40†	52	250†				
L-leucine	120†	52	125	*Carbohydrates*			
L-lysine	70	58	75	2-deoxy-D-ribose	0.5		
L-methionine	30†	15	150†	D-ribose	0.5		
L-phenylalanine	25	32	250†	glucose	1000	1000	
L-proline	40			galactose			900
L-serine	50†		200				
L-threonine	60†	48	300	*Miscellaneous*			
L-tryptophane	20†	10	20	sodium acetate	50		
L-tyrosine	40	36	300	sodium pyruvate			550
L-valine	50†	46	200†	Tween-80	5.0		
				cholesterol	0.2		
Vitamins				glutathione	0.05		
p-aminobenzoic acid	0.05			adenosine triphosphate	10		
biotin	0.01			phenol red	20	20	10–20
Ca pantothenate	0.01	1.0	1.0				
choline chloride	0.50	1.0	1.0	*Salts*			
folic acid	0.01	1.0	1.0	NaCl	6800	6800	8000
i-inositol	0.05	2.0	2.0	KCl	400	400	400
niacin	0.025			$CaCl_2$	200	200	140
niacinamide	0.025	1.0	1.0	$MgCl \cdot 6H_2O$		200	200
pyridoxal · HCl	0.025	1.0	1.0	$MgSO_4 \cdot 7H_2O$	200		200
pyridoxine · HCl	0.025			$NaH_2PO_4 \cdot H_2O$	140	140	
riboflavin	0.01	0.1	0.1	$Na_2HPO_4 \cdot H_2O$			70
thiamine · HCl	0.01	1.0	1.0	KH_2PO_4			60
vitamin A	0.10			$Fe(NO_3)_3 \cdot 9H_2O$	0.1		
ascorbic acid	0.05			$NaHCO_3$	2200	2200	

*From Lennette, E. H., and Schmidt, N. J. (eds.): Diagnostic Procedures for Viral and Rickettsial Infections. 4th ed. New York, American Public Health Association, 1969, p. 95.

†Amount of DL-form of amino acid rather than L-form.

‡Free base form.

Trypsin is ordinarily purchased as a sterile 2.5 per cent solution and diluted 1:10 with Hanks' or Earle's BSS before use. It is, however, expensive if purchased in this form, and because we are unable to filter the protein material with the equipment available, we have devised a highly unorthodox but satisfactory method for preparation from crude trypsin 1:250* or 1:300.† A 7.5 per cent (w./v.) solution in water containing 10 per cent stock antibiotic and antimycotic (v./v.) is prepared. This is centrifuged at 4° C. at 30,000 × g. for 30 minutes and the supernate removed with sterile technique. After check of the sterility it is stored frozen and is stable for at least six months. It is diluted to a final concentration of 0.25 per cent with a balanced salt solution and the pH adjusted to 7.5 to 7.6 with 8.8 per cent bicarbonate before use.

Our throat swab medium consists of 10.5 ml. each of the antibiotic and antimycotic solutions

*Difco, Detroit, Michigan.

†Nutritional Biochemicals Corp., Cleveland, Ohio.

and 79 ml. of heart infusion broth adjusted to a pH of 7.2 to 7.4. It is tubed in 2-ml. aliquots and is stable for many months when frozen.

Preparation of Specimens

Feces. A suspension is prepared by thoroughly mixing about 2 gm. of feces with 12 ml. of Hanks' BSS in a conical centrifuge tube. This can be accomplished either with wooden applicator sticks or by vigorous shaking. The material is then centrifuged at 2500 r.p.m. for 10 minutes to remove most particulate matter. Two and a half milliliters of the supernate and 0.5 ml. of the previously described antibiotic solution are mixed in another centrifuge tube and left at room temperature for 30 minutes. If a high speed refrigerated centrifuge is available, it is desirable to centrifuge at 10,000 r.p.m. for 1 hour at 4° C.; this removes material toxic to tissue cultures. If this cannot be accomplished conveniently, the material is again centrifuged at 2500 r.p.m. for 30 minutes. Aliquots of 0.25 ml. are inoculated into tissue culture tubes and the media changed 24 hours later.

Throat Swabs. Throat swabs are vigorously agitated in the previously described media, thoroughly wrung out on the side of the tube and discarded. The solution is left at room temperature for 30 minutes and 0.25 ml. aliquots placed into tissue culture tubes.

Urine. The pH of the sample is adjusted to 7.0 to 7.2 with 2.8 per cent sodium bicarbonate. If much particulate matter is present, the urine is centrifuged. Urine, 1.8 ml., is mixed with 0.2 ml. of antibiotic solution, left at room temperature for 30 minutes, and 0.25 ml. aliquots set in tissue culture tubes.

Spinal Fluid. Aliquots of 0.5 ml. of CSF are placed directly into tissue culture tubes. If the volume available is small, we set only a monkey kidney tube because the majority of isolates will be either an enterovirus or mumps virus.

Recognition of Viruses in Cell Cultures

The majority of virus isolates produce a morphologic alteration called cytopathic effect, or CPE, in the tissue cultures they infect. Although the CPE produced by a specific virus may be somewhat different in different cell cultures and in cell cultures that are rolled instead of being held in stationary racks, the CPE of the different virus groups is distinctive and permits a tentative group identification. The commonly isolated agents that produce typical CPE include the enteroviruses, cytomegalovirus, adenoviruses, respiratory syncytial virus, the herpesvirus group, and often mumps virus. Their typical morphology is illustrated in the appropriate sections of this chapter.

Some specimens, particularly feces and tissue homogenates, are toxic to tissue culture cells and can produce changes indistinguishable from CPE. This usually occurs rapidly (within 24 hours) and can be recognized by transferring a small amount of material to new cell cultures. Toxic products are diluted so that no change occurs, whereas a virus will again produce CPE.

A few viruses infect cells and produce either minimal and inconstant alterations or none at all. The majority of these are detected by a hemadsorption test in which guinea pig erythrocytes are added to cell cultures. If cells are infected the erythrocytes adhere to them, a phenomenon easily recognized microscopically. The commonly encountered hemadsorbing agents include the parainfluenza and influenza viruses and mumps virus.

Rubella virus does not hemadsorb and produces no CPE in African green monkey kidney, which is often used for isolation. Its presence is recognized by an interference test. Some of the enteroviruses (among others) that produce typical CPE in these kidney cells fail to do so if the culture has been previously infected with rubella virus. In other words, the rubella virus interferes with penetration of the enterovirus into the infected kidney cells. This test, while simple in theory, is technically demanding, and specimens for isolation of rubella virus should be sent to a reference laboratory.

Identification of an Isolate

Tissue culture techniques have made virus isolation a simple procedure, but characterization of an agent can require considerable skill and judgment. Diagnostic laboratories should attempt to identify the majority of their isolates, but the help of a reference laboratory will occasionally be required. The ability and willingness of the various state public health laboratories to provide this service varies widely.

Some viruses can be reliably identified on the basis of the cell cultures in which they replicate, whether or not they hemadsorb guinea pig erythrocytes (and if so, at what temperatures), the specimens from which they were obtained, and the type of CPE. For example, an isolate from the urine of a newborn which slowly produces discrete islands of rounded cells only in diploid human lung is safely called a cytomegalovirus. An agent from the spinal fluid of a child with mild encephalitis which produces syncytia in primary rhesus monkey kidney and hemadsorbs at both 4° C.

and room temperature can be considered a mumps virus. Other agents that may be characterized in this way include respiratory syncytial virus, herpes simplex virus, and varicella-zoster virus.

When there are multiple serotypes within a virus group, complete identification can be more difficult. For example, an isolate from feces that produces grape-like clusters of rounded cells in both primary rhesus monkey kidney and diploid human lung is probably an adenovirus. The 31 antigenic types can be subdivided on the basis of their agglutination of rat and rhesus monkey erythrocytes, but typing requires specific antisera.

In the sections that follow, identification of specific viruses is discussed in more detail.

Other Host Systems*

Embryonated eggs have a limited but definite use in the diagnostic virology laboratory. If material containing influenza virus is inoculated into the amniotic cavity of nine to 11 day old embryos, there will often be sufficient replication to detect a hemagglutinating agent in the fluid 48 hours later. While this is only presumptive evidence that a respiratory illness is influenza, the information is very useful in several clinical situations. Patients with influenza are susceptible to a variety of secondary bacterial infections, the most serious of which is staphylococcal pneumonia. A hemagglutinating agent in the sputum of an elderly or debilitated individual with a respiratory infection may warrant prophylactic antibiotic therapy. Patients on immunosuppressive drugs or receiving cancer chemotherapy are susceptible to a variety of respiratory infections, many of which respond to specific therapy. The presence of a hemagglutinating agent in sputum suggests infection with an RNA virus for which no treatment is available.

The poxviruses and herpes simplex virus produce characteristic lesions on the chorioallantoic membrane of 10- to 12-day embryos. This is sometimes useful to confirm that a generalized eruption following vaccination is due to vaccinia virus. Varicella-zoster virus produces no alterations of the chorioallantoic membrane, a fact that can be useful in distinguishing such dermal lesions from those of *herpesvirus hominis*. Finally, the characteristic pocks of herpes simplex virus are sometimes used to confirm the identity of tissue culture isolates.

*Use of embryonated eggs and suckling mice is particularly well described in S. S. Kalter's *Procedures for Routine Laboratory Diagnosis of Virus and Rickettsial Diseases.* Minneapolis, Burgess Publishing Company, 1963.

Suckling mice are required for isolation and identification of many of the coxsackieviruses A. Although these can cause a variety of syndromes, they are commonly associated with herpangina as well as hand, foot, and mouth disease. The routine inoculation of suckling mice is not recommended, but they must be used if either of these conditions is suspected.

CAPITAL AND EXPENDABLE EQUIPMENT

Capital Equipment

Our diagnostic virology is done in a separate room in the general microbiology laboratory, and the writer feels strongly that special quarters with air locks and ultraviolet lamps are not necessary. All tissue cultures should be handled as if they contain infectious agents (simian viruses are common in monkey kidney cultures), and a few virologists recommend that they be prepared and inoculated in a hood. If standard precautions for handling infectious material are observed, diagnostic virology is no more dangerous than routine medical bacteriology or mycology.* In the same vein, freezer, refrigerator, and incubator space is shared with the general laboratory. The most expensive special item of capital equipment (which has many uses in bacteriology) is either an ultra low temperature freezer (−70° C.)† or a liquid nitrogen refrigerator (−196° C.).‡ One of these is necessary for storage of stock viruses for quality control and teaching because many agents are not stable in the ordinary household freezer. If, in addition, tissue culture cells are to be stored, liquid nitrogen is necessary. Mammalian cells have metabolic activity at −70° C. and can be kept for only short periods at this temperature.

The refrigerator can be purchased with either six or 10 canisters, which are numbered. Ampules are held in lightweight aluminum canes, which we sequentially number for each canister with a small set of metal punches. Finally, we number the position of each ampule in a cane, starting from the bottom. For example, an adenovirus type 4 might be stored in canister 3, at the bottom of cane 21, and this location would be designated 3–21–1 in our file. Pyrex (or equivalent) ampules must be used and are most easily sealed with a natural gas or propane-oxygen flame. It is essential

*Arborviruses are extremely infectious, and the routine diagnostic laboratory should never work with stock cultures. These agents do not grow in the tissue cultures described but can be isolated in suckling mice.

†Revco, Inc., Industrial Products Division, Deerfield, Michigan.

‡Linde Division, Union Carbide Corp., 270 Park Avenue, New York, N.Y.

that the seal be perfect, because even a pinhole permits entrance of liquid nitrogen, which would rapidly expand when the ampule is removed and cause it to burst with some violence. In our laboratory a plastic face shield and gloves are always worn when removing ampules, which are then immediately dropped into 37° C. water in a stainless steel beaker. Despite these warnings, the equipment is easy to use, and our technologists and aides routinely replace and remove the desired ampules.

Tissue culture tubes can be held in stationary racks after inoculation with clinical specimens, but isolation of some of the more fastidious viruses is enhanced by slow rotation (12 to 15 revolutions/hour) of the tubes with a roller drum. We find it convenient to keep both inoculated and uninoculated tubes in the drum because of the ease in handling.

An inverted microscope is necessary if cells are to be propagated in bottles or grown in microtiter plates, but is not required for routine examination of tissue culture tubes.

Small and Disposable Items

Glassware used for cell culture work must be scrupulously clean, and even trace amounts of detergent can be disastrous. To avoid this, if glassware is reused it must be given multiple rinses, first in tap water and then in distilled or deionized water. Repeated autoclaving weakens glass and increases the risk of breakage, particularly when sealing tubes and bottles with rubber stoppers. For these reasons we use only disposable tubes (16 × 125 mm. heavy wall)* and bottles (clear glass Ovals from 3 to 32 oz.).† The former are available from Scientific Products (Division of American Hospital Supply Co.) and the latter from any wholesale pharmaceutical supply house. We wrap batches of the tubes in brown paper bags or aluminum foil and cover the mouths of the bottles with foil after removing the caps (which have paper liners that do not withstand autoclaving) and then autoclave the glassware *without* prior washing or rinsing. This is entirely satisfactory, the heat required to melt the glass being an excellent cleanser.

Nontoxic silicone rubber stoppers are used for tissue culture work.‡ They are boiled in 5 per cent sodium carbonate when purchased, and thereafter thoroughly rinsed after use. Storage and autoclaving of these were originally problems, which we solved by sticking the "O" stoppers (for 16-mm. tubes) into holes in serologic test tube racks (Scientific Products #B7025–2). These racks are then placed in ordinary aluminum pound cake tins, wrapped in heavy brown paper and autoclaved. When used, the tins are closed with the plastic covers designed for them. These covers cannot be sterilized, but this has been no problem. Larger stoppers (Nos. 2, 3, and 5) for bottles are individually loosely wrapped in aluminum foil and autoclaved.

*Demuth Glass Co., Demuth, Minnesota.
†Owens-Illinois Glass Co., Toledo, Ohio.
‡West Rubber Co., Phoenixville, Pennsylvania.

ADENOVIRUS DISEASES*

The initial isolation of an adenovirus was reported by Rowe and co-workers in 1953. These agents are among the most common encountered in the clinical virology laboratory. Although their name stems from the original recovery from adenoid tissue, most will be isolated from feces. Adenoviruses have been recovered from a variety of animals, and there are at least 31 different antigenic types that infect humans.

The importance of adenoviruses as a cause of illness depends on the clinical setting. In military recruits acute respiratory disease is a serious problem and epidemics are common. Symptoms are usually mild, with cough, malaise, headache, and fever. Recovery is complete and bacterial complications are rare. Most outbreaks are due to types 4 and 7. In civilian life adenoviruses are responsible for only an estimated 5 to 10 per cent of acute respiratory disease. The most common manifestation is acute pharyngitis and is usually due to type 3. The signs and symptoms include exudate on the tonsils and posterior pharynx, with fever and lymphadenopathy, which makes clinical differentiation from streptococcal pharyngitis difficult. Some cases have an associated conjunctivitis (pharyngoconjunctival fever). These usually occur in epidemics, with a characteristic triad of fever, pharyngitis, and conjunctivitis. The causative agent is often acquired while swimming.

Epidemic keratoconjunctivitis is another common syndrome due to adenovirus infection (usually type 8). There is fever, lymphadenopathy, edema of the lids, and superficial corneal opacities. These suggest the diagnosis, which may be confirmed by isolation of the virus from eye or nasal secretions obtained with a swab. Acute follicular conjunctivitis, due usually to types 3 and 7 and seen most commonly in adults, is another manifestation of ocular infection.

*The chapter on adenovirus by H. S. Ginsberg and J. H. Dingle in *Viral and Rickettsial Infections of Man*, edited by F. L. Horsfall and I. Tamm, 4th ed., J. B. Lippincott Co., Philadelphia, 1965, contains an excellent summary of the clinical syndromes and served as a reference for this section.

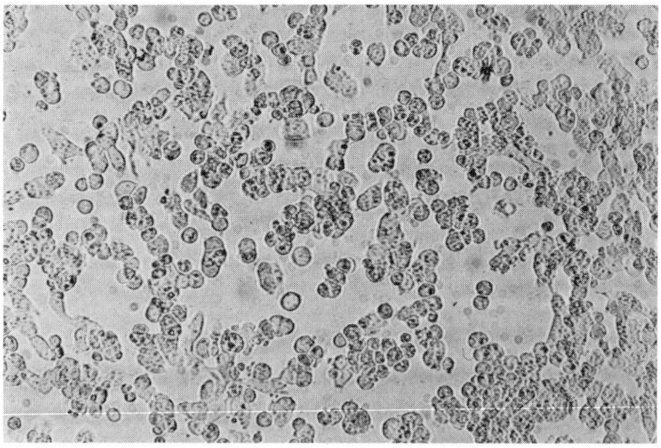

Figure 21–1. Adenovirus CPE in HeLa cells. (× 125.) (Courtesy of E. C. Herrmann, Jr., Ph.D., and T. F. Smith, Ph.D., Department of Microbiology and Immunology, Mayo Clinic.)

In respiratory infections the agent may be isolated from both the pharynx and feces, but the latter is two to three times more productive. Several studies have shown that only the lower numbered serotypes (1 to 8) are recovered from the throat, even though the higher numbered serotypes are capable of causing respiratory disease. These viruses are very hardy and are easily recovered from throat washings shipped frozen and feces mailed without refrigeration.

Primary embryonic human kidney cultures are the most sensitive for isolation. Primary monkey kidney and diploid cell strains are satisfactory. The continuous cell lines can be used, but strains of HeLa cells vary greatly in their sensitivity to these agents.

Infected cultures have a characteristic CPE, as shown in Figure 21–1. Cells become round, some swell, and they tend to clump together and form grape-like clusters. As the entire cell sheet becomes involved, many cells become detached from the tube wall. These morphologic changes develop fairly slowly, and Herrmann (1968) was able to report only 74 per cent of his isolates by the eighth day, with an accuracy of 80 per cent. The morphology may be confused with the CPE of herpes simplex virus, although this usually appears sooner. The two agents are easily separated by determination of sensitivity to lipid solvents. The adenoviruses do not contain essential lipids, and infectivity is not altered by exposure to ether or chloroform.

The adenoviruses contain both group-specific and type-specific antigens. The former is sometimes used in either a complement fixation or gel-diffusion procedure for serologic confirmation of an isolate. Neutralization of an adenovirus depends on the type-specific antigen and is used for typing. Fortunately the adenoviruses can be classified into three groups, depending on their ability to agglutinate rat and monkey erythrocytes; this somewhat simplifies the task of typing an isolate.

How much effort should a routine diagnostic laboratory expend to type an isolate before sending it to a reference facility? The clinical picture may be a clue as to the type. The vast majority of viruses (except those from epidemic keratoconjunctivitis) will be one of the first serotypes, and the majority of these are usually types 1, 2, 3 or 5. Thus, most isolates can be typed with a few specific antisera and without the use of differential hemagglutination.

The fact that adenoviruses are commonly isolated but infrequently the cause of clinical disease presents obvious problems to the clinician trying to evaluate the significance of an isolate. Unfortunately there is no easy answer. The adenovirus group-specific antigen causes antibody formation in those infected, and a complement fixation test is available and useful. An antibody rise is also seen with subclinical disease, however, and cannot be used as "proof" that an isolate is responsible for the patient's illness.

ARBOVIRUS INFECTIONS*

There are over 250 arboviruses, which share only a common mode of transmission. Many species of lower vertebrates serve as the natural hosts of these agents, which are transmitted by hemophagous vectors (usually mosquitoes or ticks). Since man is an accidental host, these illnesses are classified as zoonoses. All members of this group are ether-sensitive, RNA-containing viruses, but they have different chemi-

Clinical Virology by R. Debre and J. Celers, W. B. Saunders Co., Philadelphia, 1970, contains several excellent sections on the clinical manifestations and diagnosis of arbovirus infections and served as a reference for this material.

cal and physical properties, which has resulted in some members being classified as arenaviruses, others as togaviruses and the remainder as diplornaviruses.

The arboviruses can be divided into some 21 groups on the basis of various serologic tests, but these are not distinct and there are cross-reactions, presumably due to sharing of common antigens.

In this section we shall mention only the few viruses which are common in the United States. These are listed in Table 21-7. It must be clearly understood that the virus names listed in the table refer only to the location or host of early isolates and that today most are found in many other regions or vertebrates. For example, Western equine encephalitis is found in both wild and domestic birds and from Massachusetts to Florida. An important mission of state public health laboratories is to monitor vectors and hosts for arboviruses, and they should be consulted concerning the presence of specific agents. Arboviruses have a worldwide distribution, and health workers in other regions must be aware of many agents not encountered in North America.

The clinical manifestations of arbovirus infection can be considered under three broad and overlapping categories. Many cause an *acute febrile illness*, variously referred to as "dengue-like," "swamp fever," "summer influenza," and "three-day fever." Another characteristic picture is *hemorrhagic fever*, in which the acute febrile syndrome is associated with thrombocytopenia and bleeding into a variety of tissues. Finally, and most commonly in the United States, are the *encephalidites*, which can vary from mild to rapidly fatal.

The clinical aspects of the arbovirus encephalidites are not distinctive, and definitive diagnosis requires laboratory aid. Most cases are recognized serologically; complement fixation and hemagglutination-inhibition tests are available. Both are useful, but the latter may become positive earlier and permit definitive diagnosis within the first week of illness. The Center for Disease Control has established the following criteria for interpretation of serologic tests for the St. Louis virus:

1. Confirmed cases are those that show a fourfold or greater increase or decrease in titer between two successive serum samples from the patient by either HI or CF.
2. Titers of 1:320 or more by HI or 1:16 by CF in any single sample of serum are highly suggestive of recent infection.
3. A titer of 1:8 by CF suggests fairly recent infection. An HI titer between 1:20 and 1:160 suggests past infection, but this antibody may persist for a long time and is not necessarily indicative of recent infection.

These agents are highly infectious and clinical laboratories should never attempt isolation, which is not useful for routine diagnosis. The virus can be recovered from brain tissue in fatal cases; specimens should be frozen in dry ice and sent to a reference facility for injection into suckling mice.

Colorado tick fever (mountain fever, tick fever) is found in the western United States, its distribution corresponding to the habitat of the vector *Dermacentor andersoni*. The clinical course is usually an acute febrile illness, with headache and muscular pain three to five days after the tick bite. There are two serious complications, encephalitis and hemorrhage, which usually occur in children under the age of 10 years. The diagnosis can be made serologically, but antibody develops slowly and may not be detectable by the complement fixation test until a month or six weeks after onset of illness. Earlier diagnosis can be made by isolation of the agent from blood any time during the febrile period. This should be done only by a reference laboratory.

Table 21–7. THE COMMON ARBOVIRUSES OF NORTH AMERICA, THEIR VECTORS AND CLINICAL SYNDROMES

AGENT	VECTOR	DISEASE
Group A		
Eastern equine	Mosquito	Encephalitis
Venezuelan equine	Mosquito	Encephalitis
Western equine	Mosquito	Encephalitis
Group B		
St. Louis	Mosquito	Encephalitis
California group	Mosquito	Encephalitis
Ungrouped		
Colorado tick fever	Tick	Fever

CYTOMEGALOVIRUS DISEASES*

A historical résumé of illnesses due to the cytomegalovirus (CMV) provides an excellent sketch of how our knowledge about a viral disease increases as better methods are developed for its diagnosis. It also graphically demonstrates how a ubiquitous agent, once considered to be an uncommon cause of illness, can become an important problem when new medical and surgical frontiers are explored. Greatly en-

*J. B. Hanshaw and co-workers have written extensively on many aspects of cytomegalovirus disease. Some of the pertinent papers are in the following journals: J. Pediat. *58*:305, 1961; New Eng. J. Med. *266*:1233, 1962; *272*:602, 1965; Pediat. Clin. N. Amer. *13*:279, 1966; J.A.M.A. *201*: 725, 1967; and J. Pediat. *75*:1179, 1969. These served as references for this section.

larged cells with both intranuclear and intracytoplasmic inclusions, pathognomonic of "salivary gland virus disease" were observed in a stillborn infant in 1904. For a long time thereafter congenital disease was believed to be invariably fatal. In 1950 the suggestion was made that diagnostic cells could be found in the urinary sediment, and it was soon noted that infants with the disease may survive, although serious neurologic defects were believed common. Human CMV was first isolated in 1956. It then became apparent that congenital infection was not invariably a tragedy and that about 1 per cent of newborns, many of whom were asymptomatic, excreted the virus. Virus isolation was followed by development of serologic tests, and population surverys revealed that subclinical infection was very common, and that by age 35 over half the population had antibody to the cytomegalovirus. As renal transplantation became an accepted procedure it was found that almost three-fourths of surviving patients developed CMV infection. While usually subclinical and diagnosed by a fourfold antibody rise following surgery, occasionally there was clinical disease, usually pneumonitis, and this could be fatal. In 1965 a group of Finnish investigators found a fourfold rise in CMV antibody in a group of patients with heterophil-negative mononucleosis. The following year the same type of antibody rise was found in the postperfusion syndrome, a mononucleosis-like illness in patients undergoing open heart surgery, usually with mechanical assistance of the circulation.

Cytomegalovirus infection is a common complication of malignancy. Recent evidence also suggests that acquired CMV disease in children and adults can result in a great variety of illnesses, among which are hepatitis, interstitial pneumonitis, and acquired hemolytic anemia. Thus, in just a few years our concept of CMV disease has changed from that of an uncommon, fatal congenital infection to one that involves the vast majority of the population, usually asymptomatically but occasionally with a variety of different clinical syndromes.

Congenital Infections

Congenital CMV infection can manifest itself in several ways. The most common probably is asymptomatic and detected only by virus isolation. There are preliminary data to suggest that infants born to mothers who have CMV infection during the third trimester of their pregnancy do not develop clinical disease.

The most serious, and least common, form of illness results from generalized infection. These patients have jaundice, hepatosplenomegaly, hepatitis, neurological defects, and low birth weight.

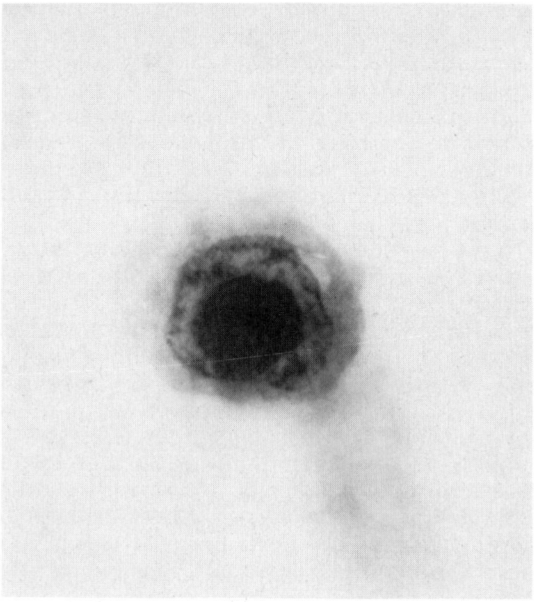

Figure 21–2. Intranuclear inclusion in a renal epithelial cell. Urinary sediment from a child with congenital cytomegalovirus disease. (From Blanc, W. A., and Goetz, R. Pediatrics 29:61, 1962.)

Some infants at birth manifest only central nervous system involvement, with microcephaly, chorioretinitis, cerebral calcification, and motor abnormalities.

Finally, symptoms may be delayed in their onset, and mental retardation, convulsions, or microcephaly are not recognized until after the neonatal period.

Laboratory Diagnosis. The most commonly requested procedure is examination of the urinary sediment for renal epithelial cells that contain the typical large intranuclear inclusions (Fig. 21–2). Unfortunately, although familiar to most clinicians and relatively easy to perform, the technique is quite insensitive. Under the *best* of circumstances, inclusion bearing cells are not found in a significant number of newborns with clinical disease proved by virus isolation. To find them at all, several facts must be kept in mind. Typically, the inclusion-bearing cells are excreted intermittently, and multiple specimens should be examined. There is rapid degeneration of epithelial cells, and urine must be processed as soon as possible after collection. A millipore filter technique is preferable and is described briefly.

1. A 25 mm. type SM plain white filter with a pore size of 5 μ is used together with the

necessary funnel, filter holder, and vacuum flask.*

2. Five milliliters or less of urine is filtered. If too much urine is filtered, the filter may clog. Be sure to leave a thin layer of urine on the filter. If the filter is allowed to dry there will be loss of cellular detail.

3. The filter is then removed and immediately placed in a cytologic fixative. Any satisfactory fixative and either hematoxylin and eosin, Papanicolaou, or Giemsa stains may be used. The original authors used 5 parts of glacial acetic acid and 95 parts of 95 per cent ethanol (or n-propanol) for at least 30 minutes as the fixative. They then stained with a regular hematoxylin and eosin technique, reducing the time to 1 minute in each stain.

The most sensitive technique for identification of congenital infection is virus isolation from the urine. To understand how this is done, some features of the virus and its excretion must be reviewed. Urine for virus isolation cannot be frozen without complete loss of infectivity; specimens stored in the refrigerator and shipped in wet ice are satisfactory for virus isolation for several days. Infants with congenital infections excrete virus for months, and all arrangements can be made for virus isolation before obtaining the specimens. The virus, which grows only in fibroblast cultures such as diploid human lung, produces a characteristic CPE which is diagnostic of cytomegalovirus. Small nests of enlarged, rounded, and refractile cells, often with brown cytoplasmic granules, are noted scattered among the normal fibroblasts (Fig. 21–3). The virus is primarily cell-associated and tends to spread to adjacent cells so that the foci of CPE enlarge slowly. Appearance of new foci and involvement of most of the monolayer can take several weeks. If such cells are fixed and stained, their nuclei contain one or several large inclusion bodies surrounded by a halo. Small intracytoplasmic inclusions are also frequently present (Fig. 21–4). These changes may appear in several days or only after weeks of incubation, depending on the titer of virus, and cell cultures should be held 30 days.

Laboratories doing only limited virus isolation with cultures obtained from autopsies are not only able to grow and identify this virus without difficulty, they will do it more rapidly than the reference laboratory which receives the chilled specimen with an unavoidable loss of titer. In contrast to clinical specimens, stock cultures of the virus are stable when frozen and can easily be obtained for study.

There are three serologic tests available for detection of CMV antibody. Unfortunately each has shortcomings, and none of them is entirely satisfactory for detection of disease. The neutralization test is usually not adequate to establish a diagnosis in a suspected case and will not be discussed. The complement fixation (CF) test is easily performed, but measures only IgG antibody. Passively acquired CF antibody in the newborn is common, and while most are in low titer, about one-third will have levels of 1:16 or greater. High titers (1:64) are suggestive but not diagnostic, because levels above 1:512 have been found without evidence of fetal involvement. Passively transferred antibody declines slowly, and persistence of a CF titer at six months of age strongly suggests CMV infection. Similarly a CF titer in an infant over two months of age that is higher than the maternal level is strongly indicative of active

*All may be obtained from Millipore Filter Company, Bedford, Massachusetts.

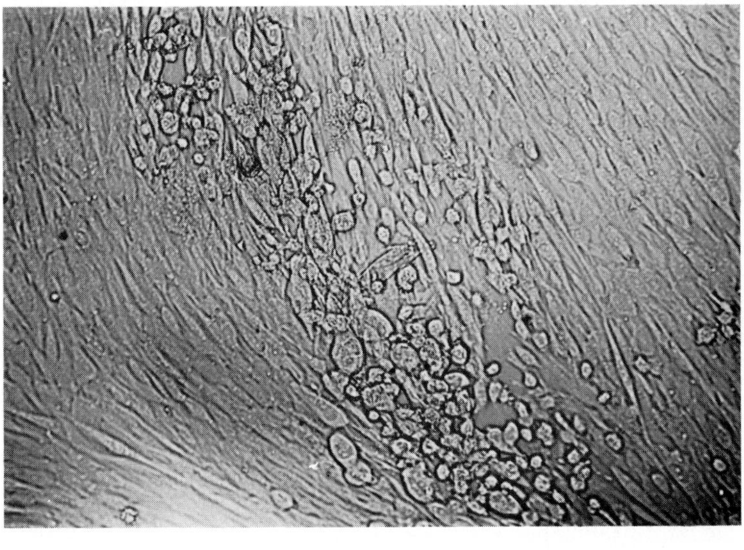

Figure 21–3. Cytopathic effect of CMV in human embryonic lung fibroblasts; focal lesion, strain C87. Unstained preparation. (× 140.) (From Lennette, E. H., and Schmidt, N. J. (eds.): Diagnostic Procedures for Viral and Rickettsial Infections. 4th ed. New York, American Public Health Association, 1969.)

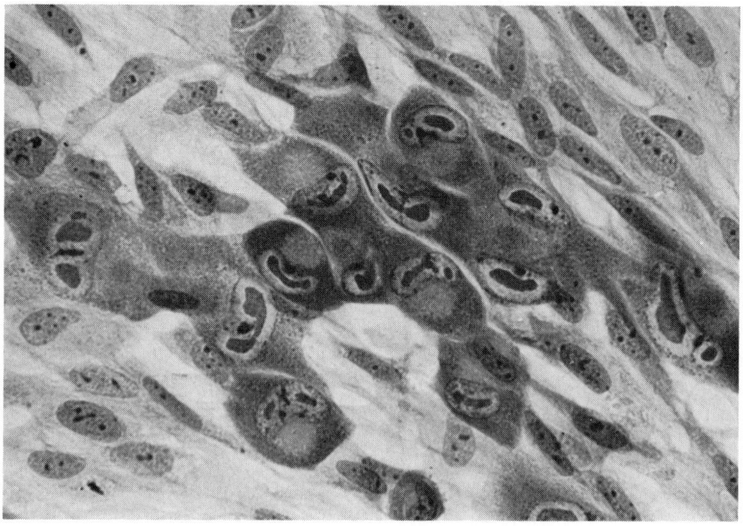

Figure 21–4. Cytopathic effect of CMV in human embryonic lung fibroblasts; strain C87. (Hematoxylin-eosin, × 560.) (From Lennette, E. H., and Schmidt, N. J. (eds.): Diagnostic Procedures for Viral and Rickettsial Infections. 4th ed. New York, American Public Health Association, 1969.)

infection. Uncommonly an infected infant will have no CF titer, so failure to detect antibody does not absolutely exclude the diagnosis.

The indirect fluorescent antibody test (IFA) for CMV is the only serologic procedure that can specifically detect IgM antibody. Since these macroglobulins do not pass the placental barrier, they are diagnostic of active disease and their detection is particularly useful in establishing the presence of congenital infection. The test can be performed on a single serum sample without having to wait (months) for a rise or fall in the titer of IgG antibody. In congenital CMV infection IgM is produced for weeks and sometimes months after birth, but older infected infants may have only IgG antibodies. Therefore, a negative test after the first year of life has little meaning. The theory of the test is illustrated in Figure 21–5, and the interested reader can consult the article by Hanshaw *et al.* (1968) for technical details. The vast majority of symptomatic newborns have IgM antibody, and absence of this macroglobulin in infants under one year of age makes the diagnosis unlikely, although a few symptomatic infants who were excreting the virus but had no IgM antibody have been observed. The situation is quite different in asymptomatic newborns who excrete CMV. The majority do not have detectable CMV IgM, but it is not yet known whether these infants are at risk from the multitude of sequelae of CMV infection.

Acquired Infections

Although the majority of CMV infections in renal transplant patients are subclinical, occasionally the laboratory may be called upon when pneumonitis develops. Lung involvement usually occurs in patients who survive at least a month after surgery and may occur in those with or without CMV antibody. Children with acute leukemia may present with high fever, cough, vomiting, diarrhea, rales, and icterus, but often the virus can be isolated from both children and adults with malignancy who have no evidence of CMV disease. Laboratory assistance may also be sought in cases with a heterophil-negative, mononucleosis-like illness, either naturally acquired or post-transfusion.*

Laboratory Diagnosis. Inclusion-bearing cells in the urinary sediment of adults with acquired CMV disease are rare, probably because they usually develop in the glomerular epithelium in contrast to disease in children, in which the

*Cytomegalovirus mononucleosis was described by Kääriäinen and co-workers: Brit. Med. J., 2:1099, 1965, and *1*:1270, 1966. Isolation of the virus from the blood is described in Blood *30*:120, 1967.

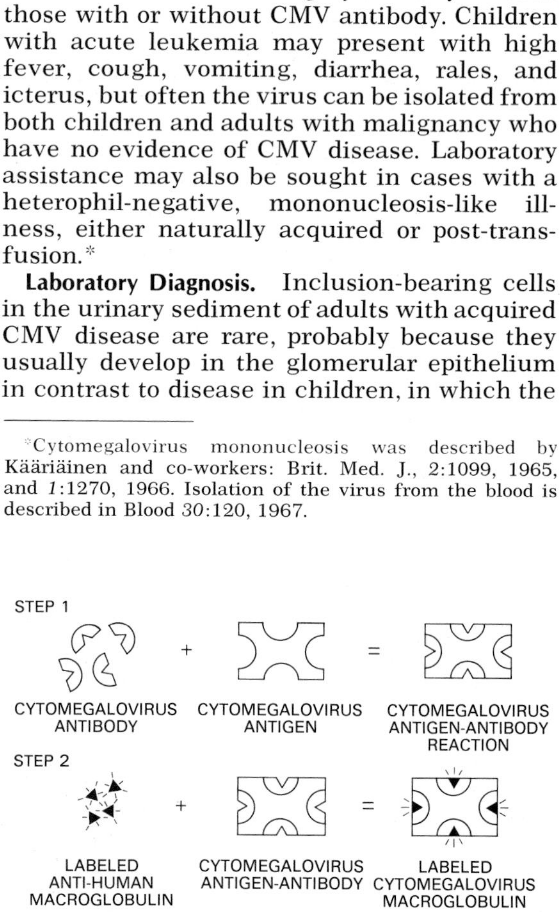

Figure 21–5. Schematic representation of the cytomegalovirus macroglobulin test. (From Hanshaw, J. B., et al.: New Eng. J. Med. *279*:566, 1968.)

inclusion bodies are found in the renal tubular epithelium. CMV can be isolated from the urine, sputum, or saliva of infected patients with a renal transplant or neoplastic disease. In patients with a mononucleosis-like illness peripheral blood leukocytes should be cultured. These can be inoculated into monolayer cultures or added to freshly trypsinized human fibroblasts.

The CF test is usually of value in all three groups of patients. It is interesting that the vast majority of transplant patients on immunosuppressives develop a rise in antibody, but an occasional patient will excrete the virus and have no detectable antibody.

HERPESVIRUS HOMINIS (HERPES SIMPLEX VIRUS DISEASES)*

Man is the natural host of *Herpesvirus hominis* and the only reservoir of infection. The host-parasite relationship is unusual because clinical disease may occur not only with the primary infection, but also with recurrent infections, generally considered to be due to reactivation of latent virus. As a general rule, symptomatic recurrent infections tend to remain localized and are usually not associated with systemic symptoms, while primary infections can be generalized and even fatal. Although most persons become infected with *H. hominis*, the majority of these infections are subclinical. Population surveys have shown that while 60 to 80 per cent of adults have antibodies against this agent, only 15 per cent have ever had clinical manifestations.

*The chapter entitled "Herpes Simplex," by J. A. Dudgeon, in Modern Trends in Medical Virology 2, by R. B. Heath and A. P. Waterson (eds.), Appleton-Century-Crofts, Inc., New York, 1970, is an excellent review and served as a reference for some of this section.

Table 21–8. SEROLOGICAL RELATIONSHIP OF *HERPESVIRUS HOMINIS* STRAINS AND ASSOCIATION WITH CLINICAL DISEASE*

SEROLOGICAL TYPE OR SUBTYPE	MAIN CLINICAL GROUP	MAIN CLINICAL MANIFESTATIONS
Type 1	Nongenital	Ulcerative stomatitis; labial; facial and corneal herpes; eczema herpeticum; meningoencephalitis
Type 2	Genital	Lesions on penis, urethra, vulvovagina; skin of buttocks; neonatal herpes

*From Dudgeon, J. A. *In* Heath, R. B., and Waterson, A. P. (eds.): Modern Trends in Medical Virology—2. London, Butterworths, 1970, p. 78.

In 1921 Lipshutz suggested that herpes febrilis and herpes genitalis were related but different entities. This caused little interest, and it was not until 1962 that the existence of two antigenic types of *H. hominis* (designated types 1 and 2) was established. This distinction is important because therapy is available and may be different for the two serotypes. The association of these with clinical disease is shown in Table 21–8. There is also some circumstantial evidence that infection with type 2 virus may be related to cancer of the uterine cervix. This is based primarily on a higher incidence of type 2 antibody in women with invasive squamous carcinoma than in matched controls. Herpetic infections chiefly involve one of five anatomical sites: (1) skin, (2) mucous membranes, (3) eye, (4) central nervous system, or (5) generalized disease; clinical manifestations depend on whether the infection is primary or recurrent. The relationships are shown in Figure 21–6.

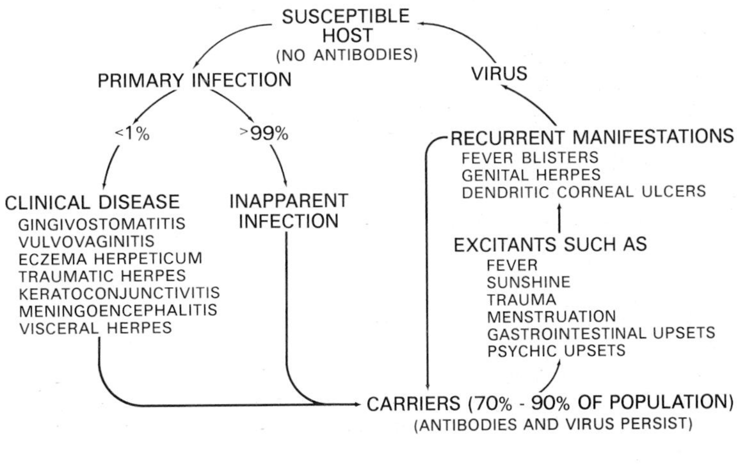

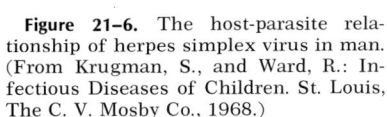

Figure 21–6. The host-parasite relationship of herpes simplex virus in man. (From Krugman, S., and Ward, R.: Infectious Diseases of Children. St. Louis, The C. V. Mosby Co., 1968.)

Skin Diseases

The commonest stigma of herpes simplex infection is the recurrent crops of vesicles that usually involve the mucocutaneous junction of the lip. These are the well known "fever blisters" or "cold sores." Laboratory confirmation is rarely required, but the virus can be isolated from vesicles for up to 48 hours after their appearance.

Eczema herpeticum (Kaposi's varicelliform eruption) is a manifestation of primary infection superimposed on atopic eczema or chronic dermatitis. The disease is characterized by the abrupt onset of high fever followed by crops of vesicles that tend to involve the previously abnormal skin. There is considerable variation in severity from mild to rapidly fatal. Lesions may resemble varicella in that they appear in several stages in an area at one time. Laboratory differentiation is simple because varicella virus grows slowly and is cell associated in contrast to the rapid appearance of CPE with *H. hominis*.

Traumatic or inoculation herpes occasionally occurs as a primary infection in either a child or adult. Lesions may develop at unusual sites following a burn or abrasion and are associated with such systemic symptoms as fever and lymphadenopathy. The vesicular lesions may resemble herpes zoster, with spread of vesicles centripetally on an involved extremity. Following recovery, vesicles or bullae tend to recur at the same site.

Mucous Membrane Diseases

Herpetic infection of the female genitalia may be either a primary or recurrent infection, and is of special interest to the pathologist for several reasons. If he is responsible for gynecologic cytology, the cellular manifestations of infection will be seen frequently. The possible association of cervical cancer and herpes genitalis has been mentioned. It must be stressed again that this is based on statistical evidence only, and the finding of infection alone on cellular smears is not an indication for cold knife conization. Generalized herpes simplex of the newborn is due to type 2 virus, which the infant acquires during his passage through the birth canal; therefore, it has been suggested that pregnant women near term with virus in the genital tract be delivered by cesarean section. A plan for the management of such pregnant patients with clinical or cytological evidence of herpes infection is outlined in Figure 21-7. This obviously can be accomplished only with laboratory assistance.

Genital infections are probably acquired by promiscuous sexual activity, and like other venereal diseases are most common in young adults who are in the lower socioeconomic groups. Ng and co-workers (1970 a and b), in a study of 256 infected women, found that 91.4 per cent were clinic patients and that 41.4 per cent were pregnant at the time of detection. Almost half these cases occurred during the third trimester or immediately post partum. Of the 252 women for whom clinical data were available, 46.8 per cent were asymptomatic and infection was usually detected by cellular studies. The remaining women had either local or constitutional symptoms, listed in Table 21-9.

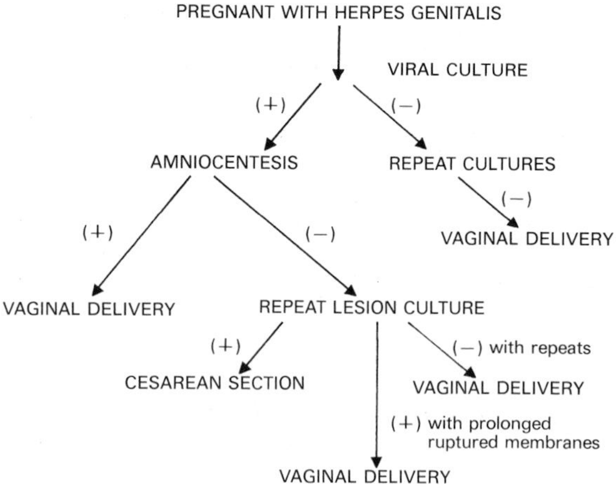

Figure 21-7. Summary of the management of patients with genital herpes infection in pregnancy based on positive (+) and negative (−) viral cultures. (From Amstey, M. S. Obstet. Gyn. 37:519, 1971.)

Cellular changes characteristic of genital herpes infection were observed in 88.7 per cent of the patients and the remainder were diagnosed by virus isolation. Primary and recurrent disease were separated by antibody titers and clinical manifestations and the cytologic features of each studied. The cytologic manifestations of herpes infection are shown in Table 21-10 and the distinguishing characteristics between primary and recurrent disease in Table 21-11 and Figures 21-8 and 21-9.

Herpes progenitalis in the male is commonly

Table 21-9. SYMPTOMS ASSOCIATED WITH HERPES GENITALIS IN 252 WOMEN*

SYMPTOMS	PATIENTS No.	PATIENTS Per Cent
Asymptomatic	118	46.8
Constitutional	37	14.7
Vaginal discharge	92	36.5
Genital pain	88	34.9
Dysuria	21	8.1
Vaginal bleeding	8	3.2

*From Ng, A. B. P., Regan, J. W., and Yen, S. S. C.: Herpes genitalis. Obstet Gynec. *36*:646, 1970.

Table 21–10. CYTOLOGIC FEATURES OF HERPES GENITALIS*

NUCLEAR FEATURES	PER CENT	S. D.
Vacuolization	10.1	7.9
"Ground glass"	67.4	16.1
Inclusions	22.5	16.9

*From Ng, A. B. P., Regan, J. W., and Lindner, E.: Cellular manifestations of primary and recurrent herpes genitalis. Acta Cytol. *14*:126, 1970.

Table 21–11. PRIMARY AND RECURRENT HERPES GENITALIS*

NUCLEAR FEATURES	PRIMARY %	RECURRENT %
Vacuolization	14.7 ± 6.9	4.7 ± 2.6
"Ground glass"	80.2 ± 9.6	52.2 ± 4.9
Inclusions	5.1 ± 3.5	43.1 ± 19.7

*From Ng, A. B. P., Regan, J. W., and Lindner, E.: Cellular manifestations of primary and recurrent herpes genitalis. Acta Cytol. *14*:127, 1970.

a recurrent disease, with clusters of vesicles on the glans and corona and sometimes on the penile shaft.

Acute herpetic gingivostomatitis is the commonest type of primary infection and is seen most often in the one to four year age group, in which it is also the commonest cause of clinical stomatitis. The gums are swollen, red, and friable and bleed easily. Early there are vesicles on the buccal mucosa, tongue, palate, and fauces, but these rapidly collapse to form grayish white 2 to 3 mm. plaques which often ulcerate before healing. Constitutional symptoms, with fever and regional lymphadenopathy, are common. The lesions of herpangina, caused by several different types of Group A coxsackieviruses, are identical in appearance, but their distribution permits clinical separation. In herpangina the gums are not involved and lesions are limited to the soft palate and anterior fauces.

Recurrent stomatitis is *not* a feature of herpetic infection, and the recurrent ulcers should be called herpetiform because the virus cannot be isolated from them and histologic studies reveal only nonspecific changes. This is in contrast to recurrent herpetic lesions of the genital mucosa.

Central Nervous System Disease

Herpes simplex virus is the commonest cause of sporadic fatal encephalitis, and

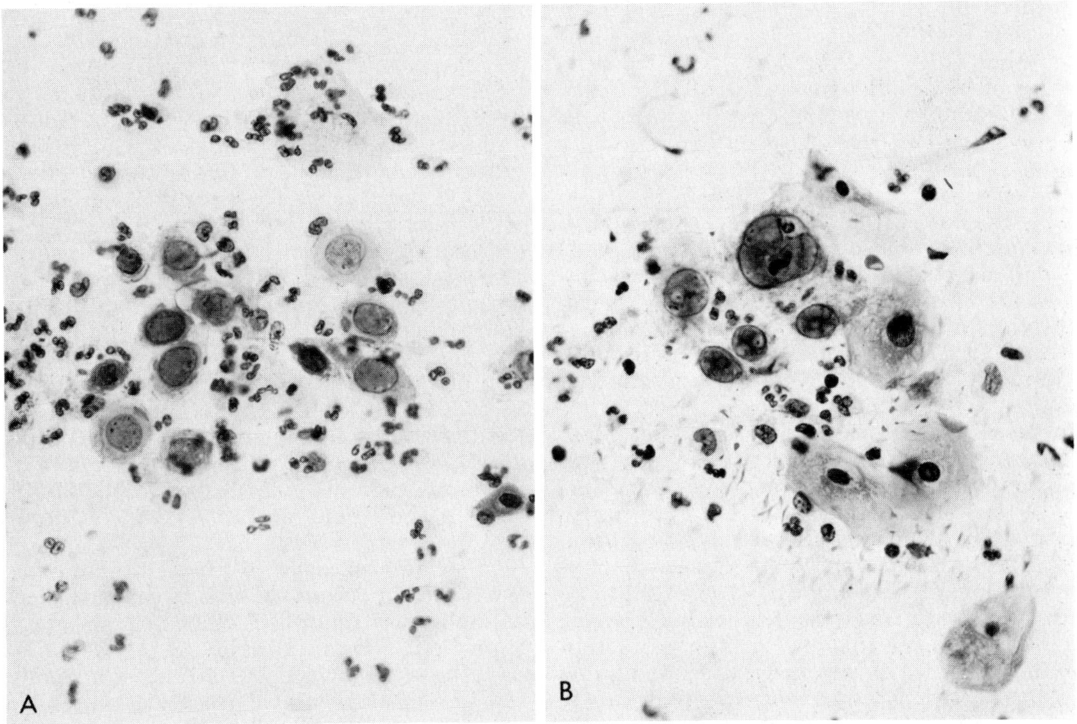

Figure 21–8. *A*, Early primary herpes genitalis. Infected squamous cells with intranuclear vacuolization and "ground glass" nuclear appearance. (× 500.) *B*, Multinucleated viral infected cells with a predominantly "ground glass" nuclear appearance. Intranuclear inclusions are identified in some of the cells. (× 500.) (From Ng, A. B. P., Regan, J. W., and Lindner, E. Acta Cytol. *14*:125, 1970.)

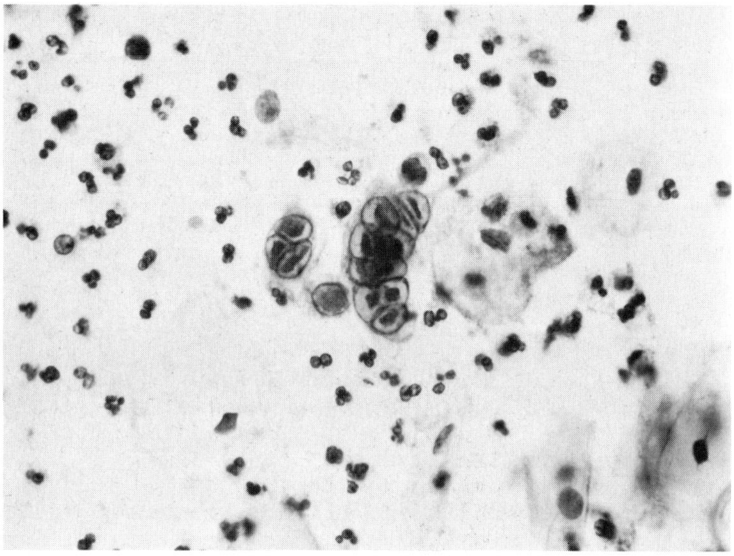

Figure 21–9. Recurrent herpes genitalis. Tight aggregates of infected cells with intranuclear acidophilic inclusions. (× 500.) (From Ng, A. B. P., Regan, J. W., and Lindner, E. Acta Cytol. *14*:126, 1970.)

patients who do survive usually have significant neurologic sequelae. The virus characteristically tends to localize in the inferomedial portions of the frontal and temporal lobes where it produces necrosis and hemorrhage. Because of this localization, disease in the adult, early in its course, may produce distinctive clinical features, with personality changes, bizarre behavior, hallucinations, and aphasia. A positive brain scan, suggestive of a mass lesion, has been described. There is some evidence that early treatment with idoxuridine may be of value, but because this drug has numerous undesirable side effects and is useful only against DNA viruses, an etiologic diagnosis before beginning therapy is highly desirable.

Laboratory methods have been reviewed in an excellent article by Johnson *et al.* (1968) and will be briefly summarized. Three techniques are available: demonstration of a significant rise in antibody titer, demonstration of Cowdry type A intranuclear inclusions, and isolation of herpesvirus hominis from the brain.

There are numerous objections to serologic methods, one of the most serious being the time required to show an antibody rise. Therapy, to be effective, must be started early; in one series death usually occurred before a convalescent serum could be obtained. Herpetic encephalitis was originally thought to be the result of primary infection with the virus, and it was believed that only primary infection resulted in a rise in antibody titer. It is now known that both these statements are false and that secondary herpes can cause a fourfold titer rise. The occurrence of herpes labialis during many systemic infections is well known and makes it apparent that a titer rise may be only an incidental occurrence with many febrile illnesses.

Because of the seriousness of the disease, and the importance of making a rapid etiologic diagnosis, open brain biopsy has been advocated. This material can be examined both for Cowdry type A intranuclear inclusions, illustrated in Figure 21–10, and the presence of *H. hominis*. If there is the characteristic localization of necrosis and the presence of typical intranuclear inclusions, a presumptive diagnosis of herpes simplex encephalitis is justified. Because the inclusions are not found in all cases due to this virus, and may be found in other diseases, neither their presence nor absence is conclusive. Absence has been reported with rapid progression of the disease and in chronic cases examined long after onset, but also in a patient dying after 12 days, a seemingly optimum time for development of inclusion bodies.

A definitive diagnosis is best made by isolation of the virus which, unfortunately, is rarely present in spinal fluid. The characteristic localization of the virus has been mentioned, and it is important that biopsies be taken from the temporal lobes. Tissue from other sites may show pathological alterations and yet not contain detectable virus.

In summary, biopsy of the temporal lobes of the brain for virus isolation is the best method of laboratory diagnosis of herpes simplex encephalitis. Immunofluorescent techniques have been described but are not yet ready for routine clinical use. Direct microscopy and identification of Cowdry type A intranuclear inclusions is good presumptive evidence. Serologic methods are of little value.

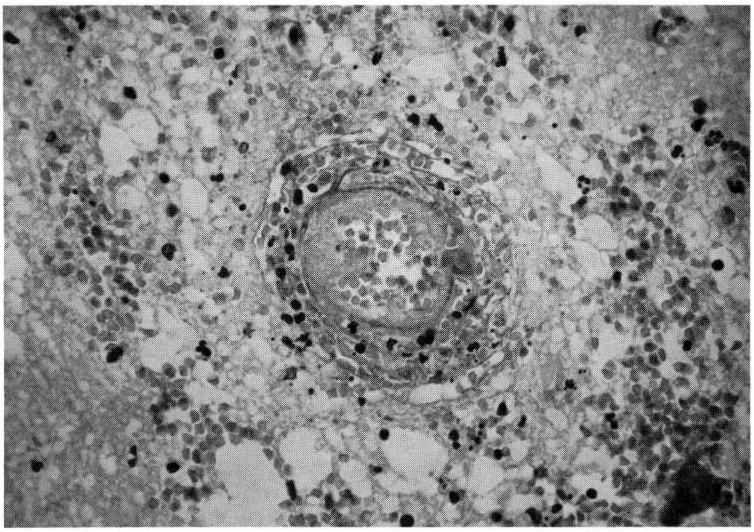

Figure 21-10. Focal hemorrhage and necrosis in the brain of a patient with fatal herpes simplex encephalitis. (Courtesy of J. Budinger, M. D.)

Generalized Infection

Disseminated herpetic infection is seen almost exclusively in the newborn infant. While transplacental viral passage may occur, the vast majority of infections are the result of passage through an infected birth canal. The typical illness begins between the fourth and seventh day, with fever or hypothermia, jaundice, and hepatosplenomegaly followed by lethargy, respiratory distress, and circulatory collapse. The outcome is frequently fatal, but mild cases have been reported.

Therapy with idoxuridine *may* be of value if the etiology can be determined rapidly. Meticulous physical examination is important, and fluid from vesicles anywhere on the body should be examined microscopically for the typical giant cells and cultured for *H. hominis*. In the absence of vesicles or stomatitis, antemortem diagnosis is difficult. Post mortem the virus can be cultured from involved organs such as the liver, and typical inclusion bodies are found in focal lesions.

Primary embryonic human kidney cells are among the most sensitive for isolation, and diploid human lung is also satisfactory. Some strains of human amnion are very sensitive, but others are less satisfactory and the use of young cultures of pooled amnion cells has been suggested. Primary monkey kidney cultures will support the growth of some genital strains but are not recommended for routine isolation. The virus grows rapidly, and CPE is usually readily apparent after 24 to 48 hours; Herrmann (1967) was able to report almost 80 per cent of his isolates by the fourth day, with an accuracy of 97 per cent. The characteristic CPE has two patterns, the more common formation of clumps of rounded

Figure 21-11. Typical CPE of H. hominis in WI-38 cells. (Courtesy of R. Martins, M.D., and W. Walker, Ph.D.)

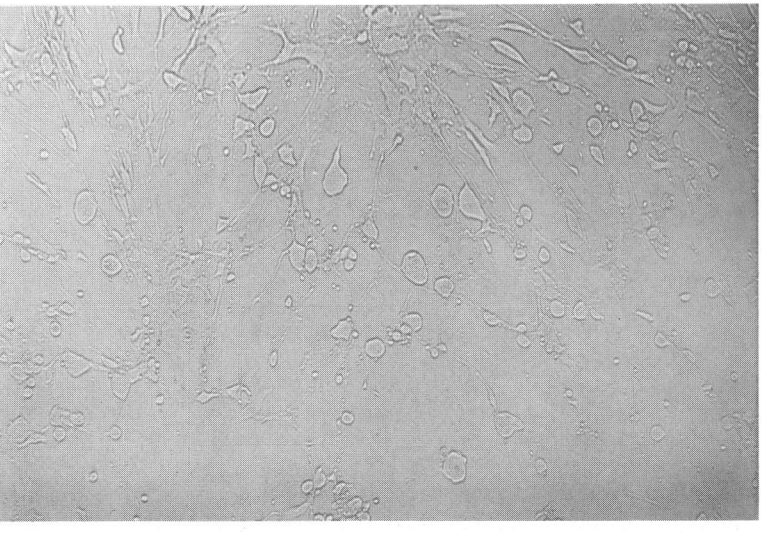

cells (Figure 21–11) and the less common development of multinucleated syncytial giant cells. The rapid development of this CPE in human kidney or lung cells together with the failure to isolate a virus in monkey kidney cultures is probably sufficient to identify an isolate from an oral or dermal lesion. A confirmatory test is based on sensitivity of the lipid-containing envelope to chloroform. To 1 ml. of tissue culture fluid from an infected culture is added 0.1 ml. of chloroform. The mixture is vigorously shaken for two minutes and the chloroform allowed to settle or the tube centrifuged, after which 0.1 ml. is transferred to a new tissue culture tube. The absence of CPE indicates chloroform sensitivity. The CPE of adenoviruses is somewhat similar, but is slower to develop, is found in monkey kidney and continuous cell lines, and is not inhibited by chloroform, differences that permit definitive separation.

LYMPHOCYTIC CHORIOMENINGITIS

Lymphocytic choriomeningitis virus is an infrequent cause of human disease; in one study it was responsible for less than 9 per cent of cases of aseptic meningitis. The clinical picture is usually that of a relatively mild aseptic meningitis which has no distinctive clinical features. The disease spectrum can, however, vary from an influenza-like illness to a fatal encephalitis.

Complement-fixing antibodies develop during the third or fourth week of illness and last about six months. Neutralizing antibodies are not present until the seventh week but persist for years.

The virus can be isolated from blood early in the initial febrile stage or from spinal fluid after onset of central nervous system symptoms. The usual tissue cultures are not satisfactory and suckling mice or young guinea pigs are often used. Virus is excreted in the urine of these animals, and care must be taken to avoid infection of other animals or the personnel responsible for their care. The virus is present in high concentrations in the brain, liver, and spleen of infected animals and can be identified by neutralization or complement fixation tests.

MUMPS

The usual clinical picture of mumps with either unilateral or bilateral parotitis is well known and does not require laboratory confirmation. There are, however, several serious complications of mumps virus infection, and these may not be preceded by parotitis. Laboratory assistance is necessary to diagnose such cases. Twenty to 30 per cent of postpubertal males with mumps develop orchitis; fortunately it is almost always unilateral. Orchitis commonly occurs during the first week of infection and is associated with systemic symptoms as well as gonadal swelling, pain, and tenderness. In about half the patients there is resultant atrophy of the testis, but, since this is unilateral, sterility is rarely a problem. Meningoencephalitis is the second most common complication. As shown in Table 21–12, mumps is by far the most commonly reported cause of encephalitis, being responsible for over 49 per cent of cases. Mumps meningoencephalitis usually follows parotitis by three to ten days and is characterized by fever, headache, nausea, vomiting, nuchal rigidity, and altered sensorium. This complication usually clears without sequelae. The spinal fluid commonly contains a lymphocytic pleocytosis, elevated protein, and normal sugar. Pancreatitis is a severe but uncommon complication, and rarely other glands such as the ovary, breast, or thyroid are involved.

Mumps virus can usually be recovered from saliva early in the course of illness and often from urine for as long as 14 days after onset of symptoms. It is frequently isolated from spinal fluid in patients with central nervous system involvement. Primary rhesus monkey kidney cell cultures are preferred for virus isolation. There is little published about the suitability of primary embryonic human kidney, but the author has had little success with it. Mumps virus usually produces characteristic CPE with large, granular syncytia, as shown in Figure 21–12. Whether or not such changes are present, a hemadsorption test is performed at five-day intervals, as described in the section on parainfluenza viruses. In one study only 73 per cent of isolates produced CPE, whereas 94 per cent hemadsorbed. An aid to presumptive identification is the increased hemadsorption at room temperature compared to 4° C. The common parainfluenza viruses (which includes type 2, the only one of the group that regularly produces CPE with syncytia that might be confused with mumps) hemadsorb best at 4° C. Definitive identification is made with a hemadsorption-inhibition test, described in the parainfluenza viruses section. Person et al. (1971) were able to report 50 per cent of isolates by the sixth day and 77.5 per cent by the tenth day. A specific report of mumps virus was made on 85.9 per cent of isolates, while a hemadsorbing agent was reported on 10.6 per cent. Incorrect reports were less than 5 per cent of the 205 isolates.

Infection with mumps virus usually results in the development of complement-fixing antibodies against two different antigens. The "S" antigen is a ribonucleoprotein. In the intact virion it is covered by the "V" antigen which is found in the envelope and is respon-

Table 21-12. ENCEPHALITIS IN THE UNITED STATES, 1961 TO 1965*†

ETIOLOGY	CASES REPORTED ACCORDING TO ETIOLOGY						PER CENT OF KNOWN CASES
	1961	1962	1963	1964	1965	Total	
Mumps	402	358	671	932	634	2997	43.2
Measles	276	337	239	300	171	1323	19.1
Varicella	75	76	84	106	112	453	6.5
Influenza	8	40	30	14	17	109	1.6
Rubella	—	—	—	59	7	66	1.0
Herpes simplex	8	—	3	6	19	36	0.5
Postvaccinal	8	7‡	3	8	9§	35	0.5
Lymphocytic choriomeningitis	3	—	2	4	8	17	0.2
Arbovirus group							
St. Louis encephalitis	42	253	19	470	58	842	18.6
Western equine encephalitis	27	17	56	64	172	336	
Eastern equine encephalitis	1	0	0	5	8	14	
California encephalitis	0	0	1	42	59	102	
Others	87	197	162	157	4	607	8.7
Total known etiology	937	1285	1270	2167	1278	6937	99.9
Total unknown etiology	1206	1125	1092	1420	1425	6268	
Per cent unknown etiology	56.2	46.7	46.2	39.6	52.7	47.5	

*From Krugman, S., and Ward, R.: Infectious Diseases of Children, 4th edition, St. Louis, The C. V. Mosby Co., 1968, p. 47.

†Compiled from annual summaries, Encephalitis Surveillance Unit, Communicable Disease Center, United States Department of Health, Education, and Welfare, Public Health Service.

‡Six postsmallpox vaccination, one postrabies vaccination.

§Eight postsmallpox vaccination, one postyellow fever vaccination.

sible for the hemagglutinating ability of the agent. Following infection, "S" antibody develops first, and an elevated "S" and normal "V" titer during the first week of an illness is presumptive evidence of mumps. Later in the illness the presence of "V" antibody at a titer above 1:32 is also suggestive evidence of mumps. Definite confirmation of infection requires a fourfold rise in antibody titer, however. "S" antibody is short-lived (several months), and immune status is evaluated only by measurement of the "V" antibodies.

It is interesting that about 25 per cent of older people have a history of mumps and are

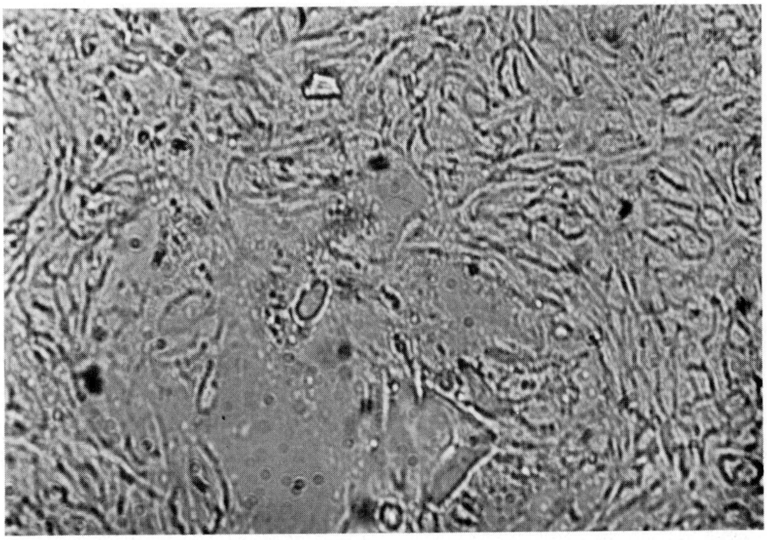

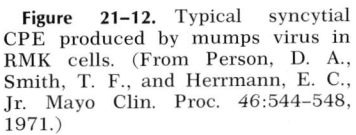

Figure 21-12. Typical syncytial CPE produced by mumps virus in RMK cells. (From Person, D. A., Smith, T. F., and Herrmann, E. C., Jr. Mayo Clin. Proc. *46*:544-548, 1971.)

presumably immune but have no detectable "V" antibody. Conversely, occasionally individuals with antibody develop clinical disease following exposure to mumps.

Because a mumps skin test may provoke complement-fixing antibodies in a patient who has never had the disease, this is not a recommended diagnostic procedure.

PICORNAVIRUS GROUP

The term picornavirus is derived from "pico" meaning small and "RNA" referring to the type of nucleic acid in the agents which constitute this large and important group. The human viruses included are shown in Table 21–13.

Rhinoviruses are distinguished from enteroviruses in several ways, the most important of which is their sensitivity to an acid pH. Infectivity of enteroviruses is not affected by a pH of 3, while that of rhinoviruses is markedly decreased. Rhinoviruses are the usual cause of the common cold in adults and will be discussed in the section on respiratory diseases.

Enteroviruses*

The characteristics of the enteroviruses are shown in Table 21–14. These agents do not share a common antigen; they are grouped together on the basis of physical and chemical properties and the fact that their natural habitat is the gut. They were originally divided into three groups on the basis of their pathogenicity in animals, but the distinctions are not sharp.† Despite this, the terms polio, coxsackie, and echo are retained because they are widely known and accepted.

*"Enterovirus infections," California Med. *103*:1–8, 1965, by D. Horstmann is an excellent and readable review that served as a reference for some of this section.

†For example, a few of the coxsackie group cause CNS disease in monkeys, and Russian workers have suggested that coxsackie A7 be renamed poliovirus type 4. Similarly, echovirus type 9 may kill baby mice and has been referred to as coxsackie A23.

Table 21–13. HUMAN PICORNAVIRUSES

	NO. OF SEROTYPES
1. Enteroviruses	
a. Polioviruses	3
b. Coxsackie A	24*
c. Coxsackie B	6
d. Echo	34*
2. Rhinoviruses	About 100

*There has recently been some reclassifying of the echo and coxsackie A viruses.

Table 21–14. CHARACTERISTICS OF ENTEROVIRUSES (POLIOVIRUS, COXSACKIE, ECHO)*

1. Transient inhabitants of the alimentary tract.
2. Multiple antigenic types.
3. Small particle size – 15 to 30 mμ.
4. Ribonucleic acid (RNA) core.
5. Lack essential lipids and therefore resistant to ether and other organic solvents.
6. Stabilized against thermal inactivation by divalent cations (Mg^{++}, Ca^{++}).

*From Horstmann, D. M.: Enterovirus infections. Calif. Med. *103*:1–8, July, 1965.

Polioviruses cause central nervous system lesions in monkeys, and the term poliomyelitis refers to the alteration in the gray matter of the spinal cord that follows infection with these agents. Poliomyelitis was recognized as a clinical entity in 1789, but the disease was not transmitted to an experimental animal (monkey) until 1909. In 1949 Enders, Weller, and Robbins discovered that poliovirus could be grown in tissue culture. For this finding they received the 1954 Nobel prize in medicine and physiology.

The coxsackieviruses are pathogenic for infant mice. The first coxsackieviruses were isolated in suckling mice from the feces of two children with paralytic disease who lived in the small town of Coxsackie, New York. This accomplishment by Dalldorf and Sickles in 1949 was the first evidence of the existence of a large group of previously unknown viruses. The numerous members of this family have been divided into two groups on the basis of the lesions produced in mice. Mice infected with group A viruses show universal destruction and acute inflammation of striated muscle and die with flaccid paralysis. Lesions are not seen in other organs. Group B viruses cause tremors, spasms, and spastic paralysis. Degeneration of skeletal muscle is focal and very limited. The interscapular fat pad shows necrosis and acute inflammation, and this is characteristic of coxsackie B infections in mice.

Echo stands for *e*nteric *c*ytopathic *h*uman *o*rphan and refers to the fact that these viruses, originally isolated from the gut of humans with no illness, produce CPE in sensitive tissue culture cells. Since adoption of the name in 1955 a number of different syndromes due to the echoviruses have been identified, and for this reason the agents are no longer "orphans."

The enteroviruses are responsible for a large number of different syndromes but few specific disease entities. A number of different viruses can cause the same clinical picture and the same virus can be responsible for a variety of different pictures. In temperate climates enteroviral illnesses have a well-defined seasonal pattern, usually being seen in the summer and fall and often in community outbreaks, with many similar cases due to one or several viruses. Virus prevalence is closely related to the standard of living. In lower socioeconomic groups 60 per cent of normal children under three years of age may be infected with an enterovirus, whereas in the middle class community (Wichita, Kansas) served by my laboratory many hundreds of fecal specimens can be cultured without isolation of a virus; when enteroviruses are isolated they usually represent a community outbreak. The viruses are highly contagious and can be spread by either the fecal-oral route or directly from pharynx to pharynx by oral secretions. Viruses can usually be isolated from the throat for at least a week, and often from feces for several weeks or longer from patients with the syndromes described below.

Neurologic Manifestations. Enteroviruses can cause aseptic meningitis, encephalitis, and paralysis. Although many different viruses are responsible for aseptic meningitis, the enteroviruses are the most common cause. Encephalitis, on the other hand, is only infrequently caused by an enterovirus (see the section on mumps for the common causes). Paralytic disease, once a common manifestation, is rare since development of effective immunization against the polioviruses. The enteroviruses usually responsible for the different neurologic syndromes are shown in Table 21–15.

The onset of aseptic meningitis may be abrupt or gradual, with headache, fever, malaise, and signs of meningeal irritation, usually a stiff neck and back, and tightness of the hamstring muscles. Coxsackieviruses A and B and a number of echoviruses are often recovered from spinal fluid, but this is rarely the case with poliovirus. Aseptic meningitis due to echo 9 or coxsackie A9 may have an associated rash, which can be similar to that seen with meningococcal meningitis. Spinal fluid cell counts usually vary between 50 and 300 per cu. mm., with lymphocytes predominating, but on occasion the cell count is over 1000 and chiefly neutrophils. The concentration of glucose is usually normal and protein slightly increased.

The coxsackie B viruses may be responsible for virulent disseminated disease in newborn infants with encephalomyelitis, pericarditis, and myocarditis that is associated with high mortality. The syndrome, which resembles that seen in suckling mice infected with a coxsackievirus B, was first described in 1952 and usually occurs in outbreaks within a nursery. While the disease may be acquired in utero, the majority of infections are acquired soon after birth.

Table 21–15. NEUROLOGIC DISEASE SYNDROMES ASSOCIATED WITH ENTEROVIRUS INFECTIONS*

SYNDROME	ASSOCIATED AGENTS
Aseptic meningitis	Poliovirus 1–3
	Coxsackie A 2, 4–11, 16–18, 22–24
	Coxsackie B 1–6
	Echovirus 1–9, 11–14, 16–19, 20–25, 30, 31
Paralysis	Poliovirus *1*†, *2*, *3*
	Coxsackie B *1*, *2*, *3*, *4*, *5*
	Coxsackie A *2*, *4*, *7*, *9*
	Echovirus *1*, *2*, 4, *6*, *9*, *11*, 13, 16, *30*
Encephalitis	Coxsackie B *5*
	Coxsackie A *2*, 4, 5, 6, 8, 9, 18
	Echovirus *9*, 14, 19
Encephalomyocarditis (neonatal)	Coxsackie B *1*, *2*, *3*, *4*, *5*

*From Horstmann, D. M.: Enterovirus infections. Calif. Med. *103*:1–8, July, 1965.

Exanthems*

The classic viral exanthems are rubeola, rubella, smallpox, and varicella. They have been well-defined illnesses for centuries and their clinical pictures and epidemiology are well known. With the development of new laboratory techniques there has been renewed interest in the exanthems, and over 40 viral types have been associated with these skin lesions in the last 25 years. The majority of these agents are enteroviruses, and the clinical features together with the associated viruses are shown in Table 21–16. Three of the more interesting will be mentioned briefly.

Hand, foot, and mouth disease is a febrile illness characterized by a maculopapular rash on the hands and feet that becomes vesicular and is associated with a vesicular oral eruption, usually on the tongue and buccal mucosa. The syndrome was first described in 1958 and is usually due to coxsackievirus A16, although A5 and A10 have been incriminated. The syndrome resembles the foot and mouth disease seen in animals, but the two viruses are serologically different. Viruses can be recovered (in suckling mice) from vesicular lesions. Although there are conflicting reports, most authors are unable to find giant cells or inclusion bodies in scrapings from the lesions.

The association of aseptic meningitis and exanthem with echo 9 has been mentioned. Apparently this agent has been the most widespread of all the enteroviruses in recent years,

*"Newer viral exanthems," Advanc. Pediat. *16*:233–286, 1969, by J. D. Cherry, is an excellent review and served as a reference for this material.

Table 21–16. CLINICAL EXANTHEMATOUS MANIFESTATIONS OF "NEWER VIRUSES"*

CLINICAL FEATURE	ASSOCIATED VIRAL AGENTS		
	Common	Occasional	Rare
Macular or maculopapular rash	Coxsackie A9, A16, B5 ECHO 4, 9, 16 *M. pneumoniae* Adenovirus 7 Measles vaccine	Coxsackie A4, A5, A10, B1, B3 ECHO 2, 5, 6, 11, 17, 25 Infectious mononucleosis Cytomegalovirus Adenovirus 2, 7a Reovirus 2 Colorado tick fever Measles†	Coxsackie A2, A7, B2, B4 ECHO 1, 3, 7, 13, 14, 18, 19, 22, 30, 33 Respiratory syncytial Adenovirus 1, 3, 4, unknown Mumps Reovirus 3
Vesicular rash	Coxsackie A9, A16	Coxsackie A4, A5, A10 ECHO 11 Herpes simplex Measles†	Coxsackie B1, B2, B3 ECHO 6, 9, 17 Mumps Reovirus 2
Petechial or purpuric rash	Coxsackie A9 ECHO 9	Coxsackie B3 Colorado tick fever Measles†	Coxsackie A4, B2, B4 ECHO 4, 7 Respiratory syncytial
Urticarial rash		Coxsackie A9	Coxsackie A16, B4, B5 ECHO 11 Infectious mononucleosis Mumps
Stevens-Johnson syndrome	*M. pneumoniae*	Herpes simplex	Coxsackie A10, A16, B5 ECHO 6 Adenovirus 7
Hand, foot, and mouth syndrome	Coxsackie A16	Coxsackie A5, A10	Coxsackie B1, B3 Herpes simplex
Roseola-like illness	ECHO 16 Measles vaccine	Coxsackie B5 ECHO 25 Adenovirus 2	Coxsackie B1 Adenovirus 1, unknown
Exanthem and meningitis	Coxsackie A9, B5 ECHO 4, 9	Coxsackie B1 ECHO 6 Colorado tick fever	Coxsackie A2, B2, B4 ECHO 11, 14, 17, 25, 33 Reovirus 2
Exanthem and pneumonia	*M. pneumoniae*	Coxsackie A9 Adenovirus 7a Measles†	ECHO 11 Adenovirus 7 Reovirus 3
Pityriasis rosea			ECHO 6 *M. pneumoniae*

*From "Newer Viral Exanthems" by J. D. Cherry in Advances in Pediatrics by Schulman (editor). Copyright © 1969 by Year Book Medical Publishers. Used by permission.
†Following inactivated measles immunization.

and in contrast to the polio and coxsackieviruses which are commonly isolated from well individuals, infection often results in clinical disease.

Coxsackievirus A9 is another common cause of aseptic meningitis with rash. In addition to the usual erythematous and maculopapular lesions, however, patients with vesicular eruptions similar to varicella have been described, and some of these have had an associated pneumonia.

Other Syndromes

In addition to neurologic manifestations, enterovirus infections can cause a variety of other illnesses, as shown in Table 21–17. We shall briefly consider the more important. There is good evidence that a coxsackie B infection is the most frequent cause of "idiopathic" pericarditis and that the myocardium is also involved in most cases. These patients present with fever and chest pain and features of either pericarditis or myocarditis may predominate. Leukocytosis due to increased neutrophils and an elevated sedimentation rate are common, and most will have an elevation of serum enzymes, most commonly lactic dehydrogenase. Viral studies should include isolation attempts from both throat swabs and feces and examination of paired sera for group B neutralizing antibodies (types 1 to 6). The height of the antibody titer bears no relation to the severity of the disease, and as has been previously mentioned, failure to demonstrate a fourfold rise does not exclude the diagnosis. An elevated titer may persist for years and permit presumptive retrospective diagnosis.

Pleurodynia (Bornholm disease, epidemic myalgia) is almost always a manifestation of coxsackie B infection and is characterized by the sudden onset of severe paroxsysmal chest pain lasting usually a week or less and ending in complete recovery. Symptoms are due to an acute myositis that may involve chest, diaphragm, and abdominal musculature. Some patients have an associated aseptic meningitis, orchitis, myocarditis, or pericarditis. Laboratory data, with the exception of viral studies, are usually normal.

Herpangina is characterized by the sudden onset of fever, vomiting, sore throat, and small vesicles or shallow ulcers on the fauces and palate. The disease is self-limiting and lasts less than a week. It is caused by a number of different coxsackie A viruses, and the diagnosis can be established by inoculation of oral or fecal samples into suckling mice. This entity is easily confused with herpetic gingivostomatitis, but the two can be distinguished on the basis of the clinical features described in the herpesviruses section. In addition, herpangina usually occurs in the summer and fall and may be epidemic in contrast to herpetic infections, which are sporadic without regard to season.

Acute lymphonodular pharyngitis is characterized by fever, sore throat, headache, and yellow or white nodular lesions on the uvula, anterior pillars, and posterior pharyngeal wall. These are composed of tightly packed lymphocytes and, in distinction to herpangina, are never vesicular. The illness can vary from four to 14 days in length and recovery is complete.

Enteroviruses are sometimes associated with both upper and lower respiratory disease in children and adults. Coxsackievirus A21 (originally called Coe virus) is an important cause of respiratory illness in military recruits.

Table 21–17. CLINICAL SYNDROMES (OTHER THAN NEUROLOGIC) ASSOCIATED WITH ENTEROVIRUS INFECTIONS*

SYNDROME	ASSOCIATED AGENTS
Minor febrile illness (nonspecific)	Polioviruses Coxsackie A Coxsackie B Echoviruses
Herpangina	Coxsackie A1, 2–4, 6, 8, 19
Acute lymphonodular pharyngitis	Coxsackie A10
Myocarditis and pericarditis in children and adults	Coxsackie B1–5
Pleurodynia	Coxsackie B1–5 Echovirus 6, 8, 9
Acute respiratory tract infections	
URI (upper respiratory illness)	Coxsackie A21, 24 Coxsackie B1–5 Echovirus 11, 20
Bronchopneumonia	Coxsackie A9 Coxsackie B4, 5
Enteritis (diarrheal disease)	Echovirus 11, 14, 17, 18 and ? others; ? Coxsackieviruses

*From Horstmann, D. M.: Enterovirus infections. Calif. Med. *103*:1–8, July, 1965.

Symptoms vary from mild upper respiratory distress to an influenza-like illness with fever, malaise, and myalgia. There is evidence that the more serious syndromes occur in those without antibody, and as the antibody titer increases the symptoms decrease. Coxsackieviruses B have been identified as a cause of mild upper respiratory disease with fever as well as pneumonia, bronchiolitis, and bronchitis in infants under two years of age. Echoviruses have also been incriminated as a cause of mild upper respiratory distress and infrequently are responsible for croup, but not pneumonia.

What is the role of enteroviruses in diarrheal disease? The etiology of most diarrhea is unknown, and in only about 15 per cent of patients have viruses been incriminated. Echoviruses 14 and 18 have been implicated in a few epidemics, but the enteroviruses are not an important cause of this malady.

Primary monkey kidney cells are the most satisfactory for isolation of enteroviruses, and all polioviruses, group B coxsackieviruses and echoviruses (with the exception of type 21) grow well. Coxsackieviruses A7 and A9 grow readily, and some of the other types may be isolated, but the majority of coxsackie A viruses are isolated in suckling mice. Those enteroviruses isolated in primary monkey kidney cultures grow in primary embryonic human kidney, which is also satisfactory for their isolation. The group B coxsackieviruses grow poorly in diploid human lung, and the echoviruses grow poorly in continuous cell lines, in contrast to the polioviruses which grow well in both types of cultures. This is useful in making a preliminary group identification of an isolate.

Enterovirus growth is usually associated with characteristic CPE; the infected cells show shrinkage, nuclear pyknosis, become refractile, and eventually fall off the glass, as shown in Figure 21–13.

There are three types of poliovirus, 24 types of group A and six types of group B coxsackievirus and 34 types of echovirus. It is obvious, therefore, that identification of an echovirus or group A coxsackievirus isolate by individual neutralization tests against the entire battery of enteroviral antisera is an almost prohibitive task. The job is simplified somewhat by using pools of antisera, as illustrated in Figure 21–14, but this is tedious and time consuming. In addition, there are technical problems that will not be mentioned, and the interested reader is referred to a review of this subject. Each laboratory must decide how to approach the problem of enterovirus identification, because only a few can keep the entire battery of antisera and do all the tests that may be necessary. Most enteroviruses are isolated during community outbreaks that are due to one or a few

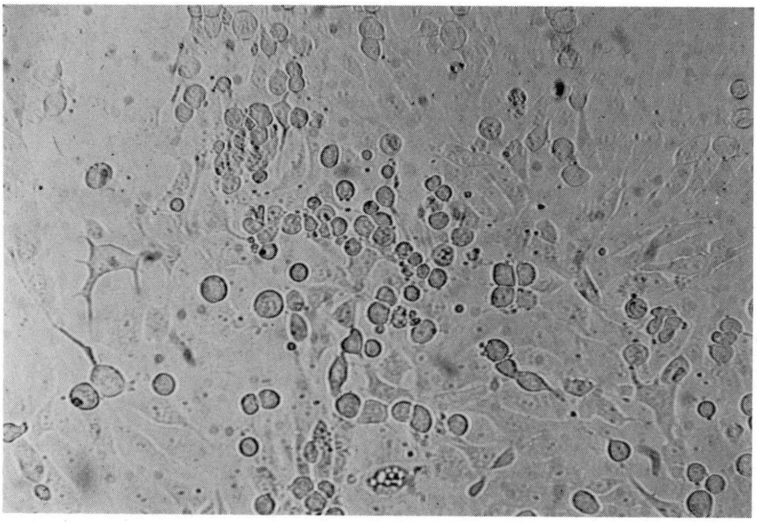

Figure 21–13. Typical CPE of enteroviruses in primary monkey kidney culture (coxsackievirus B). (× 125.) Submitted for publication to Mayo Clin. Proc. (Courtesy of E. C. Herrmann, Jr., Ph.D. and T. F. Smith, Ph.D., Department of Microbiology and Immunology, Mayo Clinic.)

different serotypes. If the isolate from an index case is identified by a reference laboratory, most subsequent isolates can easily be typed.

Serologic methods of enterovirus diagnosis present special problems. There are no group antigens shared, for example, by all the echoviruses. This means that each serum must be tested against each antigen individually, an impossible procedure unless the choice of serotypes can be narrowed by a distinctive clinical picture, isolation of an enterovirus from the patient, or presence of an epidemic of a specific viral serotype. Even if this can be done, problems remain. Antibody typically develops before the patient becomes ill, and usually the acute serum will show the maximum titer. It

Composition of serum pools

Serum pool numbers	7 ↓	8 ↓	9 ↓	10 ↓	11 ↓	12 ↓
1 ⟶	E1*	E2	E3	E4	E5	E6
2 ⟶	E7	E8	E9	Reo 1**	E11	E12
3 ⟶	E13	E14	E15	E16	E17	E18
4 ⟶	E19	E20	E21	E22	E23	E24
5 ⟶	E25	E26	E27	E28+	E29	E30
6 ⟶	E31	E32	E33	E11 prime	Cox A9	++

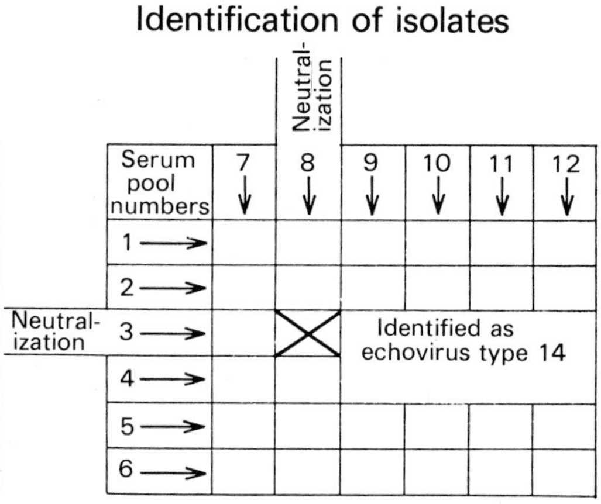

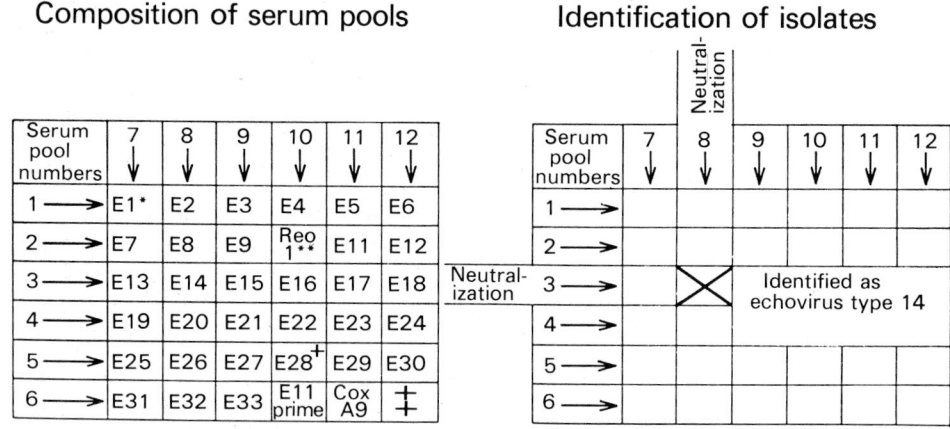

*Echovirus immune serum type

**Serum also neutralizes reovirus types 2 and 3

+Now classified as rhinovirus type la

+Immune serum to enterovirus candidate
+strains

Figure 21–14. Twelve-pool intersecting serum schema for identification of echoviruses by neutralization tests. (From Lennette, E. H., and Schmidt, N. J. (eds.): Diagnostic Procedures for Viral and Rickettsial Infections. 4th ed. New York, American Public Health Association, 1969.)

is, therefore, very difficult to be sure whether the antibody is from the present or a previous illness. To further complicate matters, cross-reactions occur and some echovirus infections may result in antibody against group B coxsackieviruses, for example.

An enteroviral isolate can be incriminated as the causative agent of illness in several ways. The recovery from spinal fluid or tissue is convincing evidence, as is demonstration of viral antigen within an anatomic lesion. Recovery of one or several serotypes from many patients with similar signs and symptoms during a community outbreak is not uncommon and relates the viruses with the illness.

POXVIRUSES*

The poxviruses include the agents of classic smallpox (variola major), mild smallpox (variola minor or alastrim), cowpox, vaccinia, and orf. Variola major is a severe disease that is endemic in many parts of the world and whose mortality may be as high as 80 per cent for the hemorrhagic form. Variola minor is due to a less virulent strain of virus and has a mortality of less than 1 per cent; it was not recognized as a distinct clinical entity until the 20th century. Cowpox is a mild infectious disease of cattle that is endemic in Europe. It was studied by Edward Jenner, who in 1798 showed that cowpox protected against smallpox. Vaccinia is a laboratory virus derived from cowpox virus that has been skin-adapted; it is used for vaccination against smallpox. Orf or contagious pustular dermatitis is a disease of sheep that is an occupational hazard to those dealing with infected animals or their carcasses.

Smallpox is so rare in the United States that routine vaccination of children is no longer recommended. We live in an era of increasingly rapid transportation, however, and endemic areas are only a few hours away by jet aircraft. The possibility always exists that a case will enter this country and a clinical laboratory will be called upon to confirm the diagnosis. Assistance may also be sought to differentiate smallpox from chickenpox or disseminated herpes simplex infection, to mention only two of many diseases with which it may be confused. A brief discussion will be given of available laboratory tests, but it must be stressed that *smallpox is a public health problem, not an individual clinical problem.* The vast majority of laboratories have had no experience in smallpox diagnosis, do not have control material available, and do not stock either the strains or antisera required for presumptive diagnosis. *If smallpox is suspected, laboratory assistance should immediately be requested from the nearest public health facility!*

The viruses of variola major and minor, vaccinia, and cowpox are distinct but antigenically closely related. They can be distinguished only after isolation on the chorioallantoic membrane of embryonated eggs or in tissue cultures of human amnion, monkey kidney, or one of the continuous cell lines. This should not be attempted in the clinical laboratory!

The presence of numerous elementary bodies in smears of skin lesions permits a tentative diagnosis of a poxvirus and rules out varicella or herpes simplex. Material is obtained by scraping papules or the bases of vesicles with a scalpel blade or needle, smeared on clean slides, and allowed to air dry. These are stained with methyl violet (Gutstein's method), silver nitrate (Morosow's silver method), or Giemsa stain.

Poxvirus antigen is present in skin lesions from any stage of the disease. It can be detected in as little as six hours by an agar gel precipitation technique. The complement fixation test is more sensitive but requires 18 to 24 hours and is technically more demanding.

Numerous serologic tests for detection of serum antibodies are available but are usually of no value until the end of the first week of illness. By this time skin lesions are usually present and the tests described previously should have been done. If the diagnosis was not suspected during the eruptive period, or in cases of "variola sine eruptione" (smallpox without skin lesions), these tests may be the only way to establish the diagnosis.

Orf is a zoonosis that in man appears as a solitary, circumscribed lesion on the hand or finger that represents the site of virus entrance (Figure 21–15). The initial lesion is an elevated erythematous spot which progresses to a weeping, ulcerated nodule in two to three weeks. A thin yellow crust forms, with a papillomatous stage. Finally, the lesion regresses to a flat red macule that eventually disappears. The illness is completely benign and lasts about 35 days. The virus is usually isolated in sheep, but has been grown in primary human amnion. Complement-fixing and neutralizing antibodies are produced, but the diagnosis is usually made from the history of exposure to infected lambs and the benign course.

*Poxvirus diagnosis is well described in both *Virus and Rickettsial Diseases of Man* by S. Bedson *et al.*, Edward Arnold, London, 1967, and *Diagnostic Procedures for Viral and Rickettsial Infections* by E. Lennette and N. J. Schmidt (eds.), American Public Health Association, New York, 1969.

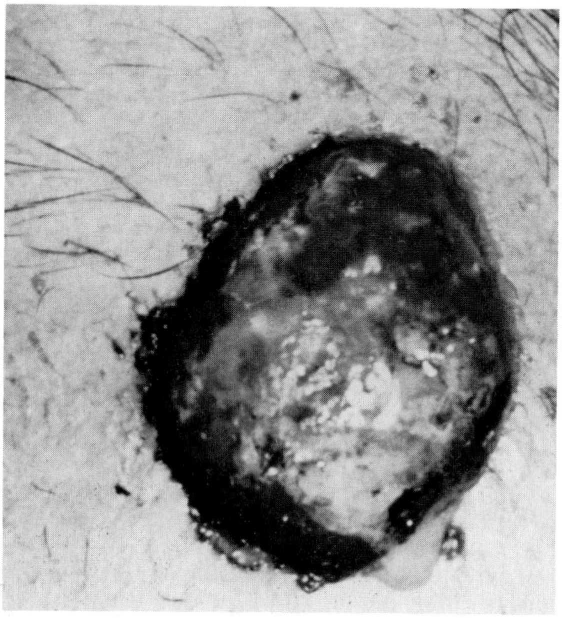

Figure 21–15. The acute stage of orf showing a nodule with a weeping, ulcerated surface. (From Leavell, U. E., et al. J.A.M.A. *204*:660, 1968.)

RABIES

Rabies has been known as a distinct illness of animals and man for many centuries. The disease has been identified in wildlife from the arctic circle to the tropics in both the Old and New Worlds. The animal reservoirs are numerous, and it is interesting that certain bats can by asymptomatic carriers for long periods of time. Most human cases follow cat or dog bites, however, and these animals are invariably symptomatic when infected.

The incubation period of human rabies can vary from 10 days to over one year, but is usually from one to three months. The frequency with which rabies develops after the bite of a rabid animal is not known, but since the disease is almost invariably fatal (the first human survival of rabies was widely heralded in the lay press in 1971), vaccine treatment is given if the offending animal cannot be found.

If the animal is available it should be observed; if no symptoms appear in seven days it is safe to assume it is not rabid. If the animal develops symptoms of rabies, it should be killed and the brain examined by the fluorescent rabies antibody test for presence of rabies virus antigen. Animals should be confined in an appropriate facility, not in a hospital or clinical laboratory, and the required tests done in a public health laboratory. Such services are universally available in the United States.

Serologic tests are used primarily to evaluate the immune status of an individual or animal and for characterization of strains of rabiesvirus. If such procedures are desired in a suspected case of rabies, the Center for Disease Control, Atlanta, Georgia, should be contacted by the appropriate state public health laboratory.

Clinical specimens for virus isolation include spinal fluid, sputum, saliva, and urine. Postmortem material should include pieces of brain about 1 cu. cm. in size from the hippocampus, thalmus, pons, cerebellum, medulla, and frontal and parietal cortex. The submaxillary salivary glands as well as pieces of lung, kidney, pancreas, and muscle should also be submitted for virus isolation. All material should be shipped frozen with dry ice. Rabiesvirus is highly infectious, and isolation should not be attempted in the clinical laboratory!

RESPIRATORY VIRUSES

Respiratory diseases are by far the commonest of human illnesses, and most have a viral etiology. The commoner syndromes, together with the causative agents, are listed in Figure 21–16, and defined in Table 21–18. The vast majority involve the upper respiratory tract and, although associated with considerable morbidity, are not usually seen by a physician because they are self-limiting and rarely fatal. Rhinoviruses are responsible for most of these infections in adults, except during epidemics when influenza virus may cause widespread upper and lower respiratory disease. The agents usually associated with lower respiratory disease in infants and children may also, on occasion, cause mild upper respiratory symptoms. Although lower respiratory disease is less common, it is more severe and more likely to require hospitalization.

In a recent study by Glezen *et al.* (1971) of over 3000 lower respiratory illnesses in children, a pathogen was identified in 28 per cent. Almost 75 per cent of these were one of four types: respiratory syncytial virus, parainfluenza viruses types 1 and 3, and *Mycoplasma pneumoniae*. The four agents tended to have characteristic clinical expressions, although all of them were responsible for the syndromes defined and could not be distinguished without laboratory aid. "Respiratory syncytial virus (RSV) was associated with bronchiolitis and pneumonia more often than any other agent. Parainfluenza (PI) type 1 was the predominant agent associated with croup. Parainfluenza type 3 was the second most common agent isolated from children with croup and was also an important cause of tracheobronchitis and

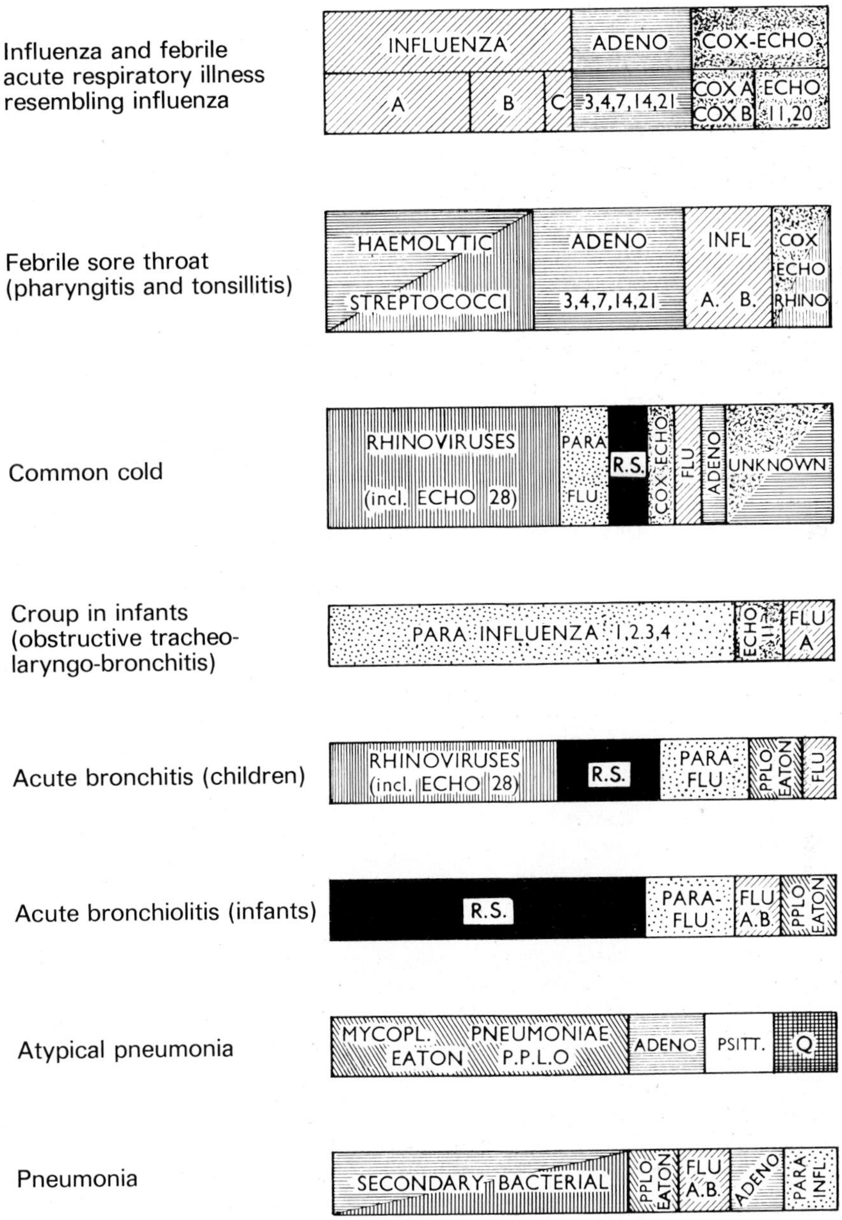

Figure 21–16. Respiratory syndromes and the causative viruses or agents. Blocks represent in width the approximate proportion of the cases due to the respective virus or agent. (From Bedson, S., Downie, A. W., MacCallum, F. O., and Stuart-Harris, C. H.: Viral and Rickettsial Diseases of Man. 4th ed. London, Edward Arnold, Ltd., 1967.)

Table 21–18. LOWER RESPIRATORY SYNDROMES AND THEIR DEFINITIONS*

SYNDROME	DEFINITION
Epiglottitis	Erythema and edema of the epiglotis with or without airway obstruction
Laryngotracheo-bronchitis (croup)	Hoarseness, cough, and inspiratory stridor with or without sufficient airway obstruction to require a tracheotomy
Bronchiolitis	Expiratory wheezing or grunting, tachypnea, air trapping, and sub-sternal retractions
Pneumonia	Râles or evidence of pulmonary consolidation on physical examination, or x-ray evidence of infiltrate or consolidation

*From Loda, F. A. *et al.*: Studies on the role of viruses, bacteria and M. pneumoniae as causes of lower respiratory tract infections in children. J. Pediat. *72* 162, 1968.

bronchiolitis. Most of the *M. pneumoniae* isolates were from children with pneumonia."

In addition to characteristic clinical syndromes, the different agents showed age and seasonal preferences. Almost 75 per cent of RSV isolates were in children under three years of age and occurred in yearly epidemics that varied in time from midwinter to early spring. PI type 1 caused biennial epidemics of croup in the autumn, most commonly in boys seven months through three years of age. PI type 3 was endemic and the least predictable.

Respiratory Syncytial Virus (RSV)

RSV is so named because its natural habitat is the human respiratory tract and it produces prominent syncytia when grown in tissue culture. From the introduction to this section it is apparent that the laboratory receiving specimens from acutely ill children will see RSV commonly. Specimens for virus isolation are usually obtained from the nose and oropharynx with a cotton swab, but virus recovery will be improved if secretions are aspirated from the nasopharynx with a No. 8 plastic disposable premature infant feeding tube with a 10-ml. syringe. Samples should be immediately transferred to throat swab media such as those previously described. RSV withstands freezing poorly, and significantly greater virus recovery will result if specimens do not have to be frozen and shipped.

RSV can be routinely isolated in either a continuous cell line or a diploid cell strain. Not all continuous cells are equally sensitive, and since these have few other uses in the diagnostic laboratory, one specifically known to be satisfactory should be obtained. HEp-2 adapted to grow in bovine serum is excellent, and tubes should be used when they contain only scattered islands of cells rather than an intact monolayer. Cell strains also vary in their sensitivity, and one obtained from autopsy material should be compared with a continuous cell line known to be satisfactory for primary isolation. CPE (Figure 21–17) is apparent sooner and is more characteristic in continuous cells than in diploid strains where syncytia may be absent and there is only destruction of

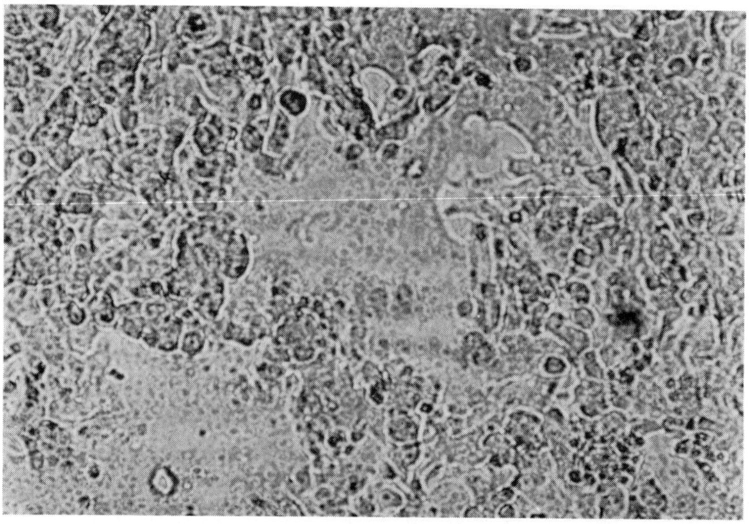

Figure 21–17. Typical RSV syncytial CPE in HeLa cells. (× 110.) (From Smith, T. F., et al. Mayo Clinic Proc. *46*:610, 1971.)

the cell sheet. Primary human and monkey kidney cells are not satisfactory for routine isolation. Horse and calf sera may contain neutralizing antibodies against RSV, and heat inactivated (56° C. for 30 minutes) fetal bovine serum is suggested.

With the exception of parainfluenza type 2, no other commonly encountered respiratory pathogen produces comparable syncytia, and this virus may be reliably distinguished from RSV by its growth in primary monkey kidney cultures and its hemadsorption of guinea pig erythrocytes. Definitive identification, if necessary, can be accomplished by neutralization, fluorescent antibody, or complement fixation tests.

Rapid diagnosis is possible with an indirect fluorescent antibody (IFA) technique. In one study, material was obtained by nasopharyngeal aspiration and examined by both virus isolation and IFA techniques. Seventy-one of 75 RSV infections (95 per cent) were diagnosed on the day of admission by the IFA method, and all were subsequently confirmed by virus isolation. Unfortunately the requisite antisera are not yet commercially available.

Influenza

Influenza is an acute respiratory disease associated with high morbidity and low mortality, except at the extremes of age and in patients with chronic debilitating illnesses. The incubation period is one to two days, with the abrupt onset of fever, headache, muscular aches, and cough. Three to four days after onset the temperature falls and recovery is rapid, although the cough may persist. Pulmonary complications during an epidemic usually occur in about 1 per cent of patients and most often are the result of secondary bacterial infection. Bronchopneumonia, lobar pneumonia, empyema, or pneumothorax may occur. A dramatic complication is the sudden onset of fulminant pneumonia with multiple pulmonary abscesses due to *Staphylococcus aureus*. In a few hours the patient becomes seriously ill with shock, cyanosis, and dyspnea and often dies.

There are three antigenically distinct types of influenza virus. Type A influenza is often associated with large epidemics that tend to occur every two to three years. Type B influenza is associated with smaller epidemics that occur every four to six years. Influenza C occurs only sporadically, and no epidemics have been documented.

There are two distinct influenza virus antigens. The soluble (S) or nucleocapsid antigen is type-specific and the envelope or V antigen is strain-specific. The division of influenza viruses into types A, B, and C is on the basis of their S antigen. Within type A the V antigen periodically changes and results in strain variation. This is clinically important because immunity is associated with V antibody, and as new strains appear there are recurrent influenza epidemics. Each year the Division of Biologic Standards of the National Institutes of Health makes an educated guess as to which strains should be included in the current vaccine. Unfortunately such a vaccine is usually ineffective during the first year's experience with a new influenza strain.

Because the antigenic structure of influenza virus periodically changes, the designation of specific strains is necessarily complex. Influenza A viruses isolated between 1933 and 1945 are designated A0, between 1946 and 1956 A1, and from 1957 until the present A2. In addition, characterization includes in order the geographic site of isolation, the strain number and year; i.e., A2/Taiwan/4/64 is the fourth strain of influenza A2 isolated on Taiwan in 1964. There are no subtypes of influenza B or C.

Throat washings or throat swabs are satisfactory for virus isolation. They should be collected as quickly as possible because the chance for virus recovery is greatly diminished after three days. Types A and B influenza viruses can be isolated both in primary rhesus monkey kidney cultures and the amniotic cavity of fertile eggs, while type C has been isolated only in eggs. Tissue culture is usually superior for type B, but there is wide variability with type A and the more sensitive system is unpredictable. The presence of a virus is established by hemadsorption in cell cultures and hemagglutination of amniotic fluid. Identification is established by complement fixation and hemagglutination tests. A flow chart for isolation and identification of influenza viruses is given in Figure 21–18.

It is apparent that isolation and complete identification of an influenza virus is not a simple task. In epidemic situations this is necessary only for recognition of index cases and is better left to public health facilities. If the laboratory serves a large number of patients with chronic diseases it may be important to rapidly identify the presence of a viral respiratory agent but not necessary to determine its antigenic composition. This is most easily accomplished by inoculation of respiratory specimens into the amniotic cavity of embryonated eggs. The presence of a hemagglutinating agent in amniotic fluid several days later is presumptive evidence of an influenza virus infection.

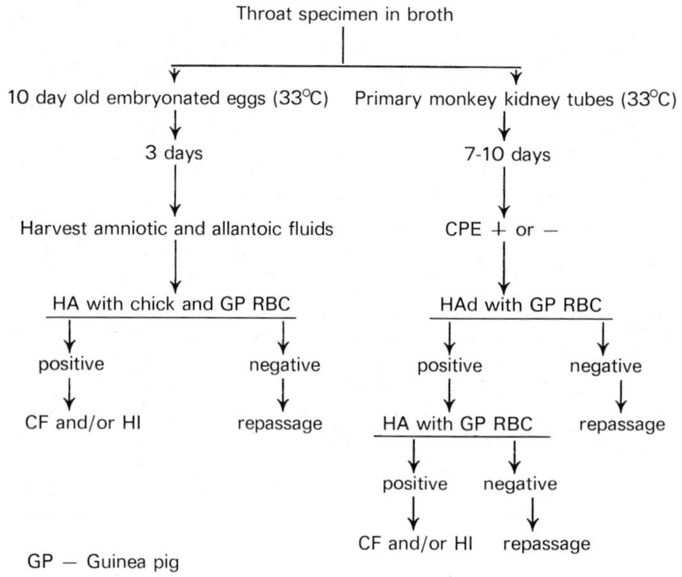

Figure 21–18. Flow chart for isolation and identification of influenza viruses. (From Lennette, E. H., and Schmidt, N. J. (eds.): Diagnostic Procedures for Viral and Rickettsial Infections, 4th ed. New York, American Public Health Association, 1969.)

Parainfluenza (PI) Viruses

There are four distinct serologic types of human PI viruses designated 1, 2, 3, and 4. Parainfluenza virus infection is very common, and most children have antibodies to these agents. By two years of age the majority of infants have antibody against type 3. Types 1 and 2 antibodies usually develop later and are common by age seven years. Type 4 virus is very infrequently encountered (13 of 399 PI isolates reported from the Mayo Clinic), and usually causes only mild upper respiratory disease. The importance of types 1, 2, and 3 as a cause of severe disease has been stressed.

Parainfluenza viruses are isolated only from throat washings or swabs, and these must be obtained as soon after the onset of illness as possible. Virus may be shed for as little as one day, although it is often recoverable during the first week of illness. If at all possible, specimens should not be frozen before culturing, but if this is not feasible they can be rapidly frozen to −60° C.

Primary rhesus monkey kidney cell cultures are preferred for virus isolation. There are several references to the use of human kidney cultures for isolation of parainfluenza viruses, particularly types 1, 2, and 3 but the author has not found these satisfactory. The virus cannot be isolated in either a human diploid cell strain or a continuous cell line. Viral inhibitors may be present in all types of serum, and cell cultures should ideally be maintained on serum-free medium for isolation.

The presence of a parainfluenza virus in tissue culture is recognized by the ability of infected cultures to hemadsorb guinea pig erythrocytes (Fig. 21–19). A 0.4 per cent red cell suspension that is stable for seven days under refrigeration is prepared in either isotonic saline or Hanks' BSS. About 0.5 ml. is added to the kidney culture tubes containing maintenance medium and these are incubated horizontally at 4° C. for 30 to 60 minutes. Types 1, 2, and 3 hemadsorb at 4° C. with reversal above 25° C. for types 1 and 3, whereas type 4 hemadsorbs at 25° to 37° C. If cultures are negative at 4° C, they should be reincubated at 25° C. for 30 to 60 minutes. Type 2 virus can be suspected from the typical syncytia produced (Fig. 21–20), but the other more common types produce either no or minimal morphologic changes and even type 2 produces hemadsorption before CPE. Hemadsorption tests should be done on the fifth day of incubation and then at 10 to 14 days. Presence of a hemadsorbing agent is reported to the physician and identified by a hemadsorption inhibition test. The time required for detection of a parainfluenza virus isolate is comparatively long because the hemadsorption tests are done only at five-day intervals. In one study only 22 per cent were reported by the fifth day and 60 per cent by the tenth day.

SV_5 (simian virus 5) is a primate myxovirus that contaminates some lots of primary monkey kidney cell cultures. It has many of the biologic properties of the human parainfluenza viruses, including the ability to hemadsorb guinea pig erythrocytes. Culture tubes can be purchased with 0.2 per cent SV_5 antisera in the medium to inhibit this agent.

A hemadsorption inhibition test for virus identification is performed by addition of antisera that have been treated with receptor-destroying enzyme and heat inactivated, to infected cell sheets that have been washed

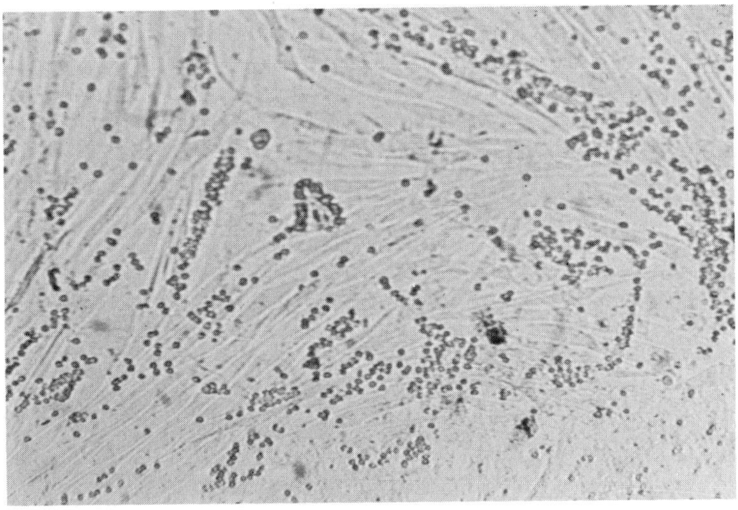

Figure 21–19. Hemadsorption with guinea pig erythrocytes in monkey kidney cells infected with parainfluenza 3. (From Herrmann, E. C., Jr., and Hable, K. A. Mayo Clin. Proc. 45:185, 1970.)

with a BSS. The cell cultures are incubated in a horizontal position at room temperature for 20 to 30 minutes and a suspension of guinea pig erythrocytes then added. The tubes are reincubated for an additional 30 minutes at the temperature of maximum hemadsorption of the original isolate. The serum which inhibits hemadsorption identifies the isolate. Isolates can also be identified by neutralization, complement fixation, and hemagglutination-inhibition tests, which may be necessary with some strains of PI type 4.

Rhinoviruses*

Rhinoviruses are the usual cause of the common cold, and over 100 serotypes have been identified. Healthy individuals and those who have recently recovered from a rhinovirus infection rarely shed these agents, and it appears that infection usually results in clinical disease. There are conflicting reports concerning the importance of these viruses in lower respiratory disease of children, but few isolations are made from hospitalized patients. The importance of these viruses in a diagnostic laboratory will depend on the type of patient from whom specimens are received. If these come only from hospitalized individuals, relatively few rhinoviruses will be encountered, but if throat swabs are received from outpatient or employee clinics, many will be isolated and must be recognized.

The highest rate of virus isolation is from specimens obtained during the first three to five days of illness, but even eight days after onset many viruses can be recovered. Nasopharyngeal washings are definitely superior

*Two monographs on the rhinoviruses are available, one by D. Hamre, S. Karger, New York, 1968, and the other by D. A. J. Tyrrell, Springer-Verlag, New York, 1968.

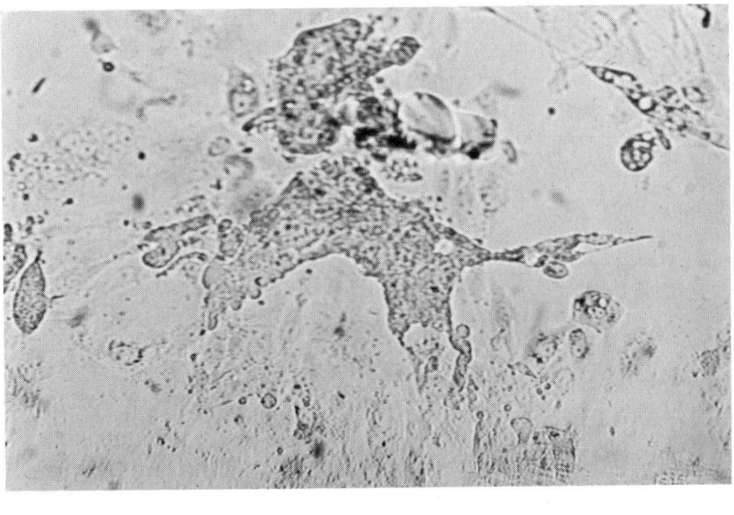

Figure 21–20. Typical syncytial pattern of cytopathic effect produced in monkey kidney cells by parainfluenza virus. (From Herrmann, E. C., Jr., and Hable, K. A. Mayo Clin. Proc. 45:184, 1970.)

to either nasal or pharyngeal swabs but are impractical for routine clinical use. Nasal swabs are preferred over either saliva or pharyngeal swabs.

Rhinoviruses have been isolated in monkey kidney (MK), human kidney (HK), and human diploid cell strains (HDCS). Some strains have been found that grow only in MK and are designated "M" strains, while others grow only in HK and are called "H" strains. This distinction, however, is related to the amount of virus present and is of limited importance. The majority are "H" strains, and MK is not recommended for rhinovirus isolation. The rhinoviruses grow particularly well in HDCS, which is the recommended cell for isolation.

There are over 100 rhinovirus serotypes, and typing of an isolate is neither necessary nor feasible. An isolate from the nose or throat can be classified as a rhinovirus on the basis of several properties. The characteristic CPE resembles that seen with an enterovirus and is shown in Figure 21–21. The isolate cannot contain essential lipids and is not inactivated by ether or chloroform. It is acid labile as determined by loss of infectivity when diluted 1:10 in a solution whose pH is between 2.0 and 2.2 and held at room temperature for two to three hours.

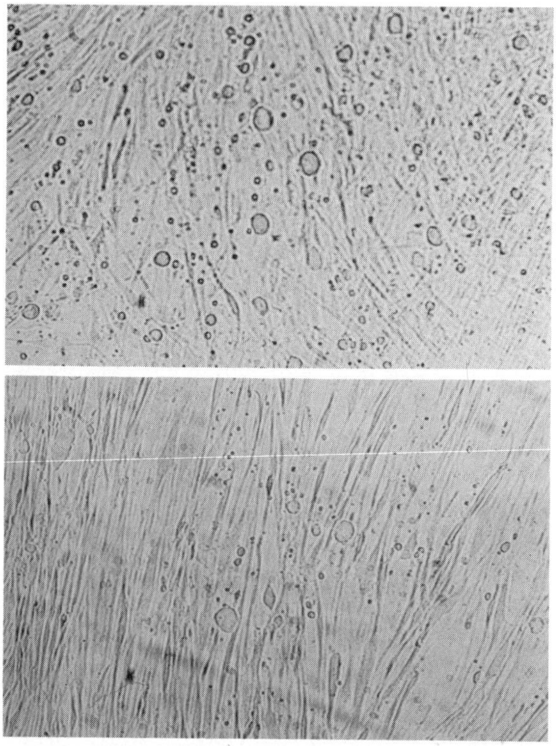

Figure 21–21. Rhinovirus CPE in WI-38 cell culture. (× 125.) (From Person, D. A., and Herrmann, E. C., Jr. Mayo Clin. Proc. *45*:521, 1970.)

In one study 73 per cent of isolates were reported within eight days even though CPE usually does not occur as rapidly as with some of the other agents commonly found in the throat. In 7 per cent of the cases the report was erroneous, the isolate originally considered to be an enterovirus or herpes simplex virus.

RUBELLA*

Rubella in both children and adults is a mild febrile exanthem that rarely produces complications and is virtually never fatal. There was little interest in laboratory diagnosis until the report by Gregg in 1941 that rubella virus is teratogenic when it infects pregnant women. Indeed, it appears that this is the only human teratogenic virus of importance. The risk to the fetus depends on how early in gestation infection occurs. The incidence of malformations ranges from about 33 per cent in the first month of gestation to 9 per cent in the third. The incidence of fetal infection, as determined by virus isolation from abortuses, varies from 47 to 90 per cent. It would appear, therefore, that infection does not always lead to clinical disease. However, it must be understood that only gross defects are detectable in the newborn. A provocative study of 22 infants born to mothers who had rubella between the 13th and 31st weeks of gestation revealed abnormalities in 15. These were more subtle (such as communication defects) than when rubella occurred earlier, and the infants had usually appeared normal at birth.

The virus was first isolated and grown in tissue culture by Weller and Neva (and by Parkman *et al.*) in 1962, and this discovery permitted the development of laboratory methods for detection of either acute or remote infection that are extremely important in clinical medicine. These will be discussed briefly.

Laboratory Procedures

Isolation of rubella virus, while not complicated, is time consuming and tedious. In primary African green monkey kidney, the established standard since 1962, no CPE is produced. Presence of virus is detected by the interference test, in which tubes are challenged with an enterovirus such as echovirus 11, coxsackievirus A9, or attenuated type 1 poliovirus 10 days postinoculation. Failure of

*The literature on rubella is enormous. An excellent source of information on this and other childhood viral diseases is *Infectious Diseases of Children* by S. Krugman and R. Ward, 4th ed., The C. V. Mosby Co., St. Louis, 1968. This served as a source of clinical information on several of the virus diseases discussed in this chapter.

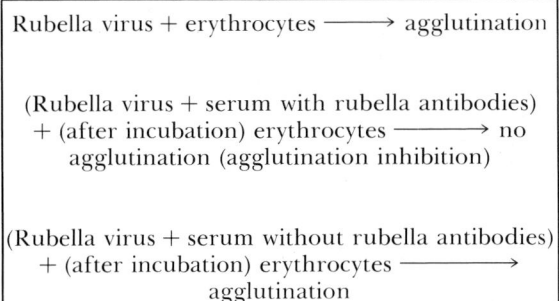

Rubella virus + erythrocytes ⟶ agglutination

(Rubella virus + serum with rubella antibodies) + (after incubation) erythrocytes ⟶ no agglutination (agglutination inhibition)

(Rubella virus + serum without rubella antibodies) + (after incubation) erythrocytes ⟶ agglutination

Figure 21–22. Theory of the HI (hemagglutination-inhibition) test for rubella.

the enterovirus to produce CPE is presumptive evidence of the presence of rubella virus. Virus isolation takes several weeks and is beyond the capability of all but the largest laboratories; fortunately it is necessary in only two situations. The infectivity of an infant with congenital rubella can be assessed only by attempted isolation of the agent from urine or pharyngeal secretions. Virus isolation from fetal tissues is the only method of establishing infection of an abortus. Virus may be present in the placenta without infection of the fetus, and care must be taken in selection of tissue for isolation.

Several serologic tests are available, and these form the basis of the laboratory diagnosis of rubella. The most widely used is the hemagglutination-inhibition (HI) test. Rubella virus will agglutinate erythrocytes from a variety of animals. If serum containing rubella antibodies is incubated with the virus prior to addition of the red cells, the ability of the virus to cause agglutination is inhibited. This is shown schematically in Figure 21–22. Kits for this test are available from a variety of manufacturers and are satisfactory if used correctly. Several comments are in order, however. Although kits are available and the procedure is simple in theory, in practice it is technically demanding. Because of the numerous controls required, the relatively short shelf life of some of the reagents, and the constant practice necessary to maintain technical proficiency, it is probably not wise to perform the test unless the laboratory volume is appreciable and the test can be done at least weekly. Serum contains nonspecific inhibitors of agglutination which must be removed. This can be accomplished in one of three ways: with kaolin, with manganous chloride and heparin, or with dextran sulfate and calcium chloride. The first of these removes antibody protein and is not acceptable; the remaining are satisfactory, but the use of manganous chloride and heparin is preferred. The interested reader should obtain the appropriate manual prepared by the Center for Disease Control and follow it EXACTLY.

The complement fixation (CF) test for rubella is straightforward and will present no problems to the laboratory familiar with this type of serologic procedure. The results of this test are usually less helpful than those from the HI test and the antigen is extremely expensive. For these reasons most clinical laboratories will not find it worthwhile to perform this procedure.

Neutralization and immunofluorescent tests have been developed but are technically demanding. They have limited usefulness in clinical medicine and will not be discussed.

Clinical Syndromes and Their Laboratory Diagnosis

Proper selection and correct interpretation of diagnostic tests requires information on previous immunization as well as an understanding of the different clinical syndromes and their patterns of antibody production and virus excretion.

Postnatal Infection. Figure 21–23 depicts the pattern of virus excretion and antibody formation in these patients. Virus may ordinarily be cultured from the blood, urine, and feces from about the seventh to the 14th day postinfection. It is present in nasal and oral secretions both during the period of viremia and for an additional seven to 14 days after termination of the viremia. HI antibody is the first to appear and can be detected about 17 days postinfection, or about the third day of the rash. It rises rapidly and reaches a plateau in about 10 days. Thereafter it may persist for many years with minimal change in titer. CF antibody does not appear until about the fourth week postinfection or the second week after appearance of the rash. It reaches a plateau in about two weeks,

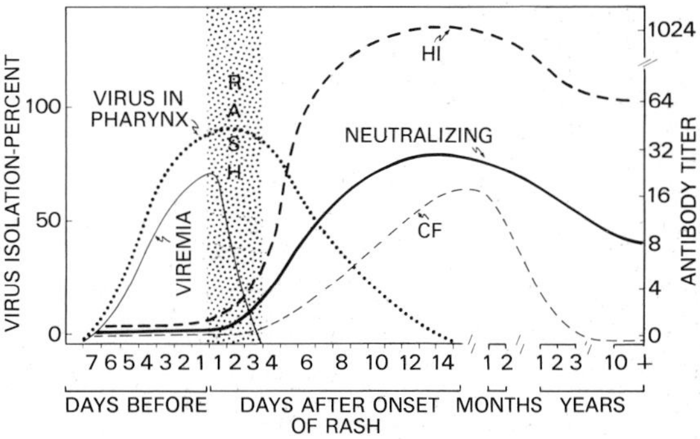

Figure 21–23. Virologic and serologic events with acute postnatal rubella infection. (From Krugman, S., and Ward, R. A.: Infectious Diseases of Children. 4th ed. St. Louis, The C. V. Mosby Co., 1968.)

and thereafter the behavior is unpredictable. Sometimes it falls to low or undetectable levels in several months, whereas in other patients it may persist for some years. The earliest rubella antibody to appear is macroglobulin (IgM) and this persists for only three to four weeks. It is then replaced by the long-lasting IgG and IgA antibodies.

The only important postnatal rubella infections requiring laboratory confirmation occur in pregnant women. Although there is evidence that reinfection with rubella virus is possible, either clinical or subclinical disease or vaccination is believed to result in antibody that effectively protects the fetus. It is, therefore, important for the laboratory to be able to identify women who have no antibody so that they may be vaccinated before marriage or immediately post partum,* and those women with antibody whose progeny will not be at risk during their intrauterine development.

Routine Evaluation of Rubella Immune Status. ANY titer detectable by the rubella HI test is considered sufficient to protect the fetus. The titers may vary widely. Following natural infection the titers may persist at levels of 1:512 or even 1:1024, but most laboratories find a mean of 1:32 or 1:64. Titers following vaccination average one-fourth to one-eighth of those following natural infection. Because of this, it would seem that screening tests for rubella antibody could be carried out only at a titer of 1:8; a prozone phenomenon has never been described with a rubella HI test. The Center for Disease Control however, recommends a short titration of at least two and preferably three tubes in screening tests. This is because the test results at a titer of 1:8 are frequently "fuzzy" (i. e., difficult to interpret), and the short titration will obviate having to repeat many tests.

Evaluation of Rubella Immune Status in the Pregnant Woman Who Has Been Exposed to Rubella. It is important to realize that many exanthems resemble rubella and that a therapeutic decision should *never* be made on clinical grounds alone! If the woman seeks advice soon after exposure or *immediately* after development of a rash, the problem is relatively simple. As we have seen, HI antibody usually does not appear before the third day of the rash or the 17th day after exposure, and any titer in a blood specimen taken before this period can be considered to indicate previous infection. It is, however, desirable to repeat the test on both the original and a second sample taken a week or two later to confirm the absence of a fourfold titer rise (which would usually indicate active disease). It must be stressed that accurate interpretation of acute and convalescent titers demands that both be obtained simultaneously during the same test run. It is, therefore, mandatory that an aliquot of the acute serum be kept either refrigerated or frozen whenever dealing with a pregnant woman exposed to rubella.

If the woman presents herself later in the course of the infection the problem is more difficult. Because of the rapidity of development of HI antibody, it may not be possible to show a fourfold rise in titer on two sera taken a week apart, and there is no way of knowing whether this antibody is from an acute or old infection. In this situation the CF test may be of value. Because this antibody appears later in the course of the infection and rises more slowly, it may be possible to demonstrate a fourfold rise of CF antibody when it is not possible with HI antibody. If the patient is not seen until two weeks after the rash, neither the HI or CF test is of value, and the only method of detecting acute infection is by examination of a single serum for rubella IgM antibody. As mentioned, this develops early and persists for only three to four weeks. Its presence, therefore, indicates acute infection.

Congenital Infection. Rubella virus can be isolated from urine, feces, nasal and oral secretions, and spinal fluid from an infected newborn. However, after a few months of life the virus is recoverable only from spinal fluid or throat swabs. Virus can be recovered from about two-thirds of infants with the disease during the first month of life, about one-third at five to seven months and only 7 per cent at one year, as shown in Figure 21–24. Isolation after 18 months is very rare. At birth the sera of infected infants contain antibodies at titers equal

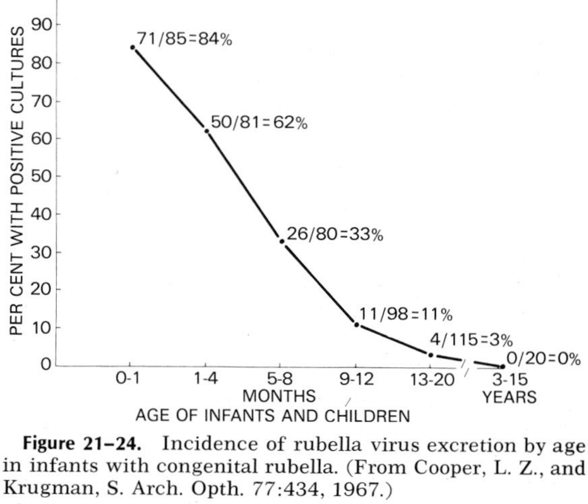

Figure 21–24. Incidence of rubella virus excretion by age in infants with congenital rubella. (From Cooper, L. Z., and Krugman, S. Arch. Opth. 77:434, 1967.)

*It is the current recommendation of the U. S. Public Health Service that women who receive vaccine not become pregnant for at least two and preferably three months. It is uncommon for women to become pregnant again within two months of delivery.

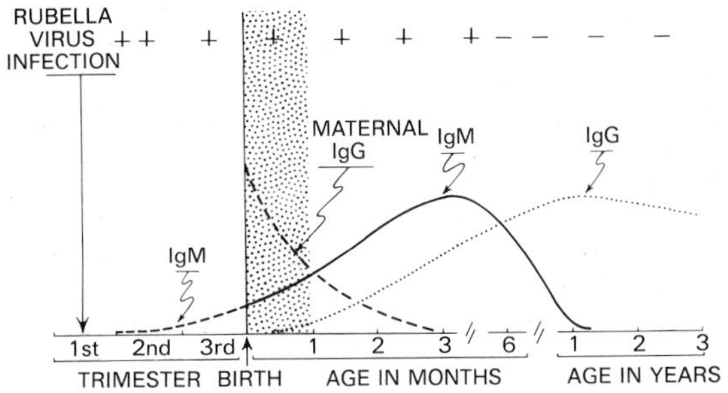

Figure 21–25. Natural history of congenital rubella. Pattern of virus excretion and antibody response. (From Krugman, S., and Ward, R. A.: Infectious Diseases of Children. 4th ed. St. Louis, The C. V. Mosby Co., 1968.)

to, or greater than, those in the maternal sera. These are both IgG of maternal origin and IgM of fetal origin. The half-life of the passively transferred maternal antibodies is one month, and persistence of titers of HI antibodies at six months is very highly suggestive of intrauterine infection. In marked contrast to the situation in postnatal rubella, the infant with congenital rubella continues to produce IgM antibodies well into the first year of life, as shown in Figure 21–25. It is apparent, therefore, that even though the infant with congenital rubella demonstrates immunological competence, it continues to excrete virus even with high titers of circulating antibodies. About 5 per cent of infants with congenital rubella do not have detectable antibodies.

Postvaccination. The sero-conversion rate of susceptible individuals following vaccination is extremely high, and virtually all develop HI antibodies. These persist for years, but at lower levels than following infection with wild virus. Since any titer is considered to confer immunity, this statistical difference is not important. However, when vaccine immune individuals are exposed to wild virus, many will have a fourfold rise in the titer of HI antibody. This is *not* associated with viremia, and available evidence suggests that the fetus would not be at risk if the person were pregnant. This dramatically illustrates the importance of an accurate history when interpreting serologic tests for rubella.

RUBEOLA (MEASLES)

Although measles has been recognized as a distinct clinical entity since antiquity, the causative agent was not isolated until 1954 by Enders and Peebles. This permitted the development of an attenuated live measles virus vaccine, which was licensed for general use in 1963. The older physicians were thoroughly familiar with this disease, but widespread use of the vaccine has greatly reduced the incidence of measles, and younger clinicians have had little experience with it. To further complicate diagnosis, atypical disease has been reported in patients immunized with inactivated measles vaccine (no longer available) two to four years previously. The spectrum of the disease was broadened in 1967 when the suggestion was made that subacute sclerosing panencephalitis is a late sequelae of measles infection. For all these reasons the laboratory diagnosis of measles is assuming increased importance.

There is generalized hyperplasia of lymphoid tissue during the prodromal period of measles, and multinucleated giant cells of the Warthin-Finkeldey type may be present. These are sometimes seen in an appendix removed from a child with measles who presents with abdominal pain before development of the rash. Similar giant cells are present in tracheal secretions in about 50 per cent of measles patients with respiratory symptoms, and their presence can be considered diagnostic. They are shown in Figure 21–26 and are distinguished from nonspecific foreign body giant

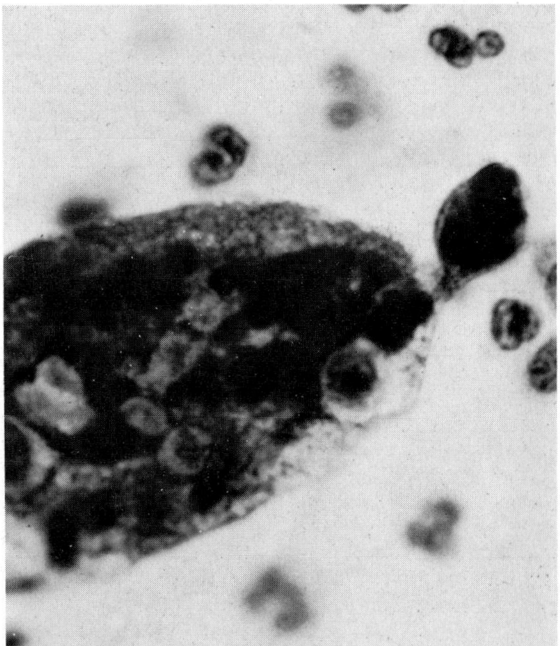

Figure 21–26. Giant cell with multiple karyopyknotic nuclei and numerous intracytoplasmic eosinophilic inclusions diagnostic of measles virus infection. (× 340.) (From Naib, Z. M., et al. Acta Cytol. *12*:168, 1968.)

cells by the variation in nuclear size and the presence of numerous acidophilic intracytoplasmic inclusion bodies.

Measles virus can be isolated from circulating leukocytes, throat swabs, conjunctival secretions, and urine in primary human or monkey kidney cultures, or in human amnion cells. Two distinct cytopathic effects are produced, the more common being the formation of syncytial giant cells with as many as 40 nuclei in one cell. The second change is alteration of the shape of the epithelial cells from polygonal to spindle or stellate in form. CPE is not apparent for five to 10 days and cultures should be held for 30 days; this limits the clinical usefulness of virus isolation. The morphology of the giant cells permits presumptive diagnosis which can be confirmed by neutralization tests.

Both hemagglutination-inhibition and complement fixation tests are available, and fourfold or greater rise in titer is suggestive of active disease.

Acute encephalitis is a serious and sometimes fatal complication of measles that occurs in about 0.1 per cent of cases. Although it usually develops from two to six days following the rash, it may occur before the rash. The pathogenesis is unknown but is believed to be an allergic type of encephalomyelitis. Virus cannot be recovered from the spinal fluid.

Subacute sclerosing panencephalitis (Dawson's encephalitis, subacute inclusion body encephalitis) was originally described in 1934. The disease is a rare and usually late complication of measles with a subacute onset. The earliest symptom is mental deterioration, which is followed by motor changes. Ultimately there is blindness and then coma and death. The disease is usually steadily progressive, although remissions have occurred. Cowdry type A intranuclear inclusions, similar to those seen in herpes simplex encephalitis, are present in neuronal and glial cells and are shown in Figure 21–27. Diagnosis is established by the presence of extremely high measles antibody titers in both spinal fluid and blood.

VARICELLA-ZOSTER (V-Z) VIRUS

Both varicella (chickenpox) and herpes zoster (shingles) are caused by the same agent, *Herpesvirus varicellae* or V-Z virus. Varicella represents the disease due to primary infection, while herpes zoster is seen in patients with partial immunity. It is believed that herpes zoster is due to activation of latent virus in much the same fashion that *H. hominis* causes recurrent skin and mucous membrane lesions. The virus is species specific (like cytomegalovirus) and cannot be propagated in experimental animals.

Varicella in children is usually a benign illness with characteristic manifestations that does not require laboratory confirmation. The disease is sometimes more serious in adults, however, and may have a fatal outcome, due usually to a diffuse interstitial pneumonitis. At autopsy focal necrosis may be present in many organs, and typical intranuclear inclusions are present. The diagnosis can be confirmed by isolation of V-Z virus from autopsy material. Encephalitis is a rare but serious complication of varicella which is fatal in about 25 per cent of the cases. It is sometimes possible to isolate the virus from spinal fluid.

Herpes zoster is characterized by a vesicular eruption which is usually unilateral and along

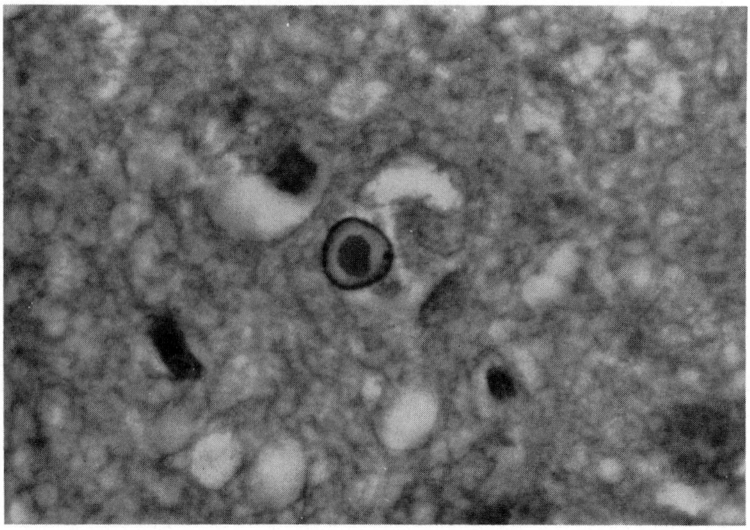

Figure 21–27. Cowdry type A intranuclear inclusion from a case of subacute sclerosing panencephalitis. (Courtesy of John Budinger, M.D.).

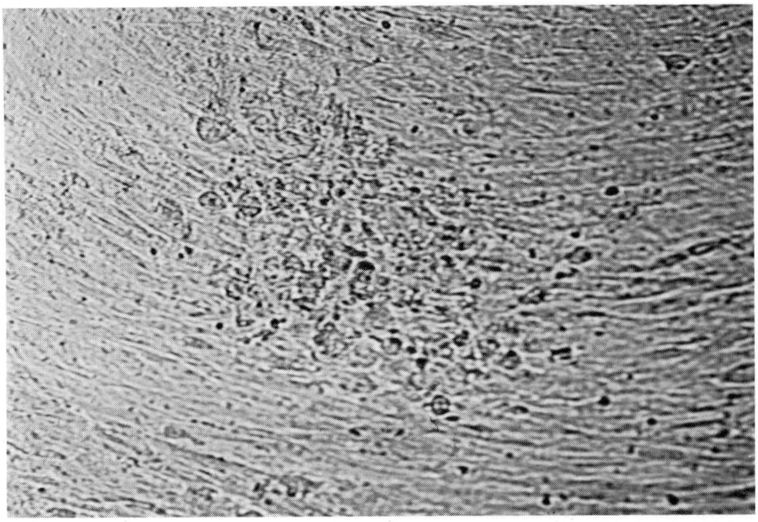

Figure 21–28. CPE of *H. varicellae*. (Courtesy of E. C. Herrmann, Jr., Ph.D., and T. Smith, Ph.D., Mayo Clinic, Rochester, Minn.)

the dermatome of a cranial, spinal, or sensory nerve. In contrast to varicella, pain and adenopathy are constant features. Virus isolation may be requested for definitive diagnosis.

Material for virus isolation is obtained from fresh vesicular eruptions; the agent is never isolated from crusted lesions or those that contain purulent material. Virus recovery is rare after the third day of illness in varicella but it may be isolated for a week or even longer from the lesions of zoster. Fluid is obtained by aspiration of vesicles and should be pooled in the throat swab media previously described. The virus is isolated only very rarely from other sites such as throat, blood, or spinal fluid.

It has been suggested that human amnion is the cell of choice for initial isolation, but there have been few studies of the susceptibility of various cell cultures. Diploid human lung is satisfactory, and embryonic human kidney is highly susceptible. Confluent cell sheets must be maintained for at least three weeks, and blind passage may be required for virus recovery. The virus is strongly cell associated, and passage must include cells as well as culture fluid. Rolled cultures apparently are preferable to stationary ones. The CPE of V-Z virus is typically focal, as shown in Figure 21–28, and there are intranuclear inclusions and syncytial giant cells. An isolate with this CPE that is from a vesicular lesion and is so strongly cell associated that it cannot be passaged with cell-free fluid alone can reliably be called V-Z virus. While the CPE of cytomegalovirus (CMV) may be similar, the green-brown pigment granules in the infected cells are lacking in cell cultures with V-Z virus. In addition, CMV does not grow in epithelial cells, is not so strongly cell associated, and is not recovered from vesicle fluid. Herpes simplex virus is easily recovered from vesicular lesions, but the rapidity of development and spread of CPE to involve the entire cell sheet and the broad range of sensitive cell cultures makes differentiation simple. The intranuclear inclusions and syncytial giant cells eliminate members of the poxvirus group.

RICKETTSIAL DISEASES*

The rickettsiae responsible for human disease are small, pleomorphic, coccobacillary forms that are a biologically distinct group of microorganisms. They resemble bacteria more than viruses in that they contain both DNA and RNA, have metabolic activity, possess cell walls, and, most importantly from the clinical standpoint, are sensitive to certain antibiotics. In contrast to both bacteria and viruses which often result in inapparent infections, rickettsial infection results in clinical disease.

The natural hosts of the rickettsiae include a variety of vertebrates and arthropods, and with the exception of epidemic typhus and trench fever (which are human diseases), man is an incidental host. Q fever is acquired by inhalation of an infected aerosol, but the other rickettsial diseases are all acquired through the bite of an insect (flea or louse) or arachnid (tick or mite). The rickettsial diseases vary from mild and self-limiting to fulminating and fatal and are common in many parts of the world. The statement has been made that more people have died of rickettsial diseases than any other illness except malaria.

*The sections on the rickettsial and bedsonial diseases in *Virus and Rickettsial Diseases of Man* by S. Bedson *et al.*, Edward Arnold, London, 1967, are excellent and served as the reference for this and the following sections.

The human pathogens can be divided into five groups on the basis of antigenic differences: the typhus group, the spotted fever group, scrub typhus, trench fever and Q fever. Information on these is summarized in Table 21–19. Although the basic lesion in all rickettsial diseases is vascular and a cutaneous eruption is present with all but Q Fever, laboratory aid is required for definitive diagnosis.

Rickettsemia occurs during the febrile period of all the diseases, and the causative agent can often be isolated by animal inoculation. These agents are highly infectious, however, and almost all laboratories working with rickettsiae have had accidental infections among employees, sometimes with a fatal outcome. Both Ricketts and von Prowazek, pioneers in the study of these agents, died from infections contracted during their investigations! Serologic tests are the most satisfactory for defining the etiology of a rickettsial disease, and clinical laboratories should not attempt to isolate an agent.

The Weil-Felix reaction is based on the development of antibodies against the nonmotile OX-19 and OX-2 strains of *Proteus vulgaris* and OX-K strain of *Proteus mirabilis* during certain rickettsial infections. Although several techniques are available, the tube test incubated at an elevated temperature overnight is preferred. Commercially available antigens differ widely, and false positive results may occur as they age; the use of known positive and negative human control sera is, therefore, very important. Paired sera should be tested together whenever possible. The usual reactions are shown in Table 21–20. False positive reactions may occur in patients with Proteus urinary tract infections, leptospirosis, Borrelia infections and severe liver disease. It must be stressed that the Weil-Felix reactions are nonspecific and not entirely satisfactory. The necessary antigens for more specific tests are not commercially available at this time, however.

Epidemic (louse-borne) typhus fever was the first rickettsial disease to be recognized. Agglutinins against Proteus OX-19 appear about seven days after onset of symptoms, at which time the titer may be as high as 1:200. Peak antibody levels occur at the end of the second week, with levels as high as 1:5000. A fourfold titer rise is considered significant, and the titer declines over several months. There is a lesser rise in the OX-2 agglutinins and none against Proteus OX-K. A complement fixation test for epidemic typhus that employs a rickettsial antigen is available and useful in three specific situations. The Weil-Felix reaction may be falsely negative in a patient previously vaccinated against epidemic typhus who develops a natural infection. A low titer of OX-19 antibody in a patient with fever may be difficult to interpret, and presence of a specific rickettsial antibody would tend to confirm the diagnosis. Finally, a specific test is required for laboratory differentiation of murine and epidemic typhus and spotted fever, all of which are associated with OX-19 antibody.

Brill-Zinsser disease probably represents an exacerbation of a latent infection with *R. prowazekii* in a patient who has had epidemic typhus previously. The disease is relatively mild, louse infestation is not necessary, and the characteristic rash is absent. Patients with Brill-Zinsser disease do not develop antibody against Proteus OX-19, but do develop very high titers of complement-fixing antibody within three to four days of onset of the disease. These are predominantly 7S in contrast to the 19S immunoglobulins initially formed during classic epidemic typhus.

Endemic or murine (flea-borne) typhus is a relatively mild disease transmitted to man by the rat flea. The causative agents of epidemic and endemic typhus are antigenically related, and recovery from one confers immunity to the other. In contrast, immunization to one does not result in protection against the other. Laboratory diagnosis is similar to that for epidemic typhus. Agglutinins against Proteus OX-19 develop but are usually present in lower titer. The complement fixation test, as indicated, is useful to distinguish epidemic from endemic typhus fever.

Scrub typhus (tsutsugamushi disease) is transmitted to man by mites which attach to the skin and then suck blood. (Tsutsugamushi means mite fever in Japanese.) The name "scrub" typhus refers to the particular type of tropical vegetation found in the Far East and Pacific areas where the disease is prevalent. In contrast to the other typhus fevers, a characteristic eschar develops at the site through which the rickettsia entered the body (mite bite). The Weil-Felix reaction is of value for diagnosis, as agglutinins develop against Proteus OX-K but not against either OX-19 or OX-2. Titers begin to rise during the second week of illness and reach a maximum early in convalescence. An indirect fluorescent antibody technique which employs smears of *R. tsutsugamushi* as antigen is available and of value.

Rocky Mountain spotted fever (RMSF) is the best known member of the spotted fever group, but there are a variety of tick fevers caused by antigenically similar agents. RMSF has been observed in almost all states of the United States and resembles typhus at the onset. The Weil-Felix reaction in this disease is variable, with high titers against either OX-19 or OX-2, sometimes against both and, on occasion, against neither. Complement fixation and rickettsial agglutination tests are available and of value.

Table 21–19. RICKETTSIAL DISEASES OF MAN*

DISEASE		GEOGRAPHICAL DISTRIBUTION	NATURAL CYCLE		TRANSMISSION TO MAN	SEROLOGICAL DIAGNOSIS	
Group and Type	Agent		Arthropod	Mammal		Weil-Felix Reaction	Complement Fixation
Typhus							
Epidemic	*R. prowazekii*	Worldwide	Body louse	Man	Infected louse feces into broken skin	Positive OX-19	Positive group- and type-specific
Brill's disease	*R. prowazekii*	N. America; Europe	Recurrence years after original attack of epidemic typhus			Usually negative	Positive group- and type-specific
Endemic	*R. mooseri*	Worldwide	Flea	Rodents	Infected flea feces into broken skin	Positive OX-19	Positive group- and type-specific
Spotted fever							
Rocky Mountain spotted fever	*R. rickettsii*	Western Hemisphere	Ticks	Wild rodents; dogs	Tick bite	Positive OX-19 OX-2	Positive group- and type-specific
Boutonneuse fever	*R. conori*	Africa; Europe; Middle East; India	Ticks	Wild rodents; dogs	Tick bite	Positive OX-19 OX-2	Positive group- and type-specific
Queensland tick typhus	*R. australis*	Australia	Ticks	Marsupials; wild rodents	Tick bite	Positive OX-19 OX-2	Positive group- and type-specific
North Asian tick-borne rickettsiosis	*R. sibiricus*	Siberia; Mongolia	Ticks	Wild rodents	Tick bite	Positive OX-19 OX-2	Positive group- and type-specific
Rickettsialpox	*R. akari*	North America; Europe	Blood-sucking mite	House mouse and other rodents	Mite bite	Negative	Positive group- and type-specific
Scrub typhus	*R. tsutsugamushi*	Asia; Australia; Pacific Islands	Trombiculid mites	Wild rodents	Mite bite	Positive OX-K	Positive in about 50% of patients
Q fever	*R. burnetii*	Worldwide	Ticks	Small mammals; cattle; sheep and goats	Inhalation of dried, infected material	Negative	Positive
Trench fever	*R. quintana*	Europe; Africa; North America	Body louse	Man	Infected louse feces into broken skin	Negative	None available

*From Lennette, E. H., and Schmidt, N. J. (eds.): Diagnostic Procedures for Viral and Rickettsial Infections. 3rd ed. American Public Health Association, New York, 1964, p. 744.

Table 21–20. WEIL-FELIX REACTIONS*

RICKETTSIAL DISEASES	MAGNITUDE OF ANTIBODY RESPONSE		
	Proteus Antigens		
	OX_{19}	OX_2	OXK
Epidemic typhus (primary)	++++	+	0
Murine typhus	++++	+	0
Rocky Mountain spotted fever	++++	+	0
and other tick-borne spotted fever group infections	+	++++	0
Rickettsialpox	0	0	0
Scrub typhus	0	0	++++
Q fever	0	0	0
Trench fever	0	0	0

*From Lennette, E. H., and Schmidt, N. J. (eds.): Diagnostic Procedures for Viral and Rickettsial Infections. 3rd ed. American Public Health Association, New York, 1964, p. 761.

Q fever in man is characterized by a pneumonitis without a rash and is contracted by inhalation of the agent instead of by the bite of an arthropod. The disease is most common among farm workers and slaughterhouse personnel who handle cattle and sheep. *Coxiella burnetii* differs from other rickettsiae in being very stable outside host cells. It is present in nasal and salivary secretions as well as in the placenta and amniotic fluid of infected animals and can remain viable in dried material for long periods of time. Infection is not associated with Proteus agglutinins so the Weil-Felix reaction is useless. The antigenic composition of the causative agent is unique, and both complement fixation and agglutination tests are available.

Trench fever is not a problem in the civilian population and was first recognized during World War I among troops in France. The causative agent is *R. quintana,* which has recently been grown on blood agar, a development that will undoubtedly raise questions about its classification.

BEDSONIA (CHLAMYDIA)

This family of microorganisms was originally considered to be viruses because they are seen as inclusion bodies in infected cells, are obligate intracellular parasites, and are about 200 $m\mu$ in diameter. However, they contain both RNA and DNA and are susceptible to some antibiotics so that they, like the rickettsia, resemble bacteria. They differ from the rickettsia in being dependent on their host for energy-rich phosphate esters such as ATP. Other differences are the presence of a heat-stable common antigen absent in rickettsia and the absence of arthropod vectors in their life cycle. There is lack of agreement on the name to be used for these agents, and some call them Bedsonia while others prefer Chlamydia.

The host range of the Bedsonia is wide and includes many species of birds as well as both small and large mammals. The clinical picture reflects the method of transmission and can vary from subclinical to fatal disease. Psittacosis is primarily an avian disease. Although the name implies that the infection is acquired from parrots, a variety of other birds have been incriminated and the terms ornithosis and psittacosis are increasingly being used interchangeably. Lymphogranuloma venereum occurs as a natural infection only in man and is transmitted by sexual intercourse. It is primarily a disease of the tropics where it is common, being exceeded in frequency only by syphilis and gonorrhea among the venereal diseases. Trachoma and inclusion conjunctivitis (TRIC) are also natural infections of man only. The former is spread by direct contact and infection is limited to the eye, while the agent of inclusion conjunctivitis can involve both the eye and the uterine cervix. It is transmitted by direct contact, venereally, and by contaminated swimming pool water (swimming pool conjunctivitis).

Bedsonia are highly infectious, and routine clinical laboratories should not attempt isolation from clinical specimens. The comments concerning the hazards of rickettsial isolation are true also for Bedsonia and should be considered before injection of clinical specimens from a particularly interesting diagnostic problem into laboratory animals. Material for isolation can be kept for several days in the refrigerator or for some weeks at −70° C.; it should be shipped packed in dry ice.

Psittacosis-ornithosis is acquired by contact with infected birds, and a history of such exposure often suggests the diagnosis. Infected birds may or may not appear ill, and healthy avian carriers are common among those who have recovered from the disease. The agent is present in bird droppings, and man is usually infected from a contaminated aerosol of fecal material. Human psittacosis usually presents as a mild respiratory infection but at times may be an acute severe or even fatal pneumonia. There is nothing distinctive about the clinical picture, and laboratory aid is essential for diagnosis.

The agent of psittacosis contains a heat-labile specific antigen as well as the group-specific, heat-stable antigen. The latter is usually used in the complement fixation test, and results must be correlated with the clinical picture. Since psittacosis and lymphogranuloma venereum present differently, this is not a problem. Normal sera may have a low antibody titer, so a level of at least 1:32 is required for presumptive diagnosis on a single serum. Demonstration of a fourfold or greater rise is much more significant, however. Antibody appears during the second week of illness and reaches a maximum level, usually between 1:64 and 1:256, in 20 to 30 days. Titers may decline in a few months following recovery or persist for years. Early antibiotic therapy may prevent a significant rise in titer and make definitive diagnosis impossible.

Lymphogranuloma venereum is characterized by the initial development of a painless, inconspicuous, self-healing, shallow ulcer which appears after an incubation period of three days to three weeks. Medical attention is rarely sought, and several weeks later the lymph nodes which drain the site of ulceration enlarge, suppurate, and may rupture through the skin. From the clinical picture it is apparent that early diagnosis is rare, and a fourfold titer rise is almost never obtained. The titer of complement-fixing antibody is almost always high when the patient is first seen and furnishes presumptive evidence of infection.

The Frei test is performed by intradermal injection of antigen and measurement of the area of induration that develops after 48 hours. The original antigen was pus from an unruptured bubo, but the bedsonia have been grown in the yolk sac of fertile eggs, and this material is purified and marketed under the name "Lygranum." The test becomes positive in from one week to six months after infection and remains positive for many years. Because the bedsonia share a common antigen, the Frei test is positive with psittacosis.

Trachoma is prevalent in Egypt, North Africa, and the Near East, and does occur in the United States. It is spread by direct contact and flourishes where personal hygiene is poor. It begins as a conjunctivitis, involving particularly the upper lids, and spreads to the cornea where vascularization and scarring result in blindness. Inclusion conjunctivitis in the adult is somewhat similar but the conjunctivitis, which has a predilection for the lower eyelids, is self-limiting and never results in blindness. Asymptomatic, venereally transmitted genital infection of the female is the source of the disease in the newborn. The purulent conjunctivitis is similar to gonococcal ophthalmitis, and laboratory aid is required for differentiation. Diagnosis is made by examination of conjunctival scrapings for intracytoplasmic inclusions as shown in Figure 21–29. These are similar in trachoma and inclusion conjunctivitis, which can be distinguished by clinical differences.

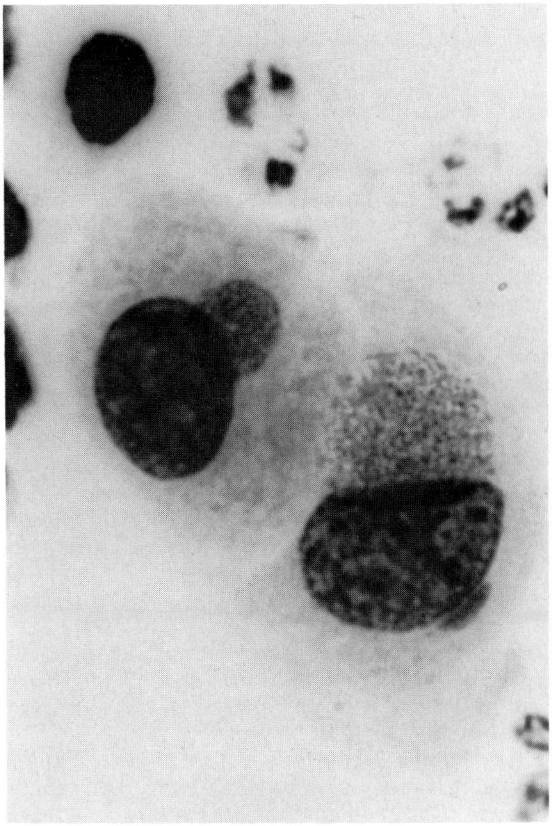

Figure 21–29. TRIC agent in conjunctival scraping. (× 1100.) (Courtesy of Z. Naib, M.D.).

DISEASES CAUSED BY MYCOPLASMAS*

This discussion of the mycoplasmas will attempt to explain what they are as well as what they are not, and why they are included (incorrectly but not without considerable historical justification) in a chapter dealing primarily with viruses.

Mycoplasmas are the smallest of the free-living microorganisms (about 200 mμ) and are capable of growth and multiplication in both liquid and solid inanimate media. Sterol is necessary for growth and replication, and most mycoplasmas contain large amounts of cholesterol (the single exception is *M. laidlawii*). They lack a cell wall and are, therefore, highly pleomorphic. Serologic and nucleic acid homology studies indicate that they are not derived from bacteria or the L-phase of bacteria.

**The Mycoplasmatales and the L-Phase of Bacteria,* by L. Hayflick (ed.), Appleton-Century-Crofts, Inc., New York, 1969, is a comprehensive book that served as a reference for this section.

L-Phase organisms are defined as independent growth variants of bacteria. They are potentially capable of reversion, but this is not demonstrable in all instances. They, too, lack a cell wall and are, therefore, pleomorphic, but they retain the ability to synthesize some cell wall components. Although the microscopic and colonial characteristics of L-phase organisms and mycoplasmas are similar, they are not related.

Contagious bovine pleuropneumonia is an important disease of cattle whose etiologic agent was isolated in 1898. Similar organisms from other animals were soon isolated and called pleuropneumonia-like (PPLO). Although bovine pleuropneumonia is caused by a mycoplasma, the terms PPLO and mycoplasma should not be considered synonymous. The correct generic name is *Mycoplasma*, and PPLO is not an acceptable alternate.

Viable organisms as small as 125 mμ that were capable of producing bovine pleuropneumonia were defined by ultrafiltration studies in 1929. On this basis the agent was considered a virus. The causative agent of primary atypical pneumonia in humans was originally isolated in embryonated eggs by Eaton, who also considered it a virus. Finally, mycoplasmas frequently contaminate the cell cultures used by virologists. For all these reasons the mycoplasmas are often considered with the viruses.

Mycoplasmas are part of the normal flora of the mouth and urogenital tract. Their role in causation of disease has been intensively studied, and they have been isolated from many different body sites such as joint fluid, blood, bone marrow, and abscesses. As might be suspected, this has resulted in an enormous amount of speculation about the importance of these agents as causes of human disease. We shall discuss briefly primary atypical pneumonia, the only illness definitely established as mycoplasmal in origin, and nongonococcal urethritis, a common venereal disease probably due to a mycoplasma.

The importance of *M. pneumoniae* has been stressed in the section on respiratory illnesses. The signs and symptoms of primary atypical pneumonia (PAP) are similar to those of pneumonias due to other causes, and definitive diagnosis is dependent on the laboratory. The distinction is important because PAP can be treated with erythromycin or a tetracycline. *Mycoplasma pneumoniae* can be isolated from throat swabs in a high percentage of cases, probably because they are quite hardy and are not killed by low temperatures. The medium required contains horse serum and yeast extract. Ideally both plates of agar medium and tubes with diphasic medium (agar overlaid with broth) should be inoculated. Growth of *M. pneumoniae* is slow (this is one of the features useful in distinguishing it from other mycoplasmas) and may not be apparent for over a month. This severely limits the usefulness of isolation as a routine diagnostic tool. A variety of serologic methods are available, but we shall consider only the two most widely used. Many patients with PAP have a high titer of cold hemagglutinins. This is not specific, and there are both false positives and negatives. Despite this, the test is useful because it is easy to perform and titers above 1:32 are uncommon in other diseases. The complement fixation test for *M. pneumoniae* pneumonia is reliable and more specific than measurement of cold agglutinins. Demonstration of a fourfold or greater rise in titer is desirable, but a titer of at least 1:16 can be considered presumptive evidence of infection. A comparison of isolation and serologic methods for the laboratory diagnosis of PAP is shown in Table 21–21.

Table 21–21. ANTIBODY RESPONSE AND *Mycoplasma pneumoniae* ISOLATIONS IN PNEUMONIA PATIENTS WITH PAIRED SERA AND THROAT SWABS*

	M. PNEUMONIAE ISOLATED (A)	M. PNEUMONIAE NOT ISOLATED (B)	PER CENT ISOLATION A (A + B) ×100
No. of patients	184	994	16
Fourfold antibody rise†	106 (58%)‡	57 (6%)§	65
No fourfold rise but acute serum titer 1:16 or greater	70 (38%)	105 (11%)	40
No fourfold antibody rise nor acute serum titer of 1:16 or greater	8 (4%)	832 (84%)	1

*From Hayflick, L. (ed.): The Mycoplasmatales and the L-Phase of Bacteria. New York, Appleton-Century-Crofts, Inc., 1969, p. 676.

†Antibody increase, as measured by CF with L-antigen. Lowest initial serum dilution tested was 1:4; a change from less than 1:4 to 1:8 was considered a fourfold antibody increase.

‡Per cent of patients with *M. pneumoniae* isolates.

§Per cent of patients without *M. pneumoniae* isolates.

Nongonococcal urethritis is a common venereal disease whose frequency rivals that of gonorrhea. In 1954 Shepard isolated a new mycoplasma strain from the genitourinary tract that was distinguished by its very tiny colony size and called a T-strain for this reason. Although it can be isolated from asymptomatic individuals, numerous workers have found it in 50 to 80 per cent of patients with nongonococcal urethritis and it probably is the cause of most cases of this illness. The classic or large colony mycoplasmas found in the GU tract are *M. hominis* and *M. fermentans*. The latter is probably a commensal, but the former has been implicated in ovarian, Bartholin, and pelvic abscesses. Its role in nongonococcal urethritis is not clear, but its frequency of isolation in this disease is no higher than in well individuals and it probably is not a urethral pathogen.

REFERENCES

Amstey, M. S.: Management of pregnancy complicated by genital herpes virus infection. Obstet. Gynec. 37:515, 1971.

Blanc, W. A., and Goetz, R.: Simplified millipore filter technique for cytologic diagnosis of cytomegalic inclusion disease in examination of urine. Pediatrics *29*:61, 1962.

Chanock, R. M., *et al.*: Myxoviruses: Parainfluenza. Amer. Rev. Resp. Dis. *88*:152, 1963.

Clarke, D. H., and Casals, J.: Techniques for hemagglutination and hemagglutination-inhibition with arthropod-borne viruses. Amer. J. Trop. Med. Hyg. 7:561, 1958.

Glezen, W. P., *et al.*: Epidemiologic patterns of acute lower respiratory disease of children in a pediatric group practice. J. Pediat. 78:397, 1971.

Gregg, N. M.: Congenital cataract following German measles in mother. Trans. Aust. Coll. Ophthal. *3*:35, 1941.

Hanshaw, J. B., Steinfeld, H. J., and White, C. J.: Fluorescent-antibody test for cytomegalovirus macroglobulin. New Eng. J. Med. *279*:566, 1968.

Hardy, J. B., McCracken, G. H., Gilkeson, M. R., and Sever, J. L.: Adverse fetal outcome following maternal rubella after the first trimester of pregnancy. J.A.M.A. 207:2414, 1969.

Herrmann, E. C., Jr.: Experience in providing a viral diagnostic laboratory compatible with medical practice. Mayo Clin. Proc. *42*:112, 1967.

Herrmann, E. C., Jr.: Experiences in laboratory diagnosis of adenovirus infections in routine medical practice. Mayo Clin. Proc. *43*:635, 1968.

Herrmann, E. C., Jr.: Efforts toward a more useful viral diagnostic laboratory. Amer. J. Clin. Path. *56*:681, 1971.

Herrmann, E. C., Jr., and Hable, K. A.: Experiences in laboratory diagnosis of parainfluenza viruses in routine medical practice. Mayo Clin. Proc. *45*:177, 1970.

Johnson, R. T., Olson, L. C., and Buescher, E. L.: Problems in the laboratory diagnosis of herpes simplex virus infections of the nervous system. Arch. Neurol. *18*:260, 1968.

Leavell, U. W., *et al.*: Orf. J.A.M.A. *204*:657, 1968.

Lennette, E. H., and Schmidt, N. J. (eds.): Diagnostic Procedures for Viral and Rickettsial Infections. 4th ed. New York, American Public Health Association, Inc., 1969.

Marshall, W. J. S.: Herpes simplex encephalitis treated with idoxuridine and external decompression. Lancet 2:579, 1967.

Melnick, J. L., and Rawls, W. E.: Herpesvirus in the induction of cervical carcinoma. Hosp. Pract. p. 37, February, 1969.

Naib, Z. M., *et al.*: Cytological features of viral respiratory tract infections. Acta Cytol. *12*:162, 1968.

Ng, A. B. P., Regan, J. W., and Yen, S. S. C.: Herpes genitalis. Obstet. Gynec. *37*:645, 1970a.

Ng, A. B. P., Regan, J. W., and Lindner, E.: Cellular manifestations of primary and recurrent herpes genitalis. Acta Cytol. *14*:124, 1970b.

Person, D. A., and Herrmann, E. C., Jr.: Experiences in laboratory diagnosis of rhinoviruses in routine medical practice. Mayo Clin. Proc. *45*:517, 1970.

Person, D. A., Smith, T. F., and Herrman, E. C., Jr.: Experiences in laboratory diagnosis of mumps virus infections in routine medical practice. Mayo Clin. Proc. *46*:544, 1971.

Rawls, W. E.: Congenital rubella: The significance of viral persistence. Prog. Med. Virol. *10*:238, 1968.

Sainani, G. S., Krompotic, E., and Slodki, S. J.: Adult heart disease due to the coxsackievirus B infection. Medicine *47*:133, 1968.

Sturdy, P. M., McQuillin, J., and Gardner, P. S.: A comparative study of methods for the diagnosis of respiratory virus infections in childhood. J. Hyg. *67*:659, 1969.

Tilles, J. G.: Status of amantadine in control of influenza (editorial). New Eng. J. Med. *285*:1260, 1971.

U. S. Department of Health, Education, and Welfare, Public Health Service: Standardized Rubella Hemagglutination-inhibition Test. Atlanta, Communicable Disease Center, 1970.

Vargosko, A. J., *et al.*: Recovery and identification of adenovirus in infections of infants and children. Bact. Rev. *29*:487, 1965.

Chapter 22

HOSPITAL EPIDEMIOLOGY

by JAMES G. SHAFFER, Sc.D.

The need for prevention of hospital-acquired infection is a recognized responsibility of the institution and its management. In its most recent specifications, the Joint Commission for Accreditation of Hospitals is highly specific in its recommendations for a Committee on Infections and on certain requirements for the establishment of policies and procedures in the hospital.

The concepts are not new since there appear in various references quotations from authorities dating back to the early 19th Century. Prominent physicians of that time recognized the dangers of exposure to infection in the hospital, although they evidently did not know how to avoid the consequences of such exposure. A number of programs were introduced to control or prevent such infections, the most notable being Semmelweis' work with puerperal sepsis. The great advances in the understanding of disease transmission that followed the work of Pasteur and Koch and the developments brought about by Lister and others in initiating antiseptic and aseptic techniques in hospital practice led to the establishment of procedures that were quite effective in the control of infection. At least within the limits of the ability to deal with the prominent disease-producing agents, it appears that infection control in the hospital in the era just preceding the introduction of antibiotics was good.

The need for further emphasis on infection control was made clear by events that began in the late 1940's, almost simultaneously with the rapid introduction of the wide spectrum antibiotics. These events were characterized by, first, the emergence of antibiotic-resistant *Staphylococcus aureus* and the occurrence of outbreaks of staphylococcal disease, particularly in nurseries; second, by the appearance of enteropathogenic *Escherichia coli* as the cause of a number of nursery outbreaks of infant diarrhea; and third, by the apparent increase in the number of postsurgical wound infections caused by *S. aureus* and other organisms, such as *Pseudomonas, Escherichia, Aerobacter,* and *Proteus.* These events have shown beyond question that there is still the critical need for the application of all techniques designed (1) to reduce the microbiological population of the hospital environment; (2) to eliminate the danger of transmission of microorganisms from one individual to another, be it from hospital personnel to patient, patient to personnel to patient, or patient to patient; and (3) to manage linens, equipment, and other inanimate objects in such a manner as to eliminate them as sources of cross-contamination. In fact, trends in the nature of the hospital population and the introduction of new procedures, such as organ transplants and treatment regimes that neutralize body defenses, indicate that a full application of infection control techniques in hospitals will become even more important in the future.

The epidemiology of the hospital situation has been modified remarkably by the introduction of the antibiotics and other therapeutic entities. These agents, along with the use of vaccines and the application of public health measures of various types, have relegated many of the highly contagious, acute, fulminating bacterial diseases to a position of somewhat minor importance. This does not mean that the organisms that caused these diseases have been eliminated, but merely that their life-threatening potential has been markedly reduced. The hemolytic streptococcus is still present in the population and occasionally breaks through to cause such diseases as scarlet fever and streptococcal sore throat. Diphtheria, typhoid fever, lobar pneumonia, and meningitis, to name a few, still occur, and it is obvious that relaxation of care in prevention, diagnosis, and treatment might lead to disaster. In fact, as previously mentioned, *S. aureus* and the enteropathogenic *E. coli* have, within recent years, provided evidence of this. The problems with *Salmonella derby* that have plagued hospitals in certain areas is further evidence of the need for constant vigilance.

Extension of the life span of the human population that has resulted from the application of the measures just outlined has had a considerable effect. This results in the development of diseases not often seen previously. Such a situation leads to the enhancement of susceptibility to microbial disease beyond that which existed in the past. Thus, the patient population of hospitals tends to contain increasing numbers of individuals of enhanced susceptibility. This must play a role in any consideration of hospital epidemiology.

THE HOSPITAL POPULATION

As indicated above, the hospital population contains a high percentage of patients who have an enhanced susceptibility to infections. This susceptibility exists in the newborn infant, the burn patient, the debilitated older patient, and those who have certain metabolic diseases, are on steroid therapy, or undergo extensive surgical procedures. Such patients provide the opportunity for numerous types of microorganisms to produce disease. Indeed, many of the bacteria associated with hospital-acquired infection are members of the normal bacterial flora of the human. These include *Proteus, Aerobacter-Klebsiella, Escherichia, Pseudomonas, Staphylococcus,* and the various intermediates of the *Escherichia-Salmonella* group. *Staphylococcus aureus* can probably be included in the normal flora, since the organism is present in the nose and/or throat of a considerable percentage of the population. It is true that there are evidently some types that are more prone to produce disease than others, but one suspects that the infected individual is more important in determining whether infection becomes disease than is the organism. The important point to emphasize here is that these organisms are constantly present in the hospital environment. They are carried by patients, visitors, and hospital personnel. In addition, numerous bacteria not generally considered part of the normal flora are carried by varying numbers of people. These include *Str. pyogenes* (hemolytic streptococcus), *D. pneumoniae* (pneumococcus), enteropathogenic *E. coli,* and various species of *Salmonella* and *Shigella.*

The hospital personnel, consisting of physicians, nurses, technicians, housekeepers, aides, orderlies, etc., although representing a normal, healthy population, carry at all times a normal flora of microbial agents. This flora may at any time be enhanced by the presence of such organisms as *Str. pyogenes, D. pneumoniae,* and *Salmonella.* Thus, the hospital personnel provide a constant potential reservoir.

In the day-to-day care of the patients, there exists a type of intimate contact between personnel and patient that does not exist in other environments, at least to the same extent. Thus, the potential for direct transmission of microorganisms from personnel to patients, patients to personnel, and patient to patient is very real.

The picture of the hospital environment as constituted by its population can be completed by considering that periodically there is introduced a patient with overt microbial disease whose contagious potential is undeniable. If poorly handled, the introduction of such a patient into a highly susceptible population could be disastrous. The number of such patients varies with the type of hospital, and the provision for isolation or segregation depends on the institution involved. Nevertheless, such provision must be made and the isolation carried through diligently.

The basic design of the internal mechanism of the epidemiology of nosocomial infection is depicted in Figure 22–1. Certain modifications of a basic epidemiologic triad have been made in this diagram. In an oversimplified manner, perhaps, there is shown here the complex interplay of the hospital population and its normal complement of microbial agents. The various viral agents, either respiratory or other, as indicated, probably fit into this pattern.

The potential for self-infection in patients is very difficult to evaluate, yet it is generally agreed that indigenous infection often affects the hospitalized individual. Each patient has a normal component of bacteria on the body surfaces, in the gastrointestinal tract, and in the upper respiratory areas. Even the best skin preparation methods may not reduce the microbial content of the skin sufficiently to prevent infection of the surgical incision in certain patients. This depends on the patient, the type of surgical procedure, and the nature of the organisms present. A temporary bacteremia may occur during and after surgery as a result of trauma of one type or another. Such a bacteremia may result in the deposition of bacteria in areas of stasis around surgical incisions. There are certainly other ways by which self-infection can occur, such as removal of an infected appendix or gallbladder or the resection of the intestine. Indeed, this is probably one of the reasons why the infection

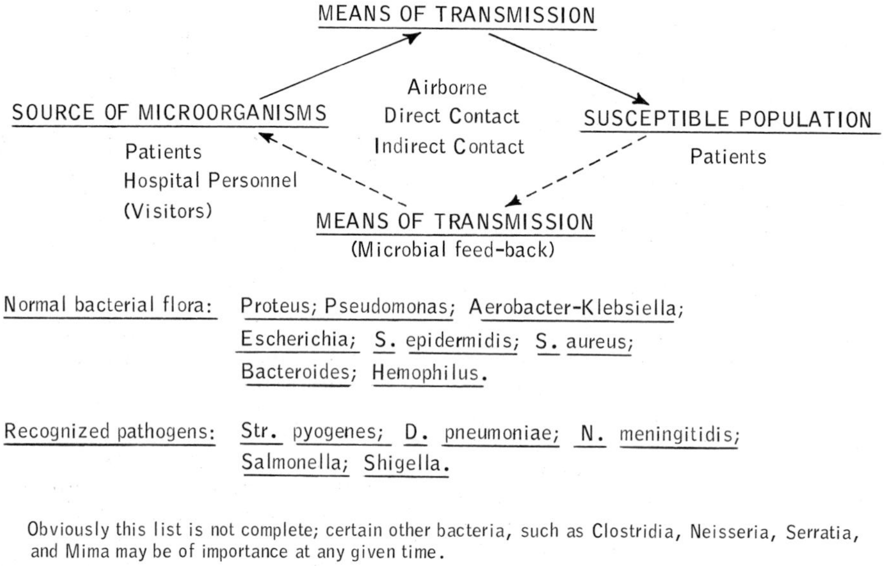

Figure 22–1. Epidemiology of hospital-acquired infection.

rate in so-called "dirty" surgery is higher than that seen in "clean" surgery.

THE HOSPITAL ENVIRONMENT

The physical environment of the hospital is a complex of areas and equipment, some of which have been termed critical, such as nurseries and operating rooms. Overall, this environment tends to become more complex all the time with the addition of new equipment and facilities. Oxygen tents, x-ray machines, physiotherapy tanks, heart-lung machines, and humidifiers are all items that need consideration. More and more hospitals are installing air-conditioning and air control devices. This has great advantage to the institution, patients, and personnel but requires careful planning and maintenance, else it may actually create infectious hazards of one type or another. Things like the location of trash and linen chutes and their design and maintenance need careful consideration.

One cannot look upon the hospital itself as a single unit in which all parts are similar. The areas vary, and the patients that occupy these areas differ in their susceptibility. The risks of the surgical patient in the operating room are not the same as those of the medical patient on the floor. In fact, the surgical patient may occupy several different environments during hospitalization and is thus exposed to different circumstances. The significance, if any, of all the variable circumstances is not yet known. In the design of studies of the hospital environment, it must be remembered that all the specific areas are related to all the other areas, and, ideally, the entire institution should be studied in such a way that specific areas can be either segregated as separate units or included in the total picture. This will be referred to later.

The microbial content of the hospital environment depends in large measure on people and their activity. Most of the organisms are those normally carried by the patients, personnel, and visitors. This determines the quality of the microbial flora at any given time. The quantity of organisms depends on a host of factors, which include the type of air control, the type of activity of the personnel, the nature of the area, and, above all, the excellence of housekeeping.

MODES OF TRANSMISSION

There has been much discussion about the means by which patients become infected in the hospital and the relative importance of the various possible routes. These routes are listed as airborne, direct contact, and indirect contact. One may make various subdivisions within some of these categories. One of the things that must be remembered is that microorganisms must have a transporting mechanism that will carry them from one place to another. Another is that there must be a sufficient number of microorganisms present for the carrying mechanism to operate. This latter is a critical issue and is a primary concern in the application of infection control programs. The relative importance of any route of transmission depends on the existing situation. It is easy to conceive of the possibility that a hospital with inadequate housekeeping and poor air control might find itself with such large numbers of airborne bacteria that the airborne route could be responsible for a considerable number of infections. On the other hand, a hospital that is immaculately clean, but in which the personnel fail to observe the necessary aseptic techniques and are careless in handling patients, might find that direct contact is of the greatest importance. Failure to properly sterilize instruments, poor technique with linens, and the careless use of instruments, e.g., failure to use a different set of instruments for each patient, would certainly encourage a belief in the importance of indirect transmission. Thus, any discussion of the relative importance of any route of infection must reckon with the conditions under which it might assume greater or lesser importance. Another important consideration involves the type of patient. The burn patient, for instance, not only presents an illustration of lowered resistance, but also may have a large burn area exposed to airborne dropout of microorganisms. Consequently, one must consider all routes of infection in designing infection control programs.

THE CONTROL OF NOSOCOMIAL INFECTIONS

Basic Organization

The epidemiologic picture presents a complex of patient, personnel, and environmental interplay in which the potential for the occurrence of endemic and epidemic infectious disease is always present. There is no body of fact on which an infection control program can be based. The principles have been known for a long time, beginning with Collins and Semmelweis and progressing through Pasteur, Lister, and others. One needs but to apply them while utilizing to the fullest extent the tools supplied by modern facilities, antibiotics, and preventive medicine.

It seems logical that the organization for infection control should conform with the basic organization of the hospital. Infection control may certainly be viewed as a part of the care of the patient in the hospital. Thus, the responsibility for this function resides with the board of trustees, since this body operates the hospital. By delegation, the responsibility for administering the infection control program becomes the duty of the administrator. In turn, the specific details devolve upon the department heads and the heads of the medical sections. Accrediting agencies

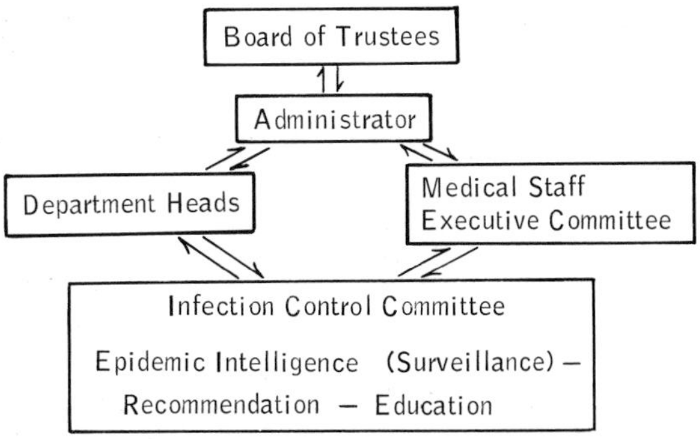

Figure 22–2. Organization and administration for control of nosocomial infection.

require that hospitals appoint an infection committee. This is an excellent requirement, and if the position and role of this committee is properly defined, it can become the hub of the program. On the other hand, if these things are not properly delineated, the committee may either be relatively useless or known only because it has a certain nuisance value.

Figure 22–2 outlines the organization of the infection control mechanism in a hospital. It will be seen that the infection control committee has three primary responsibilities: First, there is epidemic intelligence, or the establishment of a mechanism for surveillance. This is the central core of any infection control program. Without surveillance one cannot determine what problems exist and consequently what recommendations need to be made, nor can one hope to evaluate the effects of any measure that may be taken. The second responsibility is to make recommendations to the administration and medical staff on the development of rules and procedures, either of a general or corrective nature. The third is the education of the hospital personnel on the means of prevention of infection. In the latter, there is additional need to create an awareness of the hazards as outlined in Figure 22–1.

The membership of the infection control committee needs to be broad, including representatives of all groups within the hospital. The organization is shown in Figure 22–3. The participation of all groups is necessary, since this must be a broad and all-inclusive program. Infection control is, in actuality, a way of life in the hospital. Failure of one group to participate properly may have far-reaching effects.

The infection control committee must never be forced to become a legislative, policing, and judicial group. It must have the support of the policy-making and administrative arms, or it will not be an effective entity. This cannot be overemphasized.

The hospital epidemiologist can function in a variety of ways. His activities may be re-

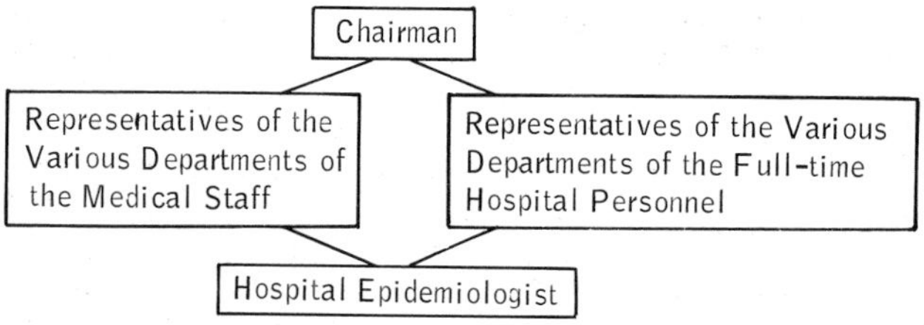

Figure 22-3. Composition of the infection control committee.

stricted to those of surveillance and consultation with the committee, or they may be broadened to include the delegation of authority by the board and/or the administrator so that he may assume some or all of the responsibility for administration of the program. This will depend on his qualifications.

The Specific Program

The actual infection control program is a multipronged endeavor. It involves, first, the establishment of a workable surveillance system, second, education of personnel regarding their responsibility and function within their daily activities, and, third, the provision of guidelines for the prevention of transmission of infection within the hospital. This latter may be subdivided into three parts—environmental control (airborne transmission), personnel (direct contact), and the management of instruments, linens, equipment, and so forth, which may be viewed as indirect contact.

Surveillance

As indicated before, the establishment of an adequate surveillance system is the keystone on which any infection control program is to be built. The adequacy of the system can be judged by the type of information it provides. It must be accurate, complete, up to date, and readily available to those who may have the need and the authority to use it at any given time.

No one surveillance program is likely to be suitable for all hospitals; thus, it is desirable to tailor the system to the size and nature of the institution. A number of different designs are in use in various hospitals and with certain variations may be applied to any hospital. Any system will require the expenditure of money, time, and effort, and the institution must be willing to provide for this in order to be successful.

A system that has been found successful in a number of hospitals requires the appointment of a surveillance officer. This individual is made responsible for daily visits to the various areas of the hospital, examination of patient records, and seeing that appropriate cultures are done and that compilation of data on the occurrence of hospital-acquired infection is accomplished. Of course, this person should work closely with the nursing staff and the physicians whose patients are involved, as well as with the infection control committee. In some hospitals a nurse has been assigned to this function, while in others a resident or attending physician may be designated to assume the responsibility.

In our experience, it has been found that, with the assistance of head nurses under the guidance from the director of nursing service, the chairman of the infection control committee, and hospital epidemiologist, and with the cooperation of the heads of the medical sections, an excellent surveillance system can be established. The head nurse and her staff are asked to consult with the physician when there is evidence of infection in any patient and suggest that a culture be done. Thus, one has a type of team approach which seems to fit with certain other modern concepts of patient care. Here, as is always the case, there is the question of defining what is to be considered infection. Space does not allow a discussion of this problem, but there are excellent presentations to be found in the references. This system has the advantage of involving a large number of personnel in the program and contributes a great deal to the degree of interest in infection control on the part of those involved. To round out this system it is necessary that the microbiology laboratory keep a continuous record of positive cultures and that, periodically, a report of findings be given to the infection control committee and the hospital epidemiologist. The frequency of this reporting depends on the circumstances. So far, it has been sufficient to have monthly reports on the surgical, medical, obstetric, and pediatric services and weekly reports on the nursery.

A useful policy was initiated some years ago in the nursery. By agreement with the department of pediatrics, the nurses were asked to assume the responsibility of doing cultures on infants where indicated, by the presence of either a pustule, a rash, or suppuration. It has provided excellent surveillance in this most critical area and on at least two occasions has revealed evidence which led to definitive improvement in technique. In both instances what might have been a situation leading to serious consequences was rapidly resolved. So far, it has not appeared to be necessary to extend this policy to the entire hospital, although certain institutions do this.

Fuerst *et al.* (1965) have described a program that not only provides surveillance within the hospital, but also relates to the community. Also, Brachman (1963) and MacPherson (1968) have commented in detail on methods of surveillance and the problems involved.

Regardless of the nature of the surveillance system that is to be established, a considerable amount of groundwork and education of the persons most intimately involved is necessary. There must be an understanding of the mechanism and the purpose of the program and the benefits to patient care that will accrue from adequate surveillance. The success or failure of any problem depends on the diligence with which those involved carry it on.

Education

The educational responsibility of the infection control committee is an essential part of a well-organized infection control program. This need not be a formal program of lectures and demonstrations, but rather a matter of establishing an awareness within the hospital of the need to prevent in-hospital infection. This can be accomplished through the key department heads who are members of the infection control committee. It has been found through experience that once the idea is presented the departments are prone to examine their own procedures and will then raise questions where uncertainty exists. When such two-way communication is established, the infection committee can act in its ideal role as an advisory group.

It should be emphasized that no individual or group of individuals such as the infection committee can solve the problems and prescribe the techniques for the various departments of the hospital. Nor can the various employees of the departments be educated and trained in this manner. Each department needs to be made aware of its responsibility, either through guidelines set up by the infection committee and approved by administration or by administrative directive made on the advice and recommendation of the infection committee.

By experience, it has been found that most if not all problems are discovered in one of two ways: either a department in the course of considering its own procedures in the light of an awareness of the modes of transmission of microorganisms discovers areas of potential danger or breaks in its procedures, or the routine surveillance system reveals evidence of a problem or indications of a potential hazard. When a department discovers a problem it may need advice, but in most cases the solution is so obvious that it can be handled internally. When a problem is indicated by surveillance, it is good practice to meet with the heads of whatever departments are involved. The evidence should be presented and the area of the problem located as nearly as the data will allow. The departments involved, after examining their procedures, are in the best position to arrive at a solution to the problem. It is significant that the most common finding involves technique in the actual performance of routine procedures. In most cases these are matters that would be recognized only by someone actually engaged in the supervision of an area. Forgetfulness about handwashing is a common observation.

There can never be any relaxation of vigilance in the infection control activity in the hospital. The infection committee through its communication mechanism can and should keep a constant flow of information circulating through the various areas of the hospital. This may be viewed as another facet of the educational function of the committee.

Prevention of Transmission

The mechanisms of transfer of microorganisms can be summarized simply as air, people, and fomites, with water and food as potential problems under specific circumstances. There is evidence to indicate that all modes of transmission play a role in the occurrence of hospital-acquired infection, but as pointed out before, the relative importance of any route will depend on a variety of factors. What is important here is the realization by hospital personnel that microorganisms do require a transporting mechanism and that prevention of such transmission requires the control of these routes.

There are some practical matters to consider in the initiation of hospital-acquired disease. One must differentiate here between infection or colonization and overt evidence of a disease process. The complex determinants that conspire to convert infection into disease are still poorly understood. In the present instance, the outcome of infection to a great extent depends upon the number and type of microorganisms implanted in or upon the patient. The debilitated patient, the one who has had a long and complex surgical procedure, the individual being given steroids, the burn patient, and the newborn infant certainly represent situations in which resistance to a given organism may be lowered. It is likely that the host is more important in determining the outcome of infection than is the organism, but all these things are relative and no real generalizations are possible. It does seem reasonable to assume that for any given patient there are a certain number of organisms of any given type which when implanted in an appropriate manner would result in the development of disease. Since one cannot eliminate microorganisms from the hospital environs, it is necessary and practical to do all possible to reduce the numbers by appropriate measures. These measures apply to environmental control (housekeeping and maintenance), personnel (personal hygiene and aseptic technique), and the handling of such items as instruments and linens.

With the development of techniques for making organ transplants, a new and revealing element has been added to the infection control problem. In order that such transplants be successful, it is necessary that immunodepressant drugs be given to the patient. This produces the extreme situation in terms of susceptibility and provides evidence that probably bears directly on the derivation of infection in other patients such as those referred to previously. The kinds of bacteria involved in post-transplant infections are the same as those found in the usual kinds of hospital-acquired infections. The most prominent of these is *S. aureus* followed by the gram-negative bacilli, such as *Proteus, Klebsiella-Enterobacter, Pseudomonas,* and so forth. Those who have studied such patients have felt that the evidence indicates most of these infections to be indigenous. In one series of 30 patients with renal transplants, it was found that 26 had some infection postoperatively. Nineteen of the 30 patients were carrying *S. aureus,* as revealed by preoperative culture. Postoperatively, 17 of these individuals developed significant staphylococcal infections. No staphylococcal infection occurred in any of the 11 patients not carrying *S. aureus* preoperatively. These findings suggest that the observed infections were indigenous. These considerations are of great importance in deciding what kinds of programs to design for these patients. Such observations suggest that such infections may become a major problem because of the highly susceptible patients who are found more and more frequently in hospitals. Obviously this is a new field and will require close observation over a period of time in order to understand the special problems involved. It is likely that these continued observations will shed more light on the problems involved with other patients.

Environmental Control and Surveillance

The potential role of airborne infection as it might apply to hospitals received renewed attention following the appearance of antibiotic-resistant *S. aureus* in considerable numbers in the hospital environment and the occurrence of numerous infections involving these organisms. There was certain evidence to indicate that, indeed, airborne transmission might be an important factor in hospital-acquired disease and there evolved the concept that hospitals tended to *develop* a "hospital flora" composed of microorganisms indigenous to the hospital. Certain types of *S. aureus* were suggested to be prone to colonize the hospital environment, and the term "hospital staphylococcus" was unfortunately introduced. The concept suggested by this term would indicate the widespread dissemination of these organisms throughout the hospital, probably by the airborne route, and indeed, studies of Walter (1960, 1963) and others would seem to confirm this. Furthermore, there was the idea that the hospital then becomes the center of dissemination of virulent staphylococci and possibly other organisms into the surrounding community. Studies by Ravenholt (1948) have shown that this does occur, although the observations of Ehrenkranz (1964) indicate that such dissemination is limited to the families of infected individuals and that widespread community involvement may be minimal. There are a number of well-documented cases in which infants who evidently became infected in the hospital transmitted the organism to other members of their family. Such observations suggest that, potentially, a hospital may become a source of dissemination of infectious agents.

The author and associates had occasion to do extensive microbiological studies in the hospital environment (Shaffer *et al.,* 1964) utilizing two contrasting hospitals, one new, modern, and air-conditioned, and the other an older hospital without the advantages of air-conditioning. No evidence was found in either hospital to indicate that there was a "hospital flora." The results of the studies indicated that the levels of bacteria in the air were most closely correlated with the excellence of housekeeping; therefore, air sampling provides an excellent means of providing quality control on this most important activity. Levels of airborne bacteria also depend on the air control system in the building. There was no evidence for any relationship between levels of airborne bacteria and the occurrence of hospital-acquired infection. Microbiological culture, however, provides an excellent means of surveillance of the environment.

To provide an adequate surveillance program, it is necessary to sample a sufficient number of sites to obtain a good assay of the total hospital situation. In one 325-bed hospital, 30 sites were sampled, and in a 185-bed hospital, 17 sites were used. The number will depend on the size and construction of the building (Shaffer *et al.*, 1965). The volume of air sampled and the frequency of sampling are also important. With the standard slit sampler, 10 to 20 cubic feet of air is probably satisfactory, although some recommend the use of high volume sampling as a routine procedure, feeling that a more accurate and meaningful result is obtained. Good discussions of the implications of these points can be found in the references. The frequency with which sampling is done will be determined by the urgency of the program. It is important to do enough samples at the outset to establish baselines and determine the normal fluctuations in airborne content of specific sites. Weekly samples for a month to six weeks will probably do this. After this preliminary period, biweekly or monthly samples are probably sufficient. Alternatively, one may start with a biweekly or monthly schedule and establish the baselines more slowly. It must be remembered that no single sample is completely definitive, since the level of airborne bacteria at any given time is subject to a number of uncontrollable influences. The medium used for air sampling is of considerable importance, and the type to be used will depend on the information desired.

Although no levels of bacteria in the air have been established as "safe" and no definitive relationship between airborne bacteria and the occurrence of in-hospital infection has been demonstrated, it does appear that it may be possible to establish some guidelines for achievable numbers of airborne bacteria. It seems entirely possible, judging from the results of extensive studies and regardless of the type of building or its location, that with good maintenance and good housekeeping one can maintain the airborne content of bacteria at an average level of between 10 and 15 bacteria per cubic foot of air in the hospital. On occasion, average levels between seven and eight have been achieved. Such levels seem to require that all conditions be favorable. In nurseries one may achieve levels of five or below. It seems that there is little to be gained by attempting to sample for specific bacteria, although our own studies with *S. aureus* have shown that, with adequate housekeeping and maintenance, levels of 1.0 to 4.0 *S. aureus* per hundred cubic feet of air can be maintained. Occasionally there have been "showers" of *S. aureus*. These are usually associated with some activity of the housekeeping or maintenance departments. On some occasions, increased levels have been associated with an infected patient who was shedding large numbers of *S. aureus* from the skin. These have never been followed by any recognizable increase in hospital-acquired infection. Attempts to sample for gram-negative organisms (e.g., coliforms, *Proteus,* and *Pseudomonas*) have failed to reveal their presence in most cases. Recently, on a number of occasions, routine air samples in specific areas have revealed the presence of *Pseudomonas* and *Mima* species. When this has occurred, investigation has revealed that a cold water type of humidifier was in use in the area. As a further check, Petri dishes were exposed over the air stream coming from the humidifier. Incubation of such plates revealed confluent growth of *Pseudomonas* and *Mima*. Extensive study of several types of cold water humidifiers has shown that with new, uncontaminated equipment, the water reservoir routinely becomes heavily contaminated with gram-negative bacteria (*Pseudomonas, Mima, Proteus,* or other genera) within a period of about 24 hours. This varies, depending on the water used in the reservoir and other factors not easy to document. Tap water in some cases is superior to distilled water, presumably because it contains some residual chlorine. The proper maintenance of cold water humidifiers to avoid this kind of contamination presents serious problems. It is not sufficient to merely clean the water reservoir and replace the water. This temporarily reduces the emission of bacteria, but in a matter of three to four hours the numbers may be back to the previous level. Thus, it is necessary to completely clean and sanitize the machine frequently, depending on the speed with which significant contamination occurs. Although it is difficult to document any relationship between these bacterial emissions and the occurrence of disease, the large numbers of potentially pathogenic bacteria sprayed into the air of a patient's room or into a hospital ward is certainly most undesirable and must constitute something of a hazard.

The determinants of airborne bacteria in the hospital are, in order of importance, housekeeping, people and their activities, and architecture, especially as it applies to air control. This refers to the more open areas of the institution, such as patient areas, corridors, and nursing stations. When one considers the more confined areas, such as operating rooms, the order of importance changes. Studies done in operating rooms indicate that here the number of people and their activities are of primary importance. The reason for this is that a relatively large number of individuals are present in a confined space, and each sheds his or her component of bacteria into the air. Certain types of equipment, such as the humidifiers referred to above, are also of importance.

By continuous air sampling in the operating room, it can be shown that the highest bacterial content occurs during the periods when there is the greatest activity. Thus, one of the ways to keep the levels lower is to control activity as much as possible and have no more than the necessary number of people present. Of perhaps just as much importance in the area of total bacterial count is the type of air control in the operating room, especially the number of air changes per hour. This is the only way to remove the bacteria that are inevitably introduced by people. Thus, care in planning and maintenance of the air control equipment in the operating room is very important. The laminar flow principle of air control has been investigated extensively in recent years and has been used successfully in operating rooms and other types of facilities to bring about and maintain low levels of airborne microorganisms. Indeed, this type of air control has been shown to be effective in achieving low levels of bacterial content even during periods of considerable activity. However, installation of the equipment is expensive, and there are still certain questions about eddies formed about objects in the path of the air flow that need investigation. There are also serious questions about the real need for such low counts except under unusual circumstances, and thus there is the question of whether one can justify the expense. Housekeeping in the operating room is of great importance, but the airborne bacterial content is not quite so definitive in determining housekeeping excellence here as it is in other parts of the hospital. Of far greater significance in this area is surface sampling of floors and other horizontal surfaces. Proper cleaning and disinfection in the operating room done at appropriate intervals is crucial to the prevention of postsurgical infections.

The significance of levels of airborne bacteria in operating rooms is not yet known, as has been indicated above. Indeed, in our experience, levels of 30 bacteria per cubic foot of air have been observed repeatedly during operations, yet infection rates have remained very low (less than 1 per cent). The Committee on Trauma, Division of Medical Sciences, National Academy of Sciences (1964), in a report on extensive studies on ultraviolet light in operating rooms, found that, although the ultraviolet lights seemed to significantly reduce the number of bacteria in the air, there was no evidence that this had any effect on the infection rate. Again, as is the case with other areas, one must assume that there are levels of bacterial contamination that would present a hazard to a particular patient, but there is no evidence to indicate what that level might be. Until such evidence becomes available, it seems logical to do all that is practically and economically possible to reduce the airborne bacterial count in operating rooms.

The source of airborne bacteria in the hospital is, of course, people, as has been indicated before. It is tempting to think that hospital employees may become infected with various types of microorganisms and, unless extremely careful, act as transmitters, contributing, as it were, to some hospital pool or flora. The extensive environmental studies referred to previously have made feasible investigation of this possibility. When *S. aureus* strains cultured from patients and from employees were compared with those found in the air, it was found that those isolated from patients in the hospital showed a much higher percentage resistant to penicillin than did those from the air or those from the employees. Indeed, in these studies, it appeared likely that the hospitalized patient might be providing the most potentially dangerous microorganisms to the hospital environment.

Surface Sampling. Although air sampling is probably the best means of maintaining environmental surveillance, the bacteriologic culture of surfaces can be very useful. Interest in surface-sampling techniques and the interpretation of the results of cultures obtained from surfaces within the hospital environment was renewed as a result of recent events to which reference has already been made. If used properly, the culture of surfaces can provide a means of evaluating the effectiveness of cleaning techniques.

Space does not allow for a detailed description of the techniques of surface sampling. These are well documented and may be found in the references. In recent years, the use of direct-contact culture with the recently developed Rodac plate or a similar technique has been increasing, mostly because of its simplicity and reproducibility when compared with the classic swab procedure.

Studies have shown that horizontal surfaces, e.g., floors, table tops, and shelves, are of more concern than vertical surfaces. Of the horizontal surfaces, floors are of the greatest importance, since they not only are subject to airborne dropout of bacteria-containing particles, but they also become heavily contaminated from the normal daily traffic of shoes, wheels, etc. It is important that the daily cleaning procedures remove this contamination effectively. Although the relation between surface contamination and air contamination is not completely understood, there is ample evidence to show that housekeeping, a large part of which is surface cleaning, does have a direct effect on the airborne content of bacteria. The data already presented in the section on air sampling supports this view.

A recent series of investigations conducted

by the Committee on Problems of Microbial Contamination of Surfaces of the Laboratory Section of the American Public Health Association has revealed the following: (1) Surface sampling, particularly on floors, with the contact agar plate is a simple and reproducible method of determining the degree of contamination present. (2) The technique can be used to evaluate the effectiveness of cleaning procedures. (3) There is great variation in the effectiveness of cleaning procedures in different hospitals.

In a cooperative study conducted in 16 different hospitals in which random sampling of a specified floor area according to the recommendations of Bond *et al.* (1963) was used, contact agar cultures were done just prior to and just after the daily mopping routine. In one hospital there were actually more bacteria cultured from the floor after mopping than were present prior to mopping, despite the fact that a good disinfectant was being used in the mop water. The results varied from this to institutions in which a 95 per cent reduction of bacterial content was achieved. At least one of the reasons for the surprising result referred to above was that the mop heads were allowed to stand in a mop closet overnight and reused without laundering and without drying. Evidently the bacterial load became so heavy, perhaps through multiplication in the wet mop heads, that even a good disinfectant could not exert its effect. In general, the hospitals with the lowest floor contamination after mopping also had the lowest contamination before mopping. Of the 16 hospitals in the program, only five showed evidence of adequate cleaning of floors. Subsequent studies by this same group (1970) have led to the recommendation of the following guidelines for effectiveness of floor cleaning procedures:

The figures are based on Rodac plate counts, average of 15 plates randomly applied in a high traffic area of about 8 square feet, immediately after cleaning, with the floor visibly dry.

GOOD	FAIR	POOR
0–25	26–50	over 50

These are quantitative figures only, and the presence of specific pathogens or opportunistic species must be interpreted separately.

In operating rooms this figure should be much lower, probably less than 5, although further study of this is necessary. It is practical to reach these figures on tile or other hard, smooth surfaces.

Surface sampling, if done properly, can be used to evaluate the efficacy of cleaning procedures. It can also be used to demonstrate to housekeeping and other personnel the presence of microbial contamination and can be very effective as a teaching device.

Thus, environmental surveillance has at least two facets – bacterial air sampling and surface culture. When used properly, such surveillance can contribute to the effective maintenance of an appropriate hospital environment.

Although it has not been possible to show a correlation between housekeeping and the occurrence of hospital-acquired infection, it does seem reasonable that there are degrees of air or surface contamination that must present a hazardous situation. Of even more importance, however, is the thought that a clean environment provides an appropriate setting in which to carry on an adequate infection control program. No doubt the psychologic effect on the personnel is, of itself, sufficient to justify establishing a suitable environmental surveillance system.

Instruments, Linens, and Other Common Items

The potential for transmission of microorganisms by improper use of instruments, linens, and other common items is obvious. Space does not allow a detailed discussion of the various problems of sterilization and disinfection of instruments, but adequate presentations are to be found in the references. Sterilization is usually accomplished by means of dry or moist heat, and it is essential that those charged with the responsibility of accomplishing this know the importance of proper packaging of items to be sterilized. They must be thoroughly familiar with the requirements for the operation of the sterilizing equipment and the technique of loading the sterilizer. Chemical indicators must be included with all items to show that proper temperatures have been attained, but one cannot depend on this as a complete control on the operation of the sterilizing equipment. In addition to the chemical indicators, it is essential that, periodically, as often as possible (daily or weekly) bacteriologic tests utilizing a standard spore preparation be used. These are available from commercial sources and are excellent when used according to directions. All autoclaves should be equipped with automatic temperature recorders, and the record sheet should be kept for reference in case problems develop.

Gas sterilization with ethylene oxide and, less commonly, betapropiolactone is being used extensively for certain items that are adversely affected by heat. When used properly, ethylene oxide has proved to be effective. There are certain requirements for humidity control that must be met in order that proper sterilization be attained with this gas. It is necessary following gas sterilization to aerate the item for a sufficient period of time to remove any residuum of absorbed gas. The time required for this aeration varies with the type of material being sterilized, and it is imperative that those using this kind of sterilization be aware of this. Thus, one is well advised to have available the proper equipment and be thoroughly familiar with its operation. Otherwise, such a measure does not accomplish its purpose. Betapropiolactone is also effective when used properly.

Disinfection and the proper use of chemical disinfectants has received a great deal of attention over the years. With the problems brought on by outbreaks of infection with *S. aureus* and other organisms, there was a rash of new disinfectant formulations. Space does not allow a review of all the types of disinfectants or formulations, except to point out that they run the gamut of phenolics, quaternary ammonium salts, iodine derivatives, long chain hydrocarbons, and so forth. They may be combined with detergents, packaged in aerosol bombs, with or without deodorants or perfumes, or put up in any manner which might appear to enhance the ease of application and the appeal as a sales item. Unfortunately the end result of such packaging may be some loss of effectiveness and an increase in cost.

Laboratories are often asked to evaluate a disinfectant. There are many pitfalls in this and before such an evaluation is attempted it is well to be familiar with the problems involved. These have been discussed very well by Spaulding (1963), Reddish (1957), and others. There are few, if any, hospital laboratories equipped to do the necessary tests. Spaulding has summarized the basic principles of selection and use of disinfectants in some detail, and thorough familiarity with such information will largely obviate the need for individual evaluation of products.

There are certain fundamentals of chemical disinfection that need to be kept in mind. The term disinfection implies that the object to be disinfected is to be rendered incapable of transmitting infection and should not be confused with sterilization, which implies destruction of all living agents. Thus, it is likely that the disinfectant will be used for a specific purpose. This must be kept in mind when the agent is chosen.

All chemical disinfectants are contact poisons and must be brought in contact with the offending bacteria in order to exert their effect. Some act by denaturing protein, others by destroying essential enzyme systems, and there are other methods as well. There is considerable variation in the speed of action of the various agents, but all require a certain minimal time for destruction of the organisms. With any given disinfectant the time required for effective action varies according to the nature of the disinfectant, the number and type of microorganisms present, the concentration of the disinfectant, the temperature, and the nature of the surface of the item being treated. The presence of proteinaceous material, dirt, or other soil may completely prevent penetration of the disinfectant, thus allowing organisms to survive. Therefore, the first step in the disinfection of any item is thorough cleaning, which accomplishes at least three things: First, it may actually remove most of the contaminating microorganisms and may, of itself, constitute an adequate or nearly adequate, disinfection; second, the removal of soil allows the disinfectant ready access to the remaining contaminants and insures its effectiveness; and third, by reducing the numbers of organisms, the time required for adequate disinfection can be considerably reduced.

The development of single-use disposable items has had a considerable effect in reducing the need for disinfection. It is certainly desirable to use these materials. But a problem arises on the matter of proper disposal of the disposables. A great deal of study will be required to determine suitable means of accomplishing this as their use increases. It is likely that most hospitals will need to study their own individual problems and facilities and use incineration, grinding, or baling as need arises.

The laundering and handling of linens need special attention. All linen when removed from the point of use should be placed in bags for transport to the sorting area. Proper surveillance of the laundry is absolutely essential to insure an adequate supply of safe linen for use in the various areas of the hospital. Periodic cultures of the various items as they come through the laundry should be done with swabbing, emulsification, or Rodac plates. Any evidence of failure to adequately remove bacterial contamination from the linen must be investigated immediately.

Personnel

The importance of personnel in the transmission of infection in the hospital has been recognized for over 100 years. This is certainly logical, since there is very intimate contact between certain hospital personnel (e.g., physicians, nurses, technicians, and therapists) and patients on a routine day-to-day basis. It is important, therefore, that all measures be taken to prevent this type of transmission.

There is general agreement that handwashing is one of the critical, if not the most critical, means of preventing person-to-person transmission of infection. Mortimer (1965) concluded from the results of a controlled study done in a nursery that handwashing was a vital part of the prevention of transmission of *S. aureus* in this area and suggested that this same consideration applied to other areas. It seems reasonable to assume that this same principle applies to organisms other than *S. aureus*.

There has been considerable concern about the possible role of carriers of potentially pathogenic bacteria in the occurrence of infection in hospitals, particularly those who carry *S. aureus* in the nose and/or throat. Numerous studies have failed to produce any definitive evidence that such carriers play a major role in the dissemination of these organisms. It is possible that these individuals contaminate their hands and transmit infection in this way; thus, handwashing, again, assumes an important role.

Skin carriers seem to present a considerable hazard, especially in those cases in which individuals shed large numbers of *S. aureus* into the environment. Such individuals may present problems of particular importance in such areas as operating rooms and nurseries. Ulrich (1965) has studied the bacterial skin flora extensively and described methods of detecting shedders. He also has discussed the possibilities of successful treatment of such shedders.

At the present time it seems there is little to be gained by doing carrier studies on hospital personnel, except under specific circumstances. Such circumstances may occur when unusual numbers of infections are observed in the hospital, particularly in surgical patients or nurseries. Any carrier survey should be done only on the advice and under the direction of a qualified epidemiologist. Otherwise, as is often the case, the results are likely to be unrewarding and will perhaps only contribute to existing confusion.

No person should be allowed on duty who has overt disease. Of particular importance are those with infected lesions of a superficial nature, particularly on the hands or other exposed area. Supervisors must be very alert to see that there is no deviation from this rule, although proper education of the employees may be more effective, since it results in voluntary compliance.

Education of personnel regarding the maintenance of appropriate personal hygiene, the necessity for using aseptic technique in all procedures, and the importance of avoiding transmission of microorganisms is one of the most important functions of an infection control program, as has been indicated above. If each employee could be trained to behave each day as if he or she were a carrier, much good would be accomplished.

Examination of Personnel. The pre-employment examination of all personnel should include a chest x-ray or tuberculin test, nose and throat cultures, and a complete stool examination, including bacterial culture and examination for ova and parasites. Ideally at least three stool examinations should be done on successive days. When shortages of laboratory personnel make it impossible to do three or more stool examinations on all employees, this may be limited to food handlers and to pediatric and nursery personnel. It is important that no person found carrying pathogenic microorganisms in the stool be put on duty in a critical area until the organisms are eradicated. It must also be remembered that carriers often either have very few organisms in the stool or shed them only periodically; hence, there is need for more than a single examination.

Following employment, periodic cultural studies on the hospital personnel are desirable. Those assigned to critical areas, such as nurseries, pediatric and obstetric services, operating rooms, and food-handling areas, should be checked more frequently than those in administrative sections, where contact with patients may not be frequent. Since the situation within a given institution is different from that in any other institution, the frequency and extent of these studies will need to be worked out to satisfy particular needs. The purposes, possible benefits, and limitations of the cultural examination of the hospital personnel must be thoroughly understood before the program is designed.

Carriers and Active Infections. The purpose of cultural examination is to discover carriers. It may be desirable to remove carriers from certain critical areas, but this may have only limited value and will depend on circumstances. A somewhat different benefit is the possibility that through these studies the personnel may be kept aware of the dangers involved and of the need for observing caution in their daily activities.

In most cases the carrier state is only transitory, especially in the nose and throat and to some extent in the intestinal tract, and a positive finding on culture signifies only that the organism was present at the time the specimen was taken. In fact, at the time the culture is examined, 24 to 48 hours after the specimen is taken, the individual may no longer be carrying the organism. In order to establish that the carrier state exists, it is necessary to do repeated cultures on all those who are positive on the first examination. Therefore, it is useless and impractical to remove individuals from duty merely on the basis of a single positive finding. This is well illustrated if one considers the situation presented by *S. aureus* in which on any given day it may be found that over 50 per cent of the personnel in a nursery or other area has positive cultures. If such a group had cultures taken on the succeeding day, undoubtedly several of those previously positive would be negative and several of those originally negative would be positive. Fortunately none of the other well-recognized pathogens induce this carrier rate, with the possible exception of *D. pneumoniae* under the most unusual circumstances.

The situation is somewhat different with the enteric pathogens, such as *Entamoeba histolytica, Giardia lamblia, Dientamoeba fragilis*, and the helminths, in which the carrier state tends to persist regularly for a long time. The same situation exists to a varying degree with enteric bacterial pathogens. Fortunately a much lower percentage of individuals normally have positive findings of enteric pathogens, and their removal from a critical area, such as a nursery, may not result in a serious depletion of personnel. All infected persons should be removed from nurseries and food-handling activities, however, especially those who have *Salmonella, Shigella*, or *E. histolytica*.

The situation with enteropathogenic *E. coli* requires special comment. Individuals who work in nurseries are evidently exposed to special risks, and a considerable number are likely to be found carrying this organism. The carrier state is not easy to eliminate, and it is impractical to remove all carriers from duty. Thus, all measures to prevent transmission are necessary.

Epidemiologic investigation of outbreaks of infection have indicated that the person suffering from an active infection is, as a rule, more dangerous than the carrier, undoubtedly because of the likelihood that the number of organisms present in the actively infected individual is much greater than in the carrier. It is thus imperative that individuals with evidence of active infection, i.e., upper respiratory infections, sore throat, ear infections, diarrhea, or infected lesions of the skin or nail bed, be discovered and removed from critical areas at the earliest possible moment. This is particularly critical in the nursery, since the newborn infant tends to be highly susceptible to infection. Daily inspection of all persons as they come on duty in operating rooms, nurseries, surgical wards, obstetric service, pediatric wards, central supply, and food-handling areas should be made by a competent and responsible individual. Bacteriologic examination is of little or no immediate help in most of these instances, except for diagnosis, since cultural results are not available for 24 to 48 hours and direct smears from lesions may be inconclusive.

It must be remembered that all infections have an incubation period and that this incubation period can be variable. For example, in newborn infants the incubation period for staphylococcal disease is said to be one to 30 days. During the incubation period for any infection, and especially in the period just prior to the appearance of symptoms, the individual may become highly infectious. Thus, the removal of an individual with clinically evident infection merely takes away a danger that has been present for an unknown period.

Obviously, then, the discovery of certain types of carriers and active cases and their removal from the environment does not eliminate the danger of nosocomial infection. There is no question, however, that these measures will reduce the risk. To further reduce the risk, and since no individual can ever with certainty be adjudged free of potentially pathogenic microorganisms, it is necessary to design and observe procedures to prevent the transmission of organisms from hospital personnel to patient and from patient to personnel. Here it must be re-emphasized that when one speaks of "potentially pathogenic" microorganisms, one refers not only to the well-recognized pathogens, but also to those organisms of the normal body flora, which, when implanted in or upon the patient whose resistance has been lowered by operation or disease, may cause serious consequences.

Maintenance of Equipment

There are certain items of equipment that need special attention. Water reservoirs of all types, such as those on oxygen equipment, are prone to become contaminated, especially with *Pseudomonas*. This can easily be prevented by cleaning these reservoirs on a daily basis. One cannot depend totally on the use of disinfectants since organisms resistant to the disinfectant in use may appear at any time. Frequent cleaning is the method of choice.

Inhalation therapy equipment is of particular importance. This equipment, used for patients who may be particularly prone to develop respiratory disease, tends to become heavily contaminated in use. The problem has been studied by Pierce and associates (1970), who have attempted to evaluate the hazard and have made recommendations for proper maintenance. Between use for patients, the equipment needs to be completely disassembled, cleaned, and disinfected. Since much of the equipment cannot be sterilized with heat, it is necessary to either use a suitable disinfectant or gas sterilization. One study which has not been published revealed that a critical point in the use of disinfectants was the rinse that was used to remove the disinfectant. This needs to be changed frequently, else it becomes heavily contaminated and recontaminates the item.

Recent events have indicated the importance of the proper management of the materials used for administering intravenous infusions. It has been shown that the sets used to give the infusion may become contaminated either as a result of long use or of improper assembly. The constant flow of bacteria-containing material then results in the development of fever in the patient, which persists until the infusion is discontinued. Of course, such introduction of bacteria may lead to various kinds of complications in debilitated patients.

All equipment such as portable x-ray machines are prone to collect dust, which may be dislodged when positioned over or near a patient. Constant attention to keeping this equipment clean is absolutely essential. Physiotherapy equipment, such as the various immersion tanks, needs to be drained, cleaned, and refilled between patients, since the warm water used routinely allows survival of most microorganisms.

Reference has already been made to the need for care and management of air control equipment. Shaffer and McDade (1962) found reservoirs of *S. aureus* in fan coil units in nurseries and patient rooms. Care needs to be used to see that such items as air filters, fan coil units, and air ducts are cleaned and kept in proper order. Routine maintenance schedules are essential in these areas.

Linen and trash chutes have received considerable attention as potential disseminators of microorganisms. There are certain basic rules that, if applied, will reduce the hazard. First, all linen must be bagged before being placed in the chute. Second, all contaminated linen must be double bagged according to accepted isolation procedures. Third, all trash must be bagged before deposit in the trash chute. This can be done easily and economically with plastic bags. Fourth, no contaminated items should be placed in the trash chute. These should be carefully bagged and transported to the sterilizer before disposal.

If all items are bagged before being placed in the chutes, much contamination of the chutes is avoided. In most cases the bags of linen are large enough to keep the chute clean and the need for further cleaning is minimal. Trash chutes should be cleaned periodically. Special devices are available which accomplish this very well.

INVESTIGATION AND FOLLOW-UP OF OUTBREAKS OF DISEASE

When an outbreak of disease occurs within any area of the hospital, extensive investigation is indicated. The microbiologist and epidemiologist play a major role in this investigation and should be consulted at the earliest possible moment, since as time passes it becomes more and more difficult to determine sources of infection. The course the investigation takes and the measures taken to prevent further spread will depend on the type of infection and the situation that exists within the area or institution involved.

One must attempt to determine whether carriers provide a continuous reservoir, whether there is a single source, such as food at a given meal, and whether there are breaks in technique in the day-to-day operation of the area involved. Information may be obtained in a number of ways, such as a careful study of the nature and occurrence of the infections and the isolation of a particular microorganism from a significant number of cases. The complete identification of the microorganism is important and can be definitive.

To take a specific example, this is perhaps the only situation in which phage typing of *S. aureus* can be justified at the present time. If, in outbreaks of staphylococcal disease, all or most cases are caused by a single phage type, the search for a source of the outbreak can be narrowed. Once the type of infection is known and its source is located, the procedure for preventing recurrences should become obvious.

The occurrence of such diseases as diphtheria and meningitis in patients occupying beds in an open ward or in other areas where other patients or hospital personnel may have been exposed also presents a problem. Here again the measures taken to prevent exposed, or possibly exposed, individuals from developing disease will depend on circumstances. The amount of help one can get from cultural studies on contacts is limited, and in most cases such studies should not be considered. Failure to culture *C. diphtheriae*, *N. meningitidis*, *Str. pyogenes*, or *H. influenzae* from the throat or nasopharynx of an individual exposed to the diseases caused by these organisms does not prove the absence of the organism. One may not have swabbed the correct area, or the organism may have been so sparse that no colonies appeared on the culture plate. Thus, the measures adopted must be determined on the basis of intimacy of contact and danger of transmission directly or indirectly to others.

The prevention of serum hepatitis is important not only in the hospital but also in doctors' offices and other places where parenteral inoculations are done. Transmission of this disease occurs when the serum of a person carrying the virus is introduced into another person. Because the most minute quantity of serum is capable of transmitting the infection, it is necessary to use extreme caution. Stylets and inoculating needles pick up enough serum to transmit the infection, and cleaning these items with alcohol between uses is not sufficient to remove or destroy the virus. Thus, when a technician is doing finger punctures, a new sterilized stylet must be used for each patient. When doing mass inoculations, such as vaccination or tuberculin testing, separate syringes and needles must be used for each individual. It is not sufficient simply to change the needle and to use the syringe for more than one inoculation. Syringes and needles must be thoroughly cleaned and sterilized between use. Disposable syringes and needles are available and should be used if possible. Transfusion is another potent source of transmission, and all possible precautions must be taken in the blood bank. No person with a history of jaundice should ever be used as a donor.

Since serum hepatitis usually has a very long incubation period, the consequences of carelessness may never come to the attention of the offending individual or institution. More recent studies indicate that serum hepatitis may also be transmitted through contact with body discharges from active cases.

THE ESSENCE OF INFECTION CONTROL IN A MODERN HOSPITAL

Modern medical care has reached a high degree of excellence, and the potential for the diagnosis, treatment, and prevention of illness is constantly improving. It would seem unfortunate if hospitals failed to utilize the utmost in diligence in the prevention of hospital-acquired infection, the occurrence of which may negate at least some of the accomplishments made possible by the techniques and treatments now available.

In the past, of necessity, isolation of the patient with infectious disease was utilized widely in the prevention of transmission of the types of highly contagious, acute fulminating diseases which were then prevalent. The problem now involves not only the transmission of disease from one patient to another, but also prevention of implantation of organisms in critical sites at critical times. Such organisms are often members of the normal body flora, and such implantation often no doubt results from faulty technique. Therefore, isolation of patients with overt microbial disease, particularly such as postsurgical wound infections, in the classic sense has only limited value. The ideal infection control program in the modern hospital requires some degree of isolation for each patient, which is accomplished by a combination of control of the environment, use of the best aseptic technique, maintenance of suitable personal hygiene by hospital personnel, and careful control of such items as instruments and linens. Indeed, if one can accomplish this, the need for isolation in the classic sense becomes limited to a certain number of special situations.

Each institution should examine its own situation and devise its policies to fit its own circumstance. This must be a continuous process, and changes should be made as indicated by surveillance, confidence in the ability to carry on appropriate procedures, and other considerations which may be peculiar to the institution.

TECHNIQUES FOR STERILITY CONTROL

The following section presents some of the most commonly requested bacteriologic checks on sterility control. In general these are methods that have been found reasonably satisfactory. In some instances other methods may be used if preferred. Whatever the technique chosen for a given determination, the advantages and disadvantages should be known. In some instances standards of acceptance must be set up by experience; in other cases they are prescribed by Public Health Service recommendations. In any case care, accuracy, and promptness must be used in doing and reporting on the studies. New methods for doing some of the tests are being developed constantly and should be adopted after proper evaluation and comparison with the older techniques.

Control of Heat Sterilization Procedures. The control of sterilization is very important, since the use of improperly sterilized equipment can lead to disastrous consequences. Detection of faulty sterilization performance can be accomplished by the use of various mechanical devices, indicators, or culture tests. Among the mechanical devices designed to eliminate the inaccuracies of human error in sterilizer operations are recording thermometers, indicating potentiometers, and automatic time-temperature controls. Properly installed, these devices undoubtedly constitute a great safety factor and a substantial saving in personnel time. Such instruments are essential for use with the newer ethylene oxide or betapropiolactone sterilizers.

The chemical or so-called "telltale" indicators are widely used but seem to suffer from a general lack of uniformity and standardization. Some indicators react to a time-temperature ratio inadequate for sterilization, or the endpoints are not sufficiently clear to permit accurate interpretation of the results (Reddish, 1957). If used, they should be placed in the center of the largest and most closely wrapped package in the load. Papers printed with chemicals that change color when adequate sterilization has presumably been accomplished are useful for some purposes but should never be used as the sole measure of control.

Culture tests are probably the methods of choice in evaluating the effectiveness of a sterilizing process. The only serious disadvantage is the delay in determining the results of culture tests.

Various types of bacterial spore preparations are now available commercially. These obviate the necessity for preparing suspensions in the individual laboratories and also have the advantage of using strains of bacteria with known thermal resistance. One type found to be convenient is a suspension of spores of *Bacillus stearothermophilus*, which is supplied in sealed ampules containing thioglycollate broth. The ampules are placed in the autoclave in the same way as other controls and simply incubated unopened at 55 to 65° C. Ampules showing no growth after 24 to 48 hours' incubation indicate that sterilization has been properly accomplished, provided the control ampule shows growth. Spore strips are also available commercially and serve nicely when used according to instructions.

Sterilization failures are the result of several factors, principally:

1. Lack of basic knowledge concerning the principles of operation and care of sterilizers.
2. Faulty equipment.
3. Failure to understand and observe the regulation of the autoclave so as to maintain a pressure of 15 to 17 lb. equivalent to 121 to 123° C.
4. Incorrect methods of packaging and wrapping material.
5. Carelessness in loading the sterilizer without due consideration of the necessity for providing for free circulation of steam throughout the load or for complete air removal.
6. Failure to time correctly the required period of exposure.
7. Failure to carry out the correct sequence of operations in the sterilizing cycle.
8. Attempts to sterilize materials that are impervious to steam, such as oils and talcum powder.

Testing for Sterility of Blood and Plasma from the Blood Bank. Plasma must be checked carefully to assure freedom from bacterial contamination. Bank blood is occasionally contaminated, even under the best of conditions, and has been shown to have caused serious or even fatal transfusion reactions.

Plasma

1. Inoculate three tubes of fluid thioglycollate medium (conforming to N.I.H. specifications) with a sample of plasma, using sterile equipment and careful technique. The volume of broth used should be at least 15 times the volume of the inoculum. Incubate the broth as follows: one tube at 37° C., one at room temperature (22 to 25° C.), and one at refrigerator temperature (5 to 10° C.).

2. Examine cultures daily for evidence of growth for at least ten days. If the test material renders the medium so turbid that bacterial growth cannot be recognized easily, transfers should be made to fresh tubes of medium at the end of three days of incubation. Gram stains and subcultures should be made if any suspicion of growth appears at the end of the incubation period. Any organism isolated should be identified as completely as possible.

Bank Blood. The organisms most likely to be found in blood that has been contaminated and their optimal temperature requirements for growth are:

Pseudomonas sp. (2 to 30° C.)
Achromobacter sp. (20 to 37° C.)
Coliform and paracolon bacilli (2 to 37° C.)
Aerobic and anaerobic diphtheroids (20 to 37° C.)
Staphylococci (30 to 37° C.)

Consequently cultures should be made at three different temperatures, as for plasma. If only one temperature is used, 32° C. is preferable.

1. Inoculate 1 ml. in each of three tubes of thioglycollate medium and add 1 ml. to the bottom of three Petri dishes. Add tubes of melted and cooled infusion or thioglycollate agar and mix with the blood. At the same time make a Gram stain of the blood.

2. The tubes and plates are incubated for at least ten days before discarding as negative. Incubate the media and examine as described previously for plasma. Identify as fully as possibly any organism isolated.

Bacteriologic Examination of Food Utensils. Bacteriologic examination of swabs taken from washed utensils is an important check on the adequacy of dishwashing techniques and apparatus. The technique consists of swabbing the essential surface of the utensils to be examined, immersing the swab in diluting fluid, and culturing by standard procedures to determine total numbers of bacteria and coliforms.

TECHNIQUE. A sterile, absorbent cotton swab is dipped in sterile buffered distilled water; the excess fluid is squeezed out against the side of the container and then rubbed briskly over the whole of the appropriate areas:

1. The inner surface of plates and bowls that would come in contact with food over an area of approximately 4 square inches.
2. The inner and outer surfaces of cups,

mugs, and glasses to a depth of 0.5 cm. below the rim.

3. The inner and outer surfaces of spoons and knives.
4. The back and front surfaces and between the tines of forks.

Each swab is used for five similar articles. Care should be taken to prevent contamination by handling during sampling.

A greater recovery of organisms can be obtained if calcium alginate swabs are used rather than cotton. The advantages are that cotton frequently contains substances that are toxic for the more fastidious strains of bacteria and also that the alginate swabs can be dissolved completely in buffered water containing sodium hexametaphosphate $(NaPO_3)_6$. In this way all the bacteria contained in the swab are liberated into the solution.

If cotton swabs have been used, the swab is broken off the wooden stick with a sterile forceps and allowed to drop into a screw-cap jar containing 10 ml. of swabbing solution.* The containers must be kept cold and should be cultured within four hours. The bottle is shaken vigorously about 50 times, and 1 ml. of buffered water is added to the bottom of each Petri dish, and a tube of 10 ml. melted and cooled plate count agar is added. The plates are incubated for 48 hours at 37° C. The results are reported as the average plate counts of organisms removed per utensil examined.

If the alginate swabs are used, two swabs should be employed for each test, one being moistened in buffered water before use and the other kept dry. The surfaces of five articles are rubbed, first with the moistened swab and then with the dry one. Both swabs are then broken off into buffered water solution. One milliliter of sterile 10 per cent sodium metaphosphate is then added, and the bottle is shaken until both swabs have dissolved. Plate counts are then done on the solutions as described previously. If desired, pour plates can be made with violet-red bile agar for coliforms or with blood agar for pyogenic cocci.

The U.S. Public Health Service standard, based on the swabbing and a standard plate count technique, allows a maximum of 100 colonies per utensil cultured. Higher counts are presumptive evidence of inadequate cleansing or antibacterial treatment or of recontamination by handling or during storage. Judgment should be made on the basis of repeated sampling.

*To 34 gm. KH_2PO_4 in 500 ml. H_2O add 175 ml. of N/1 NaOH and dilute to 1 liter with distilled water. Adjust pH to 7.2. Add 1 ml. of this stock solution to 800 ml. of distilled water. If the material to be swabbed is likely to contain residual chlorine, add 4 ml. of N/1 sodium thiosulfate to the 1 ml. of stock solution before diluting it to 800 ml.

REFERENCES

American Hospital Association: Infection Control in the Hospital. Chicago, American Hospital Association, 1970.

Angelotti, R., Wilson, L., Litsky, W., and Walter, W. G.: Comparative evaluation of the cotton swab and Rodac methods for the recovery of *Bacillus subtilis* spore contamination from stainless steel surfaces. Health Lab. Sci. *1*:289, 1964.

Bernarde, M. A.: Disinfection. New York, Marcel Dekker, Inc., 1970.

Blair, J. E., and Williams, R. E. O.: Phage typing of *Staphylococci*. Bull. WHO *24*:771, 1961.

Bond, R. G., *et al.*: Development of a method for microbial sampling of surfaces with special reference to reliability. Final report under contract PH-86-62-182. Division of Hospital and Medical Facilities, Bureau of State Services, Public Health Service, 1963.

Brachman, P.: Surveillance. *In* Proceedings of the National Conference on Institutionally Acquired Infections. University of Minnesota, Public Health Service Publication No. 1188, 1963.

Committee on Microbial Contamination of Surfaces of the Laboratory Section of the American Public Health Association: A cooperative microbiological evaluation of floor cleaning procedures in hospital patient rooms. Health Lab. Sci. 7:256, 1970.

Committee on Trauma, Division of Medical Sciences, National Academy of Sciences-National Research Council: Ann. Surg. (Suppl.), *160*:1, 1964.

Cruse, P. J. E.: Surgical wound sepsis. Canad. Med. Ass. J. *102*:251, 1970.

Dawson, F. W., Jansen, R. J., and Hoffman, R. K.: Virucidal activity of beta-propiolactone vapor. II. Effect on the etiological agents of smallpox, yellow fever, psittacosis and Q fever. Appl. Microb. *8*:39, 1960.

Ehrenkranz, N. J.: Person-to-person transmission of *Staphylococcus aureus*—quantitative characterization of nasal carriers spreading infection. New Eng. J. Med. *271*:225, 1964.

Eickhoff, T. C., Brachman, P. A., Bennett, J. V., and Brown, J. F.: Surveillance of nosocomial infections in community hospitals I. Surveillance methods, effectiveness, and initial results. J. Inf. Dis. *120*:305, 1969.

Finland, M., Jones, W. F., and Barnes, M. W.: Occurrence of serious bacterial infections since introduction of antibacterial agents. J.A.M.A. *170*:2188, 1959.

Fuerst, H. T., Lichtman, H. S., and James, G.: Hospital epidemiology—Its development and potential. J.A.M.A. *194*:329, 1965.

Hoffman, R. K., and Warshowsky, B.: Beta-propiolactone vapor as a disinfectant. Appl. Microb. *6*:358, 1958.

Holt, R. J.: Aerobic bacterial counts on human skin. J. Med. Microb. 319, 1971.

Keenan, K. M., *et al.*: Some statistical problems in the standardization of a method for sampling surfaces for microbiological contamination. Health Lab. Sci. 2:208, 1965.

King, T. C., and Zimmerman, J. M.: Skin degerming practices: Chaos and confusion. Amer. J. Surg. *109*:695, 1965.

Langmuir, A. D.: Epidemiology of airborne infection. Bact. Rev. 25:173, 1961.

Letourneau, C. V.: The committee on infections. Hosp. Manage. *89*:37, 1960.

MacPherson, C. R.: Practical problems in the detection of hospital-acquired infections. Amer. J. Clin. Path. *50*:155, 1968.

Maibach, H. I., and Hildick-Smith, G.: Skin Bacteria and Their Role in Infection. New York, McGraw-Hill Book Company, 1965.

Mortimer, E. A., Jr.: The transmission of staphylococci by the hands of personnel. *In* Maibach, H. I., and Hildick-Smith, G.: Skin Bacteria and Their Role in Infection. New York, McGraw-Hill Book Company, 1965.

Perkins, E. W.: Aseptic Technique for Operating Room Personnel. 2nd ed. Philadelphia, W. B. Saunders Company, 1964.

Pierce, A. K., Sanford, J. P., Thomas, G. D., and Leonard,

J. S.: Long-term evaluation of decontamination of inhalation-therapy equipment and the occurrence of necrotizing pneumonia. New Eng. J. Med. 282:528, 1970.
Ravenholt, R. T., and Ravenholt, O. H.: Staphylococcal infections in the hospital and community: Hospital environment and staphylococcal disease. Amer. J. Public Health *48*:277, 1948.
Recommended Procedures for Laboratory Investigation of Hospital Acquired Staphylococcal Disease. Atlanta, U.S. Public Health Service, Communicable Disease Center, 1958.
Reddish, G. F.: Antiseptics, Disinfectants, Fungicides, and Sterilization. 2nd ed. Philadelphia, Lea & Febiger, 1957.
Rifkind, D., Marchioro, T. L., Waddell, W. R., and Starzl, T. E.: Infectious diseases associated with renal homotransplantation I. Incidence, types, and predisposing factors. J.A.M.A. *189*:397, 1964.
Shaffer, J. G.: The Laboratory in Infection Control. *In* Proceedings of the National Conference on Institutionally Acquired Infections. University of Minnesota, Public Health Service Publication No. 1188, 1963.
Shaffer, J. G.: Airborne infection in hospitals. Amer. J. Pub. Health *54*:1674, 1964.
Shaffer, J. G., and McDade, J. J.: Airborne *Staphylococcus aureus*—A possible source in air control equipment. Arch. Environ. Health *5*:547, 1962.
Shaffer, J. G., and McDade, J. J.: The microbiological profile of a new hospital. I. Hospitals *38*:40, 1964a.
Shaffer, J. G., and McDade, J. J.: The microbiological profile of a new hospital. II. Hospitals *38*:69, 1964b.
Shaffer, J. G., Migit, D., and Key, I.: The microbiological profile of two hospitals of differing structures. Hospitals *39*:71, 1965.
Snyder, J. E.: Infection control. Hospitals *44*:58, 1970.
Spaulding, E. H.: Chemical Disinfection. The Becton-Dickinson Lectures on Sterilization. 1958.
Spaulding, E. H.: Principles and application of chemical disinfection. Assoc. Oper. Room Nurses J. *10*:36, 1963.
Starzl, T. E., and Putman, C. W.: Experience in Hepatic Transplantation. Philadelphia, W. B. Saunders Company, 1969, Chapter 16, pp. 329–348.
Ulrich, J. A.: Dynamics of bacterial skin populations. *In* Maibach, H. I., and Hildick-Smith, G.: Skin Bacteria and Their Role in Infection. New York, McGraw-Hill Book Company, 1965.
U.S. Department of Health, Education, and Welfare, Public Health Service: Isolation Techniques for Use in Hospitals. Public Health Service Publication #2054. Washington, D.C., U.S. Government Printing Office, 1970.
Vesley, D., and Michaelsen, G.: Application of a surface sampling technic to the evaluation of bacteriological effectiveness of certain hospital housekeeping procedures. Health Lab. Sci. *1*:107, 1964.
Walter, C. W.: The personal factor in hospital hygiene. *In* Prevention of Hospital Infection; The Personal Factor. London, Royal Society of Health, 1963.
Walter, C. W.: Evaluation of sterilizer indicators. Surgery *2*:585, 1937.
Walter, C. W., and Kundsin, R. B.: The floor as a reservoir of hospital infections. Surg. Gynec. Obstet. *111*:412, 1960.
Williams, R. E. O., and Shooter, R. A.: Infections in Hospitals: Epidemiology and Control. Philadelphia, F. A. Davis Co., 1963.

Chapter 23

SERODIAGNOSTIC TESTS FOR SYPHILIS AND OTHER DISEASES

by ALLEN L. PUSCH, M.D.

Serologic methods are used as an aid in the diagnosis of a wide variety of diseases. Classically they have been used mostly in infectious disease, but more recently serologic principles have been employed in identifying and quantitating several constituents in blood and other body fluids. Antibodies reactive with the host's own tissues (i.e., antinuclear antibody, antithyroid antibody) and the use of antibody to identify circulating substances such as carcinoembryonal antigen and immunoglobulin quantitation are examples.

This chapter will emphasize the principles and interpretations of some of the more common serologic procedures available in many general hospital laboratories. Detailed procedures are not included since these are readily available elsewhere, and most commercial manufacturers of serologic reagents include a description of methodology recommended for their product in the package insert.

A serologic diagnosis is obtained after the fact in most infectious diseases. In general, it is optimal to isolate the infectious agent from the patient. However, in several instances body sites involved by organisms are not easily reached, or the patient presents at a time when organisms may not be viable for routine cultural purposes, or the method of cultivation of the organisms is not routinely available. In such cases a serologic diagnosis may be the only one available. The optimum is to demonstrate a rise in antibody titer between two serum samples drawn at least 10 to 14 days apart (so-called acute and convalescent sera). In this situation the first sample is saved and tested together with the second sample in the same test run or batch of analyses. This is necessary to reduce spurious differences in titer resulting from day-to-day variation in the test. A two tube (or fourfold) rise in titer, and preferably greater, is considered indicative of current infection. If a patient is considered to have a chronic infection, a single antibody titer may be used. However, in such instances the single titer must be interpreted in relation to titers seen in the general population of that geographic area and in regard to the patient's past history of antigenic stimulation by infectious agents or vaccines. Cross reactions occur between antigens of several organisms and a knowledge of these specific situations is important. Titers should be measured against all the antigens that cross react, and generally that antigen giving the highest titer of antibody in the serum represents the organism evoking the antibody response.

GENERAL PRINCIPLES

In performing serologic determinations it is important to follow the procedure rigidly. A procedure should be altered only after demonstrating the modification in the method to be fully comparable, in all titer ranges, to results obtained with the original method. When using commercial reagents it is recommended that the manufacturer's instructions be followed. Each new lot of reagents should be tested in parallel with the previous lot and placed in use only if it gives results comparable to those obtained with the old standardized lot. Every test run must include known negative and positive controls, and the results for these must be consistent with previous runs in order for the present results to be acceptable.

Equipment must be kept clean and in proper working order. The temperature of refrigerators and freezers must be monitored daily. This is essential for proper specimen and reagent storage and for proper testing when 4° C. incubation is required. The water bath temperatures must be checked at the start and finish of all incubation runs with a thermometer immersed in the water. Also, water baths provide an environment in which certain bacteria and molds can multiply and possibly contaminate test tubes being incubated. Such can lead to inaccurate results.

The speed of shaking and rotating machines must be checked by hand each time they are used. The precalibrated dial on the instrument must not be considered the correct indicator of the speed. Likewise, centrifuge speeds should be checked with a tachometer and automatic pipettes checked for accuracy of volume delivery. Glassware must be chemically clean. At times pipettes and other glassware become coated with protein or other organic material; this is best removed by acid washing. Reagents must be handled properly and dating periods suggested by manufacturers properly observed. In reconstituting freeze-dried reagents always note date of reconstitution on the bottle and observe outdating instructions for reconstituted reagents.

Distilled water is used in making many reagents. The still also must be kept clean and functioning properly. Distilled water can absorb ions from various gases present in the laboratory and thus should be freshly distilled and kept in closed, hard glass containers. Chemicals used to prepare reagents, such as saline and buffers, should be of reagent grade to obtain best results. (See Chapter 9).

SEROLOGIC METHODS

There are four general classes of procedures used in the routine serology laboratory. These are: agglutination, precipitation, complement fixation (CF), and fluorescent antibody (FA). (Cytotoxic antibodies are discussed in Chapter 5.) For all practical purposes, these measure the same phenomenon, namely, a reaction between antibody and antigen. In some systems the antigen-antibody complexes give a visible indicator of a reaction, i.e., a precipitate or agglutination of particles such as bacteria. The agglutination reaction can be amplified for nonparticulate antigens by coating particles such as red cells or latex beads with the antigen. Also, the mechanics of complement fixation and fluorescent antibody procedure deal mostly in developing the indicator of the reaction. All four tests can be considered in two phases: first, the antigen-antibody reaction, and the second as an indicator that the first has occurred.

Agglutination Tests

The agglutination reactions are relatively easy to perform thanks to the wide range of commercial reagents available. However, this may lead one to forget or to overlook important variables to be controlled; namely, the concentration and pH of the buffer, the concentration of the antigen, and the time and temperature of incubation.

Particulate antigens must be well mixed and lot to lot consistency controlled by comparing density of suspensions to McFarland standards. When latex particles or erythrocytes are coated, a chemical determination of the amount of antigen is necessary. The diluent most frequently used is buffered saline of pH 7.0. The electrolytes in the diluent are essential to maintain electrostatic forces needed to promote agglutination of particles once the antigen-antibody reaction has occurred. The conditions of incubation vary with the antigen and type of particle used. In addition to the usual controls, an autoagglutination control is needed in which the antigen and diluent are mixed. If agglutination occurs in this tube, the test results are not acceptable.

Agglutination reactions can be carried out on a slide or in a test tube. With the slide procedures the antigen and appropriate dilution of patient's serum are mixed, the slide rotated or rocked back and forth for an appropriate time interval, and then observed for agglutination. Often two or three dilutions of patient serum are tested to circumvent false negative results due to a prozone effect. With the use of test tubes, serial dilutions of patient's serum are mixed with equal or constant amounts of antigen and the presence of agglutination in each tube observed. The highest dilution giving a visible reaction is called the antibody titer. It is recommended that serial dilutions start at 1:2 or a multiple of this (1:4, 1:8, and so forth) and increase by twofold dilution. This allows a better comparison of results between laboratories.

Indirect hemagglutination (IHA) methods depend upon antigens adsorbed to the surface of erythrocytes. Viral and parasitic antigens are more commonly used; other antigens, only occasionally. Erythrocytes of chickens, rabbits, sheep, or humans are used, some antigens having a greater affinity for one species than another. Polysaccharide and dipopolysaccharide antigens adsorb well to most red blood cells. However, the cells must be pretreated with tannic acid for most protein antigens to adsorb to their surface. Occasionally a patient's serum contains anti-erythrocyte antibodies which give a false positive reaction. To screen for such, a control of patient serum and antigen-free erythrocytes is needed for each patient serum tested. Prior adsorption of sera with antigen-free erythrocytes will remove such antibodies. Autoagglutination of antigen-coated erythrocyte may occur and can often be prevented by adding normal rabbit serum to the diluent.

Many soluble antigens will adsorb to the surface of latex or bentonite particles and these can then be used in slide agglutination tests. The agglutination of the gray-white particles is readily seen against a black background. The particles should be uniform in size and small enough to remain in suspension. These latex particle procedures are less sensitive than IHA, but the reagents are more easily standardized and can be stored for a longer period than antigen-coated red cells.

Precipitin Tests

In precipitin tests the antigen-antibody complexes themselves form a visible precipitate. Two methods are used: the capillary tube precipitin test and the agar double diffusion test. Soluble antigen and antiserum are run into a glass capillary tube separately so that the two liquids are in contact, or they may be mixed by rotating the tube. A precipitate forms at the interface or may settle to the bottom if the tube is upright. The agar double diffusion method is more sensitive. In this two wells in a thin sheet of agar are filled, one with antigen and the other with antiserum. The two diffuse toward each other and a precipitin line forms in the agar where the two meet if antibody is present in the serum. In some systems it takes several days for the precipitate to form. The agar diffusion system does not seem to suffer from the problems of prozone, but the capillary tube procedure does.

The agar diffusion methodology has been modified by addition of an electric current to drive the antigen and antibody toward each other. This speeds the reaction so it takes place in an hour or so and increases the sensitivity by a factor of 10. This is called counterimmunoelectrophoresis and is widely used in detection of hepatitis-associated antigen. This can be used in many different systems and requires that antigen and antibody migrate in opposite directions (i.e., toward each other) in the electrical field at the pH of the buffer used. Recent studies show this method to be useful in identifying bacterial capsular antigens in body cavity fluids such as cerebrospinal fluid; this can provide a rapid identification of the organism causing meningitis (Edwards *et al.*, 1972).

Complement Fixation Tests

The complement fixation test (CF) is a long tedious procedure that takes place in two distinct phases. The first consists of the incubation of patient's serum with the appropriate antigen to be tested and a specified amount of complement. The second phase is the indicator phase in which the presence of an antigen-antibody reaction in the first phase is indicated by the fact that complement is "fixed" to these complexes and is no longer free in the system. Red blood cells precoated with specific anti-red blood cell antibody are added to the phase 1 mixture and if any "free" complement remains it is now bound to the antibody-coated erythrocytes, causing lysis of these cells. The converse, the absence of lysis in phase 2, indicates fixation of complement and presence of antibody in the serum reactive with the antigen in the first phase of the test (Fig. 23–1).

First the complement and antibody-coated erythrocyte must be titrated against the other reagents used in the test. In addition, one must carefully control each aspect of the CF test as follows:

1. "Anticomplementary activity" of each patient's serum dilution is tested by mixing it with complement and the sensitized cells (the antigen is omitted).
2. Known negative and positive serum controls are run with antigen to demonstrate appropriate reactivity of the system and that the antigen solution does not exhibit anticomplementary activity.
3. A hemolysin control is used to demonstrate that sufficient antierythrocyte antibody is present in the system to hemolyze the red cells in the presence of complement.
4. A red blood cell control is used to demonstrate that sensitized red cells remain intact in absence of free complement.

In an effort to standardize the CF procedure, the Center for Disease Control, USPHS, Atlanta, Georgia, has recommended that one procedure be followed by all laboratories in the country. This is known as the Laboratory Branch Complement Fixation test (LBCF). Without such an effort the slight modifications in procedure in different laboratories will lead to different results on the same serum specimens.

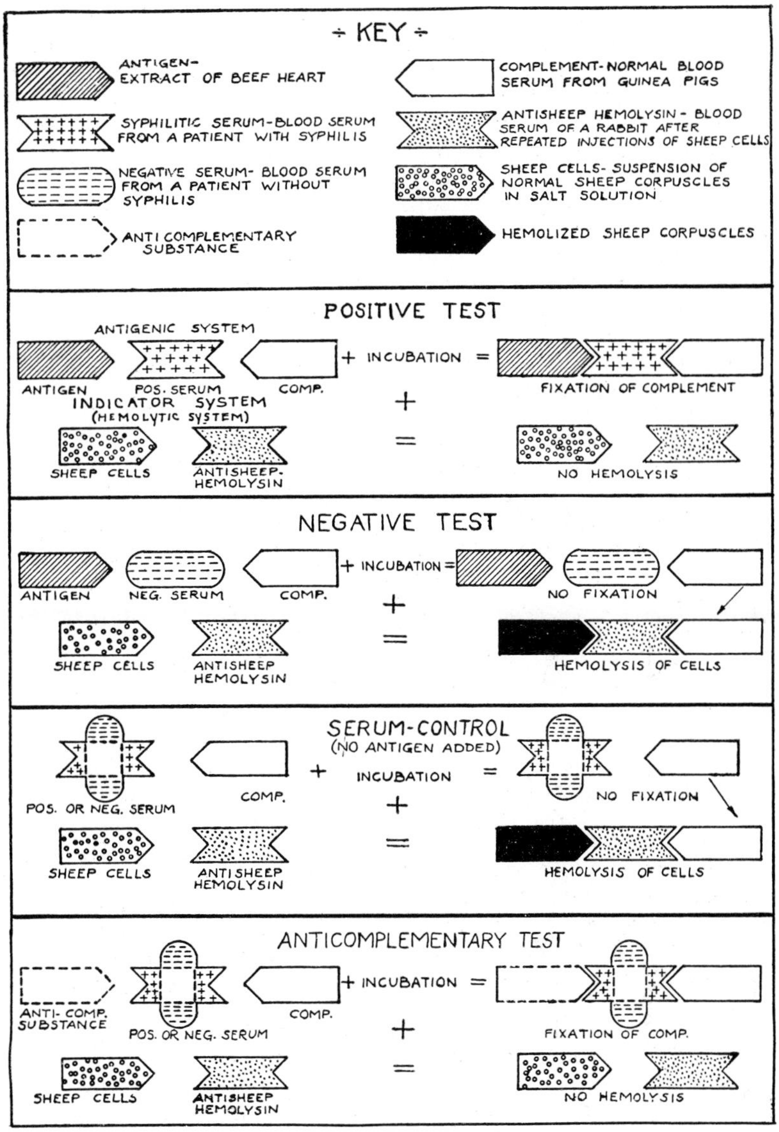

Figure 23–1. Diagram illustrating the action of the various reagents used in the complement fixation test. (From Miller, S. E.: A Textbook of Clinical Pathology. 6th ed. Baltimore, The Williams & Wilkins Company, 1955.)

Fluorescent Antibody Methods

The fluorescent antibody (FA) procedures are based upon a fluorescent dye, such as fluorescein isothiocyanate or rhodamine B isothiocyanate, being conjugated with antibody. Thus, antibody attachment to antigen can be identified under the fluorescent microscope. Goldman (1968) has described the technique and equipment in detail.

The direct FA procedure is used mostly to identify microorganisms in clinical material. The material is fixed to a microscope slide and overlaid with a specific antibody preparation in which fluorescein is conjugated to the antibody. Following incubation the conjugated antiserum is washed off and the slide examined under the fluorescent microscope. Fluorescent microorganisms (antigen) indicate the presence of reaction between the conjugated antiserum and the antigen.

The indirect FA test is used to identify the presence of antibody in a patient's serum and generally occurs in two phases: The known antigen preparation is fixed to a microscope slide. The patient's serum is laid over the antigen and allowed to incubate, and any specific antibody can attach to the antigen. The serum is then washed off the slide and the conjugated antiserum directed against human immunoglobulins is laid over the antigen. If human immunoglobulins have attached to the antigen (they will not wash off), the conjugated antihuman serum will attach to the patient's antibody and cause the antigen to fluoresce. Some workers refer to this as a sandwich technique, since the patient's antibody is layered between the antigen and the antihuman immunoglobulin. With the use of more specific conjugated antiserum (i.e., anti-IgG, anti-IgM), the immunoglobulin class of the patient's antibody can be determined.

The FA inhibition method is less frequently used. It depends upon blocking of antigenic sites by unconjugated antibody (patient's serum to be tested) so that in a second phase the specific conjugated antibody cannot bind to the antigen. Thus, presence of antibody in the patient's serum is demonstrated by the absence of fluorescence.

Nonspecific staining, autofluorescence and cross reactions are common events in FA testing and must be controlled to obtain proper results. Known negative and positive sera should be run each time also. Conjugated antisera may deteriorate upon storage, and each new lot of antisera must be checked for specificity.

The light source and its filter system must be carefully aligned for optimal fluorescence microscopy. The mercury vapor lamp delivers a greater amount of energy in the appropriate wavelength range than some other light sources such as quartz halogen or tungsten, but it is more expensive and more difficult to control. The alignment and focusing of the image of light filament must be accurate.

SYPHILIS

Syphilis is seldom diagnosed by demonstrating the organisms in a primary or secondary lesion. Either the facilities for darkfield exams are not readily available or the patient may not be aware of the primary lesion. Serology is the most common laboratory tool used in the diagnosis of this disease, and tests must be performed well. The United States Public Health Service through its Venereal Disease Research Laboratory of the Center for Disease Control has done much to improve methods and reagents available to clinical laboratories in the United States (USPHS, 1969). Furthermore, an active program of check samples is carried on through the respective state laboratories to monitor the quality of syphilis serology throughout the United States.

Syphilis serology currently consists of two general groups of procedures: (1) the nontreponemal antigen tests, of which the VDRL is the prime example, and (2) the treponemal antigen tests with the fluorescent treponemal antibody-absorbed (FTA-ABS) as the most important example. These two groups will be considered separately in greater detail.

Nontreponemal Antigen Tests

In 1906 Wassermann reported using antigen, an aqueous extract of syphilitic tissues from a human case, to demonstrate serum antibodies by CF procedure in a syphilitic patient. He presumed his antigen to consist of treponemal antigen. Thereafter, it was demonstrated that alcoholic extracts of many normal animal tissues would give the same results and, indeed, alcoholic extracts of beef heart gave the best results. This obvious nontreponemal material, called lipoidal, was rather crude and gave many nonspecific reactions. The isolation and purification of two reactive substances from beef heart muscle, namely, cardiolipin and lecithin, led to the more specific antigen used today in the VDRL test (the letters VDRL are an abbreviation for Venereal Disease Research Laboratory). This antigen consists of a proper balance of cardiolipin, purified lecithin, cholesterol, and alcohol. The antigen is standardized by adjustment of the lecithin content to give reproducible qualitative and quantitative results. The cholesterol provides adsorption centers so agglutinated particles can be visualized. The 1 per cent sodium chloride solution with phosphate buffer (pH 6.0) is also important for proper agglutination of antigen in the presence of antibody, which in this system is called "reagin."

The VDRL test was introduced in 1946 as a slide flocculation procedure. Heat inactivated (56° C. for 30 minutes) serum is mixed with antigen diluted in buffer on a rotating glass slide. The endpoint is read microscopically (100× magnification). Very rigid procedures are outlined for mixing the antigen and buffer, the size of the drops of antigen mixed with patient serum, and the speed of rotation of the slides. These must be followed strictly to obtain the greatest degree of comparable sensitivity and specificity among different laboratories. For laboratories preferring tube tests, a VDRL tube flocculation test procedure is available. The tube test is read macroscopically (USPHS, 1969).

The VDRL slide test results are graded as nonreactive (no flocculation), weakly reactive (slight flocculation), and reactive (definite flocculation). All reactive sera are serially diluted, 1:2, 1:4, and so forth, and each serum dilution tested by the VDRL slide method. The titer or highest dilution giving a reaction is also reported on all reactive sera. Rarely a patient with a high titer of reagin will have a negative VDRL on undiluted serum (prozone phenomena). If such occurs, it is usually in secondary syphilis (Sparling, 1971).

Several authors have described modifications of the cardiolipin test, mostly involving alterations in composition or preparation of antigen, sodium chloride concentration, or time of incubation. Many of these carry the name of the individual responsible for their development, such as Kline, Mazzini, Hinton, and Kahn. These procedures are no longer widely used with the exception of the Hinton test, which is used in the state of Massachusetts.

Since their inception in 1906, CF procedures have continued to be popular as confirmatory for a reactive result in the flocculation procedures. The CF methods have gone through the same evolution of antigen use, i.e., aqueous extracts of syphilitic tissue, to lipoidal, to cardiolipin, and more recently to a treponemal antigen, the Reiter protein (see later). The name Kolmer has figured prominently in CF syphilis serology. The first Kolmer modification of the Wassermann test was published in 1922 and became widely used. It underwent many modifications, the most prominent being the one-fifth Kolmer modification published in 1942. In this, one-fifth the volume of reagents are used. Generally the results of the Kolmer CF procedures and the VDRL slide test are comparable with the Kolmer procedure, being somewhat less sensitive.

Several rapid test procedures employing the cardiolipin antigen have been developed, mostly as screening procedures in "field" situations where equipment may be limited (Wallace and Norins, 1970). These are known as "rapid reagin tests" and are commercially available in kit form. As a group they are more sensitive and less specific than the VDRL, and any positive test must be followed up by a VDRL or other more specific procedure. The Rapid Plasma Reagin (RPR) test is the prototype of this group. The test is performed on unheated serum or plasma with a modified VDRL antigen containing choline chloride. Originally the test was read microscopically, but addition of charcoal particles to the antigen permits macroscopic identification of the flocculation. The RPR (teardrop) card test uses plasma from a finger-stick blood specimen, with the reaction carried out on a plastic-coated card which is rotated by hand. Another, known as the RPR (circle) card test, uses unheated serum, a plastic-coated card, and requires a mechanical rotator. The latter procedure is comparable to the VDRL qualitatively, but does not always compare quantitatively.

Treponemal Antigen Tests

In syphilis, as in all infectious disease serology, it is best to use an antigen specific for the organism thought to be infecting the patient. The TPI (*Treponema pallidium* immobilization test) was introduced in 1949 as a big step in this direction. The TPI uses as antigen a strain of live *Treponema pallidium* cultured in rabbit testis and suspended in a survival medium. The antigen is mixed with patient's serum and complement, incubated in an atmosphere of 5 per cent CO_2 and 95 per cent N_2, and then observed under the darkfield microscope to determine the proportion of treponemas immobilized relative to the controls. Sera causing immobilization are called TPI positive. This procedure has been recognized as the standard against which all other serologic tests for syphilis are measured. Unfortunately it is technically difficult and not well standardized, so the procedure varies from one laboratory to another. Only a few laboratories perform this procedure today.

In 1953 a method for preparing an antigen from the nonpathogenic Reiter treponemes, which are easily cultivated in the laboratory, was developed and widely used as a treponemal antigen, but unfortunately not *T. pallidium* antigen. This antigen was adapted to the one-fifth volume Kolmer CF procedure and designated as the KRP (Kolmer Reiter Protein) test. This procedure, more widely available than the TPI, was not completely satisfactory because only 50 per cent of sera from late syphilis give a positive test.

The FA methodology was applied to syphilis in 1957 and has led to the FTA-ABS procedure, which is highly specific and sensitive; with commercially available reagents and improvements in fluorescent microscopy, it is within the capability of most routine laboratories. The antigen consists of Nichols strain of *T. pallidium* (grown in the rabbit testis) fixed to a slide. During the development of this method a 1:5 dilution of patient serum was first used, but this gave too many false positive reactions due to nonspecific antibodies in patient sera. Continued dilution of serum to 1:200 (the test known as FTA-200) removed the nonspecific reactions, but many true positive reactions were also diluted out. Finally the fluorescent treponemal antibody-absorbed (FTA-ABS) method was developed. In this a 1:5 dilution of patient serum is absorbed with an extract of a culture of Reiter treponemes (called "sorbent") to remove the nonspecific antibodies before reacting the serum with the Nichols strain of *T. pallidium* to demonstrate specific antibodies. This procedure is equal to and at times better than the TPI in sensitivity.

The Serologic Response to Infection

The graph in Figure 23–2 is perhaps the best method to visualize and compare the incidence

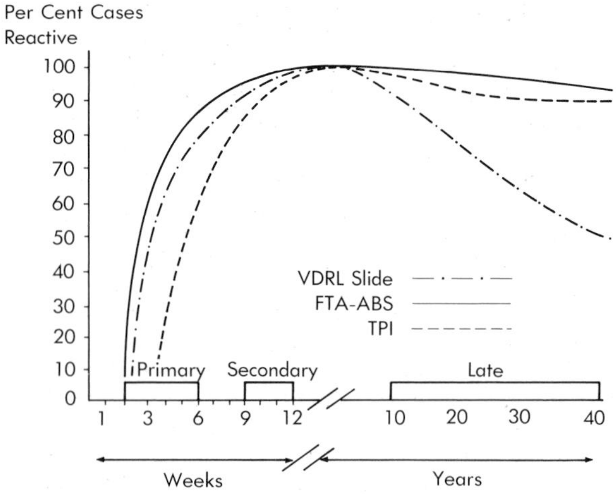

Figure 23–2. Serology of untreated syphilis.

of positive reactors with the three procedures (VDRL, FTA-ABS, and TPI) during the course of infectious syphilis. The FTA-ABS is the most sensitive in all stages but does not lend itself to screening large populations as easily as the VDRL for technical reasons. The VDRL is a good test in primary and secondary syphilis, but significantly less sensitive in late stages. However, should clinical findings be suspicious for lues and the VDRL negative, then the FTA-ABS is definitely indicated. In late syphilis it is important to note that as many as a third of the patients have a negative VDRL. Thus, if there is a clinical suspicion of late syphilis and the VDRL is negative, the FTA-ABS is again indicated. The FTA-ABS gives a significantly greater number of positive results than the TPI in primary disease (85 vs. 50 per cent) while the two are comparable in secondary lues and the TPI only slightly less sensitive in late syphilis (92 vs. 98 per cent).

The quantitative titer for the VDRL is both helpful in diagnosis and in following the course of treatment. If positive, the titers are usually low in primary syphilis, 1:32 or less, and only occasionally above 1:32. In secondary syphilis the titer is virtually always above 1:32, and in late syphilis the titers are variable. Following successful treatment the titer usually falls significantly, and if treatment is given during the primary or secondary stage the VDRL may revert to negative in a majority of cases. In late syphilis there is seldom a reversion to negative with treatment. Thus far it appears that once a patient develops a positive FTA-ABS or TPI, these remain positive regardless of therapy.

The VDRL test produces a significant number of false positive reactions. These are defined as patients whose sera give a positive VDRL reaction (usually weakly reactive or titer less than 1:8), a negative FTA-ABS and negative TPI, and who have no history or physical finding to suggest syphilis. This indicates why a positive VDRL should be followed up with a more specific test.

Of the positive VDRL's found in a laboratory, between 10 and 30 per cent may be false positives, depending on the population. These biologic false positives (BFP), as they have been called, can be separated into two groups: the acute BFP, in which the VDRL reverts to negative within six months, and the chronic BFP, in which the reaction persists for a longer time. The acute BFP is usually associated with infectious diseases such as pneumonia, tuberculosis, subacute bacterial endocarditis, chickenpox, infectious mononucleosis, scarlet fever, and atypical pneumonia; but in each of these conditions it is the rare patient who has a BFP. As much as 20 per cent incidence of BFP may occur in patients with lepromatous leprosy or those addicted to drugs. Some workers report a significant incidence of BFP in pregnant women, and others deny its existence as a result of pregnancy itself. In any regard, a patient with a positive VDRL in pregnancy, even a weak reactor, must be studied thoroughly because of the untoward effects of this treatable disease upon the fetus. The chronic BFP group has been extensively studied and there is a well-recognized association with diseases of the so-called autoimmune type, especially systemic lupus erythematosus (SLE), and with other diseases in which the patient develops hyperglobulinemia. In several patients the BFP is attributed to aging alone, with as many as 10 per cent of persons in the eighth decade having such a reaction (Sparling, 1971).

Some patients who fall into the chronic BFP group are also reported to have positive reactions with the FTA-ABS procedure but with a negative TPI and completely negative history and physical findings (Goldman and Lantz, 1971). In such rare cases the fluorescence often is weak and/or may have a beaded appearance on the treponemes instead of a frankly positive FTA-ABS reaction. This serves to emphasize that serologic results must be interpreted in light of a complete knowledge of the patient. Such reactions in the FTA-ABS have led to the USPHS to recommend that this test not be used as a screening procedure, but be used to confirm a positive VDRL or for patients with clinical signs suggesting syphilis regardless of VDRL results.

In congenital syphilis, serologic diagnosis can be a problem. IgG antibodies, which cross the placenta from the mother who has positive VDRL and FTA-ABS tests, can transfer positive reactions in these two tests to the serum obtained from the umbilical cord or from the newborn himself. A titer in cord sera significantly higher than in the mother would be suspicious for infection involving the infant. Otherwise, one can obtain serial VDRL determinations to see if the titer changes. A progressive fall in titer is expected, as passively transferred IgG is metabolized over a period of four to eight weeks, whereas the titer should stay the same or rise if the newborn is infected. Quantitative IgM levels on cord sera have been suggested as a general screen for intrauterine infection of the newborn (Alford *et al.*, 1967). Unfortunately, in cases in which the infection is subclinical or mild, the incidence of elevated total cord IgM levels is rather low, and it is in such cases that a laboratory diagnosis is important. A modification of the FTA-ABS test has been developed for use with cord or newborn sera in which specific IgM antibodies coating the treponemes are demonstrated. This requires use of a specific fluorescein-labeled antihuman IgM antiserum in place of the polyvalent antihuman immunoglobulin antiserum used in the routine procedure (Mamunes *et al.*, 1970). This approach appears to resolve the dilemma and permit early serologic diagnosis.

Examination of the spinal fluid is important in each case of syphilis, with increased cells and/or protein being highly suggestive of CNS involvement. (See Chapter 25.) However, in one series a majority of patients with clinical and serologic neurosyphilis had normal protein, and 70 per cent had normal cell counts (Hooshmand *et al.*, 1972). This points out the need for specific cerebrospinal fluid serology in neurosyphilis.

The VDRL and CF procedures performed on cerebrospinal fluid (CSF) samples have been used in the past to make the diagnosis of neurosyphilis. The use of the VDRL tube test has been limited because of the volume of CSF needed (1.0 ml.). However, a modification of the VDRL to permit testing of CSF on glass slides requires only 0.05 ml. of spinal fluid and gives results comparable to the tube test method. In Hooshmand's series, 40 per cent of the CSF VDRL's were nonreactive as contrasted to 100 per cent positive results with the FTA procedure on cerebrospinal fluid (*not* FTA-ABS as misprinted in his article [personal communication]). The FA tests for syphilis are performed differently on CSF than on serum. The FTA (unabsorbed) is the most sensitive method; however, it does give as many as 10 per cent false positive reactions in patients without syphilis, and the results must be considered in light of the serum FTA-ABS (virtually always positive in neurosyphilis) and the clinical signs. As a confirmatory test to the cerebrospinal fluid FTA, Escobar *et al.* (1970) recommend performing the FTA-ABS on the CSF using a 1:3 dilution with sorbent. If this is positive, it is diagnostic of syphilis. However, in their study only 22 per cent of patients with neurosyphilis had a positive FTA-ABS.

The false positive FTA (unabsorbed) on CSF results from contamination of CSF specimens with blood, either during the spinal tap or perhaps as the result of a disease process in which there are alterations of the blood-brain barrier such that serum proteins escape into the CSF.

SALMONELLA

The demonstration of serum antibodies directed against salmonella species is helpful in diagnosis of the typhoidal and septicemic forms of salmonellosis and may be the only positive laboratory result if cultural methods fail. In salmonella gastroenteritis serology is not helpful because titers do not rise until after clinical symptoms subside.

The demonstration of serum agglutinins to salmonella was first described in typhoid fever and is known as the Widal test. However, the incidence of infections due to *Salmonella typhi* has fallen off markedly in the United States, while the incidence of infection due to other salmonella species has increased. Thus, in present-day salmonella serum serology, antigens representative of several salmonella groups must be used. The more than 200 salmonella species isolated from humans are separated into at least 17 groups on the basis of O antigens, but fortunately 95 or more per cent of salmonella isolated from human infections fall into one of five groups. These are designated as groups A, B, C, D, and E and are

Table 23–1. THE O ANTIGEN GROUPS OF SALMONELLA USED COMMONLY

GROUP	EXAMPLES OF SALMONELLA SPECIES FOUND IN THE GROUP
A	paratyphi A
B	typhimurium paratyphi B derby san diego
C	paratyphi C cholerasuis montevideo newport
D	typhi enteritidis dublin gallinarum pullorum
E	anatum meleagridis give newington illinois senftenberg

the five O antigens routinely used for testing (Table 23–1).

The so-called H antigens are present on the flagella and are used in salmonella serology also. These antigens exist in two distinct antigenic phases on these organisms and transformation from one to the other phase occurs easily in the living bacteria under cultural conditions. Occasionally a given isolate of salmonella may exhibit antigenicity of its two phases simultaneously. These are designated as phase 1 and phase 2 H antigens. The phase 1 antigens are relatively species specific and are designated with lower case letters a through z. Phase 2 flagellar antigens are shared by several different salmonella species, are referred to as group-specific H antigens, and are designated with Arabic numerals and certain lower case letters. Most commonly four flagellar antigen preparations are used, as outlined in Table 23–2; however, these represent only a few of a long list of possible H antigens.

A third antigen, the Vi antigen or envelope antigen, is not so useful in salmonella serum serology. It is used mostly in suspected carriers of salmonella who have negative O and H titers and in whom only the Vi agglutinins may be elevated.

Titers of O agglutinins in patients with salmonella disease are elevated in 50 per cent of patients by the end of the first week, and by the fourth week 90 to 95 per cent show an elevated titer. Titers peak in the sixth week and fall to low or absent levels six months to one year later. The titers of H agglutinins rise more slowly, peak later, and may remain elevated for a few years. H agglutinins are not always demonstrable in salmonella infections; thus, the O agglutinin titer when elevated is a more reliable indicator of recent salmonella infection. Antibiotic therapy early in the disease may blunt the serum agglutinin response.

One should exercise caution in considering serologic results. Patients coming from areas where salmonella disease is endemic or who have recently received typhoid immunizations may have elevated O and/or H agglutinin titers. Indeed, titers of 1:40 or 1:80 of either are considered within the spectrum of normal. Other members of the enterobacteriaceae group of bacteria have O antigens that cross react with those of the salmonella, and infections with one of these might raise the titer. It appears that organisms other than enteric bacteria are not capable of causing false elevation of salmonella agglutinins (Kooman and Morgan, 1954). A single titer is often difficult to interpret, and paired samples taken 10 days to two weeks apart are more helpful.

The H antigen preparations consist of formalin-killed suspensions of appropriate motile isolates of salmonella. The O antigen is prepared in a similar manner from 24-hour cultures with the exception that the organisms are washed with alcohol to remove the H antigen reactivity. The antigens so prepared are used in both a rapid macroscopic slide test and in more dilute suspension in the macroscopic tube dilution procedure. The procedures are described in detail by the commercial producers of the antigens. Serum dilutions corresponding to 1:40 and 1:80 are recommended in the rapid slide procedure as a screening test, and any positives should be followed up by tube dilution titers. A hemagglutination method has been described. Antigens eluted from the bacteria can be adsorbed onto human group O red cells to give higher titers than bacterial agglutination (Neter, 1956).

Table 23–2. COMMONLY USED SALMONELLA H AGGLUTININ ANTIGENS

ORGANISM	FLAGELLAR ANTIGENS	
	Phase 1	Phase 2
S. paratyphi A	a	–
S. paratyphi B	b	1, 2
S. paratyphi C and S. cholerasuis	c	1, 5
S. typhi	d	–

BRUCELLA

Brucella organisms may be cultured from blood or tissues of persons infected. However, often the number of organisms is low, and cultural methods fail to produce the culprit; thus, a serologic diagnosis is frequently used. The most commonly used procedure is an agglutination test using either a formalin-killed or a phenolized heat-killed suspension of *Brucella abortus*. Agglutinins generated by infection with any one of the three species (*B. abortus*, *B. suis*, or *B. melitensis*) react equally well with this antigen preparation.

Two methods are used to demonstrate such agglutinins: the macroscopic slide test, and the tube dilution procedure. A titer can be determined with the slide test by mixing varying amounts of patient's serum with the antigen suspension on a glass slide. Some false positives have been noted by this method. It is suggested that the slide test be used as a screen, using dilutions of 1:40 and 1:80, and any positive reactions be followed by a tube dilution titer. Heat inactivation of patient's serum at 56° C. for 15 minutes reduces the incidence of a prozone effect in this system.

The serial tube dilution technique using saline dilutions of serum starting at 1:20 and ranging up to 1:2560 is most commonly used. The test is incubated at 37° C. for 48 hours and is read macroscopically. The prozone phenomenon is rarely noted above a 1:320 dilution of serum. Some individuals find that centrifuging the tubes just before reading the reaction increases the sensitivity. If brucellosis is specifically suspected, the tube dilution procedure should be performed regardless of the results of the slide test.

In acute brucellosis the titer begins to rise during the second week of disease and usually reaches a peak between the third and sixth week of the infection. A titer of 1:320 is considered presumptive evidence of acute active disease. Peak titers usually reach between 1:640 and 1:2560. Following recovery from active brucellosis, patients maintain a titer of 1:80 or higher for several years (usually five or more). Persons living in highly endemic areas or those working closely with animals may demonstrate titers of 1:80 without any history of active disease.

The serologic diagnosis of chronic brucellosis is more difficult. Such individuals may not demonstrate an elevated agglutinin titer unless a Coombs' technique (use of antihuman globulin) is employed with the agglutinin antigen (Kerr *et al.*, 1966). FA and CF procedures do not seem to offer advantages over the agglutinin and Coombs' procedures.

An intradermal skin test antigen has been used but does not increase the case detection rate and it, in turn, induces serum agglutinins, usually in low titer (Bradstreet *et al.*, 1970). Cross reactions occur in patients with tularemia, cholera, and proteus OX-19 infections. Individuals recently immunized against cholera also give cross reactions. Occasionally persons with healed brucellosis will experience a transient rise in agglutinin titer associated with a febrile illness. Titers may rise to 1:160 in a few days and fall to 1:20 in a week or 10 days.

TULAREMIA

An agglutination test is most commonly used in the serologic diagnosis of tularemia. The antigen consists of a formalin-killed suspension of a standard strain of the bacterium *Francisella tularensis* and is available commercially. The test can be performed on a slide, using serum dilutions, or by a tube dilution method. In the latter procedure the tubes are incubated first at 56° C. for two hours and then overnight at 4° C. "Normals" may have titers as high as 1:40. In patients with tularemia, titers of 1:80 appear during the second week of infection and rise to 1:640 and above in two to three months. Thereafter, serum titers fall off slowly and usually remain at levels of 1:80 or higher for several years and perhaps for life. Cross reactions occur with brucella and proteus OX-19 antigens, and all three should be tested to determine the most specific antigen (i.e., the one with the highest titer).

Other tests have been developed, but are not widely used. A skin test antigen (Foshay antigen) appears to react earlier in the disease, during the first week, but does not lead to increased case detection. A hemagglutination procedure using human O cells coated with *F. tularensis* polysaccharide gives higher titers than the bacterial agglutination procedure and the diagnostic (fourfold) rise in titer is observed earlier (Charkes, 1959). A cholesterol lecithin tularensis extract antigen has been used in a micro slide procedure and a macroscopic tube dilution flocculation method (Hunter, 1958).

RICKETTSIAL DISEASES

In 1916 Weil and Felix isolated a strain of Proteus from the urine of a patient with typhus and found agglutinins reactive with this same Proteus in the serum of that patient and other patients with typhus. This strain was designated OX-19 and with two later isolated strains of Proteus, designated OX-2 and OX-K, form the battery of antigens used in the diagnosis of several rickettsial diseases. This reaction is known as the Weil-Felix reaction. The results are nonspecific and are due to these Proteus strains having similar or identical antigens to those carried by the rickettsia. Being readily available, they form the most common diagnostic procedure used in the diagnosis of these diseases. Complement fixation antigens for typhus, spotted fever, and Q fever have been developed, but are not widely used. Attempting to cultivate rickettsia is dangerous for laboratory personnel and the resulting antigens are not always species specific; thus, this is not recommended for the average clinical laboratory.

The proteus antigens consist of formalin-killed saline suspensions of the bacteria. These are used in both the rapid slide agglutination and the macroscopic tube agglutination procedures. One must beware of false positive reactions resulting from nonspecific agglutination of outdated antigen. The pattern of reactions in the various rickettsial diseases is shown in Table 23–3.

In rickettsial disease such agglutinins may appear as early as the fifth or sixth day of the disease and at least by the twelfth day. The peak titers are reached in early convalescence, and in several months the titers fall to nondetectable levels. The absence of proteus agglutinins does not rule out rickettsial disease. Rickettsialpox, trench fever, and Q fever fail to generate such, and patients with Brill-Zinsser disease frequently fail to react with these antigens. Early treatment with antibiotics delays and suppresses the agglutinin response. False positive responses are seen in patients with leptospirosis, Borrelia infections, severe liver disease, and proteus bacterial infections such as in the urinary tract.

Complement fixation titers rise toward the end of the second week of disease, peak two weeks later, and then fall to negative in eight to 12 months. Such antigens are obtained by ether extraction of saline suspensions of yolk sac cultures of the respective rickettsia. Unfortunately these antigens vary considerably in respect to species and group specificity. Fluorescent antibody tests, rickettsial agglutination, hemagglutination, and neutralization tests have been used in special laboratories (Lennette and Schmidt, 1969).

ANTISTREPTOCOCCAL ANTIBODIES

The cultural documentation of group A streptococcal infection is often lacking in patients suspected of having acute glomerulonephritis or acute rheumatic fever. Because documentation of such infection is important, the serologic response to group A streptococcal (strep) infection has been extensively studied. Several streptococcal extracellular products, many of which have enzymatic as well as antigenic properties, have been identified. For many of these, the respective antibodies block the enzymatic activity, and thus reduction in activity of a standard enzyme preparation is used as an indicator of an antigen-antibody reaction. Antistreptolysin-O (ASO), antihyaluronidase (AH), antistreptokinase, antidesoxyribonuclease B (anti-DNAse-B), and anti-diphosphopyridine nucleotidase (anti-DPNase) are antibodies more often used in clinical situations.

Group A streptococcal infections are common, especially in school age children, and one

Table 23–3. SEROLOGIC REACTIONS IN RICKETTSIAL DISEASES*

GROUP	SPECIES	DISEASE	WEIL-FELIX REACTION WITH PROTEUS ANTIGENS			REACTION WITH RICKETTSIAL SOLUBLE CF ANTIGENS
			OX 19	OX 2	OX K	
Typhus	R. prowazekii	Epidemic typhus	+++	+	0	Group specific
	R. mooseri	Murine typhus	+++	+	0	
Spotted fever	R. rickettsi	Rocky Mountain spotted fever	+++	+	0	
	R. conori	Boutonneuse tick fever	+	+++	0	
	R. siberica	Siberian tick typhus	+	+++	0	Group specific
	R. australis	Queensland tick typhus	+	+++	0	
	R. ahari	Rickettsialpox	0	0	0	
Scrub typhus	R. tsutsugamushi	Scrub typhus	0	0	++++	Group specific
Trench fever	R. quintana	Trench fever	0	0	0	Species specific
Q fever	C. burnet	Q fever	0	0	0	None

*Adapted from Lennette, E. H., and Schmidt, N. J.: Diagnostic Procedures for Viral and Rickettsial Infections. 4th ed. New York, American Public Health Association, 1969.

finds significant levels of antistreptococcal antibodies in healthy individuals. The newborn has titers similar to the mother, but they fall significantly by six months of age. Streptococcal infections under age two years are uncommon, and children in this age group usually have ASO titers less than 50 units. A child in the five to 12 year age group is repeatedly exposed to streptococcus and often will have an ASO titer up to 200 units without recent infection. In adults the upper normal is slightly lower – 125 units. This same pattern is seen in all the antistreptococcal antibodies. As in other infectious diseases, paired serum samples are best; however, streptococcal serology often is not sought until the patient is well into the convalescent stage and peak titers are present. Thus, interpretation of single titers is the rule and must be made against an understanding of normal titer variation with age. The stated normal values have been obtained by measuring titers on individuals without evidence of recent streptococcal infections and arbitrarily setting the upper normal limit to include 80 per cent of the group tested (Wannamaker and Ayoub, 1960).

Streptolysin O is an oxygen labile hemolysin which is active against both human and rabbit erythrocytes. It is produced by most strains of Lancefield group A streptococci and a few strains of groups C and G. Measurement of the ASO titer has been used for decades as the single streptococcal antibody sought routinely. Antigen for the procedure is obtained from the broth of an 18-hour culture of group A streptococci mixed with dilutions of patient's serum and buffer, and incubated. Then a 5 per cent suspension of human group O or rabbit erythrocytes is added and the tubes reincubated. The endpoint is the highest serum dilution which gives no hemolysis (i.e., all streptolysin being inactivated). The reciprocal of this endpoint is referred to as "Todd units." In place of a serial twofold dilution, a more closely spaced dilution scheme is recommended using 0.1 log or one and a quarter-fold increments in dilution of the serum.

Patients with the nonsuppurative complications of streptococcal infections (e.g., acute rheumatic fever and acute glomerulonephritis) have a higher incidence of elevated ASO titers (80 vs. 60 per cent) and higher numerical titers than patients with uncomplicated streptococcal disease (Roy *et al.*, 1956). An important exception to this is in streptococcal pyoderma, in which few individuals (25 per cent) demonstrate an elevated ASO titer, even if acute glomerulonephritis occurs (Kaplan *et al.*, 1970).

Hyaluronidase is another enzyme elaborated by group A Streptococcus and demonstrating antigenic activity. The antibody titer of antihyaluronidase (AH) rises in the second week after infection and falls in three to five weeks. The antigen obtained from broth cultures is available commercially. It is mixed with appropriate serum dilutions and incubated. Then a standard amount of hyaluronate is added to each tube and reincubated; thus, any uninhibited enzyme can react with it. Finally, acetic acid is added to induce a mucin clot with any remaining intact hyaluronate. Tubes in which a clot forms are considered to contain AH. The reciprocal of the highest dilution containing a clot represents the titer of antibody.

The AH titer shows elevations in approximately 60 per cent of documented streptococcal respiratory tract infections but in a much smaller percentage of skin infections. It is less helpful alone than the ASO titer, but when used in association with the ASO, 90 per cent of persons with an antecedent streptococcal respiratory infection will show an elevated titer to at least one of the two antigens.

Streptococcal desoxyribonuclease (also called streptodornase) has proved to be an especially helpful antigen in demonstrating a serologic response to streptococcal pyoderma. Initially this antigen gave erratic results. However, once it was realized that streptococci produce at least four antigenically distinct desoxyribonucleases (designated A, B, C, and D) and that DNAse-B is the isoenzyme with the most consistent antigenicity, measurement of anti-DNAse-B titers have become very helpful.

In measurement of anti-DNAse-B titer, the patient's serum must be heat inactivated to remove its own DNAse. Appropriate dilutions of patient serum are set up and antigen derived from cultures of appropriate streptococcal strains added in standard amounts. These are incubated and then a standard solution of DNA substrate is added to each tube before reincubation. Finally, as an indicator of remaining intact DNA, 95 per cent alcohol is added, which causes highly polymerized DNA to form a mucin-like clot. Presence of a clot indicates inhibition of the enzyme DNAse-B (i.e., presence of antibody). An expression of titer similar to ASO is used.

Normal subjects have up to 250 units of anti-DNAse-B activity in their serum. The percentage of cases of acute rheumatic fever showing an elevated titer equals that of the ASO titer (80 per cent). Interestingly, fewer persons with poststreptococcal glomerulonephritis show anti-DNAse-B elevations (75 per cent) than ASO elevations (90 per cent) after streptococcal pharyngitis. This situation is reversed in glomerulonephritis following strep pyoderma, in which 60 per cent show elevated anti-DNAse-B in contrast to 25 per cent ASO elevations.

The enzyme *nicotinamide adenine dinucleotidase* (NADase) also elicits an antibody response when produced by streptococci. Anti-NADase titers are measured by determining the remaining enzyme activity after serum dilutions are incubated with a standard enzyme (antigen) preparation. The unbound NAD reacts with cyanide to form a complex that absorbs light at 340 nm. and can be measured. The anti-NADase titer rises in the same percentage of situations as does ASO titer. However, the difference between the upper normal anti-NADase titer (275 units) and the mean titer in acute glomerulonephritis (1015 units) is much greater than the respective difference in ASO titers (Wannamaker and Ayoub, 1960).

An assay for streptokinase (a plasminogen activator) antibodies has been described as an indicator of recent streptococcal infection. This is technically difficult and is seldom used.

In patients with suspected nonsuppurative sequelae of streptococcal infections, the ASO is the single most useful serologic procedure. However, a greater probability of documenting antecedent infection exists if two procedures are employed simultaneously—at least a 90 versus an 80 per cent probability. Using a third serologic procedure does not significantly increase such documentation. The AH titer is the second most commonly used procedure because of commercial availability of reagents. However, because of the added benefit of the anti-DNAse-B titer in pyoderma, this would appear to be a better second procedure.

STREPTOCOCCUS MG ANTIBODIES

When the streptococcus MG was first isolated from patients with primary atypical pneumonia and many of the patients also developed agglutinins for these bacteria, the strep MG was considered a candidate etiologic agent. Since then, these organisms have been demonstrated in normal upper respiratory tract flora of many persons, and other microbiologic agents appear as more likely etiologic agents of atypical pneumonia. However, 45 to 50 per cent of persons with clinical primary atypical pneumonia develop a rise in strep MG agglutinin titers late in their disease. Thus, it is still used as a diagnostic aid when titers are elevated. Five per cent or less of other pulmonary diseases are associated with a rise in streptococcal MG agglutinins.

In studies of strep MG agglutinins, cold agglutinins, and CF antibodies to *Mycoplasma pneumoniae* in patients with atypical pneumonia, the strep MG titers correlate best with the cold agglutinin titers (Griffin and Crawford, 1965). In all cases where strep MG and *M. pneumoniae* titers were *both* positive, the cold agglutinin titer was also positive; only a rare patient had only the strep MG titer elevated.

Attempts to demonstrate cross reactivity between antigens of streptococcus MG and *M. pneumoniae* have given conflicting results, depending on the methods used. This has been shown with the use of FA techniques, and lines of identity have been demonstrated in agar-gel precipitation studies with the two antigens and patient sera (Lind, 1968). However, not all sera from atypical pneumonia cases demonstrate this.

A washed, heat-killed suspension of an 18-hour broth culture of streptococcus MG is used as the antigen to measure agglutination titers. Titers of 1:10 may be seen in "normals," and titers of 1:20 and above are considered abnormal. In atypical pneumonia the titers to strep MG rise during the third week and peak in the fifth or sixth week. Demonstration of a fourfold rise in titer with paired serum samples is optimal.

COLD AGGLUTININS

Virtually everyone has serum antibodies that will cause agglutination of his own red cells and those of other persons at 0 to 5° C. These are known as cold agglutinins and are present in very low titer in healthy persons. In the early 1940's cold agglutinin (CA) titers above 1:32 were found associated with the clinical syndrome of primary atypical pneumonia. Also, many such patients demonstrated a fourfold rise in titer between the first and fourth weeks of the disease. After the sixth week, the titer would fall. At approximately the same time, the organism *Mycoplasma pneumoniae* was identified as a causative agent of this disease, and a rise in CA titer in this clinical setting was equated with *M. pneumoniae* infection (Chanock, 1965).

In the following two decades, better methods in viral isolation and viral serology demonstrated that influenza A, influenza B, parinfluenza, and adenoviruses can also cause the primary atypical pneumonias in which CA titer is elevated, but in these cases the titer remains static and usually does not show a fourfold rise in paired sera.

Generally a high proportion (50 to 80 per cent) of patients with atypical pneumonia have an elevated CA secondary to *M. pneumoniae* infection, especially in military and young adult populations. However, in pediatric populations with such lower respiratory tract infections and elevated CA, as few as 10 per cent will have demonstrable *M. pneumoniae* infections (Sussman *et al.*, 1966). These children have a much higher incidence of viral etiology. Considering the reverse situation, as few as one-third of individuals with documented *M. pneumoniae* respiratory tract disease will have elevated CA titers.

Cold agglutinins have blood group specificity usually for the I-i system (Race and Sanger, 1968), the CA usually reacting as anti-I. This antigen is present on virtually all human red cells following the neonatal period, but is absent from red cells obtained from umbilical cord blood. (See Chapter 5.) Absorbing sera containing elevated CA with *M. pneumoniae* reduces the anti-I titer, indicating cross reactivity between these antigens. Occasionally CA demonstrate an increased thermal range of activity which may extend up to body temperature, so the patient coats his own cells with antibody and a hemolytic anemia may develop. Patients with leukemia and lymphomas may develop a hemolytic anemia as a result of such a cold "autoantibody," the excess antibody being produced by the malignant cells.

In testing for cold agglutinins the blood sample should be kept warm, preferably near 37° C., until the cells and serum are separated. Refrigerating the sample of whole blood before separating the serum may lead to false negative results. A serial tube dilution procedure is used with fresh human group O erythrocytes as the antigen. The test incubates overnight in the refrigerator, and the presence of agglutination is determined before the cells are warmed. Following this all positive tubes are incubated at 37° C. for 30 minutes. If the agglutination is due to CA, it will disperse upon heating, whereas other antibody-mediated agglutination will not.

C-REACTIVE PROTEIN

The C-reactive protein (CRP) was first recognized in 1930 as a constituent in the serum of patients with acute pneumonia that formed a precipitin reaction with the C-mucopolysaccharide of certain groups of pneumococci. This substance also gives the capsular swelling reaction when mixed with whole organisms. CRP appears very early in several diseases, peaks in the first few days, and falls to nondetectable levels in eight to 10 days. Although it was first described associated with pneumonia, it since has been described in a wide variety of infectious diseases caused by both gram-positive and gram-negative bacteria and in noninfectious inflammatory conditions. This takes CRP out of the category of antibody and it is now classified as an acute phase reactant. A recent study suggests that CRP enhances phagocytosis of bacteria by polymorphonuclear leukocytes and that individuals incapable of mounting a CRP response may be more susceptible to bacterial infections (Gamrot and Kindmark, 1969).

CRP appears in the blood and in serous effusions. In the serum it is present in the form of a glycoprotein complex. Its molecular nature is not fully defined and its electrophoretic mobility varies, depending upon supporting medium used and pre-electrophoretic handling of the serum (Fischel, 1967). The complexed CRP travels in the alpha-globulin region. Isolated and crystallized material has been injected into animals and an antibody raised against it. This anti-CRP serum forms the basis of most laboratory methods of demonstrating its presence in patients. The capillary tube precipitin method is used and consists of observing and measuring the precipitate formed when antiserum and patient's serum are mixed within a capillary tube. This method is less sensitive, but is easier to perform than the pneumococcal capsular swelling reaction. The double diffusion in agar method is more sensitive and gives a higher percentage of positive reactions in healthy persons (usually trace reactions). Use of the quantitative radial immunodiffusion methodology has demonstrated detectable levels in many persons and allows one to show significant elevations above an upper normal range in quantitative terms. However, use of this method does require establishing an upper limit of normal.

Elevation of CRP is rather nonspecific. It is similar to the erythrocyte sedimentation rate (ESR) as a general indicator of an acute response. However, it rises faster than the ESR and returns to normal before the ESR does in many entities. In virtually all acute bacterial infections, including active pulmonary tuberculosis, some tumors, and various types of tissue destruction such as myocardial infarction, the CRP rises. However, it is most often used to monitor activity in patients with acute rheumatic fever and rheumatoid arthritis. In the former it is elevated during acute activity and falls to normal with appropriate therapy. Elevations occur in approximately 70 per cent of patients with active rheumatoid arthritis, and although the level falls with treatment it may not return to normal levels. CRP does not rise in most viral disorders and in many gastrointestinal disorders. This is most obvious in infections of the upper respiratory tract: sinusitis and streptococcal pharyngitis are associated with CRP elevations, whereas viral diseases are not.

CRP is elevated during pregnancy, appearing late in the first trimester in 15 to 20 per cent of patients and being demonstrable in about 40 per cent in the second and third trimester. In some studies the incidence of elevated CRP shoots up to 80 per cent at delivery. Between

50 and 90 per cent of women on various oral contraceptive preparations may have elevated serum CRP, as well as women with an IUD in place (Connell and Connell, 1971). Newborns and infants may also respond to acute infections with a rise in CRP, and this can serve as an indicator of infection in this age group. In normal persons in the older age groups (sixth decade and above) the incidence of positive or elevated CRP increases. Since many persons in this group may have various degenerative and/or subclinical or occult diseases, the significance of such CRP elevations is uncertain.

HEPATITIS ASSOCIATED ANTIGEN

In 1964 Blumberg found that a precipitin reaction occurred between a substance in the serum of a much transfused hemophiliac and the serum of an Australian aborigine. The material in the Australian's serum he labeled Australian antigen. This was a chance finding during a search for genetically controlled serum antigens against which frequently transfused persons often develop antibodies (Blumberg *et al.*, 1968). In a few years the presence in the serum of this antigen was demonstrated to be frequently associated with long incubation hepatitis and the name "hepatitis-associated antigen" (HAA) applied to it. Because presence of this antigen in one's serum is also associated with the ability of this individual's blood to transmit hepatitis to a recipient, blood banks have very rapidly set up facilities to screen all donors for its presence. It is estimated that 30 per cent of the donors capable of transmitting hepatitis can be identified by appropriate testing (London *et al.*, 1972), and of course continued technical refinements may permit more complete identification of such infectious donors.

Demonstration of HAA has also led to a greater understanding of the varieties of hepatitis. HAA appears to be mostly associated with the long incubation or so-called serum hepatitis. However, there are some cases of sporadic hepatitis and infectious hepatitis that have HAA in their serum, demonstrating that the agent for serum hepatitis can be transmitted by other than the parenteral route, probably by fecal oral spread. The HAA can be demonstrated in feces and urine of some hepatitis patients. Presently hepatitis is separated into long incubation and short incubation varieties, in which the incubation period is documented to correspond to the old serum hepatitis and infectious hepatitis, respectively. It can also be separated into HAA positive and HAA negative groups, but incubation times do not always correlate with this.

In most patients with HAA positive hepatitis, the antigenemia is transient, appearing during the pre-icteric phase and persisting for a few to several weeks. These patients usually recover without sequelae. Some of these patients also develop anti-HAA in their serum. A small percentage, usually less than 5 per cent, have persistent antigenemia, and a significant number of such patients go on to chronic hepatitis.

The precise nature of HAA has not been defined, but great efforts are being made to demonstrate that it is a virus. It has not yet been cultured, except perhaps in tissue cultures of liver cells from patients with hepatitis (London *et al.*, 1972). Electron microscopy (EM) studies demonstrate it to be particulate, viral-like, and appearing in three configurations: (1) small spheres 20 to 50 nm. in diameter, (2) tubular structures with the same 20 nm. short diameter, and (3) large round particles 42 nm. in diameter known as Dane particles. The Dane particles are more common in the blood of patients with chronic hepatitis, seldom seen in hepatitis patients with transient antigenemia, and not seen in healthy persons with antigenemia (Nielsen and LeBouvier, 1973). Nucleic acids are very difficult to demonstrate in association with the particle which, in turn, casts doubt on its viral nature. It has been suggested that what we see circulating are empty viral envelopes, with only one in 100,000 or so being a complete virus.

Antigenic subtypes of HAA have been described (LeBouvier, 1971). All share the basic specificity, a, which represents HAA positivity and, in addition, can be demonstrated to have one of several specificities designated b, c, d, x, and y. Recently Nielsen and LeBouvier (1973) have found different HAA subtypes to correlate with the clinical course of HAA positive hepatitis.

The first method used to demonstrate the particle was double immunodiffusion in agar. This permitted one to run controls and positively identify the precipitin band as HAA by use of lines of identity. However, this method is slow, taking anywhere from one to seven days for precipitin lines to form. Also the method is less sensitive. Complement fixation testing is more sensitive in that much higher dilutions of serum give a positive test than in double diffusion, but it appears that pick-up of carriers is not significantly increased. Also many sera of hepatitis patients demonstrate anticomplementary activity, which reduces its usefulness in such patients. Counterimmunoelectrophoresis has grown up as the most widely used method of testing in blood banks. It is rapid, requiring about one hour, significantly more sensitive, and there are a host of reagents and equipment suppliers commercially. Occasionally a prozone effect gives confusing results by this method. The most sensitive method yet devised is radioimmunoassay (RIA). This permits identification of antigen in sera up to a 1:1000 dilution of where the double diffusion method becomes negative and increases the pick-up rate of carriers by perhaps two- or threefold. Commercial reagents are available for the RIA procedure. However, this method does seem to identify antigen in more donors than are capable of transmitting hepatitis.

The flurry of reports concerning HAA and hepatitis has obscured the early studies concerning this antigen and its high incidence among certain populations in Asia and tropical countries. Up to 20 per cent of such populations demonstrate persistent antigenemia, while in Europe and North America less than 1 per cent have antigenemia. Also, in some groups it appears that antigenemia is inherited as an autosomal recessive characteristic. Persistent antigenemia is associated with certain diseases other than hepatitis such as acute and chronic lymphocytic leukemia, acute myelogenous leukemia, and mongolism. There is still much to be learned about HAA, and perhaps if the original name, Australia antigen, were retained we would be less narrow in studies of this antigen.

ANTIBODIES TO TISSUE ANTIGENS

Antibodies that react with various tissue fractions are being described with increasing frequency, and several methods of identifying these are becoming available to the general hospital laboratory as equipment and appropriate reagents become commercially available. The greatest boost to this area is the development of the FA technique and the availability of fluorescein-conjugated antihuman immunoglobulin antiserum. However, our understanding of the significance of these antibodies in the pathogenesis of disease is lagging behind our ability to demonstrate them. In most instances the presence of such antibodies is not diagnostic by itself and must be considered within the constellation of historic, physical and laboratory data for each patient. In addition, in most instances a small number of healthy, usually older persons, can be demonstrated to carry such "autoantibodies." Steffen (1970) suggests three groupings for antibodies to tissues:

Group I includes diseases associated with organ-specific antibodies. Interestingly, antibodies to several organs are present in many of these disorders, with the antibody against the organ primarily affected being in highest titer. Hashimoto's thyroiditis, pernicious anemia, idiopathic adrenal insufficiency, and ulcerative colitis are in this group.

Group II consists of the "connective tissue disorders" in which nonorgan-specific antibodies predominate. Antinuclear antibody, rheumatoid factor, and collagen antibodies appear in varying proportions in this set of diseases. The chronic liver diseases such as primary biliary cirrhosis and chronic active hepatitis are added to this group.

In Group III autoantibodies are directed against various formed elements in the circulation, i.e., antibodies to red cell antigens, leukocytes and/or platelets.

The occurrence of such antibodies in healthy relatives of patients with any of these clinical disorders raises the question of genetic predisposition toward development of these diseases. Furthermore, this must be considered in light of the possible viral particles seen with electron microscopy in a disease such as systemic lupus erythematosus (SLE) which, in turn, may somehow cause the predisposed immune system to react against "self."

SEROLOGY IN CHRONIC LIVER DISEASE

Serologic procedures have been attempted in the differentiation of various chronic liver diseases such as cirrhosis, primary biliary cirrhosis, chronic active hepatitis, and extrahepatic biliary obstruction. (Also see Chapter 13.) Various extracts and homogenates of liver tissue, sections of liver tissue, sections of other organs, and subcellular fractions of various organs have been tried. As a result, antibodies to smooth muscle, antibodies to mitochondria, and antinuclear antibodies (ANA) have been found helpful in the diagnosis of primary biliary cirrhosis and chronic active hepatitis. The antimitochondrial antibody is present in high incidence in primary biliary cirrhosis, while chronic active hepatitis demonstrates a high incidence of anti-smooth muscle antibody. In both conditions there is a moderate incidence of ANA. As shown in Table 23–4, there is a tremendous overlap in the incidence of several antibodies in these two conditions and in other liver diseases (Paronetto, 1970). A more recent report of antimitochondrial antibody in patients with extrahepatic biliary obstruction of over three months' duration brings into question the usefulness of such antibodies in making a diagnosis of primary biliary cirrhosis without first surgically exploring the biliary tract (Lam *et al.*, 1972).

Both the antimitochondrial and anti-smooth muscle antibodies can be identified by using cryostat sections of rat stomach or rat kidney as antigen and incubating with patient's serum before washing and applying the conjugated antihuman immunoglobulin antiserum and examining the preparation under the fluorescent microscope. Fluorescence of the stomach parietal cells and proximal renal tubular cells demonstrates antimitochondrial antibody. Anti-smooth muscle antibody results in stain-

Table 23-4. SERUM ANTIBODIES IN LIVER DISEASE USING FA TECHNIQUES*

	ANTI-MITO	ANTI-SMOOTH MUSCLE	ANA
Primary biliary cirrhosis	87	40	40
Chronic active hepatitis	66	85	57
Cirrhosis	0	0	7
Acute viral hepatitis	0	11	23
Extrahepatic biliary obstruction	0	11	11
Drug-induced jaundice (halothane, chlorpromazine)	69	23	0
SLE	18	12	98
Normal controls	2	6	2

*Adapted from Paronetto, F.: *In* Popper, H., and Schaffner, F. (eds.): Progress in Liver Disease. Vol. III. New York, Grune & Stratton, 1970; and Steffen, C.: *In* Stefanini, M. (ed.): Progress in Clinical Pathology. Vol. III. New York, Grune & Stratton, 1970.

ing of the muscularis of arteries in the kidney as well as the muscle coats of the stomach.

ANTIBODIES TO THYROID ANTIGENS

In various diseases of the thyroid gland antibodies to one or more tissue antigens may be demonstrated: (1) antibodies to thyroglobulin; (2) to cytoplasmic antigens; (3) to the colloid of thyroid follicles; and (4) LATS (long-acting thyroid stimulator), which is made up of IgG.

Antibodies to thyroglobulin are found in 80 per cent of patients with Hashimoto's thyroiditis and a slightly lower frequency and lower titer in thyrotoxicosis and primary myxedema. (See Chapter 10.) Patients with nontoxic goiter and thyroid carcinoma may have such antibodies (between 20 and 30 per cent of patients), but usually in low titer. Six to 15 per cent of the normal population also have these antibodies. Latex particles coated with thyroglobulin are the most widely used antigen. This antigen is intermediate in sensitivity between the precipitin methods (precipitation in liquid or agar media) and the highly sensitive passive hemagglutination procedure using thyroglobulin-coated tanned erythrocytes. In this latter procedure, titers may be very high in Hashimoto's thyroiditis, ranging from 1:2500 up to 1:2,500,000 (Anderson *et al.*, 1967).

Antibodies to cytoplasmic antigens of thyroid epithelial cells occur in similar proportions of the patient groups as do thyroglobulin antibodies. These antibodies react with the microsomal fraction of the cytoplasm and are demonstrated by FA techniques using tissue slices of thyroid glands or by CF using saline extracts of thyrotoxic glands as antigens. Sera containing these antibodies are also cytotoxic to thyroid cells grown in tissue culture.

Antibodies to thyroid colloid are demonstrated by FA techniques and were discovered when sera of Hashimoto patients negative for antithyroglobulin and antimicrosomal antibodies by CF were studied by FA (Balfour *et al.*, 1961). The FA staining pattern is distinctly different from the pattern demonstrated by antithyroglobulin antibodies.

LATS is an IgG immunoglobulin found in the serum of 60 to 70 per cent of patients with active Graves' disease. It appears to react with the cell wall of the thyroid epithelial cell, perhaps at a site similar to that at which TSH attaches. It is not clear if LATS is truly an antibody. However, because it is an immunoglobulin and reacts with the cell surface it is included here. The presence of LATS in the serum varies directly with the number of signs and symptoms of thyrotoxicosis and not with the severity of the disease. As the disease becomes inactive, the titer of LATS falls and may disappear (Volpe *et al.*, 1972).

Demonstration of thyroid antibody is most useful in the diagnosis of Hashimoto's thyroiditis where antithyroglobulin and/or antimicrosomal antibodies are present in 90 to 95 per cent of cases, and in 100 per cent if the test is for antibody to thyroid colloid. (See Chapter 10.) Thus, thyroid antibody testing is most useful in ruling out the diagnosis of Hashimoto's thyroiditis in a patient with thyroid disease. Negative results with the passive hemagglutination method, CF test for microsomal antibody, and FA testing virtually excludes this disease. On the positive side, thyroid antibodies are found in many different thyroid disorders, but the presence of a high titer is usually indicative of Hashimoto's disease or Graves' disease. Patients with pernicious anemia and miscellaneous allergic disorders have been found to have a low titer of thyroid antibodies. (See Table 23-5.)

Table 23-5. INCIDENCE OF THYROID ANTIBODIES IN VARIOUS DISEASES*

	ANTI-THYROGLOBULIN (%)	ANTI-MICROSOMAL (%)
Hashimoto's thyroiditis	80-90	80-90
Graves' disease	50-60	30-50
Primary myxedema	60	30-50
Adenomatous goiter	20-30	20-25
Thyroid carcinoma	20-30	15-25
Pernicious anemia	25	10
Allergic disorders	18	12
Healthy Individuals	6-15	6-10

*Adapted from Steffen, C.: *In* Stefanini, M. (ed.): Progress in Clinical Pathology. Vol. III. New York, Grune & Stratton, 1970; and Anderson, J. W. *et al.*: J. Clin. Endocr. *27*:937, 1967.

RHEUMATOID FACTOR

The serology of rheumatoid arthritis (RA) started in the 1930's when it was observed that approximately 50 per cent of such patients' sera would agglutinate certain strains of streptococci. In 1940 Waaler demonstrated that RA sera would agglutinate sheep red cells precoated with rabbit antisheep red cell antibodies. Rose modified this procedure in 1947 to take into account the presence of heterophil antibodies in some sera. As a result, the sensitized sheep cell test is known as the Waaler-Rose test. Subsequently, many modifications were introduced: human cells coated with rabbit antihuman erythrocyte antibody, human "Rh positive cells" coated with human anti-D (Rh_0), and small latex particles coated with human globulin (Cohn fraction II or F II). The substance in the patients' sera reacting in these procedures has been designated as RF or rheumatoid factor (Ziff, 1957) (Table 23–6).

Applications of several methods of study of gamma globulins have demonstrated RF to be a 19S or IgM immunoglobulin that reacts with gamma G immunoglobulin. A 22S globulin complex that is separable into 19S IgM and 7S IgG units has been found in sera of RA patients, suggesting that RF forms complexes in vivo. RF reacts best with altered human IgG molecules such as appear in Cohn fraction II and Fc fragments of IgG. (See Chapter 9.) It also reacts with IgG that is bound to specific antigen. RF cross reacts with rabbit immunoglobulin. That RF is a heterogeneous collection of IgM molecules is suggested by the demonstration that absorption of RF-containing sera with rabbit IgG removes only a portion of RF and that the remaining sera still reacts with human IgG (Bartfeld, 1969). The RF reacted with rabbit IgG can be recovered and demonstrated to still be reactive with human IgG. Absorption of RF-containing sera with human IgG removes all RF activity, suggesting that RF has primary specificity for human IgG. RF also reacts with immunoglobulin from different individuals with different degrees of reactivity. This is attributed to RF having varied specificity for genetically controlled sites in the IgG molecule known as Gm factors (Fudenberg *et al.*, 1972).

The ability to demonstrate RF in sera of patients with clinical RA varies with the test method and the stage of disease, with positive reactions varying from 50 to 95 per cent in different patient groups. The highest percentage of positives (up to 95 per cent) is seen in advanced disease with classic physical signs. However, in patients with atypical signs or early disease, RF may be demonstrable in only 50 to 60 per cent of cases. Furthermore, in varieties of RA, such as psoriatic arthritis and juvenile rheumatoid arthritis, as few as 10 to 25 per cent of patients yield positive results. In addition, there are a variety of diseases not associated with RA in which one finds RF activity. These are mostly inflammatory and/or chronic diseases (Table 23–7). "Normals" show a low incidence of RF (2 to 4 per cent)

Table 23–6. SPECIFICITY AND SENSITIVITY OF SEROLOGIC TESTS FOR RHEUMATOID FACTOR*

TEST SYSTEM	SPECIFICITY (%)	SENSITIVITY (%)
Perfect test	100	100
Sensitized sheep cell agglutination and sensitized human group O red cell agglutination	90	50
FII latex fixation, FII bentonite flocculation, and sensitized human D (Rho) erythrocyte agglutination	75	75

*Adapted from Cathcart, E. S.: *In* Cohen, A. S. (ed.): Laboratory Diagnostic Procedures in the Rheumatic Diseases. Boston, Little, Brown and Company, 1967.

Table 23–7. RHEUMATOID FACTOR TESTING IN VARIOUS DISEASES*

	PER CENT POSITIVE RESULT FOR RF	
	Latex Test	Sensitized Sheep Cell
Infectious Diseases		
SBE	48%	20%
Syphilis	13	5
Viral disease	15	15
Infectious hepatitis	24	20
Trypanosomiasis	27	44
Tuberculosis	11	6
Leprosy	24	15
Lung Diseases		
Bronchitis	62	18
Asthma	17	0
Asbestosis	21	
Silicosis	15	
Idiopathic pulmonary fibrosis	32	46
Miscellaneous		
Sarcoid	17	5
Multiple myeloma	18	4
Cirrhosis of liver	36	16
Sjögren's syndrome	96	74
Renal homograft	74	8
Myocardial infarction	12	20

*Adapted from Bartfeld, H.: Ann. N.Y. Acad. Sci. *168*:30, 1969; and Cathcart, E. S.: *In* Cohen, A. S. (ed.): Laboratory Diagnostic Procedures in the Rheumatic Diseases. Boston, Little, Brown and Company, 1967.

which increases with age such that persons over 60 years have a positive test incidence of 5 to 10 per cent. Because of these older groups it has been estimated that in many laboratories only half of the specimens with the positive tests for RF represent patients with RA.

The *sensitized sheep cell agglutination test* of Waaler and Rose uses sheep cells sensitized with rabbit antisheep erythrocyte immune globulin. These are reacted with heat-inactivated patient sera in a tube dilution series. Titers of 1:160 and over are considered positive for RF. This test gives few false positives (i.e., has high specificity) but is less sensitive (i.e., is positive in 50 to 60 per cent of RA patients).

The *latex fixation test* uses Cohn fraction II of pooled human serum adsorbed to latex particles as antigen. Serial twofold dilutions of patient serum in glycine buffer, starting at 1:20, are incubated with the antigen at 56° C. A positive agglutination at a dilution of 1:80 or greater is considered positive for RF. This procedure is positive in approximately 80 per cent of RA patients, but is less specific. Positive reactions in normal and in other diseases occur about twice as frequently as with the sheep cell test.

Procedures using coated bentonite particles (basically clay), charcoal, and tannic acid-treated sheep red cells have also been developed but are not widely used. Card and slide agglutination tests using globulin-coated latex or charcoal particles are available as screening tests, and if positive should be followed up with a tube dilution procedure, because false positives may occur.

ANTINUCLEAR ANTIBODY

A natural outgrowth from the demonstration of the LE cell phenomena in systemic lupus erythematosus (SLE) has been the demonstration of antinuclear antibodies in SLE and other diseases. Indeed, it is these antibodies in serum that lead to the production of the LE cell. The greatest boost to such antibody determinations has been the indirect immunofluorescent methodology. Whole nuclei of human or animal origin are used as antigen. White blood cell smears (even the patient's own will suffice) or tumor imprints are the chief human sources. Cryostat sections of liver, kidney, thyroid, or thymus represent animal sources used. Also tissue culture cells growing in monolayers are available commercially for this determination. The tissue or whole cells are fixed to the slide and then overlaid with appropriate dilutions of the patient's serum. Following incubation and washing of the slide, a solution of fluorescein-labeled antihuman immunoglobulin antiserum (reactive against all three of the main immunoglobulin classes) is laid over the cells and incubated. Finally, the preparation is examined under the ultraviolet microscope for nuclear fluorescence (Friou, 1967).

Four main patterns of fluorescence are identified which correspond to the distribution of specific antigenic components within the nuclei. These correlations can be defined by other serologic methods (i.e., complement fixation, immunodiffusion, passive agglutination, and so forth), using individual nuclear constituents as antigens. Also, there are rough correlations between the pattern and the patient's disease process. Combined or mixed fluorescent patterns occur in some sera, making such correlations difficult. However, with serial dilution of the serum, one pattern may disappear before the other at high dilutions. Those sera are thought to contain distinct antibody sets, each with separate antigen specificity.

The commonly recognized patterns are:

1. The *homogeneous* pattern gives a total nuclear fluorescence and is due to antibody directed against nucleoprotein. This pattern is most common in patients with SLE.
2. The *peripheral* pattern consists of fluorescence about the edges of the nucleus and often is described as showing a shaggy appearance. Anti-DNA antibodies cause this pattern, which tends to vary considerably with the different sources of nuclei. This pattern is also common in SLE.
3. The *speckled* pattern results from antibody directed against different nuclear antigens. Antibody against soluble material (Sm antigen), a nonchromatin antigen extracted from nuclei with dilute phosphate buffer, is found in some SLE patients. Patients with Raynaud's phenomenon and progressive systemic sclerosis may give a speckled pattern with antibody directed against nuclear material other than Sm antigen.
4. The *nucleolar* pattern is thought to result from antibody directed against a specific RNA configuration of the nucleolus or antibody specific for proteins necessary for maturation of nucleolar RNA. This pattern is seen by itself, usually in patients with progressive systemic sclerosis (Ritchie, 1970).

ANA titers and patterns may vary from laboratory to laboratory; this is probably due to differences in antigen or methodology used. To obviate this and the necessity for an ultraviolet microscope, Benson and Cohen (1970) have used horseradish-peroxidase conjugated antihuman immunoglobulin serum to label the antinuclear antibodies on cell nuclei. When the slides are finally treated with diaminobenzidine and hydrogen peroxide, the conjugate takes on a brown color which is easily visible with the light microscope. The same patterns seen with FA are identified by this method.

Other methods to demonstrate ANA using whole nuclei as antigen, such as complement fixation and antiglobulin consumption tests, are technically more difficult and not routinely used. Several different serologic reactions employing specific individual nuclear constituents as antigens, such as nucleoprotein and DNA, also have been described.

The wide range of clinical disorders and the incidence in which ANA is demonstrable is shown in Table 23–8. These are most commonly associated with connective tissue diseases, especially SLE. In SLE, the ANA is demonstrable in virtually 100 per cent of patients; if absent, the diagnosis of SLE is in doubt. Titers of ANA are highest in patients with SLE and often decrease during treatment with steroids or immunosuppressive drugs, but usually remain demonstrable in contrast to the LE cell test, which may become negative with treatment. The homogeneous pattern is the most common in SLE, followed by the peripheral pattern. The speckled and nucleolar patterns are sometimes seen in SLE, but are considered more indicative of progressive systemic sclerosis. The antinuclear factors in SLE usually belong to more than one immunoglobulin class; IgG is seen in 96 per cent of patients, IgM in 80 per cent and IgA in 50 per cent. In patients with anti-DNA antibody (a peripheral pattern), the antibodies are usually of the IgG subclasses which bind complement (IgG_1 and IgG_3). These, in turn, often correlate with the presence of lupus nephritis and the presence of DNA–anti-DNA "immune complexes" within glomeruli of such patients (Peltier and Estes, 1972). Antinuclear antibody in association with complement is also found at the dermal-epidermal junction of skin lesions in SLE patients, and gamma globulin with complement is demonstrable in vascular lesions of these patients. Such observations nominate lupus as a prime example of an immune complex disease.

Table 23–8. INCIDENCE OF ANA IN VARIOUS DISEASE STATES

	INCIDENCE OF POSITIVE ANA IN PER CENT
Connective Tissue Disorders	
Systemic lupus erythematosus	95–100
Progressive systemic sclerosis	75– 80
Rheumatoid arthritis	25– 60
Juvenile arthritis	15– 30
Felty's syndrome	100
Sjögren's syndrome	40– 75
Chronic discoid lupus	15– 50
Dermatomyositis, polymyositis	10– 30
Polyarteritis nodosa	15– 25
Rheumatic fever	0
Suspected connective tissue disease	50
Miscellaneous Diseases	
Cirrhosis of the liver	13
Posthepatitic cirrhosis	40
Lupoid hepatitis	100
Ulcerative colitis	75
Infectious mononucleosis	65
Chronic lymphatic leukemia	20
Acute leukemia, lymphatic, myelogenous	25
Waldenström's macroglobulinemia	16
Hypergammaglobulinemic purpura	65
Drug-associated	
Hydralazine	50
Procainamide	50– 77
Isoniazid R_x in tbc	20
Normals—generally	0– 4
Healthy—1st degree relative of SLE patient	30
—2nd degree relative of SLE patient	20
Patients with false positive serology	40

*Adapted from Peltier, A. P., and Estes, D.: *In* Inaachim, H. L. (ed.): Pathobiology Annual. New York, Appleton-Century-Crofts, Inc., 1972.

In adult rheumatoid arthritis the incidence of serum ANA is significantly less (25 per cent), the titers are lower, and the commonest antibody class is IgM. ANA is also found in the joint fluid of such patients. A high incidence of ANA exists in progressive systemic sclerosis (up to 87 per cent) and, interestingly, the proportion of patients with the speckled or the nucleolar pattern is highest in this group. A similar situation exists in Sjögren's syndrome, in which two-thirds of the patients' sera may have a positive ANA reaction. Chronic active hepatitis and ulcerative colitis are two additional disorders in which one encounters hyperglobulinemia and a high incidence of ANA.

The appearance of a clinical syndrome resembling SLE and an increased incidence of ANA is seen in association with certain types of drug therapy. This was first described with one of the hydrazides, i.e., hydralazine, used in antihypertensive therapy. Anticonvulsants, procainamide, and isoniazid therapy may also be associated with serum ANA reaction. The ANA is usually associated with prolonged therapy and becomes undetectable when therapy is stopped. The exact mechanism for such reaction has not been elucidated (Blomgren *et al.*, 1969).

Whenever evaluating such serologic results, one must consider the incidence of the antibody activity in sera of "normals." Generally, 1 to 4 per cent of normals can be found to have ANA activity in their serum, usually of low titer. Interestingly, the incidence increases with age such that groups over age 60 demonstrate up to 20 per cent incidence of ANA. In these groups, the antibodies are generally of IgM or IgA class and not IgG. In addition, healthy relatives of patients with SLE, progressive systemic sclerosis, and rheumatoid arthritis have an increased incidence of ANA, suggesting a hereditary predisposition to develop such antibody activity.

SEROLOGIC PROCEDURES IN PARASITIC DISEASE

The morphologic identification of parasites or their ova in feces, blood, or body tissues is the most widely available method of laboratory diagnosis of parasitic diseases. However, there are situations when the organism cannot be visualized, and in such, a serologic diagnosis is much desired. In the United States relatively few clinical laboratories perform such tests and one must rely on state laboratories, the USPHS laboratories at the Center for Disease Control (specimens must be forwarded through state laboratories), or the few laboratories that have set up specialized procedures. As more commercial reagents are perfected, such serology may become more widely available.

The proper interpretation of results of parasitic serology requires considerable understanding of the sensitivity of the test procedure, the time course in the disease when the antibodies become demonstrable, the various cross reactions possible with specific antigens, and the endemicity of the parasite in geographic areas in which the patient lives (Kagan and Norman, 1970; Miller and Brown, 1969).

Trichinosis. The bentonite flocculation and complement fixation (CF) procedures are the best all-around methods available. Unfortunately they are not consistently positive until the third week of symptoms in most patients. During the first week of disease, 25 per cent of patients give a positive test, with the incidence of a positive result rising to 90 per cent in the third week. Following this, the titers fall over a period of a few years. The commercially available latex flocculation gives similar results and is perhaps slightly less sensitive (85 per cent positive reactors by week three). False positives have been reported in periarteritis nodosa, infectious mononucleosis, typhoid fever, and tuberculosis with the flocculation procedures. A trichinella skin test antigen has been developed, but also becomes positive relatively late, and once used, can induce positive serum flocculation reactions. The FA procedure appears to yield positive results earlier in the disease.

Amebiasis. The indirect hemagglutination, agar-gel diffusion and CF methods are especially helpful in the diagnosis of hepatic amebic involvement, with 95 per cent or more of patients with amebic abscesses showing elevated serum titers. In patients with active amebic colitis, 85 per cent have demonstrated serum antibody. However, up to 6 per cent of noninfected controls have demonstrated positive reactions.

Toxoplasmosis. The Sabin-Feldman methylene blue dye test has long been used in the serologic diagnosis of toxoplasmosis but is now being replaced by the technically more simple indirect FA procedure. These two procedures give comparable results in 95 to 98 per cent of cases. Indirect hemagglutination (IHA) is another useful procedure. In both FA and IHA procedures, the titers rise early in disease and remain elevated for several years. Titers of 1:128 and below are seen in healthy controls while titers of 1:256 and above are seen in active disease, with titers usually in a range of 1:1000 in acute infections.

Table 23–9. SEROLOGIC TESTS IN PARASITIC INFECTIONS*

			PARTICLE AGGLUTINATION TESTS				
	COMPLEMENT FIXATION TEST	PRECIPITIN TEST	Bentonite Flocculation	Hemagglutination	Latex Agglutination	Cholesterol Flocculation	FLUORESCENT ANTIBODY TEST
Trichinosis	+	+	+	D	+	+	+
Echinococcosis	+	D	+	+	+		E
Schistosomiasis	+	+	D	D	D	+	+
Ascariasis/toxocariasis	E	D	+	+			
Filariasis	D		+	+			E
Cysticercosis	+	+		+			
Chagas' disease	+			+	E		D
Leishmaniasis	D			D			E
Toxoplasmosis	+			+	E		+
Amebiasis	+	+	±	+			D
Malaria	E			D	E		+

*Adapted from Kagan, I. G., and Norman, L.: *In* Blair, Lennette, and Truant (eds.): Manual of Clinical Microbiology. Bethesda, Md., American Society of Microbiology, 1970.

\+ Generally accepted, useful, routine diagnostic test.
D Used for diagnosis, but requires further development before routine use.
E Under experimental investigation.

In congenital toxoplasmosis the FA procedure is the test of choice on cord or newborn sera since IHA is often negative in these infections. An FA technique using fluorescein-conjugated anti-IgM antisera is considered diagnostic when positive on cord sera; otherwise, one must follow the regular FA titer for a month or six weeks to rule out passive transfer of maternal antibody (maternal antibody disappears with a significant fall in titer over the course of a month).

Interestingly, serum titers in toxoplasmic chorioretinitis are usually low, in the range frequently seen in healthy controls, and thus one cannot rule out such a diagnosis in the presence of a low titer.

Schistosomiasis. Cholesterol lecithin cercarial flocculation and bentonite flocculation procedures are available in this disease. Approximately 75 per cent of persons with this disease give a positive test, while up to 15 per cent of noninfected individuals also display a positive result. Thus, a positive test cannot always be considered diagnostic, but certainly designates symptomatic patients who deserve extensive studies to demonstrate the parasite in stool, urine or tissues.

Echinococcus Cysts. Echinococcus cysts occur in the liver and lung mostly as mass lesions, and a serologic diagnosis before surgery can be very helpful. The best available tests are the indirect hemagglutination and bentonite flocculation procedures, which give comparable results. It is recommended that both procedures be used. Between 80 and 90 per cent of patients with hepatic echinococcal cysts will be positive, while 30 to 50 per cent of individuals with a lung cyst react positively.

Table 23–9 lists the serologic methods available in various parasitic diseases.

REFERENCES

Alford, C. A., Schaeffer, J., Blankenship, W. J., Straumfjord, J. V., and Cassady, G.: A correlative immunologic, microbiologic and clinical approach to the diagnosis of acute and chronic infections in newborn infants. New Eng. J. Med. 277:437, 1967.

Anderson, J. W., McConahey, W. M., Alarcon-Segovia, D., Emslander, R. F., and Wakin, K. G.: Diagnostic value of thyroid antibodies. J. Clin. Endocr. 27:937–944, 1967.

Apostolov, K., Bauer, D. J., Selway, J. W. T., Fox, R. A., Dudley, F. J., and Sherlock, S.: Australia antigen in urine. Lancet *1*:1274, 1971.

Balfour, B. M., Doniach, D., Roitt, I. M., and Couchman, K. G.: Flourescent antibody studies in human thyroiditis: Auto antibodies to an antigen of the thyroid colloid distinct from thyroglobulin. Brit. J. Exp. Path. 42:307, 1961.

Bartfeld, H.: Distribution of rheumatoid factor activity in non-rheumatoid statis. Ann N.Y. Acad. Sci. *168*:30, 1969.

Benson, M. D., and Cohen, A. S.: Antinuclear antibodies in systemic lupus erythematosus; Detection with horse-radish-peroxidase-conjugated antibody. Ann. Intern. Med. 73:943, 1970.

Blomgren, S. E., Condemi, J. J., Bignall, M. C., and Vaughan, J. H.: Antinuclear antibody induced by procainamide: A prospective study. New Eng. J. Med. *281*:64, 1969.

Blumberg, B. S., Sutnick, A. I., and London, W. T.: Hepatitis and leukemia; Their relation to Australia antigen. Bull. N.Y. Acad. Med. *44*:1566, 1968.

Bodily, H. L., Updyke, E. L., and Mason, J. O. (eds.): Diagnostic Procedures for Bacterial, Mycotic and Parasitic Infections. 5th ed. New York, American Public Health Association, 1970.

Bradstreet, C. M., Tannahill, A. J., Pollock, T. M., and Magford, H. E.: Intradermal test and serological tests in suspected brucella infection in man. Lancet 2:653, 1970.

Cathcart, E. S.: Rheumatoid factors: Serologic techniques. *In* Cohen, A. S. (ed.): Laboratory Diagnostic Procedures in the Rheumatic Diseases. Boston, Little Brown and Company, 1967, pp. 96–113.

Chanock, R. M.: Medical progress: Mycoplasma infections of man. New Eng. J. Med. *273*:1199, 1257; 1965.

Charkes, N. D.: Hemagglutination test in tularemia. Results in 56 vaccinated persons with laboratory acquired infection. J. Immunol. *83*:213, 1959.

Christian, C. L.: The rheumatoid factors. J. Chronic Disease *16*:875, 1963.

Connell, E. B., and Connell, J. T.: C-Reactive protein in pregnancy and contraception. Amer. J. Obstet. Gynec. *110*:633, 1971.

Doniach, D., Walker, J. G., Roitt, I. M., and Berg, P. A.: Current concepts: Autoallergic hepatitis. New Eng. J. Med. 282:86, 1970.

Edwards, E. A., Muehl, P., and Peckinpaugh, R. O.: Diagnosis of bacterial meningitis by counterimmuno-electrophoresis. J. Lab. Clin. Med. *80*:449, 1972.

Edwards, J. M. B., Tannahill, A. J., and Bradstreet, C. M. P.: Comparison of the indirect fluorescent antibody test with agglutination, complement fixation and Coombs test for Brucella antibody. J. Clin. Path. 23:161, 1970.

Escobar, M. R., Dalton, H. P., and Allison, M. J.: Fluorescent antibody tests for syphilis using cerebrospinal fluid: Clinical correlation in 150 cases. Amer. J. Clin. Path. *53*:886, 1970.

Fischel, E. E.: The C-reactive protein. *In* Cohen, A. S. (ed.): Laboratory Diagnostic Procedures in the Rheumatic Diseases, Boston, Little, Brown and Company, 1967, pp. 70–83.

Friou, G. J.: The LE cell factor and antinuclear antibodies. *In* Cohen, A. S. (ed.): Laboratory Diagnostic Procedures in the Rheumatic Diseases. Boston, Little, Brown and Company, 1967, pp. 114–167.

Fudenberg, H. H., Pink, J. R. L., Stiles, D. P., and Wang, A. C.: Basic Immunogenetics. New York, Oxford University Press, 1972, pp. 60–76.

Gamrot, P. O., and Kindmark, C. O.: C-Reactive protein – A phagocytosis promoting factor. Scand. J. Clin. Lab. Invest. *24*:215, 1969.

George, R. B., Ziskind, M. M., Rasch, J. R., and Mogabgab, W. J.: Mycoplasma and adenovirus pneumonias. Comparison with other atypical pneumonias in a military population. Ann. Intern. Med. *65*:931, 1966.

Goldman, J. N., and Lantz, M. A.: FTA-ABS and VDRL slide test reactivity in a population of nuns. J.A.M.A. *217*:53, 1971.

Goldman, M.: Fluorescent Antibody Methods. New York, Academic Press, Inc., 1968.

Griffin, J. P., and Crawford, Y. E.: Mycoplasma pneumoniae in primary atypical pneumonia. J.A.M.A. *193*:1011, 1965.

Hooshmand, H., Escobar, M. R., and Kapf, S. W.: Neurosyphilis. A study of 241 patients. J.A.M.A. *219*:726, 1972.

Hunter, C. A., Burdorff, R., and Colbert, B.: Flocculation tests for tularemia. J. Lab. Clin. Med. *51*:134, 1958.

Kagan, I. G., and Norman, L.: Serodiagnosis of parasitic diseases. *In* Blair, Lennette, and Truant (eds.): Manual of Clinical Microbiology. Bethesda, Md., American Society of Microbiology, 1970, Chapter 51.

Kaplan, E. L., Anthony, B. F., Chapman, S. S., Ayoub, E. M., and Wannamaker, L. W.: The influence of the site of infection on the immune response to group A streptococci. J. Clin. Invest. *49*:1405, 1970.

Kerr, W. R., Coghlan, J. D., Payne, D. J. H., and Robertson, L.: The laboratory diagnosis of chronic brucellosis. Lancet 2:1181, 1966.

Kerr, W. R., Payne, D. J. H., Robertson, L., and Coombs, R. R. A.: Immunoglobulin class of Brucella antibodies in human sera. Immunology *13*:223, 1967.

Kooman, J., and Morgan, H. R.: An evaluation of the anamnestic serum reaction in certain fibrile illnesses. Amer. J. Med. Sci. *228*:520, 1954.

Kriss, J. P.: Inactivation of long-acting thyroid stimulator (LATS) by anti-kappa and anti-lambda antisera. J. Clin. Endocr. 28:1440, 1968.

Kwapinski, J. B. G.: Methodology of Immunochemical and Immunological Research. New York, Wiley Interscience, 1972.

Lam, K. C., Mistilis, S. P., and Perrott, N.: Positive tissue antibody tests in patients with prolonged extra-hepatic biliary obstruction. New Eng. J. Med. *286*:1400, 1972.

LeBouvier, G. L.: The heterogeneity of Australia antigen. J. Infect. Dis. *123*:671, 1971.

Lennette, E. H., and Schmidt, N. J.: Diagnostic Procedures for Viral and Rickettsial Infections. 4th ed. New York, American Public Health Association, 1969.

Lind, K.: Immunological relationships between Mycoplasma pneumoniae and Streptococcus MG. Acta Path. Microbiol. Scand. 73:237, 1968.

London, W. T., Sutnick, A. I., and Blumberg, B. S.: Current status of Australia antigen. *In* Ioachim, H. L. (ed.): Pathobiology Annual 1972. New York, Appleton-Century-Crofts, Inc., 1972, pp. 207–234.

Mamunes, P., Vernal, G. C., Budell, J. W., Anderson, J. A., and Steward, R. E.: Early diagnosis of neonatal syphilis. Evaluation of a gamma M- fluorescent treponemal antibody test. Amer. J. Dis. Child. *120*:17, 1970.

Messner, R. P., Laxdal, T., Quie, P. G., and Williams, R. C.: Rheumatoid factors in subacute bacterial endocarditis-bacterium, duration of disease or genetic predisposition. Ann. Intern. Med. *68*:746, 1968.

Miller, L. H., and Brown, H. W.: The serologic diagnosis of parasitic infections in medical practice. Ann. Intern. Med. *71*:983, 1969.

Neter, E., Gorzynski, E. A., Gino, R. M., Westphal, O., and Luderitz, O.: The enterobacterial hemagglutination test and its diagnostic potentialities. Canad. J. Microbiol. 2:232, 1956.

Nielson, J. O., and LeBouvier, G. L.: Subtypes of Australia antigen among patients and healthy carriers in Copenhagen. A relation between the subtypes and the degree of liver damage in acute viral hepatitis. New Eng. J. Med. *288*:1257, 1973.

Nielsen, J. O., Nielson, M. H., and Elling, P.: Differential distribution of Australia-antigen associated particles in patients with liver diseases and normal carriers. New Eng. J. Med. *288*:484, 1973.

Nilsson, L.: Comparative testing of precipitation methods for quantitation of C-reactive protein in blood serum. Acta Path. Microbiol. Scand. 73:129, 1968.

Paronetto, F.: Immunologic aspects of liver disease. *In* Popper, H., and Schaffner, F. (eds.): Progress in Liver Diseases. Vol. III. New York, Grune & Stratton, 1970.

Peltier, A. P., and Estes, D.: Antinuclear antibodies. *In* Iaachim, H. L. (ed.): Pathobiology Annual. New York, Appleton-Century-Crofts, 1972, pp. 77–109.

Race, R. R., and Sanger, R.: Blood Groups in Man. Philadelphia, F. A. Davis Company, 1968, pp. 54–55, 427–431.

Ritchie, R. F.: Antinucleolar antibodies. Their frequency and diagnostic association. New Eng. J. Med. *282*:1174, 1970.

Roy, S. B., Sturgis, G. P., and Massell, B. F.: Application of the antistreptolysin-O titer in the evaluation of joint pain and in the diagnosis of rheumatic fever. New Eng. J. Med. *254*:95, 1956.

Saxsbad, J., Nilsson, L., and Hanson, L. A.: C-Reactive protein in serum from newborn infants as determined with immunodiffusion techniques. II Infants with various infections. Acta Paediat. Scand. *59*:676, 1970.

Schmidt, P. J., Barile, M. F., and McGinnise, M. H.: Mycoplasma (pleuropneumonia-like organisms) and blood group I: Associations with neoplastic disease. Nature (London) *205*:371, 1965.

Sparling, P. F.: Medical progress: Diagnosis and treatment of syphillis. New Eng. J. Med. *284*:642, 1971.

Steffen, C.: Antibodies to tissues. *In* Stefanini, M. (ed.): Progress in Clinical Pathology. Vol. III. New York, Grune & Stratton, 1970, pp. 226–264.

Stollerman, G. H.: Streptococcal antibodies in the diagnosis of rheumatic fever. *In* Cohen, A. S. (ed.): Laboratory Diagnostic Procedures in the Rheumatic Diseases. Boston, Little, Brown and Company, 1967, pp. 168–215.

Sussman, S. J., Magoffin, R. L., Lennette, E. H., and Schieble, J.: Cold agglutinin, Eaton agent and respiratory infections of children. Pediatrics *38*:571, 1966.

Taylor-Robinson, D., Sobeslavsky, O., Jensen, K. E., Senterfit, L. B., and Chanock, R. M.: Serologic response to Mycoplasma pneumoniae infection. Amer. J. Epidemiol. *83*: 287, 1966.

U.S. Public Health Service: Standardized Diagnostic Complement Fixation Methods and Adaptation to Micro Test. Public Health Monograph No. 74. PHS Publication No. 1228. Washington, D.C. U.S. Government Printing Office, 1965.

U.S. Public Health Service: Manual of Tests for Syphilis. PHS Publication No. 411. Washington, D.C., U.S. Government Printing Office, 1969.

Volpe, R., Edmonds, M., Lamki, L., Clarke, P. V., and Row, V. V.: The pathogenesis of Graves' disease: A disorder of delayed hypersensitivity. Mayo Clin. Proc. *47*:824, 1972.

Wallace, A. L., and Norins, L. C.: Syphilis serology today. *In* Steffanini, M. (ed.): Progress in Clinical Pathology. Vol. II. New York, Grune & Stratton, 1970, pp. 198–215.

Waller, M., Toone, E. C., and Vaughan, E.: Study of rheumatoid factor in a normal population. Arthritis Rheum. 7:513, 1964.

Wannamaker, L. W., and Ayoub, E. M.: Antibody titers in acute rheumatic fever. Circulation *21*:598, 1960.

Wassermann, A., Neisser, A., and Bruck, C.: Eine seradiagnostische Reaktion bei Syphilis. Deutsch. Med. Wschr. *32*:745, 1906.

Ziff, M.: The agglutination reaction in rheumatoid arthritis. J. Chronic Dis. 5:644, 1957.

Chapter 24

THE SPUTUM

by DANIEL C. NIEJADLIK, M.D.

PHYSIOLOGY OF SPUTUM

Tracheobronchial secretions are often referred to collectively as sputum. These secretions are an inconstant mixture of plasma, water, electrolytes, and mucin. During its passage through the lower and upper respiratory tract, sputum becomes contaminated with exfoliations of the tracheobronchial tree, nasal and salivary gland secretions, and normal bacterial flora of the oral cavity.

The principal sources of tracheobronchial secretions are the mucous glands and the goblet cells. The surfaces of the trachea, bronchi, and bronchioles are lined with about equal numbers of ciliated columnar cells and goblet cells, with the goblet cells being more numerous proximally in the upper respiratory tract. Between the surface epithelial cells and the cartilaginous plates are the submucous gland cells. The goblet cells produce a thick mucin type of sputum which is diluted by a more serous mixture of acid glycoproteins, sialoproteins, and sulfoproteins secreted by the submucous glands. Both types of secretions are increased by vagal nerve stimulation and cholinergic drugs, although nerve impulses are not necessary for goblet cells to discharge their content.

Under appropriate immunologic or inflammatory stimulus, mast cells, eosinophils, and plasma cells may contribute to the secretions. An undetermined volume of the sputum occurs as a transudate from the serum in mucosal capillaries and under normal conditions appears to be quite small. With severe inflammation, though, the tracheal fluid may virtually all be a serum transudate.

The physical properties of sputum reveal the secretions to be viscoelastic, that is, some of the properties of a liquid and some of a solid. The consistency is dependent mainly on the molecular structure of the glycoproteins and on the degree of hydration. Clinicians have long recognized that patients with chronic obstructive airway disease have greater difficulty in evacuation of secretions and that rehydration is followed by easier clearing of the respiratory tract. Numerous studies have shown that unhumidified air impairs ciliary function and mucous transport by causing thicker secretions.

Chemical composition of the sputum reveals it to be composed of approximately 95 per cent water and 5 per cent total solids. The solids are primarily carbohydrates, proteins, lipids, and deoxyribonucleic acid (DNA). These solids increase in amount with increasing inflammation. The DNA originates from disrupted leukocytes, macrophages, and bronchial epithelial cells, and in some diseases such as cystic fibrosis may increase to thirty times normal levels. Numerous enzymes have been identified and studied in pathologic and normal sputum; among them are acid and alkaline phosphatase, lysozymes, DNAase, and lactate dehydrogenase.

Although large numbers of viable microorganisms are inhaled, the lower respiratory tract is maintained virtually sterile. Two mechanisms are responsible: the alveolar macrophage system, and the mucociliary system. The alveolar macrophage system will be discussed later in this chapter.

The mucociliary system provides both a mechanical removal of inhaled organisms and an antimicrobial activity in the secretions within the mucus.

The mechanical removal of inhaled organisms depends on three mechanisms to maintain a continuous outward flow of sputum. The first mechanism is the tapering of the bronchial lumen to produce a vector force directed toward the larger diameter. When sputum impinges upon the wall, this force moves the sputum forward. The second mechanism is the continuous alteration in the diameter of the bronchial lumen produced by respiration. Again, a vector force is formed which leads to the expulsion of sputum. The final and most important mechanism is the effect of the ciliary border of the respiratory epithelium. The cilia are in constant, rapid motion and carry the sputum lining the bronchi outward to the oropharynx where it is imperceptibly swallowed. Expectoration of sputum then depends on cough. Excessive mucus can inhibit the action of the cilia. Increased "thickness" is noted in response to irritation or infection, as both gland cells and goblet cells increase in activity and number.

The antimicrobial activity of the mucociliary system is composed of many factors. Lysozymes and secretory immunoglobulins are the principal secretions, with the latter the more important. Specific antibodies in the respiratory tract are predominantly dimeric IgA to which is attached an additional structure known as the secretory piece. This immunoglobulin is mostly produced locally by plasma cells in the mucosa, and the secretory piece is added by the epithelial cells in transport of the IgA across the mucosa and into the secretions. Small amounts of IgG and IgM are present, but without the secretory piece. Deficiency in either IgA production or attachment of the secretory piece significantly reduces the amount of immunoglobulin present and may render the individual more susceptible to increased infections of the respiratory tract. Also, the high or low pH of the secretions contributes to antimicrobial properties. Finally, systemically administered antibiotics diffuse into tracheobronchial secretions fairly effectively and are of importance in the laboratory when interpreting the results of a sputum culture.

SPECIMEN COLLECTION

Specimens labeled "sputum" seldom contain only lower respiratory tract secretions. Saliva, nasopharyngeal secretions, and bacteria or food particles often contaminate these specimens. Prerinsing the mouth prior to collection will remove most of these contaminants and will not affect the result of the bacteriologic examination. Sputum collection should be supervised by professional personnel familiar with the methods discussed later if proper clinical correlations are to be obtained.

For most examinations, a first morning specimen is best since it represents the pulmonary secretions accumulated overnight. Occasionally, in the presence of catarrhal states of the nasopharynx, some mucus may accumulate in the bronchi at night and contaminate the first coughed specimen.

To obtain a proper specimen, the most important step is gaining the patient's cooperation and understanding. Usually no problems are encountered in adults, but in children lack of comprehension and cooperation present a problem. To circumvent this, three different methods are widely used and advocated: In the first method a nasopharyngeal swab is obtained in children with bronchial disease and is said to be representative of the bronchial pathogens. Advocates of this method believe that the viral or bacterial pathogens affect the ciliated columnar epithelium of the nasal passages as well as the respiratory tract. In the second method a cough plate is held before the child's mouth and the child is urged to cough. The third method, the cough swab technique, is an easy procedure to do and gives the most representative, noncontaminated sputum sample. In this technique the child's mouth is held open with the aid of a tongue blade. The tongue is depressed and the visualized epiglottis is touched with a swab to induce a cough. Material from the trachea expelled from the cough deposits on the swab, and the swab is plated onto the appropriate culture medium. Contamination is avoided if the swab does not touch the nasopharyngeal walls.

In patients who are either noncooperative or unable to produce sputum spontaneously, sputum induction is becoming a popular means of obtaining specimens. Induction both promotes an increased flow of bronchial secretion and stimulates a cough.

Among the popular inductants are 10 per cent sodium chloride, acetylcysteine, and sterile or distilled water aerosols. Nebulizers are used to deliver these particles which condense on the bronchial mucosa and increase the volume of mucus present. The fine particles also have an irritant effect, causing a cough that expectorates the diluted secretions.

Sodium chloride aerosols have an additional effect, as the increased hypertonicity causes a shift in fluid from the bronchial mucosa into the lumen to further increase the volume of secretions. Distilled water and sodium chloride concentrations greater than 10 per cent are very irritating, and in patients with asthma or chronic bronchitis, bronchospasm can be worsened. Bronchodialators can be given by aerosol after the above are used. Also propylene glycol in a 10 per cent concentration is usually added to the saline solvent to increase penetration and minimize evaporation of these particles. In concentrations greater than 20 per cent, propylene glycol has an inhibitory affect on *Mycobacteria tuberculosis* by destroying or preventing its growth on culture.

Acetylcysteine and other related drugs are thought to act by breaking disulfide bonds which aid in maintaining the gel structure of mucus. Acetylcysteine is delivered by aerosol in combination with a bronchodilator; it is one of the most widely used inductants today.

The specimen should be collected in a sterile, disposable, impermeable container with a screw cap or tightly fitting cap or cork. After the patient expectorates the sputum into the container, care should be taken to see that no sputum has been smeared by the patient on the outsides of the container. The sputum specimen should be delivered to the laboratory immediately and not be allowed to stand. If 24-hour specimens are being collected for identification of tubercle bacilli or for volume measurements, a large mouth container can be used. Culturing for bacterial organisms is not recommended or suitable from these 24-hour collections.

Finally, to obtain a specimen in problem cases such as severely debilitated patients or patients with equivocal sputum culture findings, a 15-gauge needle with an intracatheter can be inserted into the trachea below the cricoid cartilage. Secretions can be aspirated with a connecting syringe or, if secretions are scant, sterile saline can be injected and reaspirated.

SPUTUM EXAMINATION

The sputum specimen should be transferred to a sterile Petri dish placed against a dark background. Disposable wooden applicator sticks are used to spread it thinly, and the specimen can be examined carefully with the naked eye or a hand lens.

Macroscopic Examination

With gross examination of the sputum the following macroscopic findings are of importance and should be noted.

Volume. Occasionally 24-hour sputum collections may be performed on patients with chronic bronchitis, lung abscesses, or bronchial asthma. The volume is used as an index of prognosis, decreasing as the patient's condition improves or increasing as his disease progresses.

Consistency and Appearance. Sputum may be described as liquid (serous), mucoid, purulent, bloody, or combinations of these, i.e., seropurulent, mucopurulent. Usually specific diseases have characteristic consistencies and appearances; e.g., in pulmonary edema, the sputum is often described as serous, frothy, and blood-tinged. In most normal sputum specimens, the appearance is clear and watery, and any opaqueness results from cellular material suspended in it. Most opaque particles are masses of pus and epithelium. Other infrequent material seen in sputum can be Curshmann's spirals, lung stones, Dittrich's plugs, caseous material, bronchial casts, or food substances. Particular attention should be paid to the examination of these opaque materials, as their presence may be the initial laboratory clue in the diagnosis of the disease.

Color. The color of sputum is determined by the material contained, and often the color can indicate the pathologic process. Sputum color, though, is an unreliable indicator of the cellular composition. A yellow color indicates pus and epithelial cells are present and is commonly seen in pneumonic processes. When coupled with a green tint, Pseudomonas may be implicated as the etiologic agent. Variation of the color red in sputum can be used as an aid in the differential diagnosis, too. Rust-colored sputum is due to decomposed hemoglobin and is seen in such diseases as pneumococcal pneumonia or pulmonary gangrene, while a bright red is found in recent hemorrhage secondary to a variety of diseases such as acute cardiac failure, pulmonary infarction, or neoplasm invading and rupturing a blood vessel. Rarely a pigmented bacteria, *Serratia marcescens*, has contributed a red tinge to sputum.

Odor. Usually no odor is present in normal and pathologic sputums, but if bacterial decomposition has taken place within the body or after expectoration, a variety of odors will be present. Suppurative conditions such as lung abscesses, cavitary tuberculosis, or gangrene produce the most putrid odors. A ruptured subphrenic or liver abscess often imparts a fecal odor.

Miscellaneous Findings. Other macroscopic findings which may be observed in sputum in certain diseases are listed below:

Cheesy Masses. These are fragments of necrotic pulmonary tissue primarily seen in such diseases as pulmonary gangrene or tuberculosis.

Bronchial Casts. These are branching tree-like casts of bronchi whose size varies with that of the bronchi in which they are formed. They are frequently composed of fibrin and are white or gray in color. At one time they were commonly seen during the consolidation stage of lobar pneumonia, but with the advent of drug therapy, they are rarely seen today. Other conditions in which they appear are fibrinous bronchitis. Their expulsion is similar to that of a foreign body, and when expelled they are so tangled they cannot be recognized until they are floated on water against a black background.

Broncholiths (Lung Stones). These are usually formed by calcification of necrotic or infected tissue within a larger bronchus or cavity. Occasionally the nidus may be a foreign body or a fungus growth. Broncholiths are rarely seen, but when present, chronic tuberculosis would be the most common cause.

Dittrich's Plugs. These are most frequently observed in putrid bronchitis and bronchiectasis. They occasionally are coughed up alone and appear as yellowish or gray caseous bodies which vary in size from the head of a pin to a navy bean. When crushed they are found to be composed of cellular debris, fatty acid crystals, fat globules, and bacteria. They appear most commonly in chronic bronchitis, bronchiectasis, and bronchial asthma.

Foreign Bodies. These consist of almost any small object a child may put into his mouth and then inhale. Among the most popular are peanuts and buttons, which are hard to visualize on roentgenographs but must be considered in a segmental pneumonia or atelectasis which does not clear on antibiotic therapy and other treatment.

Parasites. These are extremely rare in this country and thus are infrequently seen in sputum. As worldwide travel increases, the laboratory is bound to see more in the future. Among the "common" ones in this country are *Ascaris lumbricoides, Echinococcus granulosus* and *Toxocara canis.* In Japan *Paragonimus westermani,* the lung flukeworm, may be encountered, with ova found in sputum.

Microscopic Examination

After macroscopic examination is performed, all suspicious particles are transferred to a clear slide where they are examined unstained if necessary. The remaining portion of the specimen is cultured, using either the classic streak plate method or the quantitative plating method. Examination of the unstained specimen is universally neglected, yet valuable information not visualized well on a stained preparation is present. Among the more important structures to be seen are elastic fibers, Curschmann's spirals, crystals, fungi, and myelin globules. Forming the background is usually granular debris and mucus, which at times may interfere in structural visualization. Examination of the stained specimen reveals best any bacteria and cells (Fig. 24–1). When making smears, it is best to air dry the smear first, then flame it to kill all infectious organisms before applying the Gram stain. Specialized stains for specific cells or organisms can also be made at this time, e.g., Wright's stain for blood cells, buffered crystal violet for bronchial epithelial cells, Ziehl-Neelsen stain for *M. tuberculosis,* Pap smear, and so forth.

By observing the bronchial epithelial cells present it is possible to determine the adequacy of the sputum specimen. Chodosh (1970) strongly recommends that cellular morphology be the basis for a decision whether or not further tests are to be performed on the sputum. If cells characteristic of the bronchopulmonary tree are not present, then the sample should be regarded as contaminated for culture and discarded. The presence of squamous cells signifies the specimen as being more representative of the mouth pharynx than the bronchopulmonary tree.

Cells from the bronchial epithelial layer are seen in three different forms. The basal bronchial epithelial cell is usually about the size of a lymphocyte and has the greatest nuclear to cytoplasmic ratio of the three forms. Columnar bronchial epithelial cells are seen in two forms. Both forms are rectangular shaped, with one end tapered and containing a bulging nucleus. One form contains the ciliated border and is more common, while the other is the nonciliated goblet type and is infrequently seen.

The presence of the alveolar macrophage is

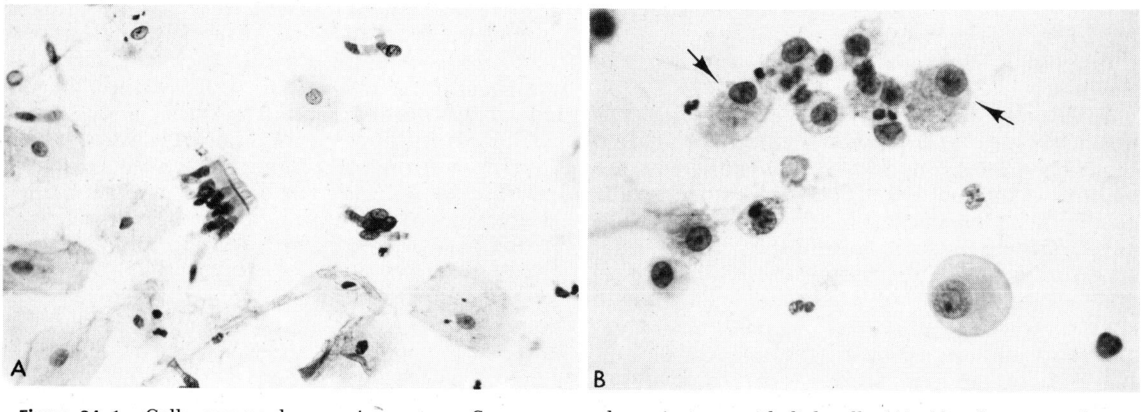

Figure 24–1. Cells commonly seen in sputum. Squamous and respiratory epithelial cells (*A*). Alveolar macrophages (arrows) and an alveolar cell (*B*). Appearance of macrophages indicates sample from lower respiratory tract. (Papanicolaou × 650.)

the best assurance that the material being examined arises from the lower respiratory tract, as macrophages have not been reported in the secretions of the upper respiratory tract. Often seen in these macrophages is anthracotic pigment, which is not of particular diagnostic importance.

Blood cells are best identified with a Wright or Giemsa strain. Neutrophils may be present as partially disintegrated cells in almost every sputum specimen, and their presence most frequently indicates a pyogenic infection. Lymphocytes are the predominant cell seen in early cases of tuberculosis. Eosinophils are found in large numbers in the sputum of patients with bronchial asthma but their presence is not pathognomonic of asthma. Erythrocytes are usually present as contaminants in all sputums, but in large numbers indicate exudation or hemorrhage.

The various bacteria seen in sputum will be discussed later in relation to the disease with which they are associated.

SPUTUM CULTURE

When culturing sputum for a possible pathogen, two methods can be used: The first is the classic technique of streaking on an agar plate. Each specimen is routinely plated in sheep blood agar, chocolate agar, MacConkeys agar, and thioglycollate broth. The plates are incubated at 39° C. for 24 hours with the chocolate and blood agar plates in a 5 per cent carbon dioxide atmosphere. Pathogens are identified and semiquantitated as to many, moderate, or few organisms present. Specific identification of all pathogens is performed by standard methods. The prime fault with this method is that culture growth depends upon where the loopful of specimen was obtained. Even in a sputum minimally contaminated with saliva, it is possible to take the specimen entirely from this contaminated area.

The second method is quantitative analysis of the organisms present. The method's hypothesis is that the organisms causing inflammation will be present in greater numbers than any other superficial contaminating organisms. Also, other problems such as overgrowth with Proteus, mixed infections, and even super infections by a single organism are easier to identify.

The reluctance to adopt the method of quantitative analysis centers about the prolonged processing of the specimen required and the numerous agar plates needed.

The superiority of quantitative methods to streak plate methods have been reported by Monroe *et al.* (1969) and Pirtle *et al.* (1969).

The following method for quantitation of sputum has been found acceptable:

REAGENTS

1. Two per cent N-acetyl-L-cysteine (NAC) prepared by adding 2 gm. of NAC to 13 ml. of 1 N NaOH and 87 ml. of buffered saline.
2. Buffered saline, 50 ml. 1 M KH_2PO_4 plus 35 ml. 1 N NaOH diluted to 1000 ml. with 0.9 per cent NaCl. Autoclave at 120° C. for 15 minutes.

TECHNIQUE

1. An equal volume of fresh 2 per cent NAC (not less than 4 days old) is added to the sputum in a graduated 50-ml. conical tube and pressed against a mechanical mixer until the sputum is completely homogenized. Final dilution is 1:2.
2. Specimen, 0.1 ml., is pipetted into 9.9 ml. of sterile buffered saline in a tube. The pipette is discarded.
3. The dilution is mixed well by pressing the tube against a mechanical mixer for at least 15 seconds.
4. With a fresh pipette, the next solution is prepared similarly and carried out to a 10^6 dilution.
5. Aliquots of 0.1 ml. of the last two dilutions (2×10^4 and 2×10^6) are plated onto sheep blood, chocolate, and MacConkey agar. With the use of a sterile loop, the material is dispersed over the entire plate. A pour plate of each dilution is also made to serve as a check for quantitation of organisms.

After 24 hours of incubation, the plates are inspected and a colony count of each bacterial species is made. All potential pathogens are identified by standard methods and quantitated by multiplying by 10 the number of pathogenic colonies observed at the highest dilution to obtain the number of organisms per ml. of sputum; e.g., $10 \times 2 \times 10^6$. A final report should include the number of pathogens isolated and identified.

MYCOBACTERIA

According to the National Tuberculosis Association, any mycobacterial disease of the lungs other than that caused by *M. leprae* can be designated as tuberculosis. In this country the etiologic agent is *M. tuberculosis* in 97 to 99 per cent of the cases, with the remaining ones caused by the atypical mycobacteria. In sputum examination no differentiation by various staining techniques can be made between *M. tuberculosis* and the atypical mycobacteria. For this reason, a culture should always be performed in a previously undiagnosed case of tuberculosis. Treatment and public health procedures are different for these organisms.

In the classic or fulminant forms of the disease, large amounts of mucopurulent sputum are raised. Evidence of pulmonary hemorrhage and particles of caseous and necrotic material are present.

Within the necrotic tissue, elastic fibers are often present. These fibers are derived from blood vessels, alveoli, and bronchi. Their presence indicates destruction of pulmonary tissue, and thus may appear in other diseases such as lung abscesses, bronchiectasis, or malignancy. Most often they are seen in advanced cases of tuberculosis. Careful selection of necrotic material will demonstrate the presence of fibers. Optimal demonstration is demonstrated by a concentration method—boiling with equal parts of 10 per cent sodium hydroxide and centrifuging. Upon examination these fibers appear as curled, slender, highly refractile, wavy fibrils of uniform diameter. Highly characteristic are the graceful curves without sharp bends.

Within the caseous material, large numbers of bacilli are usually present. Staining procedures are best performed on this material for bacillus demonstration.

The problem confronting the laboratory centers about the recognition of the disease in its early stages. To aid in the early diagnosis, efforts have centered about three parameters: (1) sputum induction and collection; (2) specimen concentration and decontamination procedures; and (3) organism demonstration by more sensitive staining techniques.

In the earliest stages of disease, sputum is present only in the morning in scant amounts and appears primarily mucoid with occasional yellow flakes. Compared to tuberculosis in later stages, the volume of sputum raised is not a criterion of the extent of pulmonary disease. To overcome this problem of small volumes, 24-hour pooled specimens and gastric lavage were collected in the past. Contamination with bacterial organisms was great. In 1966 Yue and Cohen demonstrated that sputum induction by the newer inhalation methods gave a higher recovery rate of tubercle bacilli in a single morning specimen when compared to the older methods.

With the exception of the occasional stat requests for examination of acid-fast organisms, pretreatment of sputum by digestion procedures facilitates organism demonstration by: (1) liquefying the sputum for a more even distribution of organisms; (2) lowering the specific gravity for centrifugation of the organism; and (3) decontaminating the specimen of other organisms to allow the maximal survival of the acid-fast organism.

The methods currently in use employ either sodium hydroxide, N-acetyl-L-cysteine, Zepharin-trisodium phosphate (Z-TSP), or combinations thereof. Each method has its attributes, whether in preparation time, tubercle bacilli survival, or isolation rate. Compared to sodium hydroxide and N-acetyl-L-cysteine methods, a more dependable decontamination and greater mycobacterial survival appear to be present with the Zepharin-trisodium phosphate digestion procedure.

Procedure

REAGENTS

1. Zepharin-trisodium phosphate solution, one part Zepharin (benzalkonium chloride) to 3000 parts of 24 per cent trisodium phosphate.
2. M/15 phosphate buffer, pH, 6.6, prepared with two stock solutions, each M/15.
   a. KH_2PO_4 9.08 mg./L. 630 ml. mixed with;
   b. Na_2HPO_4 9.48 gm./L. 370 ml. for a final pH of 6.6.

METHOD

1. Place an appropriate volume of specimen in a sterile 50-ml. screwcap tube and add an equal volume of Z-TSP solution.
2. Shake the specimen for 20 minutes and then leave at room temperature for an additional 30 minutes.
3. Centrifuge at 2000 r.p.m. for 20 minutes.
4. Remove supernatant fluid by aspiration or decanting.
5. Resuspend sediment in 10 to 20 ml. of M/15 sterile phosphate buffer, pH 6.6.
6. Allow to set for 15 minutes and recentrifuge for 20 minutes.
7. Remove supernatant fluid and prepare appropriate slides and media.

The slides can be stained by the auramine-rhodamine (A-R) stain and/or a modification of the Ziehl-Neelsen (ZN) method.

At present the use of fluorescent microscopy is regarded as the most reliable method for the examination of acid-fast bacilli in smears. In 1962 Traunt *et al.* described the auramine-rhodamine dye combination. Its superiority in comparison with the Ziehl-Neelsen staining procedure is due to more intensive binding of mycolic acid of the tubercle bacillus to carbol auramine than to carbol fuschin.

The auramine-rhodamine dye combination stains nonviable bacilli. Since bacilli viability is important in the evaluation of the drug effect, an acid-fast stain should be performed on all positive A-R stains. The acid-fast method stains only viable organisms.

With atypical mycobacteria, all strains of Runyon's Groups I, II, and III are auramine-rhodamine fast, while the majority of group IV do not stain by this dye technique.

Procedure (Traunt *et al.*, 1962)

REAGENTS

1. Stain:

Auramine	1.5 ml.
Rhodamine	0.75 ml.
Phenol (liquefied at 50° C.)	10 ml.
Glycerol	75 ml.
Distilled H_2O	50 ml.

2. Decolorizing solution: 0.5 per cent in 70 per cent ethanol.

3. Counterstain: 0.5 gm. potassium permanganate in 100 ml. distilled water.

TECHNIQUE

1. Heat fix slides on a slide warmer.
2. Stain for at least 15 minutes at room temperature.
3. Rinse with distilled water.
4. Decolorize with acid alcohol for 2 to 3 minutes.
5. Counterstain with potassium permanganate solution for 2 to 4 minutes.
6. Rinse, dry, and examine under the fluorescent microscope using the filter combinations suggested by Traunt.

In summary, the superiority of the A-R staining technique is attributed to the following factors: (1) the tubercle bacilli have a higher affinity for A-R dye; (2) the entire smear can be examined since the low power objective is used; and (3) the black background in fluorescent microscopy makes the bacilli stand out sharper to allow more rapid and accurate slide screening.

MYCOTIC DISEASE

The presence of mycotic organisms in sputum plays a vital role in diagnosing pulmonary lesions. Mycotic disease of the lungs often mimics either inflammatory or neoplastic disease in clinical symptoms or roentgenographic findings. If the presence of fungi in sputum is noted, valuable time is saved in the diagnosis for both the clinician and the mycologist. By recognizing characteristic morphology on sputum wet mount preparations, the mycologist can isolate and identify the organism more promptly by selecting appropriate media.

Poor communication between the clinician and mycologist often limits the effectiveness of rapid diagnosis. For example, the identification of *Actinomyces israelii* in sputum requires communication among the following: (1) clinician for the symptoms; (2) roentgenologist for evidence of pulmonary lesion; and (3) mycologist for significance of isolation. Otherwise, a possible pathogenic organism might be considered a "usual" contaminant of sputum.

A first morning specimen is preferred as it represents the overnight secretions of the tracheobronchial tree. A sterile container should be used to collect the specimen. In the laboratory the specimen should be placed in another sterile container and examined against a dark background. Fungi are usually present in tiny flecks or particles which appear yellow-gray in color and more dense than the surrounding sputum (Fig. 24–2).

A direct mount with 10 per cent sodium hydroxide should be made and examined under the low- and high-powered lens. If no fungi are found, the specimen can be concentrated by various techniques using either 4 per cent NaOH or the enzyme pancreatin. It is recommended that microscopic findings be confirmed by cultural methods. Sputum concentrate should never be cultured as this procedure kills the fungi.

Pathological Fungi

Actinomyces israelii. Although this is not a true fungi, most clinicians consider it so. *Actinomyces israelii* is a Gram-positive organism that tends to grow slowly, with branching filaments. It can be cultured from most of the human tonsils removed at routine tonsillectomy and from scrapings of gum and teeth. Why the organism becomes invasive is not known, as it is a commensal organism. It is the only species of Actinomyces which can cause pulmonary actinomycosis. In sputum *A. israelii* appears macroscopically as yellow sulfur granules, usually less than 1 mm. in diameter. Microscopically these granules appear as a mass of Gram-positive mycelial filaments surrounded by a sheath of eosinophilic material, which gives a club-shaped appearance to the ends of these filaments.

Nocardia asteroides. In pulmonary nocardiosis caused by *N. asteroides* the pulmonary lesions may resemble tuberculosis or histoplasmosis. Since treatment is radically different in all three diseases, sputum examination can play a vital role in early diagnosis. Nocardia morphology is similar to Actinomyces, but its granules, if present, lack the clubbing of peripheral filaments and are not so compact. The filaments are Gram-positive, bacilliform in shape, and in some stains are partially acid fast.

Isolation from a solitary specimen is not presumptive of the diagnosis since it may occasionally be a saprophyte in the upper respiratory tract. Its repeated presence is diagnostic of pulmonary nocardiosis.

Cryptococcus neoformans. The India ink technique is recommended for direct examination of sputum. India ink is mixed undiluted with the specimen; experience indicates the correct amount of ink to use. A negative India ink does not contraindicate performing a culture. (Most pulmonary lesions are clinically inapparent, while the disseminated lesions are more apparent and severe.)

The organism appears as a single budding blastospore, 2 to 20 μ in diameter, and is surrounded by a capsule from 3 to 5 μ in diameter.

Histoplasma capsulatum. The disease frequently starts as a flu-like syndrome; with healing, the pulmonary lesions become fibrotic and calcified, resembling healed primary tuberculosis. Occasionally the disease may become progressive and disseminated to all organs.

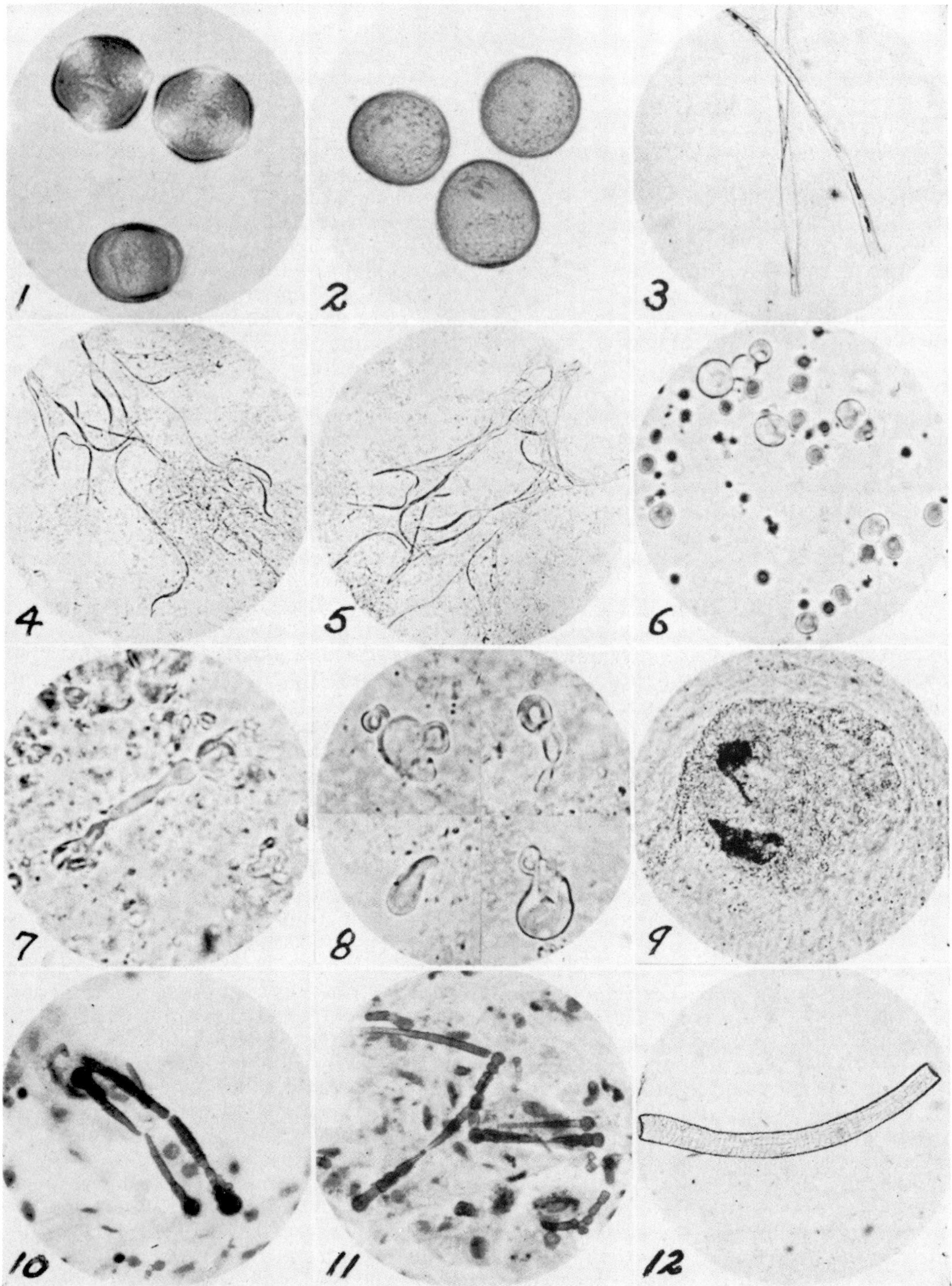

Figure 24–2. Illustrations of structures that resemble fungi found in sputum. *1*, Pollen, timothy grass (× 800). *2*, Pollen, maple (× 800). *3*, Cotton fibers (× 100). *4* and *5*, Elastic tissue (× 200). These are slender, highly refractile, wavy fibrils of uniform diameter and double contour. They may appear as single strands or in bundles and frequently show an alveolar arrangement. Their ends are often frayed or split. *6*, Fat cells (× 800). *7* and *8*, Myelin globules (× 800). Colorless globules occurring in a variety of sizes and bizarre forms. *9*, Bacterial colony (× 400). Frequently found in sputum as small, gray or yellowish granules. They consist of a mass of either cocci or bacilli. *10* and *11*, Asbestos bodies (× 800). They may occur as single structures or in small bundles and have a yellowish color. *12*, Wool fiber (× 100). (From J. M. Kurung: Amer. Rev. Tuberc., 55:387, 1947.)

Staining of sputum with either Wright's or Giemsa's stain often reveals macrophages with characteristic intracellular small yeast cells in the cytoplasm. The specimen should be cultured upon receipt, as sputum contains enzymes fungicidal for the organism.

Coccidioides immitus. The primary pulmonary disease usually has minimal manifestations. Approximately 5 per cent of patients are left with residual lesions of the lung such as nodules, abscesses, and cavities. Local destructive pulmonary lesions rarely progress to the disseminated form.

Sputum should be examined by wet direct mounts. The organism appears as a spherule, measuring 5 to 200 μ in diameter and being filled with endospores. In the chronic cavity form of the disease, hyphae may be seen.

Blastomyces dermatidis. The initial infection begins in the lungs, with subsequent hematogenous spread to other organs of the body. In direct wet mounts, the organisms appear as 8 to 15 μ in diameter sphericle cells without a capsule. Buds are attached to the mother cell by a broad base with a characteristic septum between them. No mycelium occurs in sputum.

Candida albicans. *Candida albicans* is part of the normal throat flora. With widespread antibiotic and immunosuppressive therapy there is often an overgrowth of *C. albicans.* Its appearance on repeated examination indicates it as a possible pathogen. Close communication with the attending physician is needed for proper interpretation of the results.

Candida multiply readily at room temperature, and if the sputum sits at room temperature, the overgrowth may lead to erroneous interpretation. The report should include an evaluation of the number of organisms seen per field. On direct mount the organisms measure about 4 μ in diameter, are thin walled, and may appear singly, in pairs, or in small clusters. Budding forms and pseudomycelia may be formed. The organisms stain intensely positive with Gram stain.

Aspergillus fumigatus. Like *C. albicans*, the organisms appears often as a sputum contaminant, and if demonstrated repeatedly in a specimen, it can be implicated as the principal pathogen. Again, communication is essential between the mycologist and the clinician. In pulmonary disease it can present either as an allergic bronchitis or a localized "aspergilloma."

Phycomycetes. Mucor is the most common species of the genera disease. Mucormycosis is now referred to as phycomycosis and rarely causes pulmonary lesions. When it does, it is seen usually in diabetic patients. Direct wet mounts may reveal huge hyphae, 15 μ in diameter and devoid of septa. Isolation on culture is needed for definite identification.

BRONCHIAL ASTHMA

Laboratory examination of sputum for evidence of bronchial asthma is often neglected, although characteristic patterns can be seen in sputum (Fig. 24–3). The sputum is usually white and mucoid and contains no blood or pus unless an underlying bacterial infection is present. Approximately one-third of all asthmatics will have sputum showing evidence of intercurrent respiratory infection. Some of the following findings are frequently observed in sputum.

Eosinophilia. The sputum has distinctive eosinophilic staining properties which have been attributed to the increased accumulation of serum proteins from the inflammation of the allergic reaction. This eosinophilic staining property has been used to differentiate asthma from chronic bronchitis. Also, sputum eosinophilia appears to be associated with a better response to prednisone.

Bronchial Epithelial Cells. The epithelial cells often occur singly and show hydropic degeneration, with poor definition of the original morphology. During acute exacerbations, these cells gather in larger clusters, display a vacuolated cytoplasm with ciliated borders, and are known as Creola bodies. Also present are well-preserved, hypersecretory goblet cells occurring singly or in clusters.

Blood Cells. Unless there is underlying infection, neutrophils are not present. The cell seen in greatest number is the eosinophil, both intact and degenerated. Monocytes and histiocytes appear in significant numbers during the recovery phase.

Charcot-Leyden Crystals. They are rarely found in sputum except in cases of bronchial asthma. They may be absent in fresh sputum but make their appearance if the specimen is allowed to sit. The crystals are colorless, pointed hexagons and vary greatly in size. The average length is about three to four times the diameter of a red blood cell. Often they appear needle-like. They are derived from the disintegration of eosinophils; hence, they stain strongly with eosin.

Creola Bodies. These are seen almost exclusively in the sputum of asthmatic patients and occur in approximately one-half the cases. Their appearance in large or increasing numbers is a poor prognostic sign. They are large, compact clusters of ciliated columnar cells, occasionally having vacuoles in the cytoplasm.

Curschmann's Spirals. They are found most frequently in bronchial asthma and are fairly characteristic of the disease. Occasionally they may be observed in chronic bronchitis and other respiratory diseases, but in these cases there is nearly always an underlying asthmatic tendency.

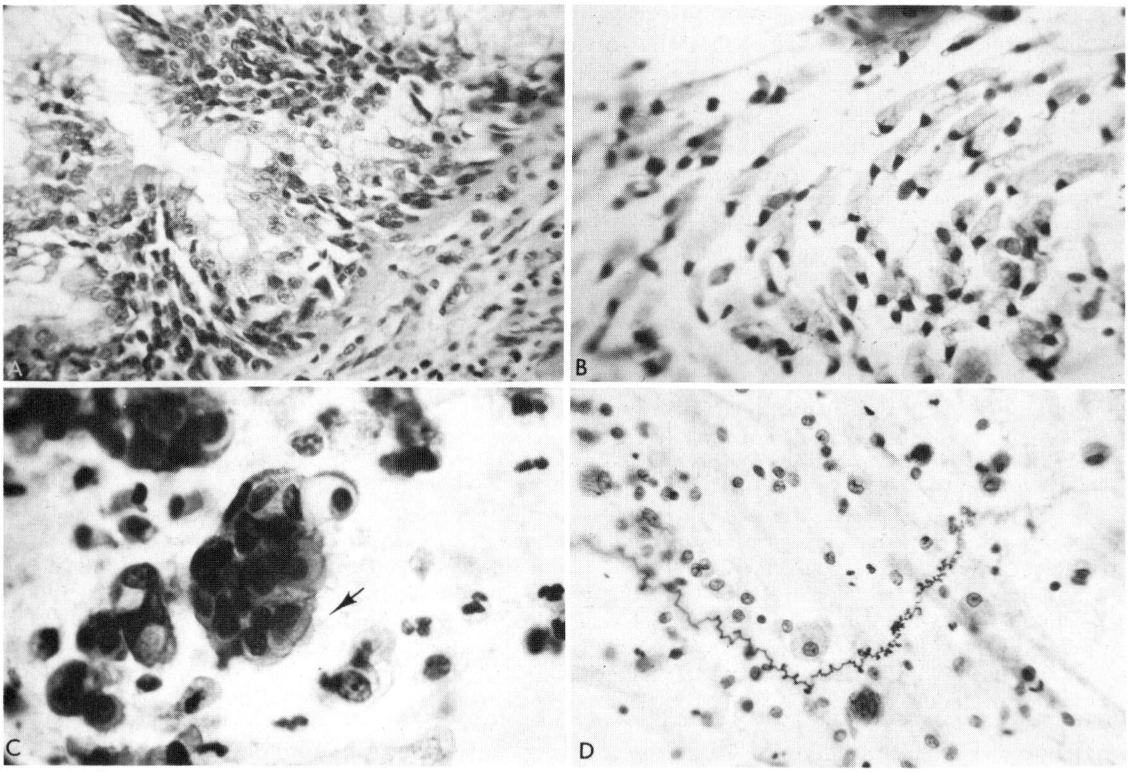

Figure 24–3. Patterns in asthma. *A*, Terminal bronchiole showing goblet cell hyperplasia (H & E stain × 650); *B*, Exfoliated goblet cells (Papanicolaou × 650); *C*, Creola body. Note presence of cilia (arrow) (Papanicolaou × 650); *D*, Curschmann's spiral. Note elongated wavy central thread. (Gram stain × 250.)

Macroscopically they can sometimes be recognized by the naked eye and appear as yellow-white, mucoid, wavy threads frequently coiled into little balls. Unraveled, their length rarely exceeds 1.5 cm. Microscopically a central thread is seen around which mucus is wrapped, supported by a fibril network. The central thread is formed by the shedding of the lining epithelium. Often embedded within the mucus are leukocytes and Charcot-Leyden crystals.

Future and promising studies center about chemical abnormalities of asthmatic sputum in the hope of improving pharmacologic approaches to asthma. Among the abnormalities identified are increased levels of sialomucins, histamine, and antitryptic activity. Clinical and laboratory application of their measurements is still in the future.

BRONCHIECTASIS

Bronchial dilatation of the saccular or cylindrical form *per se* will not cause symptoms unless a superimposed infection is present. The production of a mucopurulent sputum is one of the cardinal symptoms of this disease, and the amount expectorated varies with the posture. In the morning, production of sputum is usually the greatest, as the contents of the dilated lung sacs empty into the larger bronchi.

Characteristically, sputum is putrid, gray-green in color, and varies in volume from 50 to 250 ml. daily. Occasional blood streaking may be present. The source of this blood is usually the chronic granulation tissue of the chronically infected bronchial wall. On sitting, the sputum separates into three layers; an upper frothy layer which later subsides, a middle turbid mucus layer, and a bottom layer composed primarily of pus cells and various organisms. Closer examination of the bottom layer reveals the presence of bronchial epithelial cells, fatty crystals, various bacteria and, occasionally, Dittrich's plugs.

Dittrich's plugs are yellow-gray caseous masses which vary in size from the head of a pin to that of a navy bean. Frequently these plugs are expectorated independently from the sputum. When crushed they emit a foul odor. They are formed within the bronchi and are composed of granular debris, fatty acid crystals, fat globules, and bacteria. Occasionally elongated fatty acid crystals appear to be elastic tissue but lack the characteristic wavy appearance. The presence of elastic fibers may be used to differentiate the sputum of bronchiectasis from that of gangrene or lung abscesses. Dittrich's plugs can also be observed in bronchial asthma and putrid bronchitis.

CHRONIC BRONCHITIS

In chronic bronchitis the bronchioles as well as the bronchi may be inflamed, and the inflammatory reaction may be either cellular or catarrhal. The mildest and most frequent form of the disease in the United States is smoker's cough. Of all the criteria required to establish the diagnosis of chronic bronchitis, sputum production is accepted as the necessary minimum.

Macroscopically the sputum is tenacious, white, and mucoid in appearance. During superimposed infections, the secretions increase in volume and become purulent yellow-green in color. The average volume expectorated is about 60 ml. per day, but volumes as high as 600 ml. per day have been produced. Some clinicians use increasing or decreasing volume as a parameter in assessing the activity of the disease.

Microscopically the presence of histiocytes and monocytes can help in assessing the activity of the disease. In early chronic bronchitis, large numbers of histiocytes and monocytes indicate a stable phase, as during exacerbation these cells disappear. When entering remission again, these cells reappear. A similar pattern holds true for leukocytes and epithelial cells. In remission, a few cells are noted. The presence of necrotic tissue or elastic fibers is an ominous sign, as this indicates a superimposed severe process such as abscess formation or bronchiectasis.

Examination of the Gram stain usually reveals the presence of mixed organisms. *Haemophilus influenzae* must be diligently searched for, as it is cultured in more than 50 per cent of patients clinically ill, although 10 to 20 per cent of the patients not ill display its growth on culture.

Chemical analysis of sputum is a relatively new but promising procedure. Further clinical studies need to be performed before sound clinical applications can be construed.

Lactic dehydrogenase (LDH) activity is present in sputum. The LDH enzyme in sputum originates from serum, the inflammatory cells, and the mucosal surface. Thus, with destructive inflammatory changes in the bronchial mucosa, increased LDH activity may be expected. During exacerbation of chronic bronchitis, total LDH activity increases, with the greatest increase in the electrophoretically faster isoenzyme fractions. With improvement, the reverse is seen. When bacterial resistance to antibiotic therapy is developing, increased LDH activity may be observed before clinical deterioration. Hence, appropriate changes in antibiotics may be made sooner rather than waiting for culture or clinical changes.

DNA in sputum can be demonstrated either by fluorescent microscopy or chemical determination. It originates from disintegrated inflammatory cells and the destruction of bronchial epithelial cells. Thus, in infected secretions, DNA levels are high as a result of extensive cellular damage. Levels fall as improvement is noted.

Finally, elevated neuraminic acid levels have been measured in the sputum of patients with chronic bronchitis.

LUNG ABSCESS

Unless the abscess ruptures into a bronchus, there is little or no sputum production. Most abscesses are initiated by bronchial occlusion, either by virtue of aspirations, tumor, or foreign body occlusion. Those originating from a bacterial pneumonia usually have as their etiologic agent Klebsiella, Hemophilus, *Staphylococcus aureus*, or *Streptococcus hemolyticus* because these organisms may cause tissue necrosis.

When rupture occurs, a large amount of bloody, creamy, foul-smelling pus is suddenly and violently expectorated. Close examination reveals the presence of elastic fibers, cellular debris, and leukocytes. Usually more than one organism will be seen with Gram staining. A search for tubercle bacilli or malignant cells must also be made.

PNEUMONIA

In the early diagnosis of pneumonia a Gram stain of the sputum is perhaps the most essential examination. Proper interpretation leads to institution of appropriate therapy at a minimum of 24 hours before the results of the culture are available. However, certain hazards in the interpretation of the Gram stain are present and have been alluded to previously. Sputum should be homogenized for a more even distribution of the pathogenic organism on Gram stain.

Classically, gross examination of the sputum for certain organisms yields characteristics of certain etiologic agents. More recent work, however, has shown that the correlation is not so firm. For example, the tenacious red currant-jelly sputum characteristic of Klebsiella was not seen in any of 12 patients with Klebsiella pneumonia in a series by Tillotson and Lerner (1966).

Of the Gram-positive pneumonias, the principal pathogen is *Diplococcus pneumoniae*;

rarely are staphylococci and streptococci involved.

In pneumococcal pneumonia the character of the sputum varies with the stage of the disease. In the early stages of typical lobar pneumonia, the sputum is scanty and transparent, with occasional blood flecks. As the disease progresses to the red-hepatization stage, the sputum becomes rust red, very tenacious, and mucopurulent. Microscopic examination reveals the presence of many intra- and extracellular organisms, epithelial cells, leukocytes, and erythrocytes. During the stages of resolution, the sputum becomes more abundant and less tenacious and assumes the appearance of that seen in chronic bronchitis. The rusty character of the sputum is absent during this stage, and the reappearance of this character should alert the clinician that the disease is progressing or has involved the opposite lung. Daily sputum Gram stains should be performed on these patients for two reasons; to follow the effect of treatment on the disease, and to rule out secondary infection.

In staphylococcal pneumonia, a yellow, purulent, voluminous sputum is present. On Gram stain, large numbers of staphylococci and neutrophils are present.

The Gram-negative pneumonias are hard to diagnose initially on sputum examination. Gram stains of sputum may be confusing since morphologically similar organisms are present in normal throat flora. Almost any of the Gram-negative organisms have the potential to cause disease of the lower respiratory tract, but the more common ones are Klebsiella, Hemophilus, Pseudomonas and *Escherichia coli.* With the exception of the foul green sputum seen in Pseudomonas infections, no "classic" macroscopic findings are present in these sputums. As a group, sputums in the various Gram-negative pneumonias are purulent and foul smelling. Putrid sputums may be associated with anaerobic infections and should be cultured appropriately.

Haemophilus influenzae is often missed on Gram stain. The organism binds the safranine stain poorly and it is misinterpreted as background debris. Hemophilus is particularly important as a pathogen in adults with a diagnosis of chronic bronchitis or bronchiectasis. The methylene blue stain permits easier recognition of *H. influenzae* than does the Gram stain. If the organism suspected is *H. influenzae* and no methylene blue stain is available, 0.2 per cent fuchsin solution can be used as the counterstain instead of safranine.

PNEUMOCONIOSIS

The term pneumoconiosis refers to a fibrosis of the lung secondary to inhalation of an organic or inorganic dust. The disease is primarily occupational and its severity differs according to the type of inhaled dust.

To reach the alveoli and initiate a reaction, the particles usually have to be less than 5 μ in diameter. In the alveoli the reaction to the dust particle depends upon its composition. In general, particles are engulfed by macrophages and deposited in peribronchial lymph channels or are carried onto the regional lymph nodes. By far the commonest and severest form of pneumoconiosis in the United States is silicosis. Other types of pneumoconiosis are asbestosis, anthracosilicosis, berylliosis, bagassosis, and byssinosis. The latter two are caused by cane sugar and cotton dust, respectively.

The character and production of sputum varies with the severity and stage of the disease. Macroscopically the sputum is tenacious and can sometimes display the color of the dust inhaled. Microscopically various diagnostic features can differentiate the pneumoconiosis, but their presence is difficult to demonstrate (Fig. 24–4).

In anthracosilicosis angular black granules will be both intracellular and extracellular. Unfortunately the presence of these cells is not pathognomonic for anthracosilicosis, as similar cells with smaller carbon particles are abundant in heavy tobacco smokers and people living in highly polluted areas.

In asbestosis the presence of dumbbell-shaped abestos needles in clusters is diagnostic. They stain yellow to dark brown and measure 10 to 80 μ in size. Numerous multinucleated giant cells and histiocytes may also be observed.

In silicosis the particles are detected with polarized light. The crystals appear sharp, elongated, and fragmented. Numerous neutrophils, macrophages, and multinucleated giant cells are present.

In byssinosis polarized light should also be

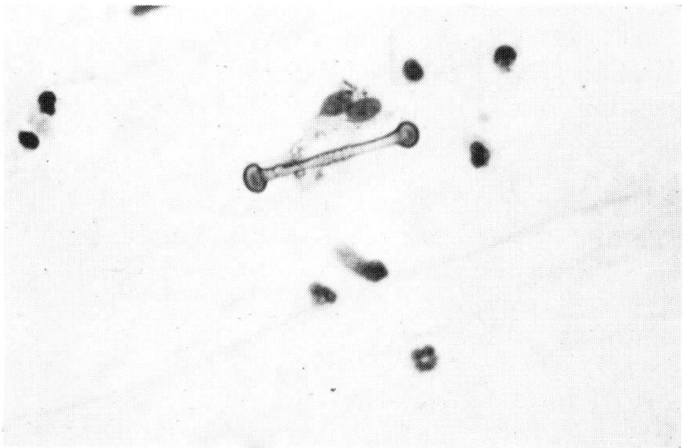

Figure 24–4. Asbestosis body from patient with pneumoconiosis; characteristics may occasionally be overlooked and considered artefact. (Papanicolaou × 650.)

used to demonstrate the crystals. They appear as rectangular, prism-shaped crystals that shine brightly with polarized light.

PULMONARY EMBOLISM

Sputum examination shortly after pulmonary infarction secondary to a blood clot reveals the presence of bright red blood in a very tenacious, mucoid background. As the infarction resolves, the sputum becomes progressively darker in color. Microscopic examination reveals erythrocytes, altered hemoglobin, and macrophages with denatured hemoglobin products in the cytoplasm. Bacteria usually start to appear at this stage as the lung is an excellent culture media.

Sputum examination in fat embolism is nondefinitive. Lipid-laden macrophages and fat droplets may be found in normal persons and especially in persons who are cigarette smokers. Endogenous fat and tobacco tar stain positive by oil red O but can be differentiated in that the tar has fluorescent properties.

HEART DISEASE

Sputum examination has characteristic findings in some types of heart disease.

In acute edema, a condition in which large amounts of serous exudate pass from the capillaries into the alveoli, the sputum is abundant, frothy, and pink. As much as 1 liter a day may be expectorated in severe conditions. Microscopically the sputum may be shown to contain numerous erythrocytes and large hyaline masses. These hyaline masses are the protein component of the serous exudate.

In mitral heart disease the sputum is tenacious and blood is present, either in streaks or in dark masses mixed with mucus.

In chronic congestive heart failure, the sputum is frothy and rust colored. Microscopic examination reveals the presence of erythrocytes and "heart failure cells." In fresh unstained sputum these cells appear as round colorless bodies filled with various-sized granules of yellow to brown pigment. This pigment may be demonstrated to be hemosiderin by staining with 10 per cent potassium ferrocyanide for a few minutes and then with 0.1 N HCl. Hemosiderin pigment stains a blue color.

PULMONARY ALVEOLAR PROTEINOSIS

In this disease a deposition of periodic acid-Schiff (PAS)-positive eosinophilic material within the alveoli occurs without serious alteration of lung structure. The disease usually pursues a chronic course ending in death but may resolve spontaneously. Diagnosis is confirmed by lung biopsy but can be made by sputum examination. Microscopic examination reveals an increase of hypertrophic, hyperplastic alveolar cells, with a granular protein deposit in the background. If formalin-fixed sections are made, PAS-positive alveolar casts with laminated bodies and acicular spaces are present.

PNEUMOCYSTIS CARINII

This infection becomes apparent clinically in patients with impaired host defenses, whether primary or secondary. With the increase in organ transplantation and immunosuppressive therapy, a greater incidence has been noted. Usually the diagnosis is made post mortem, but it can be made antemortem by histologic examination or formalin-fixed sputum. The Gomori silver stain best delineates the cysts of the organism. The cysts measure 4.5 μ in diameter and are round or cup-shaped, with a thin black wall enclosing a cylindrical or comma-shaped structure within the cyst.

GOODPASTURE'S SYNDROME

This syndrome or disease is characteristically seen in young males and usually terminates in death within two years secondary to kidney failure or pulmonary hemorrhage. Immunoglobulins appear to be deposited on the basement membranes of both lung and kidney. Sputum examination reveals the presence of large numbers of hyperplastic alveolar cells mixed with an abundance of large hemosiderin-laden macrophages.

VIRAL INFECTIONS

Viruses have been estimated to cause between 70 and 90 per cent of all respiratory infections. Six large groups of viruses are capable of causing infections, and almost all the groups include a great number of serotypes. Since the prognosis of respiratory tract infections is usually excellent, little attention has been paid to identifying the specific etiologic viral agents.

Viruses are composed of a core of RNA and DNA covered by a protein coat. All viruses require living cells for growth, and after penetration into a cell, the nucleic acid of the virus takes control of the enzymatic machinery of the infected cell, which results in multiplication of the virus and often leads to destruction of the cell. Infected cells show viral aggregates (inclusion bodies) in the nucleus (herpes simplex virus), in the cytoplasm (parainfluenza), or in both the nucleus and cytoplasm (cytomegalovirus).

Preparation of specimens for viral examination is similar to sputum cytology for malignancy. Instead of examining for malignant changes in cells, the presence of inclusion bodies is looked for.

The inclusion bodies of herpes simplex and adenovirus are intranuclear. Herpes simplex is the easier of the two to identify, and the changes involve only the young columnar or squamous exfoliated cells (Fig. 24–5). These mononuclear cells along with giant cells develop intranuclear eosinophilic inclusion bodies surrounded by a halo. Decreased nuclear basophilia is also evident in these cells except in areas where the chromatin clump has adhered to the inner surface of the nuclear membrane. In contrast to herpes simplex and other viruses, the adenovirus infection is compatible with cellular life.

Eosinophilic intracytoplasmic inclusions are seen in parainfluenza and measle viral infections, while basophilic intracytoplasmic inclusions are present in respiratory syncytial and cytomegalic viral infections.

Of these viruses, the cytomegalic viral infection is associated with the highest morbidity, and recent evidence indicates that few individuals escape infection during life. The majority of generalized severe infections occur in the newborn period and presumably originate from intrauterine infections. Infants with this disease may harbor the virus in the nasopharynx and act as a reservoir similar to infants with congenital rubella. Since prompt identification of the disease is important, rapid diagnosis can sometimes be made by obtaining sputum by tracheal aspiration. The presence of large epithelial cells with both intranuclear and intracytoplasmic inclusion bodies is diagnostic.

CYTOLOGIC EXAMINATION IN MALIGNANCY

The cytologic examination of sputum is the single most reliable method for diagnosis of early pulmonary carcinoma, having a positive yield of approximately 50 per cent as compared to 25 per cent when bronchoscopy and bronchial biopsy are performed. In combination with bronchoscopy and radiography, the number of early cases detected has significantly increased, although unfortunately the survival rate has not improved.

Since methods of specimen collection and preparation vary considerably, it is advisable to consult with the pathologist prior to specimen collection and to follow his instructions.

The commonest specimen is the single, early morning, "deep cough" sputum. These specimens should be collected on a minimum of three and preferably five consecutive mornings and submitted to the laboratory fresh without prior fixation. The fresh specimen is examined, and bloody areas and tissue flecks are selected and smeared onto a slide. Other methods of preparing smears include blenderizing, enzymatic digestion, and concentration of the sediment. Although not recommended, delineations of these methods are listed in the bibliography. The accepted criterion for a satisfactory sputum sample is the presence of alveolar macrophages. Four slides are prepared for examination and stained with the Papanicolaou stain.

If multiple sputum collections are impractical, the most reliable sputum sample is the postbronchoscopy specimen.

Central bronchogenic carcinoma gives the highest percentage positive results in sputum examination, although it is not uncommon for peripheral lesions and metastatic carcinomas to yield positive smears.

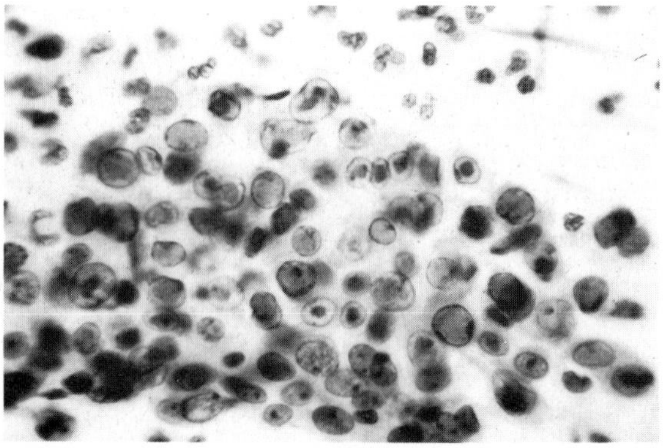

Figure 24–5. Sputum from herpes simplex pneumonia. Note presence of amphophilic intranuclear inclusion, margination of chromatin, and opaqueness of nuclei. (Papanicolaou × 650.)

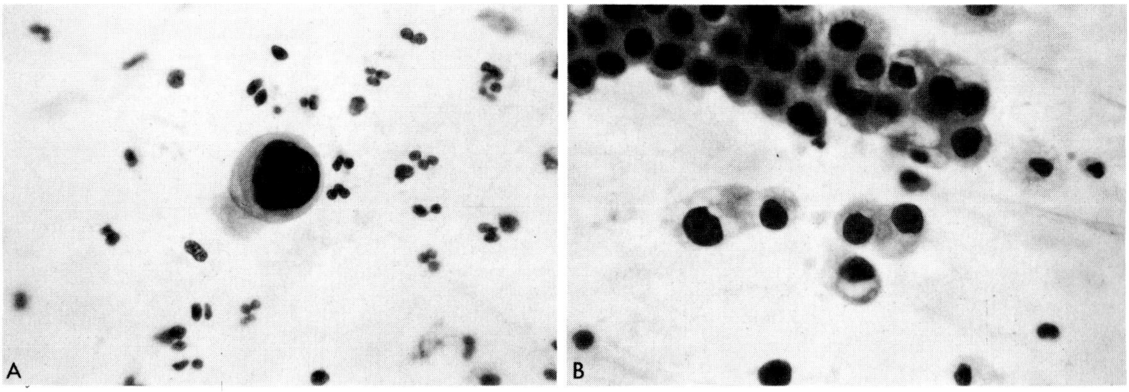

Figure 24-6. Malignant cells found in sputum. *A*, Squamous cell carcinoma, well-delineated squamous cell cytoplasm; *B*, alveolar cell carcinoma—can be confused with cells of sputum of patients with resolving pulmonary infarction. (Papanicolaou × 650.)

Interpretation of smears is difficult, as many diseases cause cellular changes mimicking carcinoma. Inflammatory pulmonary lesions, and especially tuberculosis, form atypical squamous cells which are difficult to distinguish from squamous cell carcinoma (Fig. 24-6). Pulmonary infarction, chronic bronchitis, and especially bronchial asthma may cause profound atypical terminal bronchiolar metaphasia and alveolar pneumocyte dysplasia which closely mimics pulmonary adenocarcinoma. Other diagnostic problems are caused by viral pneumonias, especially those due to herpes simplex and to cytotoxic drugs such as busulfan, cyclophosphamide, and azathioprine.

REFERENCES

Baldry, P. E., and Josse, S. E.: The measurement of sputum viscosity. Amer. Rev. Resp. Dis. *98*:392, 1968.

Bates, D. V.: Chronic bronchitis and emphysema. New Eng. J. Med. *278*:546, 600, 1968.

Bürgi, H., Wiesmann, U., Richterich, R., Negli, K., and Medici, T.: New objective criteria for inflammation in bronchial secretions. Brit. Med. J. 2:654–656, 1968.

Chodosh, S.: Examination of sputum cells. New Eng. J. Med. 282:854–857, 1970.

Darsins, E., and Pukite, A.: Cultivation of acid-fast organisms from tuberculous patients after prolonged and intensive treatment. Amer. Rev. Resp. Dis. *89*:299, 1965.

Epstein, R. L.: Sputum eosinophilia in obstructive lung disease. Ann. Intern. Med. 75:317, 1971.

Heller, C.: Fluorostaining of tubercle bacilli. Amer. Rev. Resp. Dis. *95*:1068–1969, 1967.

Joseph, S. W., and Houk, V. N.: Evaluation and application of the fluorochrome stain for microscopic detection of mycobacteria in clinical specimens. Amer. Rev. Resp. Dis. *98*:1044–1047, 1968.

Kestle, D. G., and Kubica, G. P.: Sputum collection: Early morning specimen on 24 to 72 hour pool. Amer. Rev. Resp. Dis. *94*:501, 1966.

Kubica, G. P., Dye, W. E., Cohn, M. L., and Middlebrook, G.: Sputum digestion and decontamination with N-acetyl-L-cysteine sodium hydroxide for culture of mycobacteria. Amer. Rev. Resp. Dis. *87*:775, 1963.

Kurung, J. M.: The isolation and identification of pathogenic fungi from sputum. Amer. Rev. Tuberc. 55:387, 1947.

Lauzon, R.: Sputum Bacterial Culture: Streak Plate or Quantitative Method. Masters Thesis, Department of Pathology, SUNY, Upstate Medical Center, Syracuse, New York.

Levine, I., Flief, A., Sansur, M., and Wroblewski, F.: Clinical implications of LDH activity in sputum. J.A.M.A. *207*:2436–2437, 1969.

Monroe, P. W., Muchmore, H. G., Felton, F. G., and Pirtle, J. K.: Quantitation of microorganisms in sputum. Appl. Microbiol. *18*:214, 1969.

Naib, Z. M., Stewart, J. A., Dowdle, W. R., Casey, H. L., Marine, W. M., and Nahmias, A. J.: Cytological features of viral respiratory tract infections. Acta Cytol. *12*:162–171, 1968.

Pickern, J. N.: Identification of oil red O stained granules in sputum macrophages. J.A.M.A. *215*:1985, 1971.

Pirtle, J. K., Monroe, P. W., Smalley, T. K., Mohr, J. A., and Rhoades, E. R.: Diagnostic and therapeutic advantages of several quantitative cultures of fresh sputum in acute bacterial pneumonia. Amer. Rev. Resp. Dis. *100*:831, 1969.

Sanerkin, N. G., and Evans, D. M.: The sputum in bronchial asthma: Pathognomonic patterns. J. Path. Bact. *89*:535, 1965.

Takaoski, M., and Urabe, M.: A new cell concentration method for cancer cytology of sputum. Cancer *16*:199–204, 1963.

Tappan, V., and Zolar, V.: The pathophysiology of bronchial mucus. Ann. N. Y. Acad. Sci. *106*:733, 1963.

Tillotson, J. R., and Lerner, A. M.: Pneumonias caused by Gram negative bacilli. Medicine *45*:65–75, 1966.

Traunt, J. P., Brett, W. A., and Thomas, W.: Fluorescence microscopy of tubercle bacilli stained with auramine and rhodamine. Henry Ford Hosp. Med. Bull. *10*:287, 1962.

Weller, T. H.: The cytomegaloviruses: Ubiquitous agents with protein clinical manifestations. New Eng. J. Med. *285*:203, 267, 1971.

Yeager, H., Jr.: Tracheobronchial secretions. Amer. J. Med. *50*:493–509, 1971.

Yue, W. U., and Cohen, S. S.: Sputum induction in patients with pulmonary tuberculosis by newer inhalation methods. Amer. Rev. Resp. Dis. *94*:502, 1966.

Chapter 25

CEREBROSPINAL FLUID AND OTHER BODY FLUIDS

by ARTHUR F. KRIEG, M.D.

CEREBROSPINAL FLUID

Formation, Circulation, and Composition

Cerebrospinal fluid (CSF) is formed primarily in ventricular choroid plexuses by a combination of active transport and ultrafiltration. After formation in the choroid plexuses, CSF passes through the foramina of Lushka and Magendie, circulating upward over the cerebral hemispheres as well as downward over the spinal cord and nerve roots. Absorption is chiefly through arachnoid villi into dural sinuses. A small amount of formation and absorption may occur along pial capillaries and spinal nerve roots in the subarachnoid space. Resorption, as well as formation, may occur in the choroid plexuses of patients with hydrocephalus (Milhorat *et al.*, 1970).

Concentrations of sodium, chloride, magnesium, and glutamine are greater in CSF than in plasma, while concentrations of glucose, potassium, calcium, cholesterol, uric acid, iron, thyroxine, and zinc are lower in CSF (Table 25–1). These differences may reflect: (1) formation of CSF by active transport; (2) lack of binding proteins in CSF (e.g., transferrin and thyroxine-binding globulin); or (3) cerebral metabolism (e.g., formation of glutamine). Composition of ventricular CSF differs somewhat from lumbar fluid: the former has lower protein but higher 5-hydroxyindoleacetic acid and homovanillic acid.

The concept of a blood-CSF barrier reflects the fact that different solutes diffuse at different rates between blood and CSF. The blood-CSF barrier is similar but not identical to the blood-brain barrier (Dunn and Wyburn, 1972). A few substances, such as ethyl alcohol, equilibrate very rapidly; others, such as glucose,

Table 25–1. NORMAL VALUES FOR LUMBAR CEREBROSPINAL FLUID IN ADULTS

Pressure	70–150 mm. CSF (patient lying on side)	
Volume	90–150 ml.	
Specific gravity	1.006–1.008	
Osmolality	280–290 mOsm./kg.	
Total solids	0.85–1.70 gm./dl.	
Cells	0–8 lymphocytes/cu.mm. neutrophils and erythrocytes absent	
Protein	20–50	mg./dl.
Albumin	50–70	per cent
$Alpha_1$ globulin	3–9	per cent
$Alpha_2$ globulin	4–10	per cent
Beta globulin	10–18	per cent
Gamma globulin	3–9	per cent
Fibrinogen	Absent	
Electrolytes and pH		
Sodium	144–154	mEq./L.
Potassium	2.0–3.5	mEq./L.
Chloride	118–132	mEq./L.
Carbon dioxide content	25–30	mmol.
pH	7.30–7.40	
P_{CO_2}	42–52	mm. Hg
P_{O_2}	40–44	mm. Hg
Calcium	2.1–2.7	mEq./L.
Magnesium	2.4–3.1	mEq./L.
Creatinine	0.5–1.2	mg./dl.
Cholesterol	0.2–0.6	mg./dl.
Glucose	50–80	mg./dl.
Glutamine	6–16	mg./dl.
5-Hydroxyindoleacetic acid	1.5–4.5	mg./dl.
Iron	1–2	mg./dl.
Lactate	10–18	mg./dl.
Thyroxine (total)	0.1–0.2	mg./dl.
Urea	6–16	mg./dl.
Uric Acid	0.5–4.5	mg./dl.
Zinc	2–6	μg./dl.

urea, and creatinine, diffuse freely but require several hours for equilibration; some drugs, such as penicillin and streptomycin, do not enter CSF from blood.

Lumbar Puncture

Cerebrospinal fluid is usually obtained by lumbar puncture, performed at L3–L4 or lower to avoid damage to the spinal cord. In small children and infants the conus medullaris extends lower than in adults, so puncture should be performed at L4–L5 or lower. Indications for lumbar puncture may include:

1. Detection and diagnosis of suspected meningitis, subarachnoid hemorrhage, encephalitis, central nervous system syphilis, spinal cord tumor, or multiple sclerosis.
2. Differential diagnosis of cerebral infarction vs. intracerebral hemorrhage (about 80 per cent of the latter show blood or xanthochromia in CSF).
3. Introduction of anesthetics or radiographic contrast media.
4. Treatment of elevated pressure in selected patients with benign intracranial hypertension.
5. Evaluation of blood gas and electrolyte disturbances in selected patients.
6. Removal of exudate or blood from subarachnoid space.

The procedure should be done with a stylet to avoid implantation of skin which may cause formation of dermoid cysts in the spinal canal. A manometer and three-way stopcock should be attached to the needle, so that initial pressure can be accurately measured and CSF removed under control.

Lumbar puncture carries certain risks. A mortality rate of 0.3 per cent has been reported (Marshall, 1970). If increased intracranial pressure is suspected, lumbar puncture should be performed only after careful evaluation of clinical and radiographic findings (Cole, 1969). Dangers include:

1. Production of cerebellar pressure cone in patients with increased intracranial pressure. If brain tumor is diagnosed on the basis of clinical findings, and confirmed by brain scan or arteriography, a finding of increased CSF protein adds little to the diagnosis.
2. With spinal cord tumor, progression of paresis to paralysis may follow lumbar puncture and removal of CSF. If spinal cord tumor is suspected, it is best to combine lumbar puncture with myelography, and to do both when surgical exploration can follow immediately, if needed.
3. Introduction of infection by: (a) passing the needle through superficial or deep sepsis in the lumbar region, (b) improperly sterilized equipment, or (c) poor technique.
4. Development of a dermoid tumor if no stylet is used (Marshall, 1970).
5. Postpuncture headache resulting from leakage of CSF (frequency may be decreased with small bore needle and keeping patient horizontal for 24 hours).
6. In infants, death owing to asphyxiation caused by restraint (Campbell, 1968) or tracheal obstruction from pushing the head forward (Hinterbuchner, 1968).

Elective lumbar puncture should be performed in the morning rather than late afternoon or evening:

1. If the patient is fasting, CSF glucose can be correlated with blood glucose.
2. Examination under "routine" rather than "emergency" conditions typically provides more accurate results.
3. Consultants are more likely to be available if unexpected problems arise (e.g., cerebellar pressure cone).

Lumbar puncture is not a "routine" to be performed on all patients with neurologic symptoms, but neither should it be omitted when there are clinical indications for its use.

Cerebrospinal Fluid Rhinorrhea and Otorrhea

Occasionally the question arises whether small amounts of clear fluid draining from nose or ear represent cerebrospinal fluid. It has been suggested that glucose oxidase test tape be inserted into nose or ear and left there for five minutes: a 2+ to 3+ reaction, indicating glucose present, is considered evidence of CSF rhinorrhea or otorrhea. However, over 30 per cent false positives have been reported with this technique (Kirsch, 1967), and quantitative examination for glucose should be performed. Normal concentration of glucose in nasal secretions is 10 to 25 mg. per dl. If this test is inconclusive, cotton may be placed within the nasopharynx and RISA (radioactive iodinated serum albumin) injected into the lumbar subarachnoid space; the cotton is left in place for 12 hours and then counted for gamma radiation (Brisman *et al.*, 1970).

Pressure and Dynamics

Before any fluid is withdrawn, the pressure should be measured by allowing CSF to rise in a sterile, graduated manometer tube. Normal pressure in adults is 70 to 150 mm. CSF (Table 25–1). A valid pressure reading usually cannot be obtained from adults in the sitting position.

If opening pressure exceeds 180, it is important to reassure the patient; to straighten the legs, back, and neck; and to make certain there is no breath holding or abdominal or jugular compression. If pressure then falls to normal, it is probable that the initial elevation was artefactual.

If the needle is correctly placed, minor pressure variations occur with respiration; if these are absent, incorrect placement of the needle or a block between the needle and dural sinuses may be suspected.

CSF pressure is directly related to pressure in the jugular and vertebral veins, which communicate with the intracranial dural sinuses and spinal dura. Hence, CSF pressure is decreased with circulatory collapse and increased with congestive heart failure, obstruction of the superior vena cava (superior mediastinal syndrome), straining, breath holding (due to fear), or pressure against the abdomen (e.g., obese patients in lying position). Pathologically increased pressure is usually due to inflammation of the meninges or a space-occupying lesion, such as tumor, abscess, cerebral edema, or intracerebral hemorrhage (Table 25–2).

Table 25–2. ALTERATIONS OF CEREBROSPINAL FLUID IN DISEASE*

CONDITION	PRESSURE (MM. CSF)	APPEARANCE	LEUKOCYTES PER CU. MM.	PROTEIN MG./100 ML.	GLUCOSE MG./100 ML.	CHLORIDE MEQ./LITER	COMMENT
Acute bacterial meningitis	Usually increased	Usually turbid to purulent	Increased, chiefly neutrophils (may be normal early)	Usually increased	Decreased below 40 mg./100 ml. in about 50% of cases	Slightly decreased	Gram stain reveals organisms in about 90% of cases; culture may be negative if antibiotics given
Aseptic meningeal reaction to brain abscess, epidural or subdural empyema, purulent sinusitis, etc.	Usually increased	Clear or slightly turbid	Increased, usually mononuclear cells; may be chiefly neutrophils	Normal or increased	Normal or slight decrease	Normal or slight decrease	No bacteria on Gram stain or culture
Tuberculous meningitis	Usually increased	Clear or slightly turbid; delicate clot (pellicle) may form on standing	Increased, usually with lymphocytes or mixed reaction	Increased	Decreased; usually falls progressively, often below 40 mg./100 ml.	Decreased, often under 100 mEq./liter	Organisms difficult to demonstrate by smear or culture
Aseptic meningitis due to viral meningoencephalitis (CSF findings vary in different types)	Normal or moderate increase	Clear or slightly turbid	Slight to moderate increase, chiefly lymphocytes (neutrophilic or mixed reaction in early stages)	Normal or increased	Normal or slight decrease	Normal or slight decrease	May have increased protein with normal cell count in late stages
Lead encephalopathy	Increased in about 80% of cases	Clear or slightly xanthochromic	Usually slightly increased lymphs	Normal or slight increase	Normal	Normal	Lead in CSF, blood, and urine
Multiple sclerosis	Normal	Clear	Usually normal; 30% show slightly increased lymphs	Usually normal; slight to moderate increase in about 30%	Normal	Normal	First zone colloidal gold reaction in about 50%; about 80% show increased CSF gamma globulin

Table 25–2. ALTERATIONS OF CEREBROSPINAL FLUID IN DISEASE *(Continued)*

CONDITION	PRESSURE (MM. CSF)	APPEARANCE	LEUKOCYTES PER CU. MM.	PROTEIN MG./100 ML.	GLUCOSE MG./100 ML.	CHLORIDE MEQ./LITER	COMMENT
Postinfectious encephalomyelitis	Usually increased	Clear	Usually increased (lymphs)	Normal or slight increase	Normal or slight decrease	Normal	Cell count seldom exceeds 200/cu. mm.
Polyneuritis (CSF findings vary in different types)	Normal or increased	Clear (slightly xanthochromic if marked increase in protein)	Normal	Usually increased; may exceed 500 mg./100 ml. in acute infectious polyneuritis	Normal	Normal or decreased	Protein only moderately increased in diabetic polyneuritis
Spinal cord compression due to tumor, vertebral fracture, epidural abscess, etc.	Normal or decreased (may have rapid fall on removal of CSF)	Usually clear; xanthochromic in about 40%; may show clotting if protein very high	Usually normal; about 30% show slightly increased lymphs	Increased in about 90%; may exceed 500 mg./100 ml. (Froin's syndrome)	Normal	Usually decreased	Positive Queckenstedt in about 80%
Early neurosyphilis	Normal or increased	Normal	Normal or slight increase, chiefly lymphocytes	Normal or slight increase in about 50% of cases	Normal	Normal	In early stages blood may be seropositive and CSF, sero-negative. Evaluation of CSF serology 1 to 2 years after infection may be helpful
Late neurosyphilis	Normal or increased	Normal	Slight to moderate increase, chiefly lymphocytes	Usually increased	Normal	Normal	CSF seropositive in 90%; blood often negative
Traumatic tap	Normal	Initially streaked with gross blood, clearing in subsequent tubes; no xanthochromia	Proportional to CSF RBC (see text)	Proportional to CSF RBC (see text)	Normal	Normal	About 2 WBC and 1 mg. protein added with every 1000 RBC
Subarachnoid hemorrhage	Findings similar to intracerebral hemorrhage *(vide infra)*, but usually show less fall in pressure after tap. Blood and/or xanthochromia invariably present during first week. Leukocytes may increase after 24 to 48 hours.						
Intracerebral hemorrhage	Increased in about 80%; occasionally exceeds 400 mm. CSF	Bloody or xanthochromic in about 80%	Proportional to CSF RBC (see text)	Usually increased	Normal	Normal	May have marked fall in pressure with removal of small amount CSF
Subdural hematoma	Increased in about 80%	Usually normal; may be bloody or xanthochromic if cerebral laceration also present	Normal	Normal or slightly increased	Normal	Normal	CSF findings of limited value; diagnosis confirmed by surgery

(Table 25–2 continues on the following page.)

Table 25–2. ALTERATIONS OF CEREBROSPINAL FLUID IN DISEASE *(Continued)*

CONDITION	PRESSURE (MM. CSF)	APPEARANCE	LEUKOCYTES PER CU. MM.	PROTEIN MG./100 ML.	GLUCOSE MG./100 ML.	CHLORIDE MEQ./LITER	COMMENT
Cerebral thrombosis	Usually normal; increased in about 30%; seldom exceeds 300 mm. CSF	Normal	Usually normal; slight increase in about 30% of cases	Usually normal; slight to moderate increase in about 40% of cases	Normal	Normal	Hemorrhagic infarcts due to embolism may produce bloody CSF
Brain tumor	Usually increased; may exceed 300 mm. CSF	Clear; rarely xanthochromic due to markedly increased protein	Usually normal; 30% show slightly increased lymphs	Depending on location may be normal or increased	Usually normal; decreased if malignant cells in CSF	Normal	CSF cytology may be helpful, especially with metastatic tumors
Herniated intervertebral disc	Normal	Normal	Normal	Slight to moderate increase in about 80%	Normal	Normal	May have evidence of subarachnoid block
Diffuse cerebral atrophy	Normal	Normal	Normal	Normal or slight increase	Normal	Normal	Increased CSF uric acid reported in progressive disease

*Adapted from Page and Culver: Laboratory Examinations in Clinical Diagnosis. Cambridge, Harvard University Press, 1961.

If initial pressure is over 200 mm. CSF, only 1 to 2 ml. of fluid should be removed; a 25 to 50 per cent fall in pressure after removing 1 to 2 ml. suggests cerebellar herniation or spinal cord compression above the puncture site. In such case, NO additional fluid should be removed, and the patient should be observed closely for several hours. Ordinarily three 2-ml. samples are taken in sterile tubes and labeled sequentially. Provided initial pressure is not elevated, and there is no marked fall in pressure when fluid is removed, 10 to 20 ml. CSF may be obtained without danger to the patient.

If initial pressure is normal and there is clinical suspicion of subarachnoid block, a Queckenstedt test may be performed. This should NOT be done in the presence of increased intracranial pressure! Normally if both jugular veins are manually compressed, CSF pressure rises rapidly to over 300 mm. CSF, and rapidly returns to normal when compression ceases. This effect depends on rapid transmission of pressure from the jugular veins, through dural sinuses and arachnoid villi, to intracranial CSF, which communicates through the foramen magnum with lumbar CSF.

With sinus thrombosis, obstruction at the foramen magnum, or a mass lesion in the spinal canal, the rise of CSF pressure may be decreased or delayed. This is considered a "positive" Queckenstedt test. In such cases, normal variations in pressure due to respiration will be decreased or absent, but straining or abdominal compression should result in increased CSF pressure (due to vertebral vein congestion) if the needle is correctly placed.

About 80 per cent of patients with cord compression have a positive Queckenstedt test. Lesions responsible for cord compression include herniated intervertebral disc, vertebral fracture, extradural abscess, adhesions due to pachymeningitis, and neoplasms (primary or metastatic) involving vertebrae, meninges, or spinal cord. It has been suggested that the Queckenstedt test is redundant and should be replaced by myelography (O'Reilly and Kwa, 1967).

Gross Examination

Normal CSF is crystal clear. Color should be evaluated by holding the sample beside a tube of distilled water and a clean white paper. If a pale yellow or pink color is noted, the sample should be centrifuged at high speed for at least five minutes and the supernatant examined visually. Xanthochromia (pale pink to pale orange or yellow color in supernatant) usually is graded as 1+ to 4+ and may be due to: (1) CSF protein over 100 mg./dl.; (2) traumatic tap with lysis of erythrocytes due to detergent in puncture needle or sample tube; (3) bilirubinemia (in adults conjugated bilirubin diffuses across the blood-CSF barrier, while in neonates unconjugated bilirubin may also pass); (4) intracerebral or subarachnoid hemorrhage; (5) contamination of CSF by Merthiolate used to disinfect the skin; (6) carotenemia; or (7) melanin in CSF due to meningeal melanosarcoma.

Xanthochromia of CSF usually is due to oxyhemoglobin, methemoglobin, or bilirubin. Since visual estimates of xanthochromia may vary between different observers, objective measurements have been suggested: (1) spectral absorbance scan against distilled water blank from 390 to 500 nm.; (2) "xanthochromic index" based on absorbance measurements at 415 and 460 nm. (Van Der Meulen, 1966). Although not widely used, these objective measurements of xanthochromia offer some potential advantages: (1) elimination of differences between observers; (2) estimate on relative amounts of oxyhemoglobin and bilirubin present; and (3) numerical results which may be useful in following progress of patients.

Two to 12 hours after a subarachnoid hemorrhage, pale orange xanthochromia appears in the CSF of 90 per cent of patients. Yellow xanthochromia due to conversion of hemoglobin to bilirubin develops within two to four days. The orange xanthochromia of oxyhemoglobin usually disappears in four to eight days, while yellow xanthochromia due to bilirubin typically persists for 12 to 40 days (Walton, 1956). Gross blood due to subarachnoid hemorrhage occasionally may disappear within 24 hours, but generally persists for seven to 14 days (rarely, up to 21 days).

Turbidity in CSF may result from large numbers of leukocytes or bacteria, and varies from slight opalescence typical in tuberculous meningitis to the grossly purulent appearance in some cases of pyogenic meningitis. Turbidity usually is graded from 0 (crystal clear fluid) to 4+ (newsprint cannot be seen through tube).

In addition to xanthochromia and turbidity, CSF should be grossly examined for clotting which may occur with: (1) traumatic tap, (2) markedly elevated CSF protein, or (3) moderately elevated CSF protein in association with tuberculous meningitis.

Evaluation of grossly bloody CSF is important to distinguish traumatic tap from subarachnoid hemorrhage. Crenated erythrocytes occur in both conditions and are of no diagnostic significance. Table 25–3 outlines some differences which may be helpful.

Cell Counts and Microscopic Examination

If the specimen appears clear, leukocyte counts may be performed in a hemocytometer counting chamber without diluting fluid. If the specimen appears hazy (200 to 500 white cells) or turbid (over 500 white cells), a small amount of crystal violet diluting fluid should be used (cf., section on methods).

Using nine large squares on each side of a hemocytometer, a total of $\frac{18}{10}$ cu.mm. are examined. If the "true value" is 8 cells per cu.mm., then about 16 cells will be counted.

The coefficient of variation is given by:

$$CV = \frac{100}{\sqrt{\text{no. of cells counted}}}$$

Therefore, in this example:

$$CV = \frac{100}{\sqrt{16}} = \frac{100}{4} = 25\%$$

Using a Fuchs-Rosenthal chamber (depth

Table 25–3. DIFFERENCES BETWEEN TRAUMATIC TAP AND SUBARACHNOID HEMORRHAGE

FINDING IN CSF	TRAUMATIC TAP	SUBARACHNOID HEMORRHAGE
Xanthochromia	Absent (unless CSF protein over 100 mg./dl., severe jaundice, or hemolysis due to detergent in tube)	Typically present if duration over 2–12 hours
Clotting	May occur (incubate at 37° C.)	Absent (defibrination occurs *in vivo*)
Blood staining	Typically varies from tube to tube	Usually uniform in all tubes
Pressure	Usually normal	Elevated
Repeat puncture in higher interspace	Often clear	Similar to initial tap

0.2 mm.) about 32 cells would be counted. Therefore:

$$CV = \frac{100}{\sqrt{32}} = \frac{100}{5.7} = 18\%$$

Thus, if the "true value" is 8 lymphocytes per cu.mm., one can expect ± 2 CV to equal about $\pm$ 4 cells per cu.mm.

Since so few leukocytes are counted by the chamber method, one might expect improved precision using electronic cell counters. In practice, however, variable "background counts" cause poor precision in the normal range.

Erythrocyte and leukocyte counts should be performed within 30 minutes after the specimen is obtained, because cells lyse on prolonged standing and accurate counts become impossible. Furthermore, lysis of erythrocytes will cause artefactual "xanthochromia." For this reason, physicians should be prepared to personally examine CSF samples for xanthochromia, as well as to perform the erythrocyte count, leukocyte count, Gram stain, and differential, and to plant the sample on appropriate culture media (Cole, 1969).

With traumatic tap, the CSF red cell count is occasionally used to "correct" either CSF leukocyte count or CSF protein for contamination by peripheral blood. The amount of added protein, or number of added leukocytes, may be calculated as shown in the formula below.

Thus, if serum protein is 7.0 gm./dl., peripheral erythrocyte count 4.6 million per cu.mm., and CSF red cell count 10,000 per cu.mm. (CSF very faintly blood tinged), added protein due to traumatic tap is:

protein added

$$= \frac{7000 \text{ mg./dl.} \times 10{,}000 \text{ RBC/cu.mm.}}{4{,}600{,}000 \text{ RBC/cu.mm.}}$$

$$= \frac{70}{4.6} \text{ mg./dl.} = 15 \text{ mg./dl.}$$

Therefore, 15 mg./dl. should be subtracted from measured CSF protein to obtain a "corrected" value.

It has been suggested that with traumatic tap, 15 mg./dl. should be subtracted from CSF protein for every 10,000 erythrocytes per cu.mm. Accuracy of this "correction" depends on: (1) whether the serum protein is actually 7.0 gm./dl.; (2) whether the peripheral RBC is actually 4.6 million/cu.mm.; and (3) accuracy of the CSF erythrocyte count. With high CSF erythrocyte count, inherent errors of red cell counting become important. Thus, with serum protein of 7.0 gm./dl., peripheral erythrocyte count 4.6 million per cu.mm., and CSF erythrocyte count 1.0 million per cu.mm., a 10 per cent "low" CSF erythrocyte count would have the following effect:

protein added

$$= \frac{7000 \text{ mg./dl.} \times 900{,}000 \text{ RBC/cu.mm.}}{4{,}600{,}000 \text{ RBC/cu.mm.}}$$

$$= \frac{6300}{4.6} \text{ mg./dl.} = 1370 \text{ mg./dl.}$$

But the "true" correction should be:

protein added

$$= \frac{7000 \text{ mg./dl.} \times 1{,}000{,}000 \text{ RBC/cu.mm.}}{4{,}600{,}000 \text{ RBC/cu.mm.}}$$

$$= \frac{7000}{4.6} \text{ mg./dl.} = 1522 \text{ mg./dl.}$$

Thus, a 10 per cent error in CSF erythrocyte count would cause a gross error in the "correction factor." This amount of error would be expected if 400 erythrocytes were counted in a hemocytometer:

$$CV = \frac{100}{\sqrt{400}} = \frac{100}{20} = 5\%$$

However, if an electronic cell counter were used, and 400,000 erythrocytes counted, the expected CV would be:

$$CV = \frac{100}{\sqrt{400{,}000}} \cong \frac{100}{630} \cong 0.2\%$$

If we assume $\pm$ 2CV is 1 per cent:

protein added

$$= \frac{7000 \text{ mg./dl.} \times 990{,}000 \text{ RBC/cu.mm.}}{4{,}600{,}000 \text{ RBC/cu.mm.}}$$

$$= \frac{6960}{46. \text{ mg./dl.}} = 1513 \text{ mg./dl.}$$ (quite close to the "true" value of 1522 mg./dl.)

$$\text{WBC added} = \frac{WBC_B \times RBC_O}{RBC_B} \text{ where:}$$

WBC added = leukocytes (or protein) added to CSF from traumatic tap

WBC_B = leukocyte count (or total protein) in peripheral blood

RBC_O = erythrocyte count observed in CSF

RBC_B = erythrocyte count of peripheral blood

Thus, validity of the calculated "correction factor" for CSF protein depends upon: (1) whether the CSF erythrocyte count is so low that counting errors will have little effect, or so precise that ± 2 CV is in the range of 1 to 2 per cent; and (2) accuracy as well as precision of peripheral blood erythrocyte count and total protein.

If the CSF leukocyte count is elevated (over 10 per cu.mm.) or if neutrophils (or unidentified cells) are seen in the counting chamber, a differential count, Gram stain, and culture should be performed. A rough estimate of the differential count can be obtained by classifying cells seen in the counting chamber; however, a stained film is recommended for detailed study of cellular morphology.

Many different formed elements may be identified in CSF. In early bacterial, tuberculous, or fungal meningitis, a carefully prepared and thoroughly studied Gram stain may reveal the etiologic agent. A clinical history is important; following myelography, lipid-laden macrophages and yeast-like structures may present confusing artefacts. Lipid-laden histocytes may also be seen with cerebral lipidoses, and hemosiderin-laden macrophages are often found following subarachnoid hemorrhage. In fungal meningitis due to *Cryptococcus neoformans*, the organisms may be confused with erythrocytes or lymphocytes; by mixing a small amount of India ink with CSF, the yeast cells may be recognized by budding as well as by their wide capsule (Fig. 25–1). Leukemic infiltration of meninges is not rare and may cause pleocytosis with immature "blast" forms in CSF. Primary or metastatic carcinoma may also shed malignant cells into CSF.

Primary amebic meningoencephalitis is being recognized with increasing frequency (Duma *et al.*, 1969). On wet mounts at room temperature (or on a warmed stage) amoebas can be recognized by their active movement, endoplasmic granules, vacuoles, and large central nucleolus. However, it is difficult to distinguish amoebas from mononuclear cells in the counting chamber, or on "routine" stains (Carter, 1968). The diagnosis may be suspected if there are numerous "mononuclear cells" in CSF, poor response to conventional antibiotics, and no growth on conventional culture media.

Eosinophilic meningitis (Char and Rosen, 1967) may be related to infestation with helminthic parasites, coccidioidal meningitis, rabies vaccination, or intrathecal injection of foreign protein. Observed percentage of eosinophils may vary from 10 to over 90 per cent.

The most common cellular reactions in CSF are: (1) neutrophilic reaction; (2) mixed reaction (neutrophils, lymphocytes, and monocytes); and (3) monocytic reaction (lymphocytes and/or monocytes). The type of cellular reaction – neutrophilic, mixed, or monocytic – typically depends upon nature and duration of the disease (Table 25–2).

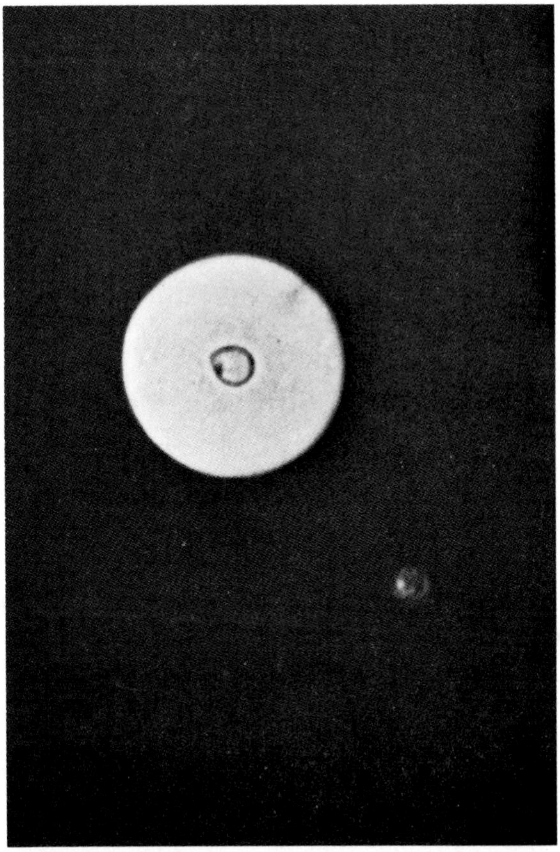

Figure 25–1. *Cryptococcus neoformans* in cerebrospinal fluid. India ink preparation; ×200. (From Anderson: The Clinical Practice of Bacteriology. Philadelphia, F. A. Davis, 1966.)

A neutrophilic reaction usually indicates meningitis due to pyogenic organisms (e.g., *Neisseria meningitidis, Haemophilus influenzae*, pneumococci, streptococci, staphylococci, or coliforms). Occasionally, moderate neutrophilic pleocytosis due to viral infection or aseptic meningeal reaction may mimic bacterial meningitis. Rarely, severe neutrophilic pleocytosis may occur with viral meningoencephalitis (Wilfert, 1969), intracerebral hematoma, fungal meningitis, following intrathecal injection of RISA (Dramov and Dubou, 1971), or following lumbar puncture with detergent-contaminated needles (Austin and Sokolowski, 1968).

A mixed reaction (neutrophils, lymphocytes, and monocytes) may occur with subacute bacterial meningitis, tuberculous or mycotic meningitis, viral meningoencephalitis, or aseptic meningeal reaction.

Monocytic and/or lymphocytic pleocytosis is typical of viral meningoencephalitis; multiple sclerosis; and tuberculous, fungal, or syphilitic meningitis. In tuberculous or fungal meningitis, histiocytes and lymphocytes with a "monocytoid" or "plasmacytoid" appearance may be present.

Microbiologic Examination

In early bacterial meningitis, the most valuable single examination is a carefully examined Gram stain of CSF, which is positive in over 90 per cent of cases. However, considerable experience is required for accurate interpretation if only a few organisms are found.

Several milliliters of CSF should be promptly cultured in order to detect fastidious organisms; this method is superior to culture from a single loop of centrifuged sediment. A combination of chocolate agar or Levinthal's transparent agar (incubated in a candle jar), thioglycollate broth, and aerobic and anaerobic blood plates should be used. Any CSF remaining after culture can be incubated at 37° C. for repeat Gram stain after four to eight hours; this is helpful if only a few organisms are noted on the initial Gram stain.

If tuberculosis is suspected, a larger volume of CSF (10 ml.) is required for adequate culture. Occasionally ventricular fluid may reveal tubercle bacilli when these are not found in lumbar CSF.

If fungus infection is suspected, in addition to an India ink preparation, CSF should be cultured on two Sabouraud agar slants incubated at 25° C., two brain-heart infusion slants incubated at 25° C., and two brain-heart infusion slants incubated at 35 to 37° C.

Recovery of virus from CSF depends to a great extent on the agent involved. Members of the enterovirus group occasionally are isolated; rarely, herpes and arbor viruses are found. In cases of known viral CNS disease, the stool is more rewarding (85 per cent positive) than CSF (10 per cent positive). However, because the CSF is normally sterile, any isolate is significant, while an isolate in the stool does not necessarily indicate that the agent is responsible for CNS disease.

Total Protein

The "normal range" for CSF protein varies according to the age of the patient and the method used. Some methods do not give comparable results since globulin gives greatest turbidity with trichloracetic acid (TCA) and albumin gives greatest turbidity with sulfosalicylic acid (SSA). The following procedures overcome this problem and can be recommended for routine use: (1) Meulemans (1960) sodium sulfate-SSA turbidometric method; (2) modifications of the Folin-Ciocalteu technique which use deproteinized CSF as a blank (Watson, 1964); (3) modified biuret reaction (Bürgi *et al.*, 1967); and (4) methods based on UV spectrophotometry at 210 nm. which remove low molecular weight nonprotein substances via gel filtration (Igou, 1967), dialysis (Pennock *et al.*, 1968), or positive pressure ultrafiltration (Werner, 1969). Agreement between these four groups of methods appears reasonably good, with a normal range of about 20–50 mg./dl. for lumbar CSF in adults. For routine laboratory work, the turbidimetric method is technically simple and appears satisfactory. Although UV spectrophotometric methods are gaining acceptance as reference procedures, it is not yet proved that this advantage offsets the complexity and cost.

The "normal range" of CSF protein appears to vary with age, but there is no universal agreement on what values should be expected. According to Bauer *et al.* (1965), normal premature infants may have CSF protein up to 400 mg./dl. Ranges for mature infants appear to be about 30–200 mg./dl. during the first six days of life, about 30–150 mg./dl. from 6–30 days, and perhaps 30–100 mg./dl. from one to six months (Watson, 1964). However, additional data is needed, and when possible each laboratory should establish its own normal range stratified by age.

Semiquantitative protein tests such as the Pandy test, zinc sulfate turbidity, Levinson test, Ross-Jones reaction, and Nonne-Apelt test are obsolete and should be replaced by accurate total protein measurement plus protein electrophoresis.

In adults, levels of 60–75 mg./dl. are considered slightly increased, levels of 75 to 150 mg./dl. moderately increased, and levels of 150 to 500 mg./dl. markedly increased. Slight, moderate, or marked increase in CSF protein may occur with any lesion causing injury to cerebral tissue or the blood-brain barrier: viral, tuberculous, mycotic, syphilitic, or bacterial meningoencephalitis; polyneuritis; intracerebral hemorrhage; degenerative disease; or aseptic meningeal reaction (Table 25–2). Brain tumors cause variable increases, depending upon their location: gliomas deep in the pons or cerebrum may be associated with normal levels, while acoustic neuromas and tumors of the corpus callosum usually cause markedly increased CSF protein. Diabetic neuropathy, myxedema, heavy metal intoxication, isopropanol intoxication, hypercalcemia, and diphenylhydantoin (Dilantin) intoxication have all been described as causes for increased CSF protein.

In general, multiple sclerosis causes minimal or no increase in CSF protein; only rarely do levels exceed 100 mg./dl. Cerebral thrombosis, subdural hematoma, and aseptic and viral meningitis usually are associated with normal CSF protein.

The term "albuminocytologic dissociation" refers to increased CSF protein with normal or near normal CSF cell count. Classically this is described in acute idiopathic polyneuritis (Guillain-Barré syndrome), but it may also occur in subarachnoid block, brain tumor, multiple sclerosis, cerebral thrombosis, and various types of polyneuritis.

The term "Froin's syndrome" refers to CSF changes which may occur with subarachnoid block at or below the foramen magnum: markedly increased total protein (often over 500 mg./dl.), xanthochromia (owing to the increased protein), and spontaneous clotting. However, these changes may be absent in some patients with subarachnoid block and spinal cord compression.

Protein Electrophoresis. Most CSF protein originates by diffusion from plasma across the blood-CSF barrier. Proteins larger than 9S do not diffuse readily, unless there is injury to the blood-CSF barrier.

The electrophoretic pattern of CSF protein is somewhat influenced by serum protein levels. Markedly increased 7S serum gamma globulin may cause diffuse or monoclonal increase in CSF protein; in myeloma the paraprotein often can be demonstrated in CSF (Frantzen *et al.*, 1969).

Two methods are commonly used for CSF protein electrophoresis: cellulose acetate and agar gel. Although unconcentrated CSF can be used (Sherwin and Moore, 1971), most procedures require concentration of 10 to 15 ml. CSF by vacuum filtration through a collodion membrane (Kaplan, 1967) or an Amicon filter (Windisch and Bracken, 1970).

CSF electrophoresis has proved especially useful as an aid to diagnosis of multiple sclerosis: increased production of IgG in areas of demyelination apparently causes increased IgG in CSF. During the very early and very late stages of multiple sclerosis, CSF gamma globulin frequently is normal; therefore, multiple determinations may be required (Schwartz *et al.*, 1970). Depending upon the stage of disease, about 60 to 80 per cent of patients with multiple sclerosis will have increased CSF gamma globulin. Fischer-Williams (1971) has suggested that electrophoretic measurement of CSF gamma globulin may be more useful than immunologic determination of CSF IgG; the former measurement probably is more easily standardized than the latter (Rowe, 1971). Although each laboratory should establish its own normal range, CSF gamma globulin levels of 10 to 15 per cent have been considered moderately elevated and levels over 15 per cent markedly elevated (Garde and Kjellin, 1971).

Agarose gel electrophoresis of CSF offers some advantage over cellulose acetate, since the former can resolve discrete pathologic gamma bands which appear in perhaps 30 per cent of patients with multiple sclerosis despite normal CSF gamma globulin (Laterre *et al.*, 1970). However, increased CSF gamma globulin and/or discrete pathologic bands in the gamma region are NOT pathognomonic of multiple sclerosis. These findings may also occur with subacute sclerosing leukoencephalitis, advanced neurosyphilis, primary laterial sclerosis, viral encephalitis, fungal meningitis, monoclonal gammopathy, and myelopathy due to vitamin B_{12} deficiency (Ivers *et al.*, 1961).

Colloidal Gold Test. Lange's colloidal gold test, introduced in 1912, is an empirical method for evaluating CSF protein fractions, and occasionally may be useful if CSF electrophoresis is unavailable.

In the Lange method, progressive dilutions of CSF are added to 10 test tubes containing colloidal gold solution. Precipitation causes the brilliant red colloidal gold color (0) to change to reddish blue (1+), purple (2+), deep blue (3+), pale blue (4+), or colorless (5+). The highest CSF concentration is reported on the left, with progressively decreasing concentrations to the right. Normal fluids cause either no reaction or slight precipitation in the middle dilutions, e.g., 0001210000.

A "first zone curve" is found in about 50 per cent of patients with multiple sclerosis, as well as in general paresis. It may also be seen in encephalitis, postinfectious encephalomyelopathy, sarcoidosis, hemorrhage, aseptic meningeal reaction, polyneuritis, and meningeal carcinoma. A typical series would be 5554210000. A "mid zone curve" or "end zone curve" is nonspecific and may be found in any CSF with high protein concentration.

It is believed that albumin tends to maintain the colloidal gold suspension and that gamma globulins facilitate precipitation. However, it is difficult to relate CSF gamma globulin levels to colloidal gold curves on a quantitative basis. A "first zone curve" suggests the possibility of multiple sclerosis or subacute sclerosing leukoencephalitis; in such cases a new sample should be obtained and sent to a laboratory which can perform CSF electrophoresis (Green, 1969).

Glucose

Normally CSF glucose is about 60 to 80 per cent of blood levels, or 50–80 mg./dl. With very high blood glucose (800 mg./dl. and over), CSF glucose is about 30 to 40 per cent of blood levels. Following an increase or decrease in blood glucose, CSF glucose undergoes a corresponding change over one to three hours. This time lag probably is related to transport of glucose across the blood-CSF barrier. Because of this relationship between CSF and blood glucose, it is desirable to obtain a blood glucose measurement one to three hours prior to lumbar puncture (Greenwald *et al.*, 1973).

It is well known that CSF glucose is decreased with meningitis and other diseases of the central nervous system. Although several explanations have been advanced, the exact mechanism is not well understood. Several factors may be involved, including impaired transfer of glucose from blood to CSF, and increased glucose utilization by brain tissue (Menkes, 1969). In some cases, increased glucose utilization by leukocytes, bacteria, or neoplastic cells may contribute.

Usually a CSF glucose under 40 mg./dl. is considered decreased. Possible causes include: (1) systemic hypoglycemia; (2) bacterial, tuberculous, or fungal meningitis; (3) meningeal carcinomatosis or leukemic infiltration; (4) sarcoidosis involving the central nervous system (Gaines *et al.*, 1970); (5) subarachnoid hemorrhage (Walton, 1956); and (6) viral meningitis, including mumps meningoencephalitis (Wilfert, 1969).

According to Feinbloom and Alpert (1969), measurement of CSF glucose has little value in diagnosis of bacterial meningitis unless pleocytosis is present: (1) low CSF glucose is nonspecific; and (2) low CSF glucose occurs in only about 50 per cent of patients with bacterial meningitis (including tuberculosis).

Enzymes

Many different enzymes have been measured in CSF, including lactate dehydrogenase (LDH), aspartate transferase (AT) or SGOT, and creatine phosphokinase (CPK).

Increased CSF LDH has been reported with both bacterial and viral meningitis (Beatty and Oppenheimer, 1968); the slow migrating isozymes LDH 4-5 typically appear in the former, and fast migrating LDH 1-2 in the latter. With bacterial meningitis, increased LDH 4-5 probably reflects participation of granulocytes in the inflammatory process. With viral meningitis, the source of LDH 1-2 is not clear; these isozymes may be derived either from plasma, erythrocytes, or brain tissue. Patients who die with bacterial meningitis have high levels of LDH 1-2, probably caused by brain damage. Increased CSF LDH also occurs with subarachnoid hemorrhage as well as primary or secondary malignancy involving the brain or spinal cord.

High levels of CSF AT have been reported with primary or secondary malignancy involving the brain or spinal cord (Davies-Jones, 1969), bacterial meningitis, intracerebral hemorrhage, and subarachnoid hemorrhage (Belsey, 1969). In bacterial meningitis, an elevated CSF AT tends to be associated with complications, while a normal CSF AT is usually found in uncomplicated cases. However, the prognostic value of CSF AT assays appears no greater than cell counts or glucose measurements.

Reports on CSF CPK have been contradictory, possibly due to the variety of methods now in use. Increased CSF CPK activity has been described in many conditions, including brain infarct, multiple sclerosis, brain tumors, demyelinating disease, and polyneuropathies (Sherwin *et al.*, 1969).

Despite considerable research, it appears that CSF enzyme measurements are relatively nonspecific; increased CSF LDH, AT, and CPK activity may occur in a wide variety of conditions.

Acid-Base Balance

Until recently CSF was believed to act primarily as a "cushion" for the brain. During the 1950's experiments revealed that respiration is stimulated by increases of CSF P_{CO_2} or [H+] and depressed by decreases in CSF P_{CO_2} or [H+]. Further studies demonstrated that CO_2 diffuses rapidly across the blood-CSF barrier, so that P_{CO_2} of CSF closely follows arterial P_{CO_2}, but diffusion of bicarbonate is much slower. Since pH of CSF depends almost entirely on the ratio $\frac{HCO_3}{P_{CO_2}}$, a high CSF P_{CO_2} causes high CSF [H+], and a low CSF P_{CO_2}, a low CSF [H+]. Thus, in respiratory acidosis or alkalosis, CSF pH tends to follow arterial pH. Attempts to correct respiratory acidosis by intravenous bicarbonate will not increase CSF pH; rather, decreased ventilation may result, causing confusion, delirium, and coma when CSF pH falls below 7.25. Correction of respiratory acidosis or alkalosis should be via pulmonary ventilation, rather than intravenous bicarbonate (Bulger *et al.*, 1966).

A recent area of interest has been the effect of CSF pH on cerebral blood flow (CBF). Normally a fall in CSF pH causes cerebral vasodilatation and increased CBF, while a rise in CSF pH causes cerebral vasoconstriction and decreased CBF. However, in traumatic brain damage, cerebral vasodilatation may cause decreased blood flow within the damaged area as a result of vasodilatation in normally reacting neighboring zones (Gordon, 1971). In patients with brain lesions, focal intracerebral metabolic acidosis usually develops; this is believed to cause spontaneous hyperventilation. The hyperventilation may reduce blood flow to normal areas and increase blood flow to damaged areas. There is some evidence that treatment with controlled hyperventilation (arterial Pco_2 levels around 25 mm. Hg) may increase blood flow to damaged areas, leading to decreased mortality in patients with brain trauma (Gordon, 1971).

Serologic Tests

The VDRL test is recommended as a well-established serologic test for syphilis using CSF. Although the Reiter protein reagent (RPR) procedure is commonly used on serum, to date there is little information on its application to CSF. According to Escobar *et al.* (1970) the fluorescent treponema antibody (FTA) test can be applied to CSF and is more sensitive than the VDRL; additional studies are needed to confirm these findings.

Latex agglutination and complement fixation tests on both serum and CSF are useful in diagnosis of cryptococcal meningitis. With the former procedure, cross reactions with rheumatoid factor may occur (Bennett and Bailey, 1971) and can be detected by appropriate controls. Charcoal particle agglutination appears more sensitive than latex agglutination and can also be used on CSF (Gordon and Lapa, 1971).

Other serologic tests have been applied to CSF on an experimental basis, including: measurement of CSF complement (decreased in patients with disseminated lupus erythematosus involving the central nervous system); measles antibody titers (suggestive evidence that measles virus is the etiologic agent in subacute sclerosing encephalitis); and identification of meningococcal antigen by counter-immunoelectrophoresis.

Miscellaneous Chemical Measurements

Alcohol. Increased CSF ethanol (measured by gas chromatography) has been used to aid in diagnosis of cryptococcal meningitis (O'Reilly and Kwa, 1967).

Biogenic Amines. A reduction in 5-hydroxyindoleacetic acid (5-HIAA) has been reported in CSF of patients with depression or Parkinson's disease (Moir *et al.*, 1970). The concentration of 5-HIAA is highest in ventricular fluid and lowest in lumbar fluid; to date, results of different studies are inconsistent.

Calcium. Concentration of CSF calcium is about 50 per cent of serum calcium and tends to reflect ionized serum calcium levels.

Chloride. Measurement of CSF chloride has been largely abandoned for clinical use.

Desmosterol. Following oral triparanol therapy, patients with brain tumors tend to have increased CSF desmosterol (Fumagalli and Paoletti, 1971). At present, this is a research technique and additional evaluation is needed.

Glutamine. Slight elevations of CSF glutamine have been described in patients with chronic hypercapnea (Jaiken and Agrest, 1969) and in those with chronic liver disease without encephalopathy (levels in the range of 22 ± 6 mg./dl.). Moderate elevations of CSF glutamine have been described in acute liver disease (Hourani *et al.*, 1971). With development of hepatic encephalopathy and progression to hepatic coma, there is a marked increase to CSF glutamine, with levels in the range of 40 ± 14 mg./dl. This appears to be a clinically useful measurement which can be performed in the average laboratory.

Lactic Acid. Increased CSF lactate may be caused by increased glycolysis or decreased oxidative respiration and is characteristic of hypoxia or tissue damage. High values may be found in many conditions, including meningitis, multiple sclerosis, brain infarct, cerebral arteriosclerosis, intracranial hemorrhage, and metastatic carcinoma. Measurement of CSF lactate may be a useful "screening test" to detect CNS disease when other laboratory findings are within normal limits (Pryce et al., 1970).

Uric Acid. Increased CSF uric acid has been reported in patients with progressive cerebral atrophy and no other abnormal CSF findings (Farstad *et al.*, 1965). However, the clinical usefulness of this measurement is not well established.

SYNOVIAL FLUID

Synovial membranes are lined by columnar cells distinguished as "A cells," "B cells," and "intermediate cells" by electron microscopy. The "A cells" may have a resorptive function; the "B cells" appear to have secretory activity (Souteyrand-Boulenger and Amouroux, 1972). These cells have no basement membrane, but are embedded in a mucopolysaccharide matrix containing hyaluronic acid. Synovial fluid (SF) is produced by: (1) dialysis of plasma across the synovial membrane, and (2) active secretion. Composition of normal synovial fluid resembles plasma ultrafiltrate, with added hyaluronic acid. However, changes in blood solute concentration require four to eight hours to affect SF levels because of slow equilibration.

Normally about 1 ml. of SF is present in each large joint: knee, ankle, hip, elbow, wrist, and shoulder. Clinical indications for aspiration include: (1) arthritis of unknown etiology, manifested by effusion; (2) possible infectious arthritis, with or without apparent effusion, to obtain material for culture; and (3) effusions of known etiology, to relieve pain, or to allow increased mobility.

During aspiration careful aseptic technique is essential, and the needle must not be passed through areas of superficial or deep sepsis. The procedure is described in textbooks of orthopedic surgery.

Since effusion often exists when aspiration is indicated, 10 to 20 ml. of fluid may usually be obtained. The specimen is collected in three or four tubes:

1. A plain tube for gross examination, evaluation of viscosity, and mucin clot test.
2. A versene (EDTA) tube for cell counts and microscopic study.
3. A sterile, plain or preferably heparinized tube (precludes clot formation) for microbiologic study.
4. Appropriate tube(s) for serologic or chemical examinations: plain tube for serologic tests or enzyme assays; heparinized tube for total protein; heparin fluoride tube for glucose.

Gross Examination, Viscosity, and Mucin Clot Test

Normal SF is crystal clear and pale yellow to colorless; newsprint may be read through the specimen in a plain tube. Clear yellow fluid is found in normal individuals as well as in traumatic arthritis, osteoarthritis, and mild rheumatoid arthritis. Turbid yellow fluid may occur with increased numbers of leukocytes, due to septic or nonseptic inflammation. Grossly milky or pseudochylous fluid may occur in chronic effusions due to rheumatoid arthritis, acute effusions due to gout, or effusions due to lymphatic obstruction (Das and Sen, 1968). Purulent fluid may occur with septic arthritis but is not present during the early stages of infection. Grossly bloody fluid occurs with hemorrhagic effusions due to trauma, hemophilia, or hemorrhagic villonodular synovitis.

If blood is noted, it is important to determine whether this is due to a traumatic tap or to previous hemorrhage. Traumatic taps typically show: blood in the initial aspirate decreasing with continued aspiration; uneven distribution or streaking of blood in the syringe; and clotting about blood streaks within 15 minutes after aspiration.

Xanthochromia in the supernatant is difficult to evaluate because a yellow color may be observed in normal as well as pathologic synovial fluid. However, a deep yellow or brown color in the supernatant may suggest previous hemorrhage.

Fluid in a plain tube should be examined after one hour for a fibrin clot; any clotting is graded as 1 to 4+ and reflects damage to the synovial membrane (usually inflammatory) which allows fibrinogen to enter the joint space.

When normal synovial fluid drips from a syringe, a tenacious "string" at least 4 cm. long forms with each drop. This provides an estimate of whether viscosity is normal, decreased (string less than 4 cm. in length), or markedly decreased (string less than 1 cm. in length). Another method for evaluating viscosity is to see how far a drop of fluid can be stretched between the thumb and index finger before breaking; fluids with very low viscosity will behave like water. Decreased viscosity reflects decreased hyaluronate in the synovial fluid.

The "mucin clot test" or Ropes' test is performed by adding 1 ml. of SF to 20 ml. of 5 per cent (v./v.) acetic acid in a small beaker. Normally a compact large clot will form, surrounded by clear solution; this is graded as "good." If a soft clot forms in turbid solution, this is graded as "fair." A friable clot with cloudy surrounding fluid is graded as "poor." No clot formation, with flakes in a cloudy suspension, is graded as "very poor." "Good" clots do not break up when agitated, while "poor" clots break up into small shreds. This procedure actually is an estimate of SF hyaluronate and not mucin, which is absent in joint fluid.

Decreased viscosity or a "poor" mucin clot test suggests alteration, destruction, or decreased production of hyaluronate due to septic or nonseptic inflammation.

Microscopic Examination

Normal synovial fluid contains fewer than 200 leukocytes per cu.mm. (Schmid and Ogata, 1965). On differential count, most of these cells are lymphocytes and monocytes, with fewer than 25 per cent neutrophils (Ropes and Bauer, 1953). The leukocyte count may be performed in a Fuchs-Rosenthal chamber using a small amount of methylene blue in saline as diluent if the fluid is clear and contains normal numbers of cells. If the fluid is grossly bloody, either 0.1 N HCl (Blau, 1971) or 1 per cent saponin in saline (Donaldson, 1972) will lyse the erythrocytes. The usual diluent for leukocyte count (1 per cent glacial acetic acid) precipitates SF hyaluronate and is unsatisfactory. If the fluid is so turbid that leukocytes are difficult to see in the counting chamber, either saline dilution or digestion with hyaluronidase (2 ml. SF incubated with 150 IU hyaluronidase for 1 hr. at 37° C.) may be helpful.

A differential count is performed on thin films stained with Wright's stain. These films may be prepared from fresh fluid at the time of aspiration, or from centrifuged sediment in the versene (EDTA) tube. The latter gives a more concentrated preparation and is easier to examine.

LE cells are frequently found in stained SF from patients with systemic lupus erythematosus; LE cells are also seen in SF from a few patients with rheumatoid arthritis (Hunder and Pierre, 1970). *In vivo* formation of LE cells in synovial fluid probably results from trauma to leukocytes. Occasionally LE cells are present in synovial fluid when the "LE clot test" is negative on peripheral blood.

Large phagocytic cells containing ingested neutrophils may be found in synovial fluid. These are sometimes called "Reiter cells" since these were first described in SF from patients with Reiter's syndrome; however, they are nonspecific and may be present in effusions of varying etiology (Cracchiolo, 1971).

A fresh wet preparation of uncentrifuged SF should be examined promptly after aspiration. A drop of SF is applied to a clean glass slide, overlaid immediately with a clean coverslip, and sealed at once with clear fingernail polish.

"RA cells" or "ragocytes" are neutrophils containing 0.5 to 1.5 μ inclusions which are easily seen with phase microscopy or Sternheimer-Malbin stain. Although present in about 95 per cent of rheumatoid joint fluids, these are NOT specific and may be found in septic arthritis, gout, and other conditions associated with increased granulocytes in SF (Sones *et al.*, 1968).

Both the fresh wet preparation and stained film should be studied for crystals, using polarized light to detect monosodium urate (MSU) or calcium pyrophosphate dihydrate (CPPD) (Good and Frishette, 1966). Examination with polarized light may be performed using an ordinary microscope: one polaroid disc is placed below the stage (in the substage condenser or over the light source) and a second disc is placed above the eyepiece. When the second disc is rotated to darken the field, monosodium urate crystals will appear birefringent and needle-like or rod shaped; calcium pyrophosphate dihydrate crystals will appear birefringent and rhomboid or rod shaped (Fig. 25–2).

Monosodium urate (MSU) crystals can be found in almost 100 per cent of fluids from acute gouty joints, in which case they are located chiefly within phagocytes. In chronic gouty arthritis, MSU crystals are found less frequently (about 75 per cent) and are mostly extracellular. Calcium pyrophosphate dihydrate (CPPD) crystals are characteristic of a disease known variously as "pseudogout," "chondrocalcinosis," and "CPPD deposition disease" (McCarty, 1970). Clinical symptoms may mimic gout, rheumatoid arthritis, or osteoarthritis; diagnosis requires demonstration of CPPD crystals in synovial fluid.

In difficult cases, use of a polarizing microscope or digestion with uricase may aid identification. MSU crystals show strong negative birefringence, and CPPD crystals weak positive birefringence.

Examination of SF for crystals presents several pitfalls: (1) oxalate used as anticoagulant may combine with SF calcium to form calcium oxalate monohydrate crystals; (2) corticosteroid esters with negative birefringence and microscopic appearance identical to urate crystals may remain in SF longer than a month following intra-articular injection (Kahn *et al.*, 1970); (3) contamination with birefringent talcum powder may prevent examination under polarized light; (4) fragments of cartilage occasionally appear in SF; and (5) cholesterol crystals may appear in SF of chronic inflammatory effusion, but form "plates" which are seldom confused with MSU or CPPD crystals.

Microbiologic Examination

Cultures for suspected bacterial, mycobacterial, or fungal infections are an essential part of SF analysis. Septic arthritis often is difficult to diagnose, since Gram stain and culture are often negative. Gram stain of SF is negative in about 50 per cent of patients with gonococcal arthritis, and culture is negative in about 75 per cent. Immediate inoculation of the sample onto chocolate agar at the bedside and use of special media for propagation of gonococcal L-forms may increase the incidence of positive cultures (Holmes *et al.*, 1971).

Chemical Examination

Normal total protein in SF averages about 2 gm. per 100 ml., with a range of 1 to 3 gm. per 100 ml. Fibrinogen normally is absent. With inflammatory joint disease (e.g., septic or rheumatoid arthritis) SF protein composition approaches that of plasma: total protein 4 to 7 gm. per 100 ml., fibrinogen present, and electrophoretic pattern similar to plasma. In most cases measurement of SF total protein gives

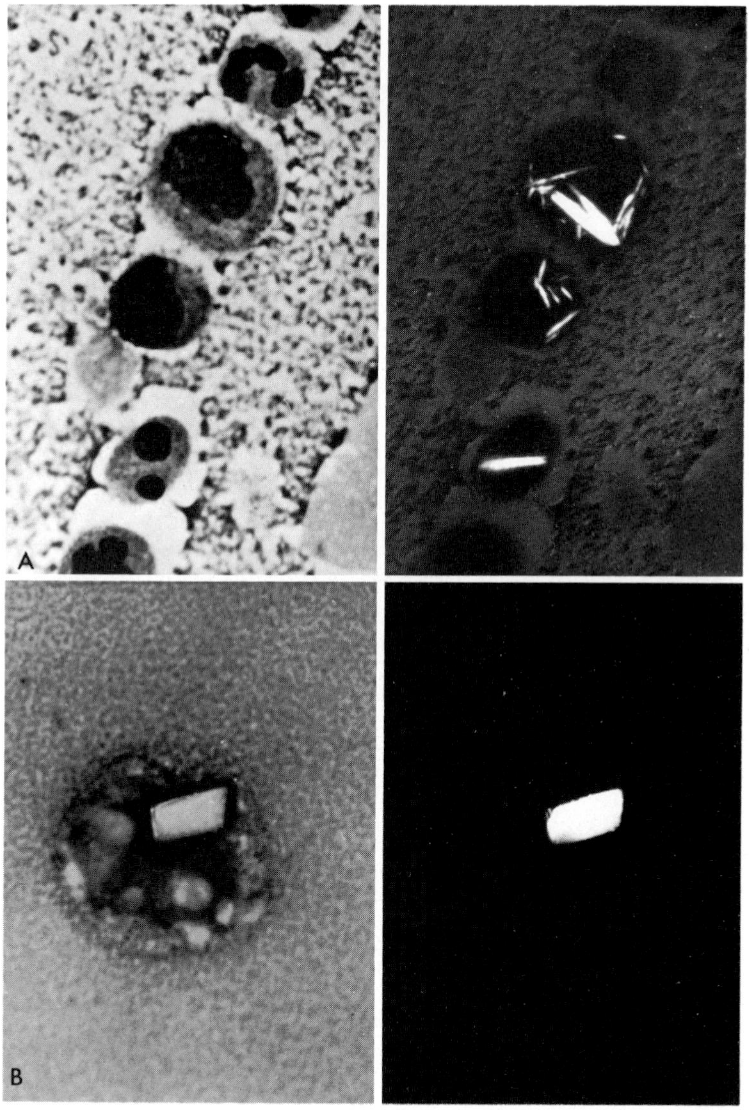

Figure 25–2. *A*, Leukocytes with uric acid crystals under normal and polarized light. *B*, Leukocyte with calcium pyrophosphate crystal under normal and polarized light. (From Good and Frishette: Crystals in dried smears of synovial fluid. J.A.M.A., *198*:80, 1966.)

information similar to the gross examination, cell count, and differential.

The difference between SF glucose and blood glucose can be useful in evaluating chronic arthritis. Normally SF glucose is about 10 mg. per 100 ml. less than blood glucose. Since equilibration between blood and synovial fluid glucose is slow, samples for SF glucose should be obtained when the patient has been fasting for eight to 12 hours and results compared with a blood glucose taken at the same time.

In noninflammatory arthritis the blood-SF glucose difference is about 10 to 20 mg. per 100 ml. With nonseptic inflammatory disease, especially rheumatoid arthritis, the difference may exceed 25 mg. per 100 ml. Although an absolute SF glucose concentration under 30 mg. per 100 ml. suggests infection (including tuberculosis), this may also be found in rheumatoid arthritis of many months' duration.

Measurements of SF enzyme activity have been studied extensively, but clinical value is not yet well established. Increased SF acid phosphatase has been reported in rheumatoid arthritis; activity apparently is normal in bacterial arthritis, osteoarthritis, and noninflammatory effusions (Beckman *et al.*, 1971). If this work is confirmed, SF acid phosphatase may be useful in distinguishing septic arthritis from atypical rheumatoid disease.

Increased SF LDH activity may occur with rheumatoid arthritis, septic arthritis, Reiter's syndrome, or gout; normal SF LDH activity is found in most patients with degenerative joint disease.

Immunologic Studies

Rheumatoid factor has been reported in SF as well as in serum of patients with rheumatoid arthritis. Some patients with sero-negative rheumatoid arthritis have a positive joint fluid; however, rheumatoid factor may also occur in SF of patients who do not have rheumatoid arthritis. Additional data are needed to establish the clinical value of this examination.

Decreased SF complement (under 30 per cent of serum level) occurs in rheumatoid arthritis and systemic lupus erythematosus. In early rheumatoid arthritis, SF complement usually is normal; with lupus, SF complement is low in almost all patients from the onset (Pekin and Zvaifler, 1970). The clinical value of this measurement is not yet well established.

Clinical Correlation

On the basis of gross appearance, viscosity, mucin clot test, cell count, microscopic study, and glucose, most fluids can be classified as noninflammatory, inflammatory, septic, or hemorrhagic (Table 25–4). Conditions associated with "Group I" changes include traumatic arthritis, osteoarthritis, neurogenic joint disease, and some cases of rheumatic fever and systemic lupus erythematosus. Conditions associated with "Group II" changes include rheumatoid arthritis, acute gouty arthritis, acute "pseudogout," Reiter's syndrome, and some cases of rheumatic fever and systemic lupus erythematosus. "Group III" SF is distinguished from "Group II" primarily on the basis of Gram stain and culture; if these are negative, diagnosis of septic arthritis may be difficult. Conditions associated with "Group IV" changes include pigmented villonodular synovitis, hemophilia, neoplasms, and some cases of neurogenic joint disease and traumatic arthritis.

Typical findings in various diseases are outlined in Table 25–5. In difficult cases, diagnosis is based on a combination of synovial fluid study, radiologic findings, and clinical course. However, some patients have monoarticular effusion with nonspecific findings in

Table 25–4. CLASSIFICATION OF ABNORMAL SYNOVIAL FLUIDS

	NORMAL	GROUP I (NONINFLAMMATORY)	GROUP II (INFLAMMATORY)	GROUP III (SEPTIC)	GROUP IV (HEMORRHAGIC)
Appearance	Clear	Clear	Turbid	Turbid	Bloody
Fibrin clot	Absent	Usually absent	May occur	May occur	Usually absent
Viscosity	High	High	Low	Low	Variable
Mucin clot	Good	Good	Fair to poor	Fair to poor	Variable
Leukocyte count (cells/cu.mm.)	< 200	200–5000	2000–100,000	20,000–200,000	200–10,000
Neutrophils (%)	< 25	< 25	> 50	> 75	> 50
Blood-SF glucose difference (mg./dl.)	< 10	< 10	>25	>25	>25
Culture	Negative	Negative	Negative	Positive*	Negative

*But may be negative.

Table 25–5. ALTERATIONS OF SYNOVIAL FLUID IN DISEASE*

	APPEARANCE	FIBRIN CLOT	LEUKOCYTES (PER CU. MM.)	NEUTROPHILS (PER CENT)	GLUCOSE† DIFFERENCE (MG./100 ML.)	MUCIN CLOT TEST	COMMENT
Normal	Clear	0	10-2000 (av. 60)	0-25 (av. 10)	0-10	Good	
Degenerative joint disease	Clear	0-2+	70-4000 (av. 700)	0-60 (av. 10)	0-10	Fair to good (usually good)	Fragments of cartilage rarely seen microscopically
Traumatic arthritis	Clear	0-1+	100-9000 (av. 1200)	0-35 (av. 10)	0-20 (av. 10)	Fair to good (usually good)	Fat droplets occasionally present
Traumatic arthritis with hemorrhage	Red	0-2+	100-9000	0-80	10-40 (av. 20)	Fair to good	30,000-6,000,000 RBC/cu. mm.
Rheumatic fever	Slightly turbid	0-3+	300-98,000 (av. 18,000)	0-98 (av. 50)	0-20 (av. 10)	Fair to good (usually good)	
Rheumatoid arthritis	Clear to turbid	0-4+	400-70,000 (av. 14,000)	0-98 (av. 70)	0-90 (av. 30)	Very poor to good (usually poor)	SF relatively normal in early stages; rarely find pseudochylous SF with birefringent cholesterol crystals in advanced disease
Gouty arthritis	Turbid	0-4+	1000-70,000 (av. 13,000)	0-98 (av. 70)	0-80 (av. 20)	Very poor to good (usually poor)	Uric acid crystals usually present
Tuberculous arthritis	Turbid	0-3+	2000-100,000 (av. 20,000)	20-96 (av. 60)	0-110 (av. 60)	Very poor to good (usually poor)	Organisms difficult to find on smear or culture; biopsy may be necessary
Bacterial arthritis	Turbid	0-4+	1000-300,000 (av. 70,000)	5-100 (av. 80)	10-120 (av. 60)	Very poor to good (usually poor)	SF may be relatively normal early in disease
Lupus erythematosus	Clear to turbid	0-2+	100-20,000 (av. 3000)	0-30 (av. 10)	10-20	Good	LE cells may be present
Pigmented villonodular synovitis	Turbid to dark red	0-3+	400-10,000	0-60	0-50	Very poor to good (usually poor)	30,000-3,000,000 RBC/cu. mm. with reddish supernatant

*Adapted from Ropes: Examination of synovial fluid. Bull. Rheum. Dis., 7(Suppl. 5): 1957.
†Difference between glucose concentration in blood (patient fasting for 12 hours prior to joint aspiration) and synovial fluid.

Type II fluid. If the condition worsens despite conservative treatment, culture for *Neisseria gonorrheae* on special media, repeated culture for *M. tuberculosis*, or even biopsy may be indicated.

PLEURAL FLUID

The pleural surfaces normally are moistened by 1 to 10 ml. of fluid derived by ultrafiltration of plasma. Normal protein concentration of this fluid is 1 to 2 gm./dl., with fibrinogen absent.

Formation of pleural fluid is influenced by: capillary wall permeability, plasma colloid osmotic pressure, and hydrostatic pressure. Plasma colloid osmotic pressure is proportional to molal concentration of protein; thus, for a given amount of protein in gm./dl., albumin exerts greater osmotic pressure than globulins. Hydrostatic pressure is related to venous pressure in the superior vena cava, innominate veins, pulmonary veins, and bronchial veins, which drain the parietal and visceral pleura.

Resorption of pleural fluid protein, as well as particulate matter and cells, is via lymphatics. The costal pleura drains anteriorly into the internal mammary system, and posteriorly into intercostal lymph nodes, while diaphragmatic and visceral pleura drain into mediastinal lymph nodes. Smaller molecules (water, electrolytes) are resorbed by capillaries as well as lymphatics, while protein is resorbed through lymphatics only (Black, 1972).

Abnormal accumulation of pleural fluid, or pleural effusion, may be caused by:

1. Increased capillary permeability due to inflammation; this typically is associated with increased pleural fluid protein (over 3 gm./dl.).
2. Decreased plasma colloid osmotic pressure due to hypoproteinemia; this typically is associated with pleural fluid protein, about 1 gm./dl.
3. Increased hydrostatic pressure due to increased systemic and/or pulmonary venous pressure, as in congestive heart failure. Concentration of pleural fluid protein is variable and depends on whether lymphatic drainage is impeded by systemic venous hypertension.
4. Decreased lymphatic drainage due to tumor, inflammation, or fibrosis involving mediastinal lymph nodes (also systemic venous hypertension; cf. above). This typically is associated with increased pleural fluid protein (over 3 gm./dl.).

Indications for thoracentesis include: (1) effusion of unknown etiology; (2) effusion of known etiology causing clinical symptoms, e.g., dyspnea; (3) intrapleural instillation of drugs for treatment of infection or malignancy; and (4) hemothorax or empyema (to prevent organization).

Complications of thoracentesis may include: (1) hemopneumothorax due to laceration of the lung by the aspirating needle; and (2) mediastinal shift or pulmonary edema, if large amounts of fluid are removed at one time (Trapnell and Thurston, 1970). To avoid potential complications, it may be desirable to: (1) use an intravenous catheter for aspiration, withdrawing the needle-stylet after the pleural cavity is entered (Van Heerden and Laufenberg, 1968); and (2) aspirate no more than 1 liter of fluid at one time.

Pleural fluid should be collected in three sterile anticoagulated tubes (EDTA or heparin) labeled sequentially. The first tube is used for culture and Gram's stain; remaining tubes are used for cell count, Wright's stain, total protein, glucose, cytology, and other studies as indicated. If malignancy or tuberculosis is suspected, it is desirable to submit several hundred milliliters of anticoagulated fluid for examination.

Gross Examination

It is important to distinguish hemorrhagic fluids from blood-tinged fluid due to traumatic tap. In traumatic tap the blood typically is nonuniform in distribution and tends to clear with continued aspiration. Xanthochromia is less helpful because pleural fluid is often yellow.

About 60 per cent of grossly hemorrhagic fluids are due to intrapleural malignancy. Other causes include pancreatitis, pulmonary infarction, pleural infection, closed chest trauma, tuberculosis, and the postmyocardial infarction syndrome (Dressler's syndrome). This last characteristically presents with hemorrhagic pericardial and pleural effusions several days to several months after myocardial infarction; etiology is not established. Occasionally transudates due to congestive heart failure or hepatic cirrhosis may appear hemorrhagic; the cause of this is unknown.

Hemothorax may be distinguished from hemorrhagic effusion by simultaneous hematocrit determinations on capillary blood and pleural fluid; with hemothorax, hematocrit of the thoracentesis fluid is similar to capillary blood.

Cloudy, turbid fluid is usually due to large numbers of leukocytes associated with septic or nonseptic inflammation.

Chronic effusions occasionally contain cellular debris and cholesterol crystals, producing a milky appearance. This type of effusion, referred to as pseudochylous, may occur with tuberculosis, rheumatoid arthritis, and other inflammatory diseases. In some cases, a "gold paint" appearance due to numerous cholesterol crystals is described.

True chylothorax, due to leakage of thoracic duct contents, is rare and is characterized by creamy fluid with the consistency of milk, which clears and decreases in volume with alkalinization and ether extraction (Table 25–6). On oral or gastric tube administration of one-quarter pound margarine and 1 gm. of lipophilic dye (D and G green No. 6, National Aniline Division, Allied Chemical Corp., 40 Rector Street, New York, N.Y.), dye will appear in true chylous fluid after 12 to 24 hours but will not appear in pseudochylous effusions (Klepser and Berry, 1954). Lymphangiography may also provide useful information. Causes for true chylothorax include trauma, lymphoma, carcinoma, benign tumors, and congenital malformations (Roy *et al.*, 1967).

The fluid should be observed for clotting, either in a plain tube or by addition of calcium chloride to an EDTA tube. Presence of fibrino-

Table 25–6. CHYLOUS AND PSEUDOCHYLOUS EFFUSIONS

	TRUE CHYLOUS EFFUSION	PSEUDOCHYLOUS EFFUSION
Appearance	Consistency and color of whole milk; may form creamy top layer on standing	Appearance varies—like milk or "gold paint" or greenish
Odor	Odorless	May be odorless or foul
pH	Alkaline	Variable
Extraction with ether after alkalinization	Clearing and decrease in volume	Does not clear completely
Microscopic examination	Lymphocytes plus fine fat droplets	Mixed cellular reaction with cholesterol crystals and fat droplets
Microbiologic examination	Sterile	Usually sterile
Etiology	Traumatic damage or neoplastic obstruction involving thoracic duct (occasionally due to tuberculous obstruction)	Chronic effusion of any cause, e.g., rheumatoid disease, tuberculosis, myxedema
Oral ingestion of lipophilic dye	Dye appears in effusion	Dye does not appear in effusion

gen suggests damage to capillary walls caused by inflammation or neoplasm.

Microscopic Examination

Leukocyte and erythrocyte counts should be performed promptly after the fluid is collected. About 10,000 erythrocytes per cu.mm. will give a pink or light red color, and over 100,000 per cu.mm. produces a grossly bloody appearance. Wright's stained films should be prepared, either from buffy coat of centrifuged sediment (if fluid is grossly bloody), from the sediment itself (if fluid is clear), or from unspun fluid (if fluid appears cloudy).

A leukocyte count over 1000 per cu.mm., or over 50 per cent neutrophils, suggests inflammation (septic or nonseptic). However, about 5 to 10 per cent of effusions due to congestive heart failure and liver disease have high leukocyte counts or numerous neutrophils with no clinical evidence of inflammatory disease.

A high percentage of lymphocytes (over 50 per cent) suggests tuberculosis, lymphoma, or carcinoma. Occasionally patients with cardiopulmonary disease, cirrhosis, systemic lupus erythematosus, infectious mononucleosis, or subacute bacterial pulmonary infection may exhibit lymphocytic effusions.

"RA cells" may be seen in rheumatoid pleural effusion but are nonspecific (Boddington *et al.*, 1971). Other findings in rheumatoid effusion include degenerating neutrophils, amorphous extracellular material, and multinucleate epithelioid cells; additional experience is needed to determine whether this combination is specific for rheumatoid pleuritis.

Eosinophilic pleural effusions are uncommon. They have been reported with convalescent pneumonia, pneumothorax, pulmonary infarction, hypersensitivity diseases (asthma, Loeffler's syndrome, periarteritis), parasitic diseases, and lymphoma (Campbell and Webb, 1964).

With granulocytic leukemia, mature neutrophils and/or immature granulocytes may be found in effusion fluid. Extramedullary hematopoiesis (due to myeloid megakaryocytic hepatosplenomegaly or other hematologic diseases) may produce young normoblasts, immature neutrophils, and megakaryocytes in pleural effusions.

Lupus erythematosus cells in pleural fluid

are uncommon but considered specific for lupus erythematosus when found (Carr *et al.*, 1970).

Chemical Examination

Pleural effusions commonly are classified as "transudates" or "exudates." Fluids with a total protein under 3 gm. per dl. are considered transudates; fluids with total protein over 3 gm. per dl. are considered exudates. Pleural transudates may result from systemic and pulmonary venous hypertension, decreased plasma colloid osmotic pressure due to hypoproteinemia, excessive negative intrapleural pressure, or transport of transudative ascitic fluid across the diaphragm into the pleural space. The protein concentration of pleural fluid in these situations may be greater than anticipated if the lymphatic system is impaired, or if complicating factors (e.g., vascular stasis) cause capillary damage and increased permeability.

Pleural exudates result from diseases which either increase pleural capillary permeability or interfere with lymphatic drainage of the pleural spaces.

Normally pleural fluid glucose is about equal to whole blood glucose. Changes in blood glucose are reflected in pleural fluid after a lag period of one to three hours. A pleural fluid glucose concentration 30 to 40 mg. per 100 ml. less than whole blood suggests bacterial infection (including tuberculosis), nonseptic inflammation (especially rheumatoid pleuritis), or malignancy. In contrast to rheumatoid disease, effusions due to systemic lupus erythematosus typically have normal glucose concentrations. In the early stages of bacterial infection, pleural fluid glucose is often normal; this measurement is most useful in evaluating chronic effusions. Etiology of low pleural fluid glucose in these conditions may be related to impaired transport of glucose, increased utilization, or both.

In effusions due to malignancy or inflammation (septic or nonseptic), pleural fluid lactate dehydrogenase (LDH) activity is usually higher than that of serum. Also, if there is hemolysis, LDH activity will be high due to release of enzyme from erythrocytes. Thus, measurement of pleural fluid LDH is nonspecific and provides little more information than cell count, total protein, and glucose.

Pleural effusion has been reported in about 6 per cent of patients with acute pancreatitis. These effusions may appear either clear or bloody and are characterized by protein greater than 3 gm./dl. plus a pleural fluid amylase activity considerably higher than that of serum amylase. Increased pleural fluid amylase may occur in other conditions, including effusions due to metastatic adenocarcinoma.

Measurements of pleural fluid pH, Pco_2, and Po_2 have been suggested as an aid in differential diagnosis (Funahushi *et al.*, 1971); a pH under 7.31 may occur with non-neoplastic inflammatory pleural effusion (empyema, rheumatoid disease, tuberculosis); a low Po_2 may occur with empyema or tuberculous effusion. Additional studies are needed to establish the value of these measurements.

Microbiologic Examination

If infection is suspected, transudates as well as exudates should be examined for bacteria by Gram stain and culture. In the early stages of bacterial infection, cultures usually are positive; later, the fluid may appear grossly purulent with positive Gram stain, but cultures may be negative because of antibiotic therapy. The incidence of positive cultures in tuberculous effusions ranges from 20 to 70 per cent; special techniques which utilize sediment from 100 to 500 ml. of centrifuged fluid may be useful. Acid-fast organisms are seldom found on smear. The possibility of tuberculosis should always be considered with idiopathic pleural effusions. If an etiology is not established, closed pleural biopsy, or even open thoracotomy, may be indicated.

Clinical Correlation

Pleural infections usually produce an exudative effusion, on the basis of increased capillary permeability. Resorption of protein by lymphatics may also be impaired as a result of pleural fibrin deposition.

Metastatic carcinoma typically causes an exudative fluid; in the majority of cases this appears due to mediastinal lymph node involvement rather than pleural metastases. About 25 to 30 per cent of such fluids are hemorrhagic.

Malignant lymphoma may cause either an exudate or transudate, depending on whether lymphatic obstruction or hypoproteinemia is the major pathologic process.

Rheumatoid arthritis almost invariably causes effusion with high protein content as a result of increased capillary permeability.

Systemic lupus erythematosus usually results in exudative fluid (increased capillary permeability), but may also cause a transudate due to congestive heart failure, nephrotic syndrome, or hepatic damage.

Congestive heart failure is a common cause of pleural effusion, typically a transudate. However, the pleural fluid may have a high protein concentration if lymphatic drainage is impeded by venous hypertension.

Chronic liver disease may cause pleural effusion by several mechanisms; the most important of these probably is transfer of fluid from the peritoneal cavity via either direct diaphragmatic defect or diaphragmatic lymphatics (Black, 1972). The latter mechanism is probably responsible for sterile pleural effusions associated with subphrenic abscess.

Pulmonary infarction is usually associated with some degree of pleuritis, and increased capillary permeability leads to exudative pleural effusion in about 50 per cent of cases. Bloody pleural fluid is found in only about 10 per cent of patients with pulmonary infarct.

Mediastinal radiation may cause pulmonary effusion with high protein content, presumably on the basis of radiation injury to lymphatics.

PERICARDIAL FLUID

Normally the pericardial sac contains 20 to 50 ml. of clear, straw-colored transudate, continually formed as a plasma ultrafiltrate, and continually resorbed by lymphatics near the base of the heart. Increased amounts of fluid produce symptoms which depend upon the rate as well as the volume of fluid accumulation. A rapid accumulation of 200 ml. may produce cardiac tamponade, while gradual accumulation of 1000 ml. or more may be relatively asymptomatic. According to well-known authorities (Hurst and Logue, 1970), indications for pericardial aspiration include: (1) acute or chronic cardiac tamponade, and (2) to confirm diagnosis and establish cause for pericardial effusion of unknown etiology.

In patients with acute tamponade, immediate aspiration is indicated; use of a sterile intracatheter unit may be safer than needle aspiration. As an elective procedure, open pericardial biopsy may be safer and more effective than blind aspiration (Kilpatrick and Chapman, 1965). Dangers of blind aspiration include: (1) cardiac arrhythmias, especially ventricular fibrillation; (2) infection of pleural spaces by purulent pericardial fluid; (3) laceration of an atrium or coronary artery; (4) pneumothorax; and (5) inadvertent injection of air into the cardiac chamber.

In many hospitals, aspiration of pericardial fluid is performed by a thoracic surgeon, with EKG, arterial pressure, and venous pressure being monitored constantly during the procedure.

At least three tubes should be obtained: EDTA tube for gross and microscopic examination, sterile plain or heparinized tube for microbiologic examination, and heparinized tube for chemical examination.

Gross Examination

Gross appearance of pericardial fluid may be normal (clear pale yellow), cloudy, blood-tinged, grossly bloody, milky (chylous or "pseudochylous"), or similar to "gold paint" (Dempsey *et al.*, 1966). Increased amounts of normal-appearing fluid may be found in congestive heart failure, early stages of inflammation, and some patients with idiopathic (?viral) pericarditis.

A cloudy appearance may be associated with septic or nonseptic inflammation (bacterial, rheumatoid, or rheumatic), as well as chronic effusions of any etiology (myxedema, postmyocardial infarction syndrome, or idiopathic). Blood-tinged pericardial fluid due to traumatic tap usually shows streaking in the syringe, and clears with continued aspiration. Grossly bloody fluid may be caused by idiopathic hemorrhagic pericarditis (?viral), postmyocardial infarction syndrome, postpericardiectomy syndrome, tuberculosis, rheumatoid arthritis, systemic lupus erythematosus, metastatic carcinoma, bacterial pericarditis, or leaking aortic aneurysm. The latter may suddenly develop into hemopericardium, with acute cardiac tamponade. Hemopericardium is characterized by a hematocrit similar to whole blood and may be simulated by inadvertent aspiration of blood from the cardiac cavity. "Milky" pericardial fluid is an unusual finding, which may be due to either true chylopericardium or chronic pericarditis from any cause (bacterial, tuberculous, fungal, rheumatoid, rheumatic, myxedema, and so forth).

Microscopic Examination

Leukocyte count and differential on Wright's stained sediment are performed routinely, using the same procedure as for cerebrospinal fluid. Increased leukocytes with a high percentage of neutrophils are characteristic of bacterial pericarditis, but may also be seen in viral pericarditis or chronic postmyocardial infarction syndrome (Soloff, 1971). A high percentage of lymphocytes suggests the possibility of tuberculous pericarditis, but may also occur in other conditions. Amebic pericarditis is rare, but may occur (Everett, 1972).

Microbiologic Examination

Cultures for bacteria, fungi, and tuberculosis should be performed in all effusions of unknown etiology. Cultures are positive in only about 50 per cent of patients with tuberculous pericarditis; hence, open pericardial biopsy with culture as well as histologic examination may be indicated when other studies are negative in chronic effusions of unknown etiology.

Chemical Examination

Pericardial effusions usually are classified as transudates or exudates, based on protein concentration, similar to pleural fluid. Transudates typically occur with congestive heart failure, hypoproteinemic states, myxedema, or viral pericarditis; however, transudates may also occur in the early stages of septic or nonseptic inflammation, and in some patients with malignant effusions. Exudates are characteristic of septic and nonseptic inflammation as well as malignancy involving the pericardium; however, high protein concentration may occur in chronic effusions of any etiology.

Measurement of glucose in pericardial fluid occasionally may be useful. Low glucose levels occur in bacterial pericarditis, as well as in nonseptic inflammation due to rheumatoid disease and malignancy.

PERITONEAL FLUID

Like pleural and pericardial fluids, peritoneal fluid is a plasma ultrafiltrate. Normally less than 100 ml. of clear, straw-colored fluid is present in the peritoneal cavity.

Indications for abdominal paracentesis may include: (1) ascites of unknown etiology; (2) symptoms, e.g., dyspnea, due to ascites; (3) possible ruptured viscus or intra-abdominal hemorrhage due to trauma; (4) acute abdominal pain of unknown etiology; (5) postoperative hypotension and pain of unknown etiology; and (6) instillation of cytotoxic drugs in ascites due to malignancy.

Several techniques for abdominal paracentesis are used:

1. Four quadrant tap with a No. 20 needle and syringe.

2. Puncture 3 to 5 cm. below the umbilicus in the midline, followed by introduction of a dialysis catheter which is manipulated into the pouch of Douglas (Gjessing *et al.*, 1972). If aspiration reveals gross blood or intestinal contents, laparotomy is performed; otherwise, washings are made using 1 liter of saline or balanced salt solution (Perry and Strate, 1972).

The chief complication of abdominal paracentesis is intestinal puncture. This may occur if there are extensive abdominal adhesions. If a catheter is used, damage to liver, spleen, or gallbladder is unlikely. Occasionally contents of the urinary bladder may be aspirated rather than abdominal fluid; distinction between ruptured urinary bladder and inadvertent aspiration of urine may be aided by chemical examination (*vide infra*).

Gross Examination

Peritoneal fluid typically appears clear and pale yellow to amber in ascites resulting from congestive heart failure, hepatic vein obstruction, cirrhosis, or nephrotic syndrome. However, a similar appearance may occur with ruptured urinary bladder. Turbid fluid suggests peritonitis due to appendicitis, pancreatitis, strangulated or infarcted intestine, torn or ruptured bowel following trauma, or primary bacterial infection. Blood-tinged or grossly bloody fluid may occur with ruptured spleen, ruptured liver, or torn mesenteric vessels due to trauma; leaking aneurysm of the aorta, the splenic or the hepatic artery; hemorrhagic pancreatitis; or peritoneal laceration following muscular effort (Deol and Updegrove, 1967). As with other body fluids, traumatic tap is characterized by streaking of blood in the syringe, and clearing on continued aspiration. Greenish (bile-stained) fluid has been described with perforated duodenal ulcer, perforated intestine, cholecystitis, perforated gallbladder, and acute pancreatitis (McCoy and Wolma, 1971). Although bile in the peritoneal cavity is usually considered to be rapidly fatal, Diamonon and Barnes (1964) state that sterile bile may be fairly well tolerated; paracentesis reveals dark green, viscid material which on chemical examination has a high concentration of bilirubin.

Rarely, milky fluid is observed and is due to chylous ascites. Causes for this condition include lymphoma, carcinoma, tuberculosis, parasitic infestation, adhesions, hepatic cirrhosis, and nephrotic syndrome (Lesser *et al.*, 1970). Oral administration of fat-soluble dye as well as chemical examination are helpful for confirmation (cf. section on pleural fluid). If surgical treatment is not indicated, elimination of dietary long-chain fatty acids will decrease accumulation of chylous fluid in abdomen, pericardium, or pleural cavity.

The presence or absence of peritoneal fluid must always be evaluated in light of other findings. Even with peritoneal catheterization and lavage, incidence of "false negatives" is about 10 per cent. Careful clinical observation (with repeated paracentesis if indicated), repeated radiographic studies, and evaluation of findings in peripheral blood are still essential.

Microscopic Examination

In peritoneal fluid or washings a leukocyte count over 500 per cu.mm. or erythrocyte count over 100,000 per cu.mm. is presumptive evidence of intra-abdominal disease. Erythrocyte counts in the 50,000 to 100,000 range are considered equivocal. Increased leukocytes, chiefly neutrophils, typically occur with acute peritonitis from any cause and may be the only evidence of intestinal rupture due to blunt abdominal trauma. The interval between peritoneal injury and initial appearance of leukocytes is usually about two hours. A high percentage of lymphocytes should suggest the possibility of tuberculous peritonitis, but may also be found with chylous ascites.

Cytologic examination of Papanicolaou-stained films as well as cell blocks should be performed if there is reason to suspect malignant effusion. The chief problem is in differentiating reactive mesothelial cells from malignant tumor cells. About 1 to 2 per cent false positives may be expected, with an overall accuracy of over 90 per cent. It is seldom possible to specify the primary site with certainty, but often a differential diagnosis can be suggested on the combined basis of clinical and cytologic findings.

Microbiologic Examination

Gram stain for bacteria is especially helpful in diagnosis of peritonitis and should be performed routinely, together with cultures, when this condition is suspected. Primary hematogenous peritonitis usually is due to gram-positive cocci, while secondary peritonitis due to gastrointestinal necrosis or perforation characteristically shows a mixed flora with many gram-negative organisms. Tuberculous peritonitis offers special difficulty in diagnosis. Cultures frequently are negative, and open biopsy with culture of tissue as well as histologic examination may be required.

Chemical Examination

Like pleural and pericardial fluids, abdominal fluids are classified as transudates and exudates. Transudates are typical of ascites due to congestive heart failure, constrictive pericarditis, hepatic vein obstruction, cirrhosis, or nephrotic syndrome. However, perhaps 30 per cent of such fluids show total protein in excess of 3 gm. per 100 ml. and must be classified as exudates. Exudates are typical of ascites due to peritonitis or malignancy involving the peritoneum; however, about 30 per cent of such cases have a total protein less than 3 gm. per 100 ml. and must be classified as transudates.

Although an acid pH of peritoneal fluid suggests perforated peptic ulcer, value of this measurement is questionable; according to Howard and Singh (1963), nearly all patients with perforated ulcers have an alkaline pH in their peritoneal fluid.

With pancreatitis, peritoneal fluid amylase is higher than serum amylase in about 90 per cent of cases. However, peritoneal fluid amylase is increased in a number of other conditions, and very high activities may occur with bowel necrosis (Mansberger, 1964).

Elevated ammonia levels in peritoneal fluid above 3 μg. per ml. are NOT found in pancreatitis, and suggest intestinal necrosis, perforation, or urinary extravasation.

Jejunal and ileal fluids have very high alkaline phosphatase activity (100 to 10,000 times serum levels); measurement of peritoneal fluid alkaline phosphatase has been suggested as an aid in diagnosis of ruptured or infarcted small intestine (Lee, 1969). However, the value of this measurement is not well established.

In effusions due to malignancy involving the peritoneum, LDH activity of ascitic fluid usually exceeds that of serum. However, elevated LDH activity is also observed with hemorrhagic peritoneal fluid or peritonitis of any etiology. Cytologic study is probably more sensitive, and certainly far more specific, than measurement of LDH activity in suspected malignant effusion.

In differential diagnosis of transudate vs. urine, simultaneous measurements of creatinine and urea nitrogen on blood and peritoneal fluid may be helpful. High levels of "peritoneal fluid" urea and creatinine with normal serum levels suggest inadvertent aspiration from the urinary bladder. High levels of "peritoneal fluid" urea and creatinine with elevated urea but normal creatinine in peripheral blood suggest rupture of the urinary bladder, since urea diffuses more rapidly than creatinine across the peritoneal surface.

TECHNICAL PROCEDURES

Cell Count on Cerebrospinal Fluid

EQUIPMENT AND REAGENTS. If available, a Fuchs-Rosenthal counting chamber (depth 0.2 mm.) is preferred. Otherwise, an ordinary hemocytometer (depth 0.1 mm.) is satisfactory.

Diluting fluid

Crystal violet	0.4 gm.
Glacial acetic acid	30.0 ml.
Distilled water q.s.	100 ml.

Acetic acid 3 per cent (v./v.)

Micro-hematocrit tubes

WBC pipettes
Saline 0.9 per cent (w./v.)

PROCEDURE. Fill WBC pipette to 0.5 mark with diluting fluid. Mix CSF well; then draw CSF to the 11 mark. This gives one part of diluting fluid in 20 parts of CSF. Mix for at least three minutes. Discard the first three drops before filling chamber; then fill both sides of counting chamber and allow cells to settle for one minute. Within the nine large squares on each side of the chamber, count: (1) polymorphonuclear leukocytes; (2) mononuclear leukocytes; and (3) unidentified cells.

CALCULATION. If the Fuchs-Rosenthal chamber (depth 0.2 mm.) is used, the total volume counted is $\frac{18}{5}$ cu.mm.

Correcting for dilution factor:

CSF volume counted

$$= \frac{18}{5} \times \frac{20}{21} = 3.43 \text{ cu.mm.}$$

If a hemocytometer chamber is used, the total volume counted is $\frac{18}{10}$ cu.mm. Correcting for dilution factor:

CSF volume counted

$$= \frac{18}{10} \times \frac{20}{21} = 1.72 \text{ cu.mm.}$$

$$\text{Cells/cu.mm.} = \frac{\text{number counted}}{\text{CSF volume counted}}$$

COMMENTS. Erythrocytes will be lysed by the diluting fluid; in order to perform a red cell count, use either undiluted CSF, or if many RBC are present, saline diluent.

The "chamber differential count" obtained by this method provides clinically useful information but should be supplemented by differential count on a stained film.

Differential Count of Cerebrospinal Fluid (Method of Skeel, Yankee, and Henderson, 1968)

EQUIPMENT AND REAGENTS
Conical centrifuge tubes (10–15 ml.)
Coverslips
Disposable pipettes
Wright's stain
Phosphate buffer, pH 7.4
Fresh serum or EDTA plasma (human)

PROCEDURE. Centrifuge at high speed in a 12-ml. conical tube 1 to 4 ml. of CSF for 10 minutes. If cell count is low, the sediment may be invisible. Carefully withdraw the entire supernatant fluid with a pipette. Add a small drop of serum to the sediment and mix gently to resuspend cells. Prepare thin films on coverslips, and air dry rapidly. Stain with equal parts of Wright's stain and buffer for five minutes (adjust time as needed for different lots of stain). Gently wash with distilled buffer and allow to dry.

COMMENTS. Morphology appears slightly more distinct than in films made without resuspending cells in human serum. Appearance of lymphocytes should be similar to peripheral blood film.

Total Protein of Cerebrospinal Fluid (Method of Muelemans, 1960)

EQUIPMENT AND REAGENTS
Spectrophotometer or nephelometer
Timer
13 × 100 mm. disposable tubes
2.0-ml. volumetric pipettes
0.5-ml. volumetric pipettes
Sulfosalicylic acid-sodium sulfate solution

Sulfosalicylic acid	30.0 gm.
Sodium sulfate	70.0 gm.
Distilled water q.s.	1000 ml.

PROCEDURE. Label three tubes "blank," "control," and "test." Into each, add as follows:

	Blank	*Control*	*Test*
SSA-SS	2.0 ml.	2.0 ml.	2.0 ml.
Saline	0.5 ml.	———	———
Control	———	0.5 ml.	———
CSF	———	———	0.5 ml.

Mix each tube by gentle inversion, and allow to stand for 10 minutes. Remix, and read against blank in spectrophotometer at 450 nm. or nephelometer.

COMMENTS. The method is linear to 130 mg./dl. If protein level is very high, dilute CSF with saline and re-run. This method is unaffected by changes in the albumin/globulin ratio, or by use of saline as a diluent; however, there is a linear relationship between turbidity and temperature, with a temperature coefficient of about 1 per cent per degree centigrade (Pennock *et al.*, 1968).

CALIBRATION CURVE. Dilutions of human serum assayed by biuret method should be used as standard. Commercially assayed reference sera or CSF may be used if assigned values are rechecked prior to use.

Cell Count on Synovial Fluid

EQUIPMENT AND REAGENTS
Either a Fuchs-Rosenthal or hemocytometer counting chamber may be used
Synovial fluid diluent–0.85 per cent sodium chloride with 0.1 per cent methylene blue
White cell and red cell pipettes
1 per cent saponin in saline or 0.1 N HCl

PROCEDURE. Thoroughly mix the anticoagulated sample of synovial fluid, and draw to the 1 mark of the white cell pipette. Draw diluent up to the 11 mark and mix thoroughly for 3 minutes. Count leukocytes and erythrocytes in the nine large squares of each chamber.

$$\text{Cells per cu.mm.} = \text{cells counted} \times \text{dilution} \times \frac{1}{\text{cu.mm. counted}}$$

If a hemocytometer chamber is used, the volume counted is $\frac{18}{10}$ cu.mm. and cells per cu. mm. = cells counted $\times 10 \times \frac{10}{18}$.

If a Fuchs-Rosenthal chamber is used, the volume counted is $\frac{18}{5}$ cu.mm.

COMMENT. If the fluid is turbid, a 1:20 dilution or 1:100 dilution may be used. For the former, draw SF to 0.5 mark of the white cell pipette; for the latter, draw SF to the 1 mark of the red cell pipette. If numerous red cells are present, these may be lysed with 1 per cent saponin in saline or 0.1 N HCl. A dilution of either 1 part synovial fluid to 100 parts saponin in saline or 1 part synovial fluid to 10 parts 0.1 N HCl should suffice to lyse the erythrocytes in grossly bloody specimens.

REFERENCES

Cerebrospinal Fluid

Austin, D. A., and Sokolowski, J. W.: Post lumbar puncture chemical meningitis. New York J. Med. *68*:2444, 1968.

Bauer, C. H., New, M. I., and Miller, J. M.: Cerebrospinal fluid protein values of premature infants. J. Pediat. *66*:1017, 1965.

Beatty, H. N., and Oppenheimer, S.: Cerebrospinal fluid lactic dehydrogenase and its isoenzymes in infections of the central nervous system. New Eng. J. Med. *279*:1197, 1968.

Belsey, M. A.: CSF glutamic oxaloacetic transaminase in acute bacterial meningitis. Amer. J. Dis. Child. *117*:288, 1969.

Bennett, J. E., and Bailey, J. W.: Control for rheumatoid factor in the latex test for cryptococcosis. J. Clin. Path. *56*:360, 1971.

Brisman, R., Hughes, J. E. O., and Mount, L. A.: Cerebrospinal fluid rhinorrhea. Arch. Neurol. *22*:245, 1970.

Bulger, R. J., Schrier, R. W., Arend, W. P., and Swanson, A. G.: Spinal fluid acidosis and the diagnosis of pulmonary encephalopathy. New Eng. J. Med. *274*:433, 1966.

Bürgi, W., Richterich, R., and Briner, M.: UV-photometric determination of total cerebrospinal fluid proteins with modified biuret reagent. Clin. Chim. Acta *15*:181, 1967.

Campbell, R. A.: Lumbar puncture in the frail infant. J.A.M.A. *204*:180, 1968.

Carter, R. F.: Primary amoebic meningo-encephalitis. J. Path. *96*:1, 1968.

Char, D. F., and Rosen, L.: Eosinophilic meningitis among children in Hawaii. J. Pediat. *70*:28, 1967.

Cole, M.: Pitfalls in cerebrospinal fluid examination. Hosp. Pract. *4*:47, 1969.

Davies-Jones, G. A. B.: Lactate dehydrogenase and glutamic oxalacetic transaminase of the cerebrospinal fluid in tumors of the central nervous system. J. Neurol. *32*:324, 1969.

Dramov, B., and Dubou, R.: Aseptic meningitis following intrathecal radioiodinated serum albumin. Calif. Med. *115*:64, 1971.

Duma, R. J., Ferrel, H. W., Nelson, E. C., and Jones, M. M.: Primary amebic meningoencephalitis. New Eng. J. Med. *281*:1315, 1969.

Dunn, J. S., and Wyburn, G. M.: The anatomy of the blood brain barrier. Scot. Med. J. *17*:21, 1972.

Escobar, M. R., Dalton, H. P., and Allison, M. J.: Fluorescent antibody tests using cerebrospinal fluid. Amer. J. Clin. Path. *53*:886, 1970.

Farstad, M., Haug, J. O., Lindbak, H., and Skaug, O. E.: Uric acid in the cerebrospinal fluid in cerebral atrophy. Acta Neurol. Scand. *41*:52, 1965.

Feinbloom, R. I., and Alpert, J. J.: The value of routine glucose determination in spinal fluid without pleocytosis. J. Pediat. *75*:121, 1969.

Fischer-Williams, M.: Cerebrospinal fluid proteins and serum immunoglobulins. Arch. Neurol. *25*:526, 1971.

Frantzen, E., Hertz, H., Matzke, J., and Videback, A.: Protein studies on cerebrospinal fluid and neurological symptoms in myelomatosis. Acta Neurol. Scand. *45*:1, 1969.

Fumagalli, R., and Paoletti, P.: Sterol test for human brain tumors. Neurology *21*:1149, 1971.

Gaines, J. D., Eckman, P. B., and Remington, J. S.: Low CSF glucose level in sarcoidosis involving the central nervous system. Arch. Intern. Med. *125*:333, 1970.

Garde, A., and Kjellin, K. G.: Diagnostic significance of cerebrospinal-fluid examinations in myelopathy. Acta Neurol. Scand. *47*:555, 1971.

Green, J. B.: The colloidal gold test of the spinal fluid. J.A.M.A. *209*:1908, 1969.

Gordon, E.: The acid-base balance and oxygen tension of the cerebrospinal fluid, and their implications for the treatment of patients with brain lesions. Acta Anaesthesiol. Scand. *39*(Suppl.):1971.

Gordon, M. A., and Lapa, B. A.: Charcoal particle agglutination test for detection of antibody to cryptococcus neoformans. Amer. J. Clin. Path. *56*:354, 1971.

Greenawald, K. A., Speicher, C. E., Evers, W., and Henry, J. B.: Glucose content in cerebrospinal fluid: A comparison with glucose levels in serum as determined by copper reduction and hexokinase methods. Amer. J. Clin. Path. *59*: 518, 1973.

Hinterbuchner, L. P.: Hazards of lumbar puncture in infants. J.A.M.A. *204*:196, 1968.

Hourani, B. T., Hamlin, E. M., and Reynolds, T. B.: Cerebrospinal glutamine as a measure of hepatic encephalopathy. Arch. Intern. Med. *127*:1033, 1971.

Igou, P. C.: An evaluation of a gel filtration-spectrophotometric method for spinal fluid protein. Amer. J. Med. Tech. *33*:354, 1967.

Ivers, R. R., McKenzie, B. F., McGuckin, W. F., and Goldstein, N. P.: Spinal-fluid gamma globulin in multiple sclerosis and other neurologic diseases. J.A.M.A. *176*:515, 1961.

Jaiken, A., and Agrest, A.: Cerebrospinal fluid glutamine concentration in patients with chronic hypercapnea. Clin. Sci. *36*:11, 1969.

Kaplan, A.: Electrophoresis of cerebrospinal fluid proteins. Amer. J. Med. Sci. *253*:549, 1967.

Kirsch, A.: Diagnosis of cerebrospinal fluid rhinorrhea; lack of specificity of the glucose oxidase test tape. J. Pediat. *71*:718, 1967.

Laterre, E., Callewaert, A., Heremans, J. F., and Sfaello, Z.: Electrophoretic morphology of gamma globulins in cerebrospinal fluid of multiple sclerosis and other diseases of the nervous system. Neurology *20*:982, 1970.

Marshall, J.: Lumbar puncture. Brit. J. Hosp. Med. *3*:216, 1970.

Menkes, J. H.: The causes for low spinal fluid sugar in bacterial meningitis: Another look. Pediatrics *44*:1, 1969.

Meulemans, O.: Determination of total protein in spinal fluid with sulfosalicylic acid and trichloracetic acid. Clin. Chim. Acta *5*:757, 1960.

Milhorat, T. H., Mosher, M. B., Hammock, M. K., and Murphy, C. F.: Evidence for choroid plexus absorption in hydrocephalus. New Eng. J. Med. *283*:286, 1970.

Moir, A. T. B., Ashcroft, G. W., Crawford, T. B. B., Eccleston, D., and Guldberg, H. C.: Cerebral metabolites in cerebrospinal fluid as a biochemical approach to the brain. Brain *93*:357, 1970.

O'Reilly, S., and Kwa, G. B.: Examination of the cerebrospinal fluid. Resident Phys. *13*:51, 1967.

Pennock, C. A., Passant, L. P., and Bolton, F. G.: Estimation of cerebrospinal fluid protein. J. Clin. Path. *21*:518, 1968.

Pryce, J. D., Gant, P. W., and Saul, K. J.: Normal concentration of lactate, glucose, and protein in cerebrospinal fluid, and the diagnostic implications of abnormal concentrations. Clin. Chem. *16*:562, 1970.

Rowe, D. S.: Measurement of concentrations of human serum immunoglobulins. Transfusion *11*:350, 1971.

Schwartz, S., Rieder, H. P., and Wüthrich, R.: The protein fractions in cerebrospinal fluid in the various states of multiple sclerosis. Eur. Neurol. *4*:267, 1970.

Sherwin, A. L., Norris, J. W., and Bulke, J. A.: Spinal fluid creatine kinase in disease. Neurology *19*:993, 1969.

Sherwin, R. M., and Moore, G. H.: Microzone electrophoresis of unconcentrated cerebrospinal fluid. Amer. J. Clin. Path. *55*:705, 1971.

Skeel, R. T., Yankee, R. A., and Henderson, E. S.: Meningeal leukemia. J.A.M.A. *205*:155, 1968.

Van Der Meulen, J. P.: Cerebrospinal fluid xanthochromia: An objective index. Neurology *16*:170, 1966.

Walton, J. N.: *Subarachnoid Haemorrhage.* Edinburgh, E. & S. Livingstone, Ltd., 1956.

Watson, D.: Modern methods for determining cerebrospinal fluid protein. Clin. Chem. *10*:412, 1964.

Werner, M.: A combined procedure for protein estimation and electrophoresis of cerebrospinal fluid. J. Lab. Clin. Med. *74*:166, 1969.

Wilfert, C. M.: Mumps meningoencephalitis with low cerebrospinal-fluid glucose, prolonged pleocytosis and elevation of protein. New Eng. J. Med. *280*:855, 1969.

Windisch, R. M., and Bracken, M. M.: Cerebrospinal fluid proteins: Concentration by membrane ultrafiltration and fractionation by electrophoresis on cellulose acetate. Clin. Chem. *16*:416, 1970.

Synovial Fluid

Beckman, G., Beckman, L., and Lemperg, R.: Acid phosphatase activity in the synovial fluid of patients with rheumatoid arthritis and other joint disorders. Acta Rheum. Scand. *17*:47, 1971.

Blau, S. P.: Leukocyte counts in synovial fluid. Ann. Intern. Med. *74*:638, 1971.

Cracchiolo, A.: Joint fluid analysis. Amer. Family Phys. *4*:8, 1971.

Das, G. C., and Sen, S. B.: Chylous arthritis. Brit. Med. J. *2*:27, 1968.

Donaldson, L. E. E.: Technique for performing white cell counts in joint fluids. Med. Lab. Technol. *29*:1, 1972.

Good, A. E., and Frishette, W. A.: Crystals in dried smears of synovial fluid. J.A.M.A. *198*:198, 1966.

Holmes, K. K., Gutman, L. T., Belding, M. E., and Turck, M.: Recovery of Neisseria gonorrheae from "sterile" synovial fluid in gonococcic arthritis. New Eng. J. Med. *284*:318, 1971.

Hunder, G. G., and Pierre, R. V.: In vivo LE cell formation in synovial fluid. Arthritis Rheumatism *13*:448, 1970.

Kahn, C. B., Hollander, J. L., and Schumacher, H. R.: Corticosteroid crystals in synovial fluid. J.A.M.A. *211*:807, 1970.

McCarty, D. J.: On the crystal deposition diseases. DM, March, 1970.

Pekin, T. J., and Zvaifler, N. J.: Synovial fluid findings in systemic lupus erythematosus (SLE). Arthritis Rheumatism *13*:777, 1970.

Ropes, M. W., and Bauer, W.: Synovial Fluid Changes in Joint Diseases. Cambridge, Harvard University Press, 1953.

Schmid, F. R., and Ogata, R. I.: Synovial fluid evaluation in joint disease. Med. Clin. N. Amer. *49*:165, 1965.

Sones, D. A., McDuffie, F. C., and Hunder, G. G.: The clinical significance of the RA cell. Arthritis Rheumatism *11*:400, 1968.

Souteyrand-Boulenger, J. D., and Amouroux, J.: Anatomy, histology, and pathology of the synovial membrane and fluid. Presse Méd. *1*:331, 1972.

Pleural Fluid

Black, L. F.: The pleural space and pleural fluid. Mayo Clin. Proc. *47*:493, 1972.

Boddington, M. M., Spriggs, A. I., Morton, J. A., and Mowat, A. G.: Cytodiagnosis of rheumatoid pleural effusion. J. Clin. Path. *24*:95, 1971.

Campbell, G. D., and Webb, W. R.: Eosinophilic pleural effusion. Amer. Rev. Resp. Dis. *90*:194, 1964.

Carr, D. T., Lilington, G. A., and Mayne, J. G.: Pleural-fluid glucose in systemic lupus erythematosus. Mayo Clin. Proc. *45*:409, 1970.

Funahashi, A., Sarkar, T. K., and Kory, R. C.: PO_2, Pco_2 and pH in pleural effusion. J. Lab. Clin. Med. *78*:1006, 1971.

Klepser, R. G., and Berry, J. F.: The diagnosis and surgical management of chylothorax with the aid of lipophilic dyes. Dis. Chest *25*:409, 1954.

Roy, P. H., Carr, D. T., and Payne, W. S.: The problem of chylothorax. Mayo Clin. Proc. *42*:457, 1967.

Trapnell, D. H., and Thurston, J. G. B.: Unilateral pulmonary edema after pleural aspiration. Lancet *1*:1367, 1970.

van Heerden, J. A., and Lanfenberg, H. J.: Simplified thoracentesis. Mayo Clin. Proc. *48*:34, 1968.

Pericardial Fluid

Brawley, R. K., Vasko, J. S., and Morrow, A. G.: Cholesterol pericarditis. Amer. J. Med. *41*:235, 1966.

Dempsey, J. J., Eissa, A., Attia, M., and Ramzy, A.: Pericardial effusion of "gold paint" appearance following myocardial infarction. Arch. Intern. Med. *118*:249, 1966.

Everett, E. D.: Pericarditis due to Entamoeba histolytica. South. Med. J. *65*:501, 1972.

Hudspeth, A. S., and Miller, H. S.: Isolated (primary) chylopericardium. J. Thorac. Cardiov. Surg. *51*:528, 1966.

Hurst, J. W., and Logue, R. B.: *The Heart.* 2nd ed. New York, McGraw-Hill Book Co., Inc., 1970.

Kilpatrick, Z. M., and Chapman, C. B.: On pericardiocentesis. Amer. J. Cardiol. *16*:722, 1965.

Soloff, L. A.: Pericardial cellular response during the postmyocardial infarction syndrome. Amer. Heart J. *82*:812, 1971.

Peritoneal Fluid

Deol, J. S., and Updegrove, J. H.: Peritoneal laceration due to muscular effort. J.A.M.A. *199*:160, 1967.

Diamonon, J. S., and Barnes, J. P.: Choleperitoneum. Amer. Surg. *30*:331, 1964.

Gjessing, J., Oskarsson, B. M., Tomlin, P. J., and Brock-Utne, J.: Diagnostic abdominal paracentesis. Brit. Med. J. *1*:617, 1972.

Howard, J. M., and Singh, L. M.: Peritoneal fluid pH after perforation of peptic ulcers. Arch. Surg. *87*:483, 1963.

Lee, Y. N.: Alkaline phosphatase in intestinal perforation. J.A.M.A. *208*:361, 1969.

Lesser, G. T., Bruno, M. S., and Enselberg, K.: Chylous ascites. Arch. Intern. Med. *125*:1073, 1970.

Mansberger, A. R., Jr.: The diagnostic value of abdominal paracentesis with special reference to peritoneal fluid ammonia levels. Amer. J. Gastroent. *42*:150, 1964.

McCoy, J., and Wolma, F. J.: Abdominal tap. Amer. J. Surg. *122*:693, 1971.

Perry, J. F., Jr., and Strate, R. G.: Diagnostic peritoneal lavage in blunt abdominal trauma. Surgery *71*:898, 1972.

Chapter 26

PREGNANCY TESTS AND CHORIONIC GONADOTROPIN ASSAYS

by ARTHUR F. KRIEG, M.D., and JOHN BERNARD HENRY, M.D.

The term "pregnancy test" is actually a misnomer; most of these procedures measure human chorionic gonadotropin (HCG) and not the presence of a fetus.

HCG is a glycoprotein produced by trophoblastic cells beginning about 10 days after conception (Wide, 1969). The structure and amino acid sequence have been elucidated recently: HCG is a dimer of molecular weight about 28,000 composed of alpha and beta subunits (Bahl *et al.*, 1972; Morgan and Canfield, 1971). The alpha subunits are nonspecific, being shared with luteinizing hormone (LH), follicle stimulating hormone (FSH), and thyroid stimulating hormone (TSH). The beta subunits are unique to HCG.

Following conception, a rapid rise in urinary HCG begins at about five weeks' gestation (five weeks after last menstrual period), with peak levels at about ten weeks' gestation. The relationship between urinary HCG, urinary pregnanediol, and urinary estriol is shown in Figure 26–1. "Weeks of gestation" refers to weeks after the last normal menstrual period rather than weeks after conception, since the latter date is difficult to determine with certainty. As placental estrogen and progesterone production increase during the second trimester, HCG levels decline. For laboratory confirmation of early pregnancy, HCG is the most logical measurement; for evaluation of fetal distress during the third trimester, estriol is more useful.

The first reliable bioassay for HCG was

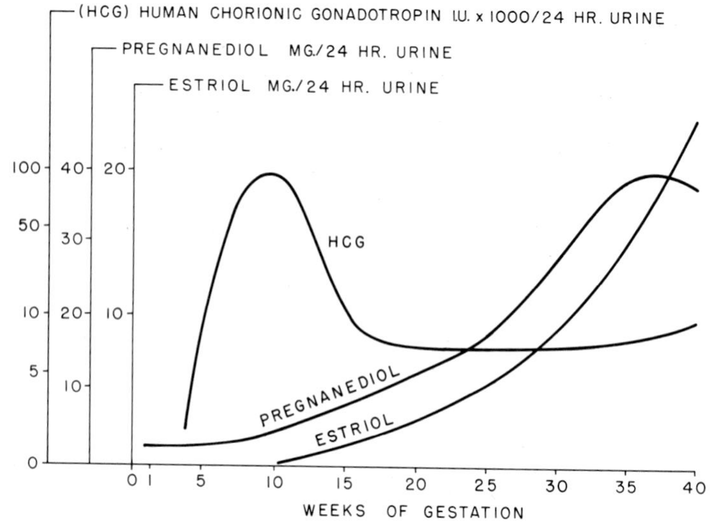

Figure 26–1. Urine levels of human chorionic gonadotropin (HCG), estriol, and pregnanediol during pregnancy.

developed by Aschheim and Zondek in 1928. Five immature female mice about 21 days old, weighing 5 to 7 gm. each, were given multiple injections of urine over a two-day period; four days after the first injection, all animals were sacrificed and their ovaries examined for corpus luteum formation. This procedure, the Aschheim-Zondek or A-Z test, is reliable, but too long and time consuming for general clinical use.

The Friedman test, developed in 1931, reduced reporting time from four days to 48 hours. A mature female rabbit is injected intravenously with urine: at 48 hours the ovaries are examined for corpora lutea and hemorrhagic follicles. False positive reactions may occur if the rabbits are not isolated for 30 days before use; if this precaution is observed, results are relatively reliable.

In 1934 Bellerby described a test using the female South African clawed toad, *Xenopus laevis*. These toads deposit eggs within 24 hours after injection with chorionic gonadotropin. Since large doses of HCG are required, concentration by alcohol precipitation or kaolin adsorption is essential for adequate sensitivity (Hon, 1961).

During 1941 Frank and Berman described their sensitive and specific rat ovarian hyperemia test. Two immature female rats weighing 45 to 60 gm. each are given two injections of urine or serum and sacrificed 24 hours later using carbon monoxide. Considerable experience is needed to evaluate the resulting ovarian hyperemia, which is due to capillary dilatation associated with thecal cell hyperplasia.

In 1948 Galli-Mainini described use of the male toad *Bufo arenarum*, while Wiltberger and Miller reported similar results with the male frog *Rana pipiens*. Four to six hours after injection with HCG, these animals release sperm which can be detected microscopically. These animals are relatively insensitive, and concentration is required for adequate sensitivity. Furthermore, sensitivity varies with the season of the year and the temperature, so frequent restandardization is necessary.

With all bioassays, drugs excreted in the urine may cause decreased sensitivity and false negative results, or even death of the test animal. Quinidine, barbiturates, laxatives, antihistamines, sulfonamides, salicylates, antibiotics, ergot, and morphine derivatives may cause interference. If possible, all medications should be discontinued by the patient for three to four days prior to bioassays. Sensitivity of the test animal may also be reduced by high concentrations of urinary electrolytes (especially potassium), bacteria, and unspecified endogenous substances, all of which may cause false negative reactions. Toxic substances may be partially or completely removed from urine by: (1) dialysis in cellophane tubing for 30 to 60 minutes under running water; (2) acidification with 0.1 N hydrochloric acid to a pH of about 6.0; (3) extraction with ether; or (4) absorption with kaolin. False positive reactions may be caused by high titers of LH and/or follicle-stimulating hormone (FSH) due to menopause or primary ovarian failure, as well as a number of drugs, especially phenothiazine derivatives such as chlorpromazine (Thorazine), prochlorperazine (Compazine), and promazine (Sparine). These drugs should be discontinued for at least 48 hours before obtaining samples for HCG measurement. False positives may also be due to ovulation induced by handling (Friedman test), or spermiation induced by epinephrine (Galli-Mainini test).

In all bioassays exact adherence to published methods is essential. Animals must be of correct age and weight, in good health, and properly cared for. Regular restandardization is needed; especially in tests using amphibians, the concentration procedure must be adjusted periodically to achieve the desired sensitivity. Considerable care and experience are required to achieve reliable and reproducible results using bioassays (Hon, 1961).

Concentration of HCG is often expressed in animal units. There are rat units, mouse units, male and female toad and frog units, and so forth. Animal units are difficult to compare. More accurate is the international unit (I.U.) of HCG, related to specific gonadotropic activity of 0.1 mg. of a dried standard kept at the National Institute for Medical Research, London. This is the amount of activity sufficient to cause cornification of the vaginal epithelium of immature rats.

In 1960 Wide and Gemzell introduced the first immunologic HCG assay, based on hemagglutination inhibition; in 1962 Robbins *et al.* described a latex particle agglutination test; more recently, radioimmunoassays have become available (Wide, 1969). The beta subunit radioimmunoassay for HCG is by far the most sensitive and specific method available. Other immunoassays, as well as bioassays, show cross reaction with LH and FSH if sensitivity is increased beyond 0.7 I.U./ml. (Varma *et al.*, 1971). Since urinary FSH and LH may reach levels of 0.6 I.U. "HCG" per milliliter during the normal menstrual cycle (at ovulation), following menopause, or with ovarian failure, most "routine" pregnancy tests have a sensitivity of about 0.7–1.0 I.U./ml.

At present, the beta subunit HCG radioimmunoassay is not used as a routine pregnancy test, but is reserved for study of patients being treated for choriocarcinoma or hydatidiform mole.

CLINICAL APPLICATIONS

The diagnosis of early pregnancy can usually be established with reasonable accuracy by careful history and physical examination two weeks after the first missed period, i.e., at six weeks' gestation. Diagnosis seldom presents any difficulty after ten weeks' gestation. Although early symptoms of pregnancy may be equivocal – early morning nausea, urinary frequency, breast tenderness, and amenorrhea – certain clinical signs are of definite value. Dilatation of superficial veins in the breasts, often the earliest sign, usually appears at six to eight weeks' gestation (Hibbard, 1971). Congestion of superficial blood vessels results in a bluish appearance of the vaginal and cervical epithelium at about the same time. The uterus and cervix become softened, and enlargement – which initially may be asymmetric – is progressive. Pulsation in the lateral fornices is noted due to dilatation and tortuosity of the uterine arteries.

During early pregnancy the more sensitive HCG assays (1 I.U./ml.) become "positive" about one week after the first missed period (five weeks' gestation), and almost invariably are positive at six weeks' gestation. Less sensitive HCG assays (5 I.U./ml.) typically become positive about three to five days later. In ectopic pregnancy, levels of urinary HCG frequently are below 1 I.U. per ml., and often below 0.3 I.U./ml. Since HCG levels below 1 I.U. per ml. are not detected by usual assays, occasionally an assay capable of detecting 0.3 I.U. per ml. (undiluted urine with UCG test kit*) may be useful despite the possibility of a false positive reaction due to cross reaction with LH. (Immediately after ovulation, increased LH may give urinary "HCG" levels up to 0.6 I.U. per ml.) Between 10 and 50 per cent of ectopic pregnancies have HCG levels less than 1 I.U./ml. (Glass and Jesurun, 1966; Kerber *et al.,* 1970); although a positive test can be helpful, LACK OF HCG, EVEN AT LOW LEVELS, DOES NOT EXCLUDE ECTOPIC PREGNANCY.

During the first trimester, quantitative HCG assay may be useful as a guide to prognosis of threatened abortion. As previously noted, peak levels of HCG normally are reached at about 10 weeks' gestation, and during normal pregnancy, "high levels" of HCG may be expected starting at the seventh week (49 days' gestation) and continuing until the thirteenth week (91 days' gestation). During this time, less than 3000 I.U./24-hr. urine is associated with inevitable abortion (Yahia, 1964). If first voided morning urine is used instead of a 24-hour collection, HCG levels under 5000 I.U./L. suggest nonviable gestation (Salzberger and Nelken, 1963). Inevitable abortion initially may present normal HCG levels, with rapid decrease over several days, and repeated assays may be useful.

Human chorionic gonadotropin levels in toxemia of pregnancy and prolonged pregnancy are not useful because of a very wide "normal range" during the last trimester. However, urinary estriol, estriol creatinine ratios, or placental lactogen (HPL) are valuable aids in monitoring fetal and/or placental malfunction during the last trimester. (See Chapter 27.)

Classically, quantitative HCG assay has been valuable in diagnosis of hydatidiform mole. Although some patients with hydatidiform mole have extremely high urinary HCG levels (up to 6 million I.U. per liter), most are in the range of normal pregnancy, and a few have relatively low levels of HCG (5 I.U. per ml.). Differential diagnosis of high HCG levels may be aided by the fact that during pregnancy sequential assays tend to follow the normal pregnancy curve, while in trophoblastic disease, repeated assays over several weeks will show irregular fluctuations. Also, in trophoblastic disease, levels of pregnanediol and estriol will be lower than would be expected for the stage of gestation (Fig. 26–1). Several pitfalls must be avoided in regard to increased HCG levels and hydatidiform mole:

1. Elevated levels may be associated with multiple pregnancies, polyhydramnios, eclampsia, and erythroblastosis fetalis during the third trimester.
2. As with other titration procedures, a variation of one tube is not significant; hence, a level given as one million I.U. per liter must be interpreted as between 500,000 (–50 per cent) and two million (+100 per cent). Repeated assays using different series of dilutions may give increased accuracy in problem cases.
3. Marked variation of HCG levels is characteristic of the third trimester; both extremely high and extremely low (500 I.U. per liter) levels may occur in normal pregnancy.

Once the diagnosis of trophoblastic disease has been made, urinary HCG levels provide an excellent indicator of response to therapy. Following expulsion of a hydatidiform mole, urinary HCG should fall to undetectable levels in seven days (the same period required for disappearance of HCG after normal term delivery). If this does not occur, the mole has been incompletely removed, or choriocarcinoma may be present.

Choriocarcinoma is a malignancy of trophoblastic tissue which in women usually develops from hydatidiform mole. In males choriocarcinoma is an unusual but highly malignant testicular tumor. In both men and women most choriocarcinomas produce either high or

*Wampole Laboratories, Stamford, Connecticut.

normal pregnancy levels of HCG; in a few cases, however, no HCG is detectable. In view of this wide range of values, it is NOT possible to accurately distinguish hydatidiform mole from choriocarcinoma on the basis of quantitative HCG assay. Ovarian and testicular teratomas, seminomas, and embryonal carcinomas have been reported with high levels of urinary HCG; such cases may be due to small foci of choriocarcinoma missed during histologic study. For this reason, HCG assays are useful in clinical evaluation of testicular tumors.

Successful treatment of choriocarcinoma is followed by progressive decrease in urinary HCG to undetectable levels. Persistent excretion is associated with incomplete removal, metastases, or recurrence; continued high levels are a poor prognostic sign.

The relationship between bioassays and immunoassays of HCG has been studied by many workers, including Hobson and Wide (1964), Borth *et al.* (1965), Tietz (1965), Driscoll *et al.* (1971), and Varma *et al.* (1971).

Apparently bioassays reflect the effect of HCG on cells, while immunoassays measure capacity to combine with antibody. Even if bioassays and immunoassays are standardized against identical reference materials, the ratio of biologic to immunologic activity (B:I ratio) varies from slightly over 1.0 during the first two months of pregnancy to slightly less than 0.5 during the second and third trimesters (Lau, 1970). Thus, during the first two months of pregnancy, levels of urinary HCG are similar when measured by bioassay and immunoassay, but during the second and third trimesters, urine HCG concentrations measured by bioassay are less than half the immunoassay values!

Patients with hydatidiform mole show a high B:I ratio, comparable to early pregnancy; it is suggested that this ratio may prove useful in diagnosis (Lau, 1970).

IMMUNOASSAYS

Most of the commonly used immunologic "pregnancy tests" are based on: (1) the presence of human chorionic gonadotropin (HCG) in urine and serum of pregnant women; and (2) the ability of HCG to stimulate production of antisera. Since 1961 a number of commercial preparations for HCG assay in urine have become available; some of these are shown in Tables 26–1 and 26–2. These procedures commonly are classified as "slide tests" and "tube tests."

Most of the presently available "slide tests" (Ortho, Hyland, Organon, Roche, and Burroughs Wellcome) are based on latex particle agglutination inhibition (Fig. 26–2). This is a two-stage procedure:

1. Anti-HCG serum is incubated with the patient's urine; if the patient is pregnant, HCG in the urine will neutralize the antiserum; if the patient is not pregnant, the antiserum will not be neutralized.

2. Latex particles coated with HCG are added; if urinary HCG has neutralized the antiserum, there will be no agglutination (posi-

Table 26–1. SLIDE TESTS FOR HCG IMMUNOASSAY

MANUFACTURER AND PRODUCT NAME	METHOD	SPECIMEN	SENSITIVITY (I.U./ml.)	COMMENTS
Burroughs Wellcome Prepurex	Latex particle agglutination inhibition	Urine	4	See Headden, 1972
Hyland HCG test	Latex particle agglutination inhibition	Urine	5–8	High incidence of false positives reported with proteinuria
Mochida Gonavislide	Latex particle agglutination (direct)	Urine	1–2	See Tamada *et al.*, 1971
Organon Pregnosticon slide test	Latex particle agglutination inhibition	Urine	2	See Lamb, 1972
Organon Pregnosticon Dri-Dot	Latex particle agglutination inhibition	Urine	1–2	See Lamb, 1972
Ortho Diagnostics Gravindex	Latex particle agglutination inhibition	Urine	3–5	High incidence of false positives reported with proteinuria
Parke-Davis Prequest	Latex particle agglutination inhibition	Urine	5–6	See Lamb, 1972
Roche Diagnostics Pregnosis	Latex particle agglutination inhibition	Urine	2	See Driscoll *et al.*, 1971
Wampole DAP Test	Latex particle agglutination (direct)	Urine; serum	2	Urine contaminated with blood reportedly does not interfere; prozone effect with high HCG concentrations

Table 26–2. TUBE TESTS FOR HCG IMMUNOASSAY

MANUFACTURER AND PRODUCT NAME	METHOD*	SPECIMEN	SENSITIVITY	COMMENTS
Ames Pretel	HCG covalently linked to RBC	Urine	2.0	
Burroughs Wellcome Prepuerin	Anti-HCG complexed with HCG on RBC	Urine	2.5	Requires longer incubation than other tube tests
Organon Pregnosticon	Lyophilized RBC	Urine	0.7–1.0	Little interference reported with proteinuria (Kerber *et al.*, 1970)
Organon Pregnosticon Accuspheres	Lyophilized RBC	Urine	0.7–1.5	Reagents premixed by manufacturer; little interference reported with proteinuria (Kerber *et al.*, 1970)
Wampole UCG	Tanned RBC	Urine; serum extract	1.0	Little interference reported with proteinuria (Kerber *et al.*, 1970); undiluted urine gives 0.3 I.U. sensitivity

*All these procedures based on hemagglutination inhibition; method refers to RBC preparation used.

tive test); if the antiserum has not been neutralized, agglutination will occur (negative test).

Two slide tests (Mochida and Wampole) are based on direct latex particle agglutination. In this one-step procedure, latex particles coated with anti-HCG serum are incubated with patient's urine: if HCG is present, the particles agglutinate (positive test); if HCG is absent, no agglutination is observed (negative test).

The presently available "tube tests" (Wampole, Organon, Ames, Burroughs Wellcome, and Roche) are based on hemagglutination inhibition. When agglutinated erythrocytes in low concentration settle in a test tube with a hemispheric bottom, they form a uniform film which covers the bottom of the tube. When unagglutinated erythrocytes settle in such a tube, they form a sharply demarcated ring or "doughnut" (Fig. 26–3). With gradually increasing agglutination, the ring increases in size, becomes very faint, and finally disappears. Salk made these observations in 1944; however, the exact mechanism is still not understood. Like latex particle agglutination inhibition, this is a two-stage procedure (Fig. 26–3):

1. Anti-HCG serum and red blood cells (RBC) coated with HCG are incubated with patient's urine; if the patient is pregnant, HCG in the urine will neutralize the antiserum; if the patient is not pregnant, the antiserum will not be neutralized.

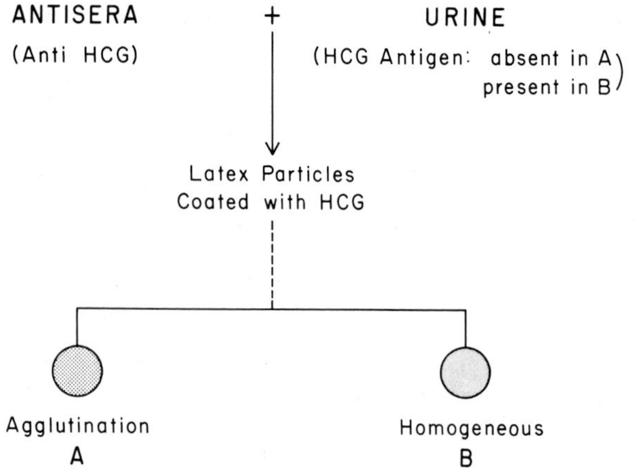

Figure 26–2.

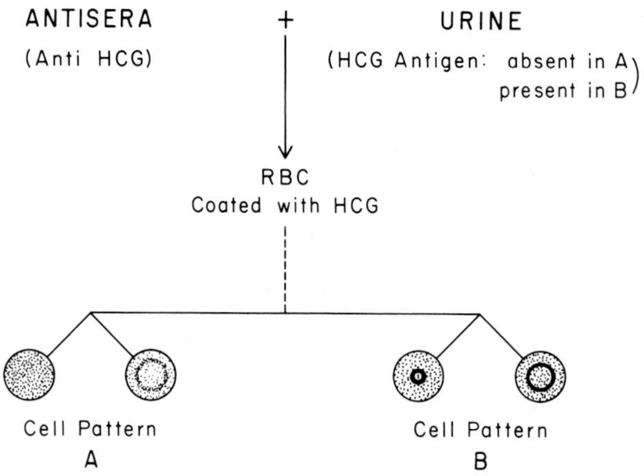

Figure 26–3.

Figure 26–2. Principle of slide latex agglutination inhibition test for human chorionic gonadotropin (HCG).

Figure 26–3. Principle of hemagglutination inhibition test for human chorionic gonadotropin (HCG). The homogeneous reaction (B) or no agglutination represents a positive pregnancy test, while the reverse indicates a negative test.

2. If urinary HCG has neutralized the antiserum, the RBC will not be agglutinated and will settle to the bottom of the tube in a "doughnut" pattern or ring of cells; if the antiserum has not been neutralized, the RBC will be agglutinated, and a diffuse mat of cells (with or without a faint ring) will form in the bottom of the tube, as noted in Figure 26–3.

Reported "accuracy" of immunologic pregnancy test kits depends upon:

1. Whether manufacturer's directions are followed carefully.
2. Proper shipment and storage of reagents.
3. Proper specimen collection, and prompt delivery to laboratory.
4. Stage of pregnancy.
5. Whether pregnancy is normal or abnormal.
6. Interfering substances in urine, including drugs, proteins, and erythrocytes.
7. Sensitivity and specificity of assay procedure.
8. Whether the user understands pitfalls of these procedures and provides a formal quality control program to:
   a. Regularly recheck sensitivity of assay system against materials which can be related to International Standard.
   b. Regularly recheck assay system against known negatives (urine from males and nonpregnant females).
   c. Regularly recheck assay system against samples with known HCG levels in ranges of two to four times the test sensitivity and one-fourth to one-half times the test sensitivity (low positive and high negative).

Unless this information is available, it is difficult to compare different reports in the literature. Lack of comparability with respect to these parameters has led to many contradictory reports, which may confuse the physician seeking information on the "best" procedure for clinical use. As with any commercially produced antisera, it is ESSENTIAL to follow EXACTLY instructions on measurement of reagents, mixing, timing, and reading results. In some cases, dilution of samples from patients over age 40 is recommended to reduce false positives due to LH. Disposable pipettes and careful rinsing of nondisposable glassware are recommended, since traces of detergent may give false positives and false negatives with slide tests (Headden, 1972) or false positives with tube tests (Hobson, 1968).

During shipment, it is possible for the antisera to be frozen or exposed to high temperature; following delivery, reagents may remain in the receiving room for weeks, or even months, before they are brought to the laboratory. And in a busy laboratory, reagents which *should* be refrigerated may occasionally be left at room temperature for prolonged periods. The resulting deterioration of antiserum typically causes *increased* sensitivity (although decreased sensitivity may be observed with direct slide tests).

In our opinion, first voided morning specimens are preferable for urinary HCG assay because: (1) these samples are more concentrated, hence false negatives are less likely than with random specimens; and (2) results expressed as I.U./L. (or I.U./ml.) are comparable to 24-hour samples, yet problems due to incomplete specimen collection are avoided. Since detergents may interfere, the specimen should be collected in a disposable urine container; if these are not available, the patient should be instructed to use a clean, thoroughly rinsed bottle, which does NOT contain traces of previous contents or detergent. It is helpful to measure specific gravity (S.G.) on all urine samples for HCG assay as an aid in interpretation of results. Dilute urine with S.G. less than 1.010 may be negative, especially prior to the sixth week of gestation; we recommend that negative assays on dilute urine be repeated on a new specimen. Prompt delivery of specimen to the laboratory is essential, since HCG may deteriorate on prolonged storage at room temperature, or even at 4° C. (Wide, 1962).

The stage of pregnancy has a marked influence on the incidence of false negatives, even if a very sensitive assay is used. Between the seventh and thirteenth weeks of gestation, even a relatively insensitive assay will be almost 100 per cent positive; if a large proportion of measurements are made before the sixth week of gestation, even the most sensitive assay may show an appreciable number of false negatives (Fig. 26–1).

Whether pregnancy is abnormal will also influence the percentage of false negatives; with ectopic pregnancy, or incomplete abortion, HCG levels frequently are low or undetectable.

Phenothiazine drugs are known to cause false positive bioassays, and apparently false positive immunoassays as well (Ravel *et al.*, 1969). Increased LH excretion has been suggested as a possible mechanism, but this is not yet established with certainty. There is evidence that promethazine (Phenergan) may inhibit agglutination, causing false positive results with tests based on hemagglutination inhibition or latex particle agglutination inhibition, but false negative results with tests based on direct latex particle agglutination (Tait, 1971).

Proteinuria in excess of 1 gm. per 24 hours may also cause false positive results on immunoassay as a result of cross reactions between antisera and urinary protein. This is not entirely related to sensitivity, since the Hyland and Ortho immunoassay systems have relatively low sensitivity, but a relatively high incidence of false positives due to proteinuria (Bell, 1969). Although highly purified HCG preparations with potency about 18,000 I.U. per mg. have been available for some time, manufacturers apparently use less purified preparations (about 6000 I.U. per mg.) and absorb the resulting antisera with normal sera or nonpregnant urine proteins. Despite the latter steps, some anti-HCG sera still react with nonspecific antigens (Horwitz *et al.*, 1971). Grossly bloody urine is also reported as a cause for false positive results.

Since the early 1960's a number of immunoassay systems for HCG have become commercially available in kit form. Although users can prepare their own reagents (Petchclai and Pongdherapol, 1970), this is seldom done in the U.S.A. For a number of reasons it is difficult to accurately evaluate relative merits of various commercial immunoassay systems based on reports in the literature:

1. Published reports are seldom comparable with respect to attention given technical details, specimen collection, stage of pregnancy, inclusion of abnormal pregnancies, and presence of interfering substances.

2. Manufacturers are constantly revising their products.

3. Different samples of a given product may give widely different results.

Tables I and II represent a composite based on our experience and reports in the literature. As previously noted, these reports often are inconsistent. According to Cabrera (1969): "Occasional bad lots of reagents . . . give very high proportions of false positives as well as false negatives. . . . The degree of deficiency (may vary) within the same lot. . . . Some boxes of a particular lot (are) unusable, while others from the same lot (are) satisfactory. . . . This unreliability . . . may result from damage . . . by extreme temperatures (during shipment). . . . It is recognized that the immunologic tests are fast and easy to perform, and possess a high degree of accuracy; . . . however, . . . many of these tests will go through periods of unreliability. . . . We strongly recommend that two . . . immunologic tests be used together. . . . Anything less is fraught with danger."

The slide tests noted in Table 26–1 are rapid and require only two minutes to perform. Sensitivity ranges from 2–8 I.U./ml. Reported incidences of false positives range from about 1 to 3 per cent, with about 2 to 6 per cent false negatives. It should be noted that the two slide tests with lowest sensitivity apparently do not have the highest specificity, but are reported to give false positives with proteinuria. One of the more sensitive slide tests (which may be used with either urine or serum) may show a prozone effect, with false negative results caused by high HCG concentrations; this may be detected if all negative results are repeated using a threefold dilution (McIssac and Karnauchow, 1971). Measurements of serum HCG by slide test are subject to prozone effect, and also to interference from elevated macroglobulin; incidence of false positives is apparently about 3 per cent, and incidence of "inconclusive" tests, about 4 per cent (Horwitz *et al.*, 1971). At present, the advantages of testing serum rather than urine do not appear to be well established.

The tube tests noted in Table 26–2 are all based on hemagglutination inhibition; most require one to two hours incubation. Sensitivity ranges from 0.7–2.0 I.U./ml. Reported incidences of false positives range from about 0.5 to 2 per cent, with about 1 to 4 per cent false negatives. The higher sensitivity is accompanied by a somewhat lower incidence of false positives than with slide tests, since the latter may be affected by proteinuria (Knight *et al.*, 1972; Bell, 1969). One of the tube tests may be used with undiluted urine to give a sensitivity of 0.3 I.U./ml.; although this may be useful to detect ectopic pregnancy and incomplete abortion, an increased incidence of false positives may be expected due to cross reactions with LH.

In addition to drugs, proteinuria, and hematuria, other causes for "false positive" results include: (1) menopause or ovarian failure (increased LH levels); (2) hydatidiform mole or choriocarcinoma; (3) ovarian cysts, teratomas, and carcinomas (? production of gonadotropin-like substances); (4) testicular seminoma, teratoma, and embryonal carcinoma (? foci of choriocarcinoma); (5) pituitary tumors and bronchogenic carcinomas (? production of gonadotropin-like substance); (6) tubo-ovarian abscess – the slide test may be positive (sensitivity about 3 I.U./ml.) with negative tube test (sensitivity about 1 I.U./ml.); the reason for this nonspecific interference is not known (Arkin and Noto, 1972); and (7) scrotal abscess – this may be due to nonspecific interference similar to that observed with tubo-ovarian abscess (Arkin and Noto, 1972).

A *minimum* quality control program for HCG assays requires that each assay be performed in duplicate using kits from two different manufacturers (Cabrera, 1969). However, this approach can detect only gross errors in reagents or technique, and discrepancies are difficult to evaluate. We recommend that, whenever possible, the user should regularly recheck sensitivity against materials which can be related to the International Standard. In our experience, manufacturers show little enthusiasm for supplying such material; however, scientists engaged in research on HCG are often willing to either: (1) assay samples from a *thoroughly mixed* pool of pregnancy urine (a liter of urine collected during the tenth week of pregnancy and frozen in aliquots will last for several years!); or (2) provide frozen or lyophilized samples of known HCG concentration, which can be used as secondary standards.

Such standards enable the user to independently check commercial reagents and to detect shifts in sensitivity which otherwise would not be apparent. It is probably unnecessary to run a "standard" with each test; a "low positive" (2-4 × test sensitivity) and "high negative" (1/4 − 1/2 × test sensitivity) probably are adequate to detect gross alterations in reagents. If the high negative becomes positive, deterioration of reagents can be suspected and further checks run against samples from males and nonpregnant females. (Male urine may react differently from nonpregnant female urine, possibly due to differences in mucoprotein content.) If the low positive becomes negative, there has been a change in test sensitivity, and recalibration (plus correspondence with the manufacturer!) is indicated.

Dilutions of HCG standard or urine samples from patients may be performed by either direct dilution or serial dilution. One may use either normal urine, phosphate buffered saline (pH 6.4) with 0.1 per cent bovine serum albumin, or phosphate buffered saline alone (pH 6.4), with reagents at either refrigerator temperature or room temperature. There is a tendency for somewhat higher values on direct dilution rather than serial dilution. This may be related either to absorption of HCG on glass during repeated transfers, or to denaturation of HCG (Tamada *et al.*, 1969).

There is a tendency for somewhat higher values when specimen aliquots are diluted with normal urine or 0.1 per cent albumin buffer, rather than buffered saline. Although the effect of normal urine is comparable to 0.1 per cent albumin, the protein content of normal urine is far less than 0.1 per cent; presumably "protective substances" other than albumin are involved. This "protective effect" of normal urine seems to vary somewhat between different individuals (Tamada *et al.*, 1969). A similar result was noted by Wide (1962), who reported that HCG dissolved in urine retained activity longer than if dissolved in saline. We have noted a tendency for HCG denaturation to proceed more slowly in concentrated solutions than in dilute preparations; perhaps HCG itself may have some degree of protective effect.

There is a tendency for somewhat higher values when specimen aliquots are diluted at "cool" temperature, rather than room temperature. Slow denaturation of HCG at room temperature may be involved.

OTHER "PREGNANCY TESTS"

A variety of colorimetric "pregnancy tests" have been described, based on the color change which occurs when urine is mixed with iodine or a halogenated cresol derivative. Although 97 per cent of pregnancy urines give a positive result with one procedure, the incidence of false positives is over 60 per cent (Schales, 1969). A commercial kit based on this principle has been shown to give over 30 per cent false negatives as well as over 30 per cent false positives (Fairweather and Cremer, 1972). In our opinion, these procedures are unsuitable for clinical use.

Various clinical tests for pregnancy have been described, based on administration of estrogen plus progesterone. In these procedures, progesterone is the key hormone; estrogen merely ensures priming of the endometrium. In a nonpregnant woman, cessation of progesterone effect is followed by bleeding. However, in pregnancy the endometrium is maintained by progesterone plus estrogen from the corpus luteum and placenta. Such tests may utilize either: (1) administration of progesterone (intramuscularly plus oral estrogen) (Graber *et al.*, 1970); or (2) oral administration of norethindrone plus estradiol (Gestest tablets, available from Squibb Pharmaceutical Co.). About 90 per cent of nonpregnant women have bleeding within five to 10 days; about 90 per cent of pregnant women have no evidence of bleeding. Although we have no personal experience with these tests, the following limitations are reported: (1) possible fetal teratogenic risk (there is no definite evidence of this in women); (2) possible thrombotic phenomena; (3) possible exacerbation of migraine, asthma, and epilepsy; (4) results may be unreliable in patients with irregular menses; and (5) contraindicated in nursing mothers, due to possible masculinizing effects of progesterone.

SUMMARY

Immunologic pregnancy tests based on detection of HCG have largely replaced bioassays for routine clinical use. Although bioassays can give good results, they require more time and attention for proper calibration and control than the immunologic methods. However, despite their speed and simplicity, HCG immunoassays DO REQUIRE careful standardization: poor results may be expected if the user does not understand the potential pitfalls and take measures to avoid them (Cabrera, 1969).

Reported accuracy of different pregnancy tests varies over a wide range; the many factors which may cause false negatives as well as false positives must be considered when evaluating reports in the literature.

REFERENCES

Arkin, C., and Noto, T. A.: A false positive immunologic pregnancy test with tubo-ovarian abscess. Amer. J. Clin. Path. *58*:314, 1972.

Aschheim, S., and Zondek, B.: Pregnancy diagnosis with urine by the demonstration of the hormone. Klin. Wschr. 7:8, 1928.

Bahl, O. P., Carlsen, R. B., Bellisario, R., Swaminathan, N.: Human chorionic gonadotropin: Amino acid sequence of the alpha and beta subunits. Biochem. Biophys. Res. Commun. *48*:416, 1972.

Bell, J. L.: Comparative study of immunological tests for pregnancy diagnosis. J. Clin. Path. *22*:79, 1969.

Bellerby, C. W.: A rapid test for the diagnosis of pregnancy. Nature (London) *133*:494, 1934.

Borth, R., Ferin, M., and Menzi, A.: Comparison of bioassay and immunoassay of human chorionic gonadotropin in urine. Acta Endocr. *50*:335, 1965.

Cabrera, H. A.: A comprehensive evaluation of pregnancy tests. Amer. J. Obstet. Gynec. *103*:32, 1969.

Driscoll, S. G., Strauss, W. F., Alba, M., Altschul, H. S., and Hager, H. J.: Evaluation of a new slide test for pregnancy. Amer. J. Obstet. Gynec. *110*:1083, 1971.

Fairweather, D. L., and Cremer, A. W.: Do-it-yourself pregnancy kit. Brit. Med. J. *1*:747, 1972.

Frank, R. T., and Berman, R. L.: A twenty-four hour pregnancy test. Amer. J. Obstet. Gynec. *42*:492, 1941.

Friedman, M. H., and Lapham, M. E.: A simple rapid method for the laboratory diagnosis of early pregnancies. Amer. J. Obstet. Gynec. *21*:405, 1931.

Galli-Mainini, C.: Pregnancy test using the male batrachia. J.A.M.A. *138*:121, 1948.

Glass, R. H., and Jesurun, H. M.: Immunologic pregnancy tests in ectopic pregnancy. Obstet. Gynec. *27*:66, 1966.

Graber, E. A., Barber, H. R. K., and O'Rourke, J. J.: A clinical test for pregnancy. Amer. J. Obstet. Gynec. *108*:991, 1970.

Headden, G. F.: An evaluation of immunological pregnancy tests. Med. Lab. Technol. *29*:332, 1972.

Hibbard, B. M.: Pregnancy diagnosis. Brit. Med. J. *1*:593, 1971.

Hobson, B. M.: Pregnancy diagnosis using the Pregnosticon haemagglutination inhibition test. J. Obstet. Gynec. Brit. Cwlth. *75*:718, 1968.

Hobson, B., and Wide, L.: The immunological and biological activity of human gonadotropin in urine. Acta Endocr., *46*:632, 1964.

Hon, E. H.: *A Manual of Pregnancy Testing.* Boston, Little, Brown and Company, 1961.

Horwitz, C. A., Polesky, H., Odenbrett, P., Gronli, M., Horowitz, A., Diamond, R., and Ward, P. C. J.: Clinical and immunologic study of a direct agglutination test for pregnancy. Amer. J. Obstet. Gynec. *111*:808, 1971.

Kerber, I. J., Inclan, P., Fowler, E. A., Davis, K., and Fish, S. A.: Immunologic tests for pregnancy. Obstet. Gynec. *36*: 37, 1970.

Knight, R. A., Kilpatrick, L., and Porter, M. M.: Evaluation of two new pregnancy tests. Amer. J. Med. Technol. *37*: 397, 1971.

Lamb, E. J.: Immunologic pregnancy tests. Obstet. Gynec. *39*:665, 1972.

Lau, H. L.: Tests for pregnancy. *In Tice's Practice of Medicine.* Hagerstown, Maryland, Harper and Row, 1970, Chapter 29.

McIsaac, S. F., and Karnauchow, P. N.: Prozone phenomenon in the direct agglutination test for pregnancy. Amer. J. Obstet. Gynec. *109*:1213, 1971.

Morgan, F. J., and Canfield, R. E.: Nature of the subunits of human chorionic gonadotropins. Endocrinology *88*:1045, 1971.

Petchclai, B., and Pongdherapol, U.: A new microhemagglutination inhibition pregnancy test. Amer. J. Clin. Path. *54*:810, 1970.

Ravel, R., Riekers, H. G., and Goldstein, B. J.: Effects of certain psychotropic drugs on pregnancy tests. Amer. J. Obstet. Gynec. *105*:1222, 1969.

Robbins, J. L., Hill, G. A., Carle, B. N., Carlquist, J. H., and Marcus, S.: Latex agglutination reactions between human chorionic gonotropin and rabbit antibody. Proc. Soc. Exp. Biol. Med. *109*:321, 1962.

Salk, J. E.: A simplified procedure for titrating hemagglutination capacity of influenza virus and the corresponding antibody. J. Immunol. *49*:87, 1944.

Saltzberger, M., and Nelken, D.: The immunologic pregnancy test. Amer. J. Obstet. Gynec. *86*:899, 1963.

Schales, O.: Chemical nature of the urinary "pregnancy test" with iodine, Clin. Chim. Acta *26*:323, 1969.

Tait, B.: Interference in immunological methods of pregnancy testing by promethazine. Med. J. Aust. 2:126, 1971.

Tamada, T., Maruyama, M., and Matsumoto, S.: Qualitative and quantitative studies on a new pregnancy test by latex direct agglutination reaction. Int. J. Fertil. *16*:101, 1971.

Tamada, T., Tsukui, Y., and Matsumoto, S.: On diluent and dilution method in hemagglutination inhibition test for human chorionic gonadotropin. Endocrinol. Jap. *16*:399, 1969.

Tietz, N. W.: Comparative study of immunologic and biologic pregnancy tests in early pregnancy. Obstet. Gynec. *25*: 197, 1965.

Varma, K., Larraga, L., and Selenkow, H. A.: Radioimmunoassay of serum human chorionic gonadotropin during normal pregnancy. Obstet. Gynec. *37*:10, 1971.

Wan, A. T.: Simple method for assay of luteinizing hormone in urine. Obstet. Gynec. *36*:88, 1970.

Wide, L.: An immunological method for the assay of human chorionic gonadotropin. Acta Endocr. *70*(Suppl.): 1962. (Vol. 4.)

Wide, L.: Early diagnosis of pregnancy. Lancet 2:863, 1969.

Wide, L., and Gemzell, C. A.: An immunological pregnancy test. Acta Endocrin. *35*:261, 1960.

Wiltberger, P. B., and Miller, D. F.: The male frog, *Rana pipiens,* as a new test animal for early pregnancy. Science *107*:198, 1948.

Yahia, C.: The quantitative toad test in normal and abnormal early gestation. Obstet. Gynec. *23*:547, 1964.

Chapter 27

AMNIOTIC FLUID AND ANTENATAL DIAGNOSIS

by ROBERT E. WENK, M.D., JERALD M. ROSENBAUM, M.D., and JOHN BERNARD HENRY, M.D.

Amniotic fluid was an untapped source of laboratory data until 1952 when Bevis suggested that it could yield information relating to hemolytic disease of the newborn. Amniotic fluid analysis subsequently proved to be more useful than maternal serum antibody titration in the management of the isoimmunization syndrome. More recently, amniotic fluid has been used to investigate other fetal disorders.

ANATOMIC AND PHYSIOLOGIC CONSIDERATIONS

The amniotic sac arises during the first week of gestation from embryonic tissues. It consists of an outer layer of mesoderm and an inner layer of ectoderm. The amniotic cavity enlarges, reflects over the embryo and its umbilical cord, and may be safely tapped (amniocentesis) by 14 weeks. At term (40 weeks), the sac contains 0.5 to 2.5 liters of fluid, which is apparently produced by cells of the fetal respiratory tract, umbilical cord and amniotic membrane. Fetal urine probably contributes little volume (Reynolds, 1969).

Normally water exchanges between the amniotic fluid and mother, between mother and fetus, and between fetus and fluid. As pregnancy advances the exchange between fetus and mother increases. In hydramnios, however, the feto-maternal exchange decreases, while the fetus increases its water contribution of fluid. The fluid, in turn, increases its contribution of water to the mother (Hutchinson *et al.*, 1959).

In effect, in the first half of pregnancy, amniotic fluid can be regarded as an extension of fetal extracellular fluid (Lind and Hytten, 1970). Rapidly developing fetal edema is therefore accompanied by acute hydramnios in disorders such as recipient-twin transfusion syndrome, hydrops fetalis, and fetal heart failure. Chronic hydramnios develops when the fetus fails to swallow fluid and is associated with a 20 per cent incidence of fetal malformations such as anencephaly or esophageal atresia. Chronic hydramnios is also associated with maternal disease (toxemia, diabetes). Oligohydramnios may be produced by chronically ill fetuses who swallow more frequently than normal. Therefore, there is often oligohydramnios in placental insufficiency or donor-twin transfusion syndrome.

At term, amniotic water is exchanged at the high rate of 500 ml. per hour; solutes in the water (1 per cent w./w.) exchange at slower rates. A rapid serial rise in osmolality sometimes occurs in diabetic mothers and predicts a grave fetal outcome (Cassady and Barnett, 1968).

The many solutes of amniotic fluid have been studied; however, further discussion is directed toward clinically relevant measurements.

HEMOLYTIC DISEASE

Sampling of amniotic fluid is now a common procedure in the isoimmunization syndrome. Although passive maternal immunization with anti-Rho(D) can effectively prevent isoimmunization in most susceptible women, sporadic cases will still occur. Severe hemolytic disease will result from untreated mothers, iatrogenic failures, sensitization by transfusion, and following abortion (Matthews *et al.*, 1969). Some of the isoimmunizations will be directed against the Rho(D) antigen, but others will involve blood group antigens such as K_1, hr′, and rh^w (Liley, 1970). The principles of management of these cases are identical to those established for Rho(D) isoimmunization.

When maternal antibodies cross the placenta to react with fetal erythrocyte antigens, hemolysis is detectable as early as 16 weeks' gestation and may progress at an increasing rate until term. As fetal hemoglobin is catabolized to bilirubin, fetal plasma carries an increased concentration of unconjugated bilirubin to the placenta. The placenta excretes the pigment unless there is feto-placental compromise. When unconjugated bilirubin increases in the fetal circulation, glucuronyl transferase activity is triggered earlier than normal so that conjugated bilirubin is detectable at 28 weeks (Brodersen *et al.*, 1967). The conjugate is not cleared by the placenta and accounts for some of the pigment (1 to 50 per cent) found in amniotic fluid. The majority of the pigment, however, is unconjugated bilirubin (Brazie *et al.*, 1966). In mild hemolytic disease, the fetus is not jaundiced *in utero*.

Principles of Amniotic Fluid Analysis in Isoimmunization Syndrome

The examination of amniotic fluid in the maternal isoimmunization syndrome is based on the fact that breakdown products of hemolysis, such as bilirubin or methemalbumin, are found in amniotic fluid. It is still unclear how these substances enter the amniotic sac.

The bilirubin pigment is apparently bound to albumin, and its concentration in the amniotic fluid is then maintained despite the rapid turnover rate of amniotic fluid water, since the turnover time for amniotic fluid protein is much longer.

A specimen of amniotic fluid may be withdrawn, filtered, and examined with a spectrophotometer. If the absorbance of the fluid is recorded continuously between 350 and 700 nm., the resulting curve can be used to detect: (1) whether or not the fluid contains bilirubin and/or other products of hemolysis, and (2) the quantity of pigment which is present.

Liley (1963) has shown that the net absorbance at 450 nm. from sensitized patients who have unaffected babies always decreases with progression of the gestation. A similar diminution in absorbance is noted in affected babies as well. Quantitative characterization of the significance of decreasing bilirubin concentration (the chief component of the 450 nm. peak) with increasing length of gestation is illustrated in Liley's prediction graph (Fig. 27–1). The slope of the boundaries demarcating three zones of the graph indicates that, at least

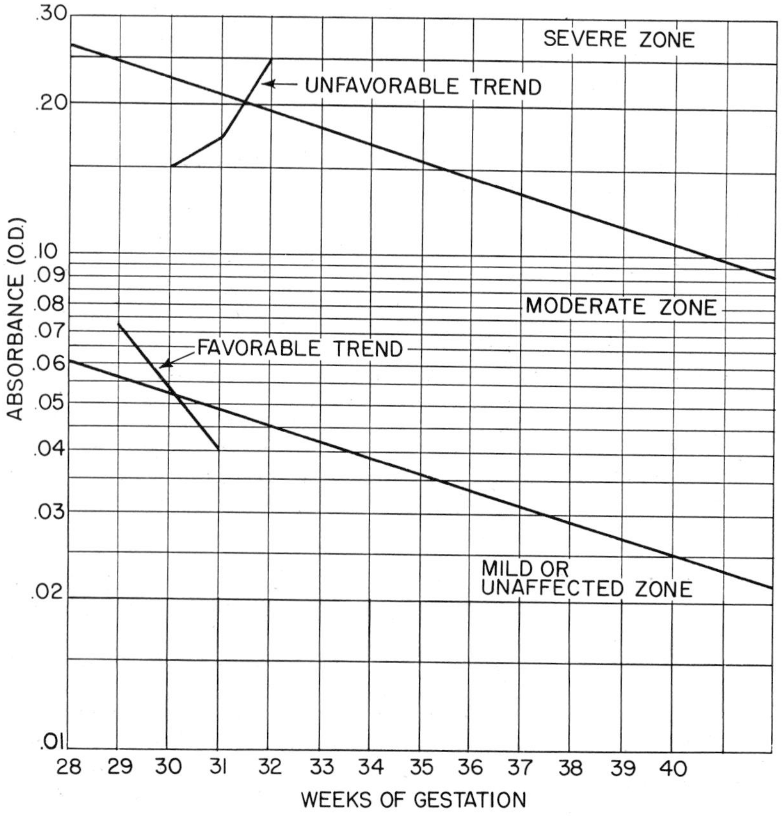

Figure 27–1. Zones indicate normal decreasing pigment concentration at 450 nm. related to duration of pregnancy. Multiple weekly scans may reveal increasing (or stationary) net absorbance (O.D.), indicating progressive hemolysis (unfavorable trend); they may also show decreasing net absorbance (O.D.), indicating regression of disease (favorable trend).

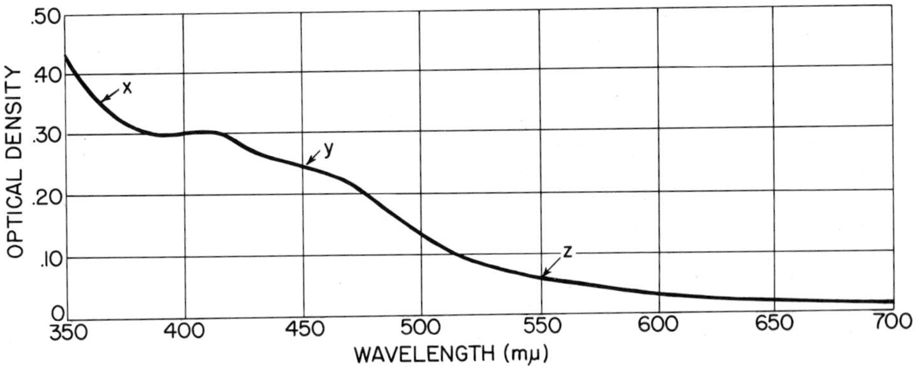

Figure 27–2. Scan of slightly abnormal amniotic fluid showing three points used in determining net optical density (see method described in text).

for bilirubin, there is a logarithmic decrease in its concentration in the amniotic fluid as pregnancy progresses. These observations may be the result of a physiological dilution of the amniotic fluid toward the end of pregnancy.

PROCEDURE. Approximately 5 ml. of amniotic fluid is collected by the obstetrician when he considers the maternal Rh antibody titer is critical, i.e., when a stillbirth or severely affected infant is anticipated (Freda, 1966a). "Critical" usually means an antibody titer of 1:16 (± 1 dilution) or higher in the antiglobulin phase. The specimen is sent in an opaque container (bilirubin is light sensitive) to a clinical pathology laboratory, where it is centrifuged at 4000 r.p.m. in the dark for 10 minutes. An additional filtration through Whatman No. 4 filter paper (in the dark) is occasionally necessary to remove turbidity. If erythrocytes are present, the sediment is submitted to the blood bank and hematology laboratories, where the cells are identified as maternal or fetal by serologic typing, Coombs antiglobulin testing, and the Betke-Kleihauer method* for identifying fetal red cells (Betke and Kleihauer, 1958). Specimens may be mailed to reference laboratories for analysis provided they are sterile, centrifuged or filtered before shipment, and sent in opaque containers.

A spectral absorption curve of clear fluid is made with a recording spectrophotometer against a distilled water blank. The absorbance (optical density, or O.D.) is recorded from the scan at three points:

1. 365 nm.: O.D. = x
2. 450 nm.: O.D. = y
3. 550 nm.: O.D. = z

The absorbance at 365 nm. and at 550 nm. is transferred from the original *linear* scan recording (Fig. 27–2) to semilog scale (ordinate, O.D. in log scale; abscissa, wavelength in linear scale), and a straight line is drawn between x and z (Fig. 27–3). Some workers do not transfer the linear scan points to semilog paper. This practice produces inaccurate net O.D. results (Nelson and Talledo, 1969). The "expected" O.D., or absorbance, is the point on the drawn line that intersects with the 450 nm. wavelength. This line represents background absorbance of normal non-bilirubin-containing amniotic fluid. Point y on the original scan is the "true O.D."

True O.D. at 450 nm. − expected O.D. at 450 nm. = net O.D. at 450 nm.

An assessment (based on net O.D.) of fetal prognosis is reported (Liley, 1963). A statement regarding fetal viability may also be reported if the net O.D. is calculated directly from the linear scan (Freda, 1966).

INTERPRETATION OF SPECTROPHOTOMETRIC TRACINGS. Although a single scan of a specimen collected from 28 to 38 weeks of gestation may be used to predict the severity of hemolytic disease in terms of cord hemoglobin, multiple sequential specimens or serial scans are most often required. The method of Liley is representative of this predictive type of interpretation. Its reliability and accuracy have been confirmed by considerable experience in many laboratories. Liley initially subdivided Rh-immunized mothers into three groups (Fig. 27–1):

1. *Small net O.D. at 450 nm.* These infants were either mildly affected or unaffected by hemolytic disease and required no transfusion.

2. *Moderate net O.D. at 450 nm.* These infants survived but often required one or more exchange transfusions.

3. *Large net O.D. at 450 nm.* These infants had grave prognoses. This zone included most stillbirths and neonatal deaths that occurred despite exchange transfusions. Subsequently,

*Blood films of fetal cells withstand acid elution and appear normal after subsequent staining. Adult hemoglobin is denatured by acid elution, so erythrocytes appear as ghosts on staining.

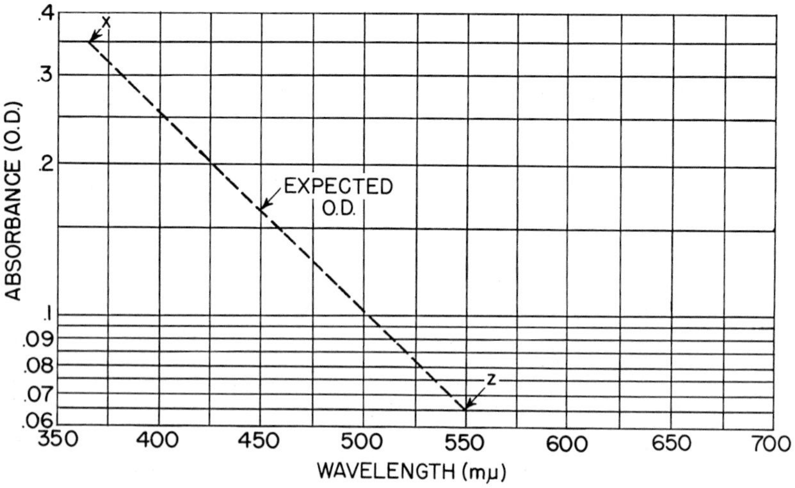

Figure 27-3. Wavelength vs. absorbance in log scale showing two points transferred from actual scan (x, z) and expected optical density (O.D.) at 450 nm.

Liley (1963) subdivided the moderate zone into halves: the upper half readings usually became worse with lengthening gestation, while the values in the lower half often improved with time. Subdivision of the severe zone into severe and very severe zones was also done (Fig. 27-4).

Predictions are valid *if the infant is delivered within one week following amniocentesis,* but the predictions are complicated by prematurity, since the date for induction of labor is preset. In other words, an infant that might be expected to do well on the basis of cord hemoglobin could do poorly because of its immaturity at the time of delivery.

Thus, this method does not incorporate the risk of prematurity in predicting fetal survival but simply permits selection of unaffected and mildly affected infants and those who are so severely affected that early delivery affords the only means of infant salvage despite the risks of prematurity.

Multiple scans beginning at 28 weeks may be used to follow the trend of hemolytic disease. If an abnormal scan is obtained initially, subsequent scans may show a reduction in severity (below that which would be expected from the diagonally sloped lines of Liley's graph). Such a favorable trend is especially apt to occur when an infant is only mildly affected. An unfavorable or stationary (horizontal) trend is likely to occur with increased hemolysis (Fig. 27-1).

Instead of predicting the severity of the disease of the newborn, it may be more valuable to correlate spectrophotometric analysis of amniotic fluid with the condition of the fetus, i.e., viability and Apgar rating (Freda, 1965). This correlation acknowledges the dangers caused by prematurity. Thus, spectrophotometric curves of amniotic fluid indicate the chances for survival of the fetus *in utero* for a given time period after amniocentesis and the chances for survival of the infant if it is delivered during this time period.

Two shortcomings may be noted in using this method. First, repeated amniocenteses, with their attendant obstetrical risks, are usually necessary, since the given "safe" time periods are brief (one to two weeks). Second, despite the advantage of setting a parameter for obstetrical management (i.e., whether to induce delivery or allow the pregnancy to continue for two weeks), the method does not make a prediction of severity of disease in terms of cord hemoglobin or number of transfusions required. It is quite disconcerting for the pediatrician caring for a severely jaundiced and anemic newborn requiring four or five exchange transfusions to recall a scan interpreted previously by the pathologist or obstetrician as showing only a slight to moderately abnormal amniotic pattern (Robertson, 1969).

Both methods of reporting may be used—permitting obstetric management and predicting the severity of hemolytic disease in the newborn (Figs. 27-4 and 27-5).

A series of representative tracings are shown to illustrate various possible interpretations.

1. Normal amniotic fluid is colorless to the naked eye. When a specimen is scanned on a recording spectrophotometer between 350 and 700 nm., a curve is obtained which relates a decrease in absorbance (O.D.) with increasing wavelength in the visible range. The curve is flat in the red (700 nm.) range of the spectrum but then becomes steeper toward the violet (short, 350 nm.) range (Fig. 27-6). A normal scan indicates either that the fetus is not afflicted with hemolytic disease or that it is mildly affected but is in no danger for the two weeks following the amniocentesis (Freda, 1966b). Cord hemoglobin, if the infant was delivered within a week, could be predicted according to the percentage probability given by Liley (Fig. 27-4).

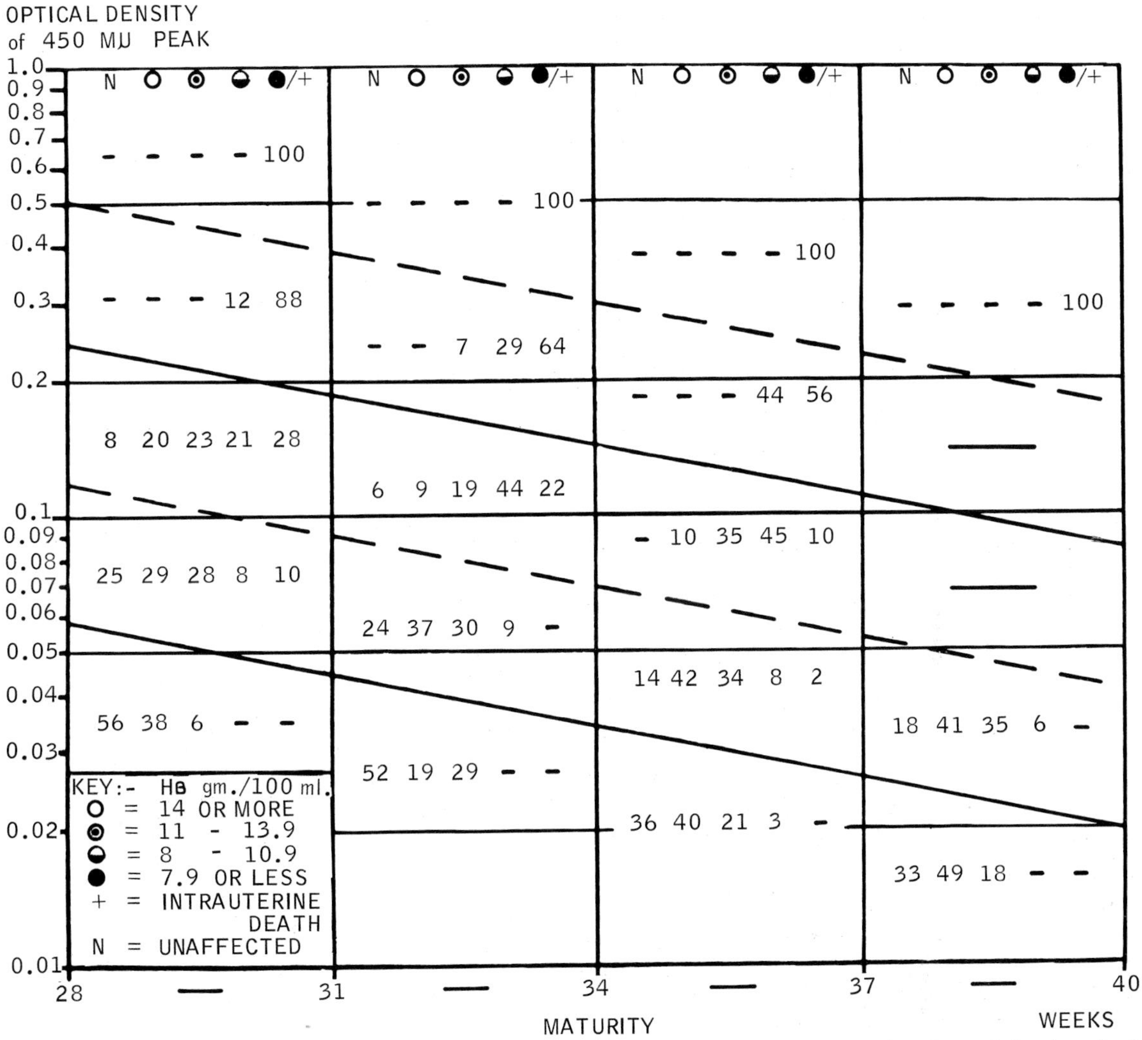

Figure 27–4. Liley prediction table. Percentage probability of the various grades of affliction for the peak size in a single specimen (From Liley, A. W.: Amer. J. Obstet. Gynec. *86*:485, 1963).

2. A slightly abnormal tracing indicates a mildly affected fetus at the time of amniocentesis; this may regress to a normal curve or may progress to a more abnormal curve in 10 days' time. The curve is characterized by an increase in absorbance above the normal scan between 375 nm. and 550 nm., with the peak of the increase occurring at approximately 450 nm.

3. Moderately abnormal tracings (Fig. 27–7) show greater increase in absorbance between 375 nm. and 550 nm. As in the slightly abnormal tracing, peak absorbance occurs at 450 nm. The latter wavelength bisects the

Grading of Abnormal Tracing	Optical Density Difference at 450 mμ
1+	0–0.2
2+	0.2 –0.35
3+	0.35–0.7
4+	0.7 and greater

Figure 27–5. Freda management table. *1+*, fetus unaffected or mildly affected at time of amniocentesis. *2+*, fetus affected but not in jeopardy. *3+*, fetus in distress. *4+*, impending fetal demise (From Freda: Progr. Hematol., 1966).

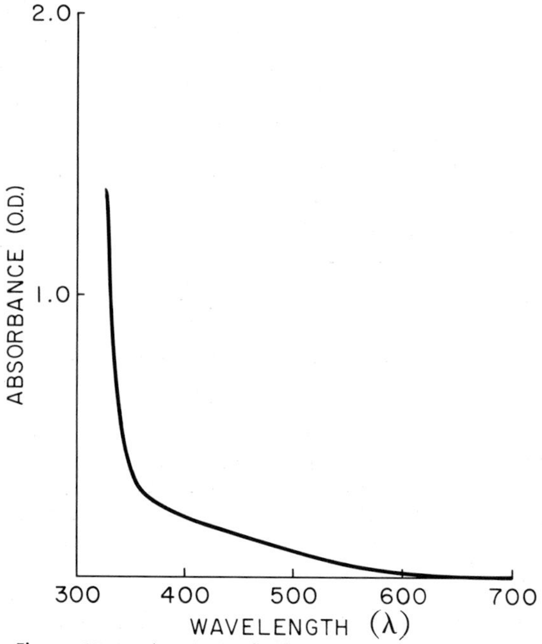

Figure 27–6. Amniotic fluid, normal scan (redrawn). Absorbance (O. D., optical density) vs. wavelength.

abnormal "bulge" in the curve. A moderately abnormal tracing usually indicates mild to moderate hemolytic disease, but severe disease is not uncommon. If the disease is severe, it is safe to allow the fetus to mature for one week (when the tracing is repeated), or the infant is delivered if it is sufficiently mature (e.g., 37 to 38 weeks). If a repeat tracing shows an unfavorable trend, delivery or intrauterine transfusion may be warranted. Working criteria for fetal transfusion have been developed for the methods of Liley and Freda (Wade *et al.*, 1969).

4. Markedly abnormal tracings show very large pigment absorbance "bulges" with peak net optical densities ranging from 0.35 to over 1.00 (3+ and 4+ of Freda). The most severely abnormal curves still retain the increased absorbance range of 375 nm. to 525 nm., but the peak absorbance is shifted from 450 nm. to a lower wavelength. This shift indicates a decrease in the pH of the amniotic fluid (normal pH 7.2), which is a sign of fetal death or impending death.

With markedly abnormal curves, due either to bilirubin pigmentation or staining by other pigments or meconium, the readings at 375 nm., 450 nm., and 550 nm. may be off scale (i.e., too high for the spectrophotometer recorder). A several-fold dilution with distilled water may be necessary to obtain the net O.D. at 450 nm. Correction for this dilution is made by calculation.

5. Bloody amniotic fluid usually results from trauma to maternal tissues. Occasionally a placental vessel on the fetal side is lacerated. Erythrocytes that escape into the amniotic fluid may be identified as fetal by antiglobulin technique, Rh typing, and the Betke-Kleihauer blood film for detecting fetal hemoglobin. Identification of fetal cells is important for three reasons: First, a second source of blood loss is established in a fetus that already has a compromising anemia. Anemia itself may be associated with hypoxic jaundice and kernicterus even with low bilirubin levels (Gartner and Bernstein, 1965). Second, it may also explain a sudden rise in maternal antibody response if the fetus bleeds into the maternal circulation. Third, escape of fetal plasma into amniotic fluid causes abnormal tracings, since the circulating plasma bilirubin of even unaffected infants is normally high.

Maternal blood distorts the normal tracing, but the scan may be interpreted unless the cell: total-fluid-volume ratio of the specimen is 0.05 or more. If the ratio is exceeded, hemolysis is usually sufficient to obscure the bilirubin absorbance peak at 450 nm. (See supplementary techniques.) The amniotic fluid curve is also distorted by maternal plasma contamination, with moderate maternal bleeding. A second clear sample should be obtained (if the hemorrhage was minor) just after the bloody tap and before diffusion has occurred in the amniotic sac. A major hemorrhage requires about two weeks to be cleared from the amniotic fluid. Major bleeding, with hemolysis of erythrocytes and release of hemoglobin, shows the three characteristic peaks of oxyhemoglobin at 415

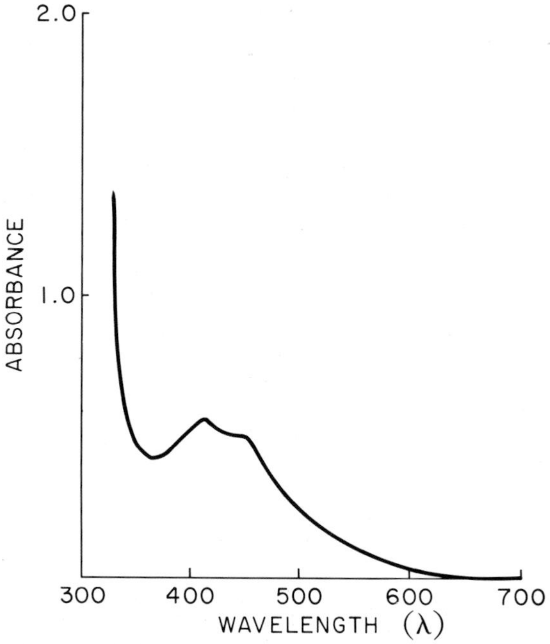

Figure 27–7. Scan of moderately abnormal amniotic fluid indicating hemolytic disease of newborn.

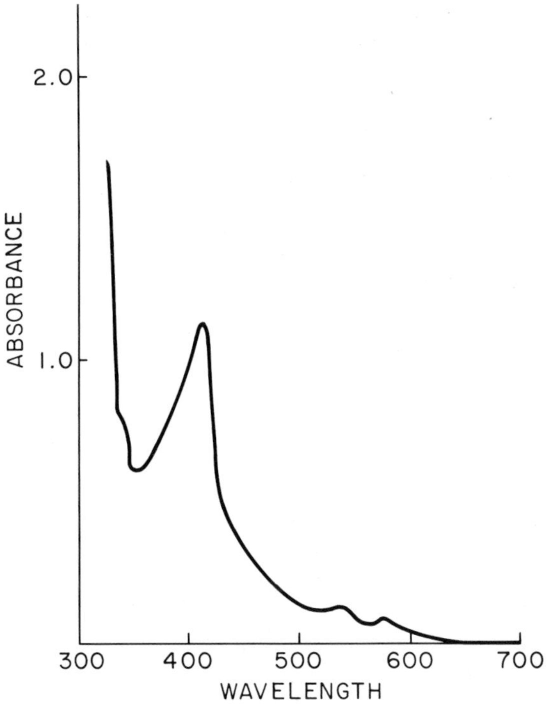

Figure 27-8. Moderate hemorrhage and hemolysis in amniotic fluid.

nm., 540 nm., and 575 nm. (Fig. 27-8). Minor bleeding may show only the Soret band at 415 nm. Generally the presence of these pigments decreases net absorbance at 450 nm., causing underestimation of fetal disease. (See supplementary techniques described subsequently.)

6. Meconium staining of amniotic fluid sample indicates fetal distress; it may or may not accompany hemolytic disease; and it may indicate related or unrelated complications of the anemia. In small quantities meconium may be identified spectrophotometrically; beginning at the red end of the spectrum, the tracing parallels that of normal amniotic fluid until about 525 nm., where it rises steadily above the baseline and reaches a peak absorbance at 405 to 410 nm. The absorbance then slowly recedes and does not return to the baseline, at 350 to 375 nm. (Fig. 27-9). Larger quantities of meconium are easily identified grossly by the turbid, dark, green-black color; however, underlying hemolytic disease is obscured. The problem is not easily resolved, because meconium contains bilirubin. Chloroform extraction of fluid stained either by meconium or hemolysis shows bilirubin pigmentation (Fig. 27-10 A). Resolution of the problem may be obtained clinically. Meconium staining early in gestation is usually not caused by, or associated with, hemolytic disease and usually clears as term approaches. Staining near term is an indication for early delivery (Liley, 1963).

7. Occasionally, in a severely affected infant, in addition to a markedly abnormal tracing, an additional peak is observed at about 620 nm. This is the absorbance peak of methemalbumin. This pigment may be better demonstrated by modifications of Schumm's test* (Fig. 27-10 *B*). In addition to the methemalbumin band at 620 nm., some of the methemalbumin may be complexed to form a hemochromogen peak at 558 nm. Presence of methemalbumin indicates massive hemolysis of long standing, depletion of haptoglobin, and a fetus that is either dead or dying.

8. The clinical pathologist should bear in mind that the obstetrician who performs amniocentesis may have technical problems in obtaining fluid when the placenta and fetus are difficult to identify and localize or when the infant is hydropic. Under these circumstances, the fluid submitted to the laboratory may not be amniotic in origin. Thus, fetal ascitic fluid, fluid from the amnion of an unaffected or affected twin, amniotic cyst fluid, and urine from the maternal urinary bladder may be aspirated.

The most common nonamniotic fluid obtained is maternal urine. The spectrophotometric tracing is similar to normal amniotic fluid, except that there is a much steeper slope

*Spectrophotometric analysis of amniotic fluid after layering with ether and shaking with ammonium sulfide.

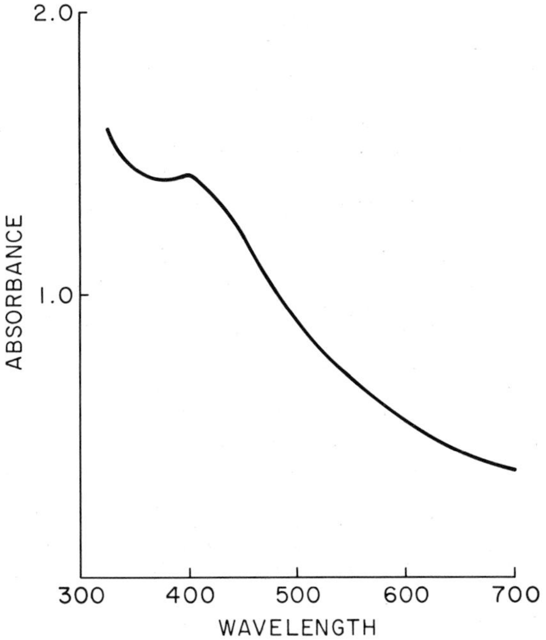

Figure 27-9. Slight-moderate staining by meconium in amniotic fluid.

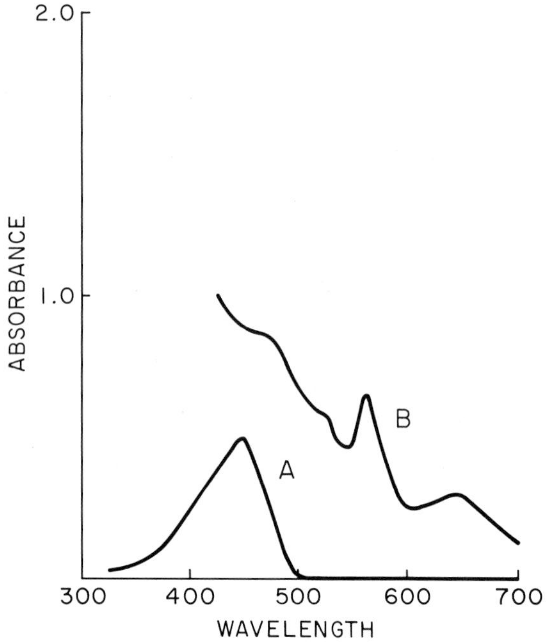

Figure 27–10. A, Chloroform solution of bilirubin (chloroform extract of meconium-stained amniotic fluid). This curve may be seen after extracting amniotic fluid in isoimmunization syndrome or in fluid containing meconium. B, Hemochromogen complex of methemalbumin (ether extraction, scan of residue – Schumm test).

to the curve. Normal maternal urine may be distinguished from amniotic fluid by urea nitrogen measurement. Urine urea nitrogen should approximate a concentration of 300 mg./dl., or higher; amniotic fluid urea nitrogen averages about 30 mg./dl.

SUPPLEMENTARY TECHNIQUES IN HEMOLYTIC DISEASE

Criteria have been suggested for obstetric decisions, e.g., when to perform first and subsequent amniocenteses, when to deliver, and when to attempt fetal transfusion. Management has usually been based on the concepts of Liley and Freda, which prove clinically satisfactory in over 95 per cent of patients (Robertson, 1969).

A major difficulty in the laboratory is contamination of aspirated fluid by blood pigments and by meconium, which obscure the bilirubin peak on spectrophotometric scan. When this occurs, a diazo chemical determination of bilirubin can be performed either by the Jendrassik-Grof procedure, which reduces interference by hemoglobin (Gambino and Freda, 1966), or a modified Malloy-Evelyn method, which eliminates methemoglobin or methemalbumin interference but not gross hemolysis. Bilirubin concentration may be converted to net O.D. for use with the Liley prediction table (Kapitulnik *et al.*, 1970).

Attempts to extract and measure bilirubin in chloroform or benzene are less precise and slower; results must often be subjectively judged with spectrophotometric tracings, gross hemolysis still interferes, and conjugated bilirubin is not measured. Extraction is not recommended.

Admittedly, spectrophotometric or chemical methods are not completely satisfactory. Variation in laboratory technique produces variable obstetric decisions. Specimens may be exposed to light, change in pH, or contain heme pigments. There are differences in instruments, standards, and methods. In fact, much of the success of current methods is directly attributable to vigorous clinical management following repeated amniocenteses rather than to the predictive value of amniotic fluid analysis, which by itself yields a 10 to 15 per cent error rate. Another source of error is varying dilution, which occurs in fluids of different patients at different gestational ages.

A spectrophotometric method has recently been developed which appears to be insensitive to heme pigments, dilution, and observer bias, but still measures bilirubin directly (Ovenstone and Connon, 1968). The method depends on deriving an optical density difference (O.D.D.) curve by subtracting the absorbance at each wavelength from the absorbance value at a wavelength 10 nm. lower. The new curve shows a bilirubin peak at 490 nm. that is proportional in height to bilirubin concentration:

$$\text{Concentration of bilirubin (mg./dl.)} = 2\ (\text{O.D.D. at 490 nm.}) - 0.04$$

More simply, a factor on a scale of 0 to 100 may be used which directly predicts fetal outcome (Connon, 1969). This "Ovenstone factor" is less than 10 in unaffected or mildly affected infants and is over 30 units in severely affected infants. The factor is calculated:

$$2.3 \times (\text{O.D.D. at 480 nm.} - \text{O.D.D. at 500 nm.})$$

The method has been reported to be most accurate and simple and does not require knowledge of gestational age (Connon, 1969).

Other improved techniques have been proposed. Bilirubin/albumin ratios may predict fetal outcome more accurately than standard methods. Ratios higher than 0.10 mg./gm. indicate severe hemolysis; ratios less than 0.05 indicate mild disease or no hemolysis. There is apparent value in measuring hemopexin/albumin ratios as well, since hemopexin binds heme released from lysed cells and then is removed by the liver. Diminished hemopexin indicates hemolysis. The albumin denominator obviates dilution errors.

At this writing, these methods appear promising, but require confirmation and more extensive trial.

AMNIOTIC FLUID AND GENETIC DIAGNOSIS

Until recently genetic counseling of prospective parents had to be based almost solely on statistical probabilities. From amniotic fluid, fetal sex and blood group can be determined, and cells of fetal origin can be obtained and used for chromosome analysis or biochemical studies. Abnormal substances in the amniotic fluid can be identified and abnormal concentrations of normal constituents detected.

At the present time there are few fetal disorders which can be diagnosed by amniotic fluid analysis. The population at risk is small and is not always available. Fluid cannot be obtained safely before 14 weeks, and analytic methods are often complex, long, or inaccurate. Treatment is not often effective; therapeutic abortion may not be acceptable to the family and must be performed before the 25th week of pregnancy. Nevertheless, amniotic cell culture technique is the most promising source of information for antenatal diagnosis and should be undertaken in a variety of obstetric situations (Jacobson and Barter, 1969).

For sex-linked disorders, determination of fetal sex by amniotic cytology should be performed by a physician who has demonstrated ability to determine the presence of Barr bodies. A male fetus is ascertained when less than 25 cells in a count of 1000 possess the sex chromatin body. The cells may be studied directly from the fluid without further culture (Fuchs, 1966). Confirmation should be obtained by study of the karyotypes of cultured amniotic fluid cells. The cells should be obtained between 15 and 18 weeks' gestation if therapeutic abortion is to be safely undertaken by 24 weeks. Precaution in technique is mandatory to prevent accidental culture of maternal cells (Littlefield, 1970).

Sex-linked disorders affect 50 per cent of male infants born to female carriers and include Duchenne muscular dystrophy, Hunter's mucopolysaccharidosis, hemophilias A (factor VIII deficiency) and B (IX deficiency), Lesch-Nyhan hyperuricemia, Fabry's lipid storage disease, Lowe's nephropathic rickets, nephrogenic diabetes insipidus, Bruton's disease (hypogammaglobulinemia), and chronic granulomatous disease.

Some chromosome abnormalities are identifiable by amniotic cell culture and karyotyping, but must be performed in laboratories which are highly proficient in these techniques. All pregnant women over 35 years old should be screened for trisomies 21, 13–15, and 18 and aneuploidies 47XXY, 47XXX, and 47XYY. Screening should also be attempted when one parent is a carrier of translocations C/E, G/G, D/G and 21/22—familial mongolisms (Milunsky *et al.*, 1970). Viral- and radiation-induced chromosome defects are also detectable antenatally in some cases (Nadler and Gerbie, 1970).

A few metabolic disorders can be diagnosed *in utero* by cytobiochemistry, but should be attempted *only in qualified laboratories* (Littlefield, 1970; Brady, 1970). Diseases which have been so identified are Tay-Sachs, Niemann-Pick, Fabry's, maple syrup urine, methylmalonic aciduria, cystinosis, metachromatic leukodystrophy, Hurler's, Hunter's, Pompe's, galactosemia, Lesch-Nyhan, lysosomal acid phosphatase deficiency, and adrenogenital syndrome.

Estimation of Gestational Age and Fetal Maturity

During the first half of pregnancy, amniotic fluid volume is proportional to fetal weight and is comparable to fetal extracellular fluid in constitution. After 20 weeks, however, the fluid becomes dilute (Lind *et al.*, 1969). Only a few amniotic metabolites consistently increase their concentrations for the duration of pregnancy. One reliable measure of gestational age is creatinine, which increases in concentration to 1.8 mg./dl. by 36 weeks (90th percentile) and to 2.0 mg./dl. by 37 weeks. Creatinine concentration does not correlate well with fetal weight, but values less than 1.5 mg./dl. are the rule when the fetus is immature; values greater than 2.0 mg./dl. indicate maturity (Begneaud *et al.*, 1969). Uric acid determinations may also be of value in assessing fetal maturity (Wolf *et al.*, 1970).

Amniotic cytology with Nile blue sulfate may be helpful in estimating gestational age. There is a rapid increase in the number of anucleate, orangeophilic cells after 35 weeks from a level of about 15 per cent or less to 30 per cent or more. Clumps of orangeophilic bodies indicate 38 weeks' gestation (White *et al.*, 1969).

In prolonged pregnancy amniotic fluid may be obtained to determine if there is oligohydramnios (by hippurate dye dilution measures). Oligohydramnios is associated with fetal distress and calls for amniotomy, measurement of fetal blood pH, and maternal estriol excretion (Beischer *et al.*, 1969).

Fetal Health and Fetoplacental Function

Decrease in maternal urinary estriol is associated with feto-placental depression. A similar, but more distinct estriol diminution may be seen in amniotic fluid (Aleem *et al.*, 1969).

The placenta and fetus are interdependent in the production of estriol. For example, the placenta contributes the major synthesized portion of pregnenolone to the fetus for conversion to 16-hydroxydehydroepiandrosterone since the placenta lacks 16-alpha hydroxylase (which is found only in the fetus). Estriol depression thus indicates early feto-placental malfunction. It now appears possible that placental reserve may be estimated by measuring estriol following stimulation by intra-amniotic injection of dehydroepiandrosterone (Hausknecht and Mandelman, 1969).

Diagnosis of Respiratory Distress

Recent studies indicate that immature fetal lung secretes the phospholipids lecithin and sphingomyelin in about equal concentrations. Since there is contact of immature pulmonary alveoli with amniotic fluid, the two lipids diffuse at equal rates into the amniotic sac. At 35 weeks of normal gestation, the lungs mature and secrete four times more lecithin (phosphatidyl choline) into amniotic fluid. The abrupt change in amniotic fluid concentration accurately indicates lung maturity when other parameters of general fetal condition are in error (Gluck *et al.*, 1971). When this technique is applied, the means are available for determining the time to induce delivery in cases of erythroblastosis, dysmaturity syndrome, in maternal diabetes, and so forth. A rapid, simple, thin-layer chromatographic method is recommended (Knieser *et al.*, 1972). Total mass of lecithin (concentration × volume of fluid) may correlate best with pulmonary maturity of the fetus (Falconer *et al.*, 1973).

Diagnosis of Neural Tube Defects

Several studies have indicated that the amniotic fluid concentration of alpha-fetoprotein is elevated when the fetus suffers from a failure of closure of the ectodermal neural tube. Alpha-fetoprotein can be quantitated immunologically. It is abnormal in cases of anencephaly, myelocele, spina bifida and other associated disorders (Allan, 1973).

Diagnosis of Ruptured Fetal Membranes

Occasionally the obstetrician is faced with the problem of deciding whether or not the amniotic sac has broken. A comparison of methods which utilize the vaginal liquid pool specimen indicates greatest accuracy in identifying released amniotic fluid by Papanicolaou staining and cytologic evaluation. If the Pap stain cannot be performed, a combination of history, alkaline pH (7.0 or greater), and positive crystallization test (amniotic fluid forms a tree-like branching pattern when a smear is air dried) are sufficient (Friedman and McElin, 1969).

REFERENCES

Aleem, F., Neill, D., and Pinkerton, J.: A method for oestriol estimation in amniotic fluid and its use in the study of normal and abnormal pregnancy. Steroids *13*:651, 1969.

Allan, L. D., Donald, I., Ferguson-Smith, M. A., Sweet, E. M., and Gibson, A. A. M.: Amniotic fluid alpha-fetoprotein in the antenatal diagnosis of spina bifida. Lancet 2:522, 1973.

Begneaud, W. P., Hawes, T. P., Mickal, A., and Samuels, M.: Amniotic fluid creatinine for prediction of fetal maturity. Obstet. Gynec. *34*:7, 1969.

Beischer, N. A., Brown, J. B., and Townsend, L.: Studies in prolonged pregnancy. III Amniocentesis in prolonged pregnancy. Amer. J. Obstet. Gynec. *103*:496, 1969.

Betke, V. K., and Kleihauer, E.: Foetaler und bleibender Blutfarbstoff in Erythrocyten und Erythroblasten von menschlichen Feten und Neugeborenen. Blut Bank *4*: 241, 1958.

Bevis, D. C. A.: The antenatal prediction of hemolytic disease of the newborn. Lancet *1*:395, 1952.

Bonsnes, R. W. L.: Composition of amniotic fluid. Clin. Obstet. Gynec. *9*:440, 1966.

Brady, R. O.: Prenatal diagnosis of lipid storage diseases. Clin. Chem. *16*:811, 1970.

Brazie, J. V., Ibbott, F. A., and Bowes, W. A.: Identification of the pigment in amniotic fluid of erythroblastosis as bilirubin. J. Pediat. *69*:354, 1966.

Brodersen, R., Jacobsen, J., Hertz, H., Rebbe, H., and Sorensen, B.: Bilirubin conjugation in the human fetus. Scand. J. Clin. Lab. Invest. *20*:41, 1967.

Cassady, G., and Barnett, R.: Amniotic fluid electrolytes and perinatal outcome. Biol. Neonatorum *13*:155, 1968.

Cherry, S. H., Kochwa, S., and Rosenfield, R. E.: Bilirubin protein ratio in amniotic fluid as an index of the severity of erythroblastosis fetalis. Obstet. Gynec. *26*:826, 1965.

Connon, A. F.: Improved accuracy of prediction of severity of hemolytic disease of the newborn. Obstet. Gynec. *33*:72, 1969.

Curl, C. W.: Immunoglobulin levels in amniotic fluid. Amer. J. Obstet. Gynec. *103*:408, 1971.

Dunstan, M. K.: Amniotic fluid volume and protein concentration in rhesus sensitized women. J. Obstet. Gynec. Brit. Comm. *75*:732, 1968.

Falconer, G. F., Hodge, J. S., and Gadd, R. L.: Influence of amniotic fluid volume on lecithin estimation in prediction of respiratory distress. Brit. Med. J. 2:689, 1973.

Freda, V. J.: The Rh problem in obstetrics and a new concept of its management using amniocentesis and spectrophotometric scanning of amniotic fluid. Amer. J. Obstet. Gynec. *92*:341, 1965.

Freda, V. J.: Antepartum management of the Rh problem. Progr. Hematol. *5*:266, 1966a.

Freda, V. J.: Recent obstetrical advances in the Rh problem. Bull. N.Y. Acad. Med. *42*:474, 1966b.

Freda, V. J., and Robertson, J. G.: Antepartum management—amniocentesis and experience with hysterotomy and surgery in utero. Jewish Mem. Hosp. Bull. (NYC) *10*:47, 1965.

Friedman, M. L., and McElin, T. W.: Diagnosis of ruptured fetal membranes, clinical study and review of the literature. Amer. J. Obstet. Gynec. *104*:544, 1969.

Fuchs, F.: Genetic information from amniotic fluid constituents. Clin. Obstet. Gynec. *9*:565, 1966.

Gambino, S. R., and Freda, V. J.: The measurement of amniotic fluid bilirubin by the method of Jendrassik and Grof, its correlation with spectrophotometric analysis. Amer. J. Clin. Path. *46*:198, 1966.

Gartner, L. H., and Bernstein, J.: Kernicterus and prematurity: Development of nuclear jaundice at relatively low serum concentrations of bilirubin. Jewish Mem. Hosp. Bull. (NYC) *10*:125, 1965.

Gluck, L., Kulovich, M. V., Borer, R. C., Brenner, P. H., Anderson, G. G., and Spellacy, W. N.: Diagnosis of the respiratory distress syndrome by amniocentesis. Amer. J. Obstet. Gynec. *109*:440, 1971.

Gorman, J. G.: Prevention of immunization to the Rh factor. Jewish Mem. Hosp. Bull. (NYC) *10*:142, 1965.

Hausknecht, R. U., and Mandelman, N.: The metabolism of intra-amniotically injected dehydroepiandrosterone as a placental function test. Amer. J. Obstet. Gynec. *104*:433, 1969.

Hutchinson, D. L., Gray, M. J., Plentyl, A. A., Alvarez, H., Caldeyro-Barcia, R., Kaplan, B., and Lind, J.: The role of the fetus in the water exchange of the amniotic fluid of normal and hydramniotic patients. J. Clin. Invest. *38*: 971, 1959.

Jacobson, C. B., and Barter, R. H.: Intrauterine diagnosis and management of genetic defects. Amer. J. Obstet. Gynec. *99*:796, 1967.

Kapitulnik, J., Kaufmann, N. A., and Blondheim, S. H.: Chemical versus spectrophotometric determination of bilirubin in amniotic fluid and the influence of hemoglobin and methene pigments. Clin. Chem. *16*:756, 1970.

Knieser, M. R., Hurst, R., and Tuegel, C. R.: Evaluation of the maturity of fetal lungs. Amer. J. Clin. Path. *58*:579, 1972.

Liley, A. W.: Errors in the assessment of hemolytic disease from amniotic fluid. Amer. J. Obstet. Gynec. *93*:485, 1963.

Liley, A. W.: Intrauterine transfusion. Jewish Mem. Hosp. Bull. (NYC) *10*:70, 1965.

Liley, A. W.: The epidemiology of severe haemolytic disease of the newborn. New Zealand Med. J. *71*:76, 1970.

Lind, T., and Hytten, F. E.: Relation of amniotic fluid volume to fetal weight in the first half of pregnancy. Lancet *1*:1147, 1970.

Lind, T., Parkin, F. M., and Cheyne, G. A.: Biochemical and cytological changes in liquor amnii with advancing gestation. J. Obstet. Gynec. Brit. Comm. *76*:673, 1969.

Littlefield, J. W.: The pregnancy at risk for a genetic disorder. New Eng. J. Med. *282*:627, 1970.

Macintyre, M. N.: Chromosomal problems of intrauterine diagnosis. Birth Defects 7:10, 1971.

Matthews, C. D., Matthews, A. E. B., and Gilbey, B. E.: Antibody development in rhesus-negative patients following abortion. Lancet 2:318, 1969.

Milunsky, A., Littlefield, J. W., Kanfer, J. N., Kolodny, E. H., Shih, V. E., and Atkins, L.: Prenatal genetic diagnosis. New Eng. J. Med. *283*:1370; 1441; 1498; 1970.

Muller-Eberhard, U., and Bashore, R.: Assessment of Rh disease by ratios of bilirubin to albumin and hemopexin to albumin in amniotic fluid. New Eng. J. Med. *282*:1163, 1970.

Nadler, H. L., and Gerbie, A. B.: Role of amniocentesis in the intrauterine detection of genetic disorders. New Eng. J. Med. *282*:596, 1970.

Nelson, G. H., and Talledo, O. E.: Amniotic fluid spectral analysis in the management of patients with rhesus sensitization. Amer. J. Clin. Path. *39*:363, 1969.

Ovenstone, J. A., and Connon, A. F.: Optical density differencing: A new method for the direct measurement of bilirubin in liquor amnii. Clin. Chim. Acta *20*:397, 1968.

Reynolds, W. A., Pitkin, R. M., and Hodari, A. A.: Transfer of iodide into amniotic fluid by the normal and nephrectomized subhuman primate fetus. Amer. J. Obstet. Gynec. *104*:633, 1969.

Robertson, J. G.: Management of patients with Rh isoimmunization based on amniotic fluid examination. Amer. J. Obstet. Gynec. *103*:713, 1969.

Wade, M. E., Ogden, J. A., and David, C. D.: Criteria for intrauterine fetal transfusion. Obstet. Gynec. *34*:156, 1969.

Wahlstrom, J., Brosset, A., and Bartsch, F.: Viability of amniotic cells at different stages of gestation. Lancet 2:1037, 1970.

Walker, A. H. C.: Liquor amnii studies in the prediction of haemolytic disease of the newborn. Brit. Med. J. *376*, Aug., 1957.

White, C. A., Doorenbos, D. E., and Bradbury, J. T.: Role of chemical and cytologic analysis of amniotic fluid in determination of fetal maturity. Amer. J. Obstet. Gynec. *104*: 664, 1969.

Wolf, P. L., Block, D., and Tsudaka, T.: Biochemical profile of amniotic fluid to assess fetal maturity. Clin. Chem. *16*:610, 1970.

Chapter 28

EXAMINATION OF SEMINAL FLUID

by DONALD C. CANNON, M.D., Ph.D.

Examination of seminal fluid is usually performed as part of a comprehensive infertility investigation involving both partners of a barren marriage. It is a laboratory procedure which has been requested with increasing frequency in the last two decades. This increased interest in seminal fluid examination is proportional both to the greater awareness on the part of the public that infertility problems may frequently be corrected and the expanded interest and diagnostic acumen on the part of physicians who must deal with this problem. As a result of its relative simplicity, semen examination is often requested before the more complicated and expensive examination of the female. Furthermore, it is now apparent that inadequacies on the part of the male contribute to a significant minority of infertility problems, estimated to be as high as 40 per cent by some investigators.

In relation to the infertility investigation, it is important to recognize the proper scope of the semen examination. Most importantly, it is but one facet of the medical examination of the male, which must also include a detailed history and general physical examination. Such specialized procedures as studies of thyroid, adrenal, and pituitary functions or testicular biopsy may also be indicated. Not only must the results of the semen examination be interpreted in light of the remainder of the medical examination of the male; the female partner must be considered as well. Indeed, it has been suggested that for purposes of the infertility investigation the male and female involved should be considered not as individuals but as a reproductive unit. An inherent limitation of the semen examination is that the standards of semen quality are the result of population studies of males from fertile and infertile marriages. Consequently the standards of semen quality are relative, not absolute indications of fertility or sterility (with the single exception of complete aspermia). Furthermore, it is usually recommended that semen examination be repeated one or more times if an abnormal result is found.

In addition to infertility studies, the clinical pathology laboratory, particularly one actively engaged in forensic studies, may frequently be requested to examine vaginal secretions or clothing stains for the presence of semen in alleged or suspected rape. Rarely, the purpose of the semen examination may be to investigate the effectiveness of vasectomy or to support or disprove a denial of paternity on the grounds of sterility.

PHYSIOLOGY OF SEMINAL FLUID

Semen is a composite solution formed by the testes as well as the accessory male reproductive organs and consists basically of spermatozoa suspended in the seminal plasma. The function of the seminal plasma is to provide a nutritive medium of proper osmolality and volume for conveying the spermatozoa to the endocervical mucus, whereupon its contribution to the fertilization process is ended. The seminal plasma may also serve to activate the spermatozoa to greater motility, although this is not certain.

The components of semen are derived from the following organs:

Testis. Spermatozoa, which comprise less than 5 per cent of the semen volume, are the only cell type present in normal semen in any appreciable number. Spermatozoa are largely stored in the ampullary portions of the vasa deferentia until released in the process of ejaculation. Spermatozoa stored in the ampullae are rather inactive metabolically because of the acid environment and diminished oxygen supply. In this location it has been estimated that spermatozoa can survive for periods of up to one month.

Seminal Vesicles. Approximately 60 per cent of the semen volume is derived from the seminal vesicles. This viscid, neutral, or slightly alkaline fluid is often yellow or even deeply pigmented as a result of its high flavin content, which is responsible for the fluorescence of semen in ultraviolet light. The seminal vesicles are the major source of the high fructose content of semen, which is the major nutrient for the spermatozoa. The importance of other components, such as the relatively high potassium and citric acid content and smaller amounts of ascorbic acid, ergothioneine, and phosphorylcholine, has not yet been established. The seminal vesicle secretion is also important in providing the substrate responsible for the coagulation of semen following ejaculation.

Prostate. The prostate contributes about 20 per cent of the volume of semen. This milky fluid is slightly acid, with a pH of about 6.5, largely as a result of its high content of citric acid, which constitutes the major anion to this component of semen. The prostatic secretion is also rich in proteolytic enzymes and acid phosphatase. These proteolytic enzymes are believed to be responsible for the coagulation and liquefaction of semen. Acid phosphatase can cleave phosphorylcholine present in the semen but the significance of this is not clear.

Epididymides, Vasa Deferentia, Bulbourethral Glands (Cowper's Glands), and Urethral Glands (Glands of Littré). Less than 10 to 15 per cent of the semen volume is contributed by these structures and little is known of their biochemical significance in man.

Fractions of Semen. The process of ejaculation results in the mixing of three distinct fractions of semen, which enter the urethra individually in rapid succession. These fractions differ as to anatomic origin and therefore also in chemical composition. The first fraction, which is of relatively slight amount, consists of a clear viscid fluid believed to originate largely or perhaps exclusively from the urethral and bulbourethral glands. The function of this component is not known with certainty, but it may be to cleanse and lubricate the urethra in preparation for the bulk of the ejaculate which is to follow. The second fraction consists largely of prostatic secretion along with most of the spermatozoa and relatively small amounts of secretions from the epididymides and vasa deferentia which have been temporarily stored in the ampullae of the vasa deferentia. The final fraction consists almost entirely of a mucoid secretion resulting from emptying of the seminal vesicles.

An understanding of the temporal sequence of mixing of the various fractions in ejaculation is important to the proper conduct of the semen examination. For example, the use of semen samples obtained from the male urethra following coitus, as recommended by some investigators, will result in a specimen which is not only nonrepresentative of the semen as a whole but is also apt to be relatively sperm poor. Furthermore, samples obtained by coitus interruptus may result in loss of part of the sperm-rich middle fraction, although it represents only a minor part of the total volume of ejaculate.

COLLECTION

It is usually recommended that the semen sample be collected following a three-day period of continence. Others have suggested that a more meaningful specimen is one collected after a period of continence equal to the usual frequency of coitus for the couple involved. Prolonged continence prior to the semen collection is to be discouraged, since the quality of the semen, especially in regard to sperm motility, may actually diminish. Regardless of what method is employed for collection, the physician will be faced with occasional patients who will not comply because of religious or esthetic standards or who are unable to cooperate because of more complex psychologic considerations. The most satisfactory specimen is that collected in the physician's office or the clinical pathology laboratory by masturbation. This allows a complete examination of the semen, particularly of the process of coagulation and liquefaction, and also eliminates the possibility of cold shock. Acceptable but somewhat less satisfactory are specimens obtained in the patient's home by coitus interruptus or masturbation and delivered soon thereafter to the laboratory. With either method, the specimen may be collected in a wide-mouth clean glass jar supplied by the laboratory (to avoid the possibility of trace amounts of detergents or other harmful contaminants) or in suitable plastic or polyethylene containers. Specimens may be collected in condoms, which are then tied and placed in a clean glass jar. Valid objections to condom collection have been expressed because of the fact that powder or lubricants applied to the condoms or other material used in their manufacture may be actively spermicidal. If the condom is used, it must first be washed with soap and water, rinsed thoroughly, and then dried completely. Plastic sheaths* have been recommended as a means

*Milex Seminal Pouch, Milex Products, Chicago, Illinois.

of avoiding the difficulties of condom collection.

In transporting specimens collected elsewhere to the laboratory, several precautions are necessary. First of all, the specimen must be received as soon as possible and in no case after more than 2 to 3 hours have elapsed following collection. It is essential that the semen specimen not be subjected to temperature extremes during delivery to the laboratory. Watson and Robertson (1966) have emphasized the importance of the container temperature at the time of collection and recommend preliminary warming to body temperature. They found maintenance of the specimen at body temperature to be particularly important until liquefaction of the coagulum is complete (about 20 minutes).

GROSS EXAMINATION

Physical Characteristics. Freshly ejaculated semen is a highly viscid, opaque, white or gray-white coagulum which may have a distinct musty or acrid odor. After 10 to 20 minutes the coagulum will spontaneously liquefy to form a translucent, turbid, viscous fluid which is mildly alkaline, with a pH of about 7.7. The pH usually does not vary greatly, although pH values of less than 7.0 are frequently associated with semen consisting largely of prostatic secretion due to congenital aplasia of the vasa deferentia and seminal vesicles (Raboch and Skachova, 1965). Increased or decreased turbidity is of little significance except when increased turbidity is the result of leukocytes associated with an inflammatory process in some part of the reproductive tract.

Viscosity can be assessed while pouring the liquefied specimen from the collection container into the glass graduate for volume measurement. The specimen of normal viscosity can be poured drop by drop. Increased viscosity is of significance if sperm motility is thereby compromised. Upon occasion, increased viscosity has been shown to be associated with poor invasion of the cervical mucus in postcoital studies and may be the only demonstrable defect in an infertile couple.

Coagulation and Liquefaction. Coagulation and subsequent liquefaction is believed to be a three-stage process (Mann, 1964): (1) Coagulation results from the formation of a fibrin clot by the action of a prostatic clotting enzyme on a fibrinogen-like precursor formed by the seminal vesicles. (2) Liquefaction is initiated by the action of fibrinolytic enzymes of prostatic origin. (3) The fibrin fragments are degraded further to free amino acids and ammonia by the action of several poorly characterized proteolytic enzymes, including an aminopeptidase and pepsin. The coagulation process has been shown to have diagnostic significance in that the semen from males with bilateral congenital absence of the vasa deferentia and seminal vesicles fails to coagulate because of the absence of the coagulation substrate (Amelar, 1962). Liquefaction should be complete within 30 minutes. It is important to distinguish persistent increased viscosity from delayed liquefaction.

Volume. The normal semen volume averages 3.5 ml., with a usual range of 1.5 to 5.0 ml. Paradoxically males associated with infertile marriages tend to have an increased rather than a decreased semen volume, which is frequently associated with a significantly diminished sperm count. Postcoital studies suggest, however, that greatly decreased semen volumes may result in poor penetration of the cervical mucus by the sperm (MacLeod, 1965). Semen volume does not vary significantly with the period of continence (MacLeod, 1951).

MICROSCOPIC EXAMINATION

Sperm Counts. Following liquefaction of the semen, the spermatozoa may be counted in a hemocytometer chamber following initial dilution in a white blood cell pipette. Mix the semen sample thoroughly and draw an aliquot to the 0.5 mark on the pipette. Dilute to the 11 mark with the following solution:

Sodium bicarbonate	5 gm.
Formalin (neutral)	1 ml.
Distilled water	100 ml.

After charging the hemocytometer chamber, 2 minutes are allowed for the immobilized sperm to settle. The spermatozoa in 4 sq. mm. (four large squares) are counted. This number multiplied by 50,000 gives the number of spermatozoa per milliliter. The entire counting procedure including the initial dilution should be repeated at least once and the results averaged.

Considerable difficulty may be encountered in diluting semen of greatly increased viscosity. Under these circumstances the counting will be facilitated if the semen is diluted 1:1 with the mucolytic agent Alevaire (Brean Laboratories, Inc.) prior to pipette dilution and the final count is multiplied by two (Amelar, 1966).

The hemocytometer method of counting sperm is relatively imprecise. Freund and Carol (1964) found that duplicate sperm counts by the same technologist varied by a mean difference of 20 per cent. For counts performed by three technicians, each of whom used duplicate pipettings on the same sample, the 95 per cent confidence limit was ± 52 per cent. In the author's experience, however, these variations seem unduly high.

The sperm count of normal semen will usually fall in the range of 60 to 150 million per ml., with a mean of about 100 million per ml. Counts of less than 20 million per ml. are usually considered to be distinctly abnormal, although successful impregnation may occur. MacLeod (1951), in studying the semen of 1000 fertile males and 800 males associated with infertile marriages, found that 5 per cent of the fertile group and 17 per cent of the "infertile" group had sperm counts in the range of 1 to 20 million per ml.

Motility. In order for the spermatozoa to penetrate the cervical mucus and subsequently migrate to fertilize the ovum in the fallopian tubes, active motility is necessary. To evaluate motility, a small drop of liquefied semen is placed on a microscope slide prewarmed approximately to body temperature and then covered with a coverslip which has been ringed with petrolatum. Motility can be evaluated by scanning several fields with the high dry objective until a total of at least 200 spermatozoa have been observed. It is essential to focus through the entire depth of a given field so as to include nonmotile sperm which may have settled to the bottom of the medium. The percentage of sperm showing actual progressive motion should be recorded. It is also desirable to render a qualitative estimate of sperm motility. Watson and Robertson (1966), for example, assign sperm to one of three categories: progressive motility, nonprogressive motility, and nonmotility. They furthermore grade those showing progressive motility according to the following code: grade I, minimal forward progression; grade II, poor to fair activity; grade III, good activity with tail movements visualized; grade IV, full activity with tail movements difficult to visualize.

Although it is frequently stated that normal semen contains more than 70 per cent or even 80 per cent motile sperm, this criterion would seem entirely too rigid in view of several large studies. For example, MacLeod and Gold (1951) found a mean of only 58 per cent motile sperm with a standard deviation of ± 16 per cent in 732 males of proven fertility. In contrast, they found a mean motility of 51 per cent ± 19 in 869 males associated with infertile marriages. These results may be somewhat low in that some specimens were evaluated as late as 5½ hours after collection. Many feel that semen should be considered abnormal if fewer than 60 per cent of spermatozoa show progressive motion in specimens examined within 3 hours of collection.

Some investigators have previously recommended motility estimates at intervals during the 24 hours following collection, e.g., 3, 6, 12, and 24 hours. The motile forms will decrease by about 5 per cent per hour after the fourth hour following collection. Thus, in a study of 100 males of proven fertility, Falk and Kaufman (1950) found the following mean values for motility: 2 to 4 hours, 61 per cent; 6 to 7 hours, 46 per cent; 12 hours, 27 per cent; 24 hours, 8 per cent. Most authorities now consider only the initial motility estimate to be of value. It has been correctly demonstrated that, since sperm must penetrate the cervical mucus within a few minutes following ejaculation (or be inactivated by the relatively low pH of the vaginal secretions), the seminal plasma is not a physiologic medium for prolonged evaluation of sperm activity. Furthermore, the metabolic activity of the sperm as well as bacterial growth will drastically alter the pH of semen after a few hours.

Sperm Morphology. Sperm morphology is evaluated by performing differential counts of morphologically normal and abnormal spermatozoa types on stained smears. Smears are prepared on clean microscope slides in a manner identical to blood films. The best stain for morphologic detail is the Papanicolaou stain (Fig. 28–1). Although somewhat complicated and time consuming, the Papanicolaou technique is to be recommended, particularly in the laboratory in which it is routinely performed by the exfoliative cytology service. It is essential that the smear be placed immediately into fixative, either 95 per cent (v/v) ethanol or 50 per cent (v/v) ethanol ether, before drying has occurred.

A method which is also satisfactory but gives somewhat poorer differentiation of sperm detail is the hematoxylin method described by Amelar (1966). In this method the film is air dried and then treated as follows: (1) 10 per cent (v/v) formalin, 1 minute; (2) water rinse; (3) Meyer's hematoxylin, 2 minutes; (4) water rinse; (5) air dry. Other staining techniques which have been recommended include Giemsa, basic fuchsin, and crystal violet. The last two named require preliminary heat fixing, which has been demonstrated to cause some degree of artifactual distortion of the spermatozoa.

At least 200 spermatozoa should be examined under oil immersion and the percentage of abnormal forms recorded (Fig. 28–2). Normal semen has fewer than 30 per cent abnormal forms. In addition to sperm morphology, the presence of red blood cells, leukocytes, and epithelial cells should be noted. Immature cells of the germinal line may appear in the semen and must be differentiated from macrophages or leukocytes. Numerous granules and globules are normally present in semen. These presumably originate from the secretion of glandular cells or perhaps from autolysis of epithelial lining cells in the accessory reproductive structures.

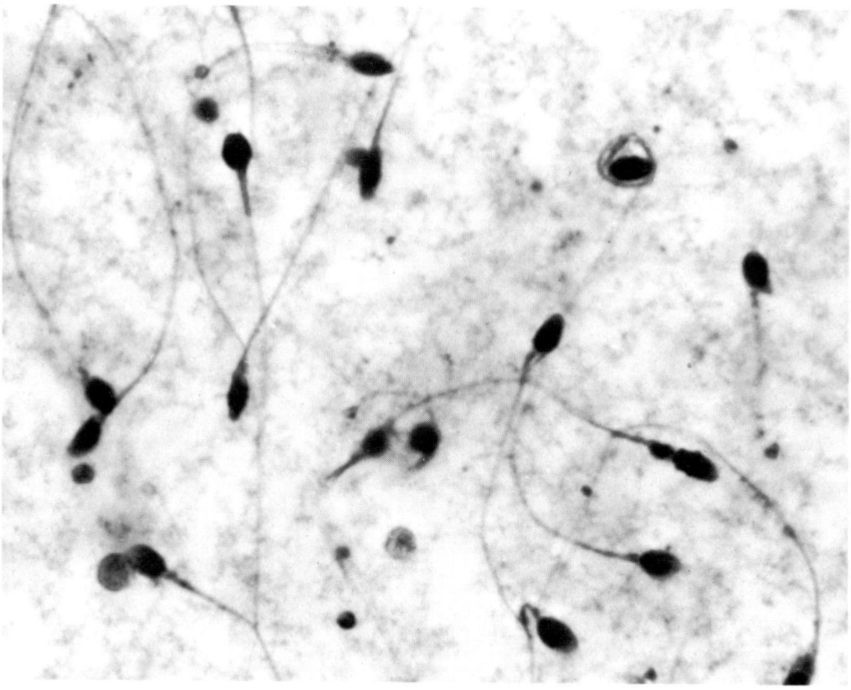

Figure 28–1. Normal spermatozoa. Papanicolaou stain; ×1580.

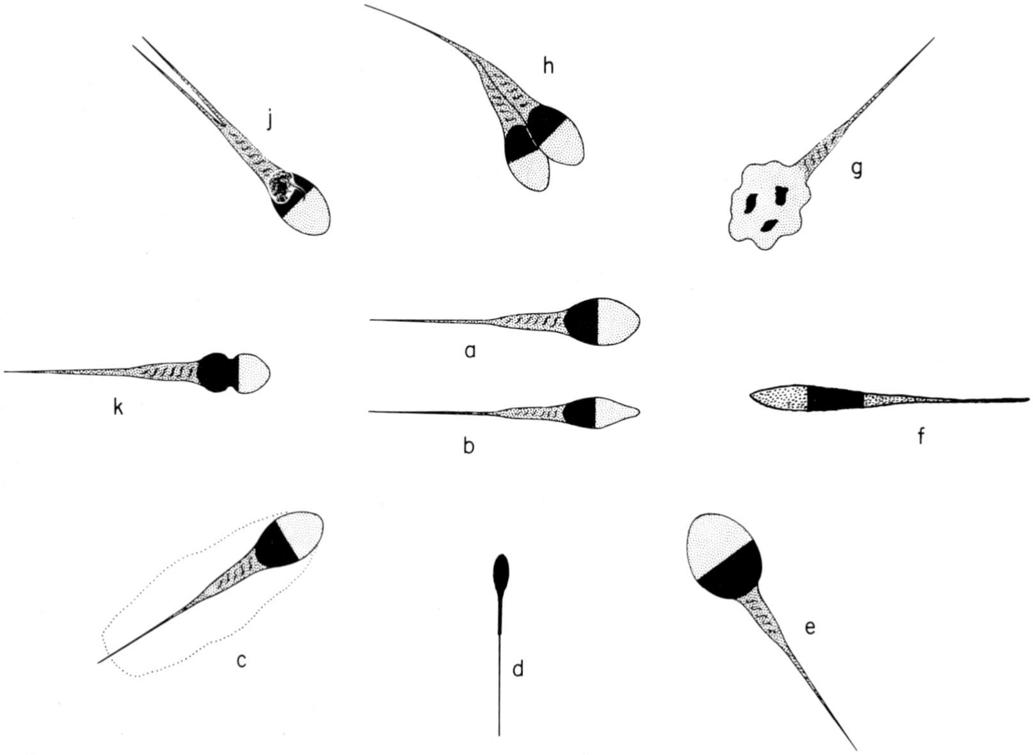

Figure 28–2. Diagrammatic representation of normal and abnormal spermatozoa. *a*, Normal, face view. *b*, Normal, lateral view. *c*, Immature spermatozoon (spermatid). *d–k*, Morphologically abnormal types: *d*, pin-head; *e*, giant head; *f*, acute tapering form; *g*, amorphous form; *h*, double head; *j*, double tail; *k*, constricted head. (Tails on all forms are disproportionately short.)

OTHER TESTS OF SEMEN

Postcoital (Sims-Huhner) Test. This test consists of the examination of cervical mucus following coitus. It is intended as a measure both of the quality of cervical mucus and the ability of the spermatozoa to penetrate the mucus and maintain activity. The cervical mucus undergoes both quantitative and qualitative changes, which are correlated with the menstrual cycle. In the ovulatory phase at midcycle, the amount of mucus is maximum while the viscosity is significantly diminished, thus facilitating penetration of the mucus by the spermatozoa. Progesterone in the secretory phase causes increased viscosity of the mucus.

During the ovulatory phase, as determined by basal temperature records, the female is instructed to report to the physician within several hours of coitus. The results of the test are constant for about 8 hours after coitus (Danezis *et al.*, 1962). The external cervical os is wiped clear of mucus. The endocervical mucus sample may be obtained by aspiration with a glass cannula attached by a rubber tube to a Luer syringe. The specimen may then be delivered to the laboratory in the syringe. The volume of mucus is measured. Following discharge into a Petri dish, its color and viscosity are noted. At midcycle the mucus should be clear and watery. One further property which is commonly evaluated is the spinnbarkeit, which refers to the tenacity of the mucus. This is tested by grasping a portion of the mucus with forceps and noting the distance which it can be drawn before breaking. A good spinnbarkeit, which should prevail at midcycle, is at least 10 cm. A drop of mucus is then placed on a microscope slide, covered with a coverslip, and examined for the presence of sperm. An estimate of the number of sperm per high-power field with percentage of motile forms should be reported. The material may also be examined for leukocytes, erythrocytes, and trichomonads.

The postcoital test typically shows better quality of mucus and better sperm penetration at the ovulatory phase than at other times in the ovulatory cycle. The degree of sperm penetration is correlated with the quality of semen as well as with the fertility of the mating, although the differences are usually not striking.

Antibodies to Spermatozoa. Recently considerable interest has focused on the occurrence of antibodies to spermatozoa, both in males with semen abnormalities and in females of infertile marriages. The extensive experimental and clinical work in this complex and as yet rather poorly understood field has recently been reviewed by Schulman (1971). Investigations thus far have established a firm immunologic basis for spermatozoal antibodies. In some species of animals there are several antigens which are specific for the sperm cell line, but information pertaining to human spermatozoa is equivocal. Various techniques have been described for detecting antibodies to spermatozoa including agglutination, immobilization, precipitation, complement fixation, passive hemagglutination, immunofluorescence, and cytotoxicity. Most of these techniques have not yet proved to be technically reliable, however, and widely variant results often occur among laboratories performing the same test.

A causal relationship between spermatozoal antibodies and disease has not been clearly established. The antibodies are found in some human males with testicular disease and also in association with autoimmune aspermatogenesis experimentally induced by immunization with spermatozoa, semen, or testicular homogenates and appropriate adjuvants. There is by no means unanimity of opinion regarding the importance of spermatozoal antibodies in the serum of females, but available evidence strongly suggests a cause and effect relationship to otherwise unexplained infertility.

Most clinical correlative studies thus far have utilized sperm agglutination tests. One of the better known albeit controversial reports is that of Franklin and Dukes (1964), who employed a straightforward agglutination reaction between serum and semen. Results were read microscopically after a 4-hour incubation at 37° C. Using this method, they were able to detect antibodies in the serum of 31 out of a group of 43 female partners of infertile marriages in which there was no other demonstrable cause for infertility in either husband or wife. In contrast, such antibodies were present in the female in only two of 35 fertile marriages. Antibodies were variously individual specific, in that they agglutinated only the husband's spermatozoa, or species specific, in that they agglutinated the spermatozoa of all males tested. The clinical importance of this test was further demonstrated by the fact that the antibody levels diminished markedly in each of 13 infertile females who were persuaded to practice continence or to restrict coitus to the use of condoms over a period of two to six months. Nine of these patients eventually became pregnant upon resumption of unrestricted coitus.

EXAMINATION FOR THE PRESENCE OF SEMEN

The clinical pathology laboratory may be requested to investigate material from the vagina or stains from clothing, skin, or hair for the presence of semen. Such cases will usually involve alleged rape or suspected sexual assault in association with homicide. In all medicolegal cases special precautions are indicated to properly identify specimens and to maintain the chain of evidence.

Obtaining the Sample. Secretions from the vagina may be obtained by direct aspiration or with saline lavage. A preliminary scan with ultraviolet light may prove helpful in selecting specific areas of clothing or other fabrics for further investigation. Semen stains frequently result in a greenish white fluorescence, although this may occur with stains from other body fluids as well. A 1 sq. cm. portion of the stained fabric should be cut out and soaked in 1 or 2 ml. of physiologic saline for 1 hour. The fluid from this washing may be subjected to further tests for semen. It is desirable to include as a control, particularly for acid phosphatase determination and the detection of blood group substances, a piece of fabric remote from the stain.

Examination for Sperm. Prior to aspiration or lavage it is desirable to prepare direct smears for Papanicolaou staining from the vagina. Alternatively, such smears may be prepared from the aspirate or lavage. Contrary to some expressed opinions, well-preserved sperm may be recovered from the vagina many hours after coitus and even from exhumed bodies, if they have been properly embalmed. Smears should also be prepared from the washings of fabric stains. The wash fluid may be first concentrated by centrifugation and a smear prepared from the sediment. Such smears may be stained with hematoxylin and eosin. The fragile tails of the sperm are frequently broken off, thus making identification somewhat more difficult.

Acid Phosphatase Determination. Acid phosphatase should be determined on the vaginal aspirate or lavage or on the wash fluid from stains. High values of acid phosphatase will render positive identification of semen even if the male involved is aspermic. Seminal fluid averages about 2500 King-Armstrong units per ml. of acid phosphatase, while other body fluids and extraneous foreign materials will have well under 5 units per ml. Acid phosphatase can be reliably determined on the wash fluid from stains which are many months old. The acid phosphatase method selected should have a high degree of specificity for prostatic acid phosphatase. (See Chapter 11.)

Detection of Blood Group Substances. In the case of positive identification of fluid or a stain as semen, the presence of A, B, or H blood group substances may be investigated. Approximately 80 per cent of individuals, those having the dominant secretor gene in homozygous or heterozygous state, will secrete the water-soluble form of blood group substances in body fluids, including semen. The identification of the specific substance is based on the ability of the semen to partially or completely neutralize the agglutinating activity of the specific antiserum. With this determination, it may be possible on occasion to demonstrate that the seminal fluid of a suspect differs from that recovered from the victim.

Florence Test. This test is a preliminary screening method and has been largely replaced by the far more dependable acid phosphatase determination. It is usually performed on stains from clothing, other fabric, or hair and depends on the presence of choline, which is found in high concentration in seminal fluid. A portion of the stained sample is extracted with distilled water by using gentle heat. Several drops of the extract are placed on a microscope slide and treated with an equal volume of a reagent composed of the following: iodine, 2.54 gm.; potassium iodide, 1.65 gm.; distilled water, 30 ml. In a positive test, rhombic or needlelike crystals of periodide of choline will be noted. The test may yield false positive results because of the high choline content occasionally found in other tissue fluids of human or animal origin.

Precipitin Test (Hektoen, 1922). This test is specific for semen of human origin and is therefore helpful in rendering positive identification of semen stains on clothing. The test requires specific antiserum obtained by immunizing suitable animals with human semen and absorbing the nonspecific antibodies with human serum. It is performed as a capillary tube precipitin reaction by overlaying the antiserum with washings from the stain.

REFERENCES

Amelar, R. D.: Coagulation, liquefaction and viscosity of human semen. J. Urol. 87:187, 1962.

Amelar, R. D.: Infertility in Men. Diagnosis and Treatment. Philadelphia, F. A. Davis Co., 1966.

Danezis, J., Sujan, S., and Sabrero, A. J.: Evaluation of the postcoital test. Fertil. Steril. *13*:559, 1962.

Falk, H. C., and Kaufman, S. A.: What constitutes a normal semen? Fertil. Steril. *1*:489, 1950.

Franklin, R. R., and Dukes, C. D.: Further studies on sperm-agglutinating antibody and unexplained infertility. J.A.M.A. *190*:682, 1964.

Freund, M., and Carol, B.: Factors affecting haemocytometer counts of sperm concentration in human semen. J. Reprod. Fertil. 8:149, 1964.

Hektoen, L.: Specific precipitin test for human semen. J.A.M.A. 78:704, 1922.

MacLeod, J.: Semen quality in one thousand men of known fertility and in eight hundred cases of infertile marriage. Fertil. Steril. 2:115, 1951.

MacLeod, J.: The semen examination. Clin. Obstet. Gynec. 8:115, 1965.

MacLeod, J., and Gold, R. Z.: The male factor in fertility and sterility. III. An analysis of motile activity in the spermatozoa of 1,000 fertile men and 1,000 men in infertile marriage. Fertil. Steril. 2:187, 1951.

Mann, T.: The Biochemistry of Semen and of the Male Reproductive Tract. London, Methuen and Co. Ltd., 1964.

Raboch, J., and Skachova, J.: The pH of human ejaculate. Fertil. Steril. *16*:252, 1965.

Schulman, S.: Sperm antibodies as a cause of infertility. CRC Critical Reviews in Clin. Lab. Sci. 2:393, 1971.

Watson, A. A., and Robertson, C. M. G.: Male infertility: A reappraisal of semen analysis. J. Med. Lab. Tech. *23*:1, 1966.

Chapter 29

CYTOGENETICS

by ROBERT R. EGGEN, M.D.

Human *cytogenetics* is the microscopic study of human chromosomes (or their counterparts in the nondividing nucleus) and correlation of abnormalities thereof with abnormalities in the patient. "Routine" laboratory procedures include sex chromatin tests and chromosome analysis (*karyotyping*). Autoradiography, meiotic karyotyping and hybridization studies are more sophisticated techniques than nonresearch laboratories will generally use.

INDICATIONS FOR CYTOGENETIC TESTING

Table 29–1 lists clinical situations in which cytogenetic testing should be used. Few laboratory tests are diagnostic in so diverse an array of diseases.

Diagnosis of Congenital Defects. It may seem redundant to recommend laboratory confirmation of a condition which appears obvious. However, there are sound reasons for studying infants with abnormalities.

For example, months may elapse before the clinical features of mongolism evolve sufficiently to allow confident clinical diagnosis. In the interim, the parents' decision whether or not to institutionalize their child must be agonizingly delayed. These same parents will also be intensely concerned that their succeeding children might also be mongols. Finally, there is the ever-present possibility that the mongol infant may in fact be a cretin (and thus can be salvaged with prompt treatment). Any of these acute problems can be resolved within a week or so with chromosome analysis.

Table 29–1. INDICATIONS FOR CYTOGENETIC TESTING

Congenital defects
Genetic counseling
Intrapartum fetal studies
Intersex
Female hypogonadism
Male hypogonadism
Sterility studies
Blood dyscrasias
Dysproteinemia
Effusions
Karyotyping tumors
Medicolegal reasons
Habitual abortion

The D-trisomy syndrome is equally illustrative of the value of cytogenetic testing. Among its clinical features are umbilical hernia, polydactylia, and hemangiomas. Any of these defects is amenable to surgical correction in an otherwise normal infant. However, the D-trisomy syndrome also embraces "hidden" central nervous system and cardiovascular defects which make surgery in an affected infant a lethal exercise. Distinction between the "otherwise normal" infant and the "hidden lethal" D-trisomy syndrome is unequivocal with chromosome analysis.

Genetic Counseling. The family to whom an abnormal child has been born has one question of paramount importance: "Will it happen again?" Many chromosomal syndromes have both sporadic and familial forms. The recurrence rates are vastly different. Parental knowledge of these differences will surely affect family planning.

A case in point is mongolism. In its sporadic form, the odds that a successive mongol child will be born to the same parents are roughly one in 80. This is in sharp contrast with the 100 per cent risk of recurrence which accompanies one variant of familial mongolism (p. 1334). Only chromosome analysis of the parents and of the affected child can make the distinction accurately.

Intrapartum Fetal Evaluation. An unborn infant can be karyotyped using cells from amniotic fluid as early as the fourteenth week of pregnancy (Jacobson and Barter, 1967). Expectant parents with an adverse family history or those who already know that they are carriers of a familial chromosome defect can be told whether their unborn child has a chromosome abnormality early enough that the pregnancy can be interrupted if necessary.

Intersex. Infants born with ambiguous genitalia present an immediate problem in sex determination which can often be solved only by cytogenetic study (either chromatin testing or karyotyping). To institute appropriate corrective measures, the true (genetic) sex must be known.

Female Hypogonadism. Ovarian deficiency often reflects a sex chromosome abnormality. Pubertal hypogonadism which has a chromosomal basis is refractory to any treatment directed to producing fertility. If the chromosome defect is discovered at the outset, the patient can be spared futile expenditure of much time and money. The only evidence of ovarian deficiency may be primary amenorrhea. Almost 30 per cent of these patients have an underlying chromosome defect.

Male Hypogonadism. The most common demonstrable chromosome abnormality of man is the form of male hypogonadism known as Klinefelter's syndrome. Cytogenetic testing provides absolute diagnosis as simply as possible.

Sterility. In both males and females, there are sex chromosomal defects which may not produce symptomatic gonadal deficiency but nevertheless render these patients sterile. A recent study of 130 males in a sterility clinic showed that almost 10 per cent had wholly asymptomatic sex chromosome defects.

Blood Dyscrasias. Some of the anemias (e.g., Bloom's and Fanconi's) and all the leukemias have interesting chromosome abnormalities in the affected cells. In chronic granulocytic leukemia the chromosomal change (the Philadelphia chromosome, p. 1336) is a real diagnostic aid. The other hematologic disorders mentioned do not require karyotyping for their diagnosis.

Dysproteinemias. Derangements of protein synthesis, either quantitative or qualitative, are usually readily identified by electrophoresis. Some dysproteinemias, however, produce paraproteins which do not migrate distinctively. The monoclonal gammopathies (e.g., Waldenström's macroglobulinemia, multiple myeloma) may be diagnosed by finding extra "W" or "MG" marker chromosomes in atypical bone marrow cells (Houston *et al.*, 1967). Generally, more conventional laboratory studies (electrophoresis, immunodiffusion) yield a diagnosis as readily.

Karyotyping Tumors. Attempts are being made to correlate the chromosome patterns of tumors with their biological behavior (benign vs. malignant; rate of metastatic spread) and to predict tumor response to varying types of treatment. At the moment, none of these investigations has reached the point of clinical application.

Study of Effusions. While microscopic study of the cells of effusions is generally satisfactory for the identification of tumor cells, there are some instances in which the cytologic findings are equivocal. In peritoneal and pleural effusions reactive mesothelial cells are often difficult to distinguish from neoplastic cells. As a rule, neoplastic cells have abnormalities of their chromosome complement which are absent from cells showing reactive dysplasia. This distinction has been used to identify neoplastic cells in effusions and is worth trying if cytologic findings are equivocal.

Medicolegal Applications. Uses for chromosome analysis can be envisioned in paternity testing, though no concrete techniques have yet been developed. Cytogenetic techniques (especially the chromatin tests) now find forensic application in identifying the sex of dismembered limbs or the sex of unknown assailants from the fingernail scrapings of victims.

Habitual Abortion. Parental chromosome defects are relatively infrequent in the genesis of habitual abortion (at least as far as present techniques allow us to discover). Nevertheless, cytogenetic testing of parents might well be advised if other avenues of investigation are unrewarding. Though parental studies are seldom very rewarding, chromosome abnormalities are forty times more common in the abortuses themselves than in liveborn infants. Many abortuses have abnormalities which have never been seen in a liveborn infant.

Cytogenetic techniques used in accord with the preceding criteria are among the most informative examinations that a clinical laboratory can perform. There is little reason for cytogenetic techniques not being available in at least one laboratory in a major metropolitan area. Mail-in techniques have made these tests available to any practicing physician.

SEX CHROMATIN TESTS

Sex chromatin tests were the first cytogenetic techniques to find practical clinical application. Mammalian sex chromatin was discovered, more or less fortuitously, in neuronal cells of cats by Barr and Bertram (1949), who later extended their investigations to humans. Initially, biopsy material was used; later Moore and Barr (1955) developed the buccal smear technique still in general use (Barr tests).

In 1954 Davidson and Smith described sex-related differences in the nuclei of polymorphonuclear leukocytes. These sex differences are simple to demonstrate, and the "drumstick" test, based upon their description, is popular.

The Barr and drumstick tests are limited to evaluating X chromosome patterns (*vide infra*). Y chromosomes can be detected in interphase nuclei by use of quinacrine staining and fluorescence microscopy. These tests are valuable screening procedures which sometimes provide enough information to make karyotyping unnecessary.

Human Sex Chromosomes. Evaluation of chromatin tests requires some understanding of the mechanisms of human sex determination. Stated simply, the X chromosome is female determining and the Y chromosome is male determining. Individuals without a Y chromosome are genetic females. Individuals with a Y chromosome are genetic males, regardless of the number of X chromosomes present. The sex chromosome pattern of the normal human female is XX—of the male, XY.

Nuclear Sex Chromatin Tests (Barr Tests). Sex chromatin (Barr body) is a mass of chromatin applied to the nuclear membrane as a (usually) planoconvex mass measuring about 1.2 by 0.7 microns (Fig. 29–1). Occasionally sex chromatin may appear to be bipartite or as an inverted pyramid with a central pale area. These are normal morphologic variants. The Barr body may be found in any nucleus with an open, vesicular chromatin pattern, e.g., the nuclei of basal layer epithelial cells.

Origin of the Barr Body. Nuclear sex chromatin is derived from one entire X chromosome. Early in the embryonic development of the normal female fetus, one member of the X chromosome pair within each cell is inactivated and becomes applied to the nuclear membrane, where it forms the sex chromatin. The single X chromosome of normal male cells does not become inactivated. Either member of the X chromosome pair may become inactivated; the process is entirely random, affecting a different X chromosome in different cells.

The inactivation of the X chromosome is reflected morphologically by *heterochromatinization*. The affected chromosome is shorter, darker, and more tightly contracted than its active counterpart. It is this shorter, darker chromosome which forms the Barr body.

If more than two X chromosomes are present in an abnormal cell, all but one of them are inactivated. Thus, the number of chromatin masses (m) expected can be predicted using the formula $m = n - 1$ where n is the number of X chromosomes in the cell.

Males, having a single X chromosome, have no chromatin mass ($1 - 1 = 0$). Normal females, having two X chromosomes, have a single chromatin mass ($2 - 1 = 1$). Triplo-X females (XXX) have two chromatin masses in some of their nuclei ($3 - 1 = 2$). The number of sex chromatin masses (Barr bodies) is wholly independent of the number of Y chromosomes present.

In sex chromatin preparations from normal women and girls, a chromatin mass will be found in about 30 per cent of nuclei. Barr bodies are probably present in all such nuclei. However, some Barr bodies will be adherent to that part of the nuclear membrane which is in the same plane as the microscopic slide and so cannot be identified with certainty. Counts of 100 per cent are not to be expected.

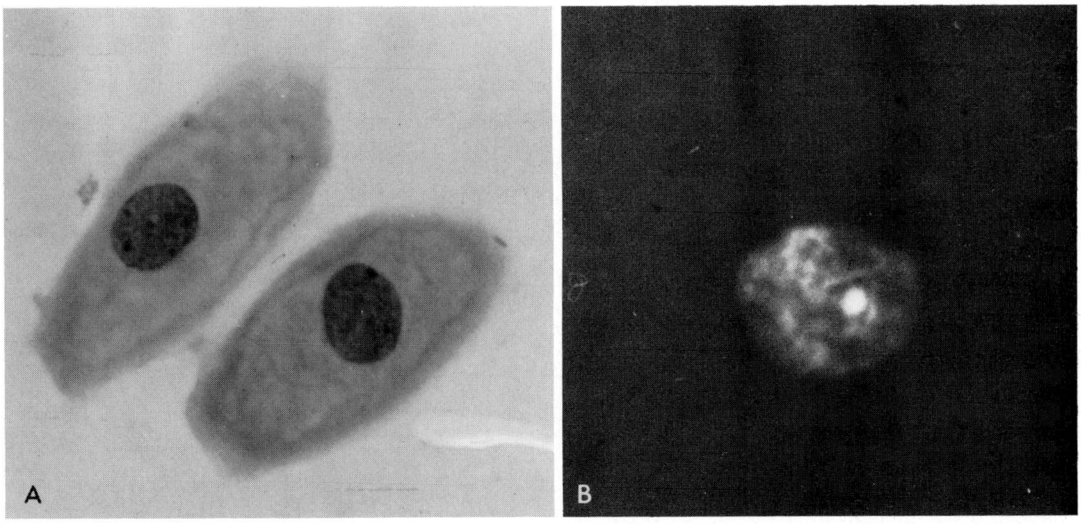

Figure 29–1. *A*, Chromatin negative (upper) and chromatin positive (lower) nuclei in a vaginal smear. (Papanicolaou stain, × 960.) *B*, Appearance of Y chromosome fluorescence in a quinacrine-stained smear using UV light source. (× 960.)

Demonstration of Sex Chromatin. Sex chromatin may be seen in any tissue which has cells with large, open nuclei. Buccal smears, vaginal smears, the epithelial cells of urinary sediment, and the cells of amniotic fluid can be used. In paraffin sections, sex chromatin can be identified in the nuclei of almost any tissue from a normal female.

Any nuclear stain will stain the Barr body. These include hematoxylin-eosin preparations and Papanicolaou stained smears as well as special stains such as orcein, cresylecht violet, thionine, Feulgen stain, the Guard stain, or carbolfuchsin.

Papanicolaou and hematoxylin-eosin stains have the advantage of general availability. However, both stain bacteria heavily, and the chromatin is stained less prominently than it is with the special stains. Orcein is a very rapid stain most easily used for temporary mounts. Orcein also stains bacteria heavily. Bacterial artefacts can be minimized with acid hydrolysis and thionine staining. However, thionine may not provide sufficiently intense staining for ease of examination.

Both Feulgen and Guard stains produce excellent preparations but are technically difficult. The Guard stain is based on the principle that Beibrich scarlet can be displaced from nuclear chromatin by fast green at a rate which is proportional to the mass of chromatin being stained. Under controlled conditions, sex chromatin, a large mass, will remain red after the rest of the nuclear chromatin has been stained green. Well differentiated Guard stains are truly beautiful, but the staining technique is sufficiently difficult that few laboratories care to use it as a routine stain.

One of the most satisfactory routine stains for sex chromatin is carbolfuchsin. Bacteria, though stained, are stained lightly and are not troublesome if hydrolysis is used. The Barr body is stained prominently (Fig. 29–1). The technique is presented in detail below.

SAMPLING. Using a metal spatula, scrape the inner surface of the cheek firmly and spread the cells obtained on a clean glass slide. Albuminized slides may be used if desired. It is important that firm pressure be used in order to dislodge deeper cells with satisfactorily vesicular nuclei. It is our practice to make two slides, scraping the same area of the cheek each time. The second scraping usually yields the more satisfactory cells. Smears should not be spread too thin; they are difficult to examine.

FIXATION. The slides should be fixed immediately, without air drying. Ninety-five per cent ethyl alcohol is the best fixative. Isopropyl alcohol or 50:50 ether:alcohol, both common fixatives for Papanicolaou smears, are almost equally satisfactory. Fixation requires a minimum of 30 minutes. Smears may be left in fixative as long as 24 hours for convenience.

PARLODION TREATMENT. Treatment of the slides with parlodion minimizes cell loss during staining.

1. Immerse slides in absolute ethyl alcohol for 3 minutes.
2. Parlodion solution, 2 minutes. Use a 0.2 per cent solution of parlodion in equal parts of absolute ethyl alcohol and ether.
3. Air dry for 15 seconds.
4. Ethyl alcohol (70 per cent), 5 minutes.
5. Distilled water, two changes of 5 minutes each.

STAINING

1. Stain in carbolfuchsin working solution for 5 to 10 minutes.
2. Immerse in 95 per cent ethyl alcohol for 1 minute.
3. Immerse in absolute ethyl alcohol for 1 minute.
4. Clear in xylol.
5. Mount in Permount or similar mounting medium.

REAGENTS

1. Carbolfuchsin stock solution:

Basic fuchsin	3 gm.
Ethyl alcohol, 70 per cent	100 ml.

The stock solution will keep for months.

2. Carbolfuchsin working solution:

Stock solution	10 ml.
Phenol, 5 per cent in water	90 ml.
Glacial acetic acid	10 ml.
Formaldehyde, 37 per cent	10 ml.

Allow to stand 24 hours before use. Make fresh working solution monthly.

Stained smears are examined with oil immersion. One hundred suitable (open and vesicular) nuclei should be examined and the percentage of chromatin-positive nuclei determined. In normal women and girls, the range of chromatin-positive nuclei is about 20 to 40 per cent. A normal range of values should be established for the individual laboratory. Smears from normal males are chromatin negative.

Reporting and Interpreting Barr Tests. Buccal chromatin tests are properly reported as either *chromatin positive* or *chromatin negative.* If more than one Barr body is present per nucleus, or if there is a strikingly lowered incidence of chromatin-positive nuclei (to less than 50 per cent of the low normal value of the laboratory), these findings should be reported.

It is an error to report these smears as "male" or "female." It is essential to remember that nonfluorescent sex chromatin tests *cannot be used to determine the true genetic sex of a patient.* The genetic sex of humans depends upon the presence or absence of a Y chromosome and *not* upon the number of X chromosomes present. Since buccal chromatin tests detect the number of X chromosomes and only inferentially indicate the presence or absence of a Y chromosome, one is *not* making a sex determination when performing a chromatin test unless the specific fluorescent stains for the Y chromosome (*vide infra*) are used. Genetic females can be chromatin negative (XO—Turner's syndrome) and genetic males can be chromatin positive (XXY—Klinefelter's syndrome).

One may also indicate the chromosome constitution which the chromatin test infers. Two alternatives are always possible and both should be mentioned. For example, "the smear is chromatin negative; this indicates a chromosome constitution of 46,XY (normal male) or of 45,X (Turner's syndrome)."

In Table 29–2 the alterations of sex chromatin patterns are classified. Particular attention is directed to the numerous artefacts to be considered.

Artefacts arise in the laboratory or reflect physiological variations of patients. Laboratory errors include false positives produced either by bacteria or by wrinkles in the nuclear membrane. Careful microscopy will readily differentiate either of these from chromatin masses.

Variation in the size of the chromatin mass is sometimes significant (*vide infra*). Assessing size alterations is not easy. Apparent variations in size follow changes in staining technique (Barr bodies appear smaller, for instance, in hematoxylin-eosin than in carbolfuchsin preparations). Variation in Barr body size may also be noted in smears from different body sites. The Barr bodies of vaginal cells are often larger than those seen in buccal smears from the same patient.

The incidence of chromatin-positive nuclei is sensitive to a variety of stimuli. Oral ingestions of antibiotics reduce the incidence of chromatin-positive nuclei in buccal smears. More important changes occur in the postpartum state when there is a depression of the incidence of chromatin-positive nuclei. The incidence of chromatin-positive cells may fall to as low as 4 or 5 per cent in both the mother and in a normal female infant; thus, the buccal smear of an infant female may be erroneously interpreted as chromatin negative in the first few days of life. The incidence of chromatin-positive nuclei rises slowly to reach normal ranges within three or four days. Chromatin testing of newborn infants should be deferred for one week.

Table 29–2. ALTERATIONS IN SEX CHROMATIN PATTERNS

Numerical alterations
Artefacts
Maternal postpartum state
First three postpartum days (infants)
Steroid and hormone therapy
Pathological alterations
Increases in males—XXY and variants
Increases in females—XXX, XXXX
Decreases in females—XO, XO/XX
Alterations in sex chromatin size
Artefacts
Oral antibiotic ingestion
Variation in cell source (buccal *vs.* vaginal)
Variation in staining procedure
Pathological alterations
Enlargement—isochromosomes of X
Diminution—deletions of X

Pathologic alterations of buccal chromatin patterns are: (1) variations in the number of chromatin masses per nucleus, (2) variations in the incidence of chromatin-positive nuclei per smear, and (3) variations in Barr body size.

Interpreting variations in the number of Barr bodies per cell is simple if the relationship $m = n - 1$ is kept in mind. Increases in the percentage of chromatin-positive nuclei per smear are rarely of significance (except in apparent males). Diminution in the percentage of chromatin-positive nuclei is usually not significant unless the percentage falls to less than half of the low normal value for the laboratory. Then sex chromosomal *mosaicism (q.v.)* is a diagnostic probability.

Alterations in the size of the sex chromatin mass reflect structural alterations of the X chromosome. These are comparatively infrequent; apparent size variation must be interpreted with great caution. Significant alteration in the size of chromatin masses will be paralleled by similar alteration in the size of polymorphonuclear leukocyte drumsticks.

Demonstrating the Y Chromosome. Chromosomal DNA binds many dyes, some of which fluoresce in ultraviolet light. The most effective of those used so far has been quinacrine (either as the hydrochloride or the mustard), which stains chromosomes distinctively (Caspersson *et al.*, 1970). The Y chromosome fluoresces especially brightly in either metaphase or interphase nuclei and is easily identified.

This simple technical procedure is worth using if the laboratory evaluates many patients with suspected chromosomal sexual deficiencies (Fig. 29–1).

1. Buccal smears obtained as previously described are fixed in 95 per cent ethyl alcohol for at least one hour.

2. Immerse slides in methyl alcohol for 3 minutes.

3. Immerse slides in three changes of ethyl alcohol (95, 70, and 50 per cent) for 3 minutes each.

4. Distilled water for 3 minutes.

5. Quinacrine hydrochloride, 0.5 per cent (aqueous), for 5 minutes. (This may be pre-

pared from either pure quinacrine hydrochloride powder or from dissolved and filtered Atabrine tablets.)

6. Two changes of distilled water, 3 minutes each.

7. Phosphate buffer (pH 5.5), 0.01 M citric acid for 3 minutes.

8. Phosphate buffer, 0.01 M (pH 7.4) for 3 minutes.

9. Mount slides in the pH 7.4 buffer and rim with clear nail polish.

10. Examine using ultraviolet light microscopy (either darkfield or incident illumination can be used).

The use of this stain in conjunction with the alkaline buffer system is a technical advance (Hollander and Borgaonkar, 1971) which makes these slides usable for a considerable time after staining.

Polymorphonuclear Leukocyte Appendages. Examination of the nuclei of polymorphonuclear leukocytes (PML) for the drumstick appendages characteristic of the female is simple. In general, the results of this test parallel those of the buccal chromatin test. The two tests are complementary rather than alternative procedures. If only a single such screening test is used, the Barr test is the more informative.

Morphology of Polymorphonuclear Leukocyte Appendages. PML of humans have a variety of distinctive appendages to their nuclei which are classified primarily as either small clubs or drumsticks. Morphologic variants of the latter include sessile nodules and balloons. (Figs. 29–2, 29–3).

SMALL CLUBS. Small clubs occur with equal frequency on the nuclei of PML from males and females. Small clubs are ovoid appendages attached to the nucleus by rather slender chromatin stalks. They are small, seldom exceeding 1 μ in diameter, though a few may approximate the size of drumsticks. The distinction between small clubs and drumsticks may be made on other morphologic grounds (Fig. 29–2). Small clubs are paler than drumsticks and usually retain a discernible internal chromatin pattern. They are equally frequent in bilobed and multilobed nuclei. Multiple small clubs may often be seen in a single cell.

DRUMSTICKS. Drumsticks are found almost exclusively on the nuclei of PML from genetic females. They are much less frequent than small clubs and are found on about 1.5 per cent (6 per 500) nuclei. Characteristically, drumsticks are large (1.5 μ) spherical bodies which stain intensely and homogeneously. Even in pale, Wright-stained smears, drumsticks are deep purple. Drumsticks are borne by slender chromatin stalks. They are infrequently seen in bilobed nuclei; their incidence increases in direct ratio with the lobe count (Arneth index). The nuclei of the PML of normal males occasionally bear one to two drumsticks per 500 PML. The incidence of drumsticks may be as low as three per 500 PML in normal women.

SESSILE NODULES AND BALLOONS. These are morphologic variants of drumsticks. Because of the spatial orientation of these bodies relative to the nucleus, they appear to lack stalks. Otherwise sessile nodules and balloons

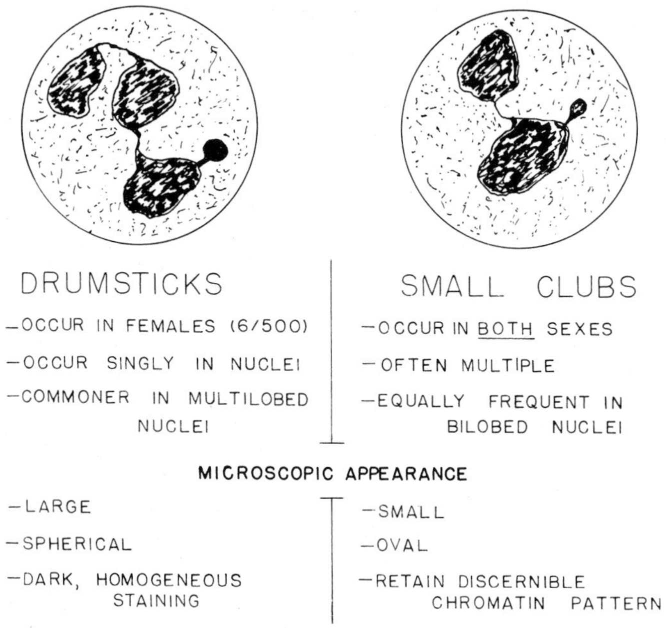

Figure 29–2. Differentiation of nuclear appendages.

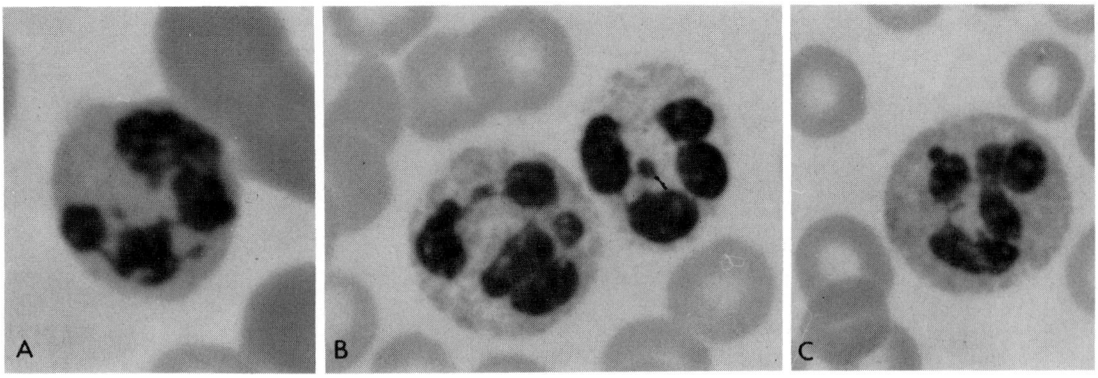

Figure 29–3. PMN leukocyte nuclear appendages. *A*, Two small clubs. *B*, The upper PMN neutrophil has a drumstick. The lower cell has both an accessory nuclear lobule and an interstitial lobe, either of which may be confused with two drumsticks. *C*, A sessile nodule and small club.

have the same morphologic features (large, spherical, and dark) as do drumsticks. When one is enumerating drumsticks, these are included in the count.

RACQUETS. Racquets differ from drumsticks in that they have a central area of pallor which gives them an appearance rather like that of a doughnut on a stick. The significance of racquets is not clear; there is no consensus as to whether they should be enumerated as drumsticks. Their frequency is so low that their inclusion or exclusion makes little appreciable difference to most counts.

Origin of Drumsticks. It is generally stated that the drumstick is the counterpart of the Barr body found in other cells, though this view is not unanimous. Whatever the origin of the drumstick, its significance is much the same as that of the Barr body. Its presence is consistent with a female karyotype.

Demonstration of Drumsticks. Drumsticks are easily demonstrated with routine blood stains such as Wright's stain. Polymorphonuclear leukocytes are enumerated until either six drumsticks have been found or 500 PML counted. These examinations can be facilitated with buffy coat preparations. The time required to make a buffy coat preparation is more than compensated by the reduced time needed to find 500 PML.

Interpretation of Drumstick Counts. Used alone, this test is only moderately satisfactory as a screen for sex chromosome defects. It is most useful in conjunction with Barr chromatin tests. The findings of the two tests should be consistent. When they are not, mosaicism may very well be present.

Structural abnormalities of the X chromosome are reflected more strikingly by alterations in the size of drumsticks than by alterations of Barr body size. This is one of the strongest points in favor of PML drumstick tests. Variations in drumstick size can be appreciated fairly easily by an experienced observer.

CHROMOSOME ANALYSIS (KARYOTYPING)

Before 1956 the chromosome number of man was thought to be 48. In 1956 Tjio and Levan modified the tissue culture techniques used to study human cells. By adding colchicine to their preparations during the last few hours of culture, they obtained large numbers of metaphase figures for study. Hypotonic treatment of the cells spread the chromosomes within the cells and made them individually distinguishable. These workers thereby demonstrated that the human chromosome number is 46.

Adoption of this technique by others led to the discovery (1959) of the chromosome anomalies of mongolism (Lejeune *et al.*, 1959) and of Klinefelter's syndrome (Ford *et al.*, 1959; Jacobs and Strong, 1959). From these beginnings cytogenetics has become a recognized laboratory diagnostic procedure.

Methods of Chromosome Analysis. Tissues with an inherently high mitotic rate or those whose cells will divide in tissue culture can be used for chromosome analysis. There are three basic techniques – immediate, ultra short and long term. Tissues with inherently active mitosis (bone marrow, tumors, etc.) can be treated directly with hypotonic solution, stained, and karyotyped immediately. The yield of mitoses can be increased by incubating such tissues with colchicine for 4 to 6 hours before the hypotonic treatment (ultra short). Other tissues are cultured until active mitosis has begun in the explants (long-term methods). Blood is most often used (Table 29–3).

Blood is easy to sample and to resample and

Table 29–3. SELECTION OF TISSUES FOR KARYOTYPING

TISSUE	ADVANTAGES	DISADVANTAGES
Peripheral blood	Easy to sample Short culture time (72 hours) *Tissue of choice for routine karyotyping*	Unicellular (lymphocytes)
Bone marrow	Ultrashort (4-hour) cultures possible Polycellular (erythroid, myeloid elements) *Tissue of choice in leukemia*	Inconvenient to sample and resample
Skin or fascia	Useful second tissue in study of mosaicism	Inconvenient to sample and resample Long culture time needed (up to three weeks)
Lymph nodes	Useful source of postmortem material Can use short term culture (72 hours)	Antemortem value only in study of lymphomas
Amniotic fluid	Intrapartum diagnosis of fetal disease	Inconvenient to sample; risk to fetus and mother; 14-day culture time

Tissues of value in specialized studies
Placental and fetal tissue—spontaneous abortions
Tumor tissue
Pleural, peritoneal fluid—differentiate neoplastic and reactive effusions
Testicular biopsies—source of human *meiotic* figures

requires only three days of culture time. Micromethods permit chromosome analysis with only finger-prick samples of blood. Only the lymphocytes reproduce in tissue culture. Polymorphonuclear leukocytes are too well differentiated to revert to mitotically active forms. Lymphocytes are very robust cells and have been successfully cultured as long as 48 hours post mortem. Their capability for survival under adverse circumstances makes them useful for mail-in methods.

Bone marrow samples may be examined within a few hours of sampling. Marrow's inherent high mitotic activity virtually guarantees that suitable metaphase figures will be obtained. Bone marrow is sufficiently inconvenient to sample that it is not recommended for routine use but is the tissue of choice when leukemia is being investigated. In bone marrow preparations, mitoses are found in both erythrocytic and leukocytic precursors.

Fetal cells in amniotic fluid can be obtained by needle puncture (amniocentesis) and used for either chromosomal or biochemical study. Fetal cells require longer culture times than blood or bone marrow—about 10 days. This technique is used to detect abnormalities in the unborn infant.

The solid tissues most commonly used are skin, fascia, and tumor tissue. Both skin and fascia are fibroblast cultures. Solid tissue cultures take several weeks and sampling is inconvenient. They are susceptible to infection and to alterations of pH and electrolyte content of the medium. The medium must be changed often. Because of such technical difficulties, solid tissue is not recommended for routine use. Solid tissue preparations are of value when searching for an elusive mosaic chromosome pattern or when the karyotype of tumors is being investigated.

Specialized techniques applied to the chromosome analysis of other tissues occasionally find application in the routine laboratory. Postmortem cultures may be the only material accessible and can be obtained successfully from either bone marrow or from lymph nodes. Placental tissue has been used in the study of habitual abortion. Testicular biopsies provide a tissue in which meiotic ("reduction" division) figures can be seen.

Blood samples yield few mitoses unless some growth-promoting factor (*mitogenic agent*) is used. *Phytohemagglutinin* (PHA) is in widest use. The mitogenic activity of PHA is mimicked by a variety of antigens (e.g., tuberculin), but only if the patient is reactive to them.

Tissue culture media are solutions of glucose, electrolytes, amino acids, and other nutrients. Antibiotics are usually added to prevent infection of the culture. Most commercial media also contain a pH indicator. Finally, a source of protein will enhance cell growth. A good source of protein is the patient's own serum in a ratio of one part of serum to four parts of medium. Some commercial media use fetal calf serum as a protein source.

Following incubation at body temperature (37° C.), the culture is harvested after cell division has been "arrested" with colchicine. Colchicine destroys the spindle apparatus of dividing cells. The spindle apparatus, a structure composed of many sticky, proteinaceous threads, drags the chromosomes to the cell poles as cell division progresses. Destruction of the spindle leaves the chromosomes scattered in the center of the cell and makes them easier to spread.

Following colchicine treatment, the cells are exposed for a short time to hypotonic solution. The cells imbibe water and swell, dispersing the chromosomes widely throughout the cell.

Among the stains used in chromosome analysis are orcein, Giemsa stain, Feulgen stain, and carbolfuchsin. Giemsa stain is probably most widely used. It stains the chromosomes deep blue to purple and is quite satisfactory for photography. Bright field oil immersion is usually used, though some prefer phase contrast.

Fluorescence microscopy using quinacrine hydrochloride (Atabrine) or quinacrine mustard-stained preparations permits more precise identification of individual chromosome pairs than routine staining with black and white photography (Caspersson *et al.,* 1970). The fluorescence quenches rather rapidly, and photography must be completed quickly. Since few laboratories are equipped for fluorescence photomicrography, this has not yet become a routine method.

Chromosomes whose heterochromatin DNA has been denatured with alkali and "annealed" in saline-citrate have "banded" Giemsa staining patterns, apparently fully as distinctive as quinacrine-fluorescence patterns (Drets and Shaw, 1971). This technique is so new that it has not yet been fully evaluated. Because it promises so simple a way to identify individual chromosomes with precision, the technique is included.

"Band" Staining of Metaphase Chromosomes

1. Immerse flame-dried slides (from step 23, in next section) in 0.07 N NaOH in 0.112 M NaCl (pH 12.0) at room temperature for 30 seconds.
2. Three 5 to 10-minute rinses in saline-citrate (S-C) solution.
3. Incubate in S-C solution at 65° C. for 60 to 72 hours.
4. Three changes of 70 per cent ethanol for 3 minutes each.
5. Three changes of 95 per cent ethanol for 3 minutes each.
6. Air dry and stain in Giemsa stain (pH 6.6).
7. Rinse in distilled water and air dry.
8. Mount in Permount.

REAGENTS

NaOH Solution: 2.8 Gm. NaOH and 6.2 Gm. NaCl in 1 L. distilled water.

S-C Solution: 105.2 Gm. NaCl and 52.9 Gm. trisodium citrate in 1 L. distilled water. Adjust to pH 7.0 with 0.1 N HCl.

Giemsa Stain: 5 ml. Giemsa stock (Curtin Scientific), 3 ml. absolute methanol, 3 ml. 0.1 M citric acid and distilled water to 100 ml. Adjust to pH 6.6 with 0.2 M Na_2HPO_4.

The banding patterns which the originators of this technique regard as characteristic for each chromosome pair are shown diagrammatically with a metaphase figure stained by this technique (Fig. 29–4).

Photography of the stained preparations demands meticulous attention to detail. Poor photographs exaggerate the inherent difficulties of karyotyping.

Chromosome Analysis with Peripheral Blood. The method detailed is only slightly modified from a method originally described by Moorehead, Nowell, Mellman, Battips, and Hungerford (1960). It is the parent method for most of the commercial "chromosome kits."

1. Using sterile precautions, collect 10 ml. of venous blood in a heparin-moistened syringe from a patient who has been fasting at least 3 hours. Morning samples are preferred.

Note: Since these cultures require three days of incubation prior to final processing, most laboratories will find it more convenient to draw blood on Monday, Tuesday, Friday, or Saturday. Samples drawn Wednesday or Thursday must be processed on Saturday or Sunday.

Bacterial contamination is a major source of culture loss. The venipuncture area should be cleaned with alcohol and allowed to dry. Those who habitually search for a suitable vein with their fingers should also clean the exploring finger.

Time is not critical. Satisfactory preparations can be obtained over a culture period of 68 to 72 hours. However, it is easier to have a patient fasting if the venipuncture is done early in the day.

Heparin is the anticoagulant of choice. EDTA and citrate may reduce the calcium concentration of the culture medium sufficiently to impair cell division. A good grade of heparin must be used – some commercially available heparin contains phenolic contaminants which cause cell death.

2. Mix the blood and heparin thoroughly. Allow the blood to stand at room temperature for 30 minutes to 1 hour. By this time, the red cells should have sedimented to the bottom of the tube, leaving a leukocyte-plasma supernatant of about 4 ml.

Note: Erythrocyte sedimentation may be accelerated in one of the two following ways: (1) Add 0.5 ml. of Phytohemagglutinin M (Difco Laboratories, Detroit) diluted to the manufacturer's specifications. (2) Centrifuge the sample gently (not over 800 r.p.m.) for 5 to 10 minutes.

3. Using a sterile pipette, transfer aliquots of the supernatant cell-plasma layer to screw-cap test tubes or culture tubes containing a premeasured amount of medium (see Reagents, p. 1318) in a ratio of one part plasma suspension to four parts of medium. It is advisable to set up duplicate cultures. The following steps in the procedure presuppose a total culture volume of 5 ml. If larger culture volumes are used, vary the proportion of reagents accordingly.

Note: Even when meticulous attention is given all phases of the technique, some cultures (about 10

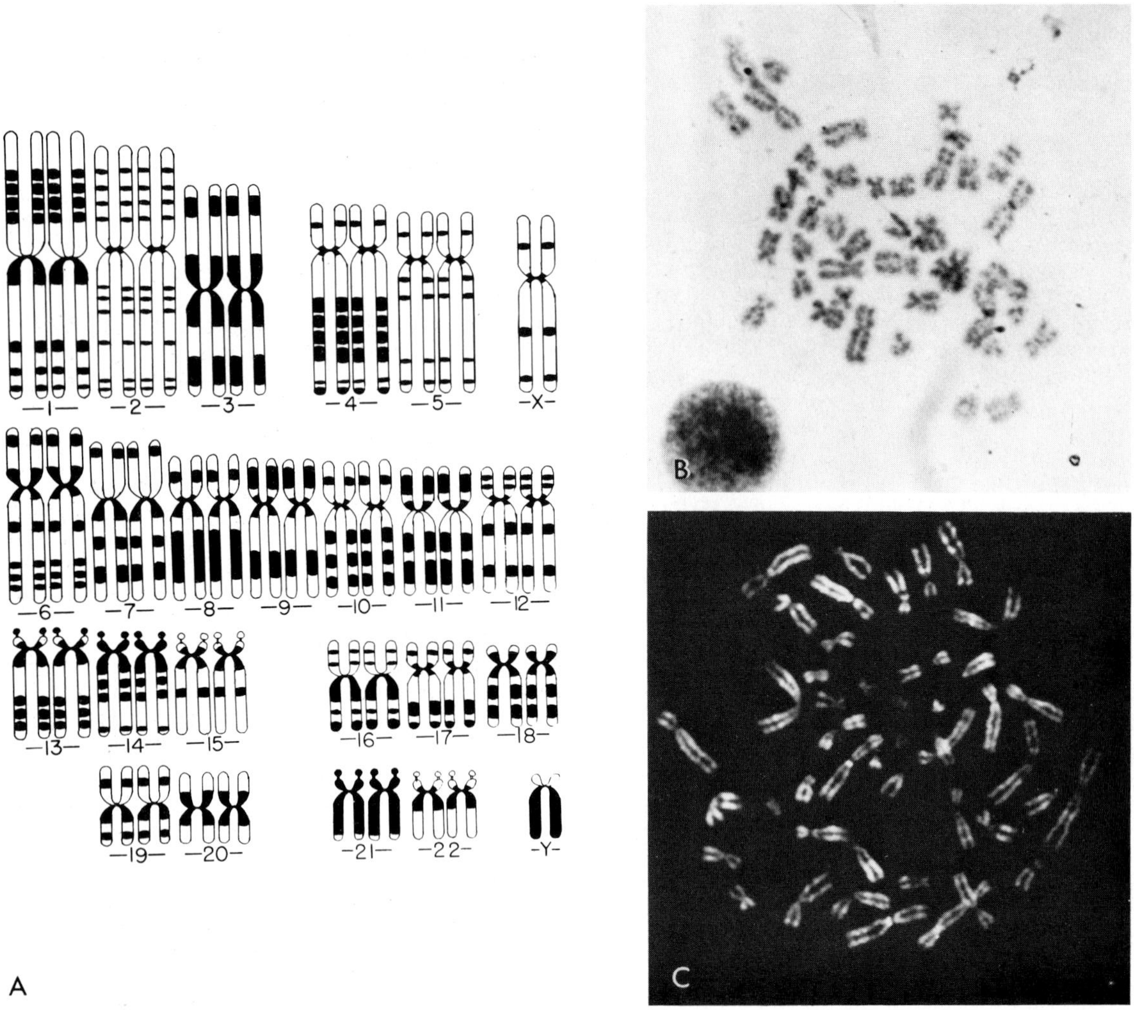

Figure 29–4. Special techniques in chromosome identification. *A*, The heterochromatin "bands" most often encountered using the differential Giemsa stain of Drets and Shaw. The number assignments are not yet "official." *B*, A differential Giemsa stain of a human metaphase. Note the punctate ("band") staining of the chromatids. *C*, A metaphase stained using the quinacrine-fluorescence technique. (Courtesy of Dr. Omar S. Alfi, Los Angeles, California.)

per cent) will fail to yield usable preparations. It is wise to advise each patient ahead of time that a call back for repeat sampling may be necessary.

Some laboratories control the leukocyte concentration of the inoculum by using hemocytometer counts and try to attain a final concentration of 3 to 5 million white cells in each ml. of culture medium. Unless the total white count is very high or there is polymorphonuclear leukocytosis, we have not found concentration of white cells to be this critical. Examination of a Wright-stained blood smear is sufficiently informative to guide the inoculum size.

When there is polymorphonuclear leukocytosis, a smaller inoculum should be used if the leukocytosis is severe. Aspiration of the uppermost layers of the cell-plasma supernatant provides a relatively higher concentration of lymphocytes than of polymorphonuclear leukocytes.

4. Cap the culture vessel tightly and incubate the culture for 72 hours at 37° C. Check the culture vessel daily for evidence of pH change or clotting. Fine fibrin clots will be found occasionally. These can be removed with *sterile* forceps and gentle agitation of the clots to dislodge adherent cells. If such small clots are left in the tube, they can be quite troublesome in later processing.

The medium recommended (see Reagents, p. 1318) contains phenol red as an indicator. Its color reactions are red to red-purple, excessive alkalinity; orange-pink to red-pink, optimum pH; and yellow orange to yellow, excessive acidity.

Note: Excessive alkalinity is rather infrequent and is most commonly a consequence of improper glassware preparation, particularly inadequate rinsing. Residual soap or detergent produces an alkaline reaction.

Excessive acidity may reflect polymorphonuclear

leukocytosis, accumulation of metabolites (CO_2 + H_2O → H_2CO_3) (larger inocula become acid rather rapidly), or bacterial contamination.

Excess acidity in the culture may be corrected by taking the following steps (in order):

A. Loosen the cap of the culture vessel for about 30 minutes (leave the vessel in the incubator). CO_2 is blown off and this simple maneuver will correct the pH of most cultures. If it does not, perform the following:

B. Add 0.1 per cent $NaHCO_3$ in sterile saline, drop by drop. Do not shake the culture vessel about too vigorously. A maximum of 8 drops in a 5-ml. culture should correct the pH. If it does not, perform the following:

C. Most cultures cannot be salvaged if the above steps are unsuccessful. Such cultures are usually contaminated. Using a sterile Pasteur pipette, aspirate a drop of the culture and do a Gram's stain. If no bacteria are present, persistent hyperacidity may reflect only a hypercellular inoculum. Add another 4 ml. of culture medium, using sterile precautions.

5. On the morning of the fourth day, after 68 to 72 hours' incubation, add colchicine or Colcemide (see Reagents, p. 1318) to the culture to produce a final concentration of not more than 1.0 μg. per ml. of culture.

6. Incubate 4 to 6 hours longer at 37° C.

7. Transfer the cultures to conical centrifuge tubes, swirling the culture gently to dislodge any cells which are adherent to the glass.

8. Centrifuge at 800 r.p.m. for 10 minutes. A firm button of cells should form at the bottom of the tube. Decant and discard the supernatant fluid.

9. Wash the cells gently, using 5 ml. of Ringer's, Hanks', or other balanced saline solution, prewarmed to 37° C. The cells can be suspended in the saline with a Pasteur pipette.

10. Centrifuge at not more than 800 r.p.m. for 5 to 10 minutes.

11. Aspirate all but 0.5 ml. of the supernatant washing saline, add 2.0 ml. of prewarmed distilled water, and incubate for 10 minutes at 37° C.

Note: The objective of hypotonic treatment is to distend the cells without rupturing them. Time, at this point, is critical. Overexposure of the cells to hypotonic solution will result in cell rupture and chromosome loss. Underexposure will leave the chromosomes clumped and difficult to enumerate.

Other hypotonic solutions can be used. Distilled water requires the least preparation.

12. Centrifuge at *not over* 600 r.p.m. for exactly 5 minutes.

Note: The total time, including centrifugation, of exposure of the cells to hypotonic solution should not exceed 15 minutes.

After hypotonic treatment, the cells are extremely fragile and all subsequent manipulation should be gentle.

13. Carefully aspirate and discard the supernatant, taking care not to dislodge the cell button. Invert and drain on filter paper or paper toweling *if* the cell button is firm enough to stand inversion.

14. Gently layer 4 ml. of acetic alcohol fixative (see Reagents, p. 1319) on the surface of the cell button, taking care not to disturb the button.

15. Let stand at room temperature for 30 minutes.

16. Gently suspend the cells in fixative, using a Pasteur pipette.

17. Centrifuge at 600 r.p.m. for 5 minutes.

18. Aspirate and discard the supernatant fixative, add 4 ml. of fresh fixative, suspend the cells by gentle agitation with a Pasteur pipette, and allow to stand another 10 minutes at room temperature.

Note: Cell clumps may form at this point. They can usually be dispersed by repeated resuspension in fresh fixative.

19. Centrifuge at 600 r.p.m. for 5 minutes.

20. Aspirate and discard the supernatant fixative. Add just enough fixative to produce a hazy suspension when the cells are resuspended (about 0.5 ml.).

21. Drop 1 or 2 drops of the cell-fixative suspension on a clean, moist glass slide that is tilted slightly.

Note: Even "precleaned" glass slides should be further cleaned before use and rinsed thoroughly in distilled water.

Slides may be moistened by storage in distilled water. Shake the excess water from the slide before use, leaving only a thin film. Another successful method is placing the slides in the freezer a few moments before use. When the slides are taken out, a thin film of water condensation will form.

The use of moist slides facilitates spreading of the smear because of the great difference in surface tension between the fixative and water.

22. Ignite the fixative by passing the slide into the flame of a Bunsen burner.

Note: This is one of several methods used for spreading and flattening the cells. Drying in a stream of warm, dry air or firm pressure with the thumbs on a wet-mounted slide may also be used. Flaming is the easiest method and gives uniform results. Squashing with thumb pressure is best used with orcein-stained wet mounts.

23. After the alcohol has burned completely, wave the slide vigorously to dry the residual acetic acid. Be sure that the alcohol has burned completely before waving the slide – alcohol has a pale flame that is difficult to see.

24. Hydrolyze in 1 N HCl at 60° C. for 15 minutes.

Note: Hydrolysis may be omitted if desired. Hydrolysis removes much of the cytoplasmic ribonucleic acid, and there is less background staining.

25. Wash in tap water and allow to dry.

26. Stain with Giemsa stain (see Reagents, p. 1319) for 15 to 20 minutes, wash slides with distilled water, and mount in Permount.

27. *Scanning.* Scan each slide using both medium-power (10 ×) and high dry (40 ×) brightfield optics. Satisfactory metaphase figures should be moderately numerous (one or two per medium-power field). Identify satisfactory metaphases with an ink dot or by recording coordinates on a graduated stage. Wide-field oculars make scanning easier.

28. *Determining modal number.* Count the chromosomes in as many well-spread and intact metaphase figures as possible. A minimum of 30 cells should be counted. Record the counts in a tabular fashion, e.g., the following:

Chromosome number	<45	45	46	47	>47
Number of cells	0	2	28	0	0

The number of chromosomes present in most cells is the *modal number.* In the example above, the modal number is 46 (normal). In trisomy, the modal number will be 47. In mosaics, two or even more modal numbers may be found.

There are almost as many counting techniques as there are people performing chromosome analysis. We have found direct counting under oil immersion very satisfactory. It is quicker and cheaper than photographic methods. One can soon acquire facility in mentally dividing the metaphase figure into imaginary geographic areas and counting the chromosomes in each.

29. *Photography.* Select "photogenic" metaphases with modal numbers for photography. A photogenic metaphase (a) has deeply stained chromosomes which are not fuzzy; (b) has a clear background; (c) has no artefacts (air bubbles, stain particles, coverglass imperfections, etc.); (d) is compact (elongated and elliptical metaphases have often lost chromosomes); and (e) shows little or no chromosome overlapping.

Illumination is critical. Kohler's illumination and brightfield optics are best. Built-in lamps provide Kohler's illumination readily. Unattached lamps and substage mirrors will also do so when properly adjusted. The technique for obtaining Kohler's illumination should be reviewed and mastered before photography is begun.

Photographs are taken with black-and-white film. The most commonly available photographic setup is the 35-mm. microscope mounted camera. The most satisfactory 35-mm. film in our hands has been Kodak High Contrast Copy (Microfile) film. With photographic equipment which permits use of larger sheet and roll films, a fine-grain and moderately high-contrast film should be selected (we prefer Kodak Panatomic-X).

Photograph quality can be improved with properly selected filters. Giemsa stains may produce a spectrum of colors ranging from deep blue to deep purple, and no single filter will be uniformly satisfactory. We alternate between a yellow and a green (Wratten 58) filter and, rarely, a red filter.

30. *Preparation of karyotype.* Eight-by-ten black-and-white enlargements are best. Cut the individual chromosomes from the photograph and arrange them according to the Denver nomenclature (see Chromosome Identification, p. 1319.)

Chromosome Analysis with Bone Marrow

IMMEDIATE METHOD. A 0.5 to 1.0 ml. aspirate of bone marrow placed directly into a prewarmed (37° C.) hypotonic solution made of one part of 0.9 per cent NaCl solution and four parts of distilled water and incubated at 37° C. for 10 minutes can then be processed as a blood sample (Steps 12 to 30, above). Metaphases will be few and far between, and screening the slides is tedious. However, culture-induced artefacts are at an absolute minimum.

ULTRA-SHORT METHOD. A 0.5 to 1.0 ml. aspirate of bone marrow placed in 5 to 10 ml. of tissue culture medium to which colchicine (1 μg./ml.) has been added is incubated at 37° C. for 4 to 6 hours and then processed as a blood sample (Steps 7 to 30, above). This is our preferred technique since it increases the number of metaphases obtained while still avoiding culture-induced artefacts as much as possible.

LONG-TERM METHOD. A 0.5 to 1.0 ml. aspirate of bone marrow is placed in 5 to 10 ml. of tissue culture medium, incubated at 37° C. for 24 hours and then processed as a blood sample (Steps 5 to 30, above). Though we still handle half of each marrow sample this way (and the other half with the ultra-short technique), we find that the yield of mitoses is only slightly greater. Some laboratories use 48- and 72-hour culture times, but we have not found these longer incubated times particularly advantageous.

Reagents for Chromosome Analysis

1. CULTURE MEDIUM. Use TC 199 (Difco Laboratories, Detroit, Michigan) or similar general purpose tissue culture medium. TC 199 is supplied in 500- and 1000-ml. bottles. To this basic medium add penicillin, 200 units per ml.; streptomycin, 100 to 200 μg. per ml.; and Phytohemagglutinin M (Difco), diluted to the manufacturer's specifications, 0.1 ml. per ml. culture medium.

2. ARRESTING SOLUTION. Use either colchicine (aqueous, for intravenous use) or Colcemid (Ciba). Each 2.0 ml. of injectable colchicine contains 1 mg. Each 2.0 ml. ampule is diluted to 100 ml. with distilled water so that each 0.1 ml. will contain 1.0 μg. of colchicine. Add 0.1 ml. of diluted solution per ml. of culture medium.

3. Fixative. Make fresh each day. Mix 15 ml. glacial acetic acid and 45 ml. absolute methyl alcohol.

This is sufficient fixative for four 5-ml. cultures.

4. Giemsa Stain. Use prepackaged stain and dilute with buffered diluent made up of Na_2HPO_4 solution (9.5 gm. per liter), 61.1 ml.; NaH_2PO_4 solution (9.2 gm. per liter), 38.9 ml.; and distilled water to make 1000 ml.

This buffer has a pH of 7.0. The usual ratio of stain to buffer is 1:20, but this will vary with different batches of stock stain.

Chromosome Analysis by Mail. Lymphocytes are sufficiently hardy to withstand mailing if temperatures are not extreme (especially freezing). Blood samples mailed in sterile heparin solution can be processed in the usual fashion when they reach the reference laboratory. To insure proper handling of the samples in transit, they should be labeled *"Perishable"* and be sent by air.

Chromosome "Kits." The time and trouble involved in making and storing large volumes of reagents may be avoided by using commercially available prepackaged kits. These are appreciably more costly per test in terms of reagent cost but their convenience more than compensates for this disadvantage. We are most familiar with the TC Chromosome Kit and the TC Chromosome Microtest Kit, available from Difco Laboratories of Detroit. These prepackaged kits have been entirely satisfactory.

Other Techniques in Chromosome Analysis. Giemsa-stained blood and bone marrow preparations are adequate to meet most clinical needs. "Band" heterochromatin staining shows every promise of becoming a routine procedure if it is proved reliable. Quinacrine-fluorescence microscopy is already a valuable research tool.

The same immediate technique described for bone marrow can be used with malignant tumors, some effusions, fetal limb buds, and testicular biopsies. Again, these tissues are utilized more in the research than in the routine clinical context. A busy cytogenetics service should be familiar with amniocentesis techniques.

Autoradiography can be used to identify some chromosome pairs more precisely. Tritium (^3H)-labeled thymidine added to culture media during the later hours of incubation becomes incorporated into chromosome segments which reproduce DNA latest. The "hot" (radioactive) late-labeling segments are identified using special photographic techniques (Schmid, 1965). It seems likely that this technique will largely be supplanted by "band" staining or by quinacrine-fluorescence studies.

Electron microscopy and scanning electron microscopy have been less informative than had been hoped. Computer-assisted chromosome analysis is much faster than cut-and-paste karyotyping but is so extremely expensive that only regional counseling centers are likely to find it practical.

CHROMOSOME MORPHOLOGY AND IDENTIFICATION

Chromosomes are studied in mitotic metaphase. By this stage of cell division, each chromosome has split longitudinally into halves (chromatids) still united at a pale area of constriction called the *centromere.* The centromere is a landmark whose position is a useful criterion for chromosome identification. Centromere positions include *metacentric* (almost centrally situated; the chromosome arms are of nearly equal length), *submetacentric* (situated eccentrically to divide the chromosome into readily distinguishable long and short arms), and *acrocentric* (the centromere is so terminally situated that the short arms are either minute or virtually indistinguishable).

Chromosomes may have areas of pallor or constriction other than the centromere (*secondary constrictions*). Some appear with sufficient constancy to aid in chromosome identification.

Any or all of the human acrocentric chromosomes may bear *satellites* on their short arms. These are either small, distinct knobs borne at the ends of slender stalks or pallid, string-like appendages. They are of little aid in identifying individual chromosomes.

Chromosome Nomenclature. Human chromosomes are classified according to a standard nomenclature formulated at a conference held in Denver in 1960. This standard (Denver) nomenclature was modified slightly at later conferences (Barnicot *et al.,* 1964; Chicago, 1966). There are 23 pairs of chromosomes in the human complement—22 pairs of autosomes and the sex chromosomes (XX in females, XY in males). The members of each individual pair are "identical" and are called *homologues.*

In a conventional karyotype, chromosomes are arranged in homologous pairs in descending order of length, and the pairs are numbered (commencing with the largest pair) as pairs 1 through 22. The X and Y chromosomes are given traditional letter designations. Human chromosomes fall into seven major groups (A, B, C, D, E, F, and G) having similar physical features (Chicago Conference, 1960).

Criteria for Chromosome Identification. Karyotypes which are being constructed in the usual diagnostic clinical laboratory context do not generally require elaborate handling. When preparing karyotypes from black-and-white photographs of Giemsa-stained preparations, these conventions should be observed:

1. The larger the chromosome, the smaller its number. The largest chromosomes are those of pair 1, the smallest those of pair 22.

2. When two pairs are of "equal" overall length, the pair with the longer short arms is given the lower number.

3. Chromosomes are oriented with their short arms uppermost.

Identification of chromosomes based upon their length and morphology (centromere position and secondary constrictions) is adequate for most clinical applications. The clinical findings in the patient generally intimate which chromosome defect is to be expected. An unusual symptom complex associated with an unusual chromosome defect may present a real challenge in chromosome identification.

In these unusual (and rather rare) cases, "band" staining, quinacrine-fluorescence microscopy or autoradiography will usually be required to reach a conclusion. Laboratories with a case load of three cases or less weekly (150 cases annually) will seldom find it practical to become adept at autoradiography or fluorescence microscopy since it is unlikely that more than one or two unusual cases will be encountered in a year.

It must be emphasized at the outset that all human chromosome pairs cannot be identified as individuals from photographs (though some very experienced investigators feel that they are able to do so). The fact that one may often be able to arrange the chromosomes of a given cell into plausible pairs does not necessarily infer that the paired chromosomes have thus been accurately "identified." A report in which each chromosome pair is assigned a number infers that identification of the constituent chromosomes has been made unequivocally. For the average laboratory, this practice reflects a good deal more optimism than scientific exactitude. The practice should be avoided (*vide infra*).

Human chromosomes can be assigned to their proper groups without difficulty in preparations of even average technical quality. The identifying features of the major groups and the chromosome pairs therein are:

Group A. Group A includes chromosome pairs 1, 2, and 3. These are the largest of the human chromosomes and have metacentric or only moderately submetacentric centromeres. Individual pairs are readily distinguishable.

PAIR 1. The largest pair of chromosomes, these are almost metacentric, though long and short arms can be distinguished by measurement. One or both members of the pair may bear a secondary constriction near the centromere in the long arm.

PAIR 2. This pair is slightly shorter than pair 1 and is easily distinguished from pair 1 by centromere position. The centromere in pair 2 is submetacentric and long and short arms are distinct. Occasionally one member of pair 2 may be slightly larger than the members of pair 1.

PAIR 3. Appreciably shorter than pairs 1 and 2, pair 3 has virtually exactly centrally situated centromeres. Long and short arms can seldom be distinguished.

Group B. Group B includes chromosome pairs 4 and 5. These are large chromosomes with strikingly submetacentric centromeres. The short arms are about one-fourth the length of the long arms. Identification of individual pairs is unreliable without special techniques. If one pair has appreciably longer short arms than the other pair, this pair should be designated pair 4. In all but exceptional preparations, these chromosomes should be identified merely as group B.

Group C. This group includes chromosome pairs 6 through 12 and the X chromosomes. In females, there are 16 (XX) group C chromosomes and in males there are 15 (XY). The chromosomes in group C are medium sized and have moderately eccentric centromeres. Only rarely can any of the pairs in the group be identified with reasonable accuracy. Pairs 6, 7, 8, and 11 tend to have more centrally placed centromeres than pairs 9, 10, and 12.

PAIR 6. If one pair is conspicuously larger than the rest of the group and its members are morphologically similar, it may be called pair 6.

PAIR 12. This is the smallest pair. They usually have the shortest short arms of the group C members.

C′(9?). Frequently one (rarely both) member of one medium-sized pair has a very conspicuous long-arm constriction. Some authors designate this as chromosome 9, while others, feeling its identity is not established, prefer the C′ designation.

CHROMOSOME X. In females one member of the X chromosome pair is readily identified through autoradiography. The other member of the X chromosome pair in females and the solitary X chromosome of males have no distinctive autoradiographic features. The X chromosome is about the size of chromosome pair 8 or 9. There are no features which identify the X chromosome readily in photographs. In some metaphases from normal females one group C chromosome will be peripherally situated in the metaphase plate, may be angulated, and may stain differently from the rest of the chromosomes. It is reasonable to call such a chromosome an X chromosome. (Presumably the position, angulation, and staining reflect the role of the chromosome in the formation of a sex chromatin mass.)

The members of this group are best identified only as group C.

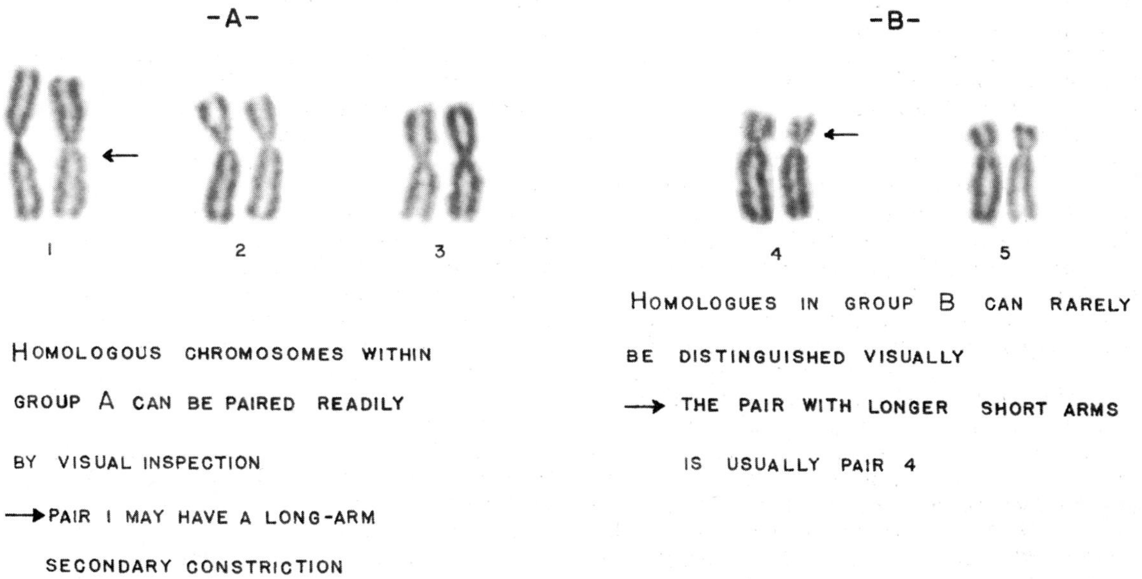

-A-
-B-
1
2
3
4
5
HOMOLOGOUS CHROMOSOMES WITHIN GROUP A CAN BE PAIRED READILY BY VISUAL INSPECTION
→PAIR 1 MAY HAVE A LONG-ARM SECONDARY CONSTRICTION
HOMOLOGUES IN GROUP B CAN RARELY BE DISTINGUISHED VISUALLY
→ THE PAIR WITH LONGER SHORT ARMS IS USUALLY PAIR 4

Figure 29–5. Identification of group A and group B chromosomes. Group A and group B chromosomes from the same cell are shown. The identification of pair 4 and of pair 5 is arbitrary (see text).

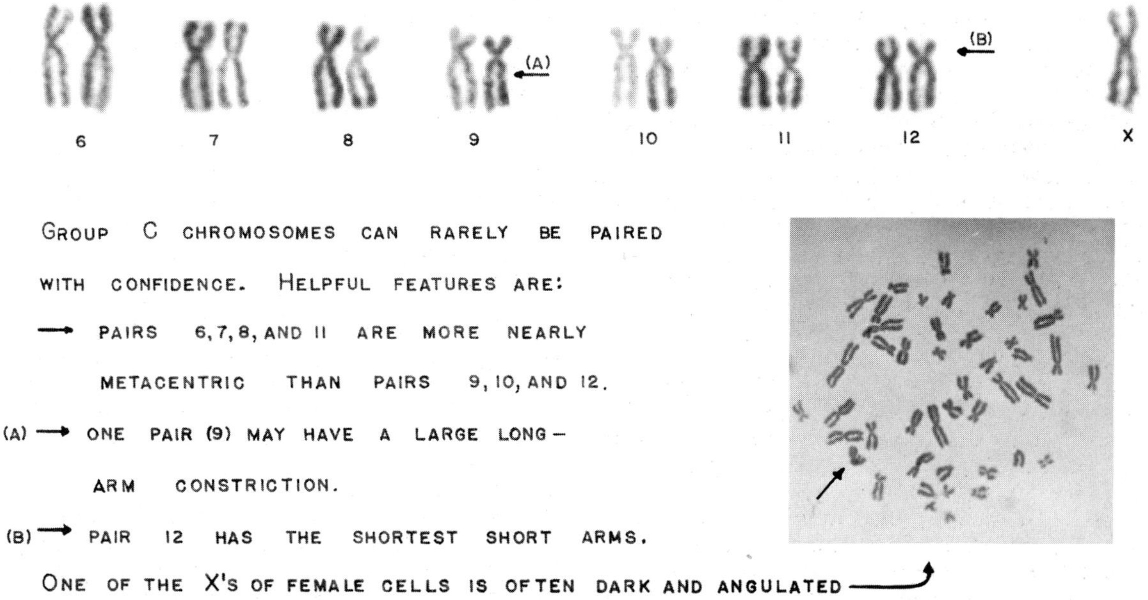

6
7
8
9
(A)
10
11
12
(B)
X
GROUP C CHROMOSOMES CAN RARELY BE PAIRED WITH CONFIDENCE. HELPFUL FEATURES ARE:
→ PAIRS 6, 7, 8, AND 11 ARE MORE NEARLY METACENTRIC THAN PAIRS 9, 10, AND 12.
(A) → ONE PAIR (9) MAY HAVE A LARGE LONG-ARM CONSTRICTION.
(B) → PAIR 12 HAS THE SHORTEST SHORT ARMS.
ONE OF THE X'S OF FEMALE CELLS IS OFTEN DARK AND ANGULATED

Figure 29–6. Identification of group C chromosomes. The presence of 15 group C chromosomes is characteristic of the male cell; females have 16. The identity of individual pairs, though made in accord with available criteria, must still be regarded as completely arbitrary. *Inset,* Metaphase plate of a normal human female cell showing a peripheral, dark, and angulated chromosome that is probably an X chromosome.

Group D. Chromosome pairs 13, 14, and 15 are the six larger acrocentric chromosomes. They have very characteristic "wishbone" or "horseshoe" configurations and have extremely short short arms. Any or all of the group may bear satellites. Autoradiography or fluorescence microscopy can distinguish the three pairs.

Ordinary photographic techniques are inadequate for the identification of individual pairs. The group should be identified only as group D.

Group E. Chromosome pairs 16, 17, and 18 are small submetacentric chromosomes. In preparations of good quality, the pairs can be readily distinguished.

PAIR 16. This is the largest pair. They have the longest short arms.

PAIR 17. The length of both the chromosomes themselves and of their short arms is intermediate between those of pairs 16 and 18.

PAIR 18. This is the smallest pair. They have very short short arms (sometimes so short as to give the appearance of acrocentric chromosomes). Distinction between pair 17 and pair 18 is sometimes troublesome.

Group F. Chromosome pairs 19 and 20 are very short, almost exactly metacentric chromosomes. Individual pairs cannot be identified. The group should be designated group F in reports.

Group G. The group includes chromosome pairs 21 and 22 and the Y chromosome. Females have four group G chromosomes; males have five. Chromosome pairs 21 and 22 are very short acrocentric chromosomes which can be distinguished as individuals only by autoradiography or fluorescence microscopy.

CHROMOSOME Y. This chromosome can be distinguished from the other group G members in good preparations. Criteria for identifying the Y chromosome in descending order of value, are: (1) the long arms of the Y chromosome tend to lie parallel rather than diverging as do those of other group G members; (2) it has a "fuzzy" appearance; (3) it generally stains differently than other group G chromosomes; (4) it is usually (not always) longer than other group G chromosomes.

Summary. Chromosome pairs 1, 2, and 3 can be identified with certainty in any satisfactory preparation. Pairs 16, 17, and 18 can be identified in good preparations, as can the Y chromosome. If autoradiography is available, individual pairs in groups B, D, and G (sometimes) and one member of the X chromosome pair in females can be identified (German *et al.*, 1966). All the pairs can be identified in good quinacrine-fluorescence preparations (Caspersson, 1970).

If photography and microscopy alone are used in chromosome analysis (karyotyping), identification of individual members of groups B, C, D, F, and G should be made only after long experience and then only if *very* good photographs have been obtained. Laboratories which do not specialize in cytogenetics should resist the temptation altogether.

CONVENTIONAL DESIGNATIONS

Conferees discussing "Standardization in Human Cytogenetics" (Chicago Conference, 1966) agreed on a conventional shorthand notation for describing karyotypes briefly. This convention has been adopted almost universally. It has this configuration:

modal number, sex chromosomes, autosome abnormalities

The sex chromosomes are designated whether normal or abnormal; the autosomes are designated only if they are abnormal. For example:

46,XX – normal female

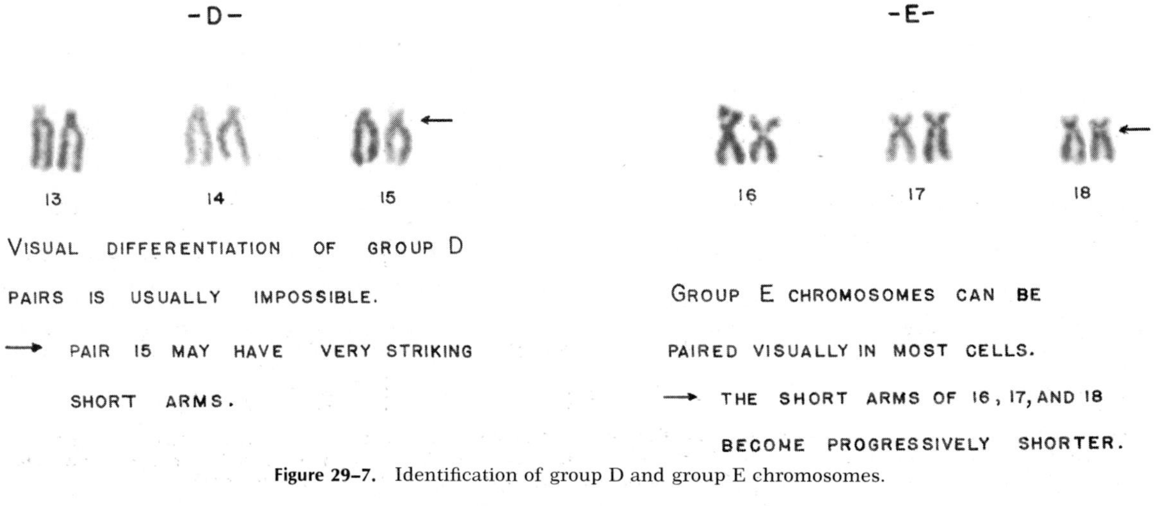

Figure 29–7. Identification of group D and group E chromosomes.

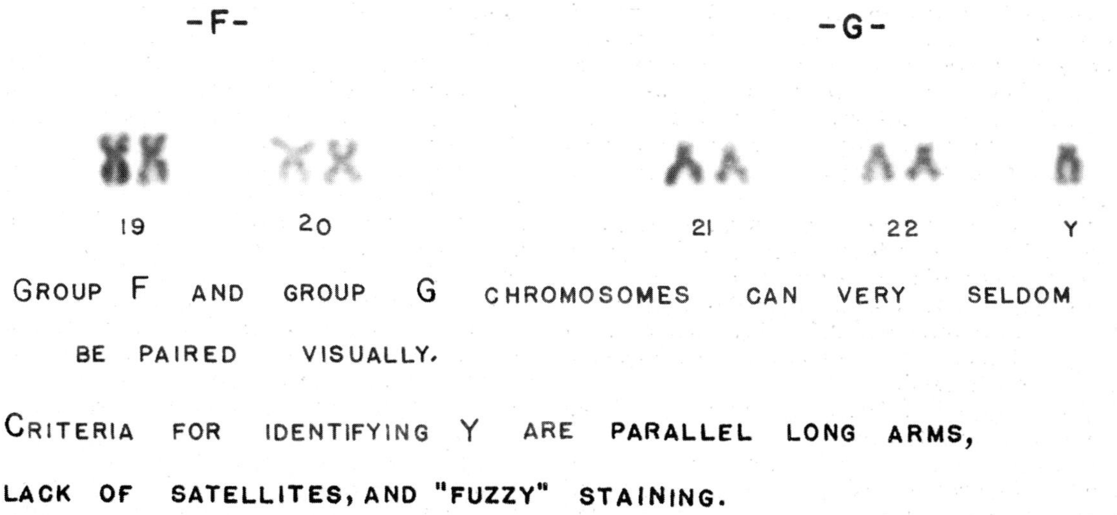

-F-
-G-
19
20
21
22
Y
GROUP F AND GROUP G CHROMOSOMES CAN VERY SELDOM BE PAIRED VISUALLY.
CRITERIA FOR IDENTIFYING Y ARE PARALLEL LONG ARMS, LACK OF SATELLITES, AND "FUZZY" STAINING.

Figure 29–8. Identification of group F and group G chromosomes. The Y chromosome is classified as a group G chromosome. Males therefore have five and females have four group G chromosomes.

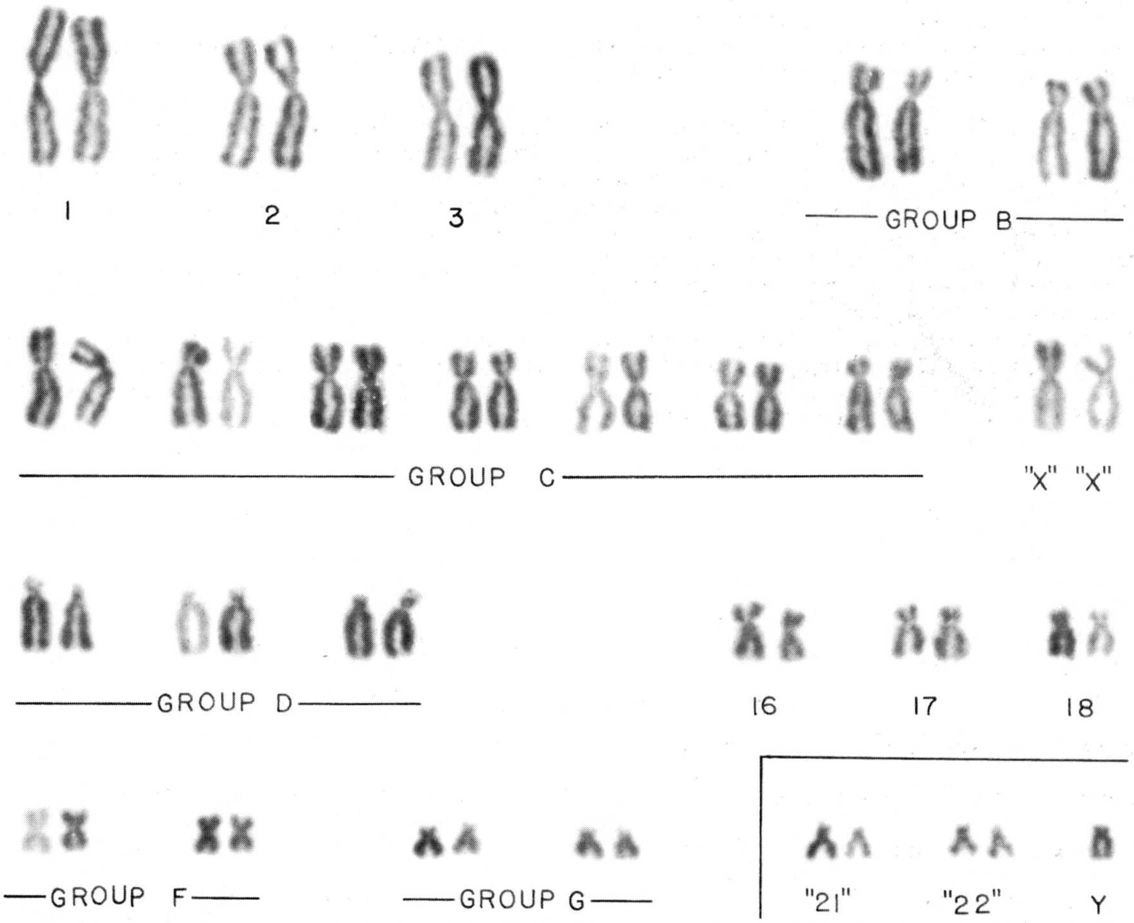

Figure 29–9. Idiogram of a normal human cell. The chromosome complement of a typical normal human female cell is shown. *Inset,* The group G chromosomes of a normal human male cell. The male karyotype differs from the female in that male cells normally have a single X chromosome and therefore have only 15 group C chromosomes.

46,XY – normal male

47,XX,21+ – female with an extra chromosome-21.

The symbols most commonly used are:

+ – increase in chromosomal material (part or all of a chromosome)

– – decrease in chromosomal material

p – short arm of a chromosome

q – long arm of a chromosome

/ – separates the stemlines of a mosaic

t – translocation. The affected chromosome arms are shown in parentheses, e.g., (DqGq). If two translocation chromosomes are present, they are both enclosed in parentheses and separated by a semicolon, e.g., t(DqGq;DpGp)

i – isochromosome

inv – inversion

r – ring

Examples:

45,X/46,XX – mosaic with an abnormal (45,X) and a normal (46,XX) stemline

46,XY,22q$^-$ – deletion of the long arm of chromosome-22 (the Philadelphia chromosome)

46,XXqi – isochromosome of the long arm of an X chromosome

45,XY,D–,G–,t(DqGq)+ – a male in whom a normal D chromosome and a normal G chromosome have been replaced by a single translocation chromosome formed by the long arms of a D chromosome (Dq) and the long arms of a G chromosome (Gq); this is the shorthand for a translocation mongolism carrier

INTERPRETING AND REPORTING CHROMOSOME ANALYSES

Specific disease-associated abnormalities are discussed later (p. 1331). Several general principles are applicable to any chromosome analysis. The most important of these is that an adequate chromosome study includes evaluation of both chromosome number *and* morphology. A count alone does not suffice; representative cells must be fully karyotyped.

Two or more cell lines with different chromosome patterns may exist in the same patient (*mosaicism*). An adequate number of cells must be examined to assure that low-incidence mosaics are not missed. Certainly no less than 15 (we routinely study 30) cells should be studied, and this number should be increased if there is the slightest suspicion that more than one cell line may be present.

Either numerical or morphologic artefacts may be encountered. Numerical artefacts are almost always chromosome losses (factitious hypoploidy) and are most likely to affect exaggeratedly elliptical, "strung out" metaphase figures. Even in good preparations, 3 to 5 per cent of cells will be nonmodal through chromosome loss. This percentage increases if excessive hypotonic treatment has been used.

Excessive exposure to colchicine (too much or too long) shortens chromosomes excessively, makes the centromeres split, and may even fragment the chromatids. The hypercontracted chromosomes may be extremely difficult to pair.

Morphologic artefacts induced by bubbles, scratches, or dye particles are easy to recognize on slides but can be most confusing if photographed. The slide should always be handy when the photos are being cut.

Differences in the rate of chromatid contraction between members of an homologous pair are rather often seen, and one chromosome may be longer and paler than its homologue. With a little practice this is not too difficult to evaluate. Oil immersion lenses which have not been especially ground for photography suffer spherical aberration, and the periphery of the field will be slightly out of focus. Chromosomes in this part of the field will be larger and paler in photographs. (Peripheral chromosomes are sometimes larger and paler than central ones even with good optics.)

Interpretation is facilitated if the clinical features of the patient are known. It should be established whether the test is being performed only for diagnosis or whether counseling is expected as well. There are many instances where adequate counseling cannot be offered if only an affected child has been examined (especially if a structural defect has been found).

As a general rule, the larger the chromosome or chromosome segment affected, the worse the defect produced will be. Gains of chromosomal material are better tolerated than losses. The X chromosome is a notable exception to these generalizations. Extra autosomes larger than those in group D have not been found (except in mosaic patterns) in living patients, nor have missing autosomes (except, rarely, from group G).

A chromosome abnormality found in all cells (*heterosomal* defect) of a patient without mental deficiency should be viewed with suspicious caution. It will almost surely be either a sex chromosome defect or a structural rearrangement of some kind. The common denominator of autosomal gains or losses (even segmental) is mental deficiency. Totally asymptomatic heterosomal chromosomal alterations can affect the Y chromosome; other asymptomatic heterosomal changes are extremely rare except as balanced exchanges (shifts of chromosomal material which do not increase or decrease the number of genes in the cell).

Deciding whether mosaicism is truly present is not easy if one stemline accounts for only 10 to 15 per cent of the total cell population. These low-incidence mosaics are not especially frequent. The criteria for identifying true mosaicism are:

1. The incidence of nonmodal cells should be greater than chance expectation (3 to 5 per cent in younger patients; up to 9 or 10 per cent in the 70 and over ages).

2. The nonmodal cells must have the same karyotype.

3. The mosaic pattern must persist on repeated examination of the same tissue and should be demonstrable in different tissues.

ETIOLOGY OF CHROMOSOME DEFECTS

Both innate physiological alterations and environmental stimuli may precipitate chromosome abnormalities. Factors which have been implicated are summarized in Table 29–4.

Intrinsic Factors. Many (probably most) human chromosome defects affect individuals who have no known exposure to noxious environmental agents. Either general physiological factors or specific inherent chromosomal vagaries are believed responsible for most chromosomal abnormalities. Obviously, exposure to adverse environmental conditions will accentuate the effects of such intrinsic factors.

Maternal Age. There is an increasing incidence of chromosome abnormalities in newborns which is directly proportional to advancing maternal age. This relationship has been demonstrated in most of the numerical abnormalities of human chromosomes; Turner's syndrome (45,X) and Klinefelter's syndrome (47,XXY) are exceptions.

There is only tenuous evidence that advancing paternal age exerts such effects. This difference is predicated upon the difference in the mechanisms by which gametes (sperms and ova) are produced. In human males a continuous supply of "new" spermatozoa is produced throughout reproductive life. In contrast, all the ova which the human female will produce are present at the time of her birth. The ova are retained in a state of suspended animation (called the *dictyotene* phase) from birth until the time of their expulsion during the course of a menstrual cycle. Thus, in the older mother the ova have remained inactive for up to 40 years. Presumably this prolonged mitotic inactivity predisposes these "old eggs" to chromosomal errors when cell division finally does occur.

The effects of aging are not unique to the germ cells. The number of nonmodal cells in cultures from younger (30 or under) adults is not usually in excess of 5 per cent. In contrast, almost 10 per cent of cells are nonmodal in the over-70 age group.

Genetic Complement. In some animals, notably Drosophila, the fruit fly, specific genes have been found which regulate cell division. Mutant forms of these genes regularly induce meiotic errors in cells which bear the mutant gene. A similar mechanism may be implicated in some of the familial chromosome defects of families in which dissimilar defects are present in different family members.

Autoimmunity. There is an unexpectedly high incidence of thyroid autoantibodies in the mothers of mongoloid children. Whether this is a direct causal relationship remains to be seen. Immunoglobulin may react with the chromosomes during cell division to make them "stickier" than normal. This, in turn, would lead to errors in mitotic and meiotic chromosome migration, with consequent numerical chromosome abnormalities.

ABO-Rh Incompatibility. In a similar vein, reports have described an incidence of maternal-fetal ABO and Rh incompatibility that is higher in families with chromosome defects than in the general population. The mechanism is much the same as that envisioned in the autoimmune states.

Chromosomal Peculiarities. Some chromosomes are more disposed to abnormal mitotic and meiotic behavior than others. While defects affecting the smaller chromosomes might appear more numerous because they are compatible with life for varying periods, some chromosomes behave sufficiently uniquely during cell division that their normal function predisposes them to accidents. Satellited

Table 29–4. ETIOLOGY OF CHROMOSOME DEFECTS

Intrinsic factors
General factors
Age – especially maternal age
Genetic complement
Autoimmune states (?)
Maternal – fetal ABO and Rh blood group incompatibility
Chromosomal factors
Nucleolus organization (acrocentric chromosomes)
Sex chromosomes
Structural abnormalities
Satellite association
Extrinsic (environmental) factors
Ionizing radiation
Drugs
Mitotic poisons (e.g., colchicine)
Radiomimetics (e.g., nitrogen mustard)
Metabolic analogs (e.g., bromouracil)
Virus infections
Chronic disease – infectious or metabolic (?)

chromosomes exhibit two peculiarities which may induce abnormalities. These chromosomes tend to lie in close association at their satellited ends (satellite association). This may reflect an increased "stickiness" at these sites which could encourage such closely apposed chromosomes to migrate together during cell division and so produce numerical abnormalities.

Secondly, the satellited chromosomes help to form nucleoli (and are therefore called the nucleolus organizers). During their association with nucleoli these chromosomes are subject to unusual mechanical stress and distortion, which may break them. Structural defects are more common in the satellited chromosomes.

The sex chromosomes are most often affected by numerical abnormalities. The X and Y chromosomes pass through the meiotic cycle slightly out of phase with the remainder of the chromosomes. This asynchrony may be responsible for their high incidence of numerical abnormalities.

Structural alterations which do not alter the total gene population of the affected cell may induce numerical abnormalities during meiosis. During meiosis the two members of each chromosome pair lie in intimate side-by-side association (*synapsis*). This chromosome pairing is exquisitely precise. Chromosomes which bear segmental rearrangements of genes must form very complex relationships with one another in order for this pairing to occur with precision. Such unusually complex figures (e.g., inversion loops, pachytene crosses) readily yield both structural and numerical accidents.

Extrinsic Factors. While the environmental factors discussed below have demonstrable effects upon chromosomes *in vivo*, the relationship of such factors to defects in the children of exposed parents remains speculative.

Radiation. X-irradiation induces chromosome fractures and structural alterations in the lymphocytes of exposed individuals. There is a progressive diminution in the percentage of affected cells from a maximum incidence about three days post irradiation. Chromosome breaks have followed both diagnostic and therapeutic x-irradiation of the spine and therapy with radioactive iodine. Parental x-ray exposure has not yet been proven responsible for chromosome defects in children. However, the known impact of x-irradiation upon human chromosomes should encourage caution in its use during the reproductive years.

Drugs. Many drugs can induce chromosome derangements both *in vitro* and *in vivo*, but no causal relationship to the birth of defective children has yet been proved. (The birth defects induced by thalidomide have not been accompanied by demonstrable chromosome alteration.) There are three main mechanisms by which drugs may affect cell chromosome patterns.

Mitotic poisons are drugs which specifically interfere with the mechanisms of cell division. Many do not act directly upon the chromosomes but upon some other cellular structure. Colchicine is a good example of such a drug; it arrests cell division by inhibiting the formation of the spindle apparatus. Colchicine added to tissue culture results in the accumulation of large numbers of cells which have reached metaphase but which can proceed no further through cell division.

Radiomimetics recapitulate the action of x-irradiation by inducing chromosome breaks and structural rearrangements. Nitrogen mustard is such a drug. Other drugs (e.g., LSD) are thought by some to have similar effects.

Analogues are compounds which have a chemical configuration sufficiently similar to that of normal molecules that they may displace normal molecules in the metabolic cycle. Bromouracil, for example, resembles uracil sufficiently closely that it may become incorporated into the RNA (ribonucleic acid) molecule as readily as uracil. However, it fails to assume the function of the uracil molecule which it replaces, and the segment of the RNA molecule into which it is incorporated becomes functionally incompetent.

Virus Infections. There is some controversy regarding the effects of virus infections upon human chromosomes. Reports of increased chromosome breakage have not been substantiated by all investigators. The impact of viral infections upon bacteria provides a model for speculating upon the effects of some viruses on human cells. Two mechanisms are particularly interesting.

Transformation is the term applied to alterations in bacterial genetic patterns which follow virus infections. In this instance the virus becomes intimately associated with the genetic material of the host bacterium and contributes its genes to the host bacterium's total gene complement (*genome*). *Transduction* is the transfer of genetic material from one cell to a second cell via a viral carrier. The added genetic material alters the hereditary patterns of the recipient second cell.

Chronic Disease. There is only inferential evidence that chronic metabolic or infectious disease predisposes to chromosome abnormalities in animals and none which suggests that such a mechanism is significant in human chromosome defects.

TYPES OF CHROMOSOME DEFECTS

There are two major types of chromosome defects—abnormalities of chromosome number (*aneuploidy*) and abnormalities of chromosome structure. These defects may affect all (*heterosomal*) or only a portion of (*mosaicism*) the body cells. Several terms unique to cytogenetics deserve definition.

The suffix *-ploidy* generally refers to variations in the number of sets of chromosomes present. Normal human cells, other than sperms and ova, have two (paired) sets of 23 chromosomes, a total of 46. This is the *diploid* (2 *n*) complement. Cells which contain a single unpaired set of chromosomes, as do sperms and ova, are *haploid (n)*. Abnormal cells may contain three (*triploid—3 n*) or even more (*polyploid*) sets of chromosomes.

Deviations from the normal complement of individual chromosomes are implied by the suffix *-somy*. Absence of a member of a chromosome pair is *monosomy;* the presence of an extra (third) chromosome is *trisomy. Polysomy* has also been found in man. A brief classification of chromosome defects is presented in Table 29-5.

Aneuploidy. Abnormalities in chromosome number arise through errors in normal chromosome migratory patterns of either mitosis or meiosis. During mitosis each chromosome splits longitudinally and the longitudinal halves of each chromosome are drawn to opposite poles of the cell by the spindle body. Here they function as new chromosomes as two new cells are formed. Chromosome splitting and migration of the halves is *disjunction*. Defects in this mechanism (*nondisjunction*) yield abnormal chromosome numbers in the two new cells formed.

Meiosis, the specialized type of cell division responsible for the formation of *gametes* (sperms and ova), differs from mitosis in that each cell divides twice and produces four new cells. These daughter cells have only a single set of unpaired chromosomes; they are haploid. Thus, during meiosis, disjunction must occur twice, and nondisjunction may affect either (or both) the first or the second meiotic division.

Nondisjunction during meiosis produces spermatozoa or ova with a numerical abnormality of chromosomes. When such gametes are fertilized, the individual produced will have a chromosome defect present in all of his body cells. A heterosomal chromosome defect implies an error during gametogenesis (Fig. 29-10).

The most significant errors of mitosis occur very early after fertilization during the one-, two-, or four-cell stages of embryogenesis. Abnormalities of mitosis yield two or even three different cell lines if the abnormal cells reproduce at about the same rate. This is the origin of *mosaic* chromosome patterns (Fig. 29-11).

Structural Defects. During cell division, nuclear chromatin condenses to form long, thread-like prophase chromosomes which move about surprisingly actively. During this time chromosomes may break, and such breaks predispose to structural rearrangements. Fractured chromosome ends are very "sticky" and have striking proclivity to unite with one another. The free ends of normal chromosomes (the *telomere* ends) are comparatively inert. They do not unite with one another nor do they unite with broken chromosome ends. Telomeres are always at the end of a chromosome and never in the middle. Consequently, any structural defect which shifts chromosomal material to a different chromosome or to a different part of the same chromosome reflects at least *two* chromosome breaks.

Single Chromosome Breaks. A fracture affecting a single chromosome may either heal (probably fairly common) or produce a structurally abnormal chromosome with two centomeres—a *dicentric*. When a fractured chromosome splits longitudinally, there is a tendency for the fractured chromatids to unite. It is this *sister strand reunion* which produces a chromosome with two centromeres. The dicentric chromosome will form a bridge between the two new cells formed. Such *anaphase bridges* may be seen after x-irradiation.

Deletions. Loss of a portion of a chromosome is called a *deletion*. It is unusual for a deletion to follow a single chromosome break. Usually, two breaks have occurred in the same chromosome and the segment between the breaks has become lost (Fig. 29-12).

Human deletions are not particularly rare. Those which have been seen often enough that distinctive defect syndromes are recognizable are 4p–, 5p– ("cat cry" syndrome),

Table 29-5. CLASSIFICATION OF CHROMOSOME DEFECTS

Aneuploidy (abnormality of chromosome number)
- Heterosomal aneuploidy (uniform aneuploidy of all cells)
  - Monosomy (absence of one member of a chromosome pair)
  - Trisomy (one chromosome present in triplicate)
  - Polysomy (four or more of the same individual chromosome present)
  - Complex aneuploidy (numerical defects of two or more individual chromosomes in the same individual)
  - Triploidy (all chromosomes present in triplicate)
- Aneuploid mosaics (two or more distinct cell populations with differing modal numbers)

Structural abnormalities
- Heterosomal structural defects
  - Translocations
  - Deletions
  - Duplications
  - Isochromosomes
  - Inversions
  - Insertions and other uncommon defects
- Structurally anomalous mosaics

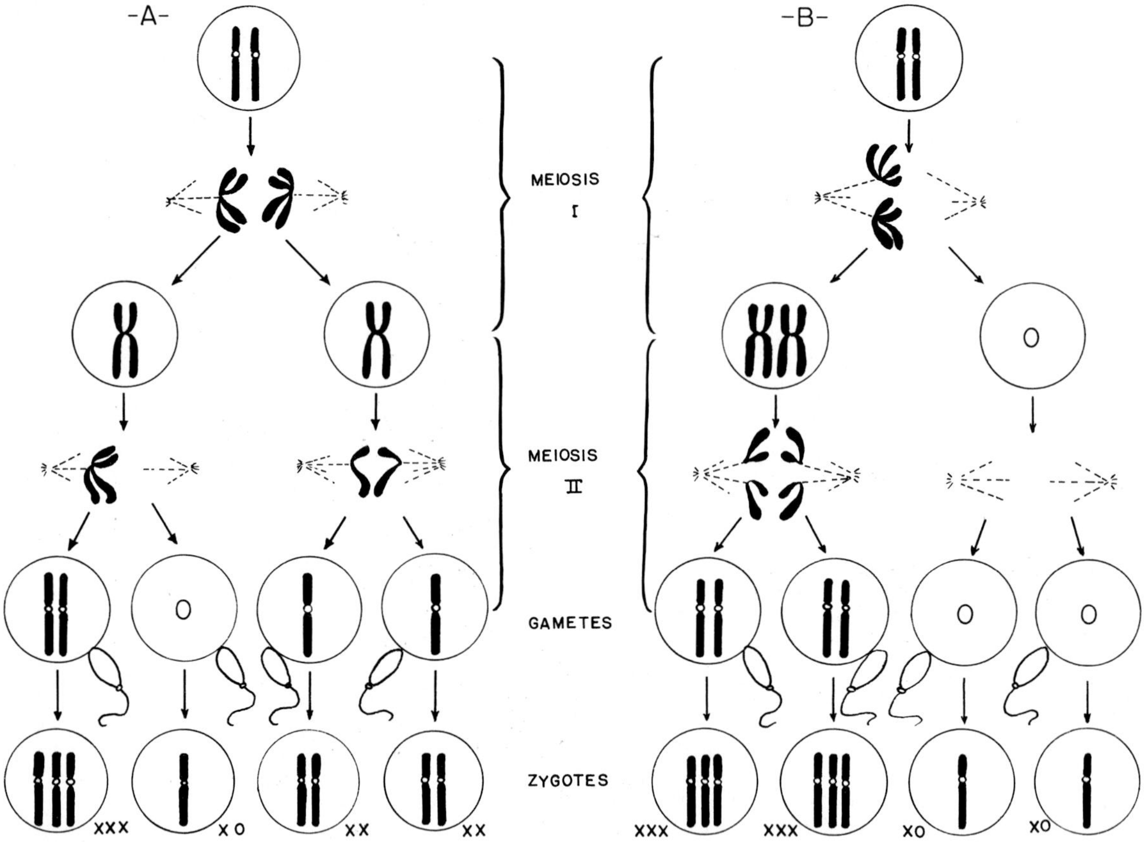

Figure 29–10. Effects of meiotic nondisjunction. *A,* Nondisjunction in Meiosis II. Half the gametes will have an abnormal chromosome complement. *B,* Nondisjunction in Meiosis I. All the gametes will have an abnormal chromosome complement.

18p–, 18q–, Xp–, Xq– and 21q– ("antimongolism"). 22q– is most often seen as the Philadelphia chromosome, though some heterosomal instances have been described.

Translocations. A *translocation* is the shift of a segment of a chromosome to a new position. Usually the term is used to imply a *reciprocal translocation,* which is an exchange of material between two nonhomologous chromosomes. Only translocations which produce morphologically unusual chromosomes can be recognized. An exchange of segments of equal length will remain unnoticed.

Human translocations most commonly affect members of the D and the G group, and the most significant are those of familial mongolism.

Transposition of chromosomal material to another site within the nucleus does not alter the total gene dosage of the affected cell. Translocations have their most significant effects upon the mechanics of meiosis. During normal meiosis, homologous chromosomes form very intimate adjacent pairs (*synapsis*). When a translocation is present, not only do the homologous segments of the translocation chromosomes pair, but pairing must also occur with homologous segments of the unaffected homologues of the translocation chromosomes. When disjunction occurs, gene distribution becomes a matter of chance. These implications are shown diagrammatically in Figures 29–13 and 29–14.

Ring Chromosomes. Ring chromosomes form when fracturing occurs simultaneously at both ends of the chromosome. The fractured ends of the middle segment may unite to form a complete ring. Ring chromosomes are not especially common but have affected the D and E groups, the X chromosome, and chromosome-5.

Isochromosomes. An *isochromosome* is one in which the arms on either side of the centromere are identical. Either long-arm or short-arm isochromosomes may form. A cell bearing an isochromosome is trisomic for the chromosome arm in the isochromosome and is monosomic for the absent arm (Fig. 29–15).

Other Defects. *Insertions* and *inversions* have been reported in man. Such reports are infrequent.

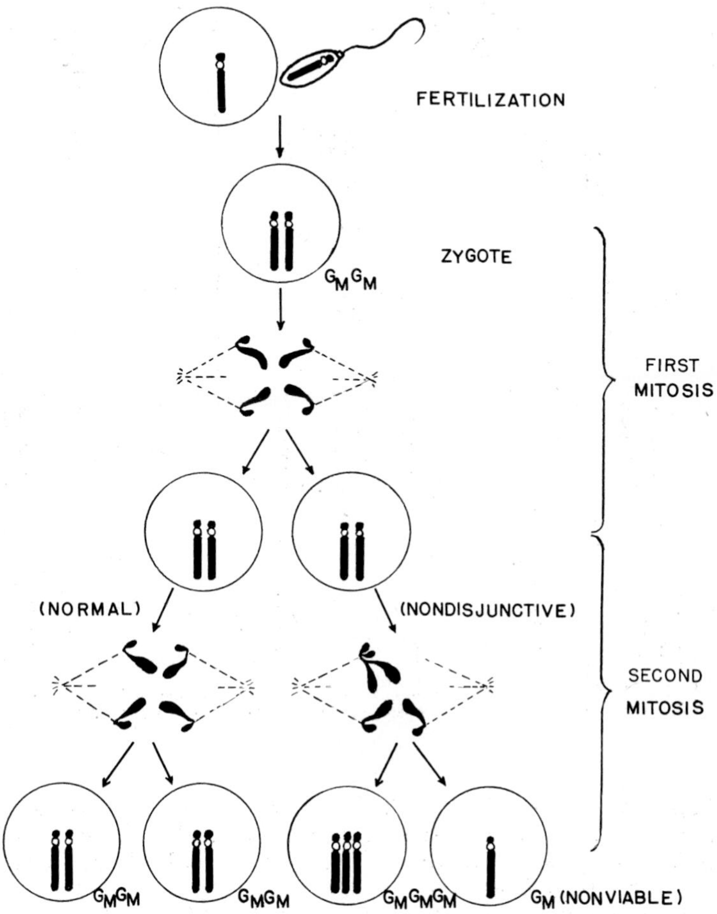

Figure 29–11. Mitotic nondisjunction. Illustration shows the origin of mosaic chromosome patterns; in this instance, the origin of mosaic mongolism is illustrated. The cell line which is monosomic for the "mongol" (G_M) chromosome does not persist.

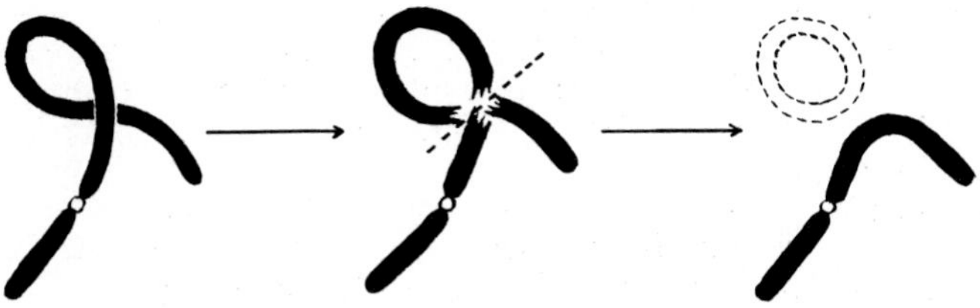

Figure 29–12. Deletion. During cell division a chromosome loops and fractures, and the isolated segment is lost.

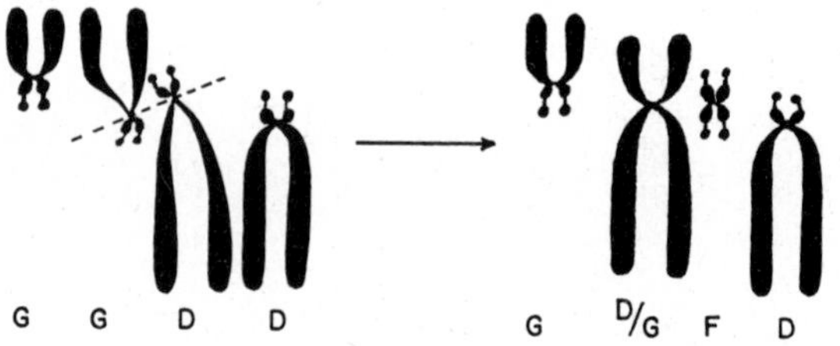

Figure 29–13. Translocation. If two adjacent chromosomes become stretched and fracture (dotted line) and the resultant fragments reunite with the "wrong" partners, a translocation is produced. In this example, formation of a D/G translocation is shown diagrammatically. The chromosome complement of the cell on the right is that of a translocation "carrier." In actual practice, the minute fragment (F) is seldom seen.

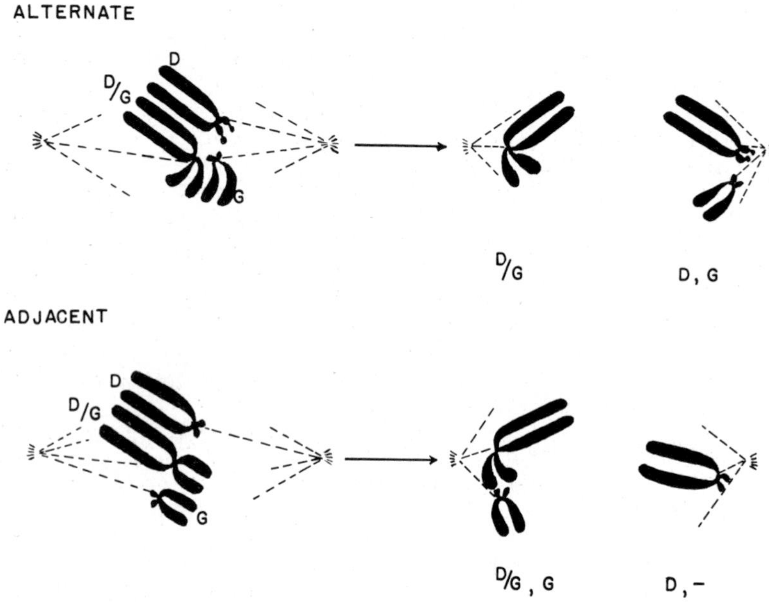

Figure 29–14. Meiosis in a translocation carrier. During meiosis, the translocation chromosome (D/G) and the homologues of the two chromosomes which formed the translocation chromosome (D and G) pair intimately as shown on the left. When the chromosomes are distributed to daughter cells as meiosis proceeds, the attachment of the spindle threads determines to which daughter cell each chromosome will travel. If the spindle attaches in an alternate fashion (*above*), one daughter cell receives the translocation chromosome and one the intact homologues. The zygotes formed when these two daughter cells are fertilized will be a carrier cell and a normal cell respectively. With adjacent spindle attachment (*below*), the translocation chromosome and one of the intact homologues go to the same daughter cell. Fertilization produces a "mongol" (D/G, D, G, G) and a nonviable zygote respectively.

Figure 29–15. Isochromosome formation. If, during cell division, a chromosome splits transversely through its centromere rather than longitudinally, as is normal, isochromosomes are formed which have two short arms and no long arm (*iso-short*) or two long arms and no short arm (*iso-long*).

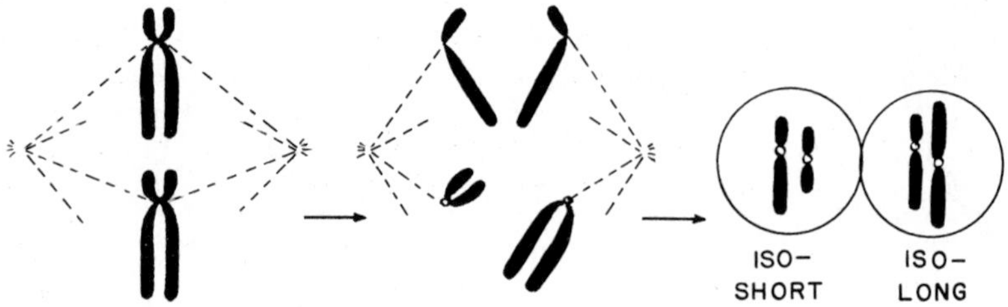

HUMAN AUTOSOMAL SYNDROMES

Human chromosomes influence either sex differentiation (sex chromosomes) or somatic development (autosomes). The autosomes are normally present as 22 pairs of "identical" (homologous) chromosomes. The human sex chromosomes are regarded as a "pair," though they are not always identical in either morphology or function (XY in males). It is most convenient to discuss autosomal and sex chromosomal defects separately.

Mongolism. If the usual signs of mongolism (e.g., epicanthal folds, simian palmar creases, high palate, and mental retardation) are present only in part, diagnosis can be very difficult since even frank clinical mongolism may not be recognized readily in early infancy (especially by the parents). Chromosome analysis resolves such dilemmas unequivocally.

Even when the diagnosis of mongolism can be made on clinical evidence alone, the family's problem is only partially resolved. Each of the chromosomal variants of mongolism (Table 29–6) has its own particular implications for the outcome of future pregnancies. Chromosome analysis offers more precise prognosis than do statistical studies alone.

Trisomic ("Sporadic") Mongolism. Trisomic mongolism is associated with the presence of an extra chromosome in group G (chromosome-21) (Fig. 29–16). The modal count is uniform and is 47. Female trisomic mongols have five instead of four group G chromosomes; male trisomic mongols have six group G chromosomes (rather than the normal five, including the Y chromosome).

Trisomy-21 is found in somewhat more than 85 per cent of mongols. Typically the affected children are born to older (35 years of age or over) mothers who have often had one or more normal children in earlier pregnancies. The probability that the next child will also be a mongol is roughly one in 80.

"Sporadic" mongolism may also affect the children of younger mothers (16 to 30 years of age). The probability of recurrence is somewhat higher in this group—about one in 40—*if both parents are normal.* Younger parents of mongol infants should have chromosome analyses performed. One or the other parent might be a clinically unrecognized mosaic mongol. When this is the case, the outlook for future normal pregnancies is less optimistic (*vide infra*).

When trisomic mongolism is found in a child, we recommend chromosome analysis of both parents (1) when the parents are young and (2) when the affected child is the firstborn child, regardless of the parents' ages. Parents in the older age group who have had previous normal children can be counseled on the basis of the chromosomal findings in the child alone.

Mosaic ("Partial") Mongolism. If a portion of the body cells are trisomic and the remainder are normal (mosaicism), the clinical features of mongolism may be moderated. Such patients have "partial," "subclinical," or *forme fruste* mongolism and may exhibit few of the usual stigmata of the disease.

The clinical significance of mosaic mongolism is twofold. First, the prognosis for the affected child is more optimistic than that of the pure trisomic form. If the percentage of normal cells is sufficiently high (over 50 per cent), the outlook for functional social adequacy is improved. The degree of mental deficiency correlates (albeit imperfectly) with the percentage of affected cells.

Second, mosaic mongols are fertile (so are some trisomic mongols) and may become parents. Since the gonads are affected by the mosaicism, the production of abnormal gametes is to be expected. Though precise estimates are impossible without gonadal chromosome analysis, on the basis of peripheral blood chromosome analysis one can predict with fair precision the probabilities that this mosaic parent will, in turn, bear a mongol child.

If, for example, the ratio of normal to abnormal cells is 1:1, roughly half the germ cells can be assumed to be abnormal as well. During meiosis the abnormal germ cells will undergo *secondary nondisjunction* and will produce equal numbers of normal and abnormal gametes.

The odds that a mosaic parent will have a mongol child in any given pregnancy may be calculated according to the formula:

$$\frac{\text{Percentage of abnormal cells/2}}{100}$$

For example, with 50 per cent of the cells abnormal, the odds that any given pregnancy will eventuate in a mongol birth are:

$$\frac{50/2}{100} = \frac{1}{4}$$

It must be emphasized that this formula is only an approximation.

Translocation ("Familial") Mongolism. The translocation chromosome associated with familial mongolism is formed when the mongol chromosome fractures at or near its centromere and becomes translocated to a recipient chromosome, which is usually a member of the D or G groups, forming (DqGq) and (GqGq) chromosomes, respectively (Fig. 29–17). The clinical features of translocation and trisomic mongolism are indistinguishable (though there are reports that some serum enzyme levels differ in the two forms). A translocation is found in less than 10 per cent of mongols.

There is a profound difference in the hereditary patterns of translocation and trisomic

Table 29–6. CYTOGENETIC VARIANTS OF MONGOLISM

CHROMOSOME ANOMALY	KARYOTYPE*	CLINICAL FEATURES	PROBABILITY OF RECURRENCE
Trisomy	47,XX,21+, or 47,XY,21+	Sporadic mongolism; older mothers with previous normal children	1:40–1:80†
Translocation:			
De novo	46,XY,D–,t(DqGq)+ or 46,XX,G–,t(GqGq)+	Affected infant has translocation; both parents have normal karyotypes	1:40–1:80
Familial	As above	Affected infant has one parent who is a carrier; recurrence risk depends on sex of asymptomatic parent: Mother (45,XX,D–,G–,t(DqGq)+) Father (45,XY,D–,G–,t(DqGq)+)	<1:3 1:12
Inevitable	46,XY,G–,t(21q21q)+	Rare familial form; if either parent is a carrier, only mongol children will be born	100%
Mosaicism	46,XX/47,XX,21+	"Subclinical" mongolism; child may have fairly high I.Q.; clinical signs sometimes minimal	>1:650‡
Normal	46,XX or 46,XY	Clinical mongolism with no karyotype abnormality (very rare)	?

*Any form may affect either sex, though only one is shown in the sample karyotypes.
†If both parents have normal karyotypes (see text).
‡Though mosaicism is a postzygotic defect, it has recurred in some families and the risk is therefore somewhat higher than random risk.

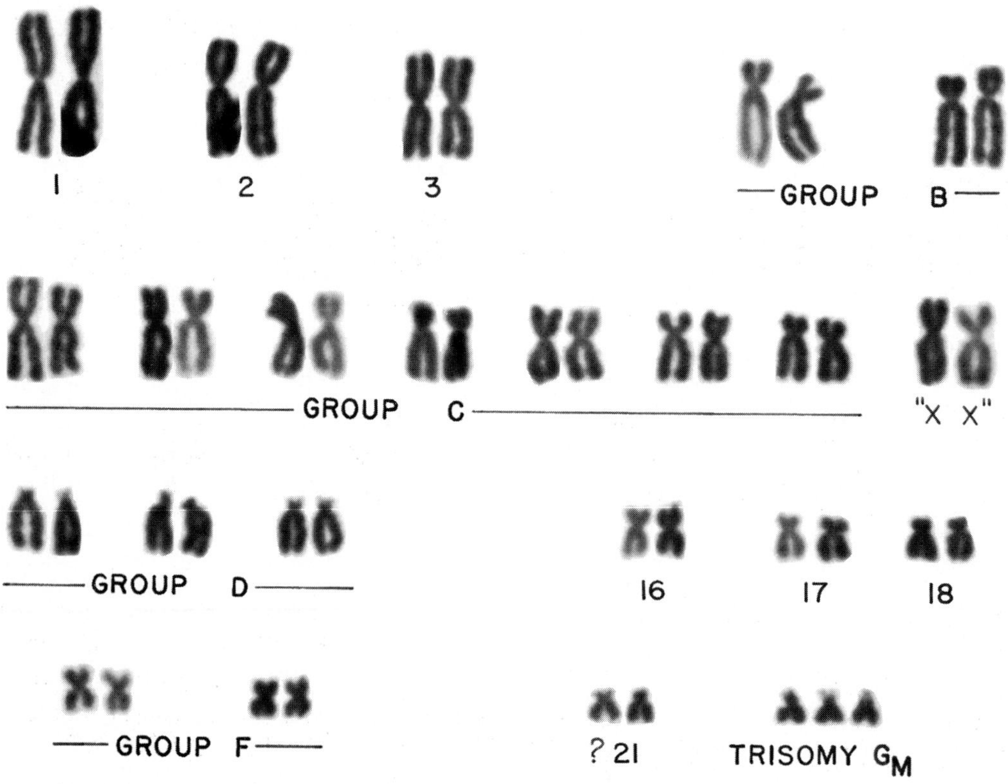

Figure 29–16. Karyotype of a trisomic mongol. There are 47 chromosomes, with an extra chromosome in group G.

mongolism. The hereditary patterns of translocations in general are similar, and the discussion of the hereditary pattern of mongolism is equally applicable to other translocations.

A (DqGq) or (GqGq) translocation chromosome bears the bulk of the functional genetic material of the two chromosomes from which it is derived. When a translocation chromosome forms, the involved cell remains genetically unaltered for all practical purposes. Such a cell (with D/G translocation mongolism as an example throughout the following discussion) has a chromosome pattern of

t(DqGq), D, G

as opposed to the normal D, D, G, G pattern. This is the pattern of cells from a "carrier." When a germ cell with such a chromosome complement forms sperms or ova, the translocation chromosome may:

1. Travel to one gamete alone:
t(DqGq), D, G ⟶ (*a*) t(DqGq) and (*b*) D, G

2. Travel with either intact homologous chromosome:
t(DqGq), D, G ⟶ (*a*) t(DqGq), G and (*b*) D, –
or
t(DqGq), D, G ⟶ (*c*) t(DqGq), D and (*d*) –, G

3. Travel with both intact homologous chromosomes:
t(DqGq), D, G ⟶ (*a*) t(DqGq), D, G and (*b*) –, –

Chromosome patterns of types 2*c*, 2*d*, 3*a*, or 3*b* have not yet been found in a human conceptus.

As far as family counseling is concerned, only four types of gametes need be considered. There is an equal chance that any one type will be formed; therefore, 25 per cent of gametes will have a chromosome pattern of t(DqGq) (1*a*, above), 25 per cent of gametes will have a chromosome pattern of D, G (1*b*, above), 25 per cent of gametes will have a chromosome pattern of t(DqGq), G (2*a*, above), and 25 per cent of gametes will have a chromosome pattern of D, – (2*b*, above).

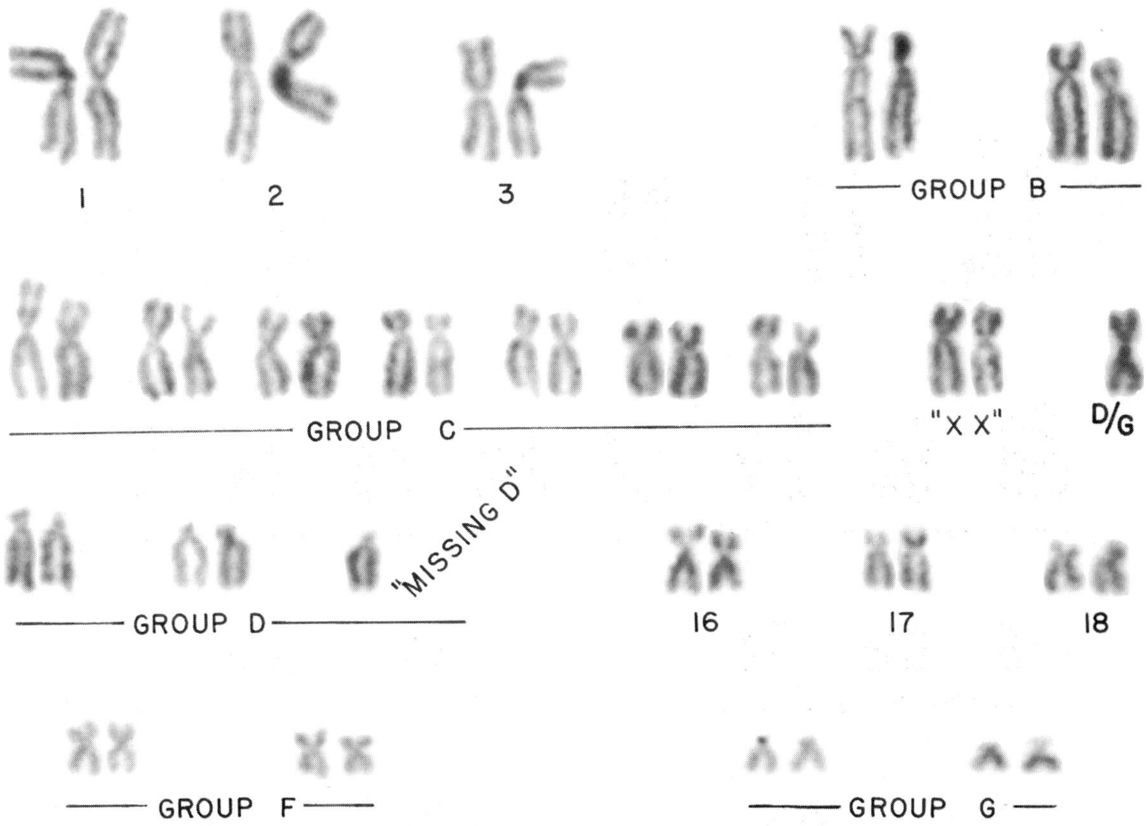

Figure 29–17. Karyotype in translocation mongolism (46,XX,D–,t(DqGq)+). There are 46 chromosomes. The D/G translocation chromosome closely resembles a group C chromosome. The clue to the translocation is the "missing D" chromosome. One might otherwise think this to be a triplo-X cell.

When these gametes are fertilized by a normal gamete (D, G), there is an equal chance that the infant will be:

t(DqGq), D, G – an apparently normal translocation "carrier."

D, D, G, G, – normal.

t(DqGq), D, G, G – translocation mongolism.

D, D, G, – – monosomy G (usually lethal).

Note that the mongol child (t(DqGq), D, G, G) has the functional genetic material of *three* G(21) chromosomes – two intact G(21) chromosomes and the G(21) chromosomal material present in the D/G translocation chromosome.

It is imperative to recognize that the foregoing discussion points out the *theoretical* expectation that mongolism will recur in families to whom a translocation mongol child has been born. Before *individual* family counseling can be offered, the karyotype of both parents should be ascertained. There are three possibilities.

PARENTS MAY BE NORMAL. Translocation chromosome patterns fairly often reflect *de novo* accidents affecting the cells of the child alone. When this is the case, the odds that mongolism will recur in a succeeding pregnancy are much the same as those in the trisomic form, i.e., about one in 80.

MOTHER MAY BE THE CARRIER. When the mother is the translocation carrier, the recurrence risk is high. In this instance there is one chance in three that the child will be normal, there is one chance in three that the child will be a carrier, and there is one chance in three that the child will have mongolism.

FATHER MAY BE THE CARRIER. Carrier fathers will sire mongol infants in about one pregnancy in 12. They are more likely to sire normal (about five in 12) or carrier (about six in 12) children.

Cytogenetic identification of translocation mongolism may be difficult. The chromosome pattern varies in the carrier and in the mongol states. *Carriers* have a modal number of 45 chromosomes. Those carrying the D/G translocation have one G chromosome "missing" and one D chromosome "missing." They also have an "extra" chromosome (the t(DqGq) chromosome) which simulates a member of the C group. Carriers of the G/G translocation have *two* chromosomes "missing" from group G and an "extra" chromosome (the t(GqGq) chromosome), which most closely resembles a group F chromosome. The G/G translocation chromosome is almost exactly metacentric.

The karyotypes of translocation *mongols* are similar to those of carriers, with the addition of one more group G chromosome. The modal number in translocation mongolism is 46. Of the two forms of translocation mongolism, the D/G variant (Fig. 29–17) is somewhat more common.

G(21)/G(21) Translocation Mongolism. A translocation which occurs between the homologous members of the "mongol" chromosome pair produces a chromosome of the type t(21q21q). An individual carrying such a translocation can bear only mongol children. When gametes are formed, a gamete will either receive the t(21q21q) chromosome or will receive no G(21) chromosomal material at all:

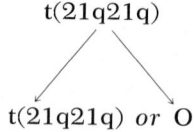

t(21q21q)

↙ ↘

t(21q21q) *or* O

When fertilized, the t(21q21q)-bearing gamete results in a mongol child. The gamete without G(21) chromosomal material will not usually produce a viable infant.

Other Forms. Mongolism has occasionally been associated with chromosome inversions and with isochromosomes. Very infrequently patients with the full clinical picture of mongolism have had no detectable chromosomal abnormalities.

Such variant patterns make family counseling very difficult, since little is known about the hereditary patterns that are to be expected.

Other Group G Abnormalities. Complete absence of one chromosome-21 ("antimongolism") is the sole example of autosomal monosomy seen in liveborn infants (Al-Aish *et al.*, 1967). Deletions of the group G chromosomes (21q– and 22q–) seem to fall into two distinct and recognizable syndromes (Warren and Rimoin, 1970). Trisomy-22 is rare, and the clinical features have been inconstant in the cases reported.

D-trisomy Syndrome. The specific complex of anomalies listed in Table 29–7 is associated with the presence of an extra member of the D group of chromosomes (seven rather than six). The modal number in affected infants is 47. The trisomic variant is the most common; mosaics and translocations are rare.

Table 29–7. MAJOR CLINICAL FEATURES OF D-TRISOMY

Mental retardation
Deafness
Low-set and deformed ears
Eye defects (microphthalmia, anophthalmia, iridic defects)
Cleft palate
Harelip
Polydactylia
Capillary hemangioma
Umbilical hernia
Cardiac defects (septal defects, patent ductus)
Abnormal appendages on polymorphonuclear leukocytes
Abnormal hemoglobin electrophoretic patterns

Table 29–8. MAJOR CLINICAL FEATURES OF E-TRISOMY

Muscular hypertonicity
Mental retardation
Micrognathia
Prominent occiput
Low-set and deformed ears
Finger overlapping (second over third)
Short, dorsiflexed great toe
Scanty subcutaneous tissue
Cardiac defects (septal defects, patent ductus)
Renal anomalies (hydroureter, horseshoe kidney)
Low birth weight

Of great clinical importance is the triad of umbilical hernia, multiple hemangiomas, and polydactylia. This triad of findings is very common in the D-trisomy syndrome and the other, more serious external findings are sometimes not well delineated. Since the three conditions mentioned are amenable to surgical correction, there may be the temptation to perform surgery on infants with these conditions. Before such surgery is undertaken, it is imperative that the D-trisomy syndrome be ruled out by cytogenetic studies.

If the D-trisomy syndrome is present, the outlook for the affected infant is hopeless. The infants rarely survive the second year. The D-trisomy syndrome is more common in female infants.

E-trisomy Syndrome. The symptom complex which comprises the E-trisomy syndrome is outlined in Table 29–8. Karyotyping usually reveals a modal number of 47 chromosomes, with an extra member in the E group. The affected chromosome is chromosome-18. Mosaic and translocation patterns are rare.

The combination of micrognathia and prominent occiput gives the affected infants a rather striking "pointed-face" appearance when the head is viewed from the side. Even more distinctive is the hand deformity which has been seen in all the infants so far investigated. The hands are clenched, and the index finger overlaps the third. The fourth finger often overlaps the fifth. The hand defect alone is sufficient indication to perform a karyotype.

The prognosis for affected infants is uniformly bad. The infants rarely survive their third year. Like the D-trisomy syndrome, the E-trisomy syndrome is more common in female infants.

E Deletion Syndromes. Both long (18q–) and short arm (18p–) deletions of chromosome-18 can be recognized from the symptoms and signs they produce. 18p– is less distinctive than the 18q– syndrome, which can be recognized by the peculiar facial changes (midface dysplasia) it induces. Both defects, in common with autosomal defects generally, produce mental deficiency (de Grouchy, 1969).

"Cat-cry" (5p–) Syndrome. The distinguishing feature of "cat-cry" syndrome is the peculiar mewing cry which these infants have. It is most remarkably cat-like in character. Affected infants have epiglottic hypoplasia, which, in addition to producing the strange cry, may predispose to accidents of swallowing.

The patients are round-faced, have wide-set eyes, and are mentally defective. Older patients (life expectancy is fairly long) develop premature graying of hair and overbite malocclusion. Their cells have 46 chromosomes and there is loss of one-half to two-thirds of the short arm of one of the B group chromosomes (5p–). The abnormal chromosome looks rather like an overlong D chromosome. The affected chromosome was identified by autoradiography (Miller *et al.*, 1969).

A similar deletion affects the other member of the B group. 4p– produces changes which are easily confused with those of 5p–. The characteristic cry is lacking. Again, mental deficiency is profound.

If either 4p– or 5p– is found in a child, the parents should have chromosome studies; parental balanced translocations are frequently encountered.

Other Autosomal Defects. There are sporadic descriptions of other autosomal defects. Many have been asymptomatic balanced chromosome interchanges. Rare instances of triploidy (69 chromosomes) and mosaic group C trisomy have been found in living patients. These rare anomalies are problems for a counselor since so little is known about their natural history.

CHROMOSOME CHANGES IN NEOPLASIA

Most malignant neoplasms have an abnormal chromosome pattern. The chromosomal defects (with the exception of the Ph^1 chromosome) are variable within the same class of tumor and within the cells of the same tumor. Chromosome analysis is not useful in identifying tumor type. The chromosome changes seem to develop at the onset of the malignancy.

Cytogenetic techniques can be used to distinguish between neoplastic and reactive mesothelial cells in pleural and peritoneal effusions. If the cells of effusions have abnormal karyotypes, it is strong evidence that the effusion is neoplastic. Full karyotypes of representative cells must be prepared. Tumor cells not infrequently exhibit "factitious euploidy" and will have a modal count of 46 chromosomes in the face of either structural or numerical chromosome abnormalities. These may be missed if only microscopic chromosome enumeration is performed.

There has not been enough success in correlating tumor chromosome patterns with their biologic behavior to make these studies useful on a day-to-day basis. Even attempts to distinguish atypical, but benign, dysplasias from early true carcinomas have not been predictable.

Philadelphia (Ph^1) Chromosome. Leukemic cells, in common with tumor cells in general, show abnormal chromosome patterns. With the exception of the chromosome changes of chronic granulocytic leukemia (CGL), the chromosome changes in leukemia are inconstant from cell to cell and are of limited differential diagnostic value.

In 1960 Nowell and Hungerford demonstrated a constant chromosome abnormality in the cells of several patients with CGL. This finding has been substantiated by several different groups and the Philadelphia (Ph^1) chromosome is generally conceded to be diagnostic of CGL.

The Ph^1 chromosome is a G(22) chromosome from which one-half to two-thirds of the long arm has been deleted. The Ph^1 chromosome is a minute acrocentric chromosome which may bear satellites. Cells bearing the Ph^1 chromosome have a modal number of 46 chromosomes. The Ph^1 chromosome is found in the myelocytic, erythrocytic, and megakaryocytic cells of patients with CGL. The Ph^1 chromosome is *not* present in lymphocytes or in other body cells.

The method of choice for demonstrating the

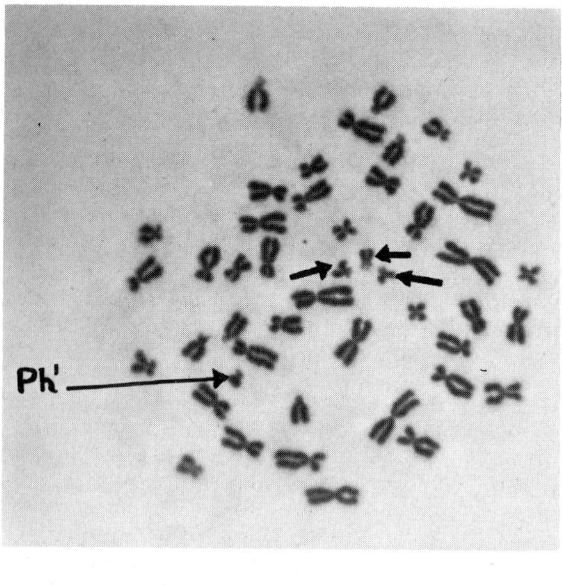

Figure 29–18. The Philadelphia (Ph^1) chromosome. Normal group G members are indicated by arrows in the metaphase figure. *Below,* The Ph^1 chromosome (second from left) is a group G chromosome from which one-half to two-thirds of the long arm has been deleted (22q–).

Ph^1 chromosome (Fig. 29–18) is marrow examination. Peripheral blood is seldom satisfactory. In CGL the peripheral blood may have few immature myelocytic elements, and in culture normal lymphocytes will frequently overgrow the few leukemic cells present. (Leukemic cells, in general, are at a selective disadvantage in tissue culture; leukemic lymphocytes are especially hard to culture.) Both a short-term and a long-term marrow culture may be prepared at the time of sampling.

Marrow culture is recommended when the differential diagnosis lies between CGL and granulocytic leukemoid reaction. Only positive findings are significant. About 15 per cent of cases of CGL are Ph^1 negative; such cases often pursue an atypical clinical course. The Ph^1 chromosome may disappear during remissions and may not be demonstrable if the CGL enters a terminal acute phase.

The Ph^1 chromosome does not appear to have any predictive value. Some reports state that the Ph^1 chromosome may appear before a diagnosis of CGL can be made on clinical or hematologic grounds. This is true enough. However, the cases in which a Ph^1 chromosome has been found have had *some* hematologic abnormality, usually a puzzling and persistent polymorphonuclear leukocytosis with some "left shift."

Monoclonal Gammopathies. Cells of the lymphocyte-plasmacyte group which produce abnormal gamma globulins (as in Waldenström's macroglobulinemia or multiple myeloma) often form cell clones bearing distinctive extra large marker chromosomes – "W" or "MG" chromosomes. These large markers resemble group A chromosomes. They are not invariably present and are not distinctive enough to make a reliable distinction among diseases of this type (Houston *et al.*, 1967).

ABNORMALITIES OF THE SEX CHROMOSOMES

The sex chromosomes are affected by numerical and structural defects more frequently than any other human chromosomes. The basic alteration in any of the sex chromosome defects is impairment of gonadal function. The degree of gonadal impairment depends both upon the magnitude of the chromosome defect and the percentage of body cells affected.

Generally speaking, loss of a sex chromosome produces much more profound derangement of gonadal function than does the presence of extra sex chromosomal material. Sex chromosome defects have clinical effects which parallel those of intrauterine castration – the more "total" the castration (i.e., the more severe the sex chromosome defect), the more nearly the patient will approach the "hypoplastic female" status.

Sex chromosome defects commonly become clinically evident at one of three following developmental periods:

At Birth. In infancy, sex chromosome defects are reflected in the clinical intersex states. In these the external genitalia are either completely ambiguous or show marked impairment of normal differentiation. A large proportion of such infants (about half) have adrenal virilism. Although this is not a chromosomally induced derangement of sex differentiation, cytogenetic studies are invaluable in its diagnosis.

The diagnostic schema which we recommend for the assessment of genital anomalies in infancy is as follows:

1. Perform a buccal chromatin test (*after* the infant is one week of age).
   A. If the infant is chromatin negative, proceed to Step 2.
   B. If the infant is chromatin positive, perform a 17-ketosteroid assay. If the 17-ketosteroid level is elevated, the infant has *adrenal virilism.* If the 17-ketosteroid level is normal, proceed to Step 2.
2. Perform a chromosome analysis. The prime purpose here is to determine the true genetic sex so that appropriate corrective measures may be taken. Occasionally a mosaic chromosome pattern will be encountered which accounts for the defects seen. One mosaic pattern which almost invariably produces genital ambiguity is 45,X/46,XY.
3. If neither chromosomal nor hormonal defects are present, proceed with other diagnostic studies. Usually surgical exploration and gonadal biopsy will be needed to resolve such cases.

The more common sex chromosome defects (45,X; 45,X/46,XX; 47,XXX; 47,XXY and 47,XYY) are rarely symptomatic in infancy—their effects are usually pubertal. An exception is 45,X (Turner's syndrome), which may produce neck webbing or edema in female infants. Even in Turner's syndrome, there is little derangement of the infant's sex differentiation.

At Puberty. Many children with sex chromosome defects develop more or less normally until puberty. In apparent females, sex chromosome defects may produce amenorrhea, masculinization, or sexual infantilism (failure of secondary sex characteristics to develop). Pubertal males usually develop the symptoms of Klinefelter's syndrome (p. 1338).

In Adults. Sex chromosome abnormalities which do not depress gonadal function to a degree which impairs pubertal sexual development may produce sterility in otherwise "normal" adults. In females the triplo-X (47,XXX) syndrome may follow this course. The mosaic variants of Klinefelter's syndrome may produce sterility in otherwise asymptomatic males. The experience of one sterility clinic, in which almost 10 per cent of male patients had an unsuspected sex chromosome defect, has already been cited.

Turner's Syndrome (Chromatin-negative Gonadal Dysgenesis). True Turner's syndrome is the most severe form of chromosomally induced gonadal dysgenesis. The gonads are "streak" gonads and are represented by minute, amorphous, fibrous structures which show no microscopic evidence of germ cell function. As often as not, the gonadal morphology is so indifferent that it is impossible to determine whether the gonad is an "ovary" or a "testis."

The chromosome complement is 45,X. There is convincing evidence that the 45,X pattern may follow the loss of either an X chromosome from a 46,XX (female) zygote or a Y chromosome from a 46,XY (male) zygote.

As might be expected, these patients develop as hypoplastic females. The patients are short phenotypic females who show no breast development, are amenorrheic, and fail to develop either pubic or axillary hair. The external genitalia are hypoplastic and the internal genitalia are hypoplastic female pelvic organs (rudimentary uterus, cervix, and fallopian tubes). Affected individuals seldom exceed 5 feet in height.

In addition to the severe sexual hypoplasia, patients with Turner's syndrome have somatic developmental defects. Their chests are broad (shield-like) and neck webbing is common. There is sometimes peripheral lymphedema in affected infants. The edema does not usually persist beyond infancy. There is also an increased incidence of coarctation of the aorta (a rare anomaly in females). Mental deficiency is not a feature of Turner's syndrome.

The diagnosis is readily made with cytogenetic techniques. Buccal and vaginal epithelial cells are chromatin negative. There are no drumstick appendages in the polymorphonuclear leukocytes. Karyotyping reveals a single population of cells with a modal number of 45 chromosomes. There are 15 group C chromosomes, and there is no Y chromosome. Other groups are normal.

45,X/46,XX (Chromatin-positive Ovarian Dysgenesis). 45,X/46,XX mosaicism is a fairly common form of ovarian dysgenesis. It arises through mitotic nondisjunction in a normal female (46,XX) zygote with proliferation of two cell lines at more or less equal rates. 45,X/46,XX may also arise following nondisjunction in a 45,X zygote. Impairment of sex differentiation is often as severe as that of Turner's syndrome, though some patients have had good secondary sex differentiation.

Generally the affected individuals are short and amenorrheic females who fail to develop adequate secondary sex features at the time of puberty. The breasts are usually hypoplastic, and axillary and pubic hair is scanty or absent.

Clinical defects common in Turner's syndrome which are rare in 45,X/46,XX mosaics are neck webbing, lymphedema, and coarctation of the aorta. The female pelvic organs are hypoplastic and the gonads are usually of the "streak" type.

The results of sex chromatin studies may be puzzling. The buccal and vaginal epithelial nuclei are usually chromatin positive (though some are chromatin negative). In chromatin-positive smears, the incidence of chromatin-positive nuclei is generally reduced. Drumstick appendages are absent or are present in lowered incidence (3 to 4 per 500 PML). Accurate diagnosis demands karyotyping.

Chromosome analysis reveals a bimodal cell population, some cells having 45 and some cells 46 chromosomes. Those with 46 chromosomes have a normal female complement of 46 XX. Those with 45 chromosomes lack one member of group C (45,X). This chromosome constitution is usually demonstrable in peripheral blood. In occasional individuals the aberrant cell line may be present in only one tissue. If clinical suspicion that mosaicism exists is sufficiently high and peripheral blood fails to reveal a mosaic pattern, skin biopsy may be necessary to prove its existence.

45,X/46,XY. 45,X/46,XY mosaicism provides one of the more dramatic examples of chromosomally induced intrauterine castration in man. Loss of a Y chromosome from a significant percentage of the cells of a genetic male results in marked impairment of testicular differentiation. This, in turn, results in arrest of Wolffian development and a "compensatory" development of Müllerian derivatives.

Most of the patients have had ambiguous external genitalia and the internal genitalia have been an admixture of male and female elements. In at least one instance the effects have been unilateral. The gonads are of the "streak" type—unrecognizable, attenuated fragments of fibrous tissue which some observers have felt resembles "ovarian" stroma.

This mosaic pattern is uncommon. The clinical sequelae are such that the abnormality is generally apparent at birth. The affected infants are chromatin negative. The polymorphonuclear leukocytes bear no drumsticks. Karyotypes reveal a bimodal chromosome count (45 and 46). The cells with a normal complement have a normal male chromosome complement (46,XY). Cells with 45 chromosomes lack a Y chromosome.

Triplo-X (47,XXX). 47,XXX (triplo-X, "superfemale") is the most innocuous of the human aneuploidies yet described. The impact of the extra X chromosome upon sexual and somatic development is inconstant. Not infrequently the defect is discovered accidentally during a family study of some unrelated chromosome anomaly. Some cases have been discovered during mass screenings of newborn infants with buccal smears.

Patients with triplo-X may be amenorrheic or hypomenorrheic, or they may have normal menses. Secondary sex characteristics usually develop normally. Some of these patients have been fertile and have had normal children. Somatic derangements are infrequent. Most often a mild degree of mental retardation has been described. Often the patients are described as being of "below average" intelligence. Since about half the population will be "below average" in mental prowess, the impact of the 47,XXX constitution upon mental development is hard to assess.

The chromosome constitution can be anticipated on the basis of buccal smear findings. The cells are chromatin positive and many have double Barr bodies. Chromosome analysis reveals a uniform cell population with 47 chromosomes. There is an extra group C chromosome (X).

The minimal impact of this chromosome defect upon its carriers has been attributed to the "inactivation" of the extra X chromosome, which then forms the inert Barr body.

Klinefelter's Syndrome (47,XXY). The most common aneuploidy of man is 47,XXY, Klinefelter's syndrome. This is also known as chromatin-positive testicular dysgenesis. The extra X chromosome present in the cells of a genetic male impairs testicular differentiation, and the affected men are sterile and are often eunuchoid in appearance. Gynecomastia and scanty hair development are common.

The condition may be diagnosed without resort to karyotyping in the straightforward case. The testes are small and firm and are insensitive. The cells of a buccal smear are chromatin positive. Drumsticks are present on the nuclei of polymorphonuclear leukocytes. Karyotypes reveal a modal count of 47 chromosomes and the cells bear an extra group C (X) chromosome.

The impact of the chromosome defect upon mental development is inconstant. Mild mental retardation is quite common, and patients with Klinefelter's syndrome are more commonly encountered in the population of institutions than in the general population. Even in those patients who are not retarded, behavioral derangements are very common.

47,XYY. Males with an extra Y chromosome are not rare. The clinical effects are rather variable, though a "syndrome" of sorts can be discerned in the many reported cases. 47,XYY males tend to be tall, aggressive, and sociopathic. Many (but scarcely all) have been found in prison populations. These patients can be fertile and sire normal children. Mental deficiency is not usual.

Testicular Feminization. Testicular feminization is not, strictly speaking, a chromosomal defect since the genetic sex (46,XY) conforms with gonadal sex (testes are present). Testicular malfunction makes these patients differentiate as girls who generally seem quite normal until puberty when they fail to menstruate and may develop deep, masculine voices and beards. The patients are chromatin-negative and have a normal male karyotype (46,XY). Accurate diagnosis is important because the malfunctioning testes should be removed. With estrogen supplementation, the patients will function as normal, though sterile, females.

Sex Chromosome Mosaicism. A tremendous variety of sex chromosome mosaics have been described. For the most part they present as variants of the gonadal dysgenesis syndromes described above, either testicular or ovarian. The clinical impact of such mosaics is very roughly proportional to the number of normal cells present. Identification of mosaic chromosome patterns requires careful karyotyping.

48,XXXY and 49,XXXXY. 48,XXXY and 49,XXXXY chromosome patterns have been seen in males who have exaggerated symptoms and signs of Klinefelter's syndrome. Generally the gonadal defects are somewhat more severe in these forms. Mental deficiency is also more common, and its severity seems to correlate with the number of X chromosomes present. In tetra-X Y, an I.Q. of less than 35 is usual.

Structural Defects of Sex Chromosomes. Both deletions and isochromosomes of the X chromosome have been described. The effects of structural defects are, in general, similar to those of X chromosome losses. Gonadal dysgenesis of variable severity results in women with structural X chromosome defects. Isochromosomes are sometimes detected by sex chromatin studies. Enlargements of either the Barr body or the drumsticks may be seen. Deletions of the X chromosome produce diminutions in the size of these structures.

The changes in karyotype depend upon the structural defect present. Isochromosomes can be identified by their configuration. They appear as exactly metacentric abnormal chromosomes. Isochromosomes of the long arm of the X chromosome resemble chromosome-3 rather closely, and the first impression is that trisomy-3 may be present. Deletions and isochromosomes do not alter the modal number of the affected cells—it remains 46.

Structural changes in the Y chromosome are reported from time to time. Deletions have variable effects. The effects may be as mild as hypospadias or as severe as clinical intersex. Increases in Y chromosome size are hard to evaluate. For the most part, they have been asymptomatic. Even the presence of an entire extra Y chromosome (XYY) often has little impact upon male differentiation.

REFERENCES

Al-Aish, M. S., de la Cruz, F., Goldsmith, L., Volpe, J., Mella, G., and Robinson, J. C.: Autosomal monosomy in man. Complete monosomy G (21–22) in a four-and-one-half-year-old mentally retarded girl. New Eng. J. Med. 277: 777, 1967.

A proposed standard system of nomenclature of human mitotic chromosomes (Report on the Denver Conference, 1960). Lancet *1*:1063, 1960.

Barnicot, N. A., *et al.*: The London conference on "The Normal Human Karyotype," August 28–30, 1963. Amer. J. Human Genet. *16*:156, 1964.

Barr, M. L., and Bertram, E. G.: A morphologic distinction between the neurones of the male and female, and the behavior of the nucleolar satellite during accelerated protein synthesis. Nature (London) *163*:676, 1949.

Caspersson, T., Zech, L., and Johansson, C.: Analysis of human metaphase chromosome set by aid of DNA-binding fluorescent agent. Exp. Cell Res. *62*:490, 1970.

Chicago Conference: Standardization in human genetics. Birth Defects: Original Article Series, Vol. II:2, 1966.

Davidson, W. M., and Smith, D. R.: A morphological sex difference in the polymorphonuclear neutrophil leukocytes. Brit. Med. J. 2:6, 1954.

Drets, M. E., and Shaw, M. W.: Specific banding patterns of human chromosomes. Proc. Nat. Acad. Sci. U.S.A. *68*: 2073, 1971.

Ford, C. E., Jones, K. W., Polani, P. E., de Almeida, J. C., and Briggs, J. H.: A sex chromosome anomaly in a case of gonadal dysgenesis (Turner's syndrome). Lancet *1*:711, 1959.

German, J. L., Miller, O. J., Rowley, J., and Schmid, W.: Notes on autoradiography. *In* Chicago Conference (op. cit.).

de Grouchy, J.: The 18p–, and 18q– and 18r syndromes. Birth Defects: Original Article Series, Vol. V.: 74, 1969.

Hollander, D. H., and Borgaonkar, D. S.: The quinacrine fluorescence method of Y chromosome identification. Acta Cytol. *15*:452, 1971.

Houston, E. W., Ritzmann, S. E., and Levin, W. C.: Chromosomal aberrations common to three types of monoclonal gammopathy. Blood *29*:214, 1967.

Jacobs, P. A., and Strong, J. A.: A case of human intersexuality having a possible XXY sex-determining mechanism. Nature (London) *183*:302, 1959.

Jacobson, C. B., and Barter, R. H.: Intrauterine diagnosis and management of genetic defects. Amer. J. Obstet. Gynec. *99*:796, 1967.

Lejeune, J., Gauthier, M., and Turpin, R.: Études des chromosomes somatiques de neuf enfants mongoliens. C. R. Acad. Sci. (Paris) *248*:1721, 1959.

Miller, O. J., Warburton, D., and Breg, W. R.: Deletions of group B chromosomes. Birth Defects: Original Article Series, Vol. V.: 100, 1969.

Moore, K. L., and Barr, M. L.: Smears from the oral mucosa in the detection of chromosomal sex. Lancet 2:57, 1955.

Moorehead, P. S., Nowell, P. C., Mellman, W. J., Battips, D. M., and Hungerford, D. A.: Chromosome preparations of leukocytes cultured from human peripheral blood. Exp. Cell Res. *20*:613, 1960.

Nowell, P. C., and Hungerford, D. A.: Chromosome studies in human leukemia. II: Chronic granulocytic leukemia. J. Nat. Cancer Inst. 27:1013, 1961.

Schmid, W.: Autoradiography of human chromosomes. *In* J. J. Yunis (ed.): Human Chromosome Methodology. New York, Academic Press, Inc., 1965, p. 91.

Tjio, J. H., and Levan, A.: The chromosome number of man. Hereditas *42*:1, 1956.

Warren, R. J., and Rimoin, D. L.: The G deletion syndromes. J. Pediat. *77*:658, 1970.

Chapter 30

CLINICAL LABORATORY COMPUTERIZATION

by ARTHUR F. KRIEG, M.D.

> "Improved service rather than time or cost savings appears to be the major advantage of the laboratory computer system. It is recommended that any system found acceptable be used "as is." If this precaution is followed, the laboratory computer "pays for itself" through cumulative summaries, improved quality control, and faster service to the physician" (Brecher and Loken, 1971).

During the early 1950's electronic data processing was restricted to a few scientists and mathematicians who had access to less than a dozen large, expensive machines that were difficult to program and maintain. However, rapid advances in computer science quickly led to decreased size, lower cost, easier programming, and improved reliability: by 1960 over 2000 computers were in use for business as well as scientific applications; by 1970 this figure exceeded 60,000 for the United States alone.

Successful commercial and scientific use led to intense interest in clinical laboratory applications during the middle 1960's. Early investigators included Williams (1964, 1967), Hicks *et al.* (1966), Rappoport (1967), and Straumfjord *et al.* (1967). This and other research on clinical laboratory computerization demonstrated many potential benefits, including: automated preparation of specimen labels, worksheets, daily logs, interim reports, and daily cumulative reports; direct acquisition of results from laboratory instruments without need for transcriptions or calculations; automated comparison of "today" vs. "yesterday" results; capture of results in machine readable form for analysis of normal range as well as clinical significance; and better use of existing personnel.

Based on these potential benefits, a wave of enthusiasm for clinical laboratory computerization developed during the middle and late 1960's. However, this potential was sometimes confused with actual capability: a newborn baby may have the potential to become an atomic scientist, but considerable time, work, patience, and expense are required to realize this goal. The potential of a computer can be achieved only via appropriate "programs" or instructions. Final results depend both on inherent ability (genetic endowment of the human, analogous to physical architecture of the machine) and training (education of the human, analogous to programming of the machine).

Both education and programming are slow, expensive, and uncertain; and in both, results may differ from the expectations of the fond parent! Too often, the warnings of Williams (1967) are not heeded:

> There are no complete . . . laboratory systems in daily operation. None meets all requirements; . . . a few are unacceptable. We . . . should avoid undertaking the development, installation, and operation of experimental (or) untried systems unless generously provided with developmental funds and staff. New manufacturers . . . entering the market . . . include a few who make exaggerated claims and misleading inferences; . . . it is advisable for the laboratory director . . . to verify . . . claims by direct inquiry to the director of the laboratory quoted. The prospective purchaser must write in detail the exact specifications of equipment and operation. Each interested company should be required to submit a proposal in writing . . . (and) include a copy of the manual . . . for laboratory personnel who will use the system. To evaluate the proposals objectively, the pathologist should visit . . . successfully automated laboratories and critically examine what has been really accomplished. The order should be written by . . . the purchaser . . . (to include) exact functional specifications of the programs, . . . an agreement concerning installation costs, evaluation period of satisfactory operation without significant failure, terms of acceptance, and provision for combining maintenance of equipment and programs. Payment . . . should not be made until the system has met all acceptance specifications.

In 1972 Rappoport summarized his observations:

> I know of several instances . . . where the reputations of laboratory physicians . . . have been shattered by failure of computerization. We have noticed an inordinate amount of uncritical enthusiasm, unwarranted optimism, and euphoric recklessness for untested and unproven methods based on . . . overly ambitious statements by vendors who promise performances which they simply cannot keep. Estimates of cost are usually unrealistically low; . . . programs . . . may be rigid, inflexible . . . and totally unacceptable for your . . . requirements.

In view of these and other warnings, it seems reasonable that users should share some responsibility for failures of clinical laboratory computerization:

> Seldom are the failures due to . . . hardware . . . (but rather) . . . the lack of well-defined goals. Organizations which would not consider buying an instrument for several thousand dollars without thorough planning . . . have embarked on . . . costly computerization programs with less forethought than that accorded minor expenditures (Editorial, American Laboratory, 1973).

However, in many cases, the potential benefits of clinical laboratory computerization have indeed been realized. Guides to planning and implementation are available (Krieg *et al.*, 1971), and in a number of laboratories, computers today are helping to provide better patient care with little or no net increase in cost.

FUNDAMENTAL CONCEPTS

Data Processing. Data processing is defined as the performance of arithmetic and logical operations on data called *"input"* to produce a specific result called *"output."* All clinical laboratories perform manual data processing; and even after computerization, some manual data processing will be required. A computer is useful in data processing ONLY if the arithmetic and logical operations can be accurately defined in advance and expressed in numeric form. Examples of clinical laboratory data processing include:

1. Deciding whether to hire a particular individual—ordinarily done by humans, since criteria usually are not easily defined in numeric form, e.g., appearance, attitude, resourcefulness, and quality and quantity of past performance.
2. Calculating protein fractions after electrophoresis—typically done by computer if available, since the arithmetic and logical operations are well defined.
3. Calculating quality control results—typically done by programmable calculator or computer, if available.
4. Preparation of daily worksheets—typically done by computer if available, since test names and workstations are easily expressed numerically.
5. Preparation of daily cumulative reports—typically done by computer if available, since most test names and results are easily expressed in numeric form.

Electronic Data Processing (EDP). EDP refers to use of a computer or programmable calculator to solve a data processing problem. *Hardware* refers to mechanical and electronic components of the computer *per se*. *Software* refers to the programs or instructions for the computer. The term *computer system* implies a combination of hardware and software designed to perform one or more specific functions.

Digital Computer. A digital computer is a device that can accept data in the form of *binary numbers* (vide infra), operate on this data according to an internally stored set of instructions, and display the results obtained by following these instructions. Figure 30–1 is a simplified block diagram outlining operation of the PDP-8, perhaps the most widely used small computer. This machine includes:

1. *Input/output devices* (I/O devices) in the form of console switches and teletype which enable an operator to give information or instructions to the computer (input) as well as receive results of the arithmetic and/or logical operations (output).
2. *Arithmetic-logic unit.*
3. *Control unit.*
4. *Memory unit.*

A photograph of the PDP-8 computer and teletype is shown in Figure 30–2. The console switches enable an operator to give instructions in binary code to the computer; results of the arithmetic and/or logical operations are displayed as binary numbers (console lights), showing the contents of each register. Entering instructions and data as binary numbers via the console switches is rather tedious; hence, a teletype is ordinarily used for most input/output (I/O) operations. Figure 30–3, a more generalized block diagram, represents a medium-sized computer system commonly used in clinical laboratories. The *central processing unit* (CPU) includes arithmetic-logic unit, control unit, and memory; attached to the CPU are a number of *peripherals*, including auxiliary memory units, I/O devices, an input device (card reader), and an output device (line printer). A photograph of the medium-sized clinical laboratory computer system at Milton S. Hershey Medical Center is shown in Figure 30–4.

In most small or medium-sized computers, an *input/output bus* (I/O bus) allows transfer of binary coded information to and from peripheral devices such as card readers, line

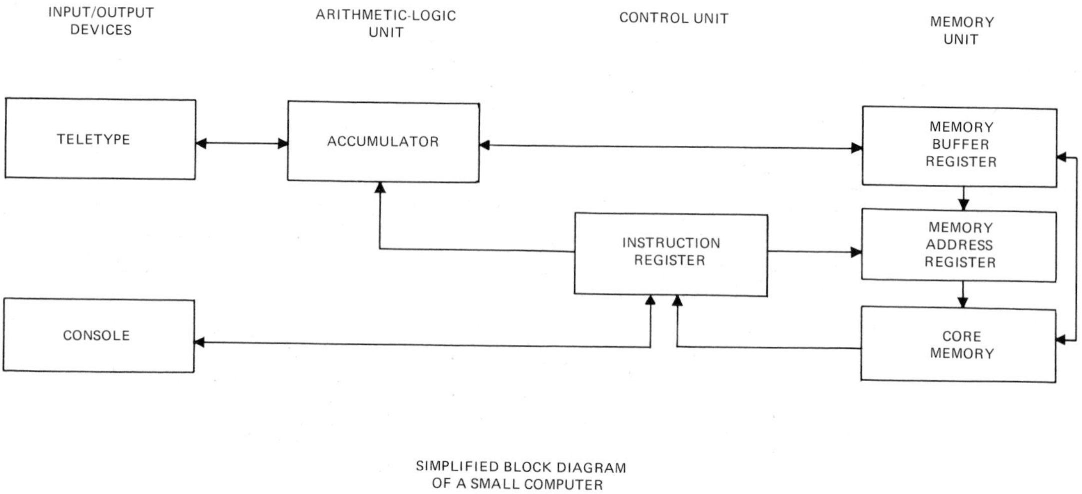

Figure 30–1. Simplified block diagram for small computer.

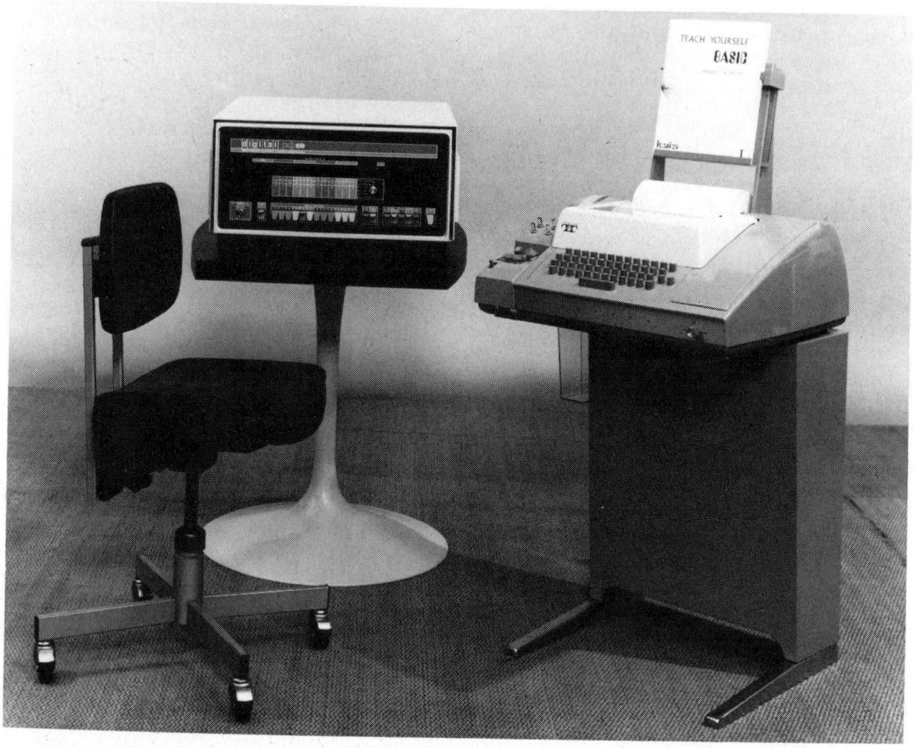

Figure 30–2. Small computer and teletype. (PDP-8, Courtesy of Digital Equipment Corp.)

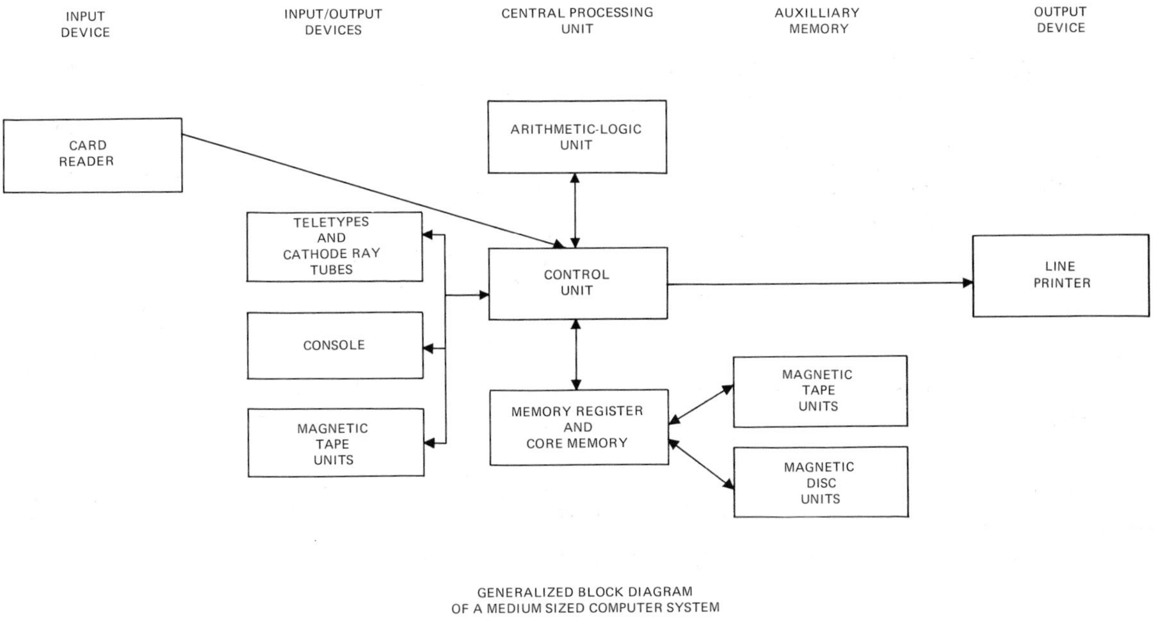

Figure 30–3. Simplified block diagram for clinical laboratory computer system.

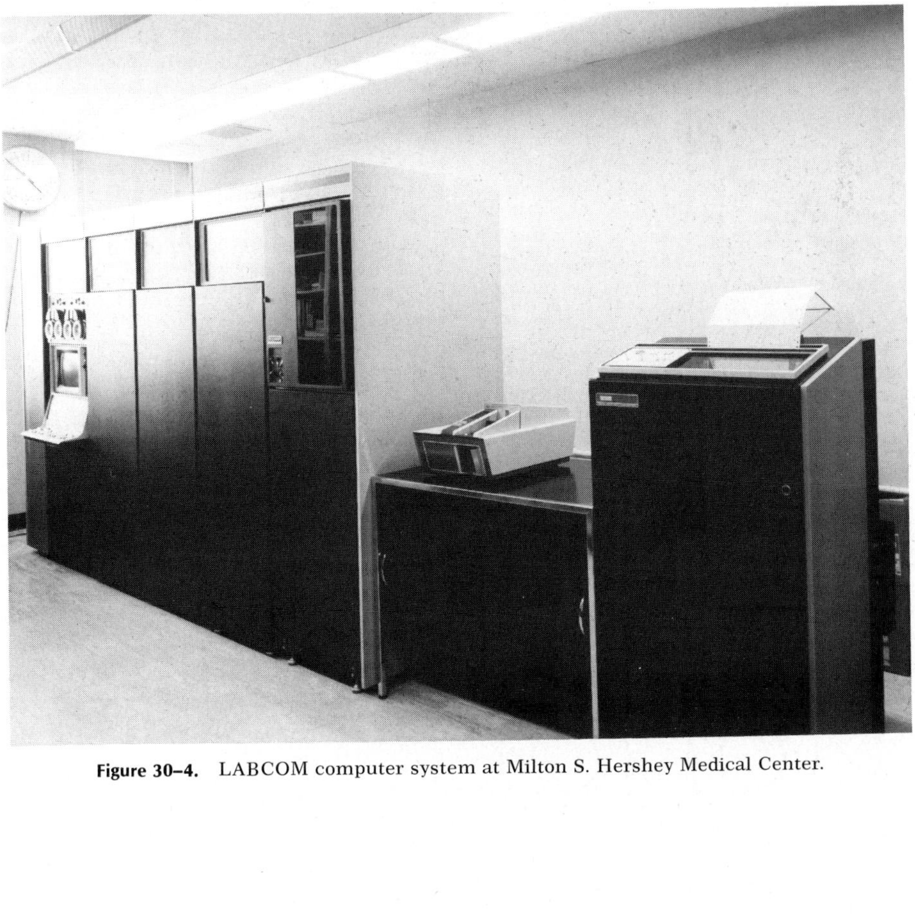

Figure 30–4. LABCOM computer system at Milton S. Hershey Medical Center.

printers, and magnetic tape units. A code associated with each block of data directs information to or from the appropriate device.

All information handled by the CPU must be in the form of *binary numbers.* This includes instructions as well as data. The decimal number 276 is based on a radix of 10, and can be represented as:

$$\begin{aligned} 2 \times 10^2 &= 200 \\ +7 \times 10^1 &= 70 \\ +6 \times 10^0 &= \underline{6} \\ \Sigma &= 276_{10} \end{aligned}$$

The *binary number* 10101 is based on a radix of 2 and can be represented as:

$$\begin{aligned} 1 \times 2^4 &= 16 \\ +0 \times 2^3 &= 0 \\ +1 \times 2^2 &= 4 \\ +0 \times 2^1 &= 0 \\ +1 \times 2^0 &= \underline{1} \\ \Sigma &= 21_{10} \end{aligned}$$

Because binary numbers are inconvenient to work with, small and medium-sized computers express binary numbers in the octal number system, with groups of three binary numbers used to represent 0 through 7:

Binary	*Octal*	*Decimal*
000 000	0	0
000 001	1	1
000 010	2	2
000 011	3	3
000 100	4	4
000 101	5	5
000 110	6	6
000 111	7	7
001 000	10	8
001 001	11	9
001 010	12	10
001 011	13	11
001 100	14	12
001 101	15	13
001 110	16	14
001 111	17	15

If you remember the binary-octal equivalents for zero through seven, it is easy to convert large binary numbers to the octal system. For example:

101	111	100	001	binary
5	7	4	1	octal

It is important to understand conversion from binary to octal, because all information in the computer is stored in binary form, all arithmetic and logical operations in the computer are performed on binary numbers, and the console lights display contents of various registers in binary form.

Information in *core memory* is stored on tiny magnetic rings, which can be magnetized in one of the two directions, clockwise and counterclockwise (Fig. 30–5). For example, if clockwise magnetization represents binary 1 and counterclockwise magnetization binary 0, then Figure 30–5 represents binary 001011, or octal 13 (13_8), or decimal 11 (11_{10}).

Each core is said to store one *bit* of information: bit is an abbreviation for *binary digit,* which can be either 0 or 1. Bits of information often are manipulated in groups called *words,* which have fixed lengths characteristic of a particular computer. Word lengths of 12, 16, 18, 32, 48, and 64 bits are commonly used. Some computers have a *variable word length*: in these machines, each word consists of 1, 2, 4, or 8 *bytes*; a byte ordinarily contains 8 bits.

Size of core memory is usually expressed in units of K words ($1\text{ K} = 2^{10} = 1024$); thus, an 8K word computer has a core storage of $8 \times 2^{10} = 8192$ separate words. This measure of memory size may be misleading unless the word length is given (e.g., 12 bits, 16 bits, 32 bits, etc.).

Core memory is often referred to as *random access storage.* Random access means that any bit of information may be retrieved as rapidly as any other bit. This can be done because each location in core storage has its own unique position or *address* (Fig. 30–6). *Access time* for information in core storage typically is on the order of a microsecond or less.

Magnetic disc memory is also referred to as random access. Information is stored in binary form as magnetized spots on a highly polished disc coated with a thin film which can be rapidly magnetized or demagnetized. Each disc is divided into concentric magnetic tracks, which are further divided into sectors. The disc rotates at high speed (typically 1800 r.p.m.), rapidly bringing each segment under a *read/write head. Moving head discs* have one read/write head, which is moved to the desired track; typical access times are in the 100 millisecond range. *Fixed head discs* have one

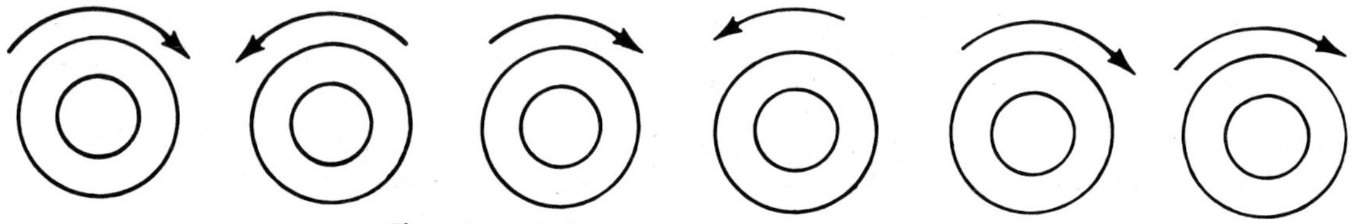

Figure 30–5. Information storage in core memory.

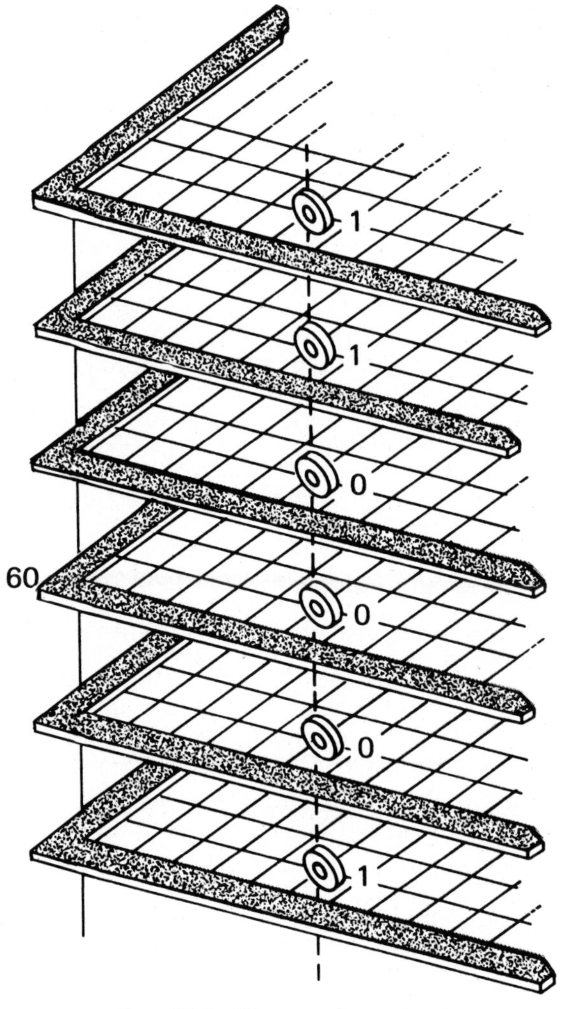

Figure 30–6. Diagram of core storage.

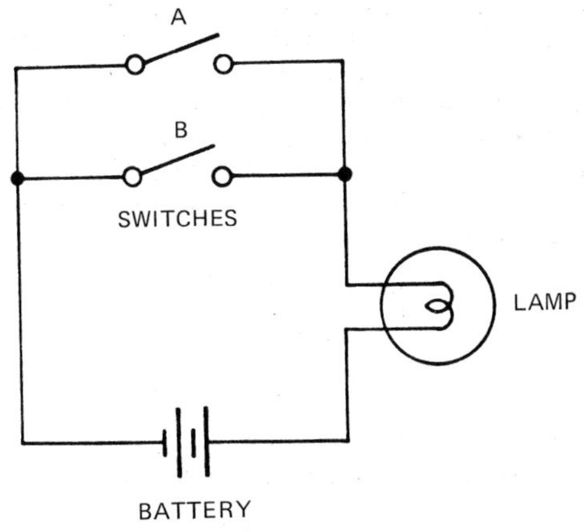

Figure 30–7. Electrical circuit to perform OR function.

head for each track; typical access times are in the 10 millisecond range. Disc capacities may range from under 50 thousand 12 bit words to over 600 million 8 bit bytes (Whitby and Lutz, 1971).

Magnetic tape memory may be *sequential* or random access. Information is stored as magnetized spots along tracks (typically seven or nine) on plastic tape coated with a thin film which can be rapidly magnetized or demagnetized. Although information stored on marked magnetic tapes (such as "LINC tapes" and "DEC tapes") is called "random access," access time varies from several tenths of a second to several seconds, depending on where information is located on the tape. However, this random access magnetic tape is considerably faster than conventional unmarked tapes, which are read sequentially, with access times ranging from several seconds to a minute or more.

Within the *registers* and *accumulators* of the CPU (Fig. 30–1), simple arithmetic and logical operations are performed by *digital logic devices,* which operate at great speed. Digital logic functions can be simulated using electrical switches and a battery, with a light bulb to indicate the output state. The input functions can be defined as open switch equal to binary 0 and closed switch binary 1; the output functions can be defined as lamp off equals binary 0, and lamp on equals binary 1. Figure 30–7 illustrates a circuit to perform the basic OR function: if A or B is closed, the lamp will light. Figure 30–8 illustrates a circuit to perform the basic AND function: if A and B are closed, the lamp will light. A third simple logic operation is NOT: if the switch is not open, the lamp will light; this is sometimes known as INVERT function. The actual electronic device used to perform a logic function is called a *gate.* Most of the complex operations performed by digital computers are based on these simple OR, AND, and INVERT functions. Symbols for these logic gates are shown in Figure 30–9. The NAND gate consists of an AND gate followed by an inverter.

The basic device used for storing information in registers or accumulators is the flip-flop, which can be constructed from gates. The most basic flip-flop is called a reset-set or RS flip-flop, which can be constructed from two

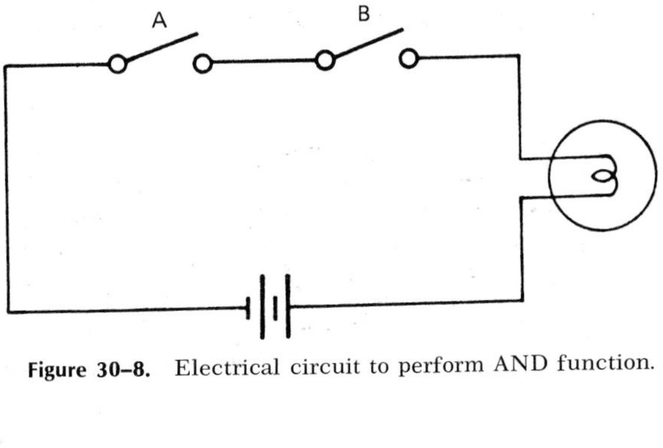

Figure 30–8. Electrical circuit to perform AND function.

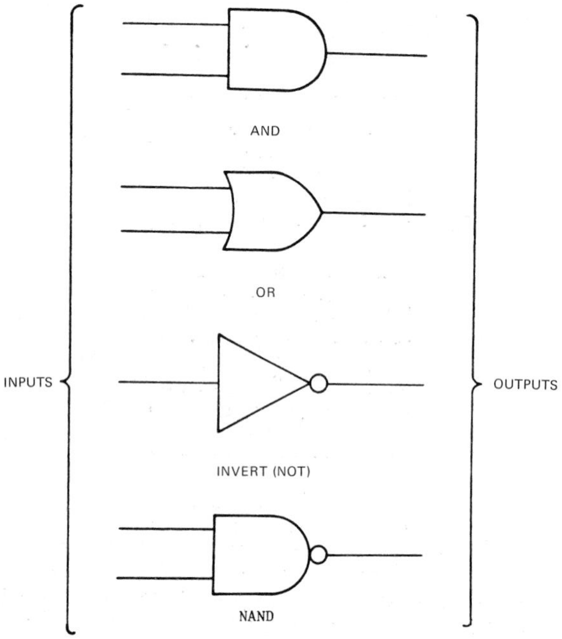

Figure 30–9. Symbols for logic gates.

cross-coupled NAND gates (Fig. 30–10). It has two inputs labeled S for set and R for reset as well as two outputs labeled O_1 and O_2. One input sets storage of a binary 1, while the other clears output and stores a binary 0. Many different logic devices are available (Digital Equipment Corporation, 1972). Operation of these devices is briefly described in the textbook by Perone and Jones (1973).

Within the arithmetic logic unit of the small computer outlined in Figure 30–1 is a register called the *accumulator* (AC), which accumulates partial sums during the execution of a program. The *instruction register* (IR) within the control unit contains the code which specifies the instructions to be executed. Data or instructions being transferred between core memory and the registers AC and IR are temporarily held in the *memory buffer register* (MB), which: (1) holds all the words that go into and out of memory; (2) sets the instruction register; (3) sets the memory address register; (4) accepts information from the accumulator; and (5) provides information to the accumulator. The *memory address register* (MA) is used to: (1) specify the address of the next instruction to be brought out of memory, and (2) hold the core memory address to which data will be sent.

The operation of a digital computer is based on accurate distinctions between:

1. The actual instructions *per se.*
2. The data to be processed according to instructions in the stored program.
3. Memory addresses which refer to locations of data and instructions stored as binary digits in core memory.

In a small computer the instructions may be limited to very simple operations such as:

Instruction	*Binary code*	*Mnemonic*
Logical AND	000	AND
Two's complement add	001	TAD
Deposit and clear the accumulator	011	DCA
Jump to subroutine	100	JMS

The AND instruction implements a bit-by-bit Boolean AND operation between contents of the accumulator and the data word specified by the instruction, with the result of this operation being left in the accumulator. A brief description of Boolean algebra is provided in the textbook *Digital Computers in Scientific Instrumentation* (Perone and Jones, 1973).

The TAD instruction performs a binary addition between the specified data word and content of the accumulator. The term "two's complement add" is used as a reminder that a special type of arithmetic called *two's complement arithmetic* must be used. A brief description of two's complement arithmetic is provided in the textbook *Digital Computers in Scientific Instrumentation* (Perone and Jones, 1973).

The DCA instruction stores the contents of AC in the location specified, destroying previous contents of this location, and setting AC to zero.

The JMS instruction enables the programmer to jump to a *subroutine* and then return to the program after completion of this task. When a particular set of instructions is used frequently (e.g., taking a square root), it is more efficient to write these as a single subroutine which can be used by many different programs.

These instructions may be used in three fundamentally different modes:

1. *Memory reference instructions,* or MRI, which operate on data stored in the machine: such instructions must tell the computer where these data are located with

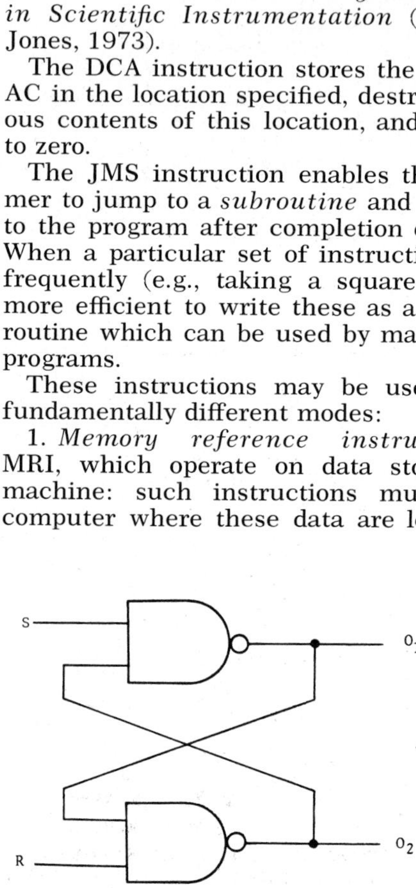

Figure 30–10. RS flip-flop.

reference to a particular location in core. A memory reference instruction refers to a location by address and causes the computer to take some specific action on the content of this location.

2. *Operate microinstructions,* which act without need for reference to a memory location. Instructions of this type are used to clear the accumulator or halt program execution.

3. *Input/output transfer,* or IOT instructions, which transfer information between a peripheral device and the computer memory.

A program may be placed in core memory by entering it via console switches; the switch register is set to binary representation of the instruction and the DEP (deposit) switch depressed. The instruction is displayed in the

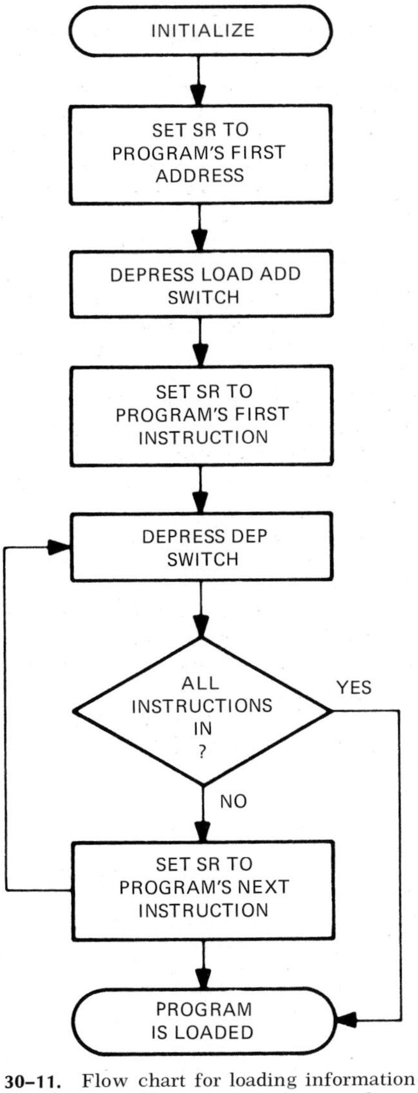

Figure 30–11. Flow chart for loading information and/or instructions into small computer via console switches. (PDP-8, Courtesy of Digital Equipment Corp.)

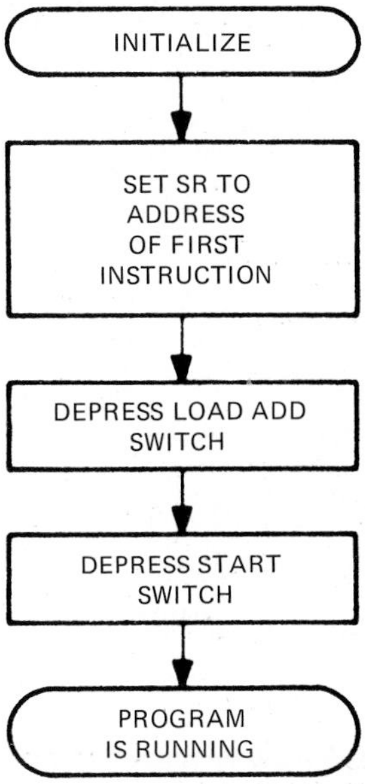

Figure 30–12. Flow chart for running program on small computer. (PDP-8, Courtesy of Digital Equipment Corp.)

MB and AC displays, while address of the memory location is displayed in the MA display. Additional instructions are loaded in the same way. This entire operation is outlined as a flow chart in Figure 30–11. To run a stored program, the binary value of the starting address of the program is entered on the switch register and the load add switch depressed, placing this address on an internal register of the control unit. On depressing the start switch, the program will be executed and the results displayed as binary numbers on the console lights. The "run" operation is outlined in Figure 30–12. However, for entering long programs, this procedure is rather tedious, and use of the teletype is far more convenient. Long programs can be rapidly entered into storage via the teletype paper tape reader, and output can be displayed in printed form as *hard copy,* rather than patterns of console lights.

Since machine language instructions are difficult to remember and use, most small computers provide a set of *mnemonics* known as *assembly language.* Assembly language instructions are translated into machine language on a 1:1 basis by a special program called an *assembler.* The binary coded machine language program produced by an assembler is known as an *object program.* To generate an object program:

1. The assembler (a binary coded machine language program) is read into memory using the teletype paper tape reader.

2. The assembly language program, prepared earlier on punched paper tape, is placed in the teletype paper tape reader.

3. The assembler is started by loading the appropriate starting address and depressing the start switch.

The assembler program will cause the assembly language program tape to read in, check for errors in format, and output diagnostic messages on the teletype. If there are no error messages, you can assume that your assembly language program has been converted to a binary code object program, which is now ready for use.

System Analysis. This refers to a systematic method for defining the steps that occur in a computer program. The same approach may also be used to study and to improve manual data processing operations (Bennington, 1972). System analysis involves:

1. A clear and accurate statement of the problem.
2. Study and flow chart present approach.
3. Develop and flow chart alternate approaches.
4. Develop and flow chart the most cost/effective solution.

Sample flow charts for some of the manual operations in the clinical hematology laboratory are shown in Figure 30–13. A complete flow chart for clinical laboratory operation would include many thousands of details, such as (1) precise morphologic criteria used to identify an "atypical lymphocyte"; (2) precise criteria used to define "few," "moderate," and "many" atypical lymphocytes; (3) precise criteria used to identify "anisocytosis;" and (4) precise criteria used to define "slight," "moderate," and "marked" anisocytosis.

The flow charts for clinical laboratory computer programs must be developed by professional computer scientists. However, the flow charts outlining operations of a clinical laboratory MUST be developed by laboratory personnel: this CANNOT be delegated to nonmedical consultants, regardless of their qualifications (Grams, 1972). It is my opinion that, when planning clinical laboratory computerization, a consultant can be most valuable in criticizing your plans *after* they have been developed in some detail. If you have spent little time or thought on planning, the recommendations developed by your consultant may not appear commensurate with his fee, which typically is $200 or $300 per day, plus travel and expenses.

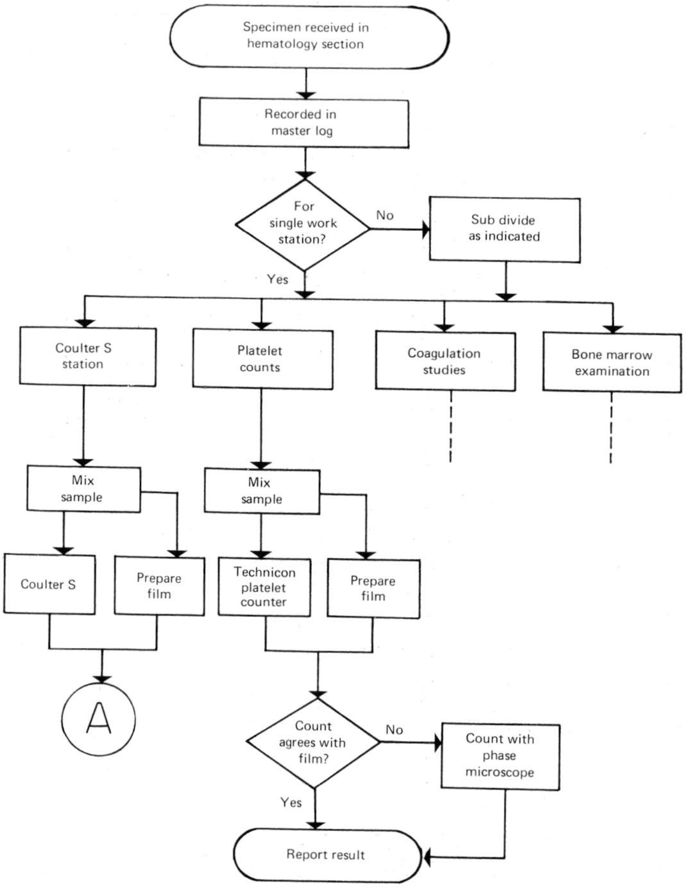

Figure 30–13. Partial flow charts for hematology section.

In my opinion an important benefit of planning for clinical laboratory computerization is that system analysis forces the laboratory director to undertake a detailed study of all operations that occur between writing a request in the order book and reporting the result. Use of systems analysis as a management tool forces the laboratory director to study the flow of specimens, service requests, worksheets, phone calls for results, and written reports in his own laboratory. Systems analysis will force the laboratory director to: (1) ask physicians and nurses, "What problems do you encounter when dealing with the laboratory?" and (2) seek cost/effective solutions to these problems. Indeed, systems analysis may force the laboratory director to reexamine roles and functions of personnel within the laboratory—including himself! A distinguished pathologist once suggested:

> By all means plan to computerize your laboratory, but first perform a careful systems analysis. Prepare flow charts, which outline the flow of specimens, service requests, worksheets, daily logs, and reports. With this information, develop an optimal manual system. Then use the manual system, and forget about computerization!

This general advice is sound, although my own decision was in favor of computerization.

Computers are characterized by:

1. Ability to perform simple operations at fantastic speed, measured in milliseconds and microseconds.

2. Ability to perform repetitive operations thousands of times with great precision, and without boredom.

3. Ability to store and retrieve large amounts of information rapidly, provided this has been coded in uniform manner.

4. Lack of intuition or judgment: a computer will do ONLY what it has been programmed to do, and no more. It is ESSENTIAL to clearly define in advance EXACTLY what should be done in EVERY situation. Unless it has received specific instructions, the computer cannot recognize inaccurate input; hence, the acronym GIGO for "garbage in—garbage out." Properly used, computers can make major contributions to improve laboratory service. But without an understanding of inherent

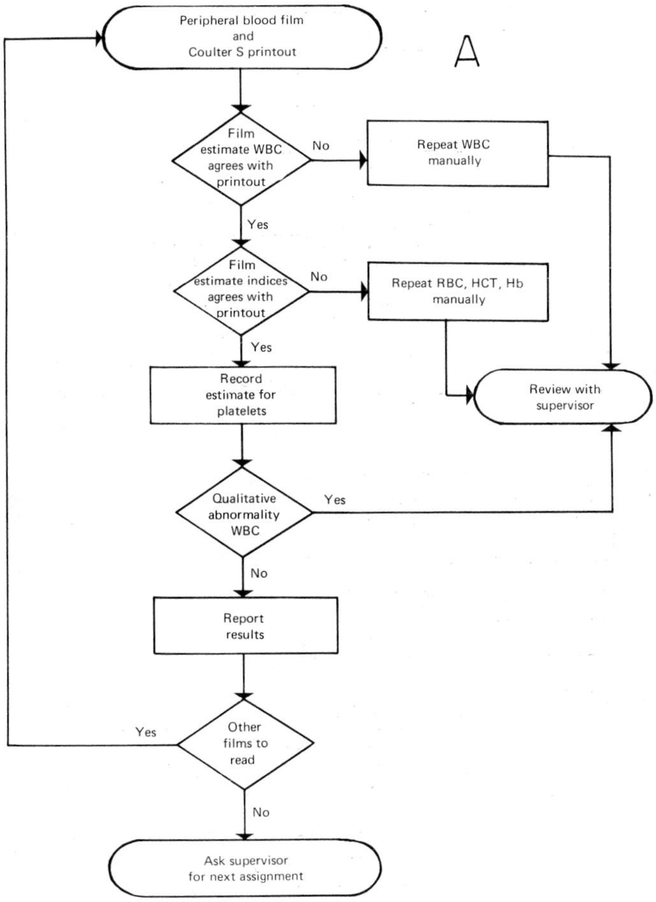

Figure 30–13. *Continued.*

limitations, and without careful planning, computerization can be a disaster, either in the clinical laboratory, or elsewhere.

APPROACHES

Although any grouping becomes somewhat arbitrary and artificial, presently available approaches to clinical laboratory computerization include:

1. Programmable calculators.
2. Shared computer systems—used to support several different services, one of which is the clinical laboratory.
3. Dedicated computer systems—used only for clinical laboratory service.

Programmable Calculators

Most laboratory calculations are relatively simple and can be performed on small programmable calculators available from several manufacturers, including Singer, Hewlett Packard, Monroe, Olivetti Underwood, Smith Corona Marchant, T and T Technology, and Wang. Some vendors provide a wide variety of programs, including calculations for serum protein electrophoresis, Beers law (concentration from per cent T), blood gases, standard deviation, serum thyroxine (competitive protein binding), T3 resin uptake, red cell indices, and radioimmunoassay. Since these commercially available programs may not be suitable for all laboratories, potential users should plan to invest a few hours in learning how to write programs. Cost of these instruments is moderate (typically under $5,000), and time saved in calculations usually justifies this investment for a busy laboratory (Knights, 1970). Small programmable calculators can be directly connected or "interfaced" to automated instruments such as the SMA 12/60, SMA 6/60, Coulter S, and dual channel AutoAnalyzer. Such systems can perform many functions, including (1) direct data acquisition from instruments, (2) automatic correction for baseline drift and sample interaction, (3) printing results on gummed labels, and (4) noting abnormal results on print-outs. Programmable calculators with interfaces for automated instruments are available from Midwest Scientific Instruments at relatively modest cost ($10,000 to $20,000). This equipment may enable small hospital laboratories to generate neatly printed cumulative reports, as well as aiding in many calculations.

Shared Computer Systems

A "shared computer system" usually implies:

1. Computer located outside the laboratory.
2. Computer used for a variety of tasks other than clinical laboratory service. An example is the IBM program package known as SLIS (Shared Laboratory Information System) used with a central hospital computer which also prepares bills, payrolls, and administrative reports. The IBM program package is more economical than writing "custom made" software, or adapting programs from some other laboratory. Although "borrowing" programs from another laboratory may appear attractive, "documentation" ordinarily is not available. Documentation refers to the information needed for a programmer to understand, use, maintain, and trouble-shoot a set of programs. Development of detailed documentation may cost almost as much as writing the programs! Without adequate documentation, it may be impossible to operate your system without a programmer who has had several years' experience with the software.

With SLIS, data from laboratory worksheets are punched into cards, repunched for verification, and then taken to the central computer for processing. Time lag between completion of laboratory work and production of a printed report usually is about two to four hours. Such systems appear attractive for several reasons: (1) there is no capital investment by the laboratory; and (2) time on the central computer may be provided with no charge against the laboratory budget. However, certain limitations often become apparent during day-to-day operation:

1. Costs may equal or exceed a dedicated laboratory system. For a 300-bed teaching hospital costs may involve $20,000 for modification of the SLIS programs, $100,000 per year for time on the central computer, and $10,000 per year for keypunching.
2. The central computer facility may be unable or unwilling to modify the SLIS software (a) to the extent required for initial operation, or (b) to provide format changes requested by the clinical staff.
3. The central computer facility may be unable to modify its schedule when there are problems in the laboratory (e.g., breakdown of the Coulter S or SMA 12/60); in some cases, data may have to be "held" until the next day.
4. The central computer facility may be unable to give high priority to production of laboratory reports; in some cases other "emergency" projects may take priority over laboratory reports.
5. The clinical staff may find that reports are delayed due to time required for keypunching (typically at least two hours).
6. The laboratory has no control over accuracy of keypunching, but will be held responsible for accuracy of the reports.
7. Technologists cannot query the computer directly for "latest" results on any given patient.

8. It may be impossible to have reports printed at a time convenient for the clinical staff.

Indeed, some laboratory directors have found the benefits of shared computer systems to be outweighed by the problems involved. Any central computer installation will be subject to pressures from many different users; in some cases it may become difficult to meet the laboratory needs for accuracy, timeliness, reliability, and response to change.

Dedicated Computer Systems

Potential problems of shared computer systems were recognized during the mid 1960's. During the past six years at least three fundamentally different approaches to dedicated clinical laboratory systems have evolved:

1. Small computer located within the laboratory, used in a batch-processing mode.
2. Large computer located outside the laboratory, used by several different laboratories in a time-sharing mode.
3. Small computer located within the laboratory used in a time-sharing mode.

"Batch processing" refers to an operation in which data are collected in "batches" prior to processing by humans or a computer. "Time sharing" refers to a computer system in which several people can use a single computer concurrently for input, data processing, and output.

There has been considerable confusion regarding the terms "off-line," "on-line," "interface," and "real time." *Off-line* implies that instructions for the computer as well as data to be processed are collected and stored on some medium such as punched cards, punched tape, or magnetic tape, which is periodically brought to the computer for batch processing at some convenient time. Turn around time may vary from several minutes to several days. *On-line* implies that the user can communicate directly with the computer at any time, typically via a typewriter terminal or similar device: in contrast to off-line operation, there is a direct line of communication between user and computer, and turn around time typically is measured in seconds. *Interface* implies that information is taken directly from an instrument without need for human intervention; this may be on-line or off-line. *Real time* implies that results of data processing are available soon enough to affect the operation, whatever it may be, that has produced the data. For administrative data or budget planning, real time might require a response time of several hours; however, for most operations in the clinical laboratory, real time will require a response time of less than a minute, and implies on-line operation with terminals and/or interfaced instruments.

The first approach – small computer located within the laboratory and used in a batch-processing mode – was developed during the late 1960's by Dr. Samuel Raymond at the University of Pennsylvania School of Medicine (Philadelphia) and Dr. David Seligson at Yale University School of Medicine (New Haven). Working independently, Dr. Raymond and Dr. Seligson developed batch-processing systems using IBM 1130 computers dedicated solely to laboratory use. Compared to large systems, the hardware cost is modest: rental for an IBM 1130 is about $25,000 per year. However, despite the low cost of hardware, several problems are present:

1. Documented programs are not available, and it would be difficult to predict accurately in advance the cost required for developing new software, or adapting present software to a new laboratory.
2. Data must be punched on cards before being entered into the computer; this may cause greater time lag between test completion and reporting than with a manual system.

A common error is to underestimate costs for software development (Krieg *et al.*, 1971); prospective users interested in the IBM 1130 should carefully evaluate these potential problems in advance.

The second approach – large computer located outside the laboratory and used by several different laboratories in a time-sharing mode – is exemplified by the Meditech system now in use at a number of hospitals. Attractive features include:

1. No capital investment by the laboratory.
2. A program "package" is available, and can be modified for individual users.

Reported costs are in the range of $30,000 per year (Hughes and Glidden, 1973). Although this approach appears interesting, I do not have detailed personal knowledge regarding advantages and limitations.

The third approach – small computer located within the laboratory and used in a time-sharing mode – is represented by systems available from Berkeley Scientific Laboratories (Clindata), Diversified Numeric Applications (Uni-Lab), Laboratory Computing Inc. (LABCOM), and Spear Medical Systems (CLAS). Most authorities agree that the average clinical laboratory SHOULD NOT ATTEMPT TO DEVELOP SOFTWARE: costs are difficult to predict and may become uncontrollable (Krieg *et al.*, 1971). Most authorities also recommend purchase of both hardware and software from a single vendor who will assume total responsibility for all aspects of operation. This does NOT necessarily imply any advantage if the hardware and software come from one manufacturer; the key issue is that a single vendor assume total *responsibility*. Typical purchase costs for these systems are in the $150,000 to $200,000 range; additional expenses will include maintenance contract (about $10,000 per year), site preparation (maximum about $5,000), and paper (about $5,000 per year). Thus, total yearly cost (lease) will be about $60,000—somewhat less than time sharing with the central hospital computer (J. Lloyd Johnson Associates, 1971). Attractive features include:

1. Under direct control of laboratory director—needs of laboratory have first priority.
2. Laboratory staff can query computer at any time for "latest" results on any given patient.
3. Reports may be printed at any time convenient to laboratory and clinical staff.
4. Automatic data acquisition from interfaced instruments.
5. Results from manual tests may be entered immediately, using terminals throughout the laboratory.
6. Vendor assumes complete responsibility for BOTH hardware and software.
7. The potential user can visit several different installations to determine in advance how the system actually operates in a routine service laboratory.
8. The vendor may assume responsibility for training laboratory staff in system operation, and may assist in installation.

These systems are often referred to as "turnkey packages"—implying that installation and implementation are comparable to turning an ignition switch. Although the vendor supplies all hardware and software as a single "package," successful planning, installation, and implementation of such "turnkey" systems are NOT simple, trivial, or automatic. Some laboratories have found no benefit from computerization and have stopped using the computer; some laboratories report moderate success; a few have experienced rapid and smooth transition to computerized operation, which provides many important advantages to the clinical staff, nursing staff, medical technologists, laboratory director, and hospital administration (J. Lloyd Johnson Associates, 1971).

In my opinion, requirements for successful installation include:

1. Advance planning by the laboratory director and his staff. There must be a clear definition of objectives, a clear understanding of what the system actually will do, a clear understanding of how the system will operate on a day-to-day basis, and a complete commitment to computerization.
2. Assistance from the vendor during planning and initial installation. The vendor must provide truly expert advice on laboratory systems analysis, truly expert training for the laboratory director and his staff prior to installation, and truly expert instruction for the "line technologists" who will operate the system on a day-to-day basis.
3. Hardware and software support from the vendor after installation. The vendor must be able to provide: (a) "hotline" telephone consultation 24 hours per day; and (b) rapid and competent service for hardware as well as software.
4. Software must be easy for the user to modify. The user should be able to freely change without reprogramming at any time: all machine readable request card formats; worksheet and daily log formats; machine readable result card formats; methods of operation for automated instruments; normal ranges; test names; English text comments; and cumulative report formats. Some components of a typical installation are shown in Figure 30–4.

PLANNING

Too often, planning for clinical laboratory computerization proceeds from the premise "we want a computer," to the argument "a computer will provide the following benefits," to the conclusion "a computer is needed in our laboratory." And too often this uncritical enthusiasm paves the way for an installation unsatisfactory to the clinical staff, medical technologists, laboratory director, and hospital administration. Although clinical laboratory computerization can be justified on an economic basis (Lame, 1972), anticipated savings may not materialize in actual practice (Brecher and Loken, 1971). In most cases, justification probably should be based on improved service rather than decreased costs.

Computerization will NOT convert a poorly organized laboratory with ineffective management into a well-organized laboratory with good leadership. Indeed, computerization usually will reveal problems which previously had escaped detection: lost billings, inaccurate assignment of hospital numbers, transcription errors, lost specimens, or failure of technologists to complete daily work. Although in some cases benefits of better management forced by computerization may be ascribed to the computer, in my opinion it is better to computerize AFTER an optimal organization has been developed. This does not necessarily imply that an optimal manual reporting system is essential prior to computerization; our own transition to computerization started with a well-organized laboratory using single sheets for reporting.

Initial planning should be oriented toward objectives. If possible, each objective should be assigned a "dollar value," related to either direct cost savings or value of improved patient care (Krieg *et al.*, 1971). Typical objectives might include:

1. Daily cumulative reports produced at any time selected by laboratory.
2. Interim reports (new results since last cumulative) produced at any time selected by laboratory.
3. Worksheets produced at any time selected by laboratory.
4. Lists of incomplete tests produced at any time selected by laboratory.
5. Printed specimen labels produced at any time selected by laboratory.
6. Ability to obtain latest results on any selected test(s) for any patient at any time in response to telephone calls.
7. Ability to enter results for a "typical" manual test within 10 seconds or less at terminals located in different sections of laboratory.
8. Ability to modify format of cumulative report from days across top of page to days along left hand margin at any time selected by laboratory.
9. Ability to freely alter test names and printing order at any time selected by laboratory.
10. Ability to record results on "industry compatible magnetic tape" for future study at any time convenient to laboratory.
11. Ability to print normal ranges stratified by age and sex on all reports.
12. Reports of results with unacceptable difference between "today" and "yesterday" printed at any time convenient to laboratory.
13. Reports of all "abnormal" results printed at any time convenient to laboratory.
14. Ability to build patient files from central hospital computer, and to perform billing on central hospital computer.

A most important factor is the expectations of the clinical staff. If the clinical staff is satisfied to personally transcribe results from individual report slips onto cumulative reports in patient charts, there may be little enthusiasm for computer printed cumulative reports—which obviously cannot be "custom made" to suit the preferences of each physician. However, if the clinical staff requires neatly printed interim and cumulative reports produced by the laboratory "on demand" in response to phone calls, and considers this service ESSENTIAL to optimal patient care, a dedicated computer system becomes most attractive. Thus, the question, "Does our laboratory need a computer?" cannot be answered on the basis of laboratory considerations alone, but only in the broader context of overall patient care. If there is no way to meet needs for patient care by improved manual reporting, computerization should be investigated. Several months should be spent on systems analysis and flow charting in all sections of the laboratory (see section on basic concepts). Computerization means extensive changes in operating procedures for laboratory supervisors, medical technologists, medical records, financial management, ward clerks, physicians, and nurses. Even if the final decision is not to computerize, the time invested in studying information flow to and from the laboratory will have been well spent. A preliminary study might include:

1. Review of relevant literature; recommended reading might include J. Lloyd Johnson Associates (1971), Krieg *et al.* (1971), and other references cited at the end of this chapter.
2. Attendance at workshops and seminars (conducted by American Society of Clinical Pathologists, BSL, IBM, LCI and Spear).
3. Advice from consultants, who may provide valuable ideas, but CANNOT reliably select "the right solution" to your problem!
4. Analysis of your present laboratory operations, to include: (a) flow charts for all sections as well as written descriptions; (b) lists of tests (both individual procedures and combinations) with normal ranges, units, test codes, prices, and workunit factors; (c) workload for each station as well as each section of the laboratory; and (d) distribution of workload throughout each day as well as throughout the week.
5. Visits to computerized laboratories.
6. Analysis of staffing pattern required for operating the new system seven days per week, 24 hours per day.

Although visits to computerized laboratories can be quite informative, this time is not always well spent. In my experience, it is helpful for several people to make the visit together and to concentrate on different areas. Comparison of computer systems in different laboratories is difficult. First, complete information will require several days to collect; the "host" laboratory can scarcely be expected to maintain a list of answers to all questions that may be asked by visitors! Second, the director of a computerized laboratory may feel obliged to defend his investment in time, effort, and dollars; he may find it difficult to point out problems, and may be tempted to "put on a good show for the visitors." Third, laboratory objectives and resources often vary widely: what is "good" in one setting may be less satisfactory in another.

Several lists of questions for vendors and users have been published (Krieg *et al.*, 1971; Beautyman, 1971). A sample list that includes questions for both vendors and users is provided at the end of this chapter. Perhaps even more important than the questions *per se* is evaluation of answers to these questions.

A key question relating to history and background information is the time required from software installation to discontinuing manual reporting. Prolonged operation "in parallel" (more than two to four weeks) suggests poor planning, poor vendor support, or both, and is extremely frustrating to staff. A second key question in this area relates to experience of the top management in the vendor's organization. If the president, director of programming, and director of systems support have had extensive clinical laboratory experience, there is some assurance that "top management" will understand your problems. A third key question is the general philosophy of the vendor: if this corresponds to the philosophy of the laboratory director, chances of success are much enhanced.

Software flexibility is especially important. It is impossible to anticipate in advance: (1) changes in instrumentation and organization that will change test combinations done at each work station; (2) new services that will be developed, and present services that will be discontinued; and (3) requests from the clinical staff for alterations in report format.

With some systems, expensive programming is required to change worksheets, test names, request card formats, result card formats, normal ranges, and the order in which test names appear on cumulative reports. With other systems, changes can be made only at specified intervals, and the user is forced to select from a set of formats prepared by the vendor. In some cases one must choose between a cumulative report with days across the top of the page and one with days along the left-hand margin. In my opinion such rigidity is unacceptable—the user should be able to freely change any of these parameters at any time and to combine days across top of page with days along left-hand margin on the same cumulative report. (Figure 30–14 shows a possible cumulative report format.)

Free text capability is NOT an acceptable substitute for software flexibility; indeed, use of free text reporting may prove a handicap rather than an advantage. Our experience is consistent with that of Whitby and Lutz (1971), who point out:

> The disadvantages of free text are very great since . . . problems arise during . . . tabulation and analysis of information within the record. Narrative recording does not assign a standard way of representing information, and it is therefore necessary to search through the record until the required item is located.
>
> Narrative form also implies the unrestricted use of synonyms and alternative forms of phrasing, so a "dictionary" is needed. Because of these objections, the use of free text . . . for computer input is usually restricted to . . . the name and address of a patient.

Input Functions. Input functions include methods for entering patient information (name, hospital number, date of birth, ward or clinic of origin, physician name) as well as service requests and results. It is essential that the system accommodate the patient hospital number—which in some institutions may be ten or eleven digits. In most cases four to six characters will suffice for a physician code. The methods used for manual entry of test results should be studied carefully: with some systems this can be done using only three key strokes for a three-digit result, while others may require ten or more key strokes to enter the same information. In my opinion, each station for result entry should provide a "hard copy audit trail," or permanent printed record of transactions at that terminal: then, if an incorrect result is entered, one can find out what happened and take measures to prevent similar errors in the future. Although some systems provide "free text" capability, my own preference is for standardized English messages, which provide greater uniformity of reports, as well as improved legibility. If you have a central hospital computer, it is almost essential that the laboratory computer accept input from this system.

Output Functions. Output functions refer to printed reports and visual displays produced by the computer. Most systems provide many different outputs. We have found the following especially useful: blood collection lists with gummed labels arranged by patient name in order of room number; worksheets; section logs; interim reports; cumulative reports; and displays of any test(s) for any patient(s) produced on demand within 30 seconds. In my opinion it is important to have the following information printed on reports: (1) normal ranges stratified by age (to the nearest month) and sex; (2) technician code; and (3) collection time. Two key questions to ask when visiting computerized laboratories are: "What complaints did you receive from clinicians regarding the new reports?" and "What complaints did you receive regarding computerized reports on outpatients?" At some installations lack of flexibility in cumulative report formats has led to many complaints from the clinical staff. And outpatient reports present a special problem, since the patients usually must be "admitted" and "discharged" from the computer on the same day. Without advance planning, there may be difficulty answering phone calls for results on an outpatient after results have been "discharged" from the computer, but not yet filed according to patient name or hospital number. Also, advance planning is required to prevent "paper build up" on charts of outpatients who receive computerized reports of prothrombin time once each week over a prolonged period. And if you have a central hospital computer, it is most

PUBLIC JOHN Q 1234567 1234 6A /6330 06/11/73 11:32 P 01

CHEMISTRY I

	GLU MG/DL	GLU1 MG/DL	2HR GLU	BUN MG/DL	BUN1 MG/DL	CR/S MG/DL	NA MEQ/L	K MEQ/L	CL MEQ/L	CO2 MM/L	PH	PCO2 MMHG	BE MEQ/L	PO2 MMHG	%O2 SAT	AIR %
05/16																
										20.	7.46	28.	2. NEG	50.	86.	ROOM
02:04P		120.			12.		143.	3.7	104.	27.						
02:04P										16.	7.43	23.	5. NEG	57.	89.	ROOM
05/17																
										23.	7.41	36.	1. NEG	62.	91.	ROOM
02:04P										24.	7.41	38.	0.	59.	91.	LABL

CHEMISTRY II

	AMY SM/UN	CA MEQ/L	CAI MEQ/L	UA MG/DL	PHOS MG/DL	CHOL MG/DL	TRIG MG/DL	BILT MG/DL	BILD MG/DL	TP GM/DL	ALB GM/DL	CPK IU/L	SGO IU/L	LDH IU/L	ALK PHOS	SGP IU/L
05/17																
07:00A				7.8												
05/19																
07:00A										7.2						

CHEMISTRY III

	MG MEQ/L	LI MEQ/L	ALBE GM/DL	ALP1 GM/DL	ALP2 GM/DL	BETA GM/DL	GAMA GM/DL	ACID PHOS	T3 %	FRT4 NG/DL	T4MP UG/DL	FE UG/DL	UIBC UG/DL	TIBC UG/DL	%SAT %
05/19															
07:00A			4.17	.28	.68	.95	1.10								

10

PUBLIC JOHN Q 1234567 1234 6A /6330 06/11/73 11:32 P 02

HEMATOLOGY I

	WBC T/UL	RBC M/UL	HGB GM/DL	HCT %	MCV FL	MCH PG	MCHC %	PLSC	NRBC	ANIS	POIK	POLY	HYPO	MIC	MAC
05/16															
02:04P	10.5	5.56	16.4	47.5	86.	29.4	34.2	N	0.	SL	N	N	N	N	N
05/17															
07:00A	6.9	5.13	15.2	42.8	84.	29.6	35.3	N	0.	N	N	N	N	N	N

DIFFERENTIAL I

	BLAS	PROM	MYEL	METM	BAND	NEUT	EOS	BASO	LYMP	MONO	ATYP LYMP	TOXI GRAN	SPHR OCYT	IRR RBC	TARG CELL	HYPR SEG
05/16																
02:04P	0.	0.	0.	0.	0.	77.	6.	0.	12.	5.	O	O	O	O	O	O
05/17																
07:00A	0.	0.	0.	0.	0.	0.	0.	0.	0.	0.	O	O	O	O	O	O

URINALYSIS

	APPR	COL	SG	PHU	BILE	ACEU	HGBF	GLUU	TPU	PKU	CYST	RED	WBCF	RBCF
05/16														
07:32P	CLR	YEL	1.025	5.0	NEG	NEG	NEG	NEG	NEG	NA	NA	NA	0.	0.

URIN MICROSCOPIC

	EPIT	BACT	MUCU	AMOR	SPER	HYL CAST	GRAN CAST	CELL CAST	RBCC CAST	WBCC CAST	WAX CAST	UACR CRYS	CAOX CRYS	TRIP CRYS	TRIC OMOS	YEST
05/16																
07:32P	O	O	1+	O	0.	0.	0.	0.	0.	0.	0.	O	O	O	0.	O

10

Figure 30–14. Sample cumulative report.

important that billing information from the laboratory system be transferable to the central machine.

Simultaneous Functions. Simultaneous functions refer to input and/or output operations which can occur "at the same time" for a given system. The effective speed of output is NOT identical to maximum speed of the printer or cathode ray tube, but depends on BOTH hardware AND software. Meaningful figures for speed of output MUST BE specified under conditions of minimum, average, and maximum anticipated workloads. Some systems with identical hardware may demonstrate markedly different speeds for printing cumulative reports and displaying "latest" results for individual patients. A few systems apparently are unable to accept input from terminals, card readers, interfaced instruments, and queries for "latest" results while printing cumulative reports.

Service and system reliability are especially important: unscheduled "down time" is highly traumatic to technologists who quickly become dependent on a system which provides collection schedules, worksheets, printed reports, and capability to respond to phone calls for latest results. In my opinion a single vendor should assume responsibility for BOTH hardware and software: lack of such unified responsibility is a major disadvantage of programs which are "home made" or "borrowed" from some other institution. In our experience one may expect minor "crashes"* perhaps once a month (system "down" for 5 or 10 minutes), and major crashes perhaps once every six months (system "down" for 5 to 24 hours). It seems reasonable to expect competent "hot line" phone service within one-half hour 24 hours per day 365 days per year, as well as a service representative available, when needed, within two to six hours. Most vendors provide a variety of service contracts: in our experience a "24-hour contract" is not needed, provided emergency service is available when needed (at additional charge). An alternative plan of manual reporting should always be ready for implementation.

Training and support provided by the vendor will largely determine speed and smoothness of transition from manual to computerized operation. User manuals should fully describe operation of all programs; in most cases this will require several hundred pages. Training programs should include factory courses for key laboratory personnel (at least one-week duration) as well as on-site training for the entire laboratory staff (should be conducted by at least three Medical Technologists with training in laboratory management as well as operation of all hardware and software). Contract negotiations are of especial importance: the recommendations of Williams (1967), as quoted in the introduction to this chapter, should be followed closely. This contract should be written BY THE USER to include performance criteria for various workload conditions which are also specified by the user. All the items noted in this discussion should be included in this contract. There should be a clear understanding in writing that no payment will be made until performance conditions are met to the user's satisfaction. If payment is made on a lease or rental basis, there should be a provision for suspending payments in event of unscheduled "down time" longer than 24 hours' duration at any time in the course of the contract. In my experience those vendors who have confidence in their product are willing to accept this type of contract.

The following questions are relevant to evaluation of electronic data processing:

A. History and Background Information
   1. How was the system selected?
   2. When was hardware installed?
   3. When was software installed?
   4. What assistance did vendor provide prior to installation? during installation?
   5. What unanticipated problems developed during and after installation?
   6. How long did the computer run in parallel with manual operation?
   7. When was manual reporting discontinued?
   8. What has been the reaction of: (a) medical technology staff? (b) clinical staff? (c) nursing staff? (d) hospital administration?
   9. What problems developed during installation? Which remain unsolved?
   10. Would you do things differently if you had the opportunity to computerize your operation at this time?
   11. What are background and history of vendor? Describe background and experience of key personnel in organization.
   12. What is general philosophy of vendor with respect to clinical laboratory computerization?

B. Software Flexibility. Which of the following changes can be made at any time by the user without reprogramming:
   1. Numbers and types of tests listed on worksheets.
   2. Test names and units.
   3. Charge codes.
   4. Test groups, e.g., organ panels.
   5. Format of machine readable service request cards.
   6. AutoAnalyzer operation (number of standards and controls).
   7. Formats of machine readable test result cards.
   8. Normal ranges.
   9. Order in which test names appear on cumulative reports.

*"Crash" means computer is nonfunctional because of hardware or software problems.

10. Cumulative report format: change from days listed across top of page to days listed down left-hand margin.

C. Input Functions
  1. Can files be built from Master Patient Index using tape or cards produced in hospital computer center?
  2. Will system accept mark sense cards as service requests? What is percentage of rejects? How many tests per card?
  3. How many digits can be used for patient hospital number?
  4. How many characters are available for physician name?
  5. How are results on manual tests entered, including leukemic differential count, abnormal red cell morphology, abnormal urinalysis, gastric analysis, synovial fluid, blood gases, and serum protein electrophoresis?
  6. Is there a "hard copy audit trail" to provide for checking whether data have been entered correctly?
  7. What problems have been encountered with interfaced instruments?
  8. Can system use mark sense cards for entry of test results? How are these cards used in practice, and what is technologist acceptance?
  9. What limitations exist for English messages? What problems are encountered in this area?
  10. Can machine readable admission, discharge, and transfer information be accepted from central computer?

D. Output Functions
  1. Which of the following are provided?
     a. Blood collection lists with gummed labels arranged by patient name in order of room number.
     b. Worksheets.
     c. Section logs.
     d. Master worksheets.
     e. Directory of patients in alphabetic order.
     f. List of incomplete results.
     g. List of abnormal results.
     h. List of tests showing greater than "x per cent" difference from previous result on file (value of "x" to be freely specified by user).
     i. Interim reports organized by ward.
     j. Daily updated cumulative reports organized by ward (specify whether access to central computer is needed and what formats are available).
     k. Reports organized by physician.
     l. Display of any specified test(s) for any patient produced in laboratory on demand within 30 seconds at any time (24 hours per day, 365 days per year).
     m. Magnetic tape with billing information for hospital computer center.
     n. Magnetic tape with test results for analysis by hospital computer center.
  2. Are normal ranges printed on reports? If so, are these automatically adjusted for age and sex?
  3. Are abnormal results automatically identified on reports?
  4. Is the responsible technician identified on reports?
  5. Is specimen collection time noted on reports?
  6. What is reaction of clinical staff to cumulative reports on inpatients?
  7. What is reaction of clinical staff to computer printed reports on outpatients?
  8. Is billing information transferable to central hospital computer?

E. Simultaneous Functions. Which of the following can be performed simultaneously?
  1. Accept data from interfaced instruments (specify number and type).
  2. Accept manual results from terminals (specify number and type).
  3. Accept manual results from mark sense card reader (specify cards per minute).
  4. Print cumulative reports (specify lines per minute under minimum, average, and peak loads).
  5. Print interim reports (specify lines per minute under minimum, average, and peak loads).
  6. Display "latest" results for any test panel on any patient on cathode ray tube (specify lines per minute under minimum, average, and peak loads).

F. Service and System Reliability
  1. Is a single vendor responsible for service and maintenance of both hardware and software?
  2. Is "hot line" phone service available 24 hours per day 365 days per year?
  3. Typically, how long a period elapses before:
     a. Telephone request for service is answered?
     b. Serviceman arrives and starts work on system?
  4. On a scale from 0 to 100, how would you grade:
     a. Telephone service?
     b. Service representatives?
     c. Interest shown by vendor in providing adequate service?
  5. What types of service contracts are available, and at what cost?
  6. During a typical six-month period, how many days of unscheduled down time have been experienced for each component of system?

G. Training and Support
  1. Does a user group exist? Is vendor responsive to suggestions made by this group?
  2. What user manuals are provided?
  3. What training programs are provided?
  4. Is full documentation of software available?
  5. How long does it take an "average" technologist to learn to use the system?
  6. What specifications is vendor willing to include in contract?

SUMMARY

During the 1960's great enthusiasm developed for clinical laboratory computerization. There were some outstanding successes, as well as a number of failures which resulted when warnings of pioneer investigators went unheeded. Approaches now available include: programmable calculators, shared computers, and dedicated computers. Dedicated computers include: small machines located within the laboratory used in a batch-processing mode; large machines located outside the laboratory used in a time-sharing mode; and small machines located within the laboratory used in a time-sharing mode. In my opinion small machines within the laboratory operating in a time-sharing mode are especially attractive, provided the user does not attempt to develop his own software, and avoids those systems that do not provide adequate flexibility. Generally acceptable alternatives include programmable calculators, large machines located outside the laboratory operating in a time-sharing mode, and shared computers. However, special conditions are required for the last approach to prove successful. There is no single "correct" approach for all laboratories.

Considerable time should be spent in planning prior to making a decision in this area. As a first step, objectives should be listed, with approximate dollar values for each. Detailed studies of the laboratory operation should be made to establish needs for improved service. A list of relevant questions should be developed before contacting vendors or visiting computerized laboratories. Even if the decision is against computerization, time spent on this project usually will result in improved service to patients.

Clinical laboratory computerization is NOT comparable to the purchase of an analytical instrument; a successful experience typically requires detailed study and planning which will include all aspects of laboratory operation as well as interfaces with the clinical staff, nursing, financial management, medical records, and central hospital computer system.

SOURCES FOR HARDWARE AND SOFTWARE MENTIONED IN THIS CHAPTER

Berkeley Scientific Laboratories (BSL), 3210 Investment Blvd., Hayward, California 94545. Clindata dedicated computer system for clinical laboratory.

Digital Equipment Corporation (DEC), Maynard, Mass. 01754. Leading manufacturer of small computers.

Diversified Numeric Applications (DNA), 9801 Logan Avenue South, Minneapolis, Minn. 55431. UNI-LAB dedicated computer system for clinical laboratory.

Hewlett Packard, 1501 Page Mill Road, Palo Alto, Calif. 94304. Programmable calculators, small computers, and peripherals.

International Business Machines (IBM), Data Processing Division, 112 East Post Road, White Plains, N.Y. 10601. Leading manufacturer of large computers.

Laboratory Computing, Inc. (LCI), 4915 Monona Drive, Madison, Wisconsin 53716. LABCOM dedicated computer system for clinical laboratory.

Medical Information Technology, Inc. (MEDITECH), 65 Rogers Street, Cambridge, Mass. Shared clinical laboratory computer system.

Midwest Scientific Instruments (MSI), 1203 Willow Drive, Olathe, Kansas 66061. Wang programmable calculator used as central processing unit for clinical laboratory information system.

Monroe International, Orange, N.J. Programmable calculators.

Olivetti Underwood, 56 Arbor Street, Hartford, Conn. 06106. Programmable calculators.

Singer Business Machines, 2350 Washington Avenue, San Leandro, Calif. 94577. Friden programmable calculators.

Smith Corona Marchant, 299 Park Avenue, New York 10017. Programmable calculators.

Spear Medical Systems, 335 Bear Hill Road, Waltham, Mass. 02154. CLAS dedicated computer system for clinical laboratory.

T and T Technology, 4820 Dale Road, McFarland, Wis. 53558. Modular data processing system for clinical laboratory.

Wang Laboratories, Inc., 836 North Street, Tewksbury, Mass. 01876. Programmable calculators with instrument interfaces available through MSI.

REFERENCES

Beautyman, W.: A check list for laboratory computer site visits. Bull. College Amer. Path. 25:228, 1971.

Bennington, J. L.: Flow charting. *In* Westlake, G. E., and Bennington, J. L. (eds.): *Automation and Management in the Clinical Laboratory.* Baltimore, University Park Press, 1972.

Brecher, G., and Loken, H. F.: The laboratory computer—is it worth its price? Amer. J. Clin. Path. 55:527, 1971.

Digital Equipment Corporation: *Introduction to Programming.* Maynard, Mass., Digital Equipment Corp., 1970.

Digital Equipment Corporation: *Digital Logic Handbook.* Maynard, Mass., Digital Equipment Corp., 1972.

Editorial: American Laboratory 5:6, 1973.

Grams, R. R.: *Problem Solving, Systems Analysis, and Medicine.* Springfield, Ill., Charles C Thomas, 1972.

Hicks, G. P., Gieschen, M. M., Slack, W. V., and Larson, F. C.: Routine use of a small digital computer in the clinical laboratory. J.A.M.A. *196*:973, 1966.

Hughes, A. C., and Glidden, H. S.: A pilot program implements laboratory computerization. Lab. Manage. *11*:46 (March) 1973.

J. Lloyd Johnson Associates: *Clinical Laboratory Computer Systems.* Chicago, College of American Pathologists, 1971.

Knights, E. M.: *Mini-Computers in the Clinical Laboratory.* Springfield, Ill., Charles C Thomas, 1970.

Krieg, A. F., Johnson, T. J., McDonald, C., and Cotlove, E.: *Clinical Laboratory Computerization.* Baltimore, University Park Press, 1971.

Lame, K. D.: Cost justification of laboratory computer systems. *In* Westlake, G. E., and Bennington, J. L. (eds.): *Automation and Management in the Clinical Laboratory.* Baltimore, University Park Press, 1972.

Perone, S. P., and Jones, D. O.: *Digital Computers in Scientific Instrumentation.* New York, McGraw-Hill Book Co., Inc., 1973.

Rappoport, A. G., Gennaro, W. D., and Constandse, W. J.: Cybernetics enters the hospital laboratory. Mod. Hosp. *118*:107, 1967.

Rappoport, A. E.: Computering without tears. In *Quality Control in Clinical Chemistry.* Transactions of the IV International Symposium, May, 1971. Bern, Switzerland, Hans Huber Publishers, 1972.

Straumfjord, J. V., Spraberry, M. N., Briggs, H. G., and Noto, T. A.: Electronic data processing system for clinical laboratories. Amer. J. Clin. Path. *47*:661, 1967.

Whitby, L. G., and Lutz, W.: *Principles and Practice of Medical Computing.* London, E. & S. Livingstone, Ltd., 1971.

Williams, G. Z.: Laboratory automation systems; availability and procurement. Bull. College Amer. Path. *21*:383, 1967.

Williams, G. Z.: The use of data processing and automation in clinical pathology. Milit. Med. *129*:502, 1964.

APPENDIX 1

CLINICAL PATHOLOGY

With continued emphasis on accuracy and precision, coupled with the increased demand for health care as well as specificity, efficiency, and economy, the number and variety of clinicopathologic measurements and examinations should increase progressively during the next decade. The full utilization of electronic data processing, with application of computers to improved and expanded automation and semiautomation, is inevitable and essential. Clinical pathology serves as a bridge between the basic sciences and the patient through the patient's physician. The selection, generation, and translation into meaningful form of basic information for diagnosis, prognosis, and management also require manpower and space. Excellence in service for patient care as a foundation for teaching and research is a philosophy that should permeate clinical pathology policies and procedures and guide their implementation. In a schematic outline these activities are shown in Table 1.

The inadequate and antiquated figure of 20 square feet per hospital bed is often cited as an approximate figure for space allocation to clinical pathology laboratories. It is more realistic, however, to define the nature and volume of workload anticipated, personnel required, and related essential activities, including research and teaching to be conducted in the area. The number of hospital admissions and categories of patients, i.e., intensive care, surgical, medical, pediatric, or psychiatric, reflects workload more accurately in terms of volume and variety. The expansion of medical care to ambulatory patients will exceed requirements for

Table 1. SCHEMATIC OUTLINE OF ACTIVITIES IN CLINICAL PATHOLOGY

	ADMINISTRATION	
	PATIENT CARE SERVICE	
Indications and Selection	Technology and Generation	Interpretation and Translation
	TEACHING	
	RESEARCH	

acutely ill hospitalized bed patients in terms of number of measurements and examinations. With this emphasis on preventive medicine and maintenance of health, clinical pathology has become an integral part of the periodic health testing; this includes more comprehensive clinicopathologic panels than the previous chemical profiles.* Furthermore, diagnostic panels that have emerged complement and supplement the health evaluation. It is therefore apparent that the yardsticks formerly useful for space allocation are no longer applicable. Outpatient or ambulatory patient workload varies from 15 to 25 per cent of total workload volume; however, these percentages of total work volume figures vary between individual sections of clinical pathology, with the highest being in chemistry, hematology, and microscopy, and the lowest in microbiology and blood bank. In some institutions the ambulatory workload approaches or is equal to inpatient (acutely ill hospital bed patient) work volume. It is a trend that will continue and must be considered in planning facilities and staff. More prompt reporting (return of ambulatory patient laboratory data) is in demand, and with increasing emphasis on ambulatory care, a more prompt turnover time should be anticipated. However, the need for additional personnel to provide such around-the-clock staffing on a full-scale basis can improve the quality of patient care remarkably. Furthermore, more and better trained registered medical technologists are now available.

In terms of working area, a work flow pattern in utilization of space is as important as the net square feet available. About 60 or 70 per cent of the allocated gross square feet will equal net square feet. Effective working area and available bench space are needed to provide optimal use of net square feet.

Trends in space utilization indicate that it is not necessary to provide gas, vacuum, and air outlets at intervals in every room. Gas outlets are needed in bacteriologic laboratories and may be limited to such areas. Vacuum is the single most useful item of the three. Air available in many institutions has insufficient pressure to use with new instruments, such as atomic absorption spectrophotometers. Portable air and vacuum units represent economy in construction, but noise resulting from their use must be controlled. Chemical and fume hoods should be carefully reviewed in terms of anticipated need and installed in areas of absolute need only; too often they just occupy space, with improper or underutilization in many laboratories.

In addition to an adequate working area, an attractive, pleasant environment with a low noise level is desirable. Intermittent background music, at least in the restrooms and lounges, has been well received by personnel. Abstinence from eating, drinking, and smoking in laboratories is important to the health and safety of personnel.

Personnel should be adequate in number to respond to peak workloads and demands as well as regular daily service anticipated. Stratification of personnel at various levels of competence and responsibility with concomitant authority should be a goal. In view of the improved manpower supply, it is possible for individuals of varying backgrounds

---

*Henry, J. B., and Arras, M. J.: An innovation in health care delivery: Organ panels. South. Med. J. 63:907–916, 1970.

in education and experience to be identified with appropriate duties and assignments to assure service of the highest quality. This necessitates job descriptions and a personnel organization that defines accountability with responsibility in terms of specific duties. An administrative manual, that is revised periodically, should incorporate such information along with general personnel policies and staffing patterns. The details will vary in different organizations, but the principles are universal. A key individual in clinical pathology is the emergence of the administrative technologist who most often has a combination background in medical technology as well as administration. This individual can facilitate communication with hospital administration and personnel, coordinate purchasing and relate to nursing as well as other key areas of the institution. Weekly scheduled meetings of the administrative technologist and on-line supervisors with pathologists enhance a smooth flow, open line of communication and quality productivity within the laboratory environment.

Expression of workload in terms of numbers of individual measurements and examinations has been and will continue to be very useful. With expansion of improved automated analytical systems and a greater utilization of simultaneous measurements (battery of tests), a more meaningful expression of workload in terms of staff, time, and space requirements is the number of specimens submitted. Despite the varied nature of the work, this index is helpful in hematology, bacteriology, blood bank, chemistry, and microscopy. This approach emphasizes the great burden of specimen processing prior to single or multiple analyses and examinations. This approach has proved valid in anatomic pathology, with expression of workload in terms of the number of surgical pathology specimens or autopsies rather than the number of tissue blocks or slides examined per specimen or autopsy. An excellent comprehensive workload reporting system has recently become available.*

As we redirect our attention to the number of blood or other specimens received for blood bank, chemistry, hematology, microbiology, and microscopy, other facets of improved patient service can be identified. Next to the number of specimens received, the time period during which they are received is important. It is more efficient to process 100 blood specimens for chemistry at 8 A.M. than to process 50 specimens received periodically throughout the entire morning. The flow of service reveals obstacles of a different nature when reviewed in this manner. Improved techniques for delivery of service are as important to clinical pathology as to other segments of medical care.

Emergency patient care service demands can be anticipated in any hospital. It is more effective and efficient to identify emergency requests in terms of patient care requirements such as the following:

Stat (immediate execution and response): A diabetic patient in coma requires *stat* glucose and pH measurements, just as a patient with meningitis requires cerebrospinal fluid cytologic, chemical, and microbiologic studies.

Expedite: Service required may be accomplished within 2 to 4 hours.

---

*A Workload Reporting Method for Clinical Laboratories. 2nd ed. Chicago, The Laboratory Management Committee, College of American Pathologists, 1972.

A serum magnesium determination may be helpful to the physician for a patient with chronic renal failure, as would a serum glutamic oxaloacetate transaminase test for a patient with hepatitis. If such an interval will not compromise patient care and will facilitate coordinated response of personnel executing a number of such determinations, it will be possible to provide a greater variety of emergency services for more patients.

Today: When a measurement or examination should be accomplished prior to a patient's discharge or transfer from the hospital, it can be performed in conjunction with regular services.

When the medical staff and house staff are advised of these types of emergency service, they can identify the specific type of emergency service required (*stat, expedite,* and *today*) when requisitions for service are initiated at other than scheduled times. This approach will not be a great burden on laboratory personnel, and when the medical staff realizes that this categorization will ensure *stat* services for those patients requiring *"stat"* work and simultaneously permit a greater variety of more accurate emergency patient care laboratory service, their endorsement is assured. Abuse of the *stat* service can be eliminated in this manner, with optimal patient care assured. A selection of emergency services should be identified with prior endorsement of the medical staff to implement this type of 24-hour service (Table 2).

Education of all personnel is a continuing process that will enhance quality and efficiency of work. All institutions should contribute to the recruitment and continuing education of personnel at all levels. Emphasis should be placed on improvement in proficiency and technical skill and personal satisfaction, with opportunities for professional advancement and recognition.

Research is important not only to satisfy the personal needs of top-flight professional people but also to improve quality of service for optimal patient care. Improvement in existing procedures, with introduction of new methods and procedures, contributes directly to improved patient care. There is no greater opportunity anywhere for clinical investigation and study of diseases than in pathology.

QUALITY CONTROL

The systematic application of quality control techniques to clinical pathology has resulted in greater reliability of the data generated. This results in improved patient care and recognition of the profession and personnel. Indeed, there is no single more important morale booster to all personnel than the knowledge that each member of the team, from glassware washer to supervisor, is contributing to the best possible service in support of patient care and promotion of health.

Quality control is also a function of general laboratory cleanliness and order, washing of glassware, method of mixing reagents, and so forth. In everything one does, one must be systematic. The importance of being methodical cannot be overemphasized. For instance, if glassware is not scrupulously washed and rinsed, residue on the glassware might interfere with microanalyses of ions or deactivate enzymes. Once a procedure is tested, it should not be changed without cause. However,

Table 2. EMERGENCY MEASUREMENTS AND EXAMINATIONS AVAILABLE 24 HOURS DAILY AND SEVEN DAYS EACH WEEK*

Blood Bank	*Microbiology*
Whole blood crossmatched	Specimens cultured
Packed red blood cells crossmatched	Gram stain CSF
Fresh whole blood crossmatched	
Albumin 25% (salt poor 100 ml.); 5% in saline (250 ml.)	*Microscopy*
Fresh frozen plasma	Urinalysis
Group, Rh, and Coombs' test	Pregnancy (HCG) test
Platelet concentration	Osmolality
Transfusion reaction evaluation	CSF cell count
Process and collect blood from donors	
Platelet-rich plasma	
Fibrinogen (dried)	
Leukocyte-poor packed cells	
Cyroprecipitate	
Commercial AHF (antihemophiliac factor)	
Plasma protein fraction	
Chemistry	
Blood amylase	
Blood total bilirubin	
Blood bromide level	
Blood carbon dioxide	
Blood chloride	
Blood glucose	
Blood pH and pCO_2, pO_2 and O_2 saturation	
Blood sodium	
Blood urea nitrogen	
Blood calcium, ionized	
B.S.P.	
Barbiturate screening	
Cardiac Injury Panel (CPK, LDH, SGOT)	
Cerebrospinal fluid glucose	
Fibrinogen	
R.B.C. potassium	
Urine sodium and potassium	
Hematology	
Hematocrit	
White cell count	
Differential count (including platelet estimate and RBC morphology)	
CBC (WBC, RBC, Hb, Hct, MCV, MCHC, scan for RBC morphology, platelet estimate, abnormal WBCs. Differential performed only if ordered or if abnormal WBC count or abnormal cells noted on peripheral blood smear scan.)	
Prothrombin time	
Partial thromboplastin time	
Thrombin time	
Platelet count	

*If any other measurements or examinations are required, consult pathologist on call.

every effort should be made to improve one's technique to achieve better efficiency and precision, but in doing so one must make changes step by step and be alert to adverse changes in precision or accuracy that may ensue.

As long as there is a human component, errors are inevitable. While it is impossible to eliminate all errors, it is realistic to strive to reduce them and more important to detect them. With detection of errors, it is possible to identify their source and causes as well as ways to eliminate or prevent them. Systematic errors can be identified and eliminated with utilization of quality control techniques.

A good quality control system will operate satisfactorily with competent and experienced personnel, but it will deteriorate promptly with deficiency of personnel and physical facilities and poor general organization. Good quality is the result of continued effort and cannot be achieved without paying the price for it. A comprehensive quality control system may increase overall costs by as much as 10 per cent, but it is the best possible single investment.

Critical selection of methods, reagents, and instrumentation to ensure accuracy, precision, specificity, and delineation of normal values are prerequisites. In order to detect errors, periodic wavelength and absorption checks of each spectrophotometer are essential. In addition to standard reference solutions for analysis, serum controls should be determined with each batch of analyses. Random unknown specimens may be split and checks on duplicate analysis evaluated daily. Assayed specimens or unknowns from interlaboratory programs should be periodically analyzed along with patient specimens. This will assure accuracy in the determination. The values obtained on controls should be recorded on a monthly quality control sheet and plotted on a Levy-Jennings type chart. (See Chapter 1.) The technologist in charge of a particular test should see that the controls are within the range of precision applicable to the test. The technologist responsible for quality control in clinical pathology should review these records, taking into consideration data from assayed controls and standards and the result of interlaboratory surveys, and institute remedial action if necessary.

A prime ingredient for good quality control is well-maintained, functioning equipment. This necessitates a routine maintenance program that is adhered to scrupulously. Such a program will eliminate a good deal of trouble-shooting and the down time this entails. It will also ensure longer service from valuable equipment.

Routine maintenance means changing manifolds, oiling motors and moving parts, cleaning filters, inspecting light sources, changing the oil in heating baths, and so on, according to a definite predetermined schedule. Frequently daily or weekly items are attended to, but those items that require less frequent servicing are neglected because responsibility for a given piece of equipment has changed. It is therefore best to have a maintenance log in which the procedures for maintenance are stated and must be initialed at the proper intervals on a calendar. Logs of this nature are available from several manufacturers for their equipment. Most equipment has recommendations for routine maintenance in an accompanying manual. This can be translated into log form. Graph paper with divisions by weeks, months, or years may be useful in setting up such logs. A maintenance log should also include details of all breakdowns, component replacements, and service calls, which can be referred to as problems arise. For larger pieces of equipment, especially when special equipment may be required to service them, service contracts should be considered.

In order to deal with maintenance, a supply of tools, oil, cleaners, volt-ohm meter, and parts must be kept available. Each piece of equipment should have an adequate stock of expendable parts and replacement parts. Service manuals frequently list what items should be stocked.

To sustain optimal service on a continuous basis, one should consider duplicate equipment in more critical areas and backup components like colorimeters, heating baths, recorders, and so forth. All backup equipment must be properly maintained. Where this is not feasible, backup manual procedures and reagents should be available. The methods employed here should ideally give values that are consistent with the normal range of the usual procedure, and expertise in these areas should not be allowed to atrophy.

The entire clinical pathology staff must be made aware of the importance of routine maintenance in achieving top laboratory performance.

Consideration in quality control must be given to progressive changes in biologic specimens, such as blood after removal from the patient, and errors in obtaining of specimen, calculation, labeling, recording, and transcription.

Of the general factors intrinsic in quality control, human factors are of paramount importance. The attitude of the director, his associates, and his supervisors will determine the attitude of the entire staff. When the patient is placed in the center of all efforts, success will be inevitable. The director should provide built-in mechanisms for protection against unreasonable demands. This is a very important factor in building and maintaining the morale of the entire staff.

Self-appraisal on the part of the medical technologist should include *ethics* (sense of responsibility), *honesty* (personal and scientific), *recognition of limitations*, and *proper attitude toward criticism.*

Regarding selection for education, the qualifications of medical technologists should include:

1. Keen mind, alertness.
2. High standards, with built-in quality control.
3. Appreciation of details and thoroughness.
4. Conscientiousness, with appreciation of responsibility and reliability.
5. Manual dexterity.
6. Initiative.

Continuing education, with a personal responsibility for self-education, is an essential attribute of the professional medical technologist. Laboratory technicians, workers, and helpers must be continually informed of the importance of their contribution and participation; specific items of cleanliness and maintenance of laboratory work areas and materials, including glassware, should be emphasized. Members of the clerical staff should likewise be advised and informed of their role in terms of contact with professional colleagues, including physicians and nurses, as well as patients and public. The extra effort by everyone, which is necessary to improve patient care, cannot be overemphasized.

An up-to-date manual of procedures is essential so that all laboratory personnel know where to find the details of a procedure. In this way, one avoids inadvertent changes in procedure owing to deletion or lapse in memory of the technologist explaining the test details to a new worker. It will deemphasize memorization and discourage shortcuts. Changes in procedure should be marked in a working manual, and these changes should be incorporated in a revised manual from time to time. Immediate notification of such changes to the entire staff should be standard operating procedure.

When the various measurements for a single specimen are completed and recorded, with duplicate checks on accurate transcription, a clinical pathologist should evaluate groups of individual measurements for correlation with the diagnosis recorded on the service request form and evaluate inconsistencies between individual components assayed. For example, total cations must be checked against total anions and discrepancies with diagnosis evaluated. Additional measurements may be selected to confirm a borderline elevation. A leucine aminopeptidase may be determined to confirm a borderline elevation of an alkaline phosphatase. Likewise, an ornithine transcarbamylase may be determined to check out an equivocal elevation of the serum glutamic oxaloacetate transaminase. Furthermore, creatinine may be measured to define a borderline elevation of blood urea nitrogen.

The final level of quality control rests with the physician at the bedside. This revolves around *confirmation request.* Whenever a measurement does not fit the clinical picture, the physician should submit a new specimen and service request with a notation reading, *confirmation request.* It is essential that such a confirmation request, with a new specimen, be brought to the attention of the clinicopathologic laboratory within 24 hours after completion of the measurement. Both new and original specimens should be analyzed concurrently and both values reported. A new specimen is essential to rule out misidentification, contamination, and so forth, inasmuch as all abnormal values should have already been repeated prior to reporting results. No charge should be made for such confirmation requests, and they should give the physician definitive information regarding the reliability of a measurement in question. There is no need for the physician at the bedside to compromise his clinical judgment or comment, "The laboratory is off today." In spite of such quality control measures, there is a possibility of random error. Since random errors are generally attributable to improper specimen identification originating on the floor or in the laboratory, where specimens may inadvertently be misplaced or misidentified, an invalid value may arise and jeopardize patient care. For this reason, we are convinced that the final level of quality control rests with the physician at the bedside. The confirmation request should eliminate any doubt in anyone's mind regarding the validity of the measurement in question.

APPENDIX 2

PHYSIOLOGIC SOLUTIONS, BUFFERS, ACID-BASE INDICATORS, STANDARD REFERENCE MATERIALS, ATOMIC WEIGHTS AND INTERNATIONAL SYSTEM OF UNITS (S.I.) AND QUANTITIES

PHYSIOLOGIC SOLUTIONS

A physiologic solution is one that contains various salts in concentrations that closely approximate the composition of fluids in the human body. The simplest of these is physiologic saline, which has the same osmotic pressure as the blood. There are more elaborate solutions, for example, to maintain tissues in a metabolically active state for longer periods of time. The table below gives formulas of solutions that are isotonic with respect to blood.

PHYSIOLOGIC SOLUTIONS

	SALINE	LOCKE'S SOLUTION	RINGER'S* SOLUTION	TYRODE'S SOLUTION
Sodium chloride	0.85 gm.	0.9 gm.	0.7 gm.	0.8 gm.
Calcium chloride		0.024 gm.	0.0026 gm.	0.02 gm.
Potassium chloride		0.042 gm.	0.035 gm.	0.02 gm.
Sodium bicarbonate		0.01–0.03 gm.		0.1 gm.
D-Glucose		0.1–0.25 gm.		0.1 gm.
Magnesium chloride				0.01 gm.
Monosodium phosphate				0.005 gm.
Distilled water	100 ml.	100 ml.	100 ml.	100 ml.

*Porter modification.

BUFFERS*

Buffers have the ability to resist changes in pH. Buffers usually consist of a weak acid and its salt or a weak base and its salt. The Hender-

*For a comprehensive discussion, including preparation of buffer solutions of a definite ionic strength, consult Roger G. Bates, *Determination of pH – Theory and Practice*. New York, N.Y., John Wiley & Sons, Inc., 1964.

son-Hasselbalch equation is useful in calculating the acid (or base) to salt ratio required to establish a desired pH from a buffer system. For example, if 1 liter of 0.1 M acetic acid buffer (total molarity of acetate ion plus acetic acid) at pH 4.90 is desired, use the expression

$$(1) \quad \mathrm{pH} = \mathrm{pK} + \log \frac{[\mathrm{A}^-]}{[\mathrm{HA}]} \quad \text{(Henderson-Hasselbalch equation)}$$

Substituting for pH = 4.90 and pK = 4.76 (for acetic acid),

$$(2) \quad 4.90 = 4.76 + \log \frac{[\text{acetate}]}{[\text{acetic acid}]},$$

$$(3) \quad \log \frac{[\text{acetate}]}{[\text{acetic acid}]} = 0.14,$$

$$(4) \quad \frac{[\text{acetate}]}{[\text{acetic acid}]} = 1.38.$$

$$(5) \quad [\text{acetate}] + [\text{acetic acid}] = 0.1\ \mathrm{M}$$

$$(6) \quad \text{and } \frac{[\text{acetate}]}{[\text{acetic acid}]} = 1.38$$

$$(7) \quad \text{or } [\text{acetate}] = 1.38\ [\text{acetic acid}]$$

$$(8) \quad 1.38\ [\text{acetic acid}] + [\text{acetic acid}] = 0.1\ \mathrm{M}$$

$$(9) \quad [\text{acetic acid}] = 0.042\ \mathrm{M} = 2.52\ \text{gm. acetic acid/liter}$$

$$(10) \quad [\text{acetate}] = 0.058\ \mathrm{M} = 4.76\ \text{gm. sodium acetate/liter}$$

Similarly, if 648 ml. of 0.025 molar diethylbarbituric acid and 10 ml. of 0.5 molar sodium diethylbarbiturate are mixed and diluted to 1 liter, the approximate pH of the solution is calculated, knowing that the pK for diethylbarbituric acid = 7.98.

$$(1) \quad \text{Molar concentration} = \frac{\text{moles}}{\text{liter}}$$

$$(2) \quad \text{liters}\left(\frac{\text{moles}}{\text{liter}}\right) = \text{moles}$$

For diethylbarbituric acid

(3) $(0.648)(0.025) = 0.0162$ moles

(4) which diluted to 1 liter = 0.0162 moles/liter

For sodium diethylbarbiturate

(5) $(0.010)(0.5) = 0.005$ moles

(6) which, diluted to 1 liter = 0.005 moles/liter

(7) $$pH = pK + \log \frac{[salt]}{[acid]} = pK - \log \frac{[acid]}{[salt]}$$

(8) $$= 7.98 - \log \frac{0.0162}{0.005}$$

(9) $$= 7.98 - \log 3.24$$

(10) $$= 7.98 - 0.51$$

(11) $$\therefore pH = 7.47$$

The maximum buffering capacity is at the pK value of the weak acid or base. For instance, for acetic acid with a pH value of 4.76, more acid will be required to change the pH of an acetate buffer from 4.76 to 4.66 than from 4.20 to 4.10. Efficient buffering capacity covers a pH range of about 1 unit on either side of the pK value of the weak acid or base. For acetic acid, this would be from about pH 3.8 to 5.8.

Sørensen's Phosphate Buffers

These buffer solutions are generally useful, since the range of the mixtures is from pH 5 to 8.

Fifteenth Molar Monobasic Potassium Phosphate Solution (KH_2PO_4). Weigh 9.0727 gm. of monobasic potassium phosphate. Dissolve it in distilled water and dilute to exactly 1 liter with distilled water. The solution must be absolutely clear and should yield no test for chloride or sulfates. Phosphate salt solutions should be kept in the refrigerator.

Fifteenth Molar Dibasic Sodium Phosphate Solution (Na_2HPO_4). Expose dibasic sodium phosphate containing 12 moles of water of crystallization to ordinary atmosphere for two weeks. It should then contain 2 moles of water of crystallization. Dissolve 11.867 gm. of disodium phosphate duohydrate in distilled water and dilute to exactly 1 liter with distilled water. The solution must be absolutely clear and should yield no test for chloride or sulfates.

SORENSEN'S TABLE OF BUFFER MIXTURES

Na_2HPO_4 SOLUTION (ml.)	KH_2PO_4 SOLUTION (ml.)	pH
0.25	9.75	5.288
0.5	9.5	5.589
1.0	9.0	5.906
2.0	8.0	6.239
3.0	7.0	6.468
4.0	6.0	6.643
5.0	5.0	6.813
6.0	4.0	6.979
7.0	3.0	7.168
8.0	2.0	7.381
9.0	1.0	7.731
9.5	0.5	8.043

Tris(Hydroxymethyl)Aminomethane Buffer*

Tris(hydroxymethyl)aminomethane buffer can be used for a pH range between 7.0 and 9.0, but its best buffer capacity is between 7.5 and 8.5. It is practically ineffective below pH 7.0 and above pH 9.0. One advantage of the buffer is its excellent stability. The buffer can be prepared by weighing the desired amount of tris(hydroxymethyl)aminomethane, dissolving it in water, and adjusting the pH to the desired value with HCl. For example, if 100 ml. of 0.05 M buffer is desired, place 0.6057 gm. of tris(hydroxymethyl)aminomethane into a 100 ml. volumetric flask. This is dissolved in approximately 50 ml. of distilled water. Add 0.1 N HCl, as indicated in the table, and fill up to the mark with distilled water. The table shows the pH values obtained when 0.6057 gm. of tris(hydroxymethyl)aminomethane dissolved in water is mixed with the indicated amounts of 0.1 N HCl and diluted to 100 ml.

*If buffers of a higher molarity are desired, the 0.1 N HCl may have to be replaced by a 1.0 N HCl.

ML. 0.1 N HCl ADDED	RESULTING pH AT 23° C.	RESULTING pH AT 37° C.
5.0	9.10	8.95
7.5	8.92	8.78
10.0	8.74	8.60
12.5	8.62	8.48
15.0	8.50	8.37
17.5	8.40	8.27
20.0	8.32	8.18
22.5	8.23	8.10
25.0	8.14	8.00
27.5	8.05	7.90
30.0	7.96	7.82
32.5	7.87	7.73
35.0	7.77	7.63
37.5	7.66	7.52
40.0	7.54	7.40
42.5	7.36	7.22
45.0	7.20	7.05

ACID-BASE INDICATORS*

An acid-base indicator is a weak acid or a weak base, the undissociated form of which has another color and constitution than the iogenic form. Color change takes place over a certain narrow range of hydrogen ion concentrations. This range is called the color change interval and is expressed in terms of pH (the negative logarithm of the hydrogen ion concentration). A great number of substances show indicator properties, although relatively few of them are practically applied for neutralization reactions and pH determinations. In general, weak acids should be titrated in the presence of indicators that change in slightly alkaline solutions. Weak bases should be titrated in the presence of indicators that change in slightly acid solutions.

The availability of precision pH meters allows titration to a selected endpoint (pH) and may replace use of indicators for several applications.

*Based on Lange, N. A.: *Handbook of Chemistry*. Revised 10th ed. New York, McGraw Hill Book Company, Inc., 1967.

ACID-BASE INDICATORS

INDICATOR	pH RANGE	QUANTITY OF INDICATOR PER 10 ML.	COLOR	
			Acid	Alkaline
Thymol blue (A)*†	1.2–2.8	1-2 drops 0.1% soln. in aq.	red	yellow
Methyl orange (B)	3.1–4.4	1 drop 0.1% soln. in aq.	red	orange
Bromphenol blue (A)†	3.0–4.6	1 drop 0.1% soln. in aq.	yellow	blue-violet
Bromcresol green (A)†	4.0–5.6	1 drop 0.1% soln. in aq.	yellow	blue
Methyl red (A)†	4.4–6.2	1 drop 0.1% soln. in aq.	red	yellow
Bromcresol purple (A)†	5.2–6.8	1 drop 0.1% soln. in aq.	yellow	purple
Bromthymol blue (A)†	6.2–7.6	1 drop 0.1% soln. in aq.	yellow	blue
Phenol red (A)†	6.4–8.0	1 drop 0.1% soln. in aq.	yellow	red
Neutral red (B)	6.8–8.0	1 drop 0.1% soln. in 70% alc.	red	yellow
Thymol blue (A)† ‡	8.0–9.6	1-5 drops 0.1% soln. in aq.	yellow	blue
Phenolphthalein (A)	8.0–10.0	1-5 drops 0.1% soln. in 70% alc.	colorless	red
Thymolphthalein (A)	9.4–10.6	1 drop 0.1% soln. in 90% alc.	colorless	blue

The letters A or B following the name of the indicator signify, respectively, that the compound is an indicator *acid* or *base*.
*For the acid range.
†Sodium salt.
‡For the alkaline range.

COMMONLY USED ACIDS AND ALKALIES*

SOLUTION	MOL. WEIGHT	SPEC. GRAVITY†	GM. PER LITER†	MOLARITY†	NORMALITY†	APPROX. NUMBER OF ML. REQUIRED TO MAKE 1000 ML. OF 1 N SOLUTION
Conc. HCl	36.46	1.19	440	12	12	83
Conc. H_2SO_4	98.08	1.84	1730	18	36	28
Conc. HNO_3	63.02	1.42	990	16	16	64
Conc. lactic acid	90.08	1.21	1030	11	11	87
Glacial acetic acid	60.08	1.06	1060	17.5	17.5	57
Conc. NH_4OH	35.05	0.90	250	15	15	67

*Commercially available.
†Figures may vary slightly according to the lot or manufacturer.

STANDARD REFERENCE MATERIALS FOR CLINICAL MEASUREMENTS*†

SRM NO.	NAME	PURITY (%)	PROPERTY CERTIFIED	AMOUNT (gm.)	DATE ISSUED
40h	Sodium oxalate	99.95	Reductometric standard	60	April 24, 1969
83c	Arsenic trioxide	99.99	Reductometric standard	75	Feb. 6, 1962
84h	Acid potassium phthalate	99.993	Acidimetric standard	60	July 9, 1969
136c	Potassium dichromate	99.98	Oxidation standard	60	March 24, 1970
186Ic	Potassium dihydrogen phosphate	99.9	pH	30	July 29, 1966
186IIc	Disodium hydrogen phosphate	99.9	pH	30	Sept. 1, 1970
350	Benzoic acid	99.98	Acidimetric standard	30	April 15, 1958
911	Cholesterol	99.4	Identity and purity	0.5	Oct. 20, 1967
912	Urea	99.7	Identity and purity	25	Sept. 24, 1968
913	Uric acid	99.7	Identity and purity	10	Sept. 24, 1968
914	Creatinine	99.8	Identity and purity	10	Sept. 24, 1968
915	Calcium carbonate	99.9	Identity and purity	20	March 4, 1969
916	Bilirubin	99	Identity and purity	0.1	March 10, 1971
917	D-Glucose	99.9	Identity and purity	25	Nov. 18, 1970
918	Potassium chloride	99.9	Identity and purity	20	Jan. 22, 1971
922	tris(Hydroxymethyl)aminomethane	99.9	pH	25	May 1, 1971
923	tris(Hydroxymethyl)aminomethane hydrochloride	99.7	pH	35	May 1, 1971
930	Glass filters for spectrophotometry		Absorbance	3 filters	Feb. 24, 1971
1571	Orchard leaves		Major and trace constituents	75	Jan. 28, 1971
2201	NaCl	99.9	pNa pCl	120	April 15, 1971
2202	KCl	99.9	pK pCl	160	May 1, 1971

*Orders and requests for information about these SRM's should be directed to the Office of Standard Reference Materials, National Bureau of Standards, Washington, D.C. 20234.

†Courtesy of W. Wayne Meinke. From Meinke, W. W.: Standard Reference Materials for Clinical Measurements. Anal. Chem. *43*(No. 6):31A, 1971.

METRIC CONVERSIONS

1 meter (m.) = 0.001 kilometer (km.)
= 10 decimeters (dm.)
= 100 centimeters (cm.)
= 1000 millimeters (mm.)
1 micron (μ) = m. $\times 10^{-6}$ = cm. $\times 10^{-4}$
1 nanometer (nm.) = 1 millimicron (mμ)* = m. $\times 10^{-9}$
= cm. $\times 10^{-7}$
1 Angstrom (A)* = m. $\times 10^{-10}$ = cm. $\times 10^{-8}$
1 gram (gm.) = 0.001 kilogram (kg.)
= 1000 milligrams (mg.)
1 gamma (γ)* = 1 microgram (μg.) = gm. $\times 10^{-6}$ = mg. $\times 10^{-3}$
1 nanogram (ng.) = gm. $\times 10^{-9}$
1 picogram (pg.) = gm. $\times 10^{-12}$
1 liter (l) = 10 deciliters (dl.)
= 1000 milliliters (ml.)
1 lambda (λ)* = 1 microliter (μl.) = liters $\times 10^{-6}$ = ml. $\times 10^{-3}$
1 meter = 39.37 inches
1 liter = 1.057 liquid quarts
1 kilogram = 2.205 pounds (avoirdupois)
1 inch = 2.540 centimeters
1 pound (avoirdupois) = 453.6 grams

*These terms are obsolete according to the Système International d'Unites (S.I.) Convention.

TEMPERATURE CONVERSIONS

CENTIGRADE	FAHRENHEIT
110°	230°
100	212
95	203
90	194
85	185
80	176
75	167
70	158
65	149
60	140
55	131
50	122
45	113
44	111.2
43	109.4
42	107.6
41	105.8
40.5	104.9
40	104
39.5	103.1
39	102.2
38.5	101.3
38	100.4
37.5	99.5
37°	98.6°
36.5	97.7
36	96.8
35.5	95.9
35	95
34	93.2
33	91.4
32	89.6
31	87.8
30	86
25	77
20	68
15	59
10	50
+5	41
0	32
−5	23
−10	14
−15	+5
−20	−4

0.54° = 1°
1° = 1.8°

To convert Fahrenheit into Centigrade, subtract 32 and multiply by 0.555.
To convert Centigrade into Fahrenheit, multiply by 1.8 and add 32.

INTERNATIONAL ATOMIC WEIGHTS OF COMMONLY USED ELEMENTS* (BASED ON CARBON-12)

	SYMBOL	ATOMIC NUMBER	ATOMIC WEIGHT
Aluminum	Al	13	26.982
Antimony	Sb	51	121.75
Arsenic	As	33	74.912
Barium	Ba	56	137.34
Beryllium	Be	4	9.0122
Bismuth	Bi	83	208.98
Boron	B	5	10.811
Bromine	Br	35	79.909
Cadmium	Cd	48	112.40
Calcium	Ca	20	40.08
Carbon	C	6	12.011
Chlorine	Cl	17	35.453
Chromium	Cr	24	51.996
Cobalt	Co	27	58.933
Copper	Cu	29	63.54
Fluorine	F	9	18.998
Gold	Au	79	196.97
Hydrogen	H	1	1.0080
Iodine	I	53	126.90
Iron	Fe	26	55.847
Lead	Pb	82	207.19
Lithium	Li	3	6.939
Magnesium	Mg	12	24.312
Manganese	Mn	25	54.938
Mercury	Hg	80	200.59
Molybdenum	Mo	42	95.94
Nickel	Ni	28	58.71
Nitrogen	N	7	14.007
Oxygen	O	8	15.999
Phosphorus	P	15	30.974
Potassium	K	19	39.102
Selenium	Se	34	78.96
Silicon	Si	14	28.086
Silver	Ag	47	107.87
Sodium	Na	11	22.990
Strontium	Sr	38	87.62
Sulfur	S	16	32.064
Thallium	Tl	81	204.37
Tin	Sn	50	118.69
Tungsten	W	74	183.85
Zinc	Zn	30	65.37

*From Lange, N. A.: Handbook of Chemistry. Revised 10th ed. New York, McGraw-Hill Book Company, 1967.

INTERNATIONAL SYSTEM OF UNITS (S.I.) AND QUANTITIES* (Prefixes for Multiples and Submultiples)

MULTIPLE	PREFIX	SYMBOL	MULTIPLE	PREFIX	SYMBOL
10^{12}	tera	T	10^{-1}	deci	d
10^{9}	giga	G	10^{-2}	centi	c
10^{6}	mega	M	10^{-3}	milli	m
10^{3}	kilo	k	10^{-6}	micro	μ
10^{2}	hecto	h	10^{-9}	nano	n
10	deca	da	10^{-12}	pico	p
			10^{-15}	femto	f
			10^{-18}	alto	a

*The *International System of Units* (S.I.) is an attempt to attain uniformity among all scientific disciplines in the expression of results from experimental data. This is the summation of a report by the Royal College of Pathologists of special interest to pathology. J. Clin. Chem. 23:818, 1970.

SPECIAL APPLICATIONS TO PATHOLOGY

Length

Basic unit is the meter (m.).

Angstrom unit should not be used. Convert to nanometers (1 A = 10^{-1} nm.).

Micron (μ), 10^{-6} m., is obsolete. Use micrometer (μm.).

Volume

Basic unit is the cubic meter ($m.^3$).

Working unit is the liter (l.), which is equivalent to the cubic decimeter ($dm.^3$).

Multiples and submultiples of the liter are to be used for all volume measurements.

Microliter (μl.) is the correct name for 10^{-6} liter; lambda (λ) for this volume is obsolete.

Mg. per cent equals mg./100 mg., not mg./100 ml.

Mass

Basic unit is the kilogram (kg.); working unit is the gram (gm.).

Multiples and submultiples are of the gram.

Microgram (μg.) is the correct name for 10^{-6} gram; gamma (γ) for this mass is obsolete.

Pressure

Basic unit is the Newton per square meter ($N/m.^2$), called alternatively the Pascal (Pa.).

Conventional units are millimeters of mercury (mm. Hg), centimeters of water (cm. H_2O).

Conversion factors (at stp): 1 mm. Hg = 133 $N/m.^2$, 1 cm. H_2O = 98 $N/m.^2$

Time

Basic unit is the second (s.). Other working units are minute (min.), hour (h.), day (d.), year (y.).

Thermodynamic temperature

Basic unit is the kelvin (K.).

Working unit for temperature is degree Celsius (° C.).

Amount of substance

Basic unit is the mole (mol.), replacing such terms as gram-molecule, gram-ion, and gram-equivalent.

Concentration is expressed as moles/liter (mol./1.), and is designated by the symbol M.

For a comprehensive review of nomenclature for quantities and units in the clinical laboratory, see R. Dybkaer's chapter in *Standard Methods of Clinical Chemistry*. Vol. 6, pp. 223–244. New York, Academic Press, Inc., 1970.

REFERENCES

Lange, N. A., and Forker, G. M. (eds.): Handbook of Chemistry. 10th ed. New York, McGraw-Hill Book Company, 1967.

Long, C. (ed.): Biochemists' Handbook. Princeton, New Jersey, D. Van Nostrand Co., Inc., 1961.

Meinke, W. W.: Standard Reference Materials for Clinical Measurements. Anal. Chem. 43:31A, 1971.

The Merck Index; and Encyclopedia of Chemicals and Drugs. 8th ed. Rahway, New Jersey, Merck & Co., Inc., 1968.

The Use of S. I. in Reporting Results in Pathology. J. Clin. Path. 23:818, 1970.

APPENDIX 3

TABLES OF NORMAL VALUES

Many of the normal values are based on the experience in the Department of Pathology, Mount Sinai Hospital, Chicago, Illinois, and the Division of Clinical Pathology, State University Hospital, State University of New York, Syracuse, New York. Actual values may vary with different techniques or in different laboratories. Appropriate chapters should be reviewed for further details pertaining to age and other variables that may yield different values.

ABBREVIATIONS USED IN TABLES

<	= less than	mI.U.	= milliInternational Unit
>	= greater than	mOsm.	= milliosmole
dl.	= 100 ml.	mμ	= millimicron
gm.	= gram	ng.	= nanogram
I.U.	= International Unit	pg.	= picogram
kg.	= kilogram	μEq.	= microequivalent
mEq.	= milliequivalent	μg.	= microgram
mg.	= milligram	μI.U.	= microInternational Unit
ml.	= milliliter	μl.	= microliter
mM.	= millimole	μU.	= microunit
mm. Hg	= millimeters of mercury		

WHOLE BLOOD, SERUM, AND PLASMA (CHEMISTRY)

TEST	MATERIAL	NORMAL VALUE	SPECIAL INSTRUCTIONS
Acetoacetic acid, qualitative	Serum	Negative	
quantitative	Serum	0.2–1.0 mg./dl.	
Acetone, qualitative	Serum	Negative	
quantitative	Serum	0.3–2.0 mg./dl.	See Chapters 2 and 9
Albumin, quantitative	Serum	3.2–4.5 gm./dl. (salt fractionation) 3.2–5.6 gm./dl. by electrophoresis 3.8–5.0 gm./dl. by dye binding	
Alcohol	Serum or whole blood	Negative	See Chapter 10
Aldolase	Serum	Adults: 3–8 Sibley-Lehninger U/dl. at 37° C. Children: Approximately 2 times adult levels Newborn: Approximately 4 times adult levels	See Chapter 14

(*Table continues on the opposite page.*)

WHOLE BLOOD, SERUM, AND PLASMA (CHEMISTRY)—*Continued*

TEST	MATERIAL	NORMAL VALUE	SPECIAL INSTRUCTIONS
Alpha-amino acid nitrogen	Serum	3–6 mg./dl.	
δ-Aminolevulinic acid	Serum	0.01–0.03 mg./dl.	
Ammonia	Plasma	20–150 μg./dl. (diffusion) 40–80 μg./dl. (enzymatic method) 12–48 μg./dl. (resin method)	Collect with sodium heparinate; specimen must be analyzed immediately
Amylase	Serum	60–160 Somogyi units/dl.	See Chapter 15
Argininosuccinic lyase	Serum	0–4 U./dl.	
Arsenic	Whole blood	< 3 μg./dl.	
Ascorbic acid (vitamin C)	Plasma Whole blood	0.6–1.6 mg./dl. 0.7–2.0 mg./dl.	Analyze immediately
Barbiturates	Serum, plasma, or whole blood	Negative	
Base excess	Whole blood	Male: −3.3 to +1.2 Female: −2.4 to +2.3	
Base, total	Serum	145–160 mEq./L.	
Bicarbonate	Plasma	21–28 mM./L.	
Bile acids	Serum	0.3–3.0 mg./dl.	
Bilirubin	Serum	Up to 0.3 mg./dl. (direct or conjugated) 0.1–1.0 mg./dl. (indirect or unconjugated) Total: 0.1–1.2 mg./dl. Newborns total: 1–12 mg./dl.	See Chapter 13
Blood gases			
pH		7.38–7.44 arterial 7.36–7.41 venous	
pCO_2		35–40 mm. Hg arterial 40–45 mm. Hg venous	
pO_2		95–100 mm. Hg arterial	
Bromide	Serum	0–5 mg./dl.	See Chapter 10
BSP (bromsulfonphthalein) (5 mg./kg.)	Serum	< 6% retention after 45 min.	See Chapter 13
Calcium	Serum	Ionized: 4.2–5.2 mg./dl. 2.1–2.6 mEq./L. or 50–58% of total Total: 9.0–10.6 mg./dl. 4.5–5.3 mEq./L. Infants: 11–13 mg./dl.	See Chapter 9
Carbon dioxide (CO_2 content)	Whole blood, arterial Plasma or serum, arterial Whole blood, venous Plasma or serum, venous	19–24 mM./L. 21–28 mM./L. 22–26 mM./L. 24–30 mM./L.	See Chapter 12
CO_2 combining power	Plasma or serum, venous	24–30 mM./L.	
CO_2 partial pressure (pCO_2)	Whole blood, arterial Whole blood, venous	35–40 mm. Hg 40–45 mm. Hg	
Carbonic acid	Whole blood, arterial Whole blood, venous Plasma, venous	1.05–1.45 mM./L. 1.15–1.50 mM./L. 1.02–1.38 mM./L.	
Carboxyhemoglobin (carbon monoxide hemoglobin)	Whole blood	Suburban nonsmokers: < 1.5% saturation of hemoglobin Smokers: 1.5–5.0% saturation Heavy smokers: 5.0–9.0% saturation	See Chapter 10

(*Table continues on the following page.*)

WHOLE BLOOD, SERUM, AND PLASMA (CHEMISTRY)—*Continued*

TEST	MATERIAL	NORMAL VALUE	SPECIAL INSTRUCTIONS
Carotene, beta	Serum	40–200 μg./dl.	
Cephalin cholesterol flocculation	Serum	Negative to 1+ after 24 hours 2+ or less after 48 hours	See Chapter 13
Ceruloplasmin	Serum	23–50 mg./dl.	See Chapter 9
Chloride	Serum	95–103 mEq./L.	See Chapter 12
Cholesterol, total	Serum	150–250 mg./dl. (varies with diet and age)	See Chapter 9
Cholesterol, esters	Serum	65–75% of total cholesterol	
Cholinesterase	Erythrocytes	0.65–1.00 pH units	
Pseudocholinesterase	Plasma	0.5–1.3 pH units 8–18 I.U./L. at 37° C.	
Citric acid	Serum or plasma	1.7–3.0 mg./dl.	
Congo red test	Serum or plasma	> 60% after 1 hour	Severe reactions may occur if dye is injected twice; check patient's record
Copper	Serum or plasma	Male: 70–140 μg./dl. Female: 85–155 μg./dl.	See Chapter 9
Cortisol	Plasma	8 A.M.–10 A.M.: 5–25 μg./dl. 4 P.M.–6 P.M.: 2–18 μg./dl.	See Chapter 11
Creatine	Serum or plasma	Males: 0.2–0.6 mg./dl. Females: 0.6–1.0 mg./dl.	
Creatine phosphokinase (CPK)	Serum	Males: 55–170 U./L. at 37° C. Females: 30–135 U./L. at 37° C.	See Chapter 14
Creatinine	Serum or plasma	0.6–1.2 mg./dl.	See Chapter 9
Creatinine clearance (endogenous)	Serum or plasma and urine	Male: 123 ± 16 ml./min. Female: 97 ± 10 ml./min.	See Chapter 3 and nomogram in Appendix 4
Cryoglobulins	Serum	Negative	Keep specimen at 37° C.
Electrophoresis, protein	Serum	*per cent* / *gm./dl.* Albumin 52–65 / 3.2–5.6 Alpha-1 2.5–5.0 / 0.1–0.4 Alpha-2 7.0–13.0 / 0.4–1.2 Beta 8.0–14.0 / 0.5–1.1 Gamma 12.0–22.0 / 0.5–1.6	See Chapter 9
Fats, neutral	Serum or plasma	0–200 mg./dl.	See Chapter 9
Fatty acids, total free	Serum Plasma	9–15 mM./L. 300–480 μEq./L.	
Fibrinogen	Plasma	200–400 mg./dl.	
Fluoride	Whole blood	< 0.05 mg./dl.	
Folate	Serum Erythrocytes	5–25 ng./ml. (bioassay) 166–640 ng./ml. (bioassay)	
Galactose	Whole blood	Adults: none Children: < 20 mg./dl.	
Gamma globulin	Serum	0.5–1.6 gm./dl.	
Globulins, total	Serum	2.3–3.5 gm./dl.	See Chapter 9

(*Table continues on the opposite page.*)

WHOLE BLOOD, SERUM, AND PLASMA (CHEMISTRY)—*Continued*

TEST	MATERIAL	NORMAL VALUE	SPECIAL INSTRUCTIONS
Glucose, fasting	Serum or plasma Whole blood	70–110 mg./dl. 60–100 mg./dl.	Collect with heparin-fluoride mixture
Glucose tolerance, oral	Serum or plasma	Fasting: 70–110 mg./dl. 30 min.: 30–60 mg./dl. above fasting 60 min.: 20–50 mg./dl. above fasting 120 min.: 5–15 mg./dl. above fasting 180 min.: fasting level or below	See Chapter 9 Collect with heparin-fluoride mixture
Glucose tolerance, IV	Serum or plasma	Fasting: 70–110 mg./dl. 5 min.: Maximum of 250 mg./dl. 60 min.: Significant decrease 120 min.: Below 120 mg./dl. 180 min.: Fasting level	Collect with heparin-fluoride mixture
Glucose-6-phosphate dehydrogenase (G-6-PD)	Erythrocytes	250–500 units/10^9 cells 1200–2000 mI.U./ml. of packed erythrocytes	See Chapter 14
γ-Glutamyl transpeptidase	Serum	2–39 U./L.	
Glutathione	Whole blood	24–37 mg./dl.	
Growth hormone	Serum	< 10 ng./ml.	See Chapter 11, pp. 702, 703
Guanase	Serum	< 3 nM./ml./min.	
Haptoglobin	Serum	100–200 mg./dl. as hemoglobin binding capacity	
Hemoglobin	Serum or plasma	Qualitative: Negative Quantitative: 0.5–5.0 mg./dl.	See Chapter 4
Hemoglobin	Whole blood	Female: 12.0–16.0 gm./dl. Male: 13.5–18.0 gm./dl.	
Hemoglobin A_2	Whole blood	1.5–3.5% of total hemoglobin	
α-Hydroxybutyric dehydrogenase	Serum	140–350 U./ml.	See Chapter 14
17-Hydroxycorticosteroids	Plasma	Male: 7–19 μg./dl. Female: 9–21 μg./dl. After 25 USP units of ACTH I.M.: 35–55 μg./dl.	Perform test immediately or freeze plasma; see Chapter 11
Immunoglobulins	Serum		
IgG		800–1600 mg./dl.	See Chapter 9
IgA		50–250 mg./dl.	
IgM		40–120 mg./dl.	
IgD		0.5–3.0 mg./dl.	
IgE		0.01–0.04 mg./dl.	
Insulin	Plasma	11–240 μI.U./ml. (bioassay) 4–24 μU./ml. (radioimmunoassay)	
Insulin tolerance	Serum	Fasting: Glucose of 70–110 mg./dl. 30 min.: Fall to 50% of fasting level 90 min.: Fasting level	Collect with heparin-fluoride mixture; see Chapter 9
Iodine, butanol extraction (BEI) protein bound (PBI)	Serum Serum	3.5–6.5 μg./dl. 4.0–8.0 μg./dl.	Test not reliable if iodine-containing drugs or radiographic contrast media were given prior to test; see Chapter 11
Iron, total Iron-binding capacity Iron saturation, per cent	Serum Serum Serum	50–150 μg./dl. 250–450 μg./dl. 20–55%	Hemolysis must be avoided

(*Table continues on the following page.*)

WHOLE BLOOD, SERUM, AND PLASMA (CHEMISTRY)—*Continued*

TEST	MATERIAL	NORMAL VALUE	SPECIAL INSTRUCTIONS
Isocitric dehydrogenase	Serum	50–250 U./ml.	
Ketone bodies	Serum	Negative	
17-Ketosteroids	Plasma	25–125 μg./dl.	
Lactic acid	Whole blood (venous) Whole blood (arterial)	5–20 mg./dl. 3–7 mg./dl.	Draw without stasis
Lactate dehydrogenase (LDH)	Serum	80–120 Wacker units 150–450 Wroblewski units 71–207 I.U./L.	See Chapter 14
Lactate dehydrogenase isoenzymes	Serum	Anode: LDH_1 17–27% LDH_2 27–37% LDH_3 18–25% LDH_4 3–8% Cathode: LDH_5 0–5%	See Chapter 14
Lactate dehydrogenase (heat stable)	Serum	30–60% of total	
Lactose tolerance	Serum	Serum glucose changes are similar to those seen in a glucose tolerance test	See Chapter 15
Lead	Whole blood	0–50 μg./dl.	See Chapter 10
Leucine aminopeptidase (LAP)	Serum	Male: 80–200 Goldbarg-Rutenburg units/ml. Female: 75–185 Goldbarg-Rutenburg units/ml.	See Chapter 14
Lipase	Serum	0–1.5 Cherry-Crandall U./ml. 14–280 mI.U./ml.	See Chapter 15
Lipids, total cholesterol triglycerides phospholipids fatty acids neutral fat phospholipid phosphorus	Serum	400–800 mg./dl. 150–250 mg./dl. 10–190 mg./dl. 150–380 mg./dl. 9.0–15.0 mM./L. 0–200 mg./dl. 8.0–11.0 mg./dl.	See Chapter 9
Lithium	Serum	Negative Therapeutic level: 0.5–1.5 mEq./L.	See Chapter 10
Long-acting thyroid-stimulating hormone (LATS)	Serum	None	See Chapter 23
Luteinizing hormone (LH)	Plasma	Male: $<$ 11 mI.U./ml. Female: Midcycle peak $>$ 3 times baseline value Premenopausal: $<$ 25 mI.U./ml. Postmenopausal: $>$ 25 mI.U./ml.	See Table 11-3, p. 704
Macroglobulins, total	Serum	70–430 mg./dl.	
Magnesium	Serum	1.5–2.5 mEq./L. 1.8–3.0 mg./dl.	See Chapter 12
Methemoglobin	Whole blood	0–0.24 gm./dl. 0.4–1.5% of total hemoglobin	
Mucoprotein	Serum	80–200 mg./dl.	
Nonprotein nitrogen (NPN)	Serum or plasma Whole blood	20–35 mg./dl. 25–50 mg./dl.	
5′Nucleotidase	Serum	0–1.6 units	See Chapter 14
Ornithine carbamyl transferase (OCT)	Serum	8–20 mI.U./ml.	See Chapter 14

(*Table continues on the opposite page.*)

WHOLE BLOOD, SERUM, AND PLASMA (CHEMISTRY)—*Continued*

TEST	MATERIAL	NORMAL VALUE	SPECIAL INSTRUCTIONS
Osmolality	Serum	280–295 mOsm./L.	See Chapter 12
Oxygen			
Pressure (pO_2)	Whole blood, arterial	95–100 mm. Hg	See Chapter 12
Content	Whole blood, arterial	15–23 volumes %	
Saturation	Whole blood, arterial	94–100%	See Chapter 12
pH	Whole blood, arterial	7.38–7.44	See Chapter 12
	Whole blood, venous	7.36–7.41	
	Serum or plasma, venous	7.35–7.45	
Phenylalanine	Serum	Adults: < 3.0 mg./dl. Newborns (term): 1.2–3.5 mg./dl.	
Phosphatase, acid, total	Serum	0–1.1 U/ml. (Bodansky) 1–4 U/ml. (King-Armstrong) 0.13–0.63 U/ml. (Bessey-Lowry) 1.4–5.5 U/ml. (Gutman-Gutman) 0–0.56 U/ml. (Roy) 0–6.0 U/ml. (Shinowara-Jones-Reinhart)	Hemolysis must be avoided; perform test without delay or freeze specimen; see Chapter 14
Phosphatase, alkaline, total	Serum	Adults: 1.5–4.5 U/dl. (Bodansky) 4–13 U/dl. (King-Armstrong) 0.8–2.3 U/ml. (Bessey-Lowry) 15–35 U/ml. (Shinowara-Jones-Reinhart) Children: 5.0–14.0 U/dl. (Bodansky) 3.4– 9.0 U/ml. (Bessey-Lowry) 15–30 U/dl. (King-Armstrong)	See Chapter 13
Phospholipid phosphorus	Serum	8–11 mg./dl.	See Chapter 9
Phospholipids	Serum	150–380 mg./dl.	See Chapter 9
Phosphorus, inorganic	Serum	Adults: 1.8–2.6 mEq./L. 3.0–4.5 mg./dl. Children: 2.3–4.1 mEq./L. 4.0–7.0 mg./dl.	Separate cells from serum promptly; see Chapter 9
Potassium	Plasma	3.8–5.0 mEq./L.	See Chapter 12
Proteins, total albumin globulin	Serum	6.0–7.8 gm./dl. 3.2–4.5 gm./dl. 2.3–3.5 gm./dl.	See Chapter 9
Protein fractionation	Serum		See Electrophoresis
Protoporphyrin	Erythrocytes	15–50 µg./dl.	
Pyruvate	Whole blood	0.3–0.9 mg./dl.	
Salicylates	Serum	Negative Therapeutic level: 20–25 mg./dl.	See Chapter 10
Sodium	Plasma	136–142 mEq./L.	See Chapter 12
Sulfate, inorganic	Serum	0.2–1.3 mEq./L. 0.9–6.0 mg./dl. as SO_4	Hemolysis must be avoided
Sulfhemoglobin	Whole blood	Negative	
Sulfonamides	Serum or whole blood	Negative	
Testosterone	Serum or plasma	Male: 400–1200 ng./dl. Female: 30–120 ng./dl.	See Chapter 11
Thiocyanate	Serum	Negative	

(*Table continues on the following page.*)

WHOLE BLOOD, SERUM, AND PLASMA (CHEMISTRY)—*Continued*

TEST	MATERIAL	NORMAL VALUE		SPECIAL INSTRUCTIONS
Thymol flocculation	Serum	0–5 units		See Chapter 13
Thyroid hormone tests	Serum	Expressed as Thyroxine	Expressed as Iodine	See Chapter 11
T_4 (by column)		5.0–11.0 μg./dl.	3.2–7.2 μg./dl.	
T_4 (by competitive binding—Murphy-Pattee)		6.0–11.8 μg./dl.	3.9–7.7 μg./dl.	
Free T_4		0.9– 2.3 ng./dl.	0.6–1.5 ng./dl.	
T_3 (resin uptake)		25–38 relative % uptake		
Thyroxine-binding globulin (TBG)		10–26 μg./dl. (expressed as T_4 uptake)		
Transaminases: GOT	Serum	8–33 U/ml.		See Chapter 14
GPT	Serum	1–36 U/ml.		
Triglycerides	Serum	10–190 mg./dl.		
Urea nitrogen	Serum	8–18 mg./dl.		See Chapter 9
Urea clearance	Serum and urine	Maximum clearance: 64–99 ml./min. Standard clearance: 41–65 ml./min. or more than 75% of normal clearance		See Chapter 3
Uric acid	Serum	Male: 2.1–7.8 mg./dl. Female: 2.0–6.4 mg./dl.		See Chapter 9
Vitamin A	Serum	15–60 μg./dl.		
Vitamin A tolerance	Serum	Fasting: 15–60 μg./dl. 3 hr. or 6 hr. after 5000 units vitamin A/kg.: 200–600 μg./dl. 24 hrs.: fasting values or slightly above		Administer 5000 units vitamin A in oil per kg. body weight
Vitamin B_{12}	Serum	Male: 200–800 pg./ml. Female: 100–650 pg./ml.		
Unsaturated vitamin B_{12} binding capacity	Serum	1000–2000 pg./ml.		
Vitamin C	Plasma	0.6–1.6 mg./dl.		Collect with oxalate and analyze within 20 minutes
Xylose absorption	Serum	25–40 mg./dl. between 1 and 2 hr.; in malabsorption, maximum approximately 10 mg./dl. Dose: Adult: 25 gm. D-xylose Children: 0.5 gm./kg. D-xylose		For children, administer 10 ml. of a 5% solution of D-xylose per kg. of body weight (see p. 914)
Zinc	Serum	50–150 μg./dl.		
Zinc sulfate turbidity	Serum	< 12 units		

URINE

TEST	TYPE OF SPECIMEN	NORMAL VALUE	SPECIAL INSTRUCTIONS
Acetoacetic acid	Random	Negative	
Acetone	Random	Negative	
Addis count	12-hr. collection	WBC and epithelial cells: 1,800,000/12 hr. RBC: 500,000/12 hr. Hyaline casts: 0–5,000/12 hr.	Rinse bottle with some neutral formalin; discard excess; see Chapter 2
Albumin, qualitative	Random	Negative	See Chapter 2
quantitative	24 hr.	10–100 mg./24 hr.	
Aldosterone	24 hr.	2–26 μg./24 hr.	Keep refrigerated; see Chapter 11
Alkapton bodies	Random	Negative	See Chapter 2
Alpha-amino acid nitrogen	24 hr.	100–290 mg./24 hr.	
δ-Aminolevulinic acid	Random 24 hr.	Adult: 0.1–0.6 mg./dl. Children: < 0.5 mg./dl. 1.5–7.5 mg./24 hr.	See Chapter 2
Ammonia nitrogen	24 hr.	20–70 mEq./24 hr. 500–1200 mg./24 hr.	Keep refrigerated
Amylase	2 hr.	35–260 Somogyi units per hour	See Chapter 15
Arsenic	24 hr.	< 50 μg./L.	See Chapter 10
Ascorbic acid	Random 24 hr.	1–7 mg./dl. > 50 mg./24 hr.	
Bence Jones protein	Random	Negative	See Chapter 9
Beryllium	24 hr.	< 0.05 μg./24 hr.	
Bilirubin, qualitative	Random	Negative	See Chapter 2
Blood, occult	Random	Negative	See Chapter 2
Borate	24 hr.	< 2 mg./L.	
Calcium, qualitative (Sulkowitch)	Random	1+ turbidity	Compare with standard
quantitative	24 hr.	Average diet: 100–250 mg./24 hr. Low calcium diet: < 150 mg./24 hr. High calcium diet: 250–300 mg./24 hr.	
Catecholamines	Random 24 hr.	0–14 μg./dl. < 100 μg./24 hr. (varies with activity)	See Chapter 11
Chloride	24 hr.	110–250 mEq./24 hr.	See Chapter 12
Concentration test (Fishberg)	Random after fluid restriction	Specific gravity: > 1.025 Osmolality: > 850 mOsm./L.	See Chapter 3
Copper	24 hr.	0–30 μg./24 hr.	
Coproporphyrin	Random 24 hr.	Adult: 3–20 μg./dl. 50–160 μg./24 hr. Children: 0–80 μg./24 hr.	Use fresh specimen and do not expose to direct light; preserve 24-hr. urine with 5 gm. Na_2CO_3; see Chapter 2
Creatine	24 hr.	Male: 0–40 mg./24 hr. Female: 0–100 mg./24 hr. Higher in children and during pregnancy	

(Table continues on the following page.)

URINE—*Continued*

TEST	TYPE OF SPECIMEN	NORMAL VALUE	SPECIAL INSTRUCTIONS
Creatinine	24 hr.	Male: 20–26 mg./kg./24 hr. 1.0–2.0 gm./24 hr. Female: 14–22 mg./kg./24 hr. 0.8–1.8 gm./24 hr.	See Chapter 9
Cystine, qualitative	Random	Negative	See Chapter 2
Cystine and cysteine	24 hr.	10–100 mg./24 hr.	
Diacetic acid	Random	Negative	
Epinephrine	24 hr.	0–20 μg./24 hr.	
Estrogens, total	24 hr.	Male: 5–18 μg./24 hr. Female: Ovulation: 28–100 μg./24 hr. Luteal peak: 22–105 μg./24 hr. At menses: 4–25 μg./24 hr. Pregnancy: Up to 45,000 μg./24 hr. Postmenopausal: 14–20 μg./24 hr.	Keep refrigerated See Chapter 11
Estrogens, fractionated Estrone (E1) Estradiol (E2) Estriol (E3)	24 hr.	Non-pregnant, mid-cycle 2–25 μg./24 hr. 0–10 μg./24 hr. 2–30 μg./24 hr.	See Chapter 11
Fat, qualitative	Random	Negative	
FIGLU (N-formiminoglutamic acid)	24 hr.	< 3 mg./24 hr. After 15 gm. of L-histidine: 4 mg./8 hr.	See Chapter 4
Fluoride	24 hr.	<1 mg./24 hr.	
Follicle-stimulating hormone (FSH)	24 hr.	Adult: 6–50 Mouse uterine units/24 hr. Prepubertal: < 10 MUU/24 hr. Post-menopausal: > 50 MUU/24 hr.	See Chapter 11 and Table 11–3
Fructose	24 hr.	30–65 mg./24 hr.	
Glucose, qualitative	Random	Negative	See Chapter 2
quantitative: copper-reducing substances total sugars glucose	24 hr.	 0.5–1.5 gm./24 hr. Average: 250 mg./24 hr. Average: 130 mg./24 hr.	See Chapter 2
Gonadotropins, pituitary (FSH and LH)	24 hr.	10–50 MUU/24 hr.	See Chapters 11 and 26
Hemoglobin	Random	Negative	
Homogentisic acid	Random	Negative	See Chapter 2
Homovanillic acid (HVA)	24 hr.	< 15 mg./24 hr.	See Chapter 11
17-Hydroxycorticosteroids	24 hr.	Male: 5.5–14.5 mg./24 hr. Female: 4.9–12.9 mg./24 hr. Lower in children. After 25 USP units ACTH, I.M.: a 2- to 4-fold increase	Keep refrigerated; see Chapter 11
5-Hydroxyindoleacetic acid (5-HIAA), qualitative	Random	Negative	Some muscle relaxants and tranquilizers interfere with test; see Chapter 2
5-HIAA, quantitative	24 hr.	< 9 mg./24 hr.	
Indican	24 hr.	10–20 mg./24 hr.	

(*Table continues on the opposite page.*)

URINE—*Continued*

TEST	TYPE OF SPECIMEN	NORMAL VALUE	SPECIAL INSTRUCTIONS
Ketone bodies	Random	Negative	Fresh, keep cool; see Chapter 2
17-Ketosteroids	24 hr.	Male: 8–15 mg./24 hr. Female: 6–11.5 mg./24 hr. Children: 12–15 yr., 5–12 mg./24 hr. < 12 yr., < 5 mg./24 hr. After 25 USP units ACTH, I.M.: 50–100% increase	Keep refrigerated; tranquilizers interfere with test; see Chapter 11
Androsterone		Male: 2.0–5.0 mg./24 hr. Female: 0.8–3.0 mg./24 hr.	See Chapter 11
Etiocholanolone		Male: 1.4–5.0 mg./24 hr. Female: 0.8–4.0 mg./24 hr.	See Chapter 11
Dehydroepiandrosterone		Male: 0.2–2.0 mg./24 hr. Female: 0.2–1.8 mg./24 hr.	See Chapter 11
11-Ketoandrosterone		Male: 0.2–1.0 mg./24 hr. Female: 0.2–0.8 mg./24 hr.	See Chapter 11
11-Ketoetiocholanolone		Male: 0.2–1.0 mg./24 hr. Female: 0.2–0.8 mg./24 hr.	See Chapter 11
11-Hydroxyandrosterone		Male: 0.1–0.8 mg./24 hr. Female: 0.0–0.5 mg./24 hr.	See Chapter 11
11-Hydroxyetiocholanolone		Male: 0.2–0.6 mg./24 hr. Female: 0.1–1.1 mg./24 hr.	See Chapter 11
Lactose	24 hr.	12–40 mg./24 hr.	
Lead	24 hr.	< 100 μg./24 hr.	
Magnesium	24 hr.	6.0–8.5 mEq./24 hr.	
Melanin, qualitative	Random	Negative	See Chapter 2
3-Methoxy-4-hydroxymandelic acid (VMA)	24 hr.	1.5–7.5 mg./24 hr. (adults) 83 μg./kg./24 hr. (infants)	No coffee or fruit 2 days prior to test; see Chapter 11
Mucin	24 hr.	100–150 mg./24 hr.	
Myoglobin, qualitative quantitative	Random 24 hr.	Negative < 1.5 mg./L.	See Chapter 2
Osmolality	Random	500–800 mOsm./L.	May be lower or higher, depending on state of hydration; see Chapters 3 and 12
Pentoses	24 hr.	2–5 mg./kg./24 hr.	
pH	Random	4.6–8.0	See Chapter 2
Phenolsulfonphthalein (PSP)	Urine, timed after 6 mg. PSP I.V.		See Chapter 3
	15 min.	20–50% dye excreted	
	30 min.	16–24% dye excreted	
	60 min.	9–17% dye excreted	
	120 min.	3–10% dye excreted	
Phenylpyruvic acid, qualitative	Random	Negative	
Phosphorus	Random	0.9–1.3 gm./24 hr.	Varies with intake
Porphobilinogen, qualitative quantitative	Random 24 hr.	Negative 0–2.0 mg./24 hr.	

(*Table continues on the following page.*)

URINE—*Continued*

TEST	TYPE OF SPECIMEN	NORMAL VALUE	SPECIAL INSTRUCTIONS
Potassium	24 hr.	40–80 mEq./24 hr.	Varies with diet
Pregnancy tests	Concentrated morning specimen	Positive in normal pregnancies or with tumors producing chorionic gonadotropin	See Chapter 26
Pregnanediol	24 hr.	Male: 0–1 mg./24 hr. Female: 1–8 mg./24 hr. Peak: 1 week after ovulation Pregnancy: 60–100 mg./24 hr. Children: Negative	Keep refrigerated; see Chapters 11 and 26
Pregnanetriol	24 hr.	Male: 1.0–2.0 mg./24 hr. Female: 0.5–2.0 mg./24 hr. Children: < 0.5 mg./24 hr.	Keep refrigerated; see Chapters 11 and 26
Protein, qualitative	Random	Negative	See Chapter 2
quantitative	24 hr.	10–100 mg./24 hr.	See Chapter 2
Reducing substances, total	24 hr.	0.5–1.5 mg./24 hr.	See Chapter 2
Sodium	24 hr.	80–180 mEq./24 hr.	Varies with dietary ingestion of salt
Solids, total	24 hr.	55–70 gm./24 hr. Decreases with age to 30 gm./24 hr.	
Specific gravity	Random	1.016–1.022 (normal fluid intake) 1.001–1.035 (range)	See Chapters 2 and 3
Sugars (excluding glucose)	Random	Negative	
Titratable acidity	24 hr.	20–50 mEq./24 hr.	Collect with toluene
Urea nitrogen	24 hr.	6–17 gm./24 hr.	See Chapter 9
Uric acid	24 hr.	250–750 mg./24 hr.	Varies with diet
Urobilinogen	2 hr. 24 hr.	0.3–1.0 Ehrlich units 0.05–2.5 mg./24 hr. or 0.5–4.0 Ehrlich units/24 hr.	See Chapter 2
Uropepsin	Random 24 hr.	15–45 units/hr. 1500–5000 units/24 hr.	
Uroporphyrins, qualitative	Random	Negative	See Chapter 2
quantitative	24 hr.	10–30 μg./24 hr.	
Vanillylmandelic acid (VMA)	24 hr.	1.5–7.5 mg./24 hr.	See Chapter 11
Volume, total	24 hr.	600–1600 ml./24 hr.	See Chapter 2
Zinc	24 hr.	0.15–1.2 mg./24 hr.	

SYNOVIAL FLUID

TEST	NORMAL VALUE
Blood-synovial fluid glucose difference	< 10 mg./dl.
Differential cell count	Granulocytes < 25% of nucleated cells
Fibrin clot	Absent
Mucin clot	Abundant
Nucleated cell count	< 200 cells/μl.
Viscosity	High
Volume	< 3.5 ml.

SEMINAL FLUID

TEST	NORMAL VALUE
Liquefaction	Within 20 min.
Morphology	> 70% normal, mature spermatozoa
Motility	> 60%
pH	> 7.0 (average 7.7)
Sperm count	60–150 million/ml.
Volume	1.5–5.0 ml.

GASTRIC FLUID

TEST	NORMAL VALUE
Fasting residual volume	20–100 ml.
pH	< 2.0
Basal acid output (BAO)	0–6 mEq./hr.
Maximal acid output (MAO) after histamine stimulation	5–40 mEq./hr.
BAO/MAO ratio	< 0.4

HEMATOLOGY

TEST	NORMAL VALUE		
Hemoglobin A_2	1.5–3.5%		
Hemoglobin F	< 2%		
Osmotic fragility	*% Na Cl*	*% Lysis (fresh)*	*% Lysis (after 24-hr. incubation at 37° C.)*
	0.20		95–100
	0.30	97–100	85–100
	0.35	90–99	75–100
	0.40	50–95	65–100
	0.45	5–45	55–95
	0.50	0–6	40–85
	0.55	0	15–70
	0.60		0–40
	0.65		0–10
	0.70		0–5
	0.75		0
Platelet count	150,000–400,000/μl.		
Reticulocyte count	0.5–1.5% 25,000–75,000 cells/μl.		
Sedimentation rate (ESR) (Westergren)	Men under 50 yrs.: < 15 mm./hr. Men over 50 yrs.: < 20 mm./hr. Women under 50 yrs.: < 20 mm./hr. Women over 50 yrs.: < 30 mm./hr.		
Viscosity	1.4–1.8 times water		

HEMATOLOGY

TEST	NORMAL VALUE	
Complete blood count (CBC)		
Hematocrit	Male: 40–54% Female: 38–47%	
Hemoglobin	Male: 13.5–18.0 gm./dl. Female: 12.0–16.0 gm./dl.	
Red cell count	Male: 4.6–6.2 × 10^6/μl. Female: 4.2–5.4 × 10^6/μl.	
White cell count	4,500–11,000/μl.	
Erythrocyte indices		
Mean corpuscular volume (MCV)	82–98 cu. microns (fl)	
Mean corpuscular hemoglobin (MCH)	27–31 pg.	
Mean corpuscular hemoglobin concentration (MCHC)	32–36%	
White blood cell differential (adult)	*Mean Per Cent*	*Range of Absolute Counts**
Segmented neutrophils	56%	(1800–7000/μl.)
Bands	3%	(0–700/μl.)
Eosinophils	2.7%	(0–450/μl.)
Basophils	0.3%	(0–200/μl.)
Lymphocytes	34%	(1000–4800/μl.)
Monocytes	4%	(0–800/μl.)
Blood volume	Male: 69 ml./kg. Female: 65 ml./kg.	
Plasma volume	Male: 39 ml./kg. Female: 40 ml./kg.	
Coagulation tests		
Bleeding time (Ivy)	1–6 minutes	
Bleeding time (Duke)	1–3 minutes	
Clot retraction	½ the original mass in 2 hr.	
Dilute blood clot lysis time	Clot lyses between 6 and 10 hr. at 37° C.	
Euglobin clot lysis time	Clot lyses between 2 and 6 hr. at 37° C.	
Partial thromboplastin time (PTT)	60–70 seconds	
Kaolin activated	35–50 seconds	
Prothrombin time	12–14 seconds	
Venous clotting time		
3 tubes	5–15 minutes	
2 tubes	5–8 minutes	
Whole blood clot lysis time	None in 24 hr.	

*See also Table 4–2.

AMNIOTIC FLUID

TEST	NORMAL VALUE: Early Gestation (Before 28 Weeks)	NORMAL VALUE: Term
Appearance	Clear	Clear or slightly opalescent
Absorbance difference at 450 nm.	< 0.05	< 0.02
Albumin	0.04 (no S.D. given)	0.05 (no S.D. given)
Bilirubin	< 0.075 mg./dl.	< 0.025 mg./dl.
Chloride	Approx. equal to serum chloride	Generally 1–3 mEq./L.; lower than serum chloride
Creatinine	0.8–1.1 mg./dl.	1.8–4.0 mg./dl. (generally greater than 2.0 mg./dl.)
Estriol	Below 10 μg./dl.	> 60 μg./dl.
Osmolality	Approx. equal to serum osmolality	< 250 mOsm./L.
pCO_2	33–55 mm. Hg	42–55 mm. Hg (increases toward term)
pH	7.12–7.38	6.91–7.43 (decreases toward term)
Protein, total	0.60 ± 0.24 gm./dl.	0.26 ± 0.19 gm./dl.
Sodium	Approx. equal to serum sodium	Generally 7–10 mEq./L. lower than serum sodium
Staining, cytologic		
Oil red O	< 10%	> 50%
Nile blue sulfate	0	> 20%
Urea	18.0 ± 5.9 mg./dl.	30.3 ± 11.4 mg./dl.
Uric acid	3.72 ± 0.96 mg./dl.	9.9 ± 2.23 mg./dl.
Volume	450–1200 ml.	500–1400 ml. (increases toward term)

MISCELLANEOUS

TEST	SPECIMEN	NORMAL VALUE	SPECIAL INSTRUCTIONS
Bile, qualitative	Random stool	Negative in adults; positive in children	
Chloride	Sweat	4–60 mEq./L.	
Clearances	Serum and timed urine		See Chapter 3
Creatinine, endogenous		115 ± 20 ml./min.	
Diodrast		600–720 ml./min.	
Inulin		100–150 ml./min.	
PAH		600–750 ml./min.	
Diagnex blue (tubeless gastric analysis)	Urine	Free acid present	
Fat	Stool, 72 hr.	Total fat: < 5 gm./24 hr. and 10–25% of dry matter Neutral fat: 1–5% of dry matter Free fatty acids: 5–13% of dry matter Combined fatty acids: 5–15% of dry matter	
Nitrogen, total	Stool, 24 hr.	10% of intake or 1–2 gm./24 hr.	
Sodium	Sweat	10–80 mEq./L.	See Chapter 12
Trypsin activity	Random, fresh stool	Positive (2+ to 4+)	
Thyroid ^{131}I uptake		7.5–25% in 6 hr.	See Chapter 11 and Fig. 11-25.
Urobilinogen, qualitative	Random stool	Positive	
quantitative	Stool, 24 hr.	40–200 mg./24 hr. 30–280 Ehrlich units/24 hr.	

SEROLOGY

TEST	NORMAL VALUE
Antibovine milk antibodies	Negative
Antidesoxyribonuclease (ADNAase)	< 1:20
Antinuclear antibodies (ANA)	< 1:10
Antistreptococcal hyaluronidase (ASH)	< 1:256
Antistreptolysin O (ASLO)	< 160 Todd units
Australia antigen	See hepatitis-associated antigen
Brucella agglutinins	< 1:80
Coccidioidomycosis antibodies	Negative
Cold agglutinins	< 1:32
Complement, C′3	100–170 mg./dl.
C-Reactive protein (CRP)	0
Fluorescent treponemal antibodies (FTA)	Nonreactive
Hepatitis-associated antigen (HAA or HBAg)	Negative
Heterophile antibodies	< 1:56
Histoplasma agglutinins	< 1:8
Latex fixation	Negative
Leptospira agglutinins	Negative
Ox cell hemolysin	< 1:480
Rheumatoid factor	
sensitized sheep cell	< 1:160
latex fixation	< 1:80
bentonite particles	< 1:32
Streptococcal MG agglutinins	< 1:20
Thyroid antibodies	
antithyroglobulin	< 1:32
antithyroid microsomal	< 1:56
Toxoplasma antibodies	< 1:4
Trichina agglutinins	0
Tularemia agglutinins	< 1:80
Typhoid agglutinins	
O	< 1:80
H	< 1:80
VDRL	Nonreactive
Weil-Felix (Proteus OX-2, OX-K, and OX-19 agglutinins)	Fourfold rise in titer between acute and convalescent sera

CEREBROSPINAL FLUID

TEST OR CONSTITUENT	NORMAL VALUE	SPECIAL INSTRUCTIONS
Albumin	10–30 mg./dl.	
Albumin/globulin ratio	1.6–2.2	
Calcium	2.1–2.9 mEq./L.	
Cell count	0–8 cells/μl.	
Chloride	Adult: 118–132 mEq./L. Children: 120–128 mEq./L.	These values are invalidated by admixture of blood
Colloidal gold curve	0001111000	
Globulins, qualitative (Pandy) quantitative	Negative 6–16 mg./dl.	See Chapter 25
Glucose	45–75 mg./dl.	See Chapters 9 and 25
Lactate dehydrogenase (LDH)	Approximately 1/10 of serum level	
Protein, total CSF ventricular fluid	15–45 mg./dl. 8–15 mg./dl.	
Protein electrophoresis		
Pre-albumin	4.1 ± 1.2%	
Albumin	62.4 ± 5.6%	
Alpha-1 globulin	5.3 ± 1.2%	
Alpha-2 globulin	8.2 ± 2.0%	
Beta globulin	12.8 ± 2.0%	
Gamma globulin	7.2 ± 1.1%	
Xanthochromia	Negative	

APPENDIX 4

DESIRABLE WEIGHTS AND BODY SURFACE AREA

DESIRABLE WEIGHTS FOR MEN AND WOMEN*
According to Height and Frame. Ages 25 and Over

HEIGHT (IN SHOES)	WEIGHT IN POUNDS (IN INDOOR CLOTHING)		
	Small Frame	Medium Frame	Large Frame
		MEN	
5′ 2″	112–120	118–129	126–141
3″	115–123	121–133	129–144
4″	118–126	124–136	132–148
5″	121–129	127–139	135–152
6″	124–133	130–143	138–156
7″	128–137	134–147	142–161
8″	132–141	138–152	147–166
9″	136–145	142–156	151–170
10″	140–150	146–160	155–174
11″	144–154	150–165	159–179
6′ 0″	148–158	154–170	164–184
1″	152–162	158–175	168–189
2″	156–167	162–180	173–194
3″	160–171	167–185	178–199
4″	164–175	172–190	182–204
		WOMEN	
4′ 10″	92– 98	96–107	104–119
11″	94–101	98–110	106–122
5′ 0″	96–104	101–113	109–125
1″	99–107	104–116	112–128
2″	102–110	107–119	115–131
3″	105–113	110–122	118–134
4″	108–116	113–126	121–138
5″	111–119	116–130	125–142
6″	114–123	120–135	129–146
7″	118–127	124–139	133–150
8″	122–131	128–143	137–154
9″	126–135	132–147	141–158
10″	130–140	136–151	145–163
11″	134–144	140–155	149–168
6′ 0″	138–148	144–159	153–173

*Prepared by the Metropolitan Life Insurance Company. Derived primarily from data of the *Build and Blood Pressure Study, 1959,* Society of Actuaries. Reproduced with permission.

NOMOGRAM FOR THE DETERMINATION OF BODY SURFACE OF CHILDREN AND ADULTS*

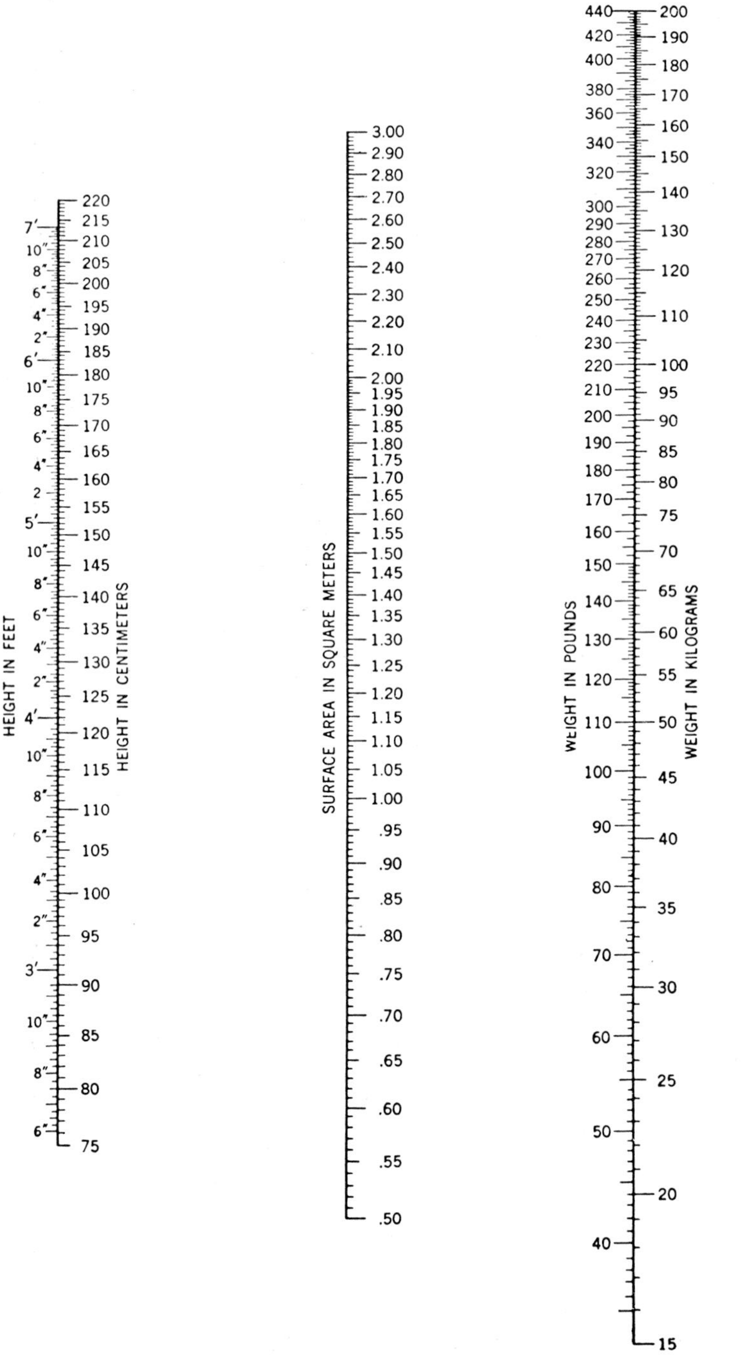

*From Boothby, W. M., and Sandiford, R. B.: Boston M. & S.J. *185*:337, 1921.

NOMOGRAM FOR THE DETERMINATION OF
BODY SURFACE AREA OF CHILDREN*

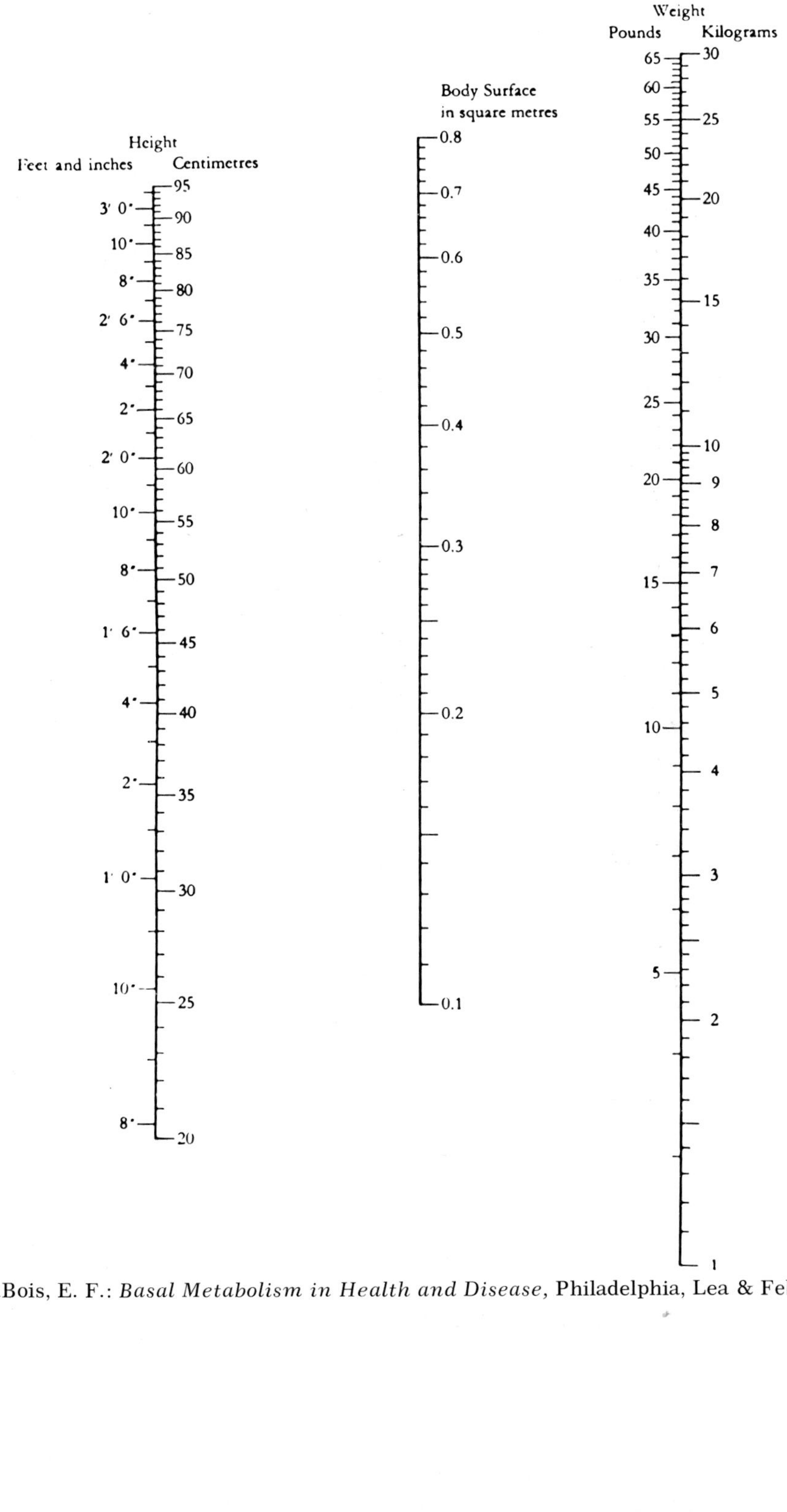

*From DuBois, E. F.: *Basal Metabolism in Health and Disease,* Philadelphia, Lea & Febiger, 1936.

INDEX

Numbers set in *italics* indicate an illustration; those set in **boldface** indicate a table.

TABLE OF FOUR

	0	1	2	3	4	5	6	7	8	9
1.0	.0000	.0043	.0086	.0128	.0170	.0212	.0253	.0294	.0334	.0374
1.1	.0414	.0453	.0492	.0531	.0569	.0607	.0645	.0682	.0719	.0755
1.2	.0792	.0828	.0864	.0899	.0934	.0969	.1004	.1038	.1072	.1106
1.3	.1139	.1173	.1206	.1239	.1271	.1303	.1335	.1367	.1399	.1430
1.4	.1461	.1492	.1523	.1553	.1584	.1614	.1644	.1673	.1703	.1732
1.5	.1761	.1790	.1818	.1847	.1875	.1903	.1931	.1959	.1987	.2014
1.6	.2041	.2068	.2095	.2122	.2148	.2175	.2201	.2227	.2253	.2279
1.7	.2304	.2330	.2355	.2380	.2405	.2430	.2455	.2480	.2504	.2529
1.8	.2553	.2577	.2601	.2625	.2648	.2672	.2695	.2718	.2742	.2765
1.9	.2788	.2810	.2833	.2856	.2878	.2900	.2923	.2945	.2967	.2989
2.0	.3010	.3032	.3054	.3075	.3096	.3118	.3139	.3160	.3181	.3201
2.1	.3222	.3243	.3263	.3284	.3304	.3324	.3345	.3365	.3385	.3404
2.2	.3424	.3444	.3464	.3483	.3502	.3522	.3541	.3560	.3579	.3598
2.3	.3617	.3636	.3655	.3674	.3692	.3711	.3729	.3747	.3766	.3784
2.4	.3802	.3820	.3838	.3856	.3874	.3892	.3909	.3927	.3945	.3962
2.5	.3979	.3997	.4014	.4031	.4048	.4065	.4082	.4099	.4116	.4133
2.6	.4150	.4166	.4183	.4200	.4216	.4232	.4249	.4265	.4281	.4298
2.7	.4314	.4330	.4346	.4362	.4378	.4393	.4409	.4425	.4440	.4456
2.8	.4472	.4487	.4502	.4518	.4533	.4548	.4564	.4579	.4594	.4609
2.9	.4624	.4639	.4654	.4669	.4683	.4698	.4713	.4728	.4742	.4757
3.0	.4771	.4786	.4800	.4814	.4829	.4843	.4857	.4871	.4886	.4900
3.1	.4914	.4928	.4942	.4955	.4969	.4983	.4997	.5011	.5024	.5038
3.2	.5051	.5065	.5079	.5092	.5105	.5119	.5132	.5145	.5159	.5172
3.3	.5185	.5198	.5211	.5224	.5237	.5250	.5263	.5276	.5289	.5302
3.4	.5315	.5328	.5340	.5353	.5366	.5378	.5391	.5403	.5416	.5428
3.5	.5441	.5453	.5465	.5478	.5490	.5502	.5514	.5527	.5539	.5551
3.6	.5563	.5575	.5587	.5599	.5611	.5623	.5635	.5647	.5658	.5670
3.7	.5682	.5694	.5705	.5717	.5729	.5740	.5752	.5763	.5775	.5786
3.8	.5798	.5809	.5821	.5832	.5843	.5855	.5866	.5877	.5888	.5899
3.9	.5911	.5922	.5933	.5944	.5955	.5966	.5977	.5988	.5999	.6010
4.0	.6021	.6031	.6042	.6053	.6064	.6075	.6085	.6096	.6107	.611
4.1	.6128	.6138	.6149	.6160	.6170	.6180	.6191	.6201	.6212	.622
4.2	.6232	.6243	.6253	.6263	.6274	.6284	.6294	.6304	.6314	.632
4.3	.6335	.6345	.6355	.6365	.6375	.6385	.6395	.6405	.6415	.642
4.4	.6435	.6444	.6454	.6464	.6474	.6484	.6493	.6503	.6513	.652
4.5	.6532	.6542	.6551	.6561	.6571	.6580	.6590	.6599	.6609	.661
4.6	.6628	.6637	.6646	.6656	.6665	.6675	.6684	.6693	.6702	.671
4.7	.6721	.6730	.6739	.6749	.6758	.6767	.6776	.6785	.6794	.680
4.8	.6812	.6821	.6830	.6839	.6848	.6857	.6866	.6875	.6884	.689
4.9	.6902	.6911	.6920	.6928	.6937	.6946	.6955	.6964	.6972	.698
5.0	.6990	.6998	.7007	.7016	.7024	.7033	.7042	.7050	.7059	.706
5.1	.7076	.7084	.7093	.7101	.7110	.7118	.7126	.7135	.7143	.71
5.2	.7160	.7168	.7177	.7185	.7193	.7202	.7210	.7218	.7226	.72
5.3	.7243	.7251	.7259	.7267	.7275	.7284	.7292	.7300	.7308	.73
5.4	.7324	.7332	.7340	.7348	.7356	.7364	.7372	.7380	.7388	.73